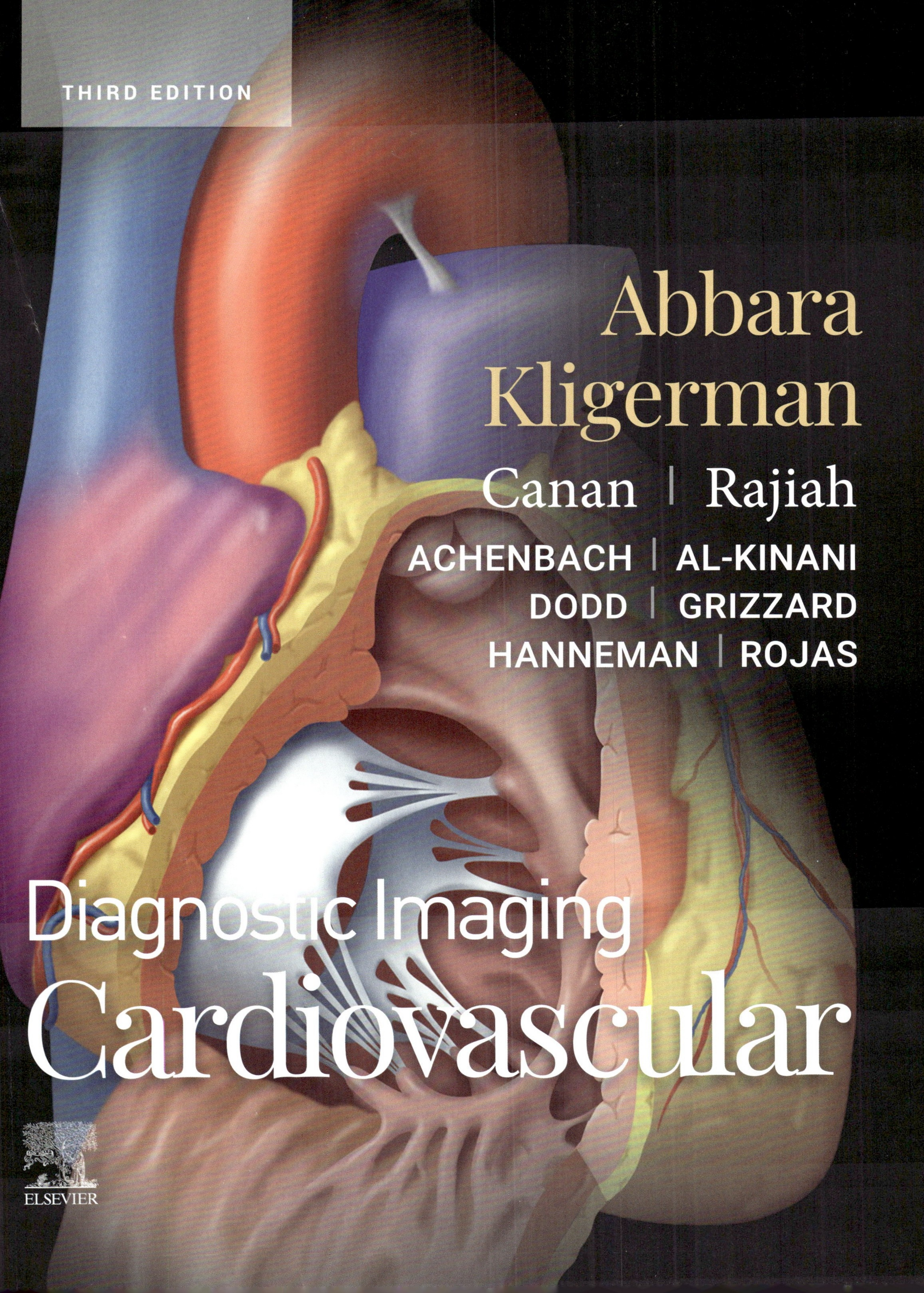

THIRD EDITION

Abbara
Kligerman
Canan | Rajiah
ACHENBACH | AL-KINANI
DODD | GRIZZARD
HANNEMAN | ROJAS

Diagnostic Imaging
Cardiovascular

ELSEVIER

Diagnostic Imaging

Cardiovascular

THIRD EDITION

Suhny Abbara, MD,
FACR, MSCCT, FNASCI
Chair, Division of Cardiothoracic Imaging
Senior Associate Consultant
Department of Radiology
Mayo Clinic
Jacksonville, Florida
Adjunct Professor
Department of Radiology
UT Southwestern Medical Center
Dallas, Texas

Seth Kligerman, MD, MS
Chairman and Professor
Department of Radiology
National Jewish Health
Denver, Colorado

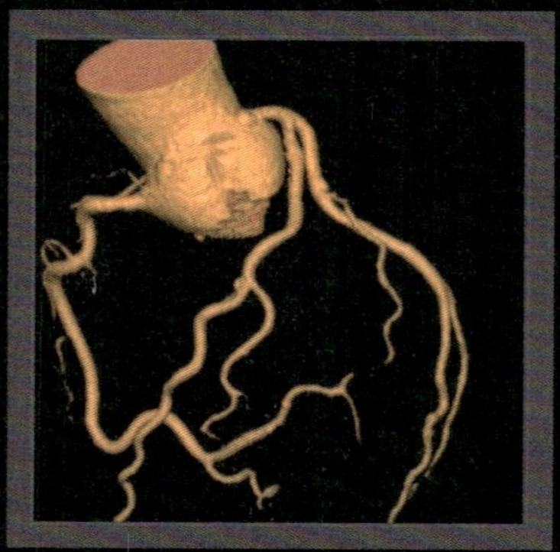

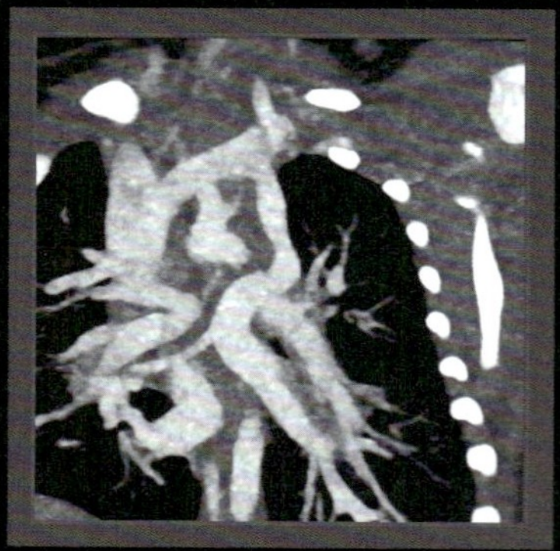

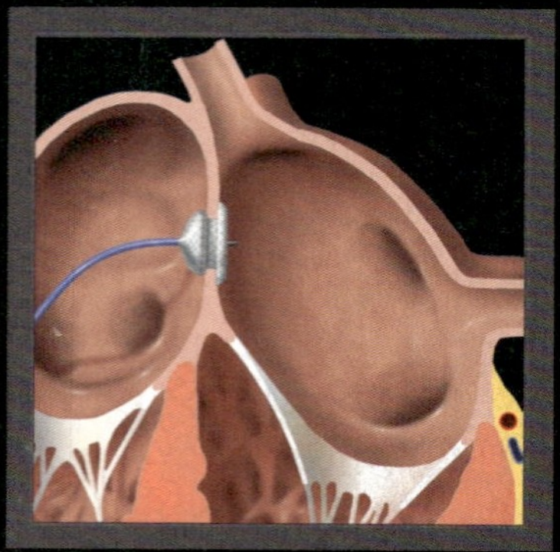

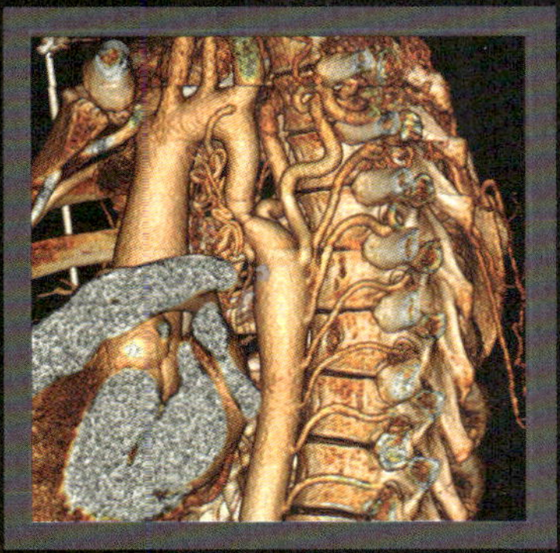 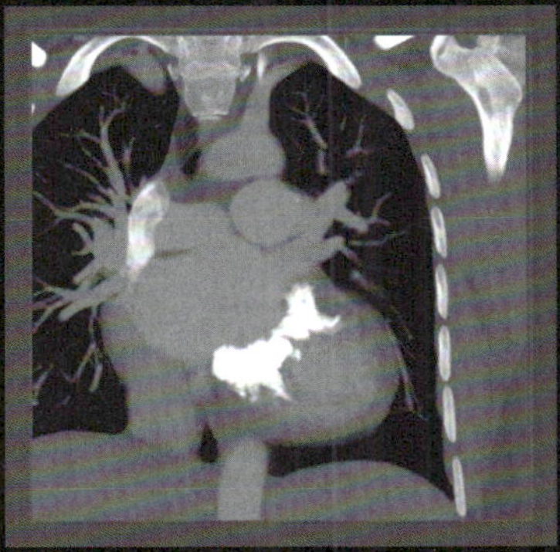 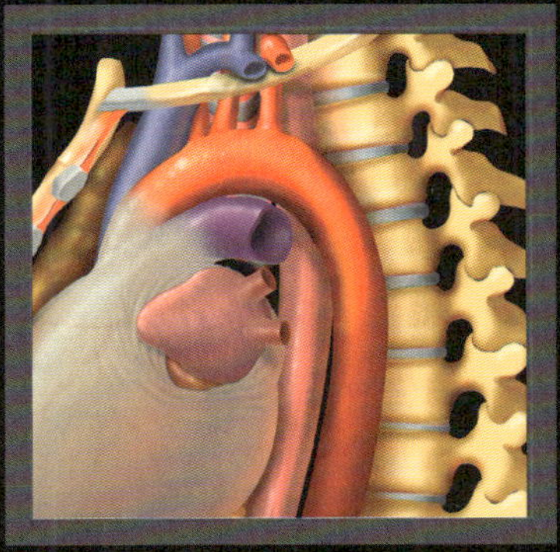

Arzu Canan, MD
Assistant Professor
Cardiothoracic Imaging
Department of Radiology
UT Southwestern Medical Center
Dallas, Texas

Prabhakar Rajiah, MBBS, MD, FACR, FRCR, FACC, FAHA, FSCCT, FSCMR
Professor of Radiology
Chair, Radiology Quality
Mayo Clinic
Rochester, Minnesota

Mortadha Al-Kinani, MD, MBChB
Fellow/Assistant Instructor of Cardiothoracic Imaging
Department of Radiology
UT Southwestern Medical Center
Dallas, Texas

Jonathan D. Dodd, MD, MSc, MRCPI, FFR(RCSI)
Consultant Radiologist
St. Vincent's University Hospital
Professor of Radiology
University College Dublin
School of Medicine &
Medical Science
Dublin, Ireland

John D. Grizzard, MD
Associate Professor
Departments of Radiology and
Internal Medicine
VCU Health Systems
Richmond, Virginia

Kate Hanneman, MD, MPH
Associate Professor
Department of Medical Imaging
University of Toronto
Toronto, Ontario, Canada

Carlos A. Rojas, MD
Chair, Division of Cardiothoracic Imaging
Associate Professor
Department of Radiology
Mayo Clinic
Phoenix, Arizona

Elsevier
1600 John F. Kennedy Blvd.
Ste 1800
Philadelphia, PA 19103-2899

DIAGNOSTIC IMAGING: CARDIOVASCULAR, THIRD EDITION ISBN: 978-0-443-28643-8

Library of Congress Control Number: 2025930222

Printed in Canada by Friesens, Altona, Manitoba, Canada

Last digit is the print number: 9 8 7 6 5 4 3 2 1

Dedications

To Amanda, Cory and Tyler, Marlene and Yasser, and Mona and Susu, with love and gratitude!

SA

I would like to dedicate this book to my family: Mom, Dad, Vickie, Elliot, David, Matthew, Maxwell, Allison, Renata, Erica, Ben, and Jack; I could not have succeeded without your support. I would like to thank my mentors Jeff, Charlie, Bob, and David; without your guidance, I would not be where I am today. Lastly, I would like to thank my dearest Elizabeth; only with your love and kindness was I able to complete this project with my sanity intact.

SK

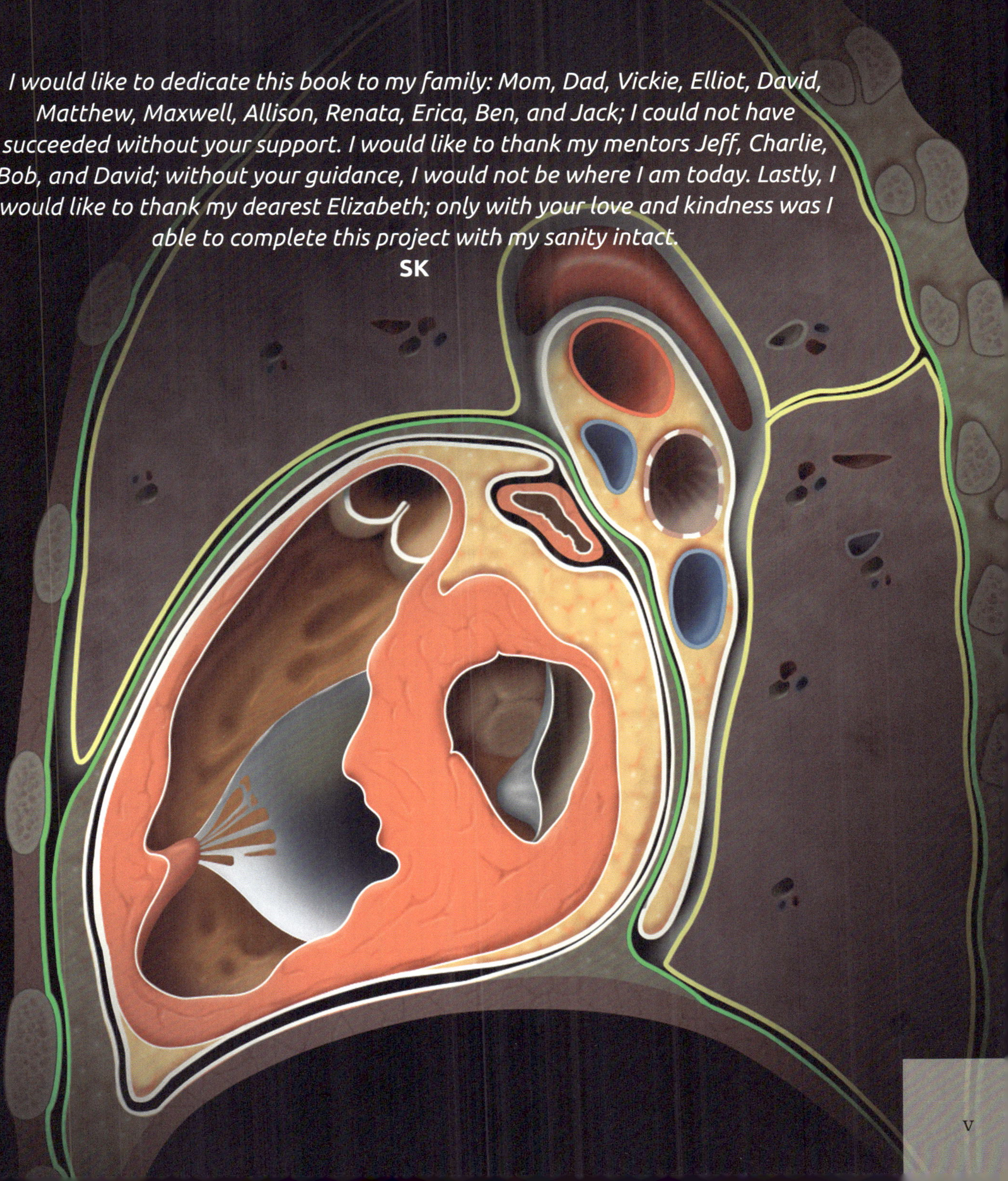

Contributing Authors

Babken Asatryan, MD, PhD, FESC
Clinical Cardiac Electrophysiology Fellow
Division of Cardiology
Department of Medicine
Johns Hopkins University
School of Medicine
Baltimore, Maryland

Benjamin Pryor Bonner, MD
Research Fellow in
Cardiovascular Imaging
Department of Radiology
Massachusetts General Hospital
Harvard Medical School
Boston, Massachusetts

Fionn Coughlan, MB, BCh, BAO (hons), FRANZCR
Advanced Cardiac Imaging
Department of Radiology
St. Paul's Hospital
University of British Columbia
Vancouver, British Columbia, Canada
Consultant Radiologist
Department of Medical Imaging
Fiona Stanley Hospital
Murdoch, Western Australia, Australia

Shane Crilly, MD
Specialist Registrar in Radiology
Department of Radiology
St. Vincent's University Hospital
Dublin, Ireland

Dominik Fleischmann, MD
Professor and Chief of
Cardiovascular Imaging
Department of Radiology
Stanford University School of Medicine
Stanford, California

Sebastian Flynn, MD
Department of Radiology
St. Vincent's University Hospital
Dublin, Ireland

Brian Gaffney, MD
Department of Radiology
St. Vincent's University Hospital
Dublin, Ireland

Brian Ghoshhajra, MD, MBA
Associate Chair of Operations
Analytics and Radiology
Academic Director of
Cardiovascular Imaging
Massachusetts General Hospital
Associate Professor of Radiology
Harvard Medical School
Boston, Massachusetts

Harold Goerne, MD
Cardiovascular Radiologist
IMSS Western National Medical Center
CID Imaging and Diagnostic Center
Guadalajara, Jalisco, Mexico

Alexander Haenel, MD
Advanced Cardiac Imaging
Department of Radiology
St. Paul's Hospital
University of British Columbia
Vancouver, British Columbia, Canada

Sandeep S. Hedgire, MD, DABAR, FSCCT
Chief of Cardiovascular Imaging
Department of Radiology
Assistant Professor
Harvard Medical School
Massachusetts General Hospital
Boston, Massachusetts

Fernando Kay, MD, PhD
Associate Professor of Radiology
Interim Division Chief of
Cardiothoracic Imaging
UT Southwestern Medical Center
Dallas, Texas

John Khoo, MBBS
Advanced Cardiac Imaging
Department of Radiology
St. Paul's Hospital
University of British Columbia
Vancouver, British Columbia, Canada

Des Killick, MB, BCh, BAO
Specialist Registrar in Radiology
Department of Radiology
St. Vincent's University Hospital
Dublin, Ireland

Tim Leiner, MD, PhD, FISMRM, FSCMR, FSCCT
Professor of Radiology
Department of Radiology
Mayo Clinic
Rochester, Minnesota

Jonathon Leipsic, MD, FRCPC, FSCCT
Professor and Head of
Department of Radiology
Professor of Medicine (Cardiology)
University of British Columbia
Vancouver, British Columbia, Canada

John P. Lichtenberger, III, MD
Professor of Radiology
The George Washington
University School
of Medicine and Health Sciences
Chief of Cardiothoracic Imaging and
Vice Chair for Education
Department of Radiology
The George Washington
University Medical
Faculty Associates
Washington, D.C.

Brent P. Little, MD
Professor of Radiology
Mayo Clinic College of Medicine
and Science
Consultant Radiologist
Division of Cardiothoracic Imaging
Mayo Clinic
Jacksonville, Florida

Andre Luppi, MD, PhD
Research Fellow in
Cardiovascular Imaging
Department of Radiology
Massachusetts General Hospital
Harvard Medical School
Boston, Massachusetts

Mohammad H. Madani, MD
Assistant Professor
Department of Radiology
University of California, Davis
Sacramento, California

Ciara Mahon, MD, MSc
Department of Cardiology
St. Vincent's University Hospital
Dublin, Ireland

Domenico Mastrodicasa, MD
Acting Instructor
Department of Radiology
University of Washington
School of Medicine
Seattle, Washington

Niall McVeigh, MD
Department of Radiology
St. Vincent's University Hospital
University College Dublin School of Medicine & Medical Science
Dublin, Ireland

Brian O'Riordan, MD
Department of Radiology
St. Vincent's University Hospital
Dublin, Ireland

Sean Quinn, MD
Department of Radiology
St. Vincent's University Hospital
Dublin, Ireland

Prajwal Reddy, MD
Assistant Professor
Department of Cardiovascular Medicine
Mayo Clinic
Jacksonville, Florida

James Ryan, MD
Department of Radiology
St. Vincent's University Hospital
Dublin, Ireland

Sachin S. Saboo, MD, FRCR, FSCMR
Cardiothoracic and Body Radiologist
South Texas Radiology Group, P.A.
San Antonio, Texas

Felipe Sanchez Tijmes, MD
Assistant Professor of Radiology
University of Toronto
Joint Department of Medical Imaging
University Medical Imaging Toronto
Toronto General Hospital
University Health Network and
Sinai Health System
Toronto, Ontario, Canada

Davis Vigneault, MD, DPhil
Department of Radiology
Stanford University School of Medicine
Stanford, California

Darragh Waters, MD
Specialist Registrar in Radiology
Department of Radiology
St. Vincent's University Hospital
Dublin, Ireland

Stefan L. Zimmerman, MD
Professor of Radiology and Cardiology
Johns Hopkins University School of Medicine
Baltimore, Maryland

Additional Contributors

Gerald F. Abbott, MD, FACR
Stephan Achenbach, MD, FESC, FACC, FSCCT
Prachi P. Agarwal, MD
Andrew Arai, MD
Aaron Auerbach, MD, MPH
Ron Blankstein, MD
Brett W. Carter, MD, CPE, CPPS
Franklin Dana, MD
Gudrun Feuchtner, MD
Sanjeev A. Francis, MD, FACC
Sherief H. Garrana, MD
Leila Rezai Gharai, MD
Robert C. Groves, MD
Mina F. Hanna, MD
Terrance Healey, MD
Sanjeeva P. Kalva, MD, FSIR, FCIRSE
Luis Landeras, MD
Jinglei Li, MD
Santiago Martínez-Jiménez, MD
Lucia Moore, MD
Arlene Sirajuddin, MD
Justin Stowell, MD
Chris S. C. Tsai, MBChB
Emily Tsai, MD
Lowie M. R. Van Assche, MD
Christopher M. Walker, MD
T. Gregory Walker, MD, FSIR
Carol C. Wu, MD
Phillip Young, MD

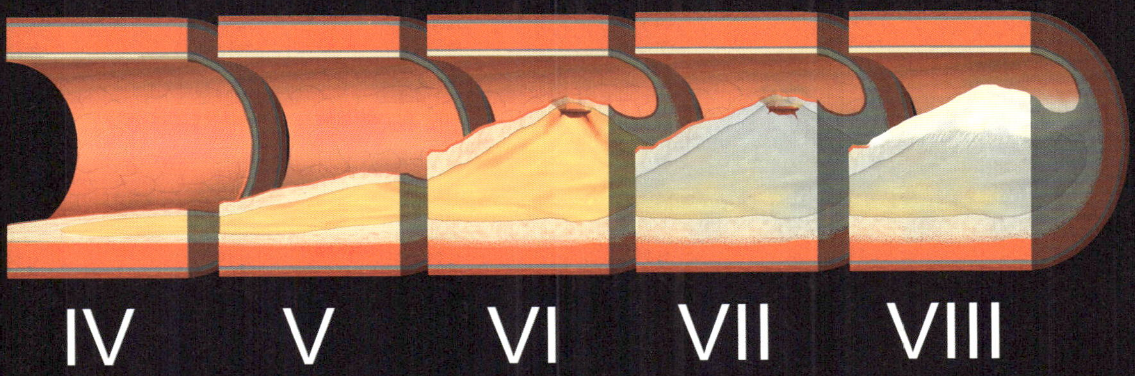

Foreword

In the dynamic and ever-evolving field of cardiovascular imaging, the 3rd edition of *Diagnostic Imaging: Cardiovascular* by Drs. Suhny Abbara and Seth Kligerman emerges as an indispensable resource for both medical professionals caring for patients with cardiovascular disease and imagers seeking to stay at the forefront of cardiovascular imaging interpretation. This comprehensive volume offers an in-depth exploration of cardiac and central vascular imaging, serving as a vital reference for cardiologists, radiologists, and trainees.

Dr. Suhny Abbara, Senior Associate Consultant and Chair of the Division of Cardiothoracic Imaging at Mayo Clinic in Jacksonville, Florida, and Dr. Seth Kligerman, Professor and Chairman of the Department of Radiology at National Jewish Health in Denver, Colorado, bring authoritative experience and expertise to this work. For nearly 20 years, as the president of the International Society for Computed Tomography and past president of the North American Society for Cardiovascular Imagers, I have been privileged to experience their development as passionate cardiothoracic imagers committed to the highest ideals of excellence in education, scientific investigation, and patient care. As leaders at the top of our field, they have assembled a veritable "who's who" of world-renowned cardiovascular imagers to author over 200 topics organized into 11 sections that encompass the breadth of cardiovascular imaging approaches and disease-based applications, richly illustrated with over 3,800 high-quality print and online diagrams, cross-sectional images, and volume renderings in this edition.

This edition is meticulously structured to cover a broad spectrum of topics essential for contemporary cardiovascular imaging. It begins with foundational chapters that delve into cardiac image acquisition techniques, postprocessing methods, and interpretation guidelines. Subsequent sections provide an in-depth exploration of cardiovascular pathologies, including coronary artery disease, cardiomyopathies, valvular disorders, pericardial diseases, cardiac neoplasms, congenital heart anomalies, and diseases of the aorta and pulmonary arteries.

In an era where technology is rapidly advancing, the authors have ensured that the content reflects the latest developments in cardiovascular imaging. This rich body of knowledge covers more than 40 topics that are entirely new to this edition. Just a few of the highlights include discussions on the growing use of AI photon-counting CT scanning, new coronary imaging guidelines for acute and chronic chest pain, the CAD-RADS 2.0 reporting system for coronary CT angiography, myocardial tissue and strain mapping, post-COVID and vaccine-related myocarditis, and 6 chapters dedicated to the recently refined 5-group clinical classification of pulmonary hypertension. These highlights provide readers with insights into the state-of-the-art and future directions of cardiac imaging.

A standout feature of this textbook is its emphasis on a multimodality approach to cardiovascular disorders. By integrating CT, MR, sonographic, and radionuclide imaging findings with clinical scenarios, the authors provide a holistic perspective that underscores the importance of a flexible approach to comprehensive cardiovascular disease assessment.

To present the breadth of richly illustrated topics within a single volume, the style is not long-form prose, but succinct paragraphs, bulleted descriptions, and tables that provide rapid access to key topics and points of emphasis within highly structured chapters organized into topic-specific sections and subsections. Rather than mired in lengthy descriptions and deep-in-the-weeds discussions of the many nuances and offshoots each topic could engender, the text is an excellent launch point for readers desiring more detail to pursue source materials and detailed scientific studies online. The benefit of this approach cannot be overstated. This modern textbook is made for the Internet age, economizing on text to maximize space available for richly presented and annotated images.

The clarity of presentation, combined with the practical focus of the content, makes this textbook an invaluable resource for both trainees and seasoned practitioners. The logical organization and comprehensive coverage ensure that readers can easily navigate through topics, whether seeking to understand basic principles or looking for detailed information on specific conditions. The inclusion of clinical pearls and diagnostic checklists further enhances its utility as a reference guide in clinical practice.

In conclusion, *Diagnostic Imaging: Cardiovascular*, 3rd edition, is a monumental contribution to the field of cardiovascular imaging. Drs. Abbara and Kligerman have succeeded in creating a resource that bridges radiology and cardiology, fostering a collaborative approach to patient care. Their dedication to advancing medical knowledge and improving clinical practice is evident throughout the pages of this textbook. As cardiovascular diseases continue to be a leading cause of morbidity and mortality worldwide, the insights and knowledge contained within this book are timely and essential.

I enthusiastically recommend this textbook to all health care professionals involved in cardiac care. May it serve as a beacon of knowledge, guiding you in your practice and inspiring excellence in diagnosing and managing cardiovascular diseases, so that you achieve the highest ideals for the health of your patients.

Geoffrey D. Rubin, MD, MBA, FACR, FNASCI

Professor and Chair of Medical Imaging
University of Arizona
Tucson, Arizona

Preface

Since the publication of the previous edition of *Diagnostic Imaging: Cardiovascular*, there have been extraordinary advancements in the field of cardiovascular medicine, making this new edition even more vital for clinicians, students, and researchers. The development of innovative treatments, significant advances in imaging technology, and the rapid expansion of scientific evidence have reshaped how we approach cardiovascular care. Cardiovascular imaging is now playing a more central role in patient management with new practice guidelines underscoring its critical importance in the diagnosis and treatment of cardiovascular disorders.

In this 3rd edition of *Diagnostic Imaging: Cardiovascular*, we are pleased to introduce Dr. Seth Kligerman as a lead author. Dr. Kligerman's deep expertise in cardiothoracic imaging and his broad clinical experience bring a valuable perspective to this edition. We have also had the privilege of working with 2 associate authors, Drs. Prabhakar Rajiah and Arzu Canan. The collaborative work of this group has been instrumental in shaping the content, and the team's insights have helped ensure that this edition remains at the forefront of cardiovascular imaging.

As with previous editions, the content of this work has been extensively revised and updated. This edition introduces several significant changes and additions. Firstly, the content has been almost entirely revamped with numerous figures updated or replaced to reflect the latest technological advancements and clinical practices. The total number of figures has now surpassed 3,800 with approximately 2,500 in the printed book and more than 1,300 additional images in the complimentary eBook version for ease of reference. Alongside these updated figures, new tables and expanded imaging galleries enhance the utility of this text.

Among the many updates, we are excited to include several new chapters that reflect the most recent developments in the field. For example, new chapters on pulmonary hypertension, CAD-RADS 2.0, and innovations in devices and procedures have been added to address the increasing complexity of cardiovascular care. These chapters represent the cutting-edge advancements in diagnosis, management, and patient outcomes, ensuring that readers are equipped with the most current information available.

Moreover, this edition incorporates detailed reviews on new imaging modalities and reporting systems and their role in diagnosing and managing cardiovascular diseases. The chapter on CAD-RADS 2.0, other new reporting standards, and chapter updates based on new guidelines for clinical management, such as the recent chest pain guideline, represent important updates and provide a more refined and clinically relevant approach to coronary artery disease risk stratification using advanced imaging techniques.

In addition, our focus on patient-centered care has led to the inclusion of sections that highlight the integration of imaging into treatment planning, the use of new devices and procedures, and the role of imaging in guiding interventions. These updates ensure that the text is not only a resource for understanding the technical aspects of imaging but also for applying this knowledge in everyday clinical practice.

This edition also benefits from the contributions of experts from both radiology and cardiology with a range of specialists who have brought their expertise in cardiac CT, MR, and related modalities to the table. I am deeply grateful to all the authors, editors, and collaborators whose contributions have made this edition possible. Their dedication, along with the exceptional support from the publishing and design teams, has been instrumental in bringing this updated edition to life.

We sincerely hope that this 3rd edition of *Diagnostic Imaging: Cardiovascular* continues to serve as an indispensable resource in your practice. Whether you are a student, clinician, or researcher, we trust that this edition will provide valuable insights, enhance your understanding, and guide your decisions in the ever-evolving field of cardiovascular medicine.

Suhny Abbara, MD, FACR, MSCCT, FNASCI
Chair, Division of Cardiothoracic Imaging
Senior Associate Consultant
Department of Radiology
Mayo Clinic
Jacksonville, Florida
Adjunct Professor
Department of Radiology
UT Southwestern Medical Center
Dallas, Texas

Seth Kligerman, MD, MS
Chairman and Professor
Department of Radiology
National Jewish Health
Denver, Colorado

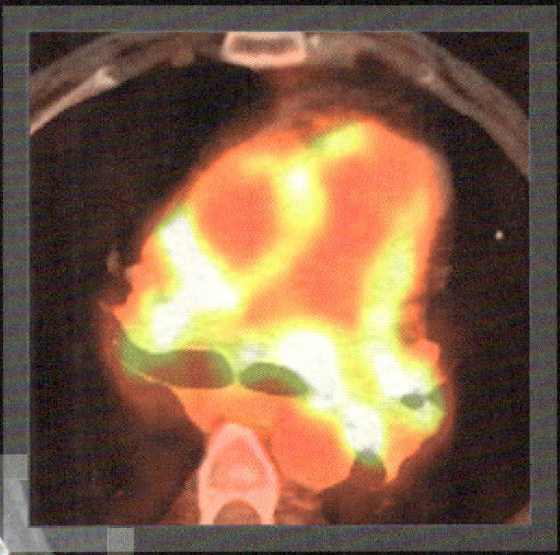

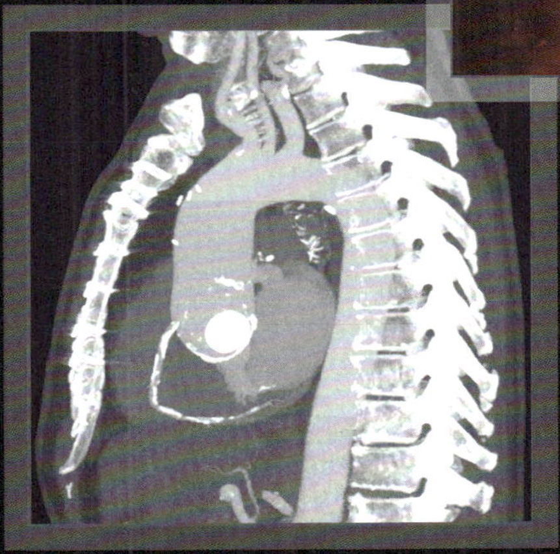

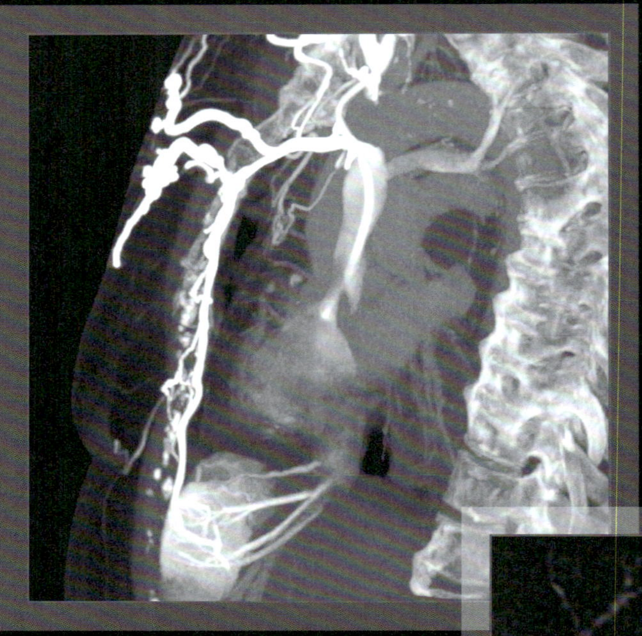

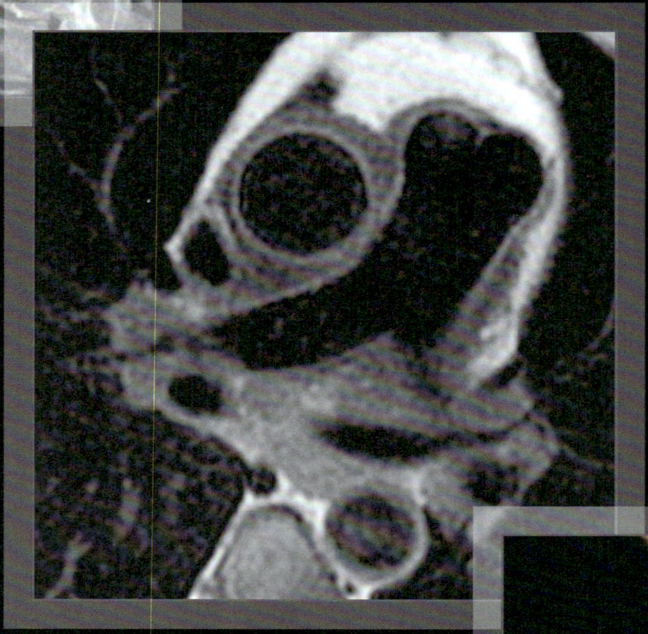

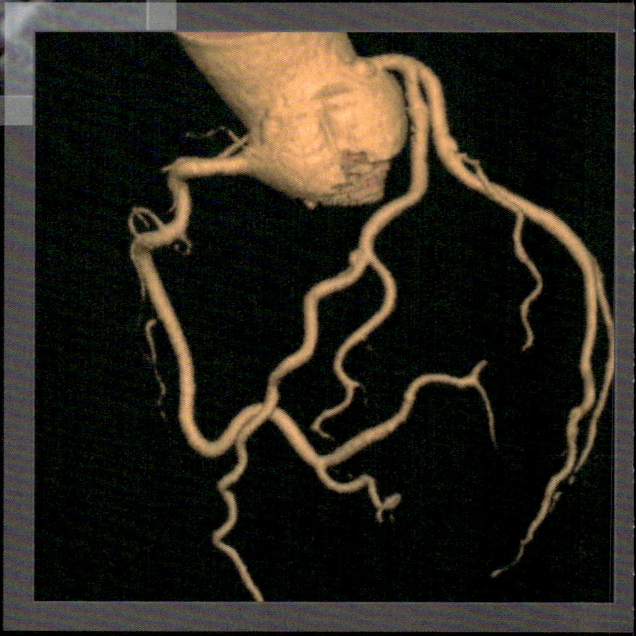

Acknowledgments

LEAD EDITOR
Nina Themann, BA

LEAD ILLUSTRATOR
Richard Coombs, MS

TEXT EDITORS
Arthur G. Gelsinger, MA
Rebecca L. Bluth, BA
Terry W. Ferrell, MS
Megg Morin, BA
Kathryn Watkins, BA

ILLUSTRATIONS
Lane R. Bennion, MS
Laura C. Wissler, MA

IMAGE EDITORS
Jeffrey J. Marmorstone, BS
Lisa A. M. Steadman, BS

ART DIRECTION AND DESIGN
Laura C. Wissler, MA
Cindy Lin, BFA

PRODUCTION EDITORS
Emily C. Fassett, BA
John Pecorelli, BS

ELSEVIER

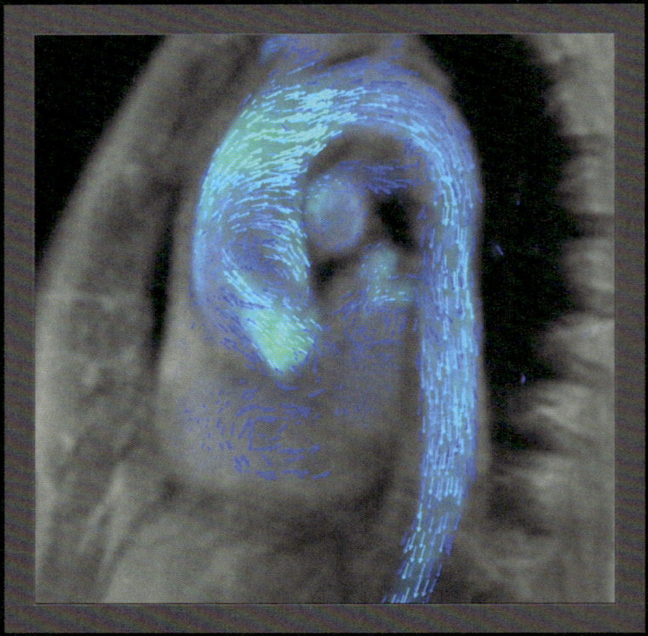

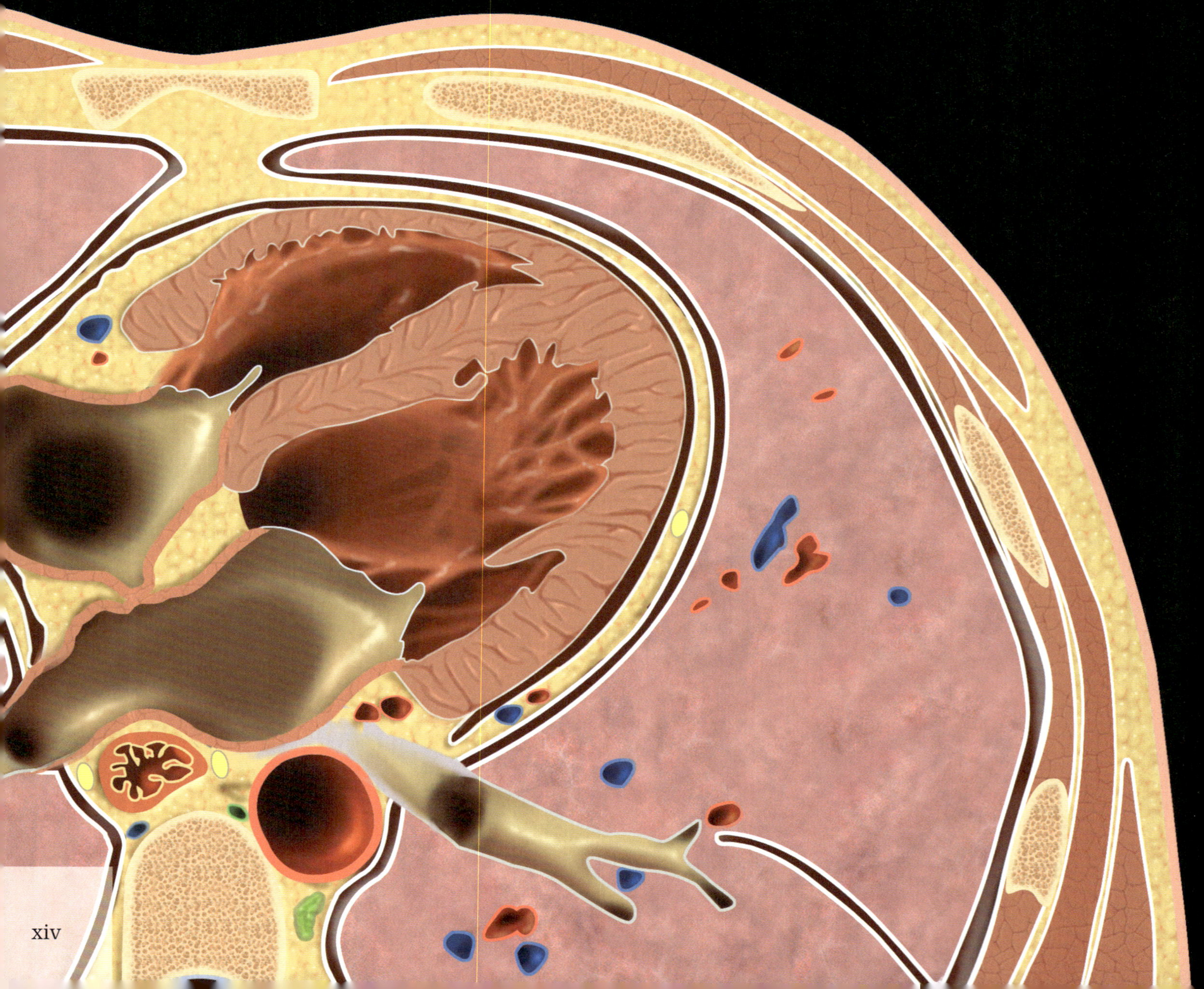

Sections

TABLE OF CONTENTS

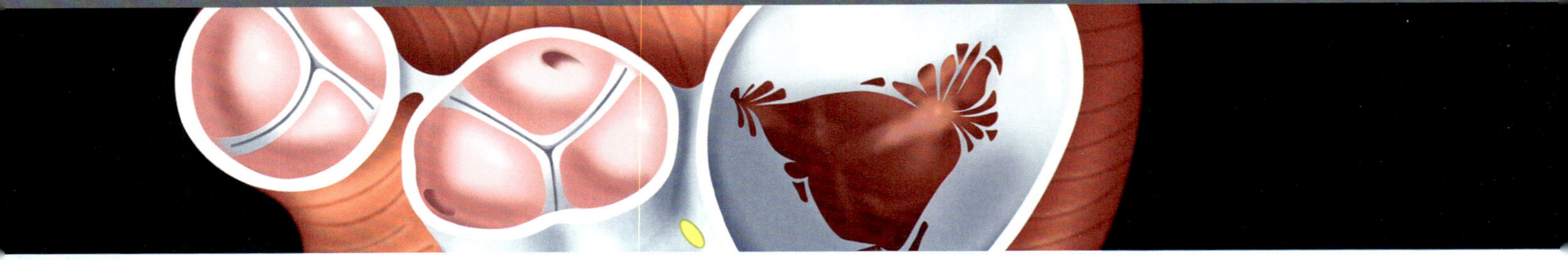

SECTION 1: INTRODUCTION AND OVERVIEW

SECTION 2: CORONARY ARTERY DISEASE

TABLE OF CONTENTS

TABLE OF CONTENTS

TABLE OF CONTENTS

TABLE OF CONTENTS

SECTION 8: INTERVENTIONAL AND ELECTROPHYSIOLOGICAL PROCEDURES

SECTION 9: AORTA

TABLE OF CONTENTS

SECTION 10: PULMONARY ARTERIES

SECTION 11: VEINS

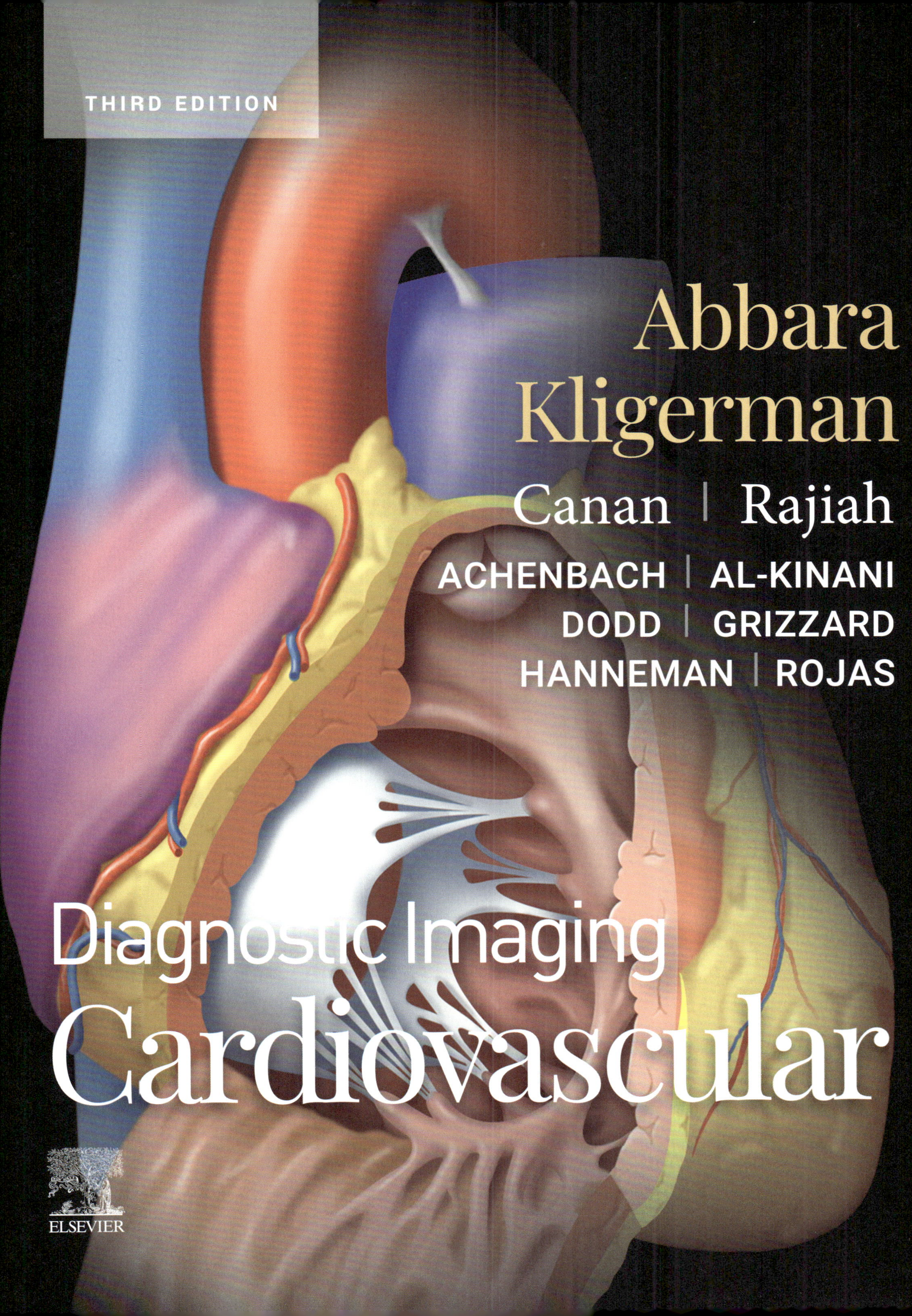

THIRD EDITION

Abbara
Kligerman
Canan | Rajiah
ACHENBACH | AL-KINANI
DODD | GRIZZARD
HANNEMAN | ROJAS

Diagnostic Imaging
Cardiovascular

ELSEVIER

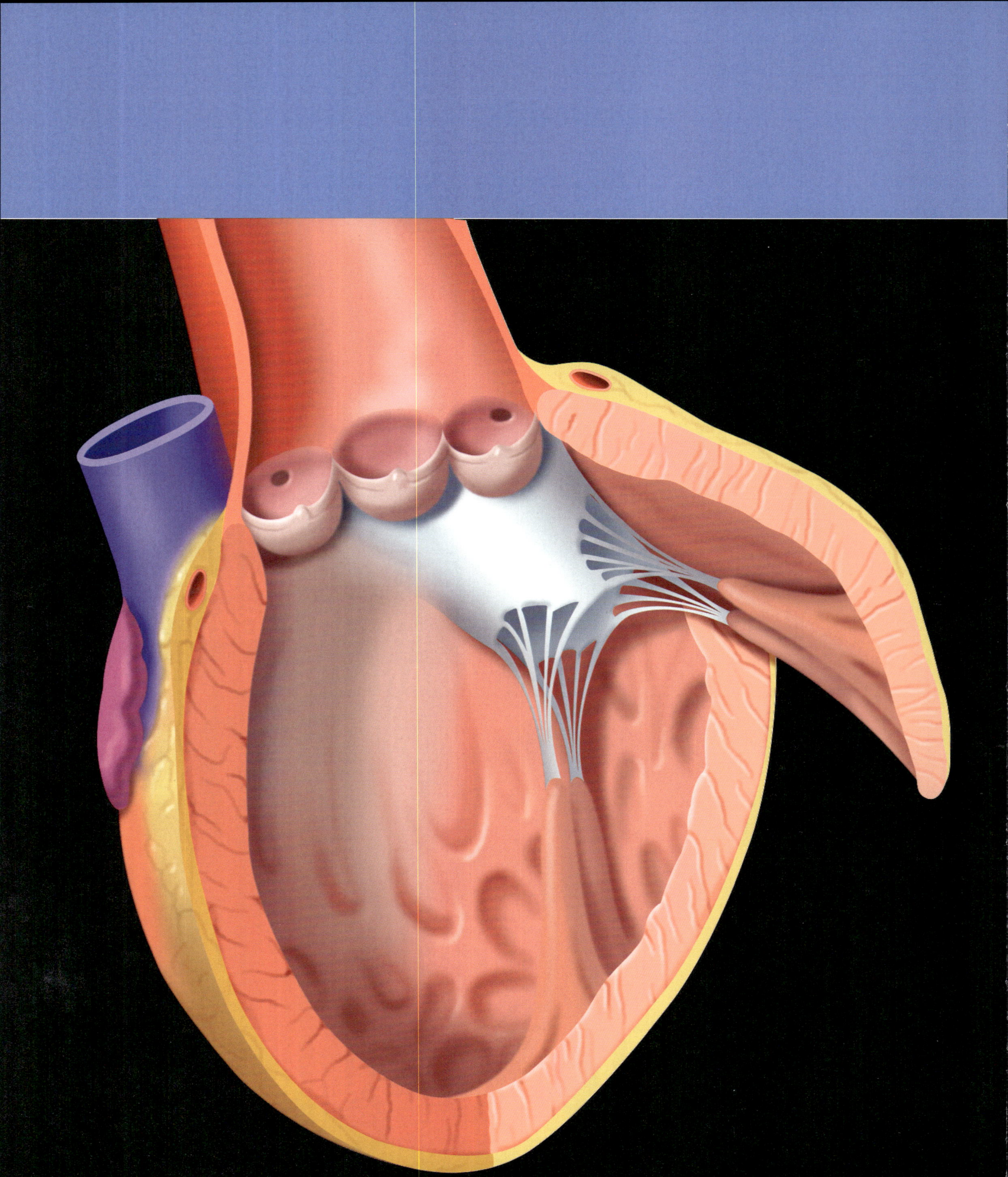

SECTION 1

Introduction and Overview

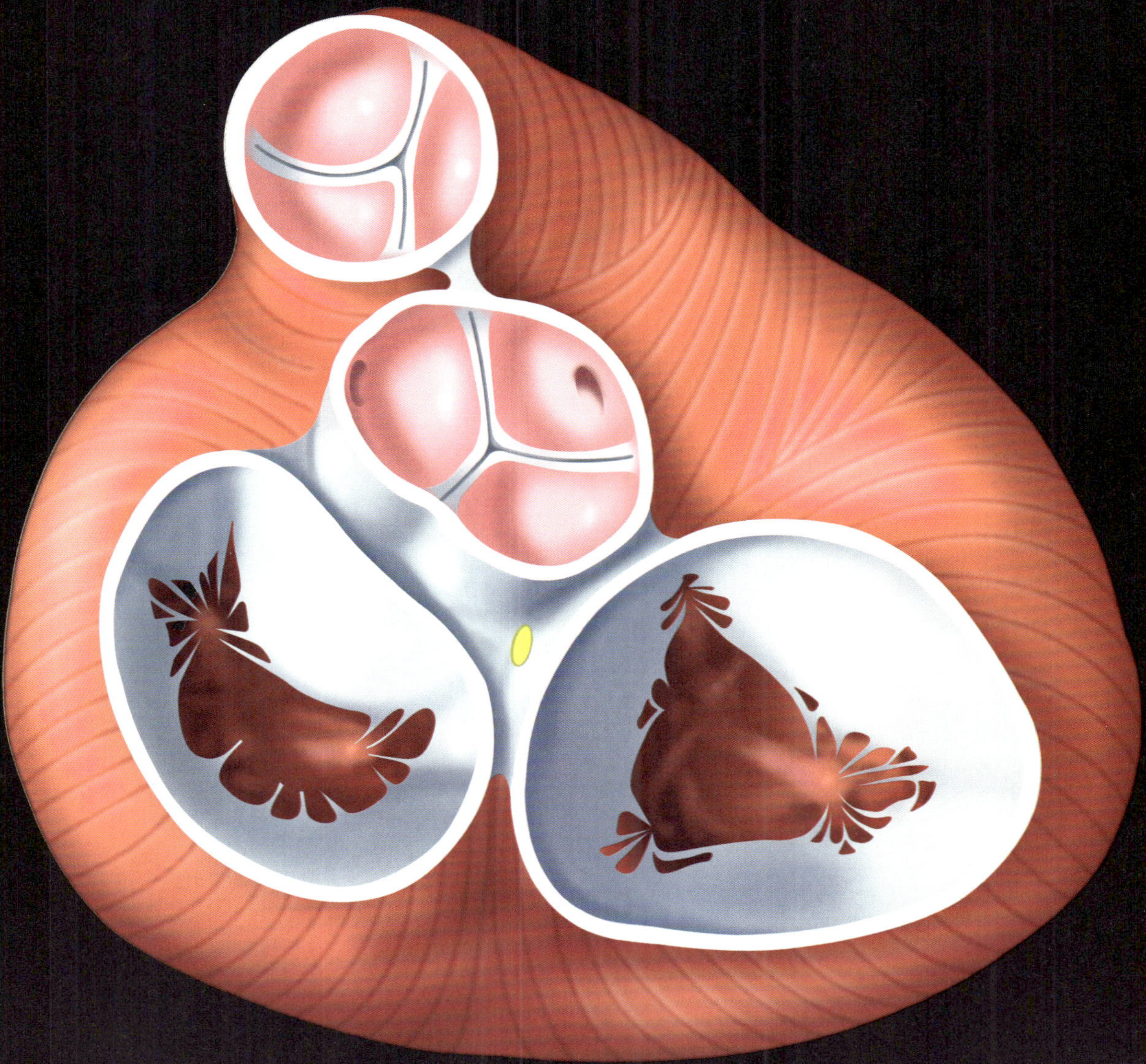

Introduction

Due to the rapid technical evolution of CT, cardiac imaging has become reliably possible, and it is an established tool for the work-up of cardiac disease. Noninvasive coronary CT angiography (CTA) in particular has tremendous clinical potential for detecting or ruling out coronary artery stenoses in some patients. Imaging of cardiac structure and function, potentially even perfusion, can be useful in selected patients. However, the spatial resolution, and especially the temporal resolution, even in the latest scanner generations, still possesses certain restrictions and can lead to artifacts and imaging limitations that must be taken into account during data acquisition and interpretation.

Imaging Protocol

Currently, 64-slice CT imaging is considered the minimum requirement for coronary artery studies. Newer technologies, such as dual-source CT and scanners that allow simultaneous acquisition of 256 or 320 cross sections, provide improved image quality, lower radiation exposure, and imaging with a smaller amount of contrast agent, and they are less susceptible to artifacts.

Patient Preparation

Even slight respiratory motion during data acquisition will cause substantial artifact on cardiac CT. Therefore, patients must be able to follow breath-hold commands and hold their breath for ~ 10 seconds. For most imaging purposes, heart rate should be regular, and if coronary CTA is attempted, heart rate should be < 65 beats/min and, optimally, < 60 beats/min. Patients therefore usually receive preprocedure medication with short-acting β-blockers that can be administered orally ~ 1 hour prior to scanning or intravenously immediately before the scan. In order to achieve coronary dilatation on CTA and thus substantially improve image quality, nitrates should be given to all patients who have no contraindications.

Contrast Injection

For contrast-enhanced imaging of the heart, 50-100 mL of iodine-based high-concentration contrast agent is injected intravenously. Recommended flow rates are 4-7 mL/s, and the contrast bolus should be followed by saline solution or a mixture of saline and contrast to improve right heart visualization. Synchronization of contrast injection and data acquisition can be achieved either through a bolus tracking method or by using a separate "test bolus" acquisition. For visualization of the coronary veins, the delay between contrast injection and the start of image acquisition must be prolonged by ~ 6-10 seconds.

Data Acquisition

Reconstructed images need to be synchronized with the heartbeat, through either retrospective ECG gating or prospective ECG triggering. Retrospectively gated scans are acquired in spiral mode and usually provide for high image quality and flexibility to choose the cardiac phase during which images are reconstructed as well as the ability to reconstruct functional data sets throughout the cardiac cycle in order to analyze cardiac function. To limit radiation exposure, the output of the x-ray tube can be modulated during the acquisition with lower output in systole and higher output in diastole. The most relevant image reconstructions are usually performed in diastole. Prospectively triggered scans are associated with substantially lower radiation exposure. Less flexibility to reconstruct data at different time instants is the trade-off for the advantage of lower dose. Scanners with 16 cm of z-axis coverage allow for the entire heart to be imaged with a single axial rotation. The scan can be acquired for a portion of or for the entire R-R interval, providing data akin to traditional prospective or retrospective studies, respectively.

Image Reconstruction and Post Processing

Although the spatial resolution of coronary CTA is now as low as 0.2 mm with newer scanner technologies, data sets for coronary artery visualization by CT consist of 0.4- to 0.75-mm thick axial slices. Useful postprocessing tools include maximum-intensity projections and multiplanar reconstructions. 3D renderings may be impressive but are not accurate for stenosis detection and play no role in data interpretation.

Coronary CT Angiography

Most cardiac CT investigations are performed to detect or rule out significant coronary artery stenosis. On CT, stenosis severity can appear to be less or more than seen on invasive coronary angiography (ICA); the typical limits of agreement are ~ ± 20%. Thus, stenoses that appear to be < 50% on CT can be assumed to be < 70% on ICA with a very high degree of certainty. In most cases, however, there is a tendency to overestimate the degree of luminal stenosis on coronary CTA as compared with catheter-based ICA.

Coronary CTA has a high sensitivity and a very high negative predictive value for the identification of coronary stenosis. Severe coronary lesions are very infrequently missed, and CTA is extremely reliable to rule out stenosis. Specificity and positive predictive value may be lower due to the tendency to overestimate stenosis and artifacts and because coronary artery stenosis does not always lead to myocardial ischemia.

The very high negative predictive value makes coronary CTA a clinically useful tool in symptomatic patients who have a lower or intermediate likelihood of coronary disease but require further work-up to rule out significant coronary stenoses. This applies both to patients with stable chest pain and to patients with acute chest pain and suspected acute coronary syndrome. Therefore, coronary CTA is listed as a class IA recommendation in the 2021 AHA/ACC chest pain guideline for patients with no known coronary artery disease in both acute and stable chest pain settings. A negative coronary CTA scan will render further testing unnecessary. Indeed, several observational trials have clearly demonstrated that when coronary CTA was negative, symptomatic patients had a very favorable clinical outcome, even without further additional testing, and downstream healthcare costs may be lower than with other diagnostic procedures.

Coronary CT Angiography and Ischemia

Coronary CTA, like ICA, is a purely morphologic imaging modality and cannot demonstrate the functional relevance of stenoses (i.e., ischemia). In the case of lesions with a borderline degree of stenosis, poor correlation of CT findings with myocardial ischemia may limit the clinical application of CTA.

However, CT-based myocardial perfusion and CT-based fractional flow reserve have been shown to be effective to predict ischemia. Based on the anatomic CT data set, computational fluid dynamics are applied to model the flow and resistance pattern and to obtain the fractional flow reserve value for all segments of the coronary artery tree. Recent Coronary Artery Disease Reporting and Data System (CAD-RADS) 2.0 recommends use of CT-perfusion or CT-fractional flow reserve (CT-FFR) to evaluate associated ischemia in patients with 50-90% stenosis or 40% stenosis with high-risk plaque features.

Imaging of Coronary Atherosclerotic Plaque

Coronary Calcification

Using cardiac CT, calcium in the coronary arteries can be detected and quantified in low radiation, nonenhanced image acquisition protocols. Tissue within the vessel wall with a CT number of ≥ 130 Hounsfield units is defined as calcified. For qualification, the Agatston score, which takes into account the area and the CT density of calcified lesions, is used. Coronary calcifications, with the possible exception of calcifications in patients with renal failure, are always due to coronary atherosclerotic plaque. The correlation between calcium and stenosis is poor. The lack of calcium therefore does not reliably eliminate the possibility of coronary artery stenosis in symptomatic individuals. On the other hand, even substantial amounts of coronary calcium are not necessarily associated with the presence of hemodynamically relevant luminal narrowing. Therefore, the detection of coronary calcium alone, even when very pronounced, should not prompt invasive coronary CTA in otherwise asymptomatic individuals. Coronary calcium is associated with individual coronary artery disease risk. In asymptomatic individuals, the absence of coronary calcium is associated with very low (< 1% per year) risk of major cardiovascular events over the next 3-5 years. Note, however, that a significantly increased risk of major cardiac events has been reported in asymptomatic subjects with extensive coronary calcification in numerous trials. For risk stratification, coronary calcium is superior to other measures of risk, such as C-reactive protein or intima-media thickness tests. A potential clinical role of coronary calcium for further risk stratification is assumed for patients who have an intermediate risk, as assessed by traditional risk factors. Coronary calcium imaging therefore can be used when a decision regarding risk-modifying treatment, such as statin therapy, hinges on additional information beyond conventional risk factor analysis. Unselected screening or patient self-referral is not recommended.

Plaque in Coronary CT Angiography

Coronary CTA allows visualization of nonstenotic coronary atherosclerotic plaque if image quality is good. With some limitations, and again under the prerequisite of excellent image quality, plaque quantification and characterization are possible. Some parameters that are readily available from CT might contribute to the detection of vulnerable plaques at an increased risk for near-term rupture. Several studies and data based on large registries have demonstrated a prognostic value of atherosclerotic lesions detected by coronary CTA both in symptomatic and asymptomatic individuals. An analysis of a clinical registry, including > 23,000 patients, confirmed the prognostic value of coronary CTA in cases where the presence of coronary stenoses and the presence of nonobstructive plaque were associated with an increased risk of mortality. However, the hazard ratio for nonobstructive plaque was relatively low (i.e., hazard ratio of 1.6 with a 95% confidence interval of 1.2-2.2). High-risk plaque features, such as low attenuation, positive remodeling, napkin ring sign, and spotty calcification, are also associated with adverse cardiovascular events. A post-hoc analysis of the SCOT-HEART study showed that major cardiovascular events are 3x higher in patients with adverse plaque features compared to ones without adverse plaque.

Noncoronary Cardiac CT

Cardiac CT permits high-resolution functional and morphologic imaging of the heart. Although cardiac CT is most frequently utilized for coronary artery imaging, it can also be useful for other applications. Cardiac CT is highly accurate in assessing left and right ventricular function. Even parameters of diastolic dysfunction can be derived from CT. Clinically, however, it will only be used if echocardiography and MR imaging fail. Morphologic imaging of the heart has applications in congenital heart disease assessing cardiovascular anatomy, vascular pathways, collaterals, and postsurgical complications, such as shunt stenosis or thrombosis.

Another application of major importance is the use of CT imaging in the evaluation of patients who are candidates for transcatheter valve replacement. Although it has started with transcatheter aortic valve replacement (TAVR), nowadays, preprocedural CT is used for transcatheter mitral, pulmonary, and tricuspid valve procedures. CT imaging permits assessment of the femoral and iliac access vessels, and CTA provides detailed measurement of aortic annulus dimensions. In fact, it has been shown that procedure success is increased, and complication rates are reduced when CT imaging is incorporated into the pre-TAVR work-up for prosthesis size selection and identification of suitable candidates. Additional preprocedural indications of cardiac CT include pulmonary vein isolation-ablation, transcatheter left atrial appendage occlusion, and left ventricular scar ablation. Furthermore, cardiac CTA can be used to assess postprocedural complications, such as prosthetic valve dysfunction, thrombus, and device migration.

Interpretation

CAD-RADS was created to provide a standardized method to improve communication between the ordering physician and reading radiologist/cardiologist. It represents the highest-grade coronary artery stenosis detected by coronary CTA, ranging from CAD-RADS 0 to CAD-RADS 5. A plaque (P) component is implemented in CAD-RADS v2 assessing and categorizing overall plaque burden: Mild (P1), moderate (P2), extensive (P3), and very extensive (P4). CAD-RADS categories can be complemented by modifiers to indicate that a study is not fully evaluable (N) or to indicate the presence of high-risk plaque features (HRP) (previously known as vulnerable plaque), ischemia (I), stents (S), grafts (G), and nonatherosclerotic causes of coronary stenosis (E). HRP consist of 2 or more the following features: Positive remodeling, spotty calcification, low attenuation (< 30 HU), and napkin-ring sign. Ischemia can be assessed by using CT perfusion &/or CT-FFR, which are recommended in patients with 50-90% stenosis or 40% stenosis with HRP. It also provides specific recommendations to facilitate further patient management depending on the nature of the chest pain and plaque burden.

Selected References

1. Canan A et al: RadioGraphics update: pictorial guide to CAD-RADS 2.0. Radiographics. 43(4):e220202, 2023
2. Cury RC et al: CAD-RADS™ 2.0 - 2022 coronary artery disease - reporting and data system an expert consensus document of the Society of Cardiovascular Computed Tomography (SCCT), the American College of Cardiology (ACC), the American College of Radiology (ACR) and the North America Society of Cardiovascular Imaging (NASCI). Radiol Cardiothorac Imaging. 4(5):e220183, 2022

CAD-RADS Classification for Patients Presenting With Stable Chest Pain

CAD-RADS	Maximum Stenosis	Interpretation	Further Cardiac Investigation	Management
0	0%: No plaque or stenosis	Absence of CAD	None	Reassurance; consider nonatherosclerotic causes of symptoms
1	1-24%: Minimal stenosis/plaque without stenosis	Minimal stenosis	None	Consider nonatherosclerotic causes of symptoms; P1: Consider risk factor modification and preventive pharmacotherapy; P2: Risk factor modification and preventive pharmacotherapy; P3 or P4: Aggressive risk factor modification and preventive pharmacotherapy
2	25-49% stenosis	Mild stenosis	None	Consider nonatherosclerotic causes of symptoms; P1 or P2: Risk factor modification and preventive pharmacotherapy; P3 or P4: Aggressive risk factor modification and preventive pharmacotherapy
3	50-69% stenosis	Moderate stenosis	Functional assessment	P1, P2, P3, or P4: Aggressive risk factor modification and preventive pharmacotherapy; other treatments (incl. antianginal therapy) should be considered per guideline-directed care; when modifier I+, consider ICA, esp. if frequent symptoms persist after guideline-directed medical therapy
4	A: 70-99% stenosis B: Left main > 50% or 3-vessel disease (≥ 70%)	Severe stenosis	A: Functional assessment or ICA B: ICA is recommended	P1, P2, P3, or P4: Aggressive risk factor modification and preventive pharmacotherapy; other treatments (incl. antianginal therapy and options of revascularization) should be considered per guideline-directed care
5	100%	Total occlusion	ICA &/or viability study	Same as CAD-RADS 4
N	Nondiagnostic study	Obstructive CAD cannot be excluded	Additional evaluation	Additional or alternate evaluation

CAD = coronary artery disease; ICA = invasive coronary angiography.

CAD-RADS Classification for Patients Presenting With Acute Chest Pain

CAD-RADS	Maximum Stenosis	Interpretation	Further Cardiac Investigation	Management
0	0%	ACS highly unlikely	No further evaluation of ACS is required; if Tn (+), consider other sources	Reassurance
1	1-24%	ACS highly unlikely	No further evaluation of ACS is required; if Tn (+), consider other sources of increased troponin	P1 or P2: Referral for outpatient follow-up for risk factor modification and preventive pharmacotherapy; P3 or P4: Referral for outpatient follow-up for aggressive risk factor modification and preventive pharmacotherapy
2	25-49%	ACS unlikely	No further evaluation of ACS is required; if clinical suspicion of ACS is high, Tn (+) or HRP features, consider hospital admission with cardiology consultation	P1 or P2: Referral for outpatient follow- up for risk factor modification and preventive pharmacotherapy; P3 or P4: Referral for outpatient follow-up for aggressive risk factor modification and preventive pharmacotherapy
3	50-69%	ACS possible	Consider hospital admission with cardiology consultation; consider functional assessment	P1, P2, P3, or P4: Preventive management, incl. aggressive preventive pharmacotherapy; when modifier I (+), consider ICA
4	A: 70-99% B: Left main > 50% or 3-vessel > 70%	ACS likely	Hospital admission with cardiology consultation A: Consider ICA or functional assessment; B: ICA is recommended	P1, P2, P3, or P4: Preventive management, incl. aggressive preventive pharmacotherapy
5	100%	ACS very likely	Hospital admission with cardiology consultation; expedited ICA and percutaneous coronary intervention if suspected acute occlusion	Same as CAD-RADS 4
N	Nondiagnostic study	ACS cannot be excluded	Additional or alternative evaluation for ACS is needed	Additional or alternative evaluation for ACS needed

ACS = acute coronary syndrome; CAD = coronary artery disease; ICA = invasive coronary angiography.

Normal Coronary Morphology

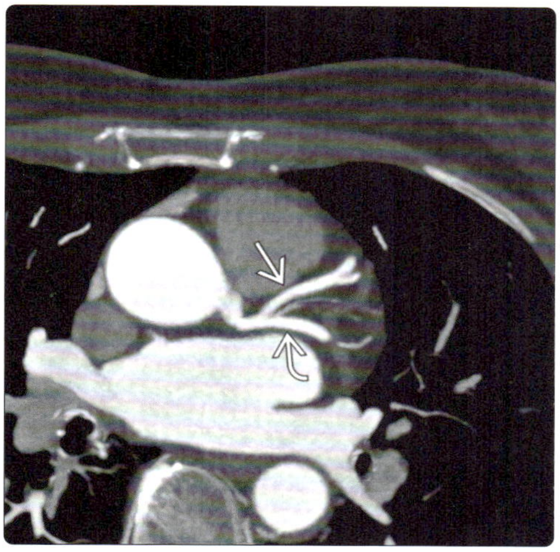

Normal Coronary Morphology

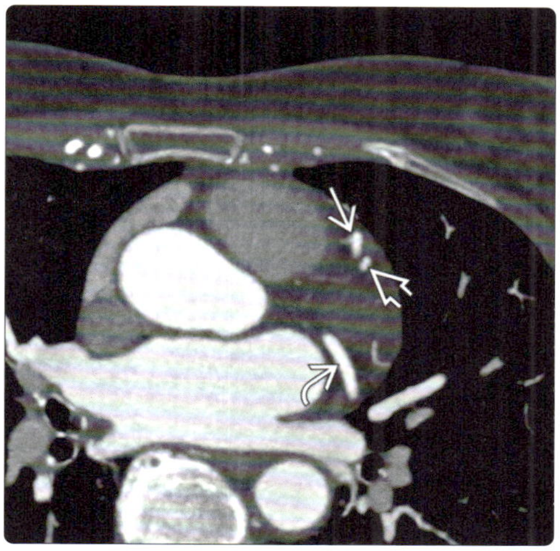

(Left) *Axial cardiac CTA 5-mm MIP at the level of the left main coronary artery shows proximal segments of the left anterior descending coronary artery and left circumflex coronary artery.* **(Right)** *Axial cardiac CTA MIP, several mm more caudally, shows cross sections of the left anterior descending coronary artery , the diagonal branch , and the left circumflex coronary artery .*

Normal Coronary Morphology

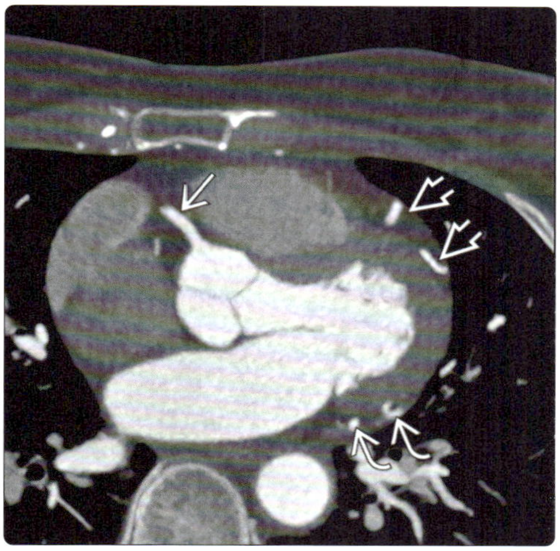

Normal Coronary Morphology

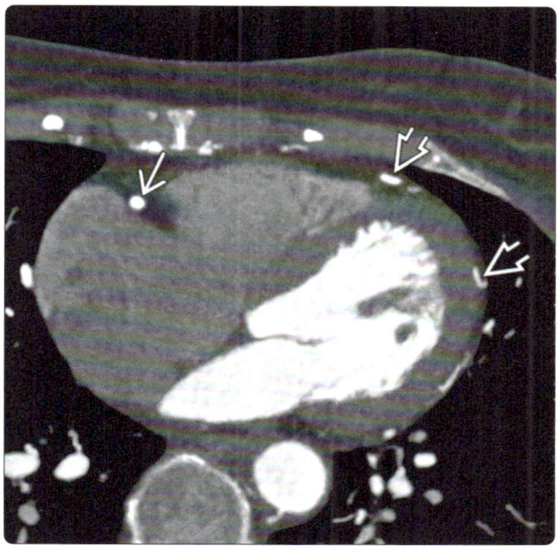

(Left) *Axial cardiac CTA thin MIP at the level of the right coronary ostium shows the proximal right coronary artery . Cross sections of the left anterior descending artery, the diagonal branch , and the left circumflex artery end branches are also seen.* **(Right)** *Axial cardiac CTA at the level of the midright coronary artery shows the right coronary artery in cross section. The end branches of the left anterior descending and left circumflex arteries are also shown.*

Normal Coronary Morphology

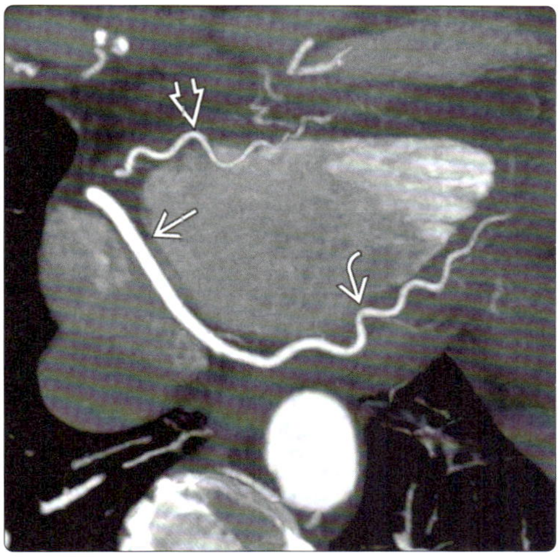

Normal Right Coronary Artery Curved MPR

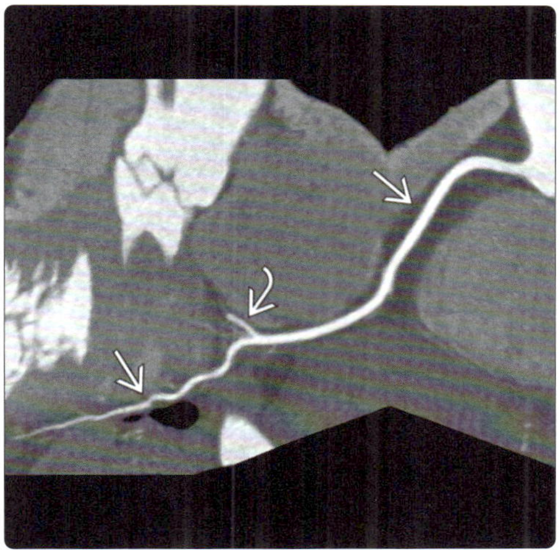

(Left) *Axial coronary CT 7-mm MIP at the level of the heart base shows the distal right coronary artery , the posterior descending artery , and an acute marginal branch .* **(Right)** *Cardiac CT curved multiplanar reconstruction shows the entire course of the right coronary artery with the proximal part of the acute marginal branch .*

Left Anterior Descending Stenosis on Angiography

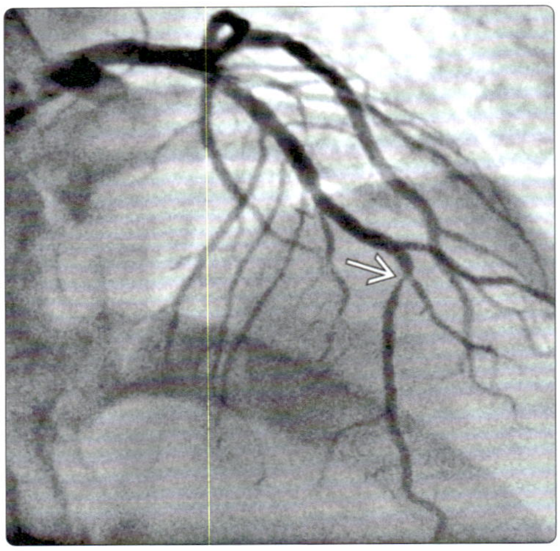

Left Anterior Descending Stenosis on CTA

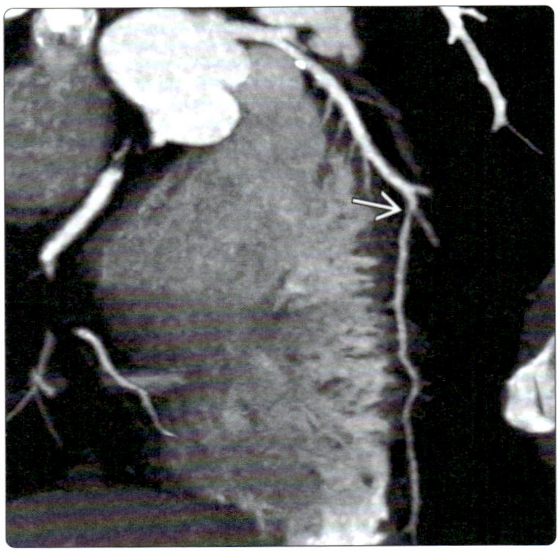

(Left) *Invasive coronary angiography shows a high-grade stenosis* *of the distal left anterior descending coronary artery after the 2nd diagonal branch.* **(Right)** *Coronary CTA curved 7-mm MIP in the same patient shows a corresponding stenosis* *of the left anterior descending coronary artery. Note the absence of calcium at the stenosis site.*

Left Anterior Descending Stenosis on VRT

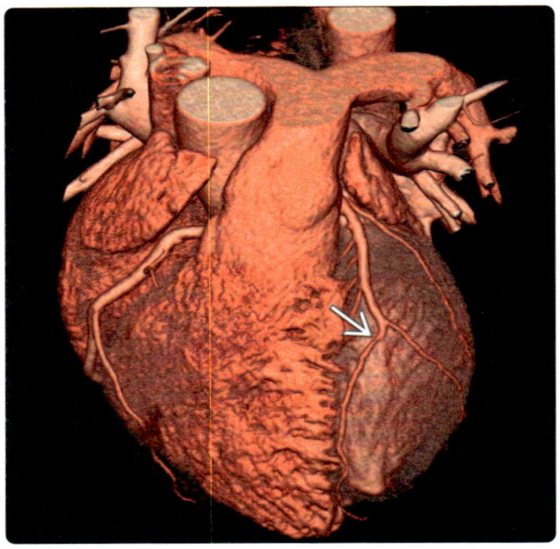

Left Anterior Descending Stenosis on VRT

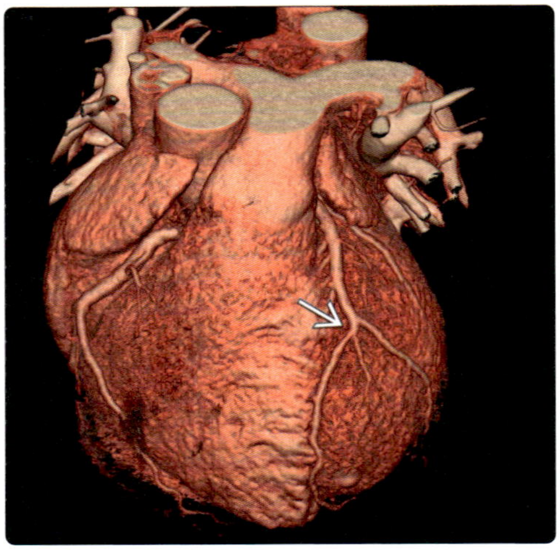

(Left) *High-threshold 3D reconstruction in the same patient shows the stenosis* . *The value of 3D reconstructions for stenosis assessment is extremely limited because the visualization of stenoses depends strongly on the manually chosen window and level settings.* **(Right)** *As this 3D reconstruction shows, the stenosis is not detectable* *with a lower threshold.*

Left Anterior Descending Stenosis on CTA MIP

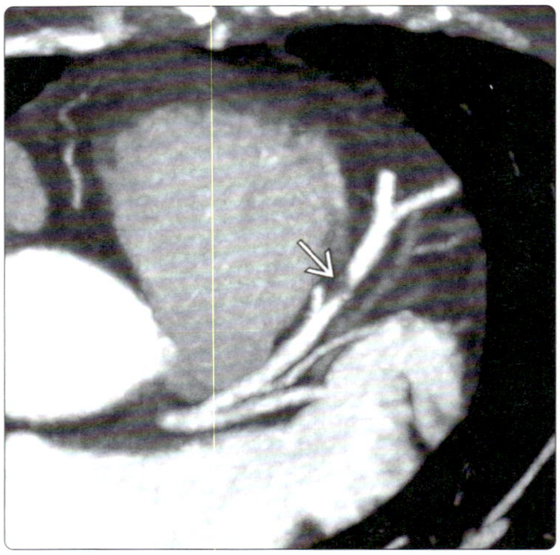

Left Anterior Descending Stenosis on Angiography

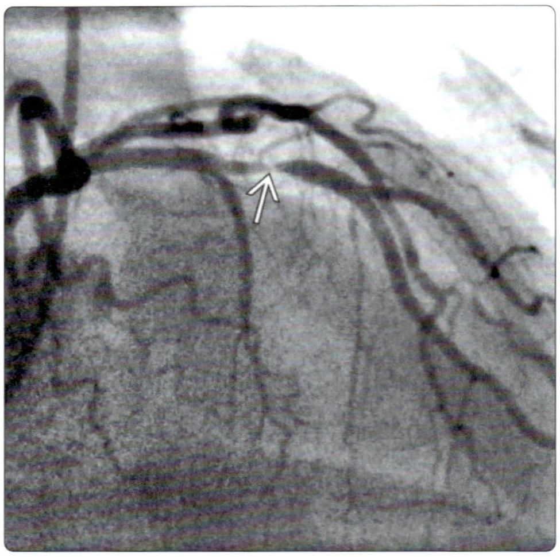

(Left) *Coronary CTA 7-mm MIP of the proximal left anterior descending coronary artery shows typical visualization of a stenosis in the midleft anterior descending coronary artery segment* . *Note the absence of calcium at the stenosis site.* **(Right)** *Invasive coronary angiogram in the same patient can be used to confirm the stenosis* *initially detected in cardiac CTA.*

Left Anterior Descending Stenosis on Curved MPR

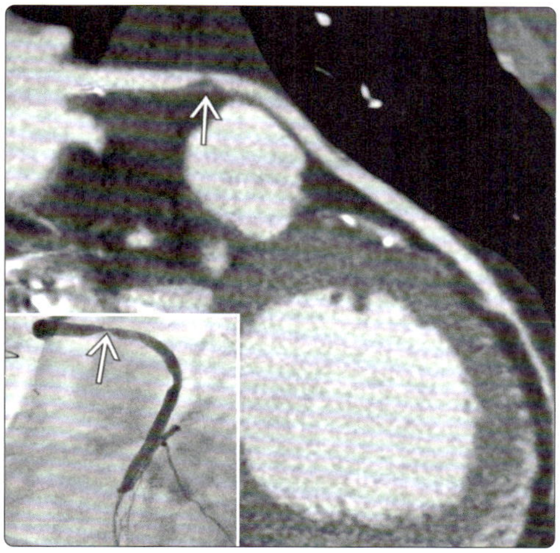

Fractional Flow Reserve CT

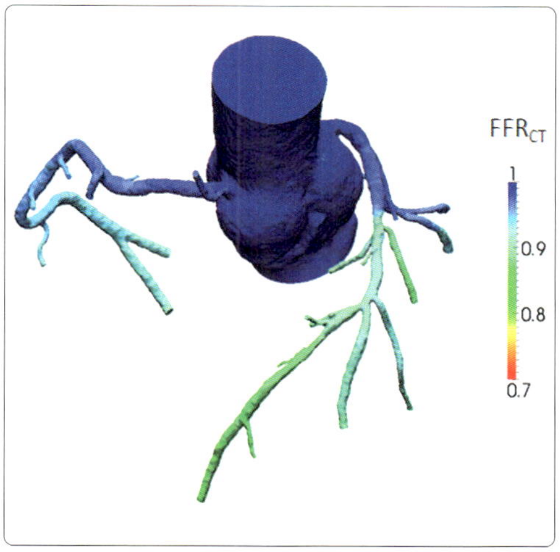

(Left) *CTA curved multiplanar reconstruction shows a venous bypass graft to the left anterior descending coronary artery with a high-grade stenosis* ➡*. Invasive coronary angiography (inset) confirms the high-grade stenosis.* **(Right)** *3D model shows simulated fractional flow reserve within the coronary tree. The color coding represents fractional flow reserve values for the respective coronary artery branch.*

Left Anterior Descending Coronary Calcifications

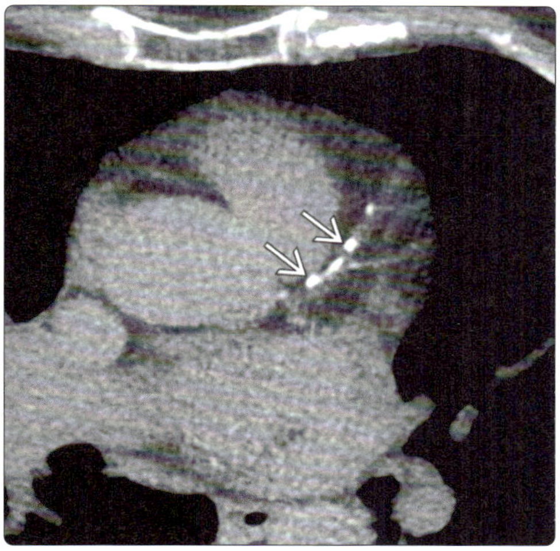

Partially Calcified Plaque

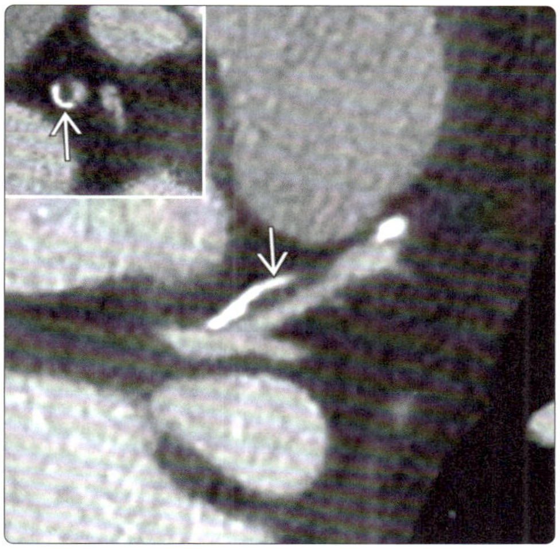

(Left) *NECT demonstrates coronary calcifications* ➡ *of the proximal left anterior descending coronary artery.* **(Right)** *CECT shows noncalcified plaque components. Here, a partially calcified plaque* ➡ *without significant luminal stenosis in the proximal left anterior descending coronary artery is present. The inset shows a cross-sectional view of the lesion. Note the low-attenuation area within the plaque due to noncalcified component.*

Functional Imaging

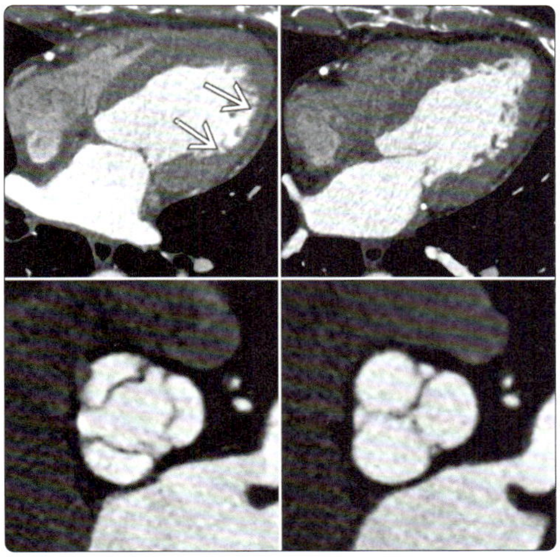

Transcatheter Aortic Valve Replacement

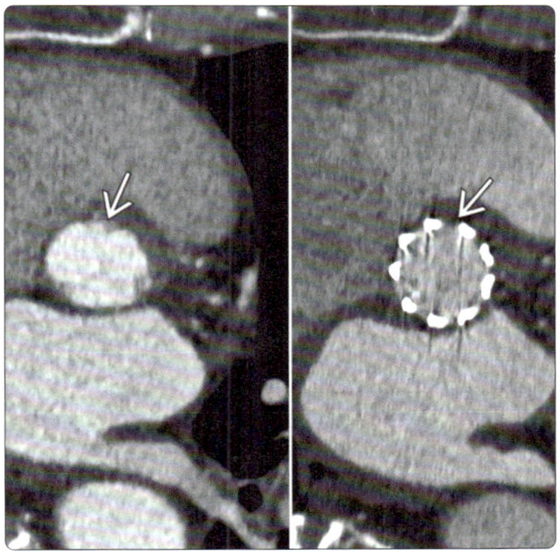

(Left) *Functional imaging via CECT (top) shows left ventricular function with a regional wall motion abnormality* ➡ *(outward motion of the lateral wall) in systole (bottom) and normal function of the aortic valve in systole (left) and in diastole (right).* **(Right)** *Aortic anulus is shown before (left) and after (right) transcatheter aortic valve replacement* ➡*. Note the oval shape prior to transcatheter aortic valve replacement, which becomes round after a valve prosthesis has been placed.*

Introduction

Cardiovascular magnetic resonance (CMR) is an important imaging modality in the evaluation of cardiovascular disorders. There have been substantial recent advances in scanner hardware, coil technology, and pulse sequence design as well as a wealth of accumulating evidence on the benefits of this technique and improved outcomes. CMR provides both morphologic and functional information and is considered the reference standard in the quantification of ventricular volumes and function. Tissue characterization is a major strength of CMR, made possible due to the use of different sequences that highlight different tissue characteristics and intravenous gadolinium-based contrast media.

CMR Techniques

Morphologic Imaging: Black-Blood Imaging

Black-blood imaging can be performed with a single-shot spin-echo sequence (fast spin-echo/turbo spin-echo/HASTE). These still-frame images are rapidly acquired in standard planes (e.g., axial) without the need for breath holding. The repetition time is typically set at 90% of R-R interval and adjusted to null the blood signal. These images are excellent for anatomic depiction of the heart and great vessels.

Higher spatial resolution black-blood images can be obtained by segmented FSE sequence with 1 breath hold per slice. Double inversion recovery (DIR), i.e., initial inversion recovery for entire imaging volume followed by a slice-selective inversion pulse, is used for robust suppression of flowing blood. These can be obtained with T1 or T2 weighting ± fat saturation. These images are used in evaluating morphology, including that of the myocardium, pericardium, and characterization of cardiac masses. T2-weighted images with fat saturation are used to evaluate regional edema in the myocardium (acute myocardial infarction, myocarditis) or arterial wall (arteritis).

T2* imaging using a multiecho gradient recall echo (GRE) sequence is an accurate technique for visualizing and quantifying cardiac iron deposition in iron overload syndromes.

Morphologic Images: Bright-Blood Imaging

Balanced steady-state free precession (bSSFP) is the sequence used for bright-blood imaging, in which the signal depends on T2:T1 ratio with blood appearing bright and the myocardium having an intermediate signal. Images can be rapidly acquired (< 300 ms per image). For morphologic evaluation, bSSFP acquired without breath holding in a single-shot mode in standard orthogonal planes. One image is typically acquired during each heartbeat (at the same cardiac phase). bSSFP sequences are very useful in the evaluation of disorders producing intraluminal abnormalities (aortic dissection).

Cine Imaging

Cine imaging with bSSFP (trueFISP, FIESTA) sequence is the workhorse of CMR with multiple images obtained at a single-slice location during different phases of the cardiac cycle and displayed as a continuous movie loop. Typically, 20-30 frames per cycle are reconstructed. Cine imaging allows qualitative and quantitative evaluation of ventricular volumes, function, thickness, and regional wall motion abnormalities. The standard cine sequence is a segmented, retrospectively ECG gated acquisition in which the data is acquired throughout the cardiac cycle and "time stamped" to allow assignment to the proper cardiac phase. Slices of 6-8 mm thickness are acquired at 10-mm intervals in the short-axis plane from the mitral valve to the apex, and standard long-axis views (2, 3, 4 chamber) are also obtained. A matrix of 256 x 256 is typically used with a spatial resolution of 1.0-1.6 mm and a temporal resolution of < 45 ms. Since the final cine image is obtained by combining data from several heartbeats, the image quality is degraded by patient's heart rate and rhythm.

In arrhythmia, prospective ECG triggering is helpful by acquiring images only for a predetermined length of time from R-wave onset. With irregular cycle lengths, the heart rate changes predominantly affect the length of diastole rather than systole. Since the terminal phase of diastole is not included, measurements of volume and ejection fraction are not accurate. If the arrhythmia is severe, or if breath holding is not possible, cine imaging can be performed in real-time mode, which operates in a single shot rather than a segmented fashion, i.e., all the data is obtained in a single cardiac cycle. The real-time sequence has lower spatial and temporal resolutions than segmented acquisition and may have blurring artifacts. Parallel imaging, compressed sensing, and spatiotemporal redundancies are other techniques used to accelerate MR imaging.

Real-time imaging is also useful in dynamic imaging, such as in the evaluation of ventricular septal changes with inspiration and expiration, which is valuable in the diagnosis of constrictive pericarditis.

Strain Imaging

Strain imaging measures the degree of deformation of a myocardial segment from its initial length. This allows evaluation of regional/segmental myocardial function, which is often abnormal in the early stages of cardiovascular disease before onset of systolic dysfunction. Dedicated sequences for MR strain include myocardial tagging, phase velocity mapping, displacement encoding with stimulated echoes (DENSE), and strain-encoded imaging (SENC). Feature tracking is a novel postprocessing technique that does not need additional sequence but evaluates strain by tracking image features in a routine cine bSSFP sequence.

Velocity-Encoded Phase-Contrast Imaging

In phase-contrast imaging, the signal intensity is dependent on the velocity of the tissue and acquired by sequential application of bipolar magnetic field gradients with opposite polarities. The opposed gradients produce a phase shift in the 1st pulse that is reversed by the 2nd pulse. Hence, stationary spins will have no net phase at the end of the sequence, whereas flowing spins will acquire a net phase shift, dependent on their velocity in the direction of flow-encoding gradients. This sequence can be used to measure velocities, pressure gradients, and flow across valves or shunts. The peak gradient can be calculated from velocity using the modified Bernoulli equation, which is $\Delta P = 4V^2$ mmHg. Flow is simply the sum of the velocities through a given area over time.

4D flow MR refers to a 3D cine (time-resolved) phase-contrast MR with flow encoding in all the 3 directions. Using computational flow dynamics (CFD), shunt, collateral and regurgitant flows can be obtained without dedicated planning, which improves workflow in congenital heart diseases. Advanced parameters, such as flow patterns and shear stress, can be evaluated.

Stress MR

MR perfusion imaging demonstrates contrast media passage during the 1st pass through the myocardium utilizing a heavily

T1-weighted inversion or saturation sequence. Images are obtained at high temporal resolution with multiple slices acquired during each heartbeat. Perfusion imaging can be used to detect myocardial ischemia or microvascular dysfunction. Stress is usually caused by pharmacologic vasodilation (e.g., adenosine or regadenoson) but some centers can perform exercise using an MR compatible ergometer. With adenosine, there is a 4x increase of blood flow downstream of normal coronary arteries, but there is no increase downstream of diseased arteries, which are already maximally vasodilated. Using dual-injection or dual-sequence techniques, myocardial flow can be quantified, which is useful in triple vessel disease and microvascular dysfunction. Perfusion imaging is also useful in the characterization of cardiac masses and intracardiac shunts.

Dobutamine stress MR is useful in evaluating inducible myocardial ischemia with a stress inducible wall motion abnormality in ≥ 1 segment or a biphasic response considered positive. It is useful in triage of intermediate coronary artery disease probability patients for invasive angiography and has a role to assess cardiac prognosis.

Late Gadolinium Enhancement

Late gadolinium enhancement (LGE) sequence is used in characterizing cardiomyopathies and masses as well as evaluating myocardial viability. Both normal and abnormal myocardium enhance immediately after contrast administration, whereas at 10-15 minutes, contrast washes out from normal myocardium, but is retained in a scar or fibrosis, which have a larger extracellular space and volume of distribution of gadolinium. The difference between normal and abnormal myocardium is optimized by using an inversion recovery sequence with GRE or SSFP readout to produce heavy T1 weighting. After magnetization is flipped to 180°, the recovery of magnetization back to baseline depends on the T1 value of tissue with a scar having shorter T1 due to gadolinium uptake, compared to longer T1 of normal myocardium. Timing the image acquisition to the inversion time at which normal myocardium is at the zero-crossing line results in maximum suppression of signal from normal myocardium and maximum conspicuity of the area of scar/fibrosis, which is above the zero-crossing line. This nulling time is obtained by using a T1 scout sequence that obtains low-resolution images at different inversion times. A phase-sensitive sequence maintains differences in magnetization at different inversion times and is not reliant on an accurate inversion time.

A standard LGE sequence can be 2D or 3D, typically acquired every other heartbeat to allow normal myocardial regions to recover longitudinal magnetization before the next inversion pulse is applied. Acquisition over multiple heartbeats takes 8-12 seconds. Single-shot LGE sequence using SSFP IR sequence is an alternative in patients with arrhythmia or poor breath holding, although they have lower contrast:noise ratio and lower sensitivity for detecting a scar. LGE sequence at a long inversion time (550-600 ms) is used in detection of thrombi, which is dark at these long inversion times, whereas masses will have some signal.

Grey or black-blood LGE has a lower signal of blood pool, which improves visualization of a subendocardial scar/fibrosis. Wideband sequence is useful in mitigating high-signal artifacts in patients with implanted cardiac devices.

Early gadolinium enhancement (EGE) is used in the diagnosis of acute myocarditis with high EGE seen in these patients due to capillary hyperemia.

Parametric Mapping

In parametric mapping, each pixel in the image represents a specific magnetic tissue property (T1, T2, T2*) derived from a corresponding set of coregistered CMR source images. T1 and T2 values are obtained by scans at different inversion times and echo times (TE), respectively. T1 mapping can be obtained before ("native") or after contrast. T2 represents decay of traverse magnetization, whereas T2* refers to decay of transverse magnetization in the presence of local field inhomogeneities. Extracellular volume (ECV) can be calculated from T1 maps using the formula (1/T1myo post- 1/T1myo native) / (1/T1blood post- 1/T1blood native) x (100-hematocrit). Synthetic hematocrit from blood T1 can also be used.

Parametric mapping allows visualization and quantification of myocardial processes, which can be intracellular (iron, glycosphingolipid), extracellular (fibrosis, amyloid), or both (myocardial infarction with intra- and extracellular edema). The values can be increased or decreased depending on the disease process, which allows evaluation of even subtle diffuse process. Native T1 also allows tissue characterization without the use of gadolinium contrast. This sequence also allows new endpoints for novel therapeutics.

Angiography

MR angiography is used for evaluation of the vasculature and is typically performed after intravenous administration of gadolinium contrast using a T1-weighted 3D spoiled gradient-echo sequence. Gadolinium shortens the T1 of tissues, and, hence, the vasculature appears bright. By appropriately timing the acquisition such that the center of the k-space is filled when the contrast is in the vessel of interest, a high-quality angiogram can be obtained. High temporal resolution angiography can be obtained by using time-resolved MRA techniques, which involve more frequent sampling of the central K-space compared to the periphery. Using blood-pool agents, such as Ferumoxytol, which have prolonged intravascular stay, allows high-resolution imaging of vasculature without concerns for missing the contrast bolus.

Angiography can also be obtained by using noncontrast MR techniques, such as 3D whole-heart navigator and ECG gated SSFP sequence. This is the primary sequence used in the evaluation of coronary arteries, particularly the proximal segments.

Standard Cardiovascular Magnetic Resonance Examination

CMR examination consists of combination of different sequences that are customized according to the clinical indication. A standard CMR examination includes cine and LGE images in the short- and long-axis planes. A stack of axial morphological dark- and bright-blood images are also obtained throughout the chest.

Selected References

1. Rajiah PS et al: Cardiac MRI: state of the art. Radiology. 307(3):e223008, 2023
2. Messroghli DR et al: Clinical recommendations for cardiovascular magnetic resonance mapping of T1, T2, T2* and extracellular volume: a consensus statement by the Society for Cardiovascular Magnetic Resonance (SCMR) endorsed by the European Association for Cardiovascular Imaging (EACVI). J Cardiovasc Magn Reson. 19(1):75, 2017

Suggested Protocols by Indication

Indication	Left Ventricle Structure/Function Cines	LGE	Morphologic Images	Perfusion Images	Other Modifications	Parametric Mapping
Infarct (chronic)	Standard	Standard: To evaluate viability	Optional	Optional: Peri-infarct ischemia	LGE at long inversion time for thrombus	
Infarct (acute)	Standard	Standard	T2: Myocardial edema, area at risk	To look for microvascular obstruction	LGE at long inversion for thrombus	
Ischemic heart disease	Standard (may perform after stress perfusion)	Done after rest perfusion images		Stress, followed by rest at 10 minutes		
Cardiomyopathy	Standard	Standard: Set to null myocardium		Not required; hypertrophic cardiomyopathy patients may show abnormal perfusion	Abnormal T1 kinetics in amyloidosis	Native T1, T2, postcontrast T1, extracellular volume
Myocarditis/ sarcoidosis	Standard	Standard: Set to null myocardium	T2: Myocardial edema	Not required	Early-enhancement imaging for capillary hyperemia	Native T1, T2, postcontrast T1, extracellular volume
Arrhythmogenic cardiomyopathy	Standard + stack of right ventricular horizontal long-axis cines of right ventricle	Standard: Set to null myocardium; inversion time for right ventricle is 20-30 s earlier than left ventricle	Evaluation for fat is no longer necessary	Not required	LGE also in right ventricular horizontal long axis for right ventricle scar	
Iron overload syndromes	Standard	Standard: Set to null myocardium	Multiecho short-axis GRE images to evaluate T2*	Not required	Postprocessing allows calculation of T2* from multiecho GRE sequence	T2* mapping: Optional native T1 mapping
Valvular disorders	Standard + high-resolution cine images through affected valve	Standard: Set to null myocardium	Aorta should be evaluated in patients with aortic valve pathology	Not required	2D phase contrast through affected valve or 4D flow through heart and aorta	Native T1, postcontrast T1, extracellular volume for fibrosis
Congenital heart disease	Standard + stack of 4-chamber and short-axis cine images through atria	Standard: Set to null myocardium	Axial, sagittal, and coronal single-shot images throughout chest	May be helpful in demonstrating shunts	2D phase contrast depending on clinical indication or 4D phase contrast through heart and aorta	
Mass	Standard	Tailored to mass	T1 and T2 images often helpful with fat suppression as needed	Very helpful in assessing lesion vascularity	LGE, long inversion for thrombus	Native T1, T2, postcontrast T1, extracellular volume, diffusion
Pericardium	Standard + real-time cine images of septum for ventricular interdependence	Standard: Set to null myocardium; pericardial enhancement in inflammation	FSE images may show pericardial thickening more clearly than HASTE or SSFP images; T2 images for pericardial edema	Not required	Tagged images may confirm abnormal adherence of pericardial layers 3D T1W volumetric images for pericardial edema/inflammation	Optional if myocardial assessment is required

Two-Chamber Image Planning

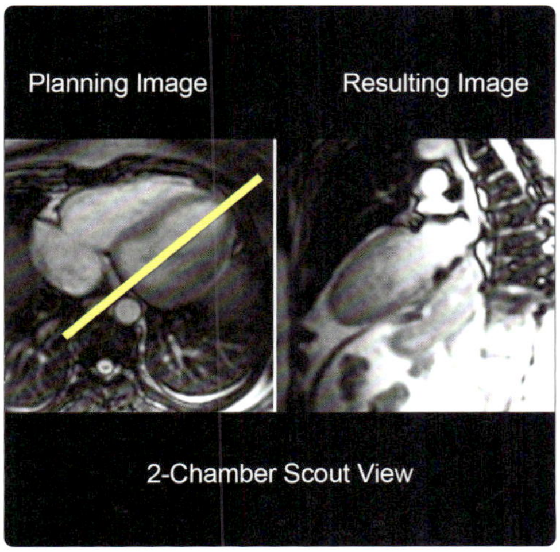

Four-Chamber Image Planning

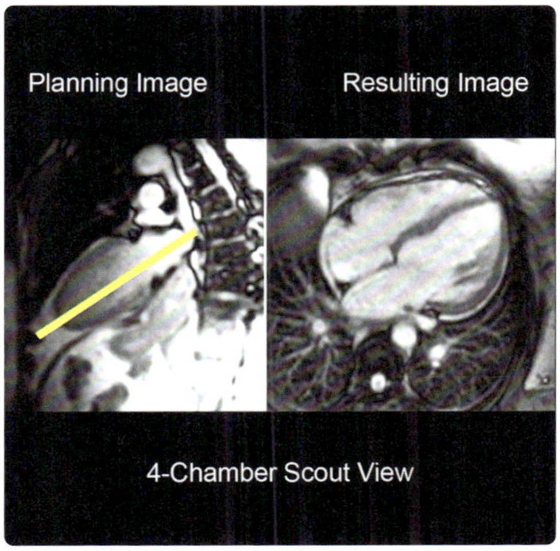

(Left) *Axial low-resolution SSFP scout image is used to begin CMR planning. To acquire the 2-chamber long-axis scout image, a line is placed bisecting the left ventricular (LV) apex and the mitral valve.* **(Right)** *Vertical long-axis (2-chamber) SSFP scout image is then used to obtain the 4-chamber scout image. The imaging plane is acquired by placing a line paralleling the long axis of the LV through the LV apex and left atrium, as shown. This results in the low-resolution 4-chamber SSFP scout image.*

Short-Axis Image Planning

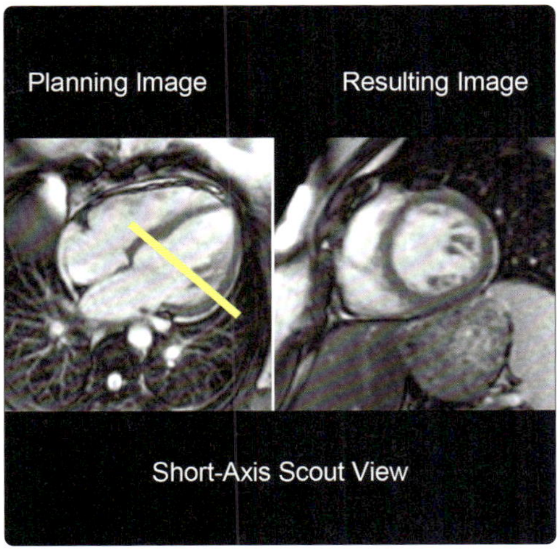

Short-Axis Cine Image

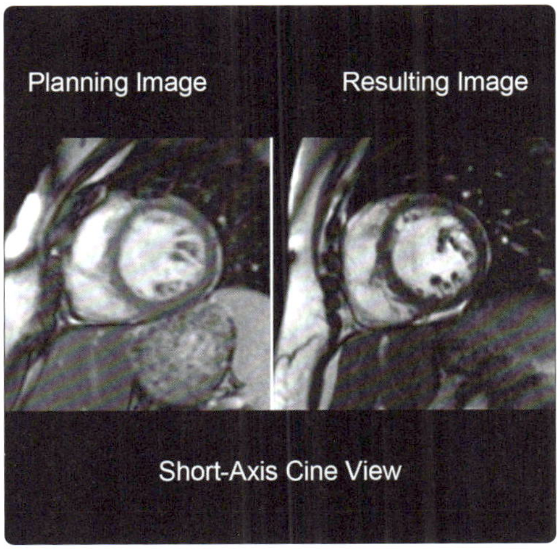

(Left) *Four-chamber SSFP scout image is used to obtain the short-axis scout image for planning the stack of short-axis cine images. The imaging plane is placed perpendicular to the septum and the lateral wall and parallels the mitral valve, as shown.* **(Right)** *Short-axis SSFP scout image is then copied to the standard, high-resolution cine SSFP technique after assuring that no wrap artifact has been produced and that the image is appropriately centered.*

Short-Axis Stack Planning

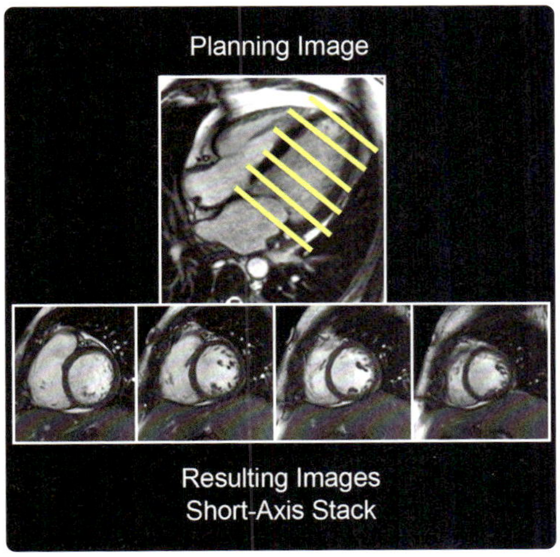

Three-Chamber Image Planning

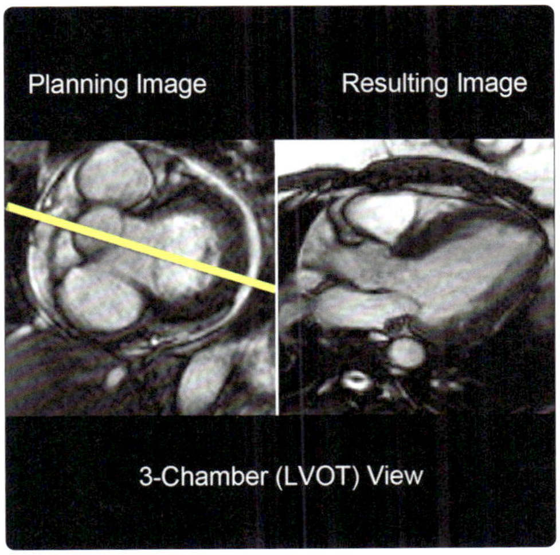

(Left) *Stack of short-axis SSFP cine MR images is then acquired from the mitral valve plane through the LV apex using their positions on the 4-chamber view to assure proper coverage. A diastolic image is used for planning as the plane of the mitral valve may move toward the apex in systole.* **(Right)** *Short-axis SSFP cine MR is used to plan the 3-chamber or LV outflow tract view (LVOT) by placing an imaging plane through the mitral valve and aortic valve, as seen on the basilar short-axis view.*

(Left) *Short-axis cine MR is used to plan the high-resolution 4-chamber cine MR by placing a line through the basal septum that is roughly perpendicular to the septum and parallel to the inferior margin of the heart. Care should be taken to avoid the inferior aspect of the aortic valve, which can be confused with a septal defect if included.* **(Right)** *Short-axis cine MR is used to plan the 2-chamber view by placing an imaging plane to bisect the anterior and inferior LV walls.*

Four-Chamber Image Planning

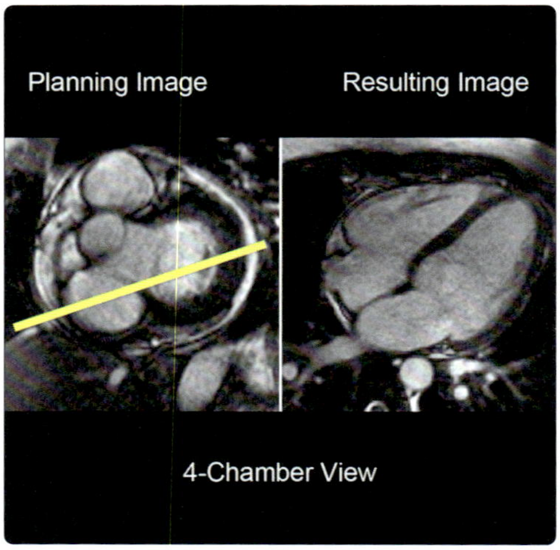

Two-Chamber Image Planning

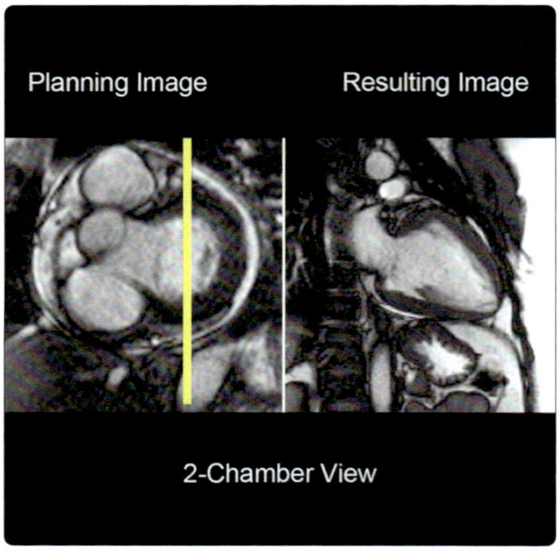

(Left) *Axial double inversion-recovery FSE (HASTE) MR in a patient with D-transposition with a systemic right ventricle shows the resultant right ventricular hypertrophy ➙. Note the excellent depiction of the myocardium and vessels.* **(Right)** *Axial SSFP single-shot MR in a patient with type A aortic dissection shows the intimal flap in the ascending ➙ and descending ➙ aorta. Note also the excellent delineation of the right inferior pulmonary vein ➙.*

Black-Blood Image

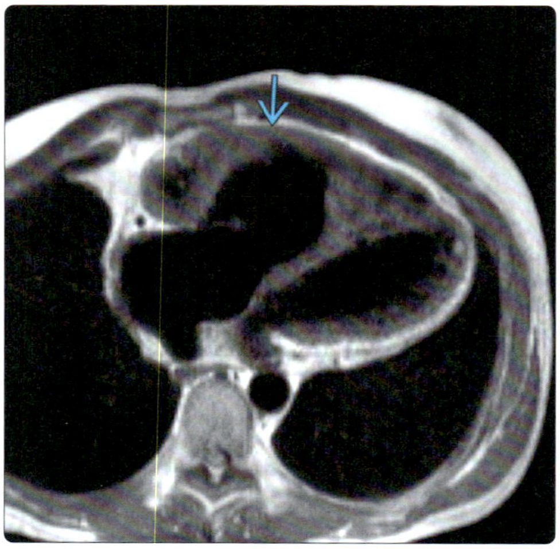

SSFP Image

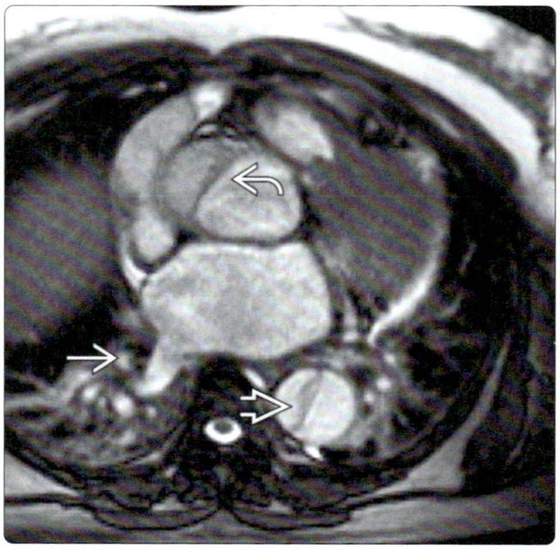

(Left) *Short-axis T1 FSE MR shows a left atrial myxoma ➙ centered in the fossa ovalis and protruding into both atria.* **(Right)** *Short-axis T2 FSE MR of the myxoma ➙ shows that it is hyperintense, indicative of its gelatinous composition. Note that this ECG gated technique results in high-resolution motion-free images that provide tissue characterization.*

Black-Blood Image in Cardiac Mass

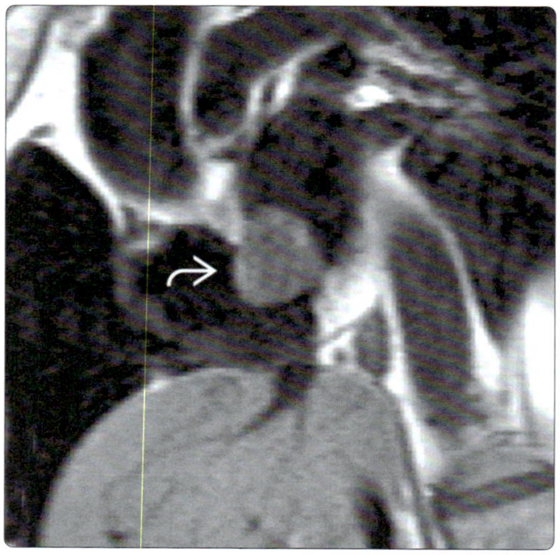

T2 FSE MR for Cardiac Mass

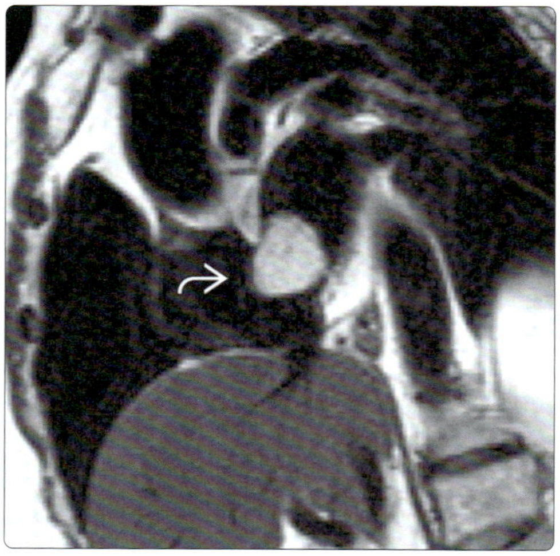

SSFP Cine Imaging

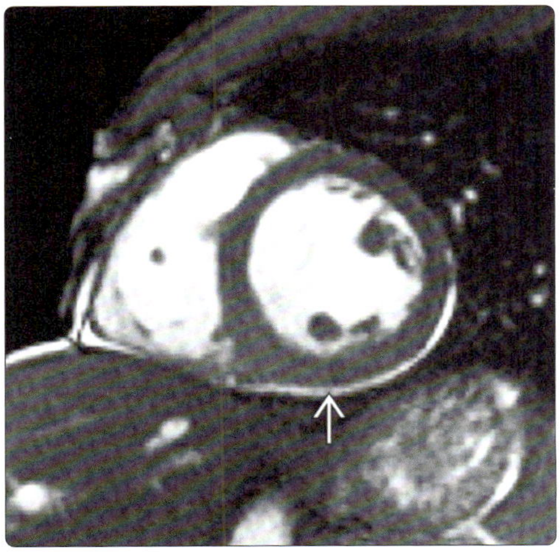

T2 FSE MR

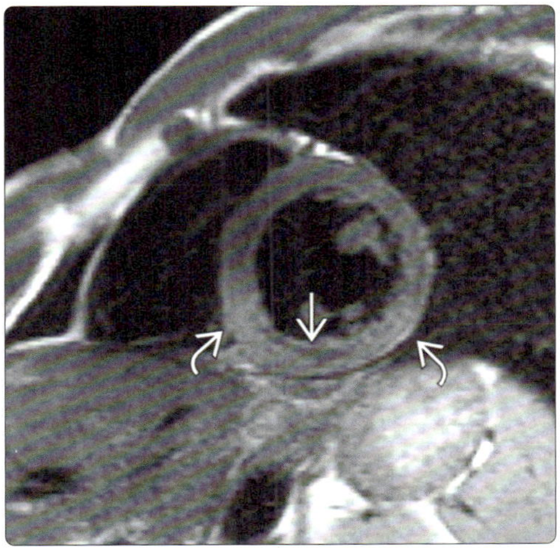

(Left) *LV short-axis SSFP cine MR in diastole shows minimal thickening of the inferior wall due to acute myocardial infarction (MI) →. The sequence shows clear contrast between the myocardium and the blood pool, facilitating volumetric analysis. Also note the subtle signal increase of the inferior wall due to edema.* **(Right)** *LV short-axis T2 FSE MR of an acute inferior MI shows increased signal in the area of infarction ↷. Note the area of decreased signal centrally → due to intramural hematoma.*

LGE MR

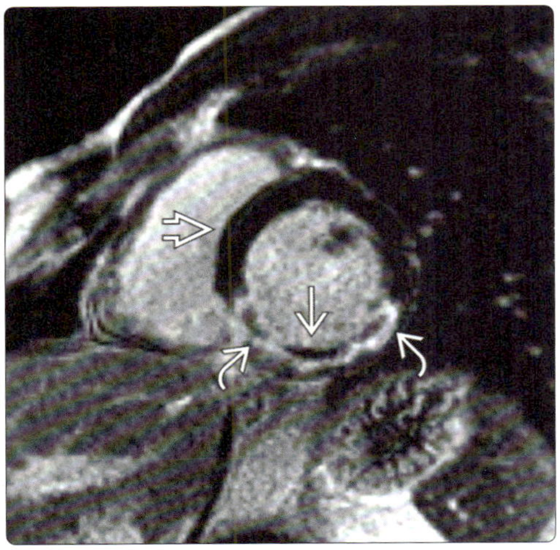

1st-Pass Perfusion MR

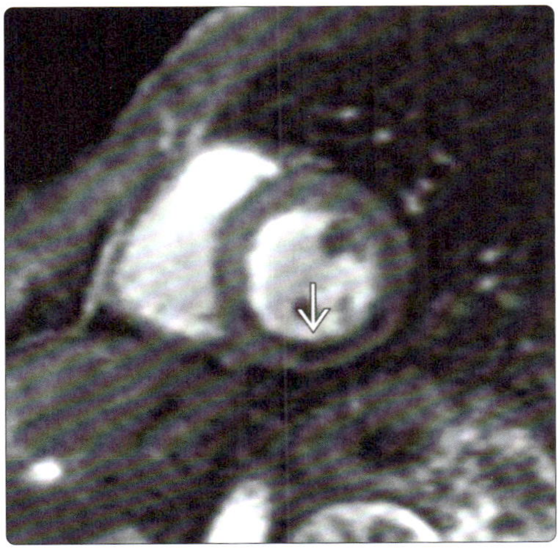

(Left) *LV short-axis LGE MR of a large inferior MI shows that the infarct is demonstrated as an area of increased signal intensity ↷, while the normal myocardium has very low signal ⇨. The low-signal foci within the area of infarction represent regions of hemorrhagic necrosis and are termed no-reflow zones or microvascular obstruction →.* **(Right)** *LV short-axis MR perfusion image of a large inferior MI shows diminished contrast uptake in the inferior wall → due to microvascular obstruction.*

LGE MR: Long Inversion Time

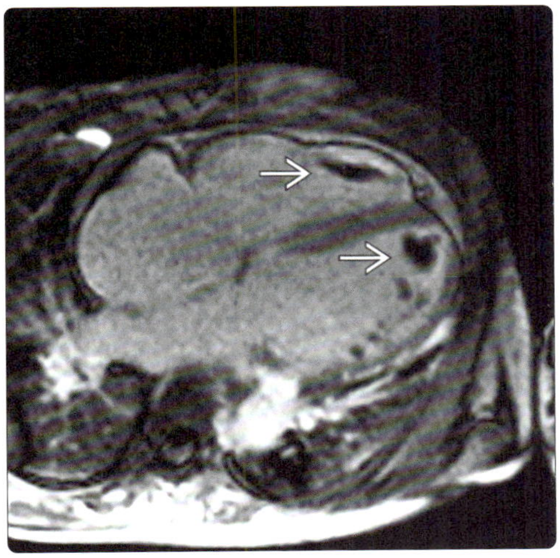

Phase-Contrast Flow Imaging

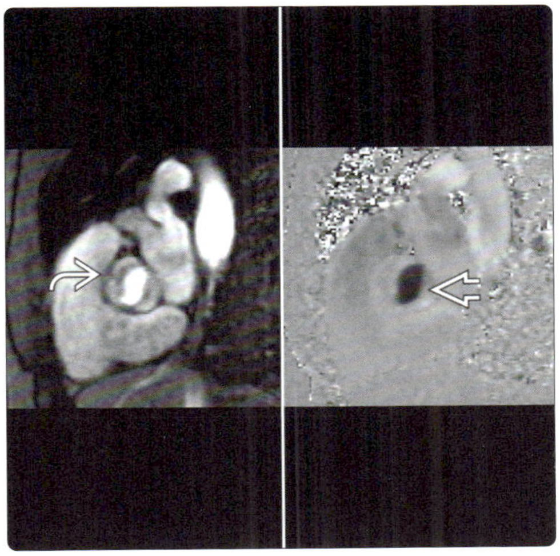

(Left) *Four-chamber LGE MR using a long inversion time (600 ms) demonstrates nonenhancing thrombi → present in both ventricles. This sequence is often helpful in characterizing thrombi, which can have a confusing etched appearance on standard LGE images.* **(Right)** *Short-axis velocity-encoded phase-contrast MR of a bicuspid aortic valve shows good delineation of the valve morphology on the magnitude image ↷, while the phase image ⇨ allows gradient and flow calculation.*

Introduction

Multimodality cardiovascular imaging is essential in the diagnosis and management of a variety of cardiovascular diseases. The development and increased adoption of cardiac computed tomography (CCT), cardiac magnetic resonance (CMR), single-photon emission computed tomography (SPECT) with a new generation of cameras, and positron emission tomography with CT attenuation correction (PET/CT) has enhanced our capabilities to evaluate many forms of cardiovascular disease. Concerning coronary artery disease (CAD) (which is the most prevalent form of cardiovascular disease), imaging can now assess a broad spectrum of diseases, ranging from the detection of preclinical atherosclerosis to advanced assessment of myocardial blood flow and viability. However, the availability of multiple testing options makes it more challenging for clinicians to select the best test for a given patient. Although the multimodality cardiac imaging approach is vital for assessing cardiomyopathies, cardiac masses, and infective endocarditis, these cases are discussed in other documents. Here, we will focus on the application of multimodality imaging in evaluating patients with known or suspected CAD and briefly review its use in valvular heart disease.

Assessment of Patients With Suspected Coronary Artery Disease

The initial approach in patients without previously diagnosed CAD relies primarily on whether they have symptoms of possible ischemic heart disease and how the results of the test may impact their management.

Asymptomatic Patients

In asymptomatic patients who do not have known CAD, routine testing is not recommended irrespective of the type of test being considered. In those who are not on any medical therapies, selective use of coronary artery calcium (CAC) testing may be considered, particularly if there is uncertainty regarding a patient's risk or the role of stain therapy. Studies have shown that the detection of coronary plaque by CAC testing is associated with intensification of both lifestyle and medical therapies.

In selected high-risk, asymptomatic patients, silent ischemia may be present; however, it is unclear if the detection of ischemia in such patients leads to any improvement in outcomes. Risk factors for silent ischemia include older age and longstanding diabetes.

Symptomatic Patients

In low-risk symptomatic patients, exercise treadmill testing (ETT), stress echocardiography, or CAC testing can all be considered if there is a need for further testing. However, there are also various emerging studies that suggest that it may be safe to defer testing in low-risk patients who have stable symptoms, especially if these are nonanginal symptoms, where the likelihood of finding any significant disease is low.

In intermediate- to high-risk patients, either anatomic testing with coronary CTA or functional testing approaches may be selected. The choice of testing will depend on local availability and expertise, the likelihood of obtaining diagnostic image quality with each test, and the anticipated impact of the test result on patient management. Patients who are not on any medical therapies may benefit from coronary CTA (or hybrid PET/CT or SPECT/CT) since the diagnosis of plaque may impact the use of downstream medical therapies and, subsequently, outcomes. On the other hand, patients who have contraindications to CTA (e.g., severe contrast reaction) should be evaluated with a functional imaging test. In patients who are already on medical therapy, functional testing may also be preferred if the main clinical question is whether there is a role for invasive angiography or coronary revascularization. In such cases, information regarding exercise capacity and exercise-induced symptoms may also be helpful in determining the potential benefit of coronary revascularization.

Assessment of Patients With Known Coronary Artery Disease

In patients with known CAD, the main clinical question is often whether they require coronary revascularization procedures. Functional testing that quantifies ischemia is preferred in this setting.

PET Myocardial Perfusion Imaging

- Offers robust attenuation correction and ability to quantify absolute myocardial blood flow (MBF)
- PET has higher diagnostic accuracy than SPECT and may be particularly useful in patients who have multivessel disease, as SPECT myocardial perfusion imaging (MPI) may underestimate severity or extent of ischemia
- When PET is used, data on MBF reserve (MBFR) adds additional prognostic value and can be used to rule out high-risk anatomy
- Specifically, normal MBFR has high negative predictive value for excluding left main or 3-vessel obstructive CAD
- Notably, information on MBFR can only be obtained during vasodilator testing
- Main limitation: Not widely available

Cardiac MR

- Accurately detects ischemia using dynamic 1st-pass perfusion imaging
- Contractile reserve can be evaluated using dobutamine MR
- Late gadolinium enhancement (LGE) can be used to evaluate for myocardial viability based on extent of scarring
- Based on patterns of LGE, cardiomyopathies can be characterized

SPECT MPI

- Widely available and can be performed during exercise or vasodilator testing
- Accuracy may be reduced in patients with multivessel disease

Coronary CTA

- Has more limited role in patients who have known CAD, particularly as native coronary arteries are more likely to have significant coronary calcifications, which may limit ability to visualize vessel lumen
- Select role in evaluating proximal large stents (≥ 3 mm in diameter)
- In patients who have undergone prior revascularization, 2 potential indications for coronary CTA exist: Evaluating proximal large stents (≥ 3 mm in diameter) and bypass grafts; development of photon-counting CT has improved image quality in patients with stents, high calcium burden or previous revascularization

Exercise Tolerance Test

- Limited by low accuracy to detect ischemia and not useful in quantifying amount of ischemia
- However, advantages include useful prognostic information, providing data on patient's functional capacity, as well as whether they develop any significant symptoms during exercise

Additional Considerations for Various Testing Strategies

Below are more specific details on various testing options, which may be useful to understand when selecting among different choices.

Exercise Testing

- ETT, stress echocardiography, SPECT MPI, and some forms of PET can be performed with exercise
- Advantages: Provide data on exercise capacity, blood pressure, and heart rate response to exercise and development of symptoms and electrocardiographic (ECG) changes with exercise
- Information on exercise capacity and symptoms may be useful when deciding on role of coronary revascularization, and thus combining data from ETT with other tests that are not performed during exercise may be beneficial
- e.g., may be useful to combined data from CTA or CAC with ETT, or, in some cases, PET or CMR with ETT

SPECT/PET

- Data derived from MPI include extent and severity of ischemia and size of infarction
- Left ventricular volumes and function can also be calculated
- Added benefit of improved spatial resolution and improved sensitivity compared to SPECT
- Furthermore, since most PET cameras also have hybrid CT, coronary calcium score can be calculated, thus providing information on burden of atherosclerotic disease
- Finally, quantification of myocardial blood flow at peak stress and rest and their ratio (MBFR) can be derived from PET/CT

Coronary CTA

- Utilization in initial assessment of patients with suspected CAD should be considered for patients at intermediate to high risk with adequate renal function who can follow breath-holding instructions
- Advantages include fast acquisition of images delineating not only anatomy of coronary tree, but also location, extent, and severity of coronary plaque
- Combination of coronary CTA (CCTA) with functional evaluation of moderate to severe stenoses using CT-based fractional flow reserve (CT-FFR) or artificial intelligence ischemia analysis (AI-IA) has been validated in a few clinical trials and registries
- Use of CT-FFR or AI-IA may increase in future, and several large comparative effectiveness studies are underway
- Functional evaluation can also be performed by using CT perfusion, which involves acquisition of images at rest and after pharmacologic stress

Stress CMR

- May be compelling in young patients in whom there is desire to avoid radiation, e.g., premenopausal women
- Usually done in combination with vasodilator or dobutamine stress testing
- MR-compatible ergometers are available in selected institutions
- In addition to assessing for presence and extent of perfusion defects, stress CMR can also provide information on left and right ventricular size and function, as well as presence of myocardial edema (via T2 imaging or T2 mapping), or myocardial fibrosis, infiltration, or scar (via LGE and parametric mapping, which can quantify myocardial T1 and extracellular volume)
- Abnormalities on LGE can help identify and differentiate ischemic from nonischemic cardiomyopathies based on pattern and distribution of LGE
- Comparable diagnostic accuracy to nuclear perfusion imaging
- Thus, stress CMR may be particularly attractive in patients who have left ventricular systolic dysfunction with possible nonischemic cardiomyopathy
- From prognostic standpoint, negative stress CMR is associated with excellent event-free survival
- Quantification of global MBFR can also be performed using stress CMR although this is not widely performed clinically and is less validated than blood flow quantification techniques used by PET MPI

Viability Testing

Viability assessment is also feasible with PET MPI. This is most commonly performed in patients with severe CAD, typically presenting with either recurrent anginal symptoms or recurrent admissions with decompensated heart failure in whom the main clinical question is whether to revascularize regions of potentially hibernating myocardium. Both scarred and hibernating myocardium will demonstrate resting perfusion defect on SPECT or PET MPI. However, the use of metabolic imaging using F-18 fluorodeoxyglucose (F-18 FDG) can identify the presence and size of hibernating myocardium. Patients with hibernating (i.e., viable) myocardium will exhibit resting perfusion defects associated with F-18 FDG uptake (mismatch pattern). In contrast, patients with scarred myocardium will have matched reduction in both perfusion and F-18 FDG uptake.

Evaluation of viability based on CMR is multiparametric and relies on combining data from LGE images, regional wall motion, and ventricular chamber size and function. The transmural extent of LGE directly correlates with the extent of scar. Studies have shown that the presence of < 25% transmural extent of LGE is associated with a high likelihood of improvement in function following revascularization, whereas segments that have > 50% transmurality are less likely to demonstrate recovery of function. Segments with transmural extent of LGE ranging between 25-50% are considered to have an intermediate likelihood of recovery of function following revascularization. In such cases, additional CMR markers can be taken into account, namely the thickness of the affected segment. It has been shown that wall thickness > 4 mm correlates with improved chance of functional recovery. Segments that are dyskinetic or aneurysmal are not considered viable. In addition, when the ventricle is severely dilated (i.e., remodeled), the likelihood of improvement in function is also reduced.

Advantages and Disadvantages of Imaging Modalities in Evaluation of Coronary Artery Disease

Modality	Advantages	Disadvantages
Coronary artery calcium	Coronary artery disease risk stratification in asymptomatic patients Correlates well with total plaque burden	Radiation Unable to detect noncalcified plaques
CCTA	Noninvasive evaluation of coronary anatomy and plaque morphology High negative predictive value for detection of coronary artery disease	Radiation Contrast administration
Cardiac MR	Viability evaluation Identification of etiology of cardiomyopathy Evaluation of valves, pericardium and heart anatomy and function Radiation free	Contrast administration
Stress echocardiography	Widely available Evaluation of valve and heart	Interobserver variability Does not visualize plaques
Exercise treadmill testing	Widely available Evaluation of functional capacity Prognostic information	Low accuracy Not useful for quantification of amount of ischemia
SPECT MPI	Widely available Prognostic information Evaluation of myocardial blood flow	Radiation Low accuracy especially in multivessel disease
PET MPI	Viability evaluation Quantification of myocardial blood flow More accurate than SPECT in multivessel disease	Radiation Low availability

Valvular Heart Disease

Multimodality imaging is vital in diagnosing, surveillance, and managing valvular heart disease. The complimentary assessment includes assessment of valve disease severity, mechanism, and its impact on the cardiac chambers using echocardiography, CCT, and CMR. Moreover, the past decade has seen rapid acceleration of transcatheter valve implantation procedures with TAVR now available for most aortic stenosis patients, including low-risk patients. The mitral and tricuspid valve interventions have seen similar innovations with transcatheter edge-to-edge repair and valve replacement. These procedures require periprocedural multimodality evaluation, in which each of the following imaging modalities plays a critical role.

Transthoracic Echocardiography

- Readily available initial diagnostic or screening test
- Quantification of valvular disease severity; valvular heart disease guidelines primarily use echocardiographic severity criteria for management decision making
- Most comprehensive hemodynamic assessment of both native and prosthetic valve function
- Identification of valvular disease mechanism may be limited by available imaging acoustic windows

Transesophageal Echocardiography

- Excellent combination of temporal and spatial resolution used in assessment of native and prosthetic valves
- Complimentary imaging to transthoracic echocardiography (TTE) with primary strength in identifying mechanism of valvular dysfunction and adjunct assessment of severity
- Transesophageal echocardiography (TEE) is used to guide transcatheter procedures
- Minimally invasive procedure that requires sedation

CCT

- Excellent spatial resolution and used for preprocedural planning for structural heart procedures; adjunct imaging can be completed for comprehensive assessment of peripheral arterial/venous access
- Prosthetic leaflets can be challenging to assess on TTE or TEE; CCT offers assessment for prosthetic thrombus or dysfunction
- It provides more comprehensive assessment of aortic root and aorta when periprosthetic injury or infection, such as pseudoaneurysm, fistula, or abscess, is suspected

CMR

- Gold standard assessment for ventricular volumes
- Adjunct assessment for valve dysfunction severity utilizing novel flow assessment techniques (4D-flow analysis)
- There is growing research into incorporating MR-derived volumes, parametric mapping, and fibrosis assessment in decision making for valve interventions

Conclusion

Significant advances in noninvasive cardiovascular imaging have occurred over the past 2 decades. Echocardiography, CCTA, CMR, and PET/CT offer complimentary assessment in various cardiovascular pathologies, including coronary artery, valvular heart disease, cardiomyopathies, cardiac masses, and infective endocarditis. However, the general practitioner needs help identifying the optimal initial and adjunct testing. As a result, multimodality imaging is a growing field that meets this clinical need and guides clinicians on the optimal imaging modality.

Selected References

1. Gulati M et al: 2021 AHA/ACC/ASE/CHEST/SAEM/SCCT/SCMR guideline for the evaluation and diagnosis of chest pain: a report of the American College of Cardiology/American Heart Association joint committee on clinical practice guidelines. Circulation. 144(22):e368-454, 2021
2. Otto CM et al: 2020 ACC/AHA guideline for the management of patients with valvular heart disease: executive summary: a report of the American College of Cardiology/American Heart Association joint committee on clinical practice guidelines. Circulation. 143(5):e35-71, 2021

CCTA in Patient With Suspected CAD

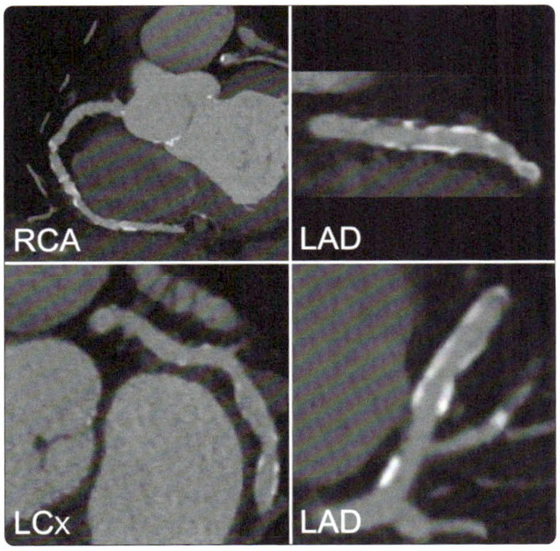

Algorithm for Noninvasive Imaging of Patients With Suspected CAD

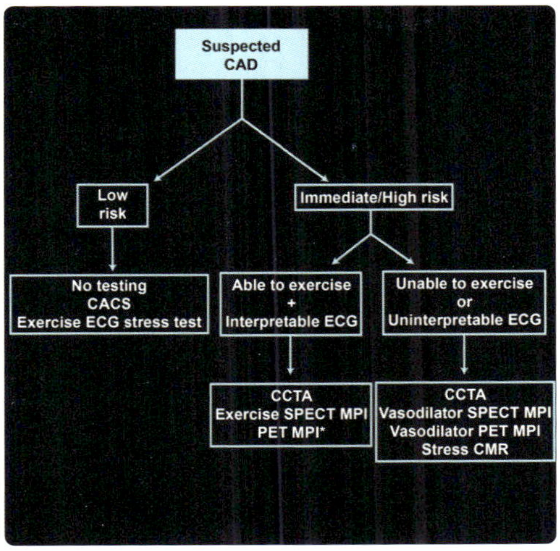

(Left) *This 52-year-old man with nonexertional chest pain and no history of CAD underwent exercise SPECT MPI, which did not reveal any perfusion defect, but he developed chest pain. CCTA revealed a large amount of predominantly calcified plaques involving all 3 coronary arteries but causing only minimal luminal stenosis (< 25%). Findings reflect high risk for adverse cardiac events, given the high burden of coronary calcifications.* **(Right)** *Algorithm for noninvasive imaging of patients with suspected CAD is shown.*

PET MPI in Patient With Known CAD

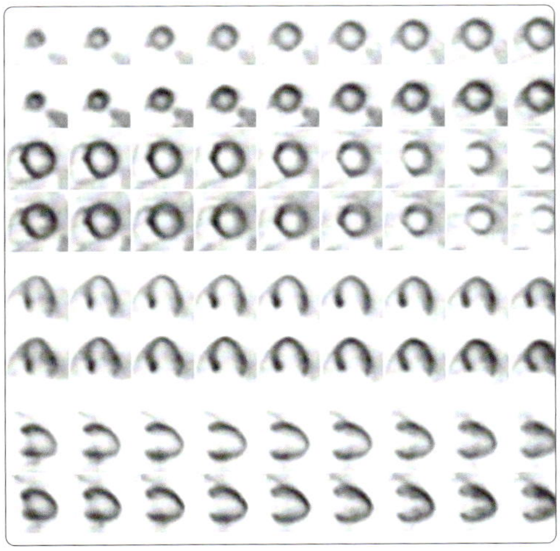

Quantitative Evaluation of MBF and MBFR

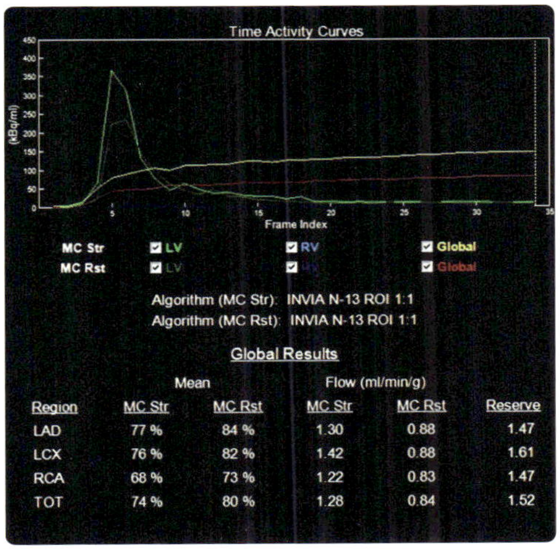

(Left) *PET MPI in a patient with a prior left anterior descending (LAD) stent reveals severe ischemia of the proximal to mid-LAD territory and mild ischemia of the mid right coronary artery (RCA)/PLV territory.* **(Right)** *Chart shows quantitative evaluation of MBF and MBFR, consistent with severely reduced peak stress MBFs of all 3 coronary arteries, most severely of the LAD and RCA. The MBFR of the LAD and RCA were also severely reduced. Of note, normal peak stress MBF is ≥ 1.8 mL/g/min, and normal MBFR is ≥ 2.0.*

Algorithm for Noninvasive Imaging of Patients With Known CAD

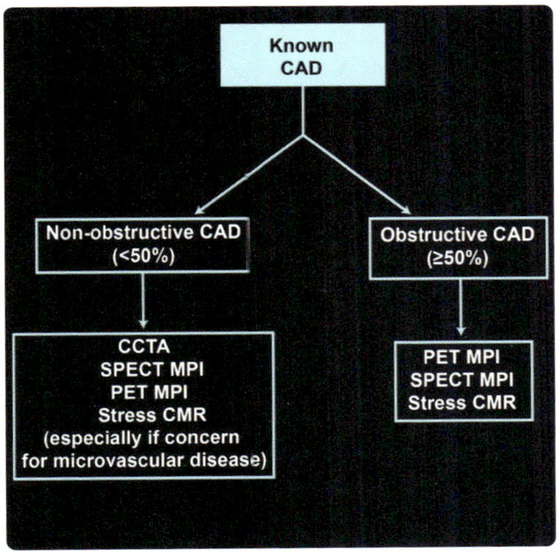

CMR in Patient With Known CAD

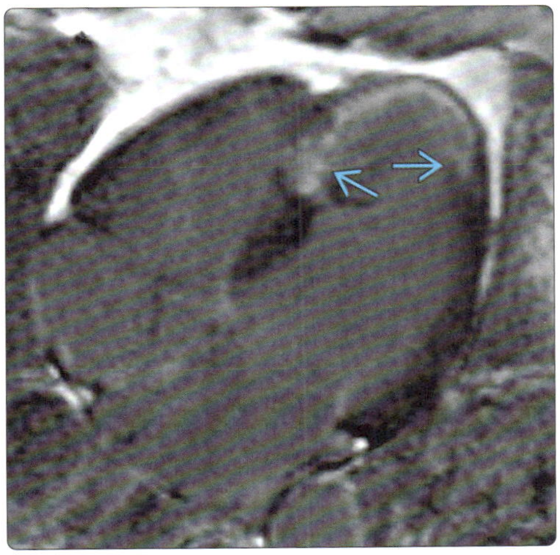

(Left) *Algorithm for noninvasive imaging in patients with known CAD is shown. The selection is made depending on the degree of stenosis.* **(Right)** *Four-chamber delayed enhancement MR shows near-transmural LGE ➔ at the mid- and apical inferoseptum, left ventricle apex, and apical lateral wall. Collectively, these findings are consistent with myocardial infarction along the distribution of the mid- to distal LAD coronary artery.*

GENERAL ANATOMY AND FUNCTION

Anatomy

- Cardiac chambers
  - **Right atrium (RA)**, **right ventricle (RV)**, **left atrium (LA)**, **left ventricle (LV)**
- Cardiac valves
  - Atrioventricular (AV) valves: Tricuspid, mitral
  - Semilunar valves: Pulmonic, aortic
- Cardiac structure
  - **Epicardium**: Serous visceral pericardium
  - **Myocardium**: Specialized cardiac muscle that forms atrial and ventricular walls
  - **Endocardium**: Thin layer of cells lining internal surfaces of cardiac chambers

Function

- Pump action
  - Delivery of deoxygenated blood to alveolar-capillary interface
  - Delivery of oxygenated blood to tissues
- Cardiac conduction system
  - **Sinoatrial node**
    - Cardiac pacemaker; atrial contraction
    - Superior end of **crista terminalis** at **superior vena cava (SVC) orifice**
  - **AV node**
    - In atrial septum, near coronary sinus orifice, close to attachment of septal cusp of tricuspid valve
    - Receives impulse generated at sinoatrial node and propagates it to ventricles
    - Produces ventricular contraction
  - **AV bundle**
    - Continuation of AV node along interventricular septum; divides into right and left bundle branches
  - **Right bundle branch**
    - Continues along right side of interventricular septum to reach subendocardial **Purkinje fibers**
  - **Left bundle branch**
    - Continues along left side of interventricular septum to apex to reach subendocardial **Purkinje fibers**

CARDIAC SHAPE AND ORIENTATION

Shape

- Pyramidal

Orientation

- Position analogous to pyramid on its side
- Apex oriented anteriorly, inferiorly, and to left

CARDIAC SURFACES

Posterior Surface (Base)

- Faces posteriorly; quadrilateral shape
- Structures: **LA**, small portion of **RA**, central **great veins**

Apex

- Faces anteriorly, inferiorly, and to left
- Structures: Inferolateral LV

Anterior Surface

- Faces anteriorly
- Structures: **RV (anterior free wall)**, portions of **RA** and **LV**

Diaphragmatic Surface

- Faces inferiorly; rests on diaphragm
- Structures: **LV**, portion of **RV**

Left Pulmonary Surface

- Faces left lung
- Structures: **LV**, portion of **LA**

Right Pulmonary Surface

- Faces right lung
- Structure: **RA**

CARDIAC SULCI OR GROOVES

General Features

- Heart divided into chambers
- Internal cardiac partitions demarcate chamber boundaries
- **Sulci**: External grooves related to internal partitions

Atrioventricular Sulcus or Groove (Coronary Sulcus)

- Surrounds heart, separates atria from ventricles
- Structures: Right coronary/circumflex branch of left coronary artery, small cardiac vein, great cardiac vein, coronary sinus

Anterior & Posterior Interventricular Sulci or Grooves

- Separate ventricles
- **Anterior interventricular groove** or **sulcus**
  - Anterior heart surface
  - Structures: Left anterior descending (LAD) coronary artery, anterior interventricular vein
- **Posterior interventricular groove** or **sulcus**
  - Diaphragmatic heart surface
  - Structures: Posterior descending (interventricular) coronary artery, middle cardiac vein (posterior interventricular vein), occasionally distal wrap-around LAD
- Anterior and posterior interventricular sulci continuous inferiorly to left of apex

CARDIAC CHAMBERS

Right Atrium

- Forms **right cardiac border** and portion of **anterior surface**
- Receives deoxygenated blood through
  - **SVC**: Superior posterior RA
  - **Inferior vena cava (IVC)**: Inferior posterior RA
  - **Coronary sinus**: Inferior posterior RA
    - **Thebesian valve**: Prevents reflux of blood back into coronary sinus from RA
  - **Thebesian veins**: Small veins that drain subendocardium
  - **Anterior cardiac vein**: Venous return from anterior RV
- Blood exits through AV **tricuspid valve**
- Structures
  - Compartmentalized by external **sulcus terminalis** cordis
    - From right of SVC to right of IVC
  - Compartmentalized by internal **crista terminalis**
    - Smooth ridge that begins at roof of atrium anterior to SVC orifice and extends to anterior lip of IVC orifice

- **Sinus of venae cavae**, posterior to **crista terminalis**
- **RA** proper
  - Anterior to crista terminalis
  - Wall covered by ridges called **pectinate muscles**
  - **RA appendage** (**auricle**)
- Vascular orifices
  - **Orifice of SVC**, **orifices** and **valves of IVC**, and **coronary sinus**
- **Interatrial septum**
  - **Fossa ovalis**: Depression in septum above orifice of IVC
  - **Limbus fossa ovalis**: Margin of fossa ovalis
  - **Fossa ovalis** marks location of primitive **foramen ovale**, which allows oxygenated blood to enter LA and bypass lungs in utero

Right Ventricle

- Forms **anterior cardiac surface** and small portion of **diaphragmatic surface**
- Structures
  - **Conus arteriosus**: Smooth-walled RV infundibulum or RV outflow tract (RVOT)
  - RV inflow tract, lined by **trabeculae carneae**, forms ridges and bridges
  - **Papillary muscles** are **trabeculae carneae** attached to ventricular surface and **chordae tendineae**; connect **chordae tendineae** to free edges of **tricuspid valve**
    - **Anterior papillary muscle**: Largest, arises from anterior ventricular wall
    - **Posterior papillary muscle**: Some chordae tendineae arise directly from ventricular wall
    - **Septal papillary muscle**: Most inconsistent
  - **Septomarginal trabecula** or **moderator band**
    - Forms bridge **between lower interventricular septum and base of anterior papillary muscle**

Left Atrium

- Forms **base** or **posterior cardiac surface**
- Structures
  - **Posterior** or **inflow portion**: Smooth-walled, receives **pulmonary veins**
  - **Anterior** or **outflow portion**: Continuous with **LA appendage**, lined by **pectinate muscles**
  - **Interatrial septum**
    - Contains **valve of foramen ovale**, prevents blood from passing from LA to RA
    - **Valve of foramen ovale** may provide passage between atria during cardiac instrumentation

Left Ventricle

- Contributions to **anterior**, **diaphragmatic**, and **left pulmonary cardiac surfaces**; forms **apex**
- Thickest myocardium
- Structures
  - Fine, delicate **trabeculae carneae**
  - Papillary muscles larger than in RV
    - **Anterior papillary muscle**
    - **Posterior papillary muscle**
  - **Interventricular septum**
    - **Thick muscular portion** forms major part of septum
    - **Membranous portion**

CARDIAC VALVES

Tricuspid Valve

- 3 cusps attached to fibrous ring
  - **Anterior**, **septal**, **posterior**
- Anatomy of right AV valve
  - Free margins attached to **chordae tendineae**
    - Cusps continuous with each other at their bases, forming **commissures**
  - **Chordae tendineae** from 2 papillary muscles attach to each cusp
- Separated from pulmonic valve by muscular ridge (crista supraventricularis)

Pulmonic Valve

- 3 semilunar cusps
  - **Left**, **right**, **anterior**
- Anatomy of semilunar cusps
  - Free edges project into lumen of pulmonary trunk forming **sinuses**
  - Each cusp has thick central focus (**nodule of semilunar cusp**)
  - Each cusp has thin lateral portion (**lunule of semilunar cusp**)

Mitral Valve

- 2 cusps attached to fibrous ring
  - **Anterior** and **posterior**, divided in 3 subdivisions each (A1, A2, A3 and P1, P2, P3; A1 and P1 are superior)
- Anatomy of left AV valve
  - Cusps continuous with each other at **commissures**
  - **Chordae tendineae** attach papillary muscles to free borders of cusps
- In fibrous continuity with aortic valve

Aortic Valve

- 3 semilunar cusps
  - **Right**, **left**, and **noncoronary** (or **posterior**)
- 3 sinuses of Valsalva
  - Right coronary artery originates from right sinus
  - Left coronary artery originates from left sinus
  - Noncoronary sinus always faces interatrial septum

HEART IMAGING

Radiography

- Analysis of cardiac borders and surfaces on PA radiograph
  - Right cardiac border: **RA**
  - Left cardiac border: **LA appendage** and **LV**
- Analysis of cardiac borders and surfaces on lateral radiograph
  - Anterior cardiac surface: **RV**
  - Posterior cardiac surface: **LA** and **LV**
- Variations in cardiac morphology
  - **Infancy**: **Prominent cardiothymic silhouette**
  - **Childhood**, adolescence, and young adulthood: **Prominent pulmonary trunk**
  - **Adulthood**: **Progressive LV configuration** with dominant left-sided structures and concavity of upper left cardiac border
- Analysis of cardiac size
  - **Cardiothoracic ratio**

- Maximum transverse cardiac diameter to transverse thoracic diameter ≤ **0.55**
- Influenced by rotation, lung volume, projection
- Analysis of individual chamber enlargement
- Analysis of abnormal cardiac density/calcification

CT/MR Anatomy

- **RA**
  - **RA appendage** (trabeculated) anterior and superior to **RV**
  - **Crista terminalis**: Vertical ridge in RA extending from superior to inferior venae cavae
- **LA**
  - Most superior & posterior cardiac chamber
  - **LA appendage** (trabeculated) anterior & superior to **LV**
  - **Smooth muscle ridge** at junction of **LA appendage** and central **left superior pulmonary vein** (**a.k.a. Coumadin ridge**)
- **Interatrial septum**
  - Thin structure, difficult identification on CT
  - Increased visibility with fat deposition
    - Fat spares **fossa ovalis** and may allow its identification
- **RV**
  - Most anterior cardiac chamber, anterior heart surface
  - Heavy trabeculations, thin wall
    - **Moderator band**: Connects anterior papillary muscle to interventricular septum near RV apex; contains right bundle branch
  - **Anterior, posterior, septal papillary muscles**
- **LV**
  - Posterior and diaphragmatic cardiac surfaces
  - Thicker than RV, less trabeculated
  - Anterior and posterior papillary muscles
- **Interventricular septum**
  - Thicker than interatrial septum
- **Valves**
  - Imaging in longitudinal and perpendicular planes
    - CECT and bright-blood cardiac MR: Thin, low-attenuation/signal structures
  - Assessment of function, morphology, calcification

CT/MR

- Assessment of cardiac chambers, valves, myocardium
  - Size, morphology, wall thickness, calcification, function
- **Short-axis view**
  - Cross section through short axis of LV cavity and bodies of papillary muscles
- **Paraseptal long-axis (2-chamber) view**
  - Display of LA and LV chambers
  - Evaluation of **mitral (left AV) valve**
  - Excellent visualization of anterior and inferior LV myocardium
- **4-chamber view**
  - Display of 4 cardiac chambers and AV valves
- **LV outflow tract view**
  - Display of LA, LV, LV outflow tract, and aorta
- **RVOT view**
  - Display of RA, RV, RVOT, and main pulmonary artery

IMAGING CLUES TO IDENTIFY MORPHOLOGIC RIGHT & LEFT VENTRICLES

Anatomic Right Ventricle

- Muscular infundibulum separates tricuspid and pulmonic valves
- Coarse trabeculae with trabeculations along interventricular septum
- Papillary muscles attached to interventricular septum and free wall
- Apical moderator band
- Septal tricuspid valve leaflet inserts more apically than matching mitral valve leaflet

Anatomic Left Ventricle

- Fibrous continuity between mitral and aortic valves
- Thin and delicate trabeculae with smooth septal surface
- Papillary muscles attached only to free walls

IMAGING CLUES TO IDENTIFY MORPHOLOGIC RIGHT & LEFT ATRIA

Anatomic Right Atrium

- RA appendage has broad opening with triangular shape
- Rule of **venoatrial concordance**
  - Chamber that receives IVC inflow is almost always morphologic RA
- Generally on same side as morphologic right trilobed lung

Anatomic Left Atrium

- Finger-like LA appendage with narrow orifice and pointed appearance
- Recently described as either of following 4 shapes: Chicken wing (48%), cactus (30%), windsock (19%), and cauliflower (3%)
- Generally on same side as morphologic left bilobed lung
- Important to not mistake normal linear pectinate muscle or Coumadin ridge for thrombus

Cardiac Fibrous Skeleton

- **Anulus fibrosus**: 4 fibrous rings between atria and ventricles
  - Points of origin of atrial (superior) and ventricular (inferior) myocardia
  - Maintain integrity of orifices
  - Traversed by **AV bundle**
  - Surround AV valves and aortic/pulmonary trunk orifices
- Interconnecting fibrous tissue
  - **Right fibrous trigone**: Between aortic and right AV rings
  - **Left fibrous trigone**: Between aortic and left AV rings

SELECTED REFERENCES

1. Haas NA et al: Normal cardiac anatomy and clinical evaluation. Adv Exp Med Biol. 1441:87-100, 2024
2. Malik SB et al: Transthoracic echocardiography: pitfalls and limitations as delineated at cardiac CT and MR imaging. Radiographics. 37(2):383-406, 2017
3. Leipsic J et al: SCCT guidelines for the interpretation and reporting of coronary CT angiography: a report of the Society of Cardiovascular Computed Tomography Guidelines Committee. J Cardiovasc Comput Tomogr. 8(5):342-58, 2014
4. Galea N et al: Right ventricular cardiovascular magnetic resonance imaging: normal anatomy and spectrum of pathological findings. Insights Imaging. 4(2):213-23, 2013

ANATOMY OF HEART SURFACES, MARGINS, AND SULCI

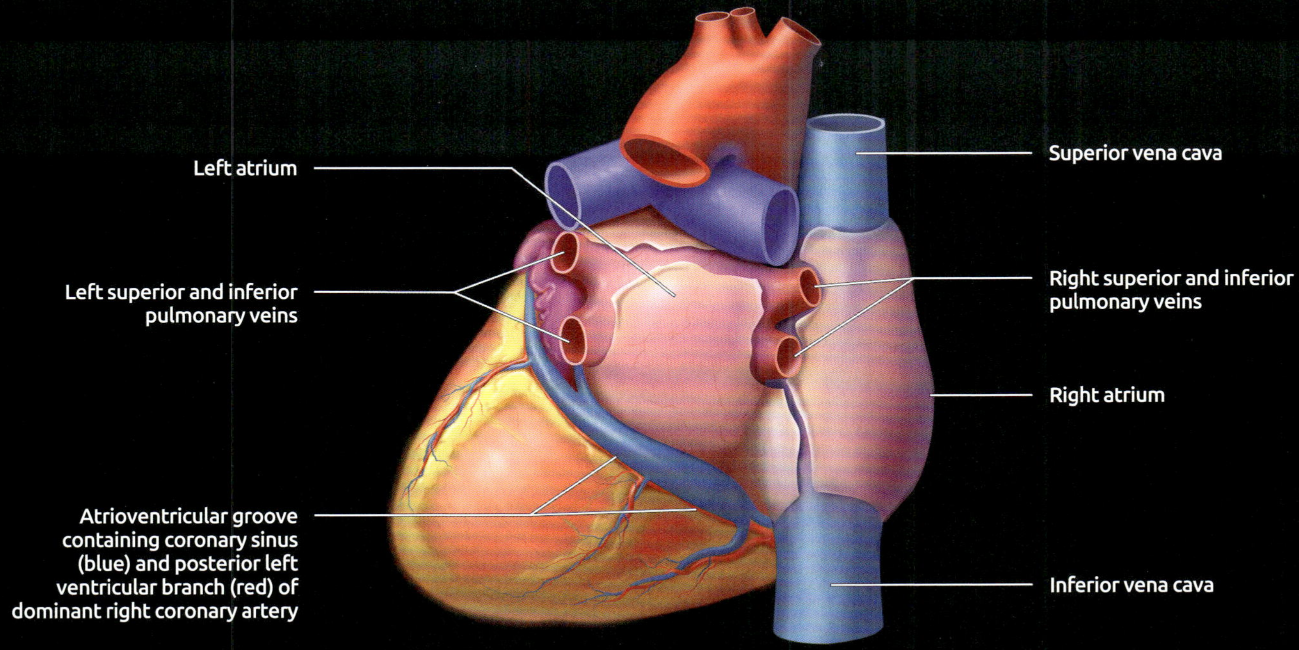

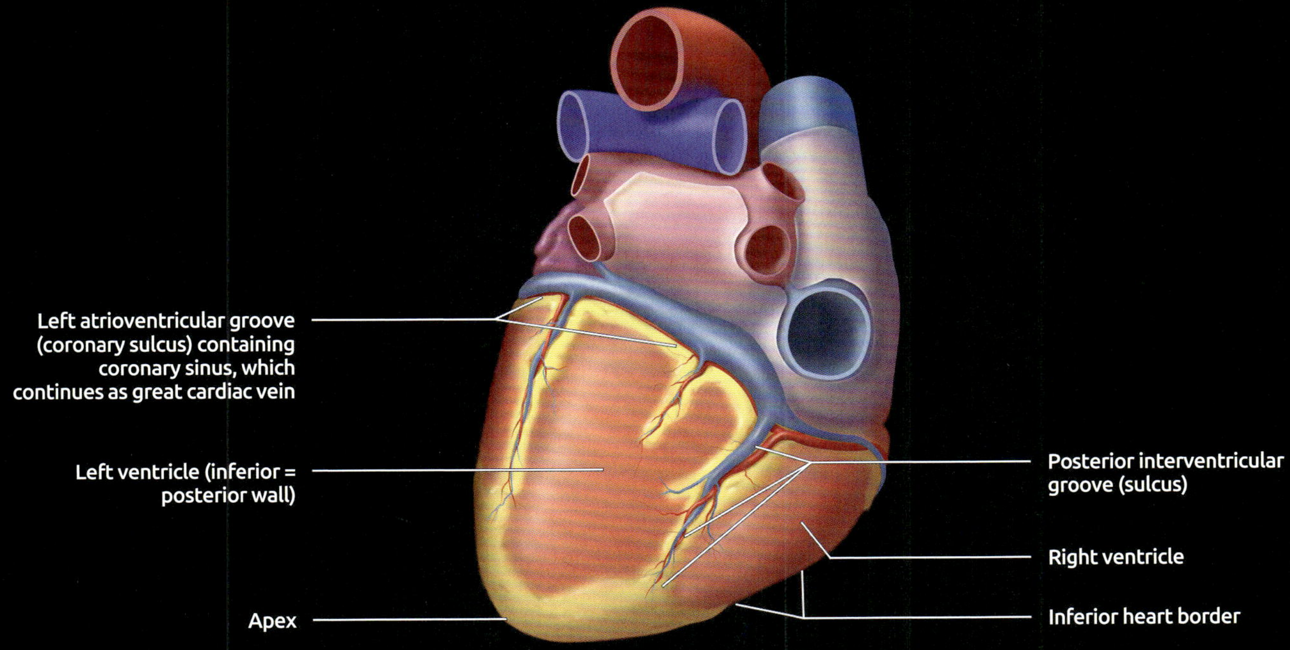

(Top) *Graphic shows the posterior heart surface, or base of the heart, which is formed by the left atrium, a small portion of the right atrium, the paired superior and inferior pulmonary veins, and the superior and inferior venae cavae, which fix the heart base to the pericardium. The left atrioventricular groove is seen at the junction of the left atrium and ventricle.* **(Bottom)** *Graphic shows the diaphragmatic heart surface, which is formed by the right and left ventricles and is separated from the heart base by the coronary sulcus (atrioventricular groove). The inferior (acute) cardiac border separates the diaphragmatic surface from the anterior heart surface. The posterior interventricular sulcus (or groove) marks the location of the interventricular septum.*

CT OF LEFT ATRIUM

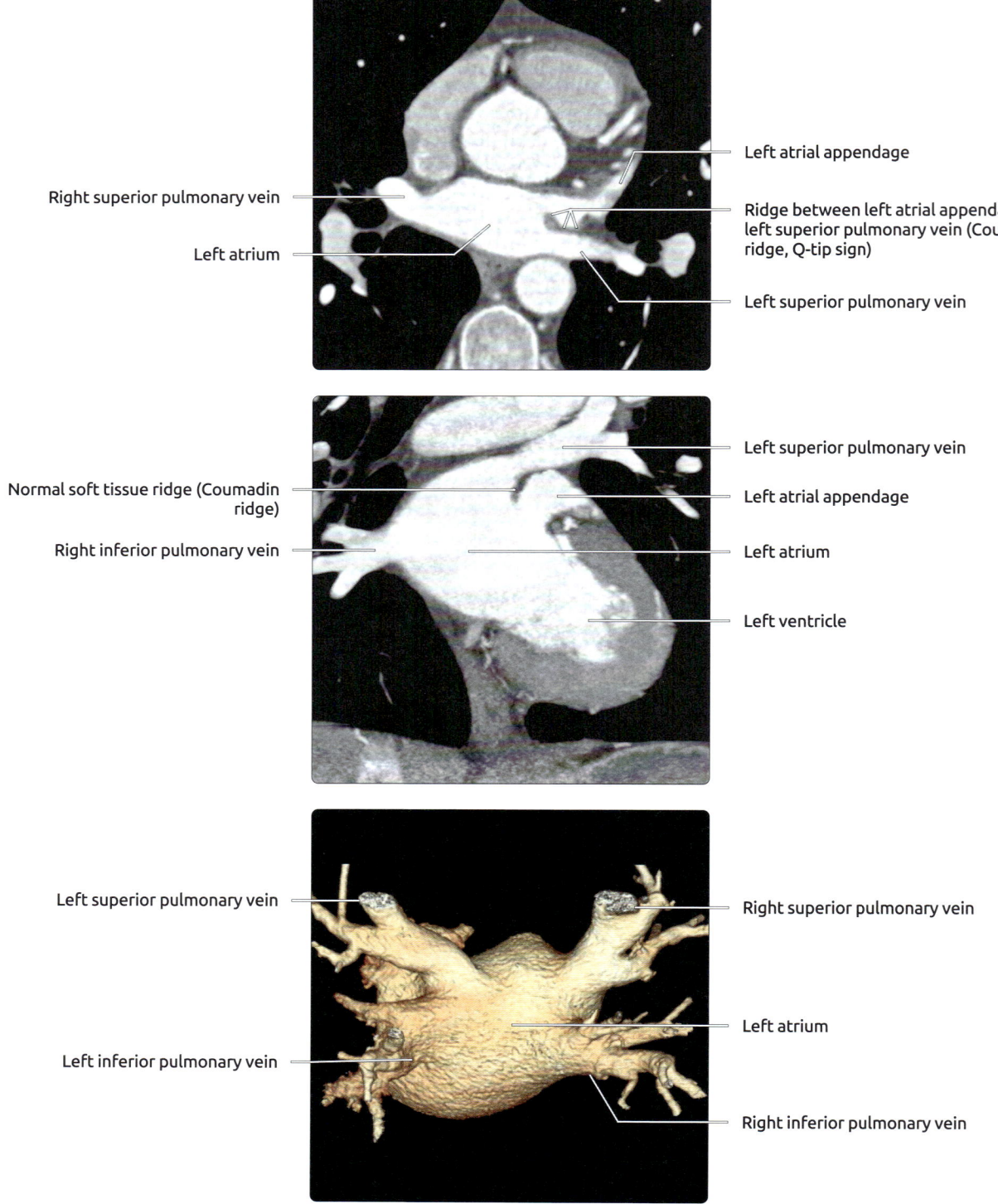

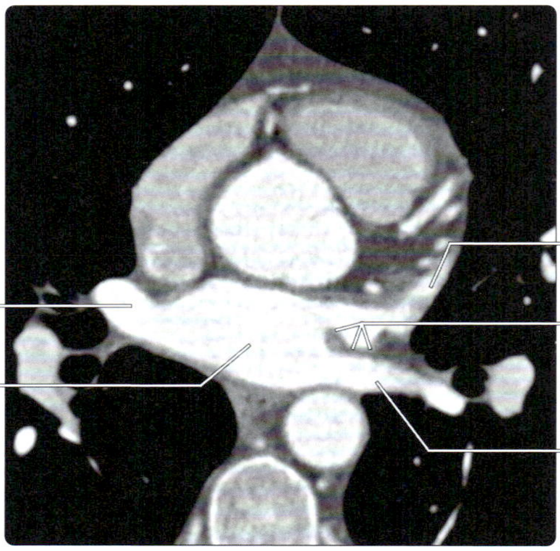

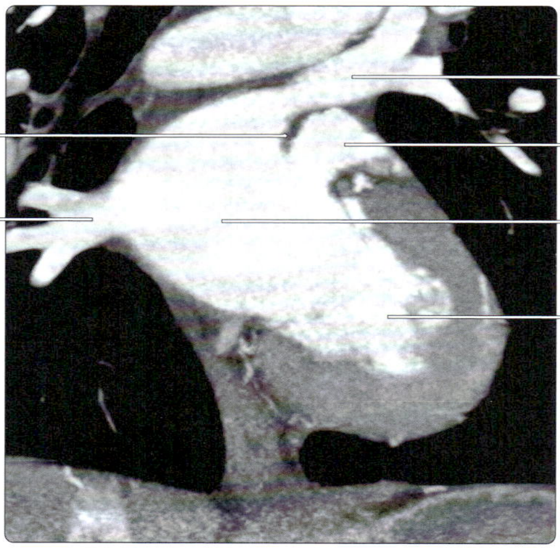

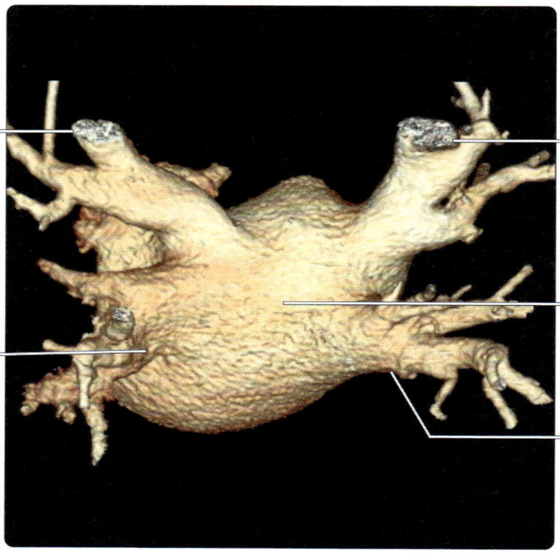

(Top) *Axial CT shows the nodular appearance of the ridge at the junction of the left atrium and left superior pulmonary vein adjacent to the left atrial appendage, which is also known as the Coumadin ridge as it can be mistaken for thrombus at transesophageal echocardiography. This image through the superior aspect of the left atrium demonstrates the constant relationship between the left superior pulmonary vein and the adjacent left atrial appendage. The left atrial appendage is always anterior and inferior to the left superior pulmonary vein.* **(Middle)** *Coronal CT through the left atrial appendage in the same patient demonstrates the normal soft tissue ridge that occurs at the junction of the left atrium with the left superior pulmonary vein adjacent to the left atrial appendage.* **(Bottom)** *Posterior 3D volume-rendered CTA shows the normal appearance of the pulmonary veins.*

CT, 4-CHAMBER VIEW

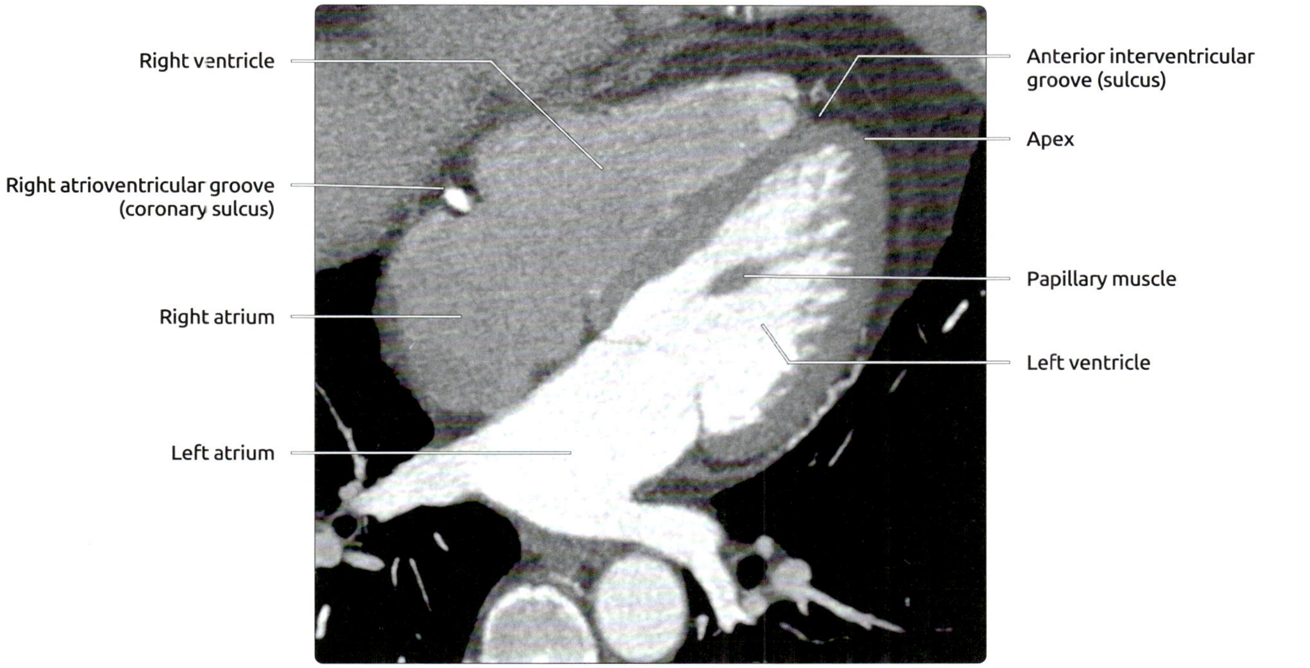

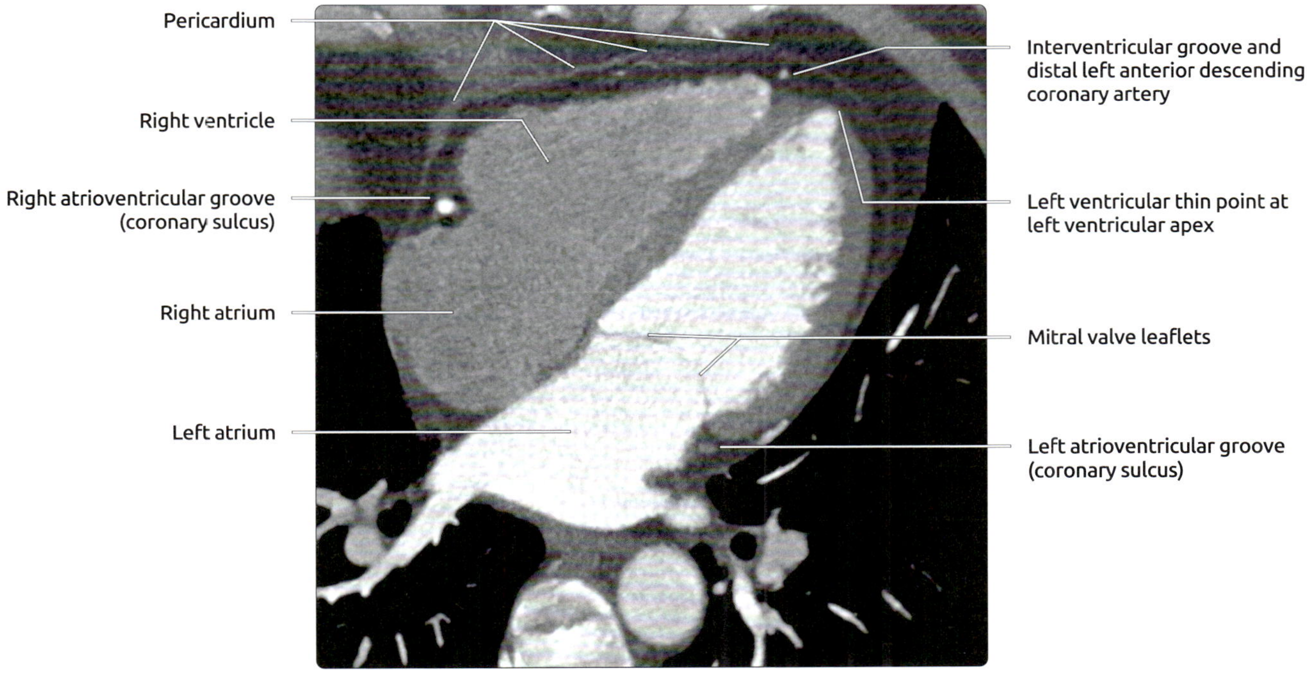

(Top) *Gated 4-chamber cardiac CECT allows simultaneous evaluation of the 4 cardiac chambers. The right chambers are projected anterolateral to the left heart chambers and are less opacified with contrast. The mitral valve leaflets manifest as thin, linear soft tissue structures between the left atrium and left ventricle.* **(Bottom)** *Gated 4-chamber cardiac CECT in the same patient demonstrates a normal mitral valve. The 4 cardiac chambers and the coronary (atrioventricular) and interventricular sulci (grooves) are demonstrated. The interventricular groove is located slightly to the right of the cardiac apex.*

CT, 2-CHAMBER VIEW

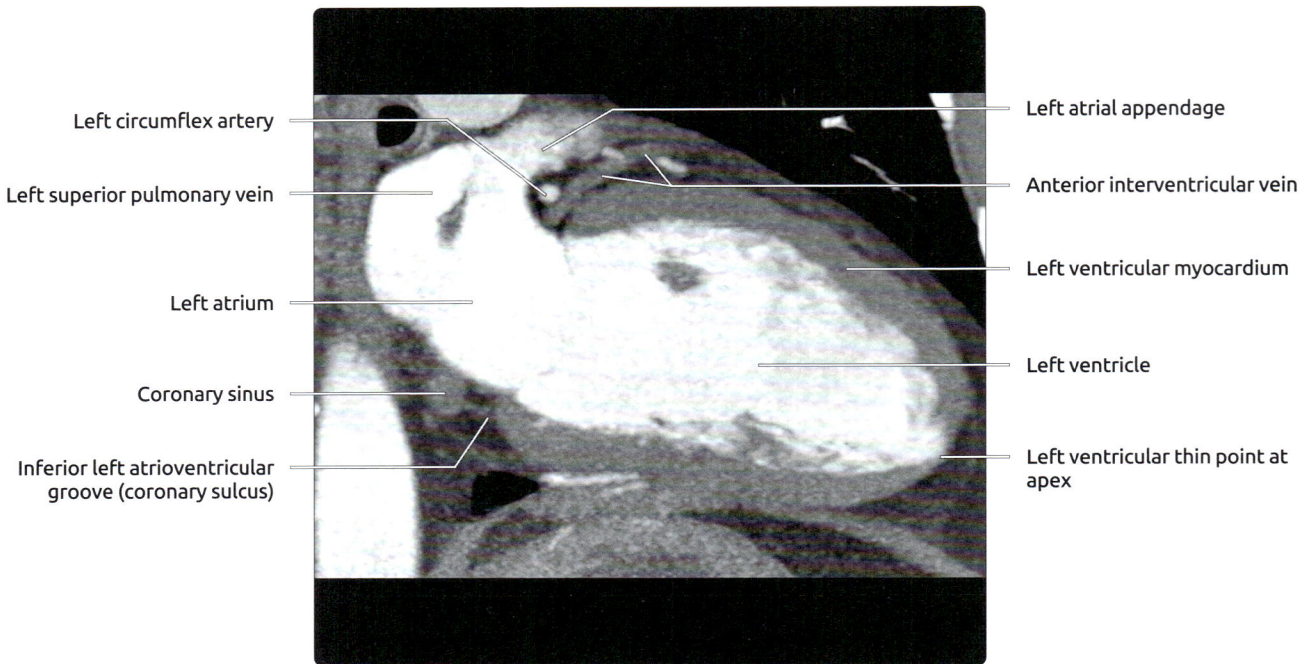

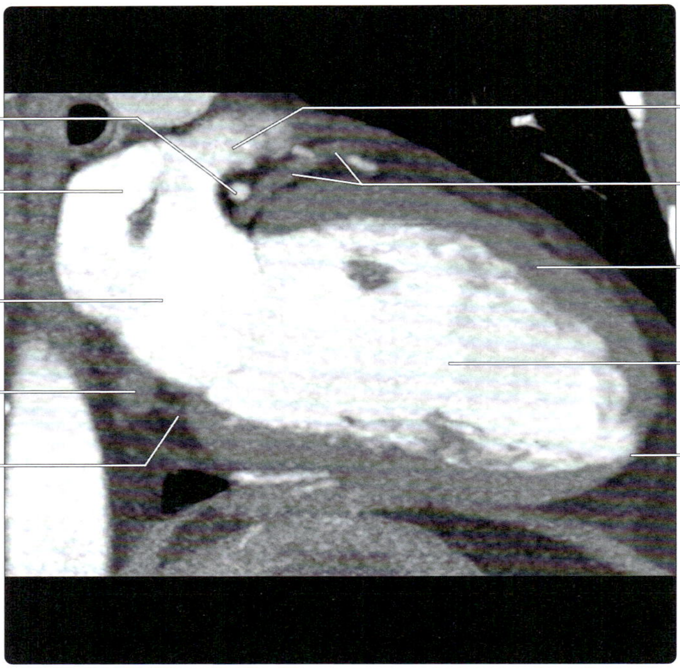

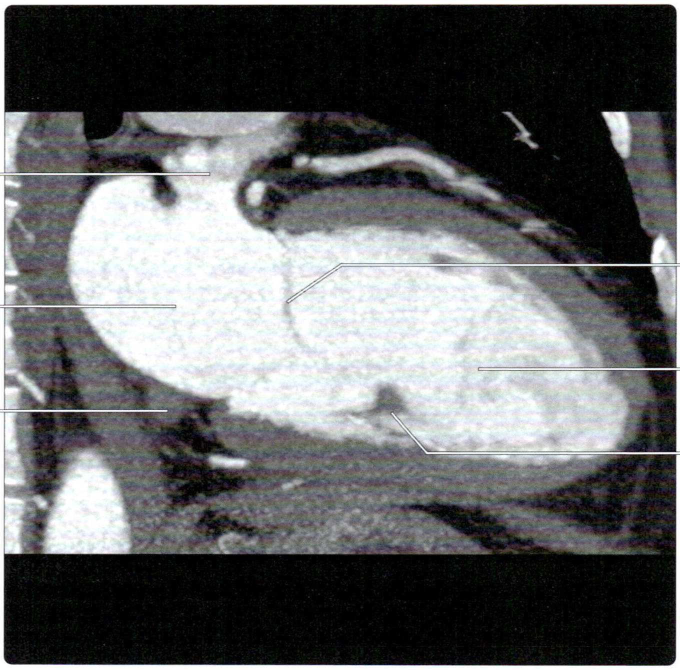

(Top) *Paraseptal long-axis (2-chamber) gated cardiac CECT shows the anatomy of the left ventricle and left atrium. Note the intimate relationship of the left superior pulmonary vein and left atrial appendage with an intervening nodular soft tissue ridge, which is also known as the Coumadin ridge. The left atrial appendage exhibits a trabeculated internal surface produced by the pectinate muscles. The left ventricle, the thickness of its wall, and its papillary muscles are well visualized.* **(Bottom)** *Paraseptal long-axis (2-chamber) gated cardiac CECT through the mitral valve obtained during systole in the same patient demonstrates coaptation of the thin anterior and posterior valve cusps. The papillary muscles manifest as rounded filling defects within the contrast-filled left ventricular chamber.*

CT, SHORT-AXIS VIEW

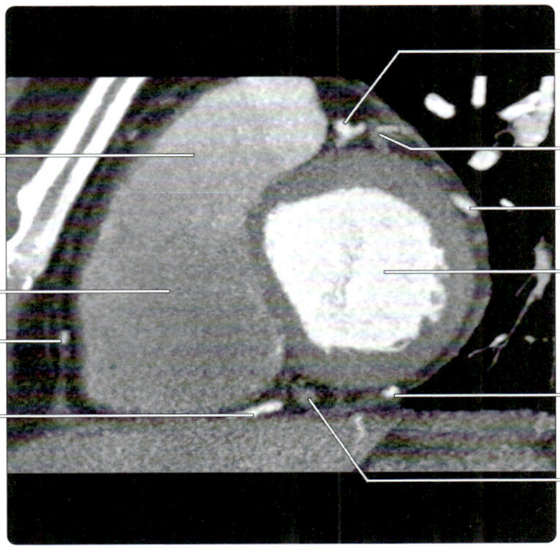

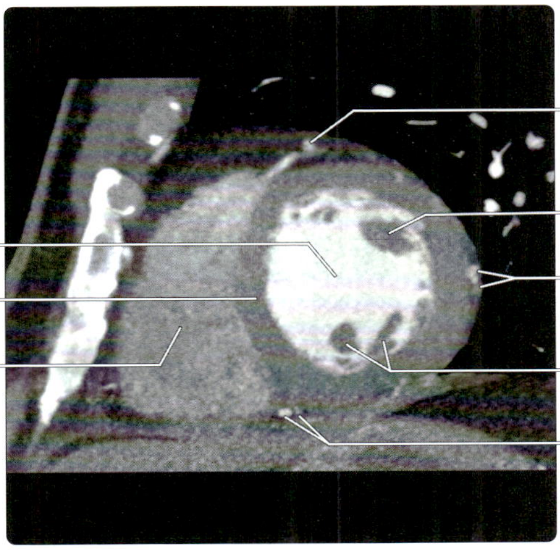

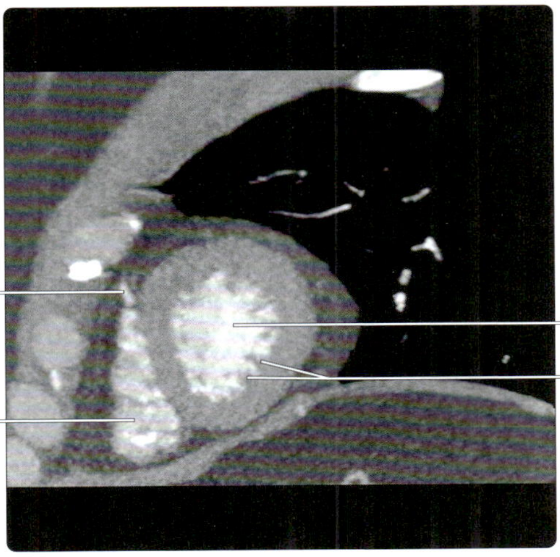

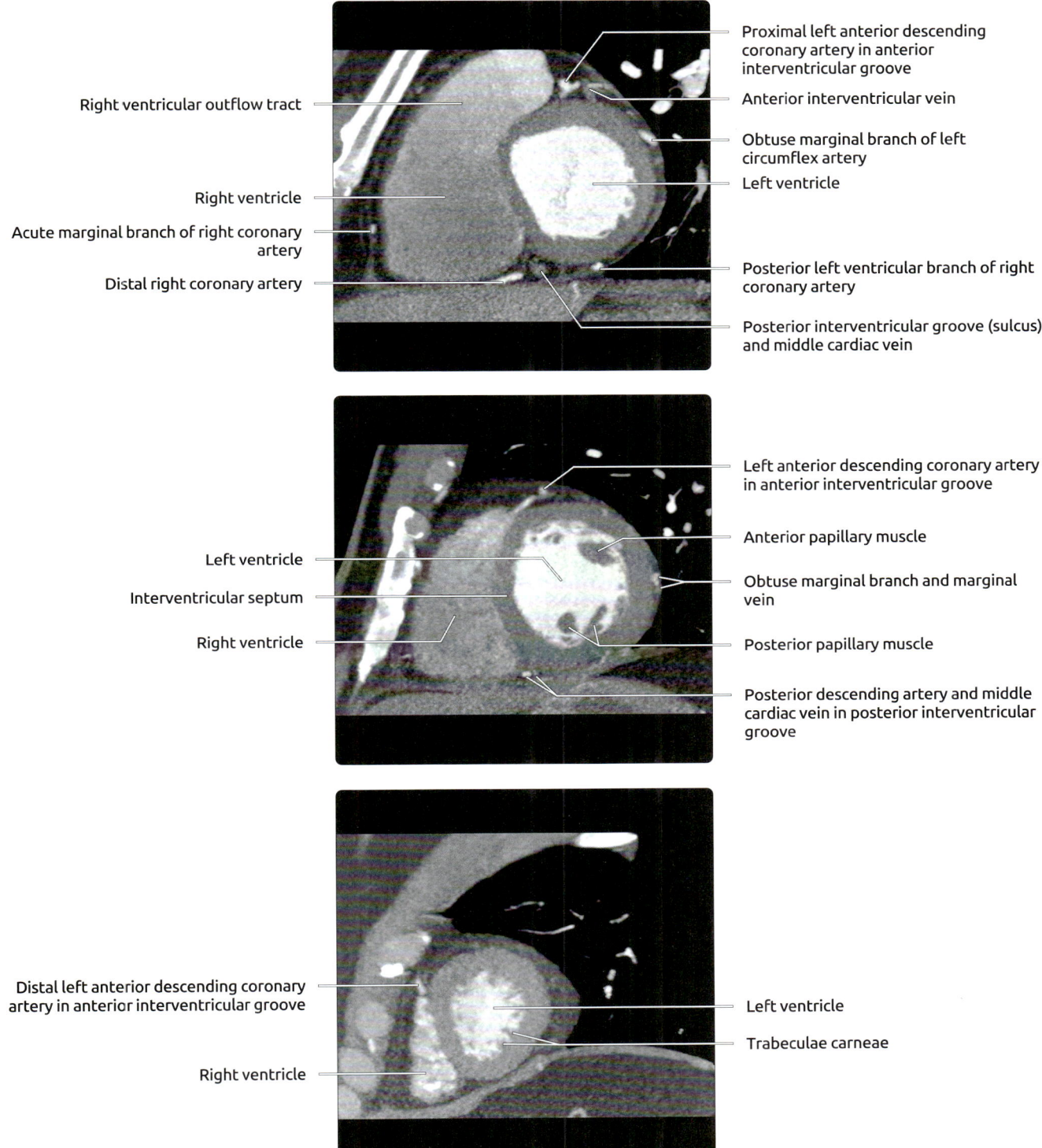

(Top) *Short-axis gated cardiac CECT shows the ventricular chambers. The right ventricle is located anteriorly and has a thin wall. The right ventricular outflow tract courses superiorly and posteriorly to give off the pulmonary trunk. The left ventricle is posterior and has a thicker myocardium than the right ventricle. The 2 chambers are separated by the interventricular sulcus (or groove).* **(Middle)** *Short-axis gated cardiac CECT through the midheart in the same patient shows the anatomy of the left ventricular chamber. The papillary muscles manifest as filling defects within the contrast-filled left ventricular lumen.* **(Bottom)** *Short-axis gated cardiac CECT obtained just medial to the left apex in the same patient demonstrates trabeculations in both ventricular chambers produced by trabeculae carneae. The right ventricle forms the anterior heart surface.*

MR OF NORMAL HEART, SHORT-AXIS VIEW

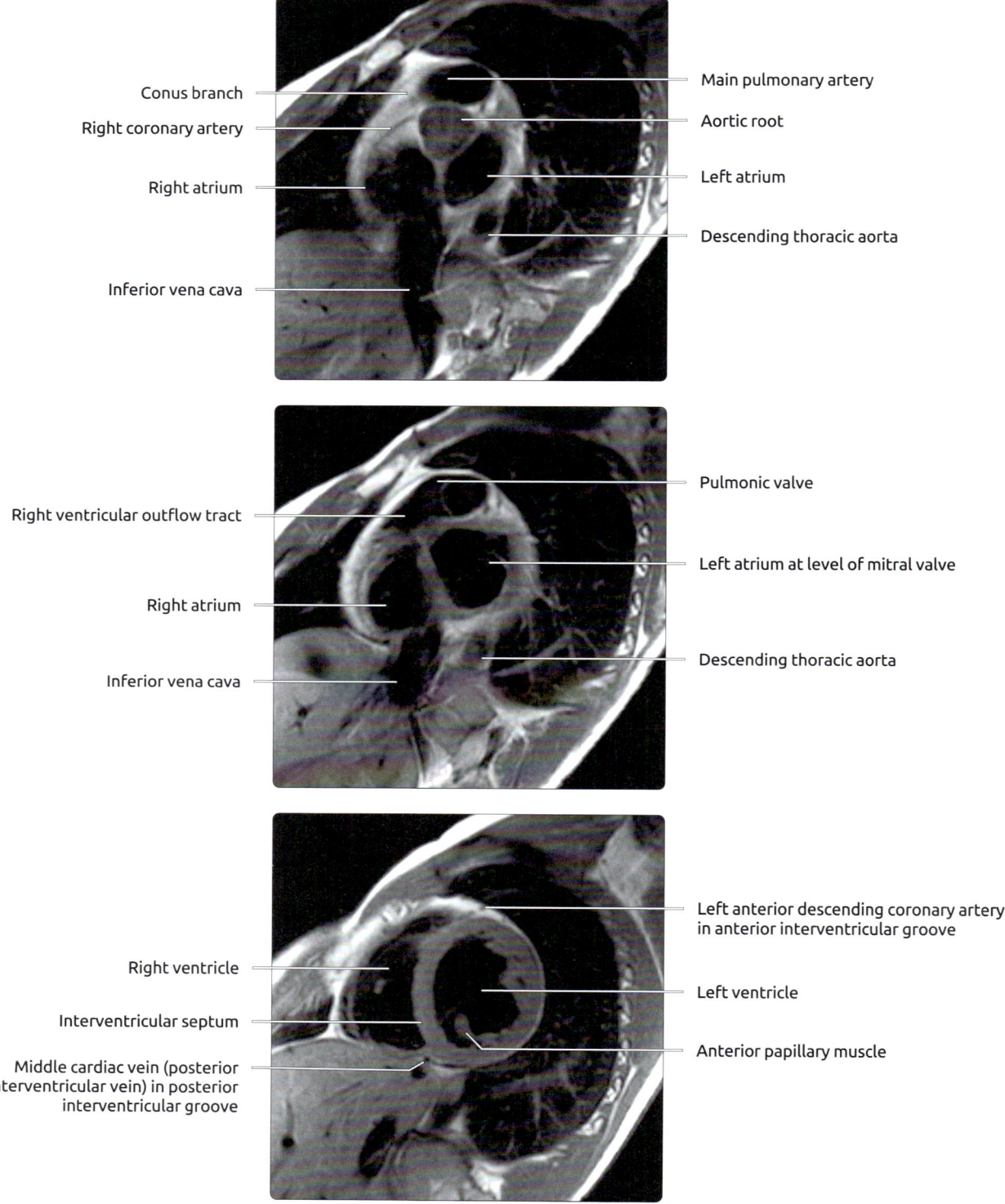

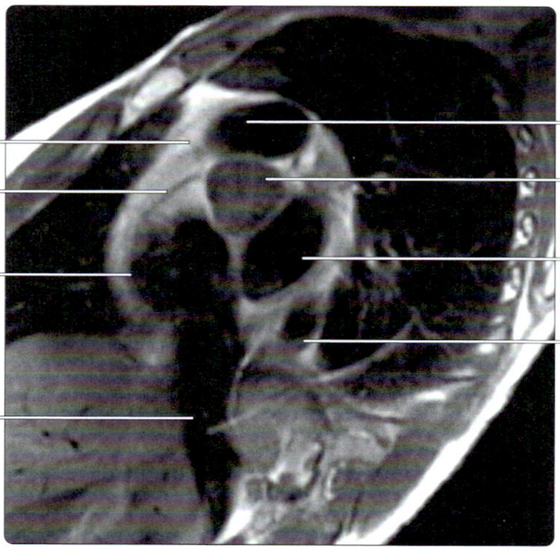

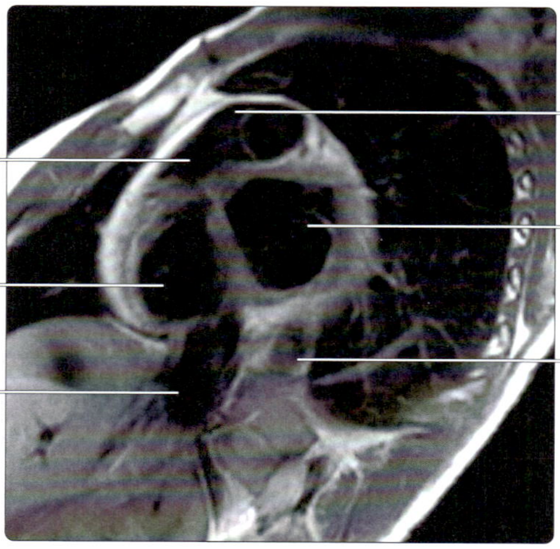

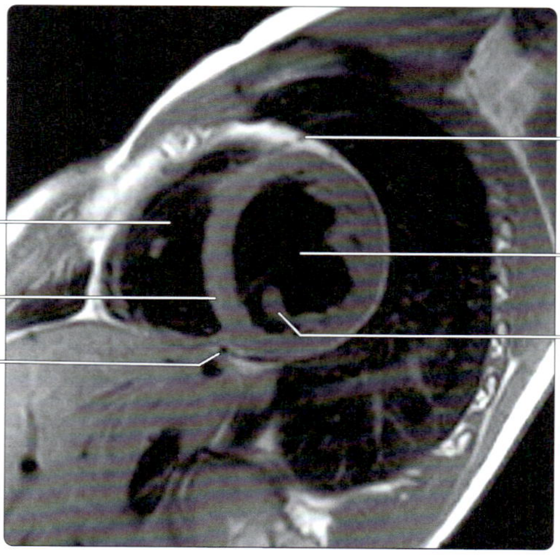

(Top) *Short-axis T2-weighted double inversion-recovery black-blood MR shows the basal aspect of the heart, which is made up of the right and left atria.* **(Middle)** *Short-axis T2-weighted double inversion-recovery black-blood MR slightly more apically in the same patient shows the pulmonic valve and right ventricular outflow tract.* **(Bottom)** *Short-axis T2-weighted double inversion-recovery black-blood MR through the midventricular level in the same patient shows a papillary muscle of the left ventricle. The midventricular level is best identified on the short-axis view by identifying the papillary muscles. The left ventricular interventricular septum is typically smooth, whereas the right ventricular interventricular septum is trabeculated.*

ANATOMY OF CARDIAC SKELETON AND HEART VALVES

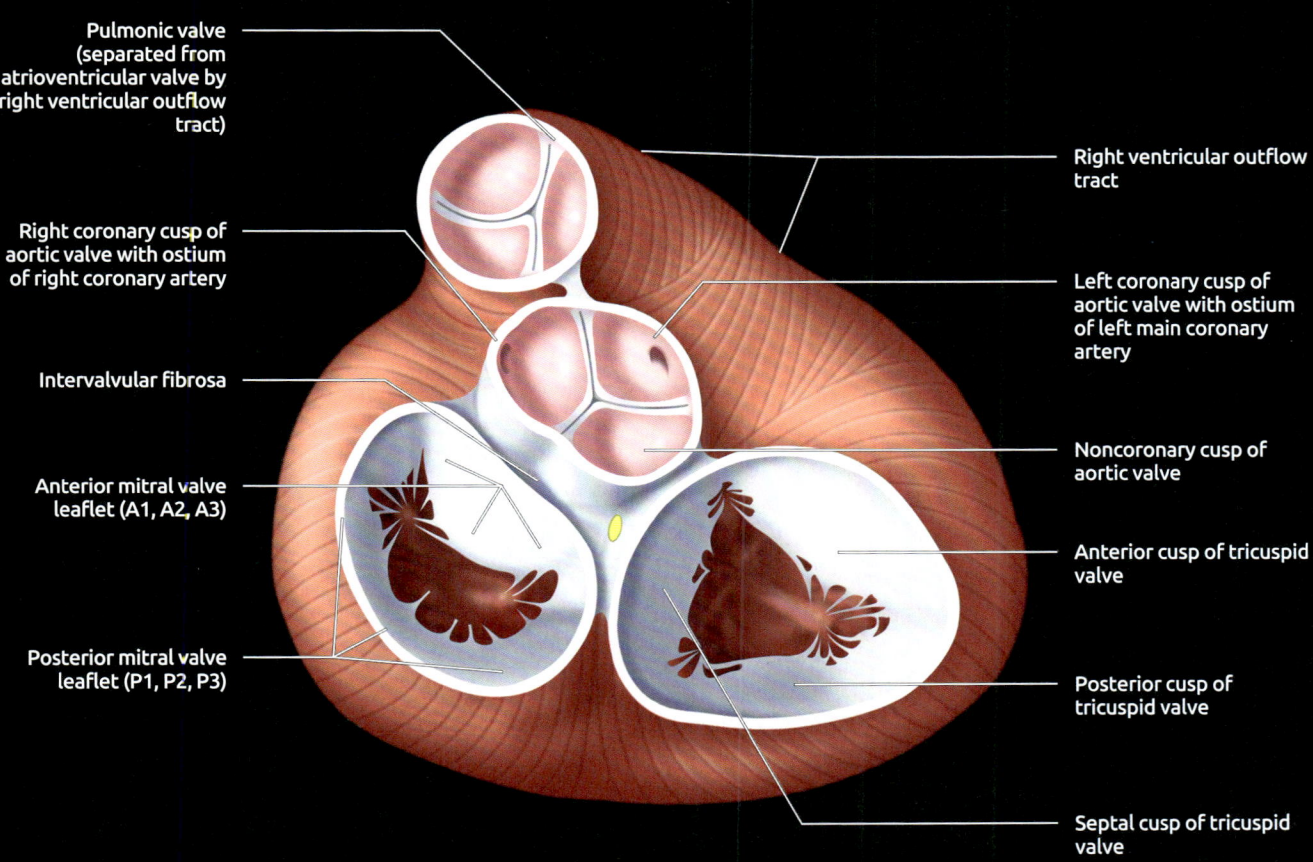

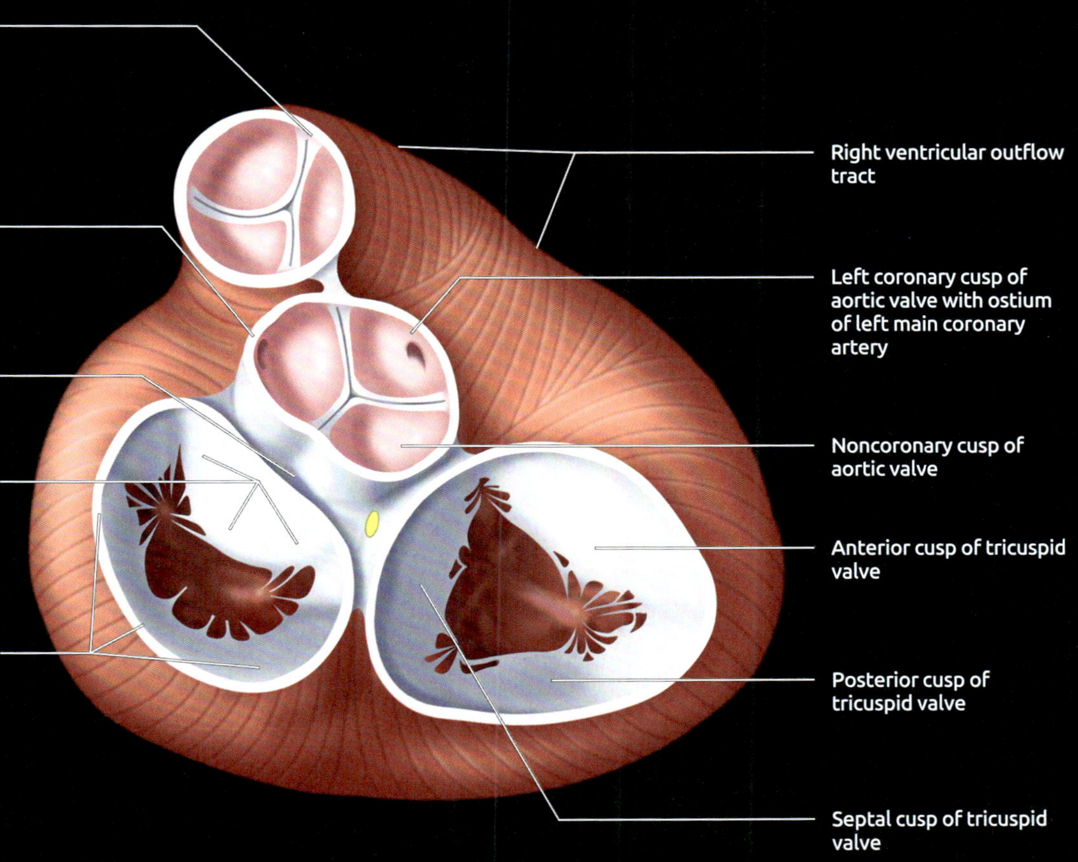

Graphic demonstrates the anatomy of the cardiac skeleton located between the atria and ventricles. The cardiac skeleton consists of thick, fibrous connective tissue and provides support for the valve orifices and the areas of attachment for the valve cusps. Here, the atria have been "removed" to expose the cardiac skeleton and heart valves seen from above. The 4 fibrous rings that surround the valves are known as the anulus fibrosus. The right fibrous trigone is the connective tissue bridge between the aortic valve and right atrioventricular (tricuspid) valve rings. The left fibrous trigone is the connective tissue bridge between the aortic valve and the left atrioventricular (mitral) valve rings. The yellow dot represents the atrioventricular bundle seen in cross section as it courses caudally from the atria to the ventricles.

ANATOMY OF LEFT HEART VALVES

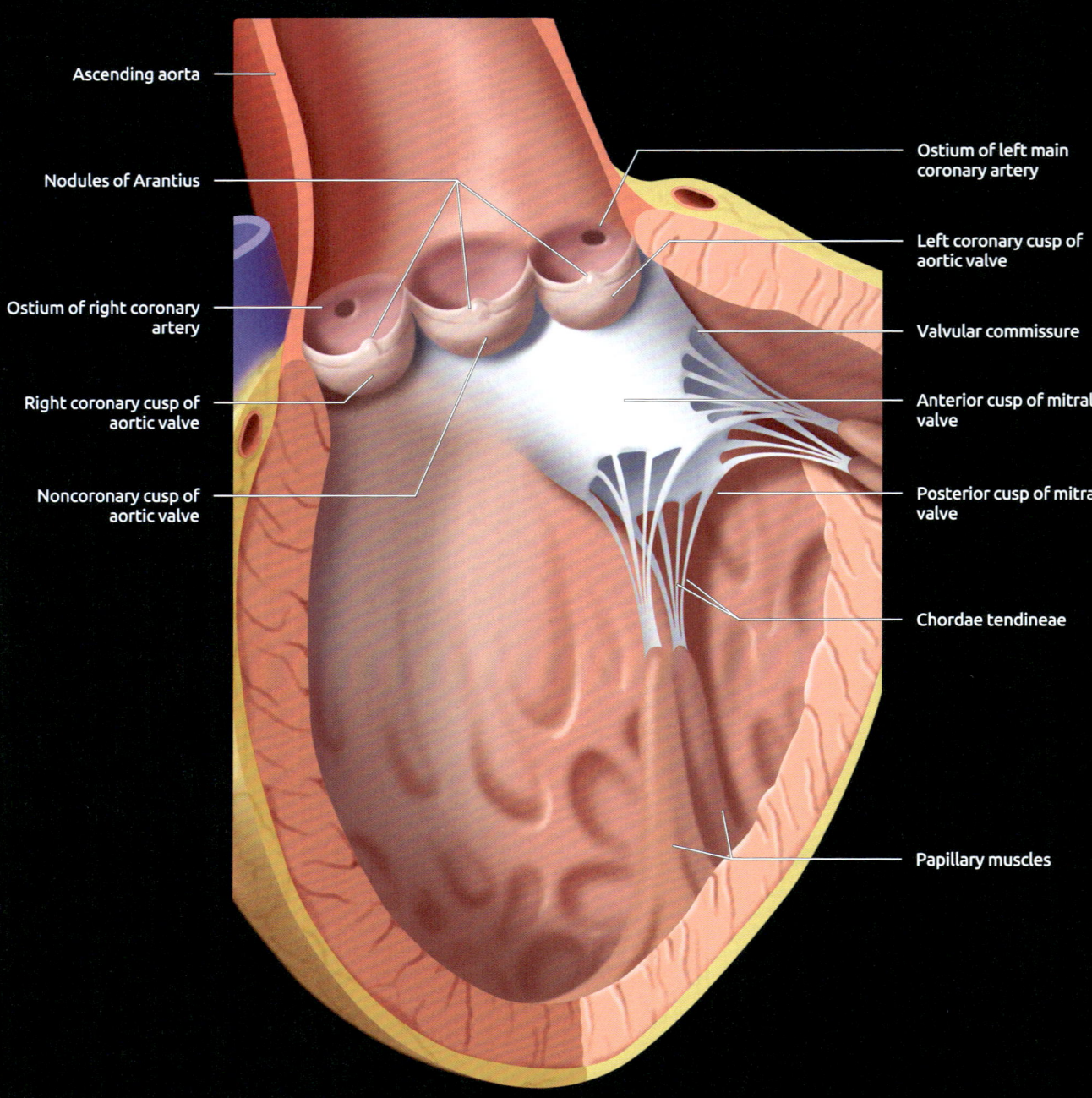

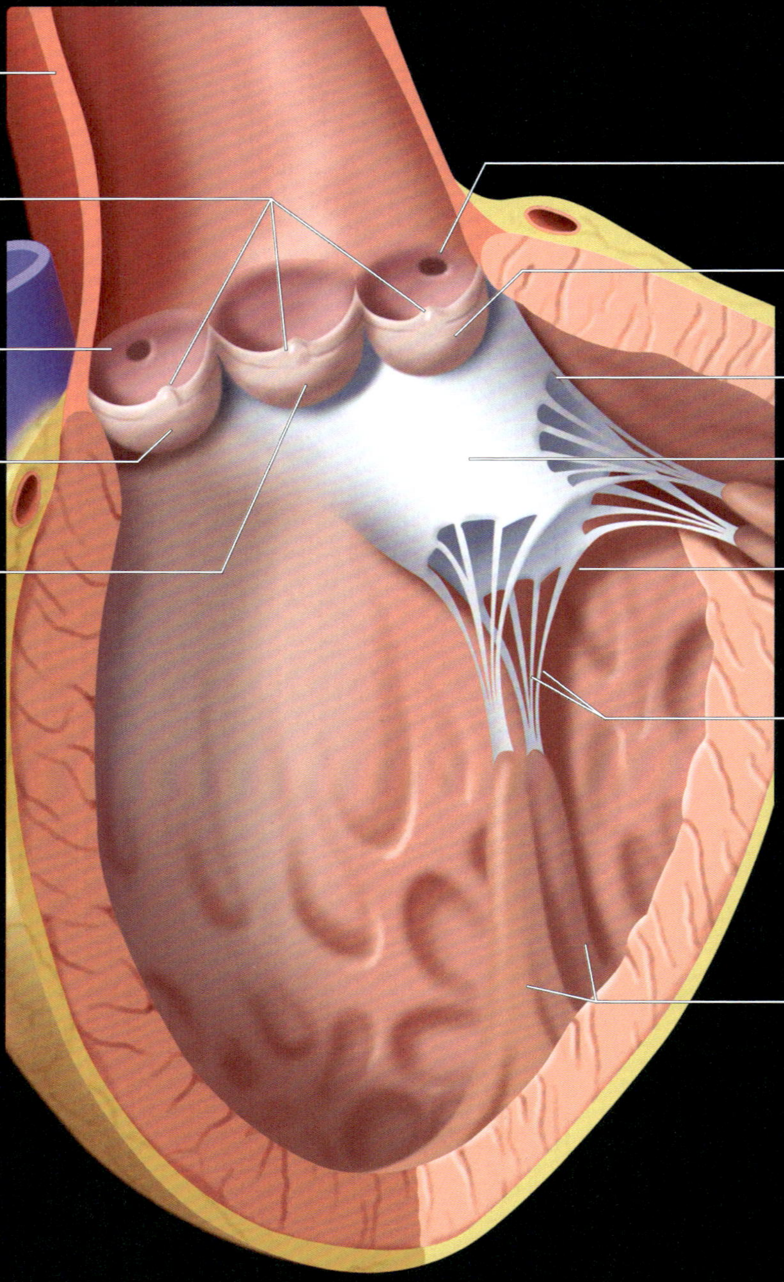

Graphic depicts the close relationship between the aortic and mitral valves. These valves are supported by fibrous valve rings connected by the left fibrous trigone. Thus, the anterior cusp of the mitral valve is closely related to the left coronary cusp of the aortic valve. The aortic valve right coronary, left coronary, and noncoronary cusps are shown. The semilunar cusps form sinuses during valve closure, which occurs by coaptation of the free cusp edges. Each valve has a fibrous nodule on the central portion of its free edge that is called the nodulus arantii. The mitral valve cusps are continuous along the left atrioventricular fibrous valve ring and are connected at the valve cusp commissures. The free edges of the mitral valve cusps attach to the anterior and posterior papillary muscles via chordae tendineae.

ECHOCARDIOGRAPHY OF AORTIC AND MITRAL VALVES

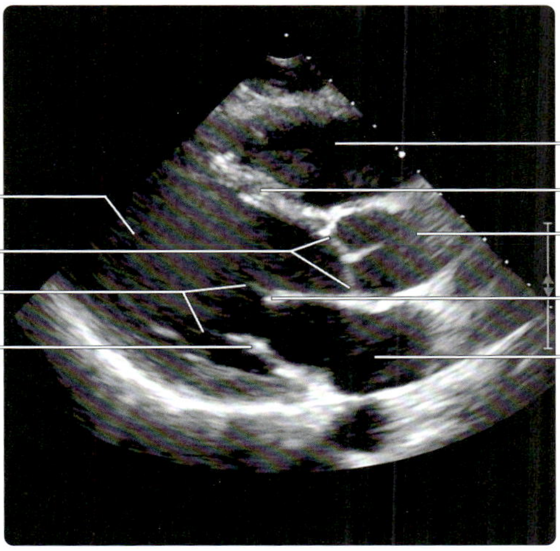

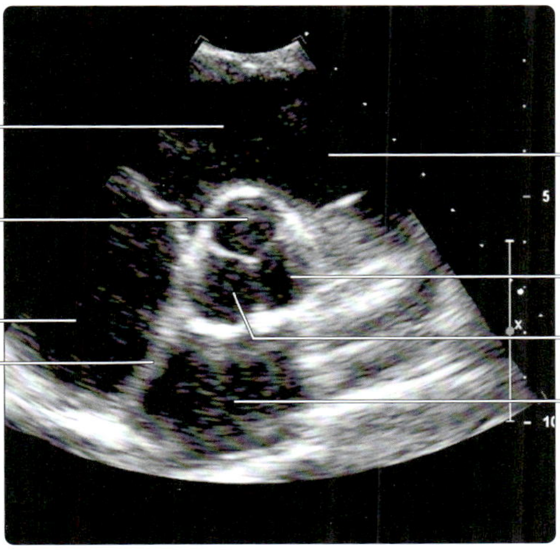

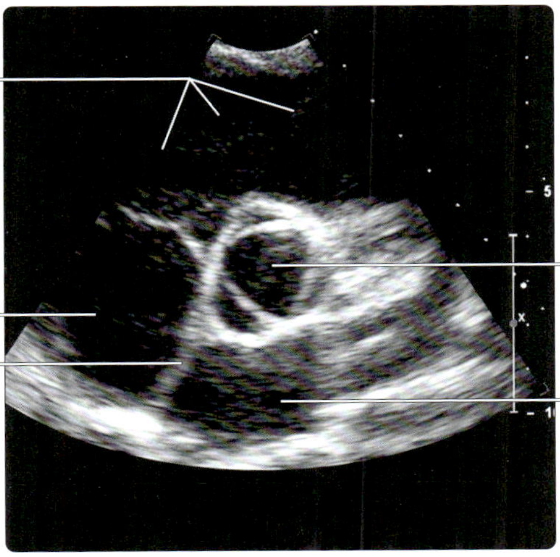

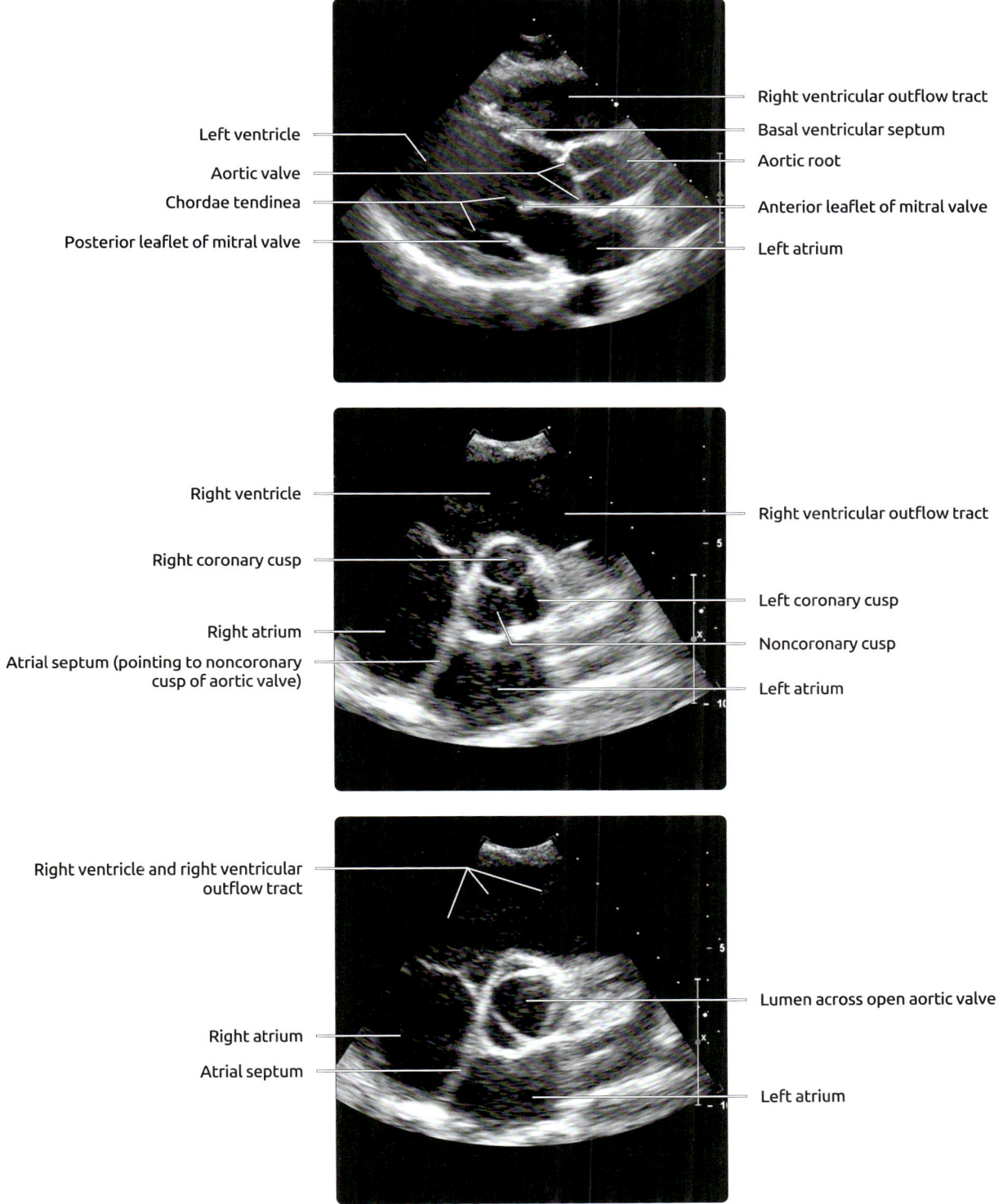

(Top) *Three-chamber transthoracic echocardiogram in diastole shows the left atrium, open mitral valve, left ventricle cavity, left ventricular outflow tract, and the aortic root with a closed aortic valve. Note that the "3rd chamber" near the probe is the right ventricle and its outflow tract.* **(Middle)** *Short-axis transthoracic echocardiogram of the closed aortic valve in diastole shows normal coaptation of all 3 cusps without regurgitant orifice. The cusps can be identified by the interatrial septum always pointing to the noncoronary cusp and by the right atrium, right ventricle, and right ventricular outflow tract "wrapping" around the right coronary cusp.* **(Bottom)** *Short-axis transthoracic echocardiogram of the open aortic valve in systole shows unrestricted opening of the cusp and confirms that it indeed has an unobstructed tricuspid configuration. Fusion along cusp edges can lead to bicuspid or unicuspid configuration and obstruction.*

ANATOMY AND CT OF LEFT HEART VALVES

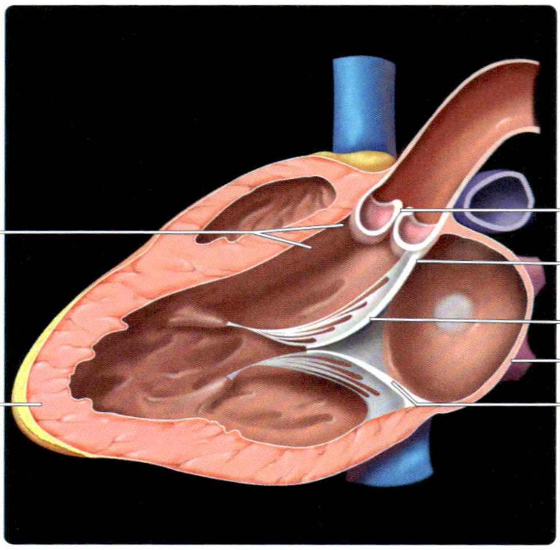

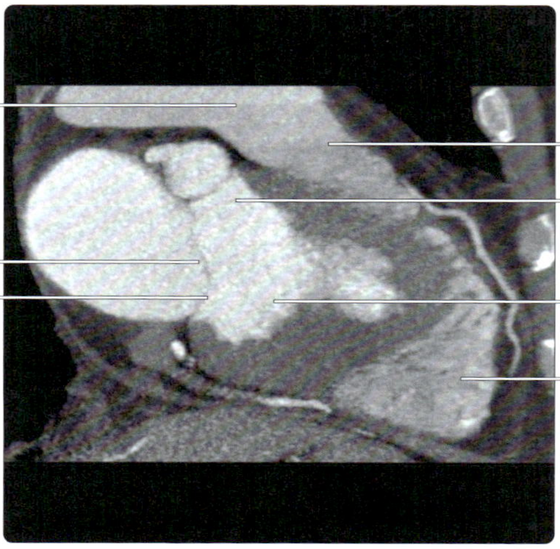

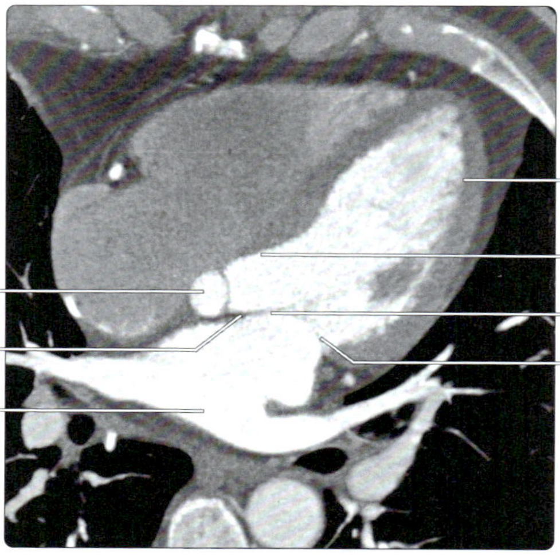

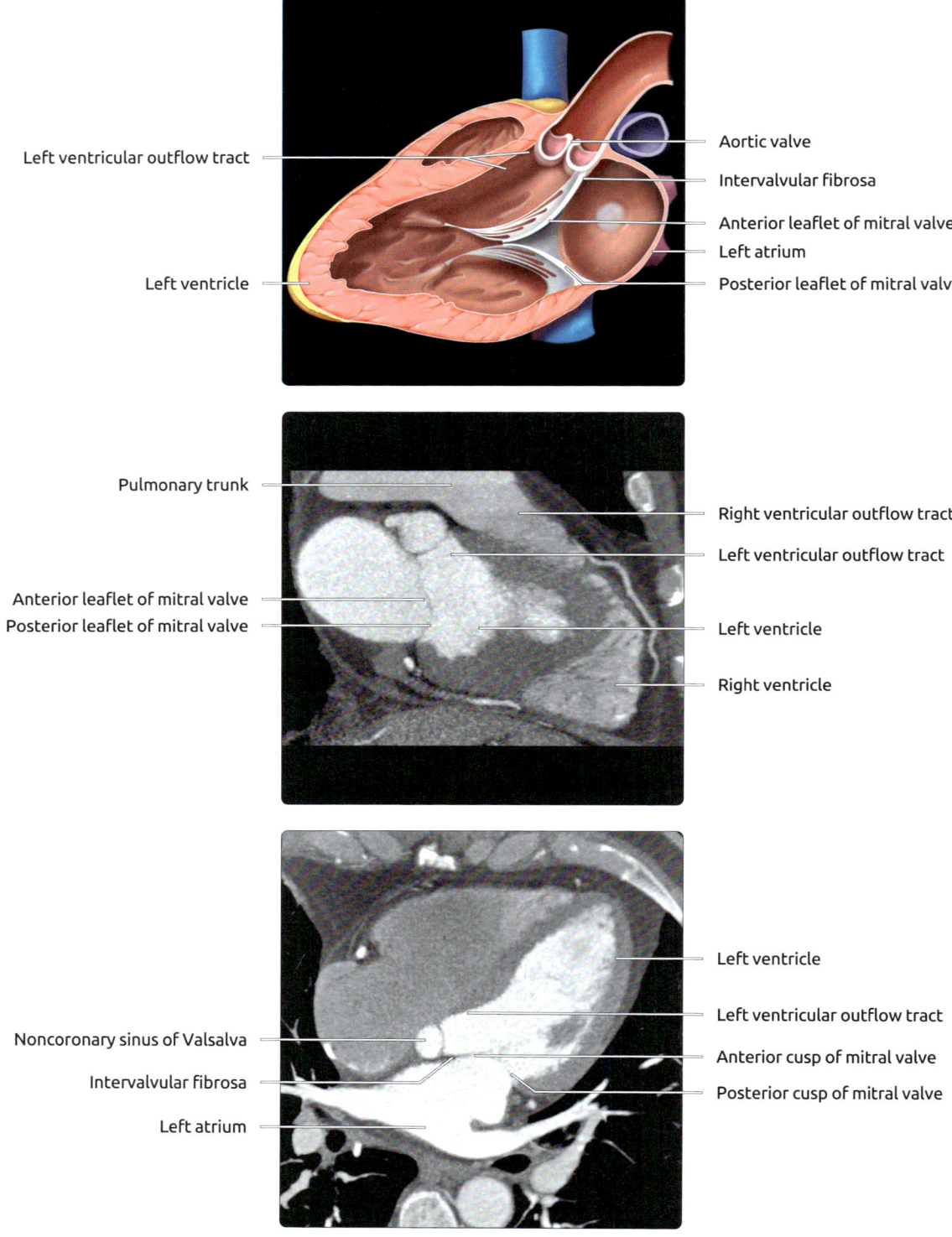

(Top) *Graphic illustrates a 3-chamber (left ventricular outflow tract) view of the heart and the relationship between the mitral and aortic valves. The fibrous rings that support these valves share a common fibrous bridge called the left fibrous trigone. The fibrous bridge forms a connection between the anterior cusp of the mitral valve and the left coronary cusp of the aortic valve.* **(Middle)** *Gated cardiac CECT demonstrates the anatomic relationship between the aortic and mitral valves. The left coronary cusp of the aortic valve shares a common fibrous attachment with the anterior cusp of the mitral valve.* **(Bottom)** *Four-chamber gated cardiac CECT demonstrates the close relationship between the anterior cusp of the mitral valve and the left coronary cusp of the aortic valve. The left coronary cusp is only partially visualized on this image.*

CT AND MR OF AORTIC VALVE

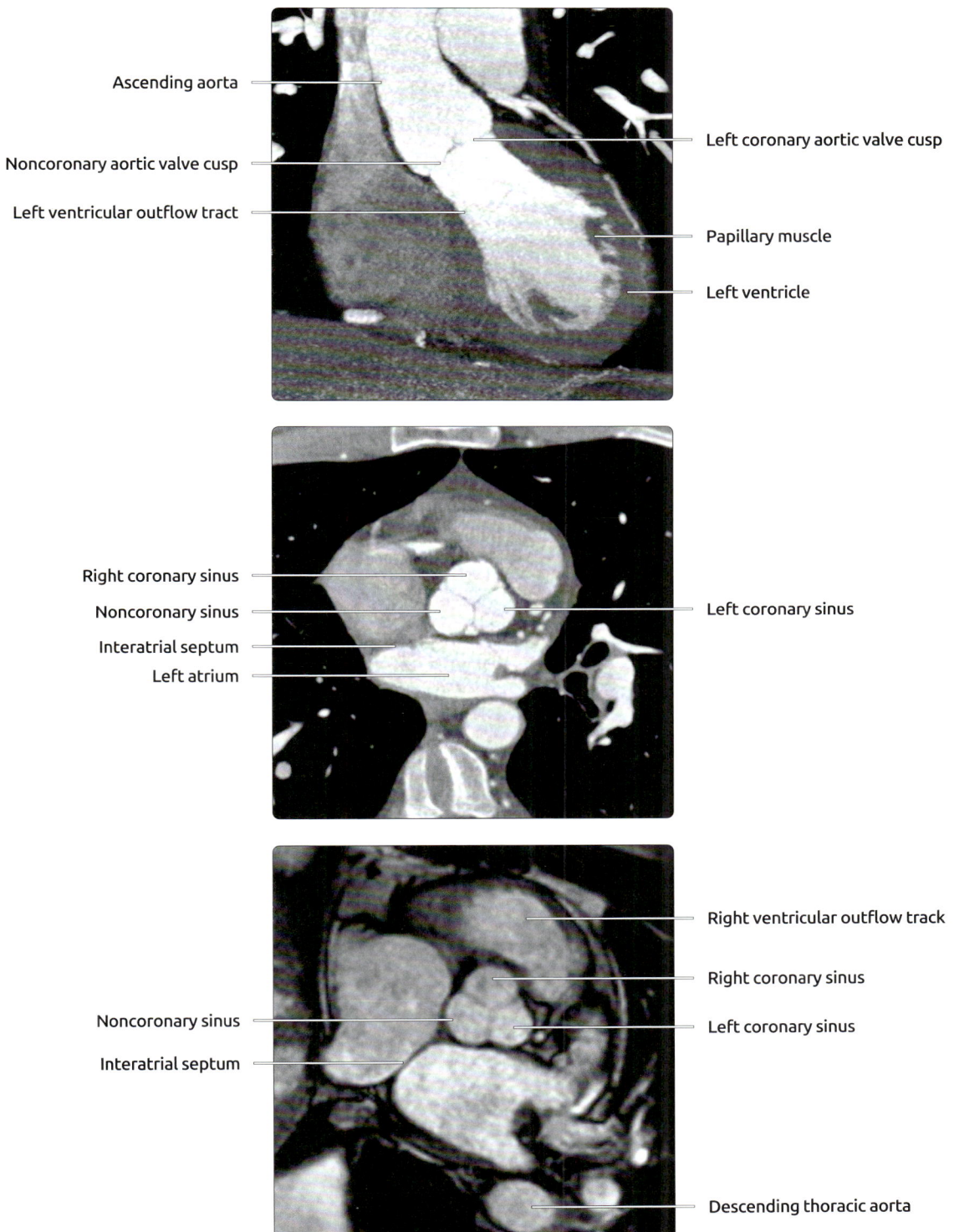

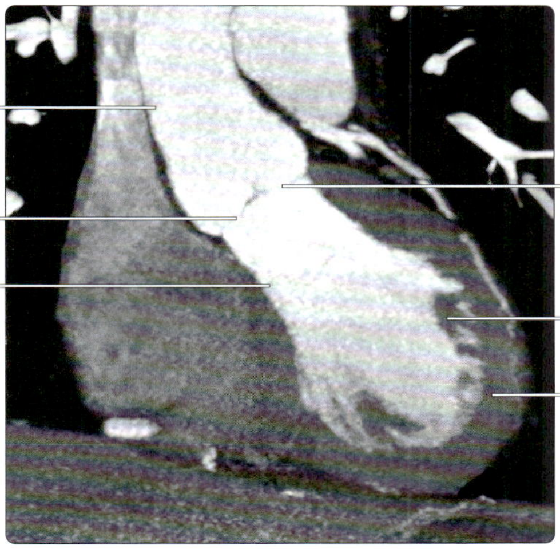

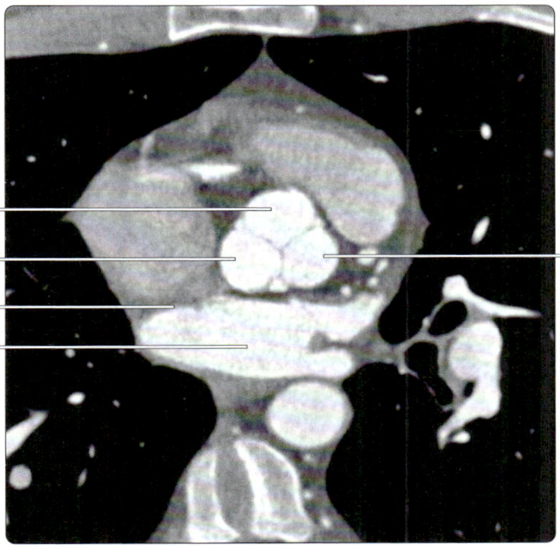

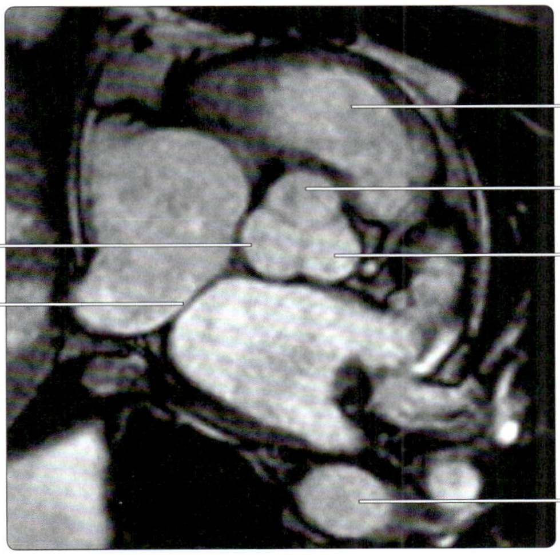

(Top) *Coronal gated cardiac CECT demonstrates the cross-sectional imaging appearance of the aortic valve. The aortic valve cusps are in coaptation, manifesting as thin, curvilinear soft tissue structures located at the apex of the left ventricular outflow tract. The sinuses of Valsalva are located above the valve cusps and are visible during diastole.* **(Middle)** *Axial gated CECT through the aortic valve in coaptation shows right coronary, left coronary, and noncoronary sinuses of Valsalva bound by the aortic wall and the corresponding valve cusps. The noncoronary sinus of Valsalva always faces the interatrial septum.* **(Bottom)** *Axial SSFP MR through the aortic valve in coaptation shows right coronary, left coronary, and noncoronary sinuses of Valsalva bound by the aortic wall and the corresponding valve cusps.*

MR, VALVE FUNCTION

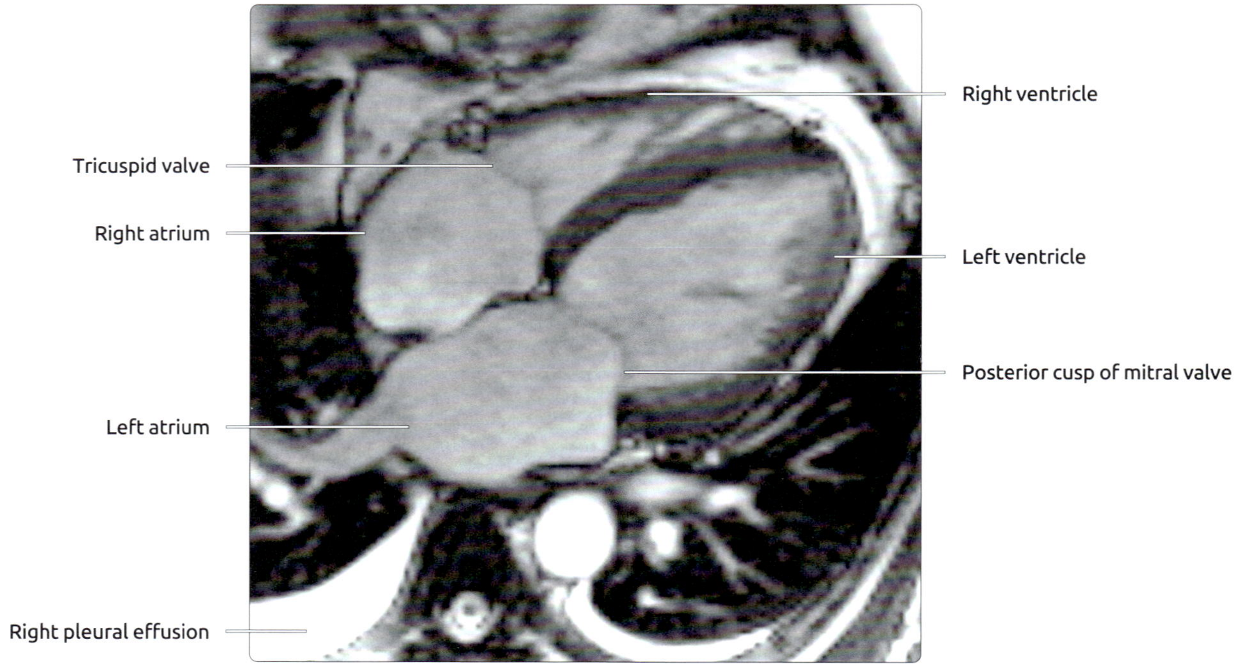

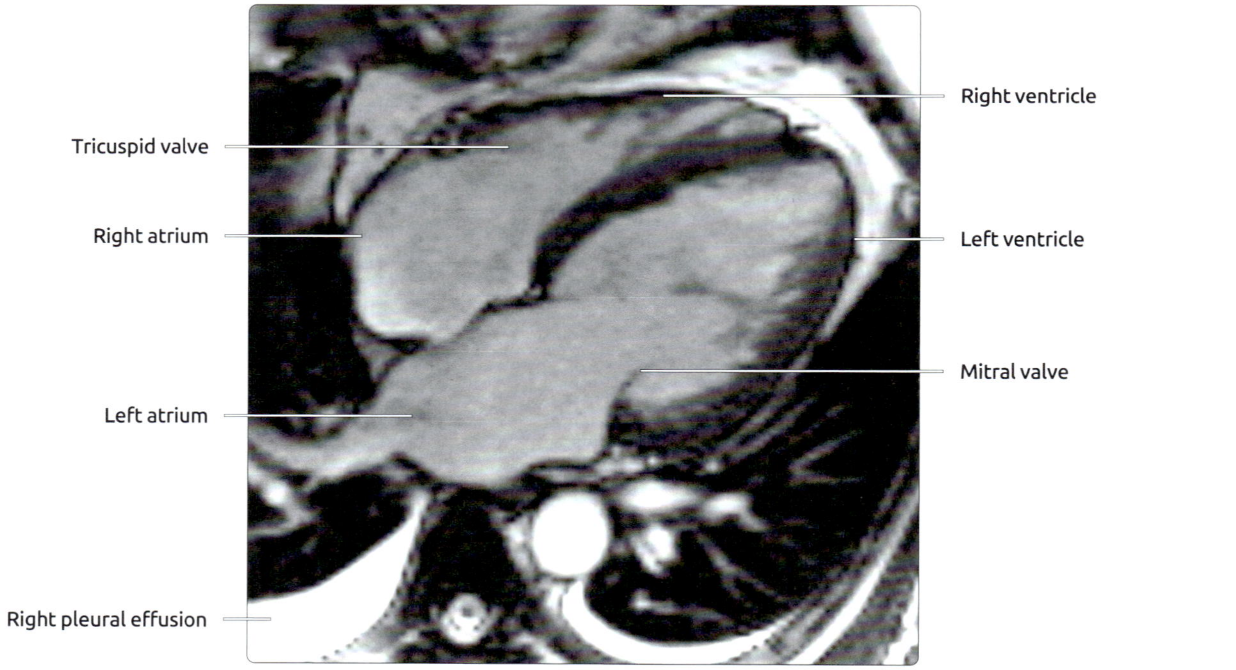

(Top) *Four-chamber gated cardiac SSFP MR through the heart demonstrates the function of the heart valves. This view, obtained during ventricular systole, shows that the atrioventricular valve cusps are coapted or closed, allowing blood to be pumped in an antegrade direction into the pulmonary and systemic arteries by the contracting myocardium without regurgitation or retrograde flow into the atria.* **(Bottom)** *Four-chamber gated cardiac SSFP MR obtained during diastole in the same patient demonstrates that the cusps of the atrioventricular valves are open, allowing blood to flow in an antegrade direction from the atria to fill the bilateral ventricles. The papillary muscles where the chordae tendineae attach are also visualized. There are small, bilateral pleural effusions, larger on the right.*

MR, VALVE FUNCTION

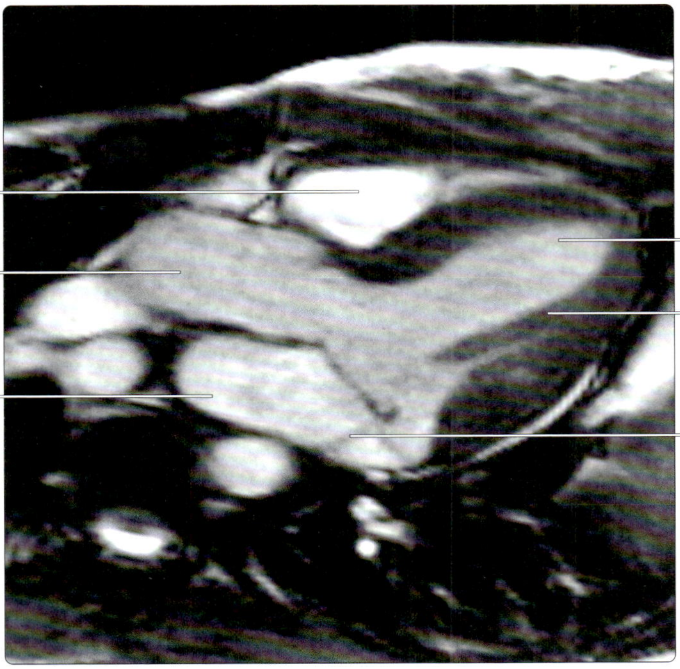

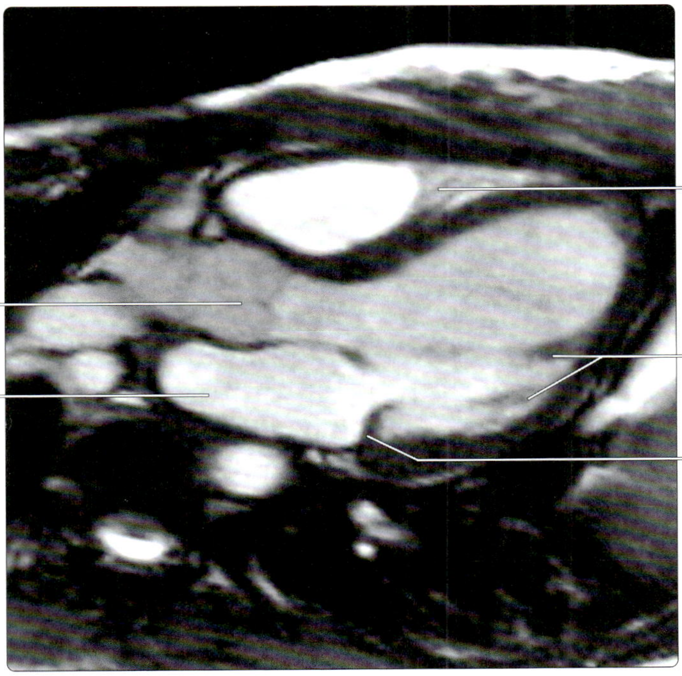

(Top) *Three-chamber gated cardiac SSFP MR demonstrates the function of the mitral and aortic valves. Left ventricular outflow tract view obtained during ventricular systole demonstrates that the aortic valve cusps are not visible at the aortic root distal to the right ventricular outflow tract, indicating that the aortic valve is open to allow antegrade flow of blood into the aorta. The mitral valve cusps are closed or coapted to prevent regurgitation of ventricular blood into the left atrium.* **(Bottom)** *Three-chamber gated cardiac SSFP MR obtained during diastole in the same patient shows that the mitral valve cusps are open to allow blood to flow into the left ventricle. The aortic valve cusps are closed, preventing retrograde flow of blood from the aorta. The papillary muscles of the left ventricle and moderator band of the right ventricle are also visualized.*

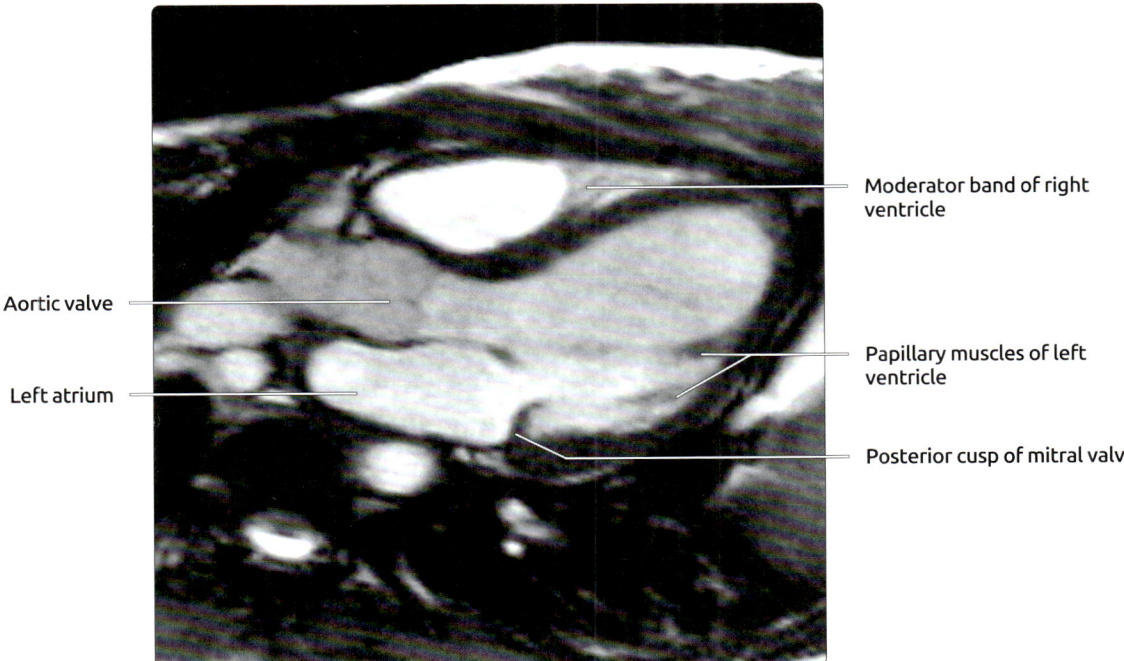

Introduction

Cardiac CT requires high spatial resolution to image small structures, high temporal resolution to image through high heart rates, and high craniocaudal (z-axis) coverage. The last several decades have witnessed several advances in cardiac CT, including scanner technology and reconstruction techniques. With each generation of technology, the acquisition speed and spatial resolution have increased, radiation and contrast doses have decreased, and new clinical applications have been developed.

Scanner Hardware

The acquisition speed of CT has progressively increased with each of the 5 generations of CT technology. Most of the current cardiac CT scanners are of 3rd-generation configuration, which has a rotate-rotate geometry with wide angular coverage and simultaneous measurements across the patient. Cardiac CT was initially performed with a 5th-generation electron beam CT, which used a stationary detector array and a stationary x-ray source. An electron gun emitted an electron beam that swept quickly across a stationery tungsten anode around the patient.

Subsequently, a spiral/helical CT was developed that allowed acquisition of volume of data in a breath hold, allowing a tube rotation time of 1 second. Current CT scanners have multiple detector rows along the z-axis (MDCT). A 64-detector scanner is considered to be a minimal requirement for good quality CT. Up to 320 detector rows are now available, which provides a z-coverage of 16 cm. These wide array or volume scanners can image the entire heart in a single heartbeat, which eliminates motion artifacts inherent in multiple heartbeat acquisitions (a major challenge in patients with arrhythmias). The gantry rotation times have also decreased with times as short as 0.25 seconds. Cardiac CT benefits from partial scan reconstruction, which uses only 180° of projection data, allowing a temporal resolution of 125 milliseconds (ms). The temporal resolution is further improved to 66 ms with a dual-source CT scanner, which has 2 x-ray tubes, and 2 detector arrays positioned 90° apart. Dual-source also has a high-pitch helical mode (pitch 3.4), which allows for a helical acquisition of the entire heart during a portion of 1 cardiac cycle, usually at end-diastole. When optimized, this allows for a significant reduction in both radiation and contrast doses. Dedicated high-resolution scanners with small detector elements are now available.

Multienergy CT

Multienergy CT (MECT) utilizes x-rays at different energy levels to differentiate and characterize materials and tissues beyond possible with a conventional single-energy CT due to differential attenuation of tissues/materials at different x-ray energies. The majority of the currently available multienergy techniques use 2 x-ray energy spectra and are appropriately called dual-energy CT. MECT techniques can be broadly classified as x-ray source based and detector based. X-ray source-based MECT techniques include dual source, rapid kVp switching, and dual spin. Dual source uses 2 x-ray sources, dual spin uses 2 consequent acquisitions at different energy levels, and rapid kvP switching switches between a low- and high-energy spectrum for each projection during gantry rotation. A split beam technique splits the x-ray beam into low- and high-energy spectra using prefiltration. Detector-based techniques include a dual-layer CT, which has 2 layers of detectors that detect low- and high-energy photons, and a photon-counting detector (PCD) CT. From this x-ray data, multiple additional MECT images are generated using either 2- or 3- material decomposition.

Virtual monoenergetic images (VMI) mimic images from a single-energy x-ray beam, which can be generated from 40-200 keV. VMI at 70 keV is equivalent to a conventional CT image obtained at 120 kVp. VMI < 70 keV are labeled low-energy VMI, which are characterized by high iodine signal. Hence, low-energy VMI are useful in low contrast-dose studies, salvaging suboptimal enhanced studies, and improving visualization of small vessels. VMI > 70 keV are labeled high-energy VMI, which are associated with lower artifacts, including beam hardening, blooming, and metallic artifacts. Iodine maps are generated by highlighting pixels that contain iodine. This can be used for characterizing lesions based on their iodine content (e.g., thrombus has no iodine content vs. slow flow with iodine content in left atrial appendage) and for evaluation of organ perfusion (e.g., myocardium, lungs). Conversely, iodine can be removed from the pixels, which generates virtual noncontrast (VNC) images. VNC can replace a true noncontrast acquisition and save some radiation dose. Further, VNC can be useful in the setting of an evaluation of a calcium score from a contrast CTA or in multiphasic vascular studies [e.g., post endovascular repair of abdominal aneurysm (EVAR]). VNC on its own or along with an iodine map can characterize some lesions, especially those which are incidentally encountered. E.g., in a postop patient, a high-attenuating cardiac/paracardiac lesion can be either calcium, hemorrhage, or surgical material, all with different management implications. High attenuation in VNC with no iodine content indicates either hemorrhage or calcium, whereas high iodine content and absence in VNC indicates contrast extravasation. A low-energy VMI and an iodine map can also be used for improving specificity and sensitivity of myocardial perfusion images by decreasing beam hardening artifact and improving visualization of perfusion defects. Myocardial extracellular volume (ECV) can also be quantified using MECT iodine map.

Photon-Counting Detector CT

PCD-CT uses a novel semiconductor detector that directly converts x-ray photons to electrical signal without generation of intermediary light signal. Each x-ray photon is assigned to a specific energy bin, which helps with multienergy imaging with improved spatial registration. The absence of septa in detectors allows smaller detector elements. Ultrahigh resolution (UHR) allows for slice thickness as low as 0.2 mm and a higher image matrix up to 1024. UHR reduces calcium blooming, which can improve assessment of heavily calcified plaques and the accuracy of stenosis quantification. Similarly, stent assessment is improved, including visualization of stent struts and improved accuracy of lumen within the stent. Therefore, UHR should provide higher diagnostic accuracy in the detection of CAD, even in a high-risk population with heavily calcified plaques and stents.

PCD-CT provides higher signal of iodine, lower noise, and lower artifacts, all of which improve the image quality with geometric radiation dose efficiency. PCD-CT allows improved multienergy binning at high temporal resolution and improved spatial and temporal alignment. All the aforementioned multienergy applications can be performed at higher quality with PCD-CT. K-edge imaging, novel contrast media (e.g., nanoparticles that target inflamed plaque), and multicontrast media (e.g., iodine and gadolinium with iodine for arterial evaluation and gadolinium for myocardial enhancement) can be used. Additionally, the multienergy mode can be combined with UHR, although the minimum slice thickness for the multienergy mode is currently 0.4 mm.

Radiation Dose Reduction Techniques

Due to the concern for the complications of radiation exposure from cardiac CT, several techniques have been developed to minimize radiation dose without compromising image quality. Using patient body habitus, the lowest possible tube voltage and tube current are selected to minimize radiation dose. Tube current can be modulated along the z-axis based on body thickness and along the R-R interval depending on the desired cardiac phase of acquisition. Beam-shaping filters and collimators also decrease radiation dose. Prospective ECG-triggered acquisition (either axial or high-pitch helical) has a lower radiation dose than retrospective ECG-based acquisition. Modern scanners use an iterative reconstruction algorithm that has significantly lower noise and artifacts than the conventional filtered back projection reconstruction. In this technique, the measured data is compared to a synthesized "forward projection" of the initial reconstructed image that follows which noise is decreased in an iterative manner. The lower noise of this technique allows low radiation dose techniques, albeit blurring at the edge of low-contrast structures.

Visualization Techniques

Visualization techniques have also developed along with advances in scanner hardware. Modern CT scanners offer isotropic spatial resolution, which benefits 3D visualization techniques, including multiplanar reconstruction (MPR), maximum-intensity projection (MIP), volume rendering (VR), and shaded surface display (SSD). These techniques allow evaluation of complex anatomy and spatial relationships with adjacent structures. MIPs project voxels with highest attenuation values through the image volume. SSD selects the superficial attenuation of voxels that are closest to the virtual viewer to generate a shaded surface. Virtual endoscopy/angioscopy is a variation of SSD that provides endoluminal views. VR uses a local lighting model and ray casting method to generate 3D from volume of data. Cinematic rendering (CR) is a recent advance in visualization, which uses a global illumination model and path tracing method to generate photorealistic images that improve assessment of complex anatomy and spatial relationships. 3D models can be used for 3D printing of personalized models of patient anatomy, which can be used for training and education of patients and physicians. Customized devices and biomaterials can be developed and bench testing of devices for surgeries or interventions can be performed.

Artificial Intelligence

Artificial intelligence (AI) algorithms enable computers to simulate human behavior with machine learning (ML) using statistical methods for optimizing performance based on experience. AI is now increasingly available and utilized in nearly every aspect of cardiac CT, beginning from selection of an appropriate protocol. AI can be used for patient positioning and determine optimal posttrigger delay after contrast material administration. AI can improve image quality by decreasing noise and artifacts and increasing spatial resolution, which can decrease acquisition time and radiation dose. AI can now perform several tasks automatically, including segmentation (coronary arteries, ventricles, myocardium, etc.) and post processing (e.g., volumetric and functional quantification). For one vendor, AI is used in computational fluid assessment to provide CT-fractional flow reserve. For another vendor, AI determines the likely presence or absence of ischemia based on quantitative measures of atherosclerosis, stenosis, and significant vascular morphology. AI can also classify atherosclerotic lesions based on the degree of stenosis, positive remodeling, and plaque characterization. Another application of AI includes quantifying opportunistic screening using data present in a CT scan, such as coronary calcium, body composition analysis, epicardial fat, liver fat, and vertebral bone mineral density.

Radiomics

Radiomics is an innovative quantitative image analysis technique that utilizes information available in images that are not visible to the eye. Radiomics uses textural information from spatial distribution of Hounsfield units and relationships. Radiomics facilitates precision medicine with personalized prognosis, risk stratification, and potentially targeted therapies. A challenge of radiomics is the variations in scan technologies and reconstruction kernels that determine the spatial resolution and noise. With the availability of AI, radiomics algorithms can potentially work across scanner models and perform evaluation very fast. Radiomics analysis of coronary artery plaques, pericoronary adipose tissue, and myocardium have been shown to provide personalized prognosis and risk stratification.

Future Applications

Phase-contrast CT is an emerging technology that utilizes organized changes in x-ray phase and refraction to generate image contrast significantly superior to current CT techniques. In ex-vivo imaging, phase-contrast CT can achieve spatial resolution ranging from 2-20 μm. Currently this technique is not feasible in humans due to the need for synchrotron, which is not widely available, high radiation doses, imaging times up to 7 hours, and reconstruction times up to 24 hours. However, this technique is expected to advance and mature to provide high-quality images of the heart.

Selected References

1. Brunet J et al: Multidimensional analysis of the adult human heart in health and disease using hierarchical phase-contrast tomography. Radiology. 312(1):e232731, 2024
2. Ayx I et al: Radiomics in cardiac computed tomography. Diagnostics (Basel). 13(2), 2023
3. McCollough CH et al: Milestones in CT: past, present, and future. Radiology. 309(1):e230803, 2023
4. Tatsugami F et al: Recent advances in artificial intelligence for cardiac CT: enhancing diagnosis and prognosis prediction. Diagn Interv Imaging. 104(11):521-8, 2023
5. Kalisz K et al: Update on cardiovascular applications of multienergy CT. Radiographics. 37(7):1955-74, 2017

(Left) *Left anterior descending (LAD) stent (top) at 0.6-mm, 0.4-mm, and 0.2-mm slice thickness shows improved visualization of struts and decreased blooming artifact with decreasing slice thickness. 0.2-mm MPR of the LAD (bottom) with multiple overlapping stents nicely shows the stent architecture with no evidence of restenosis.* **(Right)** *Sagittal oblique reconstructed CTA PCD-CT shows excellent visualization of stent struts and lumen. No significant stenosis is identified.*

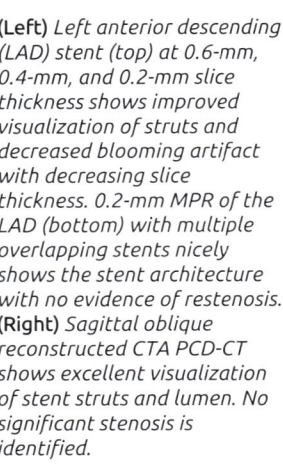

Stent Visualization With Photon-Counting Detector CT

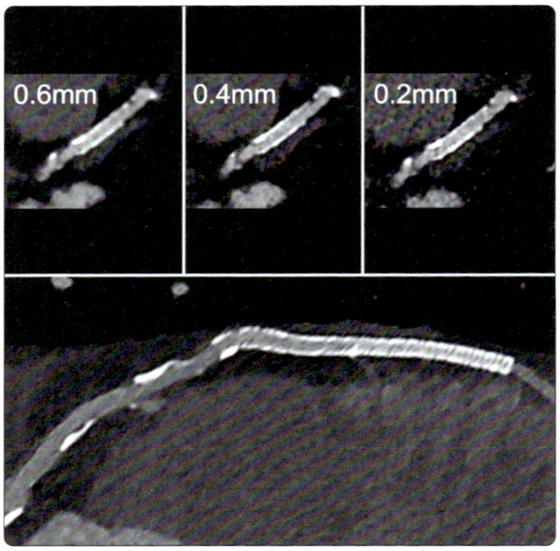

Stent in PCD-CT

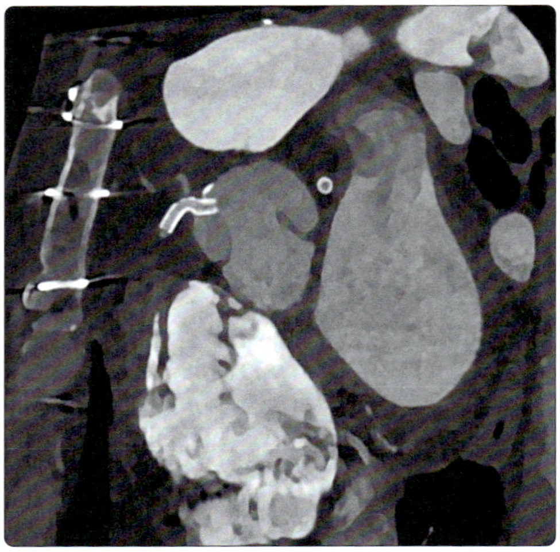

(Left) *Axial reconstructed CTA from a conventional dual-source CT scanner shows a dense calcified plaque in the midright coronary artery with calcium blooming artifact, which mimics a moderate stenosis.* **(Right)** *Axial reconstructed CTA from a PCD-CT scanner in the same patient shows improved visualization of the calcified plaque with decreased calcium blooming, which downgrades the stenosis to mild.*

Calcified Plaque Evaluation: Conventional CT

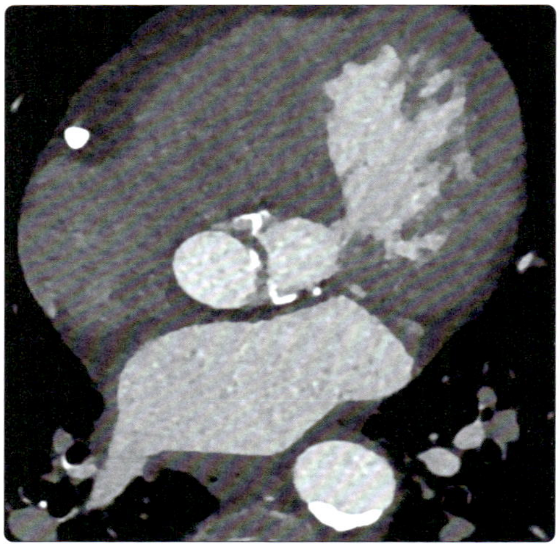

Calcified Plaque Evaluation: PCD-CT

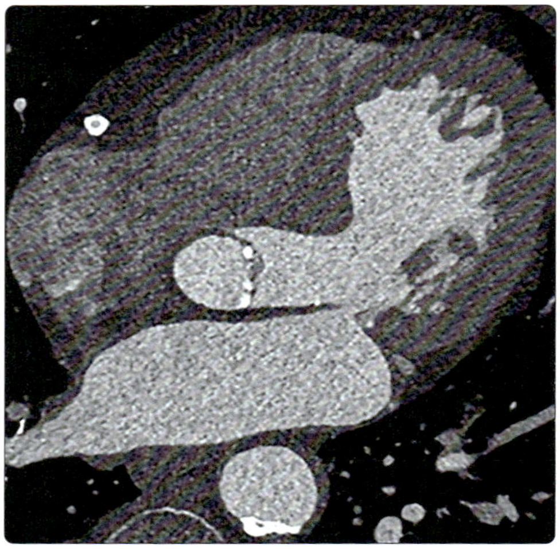

(Left) *Coronal oblique reconstructed image obtained in a PCD-CT scanner shows excellent visualization of the structure of an Amulet device placed in the left atrial appendage.* **(Right)** *Axial oblique reconstructed image obtained in a PCD CT scanner in the same patient shows excellent visualization of the structure of an Amulet device placed in the left atrial appendage.*

Device Visualization: PCD-CT

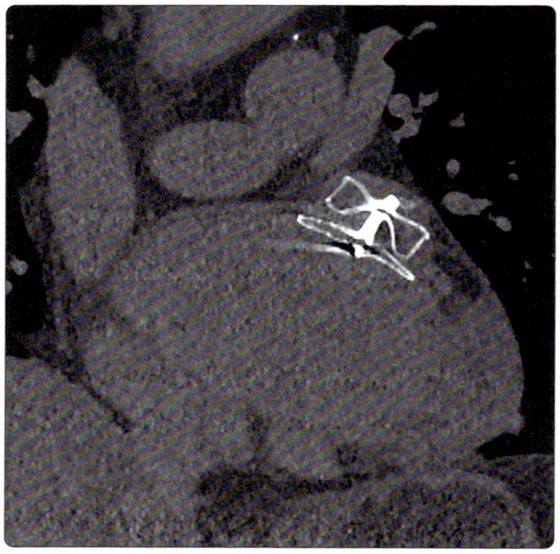

Device Visualization: PCD-CT

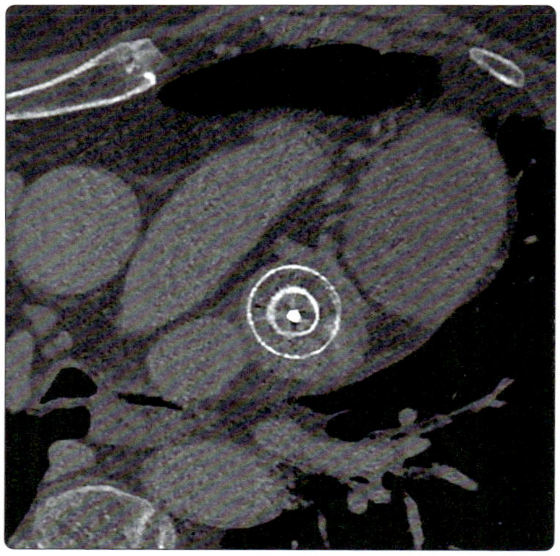

Noise in PCD-CT

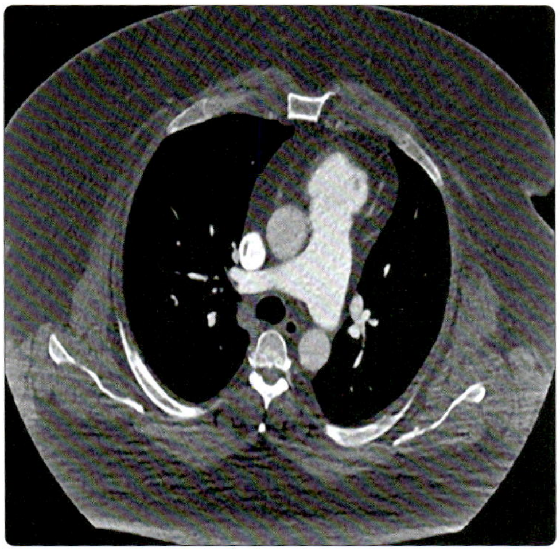

Multienergy CT

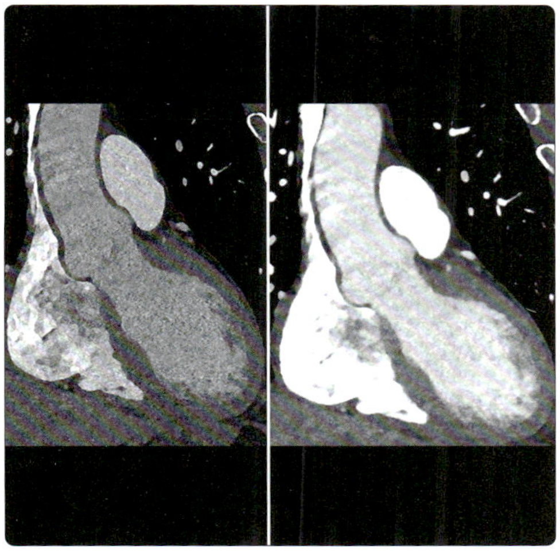

(Left) *Axial CT in a patient with a BMI > 50 shows excellent image quality with negligible noise. PCD-CT technology has low electronic noise, and, as a result, image quality is increased.* **(Right)** *CTA (left) shows poor systemic contrast opacification due to contrast extravasation. 50 keV monoenergetic image (right) shows significant improvement in the iodine signal.*

Volume Rendering vs. Cinematic Rendering

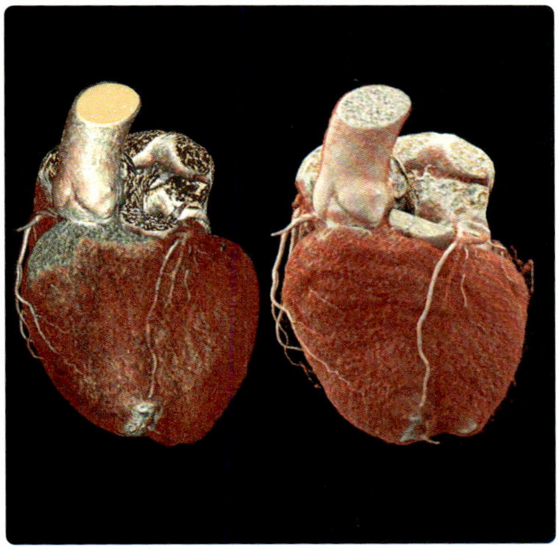

Multienergy in Left Atrial Thrombus

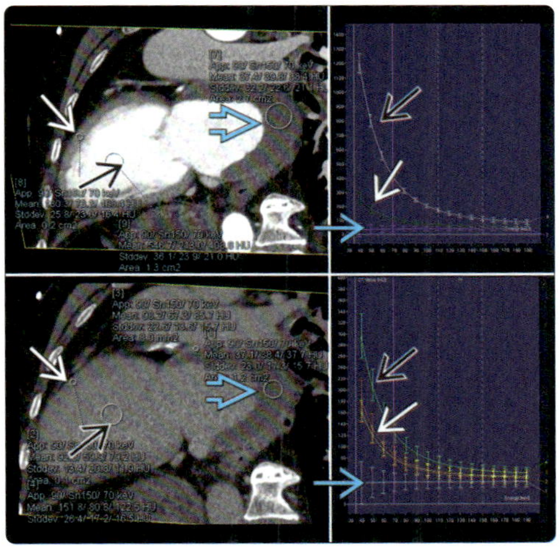

(Left) *Volume-rendered reconstruction (left) shows good details of the heart and coronary arteries, which is significantly improved using cinematic rendering (right).* **(Right)** *Arterial (top) and delayed (bottom) images show a left atrial mass ⇨ (left) with very low HU (y-axis) across the monoenergetic spectrum (x-axis) → (right), confirming thrombus. Myocardium ➔ and blood pool ⇨, which contain increasing concentrations of iodine, have a high HU at a low keV, which decreases as keV increases.*

Low Monoenergy Delayed Imaging

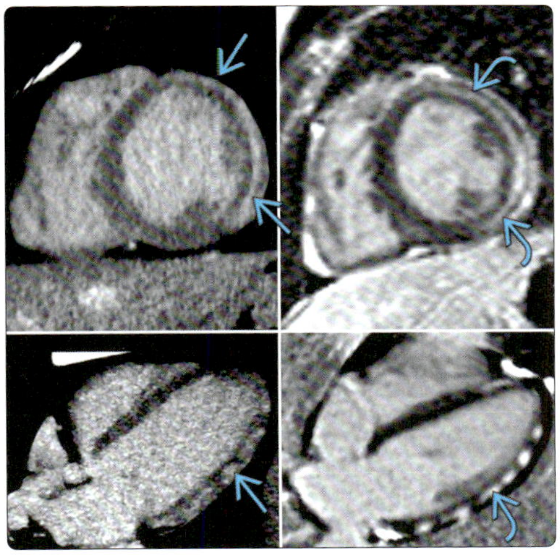

PCD-CT in Chronic Thromboembolic Disease

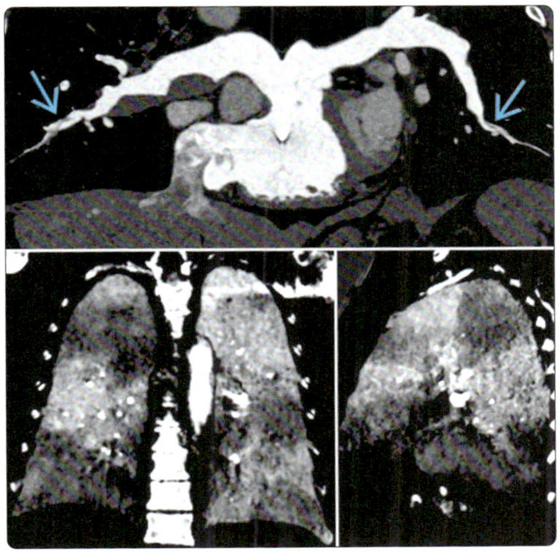

(Left) *40 keV delayed cardiac CT (left) performed 5 minutes after a coronary CTA shows subepicardial and midmyocardial delayed enhancement → due to myocarditis, which mirrors same day cardiac MR LGE ↗.* **(Right)** *0.4-mm MPR (top) shows very small distal subsegmental chronic clots → that could be easily missed with 1-mm thick slices. Coronal and sagittal iodine map images (bottom) show bilateral perfusion defects in this patient with chronic thromboembolic pulmonary hypertension (CTEPH).*

AI in Cardiac Imaging

KEY FACTS

- **Transforming cardiac imaging**: Artificial Intelligence (AI) is enhancing every step of cardiac imaging, allowing cardiac imagers to focus more on patient care and imaging interpretation rather than repetitive tasks while also providing insights that may exceed human capabilities.
- **Importance of data for training**: High-quality data is essential for training AI models, as it affects their ability to learn and generalize. Large, diverse datasets help models capture different features and patterns, while well-labeled data ensure accurate learning of input-output relationships. Balanced and augmented data further enhance model performance and reduce biases, making robust data preparation key to the success of AI algorithms.
- **Deep learning algorithms in cardiac imaging**: Multilayer neural networks are the primary AI approach for processing cardiac images, generating outputs, such as image categories, object location, and pixel labels. These algorithms learn the features of images and the relationships between features and outputs, enabling them to generalize and apply their knowledge to unseen data.
- **Radiomics in cardiac imaging**: Although still developing, AI-driven radiomics identifies quantitative features in images that highlight subtle pathologic patterns undetectable by the human eye. These insights can improve diagnostic accuracy and imaging phenotyping, potentially guiding more effective therapy.

Original Delayed-Enhancement MR

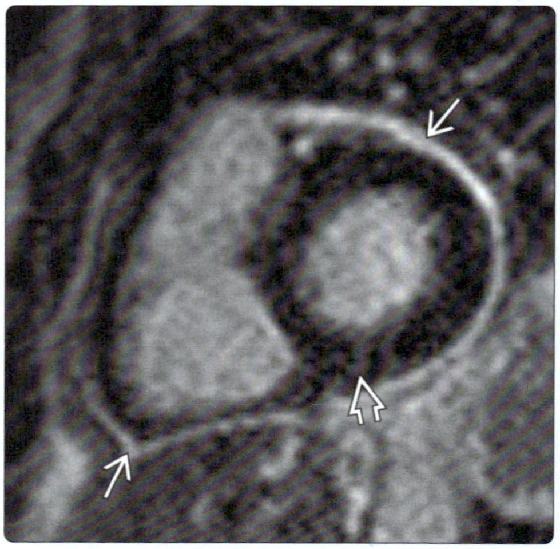

Artificial Intelligence-Enhanced MR

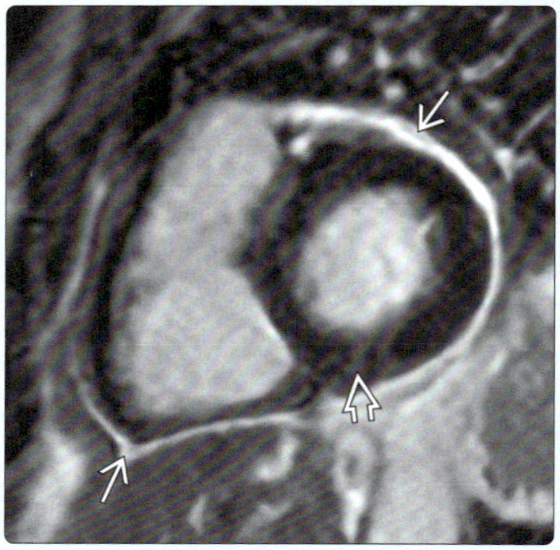

(Left) *Short-axis view of delayed-enhancement cardiac MR in a patient with pericarditis is shown. Notice the thick and enhancing pericardium. There is suspicion of late gadolinium enhancement (LGE) within the myocardium, although it could be attributed to excessive image noise.* **(Right)** *The same slice is shown after post processing with an AI enhancement tool. Note the improved imaging resolution with better definition of the pericardial thickening. Persistent LGE may suggest concurrent myocarditis.*

Automated Ventricular Segmentation (MR)

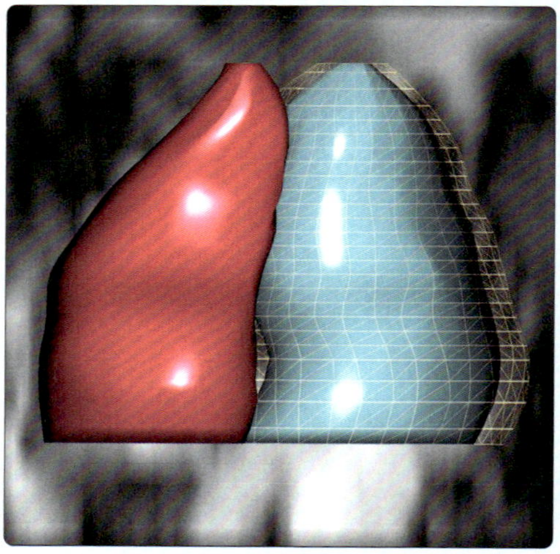

Automated Coronary Calcium Scoring (CT)

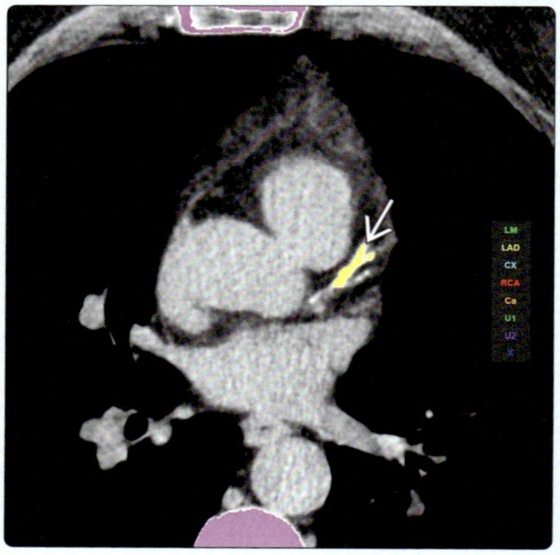

(Left) *Reconstruction shows a modified 4-chamber view with overlaid 3D models of the right ventricular cavity (red), left ventricular cavity (blue), and left ventricular epicardium (yellow mesh), all generated by an AI algorithm. These models enable the derivation of quantitative parameters for assessing ventricular function.* **(Right)** *Noncontrast axial image from a calcium scoring CT shows AI-driven automated segmentation of coronary calcium, which allows for a quicker and more consistent assessment of the risk of future coronary events.*

TERMINOLOGY

Artificial Intelligence

- Artificial Intelligence (AI) in the field of medical imaging is centered on the development of computer systems that replicate tasks usually performed by human radiologists and specialists. These tasks include analyzing imaging data, recognizing subtle patterns in scans, making informed decisions, and continuously learning from new information to improve diagnostic accuracy.

Algorithm

- An algorithm is a detailed process or set of rules used to solve a problem or accomplish a task systematically. In medical imaging, algorithms are integral for processing and interpreting data, allowing for precise calculations and improved diagnostic capabilities.

Computer-Aided Detection/Diagnosis

- Computer-aided detection/diagnosis (CAD)-T (detection) refers to software that helps cardiac imagers by identifying and highlighting areas in medical images that might need further investigation. CAD-E (diagnosis) goes beyond this by offering diagnostic support, including classifying the findings and potentially determining the likelihood of an abnormality being present.

Convolutional Neural Network

- A convolutional neural network (CNN) is a specialized deep learning algorithm that excels at processing and analyzing visual data. It consists of multiple layers, including convolutional layers, which enable the network to automatically and progressively learn spatial features from images.

Machine Learning

- Machine Learning is an AI discipline where algorithms are trained on data to autonomously make predictions or decisions, eliminating the need for explicit programming for each task. It includes techniques such as supervised learning, unsupervised learning, and reinforcement learning.

Deep Learning

- Deep Learning is a subset of machine learning that uses neural networks with numerous layers of artificial neurons to model complex patterns in data.

Model

- In the realm of AI and machine learning, a model is a mathematic representation trained on data to mirror a real world process. It is employed to make predictions or decisions when analyzing new datasets.

Radiomics

- Radiomics is a specialized area of medical research that utilizes data-characterization algorithms to extract a wide range of quantitative features from medical images. These features are then explored to construct models that may aid diagnosis, predict disease outcomes, and tailor treatments to individual patients.

Segmentation

- In medical imaging, segmentation involves partitioning an image into various sections or regions, often with the goal of isolating specific anatomic features or areas of interest, such as cardiac chambers on an MR.

APPLICATIONS

Facilitating Imaging Acquisition

- AI can streamline imaging planning in MR and cardiac CT by automating scan setup and optimizing imaging parameters. AI-driven systems can automatically adjust for scan range and slice orientation based on patient-specific factors, improving image quality, consistency, and reducing scan times.

Optimizing Imaging Quality

- AI can improve imaging quality in MR and cardiac CT by applying advanced denoising and resolution enhancement techniques in different data domains, such as K-space, sinogram space, and imaging space. These methods enhance image clarity or restore quality when faster acquisition is achieved by lowering spatial resolution or signal-to-noise ratio.

Automating Imaging Analytics

- AI can streamline imaging analytics in MR and cardiac CT by automating tasks, such as calcium scoring and cardiac chamber segmentation. This automation saves time, reduces observer variability, and enhances the consistency and accuracy of imaging analysis, enabling clinicians to concentrate on integrating imaging findings with clinical data.

Enhancing Imaging Phenotyping and Prognostication

- AI-driven radiomics enhances imaging phenotyping and prognostication in both MR and CT by extracting a vast array of quantitative features from images that go beyond standard visual assessment. These features can capture subtle patterns and textures associated with various pathologies, enabling a more detailed characterization of tissue and disease states. By integrating radiomics with advanced AI models, imaging phenotypes can be linked to specific prognostic outcomes, helping to predict disease progression and treatment response. This data-driven approach could allow for more personalized patient care, improving diagnostic accuracy and enabling targeted therapeutic strategies based on individual imaging biomarkers.

SELECTED REFERENCES

1. Morales MA et al: Present and future innovations in AI and cardiac MRI. Radiology. 310(1):e231269, 2024
2. European Society of Radiology (ESR): What the radiologist should know about artificial intelligence - an ESR white paper. Insights Imaging. 10(1):44, 2019

SECTION 2

Coronary Artery Disease

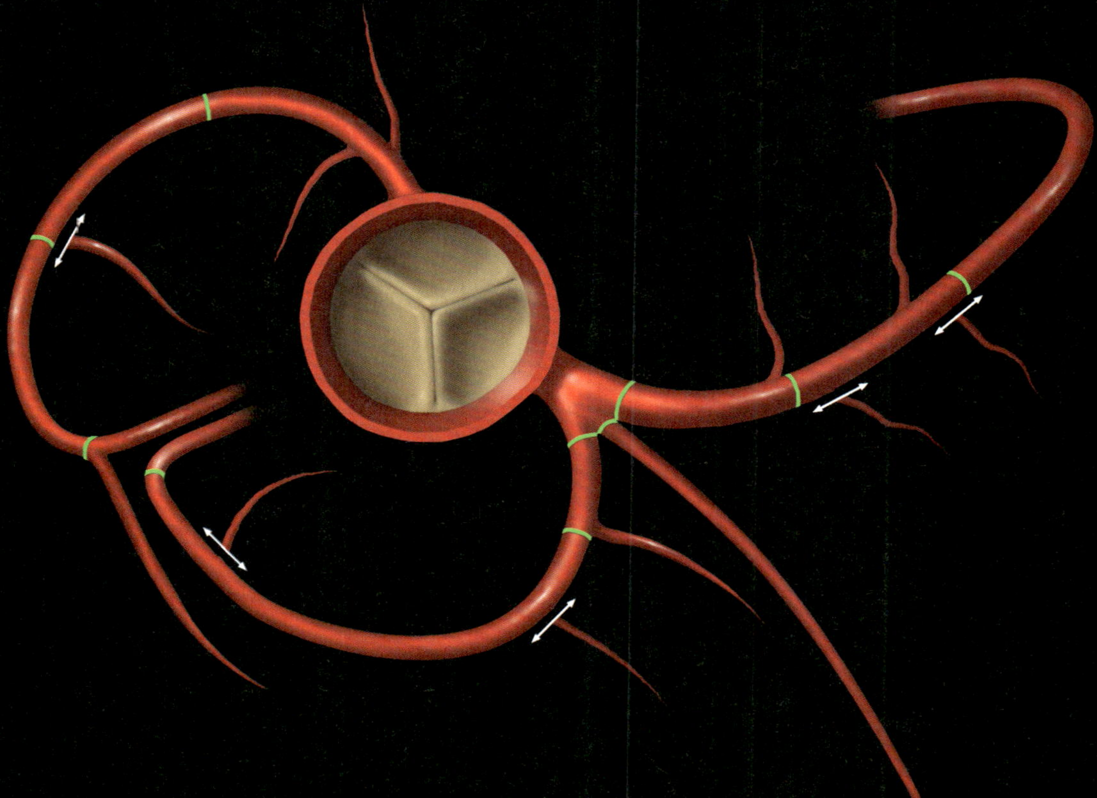

Introduction

Coronary artery disease (CAD) is a leading cause of morbidity and mortality in Western countries. The underlying pathology is the development of atherosclerotic plaque in the intima of the coronary arteries. While in most cases, coronary atherosclerotic plaque will remain clinically silent, it can clinically manifest in a number of forms, such as stable CAD, acute coronary syndrome, heart failure, and sudden cardiac death.

Clinical Manifestations of Coronary Artery Disease

Stable Coronary Artery Disease

In stable CAD, sometimes now referred to as chronic coronary syndrome, atherosclerotic plaque deposits in the coronary arteries lead to significant narrowing of the coronary lumen with subsequent obstruction of the coronary blood stream. This results in insufficient oxygen supply of the downstream myocardium during situations of increased demand (typically physical exercise). There is no close correlation between the anatomic degree of luminal obstruction and the extent of downstream ischemia at exercise, which depends on numerous factors. These include the severity and length of the lesion, the amount of dependent myocardium, the resistance of the microvasculature, and the amount of collateral flow from other coronary territories. Revascularization serves to treat symptoms and improve prognosis and is usually recommended when the amount of ischemic myocardium exceeds 10% of the left ventricular mass.

Acute Coronary Syndromes

Acute coronary syndromes have a mechanism that is different from stable CAD. Typically, the index event is the rupture (most frequently) or erosion (less frequently) of the fibrous cap of an atherosclerotic plaque. Material from within the plaque is exposed to the blood stream and leads to immediate thrombocyte aggregation so that a thrombus forms on the surface of the ruptured plaque. This thrombus can obstruct coronary blood flow, and, depending on the degree of obstruction and downstream myocardial damage, the resulting clinical manifestation is either completely silent or symptomatic in the form of unstable angina, non-ST-elevation myocardial infarction, or ST-elevation myocardial infarction. Treatment is usually emergent and includes both medication to counter thrombus aggregation and mechanical interventions to restore blood flow.

Heart Failure

Acute coronary syndromes, including myocardial infarction, can remain clinically silent; therefore, substantial damage to the myocardium can occur without the patient noticing any chest pain episodes. It is possible that heart failure with severely impaired left ventricular function is the 1st clinical manifestation of CAD, and patients with newly identified heart failure need to be worked up for the presence of coronary artery obstruction. Especially when left ventricular functional impairment is regional, CAD should be suspected.

Sudden Cardiac Death

Sudden death is a possible 1st manifestation of CAD. The underlying event is almost uniformly arrhythmia. Acute mechanical complications, such as myocardial rupture secondary to an acute myocardial infarction, are possible but exceedingly infrequent. Arrhythmia leading to sudden death is usually ventricular fibrillation. It can either occur in the context of an acute coronary syndrome or be triggered by sudden ischemia, or it can occur in patients with heart failure due to old, often previously unknown, myocardial infarction. The more pronounced the reduction in left ventricular function, the higher the risk of arrhythmic death.

Diagnostic Strategies

Stable Coronary Artery Disease

Two diagnostic strategies exist for the diagnosis of stable CAD. The underlying process is the presence of coronary stenoses that lead to myocardial ischemia. Testing can aim either at identifying the ischemic myocardium under exercise or at the direct visualization of coronary artery stenoses.

Since not all coronary stenoses cause ischemia, and since stenoses that do not cause ischemia do not require revascularization, the usual preferred approach in patients with suspected stable CAD is the noninvasive identification of stress-induced myocardial ischemia by an imaging-based stress test. Ischemia can be achieved with physical exercise (treadmill or bicycle exercise) or pharmacologic stress (dipyridamole or dobutamine to increase contractility and myocardial oxygen demand or adenosine to achieve maximum vasodilation and "steal" effects). Commonly used tests include single-photon emission computed tomography (SPECT) and positron emission tomography (PET) myocardial perfusion and metabolic imaging, stress echocardiography, and stress magnetic resonance (MR) imaging.

Direct visualization of coronary anatomy is achieved by invasive coronary angiography or noninvasively by coronary computed tomography angiography (CCTA). The 2021 American College of Cardiology (ACC)/American Heart Association (AHA) chest pain guideline endorses coronary CTA with class I indication for patients with stable chest pain and no known history of CAD. CCTA not only provides noninvasive assessment of coronary artery stenosis but also assesses hemodynamic effects of the stenosis by CT-perfusion, CT-flow fraction reserve (CT-FFR), or artificial intelligence ischemia analysis. Ischemia assessment by CCTA is also implemented into the CAD-RADS v2 as a modifier. For CT-perfusion analysis, regular coronary CTA images serve as the resting exam while postpharmacological acquisition provides the stress component of the exam. Similar to nuclear perfusion studies, any mismatch perfusion defect in the myocardium indicates ischemia along with demonstration of corresponding vessel stenosis. CT-FFR, like invasive FFR, provides hemodynamic assessment of coronary artery stenosis without the need for additional acquisition. A CT-FFR value of < 0.75 indicates the presence of ischemia. The use of CT-FFR is recommended in coronary artery stenosis between 40-90° and is especially useful for proximal vessel disease, which can be treatable with percutaneous coronary intervention (PCI). Invasive coronary angiography can be combined with measurement of the FFR, which quantifies the relationship of mean arterial blood pressure before and after stenosis during maximum vasodilation achieved by adenosine. Currently, FFR is considered the gold standard to identify myocardial ischemia, and FFR values < 0.8 indicate that the respective lesion should be revascularized.

Acute Coronary Syndromes

Acute coronary syndromes encompass a wide spectrum from unstable angina to ST-segment elevation myocardial infarction (STEMI). In STEMI, electrocardiography is the only test performed and leads to immediate coronary catheterization. In non-ST elevation acute coronary syndromes, further testing is usually performed before a decision about invasive angiography can be made. It includes laboratory testing (troponin) complemented by echocardiography to exclude differential diagnoses (acute pulmonary embolism, aortic dissection) and assess regional as well as global left ventricular function. It may also include testing for ischemia. Coronary CT angiography plays an increasingly important role to rule out CAD, endorsed as class Ia in intermediate-risk patients with acute chest pain and no known CAD by 2021 AHA/ACC Chest pain guideline. It can also be useful in patients with prior inconclusive stress testing (class 2a).

Prevention

The prevention of the 1st acute coronary event is an important goal in CAD. In individuals who are asymptomatic, the traditional risk factors, summarized, e.g., in the Framingham Risk Score, are used to estimate the risk and the necessity of risk-lowering treatment by statins, aspirin, or antihypertensive medication. It is increasingly recognized that imaging may also contribute to risk stratification (e.g., coronary calcium, coronary CTA). Presence of nonobstructive CAD, high-risk plaque features and overall plaque burden are associated with increased cardiovascular events. Additionally, visualization of presence of coronary artery plaques by calcium scoring or coronary CTA can help patients to comply with treatment plan.

Interpretation

Coronary Artery Disease Reporting and Data System

The Coronary Artery Disease Reporting and Data System (CAD-RADS) was developed to create a standardized reporting system for coronary CTA to improve communication between the provider and reading physicians. It also provides suggestions for further management on a patient basis and ultimately results in improvement to patient care.

The aim of the CAD-RADS is to create a standardized reporting system for coronary CT angiography on a patient basis to improve the communication between the providers and to facilitate the management of the patient. The CAD-RADS classification represents the highest-grade coronary artery lesion detected by CT. However, the recommendations show differences depending on the onset of the chest pain (stable vs. acute), and the stenosis grade is categorized by the same system.

- CAD-RADS 0: Absence of CAD, no plaque or stenosis (0% stenosis)
- CAD-RADS 1: Minimal nonobstructive stenosis or plaque with no stenosis (1-24% stenosis)
- CAD-RADS 2: Mild, nonobstructive stenosis (25-49% stenosis)
- CAD-RADS 3: Moderate stenosis (50-69% stenosis)
- CAD-RADS 4: Severe stenosis
- CAD-RADS 4A: 70-99% stenosis in single vessel or 2 different vessels; CAD-RADS 4B: > 50% stenosis in left main artery or 3-vessel disease (> 70% stenosis)
- CAD-RADS 5: Total occlusion (100% stenosis)
- CAD-RADS N: Nondiagnostic study; obstructive CAD cannot be excluded

All vessels > 1.5 mm in diameter should be graded for stenosis severity; the smaller vessels are not taken into account.

New in CAD RADS 2.0 is plaque quantification representing total plaque burden (P): None (P0), mild (P1), moderate (P2), severe (P3), extensive (P4).

- Visual assessment, segment involvement score (SIS), or calcium scoring may be used for quantification of plaque volume

CAD-RADS categories are complemented by modifiers to demonstrate the presence of nonevaluable segments (N), high-risk plaque (HRP), stents (S), grafts (G), ischemia (I), and nonatherosclerotic causes of coronary stenosis (E).

- N can be used as category or modifier depending on context
- If there is potentially obstructive stenosis (≥ 50% stenosis: CAD-RADS 3, 4, or 5) and, in addition, nonevaluable segment, N, should be used as modifier (CAD-RADS 4/N)
- Contrarily, if highest grade stenosis is < 50%, or there is no stenosis in diagnostic segments, and if there is at least 1 nonevaluable segment, N should be used as category (CAD-RADS N); in this situation, obstructive CAD cannot be excluded
- High-risk plaque (previously known as vulnerable plaques) have at least 2 of high-risk plaque features, which are positive remodeling, spotty calcification, low attenuation (< 30 HU), and napkin-ring sign
- Modifier I is only given if ischemia testing was performed using stress CT-perfusion or CT-FFR; it is classified as present (I+), absent (I-), or borderline (I±), and is most useful in patients with 40-90% stenosis and CAD-RADS 3 and 4
- Reversible perfusion defects or peri-infract ischemia on perfusion imaging represent ischemia (I+); CT-FFR values ≤ 0.75 are classified as ischemia positive, > 0.80 is ischemia negative, and 0.76-0.80 is borderline
- Nonatherosclerotic causes of coronary artery stenosis, such as coronary dissection, extrinsic compression or anomalous coronary artery, require use of modifier E
- If > 1 modifier is present, "/" should follow each modifier (e.g., CAD-RADS 4/S/G/V)

Further investigation and management differences are based on the clinical scenario (acute vs. stable chest pain) and total plaque volume.

Selected References

1. Antonopoulos AS et al: Preventative imaging with coronary computed tomography angiography. Curr Cardiol Rep. 25(11):1623-32, 2023
2. Canan A et al: RadioGraphics update: pictorial guide to CAD-RADS 2.0. Radiographics. 43(4):e220202, 2023
3. Writing Committee Members et al: 2021 AHA/ACC/ASE/CHEST/SAEM/SCCT/SCMR guideline for the evaluation and diagnosis of chest pain: a report of the American College of Cardiology/American Heart Association Joint Committee on clinical practice guidelines. J Cardiovasc Comput Tomogr. 16(1):54-122, 2022
4. Writing Committee et al: 2022 ACC expert consensus decision pathway on the evaluation and disposition of acute chest pain in the emergency department: a report of the American College of Cardiology Solution Set Oversight Committee. J Am Coll Cardiol. 80(20):1925-60, 2022
5. Budoff MJ et al: Ten-year association of coronary artery calcium with atherosclerotic cardiovascular disease (ASCVD) events: the multi-ethnic study of atherosclerosis (MESA). Eur Heart J. 39(25):2401-8, 2018
6. Abbara S et al: SCCT guidelines for the performance and acquisition of coronary computed tomographic angiography: a report of the society of Cardiovascular Computed Tomography Guidelines Committee: Endorsed by the North American Society for Cardiovascular Imaging (NASCI). J Cardiovasc Comput Tomogr. 10(6):435-49, 2016

Introduction

Coronary computed tomography angiography (CCTA) has become the preferred noninvasive imaging modality for the evaluation of patients with suspected coronary artery disease (CAD) since its initial introduction. Over time, advancements in CT technology, including the advent of newer scanners, such as photon-counting CT, and innovative image analysis techniques, such as CT fractional flow reserve (CT-FFR), plaque quantification, and metal artifact reduction, have significantly expanded the utility and application of CCTA. In response to these technologic advancements and the evidence derived from several prospective randomized controlled trials, several professional societies have developed guidelines, expert consensus documents, and appropriateness criteria defining the role of CCTA in the evaluation of CAD. This chapter will review the latest documents for the use of CCTA.

CAD-RADS 2.0

CAD-RADS 2.0 - 2022 Coronary Artery Disease: Reporting and Data System Expert Consensus Document of Society of Cardiovascular Computed Tomography, American College of Cardiology, American College of Radiology, and North America Society of Cardiovascular Imaging

CAD-RADS was first developed in 2016 with the goal of standardizing the reporting of coronary CTA results and enhancing communication between interpreting and referring physicians. CAD-RADS 2.0, which replaced the original version in 2022, introduced significant updates, including the assessment of plaque volume and the evaluation of myocardial ischemia (MI). CAD-RADS 2.0 comprises 4 main components: Category, plaque burden, modifiers, and management recommendations. The CAD-RADS category is a numerical system (0-5) based on the highest grade of coronary artery stenosis detected on coronary CTA, where 0 indicates no stenosis, and 5 indicates total occlusion. Additionally, a category N (nondiagnostic) can be assigned if severe stenosis cannot be excluded for any reason. A notable addition in CAD-RADS 2.0 is semiquantitative plaque assessment (P), which was not included in the original version. Plaque assessment is divided into 4 subgroups: P1 (mild), P2 (moderate), P3 (severe), and P4 (extensive). The overall plaque burden can be evaluated using coronary artery calcium scoring, segment involvement score, or visual estimation of coronary artery plaque. CAD-RADS 2.0 also includes 6 modifiers that provide additional or complementary information. The presence of a nonevaluable segment in patients with otherwise at least potentially obstructive disease (N), stent (S), and bypass graft (G) remains unchanged. The term high-risk plaque (HRP) has replaced the term vulnerable plaque, although the definition remains the same. Two new modifiers have been added in CAD-RADS 2.0: One for the evaluation of ischemia (I) and another for the presence of nonatherosclerotic causes of coronary stenosis (exception-E). Ischemia assessment is optional and can be performed using CT-FFR or CT-perfusion; if not conducted, modifier I is listed as "not tested." Based on CT-FFR or CT-perfusion results, ischemia can be classified as positive, negative, or borderline. CAD-RADS 2.0 also provides detailed guidance on further cardiac investigation and management, based on the CAD-RADS category, plaque burden, and presence of ischemia. Recommendations may vary depending on the type of chest pain (chronic vs. acute). For comprehensive details, please refer to the CAD-RADS 2.0 document.

Coronary CTA and Chest Pain

2021 AHA/ACC/ASE/CHEST/SAEM/SCCT/SCMR Guideline for Evaluation and Diagnosis of Chest Pain: Report of American College of Cardiology/American Heart Association Joint Committee on Clinical Practice Guidelines

Over the past decade, studies have consistently demonstrated the safety and accuracy of CCTA in both stable and acute chest pain settings. Consequently, the 2021 chest pain guideline outline various clinical scenarios and the appropriate use of CCTA in each context.

- For intermediate-risk patients with **acute** or **stable** chest pain and no known CAD → class I
- For intermediate-risk patients with **acute** chest pain and evidence of prior mildly abnormal stress test results (< 1 year) → class 2a
- For intermediate-risk patients with **acute** or **stable** chest pain and known nonobstructive CAD → class 2a
- For intermediate-risk patients with **acute** or **stable** chest pain, if 40-90% coronary stenosis of proximal or midvessel detected on CCTA, CT-FFR can be useful for evaluation of hemodynamical significance and guide treatment → class 2a
- For patients with prior coronary artery bypass graft (CABG) surgery presenting with **acute** chest pain and do not have acute coronary syndrome (ACS), CCTA can be obtained for evaluation of graft stenosis or occlusion → class 1
- For intermediate- to high-risk patients with **stable** chest pain after inconclusive or abnormal exercise ECG or stress imaging, CCTA is reasonable → class 2a
- For patients with **stable** chest pain and prior coronary revascularization, CCTA is reasonable to evaluate bypass graft or stent patency (stent ≥ 3 mm) → class 2a
- For patients with prior CABG surgery and **stable** chest pain who are suspected to have MI, CCTA is reasonable → class 2a
- Warranty period for negative CCTA (no plaque, no stenosis) is described as 2 years

2022 ACC Expert Consensus Decision Pathway on Evaluation and Disposition of Acute Chest Pain in Emergency Department: Report of American College of Cardiology Solution Set Oversight Committee

CCTA has been proven to be safe and effective for patients in non-high-risk groups who present to the emergency department with acute chest pain. Clinical trials and metaanalyses have demonstrated that, in low- to intermediate-risk patients, CCTA not only accelerates the time to diagnosis but also reduces the overall length of stay in the hospital or emergency department. As a result, the ACC expert consensus recommends CCTA as the preferred noninvasive test in the emergency department (when available) for patients with suspected ACS who have no known CAD. Additional patient characteristics that favor the selection of CCTA over stress testing include the absence of severe coronary artery calcification on prior chest CT, a history of normal, mildly abnormal, or inconclusive stress tests, no known contrast allergy or significant renal dysfunction, and a low likelihood of achieving high-quality stress testing or timely access to it. According to expert consensus recommendations, patients who undergo CCTA and are found to have no or nonobstructive CAD can be safely discharged from the emergency department. However, it is crucial to develop protocols for follow-up care for these patients since they may need preventive therapy and lifestyle modifications. Conversely, if CCTA reveals obstructive CAD, patients should be admitted for further evaluation and treatment.

2022 Use of Coronary Computed Tomographic Angiography for Patients Presenting With Acute Chest Pain to Emergency Department: Expert Consensus Document of Society of Cardiovascular Computed Tomography: Endorsed by American College of Radiology and North American Society for Cardiovascular Imaging

More than 10 randomized clinical trials and metaanalyses published over the past decade have established the safety of coronary CTA as the 1st-line imaging modality for low- to intermediate-risk patients presenting to the emergency department with acute chest pain. In response to these findings, the 2022 expert consensus, endorsed by SCCT, ACR, and NASCI, was developed to create a standardized practice for the use of CCTA in emergency setting. In addition to the appropriate use of CCTA in the emergency department, the document highlights the patient preparation, protocol selection, and interpretation or CCTA. In this section, we will focus on and summarize the appropriate use of CCTA. Key highlights from the expert consensus include the following:

- CCTA is the most effective imaging modality for ruling out ACS in patients who are at low to intermediate risk for ACS, specifically those with HEART scores of 1-6 and TIMI risk scores of 1-4. Patients within this risk group may present with normal or nonischemic EKG changes and either normal or equivocal baseline troponin levels or with baseline high-sensitivity troponin levels below the 99th percentile. Additionally, this group may include patients who have had inconclusive or mildly abnormal functional testing within the past year.
- CCTA is considered appropriate for patients with documented CAD and a history of prior percutaneous coronary intervention (PCI) under the following conditions: (1) The patient has a prior stent placed within a proximal coronary segment, and the stent diameter is ≥ 3 mm; (2) the patient's EKG is normal or shows nonischemic changes; (3) troponin levels are normal or equivocal.
- CCTA is appropriate in selected patients with known CAD and a history of prior CABG surgery to assess graft patency. These patients should have a normal or nonischemic baseline EKG and normal or equivocal troponin levels.
- Sequential testing with CT-FFR or stress CT-perfusion is considered appropriate in patients with 40-70% coronary artery stenosis on CCTA to assess the lesion-specific ischemia and guide the treatment.

2023 ACC/AHA/ASE/ASNC/ASPC/HFSA/HRS/SCAI/SCCT/SCMR/STS Multimodality Appropriate Use Criteria for Detection and Risk Assessment of Chronic Coronary Disease

This is a report of the appropriate use of stress testing and anatomic diagnostic procedures for risk assessment and evaluation of known or suspected chronic coronary disease (CCD) endorsed by several multidisciplinary societies. The document includes 64 clinical scenarios describing common patient encounters and highlights the appropriateness of different imaging options for diagnosis of CCD. We will focus on the ratings of CCTA, and, below, are the scenarios when it is rated as "appropriate."

- **Symptomatic patients without known CCD and no prior testing**: If anginal symptoms are likely
- **Symptomatic patients without known CCD and with prior testing**: In cases of abnormal EKG; inconclusive or abnormal exercise stress test; normal, abnormal, or inconclusive stress imaging
- **Symptomatic patients with prior MI or revascularization**: Prior MI, no revascularization, symptoms similar to prior ischemic episode &/or anginal
- **Asymptomatic patients with prior revascularization or MI**: Isolated evaluation of bypass graft patency
- **Newly diagnosed heart failure (resting left ventricular function previously assessed but no prior CAD evaluation)**: Newly diagnosed HFpEF or HFrEF or screening transplant vasculopathy
- **Evaluation of arrhythmias without ischemic equivalent (no prior cardiac evaluation)**: Prior to initiation of antiarrhythmic therapy in patients with high global CAD risk; presence of exercise-induced ventricular tachycardia (VT) or sustained VT or ventricular fibrillation

2024 Standards for Quantitative Assessments by Coronary Computed Tomography Angiography: Expert Consensus Document of Society of Cardiovascular Computed Tomography

With recent advancements in CT technology, artificial intelligence techniques, and automated postprocessing tools, the quantitative evaluation of CCTA has become increasingly accessible. Currently, commercially available softwares can provide detailed coronary artery segmentation, quantitative assessments of coronary artery stenosis and coronary artery plaque burden, and the characterization of plaque types. The recent expert consensus by SCCT seeks to establish standard definitions, CCTA techniques, and guidelines for the interpretation of these quantitative measures.

Selected References

1. Nieman K et al: Standards for quantitative assessments by coronary computed tomography angiography (CCTa): An expert consensus document of the society of cardiovascular computed tomography (SCCT). J Cardiovasc Comput Tomogr. 18(5):429-43, 2024
2. Maroules CD et al: 2022 use of coronary computed tomographic angiography for patients presenting with acute chest pain to the emergency department: an expert consensus document of the Society of cardiovascular computed tomography (SCCT): Endorsed by the American College of Radiology (ACR) and North American Society for cardiovascular Imaging (NASCI). J Cardiovasc Comput Tomogr. 17(2):146-63, 2023
3. Winchester DE et al: ACC/AHA/ASE/ASNC/ASPC/HFSA/HRS/SCAI/SCCT/SCMR/STS 2023 multimodality appropriate use criteria for the detection and risk assessment of chronic coronary disease. J Cardiovasc Magn Reson. 25(1):58, 2023
4. Cury RC et al: CAD-RADS™ 2.0 - 2022 Coronary artery disease - reporting and data system an expert consensus document of the Society of Cardiovascular Computed Tomography (SCCT), the American College of Cardiology (ACC), the American College of Radiology (ACR) and the North America Society of Cardiovascular Imaging (NASCI). Radiol Cardiothorac Imaging. 4(5):e220183, 2022
5. Writing Committee et al: 2022 ACC expert consensus decision pathway on the evaluation and disposition of acute chest pain in the emergency department: a report of the American College of Cardiology Solution Set Oversight Committee. J Am Coll Cardiol. 80(20):1925-60, 2022
6. Gulati M et al: 2021 AHA/ACC/ASE/CHEST/SAEM/SCCT/SCMR guideline for the evaluation and diagnosis of chest pain: a report of the American College of Cardiology/American Heart Association Joint Committee on Clinical Practice Guidelines. Circulation. 144(22):e368-454, 2021

CAD-RADS 2.0

KEY FACTS

DEGREE OF STENOSIS

- CAD-RADS 0 = 0% stenosis, no CAD
- CAD-RADS 1 = 1-24% luminal narrowing, nonobstructive CAD
- CAD-RADS 2 = 25-49% luminal narrowing, nonobstructive CAD
- CAD-RADS 3 = 50-69% stenosis, potentially obstructive CAD
- CAD-RADS 4A = 70-99% significant stenosis in up to 2 vessel territories
- CAD-RADS 4B = ≥ 50% stenosis in left main or ≥ 70% stenosis in all 3 vessel territories
- CAD-RADS 5 = 100% luminal occlusion
- CAD-RADS N = Noninterpretable study; obstructive disease in at least 1 segment cannot be excluded

PLAQUE BURDEN

- P1 = mild, CAC 0-100, SIS 1-2; visually: 1-2 vessels with mild plaque
- P2 = moderate, CAC 101-300, SIS 3-4; visually: 1-2 vessel with moderate plaque; 3 vessels with mild plaque
- P3 = severe, CAC 301-999, SIS 5-7; visually: 3 vessels with moderate plaque; 1 vessel with extensive plaque
- P4 = extensive, CAC > 1,000, SIS ≥ 8; visually: 2-3 vessels with extensive plaque

MODIFIERS

- N = nonevaluable segment
- HRP = replaces V; used when ≥ 2 high-risk plaque features are present
- I = used only if ischemia testing is performed (CT-FFR or mCTP)
  - I+ = positive for ischemia; I- = negative; I± = indeterminate for ischemia
- S = stent present; G = graft present; E = exceptions

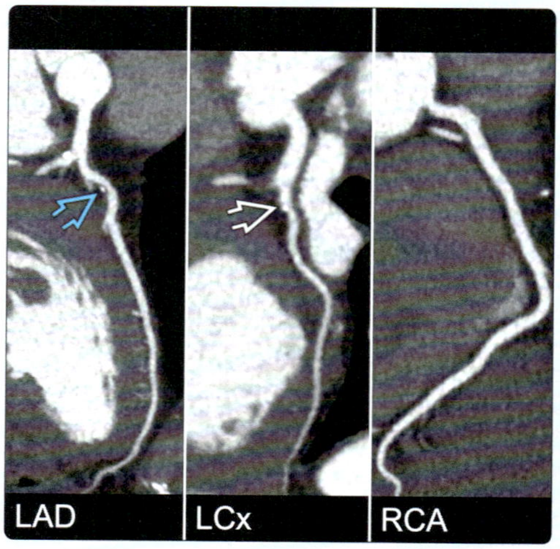

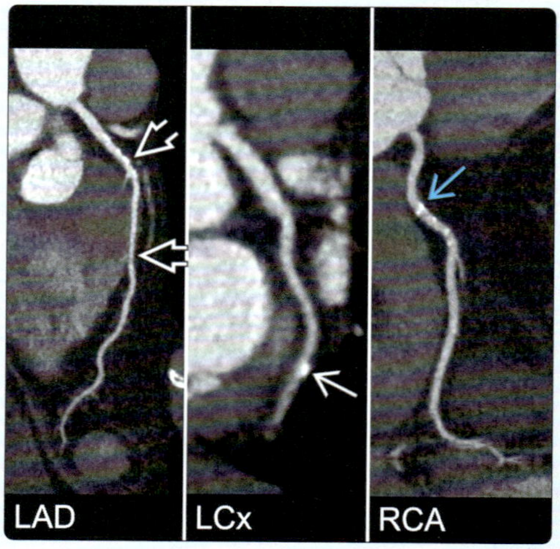

(Left) *Curved MPR CECT shows minimal stenosis (< 25%) in left anterior descending (LAD) ➔ and left circumflex (LCx) ➔ arteries, consistent with CAD-RADS 1. Visually, there is a mild amount of plaque in 1-2 vessels, consistent with P1.* **(Right)** *Curved MPR CECT shows scattered areas of calcified and noncalcified plaques in proximal and mid-LAD ➔, mid-LCx ➔, and proximal right coronary artery (RCA) ➔. Plaque burden is P2 based on visual assessment (1-2 vessels with moderate amount or 3 vessels with mild amount of plaque).*

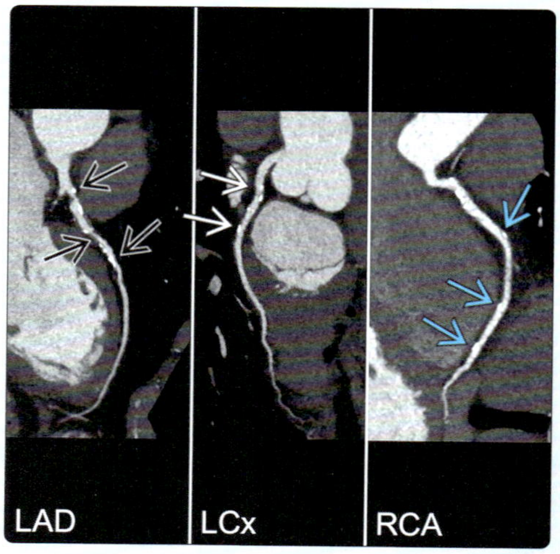

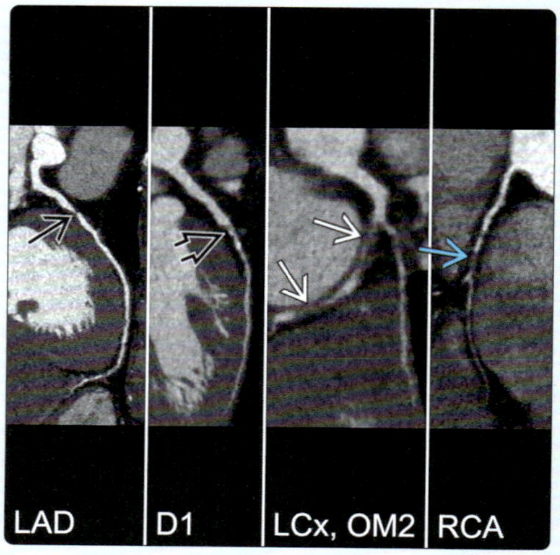

(Left) *Curved MPR CECT shows multiple areas of plaques in the proximal and mid-LAD ➔, proximal LCx ➔, and proximal, mid-, and distal RCA ➔. Calcium score is 922, consistent with P3.* **(Right)** *Curved MPR CECT shows predominantly noncalcified plaques with severe stenosis of LAD ➔, first diagonal (D1) ➔, LCx ➔, and RCA ➔. 2-3 vessels with an extensive amount of plaque are consistent with P4. It is possible that P designation can be discordant between different methods of plaque scoring.*

TERMINOLOGY

Abbreviations

- Coronary Artery Disease Reporting and Data System (CAD-RADS)

Definitions

- CAD-RADS
  - Standardized reporting system for coronary CTA
- Segment involvement score (SIS)
  - Derived from coronary CTA that represents number of coronary arterial anatomic segments exhibiting atherosclerotic plaque
- Coronary artery calcium (CAC)
  - Calcium score as determined by Agatston method
- High-risk plaque (HRP)
  - Subset of coronary atherosclerotic plaque that expresses features associated with higher risk of future adverse coronary artery events
- Computed tomography fractional flow reserve (CT-FFR)
  - Computerized estimation of fractional flow reserve based on morphology derived from coronary CTA
- Computed tomography perfusion (CTP)
  - Stress and rest myocardial perfusion using CT and usually iodinated contrast material
- CAD-RADS expresses following features in standardized manner
  - Stenosis degree
  - Plaque burden
  - Up to 6 modifiers are reported when present
    - Nonevaluable
    - HRP features
    - Ischemia [only if ischemia analysis, such as myocardial CTP (mCTP) or CT-FRR, has been performed]
    - Presence of stent(s)
    - Presence of grafts(s)
    - Exceptions (when other important features are present that are otherwise not well captured with CAD-RADS)

CLINICAL IMPLICATIONS

Purpose

- CAD-RADS 2.0 replaces initial version of CAD-RADS that was first published in 2016
- Goal is to standardize reporting of CTA results and to facilitate communication of test results to referring physicians
  - Gives suggestions for subsequent patient management
  - Meant to benefit education, research, peer review, development of AI, design of clinical trials
  - Enables quality assurance
- New major elements include plaque burden and ischemia
- Exception modifier (E) has been added to account for nonatherosclerotic obstructions, such as from intraarterial course of anomalous coronary arteries

Clinical Importance

- Management considerations
  - CAD-RADS category based on "additional cardiac investigation" and "clinical management recommendations" are provided for 2 separate clinical scenarios
    - Patients presenting with stable chest pain
    - Patients presenting with acute chest pain

DEGREE OF STENOSIS

CAD-RADS Categories

- Based on degree or severity of stenosis (0-100%)
- Ranging from 0 (0% stenosis or no stenosis) to 5 (occlusion or 100% stenosis)

CAD-RADS 0

- No atherosclerotic plaque, no stenosis
- Absence of coronary artery disease
- 0% stenosis
- Further cardiac investigation: None

CAD-RADS 1

- Minimal luminal narrowing
- Nonobstructive coronary artery atherosclerosis
- 1-24% stenosis
- Further cardiac investigation: None

CAD-RADS 2

- Mild luminal narrowing
- Nonobstructive coronary artery atherosclerosis
- 25-49% stenosis
- Further cardiac investigation: None

CAD-RADS 3

- Moderate stenosis
- Potentially obstructive coronary artery disease
- 50-69% stenosis
- Further cardiac investigation: Consider CT-FFR or mCTP or other stress testing

CAD-RADS 4A

- Significant (severe) stenosis in 1 or 2 of left anterior descending artery, right coronary artery, or left circumflex artery territories
- Likely hemodynamically significant stenosis, obstructive coronary artery disease
- 70-99% stenosis
- Further cardiac investigation: Potentially additional functional testing or invasive angiography

CAD-RADS 4B

- ≥ 50% stenosis in left main (LM) coronary artery or significant (severe) stenosis in all 3 vessel territories
- LM coronary artery obstructive disease or 3 vessel obstructive coronary artery disease
- 70-99% stenosis in all 3 vessel territories or ≥ 50% in LM
- Further cardiac investigation: Invasive coronary angiography

CAD-RADS 5

- Total occlusion or subtotal occlusion
- 100% luminal occlusion

- Further cardiac investigation: Invasive coronary angiography, functional testing, and viability assessment are all to be considered

CAD-RADS N

- Noninterpretable study with respect to coronary lumen
- Obstructive coronary artery disease in at least 1 segment cannot be excluded based on coronary CTA
- Further cardiac investigation: Additional alternative evaluation may be required

PLAQUE BURDEN

P1-P4

- Assesses amount of atherosclerotic plaque by 1 of 3 possible methods
  - Agatston method calcium score
  - CTA-derived SIS, which is sum of all segments with any type of plaque for each of 16 coronary segments (maximum score = 16)
  - Visual qualitative score created for CAD-RADS that uses estimates of amount of calcified and noncalcified plaque for each vessel
- There is no P0 because CAD-RADS 0 implies absence of plaque and absence of stenosis

P1

- Small amount of atherosclerotic plaque (mild)
- Agatston calcium score 0-100
- SIS of 1 or 2
- Visually: 1-2 vessels with mild amount of plaque

P2

- Intermediate amount of atherosclerotic plaque (moderate)
- Agatston calcium score 101-300
- SIS of 3-4
- Visually: 1-2 vessels with moderate amount or 3 vessels with mild amount of plaque

P3

- Large amount of atherosclerotic plaque (severe)
- Agatston calcium score 301-999
- SIS of 5-7
- Visually: 3 vessels with moderate amount or 1 vessel with extensive amount of plaque

P4

- Very large amount of atherosclerotic plaque (extensive)
- Agatston calcium score ≥ 1,000
- SIS of ≥ 8
- Visually: 2-3 vessels with extensive amount of plaque

MODIFIERS

Nonevaluability (N)

- 1 or more segments are not interpretable with respect to coronary lumen diameter

Ischemia (I+, I-, or I±)

- Use of modifier "I" indicates that ischemia test has been performed
- If neither CT-FFR nor mCTP have been performed, then modifier I is not used
- Modifier I is always used with either +, -, or ±
  - I+ (positive ischemia) CT-FFR < 0.75 lesion specific in vessel large enough for intervention, or mCTP shows reversible perfusion defect or periinfarct ischemia
  - I- (negative ischemia) lesion-specific CT-FFR > 0.80, or mCTP shows no ischemia or prior fixed myocardial infarct
  - I± (inconclusive for ischemia) CT-FFR 0.76-0.80, or mCTP is borderline or inconclusive for ischemia

HRP Features

- Replaces previous modifier V for vulnerable plaque
- HRP is given when at least 2 of following high-risk features are present
  - Spotty calcifications
  - Low-attenuation plaque (< 30 HU)
  - Positive remodeling
  - Napkin ring sign

Stent (S)

- Indicates presence of at least 1 coronary artery stent
- If stent exhibits significant in-stent restenosis, then stenosis degree is considered in CAD-RADS category

Grafts (G)

- Indicates presence of at least 1 coronary artery bypass graft
- If graft is present, stenosis that is bypassed is no longer considered in CAD-RADS category selection

Exceptions (E)

- Indicates nonatherosclerotic causes of coronary artery narrowing
- Examples include but not limited to
  - Anomalous coronary arteries with interarterial course and moderate stenosis
  - Coronary artery dissection
  - Coronary artery aneurysm, fistula
  - Extrinsic coronary artery compression

REPORTING OF NONEVALUABLE SEGMENTS

N as CAD-RADS Category vs. N as Modifier

- N can be used as modifier or as CAD-RADS category
  - Which one to use depends on presence or absence of potentially obstructive or obstructive disease in other segments that are evaluable
- If stenosis ≥ 50% is present elsewhere in diagnostic segment, most severe stenosis determines category (3, 4A, 4B, 5) and N is used as modifier (e.g., CAD-RADS 3/N or CAD-RADS 4A/N)
- If no stenosis ≥ 50% is present elsewhere and at least 1 noninterpretable segment is present, then category reported as CAD-RADS N

SELECTED REFERENCES

1. Canan A et al: RadioGraphics update: pictorial guide to CAD-RADS 2.0. Radiographics. 43(4):e220202, 2023
2. Cury RC et al: CAD-RADS™ 2.0 - 2022 Coronary Artery Disease - Reporting and Data System: an expert consensus document of the Society of Cardiovascular Computed Tomography (SCCT), the American College of Cardiology (ACC), the American College of Radiology (ACR), and the North America Society of Cardiovascular Imaging (NASCI). Radiol Cardiothorac Imaging. 4(5):e220183, 2022

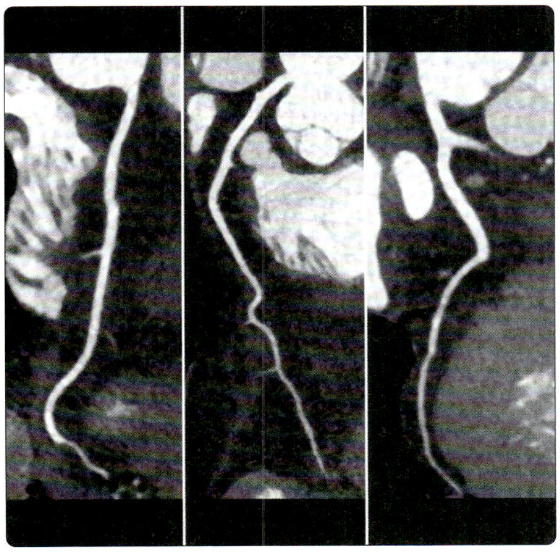

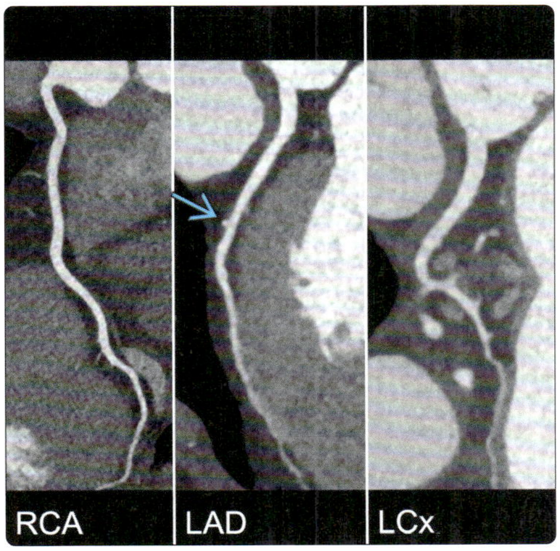

(Left) *Curved MPR CECT shows no coronary atherosclerosis in a 60-year-old patient with atypical chest pain, consistent with CAD-RADS 0.* **(Right)** *Preoperative coronary CTA in a 56-year-old patient shows a small amount of mixed plaque in mid-LAD with minimal luminal narrowing (< 25%), consistent with CAD-RADS 1. Also note slight positive remodeling of the plaque.*

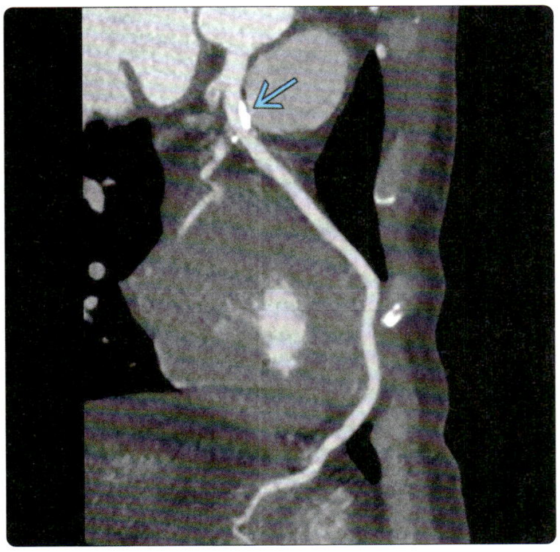

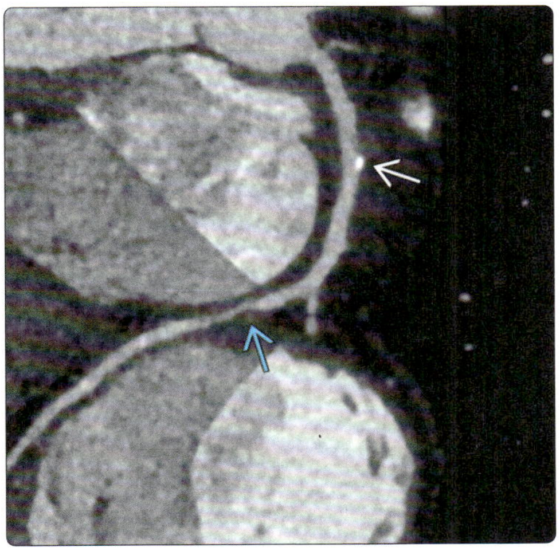

(Left) *Curved MPR CECT shows focal calcified plaque in the proximal LAD resulting in mild luminal narrowing (25-49%), consistent with CAD-RADS 2. Other coronary arteries (not shown) were without coronary atherosclerosis.* **(Right)** *Curved MPR CECT shows focal, noncalcified plaque in the distal RCA resulting in moderate stenosis (50-69%). Additional small, calcified plaque in proximal RCA results in minimal luminal narrowing. Overall, CAD-RADS category is 3 based on the most severe stenosis.*

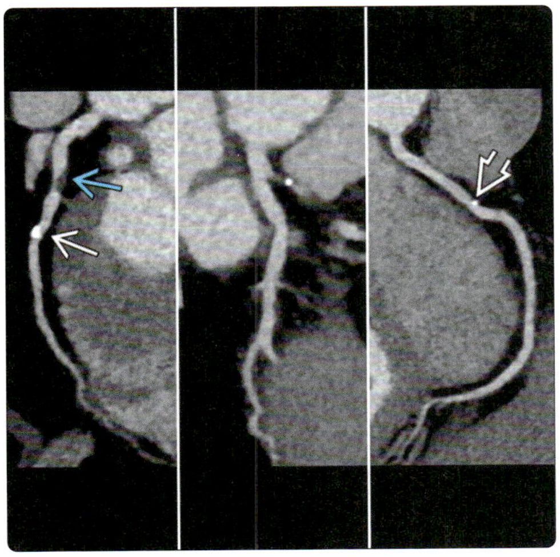

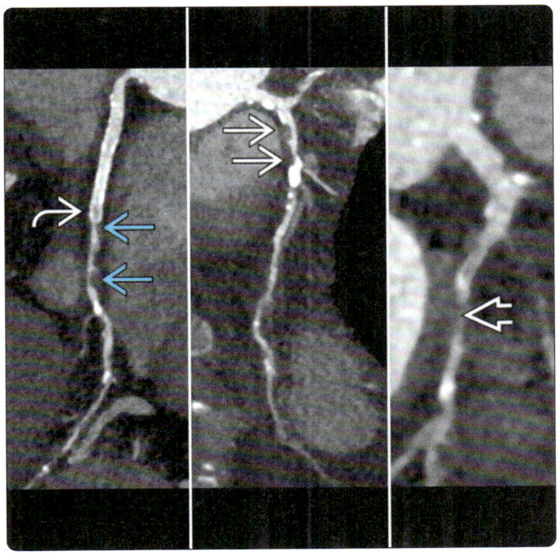

(Left) *Curved MPR CECT shows noncalcified plaque with severe stenosis (70-99%) in proximal LAD. Additional focal, calcified plaques in mid-LAD and RCA result in mild luminal narrowing. Based on the most severe stenosis in a single vessel, this is CAD-RADS 4A.* **(Right)** *Curved MPR CECT shows extensive atherosclerosis resulting in severe stenosis of mid-RCA, proximal LAD, and mid-LCx, consistent with CAD-RADS 4B. Also note coronary stent in RCA with mild luminal narrowing.*

(Left) *Axial oblique MIP CECT of the left main and LAD shows complete occlusion of LAD → after bifurcation, including the 1st diagonal branch ➡ as well. This is CAD-RADS 5.* **(Right)** *Axial oblique coronary CTA acquired during an ectopic beat shows marked motion abnormality obscuring both the LAD ➡ and LCx →, making evaluation of the vessels nondiagnostic. This would be classified as CAD-RADS N.*

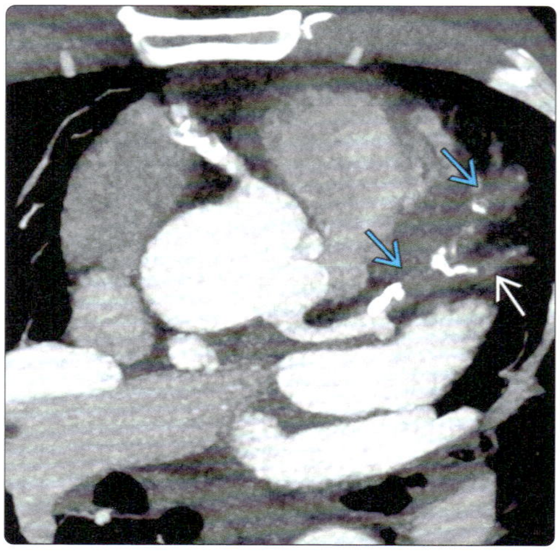

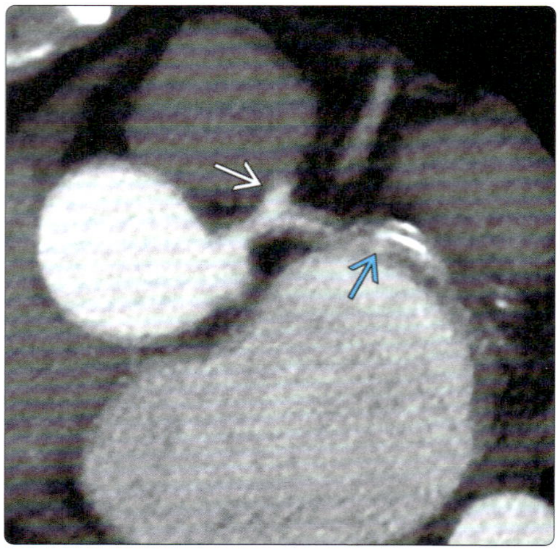

(Left) *Coronal oblique MPR CECT through the mid-LAD shows a widely patent stent →, which would be classified using the modifier S.* **(Right)** *Curved MPR CECT of a saphenous to 2nd OM bypass graft → shows widely patent graft and severe stenosis in LCx territory ➡. Additional SVG to posterior descending artery and LIMA to LAD (not shown) grafts with minimal luminal narrowing were noted. Although there is severe stenosis in native vessels, this is expected with bypass grafts. Therefore, this would be classified as CAD-RADS 1/G.*

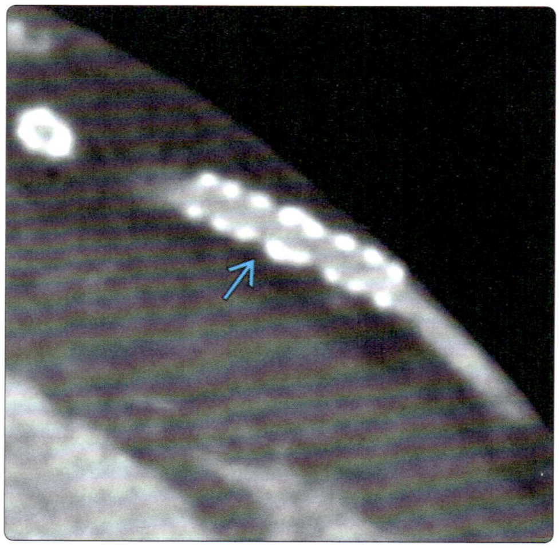

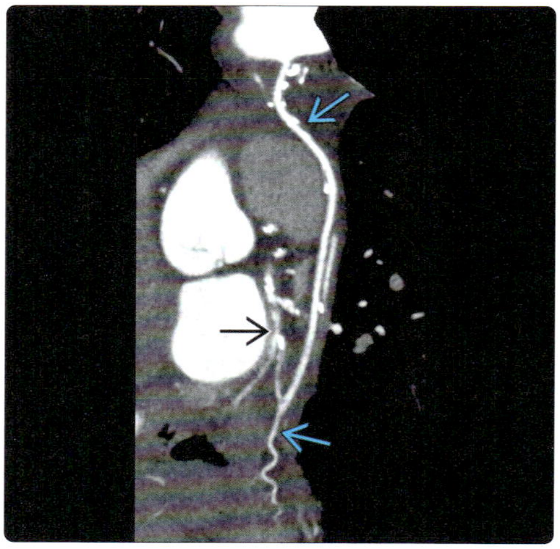

(Left) *Curved MPR CECT shows mixed plaque in the mid-RCA with positive remodeling → resulting in mild luminal narrowing. Short-axis view of plaque (inset) reveals a low-attenuation core ➡ forming napkin ring sign. Presence of positive remodeling and low attenuation indicates high-risk plaque, shown by HRP modifier.* **(Right)** *Curved MPR CECT during systole ➡ and diastole → shows substantial caliber change of mid-LAD due to myocardial bridging ➡, which is confirmed by invasive catheter angiography (systole ➡, diastole →).*

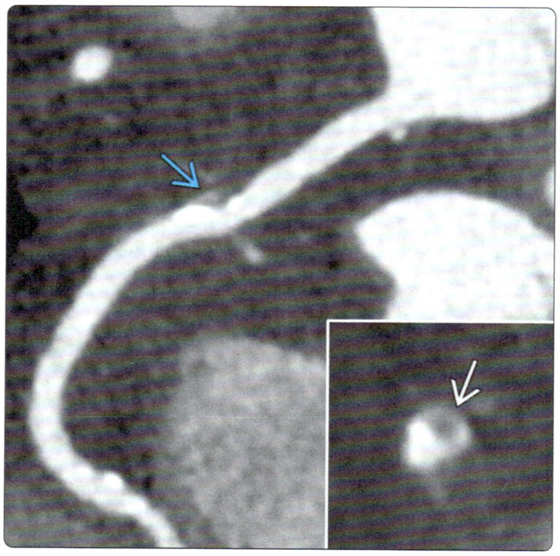

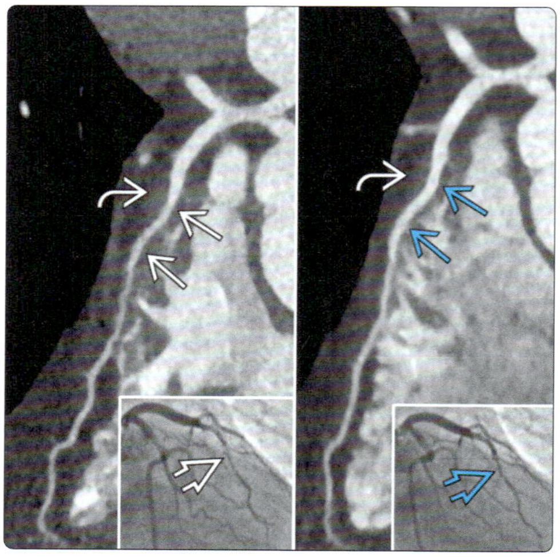

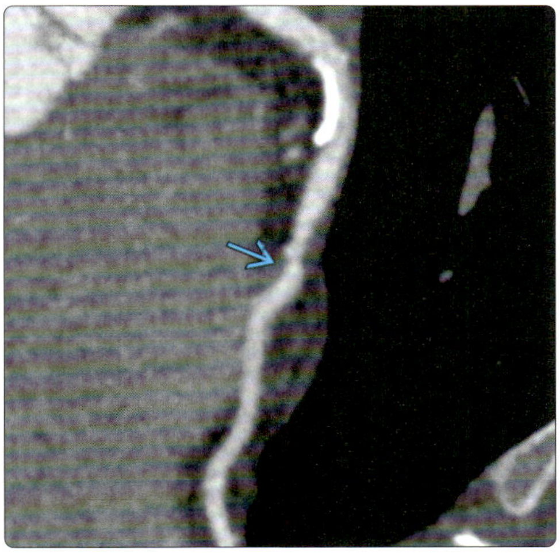

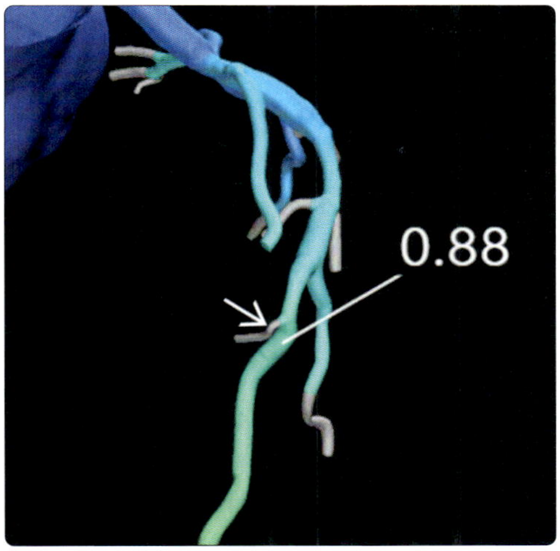

(Left) *Curved MPR CECT shows a focal moderate stenosis of the mid-LAD → of ~ 55%. This would be classified as CAD-RADS 3. The study was subsequently sent for CT fraction flow reserve analysis (CT-FFR).* **(Right)** *CT-FFR analysis shows no hemodynamically significance to the moderate mid-LAD stenosis →. This would be classified as CAD-RADS 3/I-.*

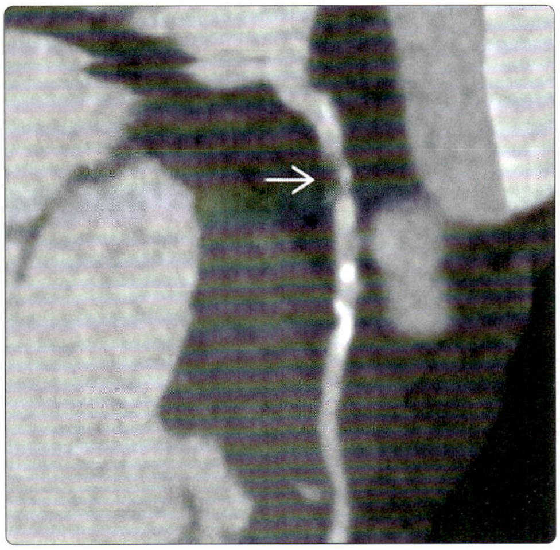

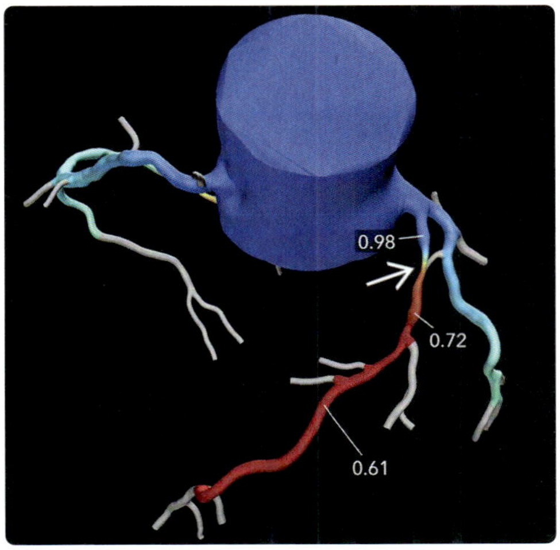

(Left) *Curved MPR CECT shows multifocal calcified and noncalcified plaques of LAD. The most proximal noncalcified plaque → results in moderate stenosis (50-69%), consistent with CAD-RADS 3. This study was subsequently sent for CT-FFR.* **(Right)** *CT-FFR analysis shows that proximal LAD stenosis is hemodynamically significant → with a value of 0.72. CT-FFR values < 0.75 receive modifier I+. This would be classified as CAD-RADS 3/I+.*

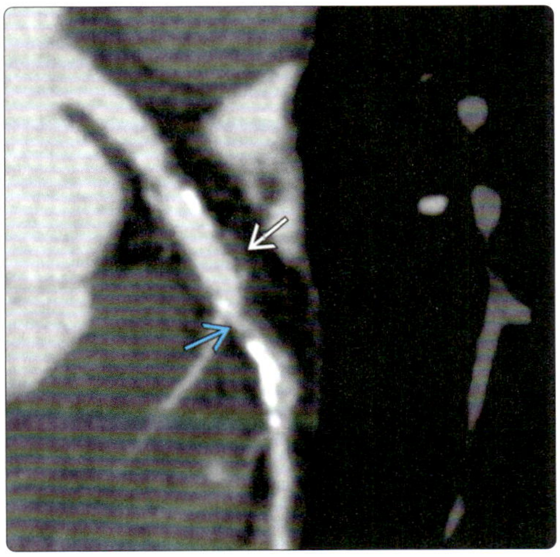

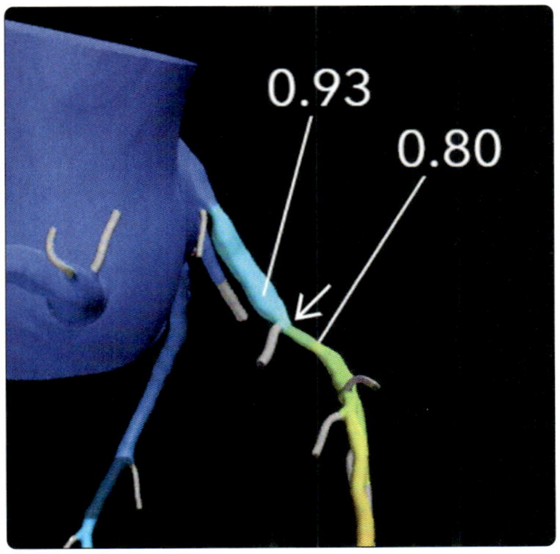

(Left) *Curved MPR CECT shows multiple areas of plaques with areas of positive remodeling →. Moderate stenosis (~ 60%) in the mid-LAD just after the 1st septal branch → leads to a CAD-RADS 3 classification. This study was subsequently sent for CT-FFR analysis.* **(Right)** *CT-FFR analysis shows that the mid-LAD moderate stenosis has a value of 0.80 →. Studies with a CT-FFR value of 0.76-0.8 are accepted as borderline and receive an I± modifier. This would be classified as CAD-RADS 3/I±.*

TERMINOLOGY

Abbreviations

- Coronary arteries and their branches
  - Left main (LM) coronary artery
  - Left anterior descending (LAD) coronary artery
    - Proximal, mid-, and distal LAD (pLAD, mLAD, dLAD)
    - Diagonal branches: D1, D2, D3, etc.
  - Ramus intermedius (RI)
  - Left circumflex (LCx) artery
    - Proximal, mid-, and distal LCX (pLCx, mLCx, dLCx)
    - Obtuse marginal branches: OM1, OM2, OM3, etc.
  - Posterior lateral branch (PLB)
  - Posterior left ventricular (PLV) branch
  - Posterior descending artery (PDA)
  - Right coronary artery (RCA)
    - Proximal, mid-, and distal RCA (pRCA, mRCA, dRCA)
    - Acute marginal (AM) branch
  - Sinoatrial node (SAN) branch
  - Atrioventricular node (AVN) branch
- Grafts
  - Saphenous vein graft (SVG)
  - Coronary artery bypass graft (CABG)
  - Left internal mammary artery (LIMA)
  - Right internal mammary artery (RIMA)
- Alternative international nomenclature
  - Ramus interventricularis anterior (RIVA) = LAD
  - Ramus circumflexus (RCx) = LCx
  - Ramus interventricularis posterior (RIVP, RIP) = PDA
  - Ramus marginalis (RM or M) = OM
  - Right posterolateral branch (RPL) = PLV branch from RCA
    - Ramus posterolateralis dexter (RPD) = PLV branch from RCA; careful not to confuse with abbreviation for right PDA (R-PDA)
  - RPD = PDA from RCA

Synonyms

- Epicardial arteries

IMAGING ANATOMY

Overview

- Major coronary arteries travel within epicardial fat of interventricular and atrioventricular grooves
- Considerable variability in size, number/location of branching vessels, and myocardial territories

ANATOMY

Left Main

- Arises from left coronary sinus
- Variable length but usually < 2 cm
- Courses behind right ventricular outflow tract between pulmonary trunk and left atrium
- LM stenosis ≥ 50% is severe
  - Stenosis of ≥ 70% is severe in all other segments
- Usually bifurcates into LAD and LCx
- Commonly trifurcates into LAD, LCx, and RI
  - RI may follow course of obtuse marginal or diagonal branch
- Rarely is absent with LM and LCx origins directly from left coronary sinus

Left Anterior Descending

- Continuation of LM
- Runs along anterior interventricular groove
- Mid-LAD occasionally dives into left ventricular myocardium, forming myocardial bridge
- Diagonal branches run diagonally and laterally over anterior left ventricular wall
  - Numbered from proximal to distal as D1, D2, D3, etc.
  - Supply anterolateral wall
- Superior septal perforator branches extend medially into interventricular septum and anchor LAD to myocardium
  - Septal perforators supply anterior 2/3 of septum
  - 1st septal perforator commonly supplies His bundle
  - Inferior septal perforators may form collaterals to PDA
- Right ventricular branches are small but may form collaterals to RCA
  - Circle of Vieussens = collateralization between branch of pLAD (left preinfundibular artery) and conus artery in setting of pLAD stenosis
- dLAD often wraps around apex and may form collaterals to distal PDA
- Segmentation
  - pLAD: End of LM to 1st large septal or D1 (1st diagonal), whichever is more proximal
  - mLAD: End of pLAD to 1/2 distance to apex
    - Some authors use origin of D2 as distal landmark
  - dLAD: End of mLAD to end of LAD

Left Circumflex

- Arises from LM at nearly perpendicular angle
- Runs around mitral anulus in left atrioventricular groove
- Obtuse marginal branches (OM1, OM2, OM3)
- Nondominant LCx often terminates as OM branch
- Native LCx distal to OM branches is often diminutive
- If left dominant, branches into PLV and PDA
- LCx and OM branches supply lateral free wall and portion of anterolateral papillary muscle
- Segmentation
  - pLCx: End of LM to origin of OM1
  - mLCx and dLCx: Distal to OM1 to end of LCx or PDA origin

Right Coronary Artery

- Arises from right coronary sinus
- Passes under right atrial appendage and descends into right anterior atrioventricular groove
- In 50%, 1st branch of RCA is conus branch
  - Alternative origin from separate ostium directly from right sinus of Valsalva
  - Conus branch supplies right ventricular outflow tract
- In 60%, SAN is next branch
  - 40% take alternative supply from LCx atrial branches
- AM branches may be large and extend to apex
- If right-dominant circulation, RCA bifurcates into PDA and PLV at cardiac crux
  - When right dominant, described as R-PDA; when left dominant, left PDA (L-PDA)

- PDA runs along posterior interventricular groove and supplies posterior 1/3 of inferior septum
- PLV courses cephalad and is usual source of AVN branch
  - AVN less commonly supplied by LCx
- Segmentation
  - pRCA: Ostium to 1/2 distance to acute margin of heart
  - mRCA: End of pRCA to acute margin
  - dRCA: Acute margin to PDA origin

Dominance

- Dominance defined by supply of PDA and PLV
- Right-, left-, and codominant coronary systems
- ~ 85% right dominant (RCA supplies PDA and PLV)
- 8% left dominant (LCx supplies PDA and PLV)
- 7% codominant (RCA and LCx share supply of PDA &/or PLV)
- Rare superdominant RCA supplies diminutive LCx territory
- Rare wraparound LAD supplies PDA

CORONARY ARTERY SEGMENTATION

Society of Cardiovascular Computed Tomography Definitions

- LM = ostium of LM to bifurcation to LAD/LCx or trifurcation to LAD/LCx/RI
- pLAD = end of LM to 1st large septal or diagonal, whichever is more proximal
- mLAD = end of pLAD to 1/2 distance to apex
- dLAD = end of mLAD to end of LAD
- D1 = 1st diagonal branch of LAD
- D2 = 2nd diagonal branch of LAD
- RI = vessel arising from LM between LAD and LCx in case of trifurcation
- pLCx = end of LM to origin of 1st obtuse marginal
- Mid- and dLCx= from 1st obtuse marginal to end of vessel or origin of L-PDA
- OM1 = 1st obtuse marginal branch of LCx
- PDA-LCx (L-PDA) = PDA from LCx
- PLB-L (L-PLB) = posterolateral branch from LCx
- pRCA = ostium of RCA to 1/2 distance to acute margin
- mRCA = end of pRCA to acute margin
- dRCA = acute margin to origin of PDA
- PDA-RCA (R-PDA) = PDA from RCA
- PLB-RCA (R-PLB) = PLB from RCA
- Alternative coronary artery segmentation
  - Original 15-segment model published via American Heart Association (AHA) committee by W. Gerald Austen in 1975
  - 28-segment model of Myocardial Infarction and Mortality in Coronary Artery Surgery Study
- Of note, some experts use 2nd diagonal branch (rather than 1/2 distance from 1st branch) to apex as landmark dividing mLAD and dLAD

NORMAL VARIANTS AND ANOMALIES

General Considerations

- Wide degree of variation with variable clinical significance
- Categorized as anomalies of origin, course, intrinsic anatomy, and termination

Anomalies of Origin and Course

- Absence of LM with separate ostia of LAD and LCx directly from left coronary sinus
- High origin of coronary ostium
  - Variably defined in literature ranging from anywhere above sinotubular junction (STJ), > 1 cm above STJ, or > 2 cm above STJ
  - Benign
- Origin from opposite, or, rarely, noncoronary cusp with anomalous course
  - Benign variants have course either retroaortic or prepulmonic/anterior to right ventricular outflow tract
  - Malignant variants have interarterial course between aorta and pulmonary artery
  - Transseptal variant, where vessel runs in myocardium just below interarterial space, is considered less malignant compared to other anomalies
- Anomalous left coronary artery from pulmonary artery (ALCAPA)
- Single coronary artery

Anomalies of Intrinsic Anatomy

- Congenital coronary ostial stenosis or atresia
- Congenital or acquired coronary ectasia or aneurysm
- Myocardial bridge
- Duplicated coronary artery

Anomalies of Termination

- Coronary-venous or coronary-cameral fistula
- Extracardiac termination

CARDIAC VEINS

- Anterior cardiac veins drain anterior right ventricular free wall, cross right atrioventricular groove, and enter right atrium directly
- Coronary sinus (largest cardiac vein at ~ 14 mm in diameter) enters right atrium near inferior vena cava inflow
  - May be complete or incomplete valve at its ostium (thebesian valve)
- Middle cardiac vein runs in posterior interventricular groove and enters coronary sinus near its ostium
- Other tributaries to coronary sinus are posterior vein of left ventricle (drains inferior left ventricular wall), marginal veins, and great cardiac vein, which runs in left atrioventricular groove
- Anteriorly, great cardiac vein becomes anterior interventricular vein, which runs parallel to LAD and receives diagonal veins

SELECTED REFERENCES

1. Abbara S et al: SCCT guidelines for the performance and acquisition of coronary computed tomographic angiography: a report of the society of Cardiovascular Computed Tomography Guidelines Committee: endorsed by the North American Society for Cardiovascular Imaging (NASCI). J Cardiovasc Comput Tomogr. 10(6):435-49, 2016
2. Leipsic J et al: SCCT guidelines for the interpretation and reporting of coronary CT angiography: a report of the Society of Cardiovascular Computed Tomography Guidelines Committee. J Cardiovasc Comput Tomogr. 8(5):342-58, 2014

AORTIC ROOT AND CORONARY ARTERIES

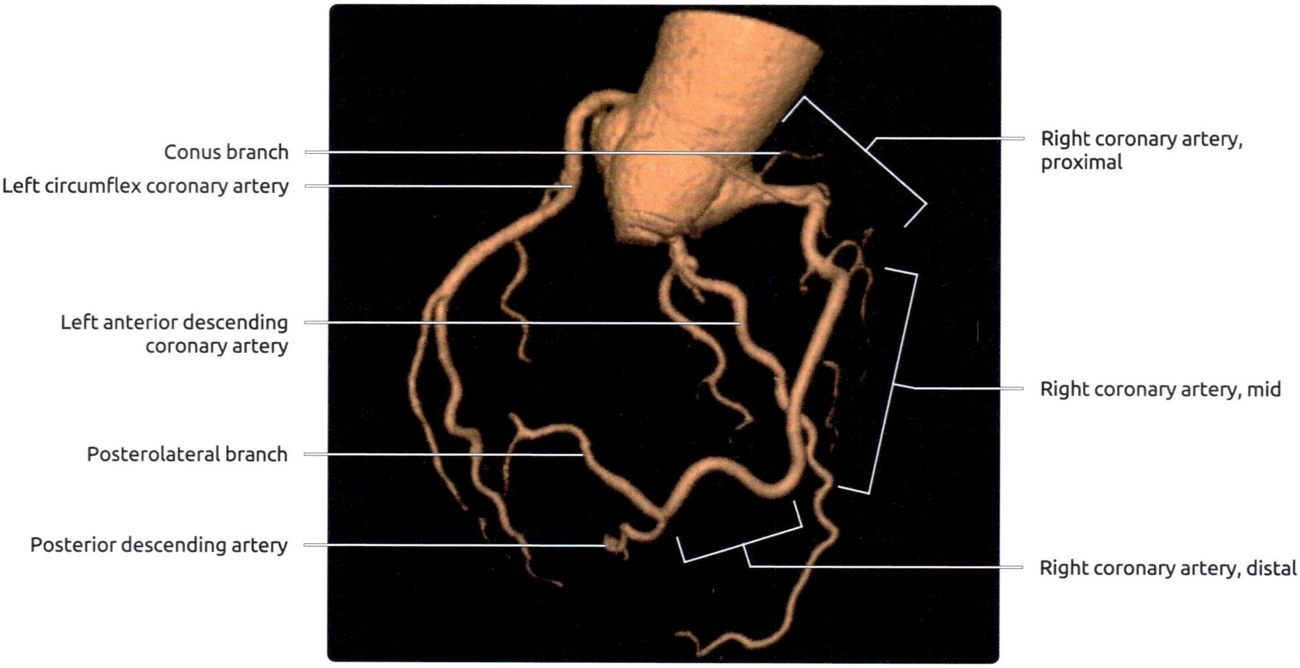

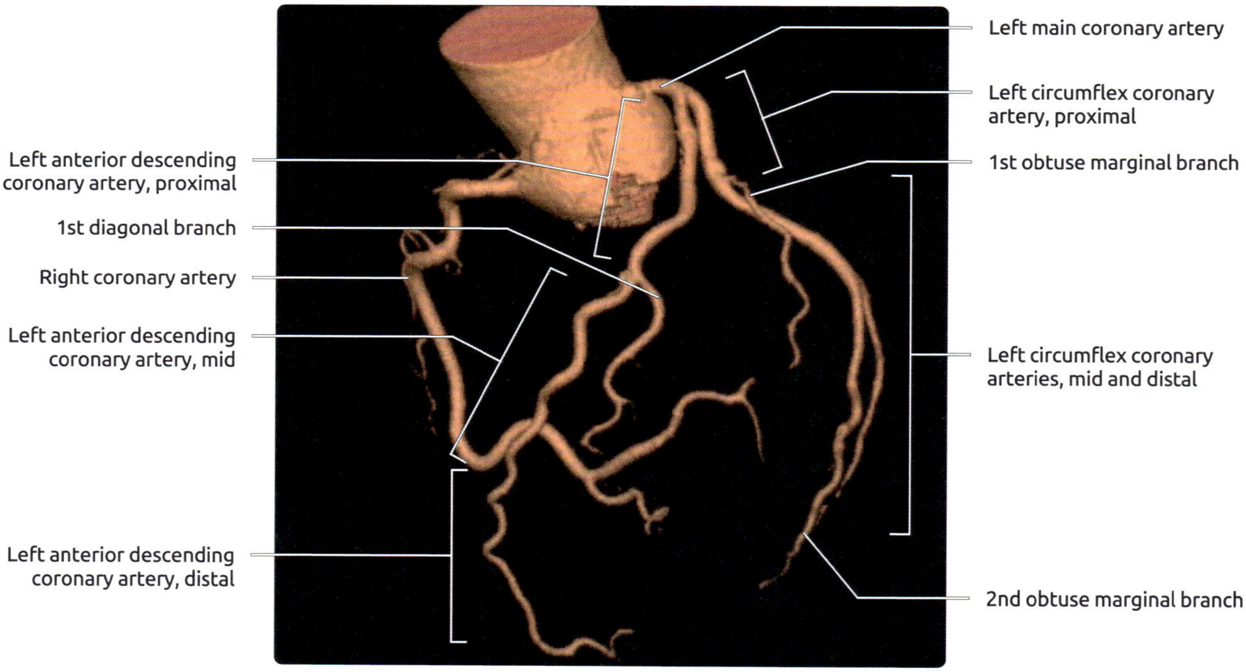

(Top) *Volume-rendered image shows the aortic root and coronary arteries, oriented to depict the right coronary artery (RCA).* **(Bottom)** *Volume-rendered image shows the aortic root and coronary arteries, oriented to depict the left coronary arteries.*

CORONARY ARTERY ORIGINS

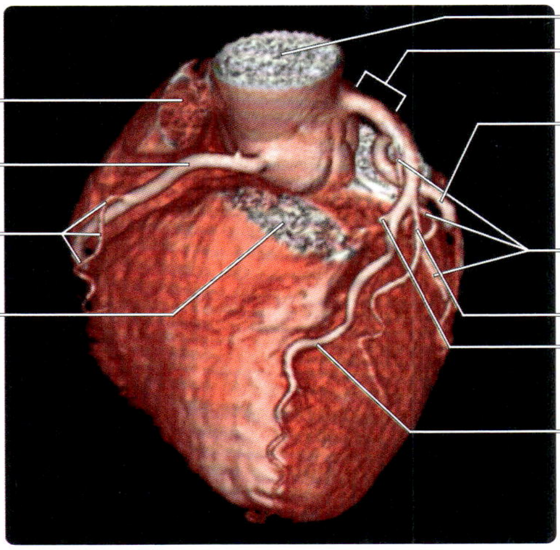

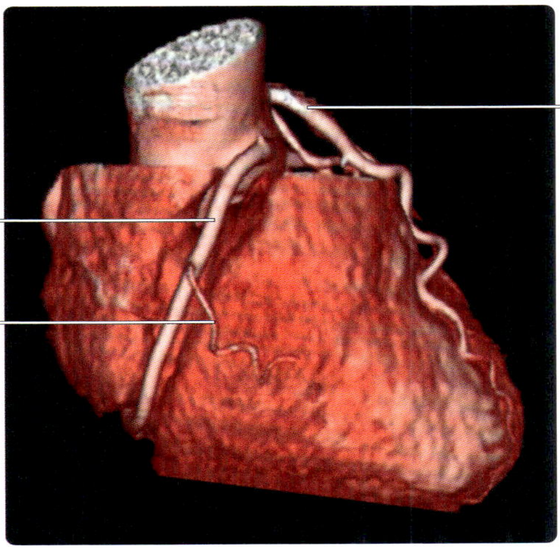

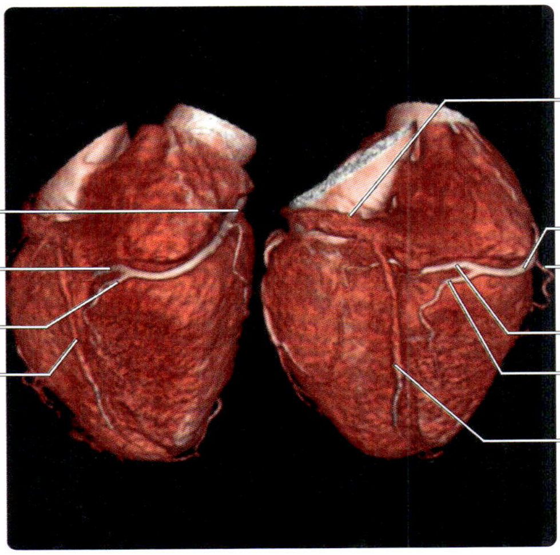

(Top) *3D volume-rendered anteroposterior image shows the coronary artery origins. The right ventricular outflow tract and atrial appendages have been excluded to depict the coronary origins.* **(Middle)** *3D volume-rendered anteroposterior image shows the coronary artery origins. The right ventricular outflow tract and atrial appendages have been excluded to depict the coronary origins.* **(Bottom)** *3D volume-rendered images show the diaphragmatic surface of the heart. In this right-dominant coronary arterial system, the RCA continues as the posterior descending artery (PDA) along the posterior interventricular groove.*

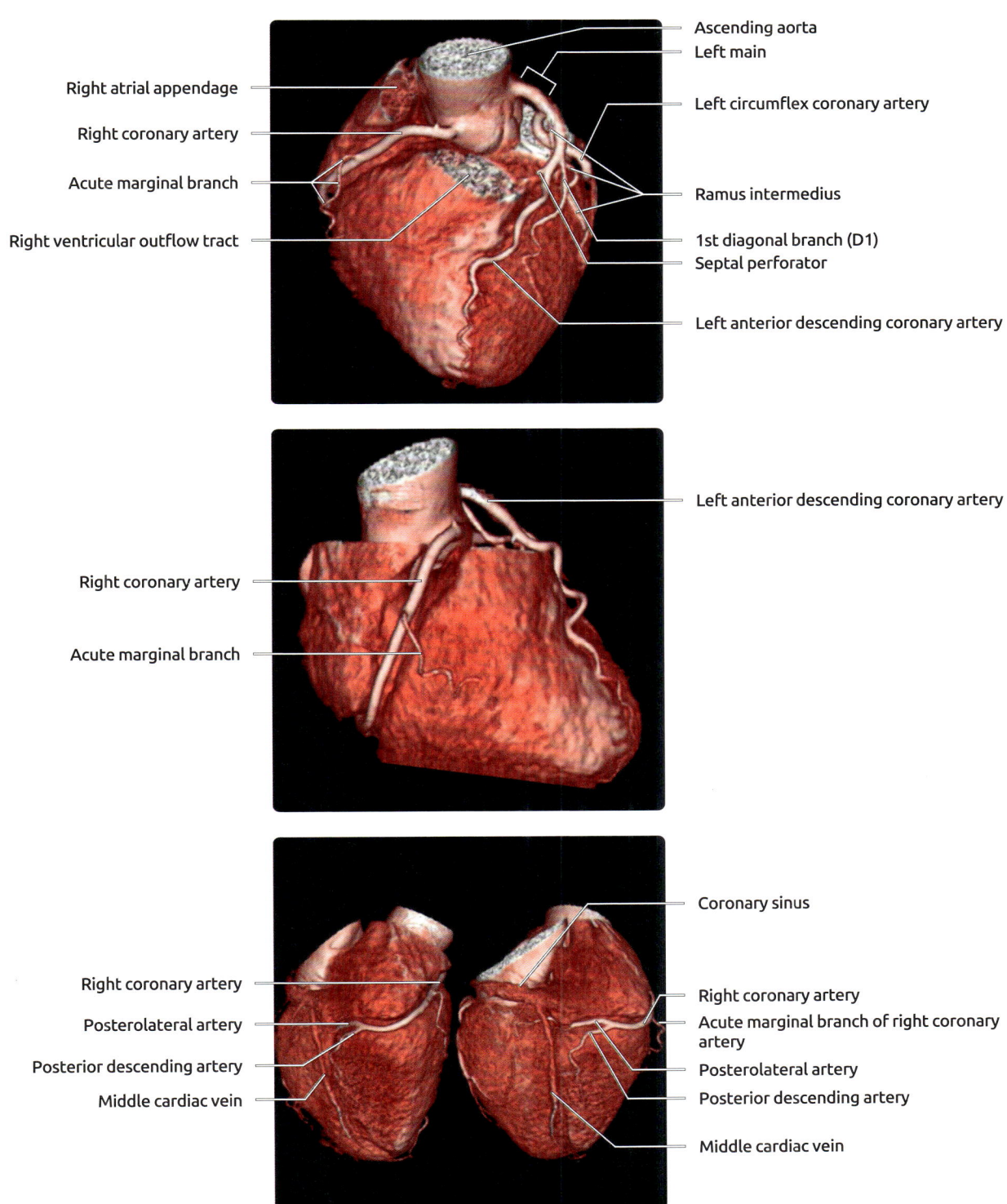

LEFT CORONARY ARTERIES

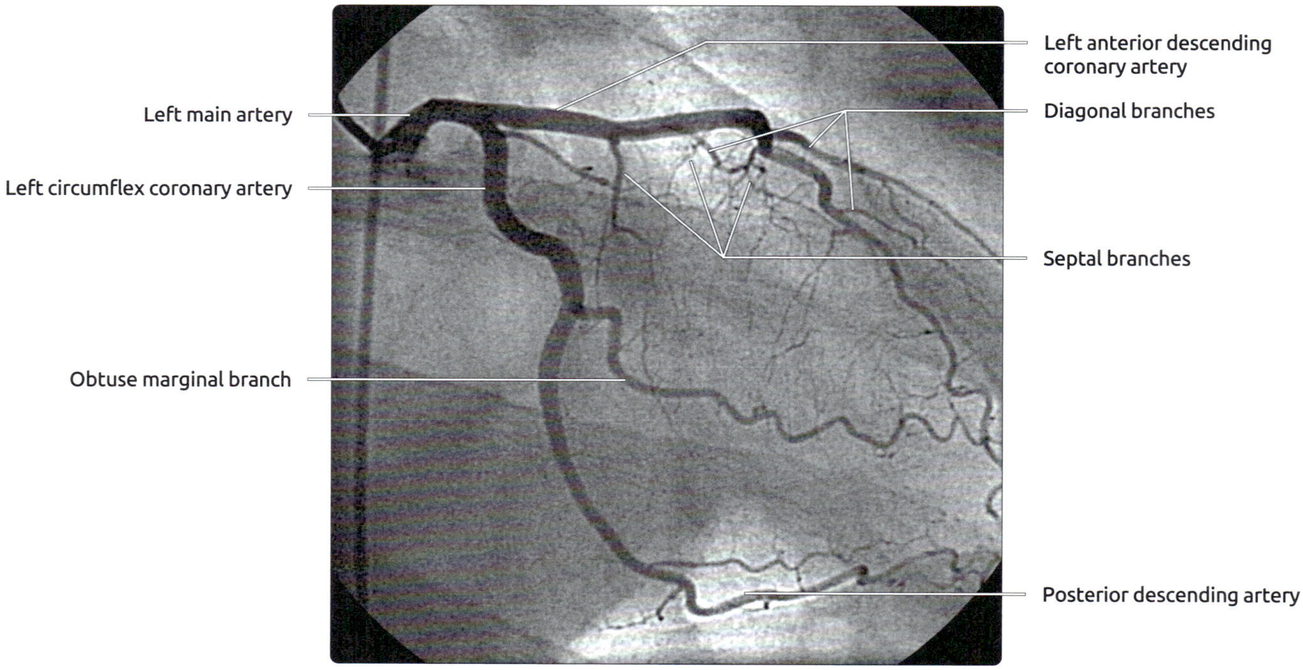

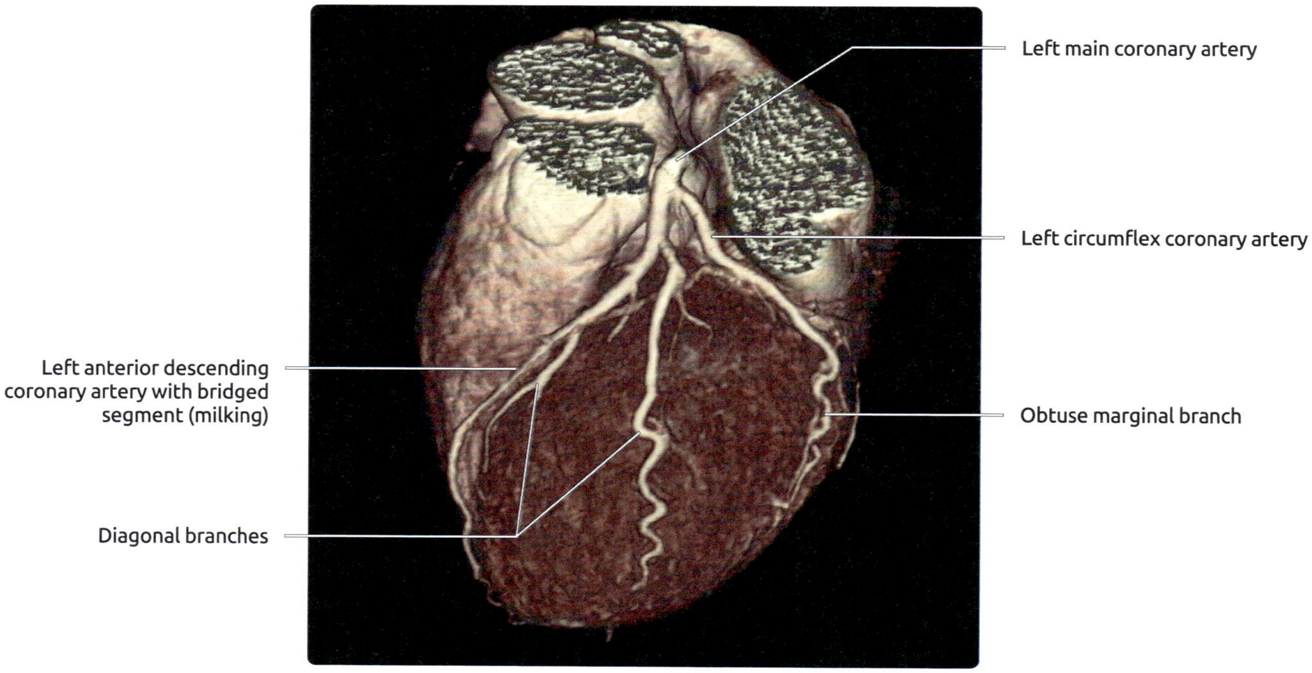

(Top) *Right anterior oblique caudal view of selective angiography shows a left-dominant coronary system.* **(Bottom)** *3D volume-rendered image shows the left coronary arteries.*

RIGHT CORONARY ARTERIES

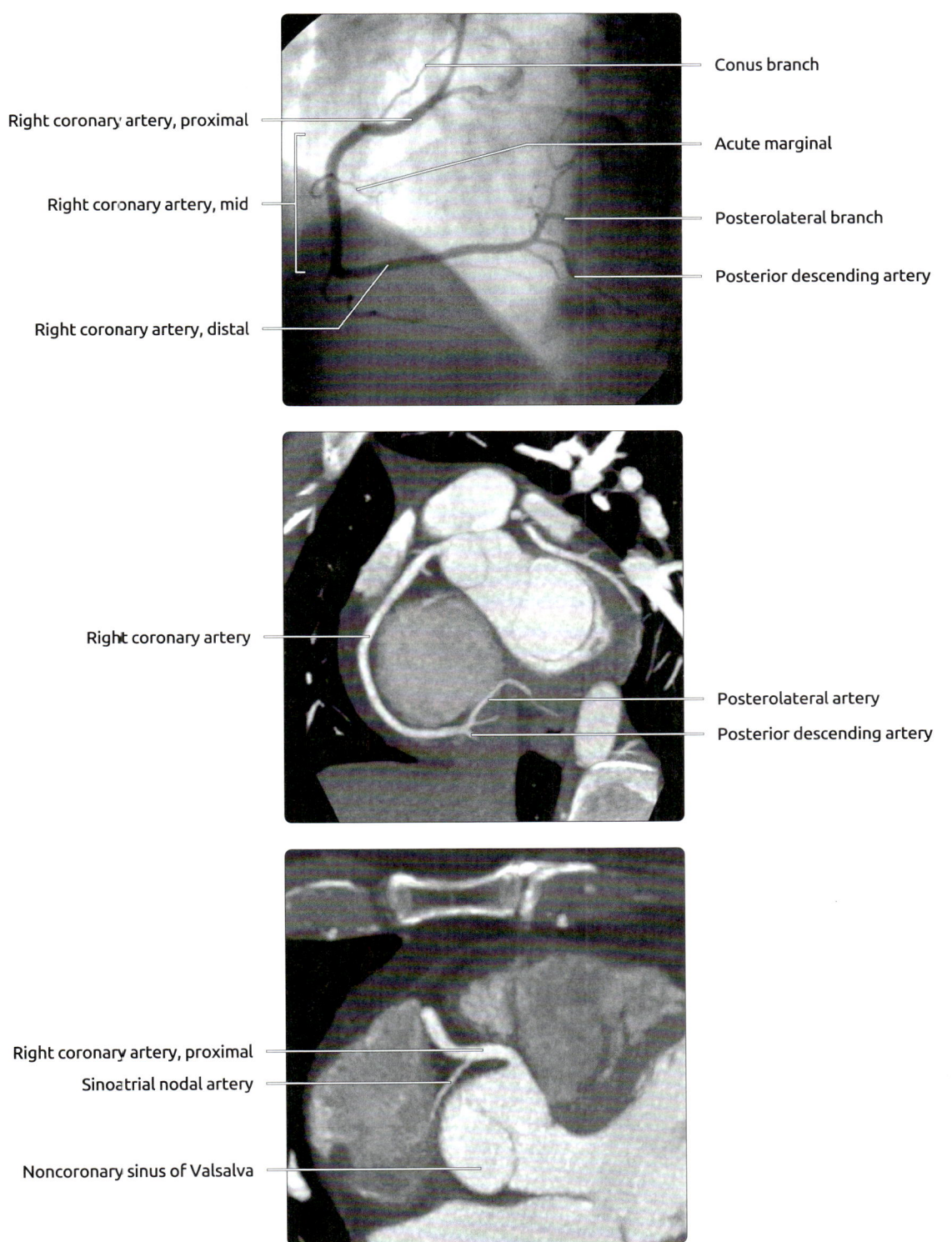

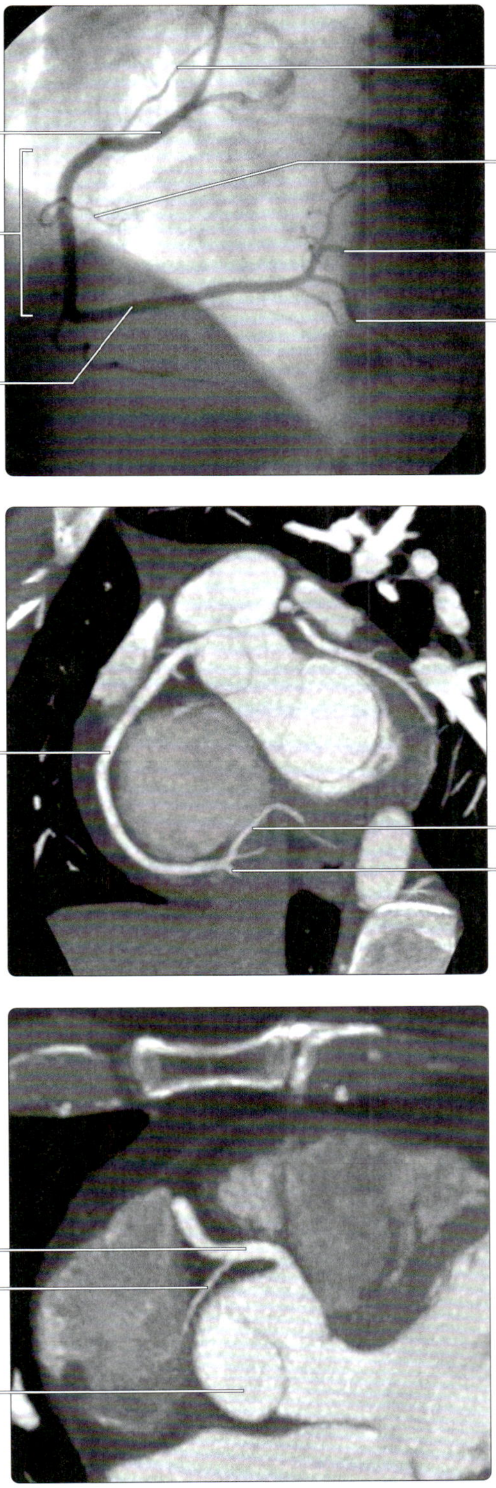

(Top) *Left anterior oblique projection shows a right-dominant coronary system.* **(Middle)** *This is a curved maximum-intensity projection (MIP) along the course of a dominant RCA. This is known as the "C view" due to the characteristic appearance of the RCA.* **(Bottom)** *Curved MIP depicts the sinoatrial artery arising from the proximal RCA, the most common variant. Less commonly, the sinoatrial artery arises from the left circumflex (LCx) coronary artery. Rarely, it may arise directly from the right coronary sinus.*

LEFT CORONARY ARTERIES

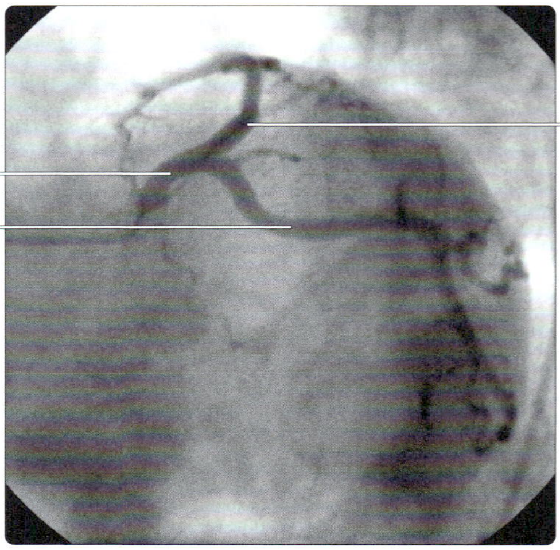

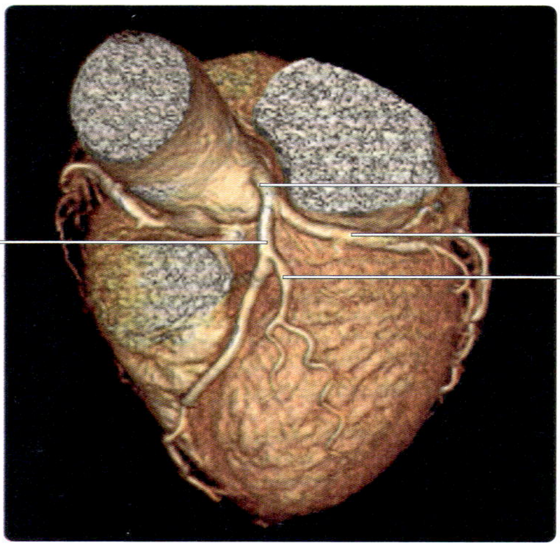

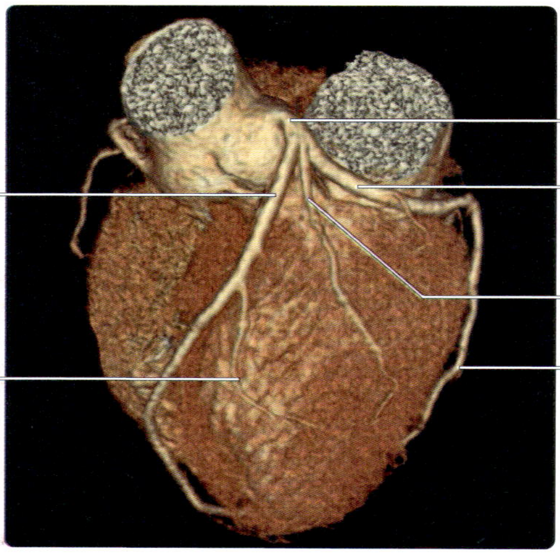

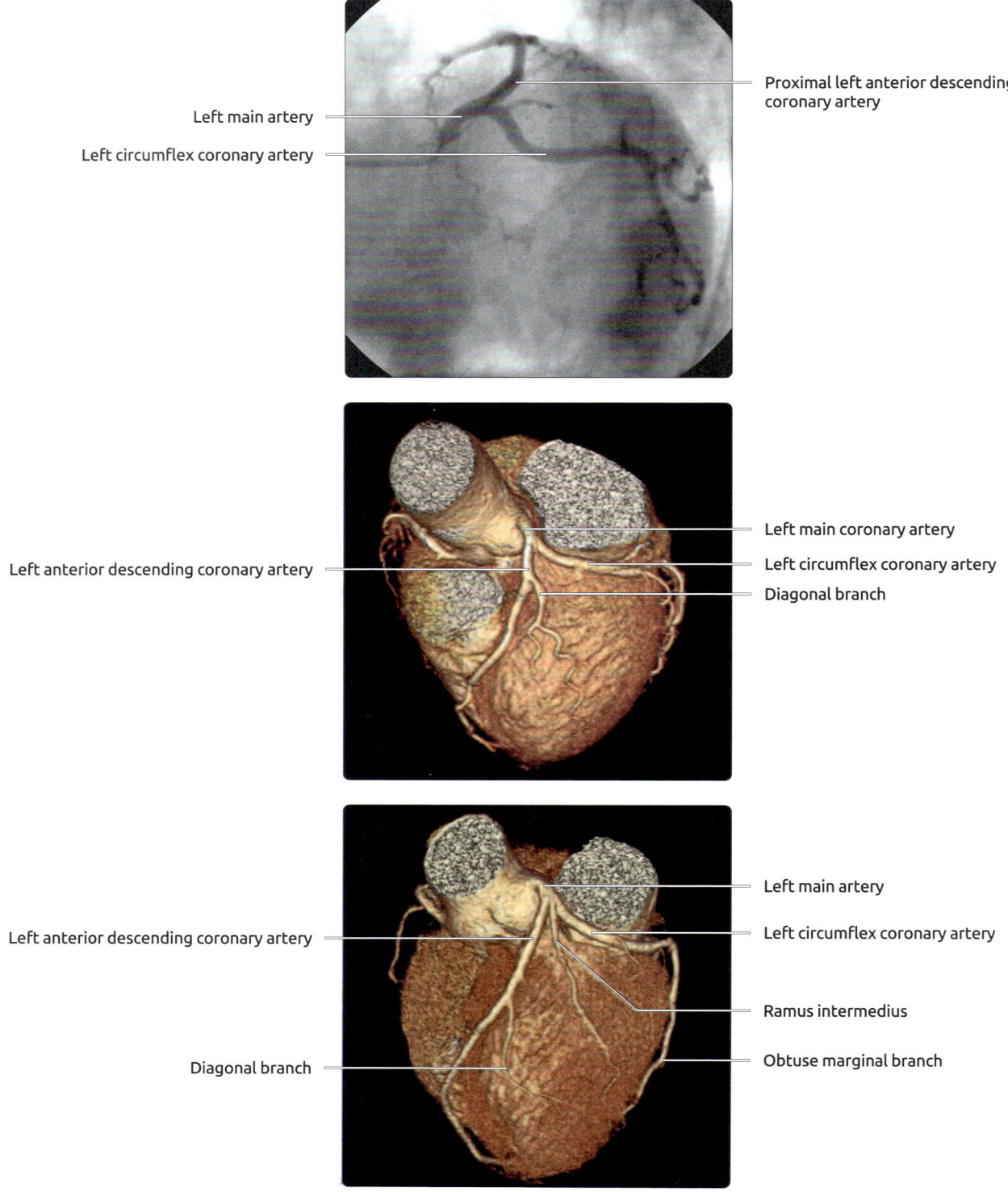

(Top) *Coronary angiogram demonstrates the course and origin of the LCx coronary artery. Left anterior oblique caudal "spider" view depicts the left main, proximal left anterior descending (LAD), and LCx coronary arteries.* **(Middle)** *3D volume-rendered image shows left main coronary artery bifurcation. The left atrial appendage has been excluded as the left main coronary artery would otherwise be hidden underneath.* **(Bottom)** *3D volume-rendered image shows the left main trifurcation into LAD, ramus intermedius, and circumflex coronary arteries.*

LEFT CORONARY ARTERIES

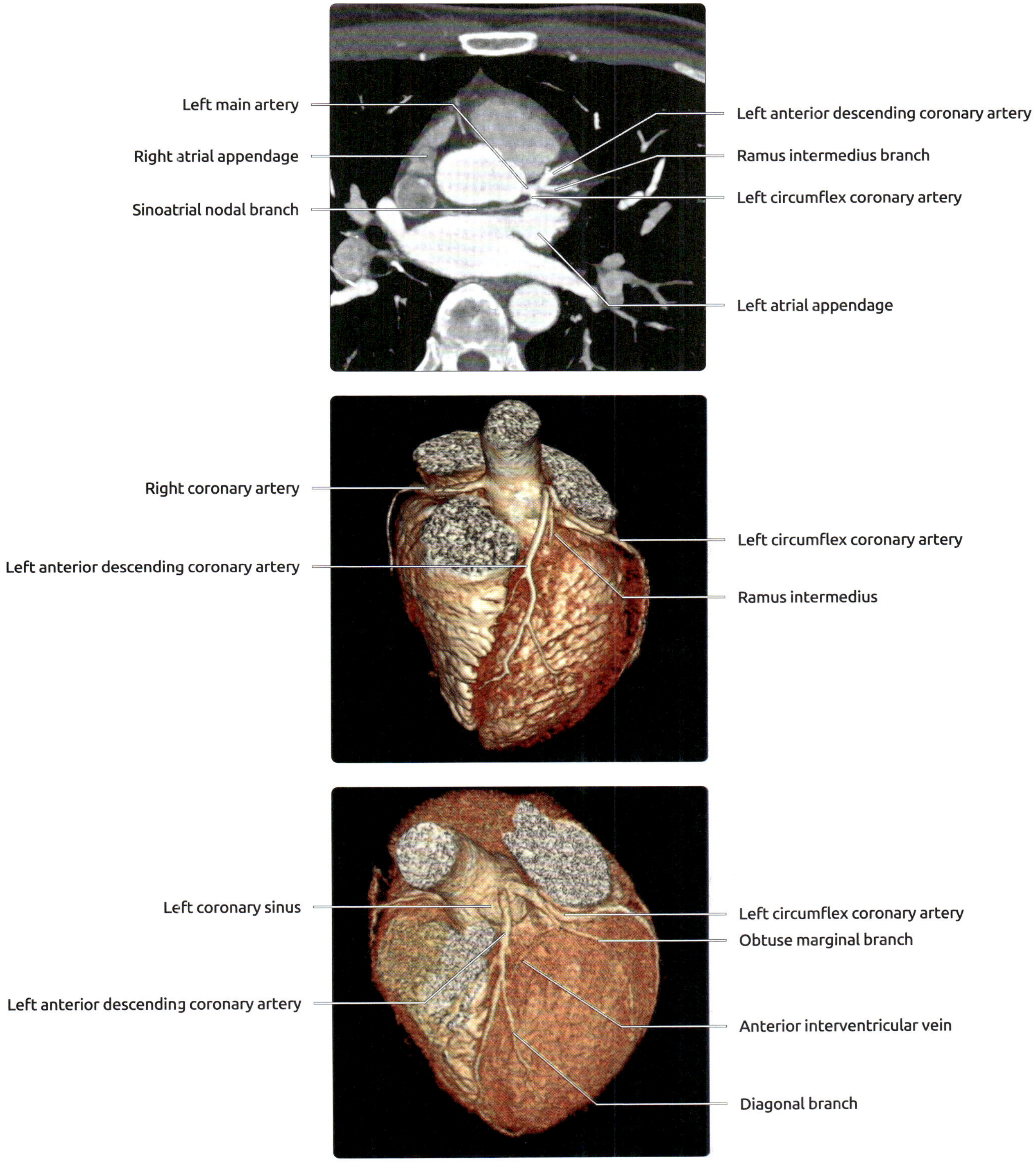

(Top) *Axial MIP demonstrates trifurcation of the left main coronary artery into LAD, ramus intermedius, and LCx branches. Here, the sinoatrial nodal artery arises from the proximal LCx, a normal variant.* **(Middle)** *3D volume-rendered image shows left main coronary artery trifurcation. The ramus intermedius most commonly courses laterally in a similar direction as the 1st diagonal but can also run parallel to the obtuse marginal arteries.* **(Bottom)** *3D volume-rendered image shows an uncommon normal variant where the left main coronary artery is absent and the LAD and LCx arise from separate ostia off the left coronary sinus.*

RIGHT-, LEFT-, AND CODOMINANT SYSTEMS

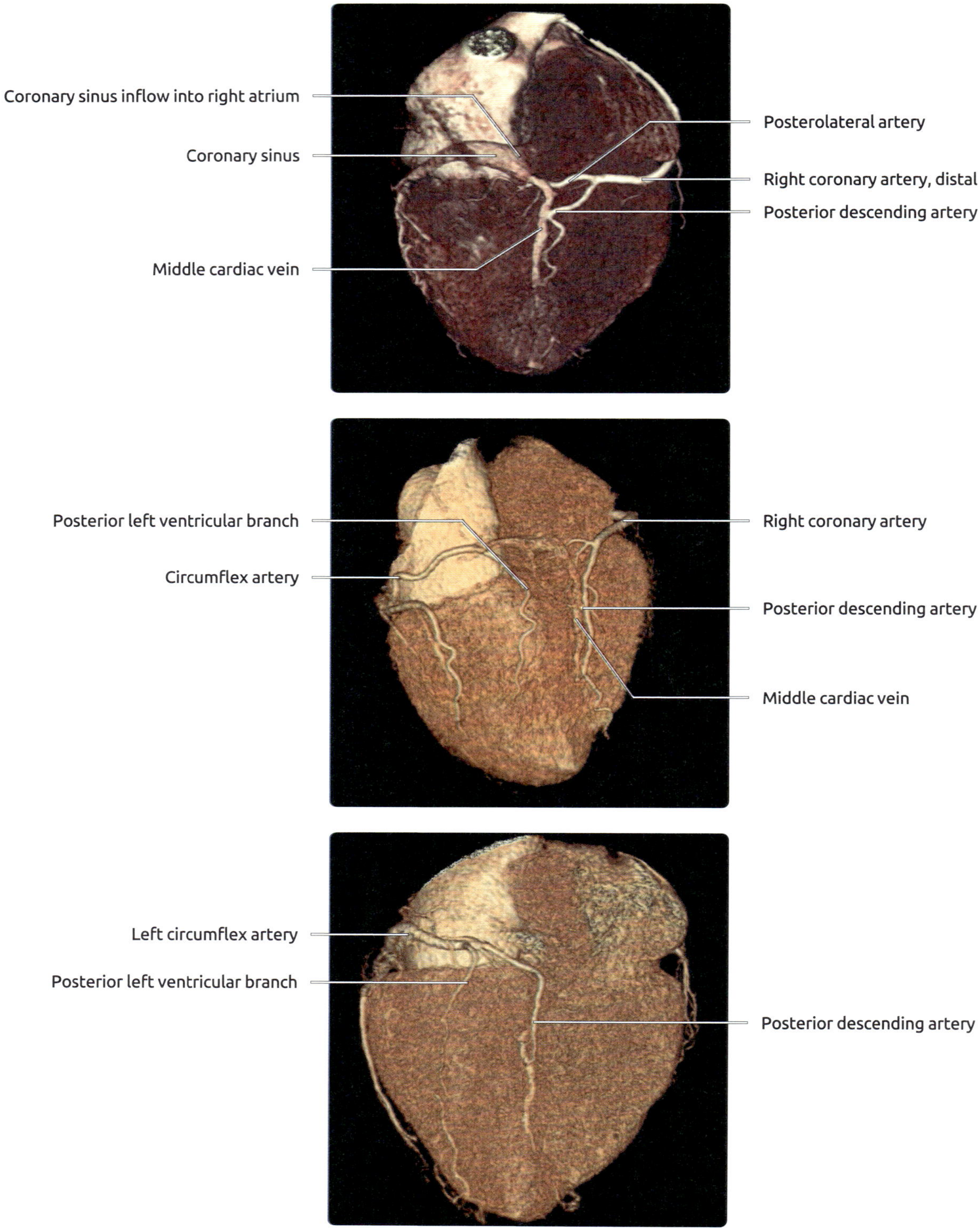

(Top) *3D volume-rendered image shows the inferior surface of the heart in a right-dominant system. Note the middle cardiac vein, which courses alongside the PDA in the posterior interventricular groove.* **(Middle)** *Codominant coronary system is shown. The posterior left ventricular (PLV) branch is supplied from the circumflex, and the PDA arises from the RCA.* **(Bottom)** *Left-dominant coronary system is shown. Both the PDA and the PLV arise from the LCx.*

CORONARY ARTERIES, ORIGINS AND COURSE

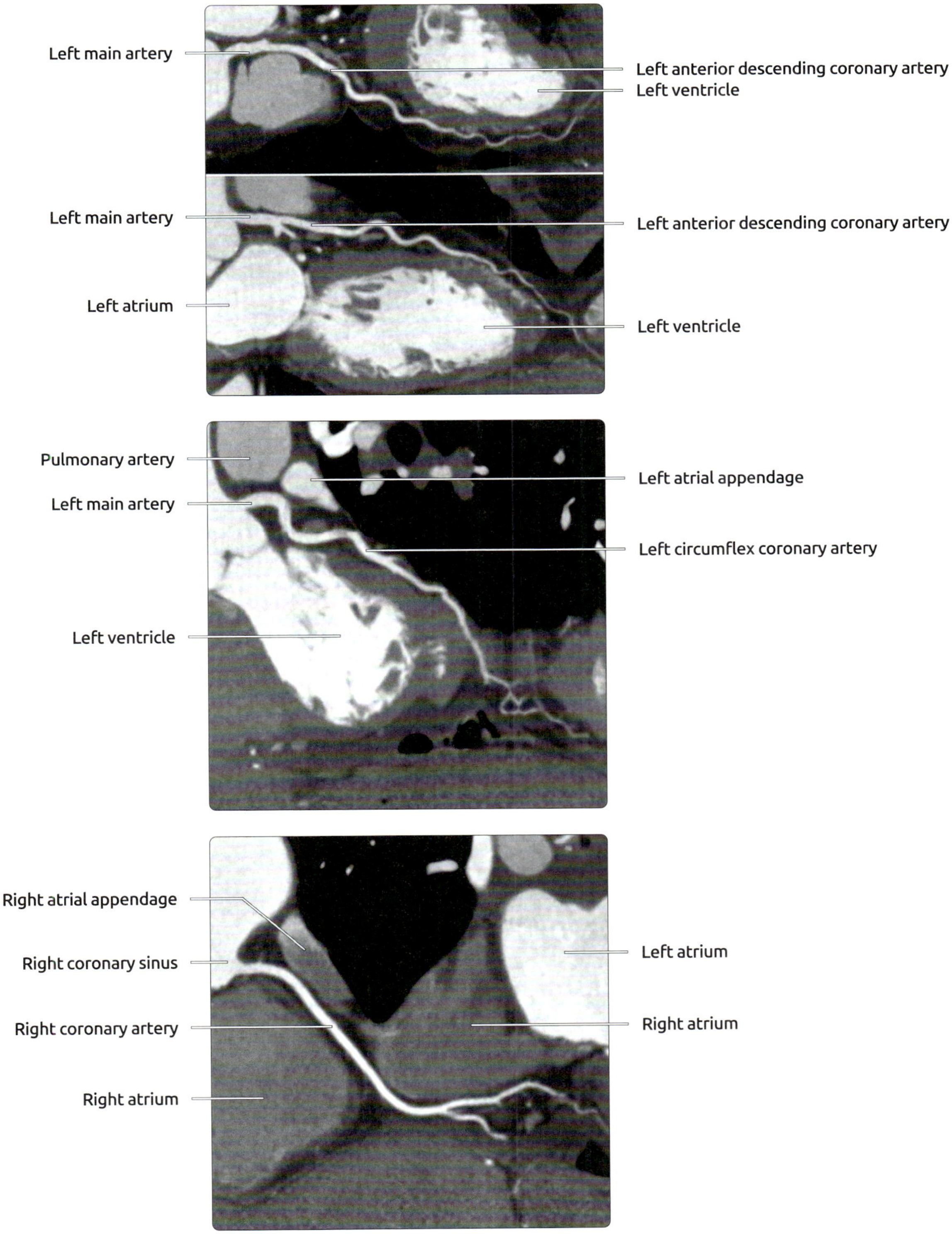

(Top) *Curved multiplanar reformation (MPR) shows the LAD coronary artery, which arises from the left main coronary artery and travels along the anterior interventricular groove.* **(Middle)** *Curved MPR shows the LCx coronary artery, which arises from the left main coronary artery and descends into the left atrioventricular groove.* **(Bottom)** *Curved MPR shows the RCA, which arises from the right coronary sinus and passes under the right atrial appendage as it descends into right atrioventricular groove.*

PERFUSION TERRITORIES

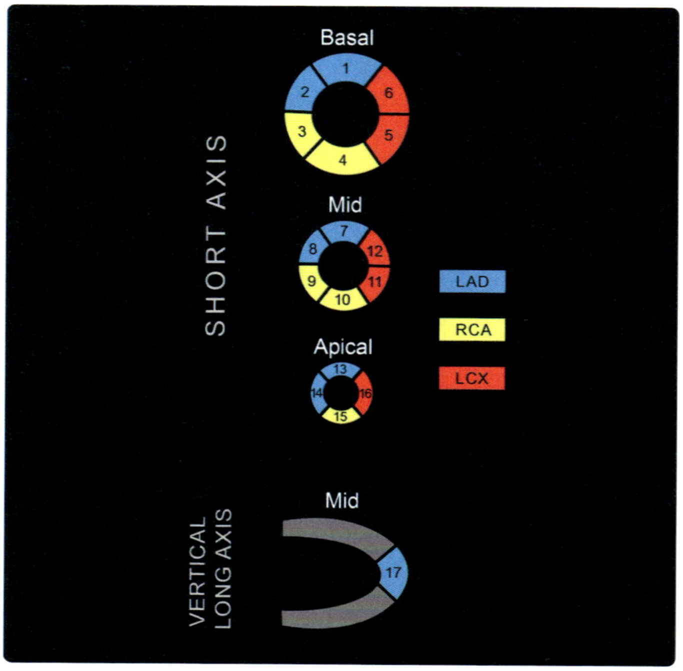

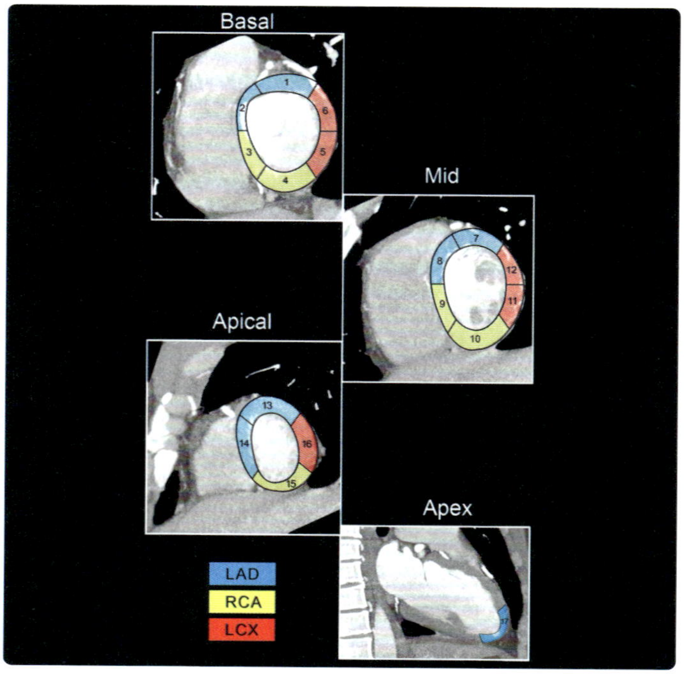

(Top) *Graphic depicts the 17 left ventricular myocardial segments with corresponding color-coded coronary artery perfusion territories for a right-dominant coronary system.* **(Bottom)** *Typically, the LAD supplies the anterior wall, anteroseptal wall, and apex. The LCx supplies the lateral wall. The RCA supplies the inferior and inferoseptal walls. Considerable normal variation exists, and these perfusion territories should be considered as a guideline rather than a rule.*

18-SEGMENT CORONARY MODEL

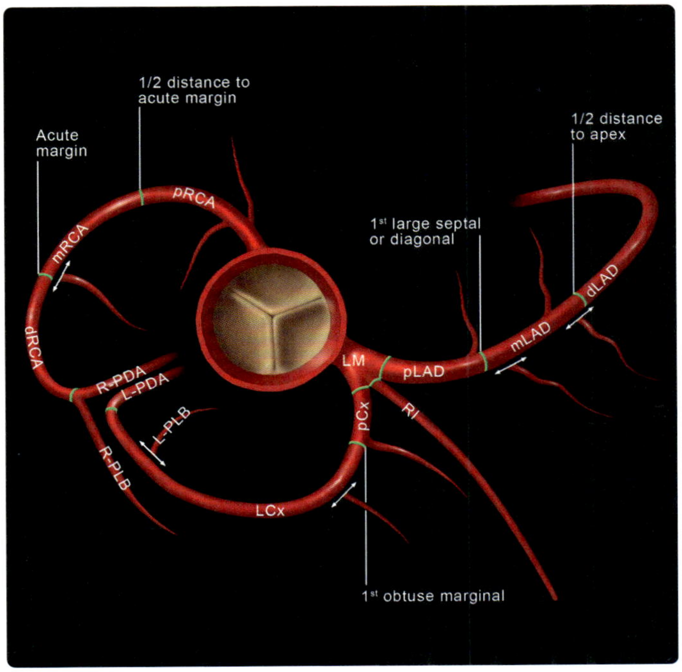

Segment	Abbreviation	Description
Proximal RCA	pRCA	RCA ostium to ½ distance to acute margin of heart
Mid RCA	mRCA	End of pRCA to acute margin
Distal RCA	dRCA	End of mRCA to origin of PDA
PDA-RCA	R-PDA	PDA from RCA
PLB-RCA	R-PLB	Posterolateral branch from RCA
Left main	LM	Ostium of LM to bifurcation or trifurcation
Proximal LAD	pLAD	End of LM to 1st large septal or diagonal, whichever is most proximal
Mid LAD	mLAD	End of pLAD to ½ distance to apex
Distal LAD	dLAD	End of mLAD to end of LAD
Diagonal 1	D1	1st diagonal branch. Subsequent diagonals D2, D3, etc.
Proximal LCx	pCx	End of LM to origin of 1st OM
Obtuse marginal 1	OM1	1st obtuse marginal branch. Subsequent branches OM2, etc.
Mid and distal LCx	LCx	Distal to OM1 to the end of the circumflex or origin of L-PDA
PDA-LCx	L-PDA	PDA from LCx
Ramus intermedius	RI	In case of LM trifurcation, vessel arising between LAD & LCx
PLB-L	L-PLB	Posterolateral branch from LCx

(Top) *Graphic depicts the Society of Cardiovascular Computed Tomography (SCCT) 18-segment coronary model, a modification of the original 1975 American Heart Association 15-segment model.* **(Bottom)** *Awareness of the differences between these 2 models is important to avoid confusion. First, ramus intermedius and left posterolateral branches have been included as the 17th and 18th segments. Second, the mid- and distal LCx are considered a single segment. Third, the boundary between the mid- and distal LAD is defined as 1/2 the distance to the cardiac apex rather than the origin of the 2nd diagonal branch. [Adapted from Raff GL et al: SCCT guidelines for the interpretation and reporting of coronary computed tomographic angiography. J Cardiovasc Comput Tomogr. 3(2):122-36, 2009.]*

Myocardial Bridge

KEY FACTS

TERMINOLOGY

- Congenital coronary anatomic variant in which segment of epicardial coronary artery takes intramyocardial course
- Most common congenital coronary abnormality
- Most common location: Midsegment of left anterior descending (LAD) coronary artery

IMAGING

- CCTA
  - Epicardial coronary artery dives into myocardium and resurfaces distally into epicardial fat
- Intracoronary US
  - Highly specific echolucent half-moon sign
- FFR does not yield significant results, but novel techniques, such as instantaneous wave-free ratio, appear to hold promise and to be more consistent with patients' symptoms and noninvasive test results

TOP DIFFERENTIAL DIAGNOSES

- Hypertrophic cardiomyopathy

CLINICAL ISSUES

- Most asymptomatic; most patients have single bridge
- Rarely, angina, arrhythmia, or sudden death; association with ischemia is controversial
  - Certain bridges (long, deep) are controversially associated with ischemia
- β-blockers and calcium channel blockers are rarely needed
- Percutaneous coronary intervention can stabilize coronary artery lumen against muscular compression (very rarely)
- Surgical myotomy in patients with significant clinical symptoms
- Coronary artery bypass graft if failure of percutaneous coronary intervention or coronary disease (extreme rarity)

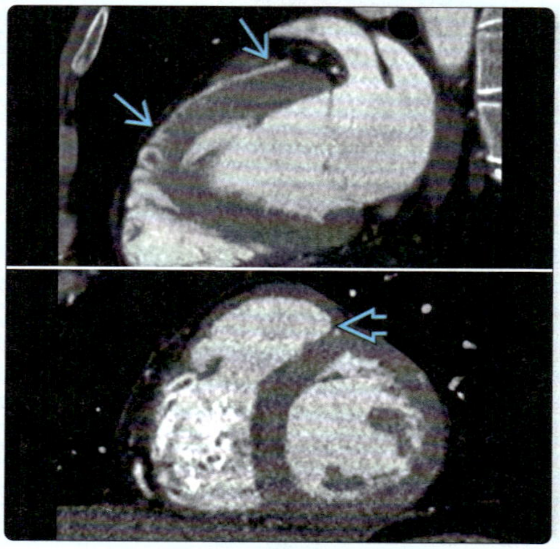
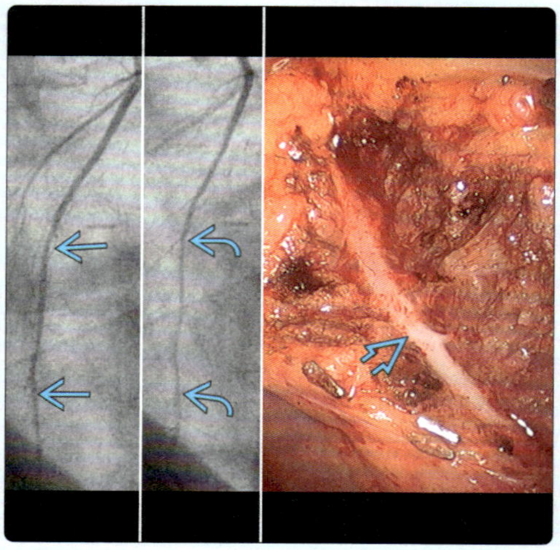

(Left) *2-chamber (top) and short axis (bottom) images in a 40-year-old man with chronic chest pain shows portions of a 7-cm long myocardial bridge of the mid- and distal LAD, which was up to 6 mm deep. The CT was otherwise normal.* **(Right)** *Angiogram of the LAD shows normal caliber during diastole (left) with milking during systole (middle) due to bridging. Due to recurrent chest pain, the patient underwent surgical myotomy (left), which shows the bridged LAD. However, this did not alleviate the patient's symptoms.*

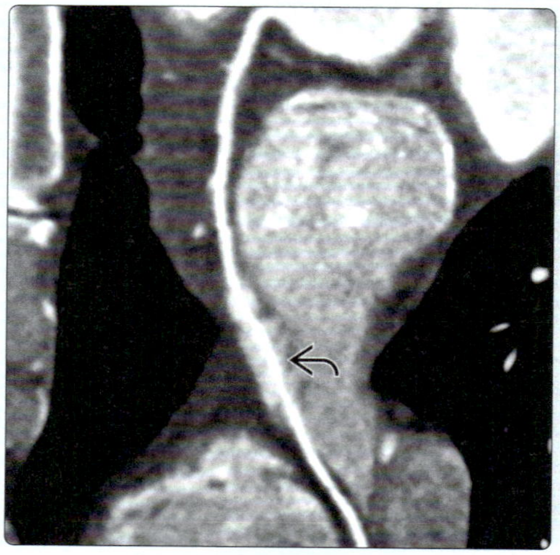
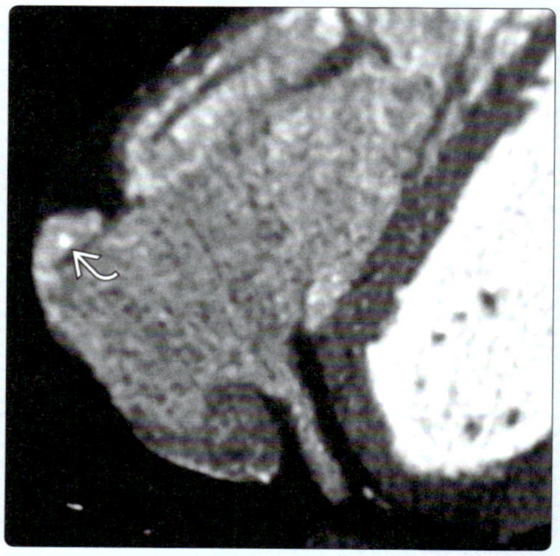

(Left) *Coronary CT curved multiplanar reformat shows a right coronary artery with a long intracavitary segment passing through the right atrium. Such appearances are difficult to depict on invasive angiography.* **(Right)** *Coronary CTA in the same patient using a cross-sectional image plane across the right coronary artery confirms the intracavitary segment within the right atrium. No stenosis of the right coronary artery was identified.*

TERMINOLOGY

Definitions

- Portion of epicardial coronary artery takes intramyocardial course and is tunneled under overlying muscular bridge

IMAGING

General Features

- Best diagnostic clue
  - Coronary artery dives into and is covered by "bridge" or layer of myocardium
- Location
  - 67-68% of myocardial bridges (MBs) located in left anterior descending (LAD) coronary artery, most commonly in proximal and mid-LAD segments; left coronary artery (40%) and right coronary artery (20%) less common
- Morphology
  - Mean depth: 2.5 mm; mean length: 19.3 mm

Imaging Recommendations

- Best imaging tool
  - Noninvasive
    - CCTA: Epicardial coronary artery dives into myocardium and resurfaces distally into epicardial fat
      - Compared with IVUS, sensitivity of 93% and specificity of 100%
  - Invasive
    - Coronary angiography: Milking effect seen allows quantification of systolic compression
    - IVUS: Echolucent half-moon sign throughout cardiac cycle
    - OCT: Fusiform signal poor with systolic compression
    - FFR: Does not yield significant result

PATHOLOGY

General Features

- Etiology
  - MB causes systolic lumen reduction (termed milking when seen on angiography)
    - Because 85% perfusion occurs during diastole, milking usually does not lead to reduced perfusion

Staging, Grading, & Classification

- Partial (~ 65%) or complete
  - "Touch-down" coronary artery: Coronary artery touches myocardium but is not fully embedded
  - Deep bridge: Typically, LAD artery deviates toward right ventricle (RV), dives into ventricular septum, with overlying longitudinal muscle bundle from RV apex
  - Coronary artery may be intracavitary, mostly if RCA bridge is in right atrium or (rarely) RV
  - Long-segment (≥ 5 mm) and deep (≥ 2 mm) MBs are potentially symptomatic compared to superficial (1- to 2-mm) MBs, which are more commonly asymptomatic
- Schwarz classification (2009)
  - Type A: Clinical symptoms but no objective signs of ischemia (incidental finding on angiography); Rx reassurance alone
  - Type B: Objective signs of ischemia
  - Type C: Altered intracoronary hemodynamics; Rx with calcium channel blockers and β-blockers

Microscopic Features

- Systolic compression of bridged segment prevents deposition of lipid molecules, leading to protection from atherosclerotic plaque
- Upstream shear wall stress predisposes to atherosclerosis upstream from bridge

CLINICAL ISSUES

Presentation

- Most common signs/symptoms
  - Most asymptomatic; most patients have single bridge; rarely, angina, arrhythmia, or sudden death; association with ischemia is controversial

Demographics

- Age
  - Congenital
  - Symptoms, if any (usually asymptomatic), may begin in 3rd decade
- Epidemiology
  - Prevalence of MBs range from 2-7% with invasive catheter angiography but higher with CCTA (19-22%) and at autopsy (as high as 45%)

Natural History & Prognosis

- Very common, and most patients are asymptomatic
- Vessels longer and deeper than 3 mm are higher risk for cardiac events

Treatment

- Asymptomatic: Often incidental finding with no Rx required; risk factor modification, antiplatelets for coexisting carotid artery disease
- Symptomatic (rare)
  - Medical: Aim to increase diastolic filling time and reduce myocardial contractility; calcium channel blockers/β-blockers improve coronary hemodynamics with decreased chronotropy and inotropy; nitrates contraindicated
  - Interventional: Stents stabilize lumen against muscular compression; superficial and shorter length MBs more amenable to PCI
  - Surgical: Very rarely if at risk of myocardial infarction; CABG if unsuccessful PCI or significant disease; myotomy involves resection of overlying muscle fibers and has been shown to increase coronary blood flow

SELECTED REFERENCES

1. Danek BA et al: Clinically significant myocardial bridging. Heart. 110(2):81-6, 2023
2. Sternheim D et al: Myocardial bridging: diagnosis, functional assessment, and management: JACC state-of-the-art review. J Am Coll Cardiol. 78(22):2196-212, 2021
3. Tarantini G et al: Unmasking myocardial bridge-related ischemia by intracoronary functional evaluation. Circ Cardiovasc Interv. 11(6):e006247, 2018
4. Cerrato E et al: What is the optimal treatment for symptomatic patients with isolated coronary myocardial bridge? A systematic review and pooled analysis. J Cardiovasc Med (Hagerstown). 18(10):758-70, 2017
5. Hostiuc S et al: Myocardial bridging: a meta-analysis of prevalence. J Forensic Sci. 63(4):1176-85, 2017

Single Coronary Artery

KEY FACTS

TERMINOLOGY

- Single coronary artery (SCA) arising from 1 coronary sinus and supplies entire heart

IMAGING

- Coronary CTA is best noninvasive imaging modality
  - Provides comprehensive assessment of coronary anatomy form origin to course and branching pattern
  - Delineate relationship with adjacent vasculature
  - Shows concurrent coronary atherosclerosis (obstructive vs. nonobstructive)
- MR can be used not only for evaluation of coronary anatomy but also for myocardial, valvular function, evaluation of LGE, or ischemia
- Echocardiogram can evaluate coronary ostia but abnormalities need confirmatory study
- Invasive angiography delineates coronary anatomy
- Most commonly used classification based on origin, branching pattern, and course of branches
  - Group I follows normal course of right or left coronary artery (RI vs. LI)
  - Group II: SCA, after arising from either cusp, gives rise to large transverse trunk that crosses to opposite site of heart
    - A: Anterior (prepulmonary); B: Interarterial; P: Posterior (retroaortic); S: Septal; C: Combined type
  - Group III: SCA arises from right coronary cusp and gives rise to separate left anterior descending and left circumflex

CLINICAL ISSUES

- Mostly incidental finding in asymptomatic patients
- Can be associated with congenital heart diseases
  - Tetralogy of Fallot, truncus arteriosus, transposition of great arteries
- Symptoms often related to underlying coronary heart disease or atherosclerotic disease

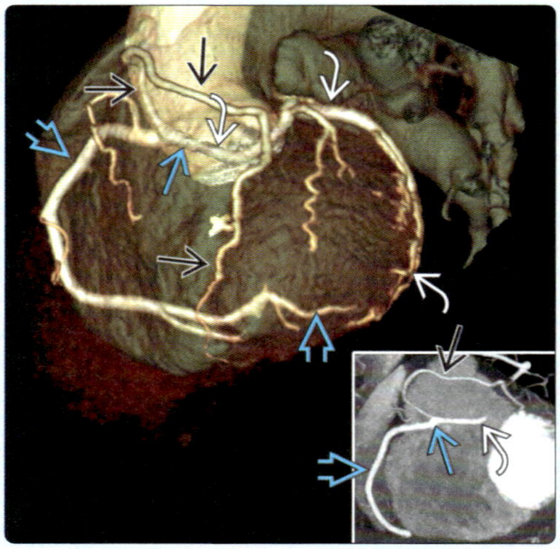
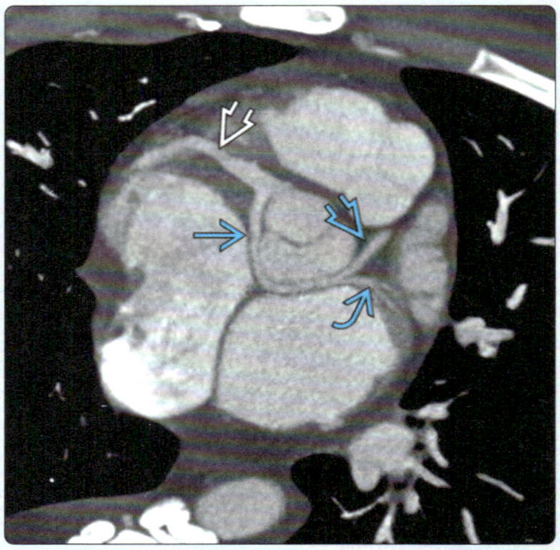

***(Left)** C-view and MIP (inset) show a single coronary artery (SCA) arising from the right sinus of Valsalva (SOV) → and trifurcating into a large right coronary artery (RCA) branch → partially supplying left circumflex (LCx) territory, a large septal branch → supplying the proximal left anterior descending (LAD) and LCx territory, and a prepulmonic branch → supplying the distal LAD territory. **(Right)** CECT shows a right SCA dividing into the RCA → and a retroaortic left main (LM) →, which divides into the LAD → and LCx →.*

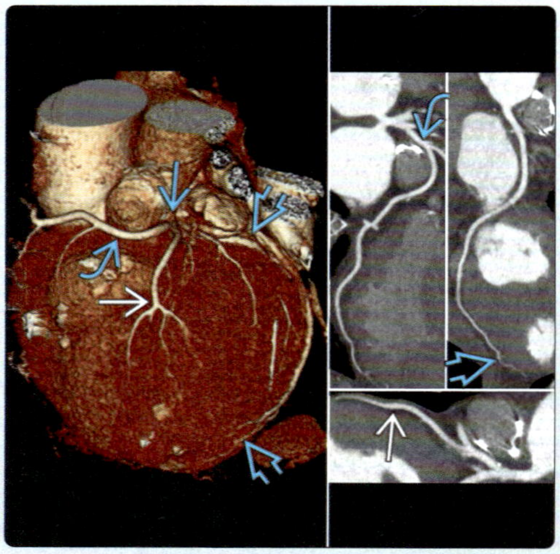
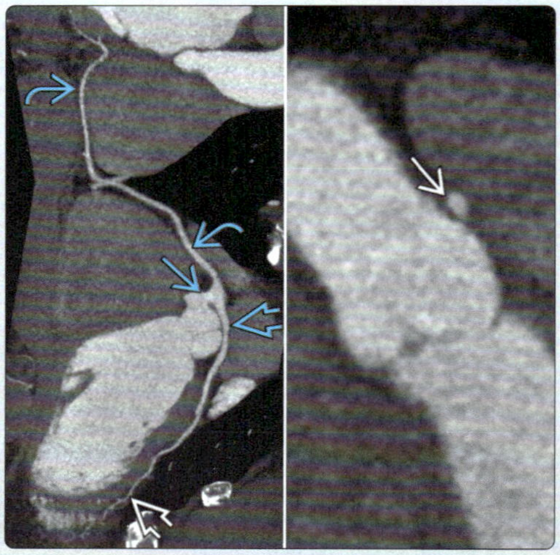

***(Left)** CECT in a Tetralogy of Fallot patient shows a left SCA → bifurcating into a dominant LCx →, which supplies much of left ventricular apex, and an anterior branch. The anterior branch bifurcates into a small LAD → and prepulmonic RCA →. **(Right)** Preablation CTA in an asymptomatic 59-year-old shows a right SCA → with an interarterial LM →, which divides into a large LAD → and small LCx (not shown). RCA → supplies much of LCx territory. Transverse CECT through the LM → shows little compression along its interarterial course.*

TERMINOLOGY

Abbreviations

- Single coronary artery (SCA)

Definitions

- SCA supplying entire coronary vasculature

IMAGING

General Features

- Best diagnostic clue
  - 1 coronary artery arising from aortic root
- Location
  - Origin could be from right or left sinus

CT Findings

- Best noninvasive modality
- Origin, course, and relationship to adjacent vasculature
- Classification based on origin, course, and branch anatomy
- Assessment of concurrent atherosclerosis

MR Findings

- No ionizing radiation but less spatial resolution that CT
- 3D whole-heart noncontrast MRA angiography
- Assess myocardial function, LGE, or perfusion abnormalities

Echocardiographic Findings

- Coronary ostia can be well visualized in many patients
- Widely available, low cost, and no radiation
- Abnormal findings should be confirmed with CT or MR

Angiographic Findings

- Identify origin and course of coronary arteries

Imaging Recommendations

- Best imaging tool
  - Coronary CTA

DIFFERENTIAL DIAGNOSIS

Anomalous Origin of Coronary Artery From Opposite Sinus

- 2 coronary arteries originate from same sinus
- Have distinct ostia

Coronary Artery Occlusion

- Normal-appearing 2 coronary ostia from each sinus
- Occluded vessel can be identified in its normal course

Left Main Coronary Artery Atresia

- Rare anomaly with absence of left main ostia
  - Flow into left circulation via collaterals from right coronary artery (RCA)
- Often symptomatic in pediatric patients with heart failure, syncope, or sudden cardiac death

PATHOLOGY

Staging, Grading, & Classification

- 3 groups based on location of ostium, anatomic distribution, and vessel course
- Group I: SCA follows normal course of right or left coronary artery
  - RI: SCA arises from right coronary cusp, follows RCA course, gives rise to obtuse marginal branches, and terminates as left anterior descending (LAD)
  - LI: SCA originates from left coronary cusp, gives rise to left circumflex (LCx) branch, courses through right atrioventricular groove, and terminates as RCA
- Group II: SCA, after arising from either of cusps, gives rise to large transverse trunk that crosses to opposite site of heart
  - Right (R) or left (L) to describe ostial location
  - Letters added at end indicates course of transverse trunk
    - A: Anterior (prepulmonary); B: Interarterial; P: Posterior (retroaortic); S: Septal; C: Combined type
- Group III: SCA arises from right coronary cusp and gives rise to separate LAD and LCx
  - LCx often retroaortic; LAD often interarterial or septal
- SCA rarely arises from pulmonary artery extremely rare

CLINICAL ISSUES

Presentation

- Most common signs/symptoms
  - Mostly asymptomatic, detected incidentally
  - Some may experience atypical chest pain, palpitation, syncope
- Other signs/symptoms
  - Mostly isolated (60%)
  - Associated with congenital heart diseases (CHDs) in 40%
    - Pulmonary atresia, tetralogy of Fallot, truncus arteriosus, transposition of great arteries
    - More likely to come to clinical attention due to CHD

Demographics

- Rare congenital anomaly, incidence <1%

Natural History & Prognosis

- Symptoms often related to underlying CHDs or atherosclerosis
- Depends on course of vasculature
- Incidental finding in vast majority of patients
- Interarterial courses often lack intramural portion
  - May be less symptomatic

Treatment

- No available guidelines for treatment or follow-up
- Concurrent atherosclerosis and myocardial ischemia may require medical treatment or revascularization

SELECTED REFERENCES

1. Bianco F et al: Echocardiographic screening for the anomalous aortic origin of coronary arteries. Open Heart. 8(1): e001495, 2021
2. Al Umairi R et al: Prevalence, spectrum, and outcomes of single coronary artery detected on coronary computed tomography angiography (CCTA). Radiol Res Pract. 2019:2940148, 2019
3. Elbadawi A et al: Single coronary artery anomaly: a case report and review of literature. Cardiol Ther. 7(1):119-23, 2018

Duplicate Left Anterior Descending Coronary Artery

KEY FACTS

TERMINOLOGY

- Rare congenital coronary artery anomaly with 2 left anterior descending (LAD) coronary arteries
  - 1 short, 1 long
- Short LAD usually originates from LAD proper and terminates in proximal anterior interventricular (AIV) groove
- Long LAD has variable origin from either left or right coronary arteries, variable course outside proximal AIV groove, and reenters distal part of AIV groove to reach cardiac apex

IMAGING

- Presence of 2 LAD: 1 short, 1 long
- Coronary CTA is ideal modality to evaluate dual LAD with comprehensive multiplanar and 3D information
- Originally 4 types reported; several recent variants have been reported
  - Type 1: Both short and long LAD originate from LAD proper
    - Long LAD descends parallel on left ventricle side of AIV groove and reenters distal AIV groove
  - Type 2: Both short and long LAD originate from LAD proper
    - Long LAD descends on right ventricle side of AIV groove and reenters distal AIV groove
  - Type 3: Both short and long LAD originate from LAD proper
    - Long LAD has intramyocardial course in septum and emerges in apical AIV groove or does not emerge
  - Type 4: Short LAD from left main coronary artery and terminates high in AIV groove
    - Long LAD originates from right coronary artery, has anomalous prepulmonic course, and reenters AIV groove
- MRA can provide comparable information, although may be limited in evaluation of distal segments

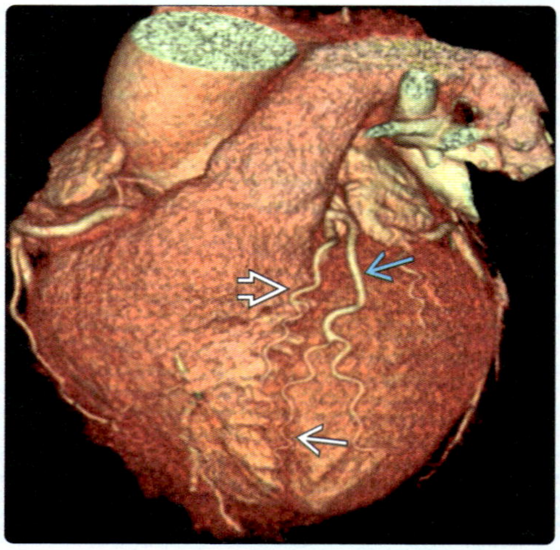

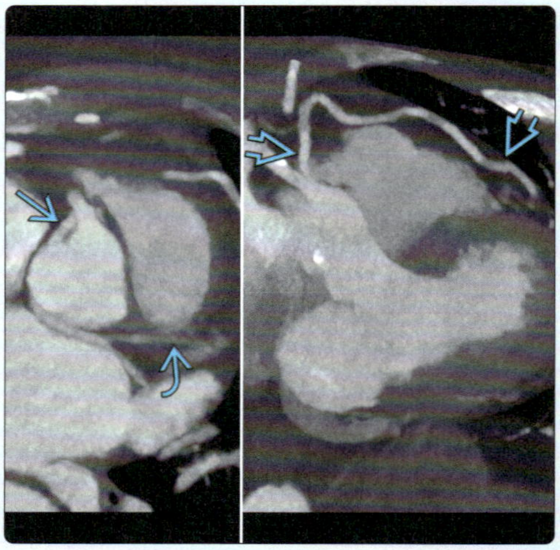

(Left) *Type 1 dual left anterior descending (LAD) shows the left main (LM) coronary artery divides into short LAD ➔ that courses in proximal anterior interventricular (AIV) groove. Proximal portion of the long LAD ➔ runs parallel to AIV groove on left ventricle side, reentering in distal AIV groove ➔.* **(Right)** *CECT MIP shows a single coronary artery with a retroaortic LM ➔ that divides into the left circumflex and a small LAD ➔ that supplies the proximal AIV. A larger prepulmonic LAD ➔ supplies mid- and distal LAD territory. (Courtesy S. Kligerman, MD.)*

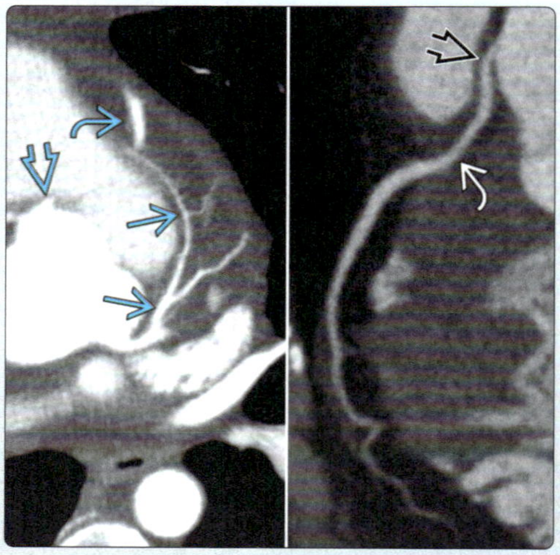

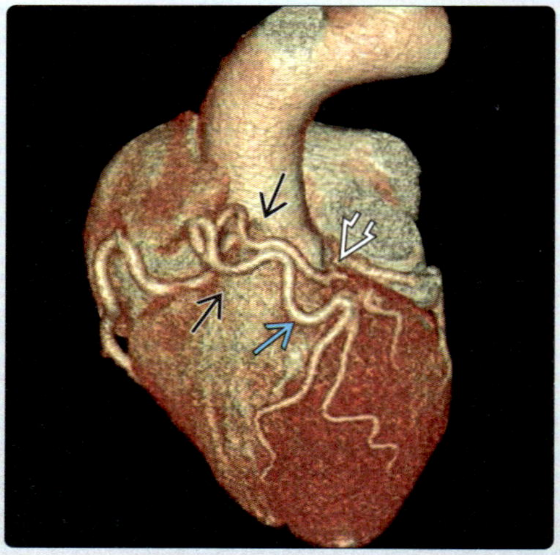

(Left) *Axial MIP (left) shows a short LAD arising from the left sinus ➔, supplying the proximal LAD territory. The ostium of a larger septal LAD from the right sinus ➔ and midportion ➔ are partially visualized. Curved MPR of the septal LAD (right) shows its ostium ➔ and transeptal course ➔. (Courtesy S. Kligerman, MD.)* **(Right)** *Coronal 3D CTA shows a prepulmonic course ➔ of the LAD that divides into a short LAD ➔, which terminates in the high AIV, and a long LAD ➔, which courses along the mid- and distal AIV groove.*

TERMINOLOGY

Abbreviations

- Duplicate left anterior descending (LAD) coronary artery

Synonyms

- Dual LAD coronary artery

Definitions

- Rare congenital coronary artery anomaly with 2 LAD coronary arteries (1 short, 1 long)
- Short LAD usually originates from LAD proper and terminates in proximal anterior interventricular (AIV) groove
- Long LAD has variable origin from either left or right coronary arteries (RCAs), has variable course outside proximal AIV groove, and reenters distal AIV groove to supply apex

IMAGING

General Features

- Best diagnostic clue
  - Presence of 2 LAD coronary arteries: 1 short, 1 long

CT Findings

- CTA findings
  - 2 LAD coronary arteries are seen: 1 short, 1 long
    - Short LAD runs in proximal AIV groove
    - Long LAD is located outside proximal AIV groove and reenters distal AIV groove
  - Type 1: Both short and long LAD originate from LAD proper; long LAD descends parallel on left ventricle side of AIV groove and reenters distal AIV groove
    - Septal perforators from short LAD; diagonals from long LAD, LAD proper, or both
  - Type 2: Both short and long LAD originate from LAD proper; long LAD descends on right ventricle side of AIV groove and reenters distal AIV groove
    - Septal perforators from short LAD; diagonals from long LAD
  - Type 3: Both short and long LAD originate from LAD proper; long LAD has intramyocardial course in septum and emerges in apical AIV groove or does not emerge
    - Septal branches from short and long LAD coronary arteries; diagonals from short LAD and LAD proper
  - Type 4: Short LAD originates from left main coronary artery (LMCA) and terminates high in AIV groove; long LAD originates from RCA, has anomalous prepulmonic course, and reenters AIV groove
    - Septal perforators and diagonals from short LAD
    - Anomalous left circumflex artery from RCA or LMCA from right coronary sinus may occur
  - Additional variants described in literature
    - Short LAD directly from left coronary sinus; long LAD directly from right coronary sinus or RCA and then intramyocardial (subpulmonic) course to reach distal AIV groove
    - Long LAD origin from main pulmonary trunk and short LAD from LMCA
      - Similar to anomalous origin of left coronary artery from pulmonary artery (ALCAPA)

MR Findings

- MR angiography can provide similar information as CTA
  - No ionizing radiation, but longer acquisition time
- Performed using 3D navigator and ECG-gated whole-heart SSFP sequence; multiplanar and 3D reconstructions

Imaging Recommendations

- Best imaging tool
  - Coronary CTA is best imaging tool
  - MR angiography can provide comparable information, although may be limited in evaluation of distal segments
- Protocol advice
  - Optimized contrast injection protocol to visualize coronary arteries, their origins and courses

DIFFERENTIAL DIAGNOSIS

Diminutive Left Anterior Descending Artery and Prominent Diagonal Branch

- LAD can be diminutive as normal variant; diagonal branch does not reenter AIV groove

Occlusion of Distal Left Anterior Descending and Prominent Diagonal Branch

- Occlusion can be visualized in CTA; diagonal branch does not reenter AIV groove

CLINICAL ISSUES

Presentation

- Most common signs/symptoms
  - Usually asymptomatic; incidental imaging finding
- Other signs/symptoms
  - Origin of long LAD from pulmonary artery: Similar to ALCAPA

Natural History & Prognosis

- Knowledge of anatomy prior to surgical revascularization
  - To revascularize correct vessel
  - To place appropriate arteriotomy
    - Exposure high in AIV groove for grafting short LAD
  - Separate grafts, if both short and long LAD coronary arteries are stenosed
    - Separate origins of septal and diagonal branches
- Erroneous interpretation of coronary occlusion in catheter angiography
  - e.g., when long LAD from RCA or pulmonary artery, short LAD can be interpreted as occluded vessel
- Incongruent wall motion abnormalities
  - Since septal and diagonals have separate origins

SELECTED REFERENCES

1. Maggialetti N et al: The role of coronary CT angiography in the evaluation of dual left anterior descending artery prevalence and subtypes: a retrospective multicenter study. J Pers Med. 13(7):1127, 2023
2. Jariwala P et al: Dual left anterior descending artery: diagnostic criteria and novel classification. Indian J Thorac Cardiovasc Surg. 37(3):285-94, 2021
3. Agarwal PP et al: Dual left anterior descending coronary artery: CT findings. AJR Am J Roentgenol. 191(6):1698-701, 2008

KEY FACTS

TERMINOLOGY

- Anomalous origin of left or right coronary artery from opposite sinus of Valsalva
- Malignant variant: Anomalous artery courses between ascending aorta and pulmonary artery-interarterial
  - Associated with increased risk for myocardial infarction or sudden cardiac death (SCD)
- Benign variant: Anomalous coronary artery courses anterior to pulmonary artery (prepulmonary), dorsal to aortic root (retroaortic), below right ventricular outflow tract through septum (subpulmonary/transseptal)

IMAGING

- Anomalous origin can be identified in invasive catheter angiography, but exact course is difficult to ascertain, even in multiple projections
- Coronary CTA is excellent for identification of anomalous coronary arteries and definition of their exact course and relationship to surrounding structures
- Coronary MRA is good for identifying origin and proximal course without use of radiation or contrast

TOP DIFFERENTIAL DIAGNOSES

- Aortic dissection
- Coronary artery stenosis or occlusion
- Coronary artery fistula
- Presence of single coronary artery

CLINICAL ISSUES

- Common symptoms: SCD, syncope, palpitation, chest pain
- Increased risk of SCD is associated with interarterial course, young age, and strenuous exertion
- Therapeutic options: Bypass surgery, surgical unroofing or reimplantation of coronaries
- Stent placement sometimes considered but value uncertain

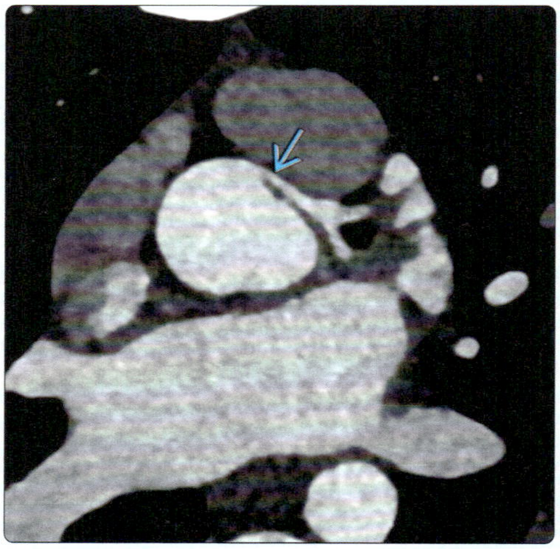
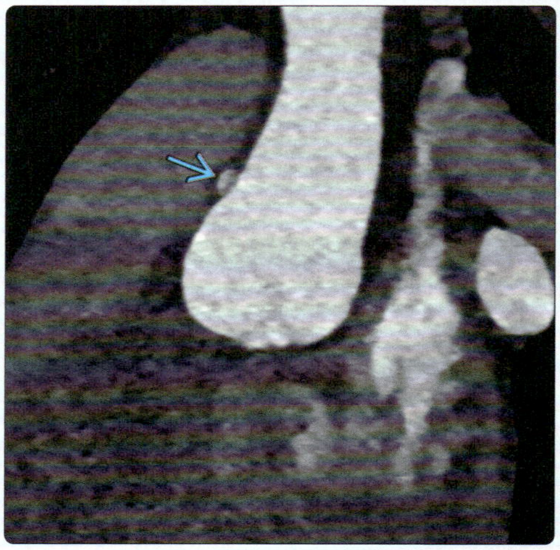

(Left) *CTA in a Marine recruit who developed syncope during a 5-mile run shows the left main (LM) coronary artery ➔ arising from right sinus of Valsalva (RSOV) with an interarterial course between aorta and pulmonary artery (PA). The proximal vessel is narrowed.* **(Right)** *Transverse CECT (same patient) shows the ovoid shape of the 3 x 2-mm proximal LM ➔ due to its intramural course in the wall of aorta. This, in conjunction with a slit-like ostium, acute angle of proximal vessel, and compression between outflow tracks, led to ischemia.*

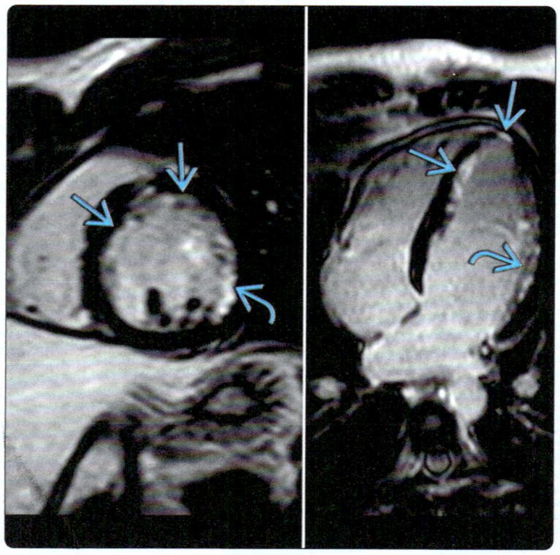
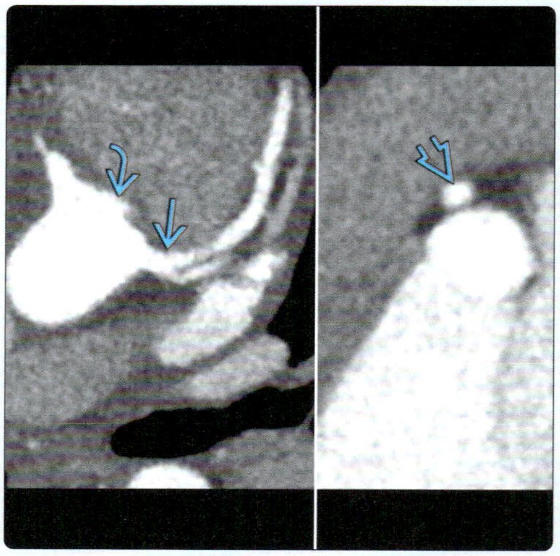

(Left) *Short-axis (L) and 4-chamber (R) delayed-enhancement MR images in the same patient soon after the CTA show subendocardial delayed enhancement in both the left anterior descending (LAD) ➔ and left circumflex (LCx) ➔ territory from the LM infarct.* **(Right)** *CTA (same patient) after an unroofing procedure shows LM arising from the left sinus of Valsalva ➔. A portion of the original LM ostium ➔ can still be seen. Transverse CTA of proximal LM ➔ shows a normal rounded contour of the vessel.*

TERMINOLOGY

Abbreviations

- Anomalous aortic origin of coronary artery (AAOCA) originating from opposite sinus

Definitions

- AAOCA arising at or above opposite sinus of Valsalva
  - AAOCA rarely may originate from noncoronary sinus
- Anomalous left coronary artery (ALCA)
  - Anomalous origin of left-sided coronary arteries [left main (LM), left anterior descending (LAD), or left circumflex (LCx)] from right sinus of Valsalva (RSOV) or very proximal right coronary artery (RCA)
  - Potentially malignant variant with LM or LAD arises from RSOV and courses between ascending aorta and pulmonary artery (PA)
    - Interarterial course with increased risk for myocardial ischemia or sudden cardiac death (SCD)
  - Benign variants: ALCA that courses outside space between aorta and PA is considered benign
  - Anomalous LCx: Originates from RCA, from common ostium with RCA, or directly from RSOV, and courses posterior and inferior to noncoronary cusp toward left side
    - LAD originates directly from left sinus of Valsalva
    - No LM coronary artery segment is present
    - Rarely, anomalous origin of LCx can be from PA
      - Associated with other major congenital cardiac defects, such as patent ductus arteriosus, aortic coarctation, and subaortic stenosis
- Anomalous RCA (ARCA)
  - Potentially malignant variant: RCA originates from left sinus of Valsalva and courses between aorta and PA (interarterial)
    - Debate concerning clinical relevance
    - Risk for SCD assumed low; may be higher if slit-like ostium, acute take-off angle, and intramural course (proximal artery within aortic wall)
  - Benign variants: RCA originates above sinotubular junction superior to right coronary cusp (common) or courses posterior and inferior to aortic root (very rare)
- Other potentially malignant anomalies include
  - Origin of left coronary artery from PA (ALCAPA) (Bland-White-Garland syndrome)
    - Extremely infrequent, usually detected in childhood
  - ARCAPA: Origin of RCA from PA

IMAGING

General Features

- Morphology
  - AAOCA originates from aorta by separate ostium, shared or common ostium, or as branch vessel
  - Anomalous artery can have 5 different courses depending on anatomic relationship of coronary artery to ascending aorta and PA
  - Potentially malignant course
    - Interarterial course; between ascending aorta and PA
      - May have intramural segment where proximal vessel runs in wall of aorta
    - Interarterial course in ALCA is rare compared to ARCA
    - Increased risk for myocardial ischemia or SCD, especially in young
    - Best detected in cross-sectional imaging
  - Benign courses
    - Prepulmonary course anterior to PA, looping around right ventricular outflow track
      - Can involve LM or just LAD
    - Transseptal course or subpulmonic course; through interventricular septum and below pulmonic valve, at level of right ventricular outflow tract
      - Most commonly involves LAD but can involve LM
      - Needs to be differentiated from interarterial course
    - Retroaortic course; behind aorta between aorta and left atrium
      - More common with LCx than LM
    - Retrocardiac course; behind left and right atria
    - Origin from noncoronary sinus
      - Extremely rare, but of doubtful clinical significance if isolated anomaly
  - Morphology of proximal vessel
    - Normal; no narrowing
    - Oval shape; narrowing < 50%
    - Slit-like; narrowing > 50%
      - High-risk feature for SCD
      - Usually associated with intramural course where coronary artery is in aortic wall
  - Take-off angle: Angle between coronary artery and aortic root wall
    - Nonacute angle: > 45
    - Acute angle: < 45
      - Assumed to be associated with increased risk of ischemia and SCD
  - Take-off level: Level of origin depending on relationship with aortic valve commissure
    - Above or below commissure
    - If course crosses commissure, marsupialization may not be feasible
    - High origin of coronary artery at level of sinotubular junction or ascending aorta
      - Most commonly involves RCA with LM or LAD being less common

Echocardiographic Findings

- Transesophageal echocardiography can identify ostia of coronary arteries, and very experienced operator can characterize their proximal course in many cases

Imaging Recommendations

- Best imaging tool
  - ECG-gated coronary CTA
  - 3D slab MRA angiogram can be considered in certain patients

CT Findings

- ECG-gated contrast-enhanced coronary CTA
  - Excellent for identification of anomalous origin of coronary arteries and definition of their exact course
  - Demonstrates anomalous vessels at high spatial and contrast resolution and depicts relationship with surrounding structures

- Volume-rendered 3D images can be helpful to demonstrate spatial relationship of aortic root and anomalous vessel
- CT-FFR
  - High-risk features (slit-like ostium, intramural course) are shown to be associated with abnormal CT-FFR results based on initial data
  - Patients with abnormal CT-FFR shown to have more angina
  - Currently not approved by FDA for use in anomalous coronary arteries

MR Findings

- Coronary MRA
  - Typically with noncontrast 3D SSFP with T2 prep, ECG, and navigator gating
    - Lower spatial resolution than CT
    - 2D sequence with breath hold is possible if limited coverage
    - Higher signal-to-noise ratio with contrast-to-noise ratio with use of intravenous contrast
  - Adequate for evaluation of anomalous origin and proximal courses
  - Long scan times limit use
    - Some sequences 5-10 minutes, image quality is not known until completed
- Additional information possible with MR
  - Function and volumes; perfusion; viability

Angiographic Findings

- Invasive coronary angiography
  - Even with multiple projections and insertion of PA catheter to delineate PA, it may not be possible to identify exact course of ALCA

DIFFERENTIAL DIAGNOSIS

Coronary Artery Stenosis or Occlusion

- Can cause ischemia and chest pain
- Anomalous vessel has to be traced back to its abnormal origin to differentiate from ostial occlusion

Coronary Fistula

- Abnormal dilated and tortuous coronary artery with normal origin
- Usually drains into right-sided cardiac chambers or PA
- ALCAPA and ARCAPA in adults are both AAOCA with fistula

Sinoatrial Node or Conus Branch

- Prominent sinoatrial nodal branch can be confused with anomalous LCx
- Prominent branches of RCA, especially conus branch, may follow course very similar to prepulmonary course of ALCA
- Best clue is identification of normal coronary arteries

PATHOLOGY

General Features

- Malignant variants: Exact mechanism of sudden death is not known
  - Most likely, ischemia and subsequent arrhythmias
  - Sudden death is related to exercise in > 50% of cases
  - Relevance of ARCA regarding SCD is not well known
- Benign variants: Not linked to SCD or ischemia

Gross Pathologic & Surgical Features

- Risk of ischemia and SCD is assumed to be associated with shear and squeezing of anomalous vessel and particularly pronounced when there is
  - Slit-like ostium, acute angle, intramural segment, compression between outflow tracks
  - Likely requires combination of multiple factors to cause ischemia and SCD

CLINICAL ISSUES

Presentation

- Most common signs/symptoms
  - Benign variant: Usually incidental finding, asymptomatic
  - Malignant variant
    - Interarterial RCA most commonly incidental finding
    - Interarterial LAD and LM more commonly present with ischemia and SCD

Demographics

- Age
  - Malignant variant: SCD rarely occurs in patients > 35 years of age
  - Benign variant: incidentally detected at any age
- Sex
  - No sex predilection
- Epidemiology
  - Present in ~ 0.3-1.6% of population
  - Malignant interarterial course of ALCA is rare compared to interarterial course of ARCA

Natural History & Prognosis

- Benign variant: Usually benign incidental finding; clinically silent with excellent prognosis
- Potentially malignant AAOCA 2nd most common cause of SCD in young athletes (5-35% of SCD)
  - Highest in young patients with interarterial LM or LAD, during or after strenuous exertion

Treatment

- Malignant variant
  - Unroofing procedure, reimplantation of coronaries above appropriate coronary sinus, or bypass
  - Treatment is indicated in patients who have demonstrable ischemia or who have survived SCD
  - Benefit is controversial in patients who are completely asymptomatic and have normal stress test results
- Benign variant
  - No treatment required

SELECTED REFERENCES

1. Gomes de Farias LP et al: Revisiting coronary artery anomalies. Radiographics. 44(8):e230145, 2024
2. Tang CX et al: Coronary computed tomography angiography-derived fractional flow reserve in patients with anomalous origin of the right coronary artery from the left coronary sinus. Korean J Radiol. 21(2):192-202, 2020
3. Agarwal PP et al: Anomalous coronary arteries that need intervention: review of pre- and postoperative imaging appearances. Radiographics. 37(3):740-57, 2017
4. Cheezum MK et al: Anomalous aortic origin of a coronary artery from the inappropriate sinus of Valsalva. J Am Coll Cardiol. 69(12):1592-608, 2017

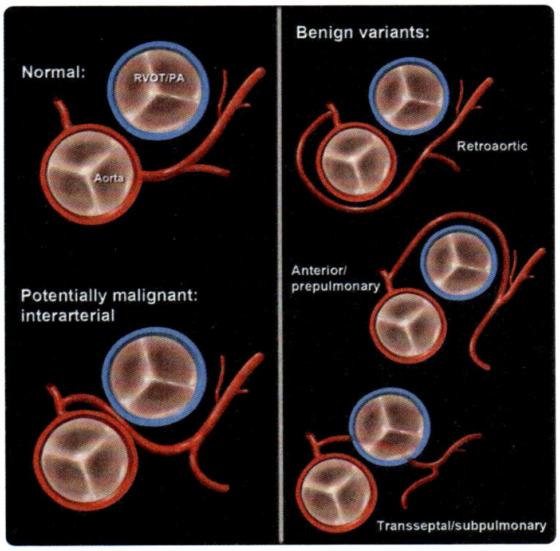

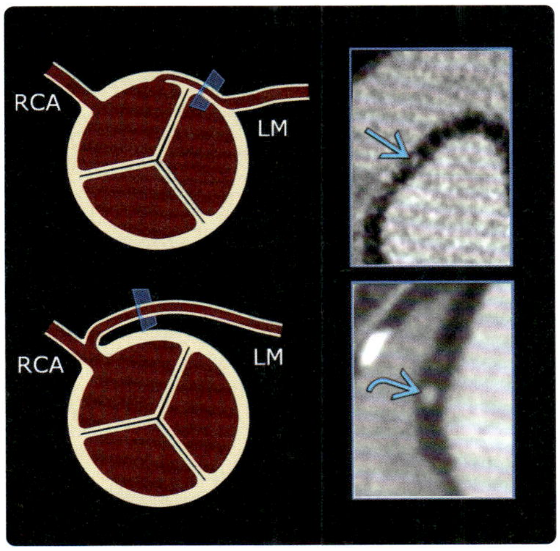

(Left) *Graphic shows normal LM coronary anatomy (top left), a potentially malignant interarterial course (bottom left), and 3 benign anomalous LM courses: Retroaortic, anterior (a.k.a. prepulmonary) and transseptal (a.k.a. subpulmonary).* **(Right)** *With an interarterial (IA), intramural (IM) course (top), the LM arises from the RSOV, and the proximal vessel runs in the wall of the aorta, which compresses it. In bottom case, LM arises from proximal right coronary artery (RCA) with an IA but no IM course with less vessel narrowing.*

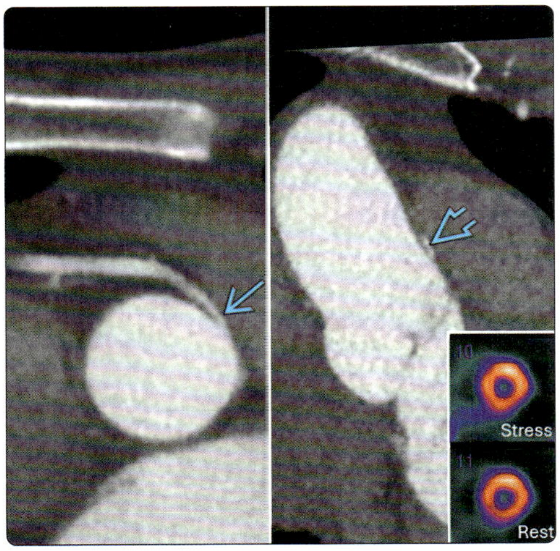

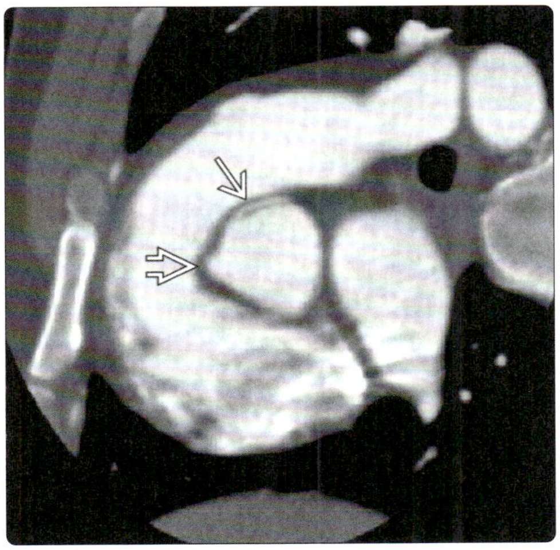

(Left) *CTA in a man with atypical chest pain shows an IA RCA arising from the left sinus of Valsalva with proximal narrowing. Transverse image shows the severe compression of the proximal RCA, measuring 5 x 1 mm. A stress test (inset) was normal.* **(Right)** *Coronary CTA shows an anomalous left coronary artery (ALCA) arising from the RSOV with an acute angle and intramural segment. A normal RCA originates from a separate ostium.*

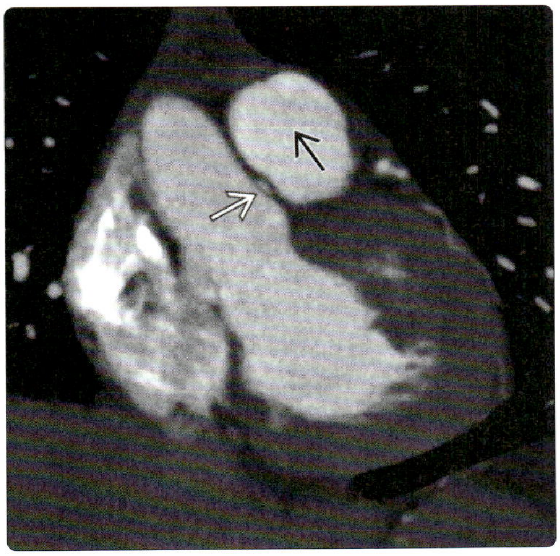

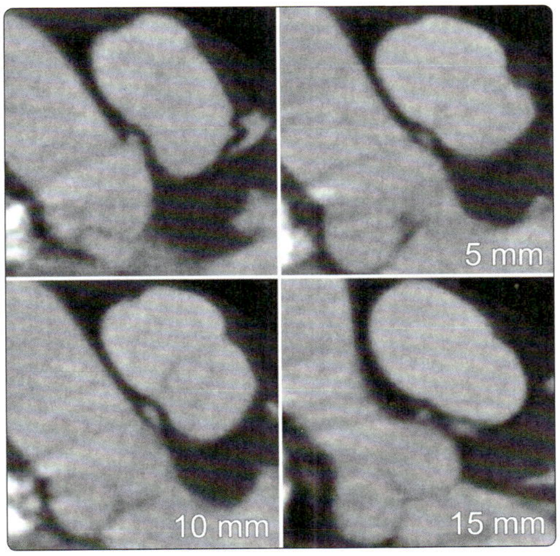

(Left) *Five-mm MIP coronary CTA in the same patient shows the slit-like appearance of the ALCA with a course between the aorta and right ventricular outflow tract (RVOT) below the pulmonic valve.* **(Right)** *Coronal CTA multiplanar reconstruction in the same patient demonstrates the length of the vessel narrowing extending from the origin to the normal caliber in distal.*

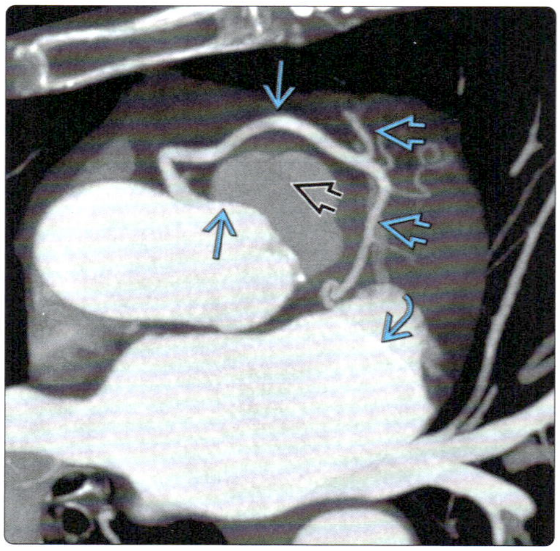

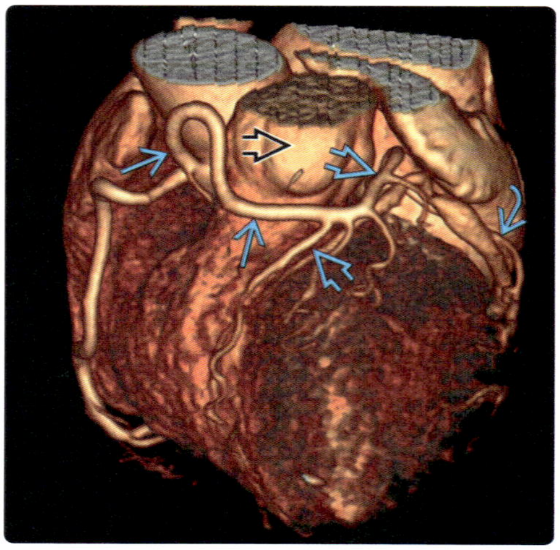

(Left) *CTA in a young woman shows the LM arising from the RSOV ➡ and coursing anterior to the PA ➡. The LM then divides into vessels supplying both the LAD ➡ and LCx ➡ territories.* **(Right)** *Volume-rendered CECT shows the prepulmonic LM arising from the RSOV ➡ and coursing anterior to the PA ➡. The LM then supplies the LAD ➡ and LCx ➡ territories. This is a benign course and requires no treatment.*

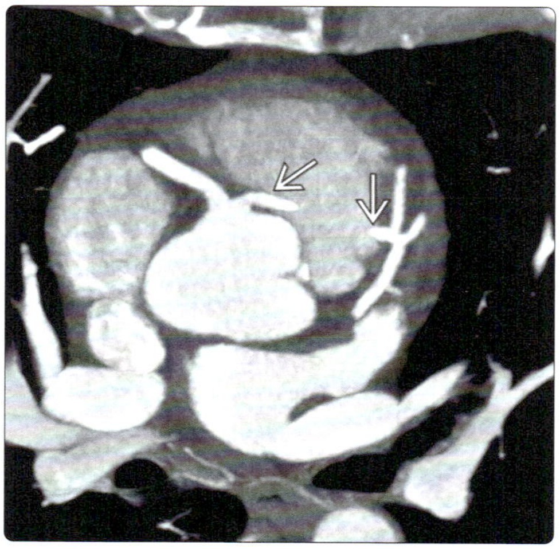

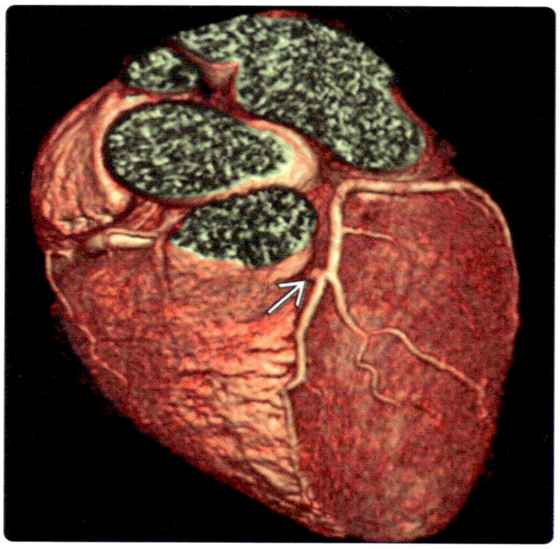

(Left) *Coronary CTA shows an anomalous LM coronary artery that originates from the RSOV and follows a course caudal to the PA, through the interventricular septum and toward the left side ➡.* **(Right)** *3D reconstruction of the same anomaly shows the LM coronary artery surfacing from below the PA ➡. The LM coronary artery then divides into LAD and LCx coronary arteries and also gives off an intermediate branch.*

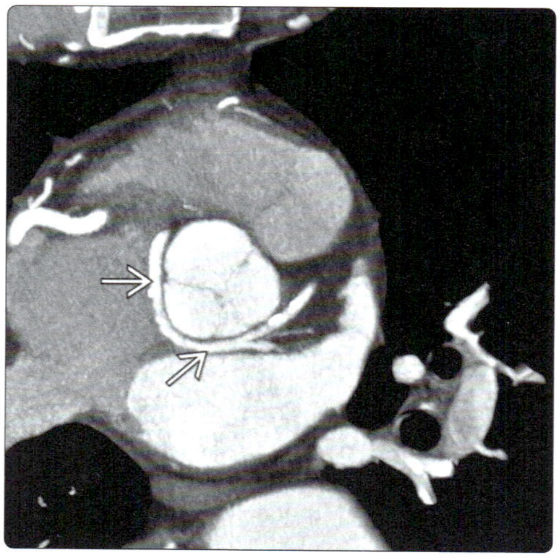

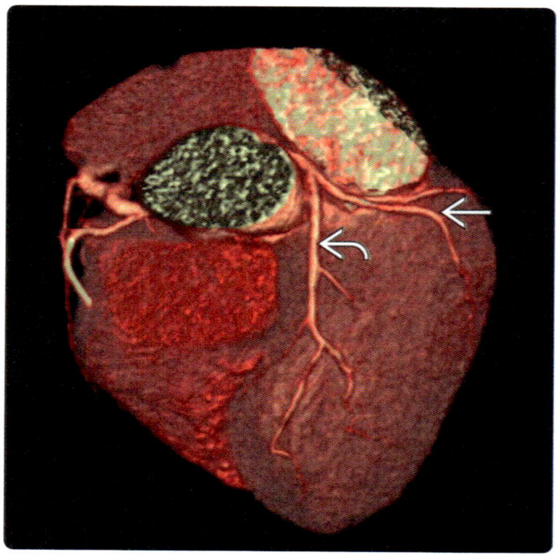

(Left) *Coronary CTA shows an anomalous LM coronary artery that originates from the RSOV or RCA (not seen here) and follows a retroaortic course dorsal to the aortic root toward the left side ➡.* **(Right)** *3D reconstruction of the same anomaly shows the retroaortic course of the LM coronary artery. The vessel then divides into LCx ➡ and LAD ➡ coronary arteries, both of which follow a normal course.*

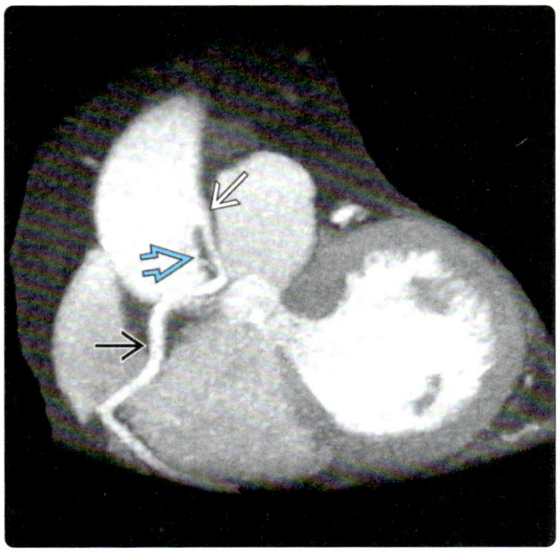

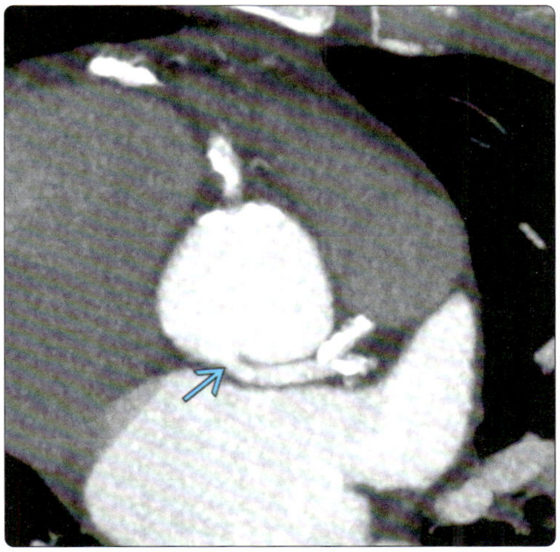

(Left) *Coronal oblique MIP shows a high origin of the RCA above the sinotubular junction , which is a benign anomaly. The artery descends into the right atrioventricular groove , which is in its normal location.* **(Right)** *MIP image from a coronary CTA in a 71-year-old man shows the ostium of the LM coronary artery from the noncoronary sinus of Valsalva . This is a very rare anomaly and likely of doubtful clinical significance in most patients.*

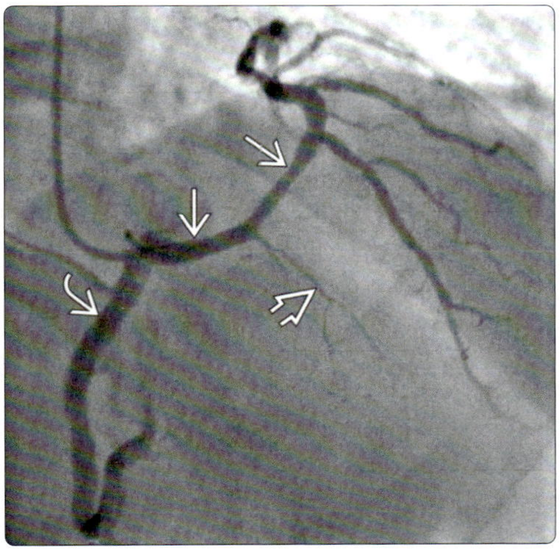

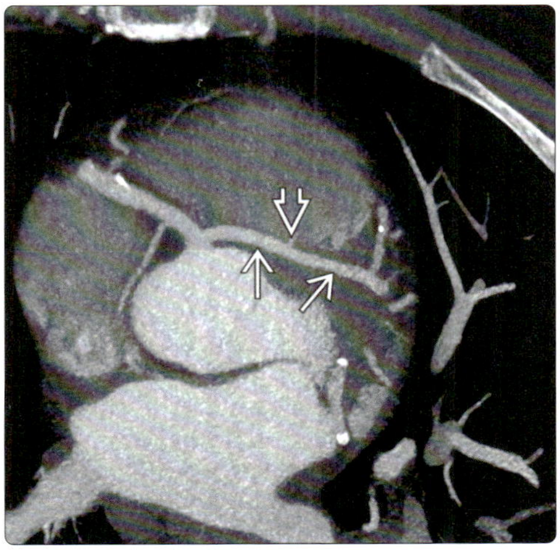

(Left) *Invasive coronary CTA of an anomalous LM coronary artery shows that the LM coronary artery originates from the same ostium as the RCA and follows a subpulmonary (or transseptal) course. This can be identified because the LM coronary artery gives rise to a small septal branch .* **(Right)** *Eight-mm MIP coronary CTA in the same patient clearly shows the subpulmonary course of the LM coronary artery and also the small septal branch .*

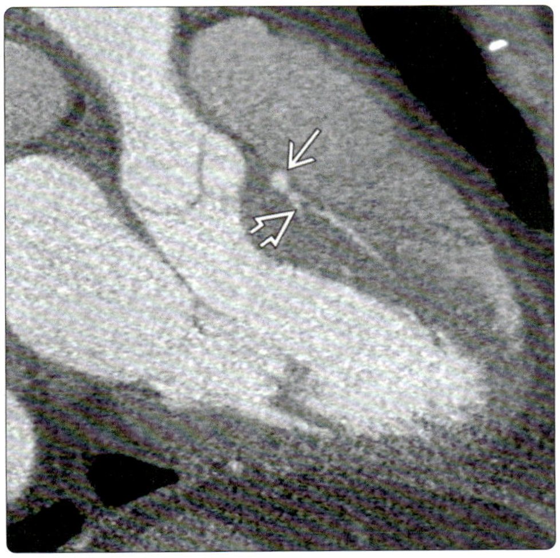

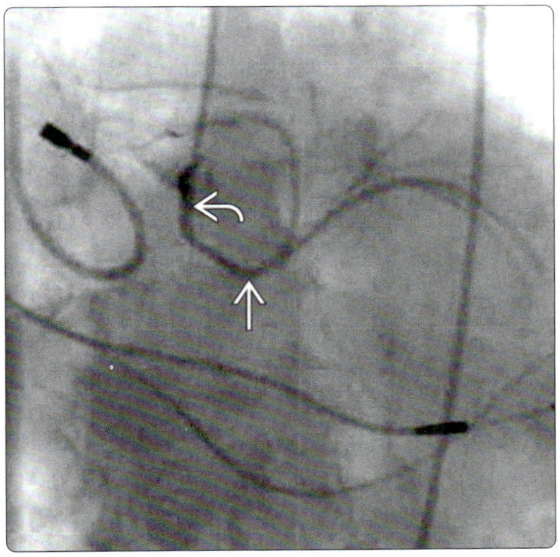

(Left) *Coronary CTA multiplanar reconstruction in the same patient shows a cross section of the LM coronary artery , which is embedded in the interventricular septum and gives rise to a small septal branch .* **(Right)** *Right anterior oblique view of a coronary catheter angiogram with selective catheterization shows an anomalous LCx with a separate origin from the right coronary cusp and a retroaortic course .*

Coronary Fistula

KEY FACTS

TERMINOLOGY

- Abnormal connection between coronary artery branch and cardiac or vascular chambers without normal transition through capillary bed of myocardium
- Synonyms: Coronary artery fistula, coronary cameral fistula

IMAGING

- Large tortuous vessel with abnormal connection to cardiac chamber, pulmonary artery, or coronary venous system
- Normal origin of coronary artery from respective sinus of Valsalva
- Cardiac gated CTA is best imaging tool
  - Ensure inclusion of top of aortic arch
  - Delineates number, size, and anatomic course of feeding vessels
  - Occasionally markedly enlarged and tortuous coronary arteries
  - Often aneurysmal dilatation immediately proximal to drainage site; distal artery is normal

TOP DIFFERENTIAL DIAGNOSES

- Anomalous coronary artery origin from pulmonary artery
- Coronary aneurysm
- Anomalous coronary artery

PATHOLOGY

- Classify according to number of feeders, origin, drainage site, and complexity
- Usually congenital malformation

CLINICAL ISSUES

- Often asymptomatic if smaller fistula without significant steal
- Prognosis is generally good, especially in smaller and moderate-sized fistula
- Treatment is often necessary only in larger or symptomatic fistulas
- Residual leakage or recanalization of treated coronary arteriovenous fistula (CAVF) in 10%

(Left) *Axial coronary CTA shows marked enlargement of the left main coronary artery. Subsequent axial images showed communication with a round aneurysm and eventual drainage into the right atrium.* **(Right)** *Axial coronary CTA in the same patient shows ectasia of the left main coronary artery. It follows an anomalous course as it drains into the right atrium.*

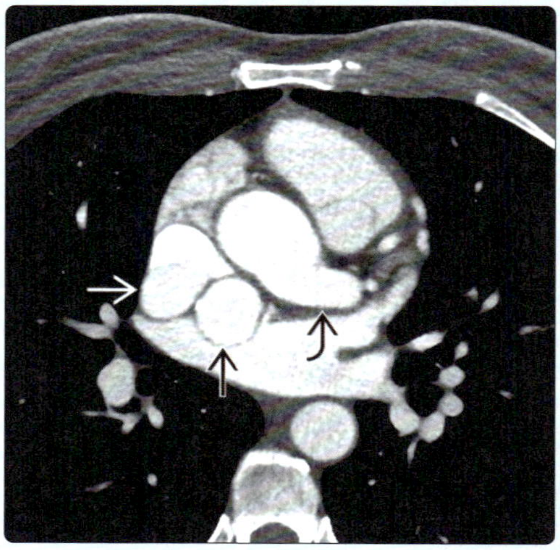

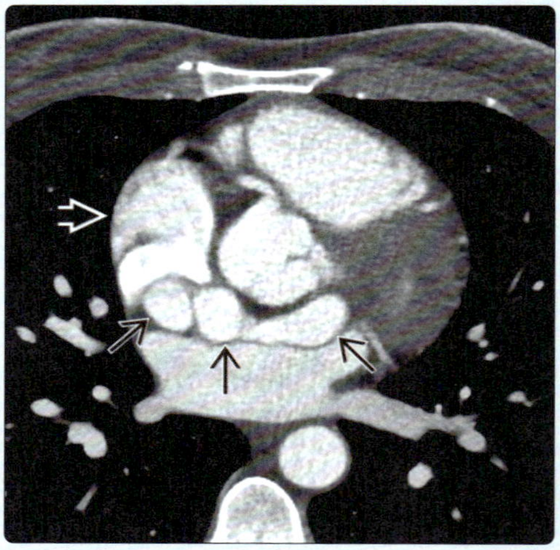

(Left) *Oblique volume-rendered CTA shows a tangle of enlarged tortuous branches from the left anterior descending artery around the anterior surface of the pulmonary trunk, consistent with a coronary-to-pulmonary artery fistula. Note vascular ring collateral coursing anterior to the pulmonary root.* **(Right)** *Coronal oblique MIP CTA shows dilated and tortuous left main and left circumflex coronary arteries. The circumflex coronary artery drains anomalously into the dilated coronary sinus.*

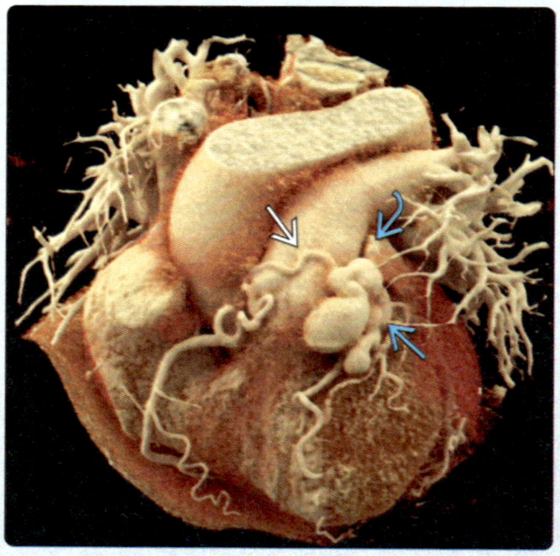

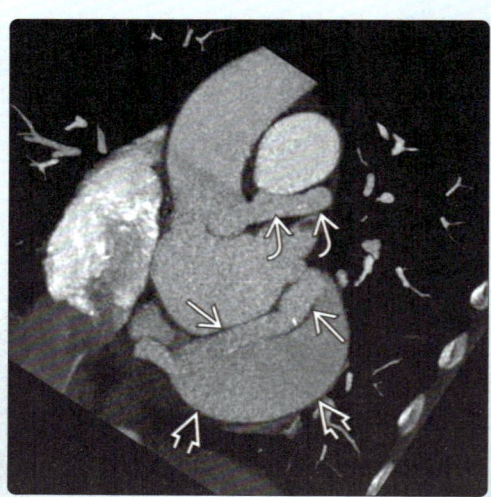

TERMINOLOGY

Synonyms

- Coronary artery fistula (CAF)
- Coronary cameral fistula
  - Abnormal direct connection between coronary artery and any cardiac chamber
- Coronary arteriovenous fistula (CAVF)
  - Connection between coronary artery and any portion of systemic or pulmonary circulation without intervening capillary network

Definitions

- Abnormal connection between coronary artery branch and cardiac or vascular chambers without normal transition through capillary bed of myocardium
  - May connect to pulmonary artery, bronchial artery, systemic veins, coronary veins, coronary sinus, atria, or ventricles
- Accounts for 0.3% of congenital heart diseases
- Usually congenital malformation (90% of cases); uncommonly develops as iatrogenic fistula after biopsy/surgery, irradiation therapy, or as traumatic fistula
- CAVFs are differentiated from anomalous coronary artery origin from pulmonary artery [Bland-White-Garland syndrome, anomalous left coronary artery origin from pulmonary artery (ALCAPA), anomalous right coronary artery origin from pulmonary artery (ARCAPA)]
  - Main difference is, in ALCAPA/ARCAPA, abnormal vessel arises from pulmonary artery, and no separate ostium from aorta is identified

IMAGING

General Features

- Best diagnostic clue
  - Large tortuous vessels with abnormal connection to cardiac chamber, pulmonary artery, bronchial artery, or coronary venous system
    - Normal origins of coronary artery from respective sinus of Valsalva
- Location
  - Usually connects high-pressure system (coronary artery) with low-pressure system; less commonly drains into high-pressure left ventricle
    - Right ventricle (41%)
    - Right atrium (26%)
    - Pulmonary artery (17%)
    - Coronary sinus (7%)
    - Other (left atrium, left ventricle, or vena cava)
  - Feeders originate from right coronary arterial system in 55%, left coronary system in 35%, and both systems or other anomalous coronary arteries in 10%
  - Within epicardial fat
    - May have feeders from bronchial or mediastinal arteries entering epicardial fat via space between pericardial reflection and great vessel wall

Imaging Recommendations

- Best imaging tool
  - Cardiac gated CTA or MRA
- Protocol advice
  - Ensure that scan is performed from top of aortic arch to avoid incomplete visualization of fistula

Radiographic Findings

- Radiography
  - Usually normal; rarely, chamber enlargement

CT Findings

- ECG-gated cardiac CT is excellent test to delineate number, size, origin, and anatomic course of feeding vessels
- Tortuous epicardial arterially enhancing vessels
  - Occasionally multiple feeders identified
- Occasional markedly enlarged and tortuous coronary arteries
- Drainage site is often identified
  - Jet of arterial density contrast into receiving chamber (lower HU) or coronary sinus may be appreciated (so-called contrast shunt sign)
- Often aneurysmal dilatation of coronary artery immediately proximal to drainage site
- Occasionally enlarged cardiac chambers, pulmonary hypertension, or ventricular hypertrophy from left-to-right shunting
- Provides overview of associated cardiac and vascular abnormalities

MR Findings

- Findings similar to CT
  - CT is superior in defining smaller feeders due to isovolumetric submillimeter spatial resolution and true volumetric imaging
- May detect late complications
  - LGE imaging is highly sensitive for nontransmural myocardial infarction

Echocardiographic Findings

- Enlarged feeding coronary artery
- Fistula drainage site demonstrates systolic and diastolic continuous turbulent flow pattern
- Microbubbles may enhance detection with color Doppler imaging

Angiographic Findings

- Delineates size and detailed anatomy of fistulous vessels
- May potentially miss feeders that arise from unexpected locations
- Often difficult to define drainage into low-pressure cardiac system
- Enables transcatheter coil embolization

DIFFERENTIAL DIAGNOSIS

Bland-White-Garland Syndrome

- Anomalous coronary artery origin from pulmonary artery
  - ALCAPA (typically)
  - ARCAPA (occasionally)
- Large left-to-right shunt and steal phenomenon leading to symptoms in infancy
  - Myocardial infarcts in infancy common
  - Dyspnea and syncope during breast or bottle feeding

Coronary Aneurysm

- No abnormal drainage into low-pressure chamber

- Absence of multiple feeders

Anomalous Coronary Artery

- Abnormal origin of coronaries from sinus of Valsalva
- No abnormal feeders

Other Causes of Coronary Artery Dilation/Aneurysm

- Kawasaki disease
  - Usually affects multiple coronary arteries
  - Coronary artery dilation or aneurysm dominates
  - Normal origin and drainage site
- Takayasu arteritis

PATHOLOGY

General Features

- Etiology
  - Usually congenital malformation
    - Persistence of embryonic intertrabecular spaces and sinusoids
  - May be iatrogenic (right ventricular biopsy, pericardiocentesis, after septal myectomy, chest irradiation, etc.) or due to trauma
  - May be complication of mycotic aneurysm

Staging, Grading, & Classification

- Classify according to number of feeders, origin, drainage site, and complexity
- Drainage site is clinically more important than origin
- Sakakibara CAF classification (classified as proximal or distal segment on basis of its origin)
  - Type A
    - Proximal artery fistula; distal coronary artery is normal in size
  - Type B
    - End-artery fistula; entire coronary artery dilated
- Classification depends on drainage site
  - Coronary cameral fistula
    - Arteriosinusoidal has indirect communication with cardiac chamber
    - Arterioluminal has direct communication with cardiac chamber
  - CAVF
    - Coronary arteries drain into any segments of pulmonary (commonly to low-pressure right side) or systemic circulation

CLINICAL ISSUES

Presentation

- Most common signs/symptoms
  - Often asymptomatic if smaller fistula without significant steal
  - Depending on size, fistula may result in
    - Arrhythmia
    - Dyspnea
    - Congestive heart failure
    - Endocarditis
    - Angina pectoris if significant steal phenomenon
    - Myocardial infarction
- Other signs/symptoms
  - In pediatric population, often manifests as cardiac murmur
    - Lower to mid left sternal border
    - Loud, superficial, and continuous murmur
    - Maximal intensity of murmur relates to shunt entry site

Demographics

- Epidemiology
  - In larger angiographic series, incidence of CAF detected during diagnostic coronary angiography is 0.1-0.3%
    - MDCT-based detection of fistulas suggests higher incidence of 0.9%

Natural History & Prognosis

- Generally good, especially in smaller and moderate-sized fistula
  - Myocardial blood flow typically not compromised
- 3-12% prevalence of infective endocarditis
- Rarely, serious complications
  - Myocardial infarction
  - Pulmonary hypertension
  - Congestive heart failure
  - Tamponade due to rupture of CAF is reported
- Rarely, spontaneous closure by thrombosis (1-2%)

Treatment

- Treatment is necessary only in larger or symptomatic fistulas
- Antibiotic prophylaxis prior to dental, gastrointestinal, or genitourinary procedures due to risk of bacterial endocarditis
- Surgical ligation
  - Carries risk of myocardial infarction
  - Useful for large CAVF, multiple terminations, large aneurysm
- Catheter-based interventions
  - Useful for proximal fistula, single drainage, older age, and absence of secondary findings requiring surgery (e.g., aortic stenosis, coronary artery bypass grafting)
  - Residual leakage or recanalization of CAVF in 10%

DIAGNOSTIC CHECKLIST

Consider

- 3D volume-rendered images are helpful in delineating anatomy and identifying feeders
- If coronary fistula is suspected, ensure that scan range is extended superiorly to include top of aortic arch
  - Otherwise, pulmonary fistula may be only partially visualized
  - Occasionally, feeders from aortic arch are present

SELECTED REFERENCES

1. Kumar R et al: Coronary artery fistula: a diagnostic dilemma. Interv Cardiol. 18:e25, 2023
2. Yun G et al: Coronary artery fistulas: pathophysiology, imaging findings, and management. Radiographics. 38(3):688-703, 2018
3. Shriki JE et al: Identifying, characterizing, and classifying congenital anomalies of the coronary arteries. Radiographics. 32(2):453-68, 2012
4. Zenooz NA et al: Coronary artery fistulas: CT findings. Radiographics. 29(3):781-9, 2009

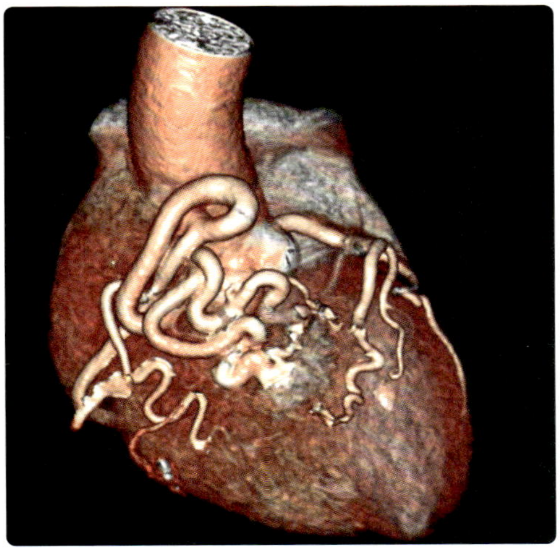

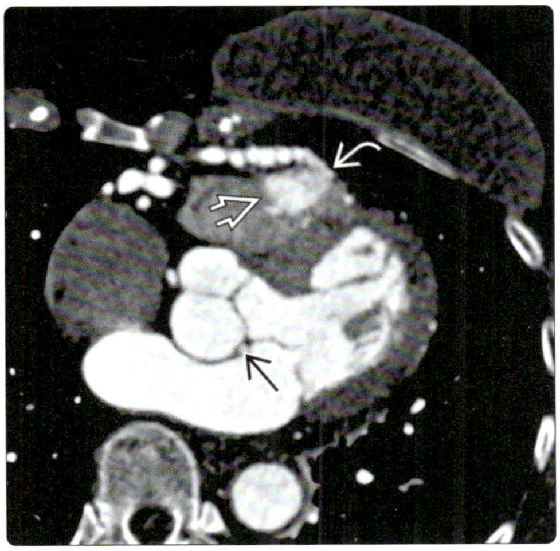

(Left) *Oblique volume-rendered cardiac CTA shows enlarged tortuous branches from the left anterior descending and right coronary arteries entering the right ventricle (RV) at its anterior surface, consistent with a coronary cameral fistula.* **(Right)** *Axial cardiac CT shows tortuous enlarged coronary artery branches at the RV anterior free wall connecting abnormally to the RV lumen →. Note high-density arterial contrast entering → the RV (contrast shunt sign). Note anomalous circumflex artery →.*

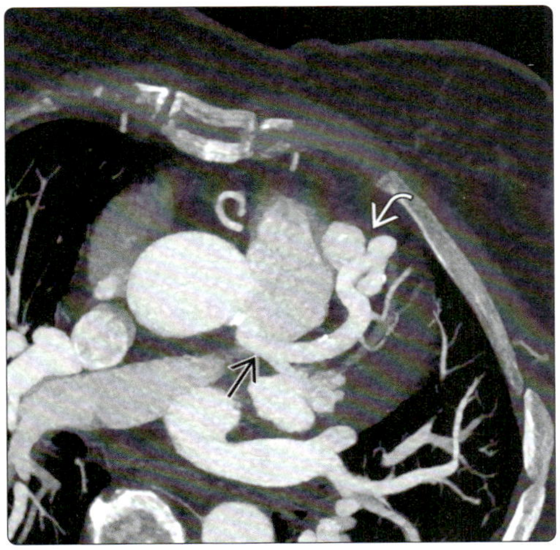

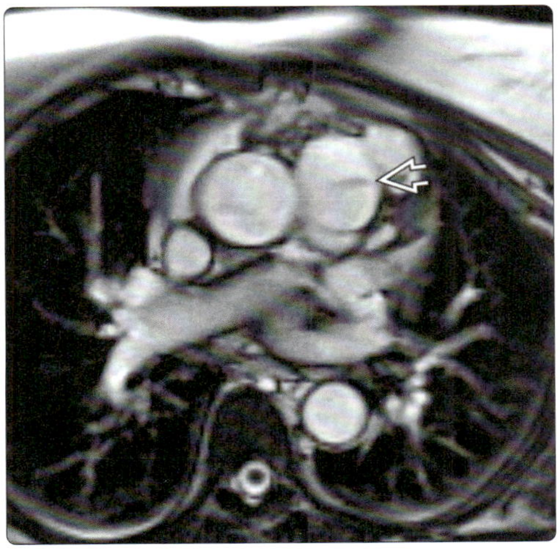

(Left) *Axial coronary CTA MIP image shows an enlarged left main coronary artery → arising normally from the aorta. Note the anomalous and tortuous vessel → arising from the proximal left anterior descending artery, which courses superiorly to drain into the pulmonary trunk.* **(Right)** *Axial SSFP MR in the same patient shows a dephasing flow jet → at the site of the anomalous connection between the left anterior descending coronary artery and pulmonary trunk.*

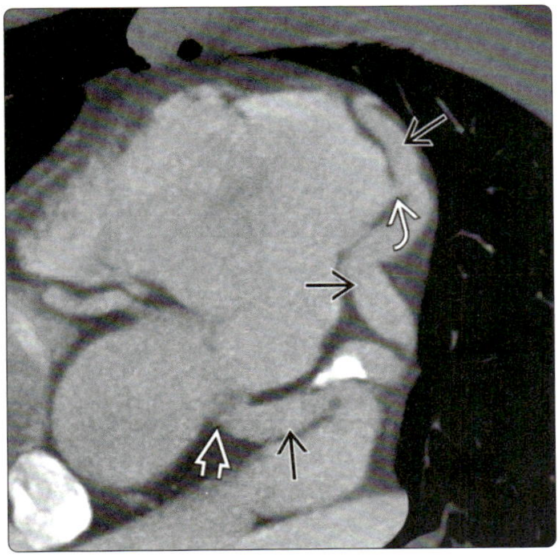

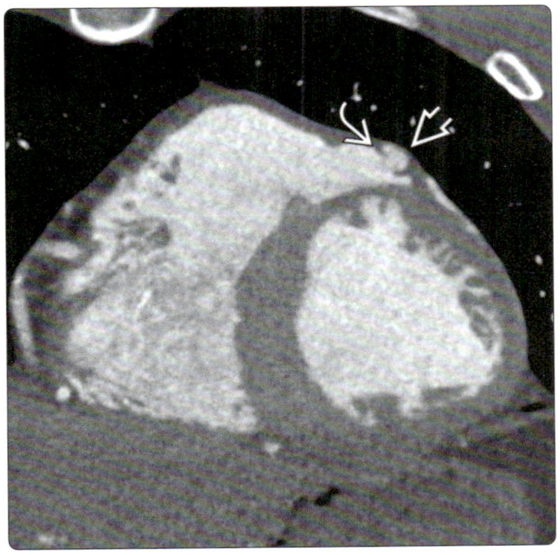

(Left) *Axial oblique MIP CTA image shows an ectatic left anterior descending artery →. An abnormal connection is present between the left anterior descending coronary artery and the RV →. The origin of the left main coronary artery is from the left sinus of Valsalva →.* **(Right)** *Modified short-axis coronary CTA in the same patient shows the enlarged left anterior descending coronary artery → and the fistulous connection → to the RV.*

Anomalous Origin of Coronary Artery From Pulmonary Artery

KEY FACTS

TERMINOLOGY

- Anomalous origin of left main coronary artery from pulmonary artery (ALCAPA)
- Endothelial bud may persist on pulmonary sinus and attach to developing left main coronary artery

IMAGING

- Left main coronary artery originates from pulmonary artery
- Best noninvasive test: Coronary CTA
  - Cardiac MR is useful alternative
- Best invasive test: Coronary angiography
- Right heart catheterizations reveal left-to-right shunt in 75% of patients
  - Average reported shunt: 1.5
- Number and extent of large collaterals arising from right coronary artery are striking features of ALCAPA

TOP DIFFERENTIAL DIAGNOSES

- Coronary fistula
- Other coronary artery anomalies [e.g., anomalous right coronary artery from pulmonary artery (ARCPA)]

CLINICAL ISSUES

- 90% of patients present in infancy with heart failure; 10% of cases reach adulthood
- Treatment
  - Infants: Establishment of dual coronary perfusion is preferred
  - Direct reimplantation of anomalous coronary artery into aorta
  - Intrapulmonary conduit from left coronary artery to aorta (Takeuchi repair)
  - Adults: Ligation of left coronary artery and bypass graft
- Many patients die from fatal ventricular dysrhythmias secondary to myocardial ischemia
- Direct reimplantation of anomalous coronary artery into aorta
- Ligation of origin of left coronary artery and bypass graft

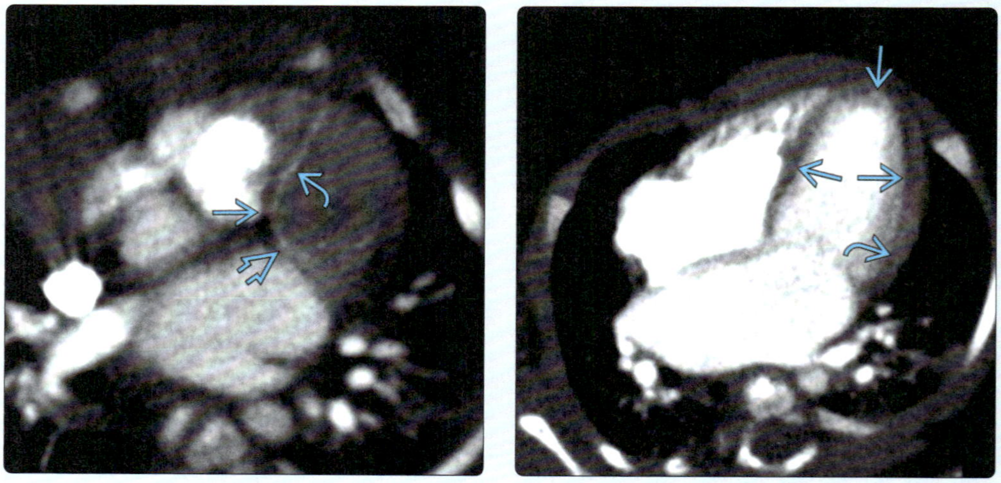

(Left) *Axial oblique CTA in a 2-month-old girl shows the left main (LM) coronary artery ➙ arising from the pulmonary artery (PA), consistent with anomalous origin of the left main coronary artery from PA (ALCAPA). The LM then bifurcates into the left anterior descending (LAD) ➙ and left circumflex (LCx) ➙ arteries.* **(Right)** *One-mm minIP CECT shows prominent left atrial ventricle dilation with diffuse subendocardial to transmural hypoperfusion in LM territory ➙. Basilar septum ➙, supplied by right coronary artery, is spared.*

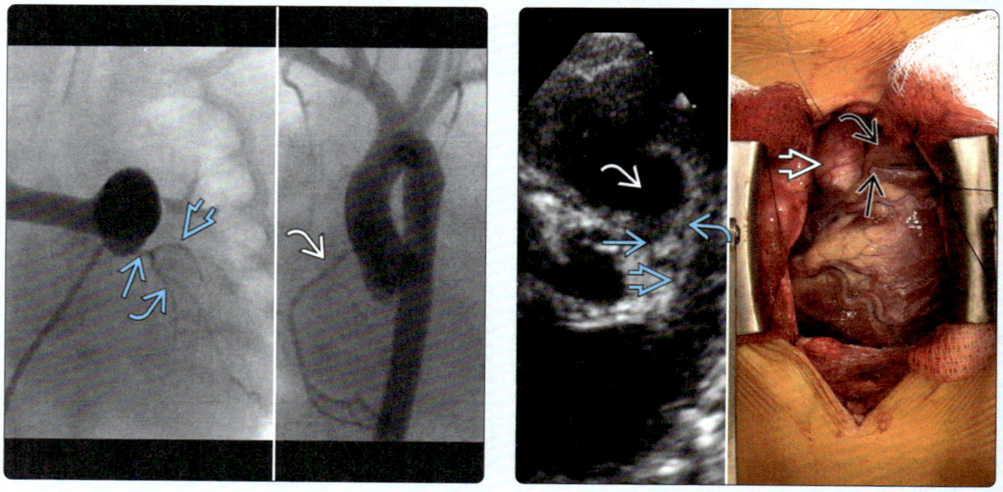

(Left) *PA injection (left) shows the LM ➙ arising from the PA and dividing into the LAD ➙ and LCx ➙. Right coronary artery injection ➙ shows no evidence of collateralization with the left-sided coronary circulation. Coronary arteries are normal in size.* **(Right)** *Echocardiogram shows the LM ➙ arising from the PA ➙ and dividing into the LAD ➙ and LCx ➙. Intraoperative photograph shows the LM ➙ arising from the PA ➙ and not the more posterior aorta ➙.*

TERMINOLOGY

Definitions

- Anomalous origin of left main coronary artery from pulmonary artery (ALCAPA)

IMAGING

General Features

- Best diagnostic clue
  - Left main (LM) coronary artery originating from pulmonary artery (PA)
- Morphology
  - In patients who survive into adulthood, size and extent of large collaterals arising from right coronary artery (RCA) are striking features

Imaging Recommendations

- Best imaging tool
  - Best noninvasive test: Coronary CTA or MR, class 1 recommendation from guidelines
    - Gated CTA better demonstrates coronary anatomy better than transthoracic echocardiography
    - Provides roadmap for repair
  - Cardiac MR
    - MRA ↓ spatial resolution better than CT but no radiation
    - Cine SSFP often shows hypokinesis in LM territory and mitral regurgitation (MR)
    - Phase contrast allows assessment of coronary steal and MR
    - LGE may show subendocardial infarcts in LM territory
  - Invasive coronary angiography
    - Right heart catheterization reveals left-to-right shunt in 75% of patients

DIFFERENTIAL DIAGNOSIS

Coronary Fistula

- Normal origin of coronary artery but abnormal distal vessel drainage site

Anomalous Right Coronary Artery From Pulmonary Artery

- Rare with older age at diagnosis
- More commonly asymptomatic or mildly symptomatic

Congenital Left Main Coronary Artery Atresia

- Extremely rare anomaly where LM has no connection to any cardiac chamber
- Survival through RCA collaterals

PATHOLOGY

General Features

- Associated abnormalities
  - Coronary steal phenomenon; myocardial ischemia; myocardial infarction; congestive cardiac failure; MR

CLINICAL ISSUES

Presentation

- Most common signs/symptoms
  - Depends on development of collaterals at early age
  - Infant type: No collaterals from RCA; myocardial infarction, congestive cardiac failure; 90% die in 1st year
  - Adult type: Collaterals from RCA; less common; presents as left ventricular dysfunction or sudden cardiac death
- Other signs/symptoms
  - Poor feeding, respiratory distress, and irritability in infants
  - Syncope and sudden death may occur due to ventricular arrhythmias

Demographics

- Age
  - 90% of patients present in infancy with heart failure
  - 10% of cases reach adulthood

Natural History & Prognosis

- During fetal/neonatal periods, ALCAPA well tolerated as pulmonary and systemic pressures equalized by patent ductus arteriosus
- Pulmonary vascular resistance nadirs ~ 2 months
  - Preferential flow away into pulmonary circulation instead of myocardium
  - If no collaterals from RCA
    - Preferential PA blood flow into lower pressure pulmonary circulation
    - Poorly oxygenated blood supplies LM
    - Myocardial ischemia/infarct with death within 1st year of life
  - If collaterals from RCA, fistula develops
    - Well-oxygenated blood flows from aorta → RCA → collaterals → left circulation → PA
    - Often asymptomatic into adulthood
    - Chronic myocardial ischemia typically leads to arrhythmias and sudden death ≈ 35 years

Treatment

- Establishment of dual coronary perfusion is preferred
  - Reimplantation of anomalous coronary artery into aorta
  - Transfer of button of PA
  - Ligation of origin of left coronary artery and bypass graft can be considered in adults
- Intrapulmonary conduit between coronary ostium in PA and aorta, using baffle (Takeuchi repair)
  - Risk of supravalvular PA stenosis

DIAGNOSTIC CHECKLIST

Image Interpretation Pearls

- Absence of left main coronary artery origin from left sinus of Valsalva differentiates ALCAPA from coronary fistula

SELECTED REFERENCES

1. Prandi FR et al: Sudden cardiac arrest in an adult with anomalous origin of the left coronary artery from the pulmonary artery (alcapa): case report. Int J Environ Res Public Health. 19(3), 2022
2. Guenther TM et al: Anomalous origin of the right coronary artery from the pulmonary artery: a systematic review. Ann Thorac Surg. 110(3):1063-71, 2020
3. Hegde S et al: Echocardiographic diagnosis of Bland-White-Garland syndrome in an asymptomatic adult. JACC Case Rep. 2(7):1021-4, 2020
4. Stout KK et al: 2018 AHA/ACC guideline for the management of adults with congenital heart disease: executive summary: a report of the American College of Cardiology/American Heart Association Task Force on clinical practice guidelines. J Am Coll Cardiol. 73(12):1494-63, 2018

Coronary Artery Aneurysm

KEY FACTS

TERMINOLOGY

- Coronary artery aneurysm: Diameter > 1.5x normal adjacent segments; width > length and involves < 50% of vessel length
- Coronary artery ectasia: Diameter > 1.5x normal adjacent segments; length > width and involves > 50% of vessel length

IMAGING

- Coronary CTA
  - Evaluation of coronary aneurysm morphology, thrombosis, dissection
  - Calcification frequently present in atherosclerosis
  - Size underestimation with mural thrombus or dissection
- MR
  - Preferred modality when surveillance required
  - Calcification difficult to detect
  - Stents and clips may degrade image quality
- Angiography: May underestimate size

TOP DIFFERENTIAL DIAGNOSES

- Coronary fistula
- Coronary pseudoaneurysm
- Coronary dissection

PATHOLOGY

- Atherosclerosis is most common cause in USA
  - Right coronary artery (RCA) is typically affected
- Kawasaki disease is most common cause worldwide
  - Left main artery is most commonly affected

CLINICAL ISSUES

- Most patients are asymptomatic
- Others have angina or acute coronary syndrome
- Treatment: Anticoagulants, antiplatelets, surgery

DIAGNOSTIC CHECKLIST

- Consider coronary artery aneurysm in patients < 20 years old with angina or acute myocardial infarction

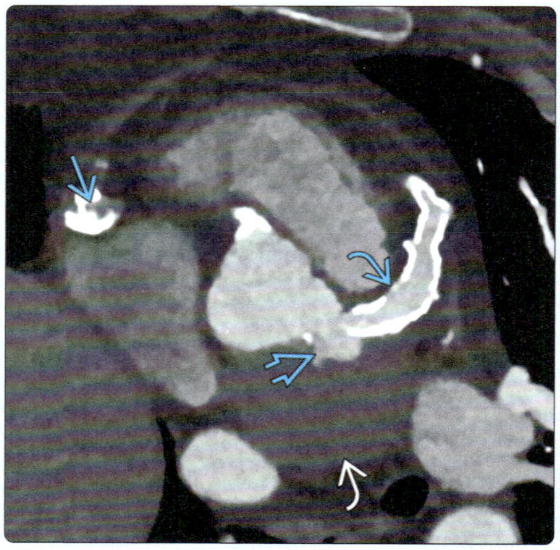
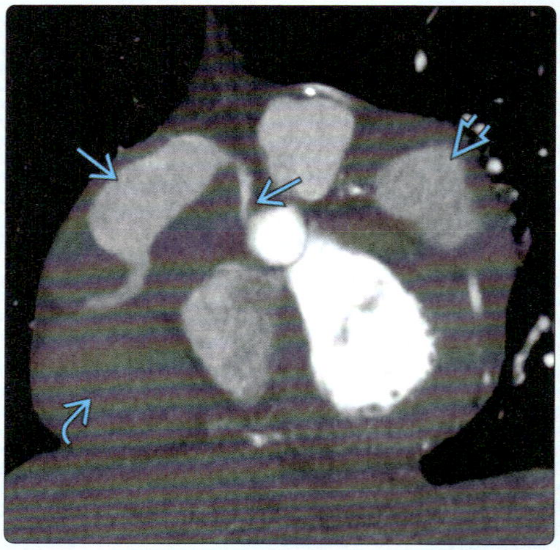

(Left) *CECT in a 72-year-old with chest pain 1 day after cardiac catheterization shows diffuse left anterior descending (LDA) artery and thrombosed right coronary artery (RCA) atherosclerotic aneurysms. There is disruption the left main wall with associated pseudoaneurysm and surrounding hematoma, likely from iatrogenic catheter injury.* **(Right)** *64-year-old man with IgG4 vasculitis has a large RCA aneurysm, which is thrombosed distally. Large left circumflex coronary artery aneurysm is partially seen.*

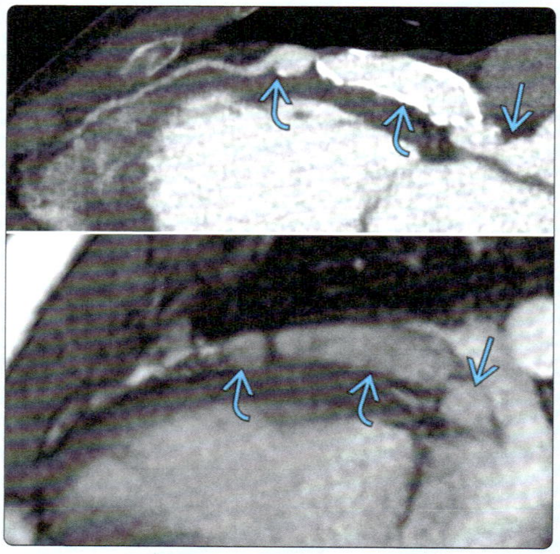
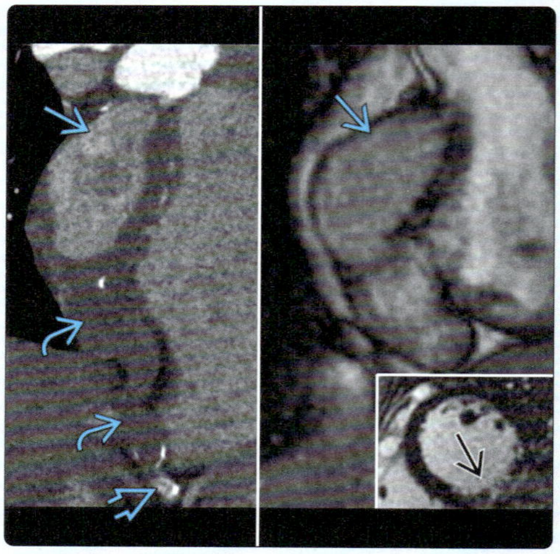

(Left) *Two-chamber images from a coronary CTA (top) and SSFP image from a cardiac MR (bottom) show an aneurysm of the left main artery and LAD artery in this 32-year-old man with Kawasaki disease.* **(Right)** *CCTA from 2019 (left) shows a large RCA aneurysm that is patent proximally but then is thrombosed. Opacification of the PDA is due to collaterals. From an MR in 2010 (right), the aneurysm is mostly patent, although there is RCA territory infarct on LGE image (inset).*

TERMINOLOGY

Definitions

- Coronary artery aneurysm: Diameter > 1.5x normal adjacent segments; width > length, involves < 50% of vessel length
- Coronary artery ectasia: Diameter > 1.5x normal adjacent segments; length > width, involves > 50% of vessel length

IMAGING

General Features

- Best diagnostic clue
  - **Dilatation of coronary artery**
- Morphology
  - Fusiform or saccular dilatation
    - May exhibit thrombus or dissection
  - Giant aneurysm > 2-15 cm in diameter in adults; > 8 mm in children

CT Findings

- Cardiac gated CTA
  - Extent and morphology of coronary aneurysm(s)
  - Delayed imaging to help differentiate between slow flow and thrombosis

MR Findings

- Available coronary angiography sequences
  - Lumen is dark on double IR-FSE
  - Lumen is bright on SSFP in absence of thrombus
- May be preferred modality when surveillance required: No use of radiation
- Calcification is difficult to detect
- Stents and clips may degrade image quality

Imaging Recommendations

- Best imaging tool
  - Gated coronary CTA is imaging modality of choice

DIFFERENTIAL DIAGNOSIS

Coronary Fistula

- Dilated vessel associated with fistula
- Coronary ectasia proximal to fistula if large shunt or steal physiology is present

Coronary Pseudoaneurysm

- Often iatrogenic

Coronary Dissection

- Common cause of myocardial infarction in younger patients
- Focal or multifocal narrowing of vessels with surrounding soft tissue

PATHOLOGY

General Features

- Etiology
  - **Atherosclerosis** is most common cause in USA
    - **Right coronary artery (RCA) is most commonly affected**, followed by left anterior descending (LAD), left circumflex, and left main coronary arteries
  - **Kawasaki disease** is most common cause worldwide
    - Coronary artery aneurysm develops in 15-25% of untreated affected children
    - May regress with treatment
    - Left main coronary artery most commonly involved
  - Large vessel vasculitis
    - 12% of Takayasu patients have coronary involvement
  - Connective tissue disease (systemic lupus erythematosus, Marfan, Behçet)
  - Other: Congenital, mycotic emboli, cocaine use

Staging, Grading, & Classification

- True aneurysm walls consist of all 3 vessel wall layers
- Pseudoaneurysms have ≤ 2 intact walls
- Coronary artery ectasia (diffuse dilation)

Gross Pathologic & Surgical Features

- Dilatation of coronary artery; may contain thrombus

Microscopic Features

- Atherosclerotic coronary aneurysms may exhibit thinning or destruction of media

CLINICAL ISSUES

Presentation

- Most common signs/symptoms
  - Most patients are asymptomatic
  - Acute coronary syndrome and heart failure may be caused by aneurysm or concurrent disease
- Clinical profile
  - Can result in thrombosis and myocardial infarction

Demographics

- Sex
  - M:F ~ 4:1
- Epidemiology
  - Present in ~ 5% of angiograms, 1.5% of necropsies

Natural History & Prognosis

- Related to severity of concomitant obstructive disease in patients with atherosclerosis
- Rupture has been reported but is rare

Treatment

- Anticoagulants, antiplatelet therapy
- **Surgical intervention if enlargement, embolization, or obstruction**
  - Bypass and exclusion of aneurysm
  - Covered stent graft
- Kawasaki disease is typically treated with high-dose intravenous γ-globulin and aspirin

DIAGNOSTIC CHECKLIST

Consider

- Coronary artery aneurysm in patients < 20 years old presenting with angina or acute myocardial infarction

SELECTED REFERENCES

1. Dimagli A et al: Coronary artery aneurysms, arteriovenous malformations, and spontaneous dissections-a review of the evidence. Ann Thorac Surg. 117(5):887-96, 2024
2. Tsujioka Y et al: Multisystem imaging manifestations of Kawasaki disease. Radiographics. 42(1):268-88, 2022

Kawasaki Disease

KEY FACTS

TERMINOLOGY

- Self-limited small and medium vessel vasculitis in young children that can lead to coronary artery aneurysms

IMAGING

- Coronary artery aneurysms in young patient with known acute illness meeting criteria of Kawasaki disease

TOP DIFFERENTIAL DIAGNOSES

- Pediatric patients and young adults
  - Noninflammatory nonatherosclerotic aneurysms
    - Marfan or Ehlers-Danlos syndrome
  - Systemic inflammatory conditions
    - Vasculitis, such as Takayasu arteritis; SLE
  - Multisystem inflammatory syndrome in children (MIS-C), associated with SARS-CoV-2 infection
- Adult patients
  - Atherosclerotic disease
  - Inflammatory or noninflammatory aneurysms

PATHOLOGY

- Small aneurysm (< 1.5x normal)
- Moderate aneurysm (1.5-4x normal)
- Giant aneurysm (> 4x normal or > 8 mm)

CLINICAL ISSUES

- Smaller aneurysms often regress
- Larger aneurysms often persist and may stenose or thrombose
  - Ischemia, infarct, or sudden cardiac death
- Treatment
  - Intravenous immunoglobulin
  - Aspirin
  - ± prednisone

DIAGNOSTIC CHECKLIST

- Echocardiography is 1st-choice imaging in children
- CT/ MR: Coronary artery evaluation after acute phase
- MR: For ischemia, infarct, microvascular dysfunction

(Left) *Coned-down PA (left) and lateral (right) chest x-rays in a 15-year-old boy with shortness of breath show a large left pneumothorax ➔. In addition, a rounded calcification in the region of the proximal left anterior descending (LAD) coronary artery ➩ is seen.* **(Right)** *Two-mm MIP of the LAD in the same patient shows a proximal 1.4-cm, partially thrombosed and calcified aneurysm ➩ with associated stenosis ➔, corresponding to the finding on CXR. A second 1.1-cm noncalcified aneurysm in seen in the mid-LAD ➔.*

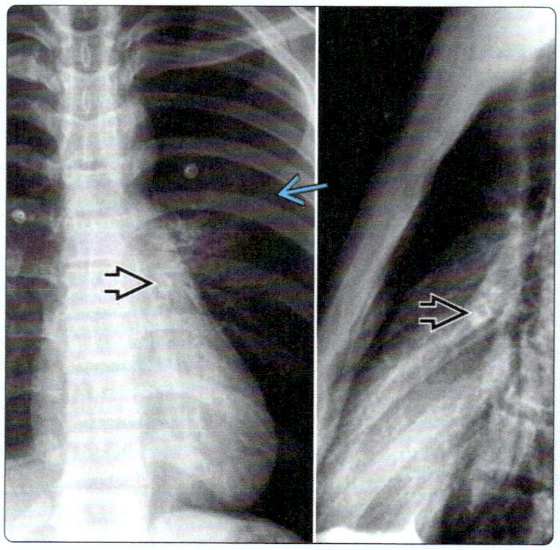

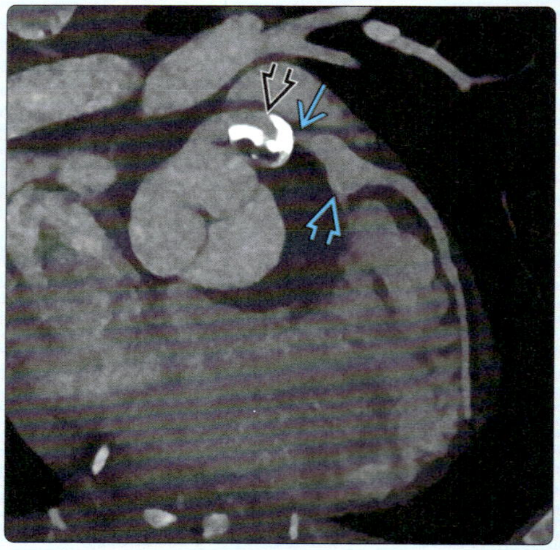

(Left) *Transverse CECT in the same patient through the giant aneurysm of the proximal LAD shows complex morphology with peripheral thrombus ➔ and both thin and chunky vascular calcifications ➩. The lumen ➡ in this region is only mildly narrowed, although there was more moderate stenosis just distal to the aneurysm (not shown).* **(Right)** *Six-mm MIP C-view of the right coronary artery (RCA) in the same patient shows a moderate-sized (7-mm) proximal coronary artery aneurysm ➔.*

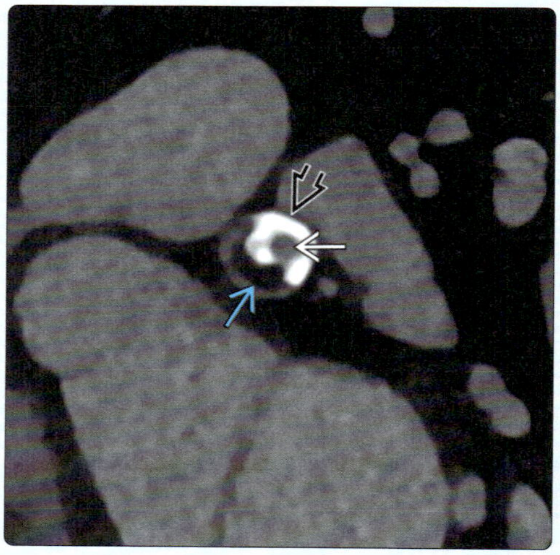

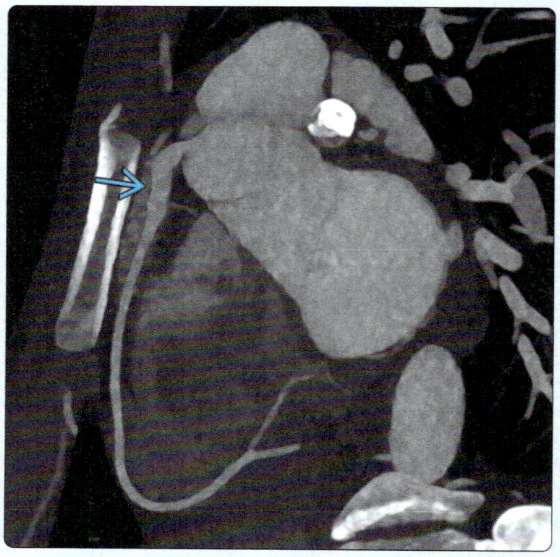

TERMINOLOGY

Abbreviations

- Kawasaki disease (KD)

Synonyms

- Mucocutaneous lymph node syndrome

Definitions

- Self-limited small and medium vessel systemic vasculitis involving arteries and veins in young children aged 6 months to 5 years that can lead to coronary artery aneurysms

IMAGING

General Features

- Best diagnostic clue
  - Coronary artery aneurysms in young patient with known history of acute illness meeting criteria of KD
- Location
  - Proximal coronary arteries
- Size
  - Small aneurysm (< 1.5x normal, < 5-mm diameter)
  - Moderate aneurysm (1.5-4x normal, 5- to 8-mm diameter)
  - Giant aneurysm (> 4x normal or > 8-mm diameter)
- Morphology
  - Single or multiple coronary artery aneurysms
  - Subacute or chronic phase: Stenosis or thrombosis

Radiographic Findings

- Calcified coronary aneurysms or stents can be seen, especially in young patient

CT Findings

- NECT
  - Calcified coronary aneurysms in child/young adult
- CECT
  - Coronary aneurysms in child/young adult
- Cardiac gated CTA
  - High spatial resolution (now as low as 0.2 mm with certain scanners)
  - Coronary artery aneurysm, thrombosis, stenosis

MR Findings

- Alternative to CTA to evaluate coronary arteries
- MR angiography
  - Contrast MRA: For aorta and large branches
  - Noncontrast MRA: For coronary arteries
    - 3D navigator sequence
- MR cine SSFP
  - Coronary aneurysms can be seen
  - Wall motion abnormalities with ischemia/infarct
  - Lower circumferential and longitudinal strain seen even with normal function in convalescent phase
  - Myocardial work index significantly decreased in KD patients ± coronary artery aneurysms
- MR perfusion
  - Myocardial ischemia seen as perfusion defect in stress images
  - Microvascular dysfunction: Diffuse subendocardial perfusion defect
    - Diminished myocardial perfusion reserve in convalescent phase, irrespective of coronary artery status
- LGE
  - Subendocardial or transmural LGE in infarct
  - Midmyocardial or subepicardial in acute myocarditis
- T2 STIR
  - Acute myocarditis: High myocardial signal due to edema
  - Edema in coronary arterial wall in acute phase
- T2 mapping
  - Global T2 values elevated in patients with acute phase KD greater than those with chronic disease
- Role of MR
  - Acute phase: Myocarditis; myocardial infarction; microvascular dysfunction; left ventricular dysfunction; coronary artery aneurysm, thrombosis, stenosis; coronary arterial wall
  - Chronic phase: Risk stratification and guiding therapy

Echocardiographic Findings

- 1st-line imaging modality
- Aneurysms in proximal coronary arteries
- May require additional imaging with gated CTA or MR as echo can miss lesions

Angiographic Findings

- Direct coronary angiography demonstrates aneurysmal dilation of coronary arteries

Imaging Recommendations

- Best imaging tool
  - Coronary CTA or MRA

DIFFERENTIAL DIAGNOSIS

Coronary Artery Aneurysms

- Atherosclerosis
  - Most common cause of coronary artery aneurysms in older patients
- Systemic inflammatory conditions associated with coronary artery aneurysms
  - Systemic lupus erythematosus (SLE)
  - Takayasu arteritis
  - Granulomatosis with polyangiitis
  - Eosinophilic granulomatosis with polyangiitis
  - Behcet disease
  - IgG4-related disease
- Noninflammatory nonatherosclerotic aneurysms
  - Marfan syndrome
  - Ehlers-Danlos syndrome
  - Loeys-Dietz syndrome
- Pseudoaneurysms
  - Iatrogenic
  - Mycotic
- Congenital

PATHOLOGY

General Features

- Etiology

- Systemic vasculitis of medium-sized arteries
  - Most common cause of acquired heart disease in children in USA
- Underlying cause unknown; may be related to abnormal antigenic immune response in genetically susceptible children
  - Multisystem inflammatory syndrome in children (MIS-C), which can affect children infected with SARS-CoV-2, shares clinical and immunologic findings with KD
- Associated abnormalities
  - Myocarditis
    - Myocarditis is more common that coronary artery involvement in KD but is usually clinically silent
  - Pericarditis
  - Valvular regurgitation
- Coronary artery aneurysms
  - Acute phase (first 2 weeks)
    - Acute necrotizing arteritis with neutrophil infiltration and luminal thrombus formation
  - Subacute phase (2 weeks to several months)
    - Vasculitis with infiltration of lymphocytes, plasma cells, and eosinophils causes aneurysm(s)
      - Peak mortality rate
  - Chronic phase (2 weeks to several years)
    - Medial thinning &/or destruction with stenosis, myofibroblastic intimal thickening, calcification, atherosclerosis, and recanalized thrombi

CLINICAL ISSUES

Presentation

- Most common signs/symptoms
  - Classic diagnosis of acute phase
    - Fever persisting for ≥ 5 days plus 4 of 5 additional findings
    - **Mucosal inflammation**
      - Cracked lips, strawberry tongue, and reddened oropharynx
    - **Bilateral conjunctival injection**
      - Reddening of eye due to dilation of blood vessels in conjunctiva
    - **Cervical lymphadenopathy**
    - **Extremity changes**
      - Redness of palms or soles, swelling of hand or feet, and periungual desquamation
    - **Polymorphous eruption**
  - Incomplete diagnosis during acute phase (~ 10%)
    - Fever persisting for ≥ 5 days with 2 or more of above findings
  - Coronary artery aneurysms
    - Usually develop 1-4 weeks after onset of acute-phase illness
  - Risk factors for coronary artery aneurysms
    - Persistent fever; anemia, hypoalbuminemia, high CRP at presentation; male; < 1 year or > 5 years of age; delay in diagnosis; no response to treatment
- Other signs/symptoms
  - May present as young patient with ischemia or infarct
  - 5% of cases of acute coronary syndrome in patients < 40 years of age due to KD

Demographics

- Age
  - Acute illness most commonly occurs from 6 months to 5 years
    - Infants < 4 months rarely affected
  - Many cases of coronary artery aneurysm in teenagers and young adults are assumed to be secondary to KD, even in absence of appropriate history
    - Other causes should be excluded
- Sex
  - M > F
- Ethnicity
  - More common in children of Asian descent

Natural History & Prognosis

- Small and moderate-sized aneurysms
  - 80% will regress (1-2 years after onset)
  - Others may evolve into stenotic lesions due to intimal thickening
- Giant aneurysms (> 4x normal size or > 8 mm)
  - Mild or no regression
  - May thrombose or rupture leading to sudden cardiac death
- Multiple aneurysms in different territories associated with lack of regression
- Acute febrile illness resolves spontaneously
- Systemic arterial aneurysms in 2%
  - In subclavian, axillary, and iliac arteries

Treatment

- Intravenous immunoglobulin (IVIG), high dose
  - Use of IVIG reduces chance of developing coronary artery aneurysms from 25% to 4%
- Aspirin
- ± prednisone

DIAGNOSTIC CHECKLIST

Consider

- Echocardiography is 1st-line imaging in children
- CT and MR useful in evaluation of coronary arteries after acute phase
- MR for noncoronary abnormalities, such as ischemia and infarct

Image Interpretation Pearls

- KD should be considered in any pediatric or young adult patient with coronary artery aneurysms

SELECTED REFERENCES

1. Hu L et al: Quantitative assessment of myocardial edema by MR T2 mapping in children with Kawasaki disease. J Magn Reson Imaging. 59(3):825-34, 2024
2. Tsujioka Y et al: Multisystem imaging manifestations of Kawasaki disease. Radiographics. 42(1):268-88, 2022
3. Wessels PA et al: A comparison of Kawasaki disease and multisystem inflammatory syndrome in children. Prog Pediatr Cardiol. 65:101516, 2022
4. Pilania RK et al: Cardiovascular involvement in Kawasaki disease is much more than mere coronary arteritis. Front Pediatr. 8:526969, 2020
5. Goh YG et al: Coronary manifestations of Kawasaki disease in computed tomography coronary angiography. J Cardiovasc Comput Tomogr. 12(4):275-80, 2018
6. Jeudy J et al: Spectrum of coronary artery aneurysms: from the radiologic pathology archives. Radiographics. 38(1):11-36, 2018

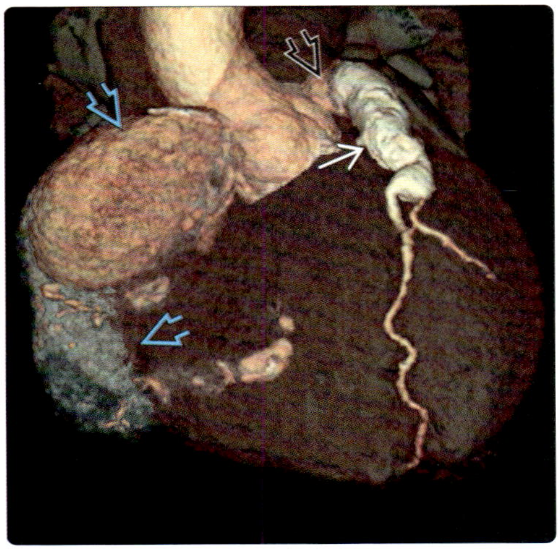

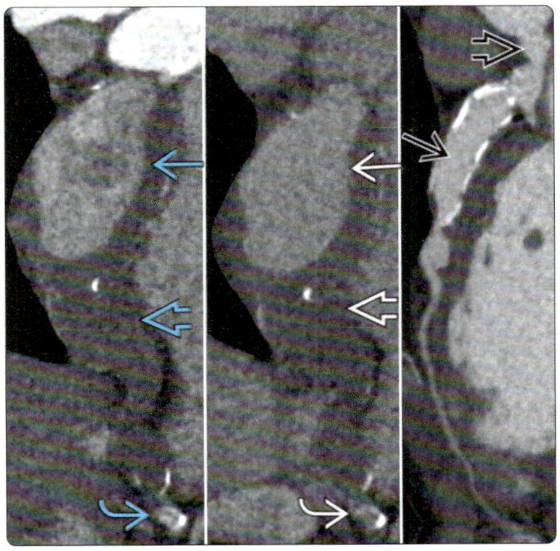

(Left) *Volume-rendered CECT in a patient with history of Kawasaki disease shows a giant, 6.1-cm diameter RCA aneurysm . A smaller, 2.2-cm aneurysm of the left main coronary artery (LMCA) extends into LAD .* **(Right)** *Curved MPR reformats of the RCA during arterial (left) and delayed (center) phases (same patient) shows slow flow in proximal RCA aneurysm , , which is thrombosed in its mid and distal portions , . Contrast is seen in PLV , , likely via collaterals. LMCA aneurysm (right) extends into LAD .*

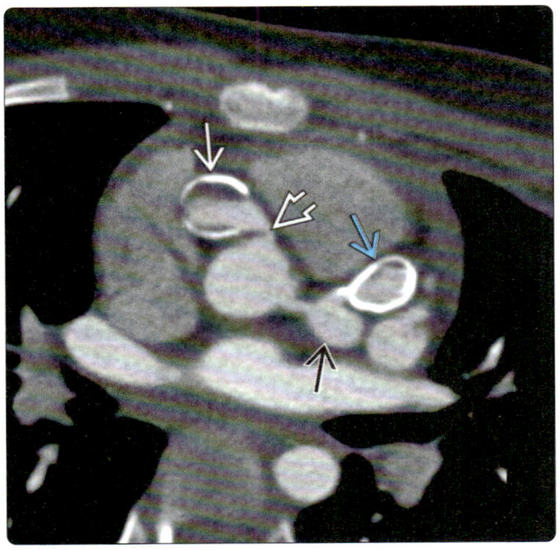

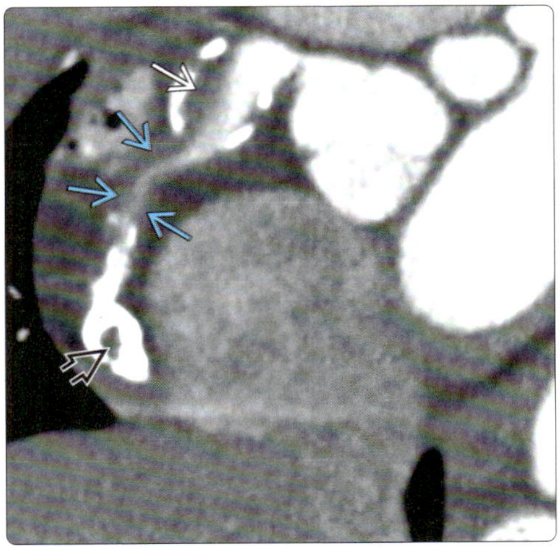

(Left) *Axial oblique CTA in a 7-year-old girl adopted from China shows giant aneurysms in the proximal LAD , left circumflex (LCx) , and RCA . The aneurysms show varying degrees of calcification and thrombus. The proximal RCA has a severe stenosis .* **(Right)** *C-view of the RCA in the same patient shows the giant proximal aneurysm . Distal to the aneurysm, the wall of the RCA is thickened , and the lumen is stenotic. Just inferior to this, there is a 2nd calcified RCA aneurysm with occlusion of the lumen.*

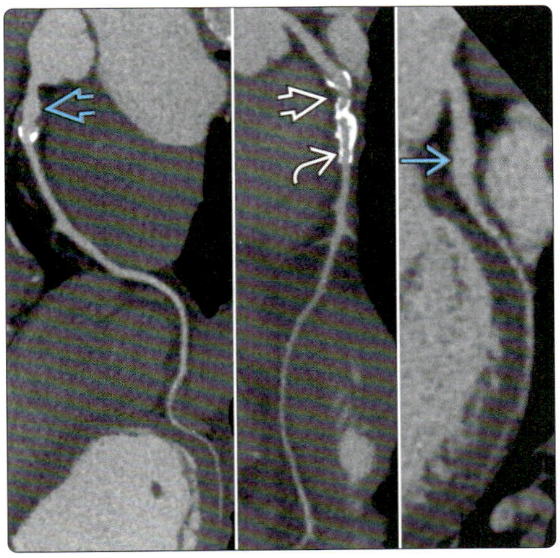

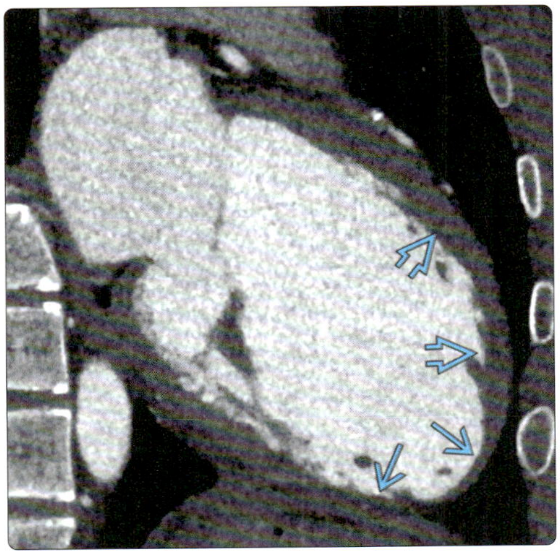

(Left) *Curved MPR images show calcified and noncalcified coronary artery aneurysms in the proximal RCA , LAD , and LCx in a 19-year-old man with a history of Kawasaki disease. There is a stent traversing part of the LAD aneurysm .* **(Right)** *Two-chamber CECT in the same patient's scan shows areas of myocardial thinning and subendocardial hypoperfusion of the mid and distal LAD territory due to prior myocardial infarction.*

KEY FACTS

IMAGING

- CTA may show vessel thickening and enhancement and caliber changes (stenosis or aneurysms); varying degree of stenosis or even occlusion are possible
- Vessel imaging can be challenging at MR
  - T2WI may show edema of vessel wall
  - T1 contrast-enhanced, black-blood sequences may reveal vessel wall thickening and enhancement

TOP DIFFERENTIAL DIAGNOSES

- Atherosclerotic coronary disease: Most common cause of coronary artery aneurysms in adults

CLINICAL ISSUES

- Clinical presentation of coronary artery vasculitis varies and commonly follows typical presentation of underlying syndrome, i.e., lymphadenopathy, hand/foot swelling, lingual erythema in Kawasaki disease (KD), abdominal pain in polyarteritis nodosa (PAN), headache or episodic blindness in giant cell arteritis (GCA)
- Worrisome findings for possible coronary involvement include episodic chest pain, shortness of breath, rhythmic irregularities on EKG, or acute changes in myocardial synchrony/wall motion on echocardiographic imaging; **it is important to note that coronary involvement may be present even if patient does not endorse or demonstrate any of these symptoms**
- **Regardless of etiology, treatment should not be delayed for imaging, as early medical intervention has been shown to reduce mortality and morbidity**

DIAGNOSTIC CHECKLIST

- Assess for other organ system involvement

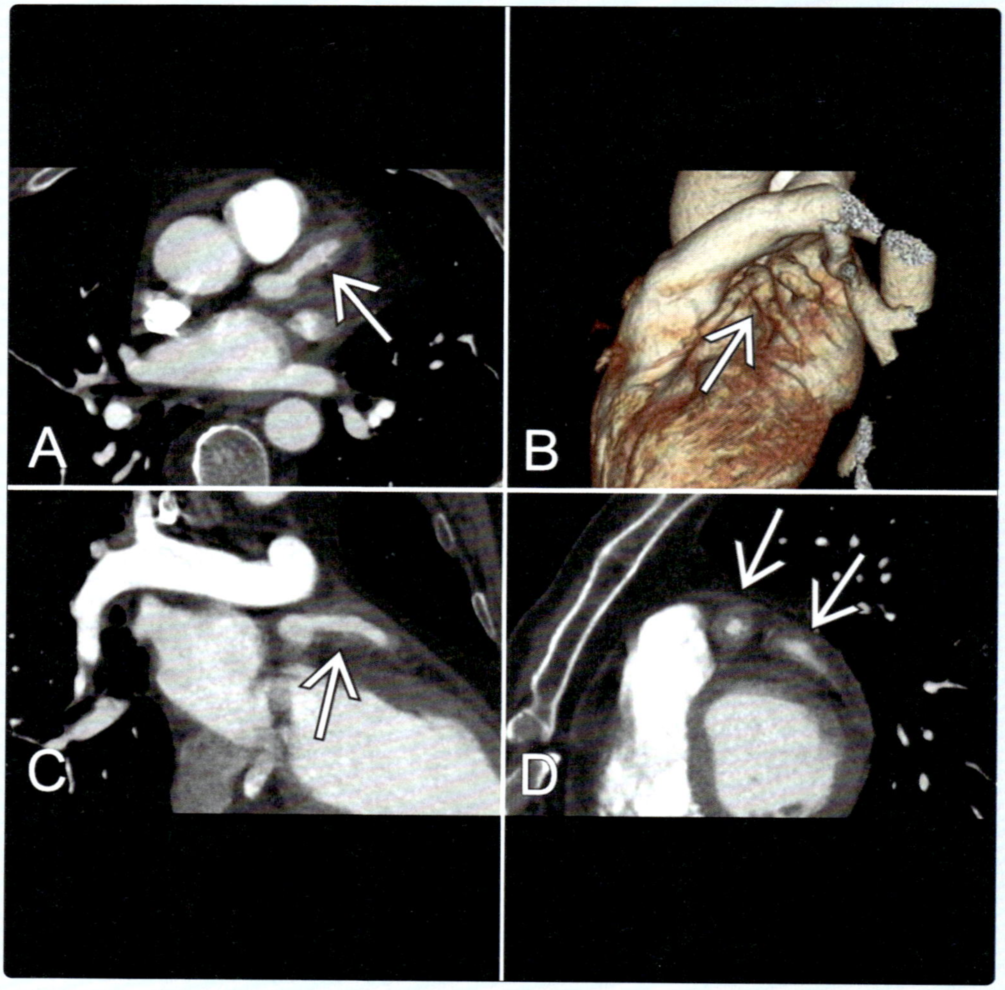

CT imaging and reconstruction of confirmed IgG4 coronary vasculitis is shown: Axial (A), 2-chamber view (B), 3D reconstruction (C), and short axis (D). Note luminal expansion and concentric wall thickening ➡ throughout the left anterior descending (LAD) coronary artery. Prominent aneurysmal dilation of the proximal LAD is visible in C.

TERMINOLOGY

Definitions

- Vasculitis: Inflammation of blood vessels

IMAGING

General Features

- Morphology
  - Wall thickening and contrast enhancement
  - Aneurysm or ectasia of ≥ 1 coronary artery
  - Regional dyskinesis or globally decreased ejection fraction

CT Findings

- Contrast CTA may show vessel thickening and enhancement and caliber changes (stenosis or aneurysms); varying degrees of stenosis or even occlusion are possible

MR Findings

- Cardiac MR evaluates effects of vasculitis on myocardium
  - Edema
  - Downstream ischemic pattern perfusion deficits
  - Scar/abnormal LCE
- Vessel imaging can be challenging in small coronary arteries with anatomic findings similar to CTA
  - T2WI may show edema of vessel wall
  - T1 contrast-enhanced, black-blood sequences may reveal vessel wall thickening and enhancement

Ultrasonographic Findings

- Transthoracic echocardiography (TTE) assessment of vessels is limited to proximal left and right main coronary arteries (any may not always be possible); TTE may reveal changes in systolic function
- US may be used to concurrently assess for extracardiac vasculitis findings, such as in the characteristic halo sign: Hypoechoic concentric thickening of temporal artery in giant cell arteritis (GCA)

Angiographic Findings

- May show luminal narrowing, ectasia, or aneurysms

Nuclear Medicine Findings

- Given anatomically broad distribution of many vasculitic syndromes, comprehensive scan coverage of PET may be particularly useful at disease onset to evaluate organ system involvement and overall disease burden
- Affected vessels are generally 18-FDG avid
- Serial scans may be useful to assess treatment response

Other Modality Findings

- Optical coherence tomography (OCT) may be useful to discriminate whether luminal stenosis seen at invasive coronary angiography (ICA) is due to plaque or mural inflammation; recent OCT study suggests that vasa vasorum proliferation may play role in healing of coronary artery aneurysms in Kawasaki disease (KD)

DIFFERENTIAL DIAGNOSIS

Atherosclerotic Coronary Disease

- Most common cause of coronary artery aneurysms in adults
- Imaging may show luminal narrowing or obstruction
- Atherosclerotic plaques with calcification
- Vessel wall thickening not typical, but mural thrombus may be present, which can be difficult to differentiate

Coronary Vasospasm

- Associated with smoking and migraine
- Transitory changes on EKG

Spontaneous Coronary Artery Dissection

- More common in women and those with connective tissue disorders
- Maintain high suspicion in previously healthy young patient with acute presentation
- CTA may show double lumen within coronary artery

Erdheim-Chester Disease

- Erdheim-Chester Disease is rare form of non-Langerhans cell histiocytosis
- May show infiltration of coronary artery vessel wall and periadventitial tissues

PATHOLOGY

General Features

- Genetics
  - Various HLA polymorphisms appear be to be associated with susceptibility to different vasculitic syndromes
- Etiology
  - In children, most commonly KD
  - Polyarteritis nodosa (PAN): Coronary artery involvement is prevalent (~ 50% of cases)
  - Takayasu arteritis and GCA
  - Eosinophilic granulomatosis (EG), IgG4 disease, Behçet syndrome, lupus, sarcoidosis, and other systemic inflammatory conditions
  - Role of pathogens: There is poorly understood but growing recognition that pathogens may represent larger role than previously appreciated
    - Hepatitis B virus and HIV are typically associated with PAN
    - Parvovirus B19 and EBV are associated more typically associated with KD
    - Streptococcus has been linked with PAN and KD
    - COVID-19: Associated with leukocytoclastic, IgA, and Kawasaki vasculitis most commonly

Microscopic Features

- KD: Necrotizing inflammation of all layers of arterial wall, largely from macrophages/monocytes
- PAN: Commonly transmural inflammation with leukocytic infiltration
- Temporal arteritis (TA): Granulomatous inflammation of medial or all layers of vessel wall with plasma cells and lymphocytes
- GCA: Intimal proliferation and medial necrosis with mononuclear infiltration and giant cells

CLINICAL ISSUES

Presentation

- Most common signs/symptoms

- Clinical presentation of coronary artery vasculitis varies and commonly follows typical presentation of underlying syndrome, i.e., lymphadenopathy, hand/foot swelling, lingual erythema in KD, abdominal pain in PAN, headache or episodic blindness in GCA
- Worrisome findings for possible coronary involvement include episodic chest pain, shortness of breath, rhythmic irregularities on EKG, or acute changes in myocardial synchrony/wall motion on echocardiographic imaging.
- **It is important to note that coronary involvement may be present even if patient does not endorse or demonstrate any of these symptoms**

Demographics

- As with its clinical presentation, demographics of coronary artery vasculitis vary following underlying condition
- KD is most prevalent in children and young adults; 15-25% of untreated KD patients develop coronary aneurysms
- TA more commonly occurs in older patients and is associated with polymyalgia rheumatica
- PAN most commonly occurs in adults with male dominance

Natural History & Prognosis

- Regardless of etiology, early identification and treatment is of paramount importance; appropriate medical management reduces risk of myocardial infarction or aneurysm rupture and reduces likelihood of relapse

Treatment

- Varies by etiology and severity of downstream myocardial injury
- In KD, intravenous immunoglobulin (IVIG) and aspirin are mainstays of treatment
  - While there has not been head-to-head study comparing IVIG and corticosteroids, there is emerging evidence, primarily from studies amongst Japanese populations, that glucocorticoids may provide additional benefit
  - They are, therefore, conditionally recommended by American College of Rheumatology in patients who are considered to be high risk for developing coronary artery aneurysms
- In PAN, initial treatment is corticosteroids; in moderate or severe cases of PAN, cyclophosphamide may be added and has shown to confer lower relapse rate and higher survival rate at 32 months
- In TA and GCA, immunosuppressive corticosteroids are typically employed
  - There is limited, but growing, evidence that biologics, such as tocilizumab, may improve outcomes
- If significant stenosis or myocardial injury is present, revascularization (surgical or percutaneous) may be considered
- **Regardless of etiology, treatment should not be delayed for imaging, as early medical intervention has been shown to reduce mortality and morbidity**

DIAGNOSTIC CHECKLIST

Consider

- Identify and treat underlying vasculitis
- Assess for other organ system involvement

SELECTED REFERENCES

1. Kakimoto N et al: Vasa vasorum enhancement on optical coherence tomography in Kawasaki disease. Pediatr Res. ePub, 2024
2. Shiono Y et al: Pathological alterations of coronary arteries late after Kawasaki disease: an optical coherence tomography study. JACC Adv. 3(6):100937, 2024
3. Frasier KM et al: Secondary vasculitis attributable to post-COVID syndrome. Cureus. 15(8):e44119, 2023
4. Katz G et al: IgG4-related disease as a variable-vessel vasculitis: a case series of 13 patients with medium-sized coronary artery involvement. Semin Arthritis Rheum. 60:152184, 2023
5. van der Geest KSM et al: Positron emission tomography imaging in vasculitis. Cardiol Clin. 41(2):251-65, 2023
6. Gorelik M et al: 2021 American College of Rheumatology/Vasculitis foundation guideline for the management of Kawasaki disease. Arthritis Care Res (Hoboken). 74(4):538-48, 2022
7. Caforio ALP: Myocarditis: endomyocardial biopsy and circulating anti-heart autoantibodies are key to diagnosis and personalized etiology-directed treatment. Eur Heart J. 42(16):1618-20, 2021
8. Khanna S et al: Coronary artery vasculitis: a review of current literature. BMC Cardiovasc Disord. 21(1):7, 2021
9. Lai J et al: Characteristics and outcomes of coronary artery involvement in polyarteritis nodosa. Can J Cardiol. 37(6):895-903, 2021
10. Miyabe C et al: Pathogens in vasculitis: is it really idiopathic? JMA J. 4(3):216-24, 2021
11. Ramdin N et al: Hidden IgG4-related coronary disease. Am J Clin Pathol. 156(3):471-7, 2021
12. Ben Shimol J et al: The utility of PET/CT in large vessel vasculitis. Sci Rep. 10(1):17709, 2020
13. Chimenti C et al: Infarct-like myocarditis with coronary vasculitis and aneurysm formation caused by Epstein-Barr virus infection. ESC Heart Fail. 7(3):938-41, 2020
14. Flossdorf S et al: Sudden death of a young adult with coronary artery vasculitis, coronary aneurysms, parvovirus B19 infection and Kawasaki disease. Forensic Sci Med Pathol. 16(3):498-503, 2020
15. Guggenberger KV et al: Imaging in vasculitis. Curr Rheumatol Rep. 22(8):34, 2020
16. Houben E et al: Predictors of fatal and non-fatal cardiovascular events in ANCA-associated vasculitis: data from the Toronto CanVasc cohort. Joint Bone Spine. 87(3):221-4, 2020
17. Norita K et al: Sudden cardiac death caused by coronary vasculitis. Virchows Arch. 460(3):309-18, 2012
18. Ward EV et al: Coronary artery vasculitis as a presentation of cardiac sarcoidosis. Circulation. 125(6):e344-6, 2012
19. Mavrogeni S et al: Detection of coronary artery lesions and myocardial necrosis by magnetic resonance in systemic necrotizing vasculitides. Arthritis Rheum. 61(8):1121-9, 2009

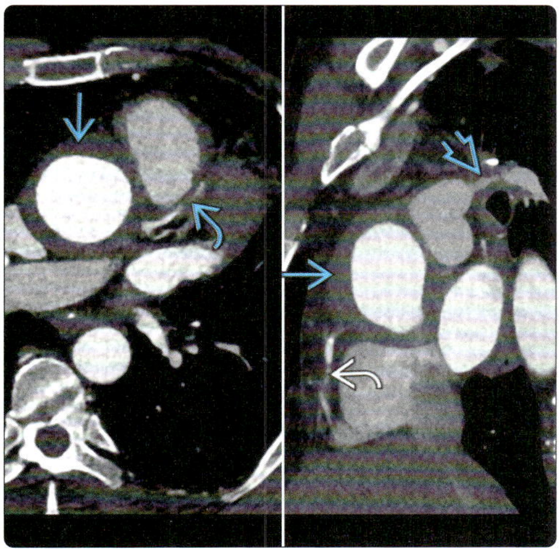

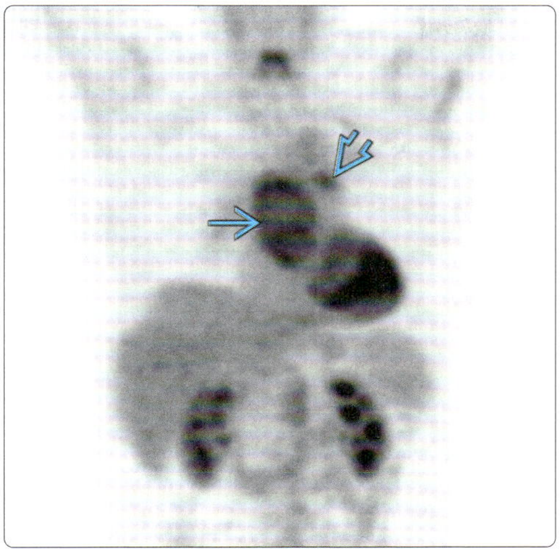

(Left) *Axial (L) and sagittal (R) oblique CECTs in a middle-aged man with history of large vessel vasculitis shows severe stenoses of LAD and right coronary artery (RCA) due to vasculitis. Marked circumferential wall thickening of aorta and severe stenosis of left pulmonary artery (PA) are also due to vasculitis. (Courtesy S. Kligerman, MD.)* **(Right)** *Frontal PET (same patient) shows marked FDG uptake in ascending aorta and left PA. More mild uptake was in LAD and RCA. (Courtesy S. Kligerman, MD.)*

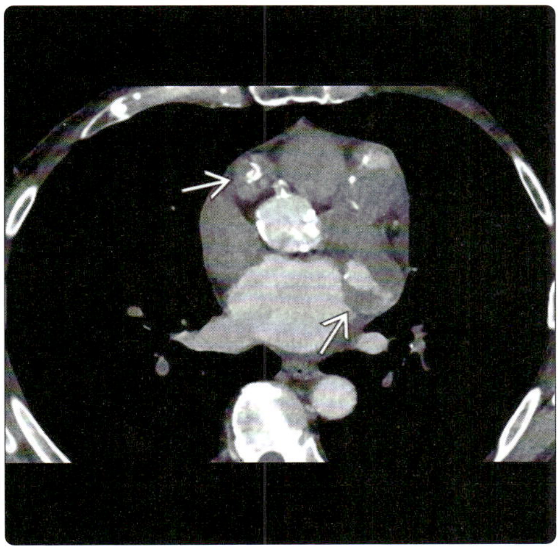

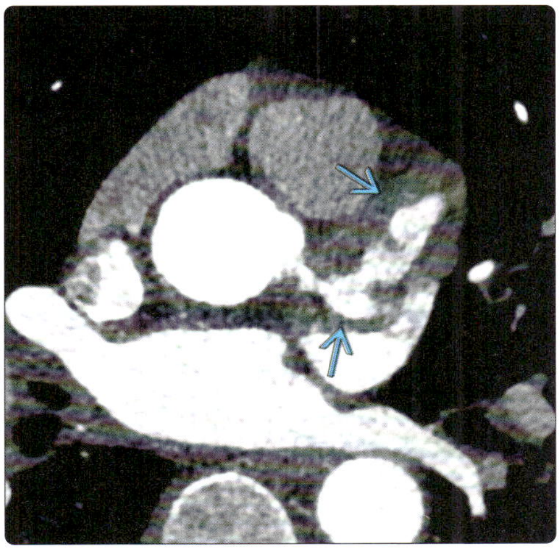

(Left) *Aneurysmal dilation of the left circumflex (LCx) coronary artery, LAD, and RCA with scattered calcifications is shown. Profound vessel wall thickening is most notable in the LCx and RCA. (Courtesy S. Kligerman, MD.)* **(Right)** *Axial coronary CT shows diffuse aneurysmal dilation of the LAD and LCx. (Courtesy S. Kligerman, MD.)*

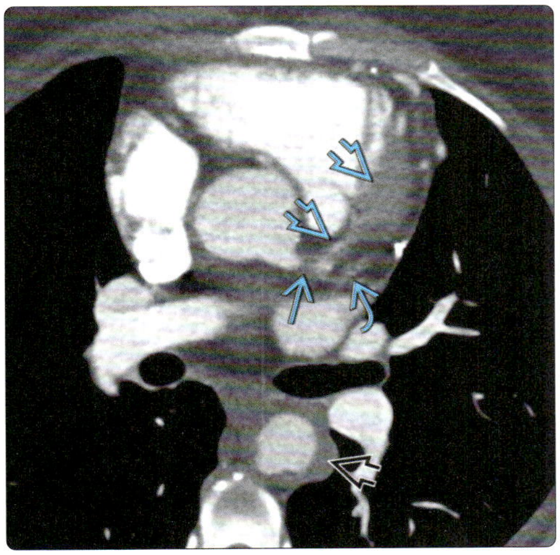

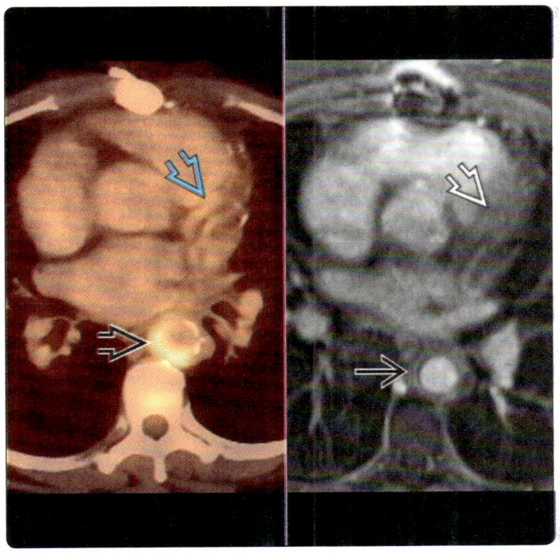

(Left) *CT in a 39-year-old woman with Takayasu arteritis shows soft tissue surrounding the left main, LAD, and LCx, leading to severe stenoses. Circumferential soft tissue encases the descending thoracic aorta. (Courtesy S. Kligerman, MD.)* **(Right)** *Axial FDG-PET (L) after coronary artery bypass grafting shows FDG uptake in the LAD and aorta due to vasculitis. Axial VIBE T1 post MR (R) shows enhancement of the soft tissue around the LAD and aorta. (Courtesy S. Kligerman, MD.)*

KEY FACTS

TERMINOLOGY

- With possible exception of patients with renal failure, who may develop medial calcification, development of coronary calcium is intimal process associated with coronary atherosclerotic plaque
- NECT imaging and quantitative software are used to determine coronary artery calcium score (CACS) (Agatston score)

IMAGING

- ECG-gated nonenhanced cardiac CT is used to detect and quantify coronary calcium
- By convention, threshold for identification of calcium is 130 HU at tube potential of 120 kV
- Identification of ≥ 3 contiguous pixels with attenuation > 130 HU in wall of coronary artery is defined as calcified coronary lesions
- Agatston score, determined from plaque area and coefficient that depends on peak CT attenuation, is widely used to quantify coronary calcium

TOP DIFFERENTIAL DIAGNOSES

- Coronary artery stent
- Mitral annular calcification
- Aortic wall calcification
- Image noise

CLINICAL ISSUES

- In asymptomatic individuals, presence and extent of coronary calcium correlate to risk of future cardiovascular events
    - Coronary calcium is therefore part of some risk assessment algorithms used to select candidates for cholesterol-lowering drug therapy
- Interscan variability is high, especially for low scores
- Repeat testing is not recommended

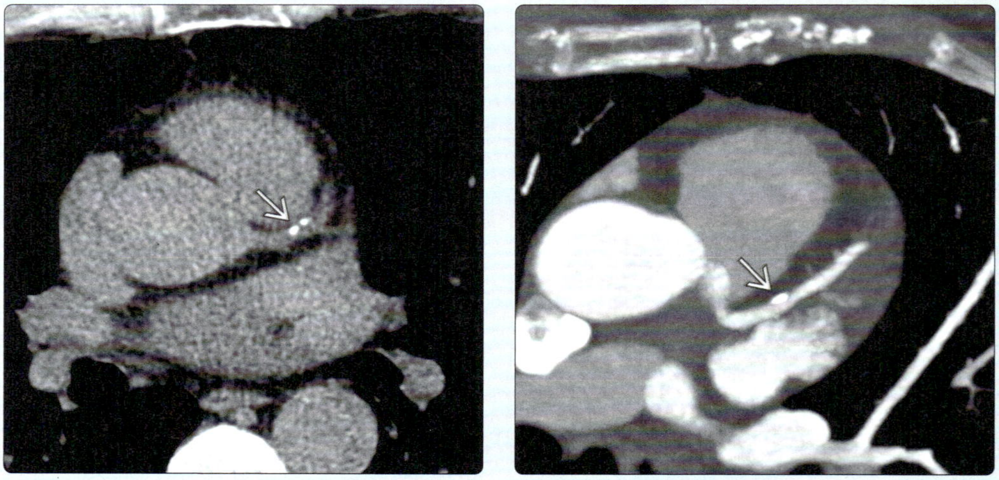

(Left) *NECT is used for visualizing coronary calcification. By international standard, 120 kV are used for acquisition, and the reconstructed slice thickness is 3 mm. Two small calcifications ➡ of the proximal left anterior descending (LAD) coronary artery are detectable.* **(Right)** *Coronary calcium is also visible on contrast-enhanced coronary CT angiography. Here, a small calcification ➡ of the proximal LAD coronary artery is present.*

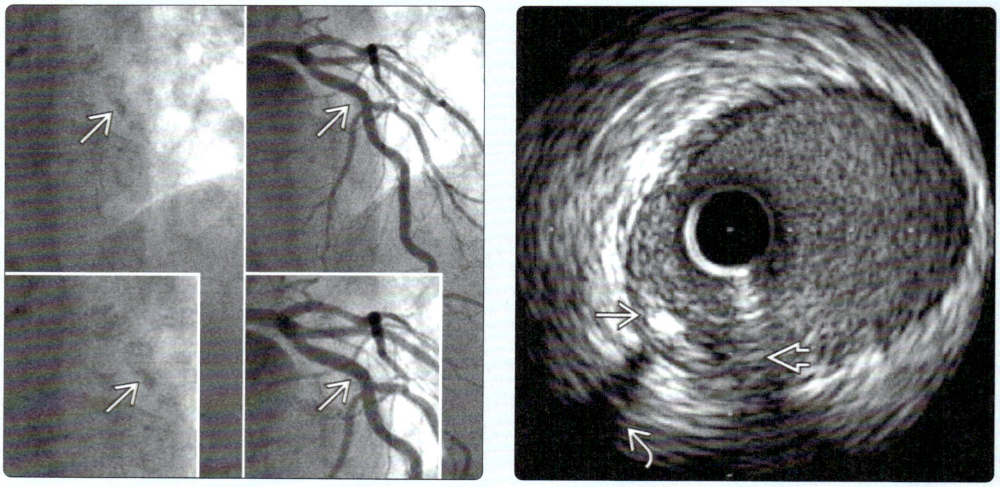

(Left) *In a fluoroscopic frame (left), calcification is detectable as a grayish shadow ➡. After injection of contrast agent (right), the calcium deposit next to the contrast-filled lumen is better visualized.* **(Right)** *Intravascular ultrasound (IVUS) is the most sensitive in vivo method for identifying coronary calcifications. They appear bright ➡ and cause shadowing ➡. The less intensive shadowing ➡ is caused by the intracoronary wire that is used to guide the IVUS catheter (present in all IVUS images).*

TERMINOLOGY

Abbreviations

- Coronary artery calcium score (CACS)

Definitions

- Deposition of calcium hydroxyapatite in coronary arteries
  - Coronary calcium is nearly always intimal process
    - Patients with diabetes and renal failure may develop medial calcification
- NECT imaging and quantitative software are used to determine CACS (Agatston score)

IMAGING

CT Findings

- NECT
  - By convention, threshold for identification of calcium is 130 HU at tube potential of 120 kVp
  - Agatston score is widely used for quantification
    - Requires reconstruction of 3-mm thick slices
    - Must have area of ≥ 3 contiguous pixels > 130 HU
      - Small calcifications may be visible but not measured
    - For each lesion, cofactor is derived from its peak attenuation
      - Cofactor 1 for 131-199 HU
      - Cofactor 2 for 200-299 HU
      - Cofactor 3 for 300-399 HU
      - Cofactor 4 for ≥ 400 HU
    - Agatston score for each plaque in each slice is product of plaque area and cofactor
    - Scores for all lesions in all slices are summarized to obtain per-vessel and per-patient Agatston scores
    - For patients aged 45-84 with no history of coronary artery bypass grafting (CABG), coronary stent, etc.
  - Alternative methods for scoring include calcified plaque volume and calcified mass (which requires phantom for reference)
  - Vast majority of published scientific literature uses Agatston score
- CECT angiography
  - Very small calcifications may be missed due to CT attenuation similar to contrast-enhanced lumen
  - Virtual noncontrast reconstructions correlate well with Agatston scores
- Nongated chest CT
  - Provides opportunistic screening by detection of incidental CAC on nongated chest CT
    - Best visualized on scanners with high temporal resolution
  - Identifies patients at risk of cardiovascular disease events and death
    - Provides opportunity for early treatment of high-risk patients and for reducing morbidity and mortality
  - Several methods can be used to categorize
    - Visual scoring method (none, mild, moderate, severe) demonstrates good correlation with Agatston score
    - Artificial intelligent algorithms for automated CAC scoring on nongated chest CTs are available and demonstrate good correlation with both visual scoring method and dedicated Agatston score

Imaging Recommendations

- Best imaging tool
  - Multidetector row CT
- Best diagnostic tool
  - Nonenhanced, ECG-gated CT imaging
  - Identification of ≥ 3 contiguous pixels with attenuation > 130 HU in wall of coronary artery is defined as coronary calcium

DIFFERENTIAL DIAGNOSIS

Coronary Artery Stent

- On NECT, coronary stent can have similar appearance to coronary calcium

Medial Calcification

- Occurs in patients with diabetes and renal failure
- Cannot differentiate with intimal calcification associated with atherosclerotic plaques
- Independent predictor of cardiovascular mortality, as it leads to ↑ vascular stiffness and ↓ compliance

Mitral Annular Calcification

- Can be misinterpreted as left circumflex (LCx) coronary artery calcification

Calcification of Aortic Sinus

- Calcification of aortic sinus near coronary artery ostium
- Can be difficult to differentiate in some cases

Image Noise

- Includes < 3 contiguous pixels

PATHOLOGY

General Features

- Calcium develops during atherosclerotic plaque development
  - Inflammation → calcium hydroxyapatite deposition
  - Processes similar to osteogenesis
- Calcification may also ↑ with plaque regression and stabilization; suggested by ↑ CAC in statin users
- Amount of calcified plaque roughly correlates to total amount of plaque
  - Calcified plaque represents ~ 20% of total plaque burden
- Atherosclerotic plaque and stenosis can occur in absence of calcium; especially in patients who are young, female, or have acute symptoms

CLINICAL ISSUES

Presentation

- Coronary calcium causes no symptoms and is present in majority of adults > 50 years of age
- In asymptomatic individuals, presence and extent of coronary calcium correlate to risk of future cardiovascular events
  - Any coronary calcium, including single focus of calcium, indicates significantly ↑ atherosclerotic cardiovascular disease risk over next 10-15 years
  - Absence of coronary artery calcium indicates < 1% risk for major adverse cardiac event in next 10 years

- Coronary calcium part of some risk assessment algorithms is used to select candidates for cholesterol-lowering drug therapy
  - Individuals with no risk factors
    - Low risk
    - Do not require further testing
  - Individuals with established cardiovascular disease or diabetes
    - High risk
    - Require lipid-lowering treatment
    - Imaging is not considered helpful for risk stratification
  - Coronary calcium is considered most useful in individuals with intermediate risk [e.g., 10-year risk of coronary artery disease (CAD) = 10-20%] according to Framingham risk score
- Typically, coronary calcium percentile is included in report
  - Puts measured amount of calcium in perspective to distribution found in individuals of same sex, ethnicity, and age class
    - Ethnicities currently limited to those who are White, Black, Chinese, and Hispanic
  - Online reference values web tool calculators are available for percentile calculation, such as from Multi-Ethnic Study of Atherosclerosis (MESA)
  - Arterial age can also be calculated from CACSs
    - Arterial age expresses estimated risk equivalent of coronary artery calcium
- **Coronary Artery Calcium Data and Reporting System (CAC-DRS)**
  - Applies to all dedicated CAC scans and nongated chest CT studies
  - Includes 4 categories (0-3) based on either Agatston score or visual assessment in case of nongated studies
  - Provides treatment recommendations based on CAC-DRS category
  - **CAC-DRS 0**: CACS 0; visually no CAC
    - Very low risk; statins generally not recommended
  - **CAC-DRS 1**: CACS 1-99; visually mild CAC
    - Mildly ↑ risk
    - Treatment: Moderate intensity statin
  - **CAC-DRS 2:** CACS 100-299; visually moderate CAC
    - Moderately ↑ risk
    - Treatment: Moderate to high intensity statin + acetylsalicylic acid (ASA)
  - **CAC-DRS 3**: CACS > 300; visually severe CAC
    - Moderate to severely ↑ risk
    - Treatment: High-intensity statin + ASA
  - Modifiers: Scoring system (Agatston = A; visual=V) and number of vessels involved (N)
    - CAC of 50 by Agatston method involving both left anterior descending and LCx coronary arteries should be reported as CAC-DRS A1/N2
- CAD Reporting and Data System (CAD-RADS) 2.0 recommends reporting of total atherosclerotic plaque burden (P); CACS can be used to quantify overall plaque burden
  - P1 (mild): CACS ≤ 100
  - P2 (moderate): CACS = 101-300
  - P3 (extensive): CACS = 301-999
  - P4 (very extensive): CACS ≥ 1,000

Demographics

- Age
  - Incidence ↑ from only small percentage in 2nd decade of life to nearly 100% by 8th decade
- Sex
  - General incidence in women is similar to that in men who are decade younger
  - Separation in prevalence with age is eliminated by age 70
- Hemodialysis patients, metabolic syndromes, and diabetes
  - Have higher incidence and absolute progression of CACS
    - Some of calcification likely medial
  - CACS is strong independent predictor of mortality

Natural History & Prognosis

- Progression of CACS is measured as percentage of baseline score
- Annual CACS progression: 14-27%; average: 24%
- Rapid progression has been connected to elevated risk for CAD events; higher risk for myocardial infarction and all-cause mortality
- Interscan variability is high, especially for low scores, and significantly limits utility of repeat testing

Treatment

- Presence of coronary calcium in conjunction with other risk factors may prompt initiation of lipid-lowering therapy
- Statins may actually ↑ CAC due to plaque stabilization and regression
- Data have shown that statins are only useful in individuals who have coronary calcium, while there was no effect on outcome in patients who did not have coronary calcium

DIAGNOSTIC CHECKLIST

Image Interpretation Pearls

- Avoid measuring plaque in aortic wall near origins of right coronary artery and left main coronary artery
- Avoid confusing mitral annular calcification with LCx coronary artery calcification
- Avoid measuring coronary artery stents as coronary artery calcification
- Be aware that motion beam-hardening artifacts may cause overestimation of calcium score
- Use thick slices (3 mm) to calculate CACS

SELECTED REFERENCES

1. Malik RF et al: Opportunistic screening for coronary artery disease: an untapped population health resource. J Am Coll Radiol. 21(6):880-9, 2024
2. Canan A et al: RadioGraphics update: pictorial guide to CAD-RADS 2.0. Radiographics. 43(4):e220202, 2023
3. Kumar P et al: Coronary artery calcium data and reporting system (CAC-DRS): a primer. J Cardiovasc Imaging. 31(1):1-17, 2023
4. Raygor V et al: Accuracy of incidental visual coronary artery calcium assessment compared with dedicated coronary artery calcium scoring. J Cardiovasc Comput Tomogr. 17(6):453-8, 2023
5. Suzuki Y et al: Coronary artery calcium score: current status of clinical application and how to handle the results. J Cardiol. 79(5):567-71, 2022
6. Hecht HS et al: CAC-DRS: Coronary artery calcium data and reporting system. An expert consensus document of the Society of Cardiovascular Computed Tomography (SCCT). J Cardiovasc Comput Tomogr. 12(3):185-91, 2018
7. Agatston AS et al: Quantification of coronary artery calcium using ultrafast computed tomography. J Am Coll Cardiol. 15(4):827-32, 1990

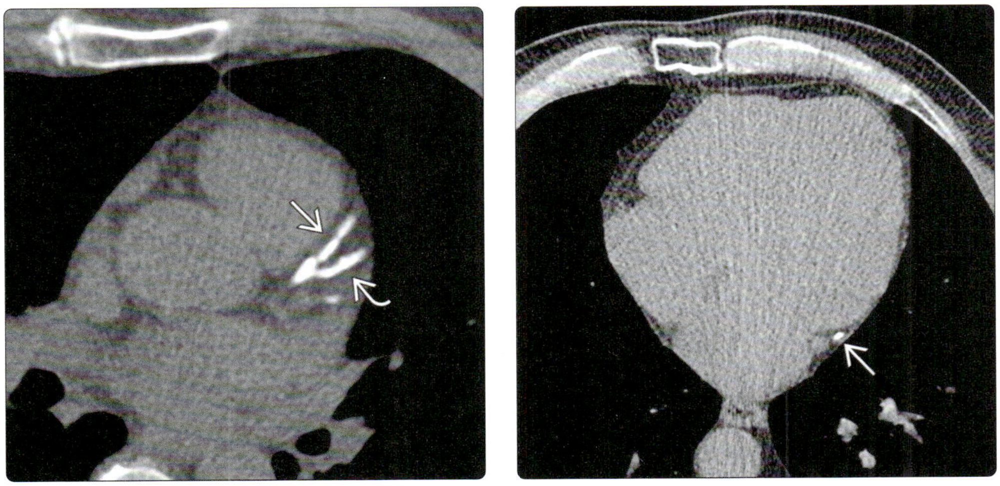

(Left) *Calcifications of the LAD coronary artery and diagonal branch are present and clearly detectable on this nonenhanced ECG-triggered CT of the coronary arteries (120 kV, 3-mm slice thickness).* **(Right)** *Calcium score CT (120 kV, 3.0-mm slice thickness) shows calcification of the left circumflex (LCx) coronary artery in the atrioventricular groove. Occasionally, beam-hardening artifact or mitral annular calcification can mimic calcification in this area.*

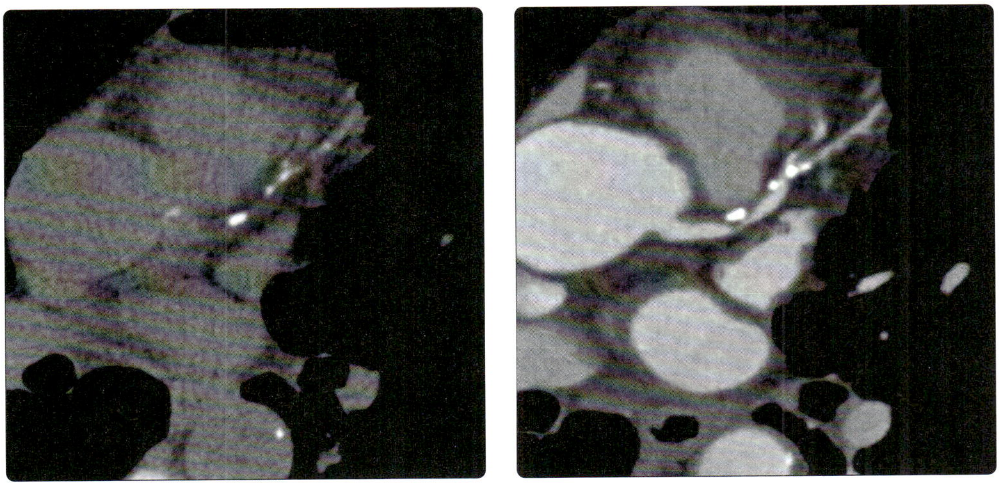

(Left) *Axial oblique NECT from a calcium score shows a moderate degree of calcium in the LAD distribution.* **(Right)** *Axial oblique CT from the contrast-enhanced portion of the study in the same patient shows a heavy burden of noncalcified atherosclerotic disease associated with the moderate calcified disease, leading to multiple areas of moderate and severe stenoses. (Courtesy S. Kligerman, MD.)*

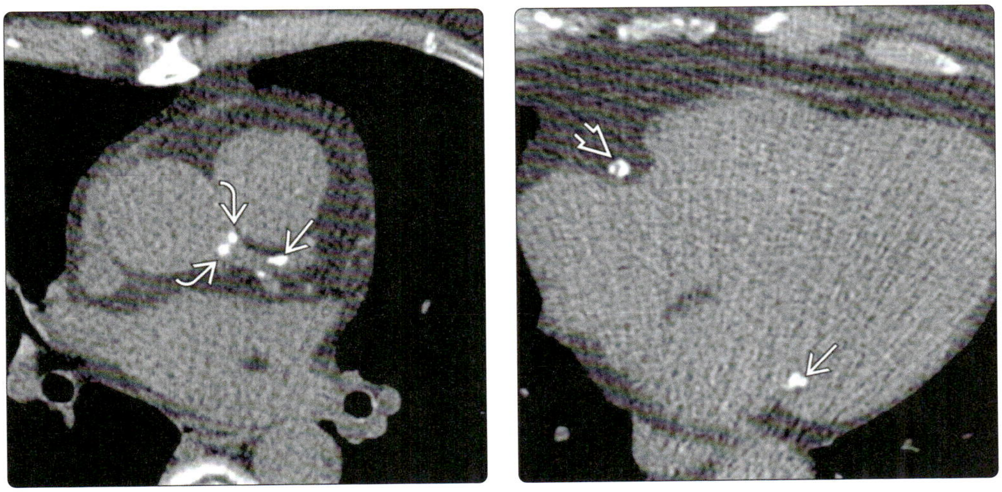

(Left) *By consensus, calcifications of the coronary ostia [here, ostium of the left main (LM)] are not included in coronary calcium evaluation. It should be mentioned in the report but not counted toward the coronary calcium score. At the LM bifurcation, calcification of LAD and LCx is present.* **(Right)** *Calcification of the mitral anulus is often present and could be misinterpreted as LCx calcification. Calcification of the midright coronary artery is present on this NECT.*

Coronary Atherosclerotic Plaque

KEY FACTS

TERMINOLOGY

- Deposit that develops in intimal layer of coronary arteries and consists of lipids, fibrous tissue, smooth muscle cells, and calcium
- Atherosclerotic plaque can develop into stenotic lesion but must not necessarily be associated with relevant reduction of coronary lumen

IMAGING

- Coronary calcium is highly specific and fairly sensitive for presence of coronary atherosclerotic plaque
- Coronary CTA can detect coronary plaque but only if image quality is optimal
- Coronary MR has potential for plaque visualization and characterization
- Invasive coronary angiography underestimates presence and extent of coronary atherosclerotic plaque and must be complemented by intravascular US for plaque assessment

TOP DIFFERENTIAL DIAGNOSES

- Myocardial bridge
- Coronary vasculopathy post heart transplant
- Vasculitis
- Spontaneous coronary artery dissection

CLINICAL ISSUES

- Most coronary atherosclerotic plaques remain clinically silent
- Sudden plaque rupture (or, less frequently, erosion) with subsequent luminal thrombosis leads to acute coronary event
- Slow plaque growth, sometimes as consequence of repeated "healed" rupture or intraplaque hemorrhage, can lead to occurrence of coronary artery stenosis and stable coronary artery disease

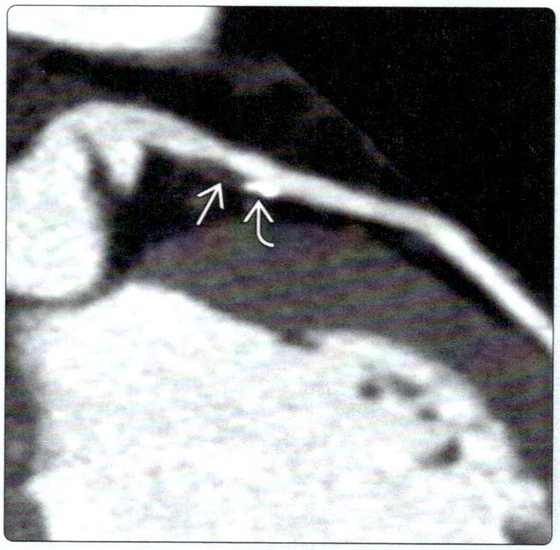
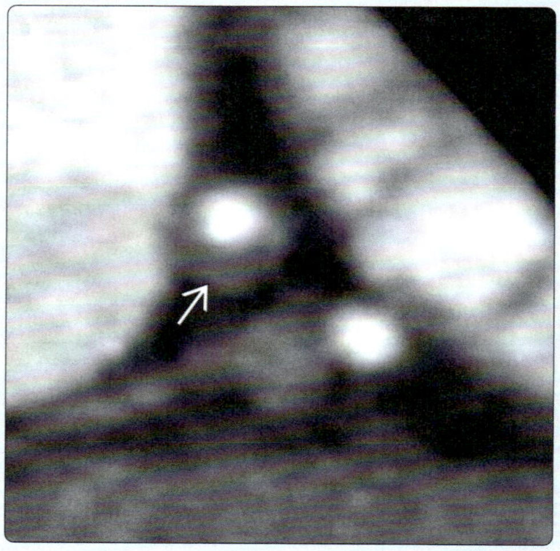

(Left) *Contrast-enhanced coronary CTA shows calcified ➡ and noncalcified ➡ components of a partially calcified atherosclerotic plaque present in the proximal left anterior descending coronary artery.* **(Right)** *Contrast-enhanced coronary CTA in the same patient shows a cross-sectional view of the proximal left anterior descending coronary artery. A noncalcified plaque ➡ is clearly detectable.*

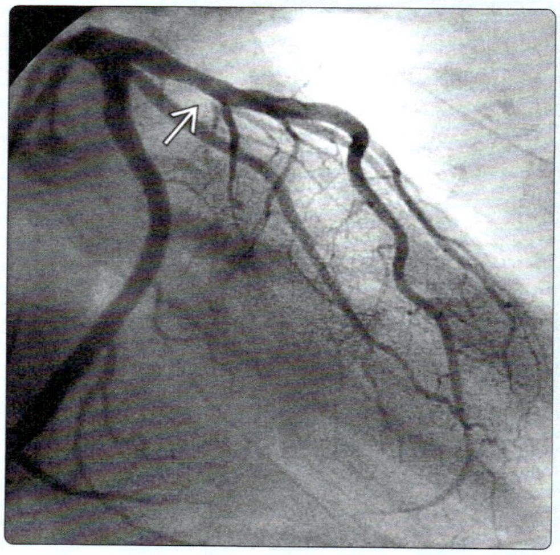
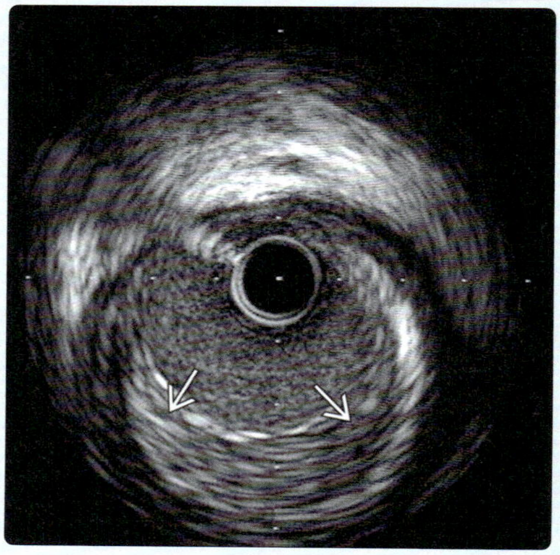

(Left) *Invasive coronary angiogram in the same patient shows an atherosclerotic plaque detected on CT. Only a very mild narrowing ➡ of the coronary artery lumen is present. Note that even a pronounced plaque is not necessarily associated with a relevant luminal stenosis.* **(Right)** *Intracoronary US of the proximal left anterior descending coronary artery in the same patient provides a cross-sectional view of the vessel and demonstrates the presence of a pronounced noncalcified coronary atherosclerotic plaque ➡.*

TERMINOLOGY

Definitions

- Deposit that develops in intimal layer of coronary arteries and consists of lipids, fibrous tissue, smooth muscle cells, and calcium
  - Necrotic core can be present, covered by fibrous cap
  - Atherosclerotic plaque can develop into coronary artery stenosis
  - Most plaques are not associated with relevant stenosis
  - Acute coronary syndromes (myocardial infarction and unstable angina) occur as result of plaque rupture with subsequent thrombosis of vessel lumen
    - Immediately before rupture, plaques are often not associated with relevant luminal stenosis

IMAGING

General Features

- Location
  - Can occur in any part of coronary arterial tree but is most frequently localized in proximal coronary segments
  - Vessel bifurcations predominantly affected
- Size
  - Plaque size is not related to degree of luminal narrowing
  - Positive remodeling occurs when vessel outwardly expands as plaque builds up in vessel wall
    - Degree of luminal narrowing therefore depends both on plaque size and on degree of remodeling
- Morphology
  - Plaques generally consist of lipid-rich necrotic core surrounded by fibrous tissue, smooth muscle cells, and calcification
    - Typically covered by fibrous cap toward vessel lumen
      - Thin, fibrous caps and large, necrotic cores are among factors that predispose plaques to rupture, which may lead to acute coronary syndrome
      - Hence, plaques with these features are called thin-cap fibroatheromas or vulnerable plaques
      - Other features associated with plaque vulnerability are plaque vascularization and macrophage infiltration of fibrous cap
    - Most acute coronary events are caused by rupture of nonstenotic plaques, because such plaques are substantially more prevalent than stenotic lesions
    - However, risk of single stenotic lesion rupturing and leading to acute event is higher than risk of single nonstenotic plaque
    - Statin therapy, over time, is shown to decrease noncalcified and increase calcified plaque components
- Plaque and stenosis
  - Not all plaques are associated with luminal stenosis

CT Findings

- NECT
  - Coronary calcium is highly specific and fairly sensitive for presence of coronary atherosclerotic plaque
  - Amount of coronary calcium correlates with overall amount of plaques
  - Amount of coronary calcium is associated with risk of future acute coronary syndromes or death
    - Coronary calcium assessment is recommended for risk stratification purposes in some asymptomatic individuals, especially when need for lipid-lowering therapy cannot be clearly determined otherwise
  - Presence of coronary calcium is not necessarily associated with luminal stenosis
- CTA
  - Can identify calcified and noncalcified plaques
  - Some CT features are associated with high-risk plaques (formerly known as vulnerable)
    - Positive remodeling
    - Low CT attenuation
    - Absence of severe calcification: "Spotty" calcification
    - Napkin-ring sign: Ring-like rim of high attenuation around central area of low attenuation
  - High image quality is required to identify and characterize noncalcified coronary plaque on CTA
- Only very small fraction of nonobstructive plaques with high-risk features detected on coronary CTA will cause coronary events in subsequent years
- Overall plaque burden (P) is currently part of **Coronary Artery Disease Reporting and Data System (CAD-RADS) 2.0**
  - Can be quantified by using different methods [Agatston score, segment involvement score (SIS) and visual assessment]
  - P1 (mild): Coronary artery calcium score (CACS) ≤ 100; SIS ≤ 2; visually 1-2 vessels with mild plaque
  - P2 (moderate): CACS 101-300; SIS 3-4; visually 1-2 vessels with moderate or 3 vessels with mild plaque
  - P3 (extensive): CACS 301-999; SIS 5-7; visually 3 vessels with moderate or 1 vessel with extensive plaque
  - P4 (very extensive): CACS > 1000; SIS ≥ 8; visually 2-3 vessels with extensive plaque
- Automated artificial intelligence (AI)-enabled plaque analysis platforms are available
  - Provides individual coronary artery and total plaque volumes including calcified, noncalcified, and low-attenuation plaque volumes
  - Strong correlation with intravascular ultrasound (IVUS)

MR Findings

- Coronary MR has potential for plaque visualization and characterization
  - Spin-echo T2WI
    - Intraplaque lipid appears hyperintense (bright)
    - Muscularis and external elastic laminae are hypointense (dark)
    - Adventitial fat (triglyceride rich) is hyperintense
  - Multispectral imaging
    - T1WI, T2WI, time-of-flight, PDWI techniques combined to identify components
    - Identify calcium, lipid, and hemorrhage
    - Plaque thickness and volume can be quantified
    - Spatial resolution is limited, and image quality is too unreliable for clinical applications
  - Coronary MRA for luminal stenosis
    - Contrast techniques are better than noncontrast SSFP
  - T2 STIR
    - Potential for detecting coronary inflammation
- PET/MR combines benefits of MR and PET

- High-risk coronary plaques in MR
  - Positive remodeling: T1 black-blood imaging
  - Angiogenesis, intraplaque hemorrhage, subclinical plaque rupture: T1 high-intensity plaque imaging
  - Large necrotic core: LGE imaging
  - Microcalcification: F-18 fluoride PET/MR
  - Macrophage infiltration: F-18 FDG PET/MR, ultrasmall superparamagnetic iron oxide (USPIO)

Echocardiographic Findings

- IVUS can detect diseased segments in angiographically normal coronaries
  - Done at time of coronary catheterization
  - Normal intima is not visible
  - Lesion extent: From lumen to external elastic lamina
  - External elastic lamina; echolucent border
  - Can differentiate calcified from noncalcified plaque
  - Detects plaque rupture and erosion with subsequent thrombus formation
  - Can guide percutaneous coronary interventions
    - Enables optimal selection of stent size
    - Prevents incomplete apposition
    - Detects dissection
  - Plaque characterization limited

Angiographic Findings

- Invasive coronary angiography (ICA)
  - Nonstenotic plaque may not be appreciable
  - Mild lumen reductions indicate plaque, but size and extent of plaque cannot be determined
  - Haziness of stenotic segment in coronary angiography suggests thrombus
  - Washed-out cavities can sometimes be detected as consequence of plaque rupture (healed rupture or plaque ulceration)
  - Can be complemented by IVUS, optical coherence tomography (OCT), or angioscopy to characterize plaque

Other Modality Findings

- OCT findings
  - Intraluminal OCT catheter placed at time of ICA
  - Examines interferogram generated by backscatter of coherent light source
  - High-resolution images; can measure on scale of μm
  - Requires blood-free vessel lumen: Contrast agent flush during OCT image acquisition
  - Penetrates only a few mm into vessel wall
  - Very infrequently used in clinical routine for plaque imaging; more frequently used in context of percutaneous coronary interventions
- Angioscopy findings
  - Optical imaging catheter is placed at time of ICA
  - Requires saline flush to clear blood from field
  - Distinguishes lesion type
    - White lesion: Thick, fibrous cap; predominantly fibrous
    - Yellow surface: Lipid-containing lesion with thin, collagenous cap; more likely to rupture
  - Not used in clinical routine

DIFFERENTIAL DIAGNOSIS

Myocardial Bridge

- Intramyocardial course of coronary artery with various degrees of systolic narrowing

Coronary Vasculopathy Post Heart Transplant

- Diffuse and concentric thickening of coronary artery wall
  - Transplant recipients are also predisposed to conventional atherosclerosis: Focal and eccentric

Vasculitis

- Mimics coronary plaque but pathologically distinct
- Extracardiac vasculature usually involved

Spontaneous Coronary Artery Dissection

- Usually isolated to single coronary artery
- Seen in younger patients, often women

PATHOLOGY

General Features

- Detection of plaque
  - Multiple stages of development: From fatty streaks to complex lesions with hemorrhage and calcification
- Histopathology features of vulnerable plaque
  - Large plaque volume; thin, fibrous cap (< 65 μm)
  - Large noncellular lipid core; cap/cap shoulder inflammation
  - Increased monocyte and macrophage content; expression of matrix metalloproteinase

CLINICAL ISSUES

Presentation

- Most coronary atherosclerotic plaques clinically silent
- Plaque rupture or erosion with subsequent luminal thrombosis leads to acute coronary event
- Slow plaque growth, sometimes as consequence of intraplaque hemorrhage or repeated "healed" rupture, can lead to occurrence of coronary artery stenosis and stable coronary artery disease

Treatment

- Lipid-lowering medication to stabilize plaque and prevent further growth
- Antiplatelet therapy (e.g., aspirin) to avoid coronary thrombosis in case of plaque rupture or erosion
  - No data to support medication if plaque is incidentally detected in noninvasive imaging
- Revascularization not justified for plaques without hemodynamically relevant stenosis

SELECTED REFERENCES

1. Narula J et al: Prospective deep learning-based quantitative assessment of coronary plaque by CT angiography compared with intravascular ultrasound. Eur Heart J Cardiovasc Imaging. 25(9):1287-95, 2024
2. Kwiecinski J et al: Noninvasive coronary atherosclerotic plaque imaging. JACC Cardiovasc Imaging. 16(12):1608-22, 2023
3. Mortensen MB et al: Impact of plaque burden versus stenosis on ischemic events in patients with coronary atherosclerosis. J Am Coll Cardiol. 76(24):2803-13, 2020
4. Williams MC et al: Coronary artery plaque characteristics associated with adverse outcomes in the SCOT-HEART Study. J Am Coll Cardiol. 73(3):291-301, 2019

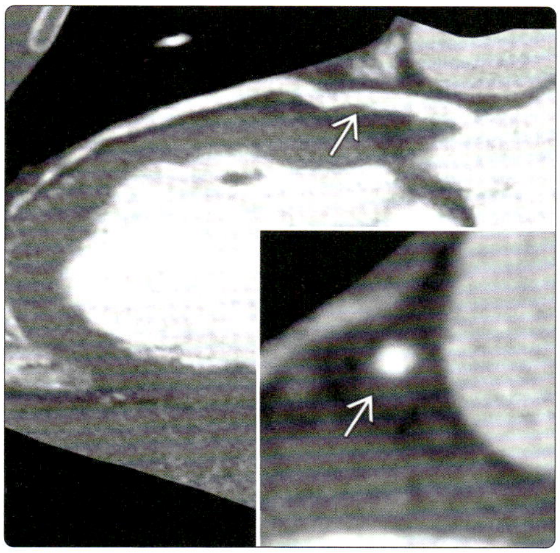

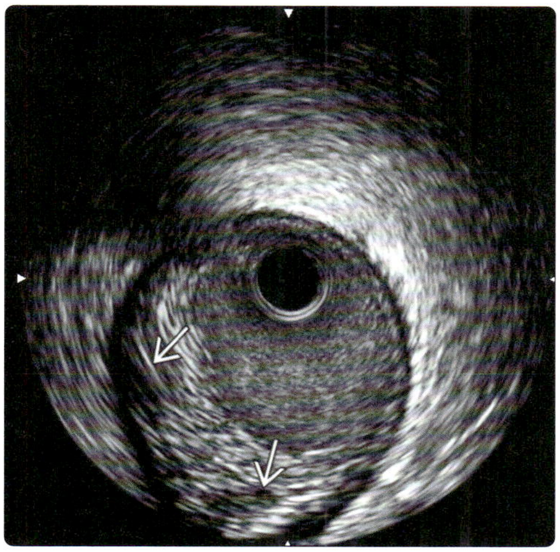

(Left) *Contrast-enhanced coronary CTA shows a completely noncalcified, nonobstructive coronary atherosclerotic plaque ➡ in the proximal left anterior descending coronary artery. The plaque is eccentric and displays positive remodeling.* **(Right)** *Intracoronary US in the same patient shows the coronary atherosclerotic plaque ➡ previously depicted by CTA.*

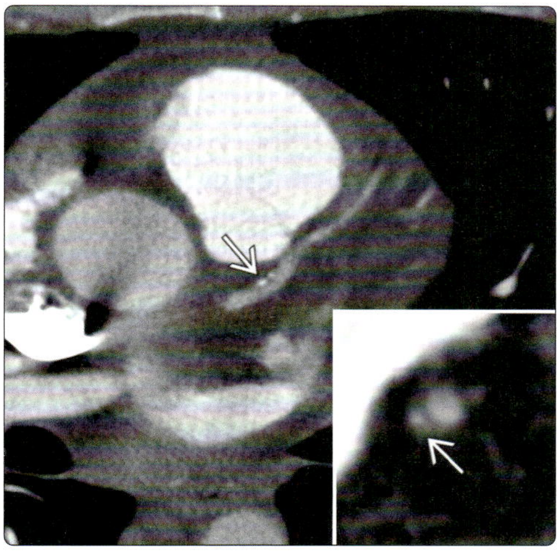

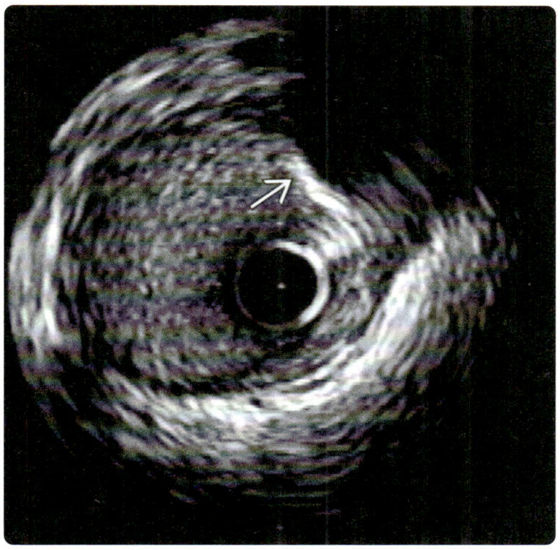

(Left) *Contrast-enhanced coronary CTA shows a partially calcified, nonobstructive coronary atherosclerotic plaque ➡ in the proximal left anterior descending coronary artery.* **(Right)** *Intracoronary US in the same patient shows the partially calcified coronary atherosclerotic plaque ➡ previously depicted by CTA. Intracoronary US is an invasive technique to detect coronary atherosclerotic plaques.*

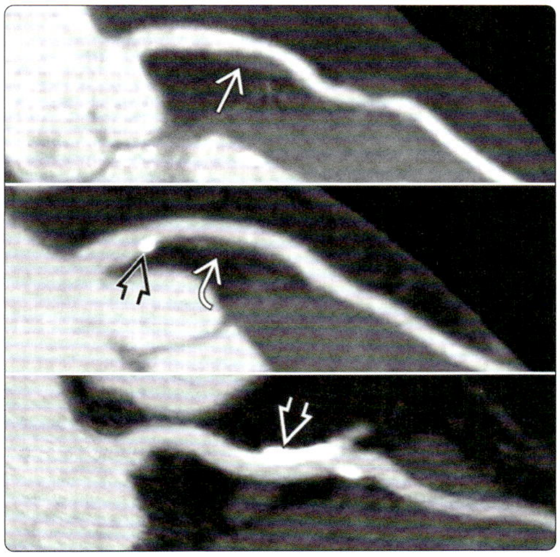

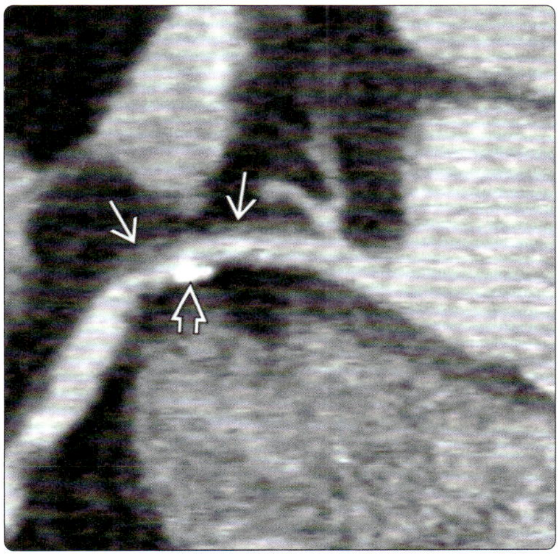

(Left) *Comparison of various types of coronary atherosclerotic plaques, as seen on CECT, shows a noncalcified plaque ➡, a partially calcified plaque with noncalcified ➡ and calcified ⇨ components, and a completely calcified plaque ➡.* **(Right)** *CTA demonstrates a vulnerable plaque ➡ with low density, positive remodeling, and spotty calcification ➡. The 4th and last criterion for vulnerable plaque is napkin-ring sign.*

(Left) *Coronary CTA demonstrates a very large, mostly noncalcified plaque ➡ of the left main and left anterior descending coronary arteries. Even large amounts of a coronary atherosclerotic plaque must not necessarily be associated with a significant luminal stenosis.* **(Right)** *Invasive coronary angiography in the same patient demonstrates absence of detectable luminal narrowing at the site of coronary atherosclerotic plaque ➡ that had been detected by CT.*

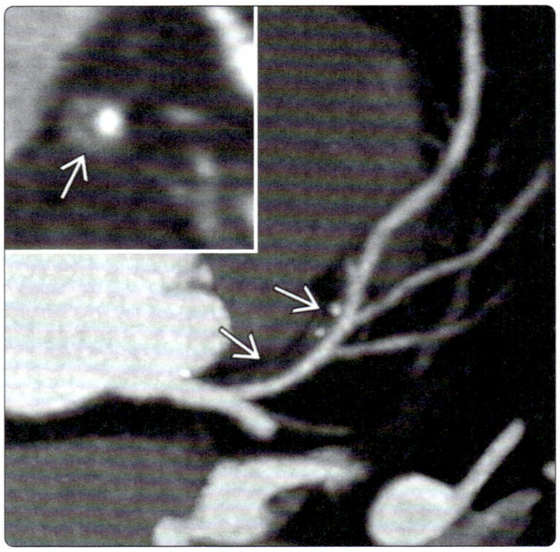

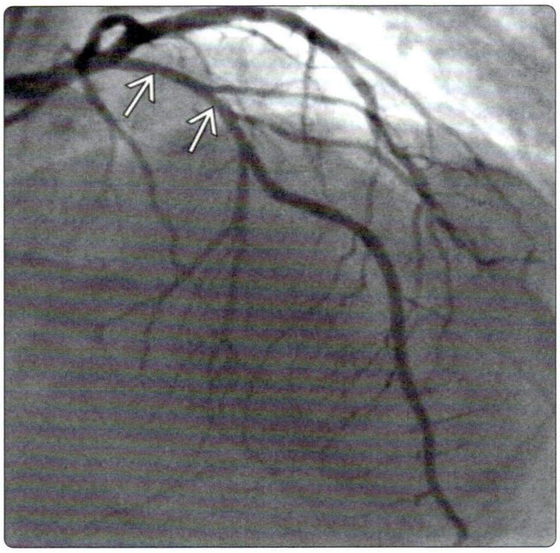

(Left) *Contrast-enhanced coronary CTA shows a transaxial image with an ulcerated plaque. A small cavity caused by a previous plaque rupture is now filled with contrast agent ➡.* **(Right)** *Invasive coronary angiogram in anteroposterior cranial projection in the same patient shows the ulcerated plaque that caused a mild to moderate coronary artery stenosis ➡.*

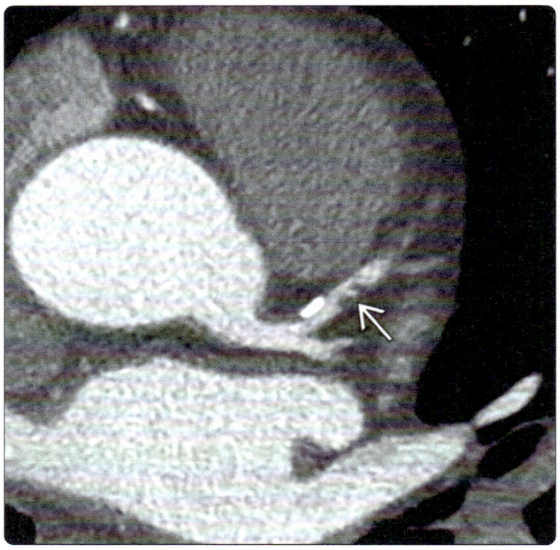

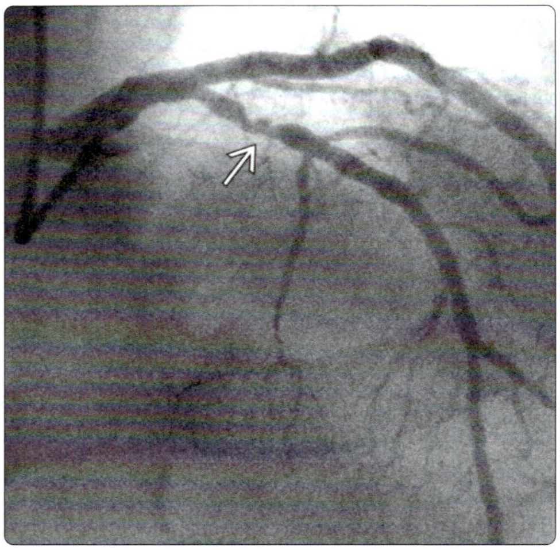

(Left) *Contrast-enhanced coronary CTA shows a curved multiplanar reconstruction of a right coronary artery (proximal and mid segments). Note the ruptured plaque, which has a large cavity filled with contrast agent ➡.* **(Right)** *Contrast-enhanced coronary CTA (oblique MIP) in the same patient shows the midright coronary artery, in which a ruptured plaque can be detected ➡. Note a smaller, calcified plaque in the proximal right coronary artery.*

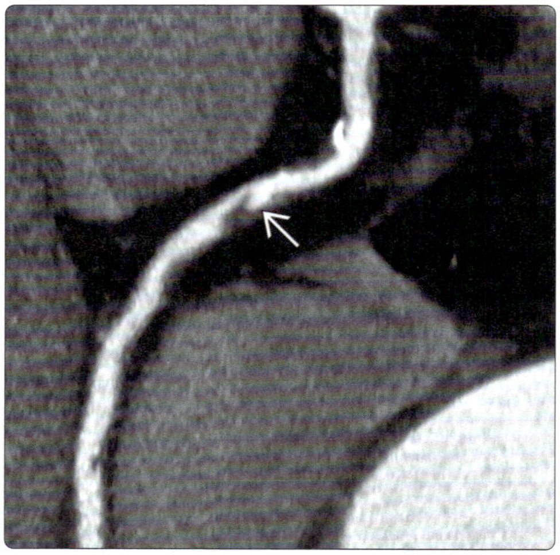

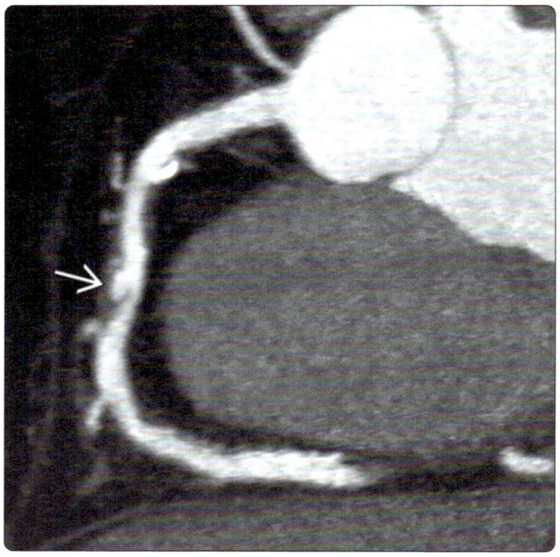

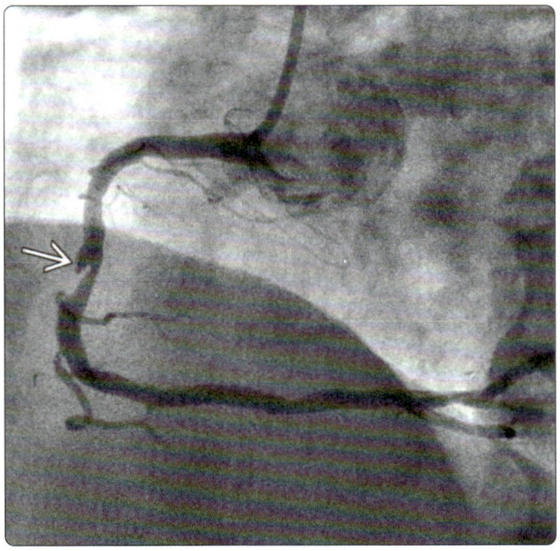

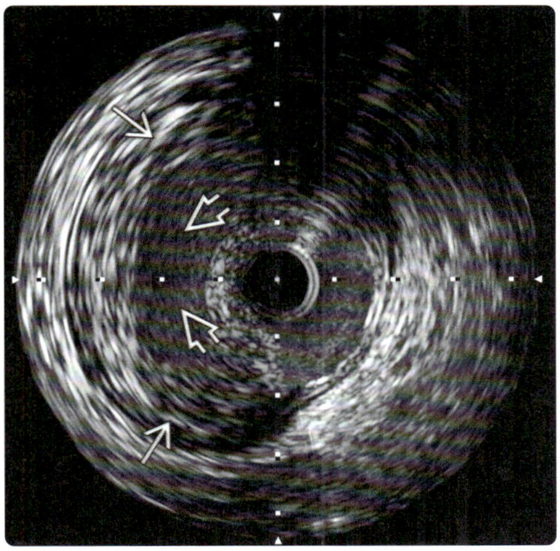

(Left) *Invasive coronary angiography in the same patient in a projection with a similar orientation shows the ulcerated portion of the plaque ➔ filling with contrast material.* **(Right)** *Intravascular US in the same patient shows an eccentric noncalcified coronary atherosclerotic plaque ➔ and, as a consequence of plaque rupture, a washed-out cavity filled with blood ➔. Acute coronary events are mostly caused by rupture of atherosclerotic plaques.*

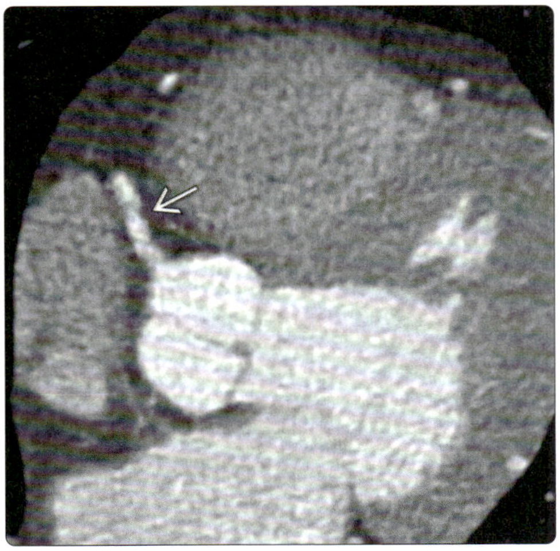

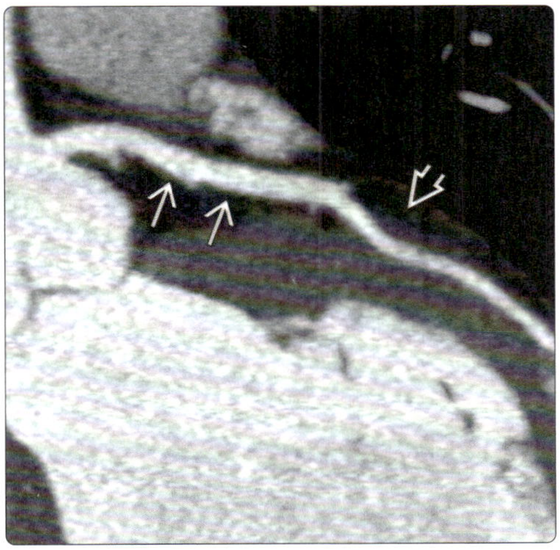

(Left) *Assessing a coronary atherosclerotic plaque via CECT can be difficult. Because of noise ➔, a noncalcified plaque can be neither reliably detected nor excluded on this image.* **(Right)** *Here, slight motion unsharpness ➔ makes it impossible to reliably detect or rule out the presence of small atherosclerotic plaque deposits. Myocardial bridging ➔ can mimic a plaque with positive remodeling.*

Different Methods to Quantify Overall Plaque Burden as Recommended by CAD-RADS 2.0

Plaque Category	Overall Plaque Burden	CAC	SIS	Visual
P1	Mild	1-100	≤ 2	1-2 vessels with mild amount of plaque
P2	Moderate	101-300	3-4	1-2 vessels with moderate amount; 3 vessels with mild amount of plaque
P3	Severe	301-999	5-7	3 vessels with moderate amount; 1 vessel with severe amount of plaque
P4	Extensive	> 1000	≥ 8	2-3 vessels with severe amount of plaque

CAD-RADS = Coronary Artery Disease Reporting and Data System; CAC = coronary artery calcium-Agatston score; SIS = segment involvement score.

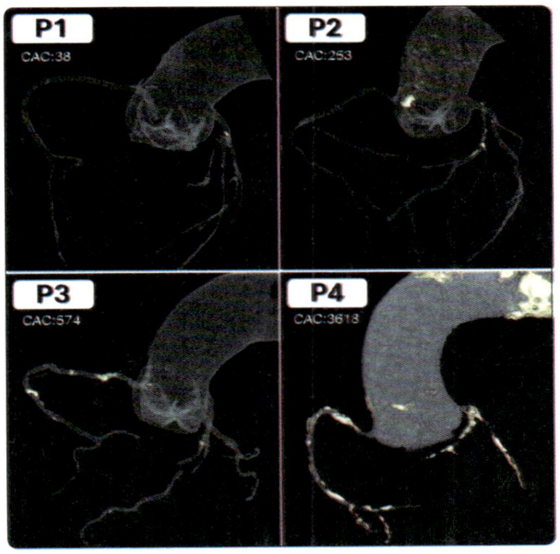

(Left) *New in CAD-RADS 2.0: Semiquantitative overall plaque burden reporting via any of the 3 methods detailed in the table. In the absence of plaque, no P modifier is required, as absence of plaque is implied in the "CAD-RADS 0" denotation.* **(Right)** *3D volume rendered images of coronary trees in 4 different patients demonstrate the distribution and amount of total plaque. The bright areas on the coronary arteries represent calcified plaques. Based on the calcium score, total plaque volume can be categorized into 4 groups; P1-P4.*

KEY FACTS

IMAGING

- **MR**: While CMR for coronary imaging is challenging due to small vessel size and motion, it offers superior soft tissue contrast, no calcium blooming, and no radiation, suggesting the potential for a future alternative to CT. Coronary MRA uses sequences like spoiled gradient-echo or SSFP with gadolinium contrast-enhancing coronary imaging. Advances in alternative contrast agents, such as albumin-binding gadolinium, are improving imaging times and plaque assessment, though MRA still lags behind CT in diagnostic accuracy.
- **CT**: Plaque analysis is most robust for epicardial vessels 2.0 mm or larger. The suggested initial settings are a window width of 800 HU and a level of 300 HU for grayscale differentiation with alternatives like 700 HU/200 HU or 740 HU/220 HU settings. A fixed 0.3-mm gap between the vessel wall and lumen is advised, along with adjusting vessel wall thresholds based on luminal intensity using a 155/65% window width/level.
- **Coronary artery calcium (CAC) scoring**: CAC scoring plays a critical role in evaluating coronary atherosclerosis, enhancing cardiovascular risk assessment, and guiding treatment decisions. This technique helps reclassify individuals at intermediate risk, confirms those at high risk, and informs the use of aspirin and adjustments in statin therapy. CAC testing supports clinical decision making by either confirming a low-risk status or indicating the need for more aggressive management strategies. Furthermore, CAC testing improves adherence to preventive therapies, optimizes risk evaluations, and reduces health care costs by enhancing medication compliance and avoiding unnecessary treatments. It is recommended that CAC scanning be repeated every 5 years for patients with a CAC score of 0, and every 3-5 years for those with a CAC > 0.

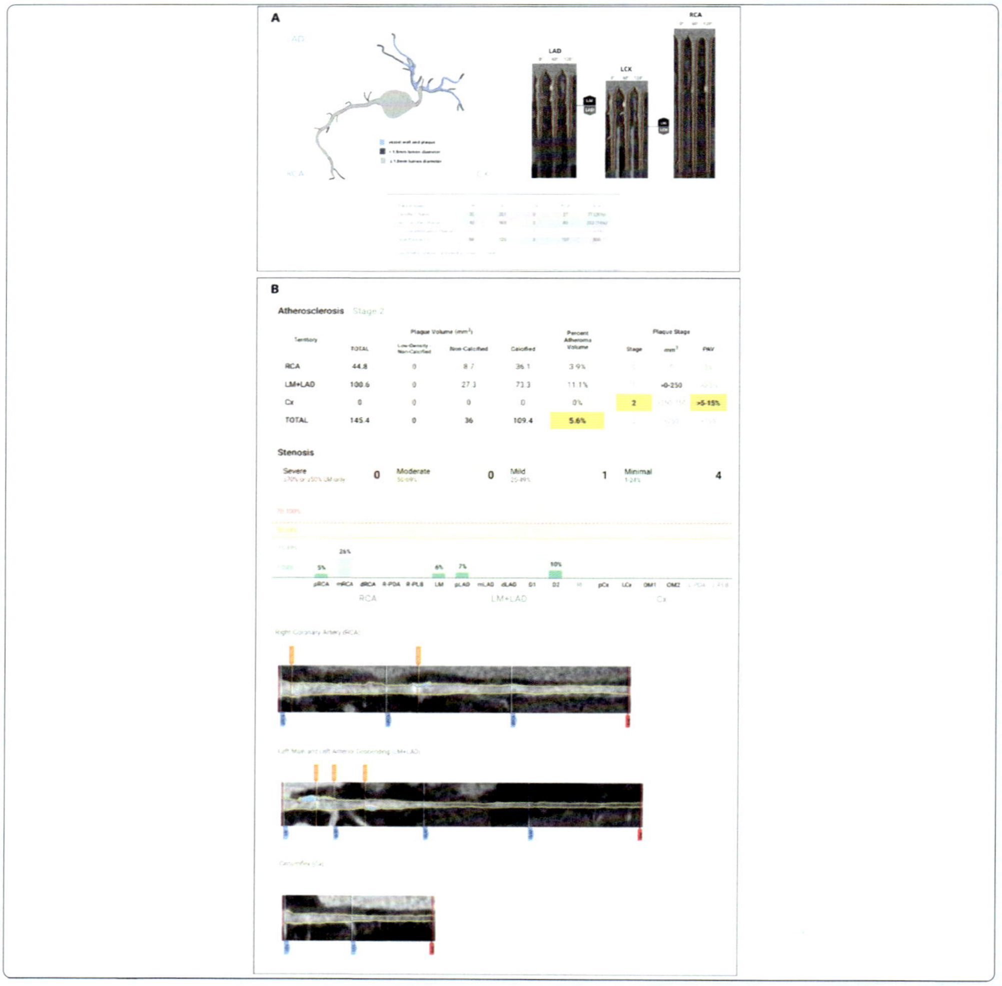

A) An overview example of what coronary artery anatomy and coronary plaque incidence rates look like is shown. B) An epidemiologic review of plaque characteristics and frequency is displayed for familiarity. At the bottom, multiplanar reformatted images demonstrate varying degrees of disease.

BACKGROUND

History of Coronary Plaque Analysis

- The risk of plaque rupture is more strongly associated with its composition than with the extent of stenosis. Pathologic studies indicate that the rupture of lipid-rich plaques, leading to thrombus formation, is the primary cause of acute coronary occlusion in 70-80% of patients with acute coronary syndrome (ACS). This occurs when a thin, fibrous cap ruptures, exposing platelets to the thrombogenic, necrotic core.
- Evolution in understanding disease progression has highlighted the importance of enhancing early detection and intervention, potentially improving outcomes through personalized preventive strategies. Recently, there has been renewed interest in noninvasive techniques, particularly CT, for the early diagnosis of coronary artery disease (CAD) and for functional assessment of stenoses, including analysis of plaque burden, morphology, and associated risk factors. This approach promotes earlier diagnosis and prevention guidance and enables noninvasive identification and prognostication of disease in populations with a higher pretest risk.
- Early studies have shown promising new tools for plaque quantitation, but also revealed wide variability in results between image acquisition and analysis techniques.

IMAGING

Computed Tomography for Asymptomatic Patients

- **Coronary artery calcium (CAC) scoring**: CAC scoring plays a critical role in evaluating coronary atherosclerosis, enhancing cardiovascular risk assessment, and guiding treatment decisions. This technique helps reclassify individuals at intermediate risk, confirms those at high risk, and informs the use of aspirin and adjustments in statin therapy. CAC testing supports clinical decision making by either confirming a low-risk status or indicating the need for more aggressive management strategies. Furthermore, CAC testing improves adherence to preventive therapies, optimizes risk evaluations, and reduces health care costs by enhancing medication compliance and avoiding unnecessary treatments. It is recommended that CAC scanning be repeated every 5 years for patients with a CAC score of 0, and every 3-5 years for those with a CAC > 0.
- **Technique**: The acquisition technique for CAC scanning involves using a CT scanner with 120 kV and 2.5- to 3-mm slice thickness. This method can be applied to both gated and nongated studies to measure the calcified plaque accurately. The CAC-Data and Reporting System (CAC-DRS) is a structured system for reporting CAC findings in noncontrast CT scans. Calcium can be assessed using the Agatston score or through visual estimation.
- **Agatston score**: Based on calcified plaque area and density, the Agatston score is used to categorize CAC risk. Scores are reported as percentiles and traditional categories are
  - 0 (very low risk)
  - 1-99 (mildly increased)
  - 100-299 (moderately increased)
  - 300-1,000 (moderate to severe)
  - > 1,000 (severely increased)
- **CAC-DRS system ranges from**
  - CAC-DRS 0: CAC score = 0 (very low risk)
  - CAC-DRS 1: CAC score 1-99 (mildly increased)
  - CAC-DRS 2: CAC score 100-299 (moderately increased)
  - CAC-DRS 3: CAC score > 300-1,000 (moderately to severely increased)
- **Visual estimation of CAC**: Visual estimation is straightforward and provides significant prognostic value, applicable to noncontrast nongated studies but not recommended for gated CAC scans. It categorizes CAC as
  - None (very low risk): CAC-DRS 0
  - Mild (mildly increased risk): CAC-DRS 1
  - Moderate (moderately increased risk): CAC-DRS 2
  - Severe (moderately to severely increased risk): CAC-DRS 3
  - Primary prophylaxis recommendations for each score
    - CAC-DRS 0: Statin not recommended (except for familial hypercholesterolemia)
    - CAC-DRS 1: Moderate-intensity statin
    - CAC-DRS 2: Moderate- to high-intensity statin + aspirin
    - CAC-DRS 3: High-intensity statin + aspirin
- When reporting the CAC-DRS, it is important to specify the scoring system used (A = Agatston or V = visual), even though the categories have the same implications. The number of vessels with CAC has prognostic value, especially in the CAC range of 1-300, and can influence treatment decisions. If the CAC-DRS grade is not 0, the N modifier should be numbered from 1 to 4.

Coronary Computed Tomography Angiography for Symptomatic Patients

- **Recommended parameters**: Plaque analysis is most robust for epicardial vessels 2.0 mm or larger. The suggested initial settings are a window width of 800 HU and a level of 300 HU for grayscale differentiation with alternatives like 700 HU/200 HU or 740 HU/220 HU settings. A fixed 0.3-mm gap between the vessel wall and lumen is advised, along with adjusting vessel wall thresholds based on luminal intensity using a 155/65% window width/level.
- Plaque analysis is validated for target heart rates of 60-80 BPM and a standard tube voltage of 100-120 kV. Modern techniques, such as dual-energy CT, spectral CT, and photon-counting CT, may add value but require independent validation. For optimal spatial resolution, it is recommended to use thin slices (< 1 mm) with a large matrix size (512 x 512) and a small field of view (≤ 20 cm). Sharp reconstruction kernels may enhance structural detail, although this could increase noise or require higher radiation exposure.

- **Technical aspects of the plaque analysis**: Motion-free images are essential for quantitative studies, achieved by selecting the fastest rotation time and using β-blockers for heart rate and rhythm control. A wider data acquisition window allows for the reconstruction of multiple cardiac phases, reducing the impact of residual cardiac motion. Plaque analysis can be manual or semiautomated, focusing on vessels with a diameter of 2.0 mm or larger due to CT resolution limits, unlike the 1.5-mm threshold used in qualitative coronary CT angiography (CCTA) evaluations. In manual plaque analysis, an expert visually identifies and measures plaques by tracing lumen and vessel boundaries, although small plaques (< 500 μm) may go undetected. A "vessel-wall" display setting, normalized for lumen attenuation, helps distinguish plaque from surrounding epicardial adipose tissue. In semiautomated plaque analysis, computer algorithms segment the vessel, lumen, and epicardial fat, identifying plaque between the vessel's outer contour and lumen, with distinctions between noncalcified and calcified plaques. Manual verification and specification of regions of interest are required. CCTA plaque volume and remodeling results strongly correlate with IV ultrasound, offering high sensitivity (93%) and specificity (92%). Semiautomated segmentation is preferred over manual methods for better reproducibility and practicality.
- Deep learning (DL) models are used for identifying plaque types, quantifying calcium scores, and performing lumen segmentation. Fully automated DL segmentation methods promise faster plaque analysis, although significant obstacles remain. In terms of nomenclature, CCTA uses "plaque" instead of "lesion," and "total plaque volume" (TPV) is preferred over "total atheroma volume" (TAV). The traditional CCTA definition of plaque is tissue measuring 1 mm^2 or more in 2 planes, distinct from the lumen and epicardial fat, whereas for automated tools, it is defined as the space between inner lumen and outer vessel boundaries filled with atherosclerotic tissue. Semiquantitative CCTA plaque analysis classifies plaques as predominantly calcified, predominantly noncalcified, or partially calcified. High-risk features include positive remodeling, napkin-ring sign, low-attenuation plaque, and spotty calcification. Measurement considerations reveal that attenuation values for noncalcified plaques vary and are influenced by contrast enhancement and reconstruction settings, with a threshold of 30 HU often used for low-attenuation plaques.
- Quantitative CCTA plaque analysis involves measuring plaque length from the proximal to the distal normal edge. Plaque tissue types are subclassified based on attenuation values, with thresholds for calcification generally set at > 350 HU. Dense, calcified plaques (> 1,000 HU) may be classified separately due to their lower risk of ACS. Low-attenuation plaques are defined by variable thresholds (30-75 HU), affected by lumen contrast enhancement. Absolute thresholds for low-attenuation plaques are not recommended; instead, scan-specific thresholds based on proximal coronary artery attenuation are advised. In specific situations, such as post revascularization, CCTA is effective in detecting in-stent restenosis (ISR) and graft disease. For bypass graft disease, CCTA accurately detects graft occlusion and is useful for assessing graft failure prevention interventions. In cases involving bifurcation lesions and chronic total occlusions (CTOs), CCTA evaluates plaque and stenosis at bifurcations and identifies total coronary occlusions with scoring systems predicting the difficulty of CTO recanalization.
- **Nonobstructive CAD**: Patients with nonobstructive CAD (1-49% stenosis) have a worse prognosis compared to those with normal CCTA, with an event rate of ~ 1.6% annually. Identifying nonobstructive plaque is crucial, and using the segment involvement score (SIS) can help assess atherosclerosis extent, with an SIS > 5 linked to higher event risk.
- **High-risk plaques**: Thin-cap fibroatheroma features, like large plaque volume and necrotic core, are key in sudden cardiac death. Atherosclerotic plaque composition is categorized by HU density: Necrotic core (-30 to 30 HU), fibro-fatty (31 to 130 HU), fibrous (131 to 350 HU), and dense calcium (> 350 HU). CCTA identifies High-risk plaque features linked to ACS. The CAD-Reporting and Data System (CAD-RADS) classification considers 2 or more of these features in a plaque to indicate higher ACS risk.
  - Positive remodeling: The outer vessel diameter is ≥ 10% the diameter of the normal adjoining segments [remodeling index (RI) > 1.1].
  - Napkin-ring sign: Low CT attenuation at the lumen's edge, surrounded by higher attenuation tissue (suggesting a circumferential necrotic core).
  - Low-attenuation plaque: Central focal area within the plaque with low CT attenuation (usually < 30 HU).
  - Spotty calcification: Calcifications < 3 mm or deposits with a length < 1.5x and width < 2/3 of the vessel diameter.
- **Prognostic**: High-risk plaque on CCTA, present in 15-34% of patients with stable chest pain, is associated with an elevated risk of major cardiac events (MACE). High-risk plaque, particularly with features such as positive remodeling and low-attenuation plaque, raises the likelihood of ACS. However, its predictive value is more effective for short-term risk and may be less robust when compared to the CAC score.

- **Quantitative measures**: Technologic progress in CCTA has introduced semiautomated and artificial intelligence (AI)-powered tools for measuring atherosclerotic plaque, with fully automated methods anticipated for future research applications. Quantitative plaque volume is a strong predictor of future CAD events, especially in ACS and MACE cases. High-risk plaque features and plaque volume are linked to ACS, independent of stenosis. Low-attenuation plaque (< 60 HU) and napkin-ring sign are key predictors of MACE, offering additional prognostic value beyond stenosis. A low-attenuation plaque burden > 4% is the top predictor of incidental myocardial infarction, particularly in nonobstructive CAD patients.
- **Limitations**: Modern CT scanners, with a spatial resolution of ~ 0.5 mm, face challenges in detecting noncalcified plaques because of the small attenuation differences with adjacent fat. There is significant variability in plaque detection compared to stenosis. While quantitative assessment of coronary plaque is possible, it is constrained by long analysis times, inconsistent software standards, and the impact of image quality and acquisition settings on plaque measurement and characterization.
- **CAD-RADS**: CCTA has progressed, and the 2022 CAD-RADS update includes CT-fractional flow reserve (CT-FFR) and myocardial CT perfusion options to enhance standardization, patient management, and communication, complementing detailed physician reports. The CAD-RADS 2.0 categories classify CAD based on stenosis severity, plaque burden, and ischemia, with modifiers for stents, grafts, and high-risk features. This system standardizes reporting to guide clinical management in both stable and acute chest pain cases.
- The CAD-RADS incorporates the "P" score to quantify the total coronary plaque burden, aiding in the assessment of disease severity and guiding treatment decisions. If there is no plaque, the notation "P0" is not necessary. The identification of the amount of plaque can be based on SIS or visual.
- **Modifiers**
  - N (nondiagnostic): Used when the scan does not provide enough information for a clear diagnosis of CAD.
  - S (stent): Indicates the presence of a coronary stent, which can affect the assessment and subsequent treatment recommendations.
  - G (graft): Applied when a coronary artery bypass graft is detected. The bypassed lesion is not considered, but the total plaque burden should also include the grafts.
  - V (vulnerable plaque): Highlights the presence of high-risk or vulnerable plaque features that increase the risk of adverse cardiovascular events.
  - I (ischemia): Shows evidence of ischemia, often identified through additional testing, like CT-FFR or myocardial perfusion imaging, impacting clinical management. I+ (ischemia positive): Used when ischemia is confirmed; CT-FFR ≤ 0.75. I- (ischemia negative): No ischemia is detected, despite any plaque or stenosis; CT-FFR (> 0.80). I+/- (indeterminate ischemia): Ischemia testing is unclear, borderline, or inconclusive; CT-FFR (0.76-0.80).
  - H (high-risk plaque): Denotes the presence of high-risk plaque features, which are associated with an elevated risk of events, such as MI.
  - E (exception): Identifies nonatherosclerotic coronary abnormalities, like dissections or aneurysms.

MR Imaging

- While cardiovascular MR (CMR) for coronary imaging is challenging due to small vessel size and motion, it offers superior soft tissue contrast, no calcium blooming, and no radiation, suggesting the potential for a future alternative to CT. Coronary MR angiography (MRA) uses sequences like spoiled gradient-echo or SSFP, with gadolinium contrast enhancing coronary imaging. Advances in alternative contrast agents, such as albumin-binding gadolinium, are improving imaging times and plaque assessment, though MRA still lags behind CT in diagnostic accuracy.
- Current guidelines recommend coronary MRA for coronary artery anomalies and aortocoronary bypass grafts, particularly due to its ability to visualize coronary ostia and aneurysms without ionizing radiation. However, MRA is less suitable for native coronary arteries due to artifacts and challenges with distal anastomosis.
- **Use of CMR to identify high-risk plaques**: CMR imaging offers several techniques for identifying high-risk plaques. One of these is the detection of positive remodeling in coronary arteries, which is accomplished by measuring the lumen diameter and plaque thickness. However, this method faces limitations due to a high rate of uninterpretable images, and the clinical significance of these findings is still under investigation.
- CMR can also be used for plaque hemorrhage and luminal thrombus detection through noncontrast T1-weighted imaging, which detects methemoglobin, a marker of fresh thrombus. This approach shows promise in identifying high-risk plaques associated with intraplaque hemorrhage and thrombus, achieving sensitivity and specificity rates around 90%. High-intensity plaques identified by this method are linked to an increased risk of cardiovascular events, making it a potentially valuable tool for predicting adverse outcomes in patients with CAD.
- For detecting inflammation and angiogenesis, CMR techniques, such as LGE and STIR imaging, are promising. LGE helps to highlight regions involved in myocardial and carotid atheroma, while STIR imaging identifies areas with increased water content, indicative of inflammation. These methods have demonstrated potential in detecting STIR signals in the culprit coronary arteries of MI patients and regions of persistent inflammation following percutaneous coronary intervention. However, further research is needed to establish their reliability in distinguishing between stable and unstable plaques.
- To assess disease activity, CMR-based tracers, like ultrasmall superparamagnetic particles of iron oxide (USPIOs) and other nanoparticles, are used to target inflammation and angiogenesis in blood vessels, providing valuable insights into atherosclerotic plaque behavior and potential therapeutic applications. Despite these benefits, implementing these technologies in coronary arteries is challenging due to strong blood-pool signals and other technical issues.
- Lastly, hybrid PET/CMR imaging, which combines the molecular imaging capabilities of PET with the superior soft tissue contrast and motion correction of CMR, holds promise for detecting high-risk atherosclerotic plaques. This approach offers advantages, such as reduced radiation exposure and enhanced image accuracy, making it potentially valuable for coronary plaque imaging and tracking disease progression.

- **AI-driven coronary plaque analysis**: This utilizes AI to analyze plaques on CT angiography (CTA) images (Fig 1). It allows the establishment of age- and sex-specific benchmarks for normal and abnormal plaque volumes across different demographics, offering a tailored understanding of patient plaque burden and improving clinical risk stratification. AI enhances risk stratification by providing precise, individualized plaque measurements, helping clinicians predict cardiovascular events, tailor preventive strategies, and define the best test methods.

Other Modalities

- **Coronary angiography**: Coronary angiography remains the gold standard for assessing CAD, primarily due to its ability to quantify the degree of obstruction within the coronary arteries. However, its capacity to determine the hemodynamic significance of these obstructions is limited, particularly in cases of stenoses ranging from 40-80%. The introduction of intravascular imaging techniques has allowed for more accurate physiologic assessment of lesions, providing a clearer understanding of their impact on blood flow.
- When it comes to assessing vulnerable plaques, the limitations of coronary angiography become more evident. While it effectively reveals luminal features, such as stenosis and large calcifications, it is unable to image the vessel wall or capture detailed plaque characteristics, such as lipid cores, plaque erosion, or inflammation. Plaque vulnerability is often associated with lipid accumulation and moderate stenosis, but the relationship between stenosis severity and plaque rupture is inconsistent across studies. Although CAC is linked to plaque rupture, angiography struggles to detect CAC reliably and differentiate between various types of calcifications. High CAC scores do indicate a greater risk of plaque rupture; however, CAC alone cannot confirm plaque vulnerability.
- Coronary angiography can identify complex atherosclerotic lesions, but it has limited sensitivity for detecting thrombi, with a detection rate of only 15-21% of cases. Additionally, the technique does not effectively capture subtle movements within the coronary arteries, such as compression-type coronary artery movement, which may contribute to plaque vulnerability and severe stenosis. Further research is needed to establish the clinical significance of these factors in predicting adverse outcomes.
- **Intracoronary testing**: These innovative techniques focus on the physiologic assessment of lesions and advanced intravascular imaging to provide a more comprehensive anatomic evaluation and improve the assessment of coronary lesions through invasive coronary angiography.
  - FFR: FFR measures the severity of coronary artery stenoses by comparing distal coronary pressure to aortic pressure during hyperemia, which is induced by a drug like adenosine. In a nonobstructed artery, the expected FFR is 1, while an FFR ≤ 0.75 is strongly associated with ischemia. Values between 0.76 and 0.80 are considered within a "gray zone."
  - Instantaneous wave-free ratio (iFR): Nonhyperemic pressure ratios (e.g., iFR) assess coronary stenosis without the need for hyperemic agents. iFR specifically measures the resting distal coronary pressure (Pd) to aortic pressure (Pa) during a specific period in diastole, known as the wave-free period. An iFR value of ≤ 0.89 indicates flow limitation and strongly correlates with an FFR of ≤ 0.8.
  - Ultrasound (IVUS): IVUS provides detailed in vivo information on plaque morphology that standard coronary angiography cannot, enhancing the assessment of CAD. It visualizes the vessel wall, helping to measure stenosis severity, detect calcification, assess remodeling, and evaluate plaque burden. IVUS distinguishes between different plaque components, such as fibrous, lipid-rich, and calcified areas, crucial for identifying high-risk plaques like thin-cap fibroatheromas that are prone to rupture. While IVUS is valuable in guiding percutaneous coronary interventions (PCI), its prognostic value in predicting future cardiovascular events is still under study.
  - Optical coherence tomography (OCT): OCT provides high-resolution imaging of coronary plaques, offering detailed visualization of the vessel wall and plaque structure. It is particularly effective in identifying features like fibrous cap thickness, lipid content, and microcalcifications, which are essential for detecting vulnerable plaques. OCT is valuable in evaluating thin-cap fibroatheromas and assessing plaque disruption or thrombus formation, aiding in the management of CAD. While it significantly improves the guidance of PCI, the long-term prognostic value of OCT in predicting cardiovascular events is still under investigation.

SELECTED REFERENCES

1. Nieman K et al: Standards for quantitative assessments by coronary computed tomography angiography (CCTA): an expert consensus document of the society of cardiovascular computed tomography (SCCT). J Cardiovasc Comput Tomogr. 18(5):429-43, 2024
2. Tzimas G et al: Age- and sex-specific nomographic CT quantitative plaque data from a large international cohort. JACC Cardiovasc Imaging. 17(2):165-75, 2024
3. Cury RC et al: CAD-RADS™ 2.0 - 2022 Coronary Artery Disease-Reporting and Data System: an expert consensus document of the Society of Cardiovascular Computed Tomography (SCCT), the American College of Cardiology (ACC), the American College of Radiology (ACR), and the North America Society of Cardiovascular Imaging (NASCI). JACC Cardiovasc Imaging. 15(11):1974-2001, 2022
4. Legutko J et al: Intracoronary imaging of vulnerable plaque-from clinical research to everyday practice. J Clin Med. 11(22):6639, 2022
5. Mintz GS et al: Clinical utility of intravascular imaging: past, present, and future. JACC Cardiovasc Imaging. 15(10):1799-820, 2022
6. Tehrani DM et al: Understanding fractional flow reserve/instantaneous wave-free ratio discordance can provide coronary clarity. J Am Heart Assoc. 11(9):e026118, 2022
7. Serruys PW et al: Coronary computed tomographic angiography for complete assessment of coronary artery disease: JACC state-of-the-art review. J Am Coll Cardiol. 78(7):713-36, 2021

CAD-RADS

	Stenosis	Investigation	Management
CAD-RADS 0	0% (no plaque or stenosis) Interpretation: Absence of CAD	None	Reassurance Consider nonatherosclerotic causes of symptoms
CAD-RADS 1	1-24% (minimal or no stenosis) Interpretation: Minimal nonobstructive CAD	None	Consider nonatherosclerotic causes of symptoms P1: Consider risk factor modification and preventive therapy P2: Risk factor modification and preventive therapy P3 or P4: Aggressive risk factor modification and preventive therapy
CAD-RADS 2	25-49% (mild stenosis) Interpretation: Mild nonobstructive CAD	None	Consider nonatherosclerotic causes of symptoms P1 or P2: Risk factor modification and preventive therapy P3 or P4: Aggressive risk factor modification and preventive therapy
CAD-RADS 3	50-69% (moderate stenosis) Interpretation: Moderate stenosis	Consider functional assessment	P1-P4: Aggressive risk factor modification and preventive therapy Consider other anginal treatments (antianginal therapy) if modifier is present; consider ICA, especially if symptoms persist after medical therapy
CAD-RADS 4	4A: 70-99% 4B: Left main > 50% or 3-vessel obstructive (> 70%) disease Interpretation: Severe stenosis	A: Consider ICA or functional assessment B: ICA is recommended	P1-P4: Aggressive risk factor modification and preventive therapy Consider other anginal treatments, including antianginal therapy and revascularization, per guidelines
CAD-RADS 5	100% (total occlusion) Interpretation: Total or subtotal occlusion	Consider ICA, functional &/or viability assessment	P1-P4: Aggressive risk factor modification and preventive therapy Consider other anginal treatments, including antianginal therapy and revascularization, per guidelines
CAD-RADS N	Nondiagnostic study	Additional or alternative evaluation may be needed	

ICA = internal carotid artery; CAD-RADS = Coronary Artery Disease Reporting and Data System.

Plaque Burden Quantification

	Amount of Plaque	Segment Involvement Score	Visual
P1	Mild	≤ 2	1-2 vessels with mild amount of plaque
P2	Moderate	3-4	1-2 vessels with moderate amount of plaque 3 vessels with mild amount of plaque
P3	Severe	5-7	3 vessels with moderate amount of plaque 1 vessel with severe amount of plaque
P4	Extensive	≥ 8	2-3 vessels with severe amount of plaque

Agatston and Visual Reporting Examples

Agatston Scoring	CAC-DRS Category
i. CAC 0	CAC-DRS AO
ii. CAC 1-99 in LM, LAD, and LCx	CAC-DRS A1/N3
iii. CAC 100 -299 in LAD, LCx, and RCA	CAC-DRS A2/N3
iv. CAC > 300 in LM, LAD, LCx, and RCA	CAC-DRS A3/N4
Visual Score	
i. CAC 0	CAC-DRS V0
ii. CAC 1 in LM, LAD, and LCx	CAC-DRS V1/N3
iii. CAC 2 in LAD, LCx, and RCA	CAC-DRS V2/N3
iv. CAC 3 in LM, LAD, LCx, and RCA	CAC-DRS V3/N4

LM = left main; LAD = left anterior descending; LCx = left circumflex; RCA = right coronary artery; CAC-DRS = Coronary Artery Calcium Data and Reporting System.

CAD-RADS 1/P1

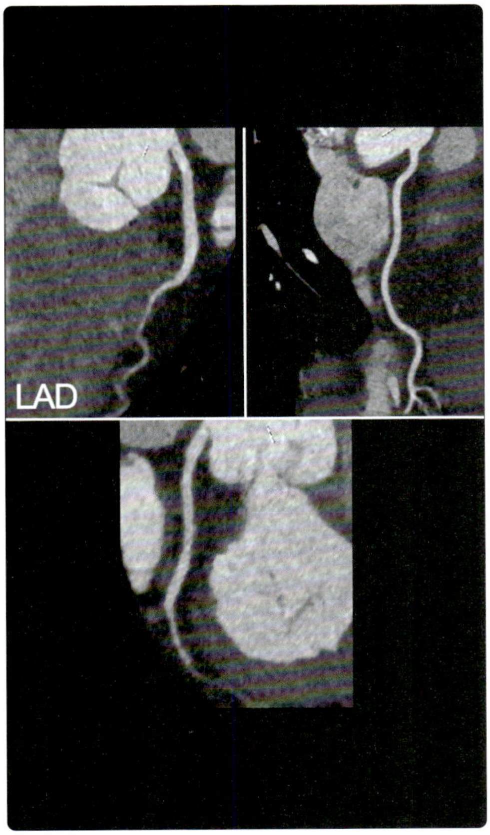

CAD-RADS 2/P2

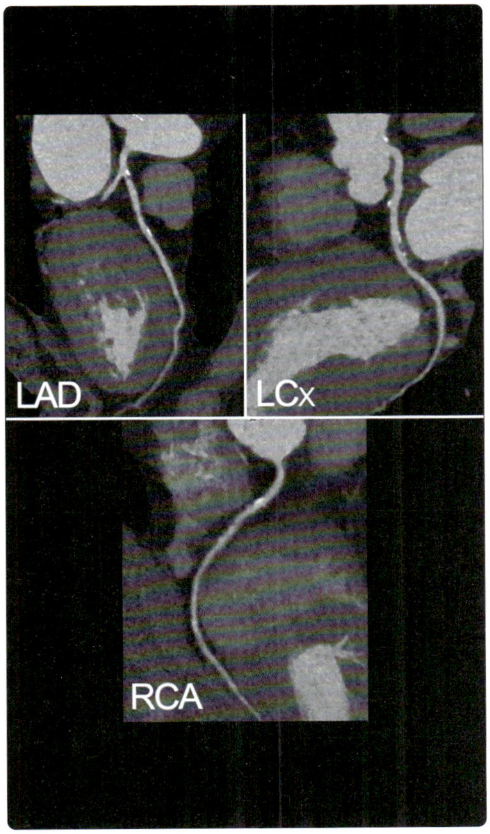

(Left) *CT angiogram images show minimal (1-24%) nonobstructive coronary artery atherosclerosis. The overall coronary artery calcium score is 0.* **(Right)** *CT angiogram shows mild (25-49%) nonobstructive coronary artery atherosclerosis. There are no significant luminal stenoses. The overall coronary artery calcium score is 170. The Agatston score for each vessel is as follows: Left main: 47 (not shown), left anterior descending (LAD): 26, left circumflex (LCx): 23, right coronary artery (RCA): 74. Overall, there is a medium amount of plaque.*

CAD-RADS 2/P3

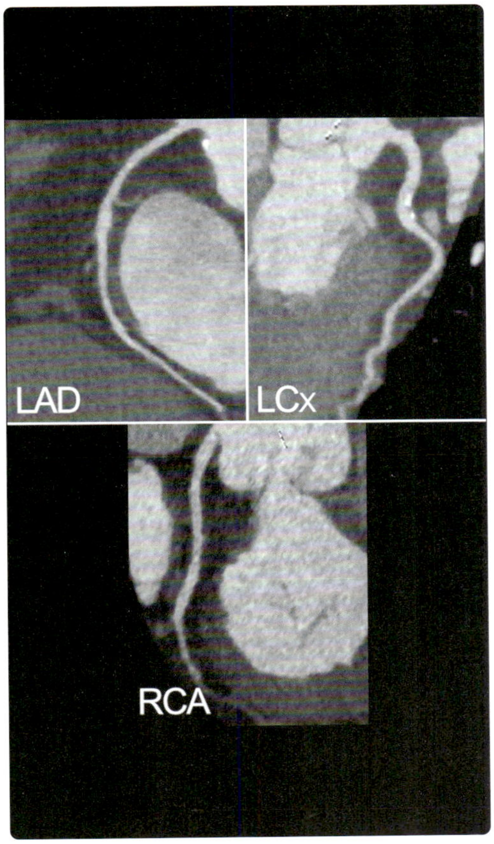

CAD-RADS 3/P4

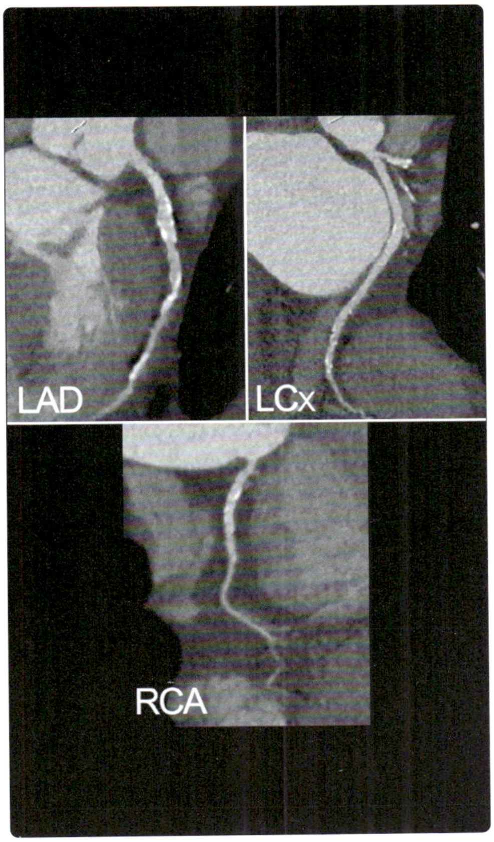

(Left) *CT angiogram shows mild (25-49%) nonobstructive coronary artery atherosclerosis. There are no significant luminal stenoses. The overall coronary artery calcium score is 393. The Agatston score for each vessel is as follows: Left main (not shown): 157, LAD: 130, LCx: 95, RCA: 11. Overall, there is a large amount of plaque.* **(Right)** *CT angiogram shows moderate (50-69%) stenosis of the mid and distal segments of the LAD coronary artery, origin of the 1st diagonal branch coronary artery, and distal LCx. The overall coronary artery calcium score is 2,486. The Agatston score for each vessel is as follows: Left main (not shown): 53, LAD: 1,415, LCx: 764, RCA: 254. Overall, there is a very large amount of plaque.*

Coronary Thrombosis

KEY FACTS

TERMINOLOGY

- Obstruction/occlusion of coronary artery by thrombus, usually due to plaque rupture

IMAGING

- Coronary angiography shows complete occlusion of coronary artery or stenosis of varying degree
  - Thrombus may be visible as filling defect or haziness if occlusion is not complete
  - Occasionally, coronary artery side branch that is completely occluded at its origin may not be visible in invasive angiography; diagnosis may be missed
- Coronary CTA shows low-density material within coronary lumen
  - Thrombus may completely occlude coronary lumen
  - Thrombus may be surrounded by contrast agent
  - Often pronounced positive remodeling (i.e., increase in coronary artery diameter) at site of thrombosis

TOP DIFFERENTIAL DIAGNOSES

- Similar imaging findings
  - Embolic coronary occlusion
  - Type III spontaneous coronary dissection
  - Stable coronary artery disease
- Similar symptoms can be seen with aortic dissection, pulmonary embolism, stress-induced cardiomyopathy, myocarditis, and pericarditis

PATHOLOGY

- Initiating event commonly break of thinned fibrous cap

CLINICAL ISSUES

- Causes acute coronary syndrome
  - ST-elevation or non-ST elevation myocardial infarction
  - Unstable angina
  - Nonobstructive plaque rupture may be asymptomatic
- High mortality if untreated
- Can occur at multiple sites in coronary artery tree

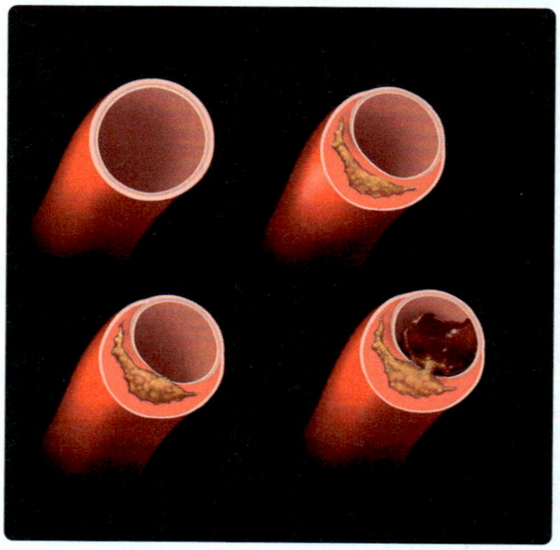

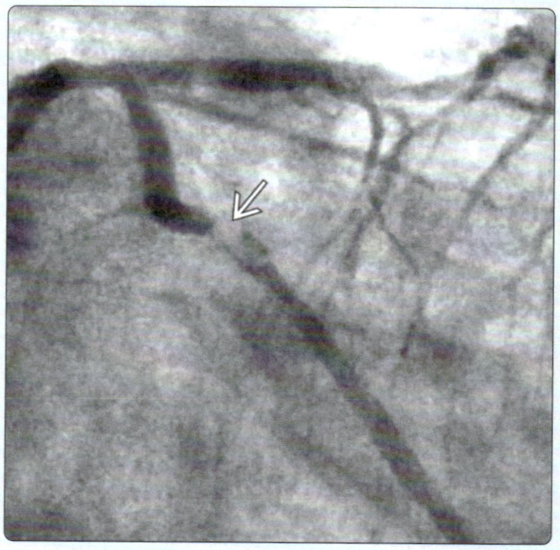

(Left) *Graphic depicts the pathogenesis of intracoronary thrombosis. Atherosclerotic plaque (top right) can develop in a normal coronary arterial wall (top left). The fibrous cap that covers the necrotic core of plaque can rupture (bottom left). When thrombogenic plaque material contacts the blood stream (bottom right), thrombosis occurs instantaneously, and an acute coronary syndrome may ensue.* **(Right)** *Invasive coronary angiogram shows plaque rupture with a subsequent thrombus ➡ in the left circumflex artery.*

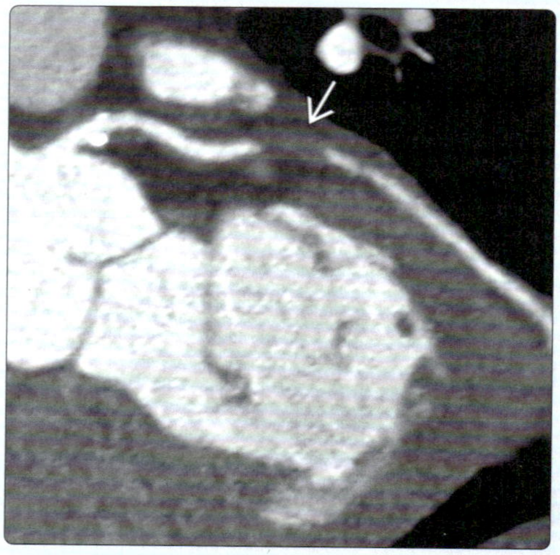

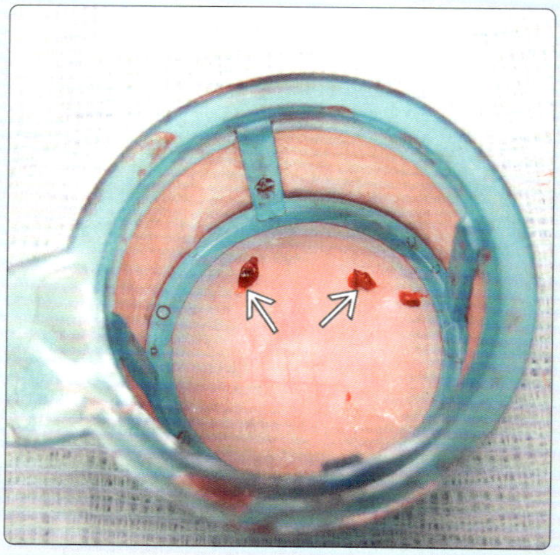

(Left) *Coronary CECT angiogram in the same patient demonstrates an acute obstructive focal lesion with an enlarged vessel diameter, the typical CT appearance of coronary thrombosis. The lumen is filled with low-density material ➡ (thrombosis).* **(Right)** *Intracoronary thrombus aspiration during an invasive coronary angiogram in the same patient produced several small thrombotic particles ➡.*

TERMINOLOGY

Definitions

- Obstruction/occlusion of coronary artery by thrombus
  - Usually consequence of plaque rupture

IMAGING

General Features

- Best diagnostic clue
  - Abrupt cutoff of coronary lumen on coronary angiography accompanied by acute symptoms
  - Thrombus may be visible as filling defect or haziness if occlusion is not complete

CT Findings

- CTA
  - Coronary CTA shows low-density material within coronary lumen
    - May completely occlude coronary lumen
    - May be surrounded by contrast agent
  - Often pronounced positive remodeling (i.e., increase in coronary artery diameter) at site of thrombosis
  - Occasionally, coronary artery side branch ostial occlusion may be missed on CTA

MR Findings

- T2WI
  - T2 hyperintensity corresponds to periinfarct myocardial edema
- LGE imaging
  - May exclude or detect and quantify transmural extent of myocardial infarction (MI) resulting from acute coronary thrombosis
- SSFP
  - Used to detect wall motion abnormality
- Direct visualization of thrombus
  - Experimental studies can visualize thrombus directly using MR
    - Nonenhanced T1 black-blood images
      - High signal due to methemoglobin within evolving thrombus or intraplaque hemorrhage
- Coronary MRA with 3D free-breathing navigator-gated sequences
  - Using fibrin-binding contrast agent, EP-2104R
  - May aid in thrombus detection in future

Nuclear Medicine Findings

- **18F-GP1 PET/CT** uses novel fluorine-18 labeled analogue of elarofiban, which is glycoprotein IIb/IIIa receptor antagonist-based radiotracer
  - 18F-GP1 binds to fresh platelet-rich thrombus
  - Single-center, observational, case-controlled study showed excellent sensitivity (100%) and specificity (80%) when used in conjunction with coronary CTA to find culprit lesions in acute MI
  - No 18F-GP1 uptake in nonculprit coronary artery lesions or additional atherosclerotic disease
  - Needs to be imaged in early stages of MI (within 7 days) to avoid false-negative results
  - Intramyocardial hemorrhage or microvascular occlusion can cause false-positive results

Intracoronary Imaging Findings

- Intravascular ultrasound (IVUS) shows characteristic hypoechogenic filling defect within coronary lumen
- Optical coherence tomography (OCT) shows irregular, hyperintense filling defect

Echocardiographic Findings

- Echocardiogram
  - Ancillary findings
    - Regional wall motion abnormality of left ventricle
    - Reduced ejection fraction
    - Hyperkinesis of remaining left ventricular walls is possible

Angiographic Findings

- Conventional
  - Coronary angiography shows complete occlusion or stenosis of coronary artery
  - Thrombus may be visible as filling defect or haziness if occlusion is not complete
- Fiberoptic angioscopy allows direct visualization of intraluminal thrombus, but it is not clinically used modality
- Occasionally, coronary artery side branch ostial occlusion may be missed on angiography

Imaging Recommendations

- Best imaging tool
  - Invasive
    - Coronary angiography, in questionable cases complemented by IVUS or OCT
  - Noninvasive
    - Coronary CTA

DIFFERENTIAL DIAGNOSIS

Embolus

- While most coronary thrombotic lesions occur as consequence of plaque rupture, embolism is potential source of thrombus

Spontaneous Coronary Artery Dissection

- Type II most common, usually long segment and multifocal
- Type I is focal lesion that can mimic plaque rupture
  - IVUS or OCT needed to confirm diagnosis
- Commonly occurs in younger patients, F > M, with arteriopathy, pregnancy, connective tissue disease, etc.

Cocaine Abuse

- Nonatherosclerotic cause of coronary artery thrombosis
- Possible consequences include dissection and plaque rupture with coronary thrombosis
- Suspect in young patients with MI

Aortic Dissection and Pulmonary Embolism

- Similar clinical presentation as acute coronary syndromes (acute chest pain)
- Similar ECG findings and increased troponins possible
- Easily differentiated with CTA

Myocarditis and Pericarditis

- Similar clinical presentation with strong, exercise-independent chest pain
- Similar ECG findings and increased troponins possible

- Invasive angiography or CT may be performed to rule out coronary obstruction
- MR may demonstrate myocarditis and pericarditis

Stress-Induced Cardiomyopathy

- Often preceded by emotional stress
- Severe wall motion abnormality in left ventricle, usually in apical region, but other regions can be affected
- Not associated with coronary obstruction
- Recedes spontaneously within several days

Kawasaki Disease

- Coronary artery aneurysms can thrombose
- Occurs in younger patients

Vasculitis (Autoimmune)

- May lead to artery occlusion ± thrombus
- Most often part of systemic disease
- Systemic lupus erythematous; rheumatoid arthritis

Takayasu Arteritis

- Most commonly large vessels (aorta and great vessels)
- Can affect coronary circulation
  - If so, coronary ostia are usually involved

PATHOLOGY

General Features

- Etiology
  - Rupture or, infrequently, erosion of coronary atherosclerotic plaque
- White thrombus (platelet rich) with secondary areas of red thrombus formation (red cells, thrombin, fibrin)
- Can occur at multiple sites in coronary artery tree
- Occasionally, thrombus can form without plaque rupture inside ectatic and aneurysmal coronary arteries

Staging, Grading, & Classification

- Coronary artery thrombosis may cause
  - Ischemia with myocardial necrosis
    - Caused by complete occlusion of coronary artery or downstream embolization of thrombotic material
    - Clinically, ST-elevation MI (STEMI) or non-ST elevation MI (NSTEMI)
  - Ischemia without myocardial necrosis
    - Due to incomplete occlusion or collaterals
    - Clinically unstable angina
  - Clinically silent

Gross Pathologic & Surgical Features

- Vulnerable plaques: Coronary atherosclerotic plaques with high likelihood to rupture and cause acute coronary event
  - Most frequently (but not exclusively) localized in proximal segments of coronary arteries

Microscopic Features

- Histologic features predisposing plaque to rupture and cause acute coronary events
  - Thin, fibrous cap (< 65 μm)
  - Large necrotic core (NC)
  - Large plaque volume and positive remodeling
    - Medial and adventitial inflammation weakens arterial wall → outward expansion (positive remodeling)
    - Increases tension on fibrous cap, which itself may be thinned due to inflammation
- Common initiating event is break of thinned fibrous cap
  - Intraplaque hemorrhage common inciting factor
    - Intraplaque hemorrhage into NC → increased pressure in NC → increased pressure on thin fibrous cap → plaque rupture
- Exposes thrombogenic plaque content to blood stream → thrombus formation

CLINICAL ISSUES

Presentation

- Most common signs/symptoms
  - Acute chest pain; dyspnea; indigestion (inferior wall infarction); arrhythmias
- Other signs/symptoms
  - Pallor
  - Diaphoresis
  - Hypotension
- Clinical profile
  - Risk factors
    - Previously known coronary artery disease
    - Older age
    - Smoking
    - Hyperlipidemia
    - Diabetes
    - Family history of premature coronary artery disease
    - Male sex or postmenopausal female sex
    - Hypertension

Demographics

- Sex
  - Mortality rate among men and women is equal
- Ethnicity
  - Coronary thrombosis with MI has higher incidence in Black population than in White population

Natural History & Prognosis

- Acute coronary syndrome has high mortality if untreated

Treatment

- Analgesia
- Antiplatelet and antithrombotic medical therapy
- Reperfusion: Interventional
  - Coronary angiography and percutaneous coronary intervention
- Medical: Thrombolysis
- Long term: Modification of cardiovascular risk factors
  - Statins
  - ACE inhibitors
  - Antihypertensive medication

SELECTED REFERENCES

1. Tzolos E et al: Noninvasive in vivo coronary artery thrombus imaging. JACC Cardiovasc Imaging. 16(6):820-32, 2023
2. Whittington B et al: Imaging of intracoronary thrombus. Heart. 109(10):740-7, 2023
3. Benjamin EJ et al: Heart disease and stroke statistics-2018 update: a report from the American Heart Association. Circulation. 137(12):e67-492, 2018
4. Goyal P et al: Cardiovascular magnetic resonance imaging for assessment of cardiac thrombus. Methodist Debakey Cardiovasc J. 9(3):132-6, 2013

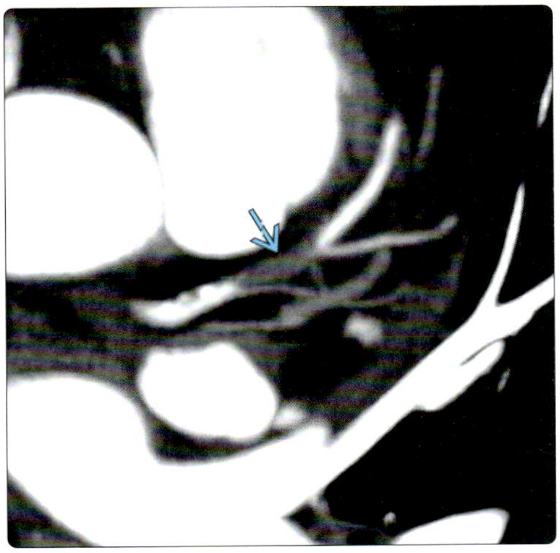

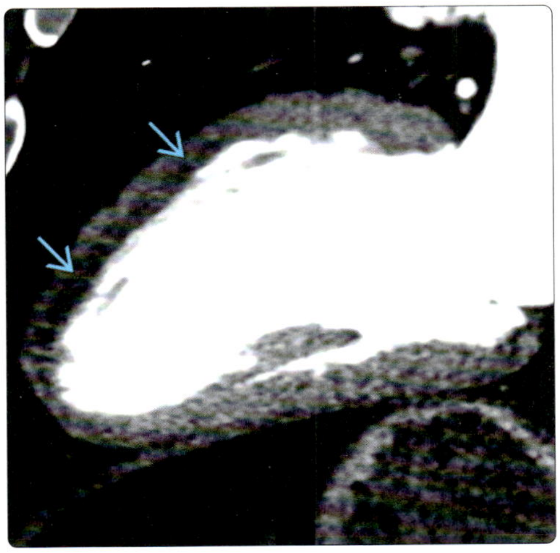

(Left) *Axial oblique MIP CECT in a 52-year-old man undergoing preoperative planning for a percutaneous coronary artery bypass grafting (CABG) procedure shows coronary thrombus in the proximal left anterior descending artery due to plaque rupture occluding the lumen.* **(Right)** *Two-chamber minIP CECT in the same patient shows subendocardial hypoperfusion in the left anterior descending artery territory due to myocardial infarction. (Courtesy S. Kligerman, MD.)*

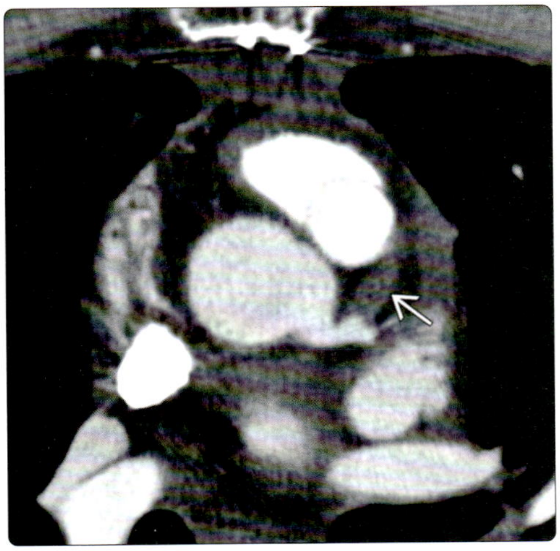

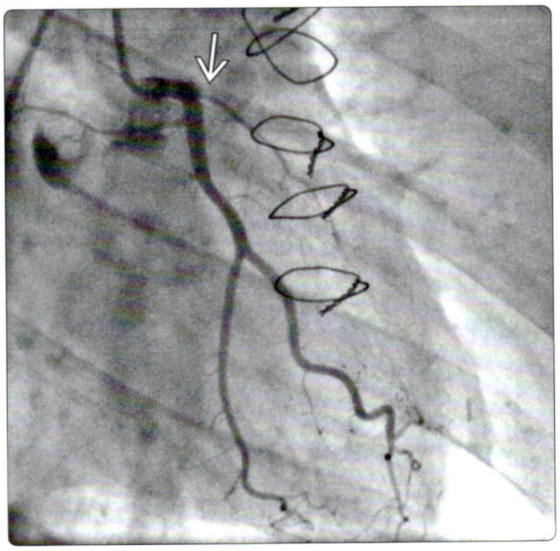

(Left) *Coronary CECT angiogram demonstrates an acute thrombotic occlusion of the ostial left anterior descending coronary artery, leading to an ST-segment elevation myocardial infarction.* **(Right)** *Invasive coronary angiogram in the same patient shows the ostial occlusion of the left anterior descending coronary artery. Only the left main and left circumflex coronary arteries are open.*

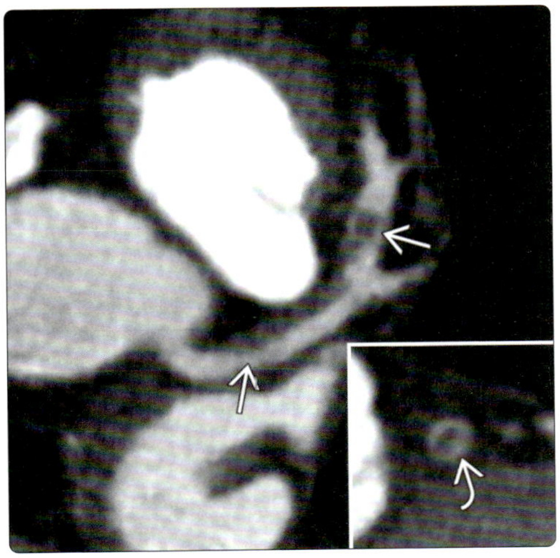

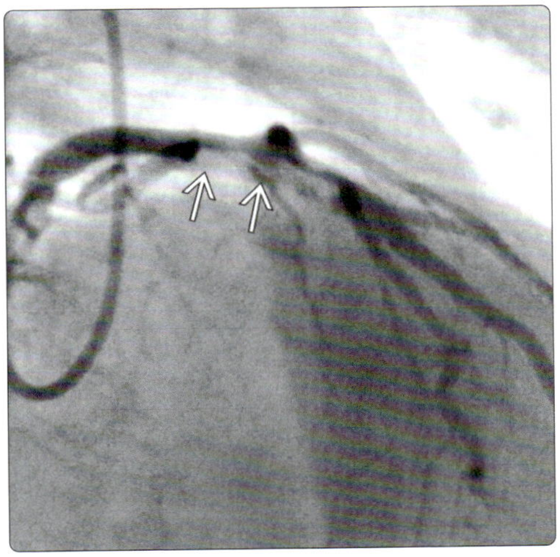

(Left) *Coronary CECT angiogram shows a large thrombus extending from the left main coronary artery to the left anterior descending coronary artery. The cross-section inset reveals the typical pattern of a central filling defect surrounded by contrast.* **(Right)** *Coronary thrombosis can lead to total vessel occlusion, as seen here in this invasive coronary angiogram showing an occlusion of the distal right coronary artery.*

Coronary Artery Stenosis

KEY FACTS

TERMINOLOGY

- Fixed obstructive coronary artery disease (CAD) that typically causes symptoms during exercise
  - Often termed stable CAD
  - More recent alternative = "chronic coronary syndrome"

IMAGING

- Testing for coronary artery stenosis
  - Direct visualization of coronary arteries (invasive angiography, coronary CT angiography)
  - Testing for ischemia (MR, nuclear medicine, stress echocardiography, CT perfusion)
- Coronary artery stenoses are traditionally assumed to be hemodynamically relevant when > 70% diameter stenosis is present (50% if left main coronary artery)
  - However, correlation between anatomic stenosis severity and hemodynamic relevance is poor
  - With exception of > 90% stenosis in left main or proximal left anterior descending (LAD), guidelines require proof of ischemia
- Choice of testing modality is influenced by patient characteristics and pretest probability of CAD
- Traditionally, guidelines mandated testing for ischemia as 1st diagnostic test in suspected CAD
  - Based on recent guidelines, coronary CT angiography is now also considered possible 1st test
  - Class Ia recommendation in intermediate-risk patients with no known CAD in setting of both acute and stable chest pain

CLINICAL ISSUES

- Common symptoms: Shortness of breath or chest, shoulder, neck, or jaw pain of tight and oppressive character, reproducible with exertion and relieved by several minutes rest or nitrates
- Treatment: Prevention of coronary artery events and symptom relief

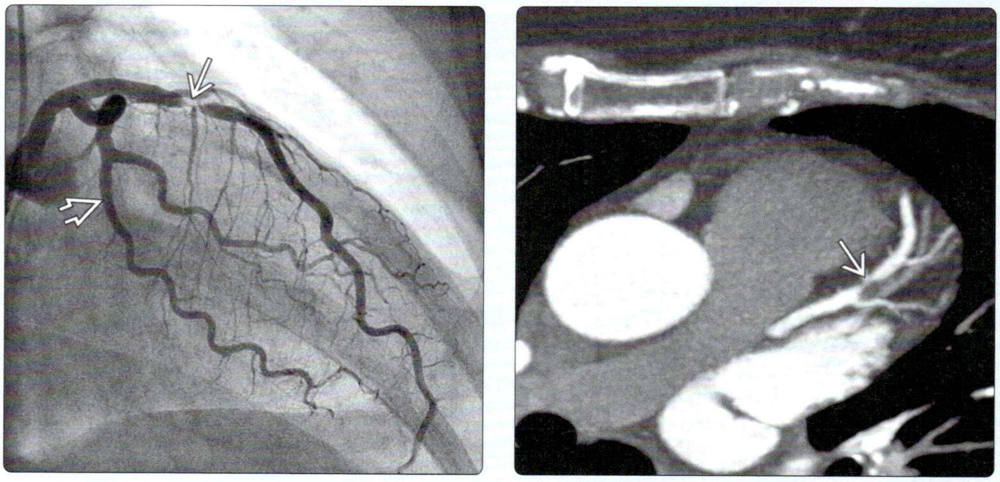

(Left) *Invasive coronary angiography of the left coronary system (left main injection) shows the left anterior descending (LAD) coronary artery with a high-grade stenosis ➡ and normal left circumflex coronary artery ⇨.* **(Right)** *Coronary CT angiography MIP in the same patient shows a high-grade stenosis of the LAD coronary artery ➡ caused by a noncalcified atherosclerotic plaque.*

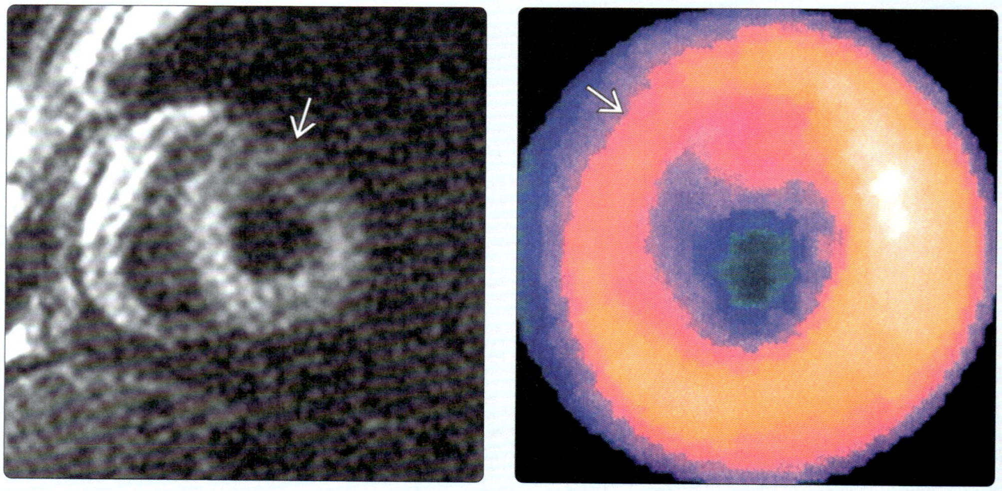

(Left) *First-pass perfusion hybrid gradient-echo-planar MR shows a perfusion defect ➡ in the anterior segment left ventricular myocardium corresponding to the LAD coronary artery vascular territory.* **(Right)** *Stress myocardial perfusion SPECT shows a perfusion defect in the anterior wall ➡, indicating a hemodynamically relevant stenosis of the LAD coronary artery.*

TERMINOLOGY

Definitions

- Fixed obstructive coronary artery disease (CAD)
  - Often termed stable CAD
  - Sometimes referred to as chronic coronary syndrome

IMAGING

General Features

- Traditionally assumed to be hemodynamically relevant when > 70% diameter stenosis is present
- Correlation of anatomic stenosis severity and hemodynamic relevance is poor
  - Fractional flow reserve (FFR) has replaced angiography as reference standard to establish significance (i.e., hemodynamic relevance) of coronary artery stenosis
  - FFR < 0.80 is considered hemodynamically significant and benefits from revascularization
  - Coronary lesions with FFR > 0.80, even if angiographically severely stenotic do not benefit from revascularization

Radiographic Findings

- Radiography
  - Coronary artery calcification may be visible in chest radiography and fluoroscopy, indicating coronary atherosclerosis

CT Findings

- NECT
  - Coronary calcium
    - Definitive for presence of coronary artery atherosclerosis but not for presence of hemodynamically relevant stenosis
    - Absence of coronary calcium makes obstructive CAD unlikely but not impossible
    - Associated with risk for future cardiovascular events in asymptomatic individuals and can be used for risk stratification
- CTA
  - 64-detector row CT is currently considered minimum standard for coronary CT angiography
  - Image interpretation may be impaired by motion artifact, large calcified plaques, and noise
  - Sensitivity for coronary artery stenosis detection is > 90%; specificity may be lower, especially in cases of impaired image quality
  - Stenosis measurement
    - Minimal: 1-24% stenosis
    - Mild: 25-49% stenosis
    - Moderate: 50-69% stenosis
    - Severe: ≥ 70% stenosis
      - ≥ 50% stenosis for left main
  - Quantified as 1 - [(luminal area stenosis/luminal area normal vessel)] x 100
    - Luminal area normal vessel: Can be single measurement or average of normal coronary artery area measured at equal distances both above and below stenosis
  - Noninvasive evaluation of FFR by computational fluid dynamics modeling (CT-FFR) may be performed as add-on test and has shown close correlation to invasively measured FFR
    - Recommended in patients with 50-90% coronary stenosis or ≥ 40% stenosis with high-risk plaque features
    - CT-FFR ≤ 0.75 indicates presence of hemodynamically significant stenosis
    - CT-FFR > 0.80 shows absence of hemodynamic significance
    - CT-FFR 0.76-0.80 is borderline
  - CT perfusion studies that include both resting and stress imaging can provide assessment of hemodynamic effect of coronary artery stenosis
    - Recommended in patients with 50-90% coronary stenosis or ≥ 40% stenosis with high-risk plaque features, similar to CT-FFR
  - Coronary Artery Disease Reporting and Data System (CAD-RADS) is used for reporting of coronary artery stenosis on CCTA

MR Findings

- Coronary MR angiography
  - Alternative to CT for evaluation of coronary artery
    - No contrast or radiation needed
    - Lumen can be assessed even in heavily calcified plaque
    - Temporal resolution can be altered using imaging parameters
  - Lower spatial resolution, long image time, and operator dependency compared to CT
    - Sensitivity and specificity: 70-90%
  - Can evaluate atherosclerotic burden in vessel wall
    - T1 MR: High-intensity plaque; LGE MR of coronary arterial wall
  - Not widely used clinically
    - Potential in future: High field strength magnets, multichannel coil, use of contrast, self navigation
- Left ventricular function at rest can be normal even in severe CAD
- Stress MR with adenosine
  - Ischemia: Defect in stress but not in rest images
  - High accuracy for identification of hemodynamically relevant stenosis
- Dobutamine stress MR and regional wall motion
  - High accuracy for identification of hemodynamically relevant stenosis
- LGE using inversion-recovery sequences
  - Scar tissue appears as bright, or hyperenhanced, myocardium
  - If typically distributed in transmural or subendocardial pattern and in vascular territory, indicative of past myocardial infarction
- MR provides multiparametric imaging: MRA, perfusion, LGE, vessel wall, function

Echocardiographic Findings

- Echocardiogram
  - Baseline study can be entirely normal; wall motion abnormalities indicate past myocardial infarction

- Stress echocardiography is most commonly performed with physical exercise or graded dobutamine stress (potential addition of atropine)

Angiographic Findings

- Invasive coronary angiography
  - Stenosis degree is usually determined by visual estimation
  - May be combined with intravascular ultrasound (IVUS) or optical coherence tomography (OCT) for more definite assessment of plaque/stenosis morphology
  - May be combined with FFR measurement to assess hemodynamic relevance

Nuclear Medicine Findings

- PET
  - Excellent for assessing perfusion, ischemia, and viability
  - Rb-82 (most frequently) or 13NH3 is used for assessment of perfusion at rest and stress
  - F-18 FDG is used for assessment of glucose utilization (viability)
- SPECT myocardial perfusion
  - Very frequently used to identify myocardial ischemia
  - Tl-201 (high radiation exposure) or Tc-99m (e.g., 99mTc sestamibi) is used as perfusion tracer
  - Comparison of physical exercise or pharmacologic stress (high-flow state) with rest (low-flow state)
  - Adenosine is most frequently utilized pharmacologic agent

Imaging Recommendations

- Direct visualization of coronary arteries: Invasive angiography, coronary CT angiography
- Testing for ischemia: MR, nuclear medicine, stress echocardiography, CT perfusion
- Choice of testing modality is influenced by patient characteristics and pretest probability of CAD
  - Traditionally, guidelines mandated testing for ischemia as 1st diagnostic test in suspected CAD
  - Recent guidelines endorse coronary CTA as Class Ia recommendation in intermediate-risk patients with no known CAD in both stable and acute chest pain settings
- Most definitive test is invasive coronary angiography combined with IVUS and FFR

DIFFERENTIAL DIAGNOSIS

Other Cardiac Disease

- Aortic stenosis, hypertrophic cardiomyopathy, hypertension, acute myocarditis, pericarditis, coronary spasm, mitral valve prolapse, syndrome X

Noncardiac Source of Symptoms

- Vascular disease: Aortic dissection or pulmonary embolism
- Gastrointestinal disease: Hiatus hernia, acid reflux, cholecystitis, or peptic ulcer
- Musculoskeletal disease: Often chest wall or shoulders

PATHOLOGY

General Features

- Etiology
  - Most common cause of stenosis: Atherosclerotic plaque
- Genetics
  - Strong genetic influence on atherosclerosis
- Atherosclerosis
  - Most important risk factors include smoking, hyperlipidemia, hypertension, diabetes, and familial history of premature CAD
  - Plaque erosion/rupture, platelet aggregation, and thrombosis lead to stenosis progression and acute coronary syndromes (myocardial infarction and unstable angina)
- Nonatherosclerotic causes for coronary artery stenosis or occlusion
  - Vasculitis, Takayasu disease, Kawasaki disease

CLINICAL ISSUES

Presentation

- Most common signs/symptoms
  - Chest, shoulder, neck, or jaw pain or shortness of breath that is reproducible with exertion
- Clinical profile
  - Risk profiling is critical part of evaluating patients suspected of significant coronary artery stenosis

Demographics

- Age
  - Likelihood of CAD ↑ with age
- Sex
  - M > F, especially at younger age
- Ethnicity
  - Blacks and Asian Indians have higher risk of CAD and higher cardiovascular mortality
- Epidemiology
  - Leading cause of mortality and morbidity in developed world

Treatment

- Prevention of coronary artery events
- Symptom relief
  - Medication: Nitrates, β-blockers, and calcium antagonists
  - Revascularization (coronary artery bypass surgery or percutaneous intervention)
    - Prognostically relevant only if > ~ 10% of myocardium is ischemic, if left main coronary artery has relevant stenosis, or if > 1 coronary artery (including proximal left main coronary artery) has hemodynamically relevant stenosis

DIAGNOSTIC CHECKLIST

Consider

- Not every stenosis necessarily causes ischemia
- Plaque burden can be extensive without relevant stenosis

SELECTED REFERENCES

1. Canan A et al: RadioGraphics update: pictorial guide to CAD-RADS 2.0. Radiographics. 43(4):e220202, 2023
2. Nørgaard BL et al: Prognostic value of coronary computed tomography angiographic derived fractional flow reserve: a systematic review and meta-analysis. Heart. 108(3):194-202, 2022
3. Nørgaard BL et al: Coronary Ct angiography-derived fractional flow reserve testing in patients with stable coronary artery disease: recommendations on interpretation and reporting. Radiol Cardiothorac Imaging. 1(5):e190050, 2019

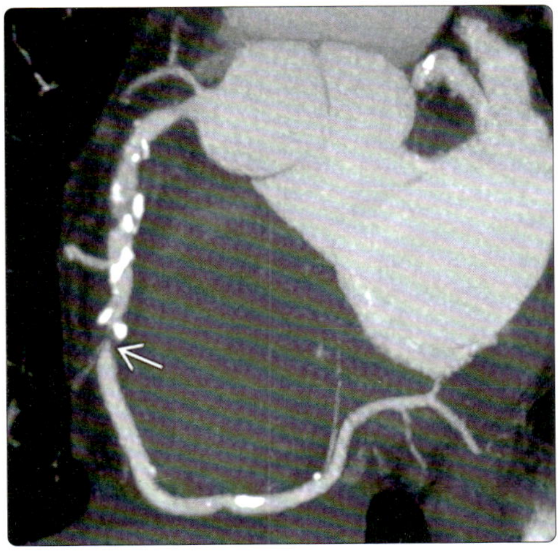

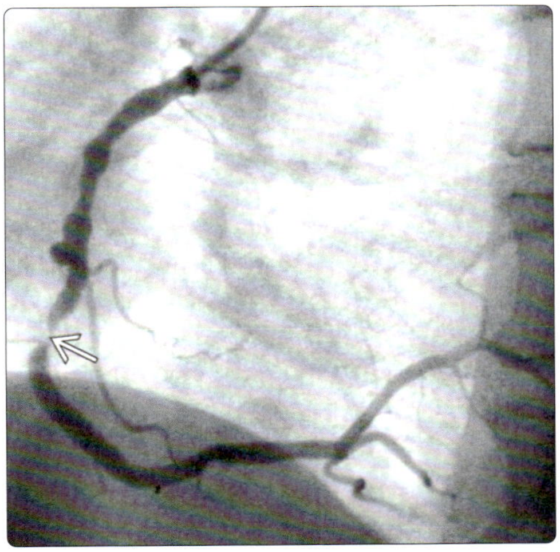

(Left) *Oblique MIP contrast-enhanced coronary CT angiography shows a high-grade stenosis* ➔ *in the midsegment of the right coronary artery (RCA). In addition, numerous calcified plaques are found along the entire course of the vessel.* **(Right)** *Invasive coronary angiography in the same patient, right anterior oblique projection, shows a high-grade stenosis* ➔ *in the midsegment of the RCA, consistent with the CT angiography findings.*

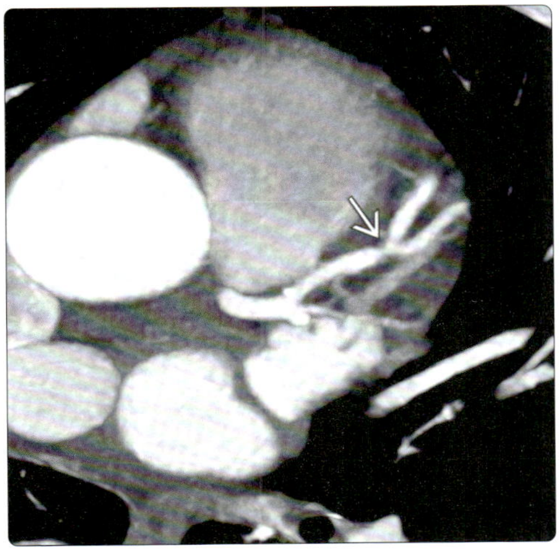

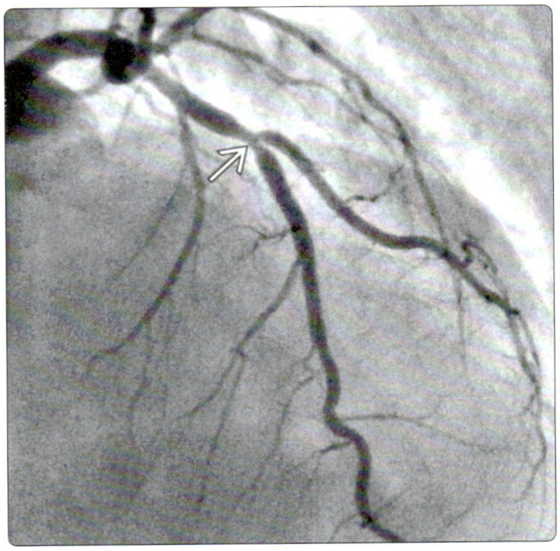

(Left) *Axial MIP contrast-enhanced coronary CT angiography shows a stenosis* ➔ *of moderate degree in the LAD coronary artery at the bifurcation to the diagonal branch.* **(Right)** *Invasive coronary angiography in anteroposterior cranial projection in the same patient shows a stenosis of moderate degree in the LAD coronary artery* ➔*. The stenosis involves the origin of the diagonal branch.*

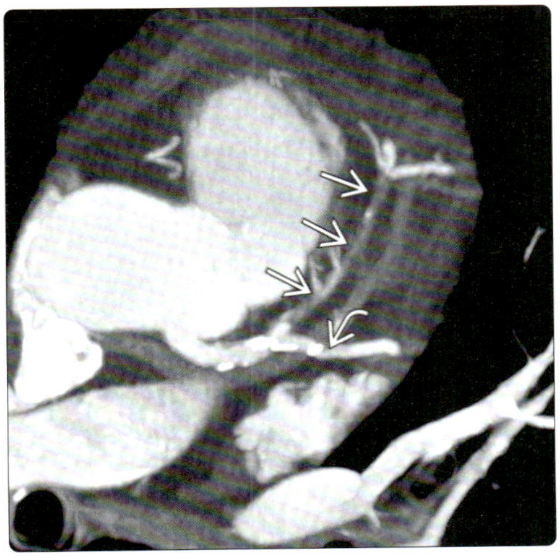

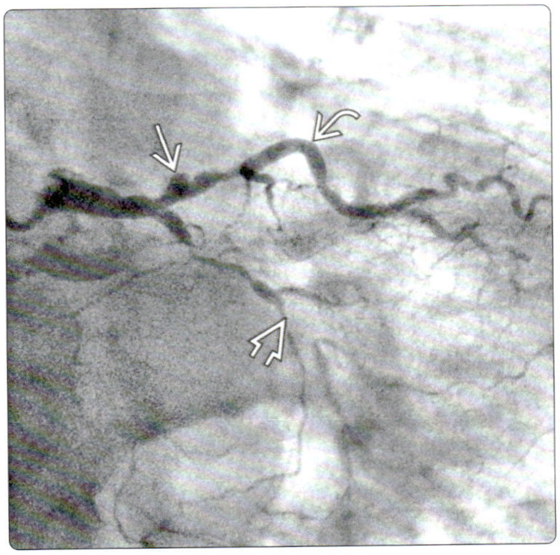

(Left) *Axial MIP contrast-enhanced coronary CT angiography shows a chronic total occlusion of the LAD coronary artery* ➔*. The vessel is occluded between the 1st* ➔ *and 2nd diagonal branches.* **(Right)** *Invasive coronary angiography in the same patient shows that the LAD coronary artery is occluded* ➔ *immediately distal to the origin of the large 1st diagonal branch* ➔*. The left circumflex coronary artery is chronically occluded* ➔*.*

(Left) *The anatomic severity and functional relevance of coronary artery stenosis do not necessarily correlate closely. Here, invasive angiography shows only mild mid LAD coronary artery stenoses* ➔, *but the corresponding invasive fractional flow reserve (FFR) using adenosine infusion has a value of 0.66, indicating hemodynamic significance.* **(Right)** *An anatomically high-grade stenosis* ➔ *in the LAD artery has an FFR of 0.95, indicating lack of hemodynamic relevance.*

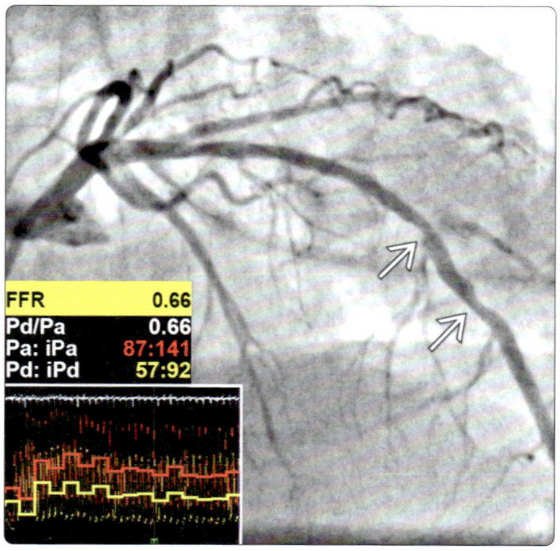

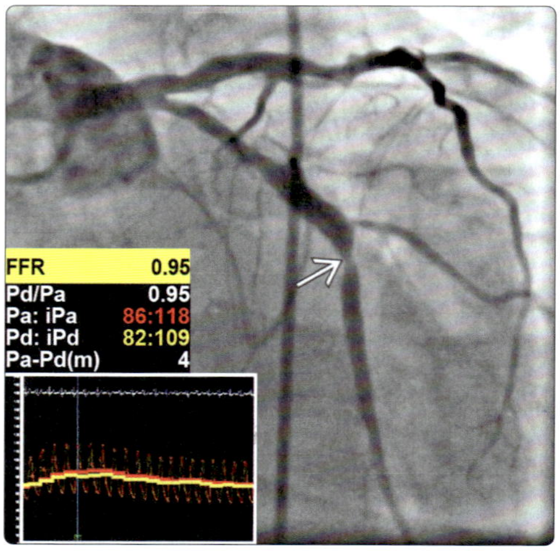

(Left) *Contrast-enhanced coronary CT angiography shows a very short, noncalcified, high-grade stenosis* ➔ *of the left circumflex coronary artery. Note that the coronary lumen within the high-grade stenosis seems completely interrupted; the residual lumen is below the spatial resolution of coronary CT angiography.* **(Right)** *Invasive coronary angiography in the same patient shows a short, high-grade stenosis* ➔ *of the left circumflex coronary artery.*

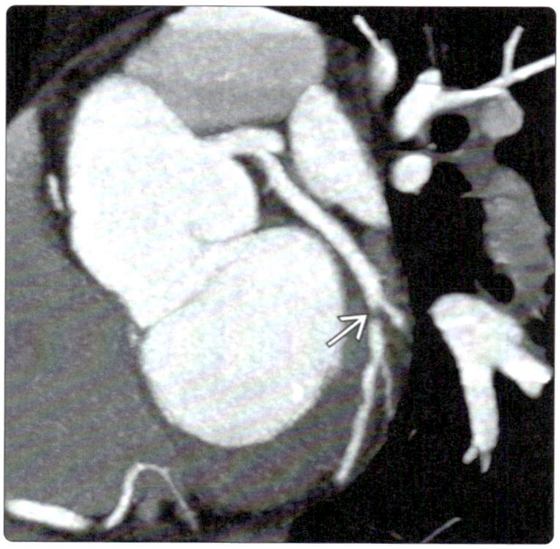

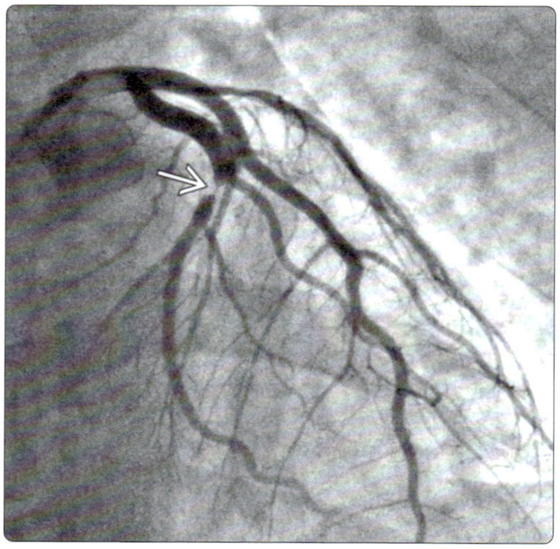

(Left) *The degree of stenosis often appears more severe in coronary CT angiography than in invasive angiography. In this example, coronary CT angiography shows a stenosis* ➔ *of the mid LAD coronary artery that appears to be moderate to high grade; the large amount of plaque and positive remodeling contribute to this visual impression.* **(Right)** *Invasive coronary angiography in the same patient shows that the degree of luminal stenosis is moderate* ➔.

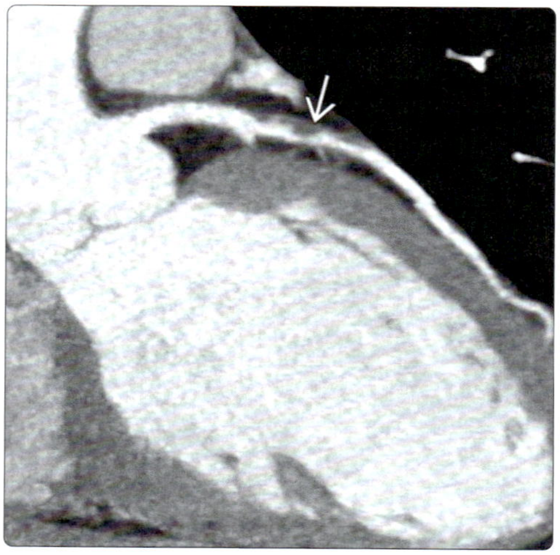

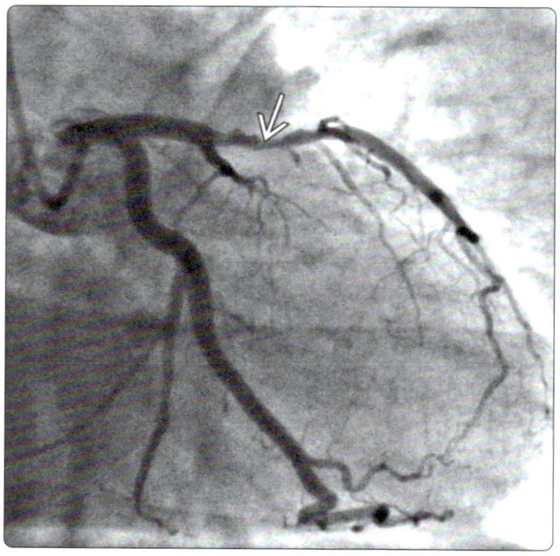

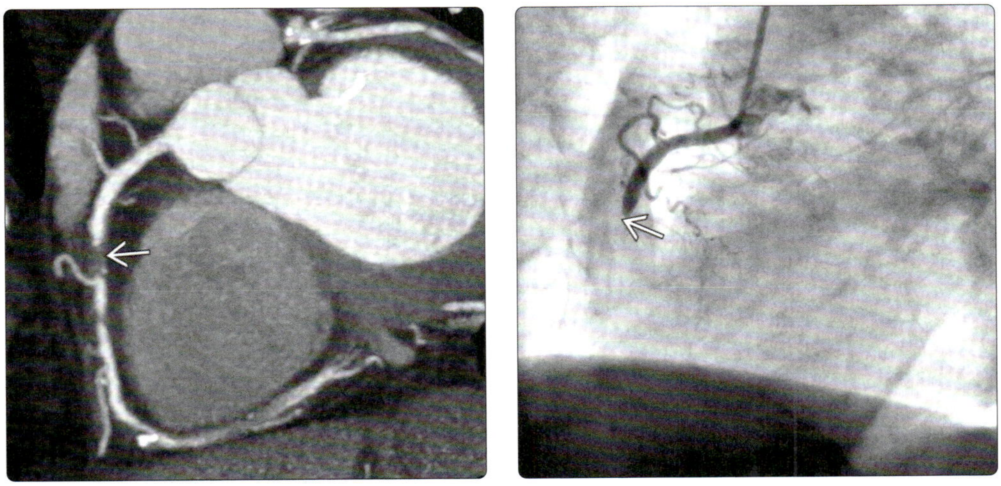

(Left) *Oblique MIP contrast-enhanced coronary CT angiography of the RCA shows a short interruption of the coronary artery lumen. Such lesions can either be high-grade stenoses or complete occlusions of a coronary artery. Distal filling may be from collaterals.* **(Right)** *Invasive coronary angiography in right anterior oblique orientation in the same patient shows a complete occlusion of the RCA.*

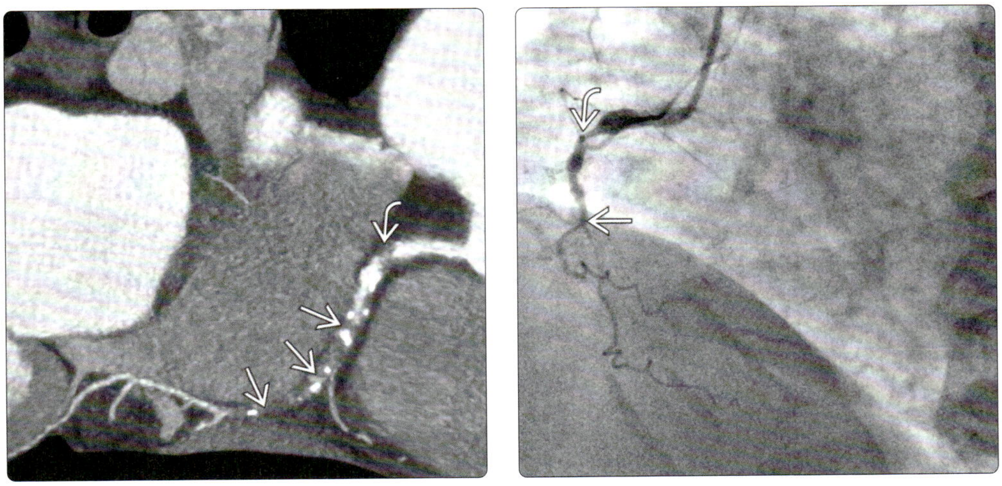

(Left) *Contrast-enhanced coronary CT angiography, curved multiplanar reconstruction of the RCA, shows a proximal high-grade stenosis followed by a long occlusion of the vessel.* **(Right)** *Invasive coronary angiography in the right anterior oblique orientation in the same patient demonstrates a short-segment, high-grade proximal stenosis followed by a total occlusion of the coronary artery.*

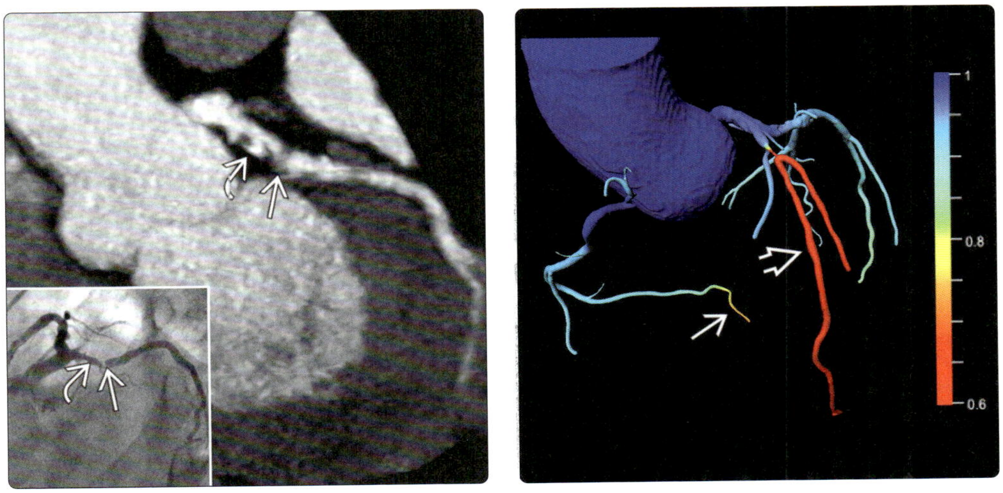

(Left) *Slight motion artifact and noise affect a partially calcified plaque that has no relevant stenosis. A subsequent short interruption of the lumen corresponds to a high-grade left circumflex artery (inset).* **(Right)** *Simulation of FFR based on coronary CTA (FFR-CT) is shown. A high-grade stenosis in the LAD causes a drop in simulated FFR to < 0.80, indicating hemodynamically relevant stenosis. In the RCA, there is a continuous and slow decrease of FFR to < 0.80 only in very distal segment. This is not considered abnormal.*

Introduction

Traditionally, clinicians investigating chest pain in the stable patient population had to decide between the mutually exclusive functional or anatomic testing. With the advent of fractional flow reserve computed tomography (CT-FFR), a unique opportunity for simultaneous functional and anatomic assessment of coronary artery disease (CAD) has been established in the noninvasive setting.

A particular advantage of CT-FFR is its ability to adjudicate lesion-specific pressure loss as with the invasive gold standard of fractional flow reserve (FFR). This ability to adjudicate anatomy and hyperemic physiology allows for the determination of lesion-specific treatment planning. Importantly, this modifies treatment decisions for most patients. It is cost-effective and improves patient outcomes.

Technology: Function From Anatomy

CT-FFR prerequisites
- Good-quality CTA data set acquired in accordance with SCCT acquisition guidelines with slice thickness of < 1 mm
- Good heart rate control and administration of nitroglycerin

CT-FFR computation process
- Determination of patient-specific anatomic model of aorta and epicardial coronaries
- Physiological boundary conditions under resting and hyperemic conditions
- Fundamentals: Allometric scaling law indicating coronary blood flow is proportional to left ventricular mass
- Murray law and Poiseuille solution: Flow rate proportional to diameter of vessel, and shear stress and inversely proportional to viscosity of blood
- Morphometry laws and fractals to further assess coronary branch flow resistance
- Boundary conditions: Cardiac output; aortic pressure and impedance; coronary microcirculation resistance is inversely related to coronary size

The computational fluid dynamics (CFD) Navier Stokes equations are based on the principles of conservation of mass and balance of momentum to derive the coronary flow and pressure. Recent advances in artificial intelligence and machine learning have enabled more rapid, reproducible, and robust coronary segmentation by iterating and improving the segmentation of the coronaries. Additionally, velocity and pressure calculations are solved by a parallel supercomputer to create a mesh of complete epicardial coronary tree.

Currently, the most commonly used and FDA-approved platform for CT-FFR is "Heartflow." Data is transferred offsite for central advanced post processing.
- Time frame from submitting data set to receiving results: 2-3 hours

Onsite vendor-based platforms are not widely available.
- Includes machine-learning-based, reduced-order models for nonstenotic regions and pressure drop models in stenotic regions

Defining Values and Standardized Fractional Flow Reserve Computed Tomography Reporting in CAD-RADS 2.0

The Coronary Artery Disease-Reporting and Data System (CAD-RADS) reporting guidelines have been updated to reflect the growing evidence of the importance of physiology in coronary revascularization decisions, and the development of noninvasive techniques that allow functional assessment. The modifier "I" indicates that an ischemia test (either CT-FFR or stress CT perfusion) has been performed.

> 0.80
- Modifier **I-** in CAD-RADS 2.0
- No lesion-specific ischemia

0.75-0.80
- Modifier **I±** in CAD-RADS 2.0
- Borderline for lesion-specific ischemia

< 0.75
- Modifier **I+** in CAD-RADS 2.0
- Lesion-specific ischemia is present

Fractional Flow Reserve Computed Tomography Case Selection

The most optimal use of CT-FFR in cases of coronary stenosis severity is between 40% and 90% (particularly CAD-RADS 3 and 4A and CAD-RADS 2 if ≥ 40% stenosis) and in locations within the proximal or midcoronary artery segments.

This approach to selecting cases for CT-FFR add-on testing holds promise for improving care through minimizing false-negatives and false-positives while enhancing clinical clarity. It is also aligned with guidance provided in the 2021 ACC/AHA Chest Pain Guideline and CAD-RADS 2.0.

Interpretation of Computed Tomography Fractional Flow Reserve

CT-FFR provides FFR values throughout the coronary tree as well as lowest CT-FFR value at distal end of each vessel analyzed. This is distinct from invasive fractional flow reserve (INV-FFR) in which pressure measurements are determined based on the operator, typically to assess pressure and flow loss across a focal lesion.
- CT-FFR value drops along length of vessel even in absence of CAD
- End-vessel CT-FFR > 0.90 in normal left anterior descending artery
- Referral to invasive coronary angiography (ICA) not recommended based on end-vessel CT-FFR
- Rather than binary classification, CT-FFR value should be interpreted as continuous variable
- Sharp drop across focal stenoses with CT-FFR value of < 0.75 more likely indicative of lesion-specific ischemia than more gradual drop with CT-FFR value of 0.75-0.80
- For borderline lesions, delta CT-FFR (translesional gradient) can be calculated as the pressure drop from 1-2 cm proximal to 1-2 cm distal to stenosis; value > 0.12 is considered significant
- Diffuse CAD, serial stenoses, small vessel:myocardium mass ratio, and inadequate nitrate response have implications on CT-FFR value
- CT-FFR value should be integrated with other CTA measures of flow reduction as well as larger clinical context of each patient to individualize decision making

Clinical Evidence

Refinements in CT-FFR technology and improved physiological modeling, particularly microcirculatory resistance, have led to an improvement in diagnostic accuracy when referenced with INV-FFR.

The diagnostic performance of CT-FFR has been established through multiple multicenter accuracy studies. The accuracy using a binary cut point of FFR is ~ 86% on a per vessel basis (PACIFIC) with a consistently excellent kappa agreement for treatment decision-making between CTA/ CT-FFR and ICA/FFR strategy (SYNTAX III, Cohen's kappa = 0.82).

In the PLATFORM trial, CT-FFR combined with CTA was compared with the usual care to determine the need for ICA. Combining CT-FFR with CTA resulted in 60% of ICA being canceled with a significant reduction in the burden of nonobstructive disease, decrease in the total number of ICA referrals, decrease in the percentage of ICA for stenoses < 50%, and from 73% to 12% with no events in those for whom ICA had been canceled through 1 year.

In clinical practice, CT-FFR has been shown as an effective clinical tool in determining whether subjects should undergo ICA or continue with medical therapy alone while enriching the population referred for ICA and achieving higher percutaneous coronary intervention (PCI):ICA ratio. Deferring ICA through a strategy of CTA and selective CT-FFR in mild to moderate stenosis (30-70%) in patients with stable chest pain has been shown by to prevent further testing in 2/3 of patients with favorable outcomes at 3-year follow-up.

ADVANCE, a large prospective multicenter international registry, assessed the real-world impact of CT-FFR. Results at 90 days revealed a change in treatment plan in 2/3 of patients as compared with CCTA alone and no MACE reported in CT-FFR > 0.80. A prospective follow-up study from the ADVANCE registry demonstrated that the prognostic value of CT-FFR can be extended to a 3-year follow-up. Importantly, CT-FFR measurements could be reliably obtained even in patients with high coronary artery calcium (CAC) scores, and the reduced risk of adverse outcomes for participants with CT-FFR values > 0.80 was maintained after adjustment for CAC score and degree of stenosis.

A metaanalysis encompassing 5,460 patients with stable CAD revealed that a negative CT-FFR result was associated with a low incidence of adverse events at 12 months and a significantly lower risk of death or myocardial infarction (MI) compared with those with a positive CT-FFR result. The CT-FFR numerical value was inversely related to clinical outcomes.

PRECISE demonstrated that customized use of CT-FFR according to patient risk status resulted in fewer invasive angiographies and greater diagnostic yield of obstructive disease without an increase in death or nonfatal MI at 1 year compared to usual care.

The FISH and CHIPS trial was designed to assess the impact of CT-FFR implementation within the NHS England on patient care. The utilization of CT-FFR resulted in a reduction in the number of cardiac downstream tests, including fewer ICAs. Concomitantly, there was an increase in the number of patients undergoing PCI, but not coronary artery bypass grafting (CABG) procedures. The all-cause mortality rates remained unchanged over time; however, the incidence of cardiovascular mortality was significantly lower in the post-CT FFR population at the 2-year mark.

In addition to its excellent diagnostic accuracy and prognostic value, CT-FFR can help to guide complex coronary revascularization decisions. A recently introduced CT-FFR planner allows for the assessment of the physiologic response to various PCI strategies through "virtual stenting." The P3 trial demonstrated that the CT-FFR planner was an accurate and precise tool for predicting FFR after PCI. Furthermore, its accuracy was found to be independent of CAD complexity and image quality.

Limitations

CTA images must pass a minimum quality score. The real-world rejection rate is ~ 5-7 %, which limits the use of this technology in some patients. This emphasizes the need to ensure that a good-quality CTA is performed.

Modest performance has been shown in nonculprit lesions in recent STEMI, likely due to small vessel volume in these patients rather than stable angina.

Additional limitations include limited use in extensive calcification, stents, and bypass grafts, cost vs reimbursement, additional costs involved in offsite transfer to specific vendors, and postprocessing time for offsite model of 2-3 hours.

Future Directions

The integration of CT-FFR findings, anatomic information, and advanced plaque characteristics derived from recently introduced artificial intelligence-enabled quantitative plaque analysis tools will facilitate the further maximization of data extraction from CCTA, thereby enhancing diagnostic accuracy, reducing interpretation time, improving clinical outcomes, and guiding treatment decisions.

Selected References

1. Douglas PS et al: Comparison of an initial risk-based testing strategy vs usual testing in stable symptomatic patients with suspected coronary artery disease: The PRECISE randomized clinical trial. JAMA Cardiol. 8(10):904-14, 2023
2. Madsen KT et al: Prognostic value of coronary CT angiography-derived fractional flow reserve on 3-year outcomes in patients with stable angina. Radiology. 308(3):e230524, 2023
3. Fairbairn TA et al: Real-world clinical utility and impact on clinical decision-making of coronary computed tomography angiography-derived fractional flow reserve: lessons from the ADVANCE Registry. Eur Heart J. 39(41):3701-11, 2018
4. Cook CM et al: Diagnostic accuracy of computed tomography-derived fractional flow reserve: a systematic review. JAMA Cardiol. 2(7):803-10, 2017
5. Gaur S et al: FFR derived from coronary CT angiography in nonculprit lesions of patients with recent STEMI. JACC Cardiovasc Imaging. 10(4):424-33, 2017
6. Lu MT et al: Noninvasive FFR derived from coronary CT angiography: management and outcomes in the PROMISE trial. JACC Cardiovasc Imaging. 10(11):1350-58, 2017
7. Nørgaard BL et al: Clinical use of coronary CTA-derived FFR for decision-making in stable CAD. JACC Cardiovasc Imaging. 10(5):541-50, 2017
8. Coenen A et al: Fractional flow reserve computed from noninvasive CT angiography data: diagnostic performance of an on-site clinician-operated computational fluid dynamics algorithm. Radiology. 274(3):674-83, 2015
9. Leipsic J et al: CT angiography (CTA) and diagnostic performance of noninvasive fractional flow reserve: results from the Determination of Fractional Flow Reserve by Anatomic CTA (DeFACTO) study. AJR Am J Roentgenol. 202(5):989-94, 2014
10. Nørgaard BL et al: Diagnostic performance of noninvasive fractional flow reserve derived from coronary computed tomography angiography in suspected coronary artery disease: the NXT trial (analysis of coronary blood flow using CT angiography: Next Steps). J Am Coll Cardiol. 63(12):1145-55, 2014
11. Taylor CA et al: Computational fluid dynamics applied to cardiac computed tomography for noninvasive quantification of fractional flow reserve: scientific basis. J Am Coll Cardiol. 61(22):2233-41, 2013

Ischemia Imaging With CT-FFR

(Left) *Double oblique reformation coronary CTA demonstrates a noncalcified plaque in the left anterior descending (LAD) coronary artery with moderate luminal stenosis* ➡*.* (Right) *Curved planar reformation in the same patient shows the noncalcified plaque in the mid LAD coronary artery* ➡ *with moderate luminal stenosis.*

Noncalcified Plaque in Left Anterior Descending Coronary Artery

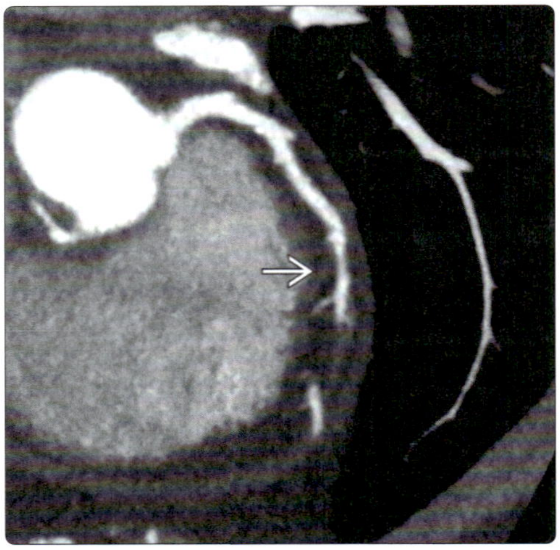

Noncalcified Plaque in Midleft Anterior Descending Coronary Artery

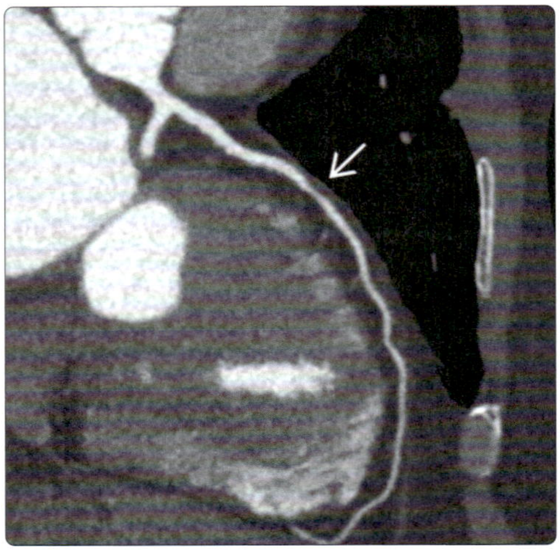

(Left) *Fractional flow reserve computed tomography (FFRCT) of the moderate LAD coronary artery lesion in the same patient demonstrates a borderline result of 0.76 for lesion-specific ischemia.* (Right) *Invasive coronary angiography (ICA) in the same patient shows moderate luminal stenosis* ➡ *of the mid LAD coronary artery with fractional flow reserve (FFR) also demonstrating a similar value of 0.77. The diagnostic accuracy of FFRCT is found to be 87% compared to invasive angiography.*

Moderate Left Anterior Descending Coronary Artery Lesion

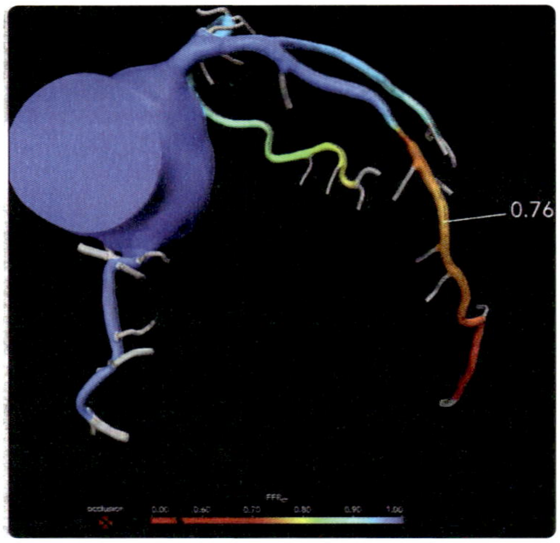

Moderate Luminal Stenosis of Midleft Anterior Descending Coronary Artery

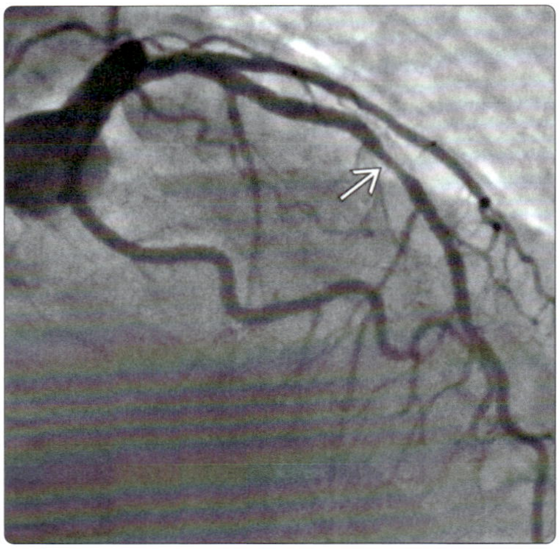

(Left) *Integration of plaque quantification and FFRCT is shown. A FFR-negative lesion was selected in the proximal LAD.* (Right) *Corresponding coronary CTA cross-sectional image with color overlay shows the automated quantitative plaque assessment based on HU attenuation (cyan = calcified plaque; pink = noncalcified plaque). The automated coronary plaque analysis of the entire coronary tree yielded a total plaque volume of 866 m³, of which 70% was noncalcified.*

Fractional Flow Reserve-Negative Lesion

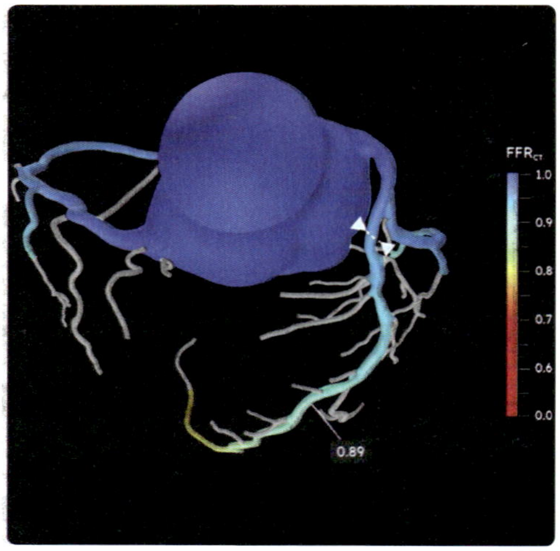

Automated Quantitative Plaque Assessment

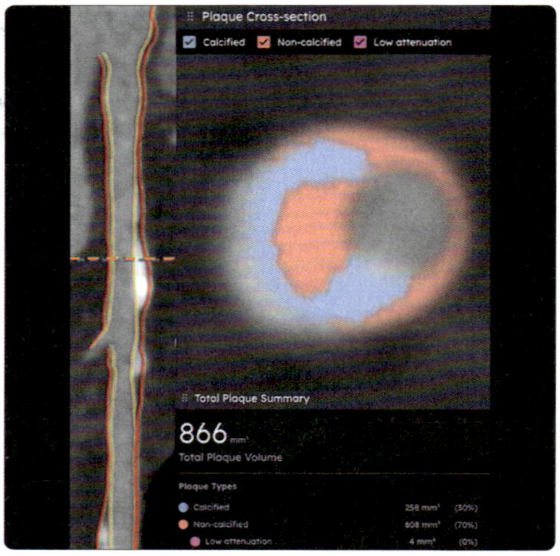

Ischemia Imaging With CT-FFR

Nonobstructive, Partially Calcified Lesion

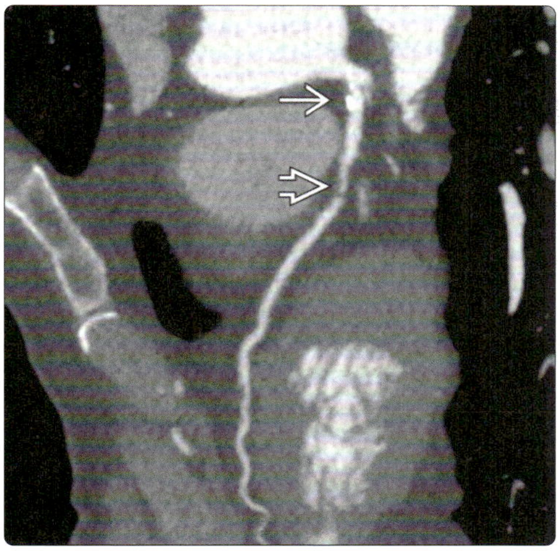

Partially Calcified Lesion

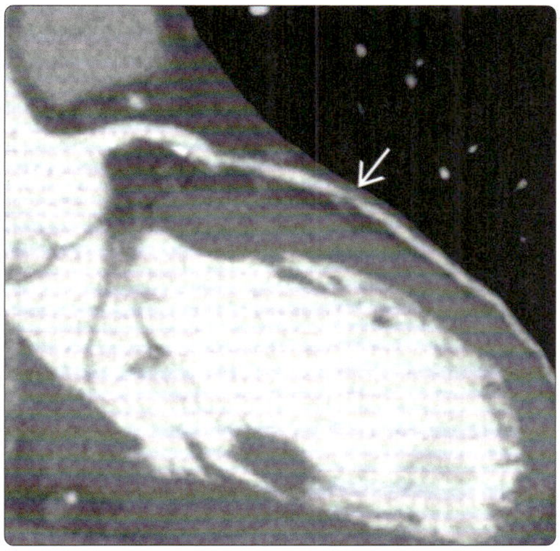

(Left) *Curved planar reformation of the LAD coronary artery demonstrates a proximal nonobstructive, partially calcified lesion* ➡ *followed by a noncalcified, moderate mid-LAD lesion* ➡. **(Right)** *Curved planar reformation of the 1st diagonal branch in the same patient demonstrates a partially calcified lesion in the midsegment of the vessel, resulting in moderate stenosis* ➡.

Moderate Noncalcified Lesion

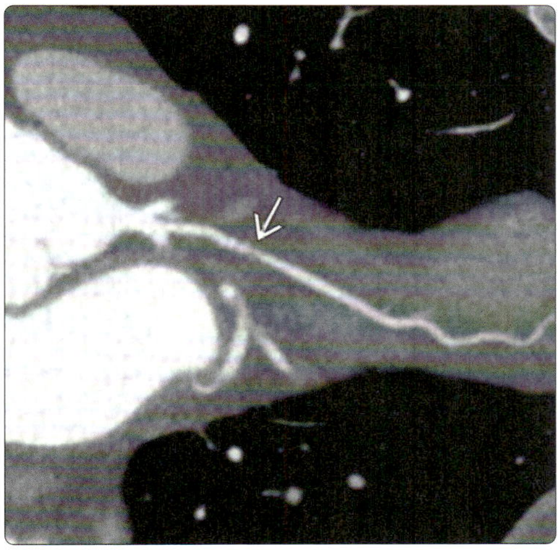

Nonobstructive, Calcified Lesion

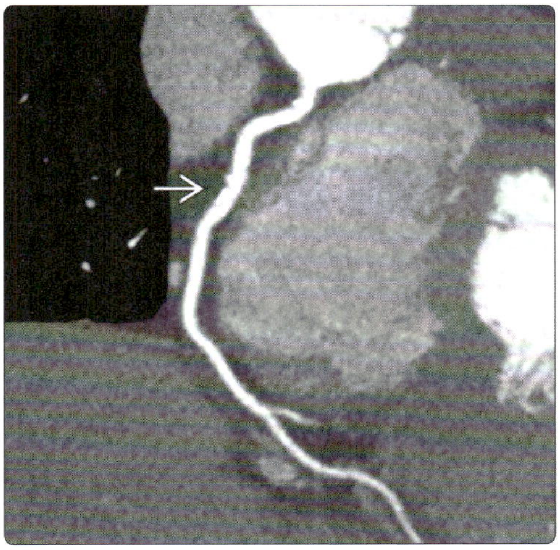

(Left) *Curved planar reformation of the 1st obtuse marginal branch in the same patient demonstrates a moderate noncalcified lesion in the midsegment of the vessel* ➡. **(Right)** *Curved planar reformation of the right coronary artery in the same patient demonstrates a nonobstructive, calcified* ➡ *lesion.*

Lesion-Specific Ischemia

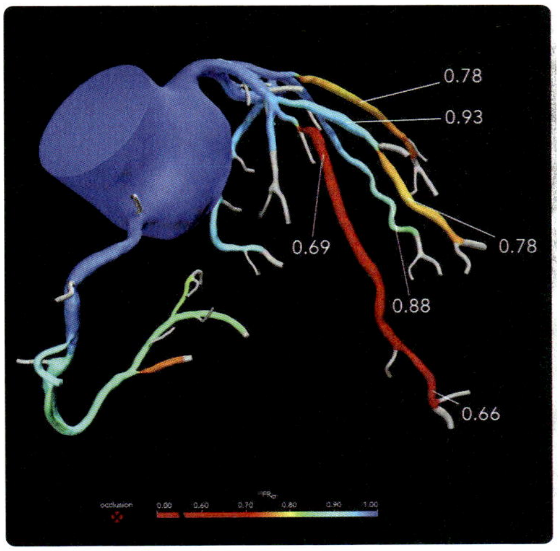

Three Lesions

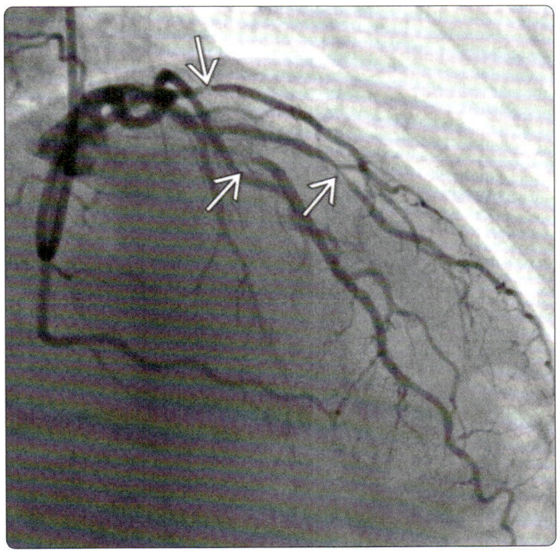

(Left) *FFRCT in the same patient demonstrates a value of 0.69 across the mid-LAD, significant for lesion-specific ischemia. In addition, borderline values of 0.78 were seen for the 1st diagonal branch and the 1st obtuse marginal. Note the normal values in the right coronary artery, indicating no significant stenosis, consistent with the CTA.* **(Right)** *ICA demonstrates the 3 lesions* ➡ *highlighted by the FFRCT.*

Introduction

Coronary CT angiography (CTA) is excellent for anatomic depiction of coronary arteries due to its high isovolumetric spatial resolution. It has a high negative predictive value for exclusion of obstructive coronary artery disease (CAD) in low- to intermediate-risk populations. However, CTA alone has limited ability to estimate the hemodynamic significance of a stenotic lesion. In addition to fractional flow reserve computed tomography (FFR-CT), CT perfusion (CTP) can provide noninvasive hemodynamic information, which helps in selecting patients that may benefit from further intervention or surgery. CTP evaluates the perfusion by the attenuation differences induced in the myocardium during the first pass of intravenously injected iodinated contrast material.

Technique & Protocol

There are multiple heterogeneous CTP techniques and protocols. Static snapshot technique is the most commonly used acquisition type, which involves a single acquisition in one point of time, typically 8-16 seconds after peak aortic attenuation. This provides only qualitative and semiquantitative information, which can be performed rapidly. In the dynamic technique, myocardium is sampled at multiple time points to generate a time attenuation curve. This allows quantitative evaluation but is associated with higher radiation dose and spatial misregistration.

CTP can be performed using either single-energy or dual-energy techniques. Dual-energy technique offers higher sensitivity and specificity, although it is not widely available. Sensitivity is increased due to improved lesion conspicuity in iodine maps and virtual monoenergetic images. Specificity is improved due to lower beam hardening artifacts in high-energy virtual monoenergetic images. Myocardial perfusion can be quantified using iodine maps.

Stress is induced using pharmacological agents, such as adenosine and regadenoson. Some centers do a stress scan first followed by a rest acquisition, which doubles as a coronary CTA study, whereas other centers do rest first. Some centers also do a delayed iodine enhancement acquisition in 10-15 minutes to look for myocardial scar similar to MR, but this technique is limited by poor contrast-to-noise ratio.

Interpretation of Findings

Qualitative analysis shows perfusion defect as a subendocardial or transmural hypoattenuating area in a vascular distribution. An ischemic defect is seen only in stress, whereas infarct is seen both in stress and rest images. Qualitative analysis is not sensitive for the detection of balanced ischemia in all 3 vascular territories since this technique relies on relative myocardial attenuation differences. Semiquantitative analysis includes transmural perfusion ratio. Quantitative analysis of myocardial blood flow (MBF) and coronary flow reserve (CFR) can be performed only in dynamic CTP technique.

A false-positive result can be seen due to beam-hardening artifact. This artifact is due to preferential initial attenuation of low-energy photons of a polyenergetic beam and manifests as a dark subendocardial defect adjacent to dense contrast in the ventricular blood pool. The use of high-energy x-ray or high-energy virtual monoenergetic images of dual-energy CT can decrease this artifact and improve specificity of CTP.

Current Evidence

CTP has higher accuracy than SPECT for predicting obstructive CAD (> 50% stenosis) on invasive coronary angiography (ICA). CTA + CTP have pooled per-vessel specificity of 93% and sensitivity of 85% for diagnosis of stenosis > 50% at ICA. CTP has been validated against nuclear medicine, MR, coronary angiography, and invasive fractional flow reserve (FFR) for evaluation of hemodynamically significant stenosis. On a per-vessel basis, CTP has a specificity of 84% and positive predictive value (PPV) of 82% with invasive FFR as the gold standard for ischemia. CTP improves the PPV and pooled specificity for lesion-specific ischemia when compared to coronary CTA alone (0.77 vs. 0.43). CTP perfusion defect and CTA stenosis > 50% is 98% specific for ischemia. A normal CTP perfusion with CTA stenosis < 50% is 100% specific for excluding ischemia. This makes CT an effective gatekeeper for ICA with a per-patient negative likelihood ratio of 0.12, which is superior to SPECT and echo and comparable to MR and PET.

CTA with CTP has a higher patient satisfaction than either CTA, CTP, MR, or SPECT alone. CTP has also been shown to be more cost-effective than SPECT with an incremental cost effective ratio per quality-adjusted life year of $3,191 for CTP compared to $3,357 for SPECT. CTP also adds an incremental prognostic value over CTA for major adverse cardiovascular events (MACE). The presence and number of perfusion defects is associated with higher risk of MACE. There is 5x reduction in downstream ICA and revascularization and low 1-year MACE by using CTP along with CTA.

CTP has a higher pooled specificity than FFR-CT (0.86 vs. 0.78) and CTA alone (0.61). CTP + CTA improves the diagnostic performance of these 2 individual techniques, whereas FFR-CT results in only a small and insignificant improvement over CTA. CTP + FFR-CT can provide complementary information with accuracy of 78% for the combination compared to 70% for individual tests. Specifically, CTP improves the accuracy of FFR-CT in intermediate range values between 0.74 and 0.85. CTP can be done in patients with heavy calcium or stents, which are typically not evaluable by FFR-CT.

Nonobstructive Coronary Artery Disease

MBF and CFR are used to evaluate epicardial disease/microvascular dysfunction, which accounts for up to 65% of patients who have nonobstructive disease in ICA (seen in 10-30% of patients with angina). Myocardial attenuation in snapshot CTP correlates with MBF measured in $^{15}O-H_2O$ PET. Early identification of these patients is important due to the associated high mortality rates, especially in women.

Limitations

CTP is not widely used since it requires additional expertise and resources, including administration and monitoring of stress agents. Additional radiation, contrast, and cost are involved. Radiation doses can be minimized by using low-kV protocols. Contraindications to adenosine include advanced heart block and asthma.

Selected References

1. Andreini D et al: Pre-procedural planning of coronary revascularization by cardiac computed tomography: an expert consensus document of the Society of Cardiovascular Computed Tomography. EuroIntervention. 18(11):e872-7, 2022
2. Tanabe Y et al: Computed tomographic evaluation of myocardial ischemia. Jpn J Radiol. 38(5):411-33, 2020

Curved MPR

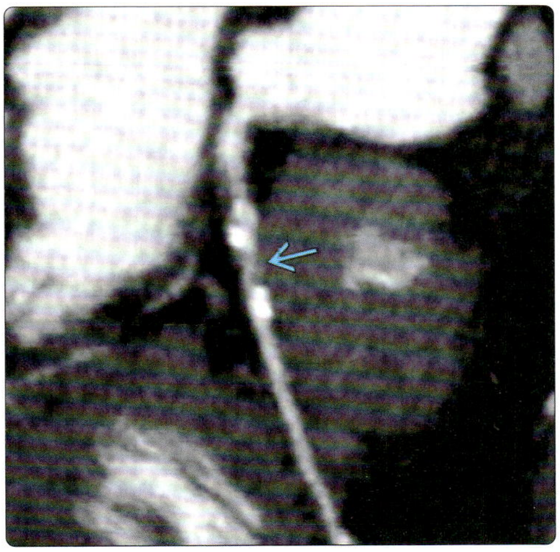

Two-Chamber CT Perfusion

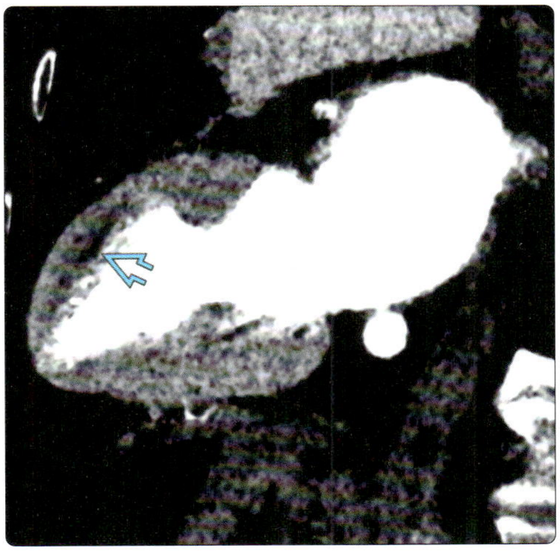

(Left) *Curved MPR of the left anterior descending artery (LAD) from a cardiac CT shows diffuse atherosclerosis of the artery. There is a noncalcific plaque in the mid LAD → with associated moderate luminal stenosis.* **(Right)** *Two-chamber CT perfusion at stress in the same patient shows a subendocardial perfusion ⇒ defect in the mid and apical anterior segments, consistent with myocardial ischemia in the LAD territory.*

Perfusion Defect

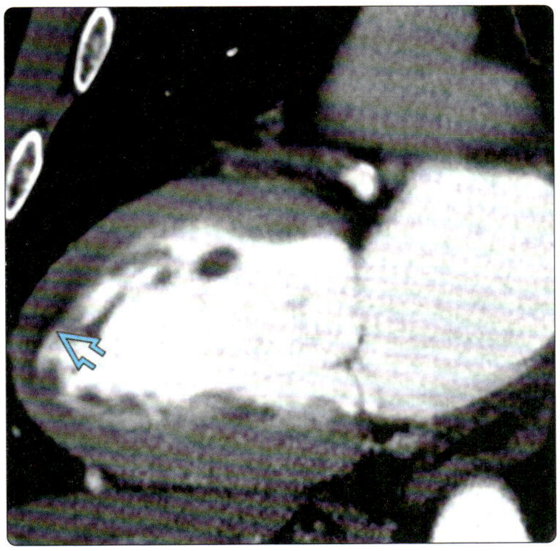

Short-Axis CT Perfusion

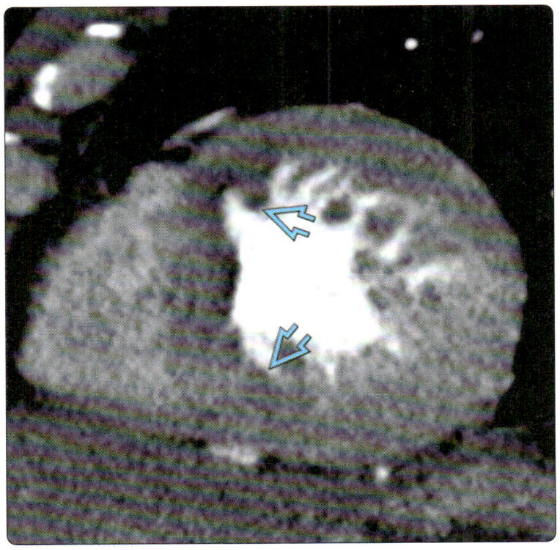

(Left) *Two-chamber CT perfusion at stress shows a subendocardial hypoattenuating area, consistent with perfusion defect ⇒ in mid and apical anterior segments and apical cap.* **(Right)** *Short-axis CT perfusion at stress in the same patient shows a hypoattenuating area ⇒, consistent with a perfusion defect in apical anterior and septal segments. CT perfusion has a high sensitivity and specificity for diagnosis of stenosis > 50%.*

Scintigraphic Perfusion

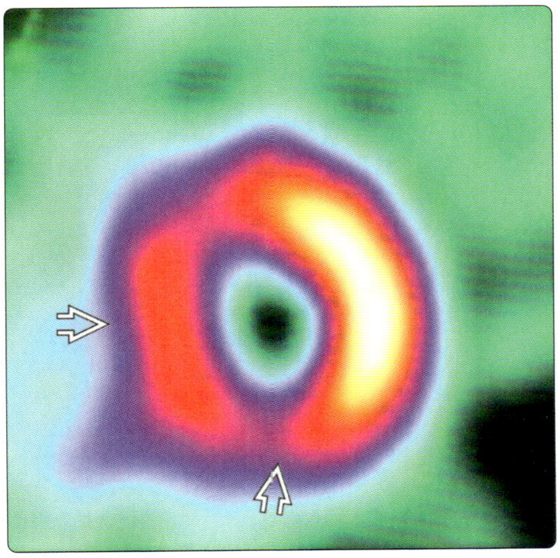

Curved Multiplanar Reformat Cardiac CT

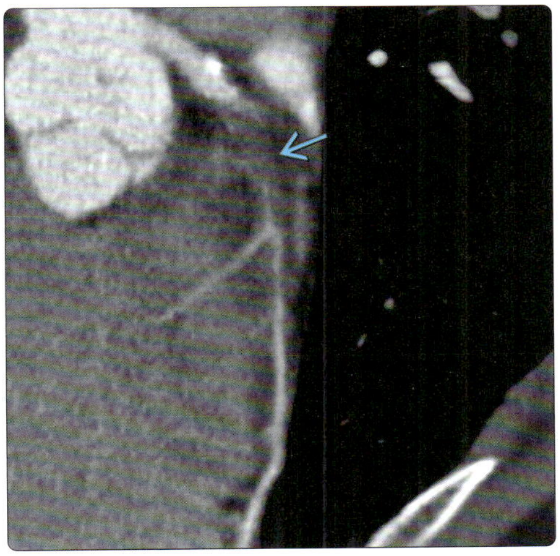

(Left) *Scintigraphic perfusion in the same patient demonstrates a perfusion defect in the apical anterior, septal, and inferior segments* ➡*. CTP has a higher accuracy than SPECT for predicting obstructive coronary artery disease (> 50% stenosis).* **(Right)** *Curved multiplanar reformat cardiac CT angiography of the LAD coronary artery in the same patient demonstrates complete occlusion of the proximal portion → of the artery.*

KEY FACTS

TERMINOLOGY

- Significant coronary artery disease
  - Fractional flow reserve < 0.8
  - ≥ 50% stenosis in left main coronary artery or ≥ 70% in other coronary arteries

ISCHEMIA IMAGING WITH MR: GENERAL CONSIDERATIONS

- CMR vasodilator stress perfusion has excellent diagnostic accuracy, has superior image resolution compared to other imaging methods, and involves no ionizing radiation

VASODILATOR STRESS AGENT PROTOCOLS

- Adenosine 140 mcg/kg/minute intravenous infusion for up to 6 minutes
- Regadenoson 0.4 mg/5mL intravenous injection followed by saline 5-mg intravenous injection
- Dipyridamole 0.56 mg/kg intravenous infusion over 4 minutes (up to maximum of 60 mg)

CMR STRESS PERFUSION IMAGING PROTOCOLS

- Quantitative perfusion imaging protocols have highest diagnostic accuracy, and methods require
  - Imaging of arterial input function and contrast dynamics in myocardium
  - Modeling of perfusion to quantify myocardial blood flow in mL/minute/g

CMR IMAGE INTERPRETATION: DETECTING OBSTRUCTIVE CORONARY ARTERY DISEASE

- Quantitative perfusion assessment is superior to qualitative assessments

IMAGING PITFALLS AND COMPLICATIONS

- Dark rim artifacts mimic subendocardial perfusion defects
- Gadolinium complications: Allergic reaction, deposition in body
- Vasodilator agent complications: Heart block, atrial fibrillation, asthma exacerbations, panic attack

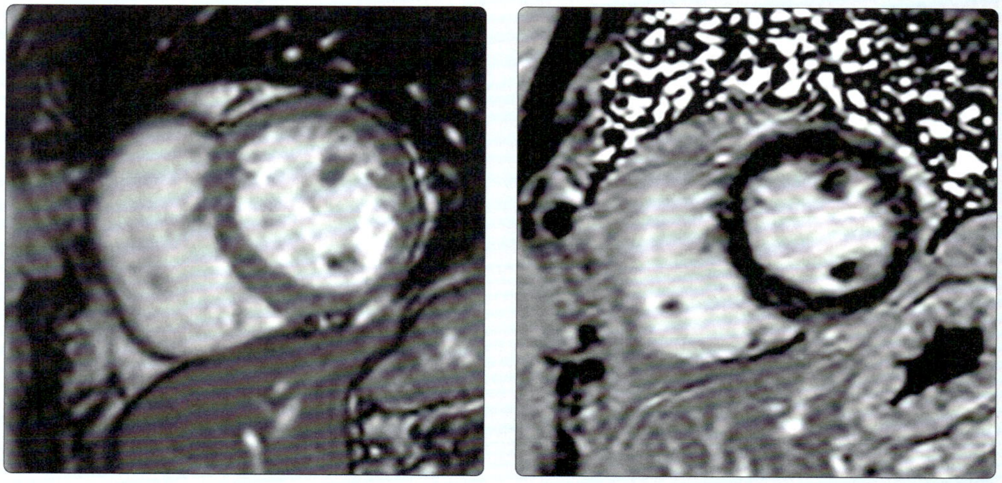

(Left) *Short-axis cine MR of the midleft ventricle in a patient with severe proximal left anterior descending coronary artery stenosis shows uniform signal intensity within the myocardium. (Courtesy F. E. Mordini, MD.)* **(Right)** *Short-axis LGE MR (midleft ventricular slice at the same level) shows no abnormal late gadolinium enhancement (LGE) to indicate myocardial infarction or fibrosis.*

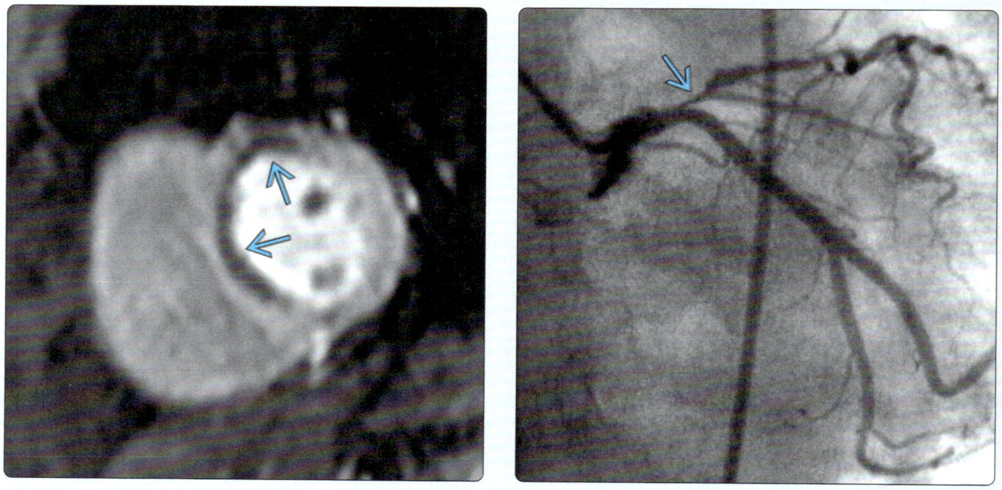

(Left) *Stress perfusion MR of the same midleft ventricular slice shows a stress perfusion defect → in the anterior and anteroseptal segments corresponding to the left anterior descending coronary artery territory.* **(Right)** *Invasive coronary angiogram shows severe stenosis of the proximal left anterior descending coronary artery →.*

TERMINOLOGY

Definitions

- **Significant coronary artery disease (CAD)**
  - Invasive fractional flow reserve (FFR) < 0.8 (arterial pressure distal:stenosis and pressure in aortic root ratio)
    - Best measure of physiologically significant CAD
  - ≥ 50% stenosis of left main coronary artery
  - ≥ 70% stenosis other coronary arteries
  - ~ 2/3 of 50-70% coronary stenoses do not cause physiologic limitations in stress perfusion

CLINICAL IMPLICATIONS

Patient Management

- Cardiac MR (CMR) stress perfusion imaging accurately rules out significant CAD and can reduce unnecessary invasive procedures

ISCHEMIA IMAGING WITH MR: GENERAL CONSIDERATIONS

CMR Vasodilator Stress Perfusion Imaging

- Excellent diagnostic accuracy for significant CAD
- Higher diagnostic accuracy than single-photon emission computerized tomography (SPECT)
- Similar diagnostic accuracy to positron emission tomography (PET)
- Evaluates cardiac function and viability in addition to myocardial perfusion
- Superior image resolution vs. SPECT and PET
- Involves no ionizing radiation

Clinical Indications for CMR Vasodilator Stress

- Known or possible stable angina in patients with either
  - Uninterpretable electrocardiogram (ECG) or
  - Inability to tolerate moderate exercise
- To evaluate physiologic significance of known coronary artery stenosis

Contraindications for CMR Vasodilator Stress

- Unstable angina or acute myocardial infarction
- Asthma/active wheezing (for adenosine, dipyridamole)
- Arrhythmias
  - 2nd- or 3rd-degree heart block
  - Sick sinus rhythm
- Critical aortic stenosis or left ventricular (LV) outflow obstruction
- Resting hypotension (systolic blood pressure < 95 mmHg)
- Caffeine within last 24 hours (relative contraindication: Possible inadequate vasodilation)
- Gadolinium allergy
- Typical contraindications to MR

VASODILATOR STRESS AGENT PROTOCOLS

Adenosine

- 140 mcg/kg/minute intravenous infusion for < 6 minutes
- Gadolinium administered ~ 3 minutes after starting adenosine
- Perfusion images obtained during gadolinium injection

Regadenoson

- 0.4 mg/5mL intravenous injection followed by saline 5-mg intravenous injection
- Gadolinium administered intravenously 70 seconds after regadenoson injection
- Perfusion images obtained during gadolinium injection
- Regadenoson reversed with aminophylline 100-mg intravenous injection after stress procedure (optional)

Dipyridamole

- 0.56 mg/kg intravenous infusion over 4 minutes (up to maximum of 60 mg)
- Gadolinium administered intravenously 4 minutes after dipyridamole
- Perfusion images obtained during gadolinium injection

CMR STRESS PERFUSION IMAGING PROTOCOLS

Typical Vasodilator Stress CMR Protocol

- **Localizer images**
- **Stress perfusion**
  - Vasodilator stress agent administered
  - Gadolinium contrast administered
    - 0.05 mg/kg dose administered at 2 mL/second (some user higher doses)
  - Perfusion images obtained during gadolinium administration
    - Adiabatic saturation recovery pulse with steady-state free precession or fast gradient-echo read out
    - 3 noncontiguous short-axis images obtained at each heartbeat, sometimes supplemented with additional 3- or 4-chamber views
    - At least 60-heartbeat acquisition duration (consider 90 beats for low ejection fractions)
- **Rest function**
  - Steady-state free precession cine
  - LV short-axis stack
  - LV 4-chamber, 3-chamber, 2-chamber views
- **Rest perfusion**
  - Gadolinium contrast administered
    - 0.05 mg/kg dose administered at 2 mL/second (some user higher doses)
  - Perfusion images obtained during gadolinium administration (same parameters as stress perfusion)
  - 3rd dose of gadolinium (0.5 mL/kg) administered after rest perfusion images obtained in preparation for LGE
- **LGE**
  - Obtained 10 minutes after rest perfusion images
  - Short- and long-axis views of LV
  - Inversion recovery fast gradient-echo sequence with inversion time set to null normal, nondiseased myocardium
    - Inversion time can be modified to null blood pool in order to increase conspicuity of small, subendocardial scars

Fully Quantitative Perfusion Techniques and Protocols

- **Requirements for quantitative perfusion**
  - Imaging arterial input function (AIF)

- Imaging contrast dynamics within myocardium
- Modeling perfusion in order to quantify myocardial blood flow (MBF) in mL/minute/g
- Common perfusion models
  - Fermi function constrained deconvolution
  - 2-compartment model
- **Quantitative perfusion methods**
  - **Low dose of gadolinium technique**
    - Allows estimation of AIF and myocardial perfusion
  - **Dual-bolus technique**
    - Uses 2 boluses of gadolinium contrast for both stress and rest (total of 4 sets of perfusion images)
      - Low-dose bolus (0.005 mL/kg) gadolinium dose allows imaging of AIF
      - High-dose bolus (0.5 mL/kg) gadolinium dose allows imaging of myocardial perfusion
      - Low-dose bolus is diluted with saline so that it is equal volume of high-dose bolus
  - **Dual-sequence technique**
    - Only 1 bolus of gadolinium contrast for both stress and rest (0.05 mL/kg) and 2 sequences run for each heartbeat
    - Saturation pulse with fast low-angle shot sequence for AIF
      - 1 low-resolution, short inversion time image obtained each heartbeat
    - Composite saturation pulse with steady-state free precession readout for myocardial perfusion
      - 3 higher resolution images obtained each heartbeat

CMR IMAGE INTERPRETATION: DETECTING OBSTRUCTIVE CORONARY ARTERY DISEASE

Qualitative Assessment

- Visual assessment of perfusion defect
  - Regions of myocardium that show lower signal intensity or slower enhancement
  - Perfusion defect must be present for 4 or more heartbeats

Fully Quantitative Assessment

- Highest diagnostic accuracy for detection of obstructive CAD
  - Superior to qualitative interpretation
- Sensitivity 87%, specificity 93%
- Validated with PET, microspheres, and coronary angiography
- Fully quantifies myocardial blood flow accurately at pixel-wise level over wide range of MBF rates
  - Quantifies MBF via Fermi function constrained deconvolution methods
  - Abnormal perfusion ≥ 50% reduction in blood flow
- Absolute stress MBFs by CMR
  - Transmural flow in nonischemic segment: 2.99 ± 0.59 mL/minute/g
  - Transmural flow in ischemic segment: 1.73 ± 0.71 mL/minute/g
  - Subendocardial flow in ischemic segment: 1.2 ± 0.53 mL/minute/g
- Myocardial perfusion reserve (MPR)
  - MPR > 1.5 = low probability of significant coronary stenosis
    - Similar to PET MPR: Abnormal < 1.5; borderline 1.5-2; normal > 2
- Fully automated quantitative perfusion now available
  - Each component of automated system extensively validated for diagnostic accuracy
  - Calculates absolute myocardial blood flows at stress and rest
  - Calculates MPR for each cardiac segment

IMAGING PITFALLS AND COMPLICATIONS

Pitfalls

- Dark rim artifact
  - Mimics subendocardial perfusion defect in septal wall
    - Seen when contrast agent bolus arrives in LV
  - Potential mechanisms leading to dark rim artifacts
    - Gibbs ringing
    - Inadequate spatial resolution
    - Motion artifact exacerbated with high heart rates
    - K-space nonuniformity
  - Distinguished from true perfusion defects by absolute myocardial blood flow calculated by fully quantitative perfusion
    - Dark rim artifact: 2.17 ± 0.61 mL/minute/g
    - True subendocardial perfusion defect: 1.2 ± 0.53 mL/minute/g

Complications

- Gadolinium
  - Allergic reaction
  - Deposition of trace amounts of gadolinium in body (no clinical correlate identified to date)
- Vasodilator stress agents
  - Heart block, atrial fibrillation, panic attack, exacerbation of asthma or emphysema (adenosine, dipyridamole)

SELECTED REFERENCES

1. Fu Q et al: Prognostic value of stress perfusion cardiac MRI in cardiovascular disease: a systematic review and meta-analysis of the effects of the scanner, stress agent, and analysis technique. Radiol Cardiothorac Imaging. 6(3):e230382, 2024
2. Sakuma H et al: Advances in myocardial perfusion mr imaging: physiological implications, the importance of quantitative analysis, and impact on patient care in coronary artery disease. Magn Reson Med Sci. 21(1):195-211, 2022
3. Holtackers RJ et al: Dark-blood late gadolinium enhancement cardiovascular magnetic resonance for improved detection of subendocardial scar: a review of current techniques. J Cardiovasc Magn Reson. 23(1):96, 2021
4. Patel AR et al: Stress cardiac magnetic resonance myocardial perfusion imaging: JACc review topic of the week. J Am Coll Cardiol. 78(16):1655-68, 2021
5. Nagel E et al: Magnetic resonance perfusion or fractional flow reserve in coronary disease. N Engl J Med. 380(25):2418-28, 2019

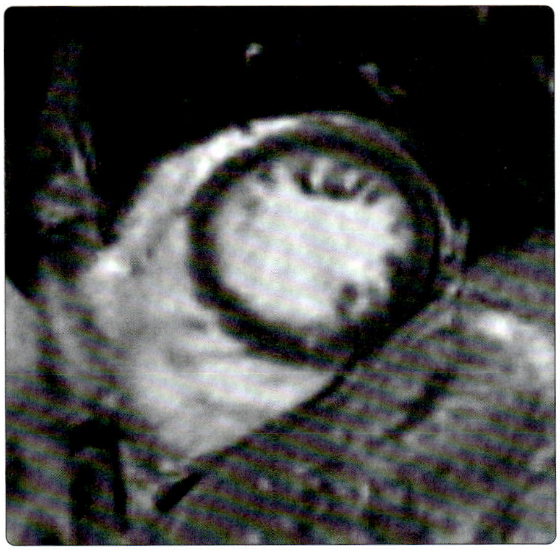

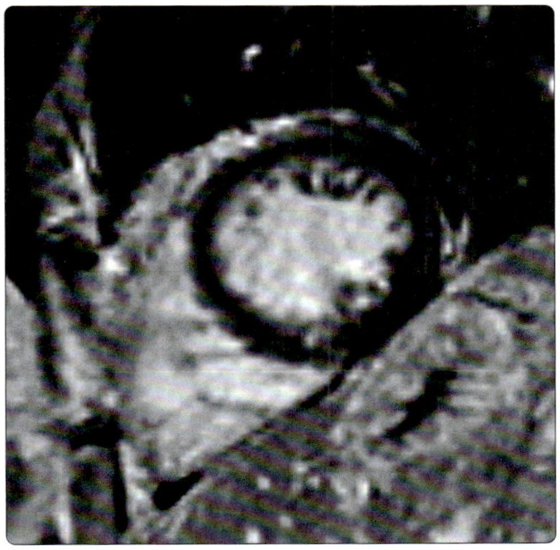

(Left) *Short-axis cine MR of the midleft ventricle in a patient with 89% stenosis of the right coronary artery on quantitative coronary angiography is unremarkable and shows uniform signal intensity of the myocardium. (Courtesy L. Y. Hsu, MD.)* **(Right)** *LGE MR of the same midleft ventricular slice of myocardium shows no enhancement to indicate myocardial infarction or other myocardial fibrosis.*

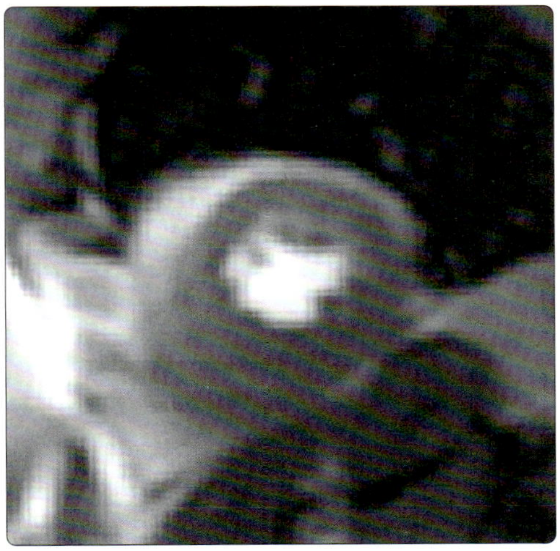

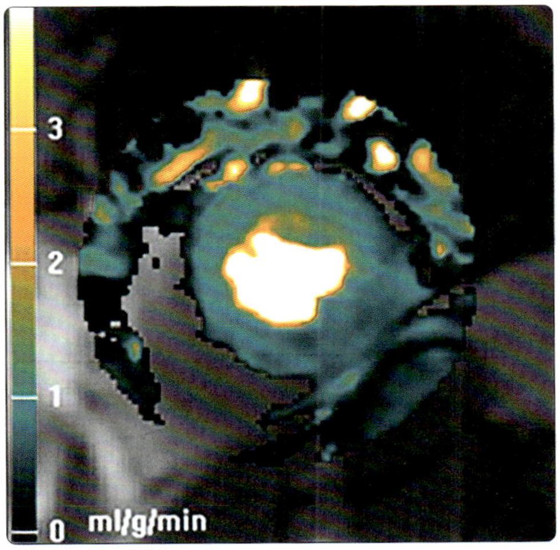

(Left) *Rest perfusion image in the same patient at same midleft ventricular slice location shows normal rest perfusion.* **(Right)** *Automated myocardial blood flow perfusion map of the same midleft ventricular slice during rest is normal.*

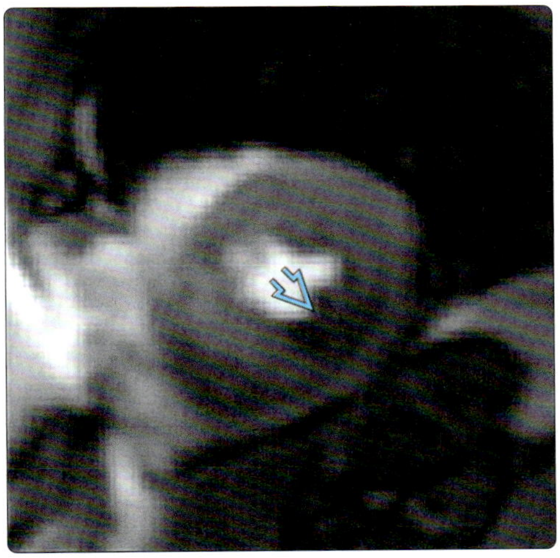

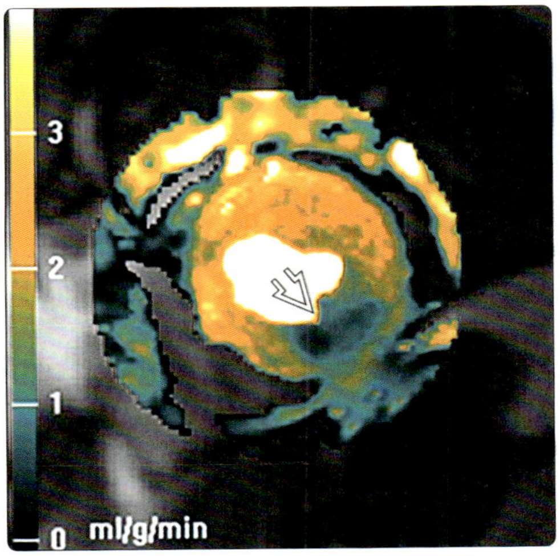

(Left) *Stress perfusion MR in the same patient at the same midleft ventricular slice location shows a severe perfusion defect within the inferior wall corresponding to the right coronary artery territory.* **(Right)** *Automated myocardial blood flow perfusion map of the same midleft ventricular slice location during stress shows a severe perfusion defect within the inferior wall.*

Coronary Embolism

KEY FACTS

TERMINOLOGY

- Part of spectrum of nonatherosclerotic cause of myocardial infarction (MI) and MI with nonobstructive coronary arteries (MINOCA)
- Dislodged thrombus, tumor, cholesterol, air, or fat obstructing coronary artery

IMAGING

- Cardiac gated CTA
  - Absence of culprit atherosclerotic lesion
  - May show subtle subendocardial perfusion defect
  - May demonstrate underlying pathology (myxoma, left atrial appendage thrombus, etc.)
  - May demonstrate patent foramen ovale (PFO), atrial septal defect (ASD), or other shunt responsible for paradoxical embolism
- MR demonstrates focal subendocardial LGE in presence of
  - PFO or ASD
  - Left atrial appendage thrombus
  - Left atrial myxoma or other mass
- SSFP cine
  - Focal wall motion abnormality with otherwise maintained global left ventricular function
- T2-weighted FSE
  - Edema adjacent to infarcted myocardium in acute setting
  - Usually larger area than infarct on LGE MR
- 1st-pass perfusion
  - Focal subendocardial perfusion defect matching LGE
- Delayed enhancement
  - Focal area of LGE based on subendocardial myocardium
- Invasive coronary angiography usually demonstrates clean coronary arteries

DIAGNOSTIC CHECKLIST

- Coronary embolus is diagnosis of exclusion
- Coronary artery disease with acute coronary syndrome and myocarditis need to be excluded

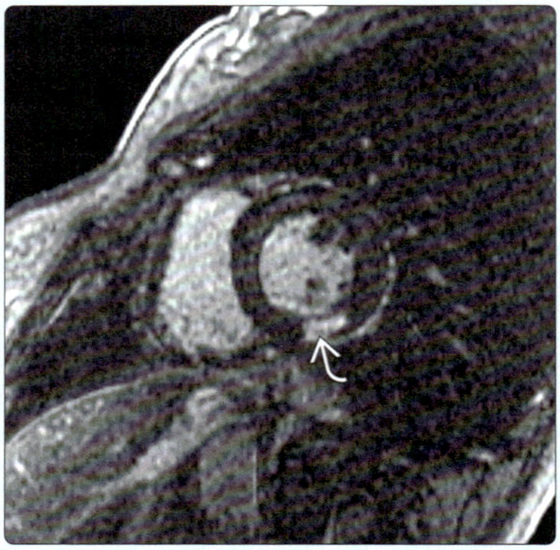
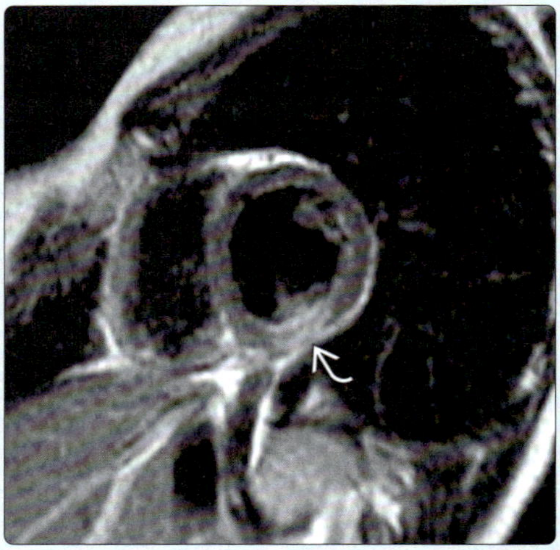

(Left) *Short-axis LGE MR 2 days after sudden onset of acute chest pain shows focal subendocardial delayed hyperenhancement ➡, nearly transmural, representing focal myocardial infarct in a subset of the right coronary artery (RCA) territory [posterior left ventricular (PLV) branch]. No other foci of delayed enhancement are present.* **(Right)** *Short-axis noncontrast T2WI FSE MR shows T2 hyperintensity ➡ larger than the infarcted myocardium seen on LGE MR, indicating periinfarct myocardial edema in a recent infarct.*

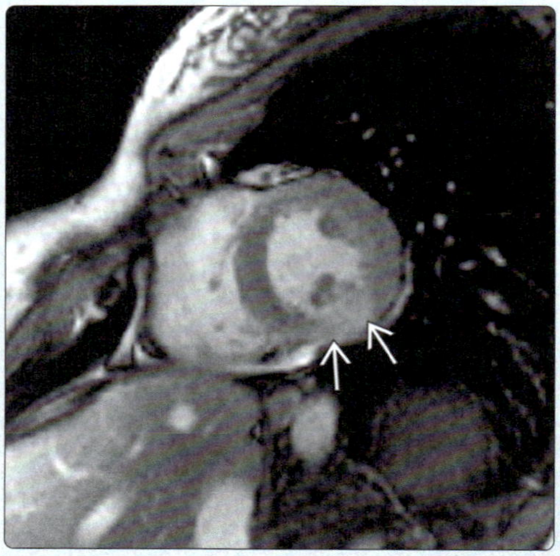
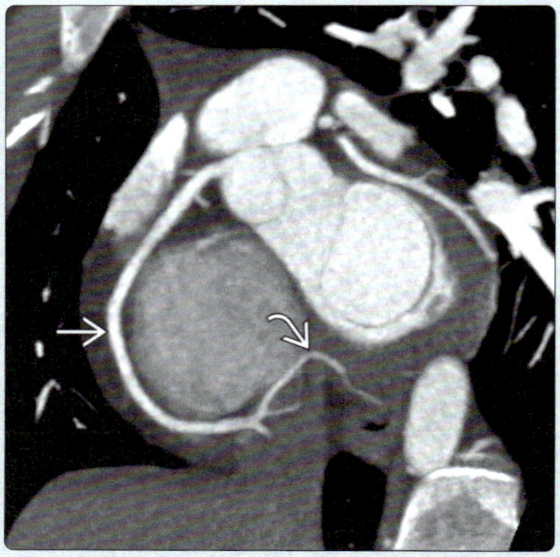

(Left) *Short-axis SSFP MR performed after contrast administration demonstrates high signal ➡ in the same location as the 1st image, which is due to a combination of hyperemic enhancement and edema. Cine images showed focal akinesis in this segment, consistent with stunned myocardium.* **(Right)** *Oblique MPR of the RCA ➡ and portion of the PLV branch ➡ shows absence of any plaque or stenosis. No culprit lesion (atherosclerotic plaque ± rupture) is identified.*

TERMINOLOGY

Definitions

- Part of spectrum of nonatherosclerotic cause of myocardial infarction (MI) and MI with nonobstructive coronary arteries (MINOCA)
- Dislodged thrombus, tumor, cholesterol, air, or fat obstructing coronary artery

IMAGING

General Features

- Best diagnostic clue
  - MR demonstrates focal subendocardial delayed hyperenhancement in presence of
    - Patent foramen ovale (PFO) or atrial septal defect (ASD)
    - Left atrial appendage (LAA) thrombus, atrial fibrillation
    - Left atrial (LA) myxoma or other mass

CT Findings

- Cardiac gated CTA
  - Absence of culprit atherosclerotic lesion
    - Often clean coronary arteries
  - May show subtle subendocardial perfusion defect
  - Regional akinesis (stunning) but maintained global function
  - May demonstrate underlying pathology (myxoma, LAA thrombus, etc.)
  - May demonstrate PFO, ASD, or other shunt responsible for paradoxical embolism

MR Findings

- SSFP white-blood cine
  - Focal wall motion abnormality with otherwise maintained global left ventricular (LV) function
  - May demonstrate edema as high signal
  - If performed after contrast, hyperenhancement may be seen
- T2-weighted FSE
  - Edema adjacent to infarcted myocardium in acute setting; usually larger area than infarct on LGE MR
- 1st-pass perfusion
  - Focal subendocardial perfusion defect matching LGE
- Delayed enhancement
  - Focal area of LGE involving subendocardial myocardium
- Parametric mapping
  - Increased native T1 values; decreased postcontrast T1; increased extracellular volume (ECV)
  - Increased T2 value in acute setting

Angiographic Findings

- Invasive coronary angiography usually demonstrates clean coronary arteries
  - May demonstrate focal intraluminal filling defect
  - Catheter-directed aspiration and embolectomy can be performed

Imaging Recommendations

- Best imaging tool
  - Cardiac MR is best modality to suggest diagnosis

DIFFERENTIAL DIAGNOSIS

Acute Myocardial Infarction Due to Atherosclerotic Coronary Artery Disease

- Associated coronary artery disease

Myocarditis

- Clean coronary arteries but elevated cardiac markers
- Myocardial edema
- Linear midmyocardial or subepicardial hyperenhancement
- Increased relative global enhancement (myocardium vs. skeletal muscle)

PATHOLOGY

General Features

- Etiology
  - LAA thrombus in setting of atrial fibrillation
    - Most common cause
  - Endocarditis, prosthetic valve thrombosis
  - Dislodged thrombus from deep venous thrombosis with presence of PFO or ASD
  - Iatrogenic: Plaque or cholesterol dislodged during coronary angioplasty
  - LA myxoma or other neoplasm
  - Fat emboli from long bone after fracture

Gross Pathologic & Surgical Features

- Usually small, focal myocardial necrosis based on subendocardial myocardium

CLINICAL ISSUES

Presentation

- Most common signs/symptoms
  - Usually atypical presentation due to small area of infarction
  - Chest pain; pain in chin, left arm, or epigastrium
- Other signs/symptoms
  - Borderline elevated cardiac enzymes

Demographics

- Epidemiology
  - Uncommon cause of acute MI (3-4%)
  - More common in young males

Treatment

- Depends on underlying cause and location of emboli
  - ASD closure device, resection of myxoma, treat deep vein thrombosis

DIAGNOSTIC CHECKLIST

Consider

- Coronary embolus is diagnosis of exclusion
  - Coronary artery disease with acute coronary syndrome and myocarditis need to be excluded

SELECTED REFERENCES

1. Monin A et al: Coronary artery embolism and acute coronary syndrome: a critical appraisal of existing data. Trends Cardiovasc Med. 34(1):50-6, 2024
2. Sucato V et al: Myocardial infarction with non-obstructive coronary arteries (MINOCA): intracoronary imaging-based diagnosis and management. J Cardiol. 77(5):444-51, 2021

Spontaneous Coronary Artery Dissection

KEY FACTS

TERMINOLOGY

- Nonatherosclerotic, nontraumatic coronary artery dissection leads to intramural hematoma, compressing lumen

IMAGING

- Involved vessels: Left anterior descending (43-60%) > left circumflex (16-38%) > right coronary artery (10-29%) > left main (0-12%)
- CTA
  - Long-segment luminal narrowing in absence of coronary artery disease in young patient
  - May show intramural hematoma/contrast within coronary artery
  - Dissection flap can occasionally be seen
- Transesophageal echocardiography
  - Assess wall motion
  - Flap may be visible with proximal dissection
- Optical coherence tomography (OCT) provides high-resolution coronary imaging but may increase risk of procedural complications
- Saw angiographic classification: Types I, II, III

TOP DIFFERENTIAL DIAGNOSES

- Coronary thrombus
- Atherosclerotic disease

CLINICAL ISSUES

- Younger patients, especially females, present with chest discomfort typically linked to acute coronary syndrome, unexplained heart failure, sudden death, or may be asymptomatic
- Conservative management preferred for stable patients due to high likelihood of spontaneous healing with careful monitoring and medical therapy
- PCI or CABG is considered for high-risk cases involving ongoing ischemia, unstable hemodynamics, or complex coronary anatomy

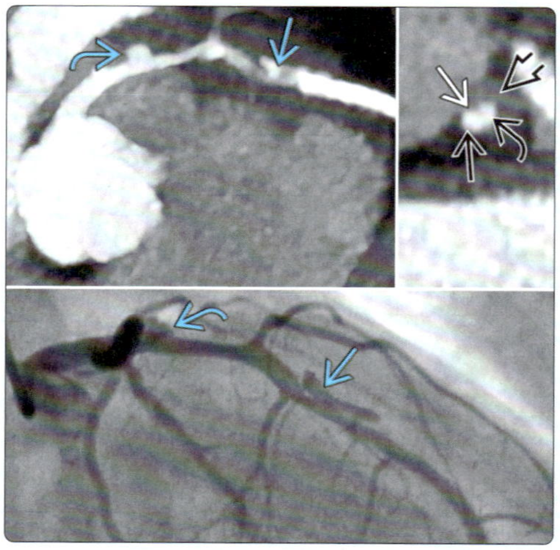

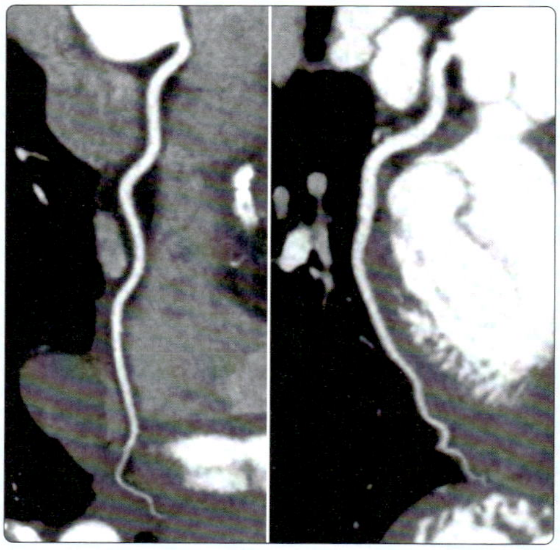

(Left) *CTA in a woman with type I SCAD during childbirth (top) shows contrast filling the false lumen (FL) in proximal* ➔ *and mid* ➔ *left anterior descending (LAD) arteries and on catheterization (bottom). Cross section through proximal LAD (top) shows true lumen* ➔ *and FL* ➔ *separated by subtle dissection flap* ➔ *with surrounding intramural hematoma* ➔. **(Right)** *MPRs of right coronary artery (L) and left circumflex (R) are normal in a woman with severe chest pain and history of genetic arteriopathy. There is no atherosclerotic disease.*

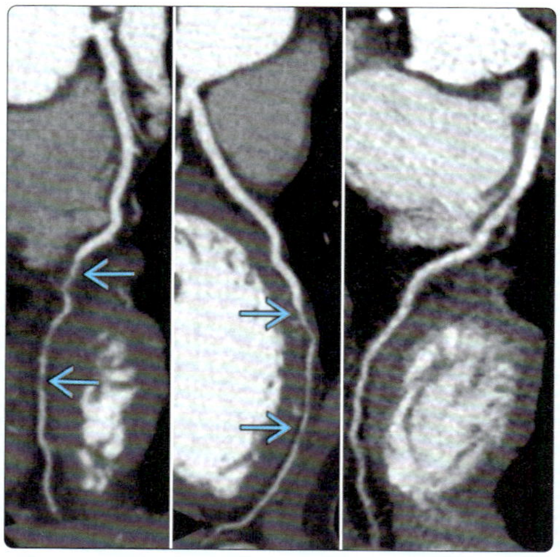

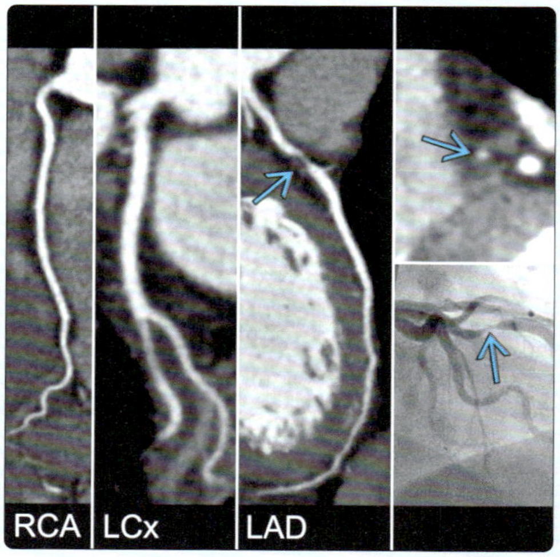

(Left) *CECT images of the LAD arteries (middle and L) show long-segment narrowing* ➔ *of the mid and distal LAD due to type II SCAD. The patient was treated conservatively. Repeat CTA (R) 3 months later shows resolution.* **(Right)** *CTA in a 41-year-old woman with ↑ troponin shows focal severe stenosis of the proximal LAD* ➔. *Coronaries are otherwise normal. It was unclear if this was due to plaque rupture or SCAD. IV ultrasound showed type III SCAD.*

TERMINOLOGY

Abbreviations

- Spontaneous coronary artery dissection (SCAD)

Definitions

- Dissection of coronary artery not related to atherosclerotic or traumatic causes
- Intramural hematoma (IMH) within arterial wall caused by hematoma separating intimal layer from other layers, resulting in lumen compression and ischemia

IMAGING

General Features

- Best diagnostic clue
  - Long-segment, often discontinuous, narrowing of single coronary artery in young patient with acute coronary syndrome
  - Dissection flap may be seen but often absent
- Location
  - Left anterior descending artery is most frequently involved (43-60%), followed by circumflex artery (16-38%), right coronary artery (10-29%), and left main (0-12%)

CT Findings

- Cardiac gated CTA
  - Best noninvasive technique for assessing SCAD
    - Normal CTA does not exclude SCAD
  - Various findings depending on type
    - Appearance similar to aortic dissection (AD) with visible dissection flap with true lumen and false lumen
      - True dissection may track retrograde to ostium and extend into aortic wall/AD
    - Appearance similar to IMH with long-segment wall thickening due to blood in media leading to vascular narrowing
    - Focal area of wall thickening with vascular narrowing often indistinguishable from focal plaque rupture due to atherosclerotic disease
    - Except for focal SCAD, both AD and IMH are often long segment and can have areas that appear normal between involved portions
  - Usually involves single coronary artery
  - Coronary artery disease often absent due to young age of patients
  - Coronary CTA excellent for SCAD follow-up
    - Aids in monitoring recurrent symptoms and detecting non-flow-limiting narrowing
  - Ancillary features include epicardial fat stranding, beading, and coronary tortuosity

MR Findings

- MR angiography
  - Lower spatial resolution than CTA and angiography: Not typically used for diagnosis; useful for serial follow-up
  - Findings similar to coronary CTA, especially in proximal coronary arteries
  - Hyperintensity reported due to IMH; neither sensitive nor specific
- Cardiac MR
  - Assesses LV function, regional wall motion abnormalities, myocardial perfusion, microvascular obstruction, infarct
  - Not initial modality for assessment of patients with SCAD

Angiographic Findings

- Intimal flap may be apparent as linear filling defect in vessel lumen
  - Linear or spiral-shaped false lumen contrast staining, may demonstrate retrograde extension into aortic wall
  - Saw angiographic classification used to classify cases
    - Type I: Multiple radiolucent lumina or arterial wall contrast staining; 2nd most common pattern
    - Type II: Diffuse stenosis that can be of varying severity and length (usually > 40 mm); most common pattern
    - Type III: Focal or tubular stenosis, usually < 20 mm in length, that mimics atherosclerosis

Intracoronary Imaging

- Can be used when angiography is not diagnostic
- Intravascular ultrasound (IVUS) or optical coherence tomography (OCT) can visualize coronary arterial wall and confirm presence of intimal flap, true and false lumina, IMH, and fenestrations
- OCT is invasive intracoronary gold standard
  - Uses light waves to image vessel wall with higher spatial resolution
  - In SCAD, complications include propagation of dissection or cannulation of false lumen
- May aid placement of stent guidewire into true lumen
- Can demonstrate contrast (hypoechogenic) or thrombus (gray echogenicity) within false lumen

DIFFERENTIAL DIAGNOSIS

Coronary Thrombus

- Less often linear and typically fill lumen, typically more mobile than dissection flap

Atherosclerotic Disease

- Type II and III SCAD can mimic atherosclerotic disease
- Clues that suggest SCAD include absence of atherosclerotic disease in uninvolved coronaries
- Many patients with SCAD are younger women with no risk factors for atherosclerotic disease

PATHOLOGY

General Features

- Etiology
  - Development of IMH between media and adventitia
    - Luminal compression and restricted blood flow may lead to infarction
  - Associated conditions of factors
    - Fibromuscular dysplasia in 25-86% of cases
    - Inherited arteriopathy or connective tissue disease in 1.2-3%
      - Ehlers-Danlos syndrome, Marfan syndrome, Loeys-Dietz syndrome
    - Exogenous hormones in 10.7-12.6%
      - Oral contraceptives, testosterone, etc.
    - Pregnancy in 2-8%
    - Multiparity in 8.9-10%
    - Systemic inflammatory disease in < 1-8.9%

- Lupus, inflammatory bowel disease, sarcoid, rheumatoid, etc.
  - Precipitating factors recalled in > 50% of patients
    - Intense physical exertion, Valsalva-like maneuvers (e.g., vomiting, childbirth), emotional stress, stimulant use, etc.

Microscopic Features

- Often normal media with IMH between media and adventitia
- Adventitial reaction progressing from acute inflammation (hours) to eosinophilic infiltration (days) and then fibroblast proliferation
  - Inflammatory infiltrate can help distinguish SCAD from iatrogenic dissections in postmortem cases
- Cystic medial necrosis can occur but uncommon

CLINICAL ISSUES

Presentation

- Most common signs/symptoms
  - Chest pain, typically in context of acute coronary syndromes (ACSs)
    - ST-elevation myocardial infarction (26-87%)
    - Non-ST-elevation myocardial infarction (13-69%)
  - ↓ left ventricular (LV) ejection fraction < 50% observed in 44-49% of cases at presentation
    - Many show improvement on repeat assessments, likely due to normalization of stunned myocardium after SCAD healing
  - Complications
    - Ventricular arrhythmias or sudden cardiac death (3-11%)
    - Cardiogenic shock (2-5%)

Demographics

- Age
  - Spontaneous-type true prevalence unknown, likely underdiagnosed
  - Younger female patients without traditional risk factors
  - Thought to make up 1-4% of ACSs, higher prevalence than previously recognized
    - May be cause of ACS in up to 35% of infarction in women ≤ 50 years of age
- Sex
  - 90% of SCAD are diagnosed in women
  - Most common cause of pregnancy-associated MI; preeclampsia appears variably related
    - Worse prognosis than nonpregnancy-associated spontaneous dissection
    - Higher association with multiparity (> ± 4 births)

Natural History & Prognosis

- Conservative management preferred for in absence of large-vessel occlusion
  - Carries risk of early ischemia, requiring close monitoring in 1st week
- SCAD progression varies
  - Isolated IMH (type II and III) is more likely to worsen early, while intimal tears (type I) might offer some protective effect
- Up to 1/2 of patients may experience SCAD progression
  - Recurrent pain may not always be ischemic
- Mortality after SCAD is low (1-2% over 1-3 years)
- 17-18% of patients experiencing new event over 3-4 years, mostly due to recurrent SCAD
  - Recurrent SCAD is new dissection in different coronary artery, separate from initial event
  - Recurrence rates range from 5% over 22 months to 15% over 27 months
- β-blockers may help prevent recurrence, particularly in managing hypertension

Treatment

- No comparative studies of treatment modalities
- Medical
  - Reports have demonstrated favorable outcomes with conservative management
    - Many small dissections will heal spontaneously
  - Focuses on managing myocardial infarction, chronic chest pain, preventing recurrence, and evaluating other vascular abnormalities, guided by registry data and expert opinion due to lack of clinical trials
- Revascularization
  - Percutaneous coronary intervention (PCI) or coronary artery bypass graft (CABG), based on coronary anatomy and expertise, is recommended for high-risk patients with persistent ischemia, recurrent chest pain, left main artery dissection, ventricular arrhythmias, or unstable hemodynamics
  - Outcomes generally worse vs. atherosclerotic disease due to weak coronary walls
    - Technical failure in 30%
  - Angioplasty: Gentle, low-caliber balloon angioplasty may restore distal flow without permanent stenting
    - Cutting balloons may reduce lumen compression in selected cases
  - Stenting considerations: Drug-eluting stents (DES) preferred over bare metal stents
  - Used if ischemia/unstable patient but no high-risk anatomy
- CABG is reserved for unstable patients, PCI failure, and high-risk anatomy left main stem, 2-vessel proximal disease, severe LV dysfunction)
  - Good acute results, but late graft occlusion is common due to native vessel healing

DIAGNOSTIC CHECKLIST

Consider

- In younger (female) patients who present with acute MI

SELECTED REFERENCES

1. Petrović M et al: Management and outcomes of spontaneous coronary artery dissection: a systematic review of the literature. Front Cardiovasc Med. 11:1276521, 2024
2. Hayes SN et al: Spontaneous coronary artery dissection: current state of the science: a scientific statement from the American Heart Association. Circulation. 137(19):e523-57, 2018

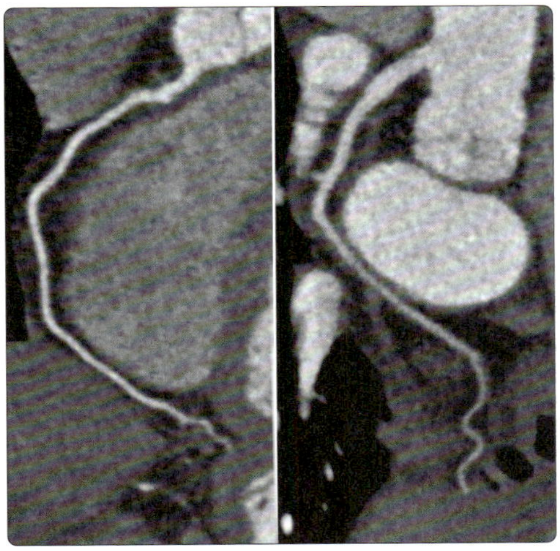

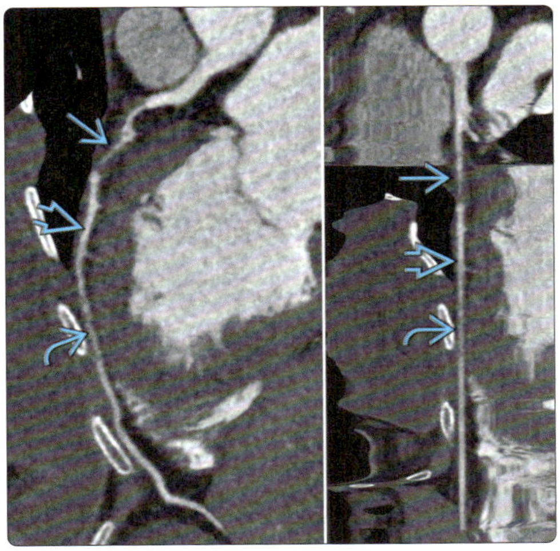

(Left) *Curved MPR images in a 29-year-old pregnant woman with severe chest pain and ↑ troponin show a normal right coronary artery (L) and left circumflex artery (R).* **(Right)** *Curved and straightened MPR images of the LAD shows severe stenosis in the proximal LAD → with mild stenosis in the mid LAD → and another focus of severe stenosis in the mid to distal LAD → due to type II SCAD.*

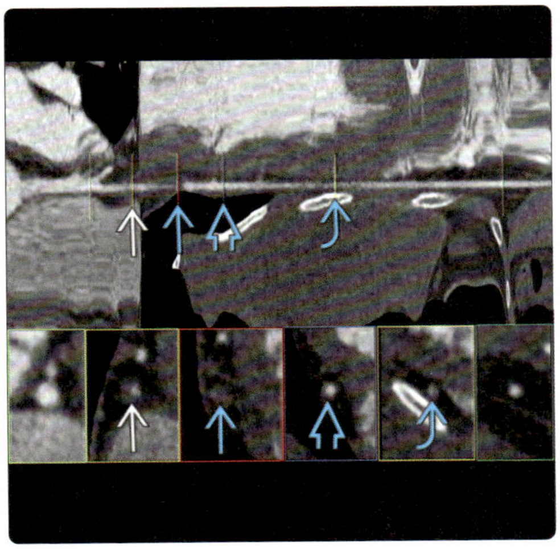

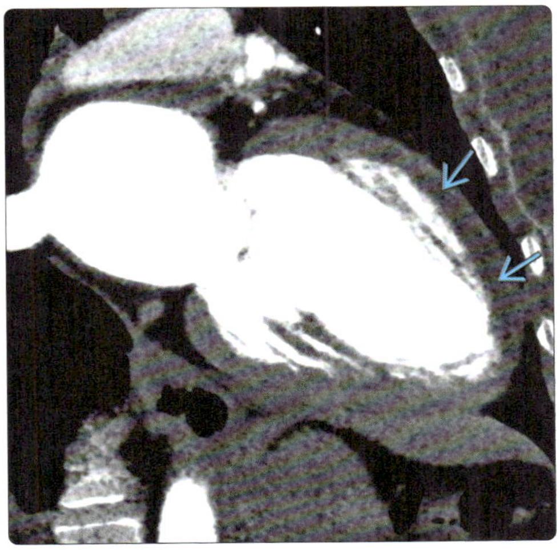

(Left) *Straightened MPR shows normal ostial LAD with an intramural hematoma (IMH) in the wall of the proximal LAD, leading to moderate → and then severe stenosis →. An IMH is seen in the wall of the proximal to mid LAD, leading to mild stenosis →. In the mid to distal LAD, IMH again leads to severe stenosis →. The very distal LAD appears normal.* **(Right)** *2-chamber minIP CECT shows anterior wall hypoperfusion → due to LAD territory infarct.*

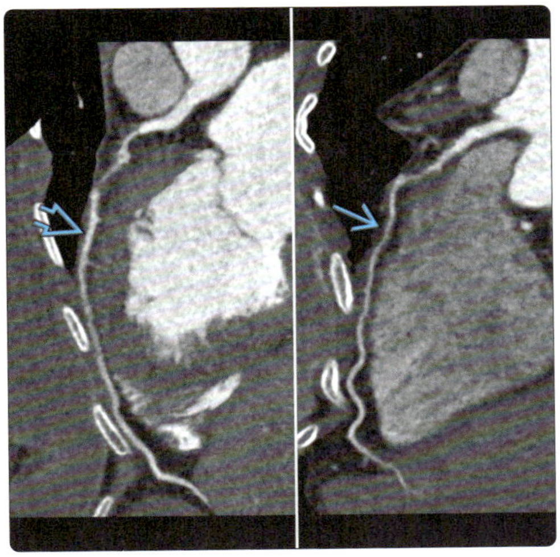

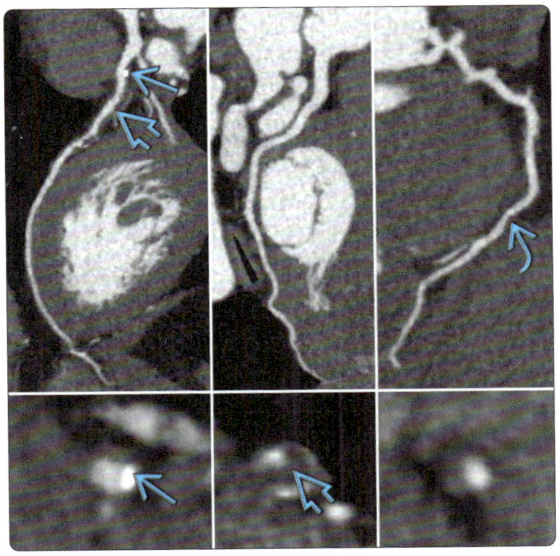

(Left) *On the initial study (L), the proximal to mid LAD → shows only mild stenosis. Repeat study 5 days later (R) shows diffuse, moderate to severe stenosis in this area → due to a worsening IMH.* **(Right)** *Coronary CTA in a 38-year-old anabolic steroid user diagnosed with SCAD shows extensive calcified and noncalcified atherosclerotic disease → in the LAD (L) with positive remodeling and low-attenuation plaque →. Atherosclerotic disease is also present in the right coronary artery →. There was no SCAD.*

Acute Myocardial Infarction

KEY FACTS

TERMINOLOGY

- Detection of rise &/or fall of cardiac biomarker values (preferably cardiac troponin) and at least 1 of following
  - Symptoms of ischemia
  - New or presumed new significant ST-segment T wave changes or new left bundle branch block
  - Development of pathological Q waves in ECG
  - Imaging evidence of new loss of viable myocardium or new regional wall motion abnormality
  - Identification of intracoronary thrombus by angiography or autopsy
- ST-segment elevation myocardial infarction (STEMI)
  - ST-segment elevation or new left bundle branch block pattern in resting ECG
  - High mortality
- Non-ST-segment elevation myocardial infarction
  - Troponin ↑, but no ST segment ↑ in resting ECG
  - Lower mortality than STEMI

IMAGING

- Coronary artery filling defect on invasive coronary angiogram in combination with wall motion abnormalities in corresponding myocardial segment and ↑ in myocardial enzymes
- **CTA**: Coronary occlusion with noncalcified material; subendocardial hypoattenuation
- **MR**
  - T2: ↑ signal intensity due to myocardial edema
  - Cine SSFP: Global/regional wall motion abnormalities, ↓ ejection fraction and ↑ ventricle volumes
  - LGE: Typical subendocardial enhancement, assessment of transmurality and viability
    - ≥ 50% → nonviable; < 50% → viable
    - Identification of microvascular obstruction and hemorrhage
  - Parametric mapping (T1, T2 mapping and extracellular volume): Diagnosis of area at risk, edema, and infarct size

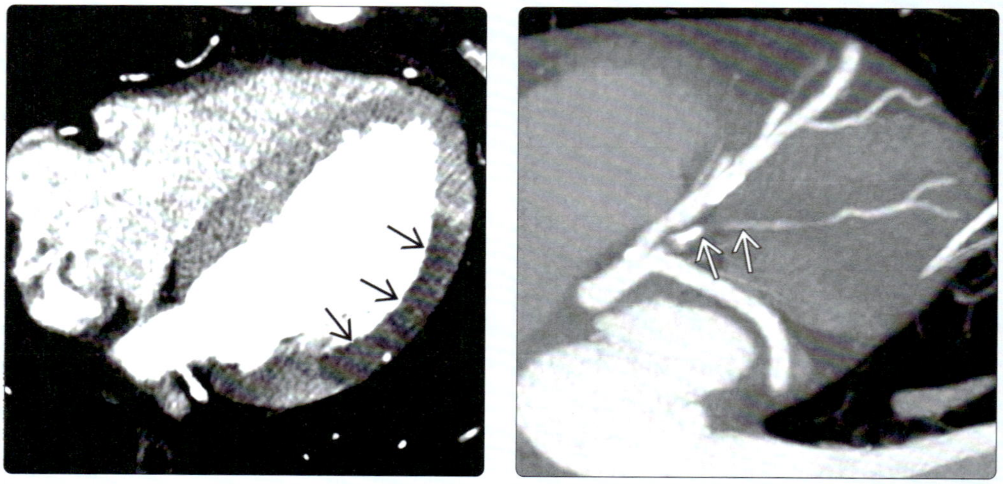

(Left) *Multiplanar CECT reconstruction (transaxial orientation; 8-mm thickness) shows clearly defined hypoperfusion of the lateral wall of the left ventricle (LV) ➔. This is the appearance of acute myocardial infarction (MI) [ST-segment elevation MI (STEMI) or non-ST-segment elevation MI (NSTEMI)] on CECT.* **(Right)** *Contrast-enhanced coronary CTA in the same patient reveals an occlusion of the intermediate branch (ramus) ➔.*

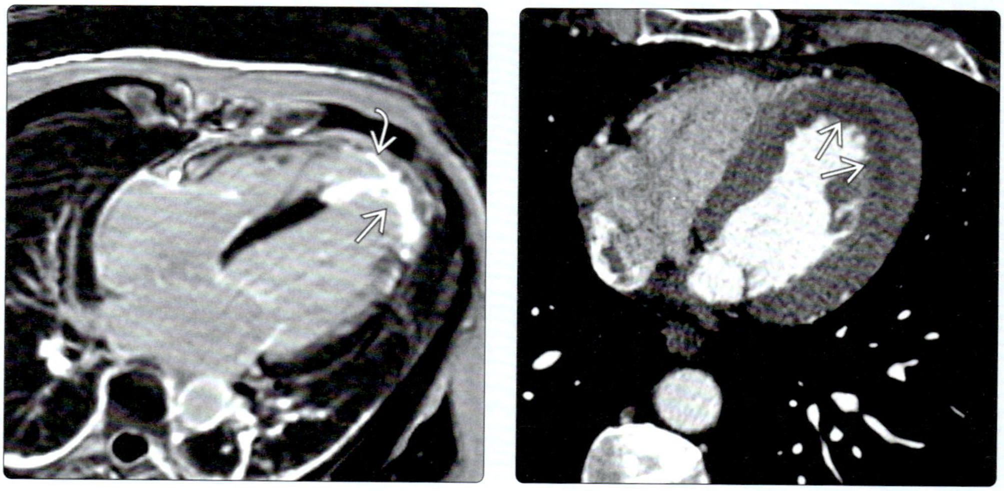

(Left) *Four-chamber LGE MR in a patient with acute chest pain shows transmural delayed hyperenhancement in the left anterior descending (LAD) coronary artery territory ➔, consistent with a transmural infarct. Note the relatively normal wall thickness, typical in the acute setting. Also, note the transmural LGE in the apical right ventricular (RV) wall ➔.* **(Right)** *Axial CT in the same patient demonstrates normal wall thickness with subendocardial low-attenuation perfusion defect ➔ in the LAD territory.*

TERMINOLOGY

Definitions

- Acute myocardial infarction (MI)
  - Rise &/or fall of cardiac biomarker values (preferably cardiac troponin) and ≥ 1 of following
    - Symptoms of ischemia
    - New or presumed new significant ST-segment T wave changes or new left bundle branch block
    - Development of pathologic Q waves on ECG
    - Imaging evidence of new loss of viable myocardium or new regional wall motion abnormality
    - Identification of intracoronary thrombus by angiography or autopsy
  - MI is acute coronary syndrome (ACS)
    - ST-segment elevation MI (STEMI)
    - Non-ST-segment elevation MI (NSTEMI)
    - Unstable angina pectoris
- 5 types of MI as per universal definition
  - **Type 1 MI**: Spontaneous MI due to plaque rupture, ulceration, or erosion, causing thrombus and myocyte necrosis
  - **Type 2 MI**: MI from imbalance between oxygen supply and demand (e.g., anemia, arrhythmia, shock)
  - **Type 3 MI**: Sudden cardiac death with symptoms of myocardial ischemia but without biomarkers or ECG confirmation before death
  - **Type 4 MI**: MI related to percutaneous coronary intervention (PCI) with subtypes 4a (post-PCI), 4b (stent thrombosis), and 4c (in-stent restenosis)
  - **Type 5 MI**: MI associated with CABG, indicated by elevated biomarkers and procedure-related complications
- MI with nonobstructive coronary arteries (MINOCA) refers to MI occurring without significant coronary obstruction and can involve atherosclerotic plaque disruption (type 1 MI), coronary spasm, or spontaneous coronary dissection (type 2 MI)

IMAGING

General Features

- **Best diagnostic clue**: Filling defect on invasive coronary angiogram + wall motion abnormalities in corresponding myocardial segment and ↑ myocardial enzymes
- **Location**: Consistent with vascular territory
  - Left anterior descending (LAD) infarction: Anterior and septal segments extending to apex or apical inferior wall
  - Left circumflex (LCx) infarction: Lateral segments of left ventricle (LV)
  - Right coronary artery (RCA) infarction (in right dominant circulation): Inferior and inferoseptal segments at base and midcavity levels; inferolateral segment involvement depending on size of PLV branch; apical involvement depending on size of PDA branch
- **Size**: More proximal lesion, larger infarct
  - More distal stenosis may be counteracted by collateral coronary arterial supply and Thebesian vein supply
- **Morphology**: Infarct starts within subendocardium and progress toward to subepicardium
  - Nontransmural infarct: Does not involve full thickness, spares subepicardium
  - Transmural infarction: Involves entire myocardial wall

Radiographic Findings

- Abnormal findings are rare in acute setting
- Pulmonary edema if heart failure ensues
- Sudden severe pulmonary edema in papillary muscle rupture with mitral regurgitation → poor prognosis

CT Findings

- CTA
  - Not typically used for diagnosis of acute MI
    - MI may be incidentally detected on CT performed for other causes, e.g., evaluation of aortic dissection
  - Coronary occlusion with noncalcified material (e.g., thrombus), often extensive positive remodeling
  - May demonstrate hypodense subendocardium in vascular territory
    - < 50% attenuation of normal myocardium
    - 5-mm thick MPR or 5-mm MIPs
  - Multiphasic cine: Assessment of ventricular global/regional function and dilation
  - Preserved wall thickness
    - Wall thinning and presence of calcification/fatty metaplasia are signs of chronic MI
  - Delayed-enhancement CT
    - May be feasible but displays poor contrast-to-noise ratio as compared with MR
    - May evaluate viability of myocardium
- CT perfusion (CTP)
  - 1st-pass perfusion at stress and rest
    - Underestimates infarct size as compared with LGE MR

MR Findings

- T2WI
  - ↑ signal intensity due myocardial edema (on T2 map or TIR)
- MR cine
  - Gold standard for functional assessment; ejection fraction, LV end-diastolic/systolic volumes, LV mass
  - ↓ regional wall motion and systolic wall thickening
  - ↓ ejection fraction, but could be preserved due to compensation from remote myocardium
  - Evaluation of RV function; prognostic indicator
- 1st-pass perfusion
  - Reduced wash-in of contrast agent (perfusion deficit) in coronary territory, involving subendocardium (both at rest and stress)
- Delayed enhancement
  - Has ability to detect 1 g of irreversibly damaged tissue
  - Demonstrate presence, location, and extension of MI
    - Normal myocardium black; infarct/ scar bright
    - Full-thickness involvement: Transmural
- Parametric mapping
  - Pre- and postcontrast T1 values are found to accurately quantify acute MI size
  - Expansion of extracellular volume (ECV) due to edema and necrosis (worse outcomes)
- **Role of MR in MI**
  - Diagnosis and differentiation of acute MI
    - In cases with subtle clinical symptoms

- Establishing diagnosis for ST elevation with normal coronary arteries on angiography (e.g., myocarditis, etc.)
- In cases with spontaneous recanalization of coronary artery stenosis; recognition of silent MI
- Has been shown to be of value in ruling out ACS, aortic dissection, acute pulmonary embolism, acute myocarditis
- Demonstrate culprit lesion in multivessel disease
- Determination of infarct age
  - Edema on T2WI or T2 mapping is seen only in acute MI
- Evaluation of reversible vs. irreversible injury
  - Salvageable area (area of edema: Area of LGE): Can be salvaged by revascularization
  - Myocardial salvage index: T2-weighted area: LGE area/T2-weighted area
- Evaluation of viability: Transmurality
  - Delayed enhancement is most accurate method
  - ≥ 50% → low likelihood of functional segmental recovery after revascularization: Nonviable
  - < 50% → high likelihood of functional segmental recovery after revascularization: Viable
- Identification of microvascular obstruction (MVO)
  - Central hypointense region within infarction (dark signal on 1st perfusion or LGE)
  - Associated with poor prognosis, adverse cardiovascular events, and adverse remodeling
- Identification of hemorrhage in core of infarct
  - Dark signal on T2 due to hemosiderin
  - Associated with adverse LV remodeling, large infarct size, ↑ LV end-systolic volume, and no improvement in ejection fraction over time
- Good modality to assess MI complications
  - Free wall rupture; ventricular septal rupture; aneurysm; pseudoaneurysm; pericarditis; pericardial effusion; thrombus; mitral regurgitation; heart failure

DIFFERENTIAL DIAGNOSIS

Chronic Myocardial Infarction

- No periinfarct signal ↑ (no edema) on T2 MR
- Thinned wall, calcification, fatty metaplasia, aneurysm

Acute Myocarditis

- Chest pain, ↑ cardiac enzymes, normal coronary arteries
- Focal edema and LGE in nonvascular territory
- Affects subepicardium rather than subendocardium

Acute Pericarditis

- Pericardial thickening, effusion and enhancement in MR

Stress-Induced Cardiomyopathy

- Reversible LV dysfunction with large apical akinesia
- Normal coronary arteries on invasive angiography
- MR: Edema may be present; no LGE typically

PATHOLOGY

General Features

- Etiology
  - Most frequent mechanism is atherosclerotic plaque rupture followed by thrombosis and acute coronary occlusion, leading to myocardial necrosis
  - Risk factors: Smoking, cholesterol elevation, diabetes, hypertension, family history

Gross Pathologic & Surgical Features

- Initiating event: Fissure in diseased plaque cap
  - Results in exposure of subendothelial matrix elements, which stimulates platelet activation/clot formation

CLINICAL ISSUES

Presentation

- Most common signs/symptoms
  - Chest tightness and pain; substernal, pressing, occasionally radiating to left arm or jaw
  - Associated with dyspnea, nausea, palpitations
  - Asymptomatic, especially in patients with diabetes
  - ECG: Typically ST-segment elevation
    - Left bundle branch block in proximal LAD infarction
    - Normal ECG does not exclude acute infarct (NSTEMI)
  - RVMI: Distended neck veins, normal lungs, hypotension; ST-segment elevation in leads V4R-V6R
- Nontransmural MI
  - May be silent or unrecognized = "missed MI"
  - Absence of Q wave on ECG, serum marker of MI, and appropriate clinical presentation
  - May result from early reperfusion that prevents transmural extension

Natural History & Prognosis

- Prognosis depends on extent of infarction and degree and location of coronary disease
- LAD infarction has higher rate of infarct expansion, aneurysm, rupture and LV thrombus
- RVMI have ↑ morbidity and mortality
  - Ventricular arrhythmias and atrioventricular conduction abnormalities
  - RV function may recover over time
- Nontransmural infarcts associated with better prognosis, less infarct expansion, lower risk of cardiac rupture

Treatment

- Medical management
  - Analgesia is managed with nitrates and opioids
  - Dual antiplatelet therapy (DAPT) is preferred
  - β-blockers: Benefit is extrapolated from earlier trials
- Reperfusion therapy
  - PCI or intravenous fibrinolytic therapy to restore flow
  - Indicated in all patients with symptoms of < 12 hours duration and persistent ST-segment elevation or (presumed) new left bundle branch block
  - Primary PCI is recommended over fibrinolysis within 120 minutes of symptom onset
- Surgical
  - CABG may be indicated in cardiogenic shock if PCI is not feasible or during repair of mechanical complications

SELECTED REFERENCES

1. Rajiah PS et al: Myocardial strain evaluation with cardiovascular MRI: physics, principles, and clinical applications. Radiographics. 42(4):968-90, 2022
2. Writing Committee et al: 2022 ACC expert consensus decision pathway on the evaluation and disposition of acute chest pain in the emergency department: a report of the American College of Cardiology Solution Set Oversight Committee. J Am Coll Cardiol. 80(20):1925-60, 2022

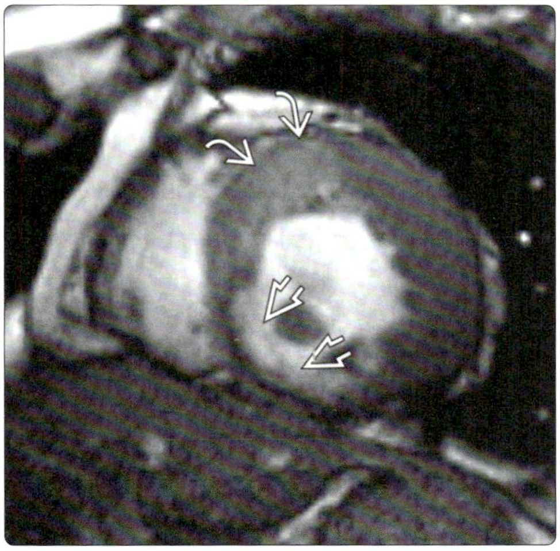

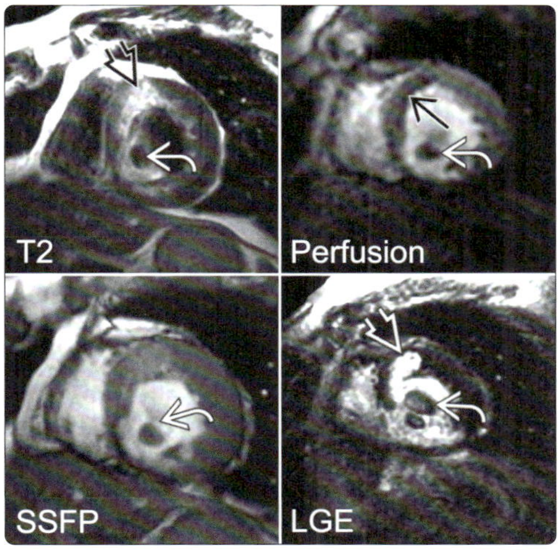

(Left) *Short-axis SSFP MR shows high signal of edema indicative of acute LAD territory MI and wall thinning with subendocardial LGE, suggestive of chronic right coronary artery territory MI. (Image obtained after Gd administration prior to LGE acquisition.)* **(Right)** *Short-axis T2 1st-pass perfusion, SSFP, and LGE MR in the same patient demonstrate edema, subendocardial perfusion defect, and LGE but a normal-thickness anteroseptal LV wall, consistent with acute MI. Note inferior chronic MI and ventricular thrombus.*

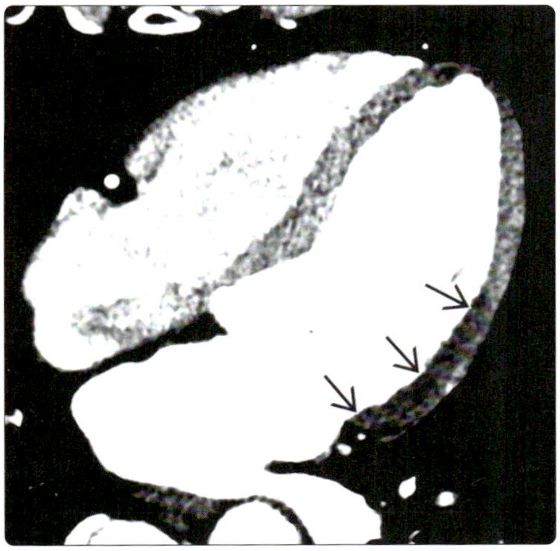

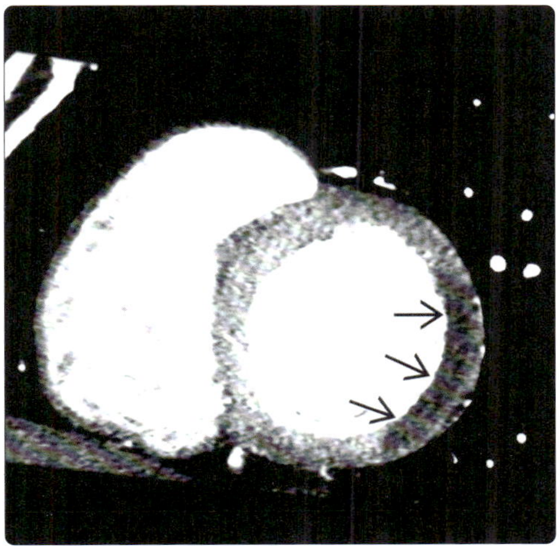

(Left) *Multiplanar reconstruction CECT (4-chamber view; 8-mm thickness) shows acute NSTEMI. Typical subendocardial hypoperfusion of the left posterolateral myocardium is seen.* **(Right)** *Short-axis CECT of the LV in the same patient shows subendocardial hypoperfusion of the left posterolateral myocardium with preserved wall thickness. Note the involvement of > 50% of the wall, suggesting low probability of functional recovery after revascularization.*

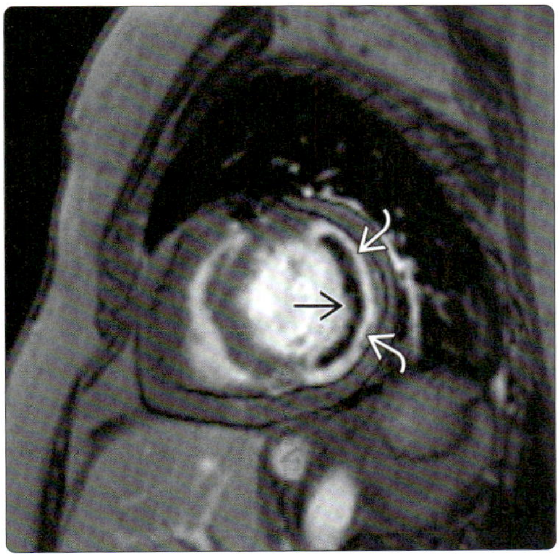

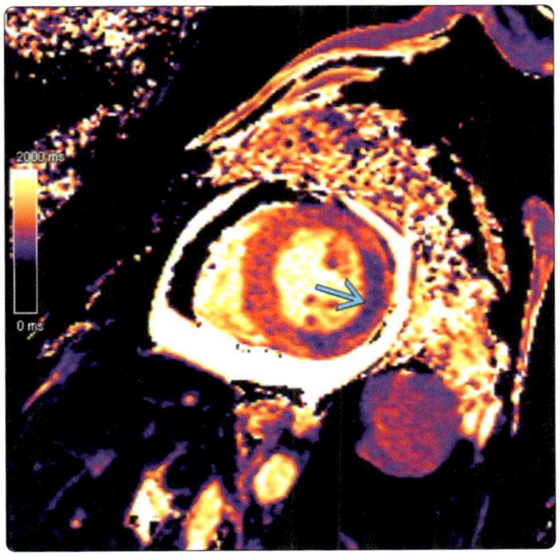

(Left) *Short-axis DE MR shows LGE within the lateral midventricle with crescentic dark areas (hypoenhancement) within the hyperenhancement, consistent with microvascular obstruction.* **(Right)** *Short-axis T1 color map in the same patient shows T1 shortening in the region of microvascular obstruction, reflecting endothelial damage, inflammation, swelling, blockage, microthrombi, and hemorrhage.*

(Left) *Black-blood short-axis T2 MR shows transmural high signal of the LV anterior ⇒ and anteroseptal ➡ myocardial segments, consistent with acute myocardial edema in the LAD vascular territory. Note anteroseptal segment hypertrophy secondary to edema.* **(Right)** *Corresponding LE MR in the same patient shows an essentially transmural infarct of the LV anteroseptal segment →. Note that the LE area is smaller than the T2 high-signal area, indicating a large area at risk on T2 sequence.*

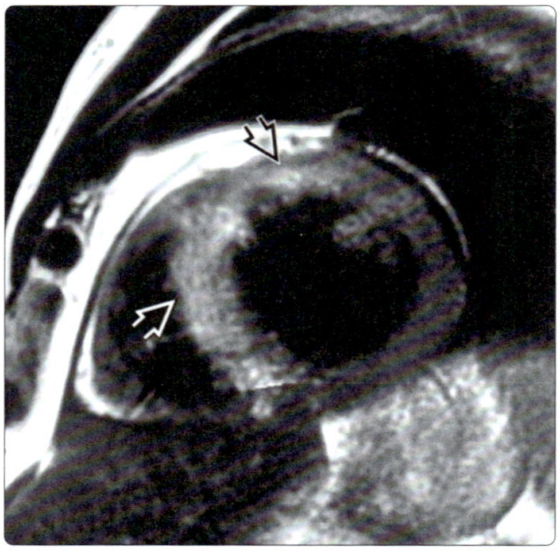

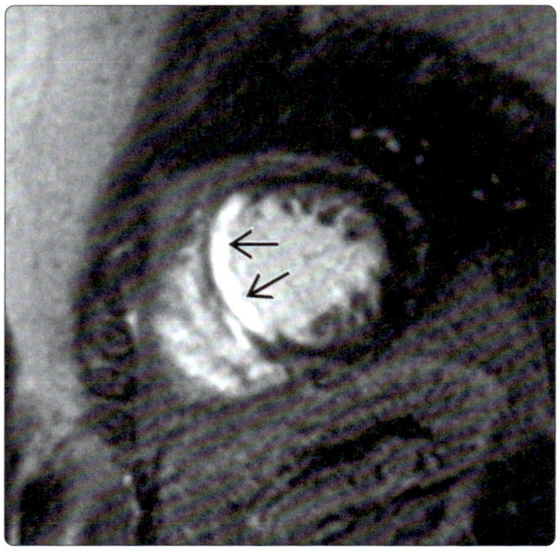

(Left) *Invasive coronary angiogram shows acutely occluded proximal segment LAD →. Note acute thrombus ⇒ in the lumen.* **(Right)** *Corresponding LE 2-chamber cardiac MR shows an extensive acute transmural infarct affecting the basal, mid, and apical anterior myocardial segments ➡ (LAD territory). Note multiple low-signal mural nodules ➡, consistent with mural thrombus. Note different location compared with microvascular obstruction, which occurs within the myocardium.*

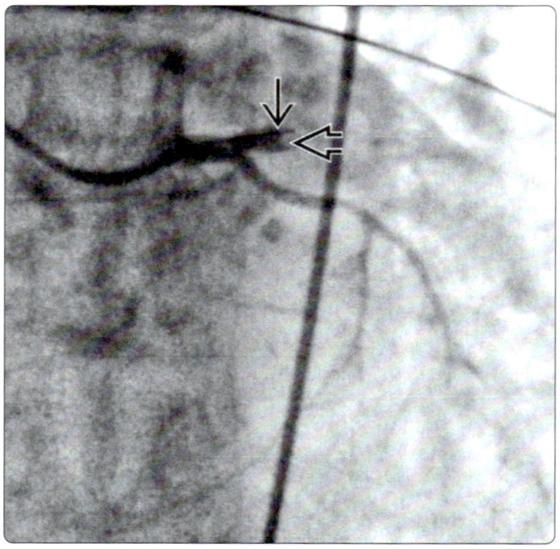

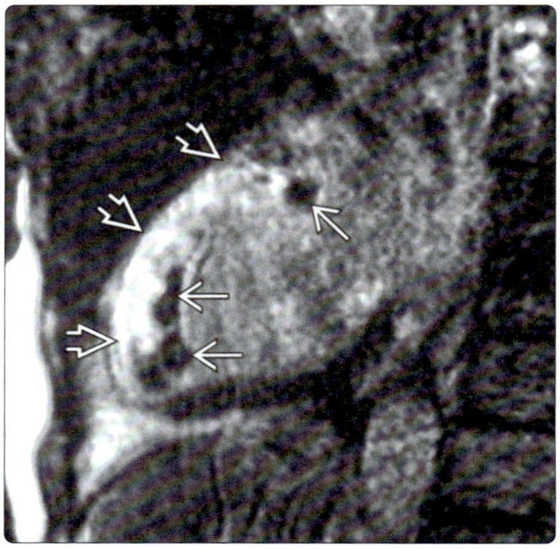

(Left) *Short-axis LGE MR shows > 50% subendocardial enhancement in the LV septum. There is nonenhancing myocardium ➡ that represents no reflow or microvascular obstruction.* **(Right)** *Short-axis LGE MR shows subendocardial enhancement → in the lateral wall of the LV. The transmurality of the enhancement is ~ 50%, suggesting a fair probability of functional segmental recovery following revascularization.*

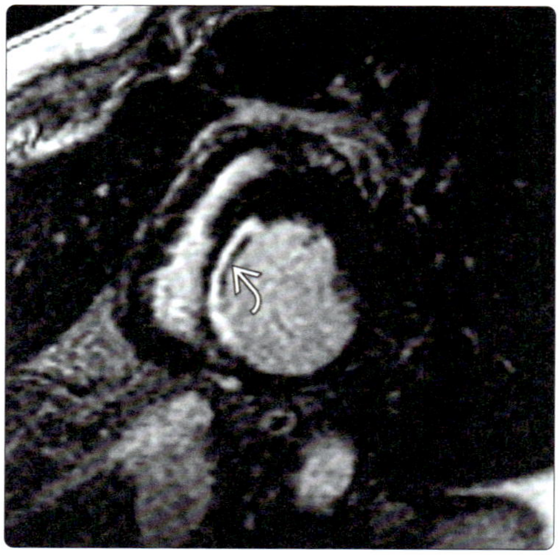

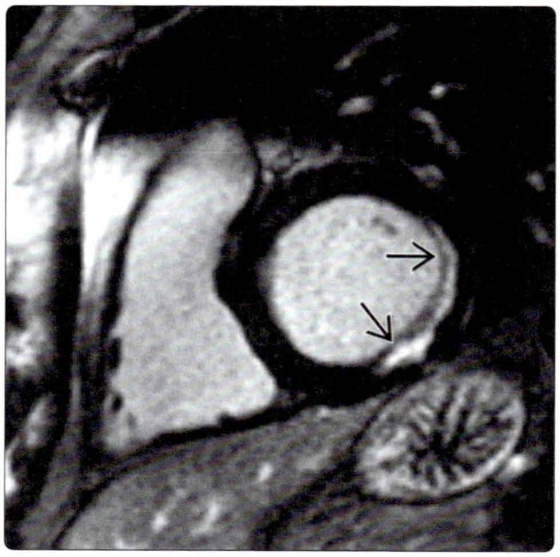

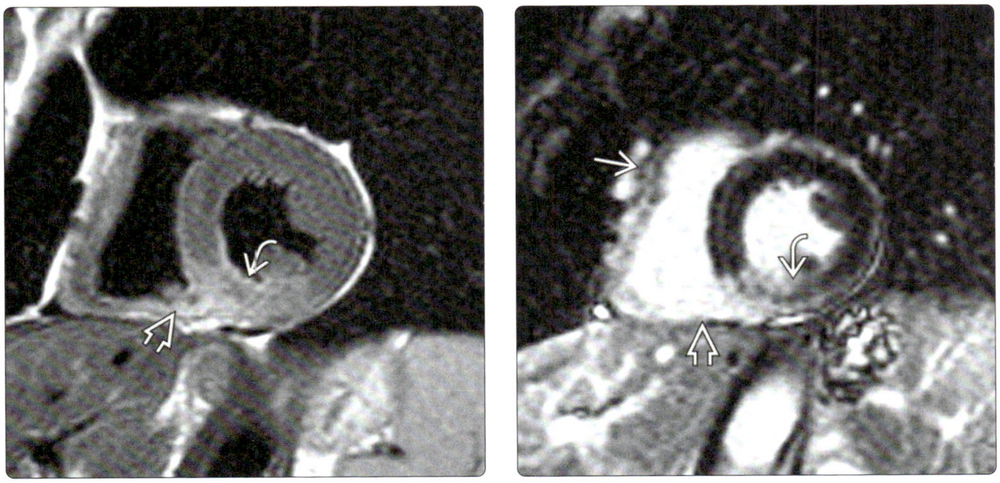

(Left) *Short-axis T2 MR of an inferoseptal and RV infarction shows abnormal increased signal of the inferior LV and inferior septum* ➔ *with extension to involve the inferior RV* ➔*, indicating that the MI is acute.* **(Right)** *Short-axis LGE MR shows abnormal enhancement signifying infarction of the inferior LV and inferior septum* ➔ *with extension to the inferior RV* ➔*. Note that the RV free wall anteriorly demonstrates no evidence of infarction* ➔*.*

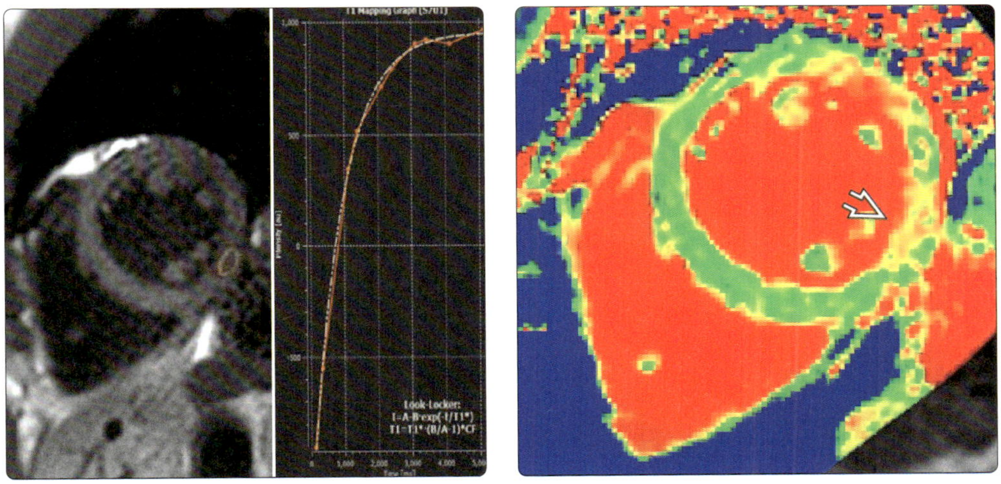

(Left) *Short-axis native T1 MR in a 57-year-old patient with acute chest pain, high troponin levels, and normal coronary arteries on invasive angiography shows elevated native T1 values (1147 ms) at the midinferolateral segment, which is also found to have severe hypokinesia.* **(Right)** *Color map of native T1 in the same patient shows the elevated T1 values at the midinferolateral* ➔ *segment compared the rest of the myocardium. Native T1 mapping allows the evaluation of the infarction size without administration of the contrast.*

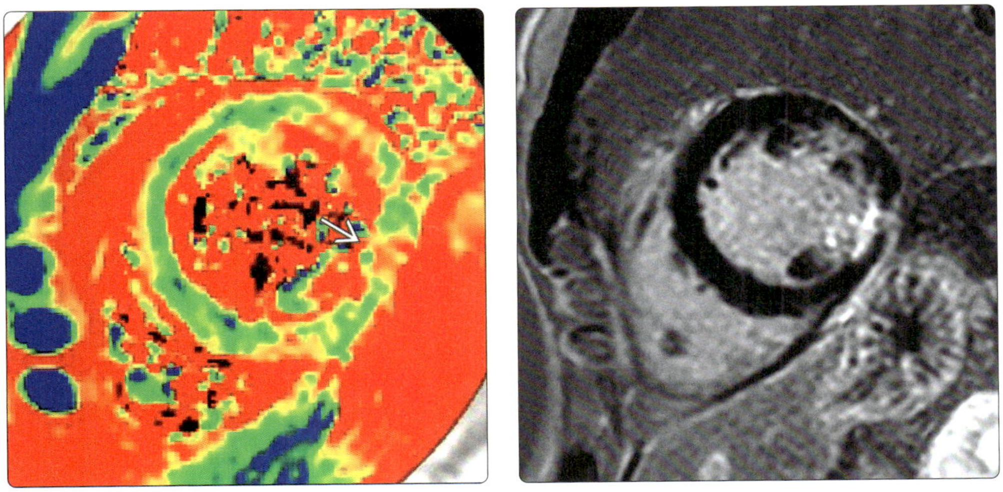

(Left) *Short-axis T2 color map in the same patient shows the high T2 values* ➔ *of the same segment, consistent with myocardial edema.* **(Right)** *Short-axis LGE MR in the same patient demonstrates the subendocardial LGE (> 50% of the wall) at the same region. Findings are consistent with acute MI in the left circumflex coronary artery territory. A near-total occlusion of an obtuse marginal branch is retrospectively identified on pre-MR angiography images, confirming MR findings.*

Chronic Myocardial Infarction

KEY FACTS

IMAGING

- LGE MR
  - Gold standard for detection of myocardial infarction and assessment of viability
- MR
  - Subendocardial LGE is present with both acute and chronic myocardial infarctions
  - Wall thinning and absent edema on T2 suggests chronicity
- CT
  - Linear myocardial calcification or subendocardial fatty metaplasia is highly specific for chronic myocardial infarction
- Complications include intraventricular thrombus and ventricular aneurysm

TOP DIFFERENTIAL DIAGNOSES

- Acute myocardial infarction
- Nonischemic cardiomyopathies
- Aneurysmal left ventricle (LV): Stress-induced cardiomyopathy, LV noncompaction, Chagas disease, diverticulum, midventricular hypertrophic cardiomyopathy
- Arrhythmogenic right ventricular dysplasia, lipomatous hypertrophy of atrial septum, tuberous sclerosis, muscular dystrophy
- Normal myocardial thinning

DIAGNOSTIC CHECKLIST

- MR
  - LGE involves subendocardium and extends outward to varying thickness, depending on infarct size
  - Absent T2 edema
  - Myocardial wall thinning and motion abnormality
- CT
  - Subendocardial fatty metaplasia and linear calcification
  - Wall thinning and motion abnormality
- Describe coronary territory and assess for culprit lesion
- Intraventricular thrombus

(Left) *Axial cardiac CT shows marked thinning and aneurysmal dilatation of the left ventricular apex, indicating remote transmural myocardial infarction in the left anterior descending coronary artery territory.* **(Right)** *Left ventricular short-axis LGE MR in a patient with remote infarct and recent onset of arrhythmias shows infarct in the right coronary artery territory with nontransmural late gadolinium enhancement. Note the transmural right ventricular infarct.*

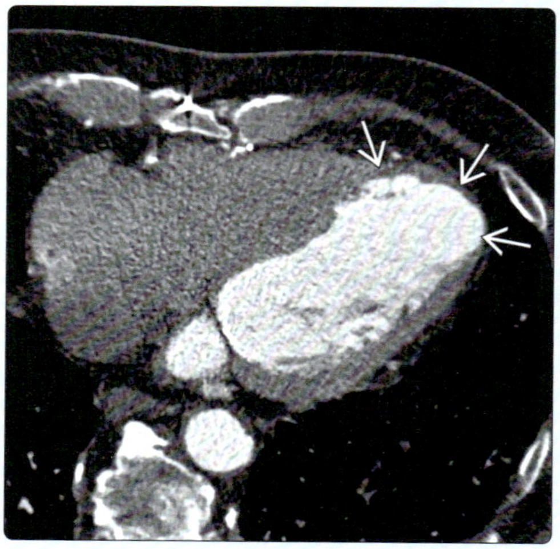

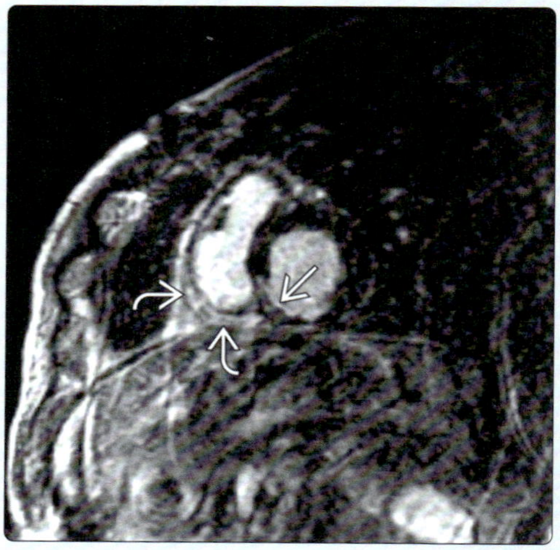

(Left) *Oblique cardiac CT shows wall thinning and transmural calcification in the right coronary artery territory, indicating remote transmural infarct in the right coronary artery territory. Note the unrelated mitral annular calcification.* **(Right)** *Axial cardiac CT shows a large lateral wall aneurysm with wall thinning, linear calcification, and mural thrombus. Note the wide neck of the aneurysm, which differentiates from pseudoaneurysm.*

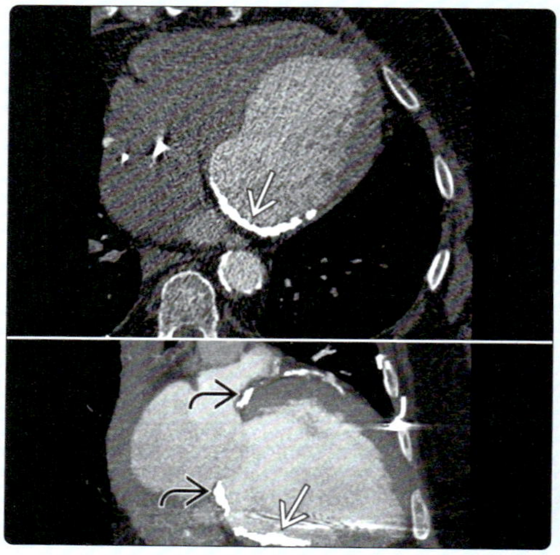

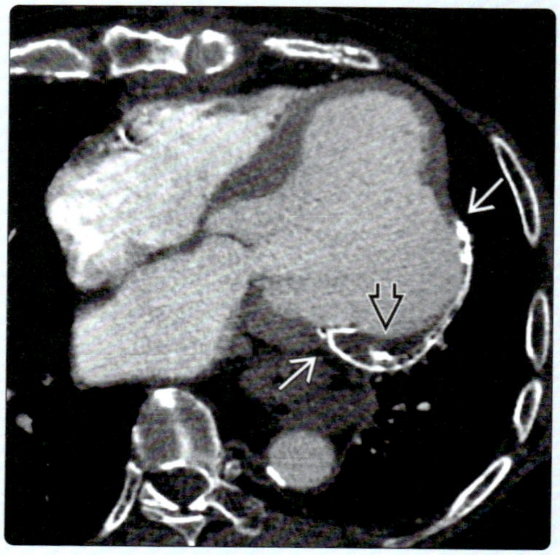

TERMINOLOGY

Synonyms

- Remote infarct

Definitions

- ≥ 8 weeks after acute myocardial infarction (MI)

IMAGING

General Features

- Best diagnostic clue
  - Linear myocardial calcification or subendocardial fatty metaplasia on CT are diagnostic of remote prior MI
  - Findings confined to coronary vascular territory
  - Myocardial thinning with hypokinesis, akinesis, or dyskinesis
  - Ventricular aneurysm or pseudoaneurysm
  - LGE on MR without T2 elevation
- Location
  - LGE or fatty metaplasia are subendocardial with varying transmurality
  - Usually confined to coronary territory (or branch territory)
- Size
  - Depends on location of culprit lesion(s)
    - More proximal culprit lesion, larger infarct territory
- General findings
  - Regional wall motion abnormality: Hypokinesis, akinesis, or dyskinesis
  - Regional myocardial thinning: From several mm to near-normal thickness

Imaging Recommendations

- Best imaging tool
  - Cardiac MR with LGE is highly sensitive and may depict small subendocardial defects
  - Linear calcification or fatty metaplasia in vascular territory on cardiac CT diagnostic of remote MI
    - Absence of these findings does not reliably exclude nontransmural chronic MI
- Protocol advice
  - T2 MR helps differentiate acute from chronic MI
    - No edema in chronic infarct

Radiographic Findings

- Radiography
  - Cardiomegaly
    - Enlarged left ventricle (LV) from aneurysm, pseudoaneurysm, or dilated LV
    - Enlarged left atrium due to functional mitral valve regurgitation or increased filling pressures
  - Myocardial calcifications indicate remote infarct

MR Findings

- MR cine
  - Akinesis, hypokinesis, or dyskinesis, depending on amount of remaining viable myocardium
  - Possible mural thrombus demonstrates absence of systolic thickening
  - Aneurysm or pseudoaneurysm may be seen
- T2WI
  - No abnormal high signal to indicate edema is seen
    - Distinguishes from acute MI, which usually has edema
  - Pericardial thickening in Dressler syndrome
- 1st-pass perfusion
  - Subendocardial perfusion defects in coronary territory, matched at stress and rest
    - Ischemia has mismatch: Defect at stress but not at rest
  - Helps delineate myocardium and mural thrombus
- LGE
  - In coronary vascular distribution
  - Always involves subendocardium and extends outward to varying thickness, depending on infarct size
  - Most sensitive test for infarcted myocardium in vivo
  - Helps differentiate myocardium from mural thrombus
  - Calcification causes signal void within LGE
  - Pericardial enhancement seen in Dressler syndrome, 2-3 weeks following MI
  - Persistent microvascular obstruction long after ST-segment elevation MI (STEMI) has negative effects of LV remodeling
- Parametric mapping
  - Native T1: Increased T1 values are seen due to presence of myocardial scar
  - Extracellular volume is increased due to scar
  - T2 values are not increased, unlike acute MI
- **MR strain imaging in MI**
  - **Tissue-tagging (TT-CMR)** and **feature-tracking CMR (FT-CMR)** are techniques used to measure myocardial strain, which includes longitudinal, circumferential, and radial strains
  - It detects early myocardial injury, aids in risk stratification, assesses viability and infarct size, and monitors function changes post percutaneous coronary intervention, coronary artery bypass grafting, or thrombolysis

CT Findings

- NECT
  - Linear low attenuation (fat density, negative HU) within LV myocardium
  - Linear calcification of myocardium
  - Enlarged LV
  - Secondary findings of sequela of chronic MI
    - Enlarged left atrium
    - Pulmonary findings of pulmonary venous hypertension
- CTA
  - Linear LV calcification or fatty myocardial infiltration in vascular territory on CT is diagnostic of remote MI
  - Typically (but not always) myocardial thinning
  - LV aneurysm
  - Thrombus seen as low-attenuation intraluminal mass: 25-80 HU
  - Radiomics models may predict adverse outcomes with incremental value over clinical and cardiac MR
- Cardiac gated CTA
  - Functional images demonstrate hypokinesis, akinesis, or dyskinesis, depending on transmurality of infarct
  - Very small remote infarcts may have normal wall thickness and normal wall motion

- Obstructive coronary artery disease in matching coronary territory
- Delayed iodine enhancement
  - Delayed enhancement of thinned wall, due to infarct
  - Not as good as MR due to lower contrast-to-noise ratio
  - Detection may be improved by using dual-energy CT

Echocardiographic Findings

- Chronic LV remodeling
  - Infarcted segment wall is thinner, and echo is more dense compared with noninfarcted segments
  - May demonstrate presence of aneurysm or pseudoaneurysm
  - Akinesis or dyskinesis of affected segments
- Functional mitral regurgitation
  - Abnormal coaptation secondary to tethering from LV dilatation/remodeling
- May detect mural thrombus

Nuclear Medicine Findings

- LV wall thinning with fixed defect
  - Akinesis in areas of fixed defects
- Visualization of right ventricle plus high lung uptake are signs of severe LV dysfunction

DIFFERENTIAL DIAGNOSIS

Acute Myocardial Infarction

- Maintained or increased myocardial thickness
- Increased T2 signal due to edema
- No fatty metaplasia, calcification, or aneurysm

Nonischemic Cardiomyopathies

- Can produce wall thinning and wall motion abnormalities, not in vascular territory
- LGE usually spares subendocardium; midmyocardial or subepicardial distribution
  - Amyloidosis can produce diffuse subendocardial LGE, not in vascular territory

Aneurysmal Ventricle

- Stress-induced cardiomyopathy
  - Follows physical/emotional stress
  - Apical ballooning, normal/hyperkinetic basal segments
  - No coronary artery disease
  - Full recovery in few weeks
- Chagas disease
  - Caused by parasite, *Trypanosoma cruzi*
  - Apical aneurysm in 50%
  - Nonischemic pattern of LGE, but no coronary artery disease
- Midventricular hypertrophic cardiomyopathy
  - May develop apical aneurysm
- Diverticulum
  - Contains all 3 layers of ventricular wall
  - Has narrow neck
  - Synchronous contraction with ventricle

Myocardial Fat

- Incidental finding in normal heart
- Arrhythmogenic right ventricular dysplasia (ARVD), lipomatous hypertrophy of atrial septum, muscular dystrophy, tuberous sclerosis, lipoma

Thinning of Myocardium

- Normal in LV apex and membranous ventricular septum

PATHOLOGY

Gross Pathologic & Surgical Features

- Thin layer of scar ± aneurysm or pseudoaneurysm
- Mural thrombus is commonly present

Microscopic Features

- Established scarring with collagen fibers

CLINICAL ISSUES

Natural History & Prognosis

- LV remodeling
  - LV dilatation
  - Increases in end-diastolic and end-systolic volumes are predictive of increased mortality
- May develop ischemic dilated cardiomyopathy
- May develop mitral regurgitation from remodeling and change of chordae tendineae geometry and resulting mitral valve malcoaptation
- May develop aneurysm or pseudoaneurysms
- May develop thrombus
  - Best evaluated on contrast-enhanced MR; detects over 2x as many thrombi as echocardiography
  - Thrombus has lower attenuation than myocardium and does not enhance on contrast-enhanced CT and MR

Treatment

- Medical treatment
- Surgical treatment
  - Coronary artery bypass grafts if viable myocardium exists
  - Dor procedure
    - Resection of aneurysm with patch aneurysmorrhaphy
  - Linear aneurysmectomy
    - Aneurysm is resected, and edges are closed in linear vertical fashion using 2 parallel layers of Teflon felt

DIAGNOSTIC CHECKLIST

Image Interpretation Pearls

- True aneurysm
  - Wide neck/base; dyskinetic
  - Low risk of rupture
- Pseudoaneurysm (false aneurysm)
  - Narrow base/neck; dyskinetic
  - Wall consists of epi-/pericardium ± thrombus
  - Higher risk of rupture

SELECTED REFERENCES

1. Chen Y et al: A coronary CT angiography-derived myocardial radiomics model for predicting adverse outcomes in chronic myocardial infarction. Int J Cardiol. 411:132265, 2024
2. Bodi V et al: Impact of persistent microvascular obstruction late after STEMI on adverse LV remodeling: a CMR study. JACC Cardiovasc Imaging. 16(7):919-30, 2023
3. Moore A et al: Chronic Infarcts and mimickers of infarcts. Radiol Clin North Am. 57(1):57-65, 2019

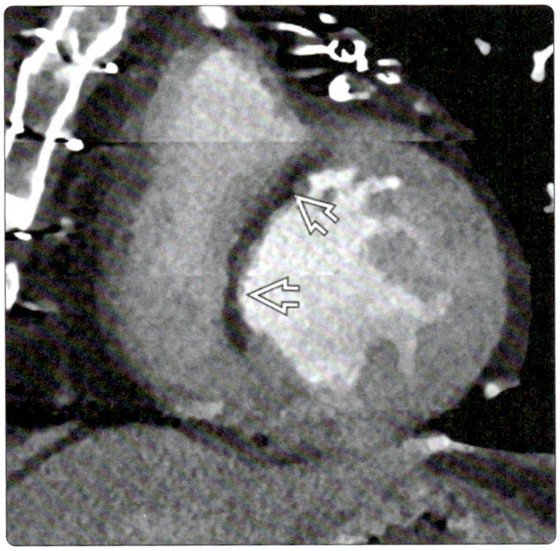

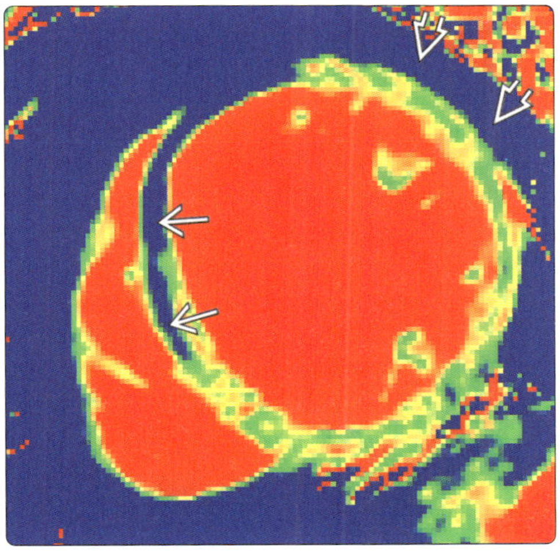

(Left) *Short-axis coronary CTA shows linear subendocardial hypoattenuation in the midseptal wall with negative Hounsfield units, consistent with fatty metaplasia from a remote myocardial infarction.* **(Right)** *Short-axis T1 color map in the same patient shows linear T1 shortening (blue) corresponding to fatty metaplasia seen in the CCTA. Note the blue color in the midseptal myocardium, which is similar to the color of the pericardial fat.*

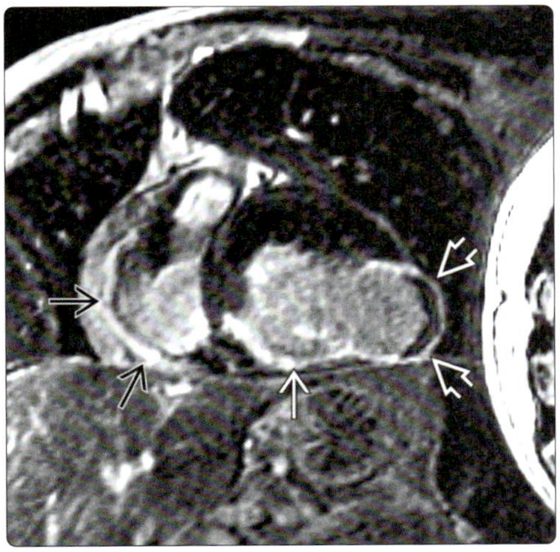

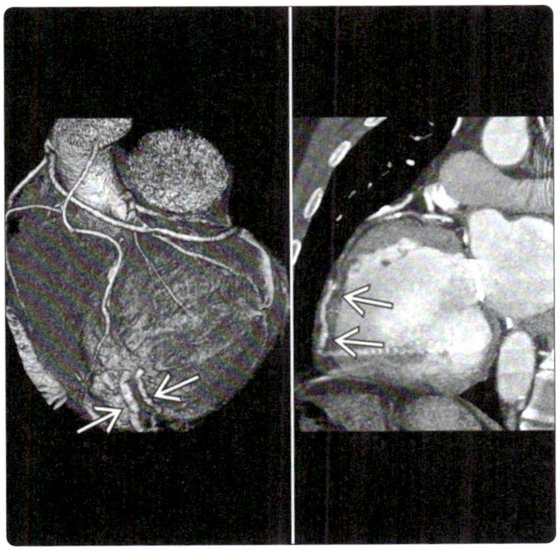

(Left) *Left ventricular short-axis delayed-enhancement MR shows hyperenhancement (infarct) of the right ventricular and left ventricular inferior and inferolateral walls, which have developed a large aneurysm. Note the unenhanced mural thrombus.* **(Right)** *Oblique cardiac CT in a patient post coronary artery bypass graft surgery and left ventricular aneurysmectomy shows 2 parallel layers of Teflon left at the resection site, indicating linear aneurysmectomy.*

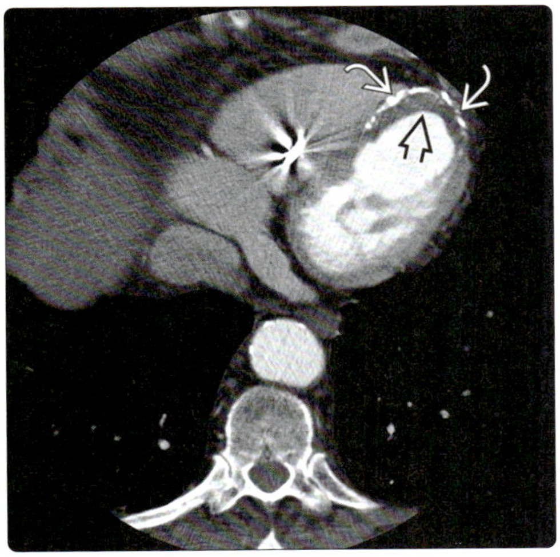

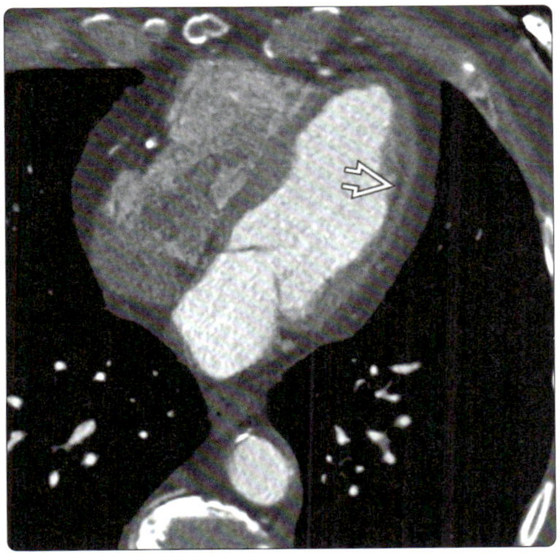

(Left) *Axial CTA shows a thinned and calcified myocardium and apical aneurysm. Note that the mural thrombus is hypodense (unenhanced) compared with the remote normal myocardium.* **(Right)** *Axial coronary CTA shows linear subendocardial fatty metaplasia but relatively preserved myocardial thickness, indicating remote nontransmural infarct in the diagonal branch or obtuse marginal branch territory. Keep in mind fatty metaplasia can also be seen in normal myocardium.*

Nonatherosclerosis Myocardial Infarction

KEY FACTS

TERMINOLOGY

- Myocardial infarction (MI) unrelated to coronary atherosclerosis
- Ischemia unrelated to coronary atherosclerosis

IMAGING

- Late-enhancement MR can demonstrate presence, location, and size of infarction
- Coronary CTA has high sensitivity (98%), specificity (88%), and negative predictive value (95-100%) for excluding coronary atherosclerosis
- Normal invasive angiogram does not mean no atherosclerotic plaque burden; CTA better at evaluating overall coronary plaque burden

TOP DIFFERENTIAL DIAGNOSES

- Acute aortic dissection, acute myocarditis, microvascular obstruction, takotsubo syndrome

CLINICAL ISSUES

- Myocardial infarction with nonobstructive coronary arteries occurs in 5-6% of MI and disproportionately affects women
- Presents with classical clinical features of atherosclerotic acute myocardial infarction
- Cardiogenic shock if large area of left ventricle is ischemic
- Lower prevalence of atherosclerosis risk factors: Smoking, cholesterol elevation, diabetes, hypertension, family history, prior angina
- Treatment depends on underlying cause
  - Standard therapy for type 1 myocardial infarction
  - Percutaneous coronary intervention/surgery is not generally used except in coronary dissection
- Compared to patients with obstructive coronary artery disease, short-term follow-up shows better prognosis, but longer term follow-up shows worse prognosis

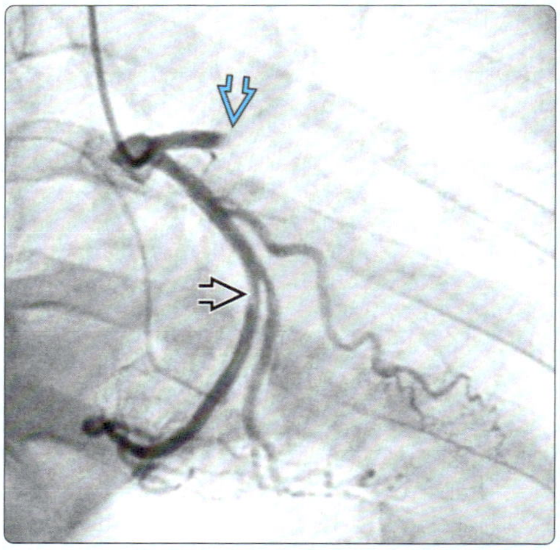
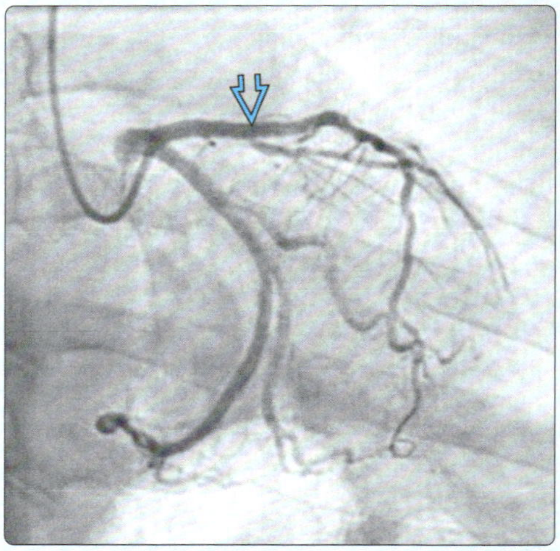

(Left) *Emergency invasive coronary angiogram in a 42-year-old man who took large quantities of cocaine and developed subsequent severe chest pain shows an acute thrombus in the proximal left anterior descending (LAD) coronary artery with an abrupt vessel lumen cutoff . Nonocclusive thrombus can also be seen in the left circumflex artery .* **(Right)** *Post angioplasty in the same patient, thrombectomy and stent insertion show a good result in opening the proximal left anterior coronary artery.*

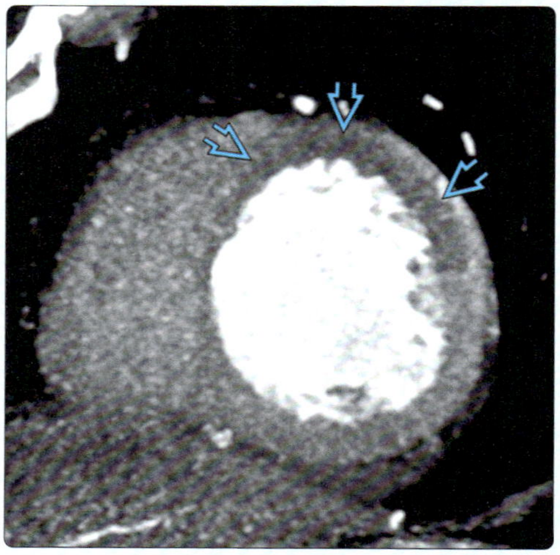
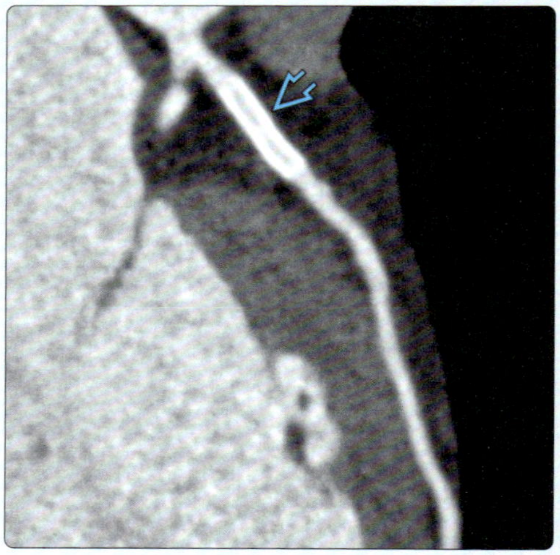

(Left) *Short-axis cardiac CTA in the same patient shows a hypodense subendocardial defect affecting the anteroseptal, anterior, and anterolateral myocardial segments in keeping with an acute cocaine-induced myocardial infarction in the LAD coronary vascular territory.* **(Right)** *Curved MPR of the LAD shows a patent stent in the proximal segment of the LAD.*

TERMINOLOGY

Abbreviations

- Myocardial infarction with nonobstructive coronary arteries (MINOCA)

Definitions

- Defined by classical criteria of myocardial infarction (MI) and absence of stenosis ≥ 50% in major epicardial artery, demonstrated on coronary CTA, and no clinically overt specific cause for acute presentation other than acute MI

IMAGING

General Features

- Best diagnostic clue
  - CTA demonstrates no evidence of coronary atherosclerosis
- Location
  - ECG and enzyme rises similar to typical acute MI
- Morphology
  - Underlying cause often difficult to elucidate
    - Cardiac CT and MR have become important tools in determining underlying cause

Radiographic Findings

- Chest radiography
  - Often normal but may show acute pulmonary edema in some settings, such as cocaine abuse

CT Findings

- CTA
  - Coronary CTA has high sensitivity (98%), specificity (88%), and negative predictive value (95-100%) for excluding coronary atherosclerosis
  - May see complications of infarction: Stunned myocardium, left ventricular thrombus, aneurysm, pseudoaneurysm rupture
  - May reveal Kawasaki disease, coronary aneurysms, and vasculitis
  - Combination of CTA with CT perfusion is fully noninvasive method that proves more sensitive and shows prevalence of MINOCA of 8%
- CT of lung and mediastinum may provide clue to underlying etiology
  - Acute pulmonary edema: ↑ ground-glass opacities and septal lines, classically seen in cocaine abuse
  - Aortic and pulmonary wall abnormalities: Thickened in vasculitis
  - Radiation: Pulmonary fibrosis, fibrosing mediastinitis
  - Pulmonary parenchymal aneurysms: Polyarteritis nodosa
  - Pulmonary embolism in thrombotic states: Systemic lupus erythematosus with antiphospholipid syndrome
  - Chest trauma: Pulmonary contusion, laceration, pneumothorax, fractured ribs
- Optical coherence tomography (OCT)
  - Can visualize coronary dissection, plaque rupture/erosion, coronary spasm, calcified nodules usually not visible on invasive angiography or IV ultrasound
  - Higher resolution but lower penetration depth, e.g., large arteries, left main stem may not be fully visualized

MR Findings

- T2WI FS
  - Myocardial edema seen in acute phase
    - T2 mapping provides quantitative assessment of myocardial edema
- T2* GRE
  - Can show arterial wall edema in large vessel vasculitis
- Delayed enhancement
  - Viability
    - Late enhancement can demonstrate presence, location, and size of infarction
  - Perfusion
    - 1st-pass perfusion (stress followed by rest) can show perfusion abnormalities, particularly in microvascular obstruction
  - Regional wall motion
    - MR is gold standard for chamber volumetrics and wall motion abnormalities
    - Standardized 17-segment AHA model utilized
    - Steady-state free precession sequence will show regional wall motion abnormality (RWMA) in infarction
    - RWMA of takotsubo cardiomyopathy is well demonstrated in MR
  - MR provided specific diagnosis in 75% of MINOCA cases; 21% were nonischemic, e.g., myocarditis (15%), takotsubo (3%)
    - Integration with OCT revealed underlying cause in 85% of cases

Echocardiographic Findings

- Echocardiogram
  - RWMAs acutely; wall thinning chronically
  - May demonstrate complications of infarction
    - Left ventricular thrombus, although cardiac MR is better

Angiographic Findings

- Invasive coronary angiography (ICA)
  - May show evidence of MINOCA, including mild narrowing (< 50%), lesions with asymmetry, narrow neck, irregular borders, haziness, or radiolucent flap
  - Many patients with apparently normal ICAs have significant coronary plaque burden with positive remodeling, and some MIs arise from lesions, causing < 50% luminal narrowing

Nuclear Medicine Findings

- PET
  - Currently regarded as gold standard for myocardial viability assessment with exception of subendocardial infarction detection

Imaging Recommendations

- Best imaging tool
  - Cardiac MR
- Protocol advice
  - (1) Careful consideration of clinical presentation, including considering alternative diagnoses, such as pulmonary embolism, sepsis, cardiac contusion, and other noncardiac causes of rise in troponin
  - (2) If MI remains clinical diagnosis of choice and there is

- Rise in troponin > 99th percentile and signs/symptoms of ischemia
- < 50% stenosis on angiography even after rereview

o Excluding nonischemic mechanisms of myocardial injury with
- CMR can exclude myocarditis, takotsubo syndrome, and cardiomyopathies; can also confirm MI

o If all of above do not point to alternative diagnoses, consider MINOCA
- Coronary vascular imaging (IV ultrasound, OCT) may show plaque disruption, coronary emboli/thrombus, spontaneous coronary artery dissection (SCAD)
- Functional assessment can show spasm, microvascular disease

DIFFERENTIAL DIAGNOSIS

Acute Aortic Dissection

- May dissect down and into coronary artery ostia

Acute Myocarditis

- Prodromal flu-like symptoms, normal invasive angiogram

Pulmonary Embolism

- Pleuritic chest pain, dyspnea, and elevated D-dimers

Takotsubo Syndrome

- "Broken heart" or "stress" cardiomyopathy

PATHOLOGY

General Features

- Etiology
  - Coronary
    - Microvascular dysfunction
      - Coronary microcirculation (vessels < 0.5 mm in diameter) is not easily visualized yet accounts for ~ 70% of coronary resistance in absence of obstructive coronary artery disease (CAD)
    - Occult plaque rupture or erosion
    - Coronary vasospasm
    - Embolization
    - SCAD
    - Hypercoagulable disorders
    - In-stent restenosis; percutaneous coronary intervention
    - Myocardial bridge
  - Cardiac: Cardiomyopathies, cardiac trauma, tachyarrhythmias
  - Extracardiac: Pulmonary embolism; supply/demand mismatch, e.g., anemia, sepsis
    - Inflammation/vasculitis

CLINICAL ISSUES

Presentation

- Most common signs/symptoms
  - Classic clinical features of atherosclerotic acute MI
    - Central, crushing chest pain, radiation to left arm classically
  - Cardiogenic shock if large area of left ventricle is ischemic
- Other signs/symptoms
  - Atypical pain in jaw, epigastrium
  - Nausea, vomiting, diaphoresis
  - No conduction disturbances
- Clinical profile
  - Lower prevalence of atherosclerosis risk factors: Smoking, cholesterol elevation, diabetes, hypertension, family history, prior angina

Demographics

- Age
  - Younger patient population with fewer risk factors for atherosclerosis except for cigarette smoking
- Epidemiology
  - 6% of acute MI patients have normal coronary arteries at autopsy

Natural History & Prognosis

- Compared to patients with obstructive CAD, short-term follow-up shows better prognosis, but long-term risk of death is similar
  - 5-year mortality is ~ 11%, and causes of death were mainly noncardiovascular; 4-year rate of major cardiac event after MINOCA is ~ 25%

Treatment

- Optimal treatment is according to underlying diagnosis and should be aimed at underlying cause
  - e.g., coronary vasodilator drugs in ventricular arrhythmia as result of refractory spasm
- Cardioprotective therapies should be considered on individual basis, e.g., recommended in plaque disruption (type 1 MI) but use in type 2 MI is uncertain
- Caution with conventional therapies, e.g., β-blockers contraindicated in coronary spasm
- Percutaneous coronary intervention/surgery only used in high-risk anatomic locations, e.g., left main artery or left anterior descending artery in SCAD or ongoing ischemia with hemodynamic instability

DIAGNOSTIC CHECKLIST

Consider

- In patients presenting with acute MI with normal coronary angiogram

SELECTED REFERENCES

1. Reynolds HR et al: Coronary optical coherence tomography and cardiac magnetic resonance imaging to determine underlying causes of myocardial infarction with nonobstructive coronary arteries in women. Circulation. 143(7):624-40, 2021
2. Schuijf JD et al: Ischemia and no obstructive stenosis (INOCA) at CT angiography, CT myocardial perfusion, invasive coronary angiography, and SPECT: the CORE320 study. Radiology. 294(1):61-73, 2020
3. Tamis-Holland JE et al: Contemporary diagnosis and management of patients with myocardial infarction in the absence of obstructive coronary artery disease: a scientific statement from the American Heart Association. Circulation. 139(18):e891-908, 2019
4. Manolis AS et al: Acute coronary syndromes in patients with angiographically normal or near normal (non-obstructive) coronary arteries. Trends Cardiovasc Med. 28(8):541-51, 2018
5. Thygesen K et al: Fourth universal definition of myocardial infarction (2018). J Am Coll Cardiol. 72(18):2231-64, 2018

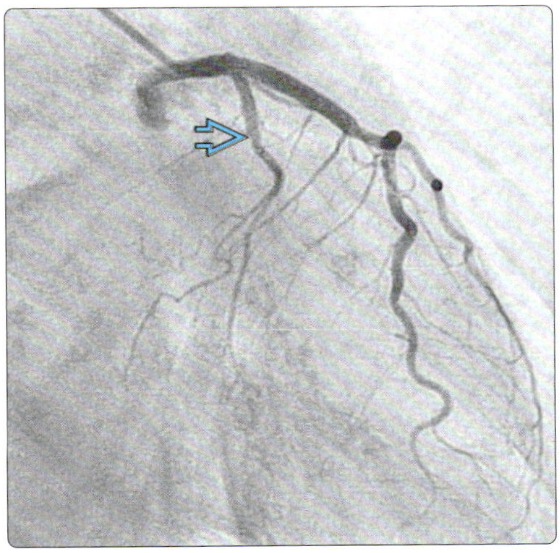

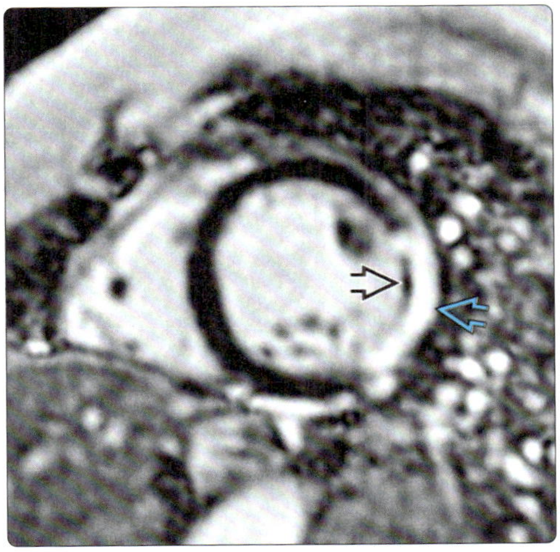

(Left) *Invasive coronary angiogram shows a normal left circumflex coronary artery* ➡. **(Right)** *Short-axis LGE image shows transmural LGE* ➡ *of the anteroseptal and inferoseptal segments, consistent with myocardial infarction in left circumflex artery territory. Note the microvascular obstruction* ➡ *within the infarct.*

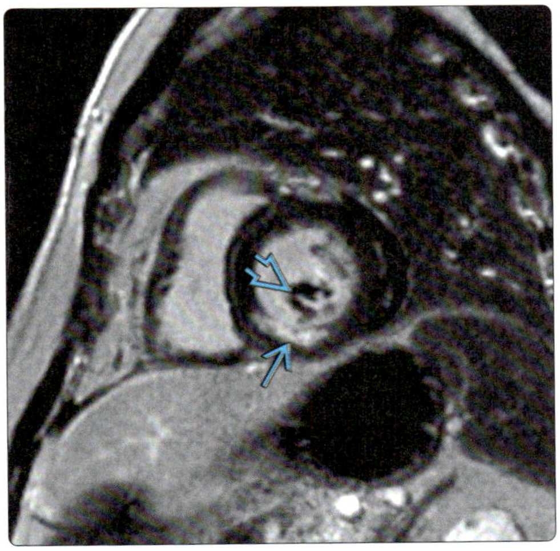

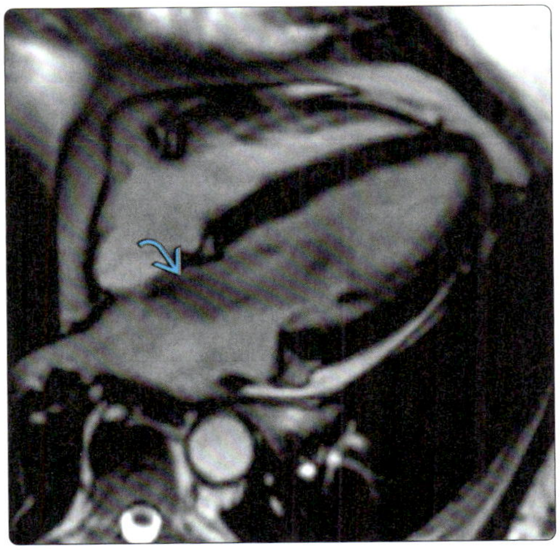

(Left) *Short-axis LGE image in a middle-aged patient shows a right coronary artery (RCA) territory infarct* ➡. *A mass is partially visualized in the left ventricle* ➡. *(Courtesy S. Kligerman, MD.)* **(Right)** *Four-chamber SSFP MR shows a large left atrial myxoma prolapsing into the left ventricle* ➡. *An embolized tumor fragment was removed from the RCA. The coronary arteries were otherwise normal. (Courtesy S. Kligerman, MD.)*

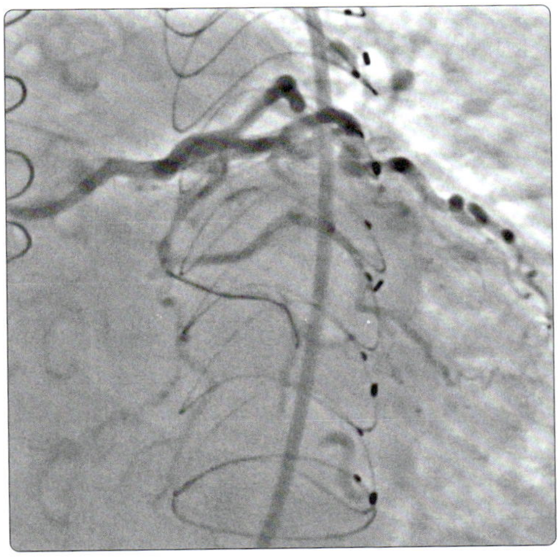

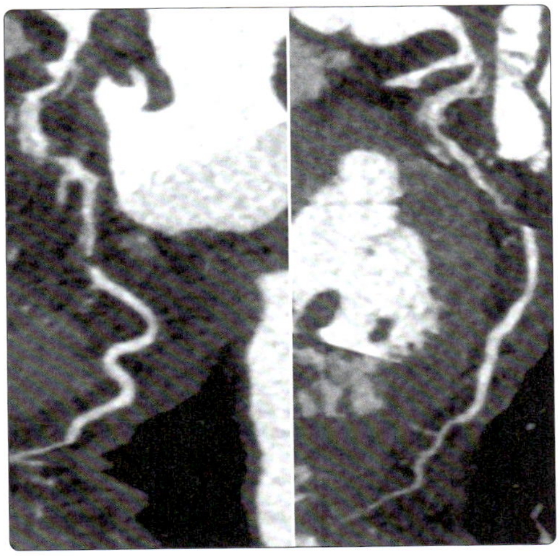

(Left) *Invasive coronary angiogram in a 59-year-old woman presenting with suspected acute coronary syndrome shows proximal stenosis and occlusion of the left posterolateral branch (suspected to be spontaneous coronary artery dissection).* **(Right)** *CT in the same patient shows an intramural hematoma and dissection starting in the left main coronary artery and extending to the mid left circumflex coronary artery. The posterolateral branch is recanalized.*

Papillary Muscle Rupture

KEY FACTS

TERMINOLOGY

- Partial or complete rupture of papillary muscle, most commonly in setting of acute myocardial infarction (MI)

IMAGING

- Flail of chordae &/or papillary muscle into left atrium along with torrential mitral regurgitation
- Transthoracic echo sensitivity of 65-85%; transesophageal echo sensitivity of 95-100%
- Right upper lobe edema is specific chest x-ray finding; mitral leaflet flail and jet of regurgitant blood is directed into right superior pulmonary vein
- CTA can provide noninvasive evaluation of coronary arteries
- MR late enhancement shows infarcted myocardium and affected papillary muscle

TOP DIFFERENTIAL DIAGNOSES

- Cardiogenic shock, chordal rupture, endocarditis

PATHOLOGY

- More commonly involves posterior papillary muscle (3x more common) with inferior MI

CLINICAL ISSUES

- Most commonly presents 2-7 days post acute MI with acute-onset chest pain and shortness of breath
- Stabilize patient with afterload and preload reduction, intraaortic balloon often required
- Once stabilized, emergency surgery essential; without surgical treatment 80% mortality
- Mitral valve repair preferable if no papillary muscle necrosis
- Recent trends for lower operative risk, particularly with associated coronary artery bypass grafting
- Substantial perioperative morbidity and mortality (35% on table mortality rate)
- 10-year survival only 35% and 10-year survival free of heart failure only 23%

(Left) *Chest radiograph shows unilateral acute pulmonary edema* ⇨ *in a patient presenting with acute myocardial infarction. The unilateral appearance is classic for severe mitral regurgitation directed into the right-sided pulmonary veins secondary to papillary muscle (PM) rupture.* **(Right)** *Corresponding chest CT in the same patient confirms nearly unilateral right-sided pulmonary edema* ➡ *with associated pleural effusions* ⇨.

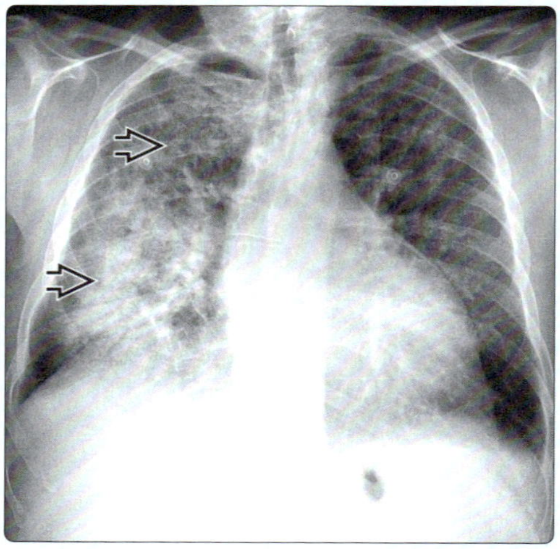

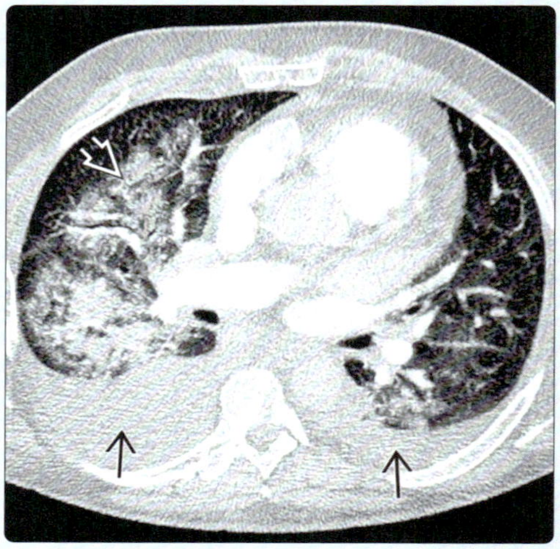

(Left) *Apical 3-chamber view transthoracic echocardiogram demonstrates a ruptured PM* ➡ *flailing in the left ventricle.* **(Right)** *Color Doppler of the mitral valve (MV) (Nyquist limit 34cm/s) on transthoracic echocardiogram demonstrates a large proximal isovelocity surface area (PISA) and effective regurgitant orifice area indicating severe mitral regurgitation.*

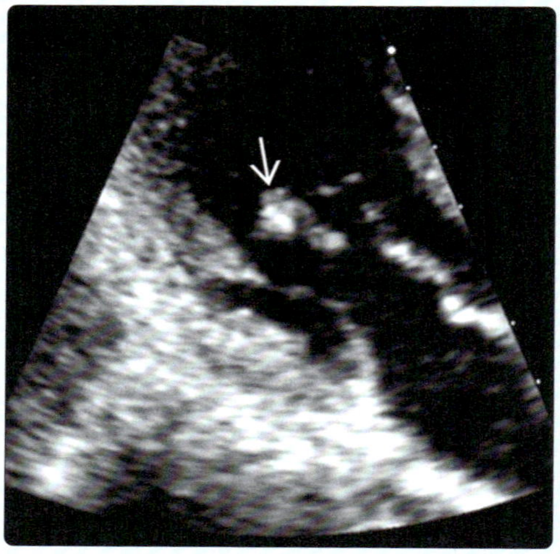

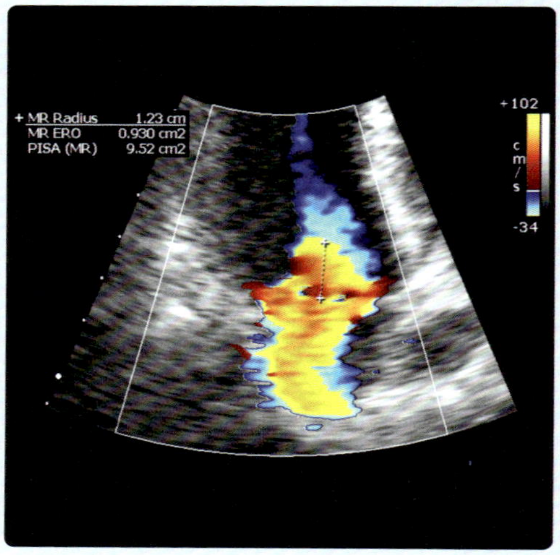

TERMINOLOGY

Definitions

- Partial or complete rupture of papillary muscle, most commonly in setting of acute myocardial infarction (MI) due to coronary artery disease

IMAGING

General Features

- Best diagnostic clue
  - Flail chordae &/or papillary muscle prolapse into left atrium (LA) along with severe mitral regurgitation
- Location
  - Posteromedial papillary muscle in 75% of cases; more prone to ischemia and rupture due to its dependence on single blood supply from posterior descending artery
  - Anterolateral muscle rupture in 25% of cases; tends to have dual blood supplies (1st obtuse marginal branch) and 1st diagonal branch (left anterior descending coronary artery)
- Size
  - Partial rupture (affecting single head) more common than complete rupture (affecting papillary muscle trunk)
- Morphology
  - Both anterior and posterior leaflets of valve are attached via primary, secondary, and tertiary chordae to both anterolateral and posteromedial papillary muscles
  - Disruption in either papillary muscle results in dysfunction of anterior or posterior leaflets

Radiographic Findings

- Radiography
  - Pulmonary venous congestion with signs of pulmonary edema
  - Asymmetric right upper lobe edema due to mitral regurgitation jet directed toward right superior pulmonary vein

CT Findings

- CTA
  - Coronary arteries can be evaluated for significant coronary stenosis
  - Myocardial perfusion defect may be detected in acute MI
  - Cine multiphasic reconstructions can show
    - Prolapse of chordae and mitral leaflet into LA
    - Global and regional left ventricular function abnormalities related to acute MI

MR Findings

- MR cine
  - Prolapse of chordae and mitral leaflet into LA and regurgitant jet
  - Global and regional left ventricular function abnormalities related to acute MI
  - Late gadolinium enhancement can quantify location and extent of MI of affected papillary muscle
    - Conventional delayed enhancement imaging underestimated prevalence of both anterior and posterior papillary muscle infarction
    - Flow-independent dark-blood delayed enhancement (FIDDLE) cardiac MR accurate in detection of papillary muscle infarction
  - Native T1 mapping can detect papillary muscle infarction without need for contrast administration

Echocardiographic Findings

- Echocardiogram
  - Transthoracic echocardiography
    - Initial cardiac modality
    - Sensitivity of 65-85%
  - Transesophageal echocardiography
    - Improves sensitivity to 95-100% due to proximity of mitral apparatus to transducer in esophageal position
    - Detached papillary muscle fragments appear as highly mobile echodensities
    - Papillary muscle head can prolapse into LA (35% of cases)
    - Mitral regurgitation, almost always severe, diagnosed by color Doppler with broad vena contracta
    - Eccentric jet with enlarged LA
      - LA can be normal in size
    - Mitral regurgitation caused by papillary muscle rupture due to MI travels in lateral (posteromedial rupture) or medial (anterolateral rupture) direction
    - Left ventricle is commonly hyperdynamic in setting of acute MI
    - Can also evaluate pulmonary artery, right heart function

Angiographic Findings

- Ventriculography
  - Severe mitral regurgitation
- Right heart catheterization can be used to differentiate ventricular septal rupture from papillary muscle rupture and associated mitral regurgitation
  - Pulmonary capillary wedge pressure in papillary muscle rupture typically very high

Imaging Recommendations

- Best imaging tool
  - Transesophageal echocardiography if patient stable

DIFFERENTIAL DIAGNOSIS

Cardiogenic Shock

- Acute MI is usually present
  - Multivessel or left main coronary disease often present
  - Usually occurs 2-7 days following MI

Chronic Mitral Regurgitation

- Myocardium usually shows marked regional wall motion abnormality
- Left ventricular remodeling changes geometry of chordae tendinea, leading to mitral valve malcoaptation
  - Lateral displacement of lateral wall changes angle of chordae (relative shortening) and results in incomplete systolic closure of posterior mitral valve leaflet
- No flail leaflet
- Lesser degree of regurgitation

Dilated Mitral Anulus

- Most commonly associated with dilated cardiomyopathy

Chordal Rupture

- Will also lead to flail leaflet
- May require transesophageal echocardiography to distinguish from papillary muscle rupture
- Lesser degree of regurgitation is sometimes noted

Endocarditis

- Vegetation may appear as mobile structure attached to regurgitant valve
- Different clinical setting, patient typically septic
- Blood cultures are helpful in diagnosis

Ventricular Septal Rupture

- Post-MI rupture of septum leading to ventricular septal defect
- No mitral valve regurgitation

PATHOLOGY

General Features

- Etiology
  - Typically acute infarction; other causes include infective endocarditis and trauma
- More commonly involves posterior papillary muscle (3x more common) with inferior MI
- Rupture most often at papillary muscle head
  - May be partial or complete
- Partial tear may also occur within body of papillary muscle
  - Higher risk of progression to complete rupture
- Typical necrosis apparent at site of rupture
- Myocardial infarct size itself may not be large
  - Incidence of mechanical complications post MI in prefibrinolytic era was as high as 6%, has significantly decreased to < 1% in reperfusion era

CLINICAL ISSUES

Presentation

- Most common signs/symptoms
  - Life-threatening condition; most commonly presents 2-7 days post acute MI
  - Acute chest pain, pulmonary edema, shortness of breath
  - Sudden onset of heart failure/cardiogenic shock
    - Systolic function is better than anticipated, or hyperdynamic, in setting of hemodynamic compromise
  - Given rapid equalization of left ventricular and left atrial pressures in patients with acute severe MR, systolic murmur on auscultation is classically absent
    - Diagnosis requires degree of suspicion and prompt evaluation with echocardiography or contrast left ventriculography
- Clinical profile
  - Risk factors include advanced age, poor nutritional status, delayed diagnosis of MI, and single vessel disease
  - Monitoring increasing trend of C-reactive protein and neutrophil:lymphocyte ratio useful in predicting development of papillary muscle rupture in setting of acute MI

Natural History & Prognosis

- Usually occurs at 1st infarct
- With early reperfusion therapy frequency of papillary muscle rupture after acute MI has decreased from 1-3% to 0.05-0.26%
- Survival rates seem related to extent of papillary muscle rupture
- Without surgical treatment, mortality can reach 80% if acute severe regurgitation
- 10-year survival only 35% and 10-year survival free of heart failure only 23%

Treatment

- Medical
  - Inotropic support
    - Afterload reduction to reduce regurgitant volume and pulmonary congestion
- Interventional
  - Coronary angiography may be helpful if patient can be adequately stabilized
  - Intraaortic balloon pump and venoarterial extracorporeal membrane oxygenation as bridge to surgery
  - Once stabilized, emergency surgery essential
  - Mitral transcatheter edge-to-edge repair is safe alternative for patients with prohibitive surgical risk
- Surgical
  - Chordal sparing mitral valve replacement or mitral valve repair (repair preferable if no papillary muscle necrosis)
    - Mitral valve repair has advantage of preserving anatomy of subvalvular apparatus and does not require long-term anticoagulation
  - Recent trends for lower operative risk, particularly with associated coronary artery bypass grafting
  - Substantial perioperative morbidity and mortality (35% on table mortality rate)
  - Mortality with surgery 40% (compared with 71% mortality with medical treatment alone)

SELECTED REFERENCES

1. Calì F et al: Transcatheter edge-to-edge mitral valve repair for post-myocardial infarction papillary muscle rupture and acute heart failure: a systematic review. Catheter Cardiovasc Interv. 102(1):138-44, 2023
2. Pambianchi G et al: Papillary muscle involvement during acute myocardial infarction: detection by cardiovascular magnetic resonance using T1 mapping technique and papillary longitudinal strain. J Clin Med. 12(4), 2023
3. Takafumi K et al: Anterolateral papillary muscle rupture predicted by post-infarction inflammatory markers. Am J Case Rep. 24:e940406, 2023
4. Murphy A et al: Mechanical complications of myocardial infarction. Am J Med. 135(12):1401-9, 2022
5. Wendell D et al: Assessment of papillary muscle infarction with dark-blood delayed enhancement cardiac MRI in canines and humans. Radiology. 305(2):329-38, 2022
6. Damluji AA et al: Mechanical complications of acute myocardial infarction: a scientific statement from the American Heart Association. Circulation. 144(2):e16-35, 2021
7. Atreya AR et al: Acute myocardial infarction and papillary muscle rupture in the COVID-19 era. JACC Case Rep. 2(10):1637-41, 2020
8. Kitada Y et al: Ischaemic papillary muscle rupture without significant coronary artery lesion. Interact Cardiovasc Thorac Surg. 29(6):971-2, 2019
9. Geis N et al: Percutaneous repair of severe mitral valve regurgitation secondary to chordae rupture in octogenarians using MitraClip. J Interv Cardiol. 31(1):76-82, 2018

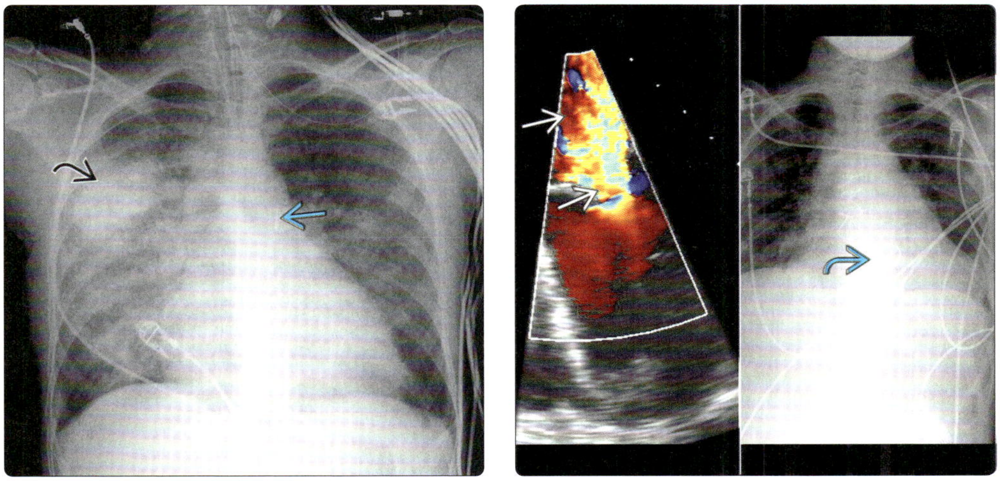

(Left) *Chest x-ray in a woman with recent right coronary artery territory infarct shows asymmetric pulmonary edema, most notably in right upper lobe . Intraaortic balloon pump has been placed. Findings are concerning for acute mitral regurgitation in the setting of a PM rupture.* **(Right)** *Echo shows severe mitral regurgitation from posterior PM rupture and flail leaflet. Jet is directed toward the right superior pulmonary vein, causing asymmetric edema. CXR 3 days later shows a bioprosthetic MV . (Courtesy S. Kligerman, MD.)*

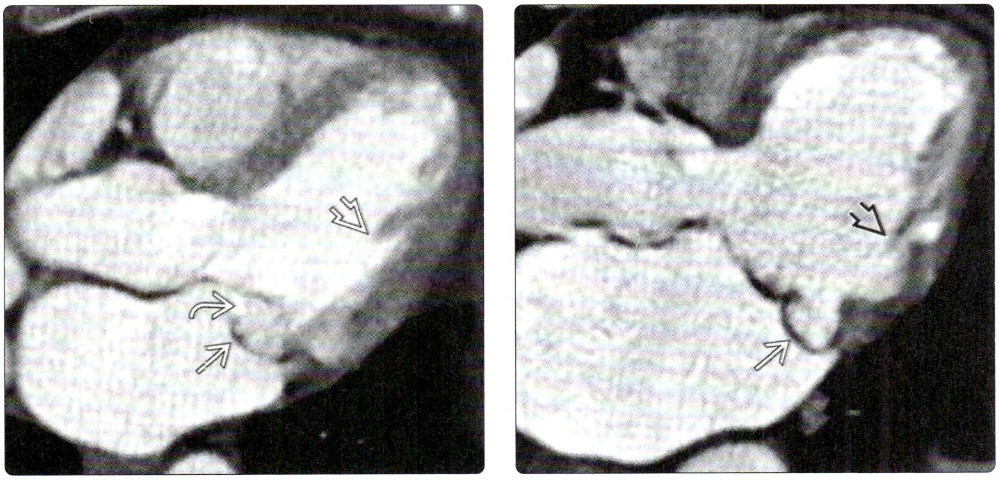

(Left) *Three-chamber coronary CTA shows a severe posterior leaflet mitral valve prolapse from an infarcted posterior PM . Note the large mitral regurgitant orifice .* **(Right)** *Three-chamber coronary CTA shows marked posterior mitral leaflet prolapse secondary to papillary head rupture in the setting of acute myocardial infarction. CTA cannot show the presence of mitral regurgitation but may show the signs of acute myocardial infarction, such as myocardial hypoperfusion or wall motion abnormality.*

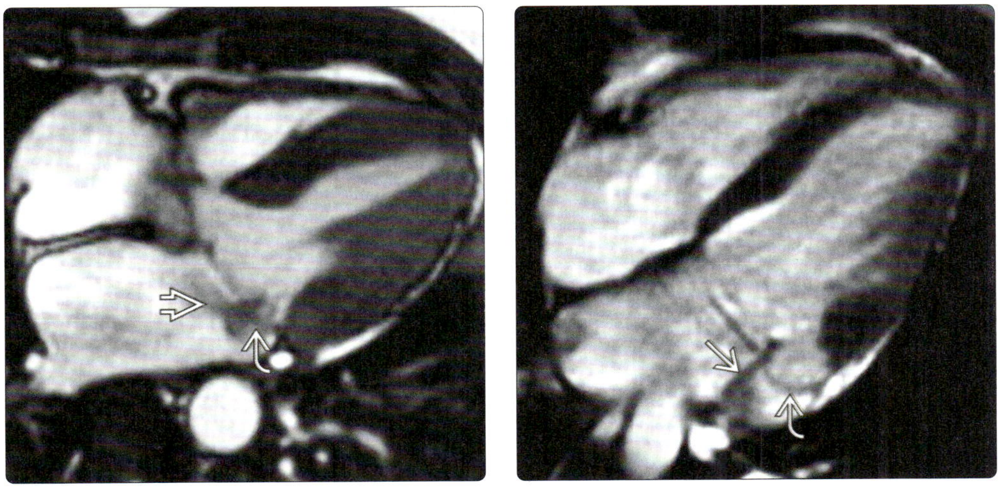

(Left) *Four-chamber SSFP cine MR shows posterior mitral leaflet prolapse secondary to a ruptured chord from the PM head. Note the jet of blood into the left atrium through the mitral valve, consistent with mitral regurgitation.* **(Right)** *Four-chamber SSFP cine MR shows posterior mitral leaflet prolapse secondary to PM rupture. Note the jet of blood into the left atrium representing mitral regurgitation.*

Postinfarction Mitral Regurgitation

KEY FACTS

TERMINOLOGY

- Ischemic mitral regurgitation (IMR) is common complication of myocardial infarction and may develop acutely or chronically

IMAGING

- Echocardiography is clinical gold standard
- Cardiac CT
  - Effective regurgitant orifice area (EROA) correlates well with echocardiography grading
  - Advantage over echocardiography: Can depict obstructive coronary artery disease
  - Calcification in papillary muscles can be hint of chronic infarction
  - Wall thinning easily identified indicating chronic infarction
- Cardiac MR
  - Steady-state free precession bright-blood sequence shows mitral regurgitant jet
  - Mitral regurgitant volume is quantified by subtracting aortic flow volume from left ventricular stroke volume
  - Late enhancement can demonstrate presence, location, and size of infarction

CLINICAL ISSUES

- Acute IMR is characterized by acute pulmonary edema, cardiogenic shock; chronic IMR is characterized by progressive heart failure
- Medical therapies for IMR have primarily aimed to prevent, delay, or revert left ventricle remodeling and heart failure
- Surgery in patients with MR is referred for coronary bypass grafts or aortic valve replacement
- Mitral valve replacement for severely symptomatic patients with chronic severe IMR and persistent symptoms despite medical therapy
- Transcatheter mitral valve therapy is evolving technology for both acute/chronic IMR

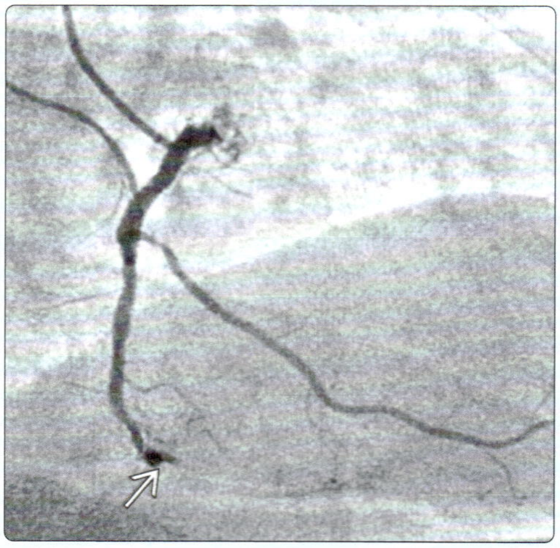

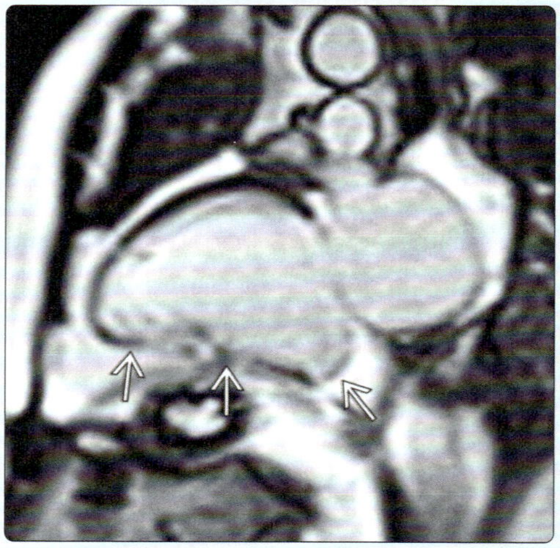

(Left) *Invasive coronary angiogram shows occlusion ➔ of the distal right coronary artery (RCA).* **(Right)** *Corresponding cardiac MR LGE 2-chamber view shows a resultant extensive inferior wall chronic myocardial infarction ➔. Note the wall thinning indicating a chronic infarct.*

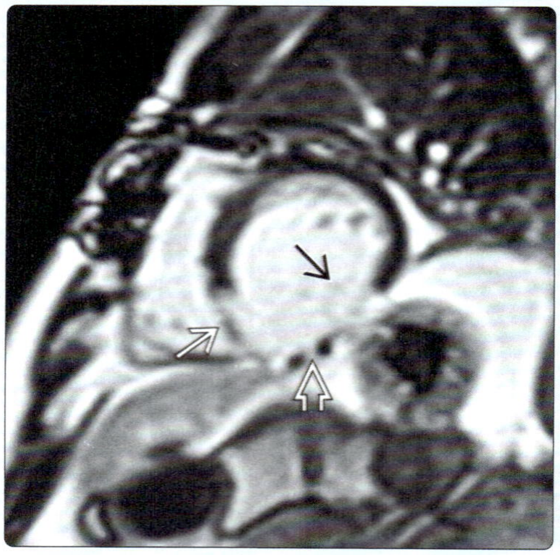

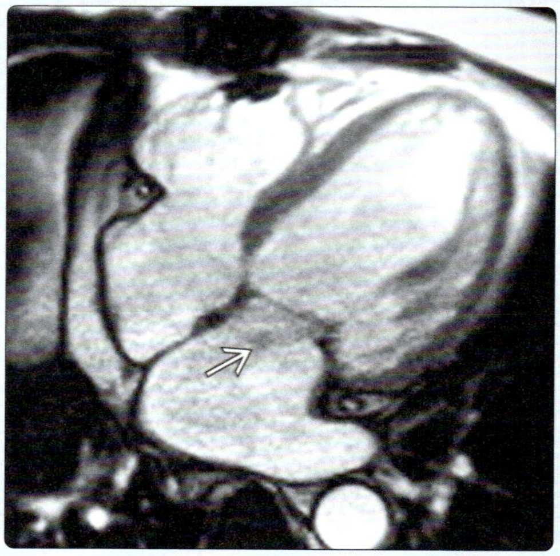

(Left) *Corresponding LGE short-axis image shows the inferior wall chronic myocardial infarction involving the inferoseptal ➔ and inferior segments ➔ in a classic dominant RCA territory. Note the posteromedial papillary muscle infarction ⇨.* **(Right)** *Corresponding SSFP 4-chamber view shows a regurgitant jet ➔ into the left atrium from the incompetent mitral valve.*

TERMINOLOGY

Definitions

- Ischemic mitral regurgitation (IMR) is common complication of myocardial infarction
  - Acute IMR is secondary to papillary muscle infarction (PMI) and rupture
  - Chronic IMR from left ventricular (LV) remodeling

IMAGING

General Features

- Location
  - Valve consists of anterior and posterior leaflets
    - Free edges are attached by multiple chordae tendineae to both papillary muscles
    - Infarcts involving posterior descending branch of dominant right coronary artery may rupture posteromedial papillary muscle
      - Anterolateral muscle less likely to rupture: Dual blood supply from left anterior descending and left circumflex coronary arteries
    - IMR is associated with significant LV remodeling, larger LV volumes, larger mitral tenting areas, larger coaptation depths, longer mitral leaflets and chords
      - Relatively new concept is that of mitral valve "plasticity," ability of mitral leaflets and chordae tendineae to elongate in response to ventricular remodeling following infarction, reduces IMR in certain patients

CT Findings

- Retrospective ECG-gated protocol
  - Motion of valve leaflets and valve plane and ventricular regional wall motion abnormalities
- Evaluation of effective regurgitant orifice area (EROA)
  - Correlates well with echocardiography grading
- Advantage over echocardiography in ability to depict obstructive coronary artery disease
- Calcification in papillary muscles can be hint of chronic infarction
- Wall thinning easily identified indicating chronic infarction

MR Findings

- Steady-state free precession bright-blood sequence shows mitral regurgitant jet
- Mitral regurgitant volume is best quantified by subtracting aortic flow volume from LV stroke volume
  - Direct quantification can be performed using PC-MR at level of mitral valve with valve-tracking algorithm
  - Can be quantified using 4D flow MR technique
- Cardiac MR LGE can demonstrate presence, location, and size of infarction
- Prevalence of lateral wall infarction is 3x higher among patients with PMI compared to patients without PMI
- Infarct distribution also impacts MR with greater MR among patients with lateral wall infarction
- Scarring of basal inferolateral segment is poor prognostic factor for mitral annuloplasty
- Tissue characterization and strain imaging have provided new insights into pathophysiology of IMR

Echocardiographic Findings

- Determination of severity of MR
  - Criteria for severe MR
  - Central jet has width > 40% of left atrial area; vena contracta ≥ 0.7 cm; systolic reversal in pulmonary veins; regurgitant volume ≥ 60 mL per beat; regurgitant fraction ≥ 50%; EROA ≥ 0.40 cm^2
- EROA can be assessed by several methods
  - 3D is superior to 2D transthoracic echocardiography
- Echogenic papillary muscles, myocardial wall thinning, and ventricular dilation
- Excellent for picking up acute papillary muscle rupture, typically associated with severe mitral leaflet prolapse

Imaging Recommendations

- Best imaging tool
  - Echocardiography is clinical gold standard, widely and acutely available
    - Indicated for baseline evaluation of LV size and function, right ventricle (RV) function, LA size, pulmonary artery pressure
  - MR is more accurate than echocardiography in assessing severity of MR
    - Useful when there is discrepancy between clinical assessment and echocardiography

DIFFERENTIAL DIAGNOSIS

Other Causes of Mitral Regurgitation

- Rheumatic heart disease
- Myxomatous degeneration, connective tissue disease
- Infective endocarditis
- Congenital mitral valve prolapse, ruptured/elongated chordae tendinea, parachute mitral valve
- Dilated cardiomyopathy (anulus)

PATHOLOGY

General Features

- Etiology
  - PMI is caused by unbalance between increased tethering forces and decreased closing forces
  - Acute IMR, papillary muscle rupture
  - Chronic IMR, LV remodeling
    - Normal valve with functional MR
    - Alteration in geometric relationship of anulus, valve leaflets, papillary muscles, and myocardium
    - Regional LV wall dysfunction tethers papillary muscles and chordae, restricting normal valve closure → regurgitation

CLINICAL ISSUES

Presentation

- Most common signs/symptoms
  - Acute IMR is characterized by acute pulmonary edema and cardiogenic shock
  - Chronic IMR is characterized by progressive heart failure
    - Dyspnea, fatigue, raised jugular venous pressure, displaced apex beat
- Clinical profile

- Risk factors: Smoking, cholesterol elevation, diabetes, hypertension, family history

Demographics

- Epidemiology
  - Occurs in 10-12% of patients with ST-elevation myocardial infarction
  - Characteristically occurs in older adult patients

Natural History & Prognosis

- Postinfarction LV is less compliant
- Dilation of left atrium and LV, pulmonary hypertension, and congestive heart failure
- If regurgitant volume > 30 mL/beat, then 5-year survival rate is 61%

Treatment

- Medical
  - To prevent, delay or revert LV remodeling and heart failure
  - Current therapies for chronic IMR have primarily targeted LV dysfunction
  - β-blockers and mineralocorticoid receptor blockers help reduce remodeling
  - ACE inhibitors or angiotensin receptor blockers reduce afterload and regurgitant volume
  - Diuretics reduce preload and regurgitant volume
- Resynchronization therapy
  - Improves LV function, reduces MR
  - Biventricular implantable cardioverter-defibrillators synchronize ventricles in those with QRS > 120 ms
- Surgery
  - For subset of patients who remain severely symptomatic despite guideline-directed medical therapy for heart failure
  - Annuloplasty in those with annular dilation, typically open procedure
  - Reimplantation of papillary muscle in selected patients
  - Reasonable to choose chordal-sparing mitral valve replacement over downsized annuloplasty repair if operation is considered for severely symptomatic patients (NYHA classes III-IV) with chronic severe IMR and persistent symptoms despite guideline-directed medical therapy for heart failure
    - Prospective randomized trial has shown that mitral valve repair is associated with higher rate of recurrence of moderate or severe MR than that associated with mitral valve replacement (58.8% vs. 3.8%) in patients with severe, symptomatic IMR without difference in mortality rate at 2-year follow-up
- Interventional
  - Transcatheter mitral valve therapy is evolving technology for both acute/chronic IMR
    - EVEREST II trial showed significantly reduced MR, improved clinical symptoms, and decreased LV dimensions at 12 months in high-surgical-risk cohorts with grades 3-6 MR
    - Valve-in-valve therapy is currently being evaluated for failed bioprosthetic mitral valve replacements, good early reports, larger trials awaited
  - In acute setting of papillary muscle rupture, several centers are reporting good early results from use of MitraClip as percutaneous transcatheter option in carefully selected patients unable for open surgical repair
  - In patients with annular dilation, new technique device offers percutaneous annuloplasty system rather than open surgery; larger trials are awaited; initial reports favorable

SELECTED REFERENCES

1. Kwon DH et al: Cardiac MRI-enriched phenomapping classification and differential treatment outcomes in patients with ischemic cardiomyopathy. Circ Cardiovasc Imaging. 17(4):e016006, 2024
2. Gomez-Polo JC et al: Post-infarct mitral insufficiency: when to resort to reparative surgery, when to the mitral clip. Eur Heart J Suppl. 24(Suppl I):I104-10, 2022
3. Marsit O et al: Effects of cyproheptadine on mitral valve remodeling and regurgitation after myocardial infarction. J Am Coll Cardiol. 80(5):500-10, 2022
4. Otto CM et al: 2020 ACC/AHA guideline for the management of patients with valvular heart disease: executive summary: a report of the American College of Cardiology/American Heart Association Joint Committee on Clinical Practice Guidelines. Circulation. 143(5):e35-71, 2021
5. Zhang C et al: Predictors of moderate to severe ischemic mitral regurgitation after myocardial infarction: a cardiac magnetic resonance study. Eur Radiol. 31(8):5650-8, 2021
6. Cavalcante JL et al: Prognostic impact of ischemic mitral regurgitation severity and myocardial infarct quantification by cardiovascular magnetic resonance. JACC Cardiovasc Imaging. 13(7):1489-501, 2020
7. Chew PG et al: Multimodality imaging for the quantitative assessment of mitral regurgitation. Quant Imaging Med Surg. 8(3):342-59, 2018
8. Sandoval Y et al: Contemporary management of ischemic mitral regurgitation: A Review. Am J Med. 131(8):887-95, 2018
9. Uretsky S et al: Use of cardiac magnetic resonance imaging in assessing mitral regurgitation: Current evidence. J Am Coll Cardiol. 71(5):547-63, 2018
10. Ávila-Vanzzini N et al: Clinical and echocardiographic factors associated with mitral plasticity in patients with chronic inferior myocardial infarction. Eur Heart J Cardiovasc Imaging. 19(5):508-15, 2018
11. Nishimura RA et al: 2017 AHA/ACC Focused Update of the 2014 AHA/ACC guideline for the management of patients with valvular heart disease: a report of the American College of Cardiology/American Heart Association Task Force on Clinical Practice Guidelines. Circulation. 135(25):e1159-95, 2017
12. Michler RE et al: Two-year outcomes of surgical treatment of moderate ischemic mitral regurgitation. N Engl J Med. 374(20):1932-41, 2016
13. Nickenig G et al: Treatment of chronic functional mitral valve regurgitation with a percutaneous annuloplasty system. J Am Coll Cardiol. 67(25):2927-36, 2016
14. Glower DD et al: Percutaneous mitral valve repair for mitral regurgitation in high-risk patients: results of the EVEREST II study. J Am Coll Cardiol. 64(2):172-81, 2014
15. O'Gara PT et al: Transcatheter therapies for mitral regurgitation: a professional society overview from the American College of Cardiology, the American Association for Thoracic Surgery, Society for Cardiovascular Angiography and Interventions Foundation, and the Society of Thoracic Surgeons. J Am Coll Cardiol. 63(8):840-52, 2014
16. Beaudoin J et al: Late repair of ischemic mitral regurgitation does not prevent left ventricular remodeling: importance of timing for beneficial repair. Circulation. 128(11 Suppl 1):S248-52, 2013
17. Chinitz JS et al: Mitral apparatus assessment by delayed enhancement CMR: relative impact of infarct distribution on mitral regurgitation. JACC Cardiovasc Imaging. 6(2):220-34, 2013
18. Arnous S et al: Quantification of mitral regurgitation on cardiac computed tomography: comparison with qualitative and quantitative echocardiographic parameters. J Comput Assist Tomogr. 35(5):625-30, 2011
19. Killeen RP et al: Chronic mitral regurgitation detected on cardiac MDCT: differentiation between functional and valvular aetiologies. Eur Radiol. 20(8):1886-95, 2010

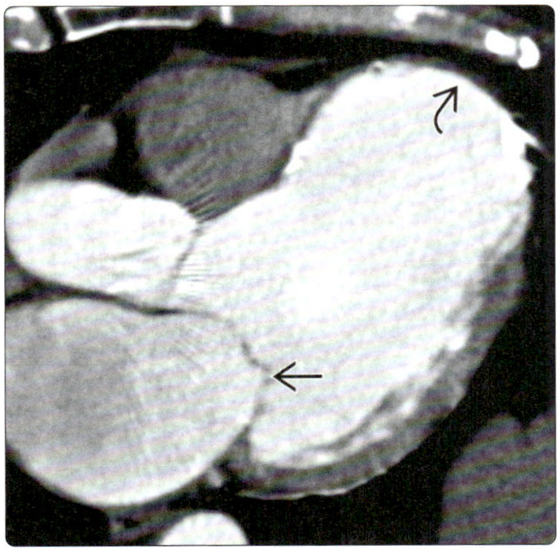

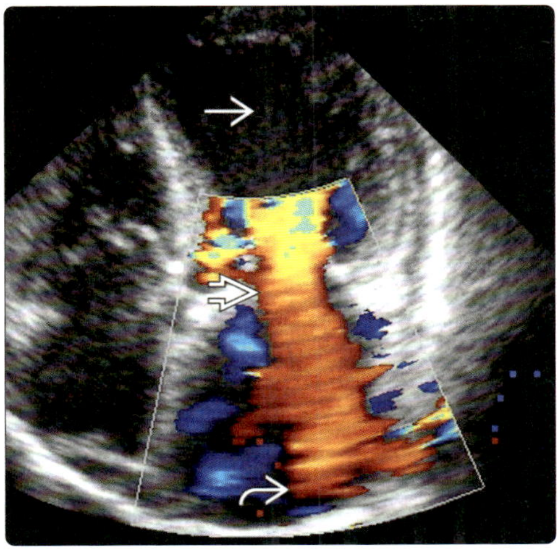

(Left) *CTA shows LV and mitral annular dilation with incomplete coaptation of mitral valve leaflets, consistent with mitral regurgitation. Note the LV dilation, large apical chronic myocardial infarction with severe wall thinning, aneurysmal formation, and wall calcification.* **(Right)** *Corresponding echocardiogram 4-chamber view confirms a dilated LV post infarction with severe mitral valve regurgitation with the jet reaching the posterior wall of the dilated left atrium.*

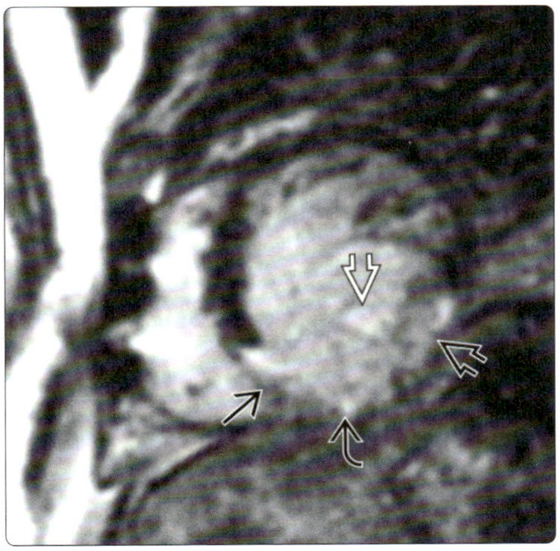

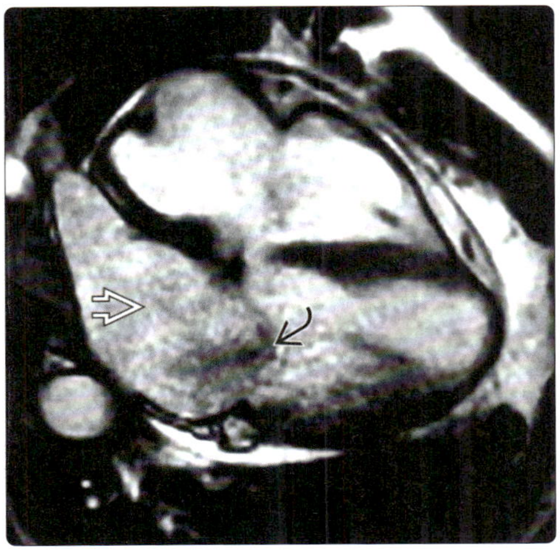

(Left) *Chronic transmural infarct involves the inferoseptal, inferior, and inferolateral segments, involving a dominant RCA system and a large posterolateral ventricular branch of the RCA. Note the infarcted posteromedial papillary muscle.* **(Right)** *Corresponding cine MR shows a regurgitant jet from secondary mitral regurgitation related to tethering of the posteromedial papillary muscle from the infarct. Note the enlarged left atrium.*

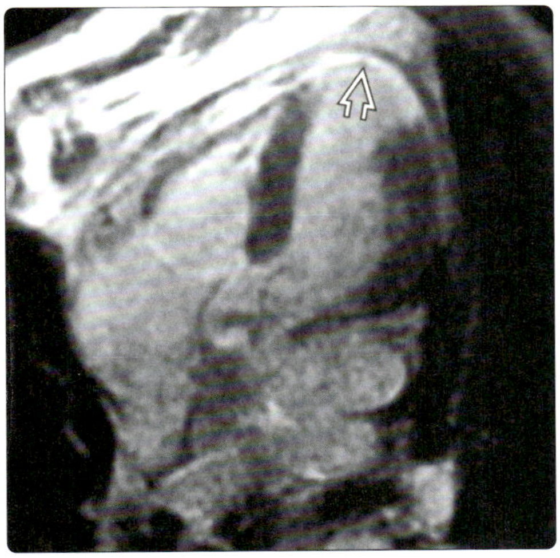

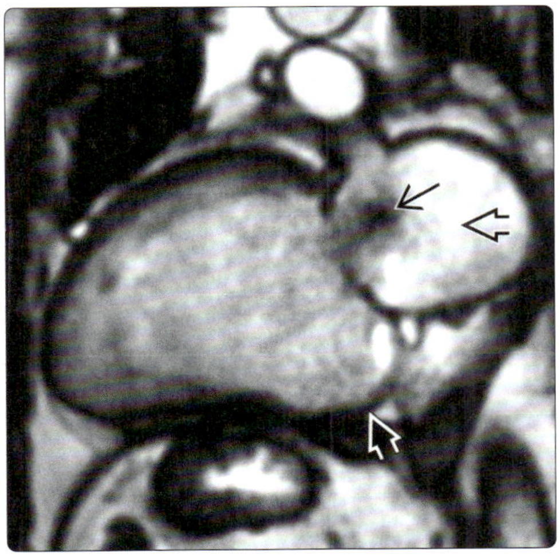

(Left) *Four-chamber delayed enhancement MR shows transmural LGE at the apex of the LV involving the septal, inferior, and lateral segments. Associated wall thinning of these segments is suggestive of chronic infarct.* **(Right)** *Corresponding 2-chamber cine MR shows a large regurgitant jet from secondary mitral regurgitation back into a dilated left atrium. Note the wall thinning of the inferior myocardial segment at the basal level indicating a further infarct.*

Left Ventricular Free Wall Rupture

KEY FACTS

TERMINOLOGY

- Rupture of left ventricular myocardial wall with ensuing communication between left ventricular cavity and pericardial space
  - Usually seen in setting of acute myocardial infarction
  - Often accompanied by acute hemodynamic deterioration or electromechanical dissociation
  - May be contained if inflammatory pericardium seals rupture

IMAGING

- Sudden development of hemopericardium seen on echocardiography, CT, and MR
- Accompanying wall motion abnormality in respective myocardial segment
- Size of defect is very variable

TOP DIFFERENTIAL DIAGNOSES

- Pericardial effusion
- Hemopericardium
- Pericardial hematoma
- Left ventricular pseudoaneurysm following surgical heart valve replacement
- Left ventricular aneurysm following myocardial infarction

CLINICAL ISSUES

- 3 forms of presentation
  - Acute rupture: Acute tamponade with sudden electromechanical dissociation or severe hypotension
  - Subacute rupture: Moderate to severe pericardial effusion with tamponade and hemodynamic compromise with modest or progressive hypotension or without tamponade
  - Chronic: Incidental detection of contained rupture in long-term interval following myocardial infarction
- Symptoms: Chest pain, syncope, or may be asymptomatic if contained rupture

(Left) *Pathology specimen shows a noncontained rupture of the anterior wall after myocardial infarction (MI). Note the slit-like rupture ➡ and thrombi ➡ due to the resulting hemorrhagic pericardial effusion. In most cases, noncontained rupture of the left ventricular (LV) wall leads to instant pericardial tamponade and death.* **(Right)** *CECT 4 days post MI shows a narrow-neck tear through the LV anterior wall ⇗ with adjacent pseudoaneurysm ⇨ and surrounding hemopericardium ⇨. (Courtesy S. Kligerman, MD.)*

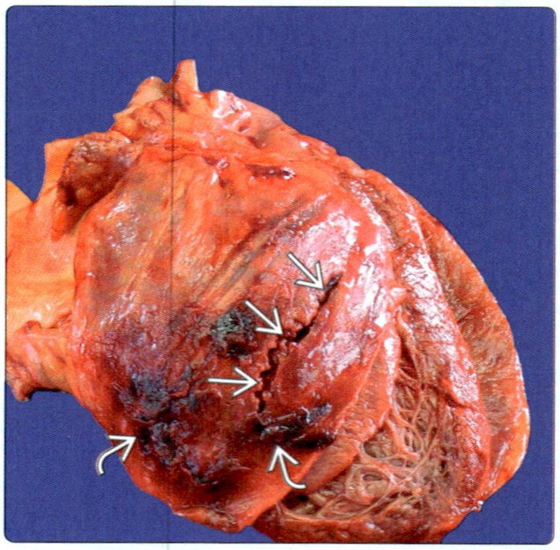

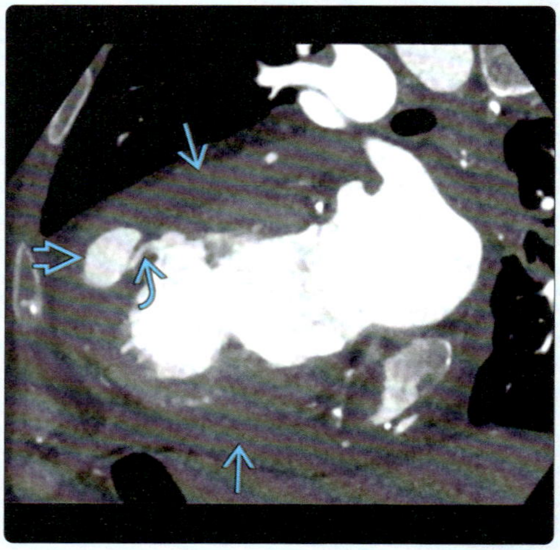

(Left) *Short-axis reformat cardiac CECT shows a small, contained rupture of the lateral wall of the left ventricle in a patient with myocardial infarction secondary to occlusion of the left circumflex coronary artery ➡.* **(Right)** *Bright-blood MR in the same patient also shows the contained rupture ➡. Note the significantly lower spatial resolution of MR as compared with CT.*

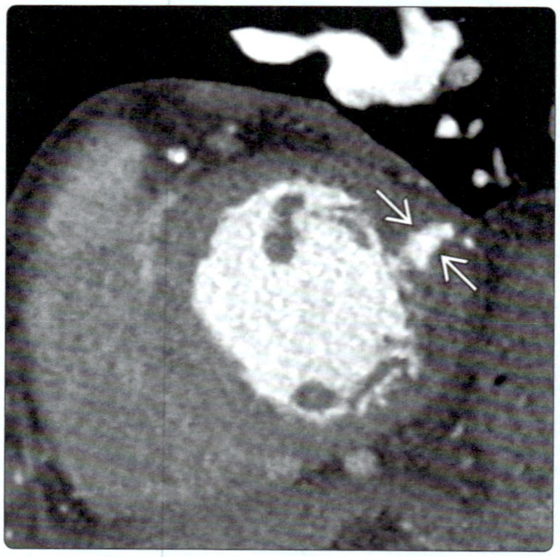

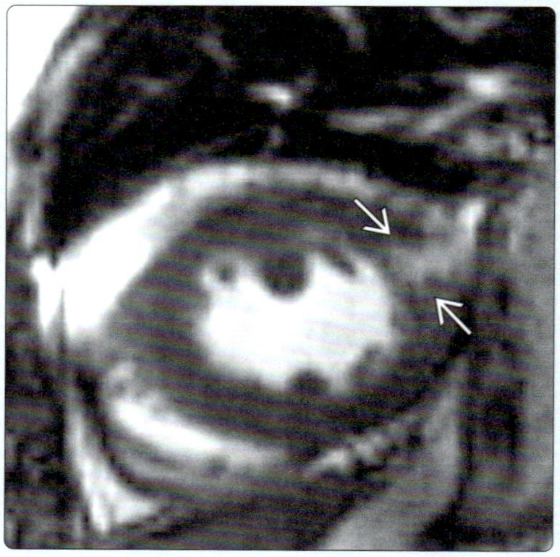

TERMINOLOGY

Definitions

- Rupture of left ventricular myocardial wall with ensuing communication between left ventricular cavity and pericardial space
  - Usually seen in setting of acute myocardial infarction
  - Often accompanied by acute hemodynamic deterioration or electromechanic dissociation

IMAGING

General Features

- Best diagnostic clue
  - Sudden development of hemopericardium
  - Left ventricular (LV) wall motion abnormality

Radiographic Findings

- Radiography
  - Chest radiography findings
    - May be normal
    - Flask-shaped heart, typical of pericardial effusion

CT Findings

- Varying degree of hemopericardium
- Discontinuity of left ventricular myocardium
- Myocardial akinesis or dyskinesis
- Classically, teaching is that pseudoaneurysms have narrow neck and are more common in posterior and lateral segments

MR Findings

- Cine: Hypokinesis or akinesis of free wall
- LGE may demonstrate loss of continuity of myocardium with irregular margins
  - Hematoma, thrombus, or fluid in pericardial space
  - Transmural LGE may be seen

Echocardiographic Findings

- Echocardiogram
  - 2D echocardiography
    - Varying degrees of pericardial effusion
    - Typical flap-like dyskinesis of myocardial segment
    - Often accompanied by left ventricular thrombus
- Color Doppler
  - May infrequently be able to demonstrate communication between left ventricle and pericardium, depending on size and extent of defect

Angiographic Findings

- Left ventricular angiography
  - Regional wall motion abnormality
  - Potentially, communication between left ventricle and pericardial space

DIFFERENTIAL DIAGNOSIS

Pericardial Effusion

- Infection, inflammation, uremia

Hemopericardium

- Acute aortic dissection, trauma, neoplasm, consequence of cardiac surgery

Postsurgical Left Ventricular Pseudoaneurysm

- Due to dehiscence following surgical aortic valve or mitral valve replacement

Left Ventricular Aneurysm

- Typically have wide neck
- More common in apex and anterior segments
- Pseudoaneurysms can have similar appearance

PATHOLOGY

General Features

- Associated abnormalities
  - Hemopericardium
- Acute myocardial infarction

Staging, Grading, & Classification

- 3 typical variants of rupture defect
  - Slit-like: Early infarct
    - Seen within 12 hours of infarction
    - Associated with delayed thrombolysis (> 12 hours after infarction)
  - Erosion at borders of infarct
    - Extension of infarct, intermediate in timing
  - Expansion of infarct
    - Large infarction, late-appearing

Gross Pathologic & Surgical Features

- Contained ventricular rupture with blood &/or thrombus in pericardial space

CLINICAL ISSUES

Presentation

- Most common signs/symptoms
  - Chest pain, syncope, or may be asymptomatic if rupture is contained
- Clinical profile
  - Occurs early (< 48 hours) or late (2-7 days) post infarction

Demographics

- Age
  - Generally > 60 years (median: 65-70 years)
- Epidemiology
  - < 1% of all patients with acute myocardial infarction

Natural History & Prognosis

- Very high mortality unless contained rupture

Treatment

- Emergent surgical repair may be attempted
  - High long-term survival rate if surgery is successful
  - Off-pump sutureless repair is promising for left ventricular free wall rupture
- Conservative approach may be preferable in patients with contained rupture, lack of severe hemodynamic compromise, and comorbidities

SELECTED REFERENCES

1. Makhoul M et al: Sutureless repair of subacute left ventricular free wall rupture. Ann Cardiothorac Surg. 11(3):299-303, 2022
2. Formica F et al: Postinfarction left ventricular free wall rupture: a 17-year single-centre experience. Eur J Cardiothorac Surg. 53(1):150-6, 2018

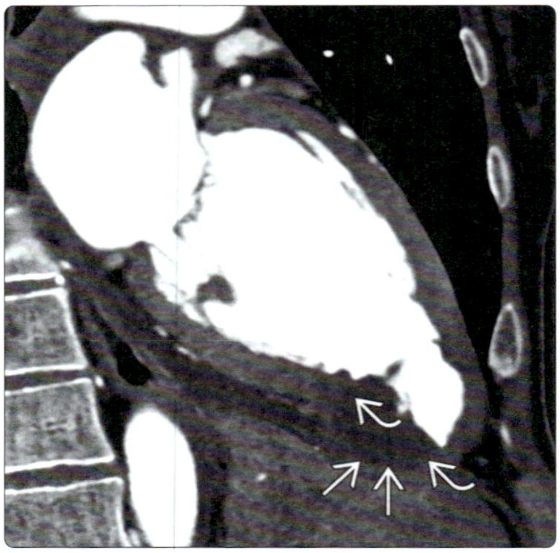

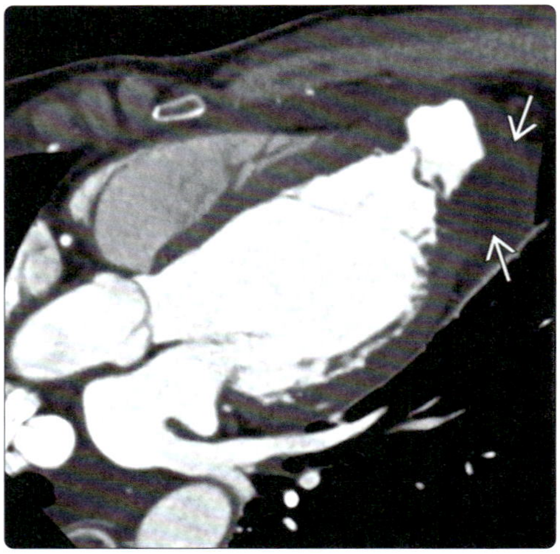

(Left) *Long-axis parasagittal CECT of the left ventricle demonstrates a contained rupture of the LV apex that is filled with thrombotic material. The presenting symptom in this patient was a stroke.* **(Right)** *Four-chamber CECT reformat in the same patient also demonstrates the contained rupture at the apex and reveals a thrombus.*

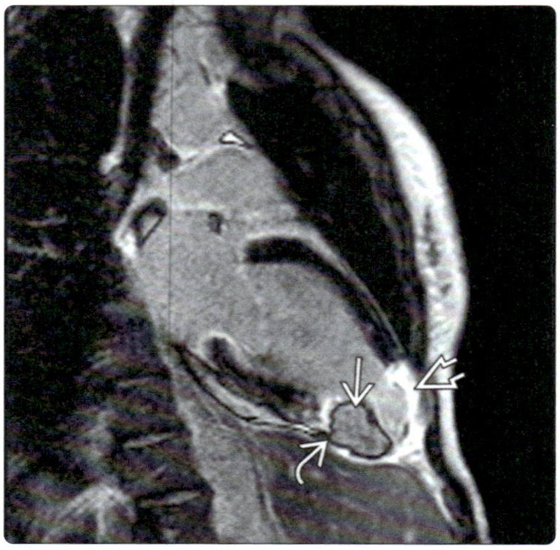

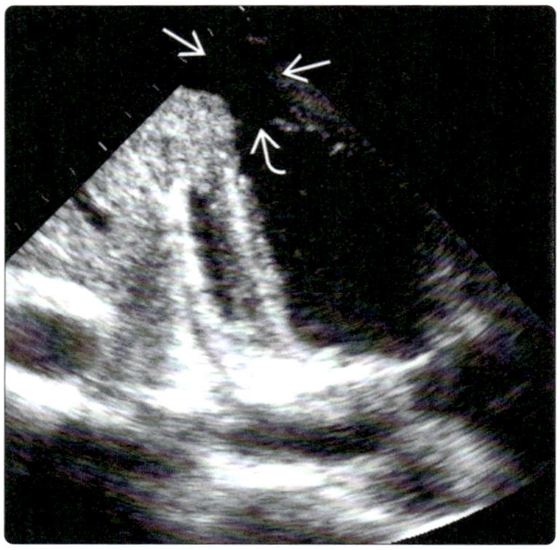

(Left) *LGE MR in the same patient shows transmural apical delayed hyperenhancement consistent with infarct and thrombus. Discontinuation of the enhanced myocardium suggests the presence of a contained rupture.* **(Right)** *Modified parasternal long-axis transthoracic echocardiogram in the same patient shows the rupture in the apical region of the left ventricle and blood extending beyond the wall (pseudoaneurysm).*

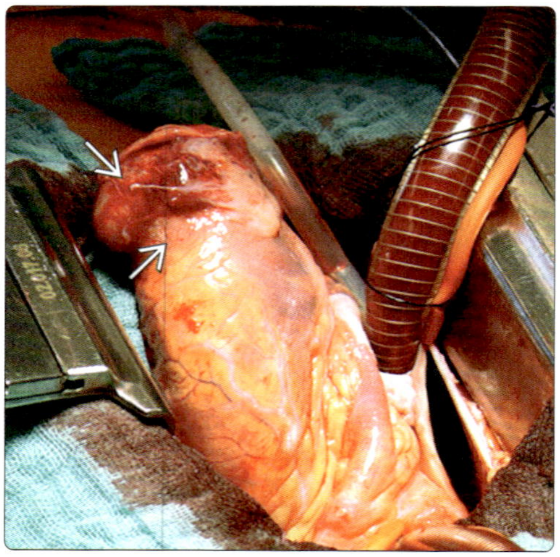

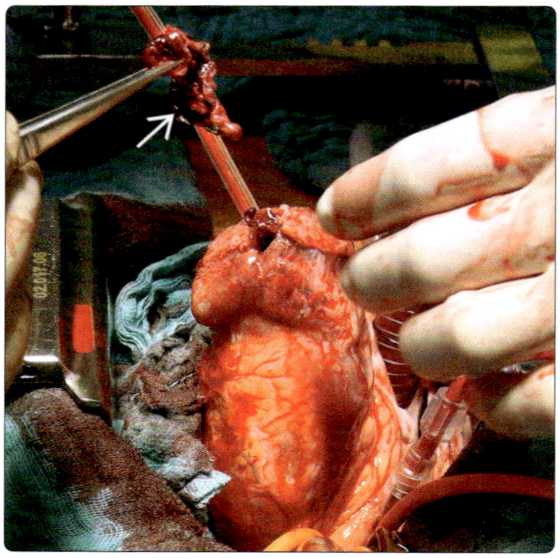

(Left) *Intraoperative photograph of the exposed heart in the same patient shows the rupture and thrombotic material contained by inflamed epicardium. The grayish shade of the epicardium (usually clear) indicates postinfarct pericarditis, which is a prerequisite to having enough adhesions to prevent tamponade in case of rupture.* **(Right)** *Clinical photograph in the same patient shows the thrombus removed from the pseudoaneurysm after the surgeon opened the latter.*

Left Ventricular Free Wall Rupture

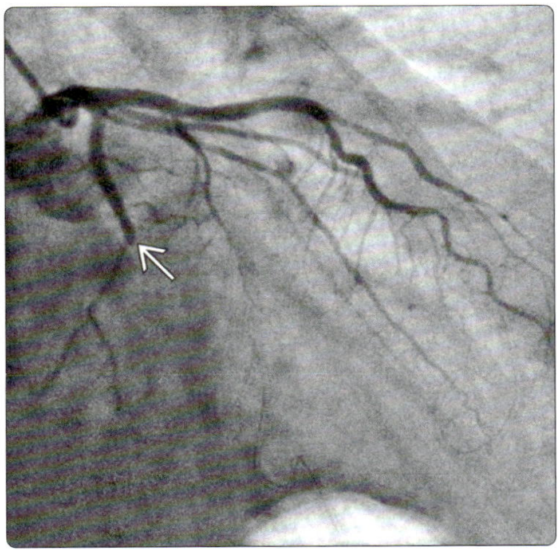

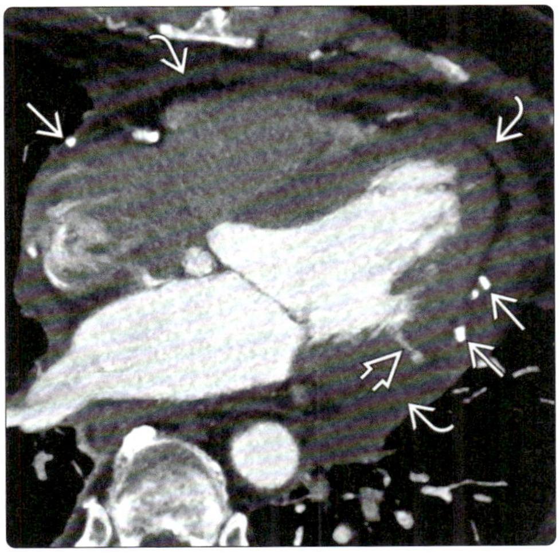

(Left) *Coronary angiography shows occlusion of the left circumflex coronary artery* . **(Right)** *CECT in the same patient shows a very small free-wall rupture in the posterolateral region of the left ventricle , which is supplied by the occluded circumflex artery. A small pericardial effusion is present. Within the effusion, several cross sections of a pigtail catheter are visible. The catheter has been placed percutaneously for drainage of the effusion.*

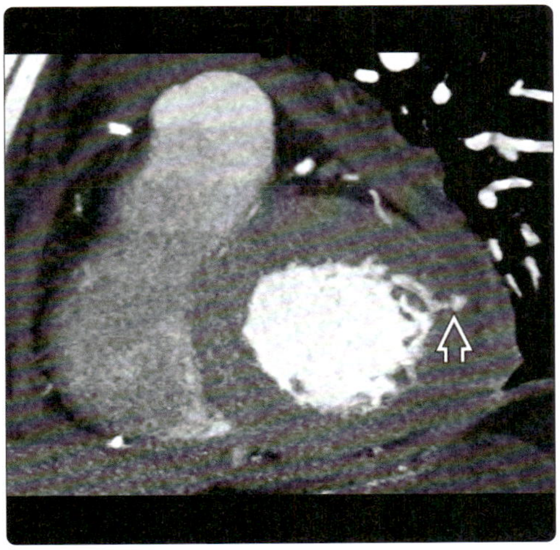

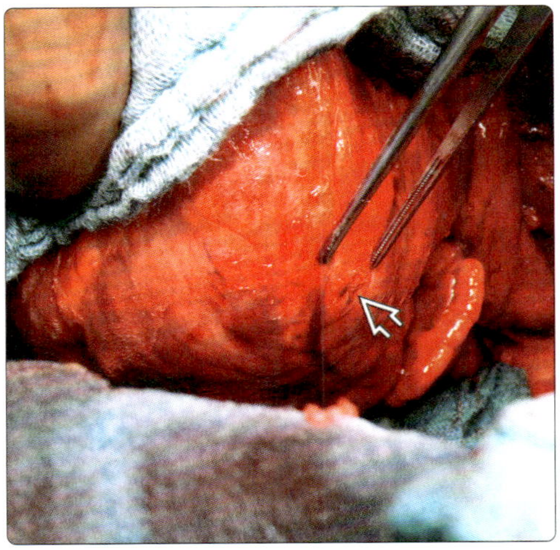

(Left) *Short-axis CECT reconstruction of the left ventricle in the same patient shows contrast extending radially through the posterolateral left ventricular wall, consistent with a small rupture* . **(Right)** *Intraoperative photograph in the same patient shows the very small perforation of the LV lateral wall , confirming LV free-wall rupture.*

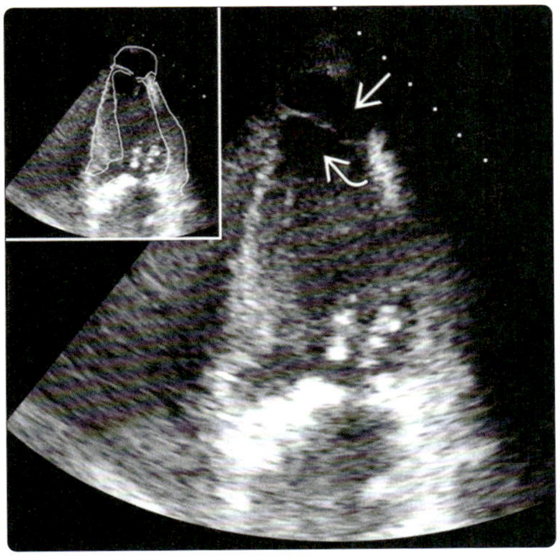

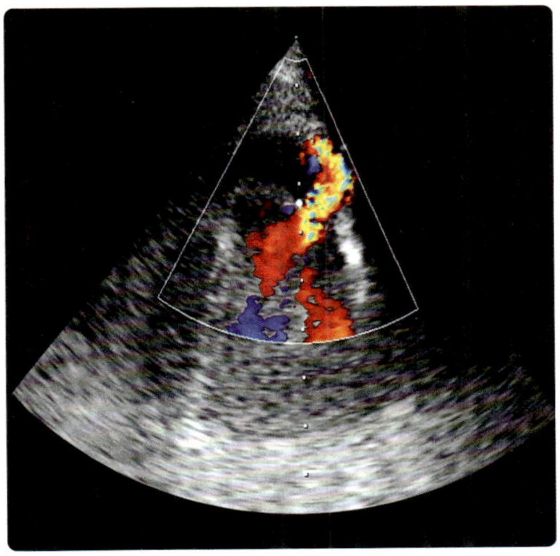

(Left) *Echocardiography 1 year after transapical aortic valve replacement shows a contained rupture of the LV apex. Note the blood-filled cavity that has ensued. The site of rupture is in the apical myocardium . Contours have been redrawn (inset) for better visualization.* **(Right)** *Color Doppler flow signal in the same patient shows the communication between the LV cavity and the contained rupture.*

Ventricular Septal Rupture

KEY FACTS

TERMINOLOGY

- Abnormal communication between right and left ventricles following acute myocardial infarction
  - Typically diagnosed 2 days after infarct
  - Results in left-to-right shunt, which is often severe and frequently leads to cardiogenic shock

IMAGING

- Echocardiogram (best imaging tool)
  - New ventricular septal defect with pattern of right ventricular overload
  - Left-to-right shunt in Doppler echocardiography
- Chest radiography: Biventricular enlargement, pulmonary edema
- Cardiac gated CTA: May show focal defect involving ventricular septum with areas of myocardial thinning, hypokinesis, or akinesis adjacent to defect
- Cardiovascular MR: Provides anatomic detail and shunt quantification

TOP DIFFERENTIAL DIAGNOSES

- Congenital ventricular septal defect
  - Not preceded by myocardial infarct
- Contained rupture of left ventricle
  - Not associated with left-to-right shunt

CLINICAL ISSUES

- Sudden chest pain and deterioration of hemodynamics after acute myocardial infarction
- Immediate placement of intraaortic balloon pump or microaxial pump to decrease left ventricular afterload
- Very high mortality when untreated
- Treatment options include surgery and interventional closure
- Mortality remains high, even when defect closure is attempted

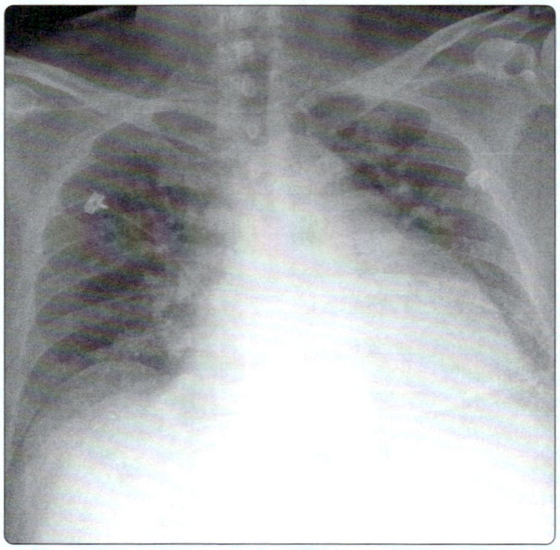
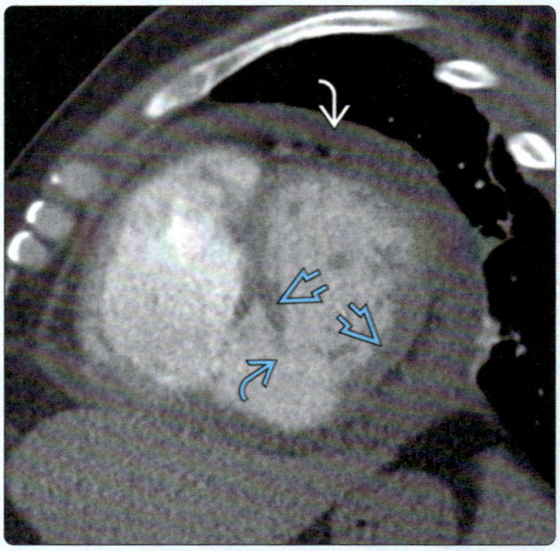

(Left) *AP radiograph in a 64-year-old man with right coronary artery territory myocardial infarct 4 days prior shows marked enlargement of the cardiac silhouette and pulmonary edema.* **(Right)** *Short-axis CT shows a large ventricular septal rupture (VSR) involving the inferior and inferolateral segments at the base. The rim of infarcted tissue is hypoperfused, and there is a small amount of hemopericardium.*

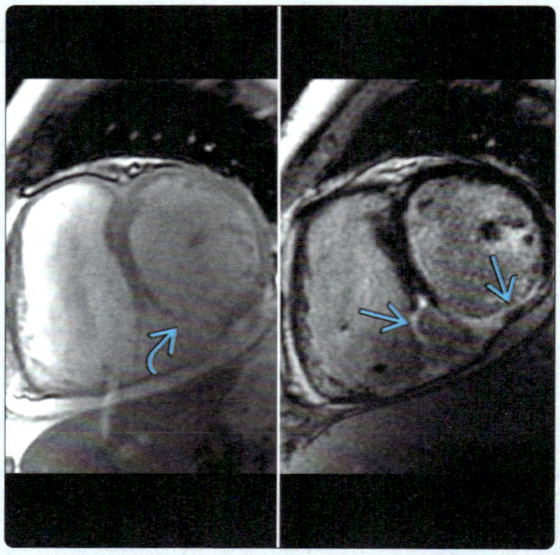
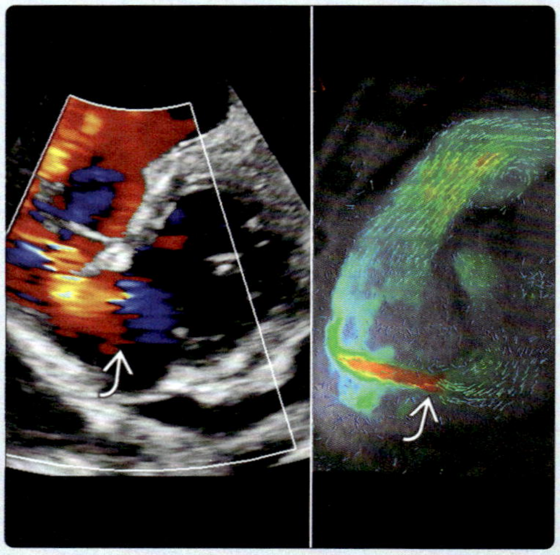

(Left) *Short-axis SSFP cine MR (left) shows the large VSR. PSIR delayed enhancement image (right) shows the VSR and surrounding infarcted tissue, a portion of which dangles into the VSR.* **(Right)** *Modified short-axis images from an echocardiogram (left) and 4D flow MR (right) show left-to-right flow across the VSR with a Qp:Qs of 3.1. The patient was referred for surgical repair.*

TERMINOLOGY

Synonyms

- Postinfarct ventricular septal defect (VSD)

Definitions

- Abnormal communication between right and left ventricles
  - Generally following acute myocardial infarction

IMAGING

General Features

- Location
  - Anterior myocardial infarction
    - Generally involves apical portion of septum
    - Usually simpler, discrete communication across septum
  - Inferior myocardial infarction
    - Generally involves inferoposterior septum
    - Potentially more complex rupture with irregular, serpiginous tracts through myocardium
- Size
  - Few mm to several cm
- Morphology
  - Defect in ventricular septum
  - Size of infarct in part determines prognosis

Radiographic Findings

- Radiography
  - Chest radiography findings
    - Biventricular enlargement
    - Pulmonary congestion

CT Findings

- CTA
  - Gated study demonstrates focal defect involving ventricular septum with areas of myocardial thinning, hypokinesis, or akinesis adjacent to defect

MR Findings

- Cine SSFP
  - Visualizes anatomy of defect
    - Peridefect hypokinesis or akinesis on cine imaging
- Flow imaging: To quantify shunt using Qp:Qs
- LGE: Transmural hyperenhancement surrounding septal defect may be seen

Echocardiographic Findings

- Echocardiogram
  - New VSD apparent on echocardiogram
  - Pattern of right ventricular overload
  - Wall motion abnormalities corresponding to infarction
- Color Doppler
  - Left-to-right shunt

Angiographic Findings

- Coronary angiography demonstrates occlusion of infarct vessel
- Left ventriculography demonstrates left-to-right shunt

Imaging Recommendations

- Best imaging tool
  - Doppler echocardiography

DIFFERENTIAL DIAGNOSIS

Congenital Ventricular Septal Defect

- Not preceded by myocardial infarct

Contained Rupture of Left Ventricle

- Not associated with left-to-right shunt

PATHOLOGY

General Features

- Etiology
  - Complication of anterior or inferior myocardial infarction
  - Occurs 1-5 days post myocardial infarction with median time of diagnosis 2 days
- Necrosis of ventricular septum
  - Direct communication across septum, usually at ventricular apex for anterior infarction
  - Often dissection of right ventricular free wall with complex communication to right ventricular cavity for inferior infarction
- Based on location 3 types: Anterior, posterior, and apical
  - Anterior and apical are mostly seen in anterior myocardial infarction
  - Posterior rupture is more common in right coronary artery territory infarct and associated with higher incidence of biventricular dysfunction

CLINICAL ISSUES

Presentation

- Most common signs/symptoms
  - Recurrent chest pain after infarction
  - Shortness of breath
  - Heart failure and hypotension

Demographics

- Epidemiology
  - 0.25% of acute myocardial infarcts

Natural History & Prognosis

- Invariably fatal if untreated
- Surgical treatment is also associated with high mortality

Treatment

- Medical therapy to reduce afterload using intraaortic balloon pump or microaxial pump
- Interventional occlusion of VSD can be attempted
- Surgical treatment has high perioperative risk
  - Pericardial patch ± infarct resection

SELECTED REFERENCES

1. Cubeddu RJ et al: Ventricular septal rupture after myocardial infarction: JACC focus seminar 3/5. J Am Coll Cardiol. 83(19):1886-901, 2024
2. Rodríguez-Zanella H et al: Multimodality imaging with 3D echocardiography transillumination and 3D CT rendering for a ventricular septal rupture's morphological analysis. Eur Heart J Cardiovasc Imaging. 23(2):e92, 2022
3. Gattani R et al: Multimodality imaging assessment of ventricular septal rupture and intramyocardial dissecting hematoma post late-presenting acute myocardial infarction. Circ Cardiovasc Imaging. 14(10):e013185, 2021
4. Gong FF et al: Mechanical complications of acute myocardial infarction: a review. JAMA Cardiol. 6(3):341-9, 2021
5. Ronco D et al: Surgical treatment of postinfarction ventricular septal rupture. JAMA Netw Open. 4(10):e2128309, 2021

KEY FACTS

TERMINOLOGY

- Akinetic or dyskinetic segment of well-demarcated, thin, scarred myocardium resulting from transmural myocardial infarction (MI)

IMAGING

- Chest radiography
  - Usually shows enlarged cardiac silhouette
- Nonenhanced CT
  - Linear calcifications of infarcted myocardial wall
- Contrast-enhanced CT
  - Thinned and scarred myocardium
  - Left ventricular apical filling defect consistent with mural thrombus
- CT angiography
  - Severe coronary artery disease
- MR imaging
  - SSFP cine imaging will show aneurysms as regions of wall thinning and motion abnormality
  - LGE: Transmural hyperenhancement = scar
    - LGE MR detects associated thrombi with 2x greater sensitivity than echocardiography; longer inversion times can help differentiate thrombi from other filling defects
  - 1st-pass perfusion: Thrombus may be seen as nonenhancing mural mass
- Echocardiographic findings
  - Excellent method to detect aneurysm
  - Spontaneous echo contrast (smoke) suggests slow flow in aneurysm and increased likelihood for thrombus formation

TOP DIFFERENTIAL DIAGNOSES

- Pseudoaneurysm
- Chagas disease
- Takotsubo cardiomyopathy
- Sarcoidosis

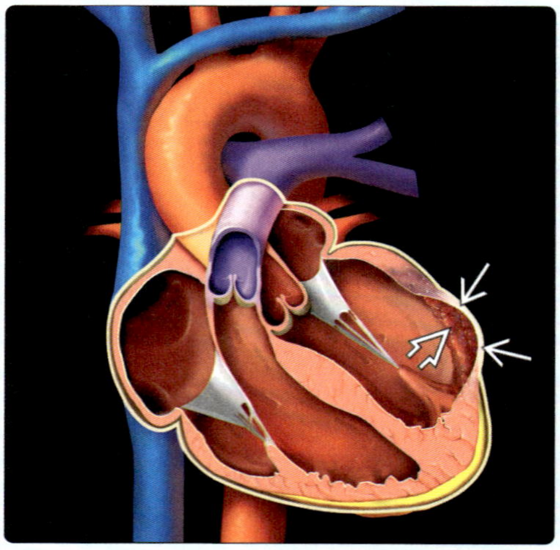

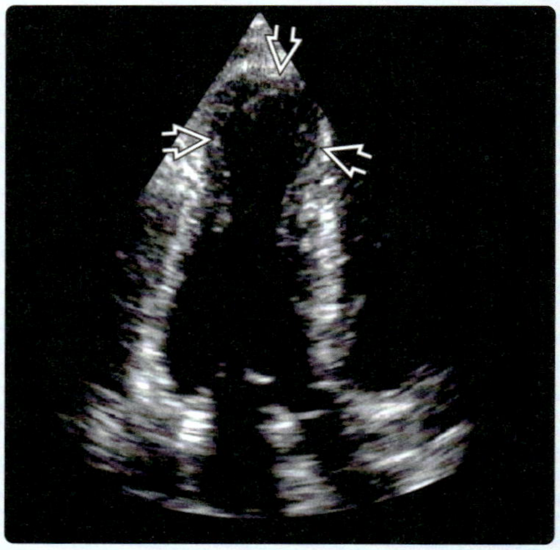

(Left) *Graphic shows a mid to apical anterolateral wall aneurysm ➾. Note thinning and fibrosis of the myocardium and outward bulge of the wall. Also, a mural thrombus ➾ is layered against the aneurysm wall.* **(Right)** *Three-chamber transthoracic echocardiogram shows that a myocardial infarction in this patient has resulted in formation of an aneurysm at the left ventricular apex. Note the outward bulge of the apex ➾ on this diastolic image.*

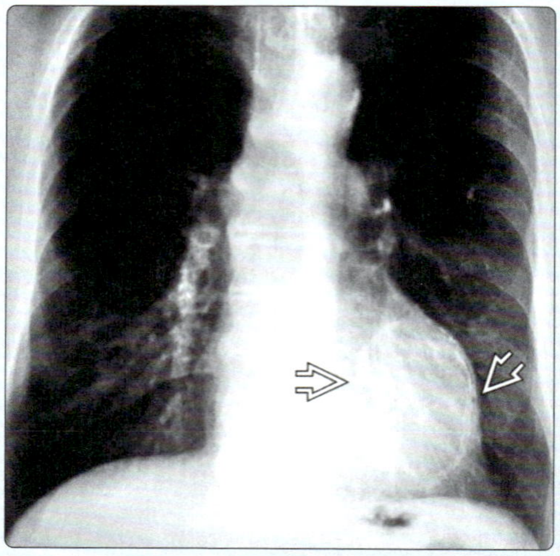

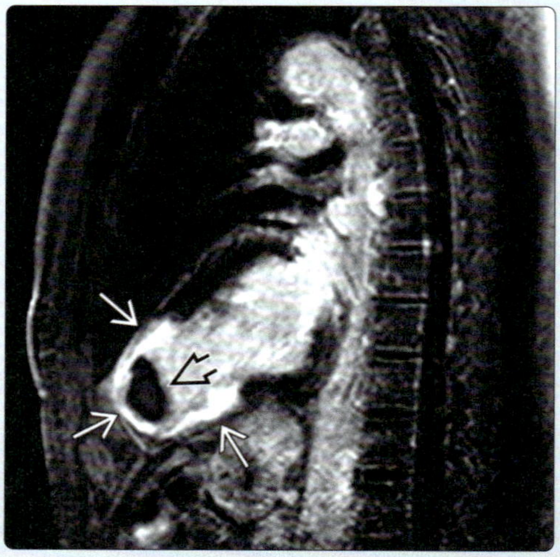

(Left) *PA radiograph shows circumscribed curvilinear calcification ➾ at the cardiac apex corresponding to the expected location of the left ventricle (LV). This represents a left anterior descending (LAD) coronary artery territory LV true aneurysm.* **(Right)** *Two-chamber LGE MR shows transmural late enhancement of the thinned, ballooned anterior and apical myocardium ➾ signifying an extensive scar. There is a large, nonenhancing thrombus at the apex ➾. MR is 2x more sensitive than echo for detecting thrombi.*

TERMINOLOGY

Definitions

- Akinetic or dyskinetic segment of well-demarcated, thin, scarred, and fibrotic myocardium resulting from healed, remodeled, transmural myocardial infarction (MI)

IMAGING

General Features

- Best diagnostic clue
    - Focal contour bulge of left ventricle (LV) present in diastole that worsens in systole (dyskinesia) on cine imaging (CMR, ECG, angiography, gated CT)
- Morphology
    - Differentiated into true and false aneurysms (pseudoaneurysms)
        - True aneurysms have residual layer of myocardium present
            - Most often involves anterior wall and apex [left anterior descending (LAD) coronary artery territory]
            - Opening or mouth of aneurysm is as wide or wider than periphery
            - Rarely rupture
        - False aneurysms (pseudoaneurysms) represent contained ruptures of myocardium held together by pericardium/pericardial adhesions
            - Most often involve inferobasal or inferolateral walls
            - Opening or mouth of aneurysm is smaller than periphery (reflecting its nature as contained rupture)
            - Have significant risk of complete rupture with tamponade

Radiographic Findings

- Radiography
    - Enlarged cardiac silhouette
        - Occasionally can identify aneurysm as definable outpouching
        - Aneurysm-associated calcifications may be visible on frontal and lateral CXR
            - Curvilinear calcifications confined to LV
            - If calcifications extend beyond LV, they are likely pericardial calcifications

CT Findings

- NECT
    - Aneurysmal remodeling of LV and calcifications of infarcted myocardial wall (only in chronic MI)
        - Mural thrombus may calcify
- CECT
    - Thinned and scarred myocardium is easily detected
    - Frequently accompanied by LV apical filling defect, consistent with mural thrombus
- CTA
    - Coronary CTA usually shows > 70% stenosis (often total occlusion) of artery supplying aneurysmal segment
        - Dyskinesia is apparent on multiphase ECG-gated (cine) reconstruction
- Dual-energy CT
    - Low or no iodine uptake in thrombus in iodine maps; can identify residual myocardial perfusion defects

MR Findings

- SSFP cine
    - LV aneurysm is visible as area of wall thinning and dyskinesia; can identify thrombi as filling defects within aneurysm
    - Accurately quantifies LV volumes, mass, and wall thickness
- Delayed enhancement
    - Transmural LGE of aneurysm wall secondary to scar/fibrosis
        - Such segments are not viable and will not recover function if revascularized
    - Will demonstrate any associated thrombus as intracavitary focus of low signal intensity
        - Thrombi are often attached to areas of transmural late enhancement (infarct)
        - Most easily visualized using LGE MR with long inversion time (~ 600 ms)
- 1st-pass perfusion
    - Aneurysm with perfusion defect secondary to coronary artery occlusion
    - Thrombus can be detected as nonenhancing mural mass

Echocardiographic Findings

- Echocardiogram
    - Excellent method to identify aneurysm and wall motion abnormalities
    - Can demonstrate thrombus in aneurysm
        - Less sensitive than contrast-enhanced MR for thrombus detection (misses ~ 50% of thrombi found on MR), particularly apical thrombus
    - Spontaneous echo contrast ("smoke") within aneurysm suggests slow flow and increased likelihood for thrombus formation

Angiographic Findings

- Coronary angiogram will usually show occlusion of infarct-related artery
    - Typically few or absent collaterals
- Left ventriculogram
    - Detects wall motion abnormality in aneurysmal segment
    - May detect thrombi as filling defects but is much less sensitive than MR

Nuclear Medicine Findings

- Radionuclide scintigraphy findings
    - Fixed perfusion defect in aneurysmal segment with abnormal wall motion

DIFFERENTIAL DIAGNOSIS

Pseudoaneurysm

- Contained rupture of myocardium lacking myocardial wall
- Narrow neck with wider base along retaining pericardial surface
- Typically, basal inferior or lateral LV segments

Sarcoidosis

- Coalescent granulomas can result in aneurysm formation
    - Tends to involve inferolateral wall at basal level

Takotsubo Cardiomyopathy

- Hallmarks are absence of coronary artery disease and recovery of wall motion
  - Apical "ballooning" on cine images with no abnormal LGE
  - May show edema at T2-weighted imaging and elevated T2 relaxation times at T2 mapping

Chagas Disease

- Apical aneurysm (vortex lesion) is classic lesion of advanced disease

Diverticulum

- Congenital outpouching of LV containing all 3 layers of muscle
- Contracts synchronously with LV
- Associated with thoracoabdominal malformations

Myocardial Crypt

- Narrow, deep, blood-filled fissures in LV wall, extending over > 50% of LV myocardial thickness; only visible in diastole; obliterate in systole
  - Blood-filled fissure extending over < 50% of LV wall thickness = recess
- Phenotypic variation seen in hypertrophic cardiomyopathy (HCM)

Double-Chambered Left Ventricle

- Very rare congenital disease where LV is divided by abnormal myocardial tissue

PATHOLOGY

General Features

- Transmural infarct
  - 70-85% located in anterior and apical walls due to LAD occlusion and lack of collaterals
  - 10-15% involve inferobasal walls due to right coronary artery occlusion
- Size can vary; generally, 1-8 cm in diameter

Microscopic Features

- Early phase demonstrates coagulative myocardial necrosis with inflammation
- Gradual replacement with scar tissue (fibrosis)
- Border zone between aneurysm and normal myocardium has patchy fibrosis and abnormal myocardial fiber arrangement
  - Potential for arrhythmogenic substrate

CLINICAL ISSUES

Presentation

- Most common signs/symptoms
  - History of MI is virtually always present
  - Persistent ST elevation after MI
  - Frequently asymptomatic; can present with transient ischemic attack or ischemic stroke
- Other signs/symptoms
  - Cardiac enlargement with diffuse dyskinetic apical impulse
  - Extra heart sounds (S3 and S4) from blood flow into dilated, stiffened cavity
  - Mitral regurgitation due to altered ventricular geometry
- Clinical profile
  - Heart failure and angina
    - Systolic bulging of aneurysm "steals" part of LV stroke volume
      - Leads to reduction in cardiac output, which triggers further adverse remodeling
  - Ventricular arrhythmias
    - 2 mechanisms for arrhythmias and sudden cardiac death
      - Further myocardial ischemia leading to ventricular tachycardia or fibrillation
      - Reentrant tachycardias from border zone
  - Systemic embolization of intracardiac thrombus
  - Ventricular rupture is rare with true aneurysms

Demographics

- Epidemiology
  - Incidence is ~ 5-10% in patients who present with ST elevation MI
    - Recent improvements in revascularizations and post-MI medical therapy have resulted in decrease in development of LV aneurysms

Natural History & Prognosis

- Natural history of LV aneurysms varies with extent of underlying infarction
- Presence of aneurysm indicates poor prognosis
  - 6x higher mortality than in postinfarction patients without aneurysms

Treatment

- Medical therapy
  - Afterload reduction with ACE inhibitors
  - Heart rate and blood pressure control with β-blockers
  - Anticoagulation with warfarin
    - After large anterior MI with significant LV dysfunction
    - Documented thrombus in aneurysm
- Surgical therapy: Aneurysmectomy
  - ACC/AHA class IIa recommendation in patients with LV aneurysm with intractable ventricular arrhythmias &/or heart failure despite catheter-based or medical therapy
  - Systemic embolization in patients who cannot take warfarin
- Percutaneous therapy
  - Percutaneous ventricular restoration, e.g., parachute device
    - Isolation of dysfunctional region of LV
  - Endocardial mapping with endocardial resection/ablation can be performed to control intractable ventricular arrhythmias in border zones

DIAGNOSTIC CHECKLIST

Consider

- LV aneurysms in all patients with transmural MI and LV dilation and systolic dysfunction

SELECTED REFERENCES

1. Kim SJ et al: Surgical repair of postinfarction left ventricular pseudoaneurysm. Tex Heart Inst J. 51(2), 2024
2. Tassetti L et al: Multimodality imaging approach in diagnosis and management of post-infarctual evolving left ventricular pseudoaneurysm. Eur Heart J Cardiovasc Imaging. 25(10):e257, 2024

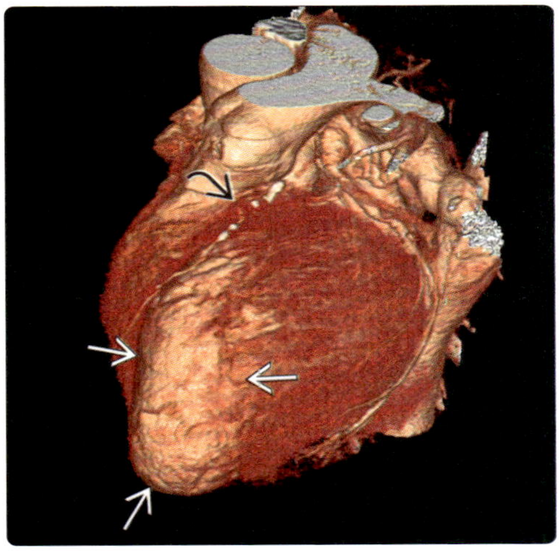

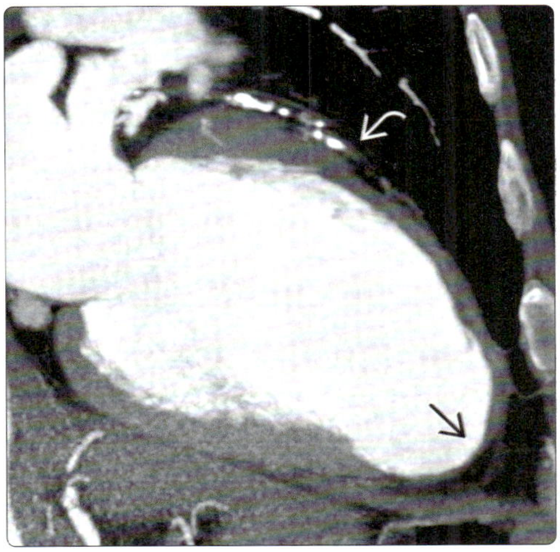

(Left) *Left anterior oblique 3D reconstruction coronary CTA shows extensive calcification and occlusion of the proximal LAD, which has resulted in a large apical aneurysm. Note the broad-based outpouching of the aneurysm, which has the location and morphology associated with true aneurysms.* **(Right)** *Vertical long-axis (2-chamber) coronary CTA shows occlusion of the proximal LAD and apical aneurysm with thinned myocardium and subendocardial hypoattenuation.*

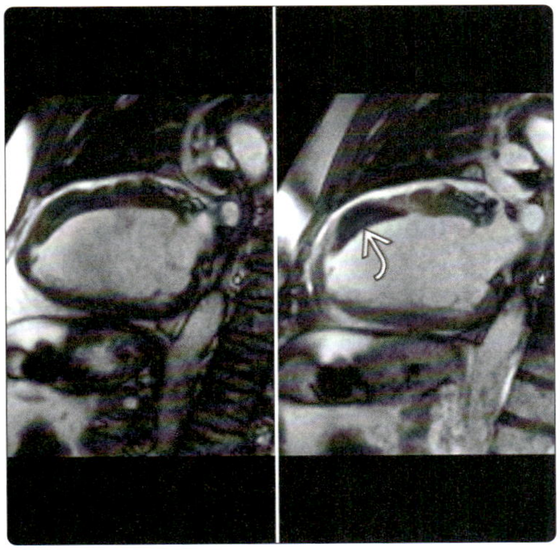

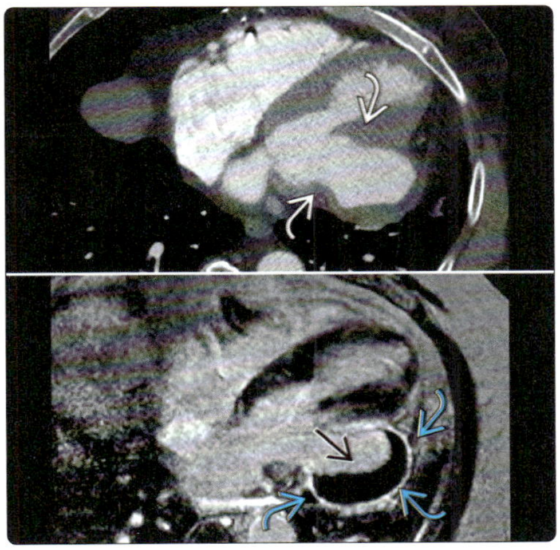

(Left) *Two-chamber cine MR before (left) and after (right) contrast show mural thrombus lining a true aneurysm of the anterior wall. It is not seen on the precontrast image, as the thrombus is isointense to myocardium.* **(Right)** *Axial CECT (top) and LGE MR (bottom) demonstrate a pseudoaneurysm of the lateral basal wall. Note that the neck of the lesion is smaller in diameter than the base. MR shows the marginal enhancement and lining thrombus with greater clarity than CT.*

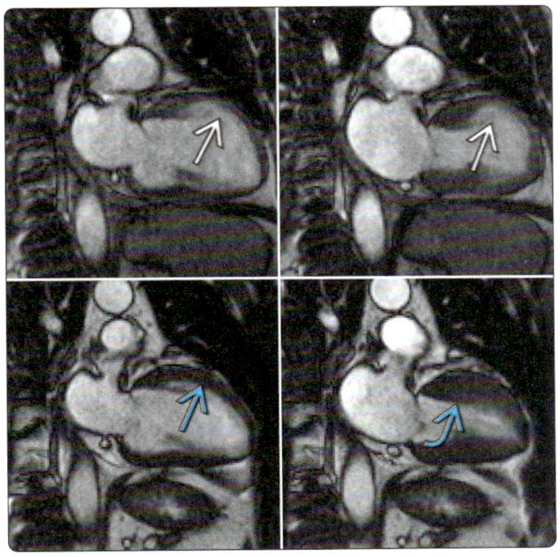

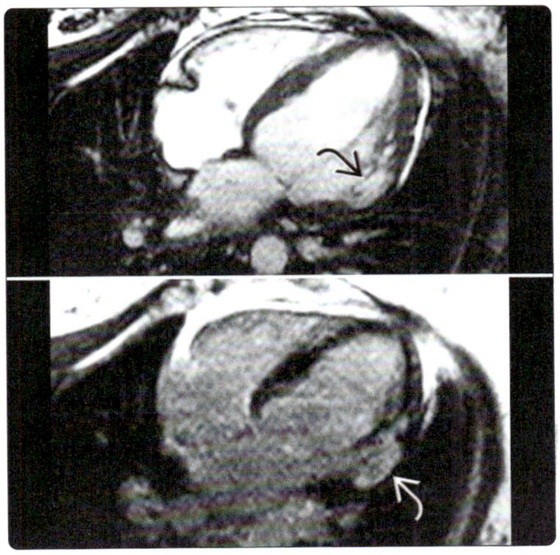

(Left) *Top row diastolic (left) and systolic (right) images show thinning and dyskinesia of the hibernating anterior wall. Bottom row postrevascularization images show recovery in diastolic thickness and systolic contraction. Hibernating myocardium remains viable and can show significant recovery if revascularized.* **(Right)** *Four-chamber cine MR cine (top) and LGE (bottom) in a patient with sarcoidosis show aneurysm formation of the basal lateral wall. Note abnormal enhancement on the LGE image.*

Postinfarction Left Ventricular Pseudoaneurysm

KEY FACTS

TERMINOLOGY

- Rupture of left ventricular wall contained by epicardium or pericardium
- Discontinuation of left ventricular endocardium and myocardium in pseudoaneurysm, whereas true aneurysm wall consists of all 3 myocardial layers

IMAGING

- Visualization of morphology on echocardiography, MR, CT, and left ventriculography
- Typically, there is area of dyskinesis (outward movement in systole)
- Neck is often narrower than aneurysmal sack
- Difficult to differentiate from true aneurysm
- Discontinuation of myocardium can sometimes be detected on CT, MR, and echocardiography
- Mural thrombi may be present

TOP DIFFERENTIAL DIAGNOSES

- True aneurysm
- Diverticulum
- Other fluid-filled structures (e.g., pericardial cyst)

CLINICAL ISSUES

- Myocardial infarction is most frequent cause
- Valvular surgery, especially mitral valve surgery, is 2nd most frequent cause
- Pseudoaneurysms may occur in apical region after transapical aortic valve replacement
- High rate of spontaneous rupture
- Clinically silent course is possible
- Only 3% present as sudden death
- Prompt surgical intervention is required
- Conservative treatment if high surgical risk or stable over long time period

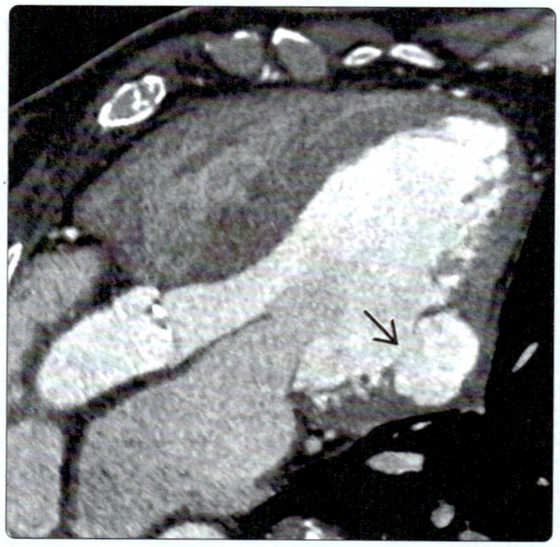

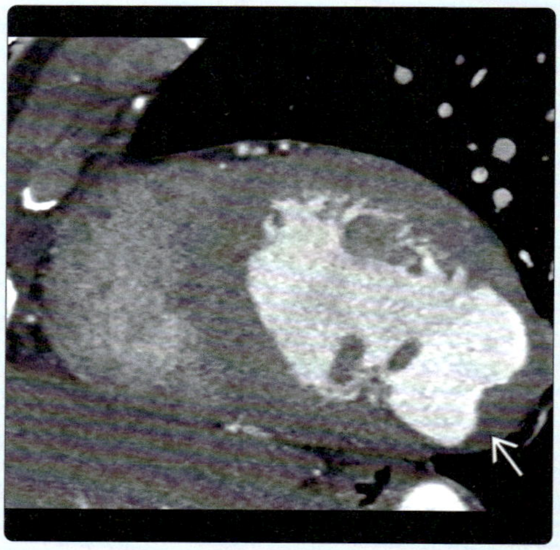

(Left) *Contrast-enhanced CTA shows a small left ventricular pseudoaneurysm → in the posterolateral wall. The neck of a pseudoaneurysm is typically narrower than the aneurysmal sac, but it is usually not possible to unambiguously differentiate pseudoaneurysms from true aneurysms of the left ventricle.* **(Right)** *Short-axis CTA of the left ventricle shows the same pseudoaneurysm →. Most often, a left ventricular pseudoaneurysm is a consequence of myocardial infarction.*

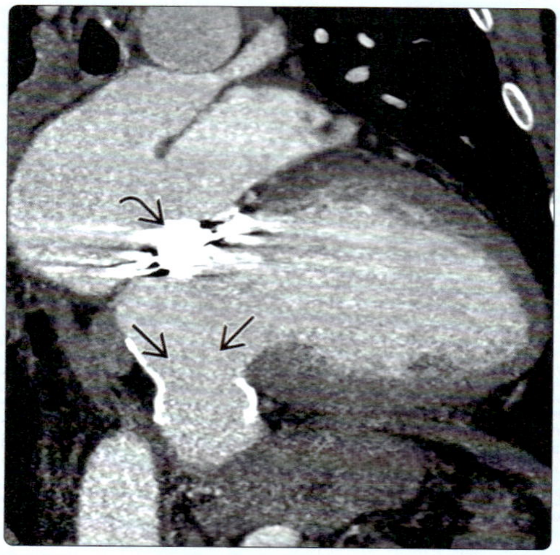

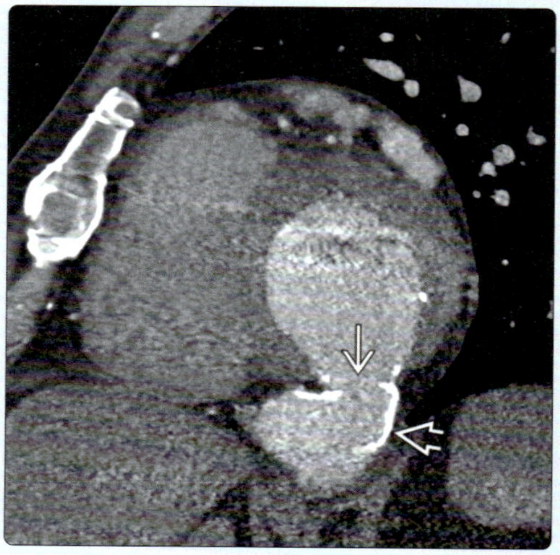

(Left) *Left ventricular pseudoaneurysms can also be the consequence of cardiac surgery, especially mitral valve replacement, as seen in this example of a pseudoaneurysm → in the inferior wall secondary to mechanical mitral valve replacement. Note mitral valve prosthesis →.* **(Right)** *Short-axis CECT clearly shows the narrow neck of the pseudoaneurysm →. The walls of the pseudoaneurysm are partly calcified →.*

TERMINOLOGY

Definitions

- Myocardial rupture contained by pericardial adhesions

IMAGING

General Features

- Location
  - More common with inferior wall myocardial infarction (MI)
- Morphology
  - Wall is composed of organized hematoma and pericardium; no myocardial tissue

Echocardiographic Findings

- Color Doppler
  - Hallmark Doppler finding is bidirectional flow into and out of pseudoaneurysm (to-and-fro murmur)

MR Findings

- SSFP cine
  - Detection, characterization, and sizing of pseudoaneurysm
    - Narrow neck of pseudoaneurysm
      - Ratio of neck width:maximal internal diameter < 1.0 (usually 0.25-0.5)
  - Dyskinetic or akinetic movement with cardiac cycle
  - Postinfarction left ventricular pseudoaneurysm often displays abrupt myocardial "cutoff" vs. gradual wall tapering in true aneurysm
  - May demonstrate small pericardial effusion
- Delayed enhancement
  - No intact myocardial wall or enhancement
  - Marked delayed enhancement of pericardium
    - Not limited to area adjacent to infarction, but involves remote areas
    - Likely pericardial inflammatory reaction to blood released during rupture
  - Thrombus is seen as nonenhancing area within aneurysm

CT Findings

- Cardiac gated CTA
  - Identifies pseudoaneurysm by location and neck that is narrower than pseudoaneurysm sac
  - Abrupt discontinuation of ventricular wall may be appreciable
  - May demonstrate small pericardial effusion

Imaging Recommendations

- Best imaging tool
  - Cardiac MR
- Protocol advice
  - Cine and delayed enhancement

DIFFERENTIAL DIAGNOSIS

True Aneurysm

- Thinned, akinetic/dyskinetic myocardium forming outpouching
  - All 3 myocardial layers are present, showing thinned and enhancing myocardium due to infarction
- Wide neck (ratio of neck:internal diameter of 0.9-1.0)
- More common in anterior wall and apex
- Often, it is challenging to distinguish from pseudoaneurysm
- Does not tend to rupture, especially in chronic stages

Muscular Diverticulum

- Contains all 3 cardiac layers
- In apical region; tubular with narrow neck
- Contract synchronously with myocardium

Double-Chambered Left Ventricle

- Thick, membranous structure divides left ventricle
- Wide communication with left ventricular chamber
- Distal chamber has all 3 layers
- Usually have associated cardiomyopathy
- Hypokinesis may be seen in distal chamber

Epicardial Cyst

- Multiloculated cyst in epicardium
- Communicates with left ventricle cavity through narrow channels opening into intratrabecular spaces

PATHOLOGY

General Features

- Etiology
  - Post-MI is most likely
    - Inferior and lateral wall infarctions lead to pseudoaneurysms 2x as often as anterior infarcts
  - Cardiac surgery is 2nd most common cause of pseudoaneurysm
    - Mitral valve replacement and aneurysmectomy
    - Transapical aortic valve replacement
  - Trauma accounts for ~ 7% of cases

CLINICAL ISSUES

Presentation

- Most common signs/symptoms
  - Often clinically silent (asymptomatic)
  - Chest pain and dyspnea in case of impaired left ventricular function
  - Syncope can occur
  - Stroke may be caused by thrombi in pseudoaneurysm
  - To-and-fro murmur may be detectable in up to 2/3 of patients
  - Often accompanied by ST-segment elevation on ECG

Natural History & Prognosis

- 30-45% of untreated pseudoaneurysms result in rupture, irrespective of their age

Treatment

- Prompt surgical intervention
- Conservative if high surgical risk or stable over long time period

SELECTED REFERENCES

1. Hassani C et al: Cardiac outpouchings: practical approach to normal variants and pathologic conditions at CT and MRI. Radiographics. 43(5):e220063, 2023
2. Kim JY et al: Epicardial cyst originating from right ventricle. Korean J Thorac Cardiovasc Surg. 46(2):138-41, 2013
3. Rajiah P et al: MR imaging of myocardial infarction. Radiographics. 33(5):1383-412, 2013

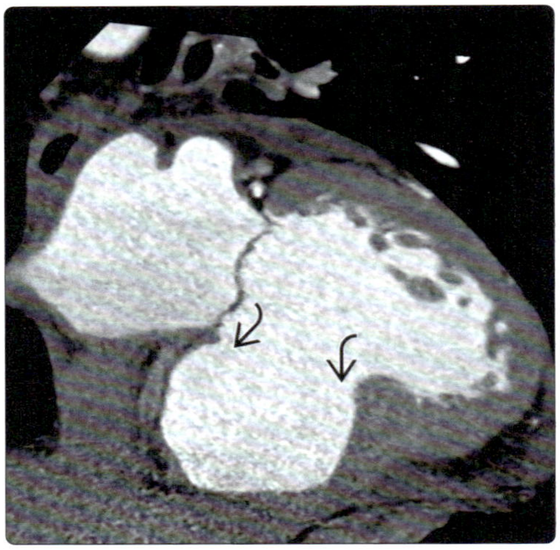

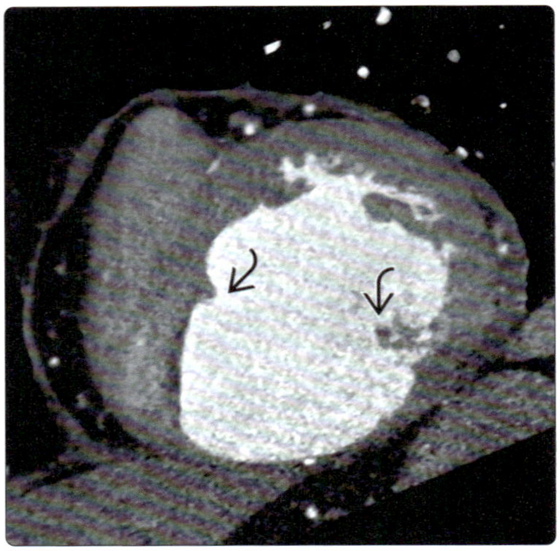

(Left) *CECT shows a large inferior left ventricular pseudoaneurysm secondary to a myocardial infarction. The rim of healthy myocardium* → *and the fact that the neck is narrower that the aneurysmal sac are clearly demonstrated. This makes pseudoaneurysm highly likely, but it is not an absolute proof.* **(Right)** *Short-axis CECT in the same patient clearly demonstrates the rim of healthy myocardium at the neck of the aneurysmal sac* →*, which suggests a pseudoaneurysm rather than a true aneurysm.*

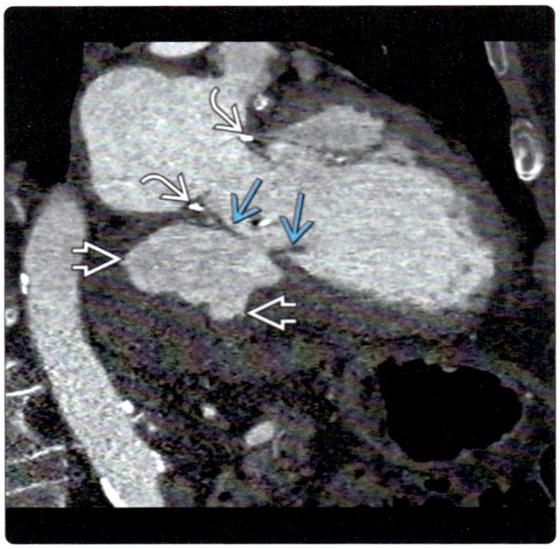

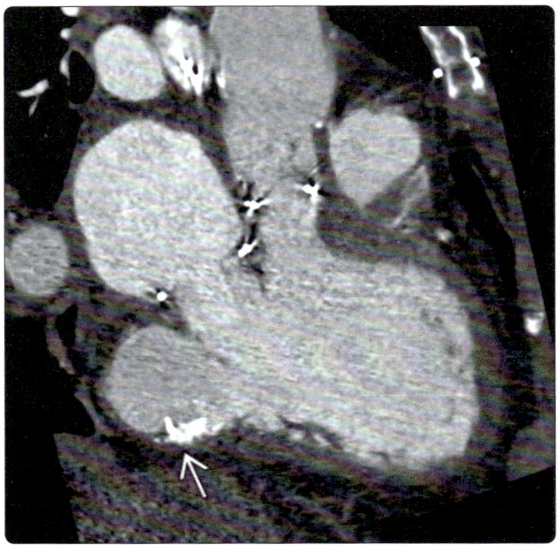

(Left) *Two-chamber CECT shows a pseudoaneurysm of the basal inferior wall* → *complicating mitral valve surgery. The narrow neck of the pseudoaneurysm and the rim of myocardial tissue* → *are clearly seen. Small metallic structures represent cross sections of the mitral valve prosthesis* →*.* **(Right)** *Three-chamber CECT in the same patient shows the pseudoaneurysm with calcification* →*. Along with the mitral valve, the aortic valve has also been replaced by a bioprosthesis.*

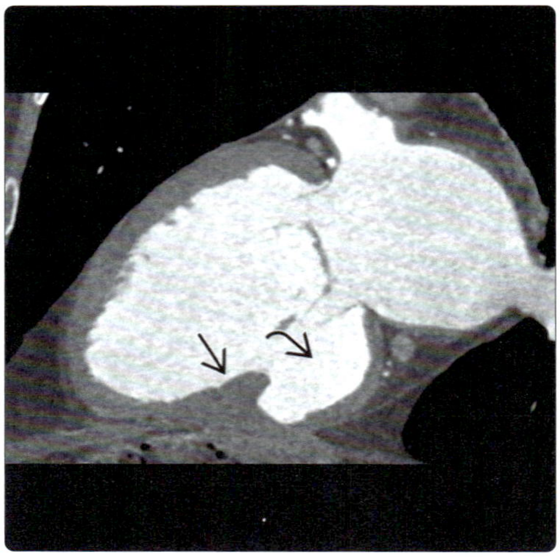

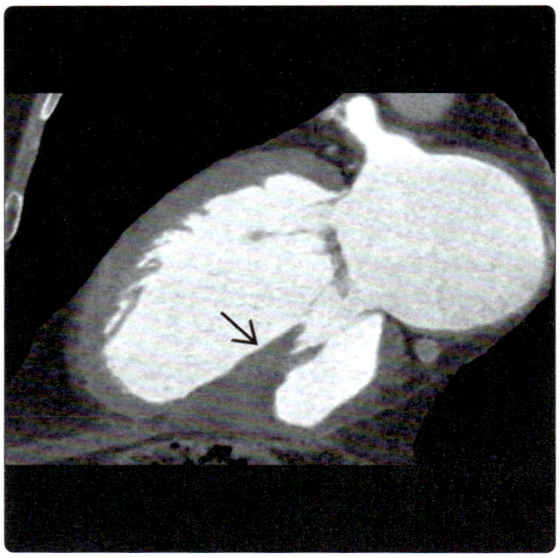

(Left) *Image orientation and anatomic circumstances can create the impression of a narrow neck, making it an unreliable criterion to differentiate pseudoaneurysms from true aneurysms, in which the entry is presumably the widest point. Here, the entry appears narrower than the aneurysmal sac* → *due to submitral apparatus (papillary muscle and chordae)* →*.* **(Right)** *10-mm thickness MinIP in the same patient clearly shows that the impression of a narrow neck is caused by the papillary muscle* →*.*

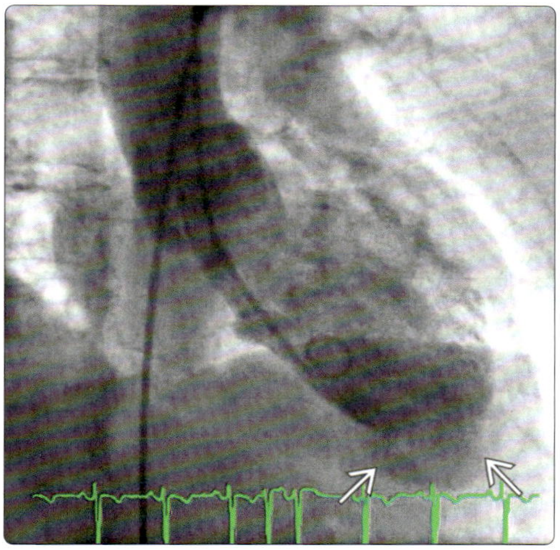

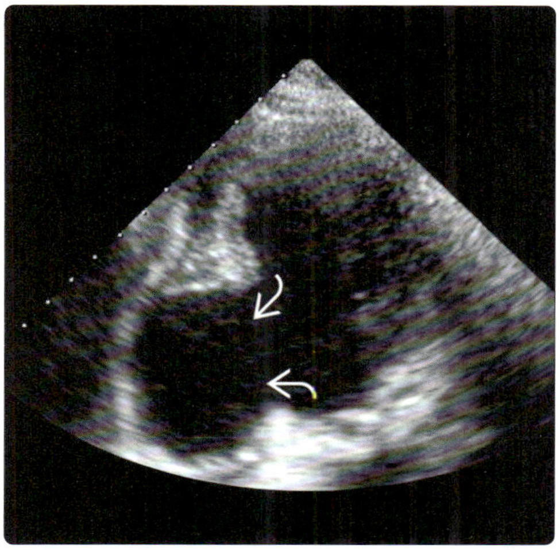

(Left) *Left ventriculography shows aneurysmal bulging at the inferior side of the left ventricular apex. The presence of a narrow neck makes a pseudoaneurysm possible, but it cannot be definitely proven. Analysis in motion would typically show outward-directed movement during systole.* **(Right)** *Echocardiogram shows a large inferobasal pseudoaneurysm with a neck that is narrower than the diameter of the aneurysm.*

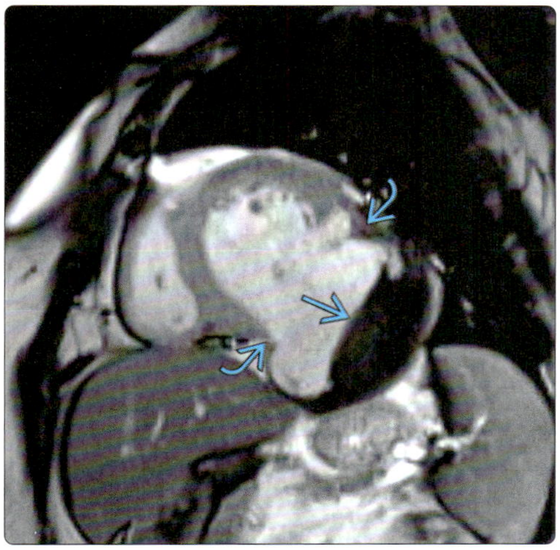

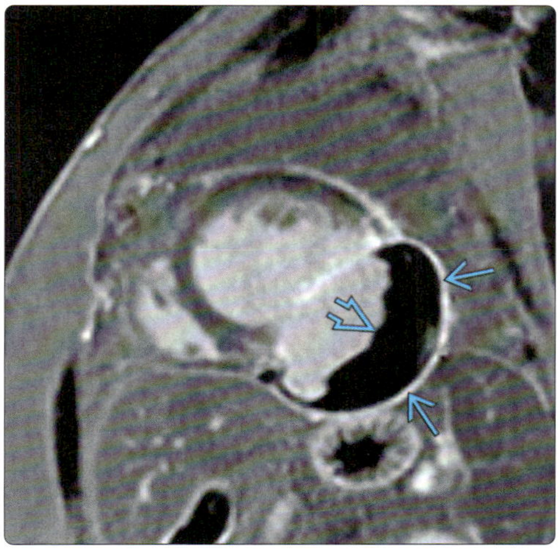

(Left) *Short-axis SSFP CMR shows a large outpouching in the inferolateral segments with a neck that is narrower than the aneurysm diameter. There is apparent abrupt discontinuity of the myocardium ("myocardial cutoff") and a large mural nonenhancing mass consistent with thrombus.* **(Right)** *PSIR MR shows LGE and marked thinning of the wall of the pseudoaneurysm. Dark nonenhancing tissue is pasted against the thinned wall is mural thrombus.*

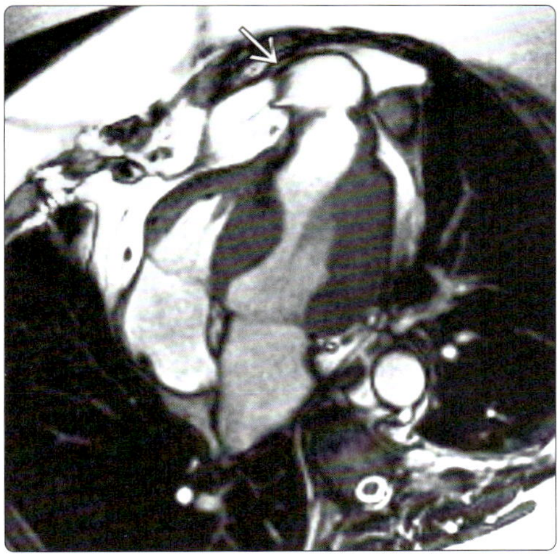

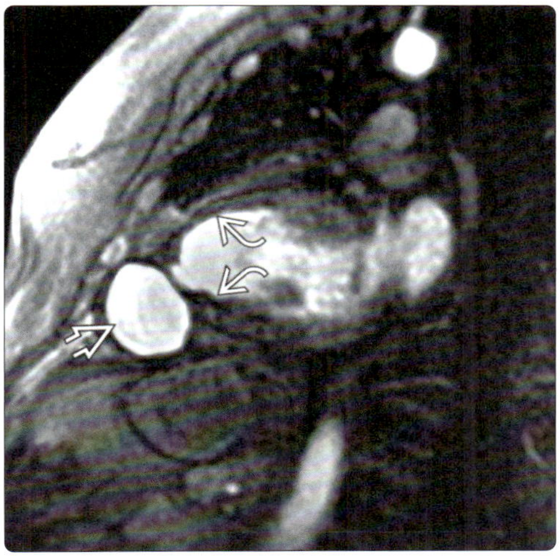

(Left) *Four-chamber cine MR shows a rare case of a left ventricular apical pseudoaneurysm contained by the pericardium. This location rarely harbors pseudoaneurysms but is frequently affected by true aneurysms.* **(Right)** *Two-chamber MR perfusion shows gadolinium filling the apical pseudoaneurysm. There are also perfusion defects in the anterior and inferior apical left ventricular walls.*

Postangioplasty Restenosis

KEY FACTS

TERMINOLOGY

- Recurrent narrowing of treated segment of coronary artery after either balloon angioplasty or percutaneous coronary intervention

IMAGING

- Coronary artery stenosis in previously ballooned segment
- Invasive coronary angiography superior to CTA for stenosis quantification
  - Evolving technologies using dual-source CT, ultrahigh resolution deep learning image reconstructions, and photon-counting CT are improving image quality and artifact
- Emerging use of bioresorbable stents may solve several of these issues since struts are made of resorbable polymer

TOP DIFFERENTIAL DIAGNOSES

- Coronary artery stenosis, stent thrombosis

PATHOLOGY

- In-stent restenosis (IRS) is attributable to neointimal hyperplasia
  - Compared with bare metal stent (BMS), drug-eluting stent (DES)-associated ISR tends to be focal, particularly at stent edge or areas of stent fracture
- Balloon angioplasty is associated with vascular injury and healing → tissue ingrowth and resultant restenosis

CLINICAL ISSUES

- Restenosis after balloon angioplasty occurs in up to 50% of patients
- ISR occurs in up to 30% of BMSs and up to 10% of DESs
- **Treatment**
  - Interventional: Stent placement is preferred over balloon angioplasty in patients with ISR; DES is superior to other treatments

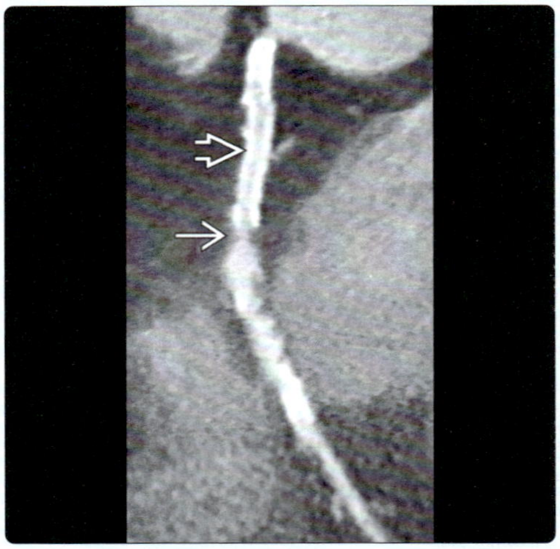

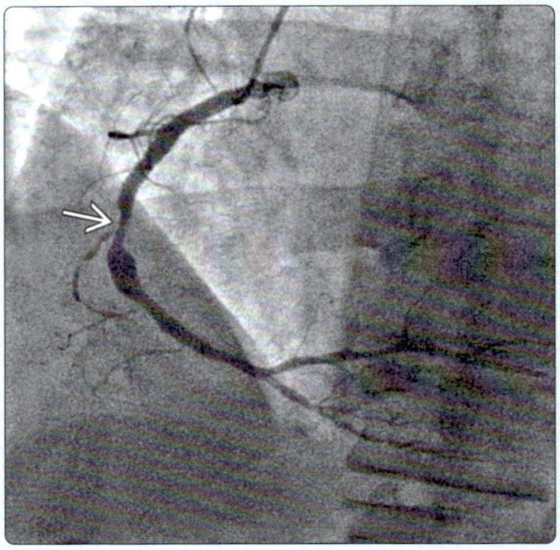

(Left) *Curved multiplanar coronary CTA in a 62-year-old man who presented with recurrent chest pain shows a drug-eluting stent ➡ in the proximal right coronary artery and a severe stenosis ➡ from noncalcified plaque just distal to the stent.* **(Right)** *Subsequent invasive coronary angiography several weeks later in the same patient confirmed an obstructive stenosis ➡ that had elongated in the interim just distal to the stent.*

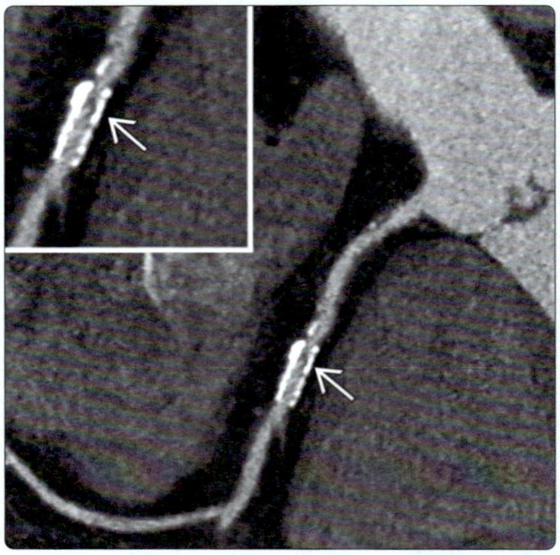

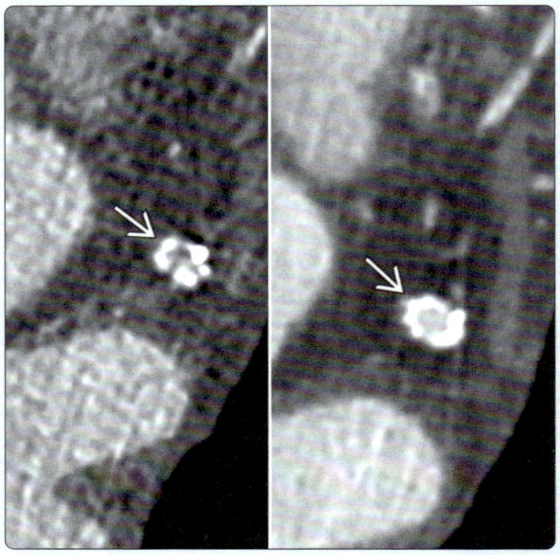

(Left) *Coronary CTA shows a false-positive finding within a coronary artery stent implanted in right coronary artery. Loss of signal intensity within the stent suggests focal high-grade in-stent restenosis (ISR) ➡. Invasive coronary angiography (not shown) showed no significant in-stent stenosis.* **(Right)** *Motion artifacts often cause false-positive findings on coronary CTA. Here, the same stent ➡ is shown in a systolic (left) and diastolic (right) reconstruction. Slight motion in systolic reconstruction causes the impression of ISR.*

TERMINOLOGY

Definitions

- Recurrent narrowing of coronary artery treated by either balloon angioplasty or percutaneous coronary intervention (PCI)
- PCI first introduced in 1970's with concept of "plain old balloon angioplasty" (POBA) without stenting
  - POBA use was limited because of early complication of vascular recoil property and restenosis after balloon deflation, which led to invention of bare metal stents (BMSs)
  - Long-term, in situ BMSs can induce wall stress, endothelial discontinuity, and fibrin deposition promoting myofibroblast migration, leading to in-stent restenosis (IRS)
  - By combining metallic stent platform with polymer releasing antiproliferative drug, drug-eluting stents (DESs) significantly improved efficacy of PCI by suppressing formation of neointimal hyperplasia (NIH) and reducing risk of ISR
- High pressure balloon angioplasty still has important role in treating DES-ISR due to underexpansion

IMAGING

General Features

- Best diagnostic clue
  - Reduction in treated coronary lumen

CT Findings

- CTA
  - Coronary artery stenosis in previously treated segment
  - Shows low-density material in stent lumen; evaluation of coronary stents > 3 mm is more accurate
  - Improved image quality can be obtained by using
    - Dual-energy CT (high-energy virtual monoenergetic images); higher tube potential (e.g., 140 kVp)
    - Decreased slice thickness; iterative reconstruction; sharper reconstruction filters; increased display window width
    - Photon-counting CT: Decreases blooming artifacts related to stent frame, increases image sharpness, and provides thinner slices
  - CT techniques for improved evaluation: Higher tube potential

Angiographic Findings

- Invasive coronary angiography: Diffuse or focal lesion; may show evidence of associated vessel wall dissection
  - Superior to CTA for smaller stents
- Intravascular ultrasound (IVUS) to evaluate ISR severity and location is well established
- Optical coherence tomography has higher resolution, adding insight to neointimal composition
- Fractional flow reserve increasingly used to assess hemodynamically significant restenosis; if > 0.8, appears safe to defer revascularization

PATHOLOGY

General Features

- Etiology
  - Balloon angioplasty is associated with vascular injury and healing → tissue ingrowth and resultant restenosis

Staging, Grading, & Classification

- ACC/AHA lesion classification: Low, moderate, and high risk of failure based on morphologic patterns

CLINICAL ISSUES

Presentation

- Most common signs/symptoms
  - Most often asymptomatic but can represent with typical ischemic symptoms, infarction, or heart failure

Demographics

- Epidemiology
  - Restenosis after balloon angioplasty occurs in up to 50% of patients
    - Stent placement is currently preferred to balloon angioplasty due to high risk of restenosis
  - Clinical predictors of restenosis: Diabetes mellitus, chronic kidney disease, older age, female sex
  - Anatomic factors: Calcified lesions, bifurcation lesions, ostial lesions, PCI of chronic total occlusions or saphenous vein grafts

Treatment

- Medical
  - Little evidence to support medical treatment, dual antiplatelet therapy after DES implantation, and lipid control conventionally
- Interventional
  - Stent placement is preferred over balloon angioplasty in patients with obstructive coronary artery disease
  - Historically, ISR balloon angioplasty achieved adequate luminal gain through tissue compression and previous stent expansion but fell short due to recoil and tissue reprotrusion into lumen soon after treatment
- Surgical
  - Coronary bypass for severe stenoses not amenable to percutaneous treatment or for multivessel disease

SELECTED REFERENCES

1. Chhabra L et al: Angioplasty. StatPearls. 2024
2. Qin L et al: Improvement of coronary stent visualization using ultra-high-resolution photon-counting detector CT. Eur Radiol. 34(10):6568-77, 2024
3. Giustino G et al: Coronary in-stent restenosis: JACC state-of-the-art review. J Am Coll Cardiol. 80(4):348-72, 2022
4. Latina J et al: Ultra-high-resolution coronary CT angiography for assessment of patients with severe coronary artery calcification: initial experience. Radiol Cardiothorac Imaging. 3(4):e210053, 2021
5. Andreini D et al: CT perfusion versus coronary CT angiography in patients with suspected in-stent restenosis or CAD progression. JACC Cardiovasc Imaging. 13(3):732-42, 2020
6. Shlofmitz E et al: Restenosis of drug-eluting stents: a new classification system based on disease mechanism to guide treatment and state-of-the-art review. Circ Cardiovasc Interv. 12(8):e007023, 2019
7. Vos NS et al: Paclitaxel-coated balloon angioplasty versus drug-eluting stent in acute myocardial infarction: the REVELATION randomized trial. JACC Cardiovasc Interv. 12(17):1691-9, 2019
8. Dai T et al: Diagnostic performance of computed tomography angiography in the detection of coronary artery in-stent restenosis: evidence from an updated meta-analysis. Eur Radiol. 28(4):1373-82, 2018
9. Patel S et al: Drug-eluting balloons with provisional bail-out or adjunctive stenting in de novo coronary artery lesions-a systematic review and meta-analysis. Cardiovasc Diagn Ther. 8(2):121-36, 2018

KEY FACTS

TERMINOLOGY

- Stenosis > 50% diameter reduction of coronary artery lumen inside or at edges of implanted stent
  - Focal in-stent restenosis (ISR): Short stenosis anywhere within stent
  - Diffuse ISR: Stenosis along entire length of implanted stent

IMAGING

- Identification of in-stent stenosis by coronary CTA is problematic and prone to false-positive results
- Stents ≥ 3.0 mm in diameter are easier to assess on CT angiography for ISR than smaller ones
- Since left main (LM) coronary artery is larger caliber vessel and displays relatively little motion artifact, CT angiography is relatively reliable to exclude in-stent stenosis in LM stents
- Photon-counting CT can provide assessment of coronary stents and ISR with high accuracy

TOP DIFFERENTIAL DIAGNOSES

- De novo coronary artery stenosis
- Stent thrombosis

CLINICAL ISSUES

- Factors that influence restenosis include stent type, length, and diameter
- Has become very infrequent with modern drug-eluting stents and more elaborate lesion preparation during percutaneous coronary intervention
- Small-diameter stents, long lesions, ostial lesions, and bifurcation lesions have higher rates of restenosis
- More frequent in patients with diabetes
- Risk for stent thrombosis is likely mediated by polymer that carries antiproliferative drug, not by drug itself

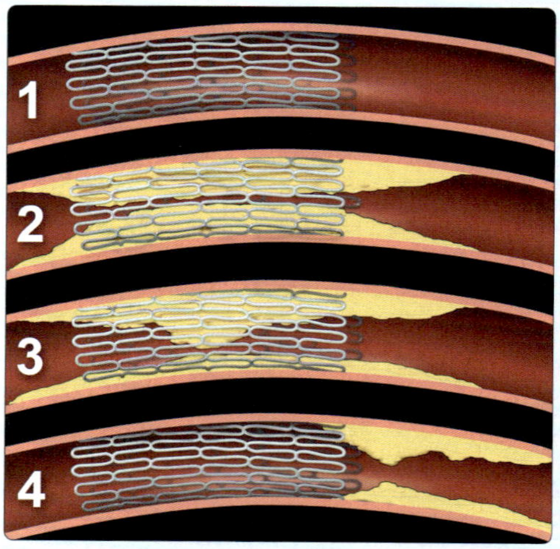

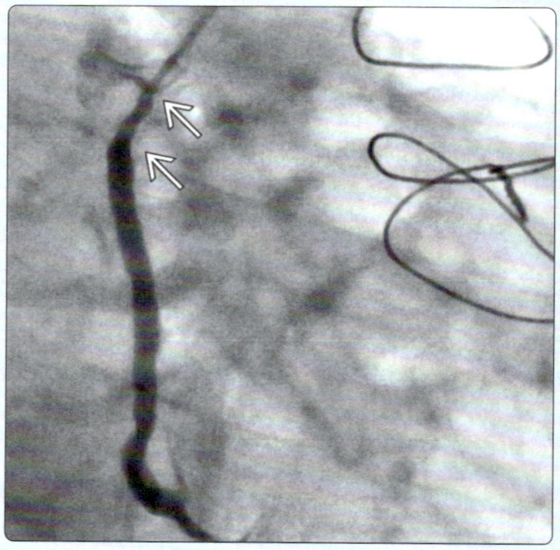

(Left) *Graphic shows the (1) normal appearance of a coronary artery stent; (2) diffuse in-stent restenosis (ISR), which is typically rather concentric (most frequent type); (3) focal ISR with a short lesion within the stent (less frequent type); and (4) new lesions (de novo stenoses) that may develop outside the stent.* **(Right)** *Invasive coronary angiogram shows diffuse ISR of a stent placed in the ostial segment of an aortocoronary bypass graft. Note the beginning and end of the stent ➡.*

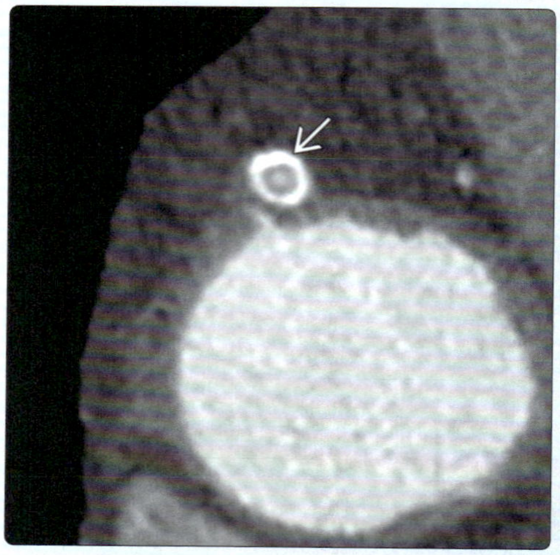

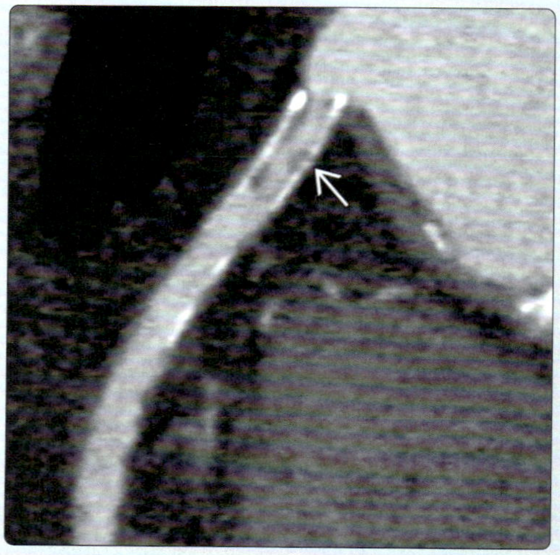

(Left) *Contrast-enhanced coronary angiogram in the same patient demonstrates a cross section of the stent ➡. Concentric in-stent stenosis and a narrowed lumen are visible.* **(Right)** *Multiplanar reconstruction of a contrast-enhanced coronary angiogram in the same patient shows a longitudinal view of the stent with diffuse ISR over the entire length of the implanted stent ➡.*

TERMINOLOGY

Abbreviations

- In-stent restenosis (ISR)

Definitions

- Diameter reduction of coronary artery lumen inside or at edges of implanted stent
- 2 different morphologies
  - Focal ISR: Short stenosis anywhere within stent
  - Diffuse ISR: Stenosis along entire length of implanted stent

IMAGING

CT Findings

- CTA
  - Coronary CTA
    - Metal stent structure is prone to cause artifacts and increase false-positive results regarding ISR
      - Blooming artifact due to partial volume effects makes stent struts appear thicker and lumen look smaller
      - Beam hardening and motion artifacts cause areas of hypoattenuation inside stent lumen and mimic stenoses
      - Photon starvation effects
      - ~ 12 % of coronary stents cannot be imaged with diagnostic quality
    - Image reconstruction should be performed with sharp (high-resolution) kernels and thinnest possible slice thickness to improve interpretability
    - Stent size is major determinant of interpretability by CT
      - Stents ≥ 3 mm in diameter are more likely assessable for ISR than are smaller ones
      - Multidetector CT is relatively reliable in excluding in-stent stenosis in left main coronary artery and proximal stents
    - Continued improvement in cardiac CTA technologies has improved accuracy for assessing ISR
    - Recent advances in CT technology may improve visualization of stent and stenosis
      - Photon-counting detector CT (PCCT): Semiconductor materials convert x-rays directly into electrical signal pulses
      - Ultrahigh resolution images as low as 0.2 mm improve assessment of ISR by improving spatial resolution, decreasing artifacts, and increasing image sharpness
      - For stenosis > 50%, reported sensitivity, specificity, and accuracy of PCCT is 100%, 92%, and 93%
      - Dual-energy CT: High-energy virtual monoenergetic images can decrease metallic artifact but also decrease contrast attenuation
      - Iterative reconstruction algorithms can reduce noise associated with stents
    - Bioabsorbable scaffolds were developed as alternative to conventional stents made of metal
      - Bioabsorbable material (e.g., polylactic acid) may be nonradiopaque and not visible on CT
      - Such scaffolds typically have metal markers at either end
      - Clinical use has been interrupted due to high rates of scaffold thrombosis

MR Findings

- MRA
  - Direct visualization of in-stent lumen is not possible because metallic stents cause susceptibility and radiofrequency artifacts on MRA, which lead to local signal void
  - Stress MR and MR myocardial perfusion imaging can be used to detect hemodynamically relevant ISR

Angiographic Findings

- Conventional
  - Quantitative coronary angiography is clinical gold standard for detecting ISR and determining degree of stenosis
  - Intravascular ultrasound (IVUS) may be useful adjunct
  - Optical coherence tomography (OCT) is optimal method to assess stent expansion, malapposition, and stent fracture, but it is infrequently applied

Nuclear Medicine Findings

- SPECT/ET stress perfusion imaging show mismatched perfusion in hemodynamically relevant in-stent stenosis

DIFFERENTIAL DIAGNOSIS

De Novo Coronary Artery Stenosis

- New coronary stenosis in segment not previously treated by stent implantation
- Exact position of previously implanted stents can (infrequently) be difficult to identify in invasive coronary angiography
  - Therefore, it is occasionally impossible to differentiate in-stent stenosis from de novo stenosis

Stent Thrombosis

- Sudden narrowing of stent lumen due to thrombus formation
  - Acute: < 24 hours of stent placement
  - Subacute: 1-30 day(s) after stent placement
  - Late: > 1 month to 1 year after stent placement
  - Very late: ≥ 1 year after stent placement
- Usually complete occlusion with consequence of ST-segment elevation myocardial infarction
- High mortality
- More frequent if stent implantation is not followed by dual antiplatelet therapy (DAPT)
- Early generation drug-eluting stents were more frequently affected than bare metal stents
- Modern drug-eluting stents are less frequently affected than bare metal stents

Post-Stent Aneurysm

- Coronary aneurysm after stent implantation is extremely rare complication
- Aneurysm could result from inflammation due to hypersensitivity reaction to metal, or, in drug-eluting stents, to drug or polymer that carries drug

- Multiple small aneurysms after stent implantation sometimes referred to as "evaginations"

PATHOLOGY

General Features

- Etiology
  - Multiple risk factors for ISR
    - Long total stent length
    - Small stent diameter
    - Diabetes
    - Ostial location
    - Stent location in left main coronary artery
    - Bifurcation
- Neointimal proliferation from arterial damage
  - Generally diffuse process but may be focal
- Macrophage accumulation with cellular proliferation
- In-stent stenosis usually occurs within first 6 months of coronary stent placement

Staging, Grading, & Classification

- 4 described patterns of ISR
  - Pattern I
    - Focal lesion (< 10-mm length) within stent
  - Pattern II
    - Diffuse lesion (> 10-mm length) within stent
  - Pattern III
    - Stenosis (> 10-mm length) extending outside stent
  - Pattern IV
    - Totally occluded stent

Microscopic Features

- Pathophysiology of ISR is multifactorial and comprises
  - Inflammation
  - Smooth muscle cell migration and proliferation
  - Extracellular matrix formation
  - All mediated by distinct molecular pathways

CLINICAL ISSUES

Presentation

- Most common signs/symptoms
  - Recurrent angina is most likely symptom and develops within first 6 months of stent placement
    - After 1 year, recurrent angina is more likely due to progression of nonculprit lesions
  - ISR may be completely asymptomatic
- Other signs/symptoms
  - Acute myocardial infarction is unlikely to result from restenosis
    - This presentation is more likely to result from acute stent thrombosis
    - Mechanism (thrombus formation rather than neointimal proliferation) is different from ISR

Demographics

- Epidemiology
  - Bare metal stents
    - At 1 year, target lesion or target vessel revascularization is performed in 12-14% of cases
      - Factors that influence restenosis include stent type, stent length, and stent diameter
      - Small vessels, long lesions, ostial lesions, and bifurcation lesions have higher rates of restenosis
      - Diabetes predisposes patients to ISR
  - Drug-eluting stents
    - Markedly reduce incidence of ISR and rate of target vessel revascularization
      - Early generation drug-eluting stents were more frequently affected than bare metal stents
      - Modern drug-eluting stents are less frequently affected than bare metal stents

Treatment

- Prevention
  - Adequate stent deployment and expansion
  - Use of drug-eluting stents
- Repeat percutaneous coronary intervention
  - Repeat stenting or treatment with drug-eluting balloon is currently preferred approach for treating restenosis
  - Bypass surgery may be necessary
  - IVUS guidance and OCT are helpful in evaluating restenotic stent as well as persistent areas
  - Due to high rates of subsequent stent thrombosis, radiotherapy is no longer used to prevent or treat ISR

DIAGNOSTIC CHECKLIST

Consider

- Testing for in-stent stenosis can be through angiography (direct stent visualization) or testing for ischemia (clinically recommended approach)
- Invasive angiography and IVUS are reference standards for determining severity of in-stent stenosis and planning intervention
- Fractional flow reserve (FFR) or AI ischemia analysis may be useful to evaluate hemodynamic consequence of ISR (presence of absence of ischemia)
  - Not FDA approved for ISR
- Improved CTA technologies have led to continued improvements in accuracy for ISR
  - False-positives for ISR > false-negatives
  - Photon-counting CT with 0.2-mm spatial resolution improved ISR assessment with increased accuracy compared to energy-integrated detectors

SELECTED REFERENCES

1. Hagar MT et al: Ultra-high-resolution photon-counting detector CT in evaluating coronary stent patency: a comparison to invasive coronary angiography. Eur Radiol. 34(7):4273-83, 2024
2. Qin L et al: Improvement of coronary stent visualization using ultra-high-resolution photon-counting detector CT. Eur Radiol. 34(10):6568-77, 2024
3. Hagar MT et al: Accuracy of ultrahigh-resolution photon-counting CT for detecting coronary artery disease in a high-risk population. Radiology. 307(5):e223305, 2023
4. Latina J et al: Ultra-high-resolution coronary CT angiography for assessment of patients with severe coronary artery calcification: initial experience. Radiol Cardiothorac Imaging. 3(4):e210053, 2021
5. Rajagopal JR et al: Evaluation of coronary plaques and stents with conventional and photon-counting CT: benefits of high-resolution photon-counting CT. Radiol Cardiothorac Imaging. 3(5):e210102, 2021
6. Dai T et al: Diagnostic performance of computed tomography angiography in the detection of coronary artery in-stent restenosis: evidence from an updated meta-analysis. Eur Radiol. 28(4):1373-82, 2018
7. Mannil M et al: Photon-counting CT: high-Resolution Imaging of Coronary Stents. Invest Radiol. 53(3):143-9, 2018

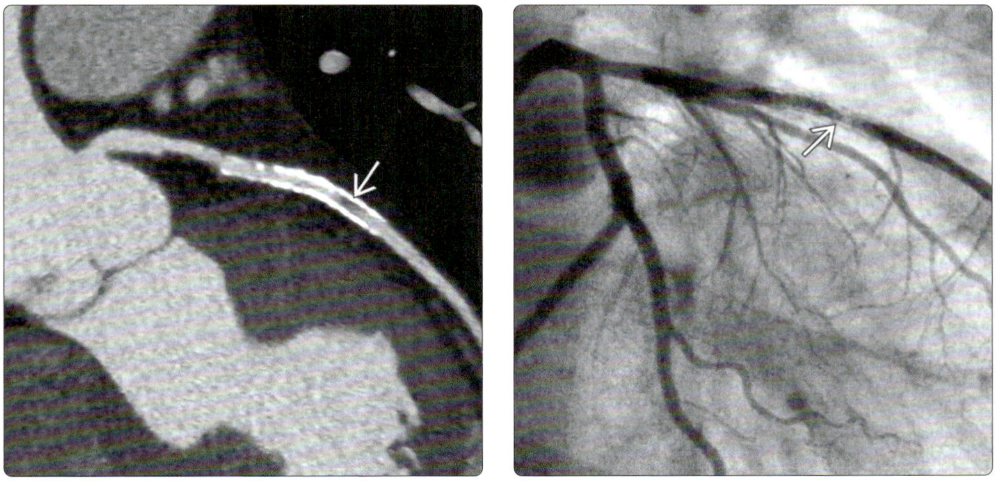

(Left) *Coronary CECT angiogram demonstrates focal in-stent stenosis* ➡ *of a coronary artery stent in the proximal left anterior descending (LAD) coronary artery.* **(Right)** *Invasive catheter-based coronary angiography in the same patient shows the short, focal in-stent stenosis* ➡*, although it is not always possible to see the stent itself in invasive coronary angiography.*

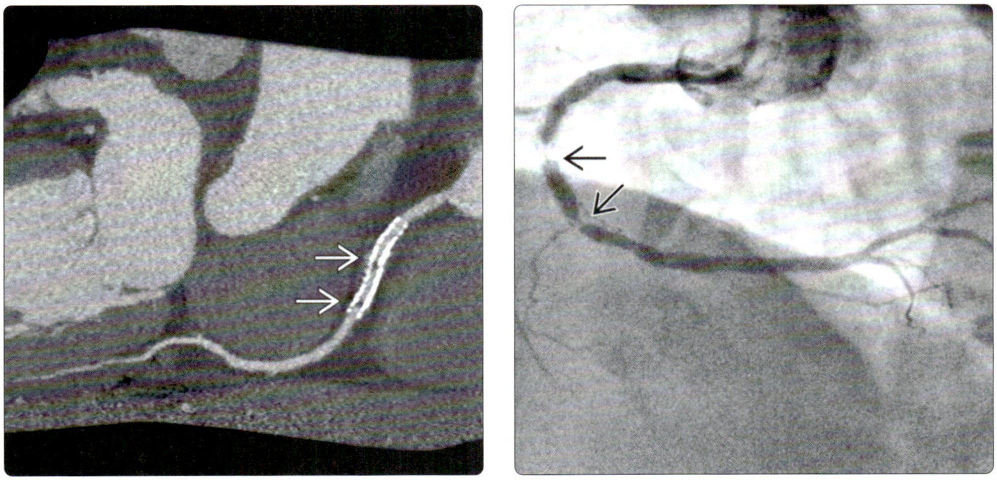

(Left) *Coronary CECT angiogram shows that 2 focal in-stent stenoses are present in a long-stented segment of the right coronary artery* ➡*. This finding is rather unusual.* **(Right)** *Invasive catheter-based coronary angiography in the same patient also demonstrates that 2 focal restenoses* ➡ *are present in the stent of the proximal and midportions of the right coronary artery.*

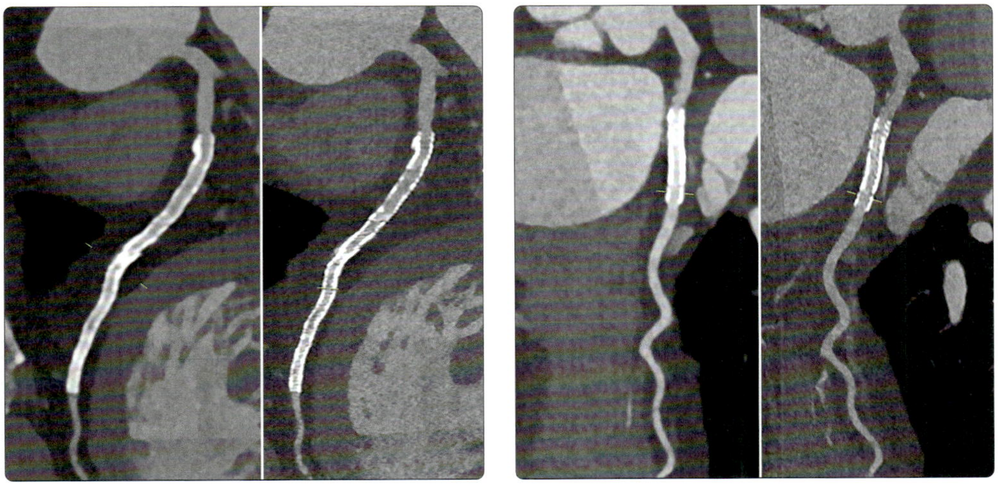

(Left) *Curved MPR images of the LAD show overlapping stents. Note improved sharpness and decreased blooming of the stent on the ultrahigh resolution image (R) at 0.2 mm, allowing better visualization of the lumen.* **(Right)** *Curved MPR of the left circumflex shows a patent stent. Although the lumen is visible on conventional CT (L) at 0.6-mm slice thickness, ultrahigh resolution (R) with 0.2-mm slice thickness provides a sharper image with less blooming and better visualization of neointimal hyperplasia.*

KEY FACTS

TERMINOLOGY

- Acute saphenous vein or atrial graft failure due to subtotal or total occlusive thrombosis
  - In early (< 1-month) postoperative period, acute thrombosis is dominant etiology
  - Thrombosis, intimal hyperplasia, and accelerated atherosclerosis contribute to graft failure in acute, subacute, and late postoperative periods, respectively

IMAGING

- Invasive coronary angiography
  - Can demonstrate graft occlusion, but grafts can be difficult to locate
- CTA
  - High accuracy for bypass graft occlusions
  - May show only smooth, small focus of contrast outpouching at aortic root in chronic setting
  - May demonstrate complete absence of luminal contrast in total occlusion with low-density luminal material (thrombus)

TOP DIFFERENTIAL DIAGNOSES

- Coronary artery stenosis
- Coronary artery bypass graft atherosclerosis
- Perioperative infarction

CLINICAL ISSUES

- Recurrent angina is most common presentation
- Perioperative antiplatelet therapy can reduce early thrombosis and graft failure
- Drug-eluting stents and bare metal stents may be used for saphenous vein graft interventions
- Use "no-touch" technique for harvesting grafts, preventing disruption to endothelium
- Cardiac CT detects 7-15% of patients have postoperative graft failure within 1st week

(Left) *Cardiac CT shows an occluded saphenous vein graft to a diagonal branch with an abrupt cutoff indicating thrombosis.* **(Right)** *3D color-rendered volumetric reformat image shows the occluded graft as a button arising from the ascending aorta. 3D reformats can be very useful for assessing the orientation and configuration of the occluded grafts that are being considered for revascularization or redo coronary artery bypass graft (CABG).*

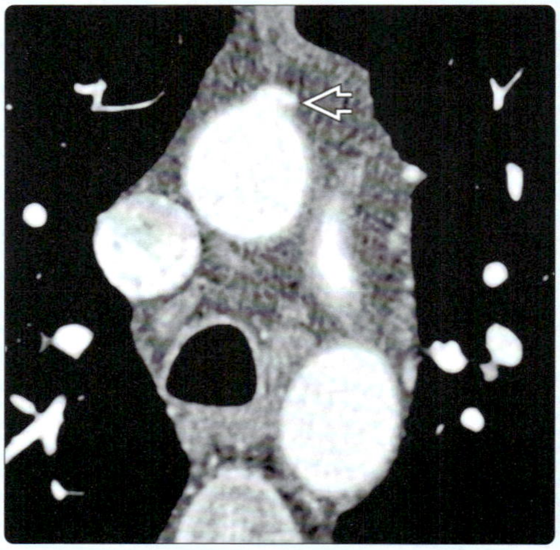

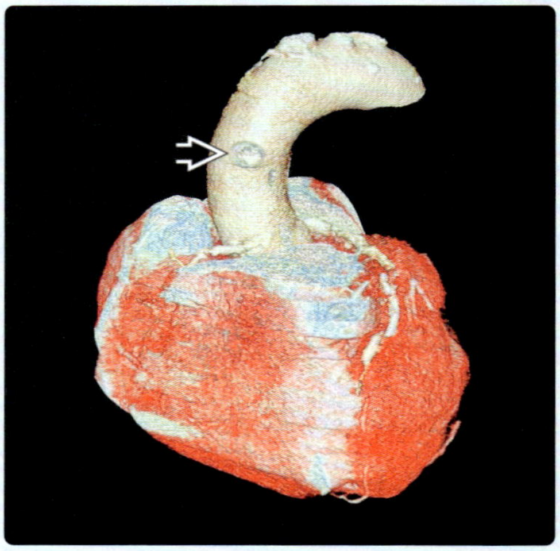

(Left) *Cardiac CT shows a totally occluded saphenous vein graft to the distal right coronary artery. Note the occluded button-like appearance arising from the ascending aorta characteristic of occluded venous grafts.* **(Right)** *Corresponding cardiac MR LGE 2-chamber view shows a chronic myocardial infarction in the inferior wall. Such a transmural infarct makes revascularization of the thrombosed graft or redo graft unlikely to result in patient-improved outcomes.*

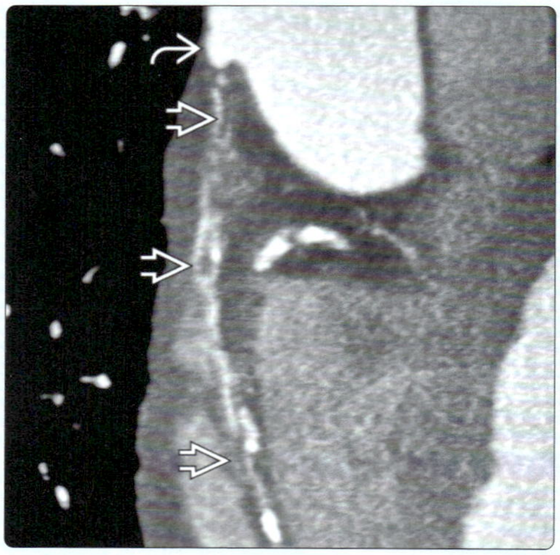

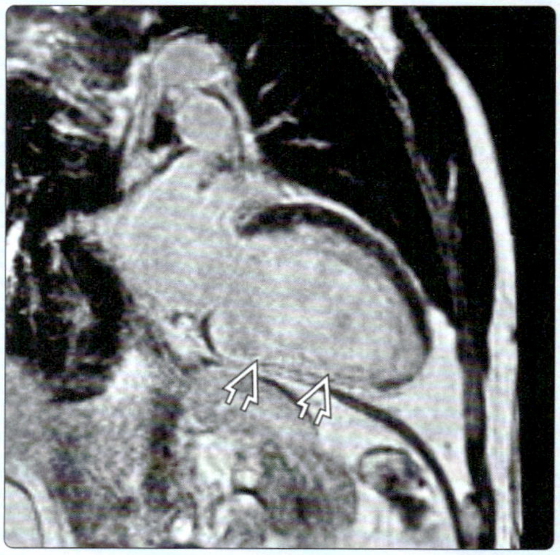

TERMINOLOGY

Abbreviations

- Coronary artery bypass graft (CABG)

Definitions

- Saphenous vein graft (SVG) failure due to subtotal or total occlusive thrombosis
  - Thrombosis, intimal hyperplasia, and accelerated atherosclerosis contribute to graft failure in acute, subacute, and late postoperative periods, respectively
  - In early (< 1-month) postoperative period, acute thrombosis is dominant etiology
    - Technical failure may contribute
- Left internal mammary or other arterial graft failure less common

IMAGING

General Features

- Best diagnostic clue
  - Acute/subtotal/total occlusion of saphenous vein or arterial graft by thrombus
    - Invasive coronary angiography is traditional gold standard but is invasive
    - CTA is excellent for graft depiction
- Location
  - Aortocoronary reversed SVGs
  - Left internal mammary artery graft
    - Other arterial grafts less commonly employed
- Morphology
  - Low-density material within graft lumen
    - May also demonstrate graft expansion
    - Absence of contrast in lumen

CT Findings

- NECT
  - May demonstrate material of slightly increased density within occluded graft lumen
- CTA
  - Provides high-quality images of bypass graft occlusions
  - May demonstrate complete absence of luminal contrast in total occlusion with low-density luminal material (thrombus)
  - May demonstrate crescentic rim of contrast in subtotal occlusion
  - May demonstrate expansion of vein graft
  - Smooth, broad-based area of contrast outpouching at aortic anastomosis may be best clue
    - Beware: Aortic cannulation sites can mimic outpouching at occluded graft anastomosis
  - Problems with CTA graft evaluation
    - Difficulty in evaluating native coronary arteries (usually heavily calcified)
    - Clips adjacent to left internal mammary artery can cause beam hardening artifact
    - Longer range required to include left internal mammary artery origin results in higher radiation dose
    - Anastomosis can be difficult to evaluate

MR Findings

- MRA
  - 3D gadolinium-enhanced MR techniques are more sensitive than 2D gradient-echo or spin-echo techniques for detecting graft occlusion
    - Sensitivity = 85%; specificity = 94%
  - Respiratory navigating markedly improves image quality but is time-consuming
  - Occluded grafts are absent; correlation with operative notes is crucial
    - May demonstrate small, smooth outpouching of contrast at aortic anastomosis

Angiographic Findings

- Invasive coronary angiography
  - Can demonstrate graft occlusion, but grafts may be difficult to locate
  - Can be time-consuming

Nuclear Medicine Findings

- PET
  - Myocardial perfusion imaging (MPI) with 82-rubidium
    - 82-rubidium PET has increased sensitivity (90% vs. 85%) and specificity (88% vs. 85%) over SPECT MPI
  - Viability imaging with F-18 FDG
    - F-18 FDG viability imaging can be combined with resting 82-rubidium PET perfusion scan to assess for perfusion/viability mismatch
- SPECT
  - Tc-99m sestamibi
    - Reduced tracer uptake in ischemic areas corresponding to areas of decreased perfusion/infarction

Imaging Recommendations

- Best imaging tool
  - Coronary CTA (noninvasive, fast, highly sensitive/specific)
  - Coronary angiography
    - Traditional gold standard but time-consuming
    - May not locate all grafts
- Protocol advice
  - Include takeoff of left internal mammary artery from subclavian artery to avoid missing left internal mammary artery ostial stenosis or subclavian artery stenosis proximal to left internal mammary artery origin

DIFFERENTIAL DIAGNOSIS

Coronary Artery Stenosis

- New stenosis on native coronary arteries

Coronary Artery Bypass Graft Atherosclerosis

- Within 1st postoperative year, often due to perianastomotic narrowing (especially in first 3 months)
- After 1st postoperative year, typically due to atherosclerosis within native coronary vessels or grafts

Perioperative Infarction

- Seen especially in left main stenosis and triple vessel disease

PATHOLOGY

General Features

- Etiology

- Endothelial injury
  - Direct physical trauma during surgery
  - Leukocyte response
  - Ischemia of wall after loss of vasa vasorum
  - Risk factors, such as smoking, elevated low-density lipoprotein cholesterol
- Low SVG flow
  - Small luminal size of recipient artery
  - Diseased native artery distal to anastomosis
  - Bypass of nonhemodynamically significant lesion (< 70% stenosis) due to competitive flow from native vessel
- Development of local atheroma within vein graft
- Technical factors
  - Narrow distal anastomosis
  - Insufficient/excessive graft length
  - Mismatched size of graft to recipient artery
  - Angle of graft to aorta < 90° can lead to kinking
- Resistance to antiplatelet agents

- Loss of endothelium with accumulation of fibrin
- Adherence of platelets and WBCs
- Thrombus occluding vessel lumen, especially at sites of anastomosis

Gross Pathologic & Surgical Features

- Atherosclerosis is diffuse and concentric
- Lesions are friable and fragile
- Prone to atherosclerotic embolism, particularly during reoperation

Microscopic Features

- Fibrous cap is absent or weak and thin
  - Foam cells and lipid debris are exposed to bloodstream
- Infiltrate of inflammatory cells and lipid-laden multinucleate giant cells

CLINICAL ISSUES

Presentation

- Most common signs/symptoms
  - Recurrent angina (most common presentation)
  - Myocardial infarction
  - New/worsening heart failure
  - Arrhythmias
  - Sudden death

Natural History & Prognosis

- 10-year patency of SVG ~ 68%
  - Early vein graft failure most commonly due to thrombosis occurs in as many as 18% of cases
  - Vein graft failure is associated with worse clinical outcomes
- 10-year patency left internal mammary artery closer to 90%

Treatment

- Medical
  - Perioperative antiplatelet therapy can reduce early thrombosis and graft failure
  - Lipid lowering can attenuate process of atherosclerosis in vein grafts
- Interventional
  - Balloon angioplasty: Unsatisfactory restenosis rate of at least 45%
  - Drug-eluting stents and bare metal stents may be used for SVG interventions
  - Therapeutic US thrombolysis in setting of acute coronary syndrome has been evaluated but leads to increased incidence of ischemic complications
- Surgical
  - Avoid endothelial injury during harvesting
  - Use "no-touch" technique for harvesting grafts, preventing disruption to endothelium
    - Involves removing pedicled SVG with perivascular tissue intact, thus avoiding direct contact
  - Avoid excessive manual distension
  - Some use α-adrenergic antagonist solutions to minimize vasospasm

DIAGNOSTIC CHECKLIST

Consider

- In patients presenting again with angina post CABG
- Obstruction/occlusion in grafts or native vessels

SELECTED REFERENCES

1. Chamberlin JH et al: Non-contrast computed tomography findings for identification of chronically occluded coronary artery bypass grafts. Acta Radiol. 64(10):2722-30, 2023
2. Harik L et al: Graft thrombosis after coronary artery bypass surgery and current practice for prevention. Front Cardiovasc Med. 10:1125126, 2023
3. Károlyi M et al: Routine early postoperative computed tomography angiography after coronary artery bypass surgery: clinical value and management implications. Eur J Cardiothorac Surg. 61(2):459-66, 2022
4. Lawton JS et al: 2021 ACC/AHA/SCAI guideline for coronary artery revascularization: executive summary: a report of the American College of Cardiology/American Heart Association Joint Committee on Clinical Practice Guidelines. Circulation. 145(3):e4-17, 2022
5. Brilakis ES et al: Drug-eluting stents versus bare-metal stents in saphenous vein grafts: a double-blind, randomised trial. Lancet. 391(10134):1997-2007, 2018
6. Jungmann F et al: Multidetector computed tomography angiography (MD-CTA) of coronary artery bypass grafts - update 2017. Rofo. 190(3):237-49, 2018
7. Zhao Q et al: Effect of ticagrelor plus aspirin, ticagrelor alone, or aspirin alone on saphenous vein graft patency 1 year after coronary artery bypass grafting: a randomized clinical trial. JAMA. 319(16):1677-86, 2018
8. Lee M et al: Current state of the art in approaches to saphenous vein graft interventions. Interv Cardiol. 12(2):85-91, 2017
9. McKavanagh P et al: Management and prevention of saphenous vein graft failure: A review. Cardiol Ther. 6(2):203-23, 2017
10. Arampatzis CA et al: Graft failure prior to discharge after coronary artery bypass surgery: a prospective single-centre study using dual 64-slice computed tomography. EuroIntervention. 12(8):e972-8, 2016
11. Chan M et al: A systematic review and meta-analysis of multidetector computed tomography in the assessment of coronary artery bypass grafts. Int J Cardiol. 221:898-905, 2016
12. Gabriel J et al: Should computed tomography angiography supersede invasive coronary angiography for the evaluation of graft patency following coronary artery bypass graft surgery? Interact Cardiovasc Thorac Surg. 21(2):231-9, 2015
13. Heye T et al: Computed tomography angiography of coronary artery bypass grafts: robustness in emergency and clinical routine settings. Acta Radiol. 55(2):161-70, 2014
14. Hillis LD et al: 2011 ACCF/AHA guideline for coronary artery bypass graft surgery: executive summary: a report of the American College of Cardiology Foundation/American Heart Association Task Force on Practice Guidelines. Circulation. 124(23):2610-42, 2011. Erratum in: Circulation. 124(25):e956, 2011. Circulation. 126(7):e105, 2012
15. Gluckman TJ et al: Effects of aspirin responsiveness and platelet reactivity on early vein graft thrombosis after coronary artery bypass graft surgery. J Am Coll Cardiol. 57(9):1069-77, 2011
16. Fitzgibbon GM et al: Coronary bypass graft fate and patient outcome: angiographic follow-up of 5,065 grafts related to survival and reoperation in 1,388 patients during 25 years. J Am Coll Cardiol. 28(3):616-26, 1996

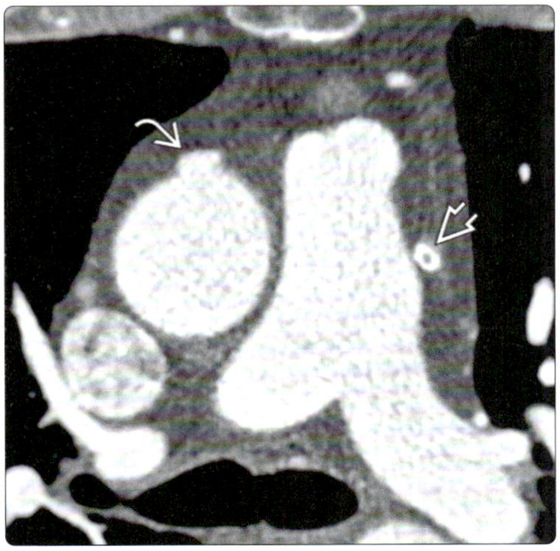

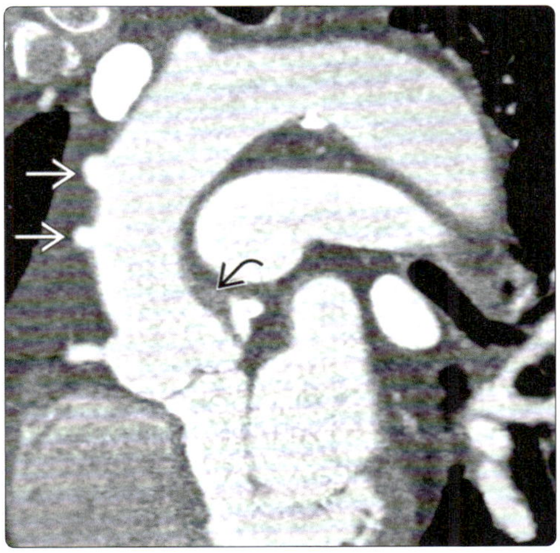

(Left) *Coronary CTA shows an occluded graft to an obtuse marginal branch. Occluded vein grafts have a characteristic button appearance* ➡ *off the aortic wall when they occlude. Note the occluded stent* ➡ *in a vein graft to a diagonal branch.* **(Right)** *Corresponding coronal oblique coronary CTA shows both grafts with a button appearance* ➡ *typical of occluded vein grafts. Note left aortic cusp focal dissection* ⇨ *from an attempted left main stent procedure.*

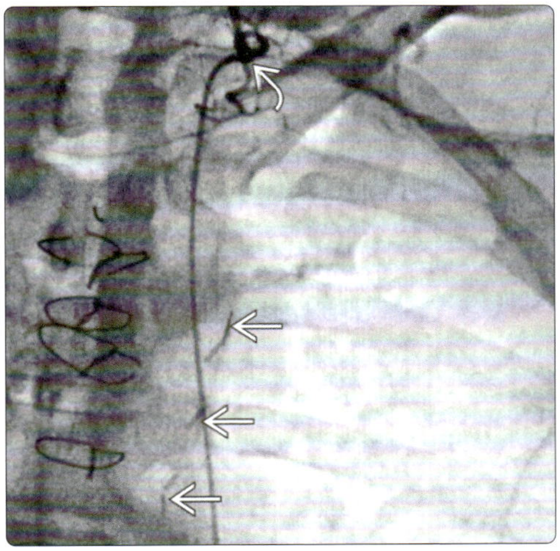

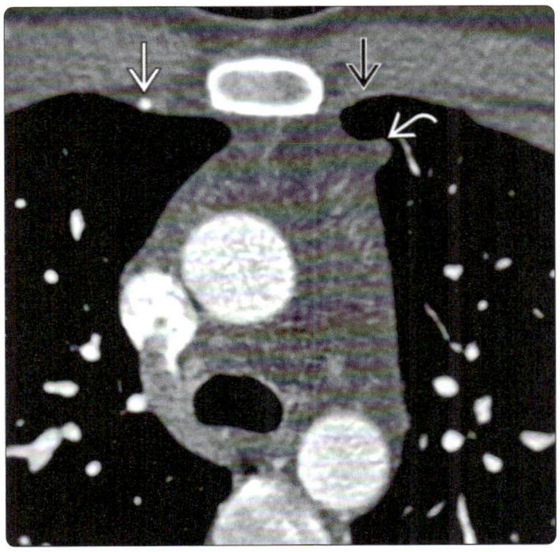

(Left) *Coronary angiogram in a 76-year-old man with a history of CABG 12 years prior shows the tip of a catheter in the subclavian artery at ostium of the left internal mammary artery (LIMA) ostium* ➡ *and no contrast in expected path of LIMA outlined by surgical clips* ➡*.* **(Right)** *Axial coronary CT (same patient) shows the LIMA graft* ➡ *is occluded throughout its length. Note that LIMA is absent from its normal anterior chest wall position* ⇨*. The normal position of the right internal mammary artery (RIMA)* ➡ *excludes a RIMA graft.*

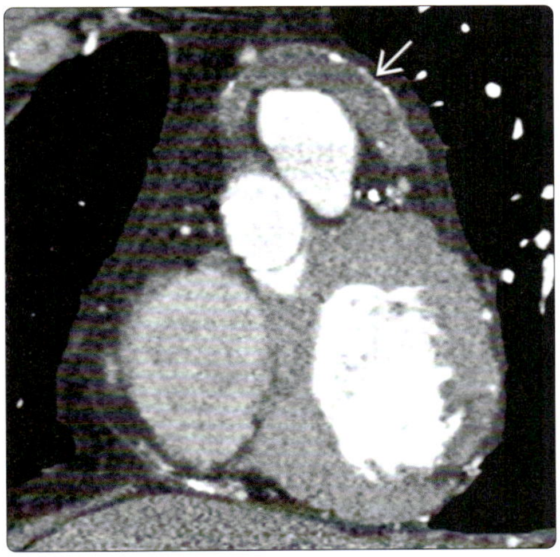

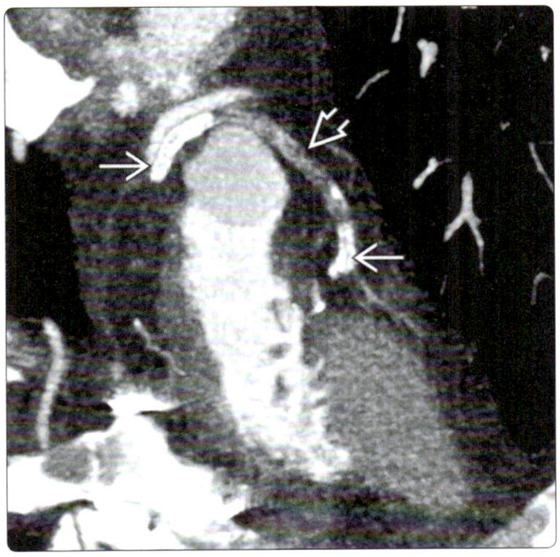

(Left) *Coronary CTA in a 68-year-old man with recurrent angina shows a thrombosed, occluded, and expanded saphenous vein graft* ➡ *to an obtuse marginal branch.* **(Right)** *Coronary CTA shows 2 stents* ➡ *placed across the proximal and midgraft stenosis. Both stents and graft are now completely occluded by a thrombus* ➡*. CTA is the noninvasive imaging modality of choice for detection of coronary bypass graft occlusion.*

Post-CABG Atherosclerosis

KEY FACTS

TERMINOLOGY

- Postoperative atherosclerotic disease of bypass grafts or native coronary arteries
- SYNTAX score II: Combines anatomic SYNTAX score and 7 independent clinical predictors for 4-year all-cause mortality in patients undergoing either surgical or percutaneous revascularization

IMAGING

- Invasive coronary angiography: Clinical gold standard
  - Demonstrates degree of luminal stenosis or occlusion
- High accuracy of MDCT for graft stenosis/occlusion
- CTA enables assessment of severity of coronary lesions, length of lesion, diffuse character of lumen reduction, tortuosity of target vessel, and degree of coronary calcification
- Allows assessment of left internal mammary artery origin and coronary arteries while maintaining low overall radiation dose
- Compared to CTA alone, addition of CT myocardial perfusion (CT-MPI) imaging improves diagnostic accuracy for functional assessment of coronary artery disease
- Photon-counting CT improved spatial and contrast resolution for graft assessment with lower radiation dose

CLINICAL ISSUES

- Angina recurs in 15-20% of patients during 1st year postop
- 10% of all grafts fail early (within 1 month) due to thrombotic occlusion
- Cumulative graft failure rate of 50% at 10 years postop
- Graft failure rate of 10% at 10 years postop
- State of distal vasculature influences bypass graft patency

DIAGNOSTIC CHECKLIST

- Post coronary artery bypass graft (CABG) atherosclerosis in patients with recurrence of angina postoperatively

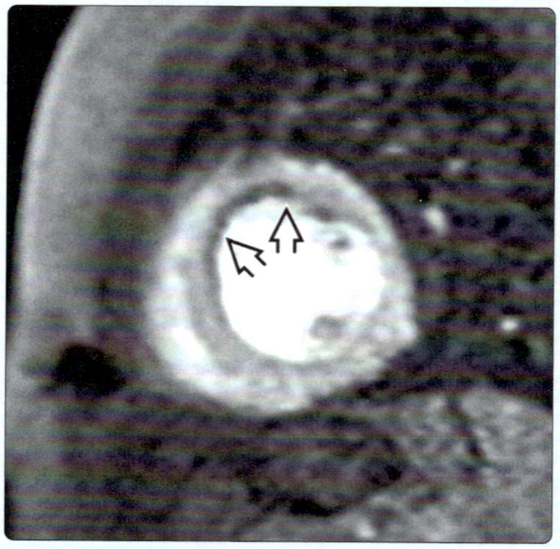
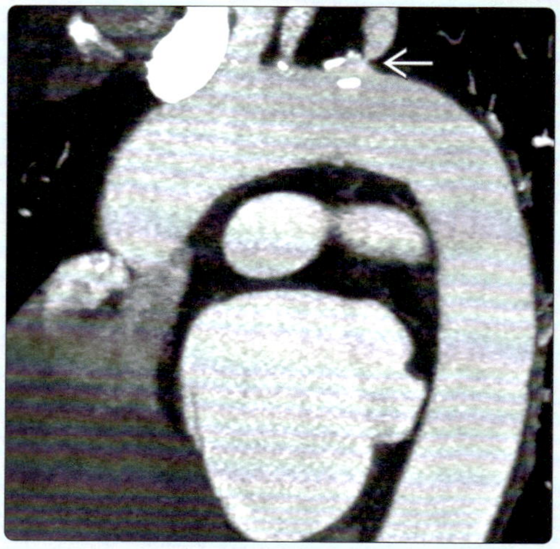

(Left) *Stress adenosine perfusion cardiac MR demonstrates a subendocardial perfusion defect ⇨ in the left ventricular midanterior and anteroseptal segments in the left anterior descending artery vascular territory.* **(Right)** *Corresponding coronary CTA demonstrates the underlying etiology for the recurrent chest pain and inducible ischemia. High-grade stenosis is identified on the left subclavian artery origin from the aortic arch ➡, resulting in poor left internal mammary artery (LIMA) perfusion.*

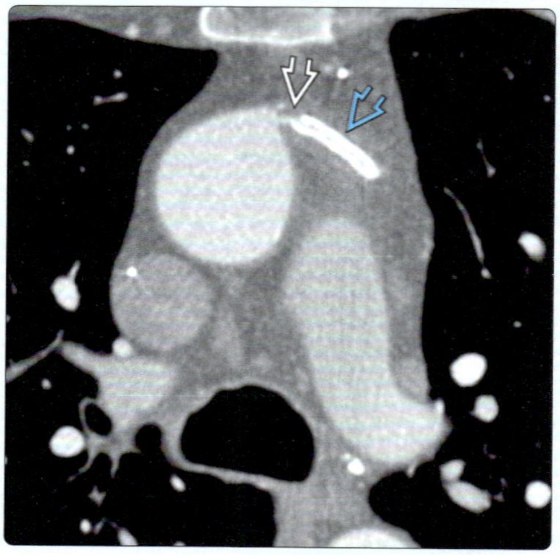
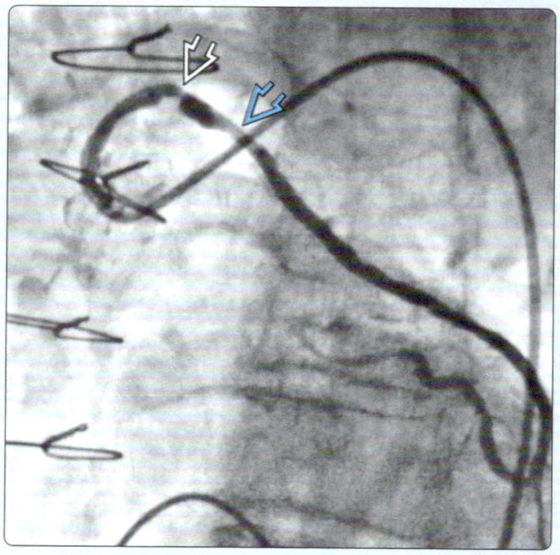

(Left) *Post coronary artery bypass grafting (CABG) cardiac CT shows a patent stent ⇨ in a saphenous graft to a diagonal branch. However, note obstructive stenosis from mixed plaque proximal to the stent ➡.* **(Right)** *Corresponding invasive coronary angiography 3 months later shows in-stent restenosis ⇨ and progression in obstructive plaque proximal to the stent ➡.*

TERMINOLOGY

Abbreviations

- Coronary artery bypass graft (CABG)

Definitions

- Postoperative atherosclerotic disease of bypass grafts or native coronary arteries

Scoring systems

- SYNTAX score II: Combines anatomic SYNTAX score and 7 independent clinical predictors for 4-year all-cause mortality in patients undergoing either surgical or percutaneous revascularization
  - Prediction model updated as SYNTAX score 2020, which could predict 5-year MACE and 10-year all-cause mortality based on cross validation in SYNTAX trial and external validation in FREEDOM, BEST and PRECOMBAT trials

IMAGING

General Features

- Best diagnostic clue
  - Stenosis or occlusion of graft or native coronary artery on coronary angiography or cardiac CT
- Location
  - Bypass conduits may include
    - Left or right internal mammary artery
    - Radial artery segments
    - Autologous reversed saphenous veins grafts
  - Arterial conduits are preferred, but saphenous vein grafts commonly required for complete revascularization

CT Findings

- CTA
  - High accuracy of MDCT for graft stenosis/occlusion
    - CTA enables assessment of severity of coronary lesions, length of lesion, diffuse character of lumen reduction, tortuosity of target vessel, and degree of coronary calcification
    - Only noninvasive tool capable of robustly imaging coronary atherosclerotic plaque that leads to myocardial infarction (MI) and angina pectoris
  - Prospective ECG-triggered or retrospectively ECG-gated, tube-modulated imaging allows high-quality images of arterial and venous bypass grafts
  - Photon-counting CT improved spatial and contrast resolution for graft assessment with lower radiation dose
    - High-pitch prospective or nongated high-pitch acquisition covering entire thorax followed immediately by prospectively triggered or retrospectively gated acquisition of heart only
    - Allows assessment of left internal mammary artery origin and coronary arteries while maintaining low overall radiation dose
  - Superior to invasive angiography for true diameter measurements of grafts as mural thrombus is visible
    - Aneurysm size is often underestimated on angiography
  - Cardiac CTA with sagittal reconstructions and 3D reconstructions best demonstrate relationship and proximity of grafts to sternum and sternal wires prior to redo sternotomy
  - May demonstrate subendocardial fatty metaplasia or hypoattenuation in areas of prior infarct
  - Compared to CTA alone, addition of CT myocardial perfusion (CT-MPI) imaging improves diagnostic accuracy for functional assessment of coronary artery disease (CAD)
    - CT-MPI preferred in patients with extensive coronary calcification, chronic occlusions, and in those with previous revascularization
    - CT-MPI can follow positive CTA to assess functional severity of coronary lesions with benefit of direct spatial correlation of stenotic branches and their dependent myocardium
  - FASTTRACK CABG trial: CABG-guided by CCTA is feasible and has acceptable safety profile in selected population of complex CAD

MR Findings

- MRA
  - Metallic clips in grafts constitute most common limitation of coronary bypass MRA
    - Lower spatial resolution compared to CT
    - Limited visibility of stent lumen due to radiofrequency shielding effects
  - 3D gadolinium-enhanced techniques are more sensitive than 2D gradient-echo or spin-echo techniques
- MR cine
  - Global and regional ventricular function can be assessed with steady-state free precession sequences
- Delayed enhancement
  - Depicts volume of infarcted tissue

Echocardiographic Findings

- Echocardiogram
  - Transthoracic Doppler echo has high accuracy for detecting left internal mammary artery graft stenosis

Angiographic Findings

- Invasive coronary angiography the clinical gold standard
  - Demonstrates degree of luminal stenosis or occlusion
  - Finding and cannulating the coronary graft ostium can be challenging and may preclude assessment
- Intravascular ultrasound (IVUS) used to characterize plaque morphology and composition

Nuclear Medicine Findings

- PET
  - Myocardial perfusion imaging (MPI) with 82-rubidium
    - 82-rubidium PET has increased sensitivity (90% vs. 85%) and specificity (88% vs. 85%) over SPECT MPI
  - Viability imaging with 18-F FDG
    - 18-F FDG viability imaging can be combined with resting 82-rubidium PET perfusion scan to assess for perfusion/viability mismatch

Imaging Recommendations

- Best imaging tool
  - Invasive: Invasive coronary angiography
  - Noninvasive: Cardiac CT

DIFFERENTIAL DIAGNOSIS

Graft Thrombosis

- Occurs in early postoperative period
- May occur in absence of graft atherosclerotic disease

Subclavian Artery Stenosis Proximal to Left Internal Mammary Artery Origin

- May have same effect as left internal mammary artery stenosis

PATHOLOGY

General Features

- Etiology
  - Neointimal hyperplasia predominates in 1st year post CABG
    - Progressive intimal thickening and superimposed atheromas can result in significant luminal narrowing and reduction in coronary blood flow, resulting in recurrent symptoms
  - Accelerated atherosclerosis
    - Progression of atherosclerosis in native coronary arteries proximal to grafts
    - Patients with diabetes have higher whole plaque volume and calcified plaque progression than nondiabetics
  - Multiple factors contribute to pathogenesis of atherosclerosis and its complications, including endothelial dysfunction, inflammatory and immunologic factors, plaque rupture or erosion, and traditional risk factors of hypertension, diabetes, dyslipidemia, and smoking

CLINICAL ISSUES

Presentation

- Most common signs/symptoms
  - Angina recurs in 15-20% of patients during 1st year postop
    - Subsequent recurrence ~ 4% per year
    - SYNTAX trial comparing CABG with percutaneous coronary intervention (PCI) showed that repeat CABG was required in 1% of patients originally assigned to CABG group

Natural History & Prognosis

- Vein grafts are most often used but subject to graft disease and reduced long-term patency compared to arteries
- Saphenous veins grafts
  - 10% of all grafts fail early (within 1 month) due to thrombotic occlusion
  - 15% fail within 1 year due to intimal thickening
    - Main determinants of failure within 1 year include small vessel diameter, reduced wall motion of vessel-dependent myocardial region, and right coronary as target vessel
  - 25% fail in subsequent years due to accelerated atherosclerosis
  - Cumulative graft failure rate of 50% at 10 years postop
- Arterial grafts
  - Graft failure rate of 10% at 10 years
  - Left internal mammary artery provides highest 10-year patency rate, improved survival, and greatest freedom from cardiac events
- Distal vasculature
  - State of distal vasculature influences bypass graft patency
  - Highest graft patency rates in
    - Native vessels distal to graft with diameter > 1.5 mm
    - Large distal vascular territory
    - Free of atheroma obstructing > 25% of native distal vessel
- Rate of progression of disease in native vessels is highest in arterial segments with already established disease
  - 3-6x higher rate of progression in grafted vs. nongrafted vessels
  - Lesions in native vessels that are long (≥ 10 mm) and > 70% stenosed are at greatest risk of occluding

Treatment

- Medical
  - Antiplatelet therapy can reduce graft failure
  - Lipid-lowering therapy can attenuate process of atherosclerosis
  - β-blockers if history of MI or reduced ejection fraction
- Interventional
  - Stenting is preferred over balloon angioplasty
  - Drug-eluting stents preferred
- Surgical
  - Redo bypass surgery

SELECTED REFERENCES

1. Serruys PW et al: Coronary bypass surgery guided by computed tomography in a low-risk population. Eur Heart J. 45(20):1804-15, 2024
2. Mézquita AJV et al: Clinical quantitative coronary artery stenosis and coronary atherosclerosis imaging: a consensus statement from the Quantitative Cardiovascular Imaging Study Group. Nat Rev Cardiol. 20(10):696-714, 2023
3. Andreini D et al: Pre-procedural planning of coronary revascularization by cardiac computed tomography: an expert consensus document of the Society of Cardiovascular Computed Tomography. EuroIntervention. 18(11):e872-87, 2022
4. Omer S: Commentary: saphenous vein graft patency after coronary artery bypass grafting. It's all about getting the basics right. J Thorac Cardiovasc Surg. 163(3):1040-1, 2022
5. Pontone G et al: Clinical applications of cardiac computed tomography: a consensus paper of the European Association of Cardiovascular Imaging-part II. Eur Heart J Cardiovasc Imaging. 23(4):e136-61, 2022
6. Abazid RM et al: Coronary artery calcium progression after coronary artery bypass grafting surgery. Open Heart. 8(1), 2021
7. Dimitriadis S et al: Secondary prevention medications post coronary artery bypass grafting surgery-a literature review. J Cardiovasc Pharmacol Ther. 26(4):310-20, 2021
8. Caliskan E et al: Saphenous vein grafts in contemporary coronary artery bypass graft surgery. Nat Rev Cardiol. 17(3):155-69, 2020
9. Stuijfzand WJ et al: Stress myocardial perfusion imaging vs coronary computed tomographic angiography for diagnosis of invasive vessel-specific coronary physiology: predictive modeling results from the computed tomographic evaluation of atherosclerotic determinants of myocardial ischemia (CREDENCE) Trial. JAMA Cardiol. 5(12):1338-48, 2020
10. Patel MR et al: ACC/AATS/AHA/ASE/ASNC/SCAI/SCCT/STS 2017 appropriate use criteria for coronary revascularization in patients with stable ischemic heart disease: a report of the American College of Cardiology Appropriate Use Criteria Task Force, American Association for Thoracic Surgery, American Heart Association, American Society of Echocardiography, American Society of Nuclear Cardiology, Society for Cardiovascular Angiography and Interventions, Society of Cardiovascular Computed Tomography, and Society of Thoracic Surgeons. J Am Coll Cardiol. 69(17):2212-41, 2017

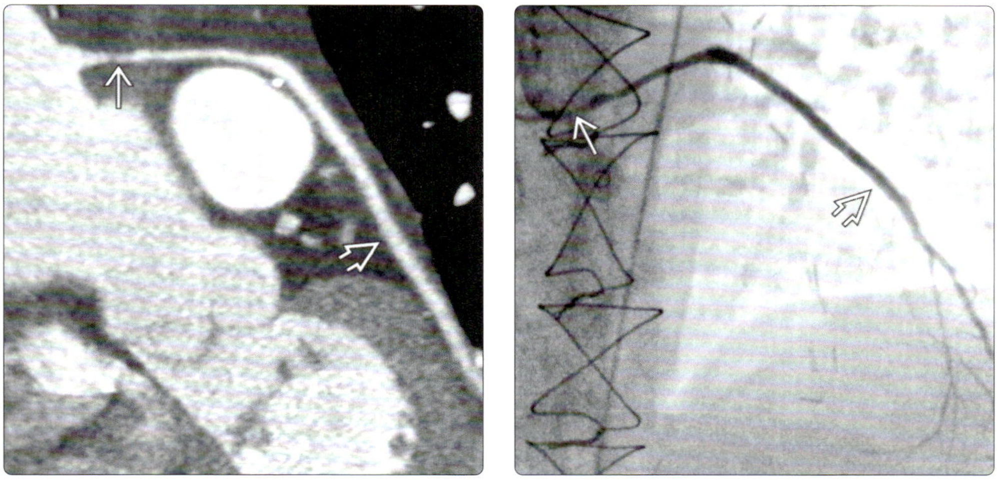

(Left) *Coronary CTA in a 72-year-old man 10 years post CABG shows that the venous graft to the obtuse marginal branch has a noncalcified plaque, causing stenosis of the proximal portion → of the graft. The remainder of the graft is widely patent →.* **(Right)** *Subsequent invasive angiogram confirms obstructive lesion → in the proximal portion. Also, the remainder of the graft is widely patent →. This patient subsequently underwent percutaneous coronary intervention to the graft.*

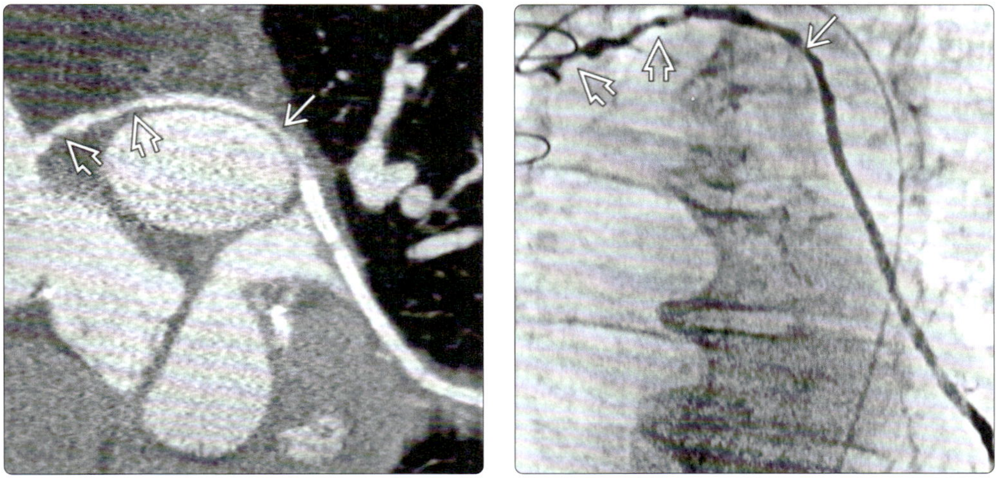

(Left) *Coronary CTA in a 78-year-old man with recurrent chest pain 15 years post CABG shows mild to moderate diffuse atherosclerosis → in the proximal portion of a vein graft to a diagonal branch and an obstructive stenosis → in the proximal midportion. Note 4 stents more distally, all of which appear patent.* **(Right)** *Subsequent corresponding invasive angiogram confirms diffuse disease in the proximal portion → of the vein graft and an obstructive lesion in the proximal midportion →.*

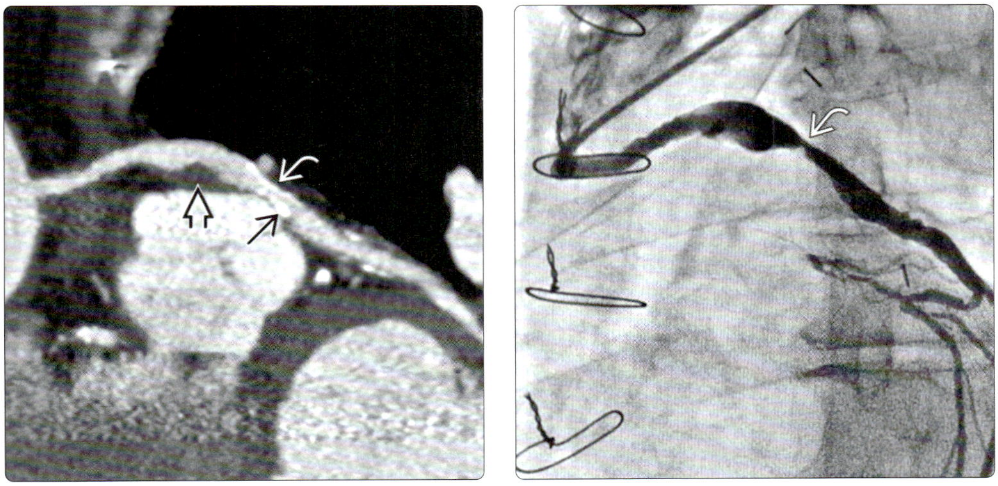

(Left) *Coronary CTA in a 63-year-old man with recurrent chest pain 9 years post CABG shows diffuse atherosclerosis scattered throughout this vein graft to an obtuse marginal branch. Note calcified → and noncalcified → plaques. Obstructive stenosis → is noted in the midportion.* **(Right)** *Subsequent corresponding invasive angiogram confirms an obstructive stenosis → in the midportion of the graft. Note that the plaque burden is underestimated on the invasive angiogram.*

Post-CABG Aneurysm

KEY FACTS

TERMINOLOGY

- Aneurysm of saphenous vein bypass graft after surgery

IMAGING

- Aneurysmal dilation of saphenous vein bypass graft
- Average size is 6 cm but may measure 16 > cm
- Best visualized on ECG-gated cardiac CTA
- Consider both systemic arterial and venous phases to differentiate slow flow from thrombus

TOP DIFFERENTIAL DIAGNOSES

- Saphenous vein graft pseudoaneurysm (SVGPA)
  - Occurs at anastomotic sites
  - Classically occurs within few months of surgery
  - Much less common than saphenous venous graft aneurysm (SVGA)
- Coronary artery aneurysms

PATHOLOGY

- Secondary to accelerated atherosclerosis of vein graft

CLINICAL ISSUES

- Patients often asymptomatic
- Can become symptomatic; ischemia or infarct due to thrombosis; worsening heart failure due to thrombosis or fistulization

DIAGNOSTIC CHECKLIST

- Rounded mass on chest radiograph in anterior mediastinum in patient who is post CABG should raise concern for SVGA
- Although ECG-gated study is preferred method to evaluate SVGA, Dx can be made on both routine contrast and noncontrast CT studies

SCANNING TIPS

- If there is concern for SVGA, perform ECG-gated CTA through entire thorax

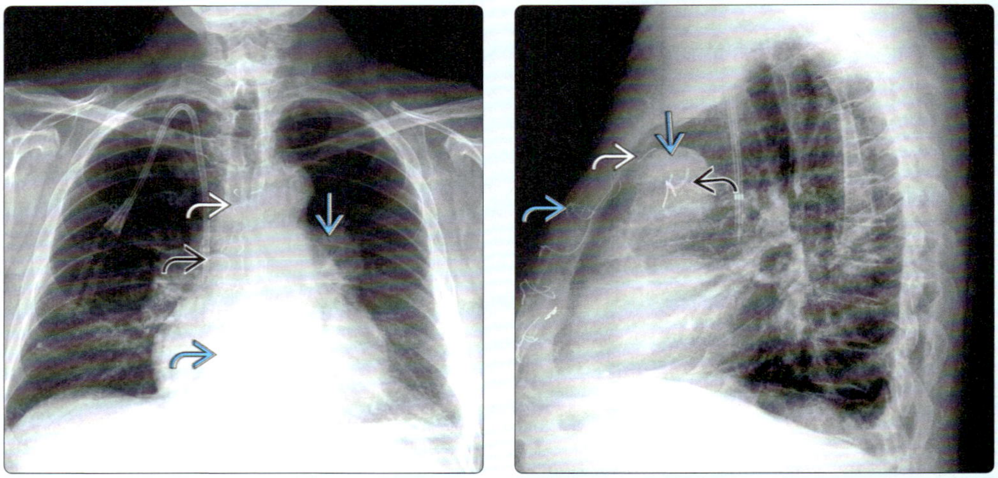

(Left) *PA radiograph in a 73-year-old man shows an ovoid anterior mediastinal mass to the left of and anterior to the main pulmonary artery ➔. There are findings of prior coronary artery bypass grafting (CABG), including median sternotomy wires ➔, some of which are fractured ➔. C-shaped markers ➔ denoting the site of bypass grafts are also seen.* **(Right)** *Lateral radiograph in the same patient again shows the main pulmonary artery ➔, sternotomy wires ➔ (some fractured ➔), and site of the bypass grafts ➔.*

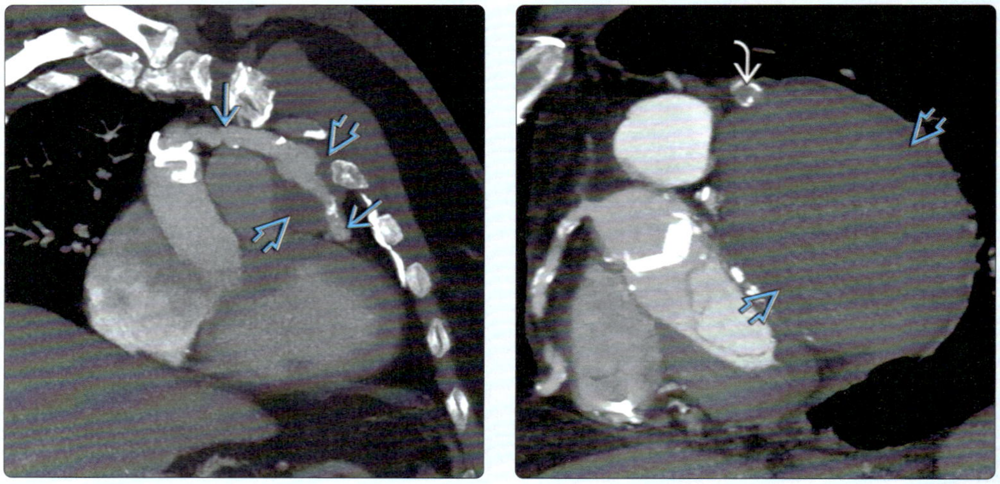

(Left) *Coronal oblique MIP CECT in the above patient shows an aneurysmal saphenous vein to obtuse marginal graft ➔. In its midportion, there is a partially thrombosed, 6-cm, rounded graft aneurysm ➔. The graft was occluded distally.* **(Right)** *Coronal oblique MIP CECT in an 81-year-old man with a history of 3-vessel CABG shows a 12-cm thrombosed saphenous vein bypass graft aneurysm (SVGA) ➔. The more proximal graft is mildly dilated and also thrombosed ➔. The SVGA causes mass effect on the left ventricle.*

TERMINOLOGY

Abbreviations

- Coronary artery bypass grafting (CABG)

Synonyms

- Saphenous venous graft aneurysm (SVGA)

Definitions

- Aneurysm of saphenous vein bypass graft after coronary artery bypass surgery

IMAGING

General Features

- Best diagnostic clue
  - Aneurysmal dilation of saphenous vein bypass anywhere along its course from its origin to termination
- Location
  - Along course of saphenous vein bypass grafts arising from ascending aorta
    - Right coronary artery and left circumflex territory most common involved as saphenous vein grafts (SVGs) commonly used to bypass
    - Left anterior descending bypass usually via left internal mammary artery (LIMA) graft
  - True aneurysm of LIMA graft very rare; related to surgical trauma or technical error at anastomosis
- Size
  - Size definition of SVGA varies
    - Minimal size criteria: No set definition
      - Some authors use 1.5x normal size of SVG; others use 2 cm
    - Maximum size: Case reports > 16 cm
- Morphology
  - Various morphologies, including focal rounded aneurysm to diffuse aneurysmal dilation of graft

Radiographic Findings

- Usually rounded mass in anterior or middle mediastinum
- Findings of prior CABG surgery

CT Findings

- Nongated CT
  - SVGA can be seen in routine noncontrast or contrast CT scan without ECG gating
  - Any mass in region of saphenous vein bypass graft in post-CABG patient should raise suspicion of SVGA
- Cardiac gated CTA
  - Aneurysmal dilation of saphenous vein bypass graft along course of vessel
    - Graft may maintain patency even with giant aneurysm
    - Areas of thrombosis often seen even in small SVGAs
    - Consider both systemic arterial and venous phases
      - Helps differentiate between slow flow in SVGA vs. thrombus
  - Distinction between SVGA and SVG pseudoaneurysm (SVGPA) on imaging is not always clear
    - Typical timing and location are different
      - SVGPAs occur at proximal and distal anastomotic sites day to months after surgery
      - SVGAs occur in midsubstance of vein graft many years after surgery
  - Fistulas can occur between SVGA and adjacent mediastinal structures

MR Findings

- SSFP
  - Lumen: High signal
  - Thrombus: Intermediate signal
- T1W and T2W
  - Lumen: Low signal
  - Thrombus: Intermediate to high signal
- T1W+
  - Lumen enhances while thrombus does not

Imaging Recommendations

- Best imaging tool
  - ECG-gated cardiac CTA
- Protocol advice
  - If SVGA is expected, scan entire chest
    - Graft origin is from ascending aorta, not aortic root
    - Lesions can be large and can extend high into chest
  - Recommend delayed scan to better differentiate mural thrombus from slow flow

DIFFERENTIAL DIAGNOSIS

Saphenous Bypass Graft Pseudoaneurysm

- Differentiation between SVGA and SVGPA on imaging is not always easy
  - Occurs at anastomotic sites
  - Classically occurs within few months after surgery
    - However, some cases can occur years after CABG
  - Imaging features of SCGA and SVGPA can overlap
  - Certain pathologic features can overlap
    - Destruction of media is hallmark of pseudoaneurysm
    - Since venous media is very thin, true aneurysms may show complete absence of media on pathology
- SVGPA is much less common than SVGA; SVGPA:SVGA 1:6 ratio

Coronary Artery Aneurysm

- May be difficult to distinguish on nongated studies

DIAGNOSTIC CHECKLIST

Image Interpretation Pearls

- Rounded mass on chest radiograph in anterior mediastinum in patient who is post CABG should raise concern for SVGA
- Although ECG-gated study is preferred method to evaluate SVGA, diagnosis can be made on both routine contrast and noncontrast CT studies

SELECTED REFERENCES

1. Lawani O et al: Incidental finding and endovascular repair of a left internal mammary artery aneurysm following a multivessel coronary artery bypass graft. Case Rep Cardiol. 2021:8831235, 2021
2. Vinciguerra M et al: Management of patients with aortocoronary saphenous vein graft aneurysms: JACC state-of-the-art review. J Am Coll Cardiol. 77(17):2236-53, 2021
3. Ramirez FD et al: Natural history and management of aortocoronary saphenous vein graft aneurysms: a systematic review of published cases. Circulation. 126(18):2248-56, 2012

Coronary Dissection, Secondary/Iatrogenic

KEY FACTS

IMAGING

- National Heart, Lung, and Blood Institute (NHLBI) classification system for coronary artery dissections is divided into types A-F, based on angiographic appearance
- Possible ECG-gated CTA findings include
  - False lumen or intramural hematoma with vascular narrowing
  - Adjacent soft tissue stranding
  - Signs of trauma or type A dissection
- MR is not primary modality for diagnosing secondary coronary artery dissection
  - Can assess extent of injury of myocardial injury
  - T2 cardiac MR mapping with T2 value of < 20 ms and associated myocardial hemorrhage may be used to detect intramural hematoma
- Traumatic: Left anterior descending artery is often affected due to its proximity to chest wall
- Iatrogenic: Right coronary artery is most affected (84-87%)
- Propagation of type A dissection in coronary arteries ranges from 5-11%

PATHOLOGY

- Pathology depends on etiology; all can lead to coronary occlusion, infarct, and sudden cardiac death

CLINICAL ISSUES

- Mortality depends on underlying cause; up to 40% with type A dissections involving coronary arteries and much lower with iatrogenic causes
- Conservative management suitable for asymptomatic patients with minor, stable dissections (NHLBI types A-B)
- Includes β-blockers and antiplatelet therapy
- May be asymptomatic
- Can be complicated by myocardial infarction or fistulas (coronary arteriovenous fistula or coronary cameral fistula)
- Percutaneous coronary intervention: Required for severe dissections (NHLBI types C-F) or those with compromised blood flow

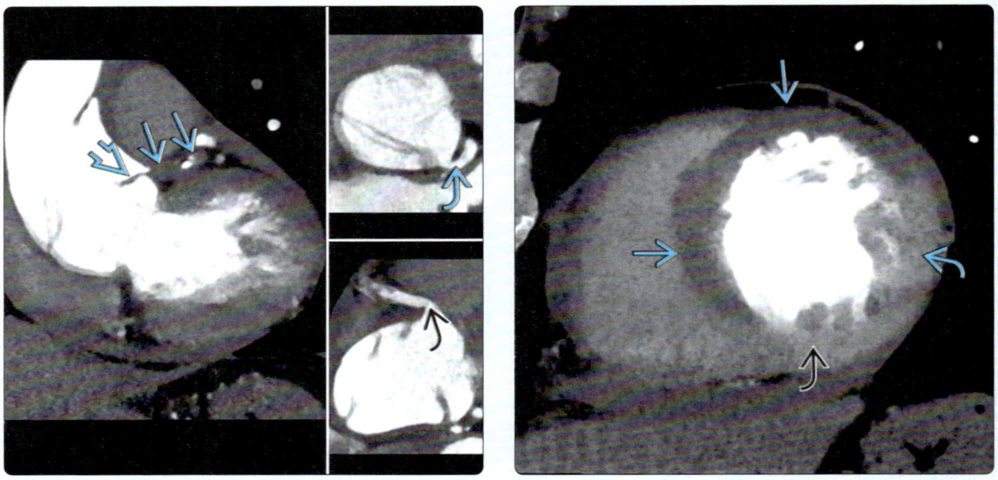

(Left) *ECG-gated CTA shows a type A dissection. The intimal flap occludes what appears the be the left main coronary artery, which would be fatal. However, the patient has a variant where the occluded left anterior descending (LAD) (left) and patent left circumflex (LCx) (top right) have separate origins from the left sinus of Valsalva. The right coronary artery (RCA) (bottom right) is also patent.* **(Right)** *CECT shows LAD territory transmural infarct. The LCx and RCA territories are normal. (Courtesy S. Kligerman, MD.)*

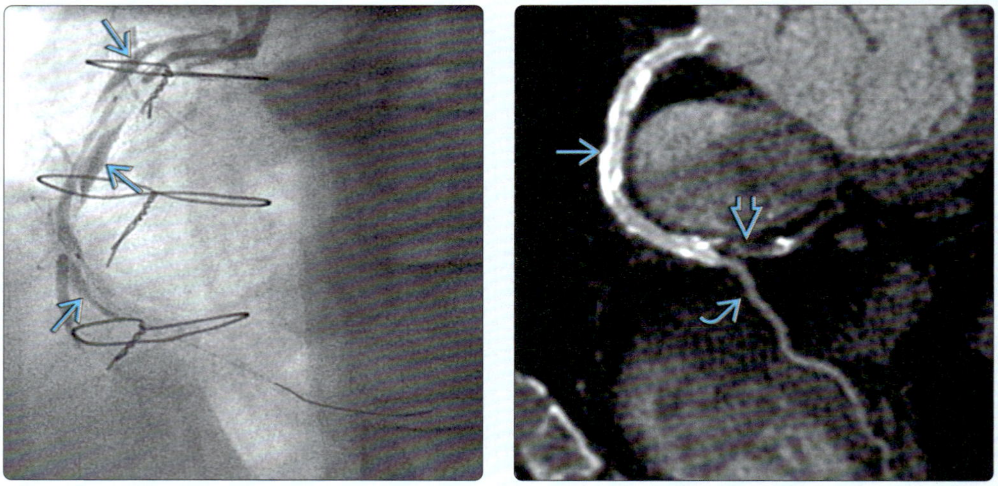

(Left) *Catheter angiogram of the RCA shows a very large spiral dissection involving the proximal, mid-, and distal RCA with contrast staining within the vessel wall. The dissection was treated with multiple overlapping stents.* **(Right)** *C-view of the RCA from a CTA shows the multiple overlapping stents. While the patent ductus arteriosus is patent, the posterior lateral branch is occluded. (Courtesy S. Kligerman, MD.)*

TERMINOLOGY

Definitions

- Dissection of blood between medial and adventitial layers of coronary artery secondary to trauma, intervention, or propagation of type A dissection

IMAGING

General Features

- Best diagnostic clue
  - Secondary/false lumen
  - Abrupt luminal narrowing
  - Intramural hematoma
  - Intimal tear
  - Persistent contrast staining
  - Compressive effect of hematoma
- Location
  - Traumatic: Left anterior descending (LAD) artery is often affected due to its proximity to chest wall
  - Iatrogenic: Right coronary artery (RCA) is most affected
  - Propagation of type A dissection: RCA > left main (LM)

CT Findings

- Possible findings include
  - False lumen or intramural hematoma
  - Narrowing or occlusion of lumen
  - Nearby soft tissue stranding
  - Rarely, hypoattenuating flap with contrast in vessel wall
- Types of luminal stenosis
  - Abrupt stenosis: Diameter reduction > 50% over 0.5 mm
  - Gradual stenosis: Diameter reduction > 50% over 5 mm
  - Dissection flap's extension varies
    - Class I: Reaches ipsilateral sinus of Valsalva
    - Class II: Reaches both sinus of Valsalva and tubular aorta (≤ 4 cm)
    - Class III: Extends to ascending aorta (> 4 cm)
- Additional findings
  - Soft tissue stranding in epicardium
  - Myocardial perfusion defects and wall motion abnormalities
  - Type A dissection
    - In setting of type A dissection, recommend ECG-gated CTA to visualize coronary arteries
    - Can be due to propagation of type A dissection into coronaries or propagation of coronary dissection into aorta
  - Findings of chest wall trauma

MR Findings

- MR is not primary modality for diagnosing secondary coronary artery dissection, but it is valuable for evaluating extent of injury and provides consistent functional quantification
- Can measure myocardial blood flow conditions through 1st-pass perfusion or arterial spin labeling
- T2 cardiac MR mapping with T2 value of < 20 ms and associated myocardial hemorrhage may be used to detect intramural hematoma
- Diagnostic indicators, suggesting infarction
  - Abnormal wall motion
  - Edema
  - Abnormal perfusion
  - LGE

Echocardiographic Findings

- Assessment of wall motion abnormalities associated with ischemia and infarct
- Intimal flap map be visible in proximal coronary dissection

Angiographic Findings

- Iatrogenic coronary dissections are often caused by cardiac catheterization and usually treated during same examination
- Appears as luminal haziness, linear dissection, extraluminal contrast staining, spiral dissection, reduced flow, or total blockage
- National Heart, Lung, and Blood Institute (NHLBI) classification system for coronary artery dissections is divided into types A-F based on angiographic appearance
  - Type A: Radiolucent areas within coronary lumen during contrast injection with minimal or no persistence of contrast after dye has cleared
  - Type B: Parallel tracts or double lumen separated by radiolucent area during contrast injection with minimal or no persistence after dye clearance
  - Type C: Contrast appears outside coronary lumen
  - Type D: Long spiral dissections
  - Type E: Dissections associated with thrombus
  - Type F: Dissections leading to total occlusion of coronary artery without distal anterograde flow
- Risk of arterial closure
  - Type A: < 3%; type B: 3.1%; type C: 9.7%; type D: 30.3%; type E: 38.9%; type F: 68.6%
- Can propagate proximally to involve aorta

Other Modality Findings

- Intracoronary imaging is gold standard for confirming coronary dissection, even if coronary angiography results are normal
- Intravascular ultrasound (IVUS) and optical coherence tomography (OCT) help distinguish between plaque rupture, thrombus, dissection, and external compression, aiding in identifying cause of coronary artery occlusion and guiding best management strategy
- Upon detection of dissection, further antegrade injections are avoided; hemodynamic support is provided, guide catheter is carefully positioned, and stent implantation is performed following placement of nonhydrophilic guidewire in true lumen

Imaging Recommendations

- Best imaging tool
  - Cardiac catheterization

DIFFERENTIAL DIAGNOSIS

Spasm

- Associated with cigarette, stimulant use, medications, stress
  - No ischemic changes on resting EKG
  - No stenosis on CTA

Coronary Artery Atherosclerotic Disease

- If true and false lumens are not visible, can appear similar to atherosclerotic disease with plaque rupture
- Histories often different
- Presence of calcified and noncalcified plaque along area of narrowing may help differentiate

Spontaneous Coronary Artery Dissection

- Younger patients with no risk factors for coronary artery disease
- Common causes include fibromuscular dysplasia (FMD), genetic arteriopathies, pregnancy, systemic inflammatory conditions
- Often precipitated by physical or emotional stress
- Different patient histories

PATHOLOGY

General Features

- Etiology
  - Iatrogenic
    - Coronary procedures, such as percutaneous coronary intervention (PCI), atherectomy, or coronary angiography
      - Prevalence of 0.04% in diagnostic and 0.12% in therapeutic procedures
    - Less frequently linked to cardiac surgery and radiofrequency ablation
    - Catheter- or balloon-induced injury of endothelium leads to dissection of blood into vessel
  - Blunt chest trauma
    - Very rare with incidence of 0.1% following blunt chest trauma
    - History is key to making diagnosis
    - Likely related to
      - Rapid deceleration → ↑ endothelial shear forces on LAD
      - Severe stress on body → ↑ catecholamine levels → ↑ acute ↑ in coronary blood pressure
  - Propagation of type A dissection in coronary arteries ranges from 5-11%
    - Remember that iatrogenic coronary dissections can propagate into aorta as well
  - Risk factors
    - Catheter trauma: Caused by diagnostic or guiding catheters during PCI, either intentionally for device support or unintentionally due to traction forces when withdrawing intracoronary devices
    - Radial access procedures: Requires aggressive catheter manipulation for engagement and alignment
    - Patient factors: Heavy atherosclerotic burden, especially in LM; patients with underlying connective tissue disorders, FMD, arteriopathy
    - Additional risk factors: Improper catheter positioning, overinflation of angioplasty balloons, use of oversized or stiff guidewires, rotational and orbital atherectomy

CLINICAL ISSUES

Presentation

- Most common signs/symptoms
  - Ranges from asymptomatic to sudden cardiac death

Demographics

- Traumatic coronary artery dissection
  - Demographic data are scarce
  - In posttraumatic myocardial infarction patients
    - Traffic accidents most common followed by sports injuries, falls, fights, and being kicked by animals
    - 83% were male
    - 82% of patients < 45 years old
    - Diagnosis often missed
- Iatrogenic coronary artery dissection
  - Average age: 64 years
  - Women > men

Natural History & Prognosis

- Can be complicated by myocardial infarction or fistulas (coronary arteriovenous fistula or coronary cameral fistula)
- High mortality rate with type A dissection involving coronaries
  - As high as 40% in old large multicenter Japanese study
- 6% mortality with catheter-induced coronary dissection

Treatment

- Conservative management
  - Suitable for asymptomatic patients with minor, stable dissections (NHLBI types A-B)
  - Includes β-blockers and antiplatelet therapy
- PCI: Required for severe dissections (NHLBI types C-F) or those with compromised blood flow
- Coronary artery bypass grafting (CABG): Considered when true lumen wiring is unsuccessful during PCI
- In cases of aortic root dissections
  - Small dissections (limited to sinus of Valsalva or up to 4 cm in ascending aorta) can be managed conservatively
  - Large dissections involving supraaortic vessels, aortic valve, or causing hemodynamic collapse requiring surgical intervention

DIAGNOSTIC CHECKLIST

Consider

- Blunt chest trauma
  - New electrocardiographic changes
  - Normal electrocardiogram with elevated troponin
- After coronary procedures
  - History of vessel trauma from catheters
  - Use of PCI devices, such as balloons and stents
- Type A dissection
  - Recommend ECG-gated CTA to assess coronary ostia

Image Interpretation Pearls

- Assess for secondary lumen, abrupt luminal narrowing, intramural hematoma, intimal tear

SELECTED REFERENCES

1. Chen Y et al: Preoperative diagnostic value of coronary CT angiography in acute Stanford type A aortic dissection involving the coronary arteries. Clin Radiol. 79(1):e57-64, 2024
2. Page E et al: Incidence, treatment and outcomes of coronary artery dissection during percutaneous coronary intervention. J Invasive Cardiol. 35(7):E341-54, 2023

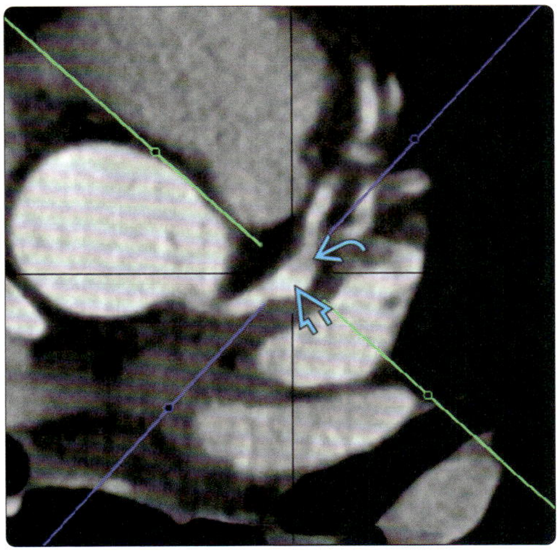

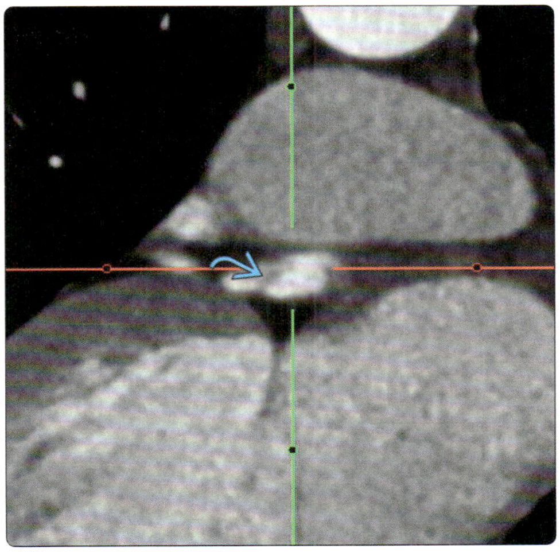

(Left) *Axial CTA in a patient with a history of blunt force trauma shows focal dilation of the left main coronary artery with a subtle dissection flap.* **(Right)** *Oblique view of the left main dissection in the same patient shows the dissection flap as the hypoattenuating band within the vessel.*

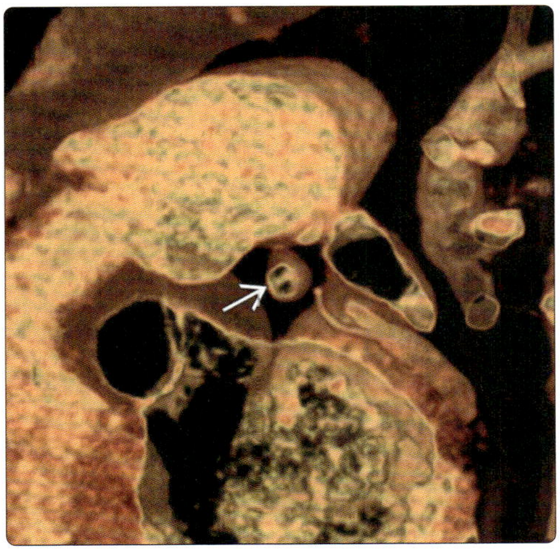

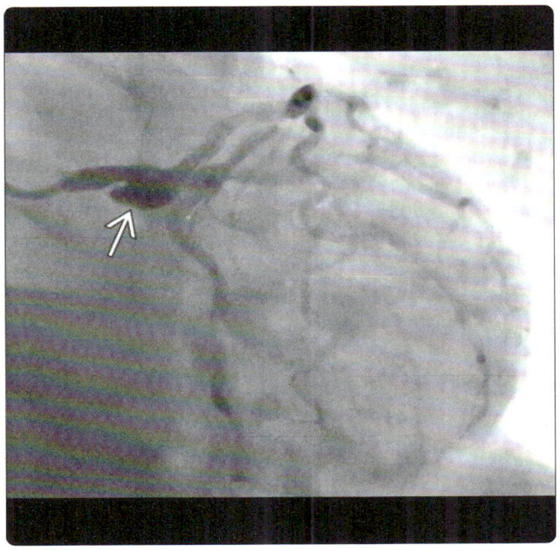

(Left) *3D reconstruction of the CTA in the same patient clearly shows the double lumen left main coronary artery due to traumatic dissection.* **(Right)** *Coronary angiogram of the left main dissection in the same patient shows contrast filling the false lumen.*

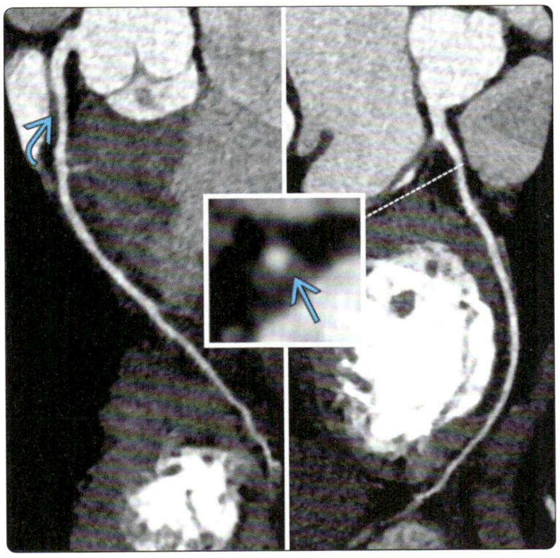

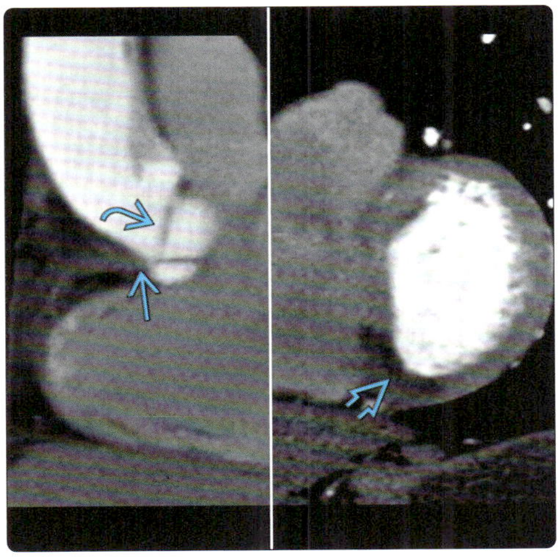

(Left) *CTA reveals focal narrowing of LAD in a 47-year-old with ↑ troponin following a motor vehicle accident. Transverse view (inset) of the narrowed LAD shows surrounding soft tissue thought to represent an intramural hematoma.* **(Right)** *Coronal oblique CECT shows a type A dissection involving the aortic root with an intimal flap extending into the RCA ostium and subsequent RCA occlusion. Short-axis image of the heart shows the transmural infarct in the RCA territory. (Courtesy S. Kligerman, MD.)*

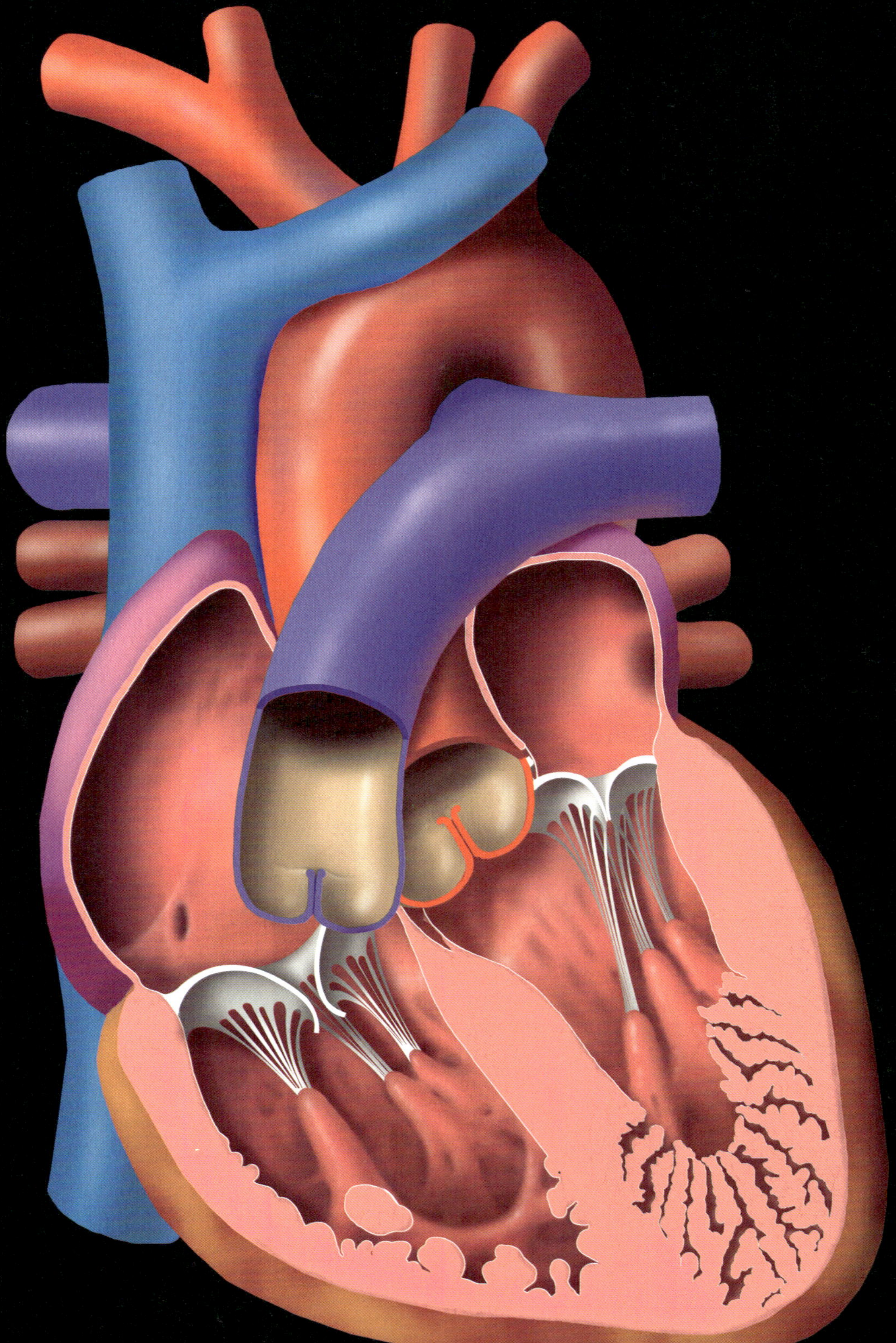

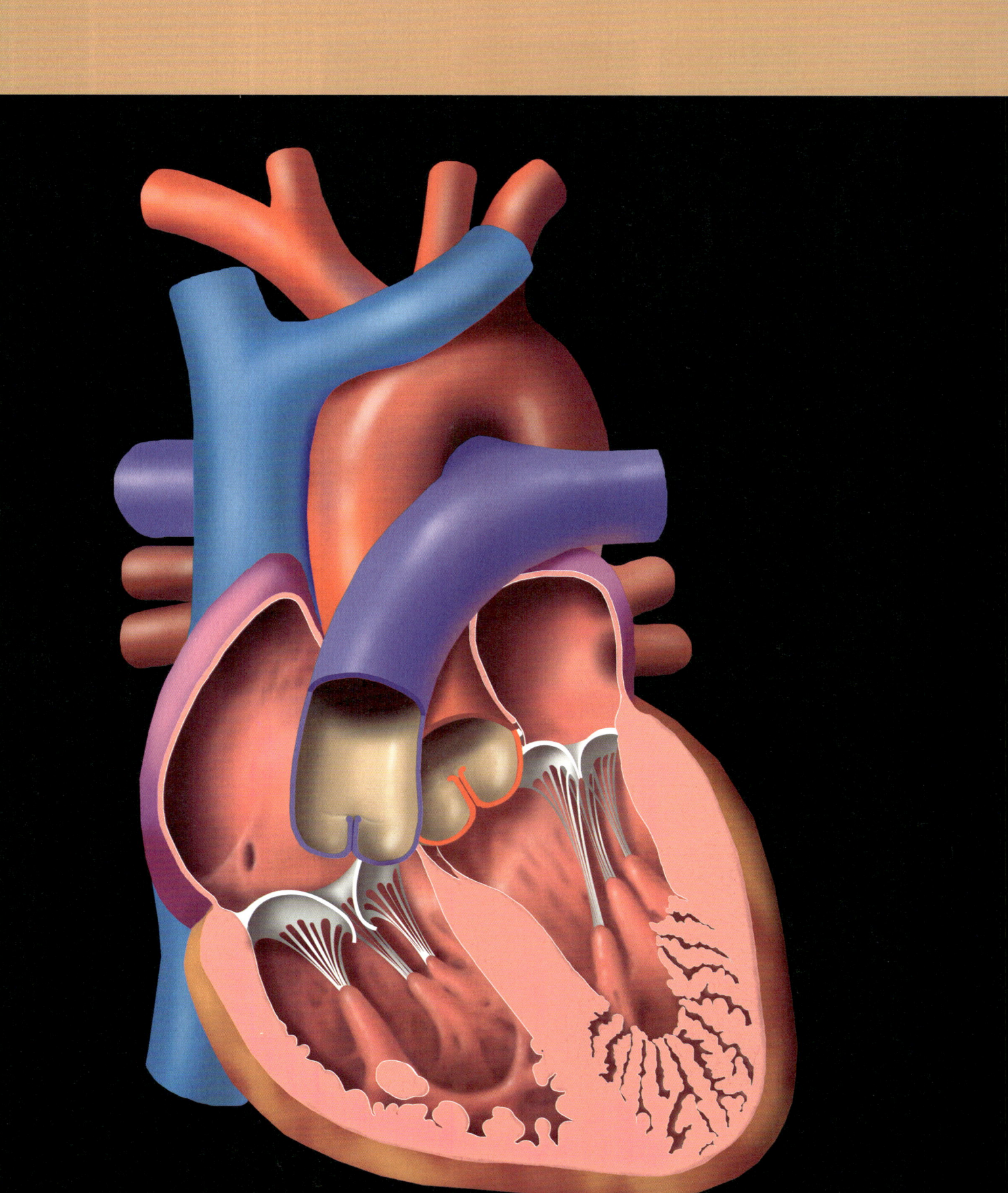

SECTION 3

Heart Failure and Cardiomyopathies

Introduction

Heart failure (HF) is a pathophysiologic state in which abnormality of cardiac function is responsible for failure of the heart to pump blood at a rate commensurate with the requirements of the metabolizing tissues. The cardinal manifestations of HF are dyspnea and fatigue resulting in exercise intolerance and fluid retention and leading to pulmonary congestion and peripheral edema.

Prevalence

HF is increasing in prevalence. Nearly 6.5 million adults in the USA are estimated to have HF, and, every year, 960,000 are newly diagnosed. An estimated 23 million people are affected by HF worldwide with the prevalence of symptomatic HF ranging between 0.4-2.0%. HF is more prevalent in men and with increasing age.

Importance

HF causes more deaths than all forms of cancer combined. The 5-year mortality rate for a patient diagnosed with HF is 50%.

Pathophysiology

Preserved Ejection Fraction vs. Reduced Ejection Fraction

HF is often classified based on left ventricular ejection fraction (LVEF). HF with preserved ejection fraction (HFpEF) is defined as HF with LVEF ≥ 50% with evidence of elevated left ventricular filling pressure. In HF with a midrange ejection fraction (HFmEF), LVEF is 41-49%. Finally, HF with reduced ejection fraction (HFrEF) has LVEF ≤ 40%. The diagnosis of HFpEF can be challenging because symptoms are nonspecific and can be seen with other noncardiac conditions. Transthoracic echocardiogram (TTE) remains the principal diagnostic tool. The use of invasive hemodynamic testing and evaluation of coronary arteries is often advocated to reliably diagnose HFpEF. Less common diseases, including restrictive cardiomyopathies that result in HFpEF, can be evaluated by CMR. The use of stress CMR diagnosed new significant pathology in 27% of patients with HFpEF.

Left vs. Right Heart Failure

Left HF refers to the signs and symptoms of elevated pressure and congestion in the pulmonary veins and capillaries as well as low systemic cardiac output. Right HF refers to the signs and symptoms of elevated pressure and congestion of the systemic veins and capillaries, as characterized by jugular vein engorgement and hepatic congestion.

Systolic vs. Diastolic Heart Failure

In systolic dysfunction, the left ventricle appears large, dilated, and eccentrically hypertrophied, and the cardiac output is limited by impaired systolic ejection fraction. In diastolic dysfunction, the left ventricle typically appears thickened with a normal to small cavity in which filling is limited because of abnormal left ventricular compliance.

Treatment

The American College of Cardiology/American Heart Association Heart Failure Guidelines (2022) provide detailed information regarding the management and prevention of HF.

Imaging/Assessment Techniques

Different techniques are available to evaluate patients with HF; underlying clinical circumstances determine which test is most appropriate.

Electrocardiogram

An electrocardiogram (EKG) is used to detect many myocardial abnormalities, such as arrhythmias, previous myocardial infarction (MI), or ventricular hypertrophy. A normal EKG indicates HF from structural heart disease is unlikely, but its positive predictive value is low.

Chest Radiograph

Chest radiography (CXR) is used to evaluate the overall cardiac size and to check for signs of HF, such as pulmonary vascular congestion, pulmonary edema, and pleural effusions. CXR is also used to exclude other causes of dyspnea (cardiovascular pericardial calcifications, coronary calcifications, noncardiac pneumonia, lung carcinoma, etc.). Although echocardiography has largely replaced CXR as a method to determine heart dimensions and function, radiography is often used to monitor acutely ill patients and their responses to therapy. In patients with decompensated HF, CXR may show cephalization of pulmonary blood flow, interstitial or alveolar edema, effusions, and increased vascular pedicle width. Clearing of these findings on follow-up CXR is indicative of a response to therapy.

Echocardiography

2D transthoracic echocardiography and Doppler US are strongly recommended as a 1st-line technique for imaging patients with new-onset HF. It provides extensive information about the etiology and severity of HF, as it can accurately assess chamber dimensions, ventricular function, valvular stenosis or regurgitation, and systolic/diastolic function (filling pressures and patterns).

Four-chamber dilatation suggests a nonischemic etiology, whereas regional wall motion abnormalities may suggest an ischemic etiology. Other diagnoses may present with classic findings. For example, cardiac amyloidosis may present with biventricular thickening, small chamber size, restrictive physiology, and "sparkling" echogenicity. Similarly, hypertrophic cardiomyopathy can present with systolic anterior motion of the mitral valve, outflow tract obstruction, and asymmetric septal hypertrophy. Serial echocardiography is reasonable in patients with ST-segment elevation MI (STEMI) to reevaluate cardiac function during recovery when results are utilized to guide therapy.

Single-Photon Emission Computed Tomography

Single-photon emission computed tomography (SPECT) is not primarily used to determine left ventricular systolic function unless the relevant parameters are quantified from a myocardial perfusion assessment. Gated SPECT improves accuracy and provides information on left ventricular volumes, LVEF, and motion abnormalities. SPECT can also be used for evaluation of myocardial ischemia.

Radionuclide Ventriculography

Radionuclide ventriculography (RNV) is a planar technique useful for assessment of volumes in patients with significant wall motion abnormalities or distorted geography. Though used less often, RNV is an alternative to evaluate cardiac function. Quantitative assessments are reproducible, and serial measurements have been used to track efficacy of therapies in patients with HF.

Computed Tomography

CT can provide an accurate assessment of cardiac structure and function, though it is slightly less accurate than MR. CT has very high spatial resolution and is particularly useful for noninvasive evaluation of the coronary arteries. Coronary CTA can be used to exclude ischemic etiology in new-onset HF. One advantage of CT over echocardiography is the ability to detect pericardial calcification, as may be seen with constrictive pericarditis. CT is often used to exclude other etiologies for dyspnea, such as pulmonary embolism.

Cardiac Catheterization

Cardiac catheterization can accurately assess the overall cardiac function and hemodynamics and serves as the gold standard for the evaluation of the suspected obstructive coronary artery disease (CAD). Cardiac catheterization is also the gold standard for the evaluation of many valvular disorders (e.g., aortic stenosis, pulmonic stenosis).

Coronary catheterization should be performed in patients presenting with HF who have angina or significant ischemia, unless the patient is not eligible for revascularization of any kind (class 1, level B recommendation). Coronary catheterization is reasonable for patients with HF who have angina without evaluation of their coronary anatomy and who have no contraindications to coronary revascularization (class 2a, level C recommendation). Coronary catheterization is also reasonable in patients with new-onset HF without angina but with known or suspected CAD (class 2a, level C recommendation).

Magnetic Resonance Imaging

Magnetic resonance (MR) imaging is considered the reference standard for volumetric analysis and cardiac function due to high accuracy and reproducibility. MR can also assess myocardial perfusion, viability, and fibrosis, which can be very useful in identification of the etiology and facilitate prognosis in patients with HF. Stress perfusion CMR precisely diagnoses CAD with higher accuracy than SPECT imaging. Parametric techniques, such as T1 and T2 mapping and extracellular volume fraction, help in identification of diffuse fibrosis. Newer tissue-tracking techniques using CMR allow for evaluation of various forms of myocardial strain, including longitudinal strain. Abnormalities in longitudinal strain can allow for earlier detection of myocardial dysfunction, provide prognostication at all stages, and assess therapeutic effects.

Determining Etiology of Heart Failure

In patients with HF, it is important to determine the etiology in order to provide appropriate treatment and prognostic information. Even when patients still have normal systolic function, early diagnosis may allow for preventative measures that can change the natural history of the disease. The basic differentiation between ischemic and nonischemic cardiomyopathies is important and useful because this classification directly affects patient management.

LGE Magnetic Resonance

LGE MR is useful for detecting acute and chronic MI, predicting functional improvement after revascularization, and characterizing an extensive array of nonischemic cardiomyopathies. The use of LGE in the setting of HF is based on the understanding that rather than simply measuring viability, this technique also reveals the presence and patterns of hyperenhancement, which yield significant additional information. A systematic approach for interpreting LGE MR in patients with HF has been proposed. This approach is based on 4 steps.

Step 1: Assess the severity and regionality of left ventricular dysfunction, chamber size, wall thickness, and valvular function using cine CMR.

Step 2: Determine the presence or absence of hyperenhancement. In patients with severe ischemic cardiomyopathy, almost all patients have prior MI. This means that if patients with severe cardiomyopathy do not have hyperenhancement, the diagnosis of nonischemic cardiomyopathy should be strongly considered. Common conditions in which hyperenhancement is often absent include idiopathic dilated, alcoholic, Takotsubo, and peripartum cardiomyopathies.

Step 3: If hyperenhancement is present, the location and distribution of hyperenhancement should be classified as a CAD or non-CAD pattern. Understanding the physiology of ischemic injury, which progresses as a wavefront phenomenon from subendocardium to epicardium, is fundamental to distinguishing between these patterns. Hyperenhancement patterns that spare the subendocardium and are limited to the mid- or epicardial portion of the left ventricle are generally considered non-CAD patterns.

Step 4: If hyperenhancement is present in a non-CAD pattern, further classification is possible. There are now abundant data indicating that certain nonischemic cardiomyopathies have a predilection to produce specific LGE patterns. For example, in patients with left ventricular hypertrophy, the presence of midwall hyperenhancement in 1 or both junctions of the interventricular septum with the right ventricular free wall is highly suggestive of hypertrophic cardiomyopathy, whereas midwall or epicardial hyperenhancement in the inferolateral wall is consistent with Anderson-Fabry disease. It appears that a broad stratification into a limited number of common LGE MR patterns is possible.

Summary

Imaging Plays Important Role in Evaluation of Heart Failure

Diagnosis of HF is based on clinical features with TTE and CXR as supplementary tools.

In differentiating HFrEF from HFmEF and HFpEF, LVEF can be quantified using TTE and, in difficult or indeterminate cases, MR.

Establishing the etiology of HF: Ischemia as an etiology can be evaluated using anatomic techniques, such as coronary CTA and invasive angiography, or with functional techniques, such as stress echo, nuclear medicine (SPECT/PET), or MR. Further characterization of ischemic and nonischemic etiologies can performed using LGE MR, which shows different patterns of LGE.

Selected References

1. Heidenreich PA et al: 2022 AHA/ACC/HFSA guideline for the management of heart failure: a report of the American College of Cardiology/American Heart Association Joint Committee on Clinical Practice Guidelines. Circulation. 145(18):e895-1032, 2022
2. Argulian E et al: Advanced cardiovascular imaging in clinical heart failure. JACC Heart Fail. 9(10):699-709, 2021
3. Expert Panel on Cardiac Imaging et al: ACR appropriateness criteria suspected new-onset and known nonacute heart failure. J Am Coll Radiol. 15(11S):S418-31, 2018
4. Kanagala P et al: Diagnostic and prognostic utility of cardiovascular magnetic resonance imaging in heart failure with preserved ejection fraction - implications for clinical trials. J Cardiovasc Magn Reson. 20(1):4, 2018
5. Messroghli DR et al: Clinical recommendations for cardiovascular magnetic resonance mapping of T1, T2, T2* and extracellular volume: a consensus statement by the Society for Cardiovascular Magnetic Resonance (SCMR) endorsed by the European Association for Cardiovascular Imaging (EACVI). J Cardiovasc Magn Reson. 19(1):75, 2017
6. Patel AR et al: Role of cardiac magnetic resonance in the diagnosis and prognosis of nonischemic cardiomyopathy. JACC Cardiovasc Imaging. 10(10 Pt A):1180-93, 2017

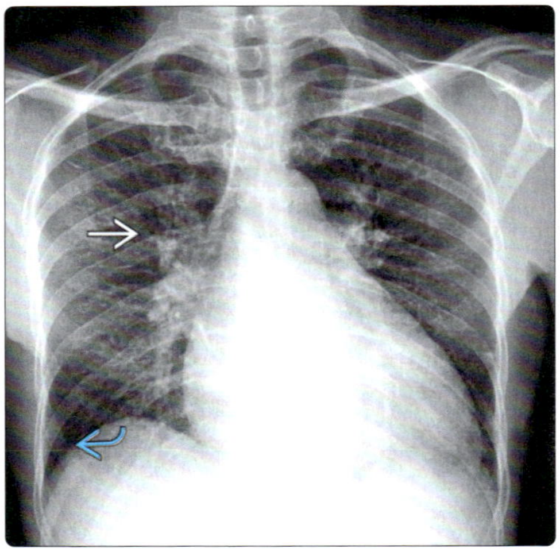

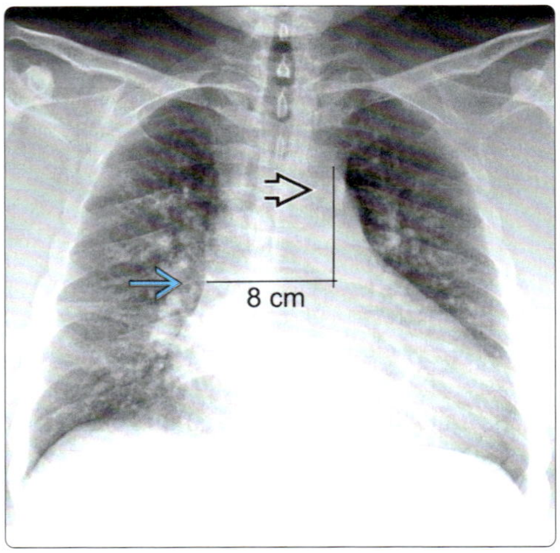

(Left) *Frontal view shows an enlarged cardiac silhouette, peribronchial cuffing →, and Kerley B lines ↩ (peripheral, short, horizontal lines perpendicular to pleural surface representing fluid within interlobular septa).* **(Right)** *Cardiomegaly, diminished clarity of pulmonary vasculature, and widened vascular pedicle are shown. A vertical line is drawn distal to the origin of the left subclavian artery ⇨, and the vascular pedicle width is measured across from where the superior vena cava meets right mainstem bronchus →.*

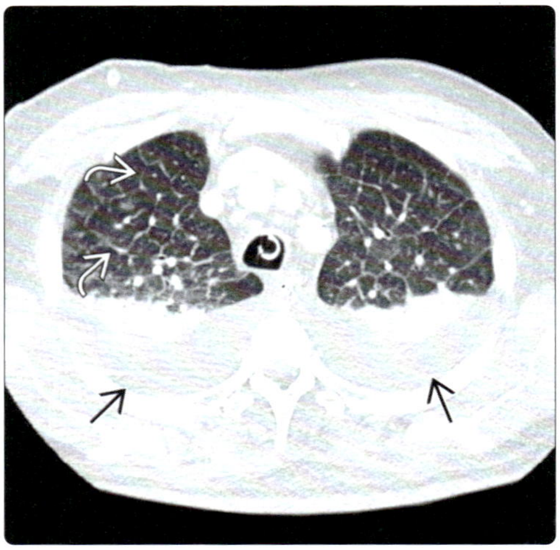

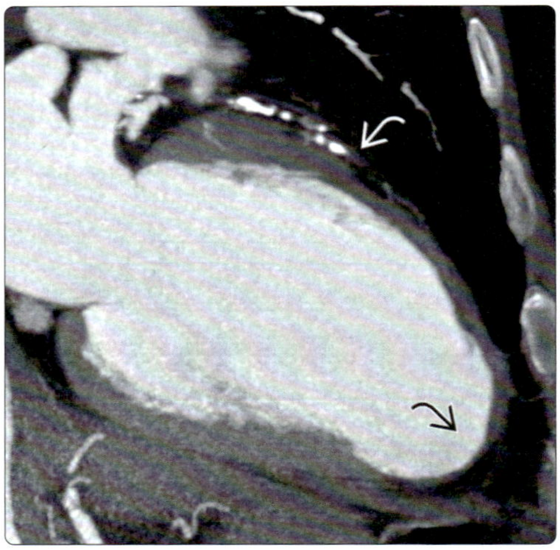

(Left) *Axial CECT shows findings of left ventricular failure with prominent smooth interlobular septal lines ↪ outlining the secondary pulmonary lobules and bilateral pleural effusions → evident.* **(Right)** *Vertical long-axis (2-chamber) coronary CTA shows occlusion of the left anterior descending coronary artery ↪ with resultant apical infarction and aneurysm formation ↪ that caused the patient's heart failure.*

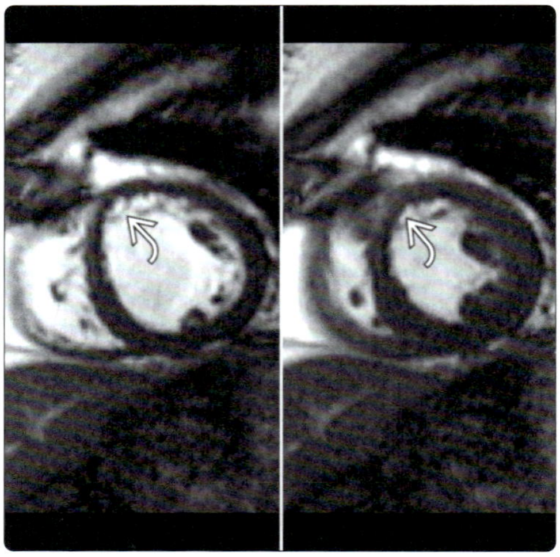

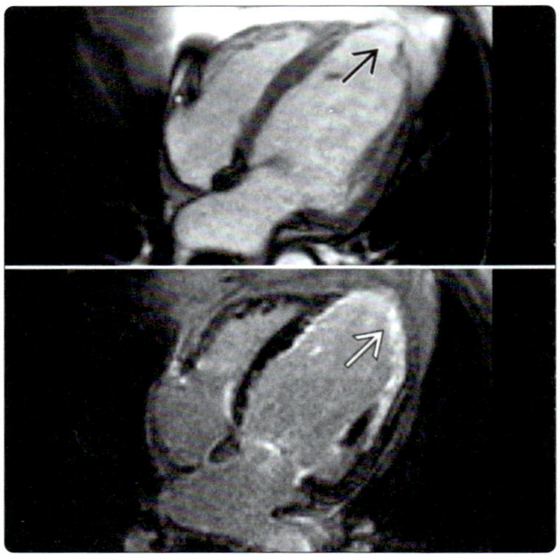

(Left) *Short-axis MR cine in diastole (left) and systole (right) demonstrates an area of wall thinning involving the anterior and anteroseptal walls ↪. Note the lack of change between systole and diastole, which is indicative of impaired wall motion.* **(Right)** *Four-chamber view cine SSFP (top) and LGE MR (bottom) show findings of prior apical infarction evident as thinning → on cine and as abnormal enhancement → on the LGE image. The apex was dyskinetic as well, further impairing cardiac output.*

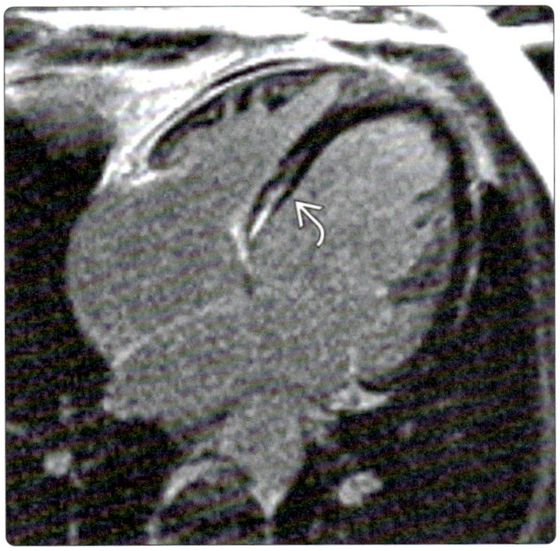

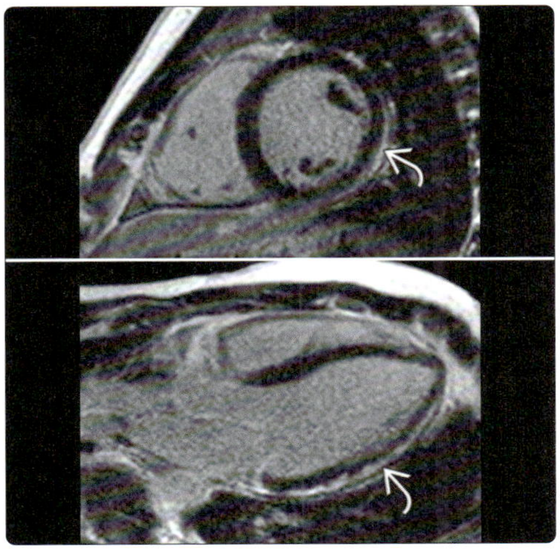

(Left) *Four-chamber view LGE MR from a patient with dilated nonischemic cardiomyopathy shows a midwall stripe pattern of uptake* ➔. *This is clearly different from an ischemic (subendocardial) pattern, which allows this entity to be differentiated from ischemic cardiomyopathy.* **(Right)** *Short-axis LGE (top) and LVOT LGE MR (bottom) of a patient with viral myocarditis show epicardial enhancement* ➔ *in a noncoronary distribution.*

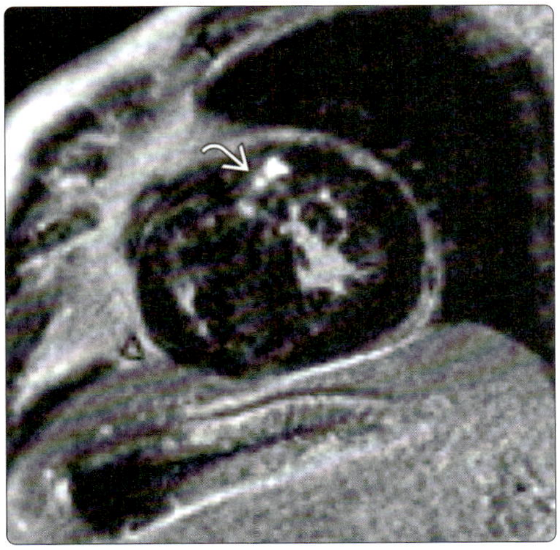

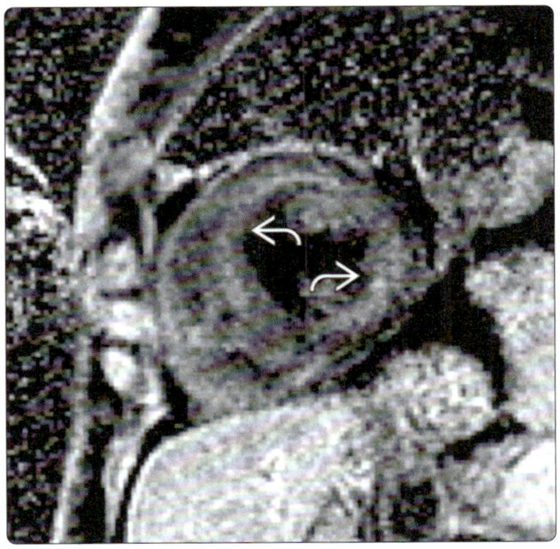

(Left) *Short-axis LGE MR of a patient with the asymmetric septal variant of hypertrophic cardiomyopathy demonstrates abnormal enhancement of the right ventricular insertion site* ➔ *upon the septum. This pattern is common in hypertrophic cardiomyopathy and clearly differs from a coronary injury pattern.* **(Right)** *Short-axis LGE MR from a patient with amyloidosis shows the typical diffuse subendocardial pattern of enhancement* ➔ *seen in this disorder. Note the dark appearance of the blood pool.*

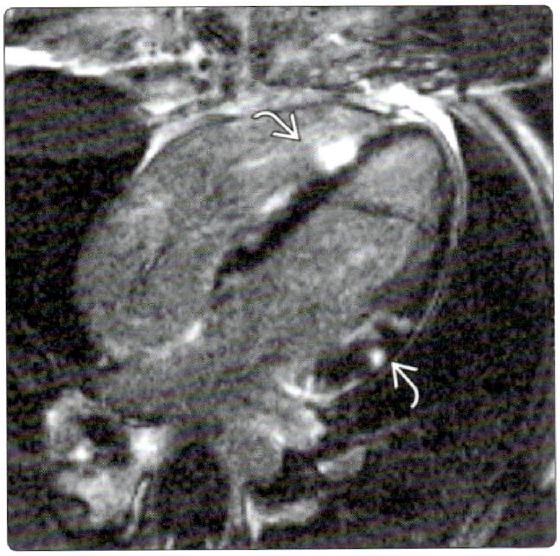

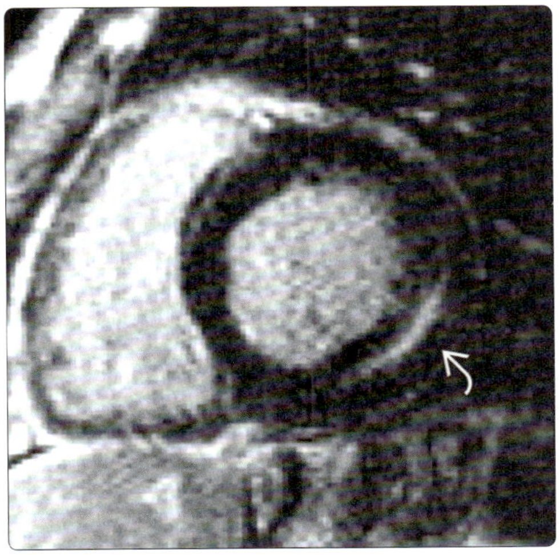

(Left) *Four-chamber view LGE MR from a patient with cardiac sarcoidosis shows patchy foci of abnormal enhancement* ➔ *in the septum and lateral wall in a noncoronary artery pattern.* **(Right)** *Short-axis LGE MR of a patient with Fabry disease shows characteristic concentric thickening as well as abnormal subepicardial enhancement of the basal inferolateral wall* ➔ *with subendocardial sparing, which differentiates this from the coronary artery disease pattern.*

KEY FACTS

TERMINOLOGY

- Right ventricular (RV) dysfunction that results in 1 or both of following
  - Inadequate RV systolic forward flow to maintain normal cardiac output
  - Diastolic filling impairment that results in abnormally high venous filling pressures
- Most often due to either left heart failure or pulmonary hypertension (PH)

IMAGING

- Echocardiography is best screening tool; MR provides best noninvasive evaluation of RV function
- Right heart catheterization is best differentiator of causes of PH
- CXR: Signs of underlying PH, including dilated main and hilar pulmonary arteries, may be seen on frontal and lateral views
  - RV enlargement is demonstrated as increased filling of retrosternal clear space on lateral view
- CT/MR: Contrast refluxing into enlarged hepatic veins indicates diastolic impairment or tricuspid regurgitation
- Cine MR: Gold standard for assessing RV volumes and RV ejection fraction
- LGE imaging: Shows enhancement at sites of RV insertion in septum
- Acute right heart failure may be seen with massive pulmonary emboli

TOP DIFFERENTIAL DIAGNOSES

- Isolated left heart failure
- Constrictive pericarditis
- Atrial septal defects/partial anomalous pulmonary venous return
- Pulmonic stenosis
- Noncardiogenic edema

(Left) *Posteroanterior (left) and lateral (right) radiographs in a patient with idiopathic pulmonary arterial hypertension (PAH) demonstrate marked enlargement of the main and hilar pulmonary arteries. Note that the heart size is normal on the frontal image and that the significant right ventricular (RV) enlargement is only apparent on the lateral view.* **(Right)** *Coronal CECT of PAH and RV overload demonstrates enlarged pulmonary arteries and reflux of contrast into the hepatic veins.*

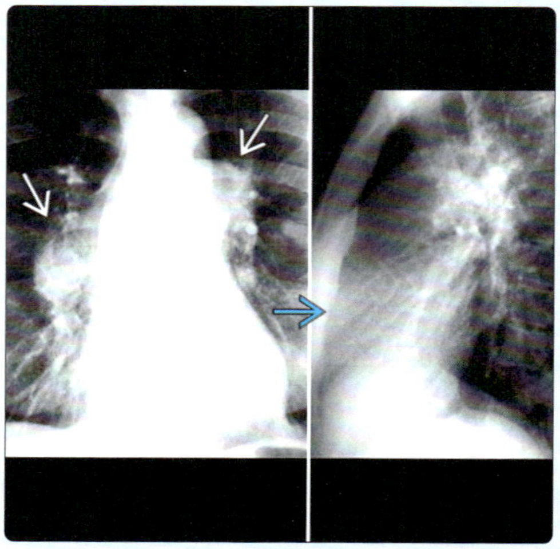

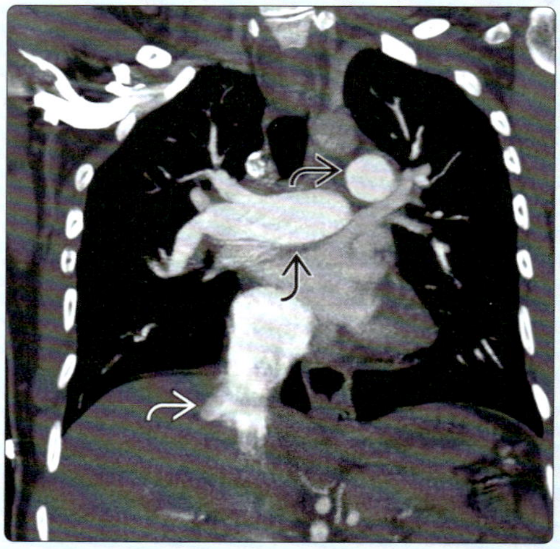

(Left) *Axial CECT in a patient with PAH shows an enlarged RV and right atrium (RA) and ventricular septal bowing to the left, indicative of elevated RV pressure.* **(Right)** *Four-chamber cine MR (top) and LGE MR (bottom) in a patient with biventricular enlargement and failure due to ischemic cardiomyopathy show extensive abnormal LGE of the left ventricular (LV) apex, consistent with prior infarction. Most cases of right heart failure result from left heart failure.*

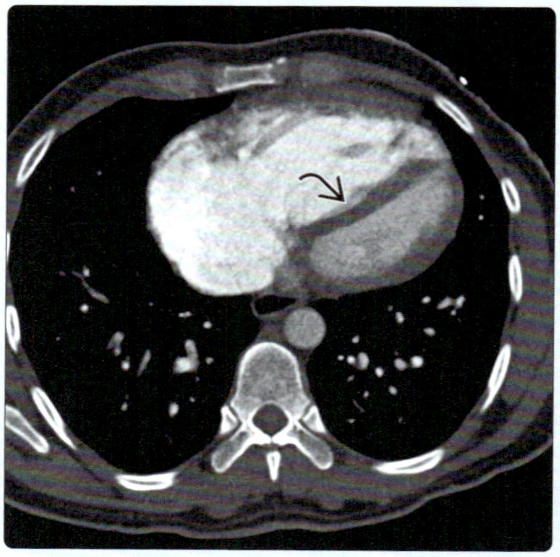

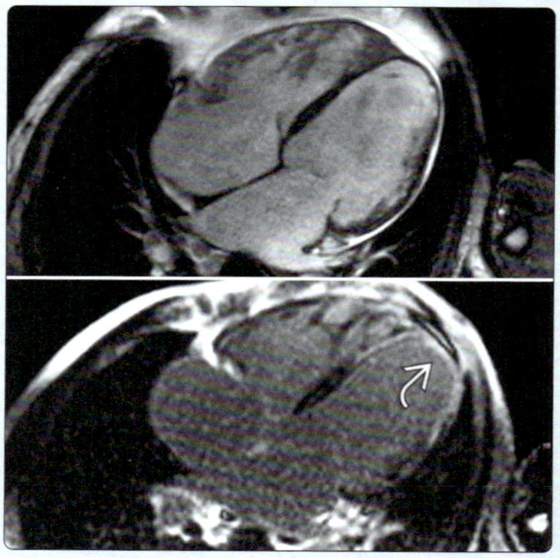

TERMINOLOGY

Abbreviations

- Right heart failure (RHF)

Definitions

- Right ventricular (RV) dysfunction that results in inadequate RV systolic forward flow to maintain normal cardiac output, diastolic filling impairment leading to abnormally high venous filling pressures, or both
  - Forward and backward components of RHF often coexist but manifest differently
    - Forward failure manifests as decreased RV ejection fraction (RVEF), increased pulmonary circulation time, decreased pulmonary artery (PA) velocity
    - Backward failure results in peripheral edema, hepatic congestion, ascites, pleural effusions
- Most often due to either left heart failure (LHF) or pulmonary hypertension (PH)
- Often from PH resulting in maladaptive RV hypertrophy and later failure
  - Cor pulmonale = RV failure due to pulmonary parenchymal or vascular disease
  - Acute RHF may be seen with massive pulmonary emboli
- RHF occurring without LHF is identified when abnormally high right atrial pressures are accompanied by normal capillary wedge pressures

IMAGING

General Features

- Best diagnostic clue
  - Impaired RV function (estimated by RVEF)
    - MR is gold standard for measurement of RV function, volumes, and mass
      - Alternatives include echocardiography and nuclear scintigraphic techniques
- Size
  - Abnormal RV enlargement; RV diameter > corresponding left ventricular diameter at same level
- Morphology
  - Increase in RV sphericity is often seen as RV enlargement progresses

Radiographic Findings

- Radiography
  - RV is not usually evident on frontal radiograph
    - Widening of vascular pedicle is often apparent, indicating central venous engorgement
      - Azygos vein may become prominent
  - RV enlargement is demonstrated as increased filling of retrosternal clear space on lateral view
  - Signs of underlying PH, including dilated main and hilar PAs, may be seen on frontal and lateral views
  - As RHF and LHF frequently coexist and are often causally related, signs of LHF may be present
    - Cardiomegaly, vascular redistribution, and interstitial and alveolar edema

CT Findings

- NECT
  - Coexisting or causative lung disease (severe fibrosis, emphysema, etc.) is usually readily apparent
  - Dilated inferior vena cava (IVC), ascites, peripheral edema, and anasarca may be seen
- CECT
  - Retrospectively gated cardiac CT can demonstrate decreased RV function
  - Enlargement of right-sided structures (RV, right atrium, and systemic veins) is often seen with systolic dysfunction
  - Contrast refluxing into enlarged IVC and hepatic veins may indicate diastolic impairment or tricuspid regurgitation
  - Underlying PH (when present) causes dilatation of main and hilar PAs
  - CT pulmonary angiography may show pulmonary emboli &/or findings suggestive of chronic pulmonary thromboembolic disease

MR Findings

- MRA
  - Chronic PH results in dilatation of main and hilar PAs
  - Perfusion defects may be seen in lungs
- MR cine
  - RV systolic function is typically decreased
  - Impaired diastolic function can be evaluated using through-plane flow studies of tricuspid and mitral valves
  - Radius of septal curvature during systole can be used to estimate relative PA and aortic pressures
    - Progressive flattening with greater degrees of PH
  - Flattening of septum during diastole usually due to increased RV volumes
  - Right atrial pressure is estimated by size of IVC
  - Morphologic abnormalities (e.g., arrhythmogenic cardiomyopathy, congenital heart diseases) and valvular abnormalities (tricuspid/pulmonic regurgitation) can also be assessed
- Delayed enhancement
  - Enhancement is often noted at sites of RV insertion in septum
  - Myocardial infarction: Subendocardial or transmural LGE in vascular territory in left ventricle/RV
  - Different patterns of LGE in nonischemic cardiomyopathies
- Normal RV functional parameters
  - RV end-diastolic volume index: 82 ± 21 ml/m2 (men); 70 ± 17 ml/m2 (women)
  - RV end-systolic volume index: 34 ± 11 ml/m2 (men); 37 ± 11 ml/m2 (women)
  - RV free wall mass: 41 (men), 35 (women) ± 8 gm; (21± 4 gm/m^2)
  - RVEF: 56% ± 6%
  - RV stroke volume index: 42 ± 11 ml/m2 (men); 45 ± 12 ml/m2 (women)
- Phase-contrast imaging
  - Provides velocity and flow information; noninvasive hemodynamics
  - RA pressure can be indirectly estimated from superior vena cava
- Strain imaging
  - Early detection of RV functional abnormalities

- Feature tracking can be performed from routine cine images

Echocardiographic Findings

- Echocardiogram
  - Common screening technique for PH and congenital heart disease
    - RV systolic pressure (which reflects PA pressure) is calculated by measuring tricuspid regurgitant jet velocity
    - Decreased RV outflow tract acceleration time
    - Dilated IVC and hepatic veins
- Pulsed Doppler
  - Tricuspid plane systolic excursion and peak velocity of D wave correlate well with RVEF

Angiographic Findings

- Conventional right heart catheterization (RHC) is gold standard for diagnosis of PH
  - PH: Systolic pressure > 20 mmHg (at rest)
  - PA hypertension (PAH) is present when pulmonary vascular resistance > 2 Woods units, and pulmonary capillary wedge pressure (PCWP) ≤ 15 mmHg
  - Left ventricular dysfunction is evaluated by PCWP measurement

Imaging Recommendations

- Best imaging tool
  - Echocardiography common screening tool
  - MR provides best noninvasive evaluation of RV function and volumes
  - RHC is best differentiator of causes of PH

DIFFERENTIAL DIAGNOSIS

Isolated Left Heart Failure

- Acute or chronic left heart dysfunction may result in RHF

Constrictive Pericarditis

- Produces similar clinical findings (dilated IVC, leg edema, hepatic congestion)
- Distinction from RHF can be made with MR
  - Recognized by abnormal pericardial thickening (> 4 mm) and adhesions between layers
    - Constriction can occur without pericardial thickening
  - "Septal bounce" noted on cine imaging suggests altered hemodynamics
    - Real-time cine imaging during deep inspiration showing septal inversion directly demonstrates abnormal hemodynamics

Atrial Septal Defects/Partial Anomalous Pulmonary Venous Return

- Typically, produce enlargement of right atrium and RV, but function is preserved

Congenital Pulmonary Stenosis

- Produces RV hypertrophy and PA enlargement
  - Left PA is often larger than right PA due to direction of flow jet

Noncardiogenic Edema

- End-stage liver disease with ascites and pleural effusions, renal disease

PATHOLOGY

General Features

- Etiology
  - Most common cause is LHF (myocardial infarction, ischemic cardiomyopathy, etc.)
  - PH is 2nd most common cause
  - Volume overload: Valvular dysfunction (tricuspid regurgitation, pulmonary insufficiency) or shunts (atrial septal defects, partial anomalous pulmonary venous return)
  - Congenital heart disease
  - Primary RV cardiomyopathy/infarction

Staging, Grading, & Classification

- Class I: No limitation during ordinary activity
- Class II: Slight limitation by shortness of breath ± fatigue during moderate exertion
- Class III: Symptoms with minimal exertion that interfere with normal daily activity
- Class IV: Inability to carry out physical activity; patients typically have marked neurohumoral activation, muscle wasting, and reduced oxygen consumption

Gross Pathologic & Surgical Features

- RV is often dilated and hypertrophied

CLINICAL ISSUES

Presentation

- Most common signs/symptoms
  - Fatigue, lethargy, and dyspnea
  - Lower extremity edema, ascites, and weight gain are seen in chronic RHF
  - Symptoms reflect underlying illness precipitating RHF (COPD, pulmonary embolism, etc.)
- Other signs/symptoms
  - Loud P2 on auscultation indicates PH

Demographics

- Epidemiology
  - Commonly result of LHF
  - Major source of morbidity and mortality

Natural History & Prognosis

- Outcome of RHF most often depends on prognosis of underlying left heart dysfunction or precipitating pulmonary disease

Treatment

- Patients with LHF: Standard CHF therapy with diuretics, afterload reduction, ACE inhibitors, β-blockers
- Patients with cor pulmonale: Treatment of underlying lung disease, hypoxia (oxygen therapy)
- Patients with PAH: Endothelin receptor antagonists (bosentan), phosphodiesterase inhibitor (sildenafil), prostacyclin analogues, inotropes

SELECTED REFERENCES

1. Addetia K et al: Normal values of three-dimensional right ventricular size and function measurements: results of the World Alliance Societies of Echocardiography study. J Am Soc Echocardiogr. 36(8):858-66.e1, 2023
2. Houston BA et al: Right ventricular failure. N Engl J Med. 388(12):1111-25, 2023

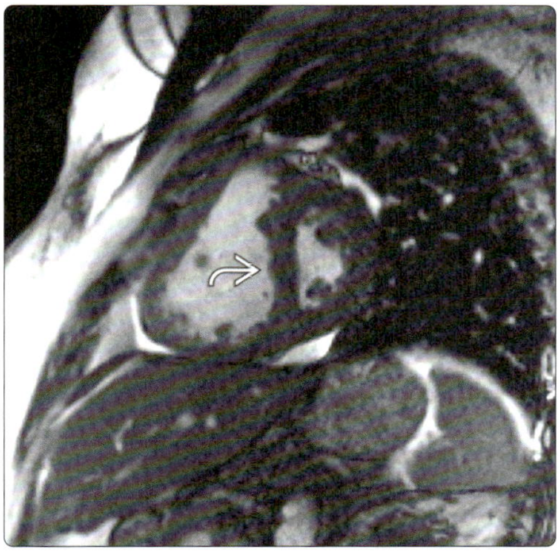
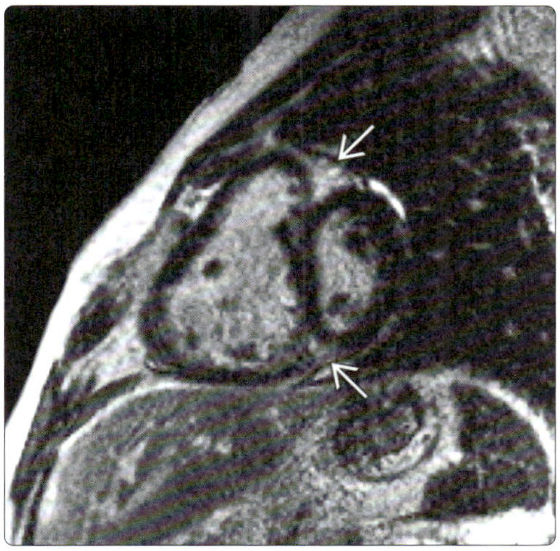

(Left) *Short-axis systolic cine MR in a patient with severe pulmonary hypertension associated with extensive fibrotic lung disease (cor pulmonale) shows systolic flattening of the septum, indicating equilibration of pulmonary and systemic pressures. The radius of septal curvature on MR cine images correlates with pulmonary artery pressures.* **(Right)** *Short-axis LGE MR in the same patient shows typical abnormal enhancement at the RV insertion sites on the septum.*

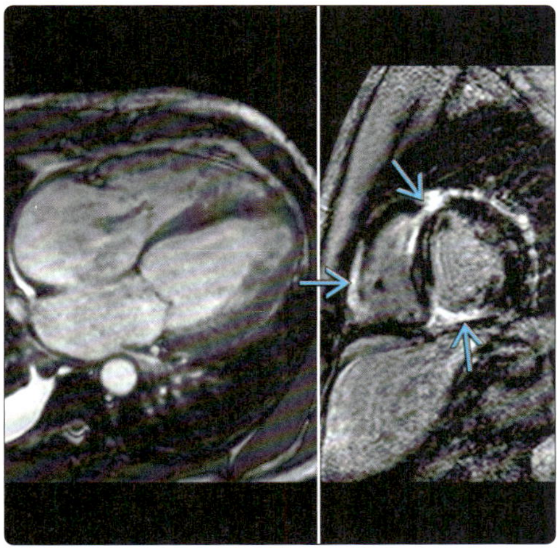
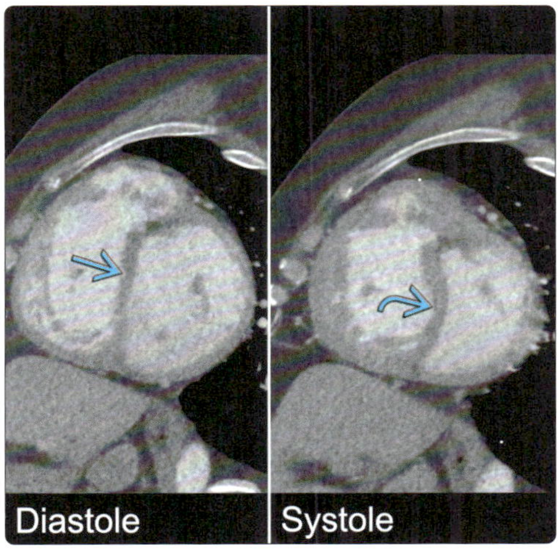

(Left) *End-systole SSFP MR (left) shows poor biventricular function. The LV ejection fraction (EF) = 21% and the RVEF = 24%. Short-axis LGE MR (right) shows extensive biventricular subepicardial to transmural delayed enhancement due to biopsy proven sarcoidosis.* **(Right)** *Patient with D-transposition status post atrial switch shows diastolic flattening of the interventricular septum due to elevated RV volumes. During systole, there is septal inversion due to elevated RV pressures.*

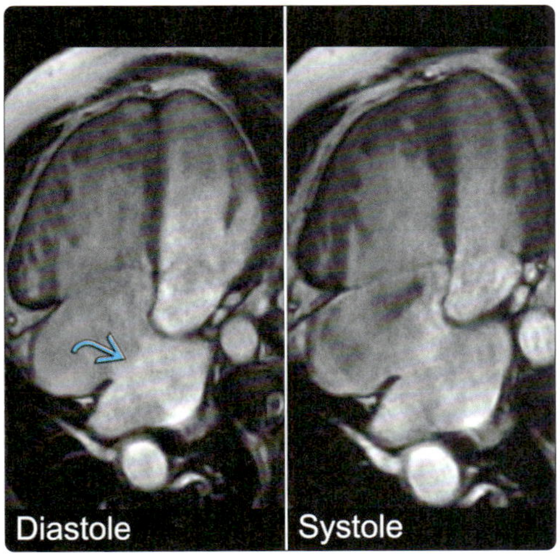

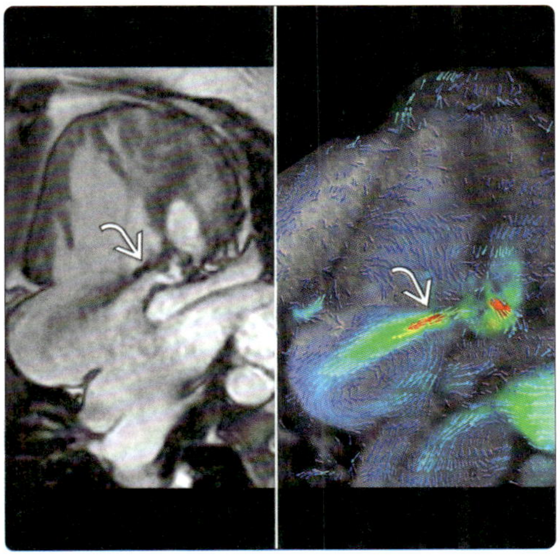

(Left) *SSFP MR images in the same patient (atrial baffle) show severe RV hypertrophy and dilation with septal flattening and inversion during diastole and systole, respectively. The RV end-diastolic volume was 271 ml/m2 and the RVEF was 23%. The RV is ill-suited to handle systemic arterial pressures, leading to RV failure in these patients.* **(Right)** *In the same patient, a Gerbode defect between the LV outflow tract and RA also contributed to RV failure.*

Left Heart Failure

KEY FACTS

TERMINOLOGY

- Pathophysiologic state in which left ventricle is unable to pump blood at rate sufficient to meet oxygen needs of end organs

IMAGING

- Radiography
  - Enlarged cardiac silhouette with pulmonary edema and pleural effusions
  - Increased pulmonary artery:bronchus ratio
  - Kerley B lines
- CT
  - Thickening of interlobular septa
  - Bronchovascular bundle thickening
  - Ground-glass opacities
  - Enlarged hilar nodes
- CTA
  - May demonstrate underlying cause of congestive heart failure (CHF)
- MR cine
  - Decreased stroke volume and ejection fraction
- LGE MR
  - Used to identify viable and nonviable myocardium
  - May demonstrate ischemic or nonischemic etiology of CHF
- Stress cardiac MR for detection of coronary artery disease
- MR also used for prognosis, risk stratification, and monitoring therapy
- Echocardiography
  - 1st-line diagnostic test in evaluation of heart failure per ACC/AHA guidelines
- Decreased ejection fraction with systolic dysfunction
- Decreased compliance with diastolic dysfunction

TOP DIFFERENTIAL DIAGNOSES

- Noncardiogenic pulmonary edema
- Pericardial effusion

(Left) *PA radiograph of a patient with left heart failure shows cardiomegaly (with an enlarged cardiothoracic ratio), cephalization of pulmonary blood flow, and interstitial edema. Kerley B lines and small pleural effusions ➔ are also apparent.* **(Right)** *Coronal reformat CECT in a patient with left ventricular (LV) failure shows prominent interlobular septal lines in the upper lobes bilaterally ➔, demarcating the secondary pulmonary lobules. These reflect the presence of interstitial edema with lymphatic distention.*

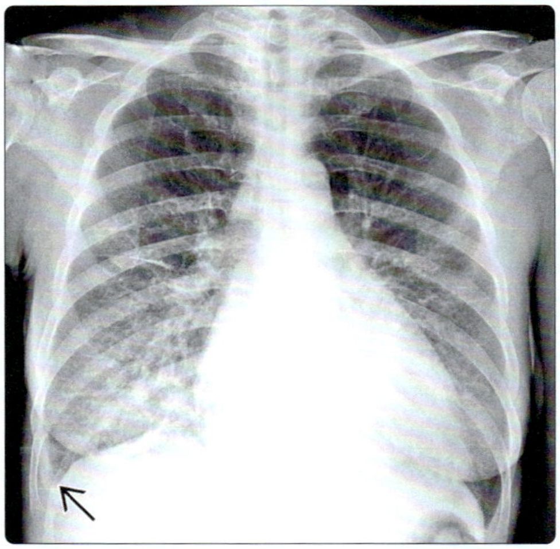

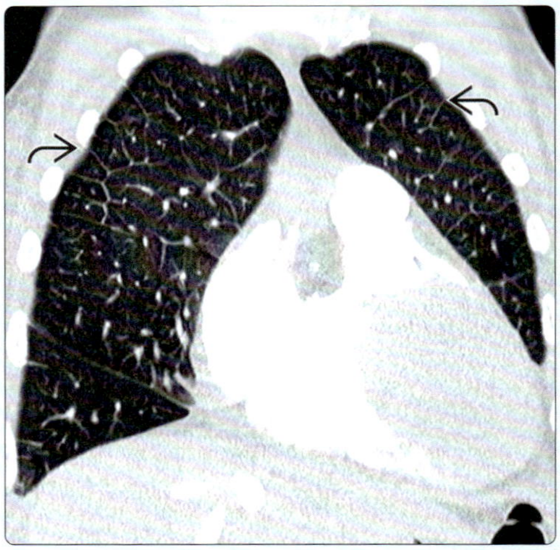

(Left) *Axial CECT in a patient with LV failure demonstrates an abnormal pulmonary artery:bronchus ratio ➔ with the arterial branch clearly larger than the adjacent bronchus. The faint ground-glass opacities ➔ noted represent alveolar edema. Small pleural effusions ➔ are also noted.* **(Right)** *Axial CECT shows bilateral pleural effusions ➔, interstitial edema with bronchial cuffing ➔, and a dilated LV with subendocardial rest perfusion defect ➔ in a patient with LV failure due to ischemic cardiomyopathy.*

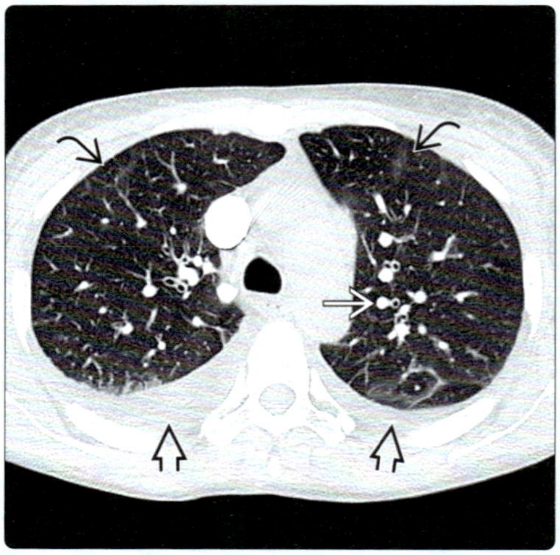

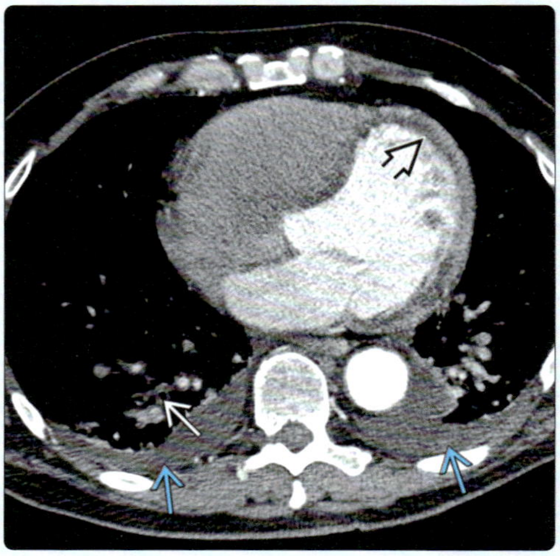

TERMINOLOGY

Synonyms

- Left ventricular (LV) failure
- Congestive heart failure (CHF)
  - CHF often used interchangeably with LV failure: LV failure should be differentiated from biventricular and right ventricular (RV) failure

Definitions

- Pathophysiologic state: Abnormality of myocardial function responsible for failure of heart to pump blood at rate commensurate with requirements of metabolizing tissues during ordinary activity
- HF with reduced ejection fraction (EF) (HFrEF; previously known as systolic HF): Decrease in myocardial contractility
- HF with preserved EF (HFpEF; previously known as diastolic HF): LVEF is preserved; there is usually abnormal decrease in LV diastolic distensibility

IMAGING

General Features

- Best diagnostic clue
  - Cardiomegaly with pulmonary venous hypertension (Kerley lines, redistribution, pulmonary edema, effusion) on chest radiograph

Radiographic Findings

- Radiography
  - Chest radiograph demonstrates enlarged cardiac silhouette with pulmonary edema and, possibly, pleural effusions
    - Cardiothoracic ratio > 0.50 (transverse diameter of cardiac silhouette divided by that of inner rib cage at diaphragms) neither sensitive nor specific for cardiomegaly
  - Rough correlation of pulmonary capillary wedge pressure with chest radiograph findings
    - Pulmonary venous redistribution (larger apical veins, smaller basal veins): Pulmonary venous pressure = 18-23 mmHg
    - Kerley B lines: Pulmonary venous pressure = 20-25 mmHg
    - Alveolar edema with "butterfly" or "batwing" distribution ± effusions: Pulmonary venous pressure > 25 mmHg
  - Azygos, superior vena cava, and inferior vena cava distention if biventricular or RV failure

CT Findings

- NECT
  - Readily apparent cardiomegaly
    - Coronary calcifications signifying coronary artery disease may be seen in ischemic cardiomyopathy (ICM)
  - Increased pulmonary artery:bronchus ratio
  - Mildly enlarged hilar nodes = reactive
- HRCT
  - Thickening of interlobular septa
  - Bronchovascular bundle thickening
  - Ground-glass or airspace opacities, most prominent in dependent portions of lungs
- Cardiac gated CTA
  - May demonstrate underlying cardiac cause of failure
    - Myocardial infarction (thinning, calcification, fatty metaplasia, subendocardial perfusion defects)
    - LV dilatation indicating dilated cardiomyopathy
    - Mitral valve disorders
    - Coronary artery disease
- Delayed enhancement CT
  - Different patterns of delayed enhancement may be seen similar to LGE MR
  - Improved detection with dual-energy CT
- Extracellular volume
  - Increased extracellular volume can be seen in single- or dual-energy CT technique; correlates with MR

MR Findings

- Functional findings are similar to those of echocardiography, but MR is more precise in quantifying myocardial functional parameters (e.g., stroke volume, EF) and ventricular sizes
  - Some cardiomyopathies can be distinguished based on morphology, e.g., hypertrophic cardiomyopathy (HCM), Takotsubo, LV noncompaction, congenital heart disease
- LGE MR may also be used to identify viable and nonviable myocardial tissue
- LGE MR can often distinguish dilated non-ICM (NICM) from ICM
  - Patients with significantly reduced LVEF (< 35%) due to ICM will almost always have discernible foci of abnormality on LGE MR
  - Patients with dilated NICM usually show normal LGE MR pattern (60%) or midwall stripe pattern (28-30%) different from ICM
- May demonstrate and characterize other nonischemic causes of LV failure: HCM, infiltrative cardiomyopathies (e.g., amyloid), myocarditis, Takotsubo disease, etc.
  - Different patterns of LGE seen in nonischemic disorders
  - Midmyocardial (linear, patchy), subepicardial, RV insertion points, diffuse subendocardial
  - Presence and amount of scar is adverse prognostic indicator
- Viability on LGE MR may be used to predict response to β-blocker therapy and revascularization
- Stress CMR imaging, using vasodilator stress agent, has emerged as useful tool in assessment of physiologic significance of coronary artery disease in symptomatic intermediate- to high-risk patients
- Parametric mapping
  - Native T1 mapping is useful in early identification of fibrosis, particularly diffuse fibrosis: Increased T1
  - Extracellular volume is increased in fibrosis; calculated from pre- and postcontrast T1 along with hematocrit
  - T2 value is increased in myocardial edema
- MR may be used for prognostication, risk stratification, and to monitor therapy

Echocardiographic Findings

- Echocardiogram
  - Echocardiography with Doppler flow imaging is considered most useful diagnostic test in evaluation of heart failure patients (per ACC/AHA Chronic Heart Failure Evaluation and Management Guidelines)

- Determination of LV function
- Abnormalities of pericardium, myocardium, and valves
- Findings vary depending on etiology
- Decreased EF with systolic dysfunction
- Decreased compliance with diastolic dysfunction

Nuclear Medicine Findings

- Radionuclide ventriculography is alternative diagnostic test to evaluate LV function (ACC/AHA CHF Guidelines)

Imaging Recommendations

- Best imaging tool
  - MR is best means of distinguishing ischemic from NICM
    - MR can also characterize different types of cardiomyopathies

DIFFERENTIAL DIAGNOSIS

Noncardiogenic Pulmonary Edema

- Acute respiratory distress syndrome
- Neurogenic pulmonary edema
- May closely resemble CHF, but heart size is usually normal, and effusions are usually absent

Pericardial Effusion

- Enlarged cardiac silhouette on chest radiograph
- May have clear lungs

PATHOLOGY

General Features

- Etiology
  - Causes of CHF
    - Myocardial ischemia/infarction
    - NICM (dilated, restrictive/infiltrative, hypertrophic, noncompaction)
    - Myocarditis
    - Arrhythmias
    - Congenital heart disease
    - Valvular heart disease
    - High-output states
      - Anemia, valvular heart disease, papillary muscle rupture, thyrotoxicosis
      - Vein of Galen aneurysm/other congenital arteriovenous fistulae in neonates
- Genetics
  - Dilated and hypertrophic cardiomyopathies are known to show some familial inheritance pattern (e.g., muscular dystrophies)

Staging, Grading, & Classification

- New York Heart Association (NYHA) classification
  - Class I: No limitation during ordinary activity
  - Class II: Comfortable at rest; slight limitation by shortness of breath, palpitation, dyspnea, or angina during ordinary physical activity
  - Class III: Comfortable at rest; symptoms with minimal exertion that interfere with normal daily activity
  - Class IV: Unable to carry out any physical activity; patients typically have marked neurohumoral activation, muscle wasting, and reduced peak oxygen consumption

Gross Pathologic & Surgical Features

- Areas of infarcted myocardium in ischemic systolic dysfunction
- Variety of other pathologies in alternative types of cardiac dysfunction

Microscopic Features

- Infarcted areas of myocardium in ischemic heart failure
- Infiltrating diseases in restrictive cardiomyopathy

CLINICAL ISSUES

Presentation

- Most common signs/symptoms
  - Dyspnea on exertion/shortness of breath at rest
  - Jugular vein distention
  - Pulmonary rales/cough
  - Orthopnea
  - Tachycardia
- Other signs/symptoms
  - Nocturia/paroxysmal nocturnal dyspnea
  - Fatigue
  - Cerebral symptoms: Confusion, memory loss
  - Pleural effusions

Demographics

- Age
  - Can affect any age; more common in older adults
- Epidemiology
  - Among leading causes of death in USA

Natural History & Prognosis

- Prognosis worsens with increasing NYHA class

Treatment

- Diuretics, ACE inhibitors, β-blockers, and inotropic agents are commonly used
- Treat underlying coronary disease

DIAGNOSTIC CHECKLIST

Consider

- Pulmonary venous redistribution and azygos vein diameter may not be evaluable on nonupright radiographs

Image Interpretation Pearls

- RV or biventricular failure can be differentiated from LV failure by presence (RV failure) or absence (LV failure) of distended systemic veins (e.g., inferior vena cava, superior vena cava, azygos vein) on CXR, CT, or MR

SELECTED REFERENCES

1. Del Torto A et al: Advances in multimodality cardiovascular imaging in the diagnosis of heart failure with preserved ejection fraction. Front Cardiovasc Med. 9:758975, 2022
2. Di Cesare E et al: Multimodality imaging in chronic heart failure. Radiol Med. 126(2):231-42, 2021
3. Messroghli DR et al: Clinical recommendations for cardiovascular magnetic resonance mapping of T1, T2, T2* and extracellular volume: a consensus statement by the Society for Cardiovascular Magnetic Resonance (SCMR) endorsed by the European Association for Cardiovascular Imaging (EACVI). J Cardiovasc Magn Reson. 19(1):75, 2017

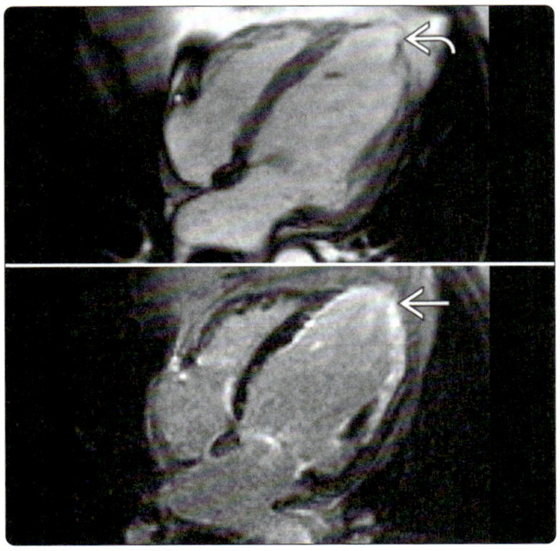

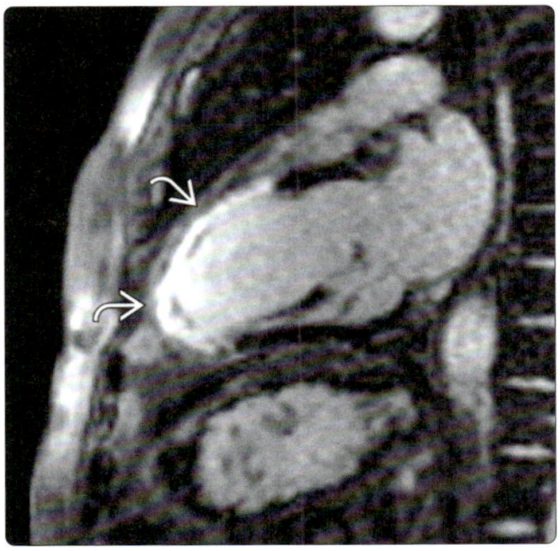

(Left) *Four-chamber cine (top) and LGE (bottom) MR images in a patient with ischemic cardiomyopathy show thinning and dilatation of the LV apex due to prior myocardial infarction, as demonstrated by transmural enhancement on LGE MR.* **(Right)** *Vertical long-axis (2-chamber) LGE MR in a patient with ischemic cardiomyopathy demonstrates an anterior wall infarction noted by extensive subendocardial enhancement of the anterior wall and apex. The infarction is in the left anterior descending (LAD) territory.*

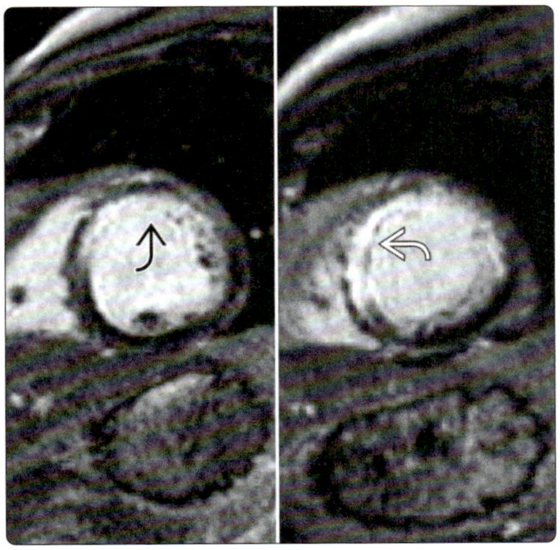

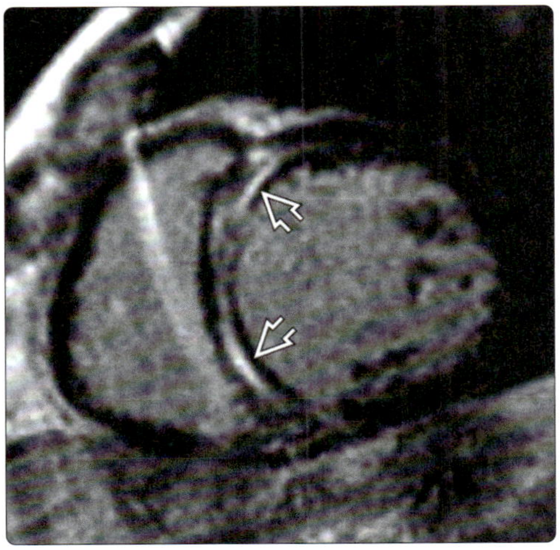

(Left) *Short-axis LGE MR images at midventricular (left) and apical (right) levels show subendocardial enhancement of the anterior wall and transmural enhancement of anteroseptum, signifying LAD territory infarction.* **(Right)** *Short-axis LGE MR in a patient with dilated nonischemic cardiomyopathy demonstrates a linear stripe of hyperenhancement that is limited to the midwall of the interventricular septum. This pattern is clearly different from an ischemic pattern, which would involve the subendocardium.*

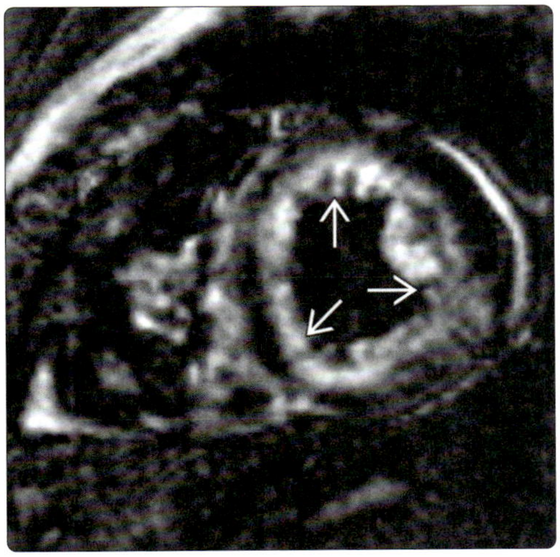

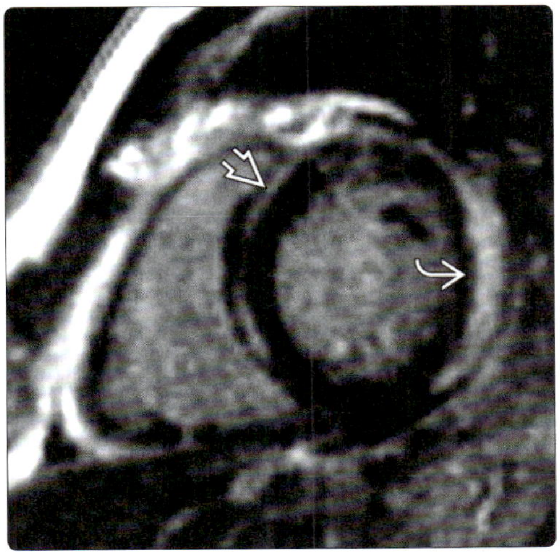

(Left) *Short-axis LGE MR in a patient with congestive heart failure shows diffuse LGE affecting the endocardial 1/2 of the myocardium throughout the entire left ventricle, consistent with cardiac amyloidosis.* **(Right)** *Short-axis LGE MR in a patient with new-onset heart failure due to viral myocarditis shows 2 regions of hyperenhancement: A linear midwall stripe in the interventricular septum and a large confluent region affecting the epicardial 1/2 of the LV lateral wall.*

Left Ventricular Hypertrophy

KEY FACTS

TERMINOLOGY

- ↑ in left ventricular (LV) wall thickness &/or myocardial mass due to ↑ cardiac myocyte size

IMAGING

- Echocardiogram is often initial imaging test for evaluation of LV morphology and function
  - ↑ myocardial mass; ↑ wall thickness
  - Assessment of LV wall thickness (LVWT) can be limited if images are of poor resolution (i.e., limited acoustic windows)
- Cardiac MR is useful if there are equivocal findings on echocardiography
- MR used for establishing diagnosis, determining LV geometry, establishing etiology, quantification, risk stratification, serial follow-up, treatment response

PATHOLOGY

- Primary causes (due to genetic factors)
  - Hypertrophic cardiomyopathy
- Secondary causes
  - Hypertension, aortic stenosis, obesity, athlete's heart
- Characterization of hypertrophy
  - Concentric hypertrophy: Uniform ↑ in wall thickness; different thresholds for men and women
  - Asymmetric hypertrophy
  - Eccentric hypertrophy: Normal or reduced wall thickness with ↑ LV cavity size

CLINICAL ISSUES

- Population studies estimate prevalence of LV hypertrophy (LVH) of 15-21%
- LVH is independent predictor of cardiac mortality regardless of underlying etiology

DIAGNOSTIC CHECKLIST

- Consider hypertrophic cardiomyopathy or infiltrative heart disease in patients without significant hypertension or valvular heart disease

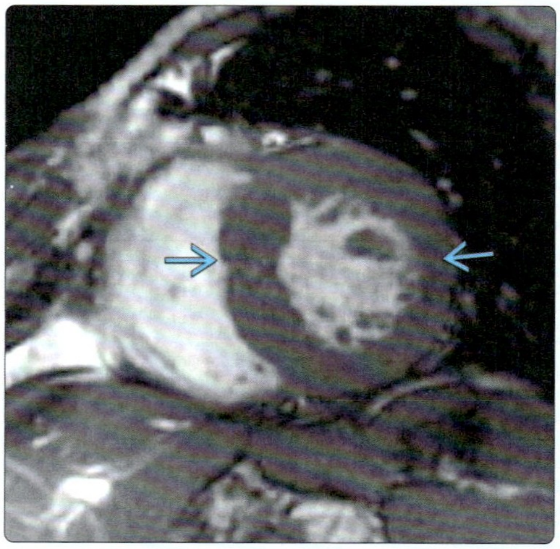
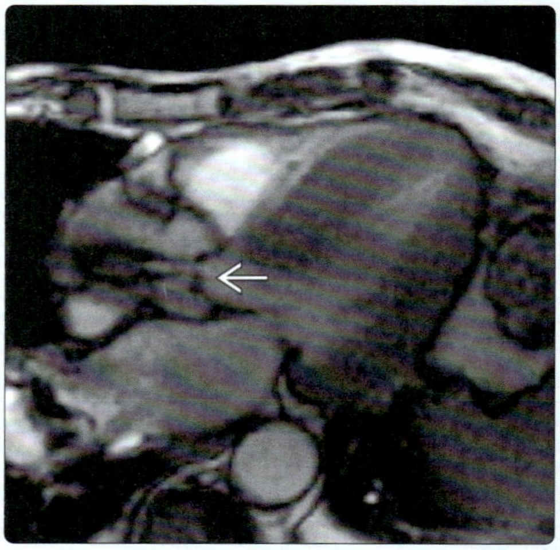

(Left) *Short-axis MR cine shows moderate concentric left ventricular hypertrophy* → *in an older adult man with heart failure and aortic stenosis.* **(Right)** *Three-chamber view MR cine in the same patient shows a thickened aortic valve with restricted leaflet excursion and an associated dephasing artifact due to turbulent flow across the aortic valve* ➡. *Late gadolinium enhancement images (not shown) did not reveal evidence of focal fibrosis or scar to suggest an infiltrative process, such as amyloidosis.*

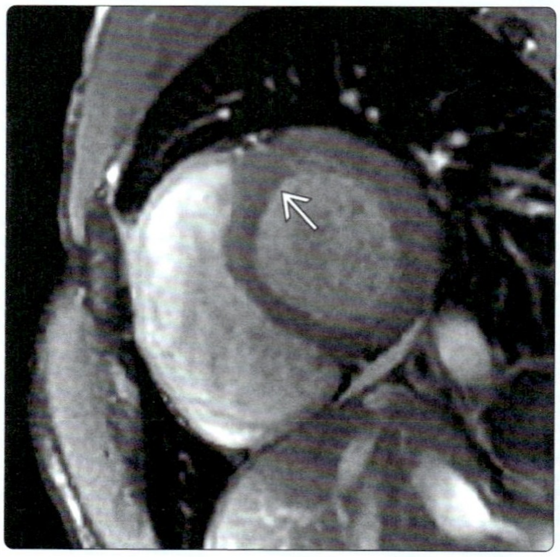
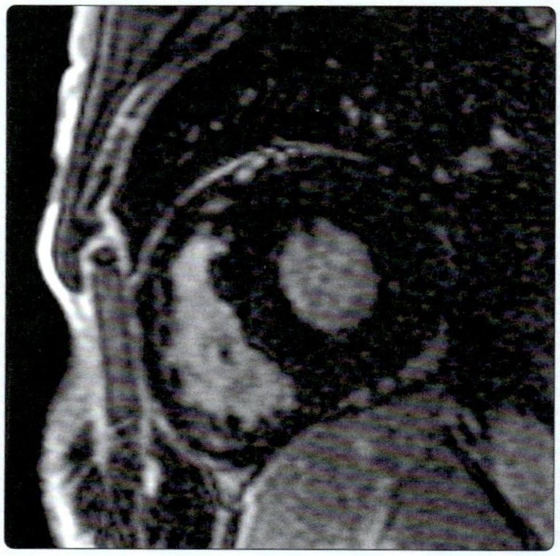

(Left) *Short-axis MR cine in a 16-year-old athlete who had a borderline echocardiogram after an abnormal electrocardiogram (ECG) shows mild upper septal hypertrophy with a maximal wall thickness of 14 mm* ➡. **(Right)** *Short-axis LGE MR from the same patient shows no evidence of focal fibrosis or scar. The differential for these findings includes physiologic remodeling from exercise (athlete's heart) or mild neutral subtype hypertrophic cardiomyopathy.*

TERMINOLOGY

Abbreviations

- Left ventricular hypertrophy (LVH)

Definitions

- ↑ in left ventricular (LV) wall thickness &/or myocardial mass due to ↑ in cardiac myocyte size

IMAGING

MR Findings

- ↑ myocardial mass
  - 95% limits of normal ranges for LV mass (indexed by BSA) with cardiac MR; papillary muscles included in LV blood pool
    - Males: 57-152 g (36-75 g/m²); mean: 105 g (mean index: 56 g/m²)
    - Females: 43-103 g (30-59 g/m²); mean: 73 g (mean index: 45 g/m²)
- ↑ wall thickness
  - Normal ranges for end-diastolic LV wall thickness (LVWT) (+/- 2 SD from mean) = 4-12 mm (males); 3-10 mm (females)
    - Mild LVH: 1.2-1.4 cm
    - Moderate LVH: 1.5-1.9 cm
    - Severe LVH: ≥ 2 cm
- Morphologic types of LVH
  - **Concentric hypertrophy**
    - ↑ LVWT and mass
    - Relative wall mass (RWM) = LV mass (LVM)/LV end-diastolic volume
      - Normally > 1.16
    - Normal septal:lateral wall ratio (SLR), normally 1
  - **Asymmetric hypertrophy**: ↑ LVWT, LVM, RWM, SLR
  - **Eccentric hypertrophy**: ↑ LVM, ↓ RWM, normal SLR
- Multiple MR sequences are available
  - Cine-balanced steady-state free precession (SSFP): For qualitative and quantitative evaluation
  - Strain imaging: For quantification of regional myocardial function
  - LGE: For tissue characterization and establishing etiology; adverse prognosis
  - T1 mapping: Detection of diffuse fibrosis, amyloid
  - Flow sequences: Quantification of valvular lesions, coarctation, and shunts
- MR used for establishing diagnosis, determining LV geometry, establishing etiology, quantification, risk stratification, serial follow-up, treatment response

CT Findings

- Cardiac gated CTA
  - Can demonstrate ↑ wall thickness and myocardial mass if end-diastolic images are obtained
  - Used only when MR is contraindicated or has artifacts

Imaging Recommendations

- Best imaging tool
  - Echocardiography is often most accessible and practical initial test
  - MR is useful if there are equivocal echo findings or to evaluate for specific etiologies, such as hypertrophic or infiltrative cardiomyopathy

DIFFERENTIAL DIAGNOSIS

Infiltrative Cardiomyopathy

- Patterns of LGE help in diagnosis

PATHOLOGY

General Features

- Etiology
  - Primary causes (due to genetic factors)
    - Hypertrophic cardiomyopathy
  - Secondary causes
    - Hypertension: Most common cause of LVH
    - Aortic stenosis, coarctation, subaortic membrane, obesity, athlete's heart

Microscopic Features

- ↑ in myocyte size

CLINICAL ISSUES

Presentation

- Clinical profile
  - LVH on ECG
  - Hypertension
    - Systolic blood pressure ≥ 130 mmHg; diastolic blood pressure ≥ 80 mmHg

Demographics

- Epidemiology
  - Population studies estimate prevalence of LVH of 15-21%
  - ~ 46% of adults in USA have hypertension based on 2017 ACC/AHA guidelines

Natural History & Prognosis

- LVH is independent predictor of cardiac mortality, regardless of underlying etiology

Treatment

- Targeted to underlying cause

DIAGNOSTIC CHECKLIST

Consider

- Consider hypertrophic cardiomyopathy or infiltrative heart disease in patients without significant hypertension or valvular heart disease

SELECTED REFERENCES

1. Kawel-Boehm N et al: Reference ranges ("normal values") for cardiovascular magnetic resonance (CMR) in adults and children: 2020 update. J Cardiovasc Magn Reson. 22(1):87, 2020
2. Fulton N et al: Utility of magnetic resonance imaging in the evaluation of left ventricular thickening. Insights Imaging. 8(2):279-93, 2017

Right Ventricular Hypertrophy

KEY FACTS

TERMINOLOGY

- Increased right ventricular (RV) wall thickness &/or myocardial mass

IMAGING

- Increased RV wall thickness (> 5 mm)
- Increased RV mass
- Echocardiography is often initial imaging test
  - RV systolic pressure can be estimated by measuring peak velocity of tricuspid regurgitant jet by Doppler
- Cardiac MR is gold standard for quantitative assessment of RV size and function
  - LGE at anterior and posterior RV insertion sites in cases of RV pressure overload
  - Pulmonary artery dilatation if there is pulmonary hypertension
- Cardiac CT
  - RV wall thickness, mass, and volumes can be measured if end-diastolic images are acquired

TOP DIFFERENTIAL DIAGNOSES

- Infiltrative cardiomyopathy
- Cardiac sarcoidosis
- Athlete's heart
- Pulmonary hypertension

PATHOLOGY

- RV pressure overload
  - Congenital heart disease
  - Primary pulmonary hypertension
  - Secondary pulmonary hypertension
    - Acquired heart disease, especially left ventricular dysfunction; valvular heart disease; chronic pulmonary embolism; chronic obstructive pulmonary disease; chronic interstitial lung disease
- Hypertrophic cardiomyopathy
- Athlete's heart

(Left) *Short-axis MR cine of a 37-year-old man with D-transposition of the great arteries, who underwent a Mustard atrial switch procedure as an infant, shows significant right ventricular hypertrophy ➔ with a D-shaped septum or left ventricle during systole, consistent with RV pressure overload ➔. The RV is connected to the aorta and is therefore the systemic ventricle.* **(Right)** *Axial cardiac CT from the same patient shows significant hypertrophy of the RV free wall ➔.*

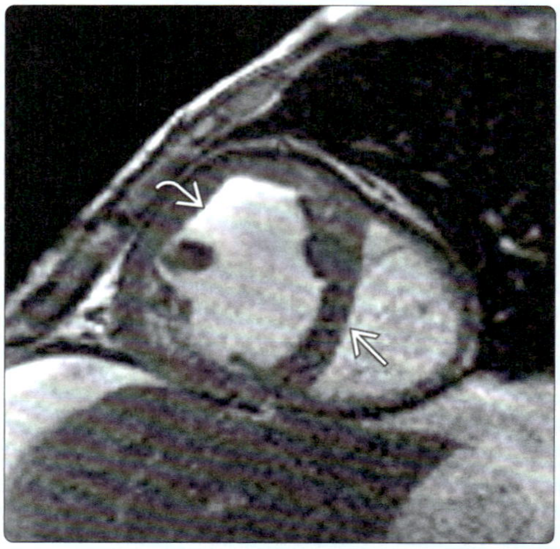

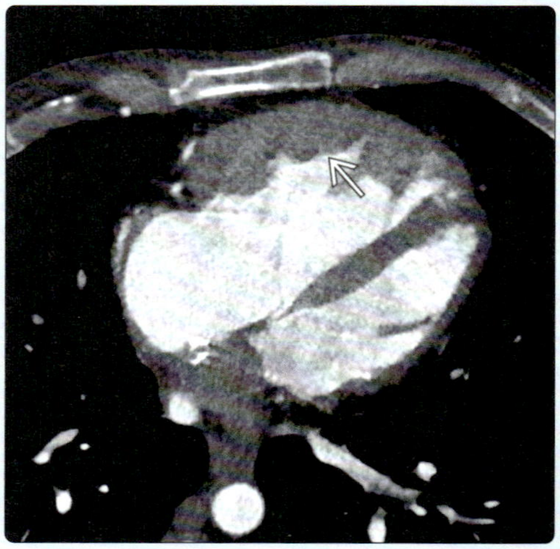

(Left) *RVOT MR cine from a 34-year-old man with congenital pulmonic stenosis shows thickening of the pulmonic valve with associated dephasing artifact due to pulmonic stenosis ➔.* **(Right)** *Short-axis LGE MR in the same patient shows 2 foci of LGE involving the anterior ➔ and inferior ➔ septa at the RV insertion sites. This pattern of LGE can be seen with RV pressure overload. Due to progressive dyspnea, the patient underwent balloon valvuloplasty.*

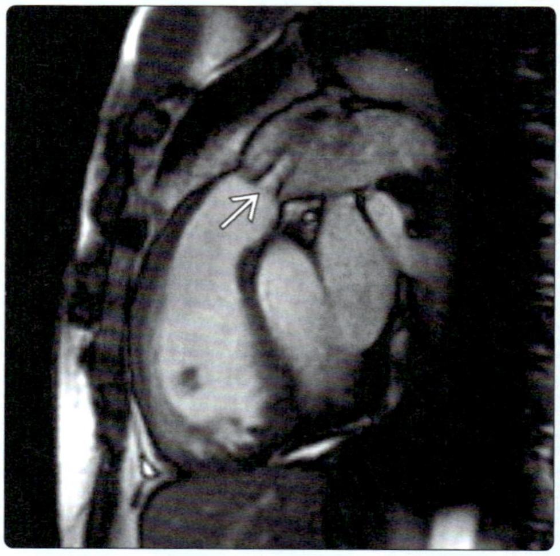

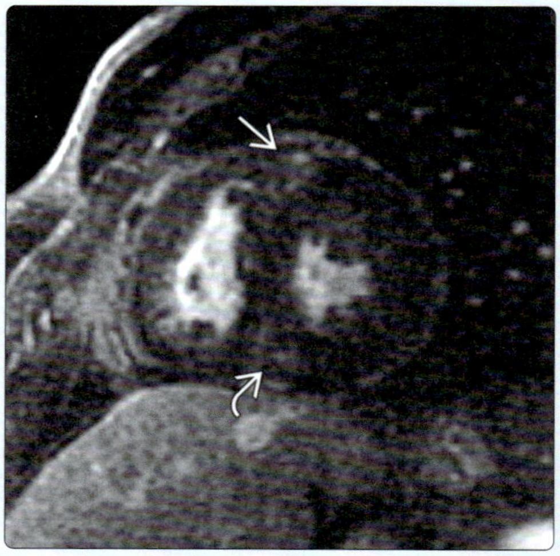

TERMINOLOGY

Abbreviations

- Right ventricular hypertrophy (RVH)

Definitions

- Increased RV wall thickness &/or myocardial mass

IMAGING

Radiographic Findings

- Radiography
  - Diminished retrosternal clear space on lateral radiograph and elevation of cardiac apex

Echocardiographic Findings

- Echocardiogram
  - Increased RV wall thickness
  - RV mass can be difficult to measure using conventional echocardiography
    - May be more accurately measured by 3D techniques
  - Evidence of RV pressure overload if there is concomitant pulmonary hypertension
    - RV systolic pressure can be estimated by measuring peak velocity of tricuspid regurgitant jet by Doppler
    - D-shaped septum during systole can be seen with RV pressure overload
  - Right atrial pressure (P right atrium) can be estimated by size of inferior vena cava (IVC)
    - Normal IVC: 1.5-2.5 cm, 5-15 mmHg
    - Dilated IVC: > 2.5 cm, 15-20 mmHg
    - Dilated, enlarged hepatic veins: > 20 mmHg

MR Findings

- Increased RV wall thickness (> 5 mm)
- Increased RV mass
  - Normal values (papillary muscles included in RV blood pool)
    - Males: 95% lower-upper limit = 17-54 g; mean: 36 g (10-28 g/m^2; mean 19 g/m^2)
    - Females: 95% lower-upper limit = 13-48 g; mean: 30 g (7-28 g/m^2; mean 17 g/m^2)
- LGE at anterior and inferior RV insertion sites in cases of RV pressure overload
- Pulmonary artery dilatation if pulmonary hypertension

CT Findings

- Cardiac gated CTA
  - RV wall thickness, mass, and volumes can be measured if end-diastolic images are acquired

Imaging Recommendations

- Best imaging tool
  - Echocardiography is often initial imaging test
  - Cardiac MR is gold standard for quantitative assessment of RV size and function
- Protocol advice
  - Cardiac MR
    - Steady-state free precession (SSFP) for qualitative and quantitative analysis of RV volumes and mass
    - LGE may show patterns of fibrosis indicative of RV pressure overload or may suggest alternative etiology

DIFFERENTIAL DIAGNOSIS

Infiltrative Cardiomyopathy

- Typically associated with increased left ventricular wall thickness &/or atrial wall thickening
- May show diffuse or focal late contrast enhancement

Cardiac Sarcoidosis

- May be associated with increase in left or RV wall thickness
- May show various patterns of late contrast enhancement
- Mediastinal adenopathy may be present

Athlete's Heart

- Endurance athletes may have RV elongation and dilatation
- Isometric activities (i.e., weightlifting) typically do not cause changes in RV morphology

Noncompaction

- Prominent RV trabeculations
- Prominent 2-layered structure; deep intertrabecular spaces communicating with RV; thickness of noncompacted RV > 75%

PATHOLOGY

General Features

- Etiology
  - RV pressure overload
    - Congenital heart disease
      - Tetralogy of Fallot; transposition of great vessels
    - Pulmonary hypertension (WHO groups I-V)
  - Hypertrophic cardiomyopathy (HCM)
    - RV involved in 33% of HCM patients
    - Contiguous to septum or focal apical thickening

CLINICAL ISSUES

Presentation

- Clinical profile
  - Symptoms depend on underlying etiology and can include exertional dyspnea, chest pain, and lightheadedness
  - RVH on ECG
  - Right-axis deviation on ECG

Treatment

- Depends on underlying etiology
  - Pulmonary hypertension: Vasodilators
  - Congenital heart disease: Surgical or percutaneous therapy depending on nature of anatomic defects, symptoms, and associated impact on RV size or function
  - Left-sided heart disease: Medical &/or surgical therapy as indicated

SELECTED REFERENCES

1. Kawel-Boehm N et al: Reference ranges ("normal values") for cardiovascular magnetic resonance (CMR) in adults and children: 2020 update. J Cardiovasc Magn Reson. 22(1):87, 2020
2. Foschi M et al: The dark side of the moon: the right ventricle. J Cardiovasc Dev Dis. 4(4):18, 2017
3. Galea N et al: Right ventricular cardiovascular magnetic resonance imaging: normal anatomy and spectrum of pathological findings. Insights Imaging. 4(2):213-23, 2013

Pulmonary Venous Hypertension/Pulmonary Edema (Cardiogenic)

KEY FACTS

TERMINOLOGY

- Pulmonary venous hypertension (PVH) = elevated left atrial and ventricular filling pressures → increased pulmonary venous pressure
- Cardiogenic pulmonary edema = PVH → elevated pulmonary capillary pressure → increased transudation of fluid into lung's interstitial and alveolar spaces

IMAGING

- Radiography
  - Vascular indistinctness
  - Fissural and bronchial wall thickening
  - Kerley B lines
  - Consolidation or hazy opacities
  - Cardiomegaly
  - Pleural effusion
- CT
  - Thickening of septa and fissures
  - Thickening of peribronchovascular interstitium
  - Centrilobular or patchy ground-glass opacities
  - Consolidation
  - Cardiomegaly
  - Pleural effusions
  - Increased attenuation or haziness of mediastinal fat
  - Mediastinal lymph node enlargement, often low attenuation

TOP DIFFERENTIAL DIAGNOSES

- Interstitial edema: Lymphangitic carcinomatosis
- Alveolar edema: Pneumonia, hemorrhage
- Interstitial and alveolar edema: Alveolar proteinosis

CLINICAL ISSUES

- Dyspnea; orthopnea; paroxysmal nocturnal dyspnea
- B-type natriuretic peptide (BNP); 90% accuracy

DIAGNOSTIC CHECKLIST

- Prior studies helpful in detection of early findings

(Left) *PA chest radiograph in a patient with mitral valve disease shows pulmonary venous hypertension manifesting with vascular redistribution. The upper lung zone vessels* ➔ *are larger than those in the lower lung.* **(Right)** *PA chest radiograph in chronic left ventricular failure shows pulmonary venous hypertension manifesting with enlargement of upper lobe pulmonary vessels* ➔*, which are much larger than adjacent bronchi. Note that a dilated azygos vein* ➔ *indicates biventricular failure.*

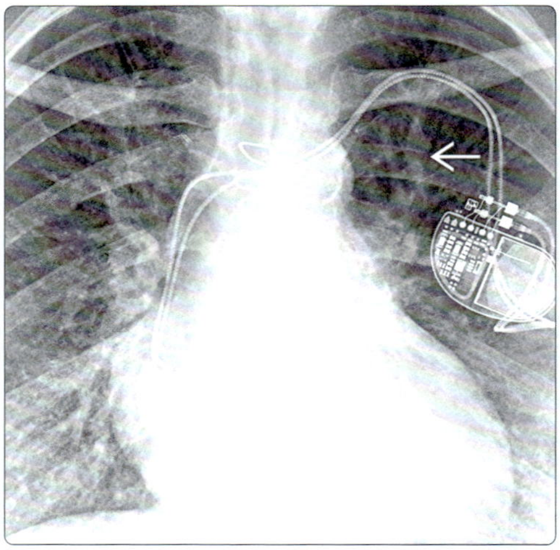

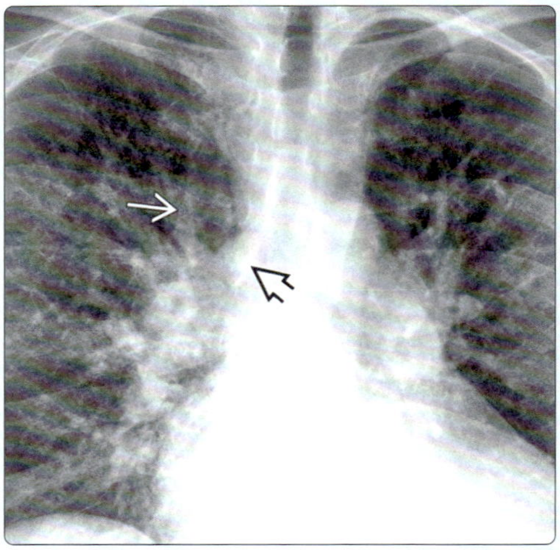

(Left) *PA chest radiograph shows numerous short lines perpendicular to the pleura (Kerley B lines)* ➔ *representing thickened interlobular septa.* **(Right)** *Coronal reformat CECT in a patient with interstitial edema demonstrates thick interlobular septa* ➔ *and thick interlobar fissures* ➔ *secondary to edema of the subpleural interstitium. Subpleural edema may precede septal thickening and peribronchial cuffing as a manifestation of interstitial edema.*

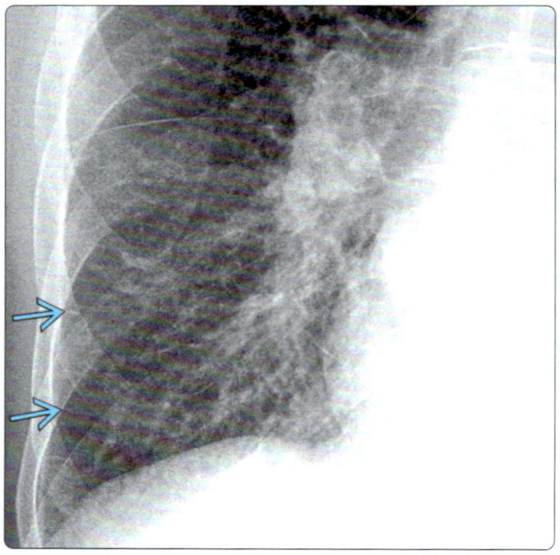

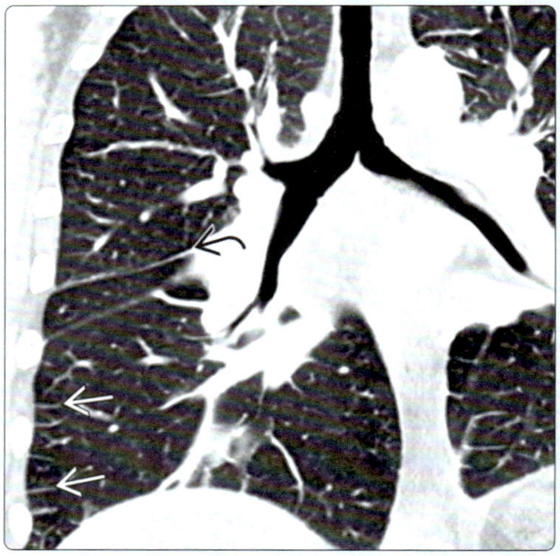

TERMINOLOGY

Synonyms

- Hydrostatic pulmonary edema

Definitions

- **Pulmonary venous hypertension (PVH) = elevated left atrial and ventricular filling pressures → increased pulmonary venous pressure**
- Cardiogenic pulmonary edema = PVH → elevated pulmonary capillary pressure → increased transudation of fluid into interstitial and alveolar spaces of lung

IMAGING

General Features

- Best diagnostic clue
  - Pulmonary venous redistribution
  - Smooth interlobular septal thickening
  - Kerley B lines (interstitial edema)
  - Perihilar consolidation (alveolar edema)
  - Cardiomegaly; pleural effusions

Radiographic Findings

- **PVH**
  - **Vascular redistribution** or cephalization
    - Size of upper lobe veins ≥ size of lower lobe veins (reversal of normal)
      - Based on radiograph taken in upright standing position
      - May be seen in supine position without PVH
    - Pulmonary arteries:bronchus diameter ratio in upper lung zone > lower lung zone
      - Based on diameter of end-on pulmonary arteries and adjacent bronchus
- **Interstitial edema**
  - **Perihilar haze** or **vascular indistinctness**
    - Blurred or indistinct vessel wall margins
    - Comparison with previous radiograph helpful
  - **Subpleural edema**: Fluid in subpleural interstitium
    - Thickening of interlobar fissures
    - Increased density parallel to chest wall
      - Can mimic pleural effusion or extrapleural fat
  - **Peribronchial thickening** (peribronchial cuffing): Fluid in peribronchovascular interstitium
    - Increased thickness of airway walls
    - Posterior wall of bronchus intermedius on lateral radiograph > 3 mm
  - **Septal thickening**
    - **Kerley A lines**
      - Distention of anastomotic channels between peripheral and central lymphatics
      - Central linear opacities radiating from hila
      - Length ≤ 4 cm
    - **Kerley B lines**
      - Thickened, edematous interlobular septa
      - Basilar peripheral horizontal thin lines; perpendicular to pleura
      - Length < 1 cm
- **Alveolar edema**
  - **Consolidation and hazy opacity**
    - Poorly marginated; usually bilateral but often asymmetric
    - Predilection for right lung if unilateral
      - Preferential involvement of right upper lobe in mitral regurgitation
    - Bat-wing pattern
      - Central perihilar opacity with sparing of periphery, < 10% of cases
    - Distribution affected by underlying lung disease
      - Greater involvement of lower lung zone in patients with upper lung zone emphysema
    - Distribution changes with gravity
      - Increased opacity in dependent portion of lung if patient remains in same position for few hours
- Associated findings
  - **Cardiomegaly**
    - Transverse cardiac diameter > 1/2 transverse thoracic diameter
  - **Pleural effusion**
    - Most commonly bilateral, but unilateral can occur
    - Meniscus sign
    - Blunt costophrenic angle
    - Lateralization of apparent dome of diaphragm on frontal radiograph: Subpulmonic effusion
    - Fissural **pseudotumor**: Fluid within interlobar fissure
  - **Widened vascular pedicle**
    - Marker of **increased central venous pressure** and circulating blood volume
    - Vascular pedicle width measurement = horizontal distance between right and left margins
      - Right margin: Superior vena cava interface where it crosses right mainstem bronchus
      - Left margin: Lateral border of left subclavian artery as it arises from aorta
      - Varies with body habitus, mediastinal fat
      - Measures **up to 58 mm in normal subjects**
  - Dilated azygos vein
    - Seen end-on at right tracheobronchial angle
    - > 1 cm on upright radiograph considered dilated
      - Indicates systemic venous hypertension/right ventricular failure
- Temporal relationship of cardiogenic edema
  - Unpredictable sequence of findings
    - Interstitial edema may not follow PVH
    - Alveolar edema may not follow interstitial edema
  - Imaging findings may manifest before clinical signs
  - Interstitial edema resolves in hours to days
  - Radiographic improvement may lag behind clinical course

CT Findings

- PVH
  - Cardiomegaly with dilated left atrium
  - **Vascular engorgement**
- Interstitial edema
  - Smooth thickening of interlobular septa and interlobar fissures
    - Rarely nodular; caused by focally dilated venules (venous lakes), resolves with clearing of edema
  - Thickening of peribronchovascular interstitium

  - Generalized increase in attenuation of lungs
- Alveolar edema
  - Ground-glass opacity or consolidation
  - Centrilobular ground-glass nodules
  - Distribution
    - Diffuse or patchy
    - Bilateral perihilar; bat-wing pattern
  - Findings of interstitial edema can also be seen in setting of alveolar edema
- Associated findings
  - Pleural effusions
  - Mediastinal lymph node enlargement, often low attenuation
  - Increased attenuation and haziness of mediastinal fat

Imaging Recommendations

- Best imaging tool
  - Chest radiography; prior studies are helpful in detection of early findings

DIFFERENTIAL DIAGNOSIS

Resemble Interstitial Edema

- Lymphangitic carcinomatosis
  - Usually known malignancy
  - Nodular or irregular interlobular septal thickening; can also be smooth
  - Patchy and asymmetric distribution more common than diffuse
  - ± lymphadenopathy and pleural effusion
- Erdheim-Chester disease
  - Rare disease
  - Thickening of interlobular septa and interlobar fissures
  - ± sclerotic skeletal lesions

Resemble Alveolar Edema

- Permeability edema
  - Gravity-dependent density gradient with dense consolidation in posterobasal segments
  - Absence of cardiomegaly or widened vascular pedicle
  - Septal lines and bronchial wall thickening are less common than in cardiogenic edema
- Pneumonia
  - Signs and symptoms of infection
  - Focal or multifocal consolidation and ground-glass opacities
    - Usually evolve less rapidly than in pulmonary edema
- Pulmonary hemorrhage
  - Consolidation and ground-glass opacities
  - Centrilobular nodules

Resemble Interstitial and Alveolar Edema

- Pulmonary alveolar proteinosis
  - Crazy paving pattern on CT
  - No cardiomegaly or pleural effusion

PATHOLOGY

General Features

- Etiology
  - Left ventricular dysfunction
    - Uncontrolled hypertension
    - Arrhythmias
    - Myocardial infarction or ischemic cardiomyopathy
    - Dilated cardiomyopathy
  - Fluid overload
  - Valvular disease
    - Mitral regurgitation or stenosis
    - Aortic regurgitation or stenosis

Microscopic Features

- Widening of peribronchovascular interstitium and interlobular septa
- Lymphatic distention
- Increased alveolar wall thickness
- Fluid-filled alveoli

CLINICAL ISSUES

Presentation

- Most common signs/symptoms
  - **Dyspnea**; orthopnea; paroxysmal nocturnal dyspnea
  - Diaphoresis
  - Tachypnea; tachycardia
  - Jugular vein distention
  - Basilar rales
- Other signs/symptoms
  - Pink, frothy sputum; cough
- Clinical profile
  - **B-type natriuretic peptide (BNP)**
    - Serum level used for diagnosing congestive heart failure
    - Produced as response to ventricular stretch/strain
    - 80-90% accuracy; 96% negative predictive value
  - **Pulmonary capillary wedge pressure (PCWP)**
    - Evolving role for use of pulmonary artery catheterization
      - Rate of adverse complications: 5-10%
      - Randomized studies did not show mortality benefits

Natural History & Prognosis

- Acute or insidious course
- Prognosis depends on severity and reversibility of underlying hemodynamic dysfunction

Treatment

- Preload and afterload reduction
- Intraaortic balloon pump
- Ultrafiltration

DIAGNOSTIC CHECKLIST

Consider

- Appearance of cardiogenic edema is affected by anatomic abnormalities, especially emphysema

SELECTED REFERENCES

1. Donuru A et al: Uncommon causes of interlobular septal thickening on CT images and their distinguishing features. Tomography. 10(4):574-608, 2024
2. Tsuchiya N et al: Imaging findings of pulmonary edema: part 1. Cardiogenic pulmonary edema and acute respiratory distress syndrome. Acta Radiol. 61(2):184-94, 2020
3. Assaad S et al: Assessment of pulmonary edema: principles and practice. J Cardiothorac Vasc Anesth. 32(2):901-14, 2018

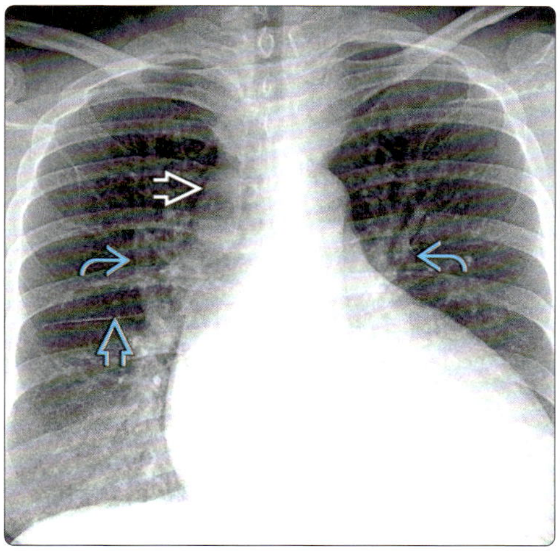

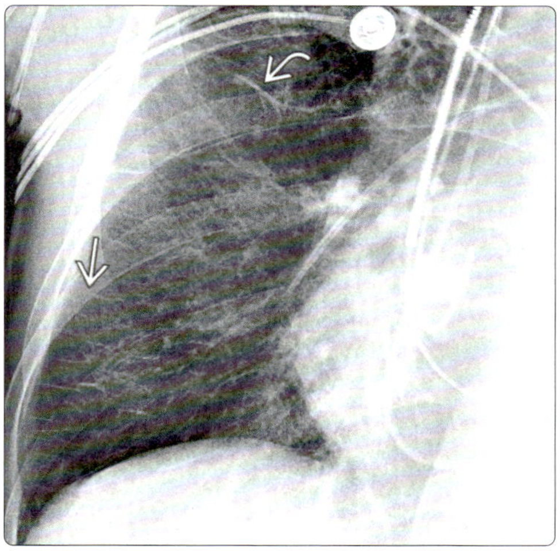

(Left) *PA chest radiograph shows vascular redistribution in pulmonary venous hypertension. Upper lobe vessels* *are larger than adjacent bronchi and lower lobe vessels. Note enlarged cardiac silhouette and azygous vein* *and thickening of a minor fissure*. **(Right)** *Coned-down AP chest radiograph in a patient with interstitial pulmonary edema shows several horizontal peripheral short lines, consistent with Kerley B lines*, *as well as longer oblique radial lines that represent Kerley A lines*.

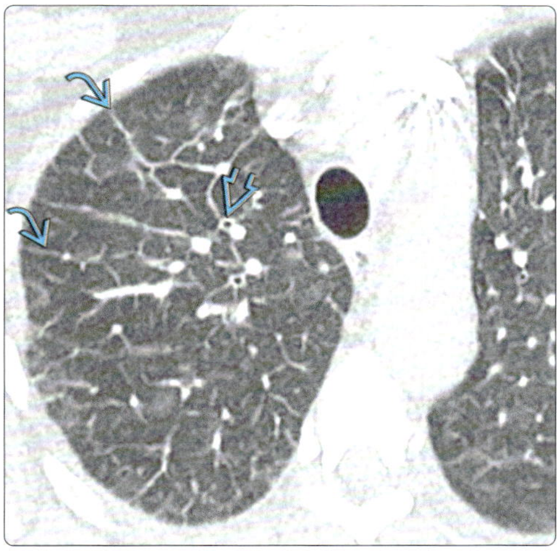

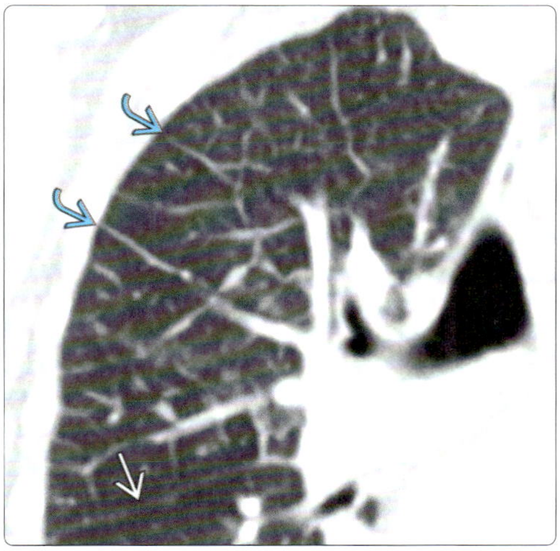

(Left) *Axial NECT shows diffuse smooth thickening of the interlobular septa* *representing interstitial pulmonary edema. Note bronchial wall thickening* *representing edematous peribronchovascular interstitium.* **(Right)** *Coronal NECT in the same patient shows diffuse smooth thickening of the interlobular septa* *and thickening of the right minor fissure*. *The subpleural interstitium courses along the interlobar fissures and is thickened in interstitial edema.*

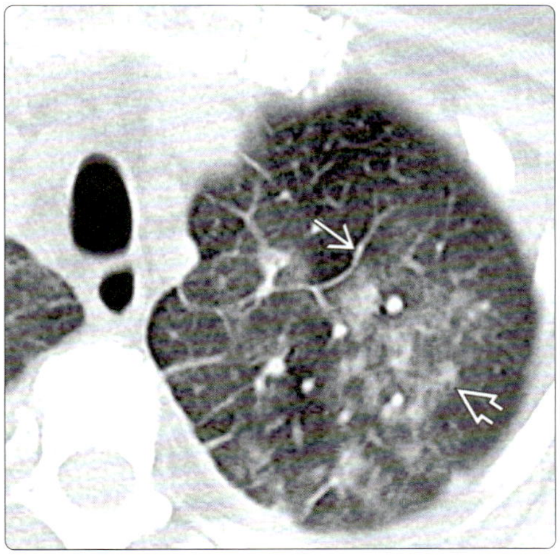

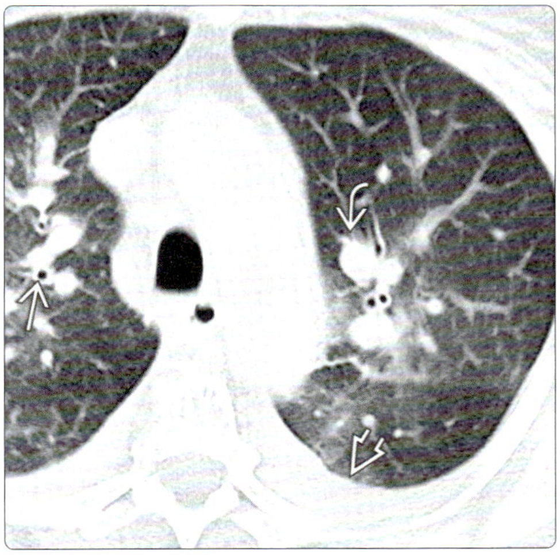

(Left) *Axial NECT (lung window) in a patient with pulmonary edema shows centrilobular ground-glass opacities* *and smooth thickening of interlobular septa*, *consistent with alveolar and interstitial edema. Note the patchy distribution of opacities and coexistence of normal and thickened interlobular septa.* **(Right)** *Axial NECT (lung window) in the same patient shows bronchial wall thickening*, *enlarged central pulmonary vessels*, *and small bilateral pleural effusions*.

Introduction

Cardiomyopathy refers to a primary disease of the myocardium that can result in systolic &/or diastolic dysfunction and manifest in congestive heart failure. The WHO classification of cardiomyopathies includes etiologies, such as ischemic, nonischemic, restrictive, hypertrophic, inflammatory, valvular, hypertensive, and metabolic. The accurate identification of the cause of the cardiomyopathy has important implications for prognosis and treatment. Noninvasive cardiac imaging is a critical part of the evaluation of patients with cardiomyopathy. Echocardiography is often the primary modality used in the initial evaluation of patients with heart failure, though its ability to accurately characterize myocardial tissue and determine the underlying etiology is often limited. Advanced imaging modalities, such as cardiac MR, cardiac CT, and cardiac PET, are increasingly used in the diagnostic evaluation of cardiomyopathies. With increased attention on the cost and cost effectiveness of cardiac imaging, there will be increased scrutiny on the evidence base supporting the clinical utility of these imaging techniques. The following is a brief summary of the evidence supporting the use of advanced imaging modalities, such as cardiac MR and cardiac CT, for the evaluation of various cardiomyopathies.

Ischemic Cardiomyopathy

Cardiac MR with late gadolinium enhancement (LGE) has become the gold standard for the noninvasive detection of myocardial infarction owing to its superior spatial resolution and signal-to-noise contrast ratio when compared with other modalities, such as echocardiography and nuclear imaging. Many publications note that the presence of myocardial infarct as detected by cardiac MR is associated with a worse prognosis with regard to major adverse cardiac events. In the ICELAND MI study, the prevalence of unrecognized myocardial infarction by cardiac MR was greater than the prevalence of recognized myocardial infarction and was independently associated with mortality. Whether the detection of subclinical myocardial infarction by cardiac MR leads to improved outcomes requires additional clinical trials.

In the evaluation of a newly diagnosed cardiomyopathy, one of the first considerations is the presence of obstructive coronary artery disease. There are several modalities for the detection of obstructive coronary artery disease. Exercise treadmill testing, nuclear stress testing, and stress echocardiography have been in widespread use for decades. Stress perfusion by cardiac MR and cardiac CT have demonstrated excellent diagnostic and prognostic utility across a range of clinical indications. In the evaluation of newly diagnosed heart failure, the most recent (2018) criteria for cardiac CT give an appropriate grade for the use of cardiac CT in the evaluation of patients with heart failure of uncertain etiology.

In patients with ischemic cardiomyopathy, the role of revascularization is controversial given the results of the STICH study, which showed similar outcomes in patients undergoing surgery compared with medical therapy. Viability was included as a substudy, though it did not include cardiac MR or cardiac PET, i.e., modalities that may perform better when compared with echocardiography or thallium imaging. Prior data from Kim et al showed that the degree of transmural enhancement is associated with the likelihood of segmental functional recovery after revascularization. Data from Ling et al show that, in patients with hibernating myocardium, there may be a survival benefit from revascularization with PET. A metaanalysis (Allman et al) investigating the impact of revascularization after myocardial viability testing on patient long-term prognosis by analyzing 24 studies with > 3,000 patients showed a strong association between myocardial viability and improved survival after revascularization. Despite controversy regarding viability testing, it is still used in clinical practice to enforce a decision-making process regarding revascularization in patients with high surgical risk or complex medical history.

Nonischemic Dilated Cardiomyopathy

Using registry data from EuroCMR, Bruder et al (2009) demonstrated that cardiac MR had a direct impact on diagnostic and therapeutic management in ~ 2/3 of a large cohort of patients. In addition, a new diagnosis was provided by cardiac MR in ~ 9% of the cases. In this cohort study, ~ 1/3 of patients underwent evaluation for cardiomyopathy &/or myocarditis. In addition to the diagnostic yield of cardiac MR, there is growing evidence of the prognostic value in various cardiomyopathies. Gulati et al reported in a prospective longitudinal study of 472 patients with dilated cardiomyopathy that the presence of myocardial fibrosis by LGE was an independent predictor of mortality and sudden cardiac death. The utilization of LGE imaging results in an additional 19% of patients receiving implantable cardioverter-defibrillators (ICDs) and 11% avoiding ICD. LGE is superior to conventional parameters, such as ejection fraction, in predicting adverse outcome, even in asymptomatic or mildly symptomatic patients.

The use of ICD and cardiac resynchronization therapy (CRT), a.k.a. biventricular pacing, has been shown to improve the survival in patients with both ischemic and nonischemic cardiomyopathies. Despite this clear benefit, appropriate patient selection remains a challenge. In the case of ICDs, current guidelines use left ventricular ejection fraction (LVEF) to predict who would benefit, though ejection fraction is not a good predictor of an individual's risk of sudden cardiac death. A metaanalysis by Scott et al shows that the extent of LGE is strongly associated with the risk of sudden cardiac death in patients with low ejection fraction and may prove to be useful in selecting patients for ICD therapy. The heterogeneity in risk of sudden cardiac death was highlighted in the DANISH study, which did not show a benefit to prophylactic ICD implantation in patients with a nonischemic cardiomyopathy. A consistent finding has been the association of fibrosis (assessed by LGE or T1 mapping) and increased risk of major adverse cardiac events. Additional prospective clinical trials are necessary to determine whether an imaging-guided strategy will lead to a more individualized approach with regard to ICD device therapy. Similarly, with CRT, it is recognized that the nonresponse rate can be as high as 40%. Various echocardiographic techniques, such as M-mode, tissue Doppler imaging, speckle tracking, and 3D imaging, have been used to quantify the degree of myocardial dyssynchrony by measuring myocardial strain. Similarly, techniques in cardiac MR and CT can also measure the degree of dyssynchrony. At this time, however, no imaging technique has been shown to adequately predict response to CRT. The EuroCRT trial, which is an international observational study on multimodality imaging and CRT, should help clarify the role of multimodality imaging in predicting response to CRT.

Hypertrophic Cardiomyopathy

In a review of the performance of cardiac MR in hypertrophic cardiomyopathy, Noureldin et al report that echocardiography may underestimate the degree of wall thickness and may be limited in specific patterns of hypertrophy, such as apical hypertrophic cardiomyopathy. Many hypertrophic cardiomyopathy centers now routinely use cardiac MR for the diagnosis and evaluation of hypertrophic cardiomyopathy.

Several groups have reported the presence of LGE in hypertrophic cardiomyopathy and its association with adverse events. Noureldin et al reported a 65% combined incidence of LGE in hypertrophic cardiomyopathy from 18 studies. Similarly, Green et al reported in a metaanalysis of 1,063 patients that the prevalence of LGE was 60% and was associated with risk of cardiac death and all-cause mortality.

Chan et al reported on the prognostic value of quantitative LGE on the risk of sudden cardiac death. Based on this growing evidence base, the assessment of LGE is now a standard of care for most patients with hypertrophic cardiomyopathy. T1 mapping to measure diffuse fibrosis is the subject of active research, but, at present, the clinical utility remains unclear.

Cardiac Sarcoidosis

In patients with sarcoidosis, cardiac involvement is the leading cause of death, highlighting the importance of accurate diagnosis. Patel et al demonstrated that, in a cohort of 81 patients, 26% had cardiac involvement by LGE compared with only 12% using Japanese Ministry of Health criteria; in addition, LGE was associated with an increased risk of cardiac events. Similarly, Greulich et al demonstrated that the presence of LGE is the best independent predictor of potentially life-threatening arrhythmias and that the absence of LGE is associated with a very low event rate.

Coleman et al performed a metaanalysis confirming that the presence of LGE in patients with sarcoidosis is associated with an increased risk of arrhythmogenic events as well as all-cause mortality. Good response to treatment was shown in patients who had a lower amount of LGE at the initiation of therapy than those with severe LGE.

The type and location of LGE could vary in cardiac sarcoidosis with midwall and subepicardial being the most common types and basal septal and lateral wall being the most common locations. The hook sign (LGE in superior right ventricle insertion point extending into the right ventricle wall) is highly characteristic of cardiac sarcoidosis with > 90% likelihood.

Additionally, T2WI (T2 parametric mapping, triple IR) can demonstrate myocardial edema/inflammation.

Amyloidosis

Historically, the diagnosis of cardiac amyloid relied on endomyocardial biopsy. Cardiac MR now allows for the use of a noninvasive method that performs better than echocardiography alone. Syed et al performed cardiac MR with LGE in 120 patients with systemic amyloidosis. Of those with histologically confirmed cardiac amyloidosis, abnormal LGE was present in 97%. Of those without known cardiac amyloidosis and a normal wall thickness on echocardiography, 47% had abnormal LGE, suggesting a greater sensitivity of cardiac MR. LGE was also associated with clinical markers of poor prognosis. MR can also potentially distinguish the different types of amyloidosis with more extensive left ventricular thickening, left ventricular mass, LGE, and low ejection fraction with transthyretin (TTR) type than primary or light chain (AL) type. 90% of transthyretin amyloid (ATTR) shows transmural enhancement compared to 37% in AL. Right ventricular LGE was seen in 100% of ATTR and 72% of AL type.

Banypersad et al and Mongeon et al describe methods of calculating the extracellular volume (ECV) fraction using T1 mapping techniques. These techniques are more sensitive to diffuse myocardial processes, such as cardiac amyloidosis. Mongeon et al demonstrated that patients with cardiac amyloidosis have a significantly elevated ECV fraction compared with controls. Banypersad et al showed that ECV measurement is higher even in patients without focal LGE, suggesting that this may be a more sensitive diagnostic technique. Recent research demonstrates the prognostic value of LGE and T1 mapping and the utility in tracking response to therapy.

Myocarditis

Since 2009, Lake Louise criteria (LLC) (early global relative enhancement, myocardial edema by T2, and LGE) has been used to diagnose acute myocarditis on MR. Advances in cardiac MR and the use of novel techniques, such as parametric imaging and ECV, resulted in revision of the LLC in 2018. The revised LLC consists of 2 main criteria: (1) T1-based (increased native T1, ECV, or presence of LGE) and (2) T2-based criterion (increased T2 parametric mapping or high signal on T2WI or high T2 signal intensity ratio). The presence of at least 1 T1- and T2-based criterion is required for MR diagnosis of acute myocarditis. Compared to the original LLC, the 2018 LLC demonstrates higher sensitivity (87.5% vs. 72.5%) and accuracy (90.9% vs. 81.8%).

LGE is associated with increased all-cause and cardiac mortality, independent of clinical presentation. In a metaanalysis by Georgiopoulos et al, patients with LGE have 3x higher risk for combined endpoint. Regarding the LGE, the ITAMY study showed that anteroseptal location and midwall LGE are associated with worse outcomes. Furthermore, an ECV > 35%, even after adjusting for LGE and LVEF, is an independent marker of MACE. Recent small studies also showed association between native T1 and T2 mapping and major advance cardiovascular events in patients with myocarditis.

Although cardiovascular magnetic resonance (CMR) feature tracking strain analysis does not provide a direct assessment of myocardial inflammation, it can be used for assessment of left ventricular dysfunction. When CMR strain is combined with T1 or T2 mapping, diagnostic accuracy is higher compared to LLC alone with an area under curve (AUC) of 0.98. However, larger trials are needed to establish its clinical use in daily practice.

Left Ventricular Noncompaction

Left ventricular noncompaction is a genetic cardiomyopathy characterized by an increase in the noncompacted myocardial layer and can lead to heart failure, arrhythmias, and embolic complications. The currently used cardiac MR criteria for left ventricular noncompaction (noncompacted:compacted ratio of > 2.3 in diastole) was first described by Petersen et al in 2005 in a study including 7 patients with established left ventricular noncompaction compared with healthy controls, athletes, and patients with aortic stenosis, hypertrophic

LGE Patterns on Cardiac MR

LGE Patterns	Description	Associated Diseases
Ischemic		
Subendocardial	Involves only subendocardium	Ischemic cardiomyopathy
Transmural	Involves entire myocardial wall	Ischemic cardiomyopathy
Nonischemic		
Diffuse subendocardial	Diffuse involvement of subendocardial myocardium; spares subepicardium	Amyloidosis Systemic sclerosis
Midwall: Linear	Linear hyperenhancement within myocardial wall; spares subendocardium and subepicardium	Idiopathic dilated cardiomyopathy (typically septum) Myocarditis Sarcoidosis Anderson-Fabry disease Chagas disease
Midwall: Patchy	Patchy enhancement in midmyocardium; may be at right ventricular insertion sites or randomly distributed	Hypertrophic cardiomyopathy Right ventricular pressure overload (pulmonary HTN, congenital heart disease)
Subepicardial	Linear subepicardial enhancement; spares subendocardial myocardium	Sarcoidosis Myocarditis Anderson-Fabry disease Chagas disease

cardiomyopathy, and dilated cardiomyopathy. Concern about the specificity of these criteria emerged given the small size of this study. Kawel et al reported on the prevalence of an elevated ratio in the large, population-based Multi-Ethnic Study of Atherosclerosis (MESA) cohort. In a group of 323 adults without cardiac disease or hypertension, 43% had at least 1 myocardial segment with a noncompacted:compacted ratio > 2.3, while 6% had > 2 segments. The most common location of prominent trabeculations in this healthy cohort was the apical lateral and midanterior segments. There was a negative correlation between the noncompacted:compacted ratio and ejection fraction and a positive correlation with left ventricular end-diastolic and end-systolic dimensions.

Arrhythmogenic Right Ventricular Cardiomyopathy

Arrhythmogenic right ventricular cardiomyopathy (previously referred to as arrhythmogenic right ventricular dysplasia) is a genetic condition characterized by fibrofatty replacement of the right ventricle (and, rarely, of the left ventricle) that can increase the risk of sudden cardiac death. In 2006, Marcus et al reported the revised task force criteria for arrhythmogenic right ventricular cardiomyopathy, which emphasizes a major regional right ventricular wall motion abnormality with associated right ventricular dilatation &/or dysfunction. Of note, the presence of intramyocardial fat by T1 imaging is not part of the imaging criteria. Studies have shown a variable prevalence of intramyocardial fat with Tandri et el reporting ranges from 22-100% depending on the cohort and technique utilized. The limited spatial and contrast resolution can be particularly challenging when trying to distinguish intramyocardial fat from epicardial fat with the thin-walled right ventricle. Vermi et al examined the performance of the revised criteria compared with the older criteria in a cohort of 294 patients who underwent cardiac MR. They found that the new imaging criteria were associated with a lower sensitivity and maintained a high specificity. It is important to note that a diagnosis of arrhythmogenic right ventricular cardiomyopathy requires a combination of clinical and imaging criteria.

Iron Overload Syndromes

In iron overload syndromes, such as thalassemias, the leading cause of death is often cardiac, highlighting the importance of reliable noninvasive methods for quantification of myocardial iron content. In 2001, Anderson et al reported the utility of myocardial T2*, which is now widely used for measuring myocardial iron content. Multiple studies have shown the improvement in T2* and LVEF with initiation of chelation therapy. Modell et al demonstrated that the use of cardiac MR was associated with improved survival of patients with thalassemia major in the United Kingdom, marking one of the few scenarios where a cardiac imaging strategy has been shown to correlate with improved survival.

Cost Effectiveness

Given the economic climate within the United States and in many nations across the world, there is increased pressure to demonstrate the cost effectiveness of a particular imaging technique and the associated impact on patient outcomes. Carefully conducted clinical trials can be costly, and retrospective analyses can be limited given the challenges in modeling downstream decision making after an imaging test.

Selected References

1. Pöyhönen P et al: Cardiac magnetic resonance in giant cell myocarditis: a matched comparison with cardiac sarcoidosis. Eur Heart J Cardiovasc Imaging. 24(4):404-12, 2023
2. Shrivastav R et al: Evaluation and management of cardiac sarcoidosis with advanced imaging. Heart Fail Clin. 19(4):475-89, 2023
3. Eichhorn C et al: Multiparametric cardiovascular magnetic resonance approach in diagnosing, monitoring, and prognostication of myocarditis. JACC Cardiovasc Imaging. 15(7):1325-38, 2022
4. Heidenreich PA et al: 2022 AHA/ACC/HFSA guideline for the management of heart failure: a report of the American College of Cardiology/American Heart Association Joint Committee on Clinical Practice Guidelines. Circulation. 145(18):e895-032, 2022
5. Gräni C et al: Incremental value of extracellular volume assessment by cardiovascular magnetic resonance imaging in risk stratifying patients with suspected myocarditis. Int J Cardiovasc Imaging. 35(6):1067-78, 2019

Ischemic LGE Patterns

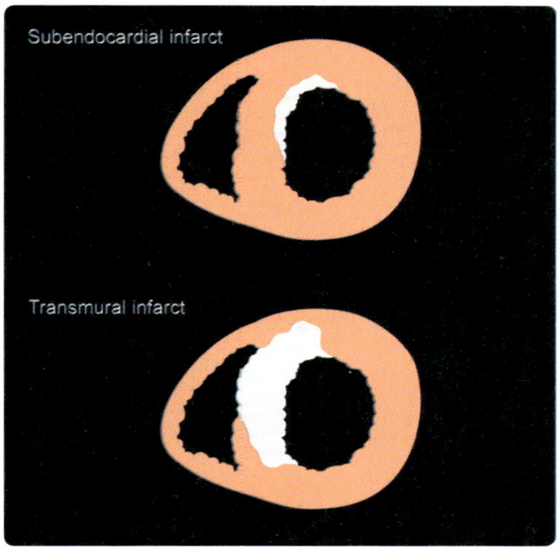

Ischemic Cardiomyopathy

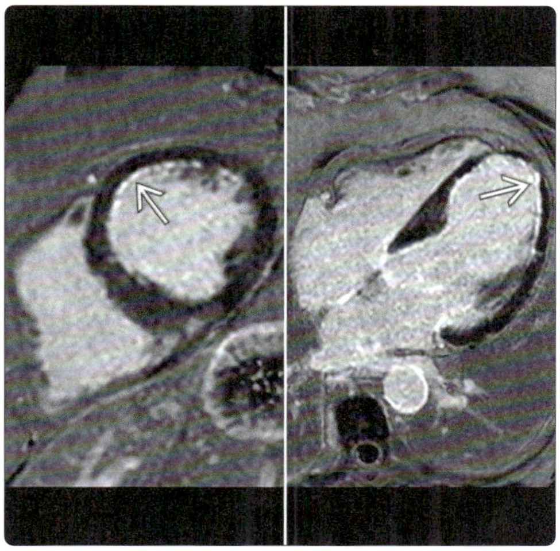

(Left) *Graphic shows LGE patterns in infarcts (both abutting endocardium).* **(Right)** *Short-axis (left) and 4-chamber (right) delayed-enhanced MR in known total occlusion of left anterior descending (LAD) coronary artery show subendocardial LGE ➡ in the mid- and apical anterior segments, consistent with LAD territory infarct. The involvement of < 50% of the myocardium indicates viability.*

Ischemic Cardiomyopathy

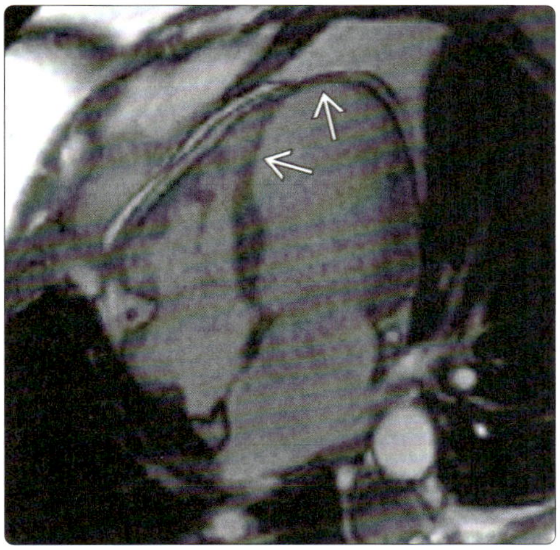

Ischemic Cardiomyopathy

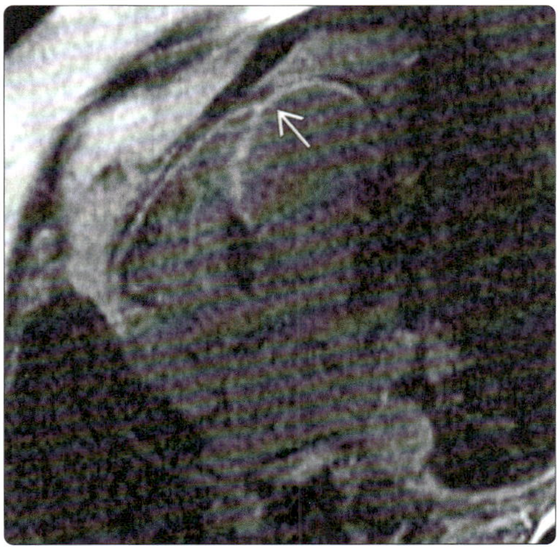

(Left) *Four-chamber cine MR shows a large area of wall thinning and severe hypokinesis/akinesis involving the mid- to distal septum and apex ➡.* **(Right)** *Four-chamber LGE MR shows a large, nearly transmural infarct ➡ affecting mid-LAD territory. Cardiac catheterization revealed chronic total occlusion of the LAD. Given the transmural extent of LGE (> 50%) and the low likelihood of segmental functional improvement with revascularization, the patient was medically managed.*

Nonischemic LGE Patterns

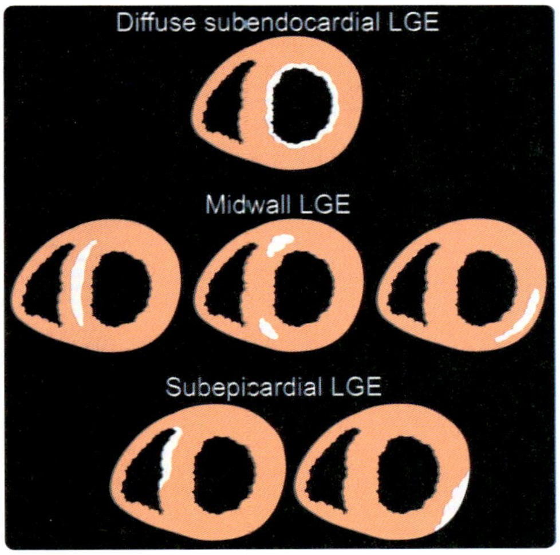

Cardiac Amyloidosis

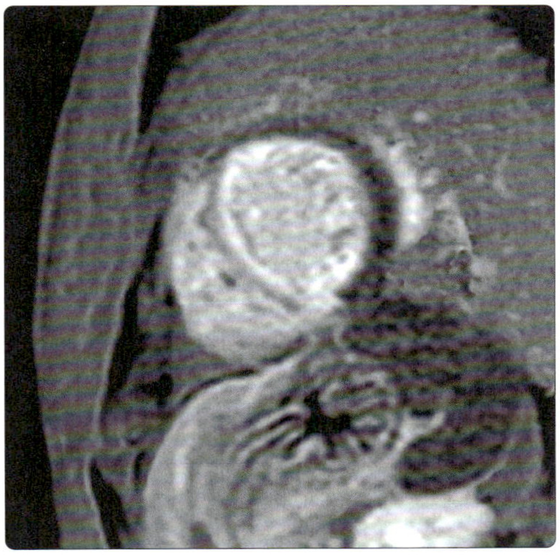

(Left) *Diffuse subendocardial LGE is seen in amyloidosis; septal midwall LGE in dilated cardiomyopathy and myocarditis; patchy midwall LGE at RV insertion sites in hypertrophic obstructive cardiomyopathy, pulmonary hypertension; lateral midwall or subepicardial LGE in sarcoidosis, myocarditis, Fabry and Chagas disease.* **(Right)** *Short-axis LGE MR shows diffuse subendocardial LGE in a patient with suspected amyloidosis. Parametric T1 mapping shows elevated T1 values (1,215 ms), also consistent with amyloidosis.*

Nonischemic Dilated Cardiomyopathy

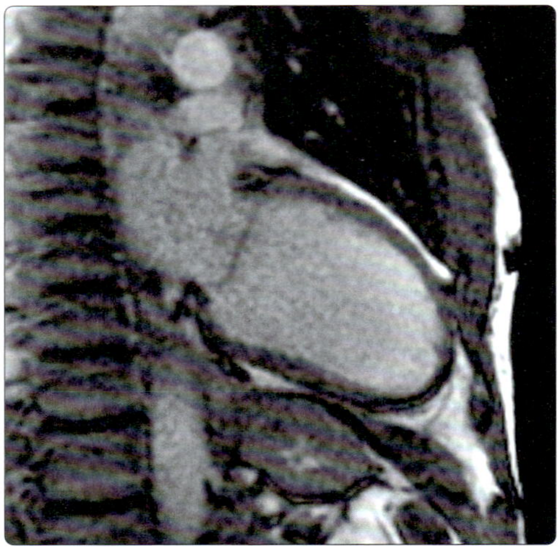

Nonischemic Dilated Cardiomyopathy

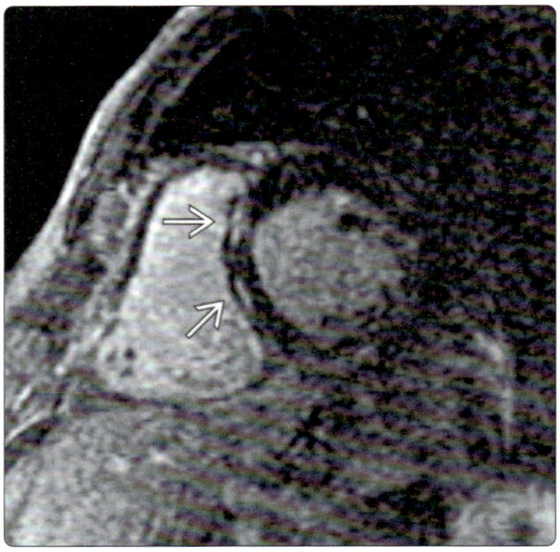

(Left) *Vertical long-axis (2-chamber) cine MR shows severe left ventricular (LV) systolic dysfunction [LV ejection fraction (LVEF) = 30%] in a patient presenting with sustained ventricular tachycardia (VT).* **(Right)** *Short-axis LGE MR shows a linear pattern of midwall late enhancement involving the midanteroseptum and inferoseptum ➡. This pattern is consistent with a nonischemic dilated cardiomyopathy and has been shown to be an independent predictor of outcomes, including all-cause mortality.*

Hypertrophic Obstructive Cardiomyopathy

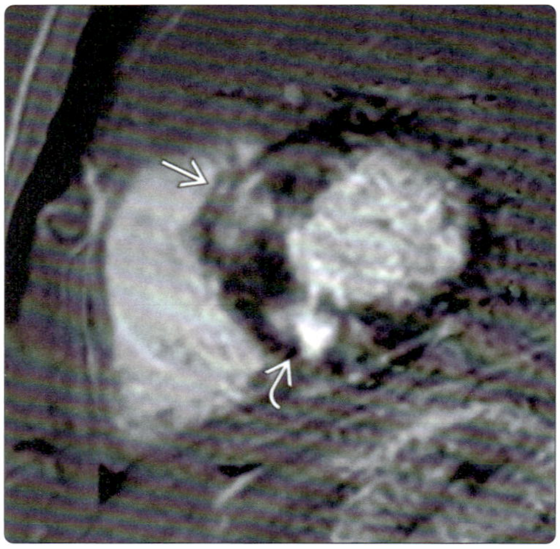

Muscular Dystrophy

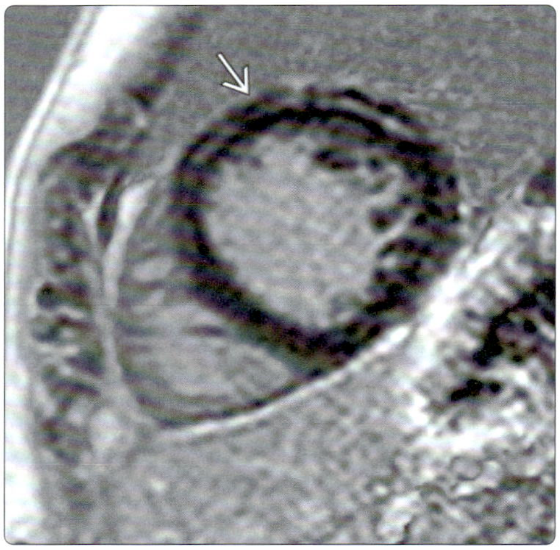

(Left) *Short-axis delayed-enhancement MR in a patient with nonsustained VT shows patchy midwall LGE in the anterior ➡ and inferior ➡ RV insertion sites. Asymmetric septal thickening and LV outflow tract obstruction (not shown) are noted. Findings are consistent with asymmetric hypertrophic obstructive cardiomyopathy.* **(Right)** *Short-axis delayed-enhancement MR in a 23-year-old patient with Becker muscular dystrophy demonstrates linear midwall LGE ➡ in the anterior and lateral segments, indicative of nonischemic cardiomyopathy.*

Myocarditis: LGE

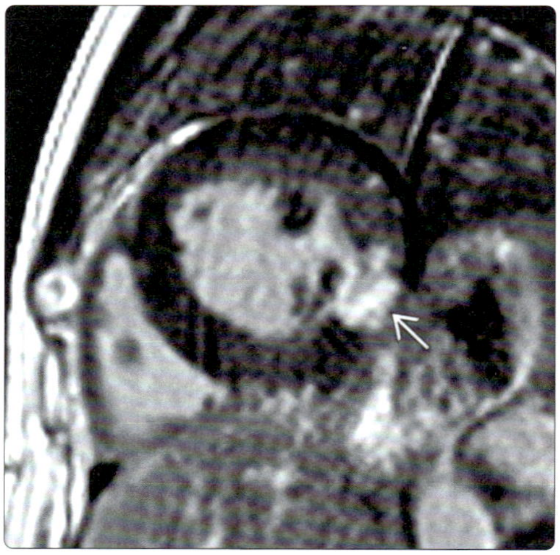

Myocarditis: T2

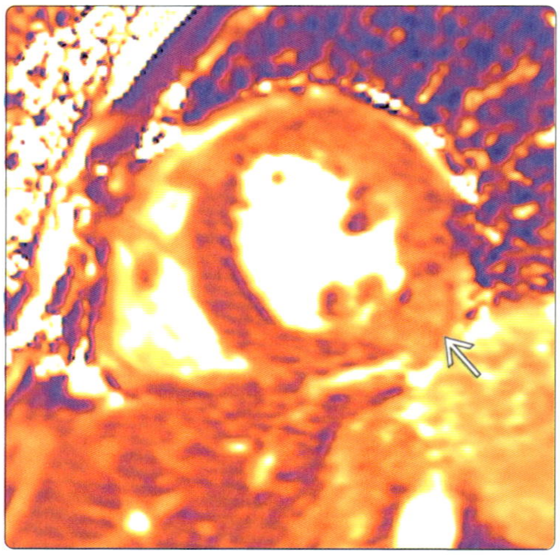

(Left) *Short-axis phase-sensitive inversion recovery image in a patient with suspected myocarditis shows focal transmural enhancement in midinferolateral wall ➡.* **(Right)** *T2 parametric map in the same patient shows focal T2 elevation ➡ in the midinferolateral wall corresponding to the area of LGE. The presence of LGE and elevated T2 meet the 2018 Lake Louise criteria for the diagnosis of acute myocarditis.*

Cardiac Sarcoidosis: SSFP

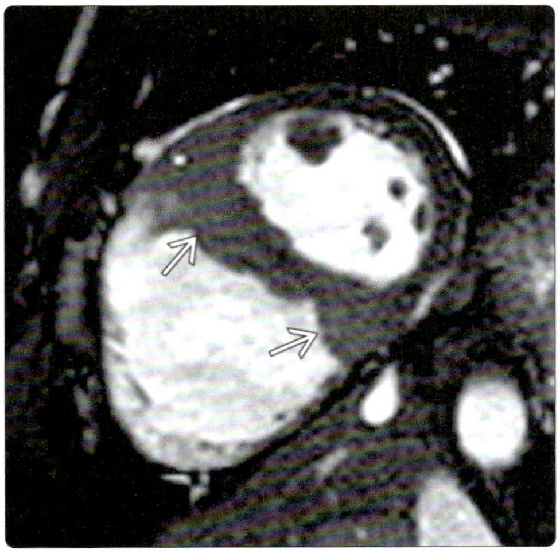

Cardiac Sarcoidosis: Triple Inversion Recovery

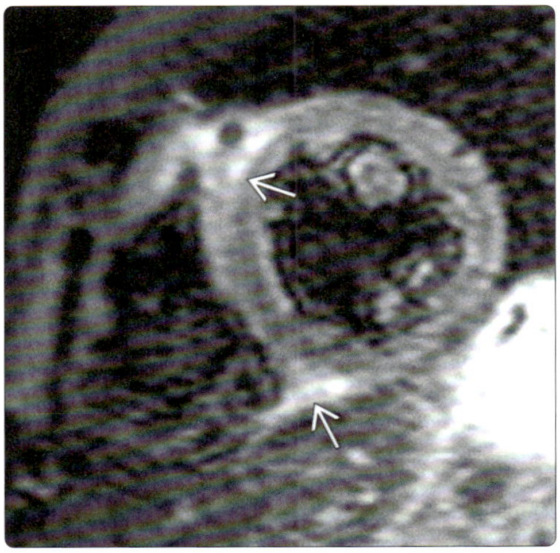

(Left) *Short-axis cine in a patient with cardiac sarcoidosis shows irregular thickening → of the interventricular septum. Additional areas of wall thickening are also noted in the RV free wall (not shown).* **(Right)** *Short-axis triple inversion recovery image in the same patient shows increased signal intensity →, indicating the presence of myocardial edema/active inflammation.*

Cardiac Sarcoidosis: LGE

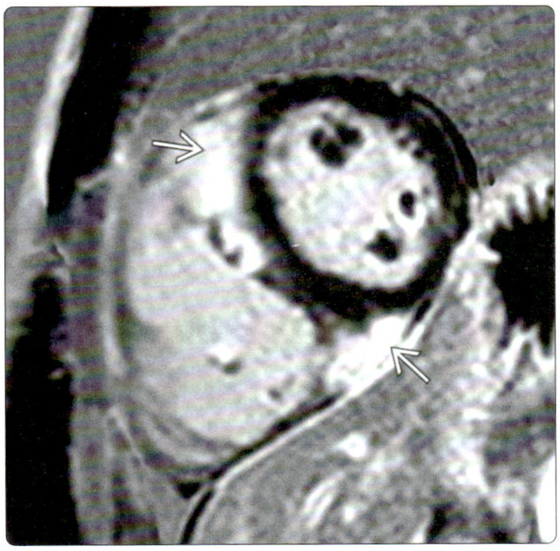

Cardiac Sarcoidosis: PET/CT

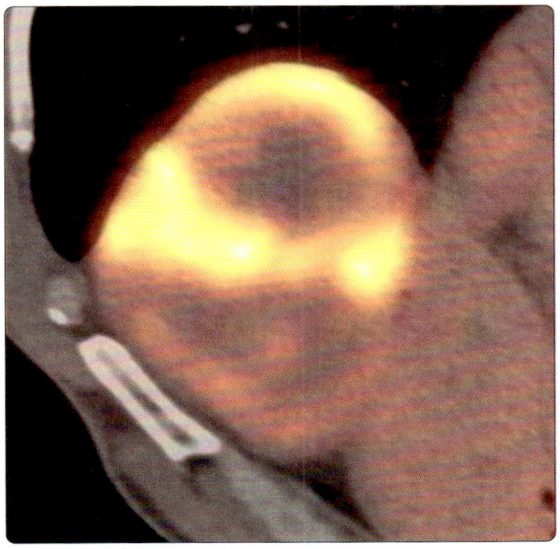

(Left) *Short-axis phase-sensitive inversion recovery image in the same patient demonstrates dense subepicardial enhancement → along the interventricular septum, especially involving RV insertion sites, and corresponding to areas of wall thickening.* **(Right)** *F-18 FDG PET/CT in the same patient reveals increased FDG uptake in the same region. PET/CT can be used for the evaluation of active inflammation and treatment response in cardiac sarcoidosis.*

Left Ventricular Noncompaction

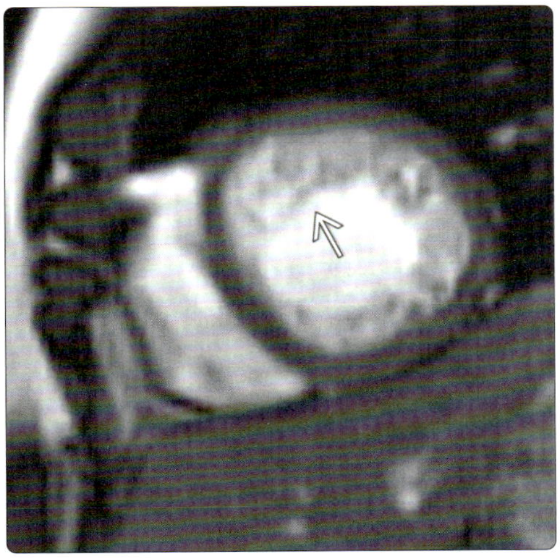

Left Ventricular Noncompaction

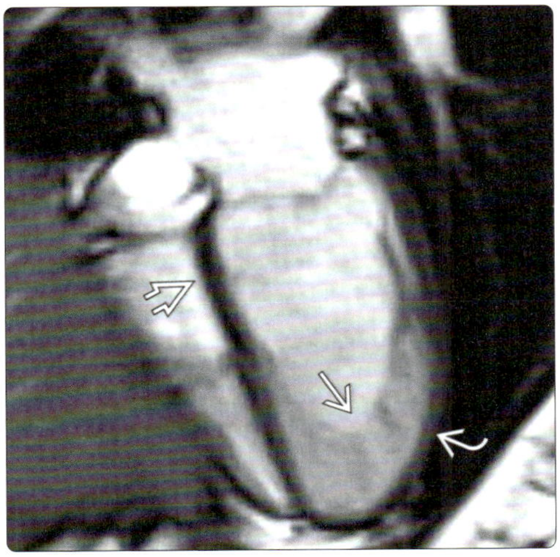

(Left) *Short-axis SSFP cine MR in diastole demonstrates the increased trabeculation → in all apical segments. The noncompacted:compacted ratio of myocardium is 4, consistent with LV noncompaction.* **(Right)** *Four-chamber SSFP cine MR in diastole in the same patient demonstrates the increased trabeculation → involving only the mid- and apical segments. Note the normal basal segments with relatively thick myocardium → compared to affected segments →.*

Normal Values for T1, ECV, T2, and T2*

Parameter	Normal Range at 1.5T	Normal Range at 3.0T
Native T1	Mean: 972-989 ms; LL-UL: 885-1,073 ms	Mean: 1097-1,197 ms; LL-UL: 964-1,290 ms
ECV	Mean: 23-26%; LL-UL: 17-32%	Mean: 25-26%; LL-UL: 16-36%
T2	Mean: 51-56 ms; LL-UL: 42-65 ms	Mean: 45-52 ms; LL-UL: 37-58 ms
T2*	> 20 ms	N/A

LL-UL = lower limit-upper limit (defined as 2 SD below or above mean; values are vendor dependent).

Data from Kawel-Boehm et al. J Cardiovasc Magn Reson. 22:87, 2020

Terminology

Myocardial tissue mapping refers to quantification of intrinsic tissue parameters T1, T2, T2*, and several other less well-known parameters.

Abbreviations

- Extracellular volume fraction (ECV)
- Left ventricle (LV)
- Contrast media (CM)
- Shortened modified Look-Locker inversion recovery (ShMOLLI)
- Modified Look-Locker inversion recovery (MOLLI)
- Shortened modified Look-Locker inversion recovery

Synonyms

- T1/ECV/T2/T2* mapping
- Parametric mapping
- T1 relaxation time = spin-lattice relaxation time
- T2 relaxation time = spin-spin relaxation time

Definitions

T1 is the time constant in ms representing the recovery of longitudinal magnetization (spin-lattice relaxation).

- Native T1 is T1 value acquired without stress or administration of contrast material

ECV is derived from pre- and postcontrast measurements of T1 relaxation times of the LV myocardium and the LV blood pool (expressed as percentage).

- Reflects size of myocardial extracellular space
- Based on concentration of CM in myocardium:plasma part of blood pool ratio
- Calculated by formula: Myocardial ECV = (1 - hematocrit) × (ΔR1myocardium/ΔR1blood pool); R1 = 1/T1
- Synthetic ECV refers to process of calculating hematocrit from blood T1 measurements instead of by blood sampling

T2 is the time constant in ms representing the decay of transverse magnetization (spin-spin relaxation).

T2* (T2 'star') is the time constant in ms representing the decay of transverse magnetization due to local field inhomogeneities.

Mapping is distinguished from quantification or relaxometry by presenting both the parametric values and their spatial relationship on a pixel-by-pixel matrix, the "map."

- Advantages of mapping include enabling visualization and quantification of disease independent of its distribution within myocardium, whether it is focal or diffuse; this is advantageous because diffuse myocardial disease can be difficult to detect or quantify with conventional CMR techniques

Imaging Protocols

Parametric mapping protocols typically consist of basal, mid-, and apical short-axis and 4-chamber long-axis acquisitions.

T1 mapping can be performed with different pulse sequences, such as MOLLI or ShMOLLI, depending on the field strength, vendor, scanner model, and software version.

ECV mapping necessitates coregistered native and postcontrast T1 maps. Postcontrast images are typically acquired 10-30 minutes post injection.

T2 mapping is mainly performed with a balanced steady-state free precession or gradient-echo sequences.

T2* mapping is best performed at 1.5T field strength, using a multiecho sequence with at least 8 echoes.

Parametric maps can be calculated on the MR scanner &/or by using dedicated postprocessing software.

Clinical Indications

Native T1 mapping is particularly useful to detect changes in the myocardium due to infiltrative disease (amyloid, Anderson-Fabry) and acute myocardial injury (edema and necrosis).

Postcontrast ECV mapping is particularly useful to quantify conditions that diffusely expand the myocardial extracellular space, such as amyloid and myocardial fibrosis.

T2 mapping is particularly useful for the detection of myocardial edema.

T2* mapping is particularly useful for detection of iron overload.

- T2* values between 10-20 ms indicate iron overload
- T2* values < 10 ms indicate severe iron overload

Normal Values

It is recommended to obtain local reference ranges for native T1 and T2 mapping from a cohort of healthy subjects.

- Normal values derived from literature listed in table

Clinical Implications

Myocardial tissue mapping can provide important information regarding the presence and severity of both focal and diffuse myocardial abnormalities that may not be readily detectable using other MR pulse sequences.

Suspected or known infiltrative diseases, myocardial edema, and iron overload assessment are the main clinical indications.

Multiparametric myocardial assessment has been used to examine a number of subclinical conditions. For example, it has been studied in COVID-19-recovered individuals and showed that recovered patients are more likely to have signs of myocardial injury than healthy controls.

Selected References

1. Muser D et al: Clinical applications of cardiac magnetic resonance parametric mapping. Diagnostics (Basel). 14(16), 2024
2. Mojica-Pisciotti ML et al: CMR findings in COVID-19 recovered patients: a review on parametric mapping, feature-tracking, and LGE. Rev Cardiovasc Med. 23(11):355, 2022
3. Nakou E et al: Cardiovascular magnetic resonance parametric mapping techniques: clinical applications and limitations. Curr Cardiol Rep. 23(12):185, 2021
4. Ferreira VM et al: CMR parametric mapping as a tool for myocardial tissue characterization. Korean Circ J. 50(8):658-76, 2020
5. Messroghli DR et al: Clinical recommendations for cardiovascular magnetic resonance mapping of T1, T2, T2* and extracellular volume: a consensus statement by the Society for Cardiovascular Magnetic Resonance (SCMR) endorsed by the European Association for Cardiovascular Imaging (EACVI). J Cardiovasc Magn Reson. 19(1):75, 2017

T1 Mapping in Amyloid

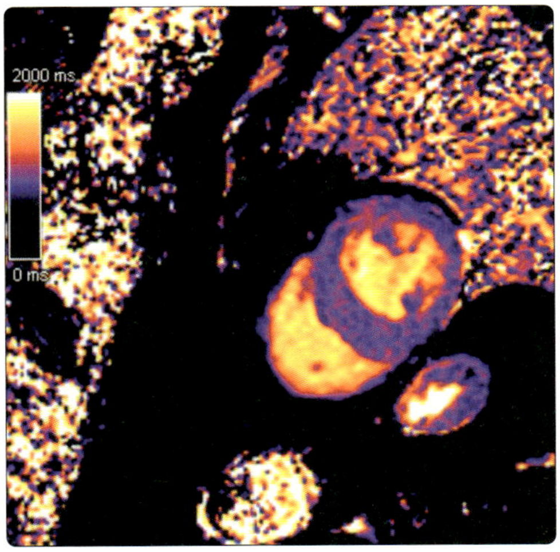

T2* Mapping in Iron Overload

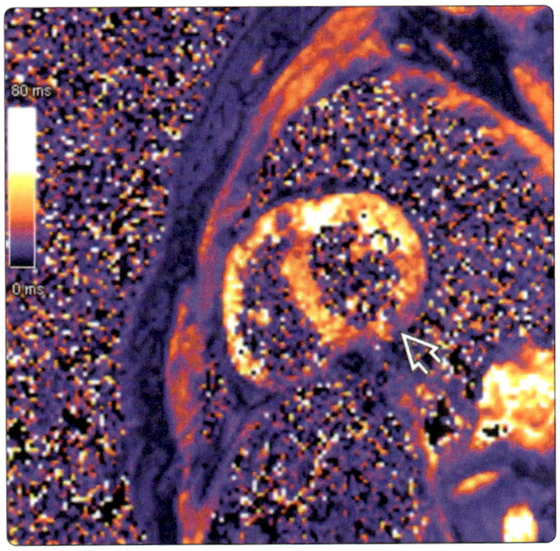

(Left) *Midventricular T1 map in a patient with proven myocardial amyloidosis is shown. Images were obtained on a 1.5T scanner. Native T1 of the thickened septum was 951 ms (blood pool: 1738 ms); postcontrast myocardial T1 was 222 ms (blood pool: 171 ms). Same-day hematocrit was 39%, yielding an elevated extracellular volume fraction of 40%. Note absence of overt focal abnormalities.* **(Right)** *T2* mapping shows mildly decreased T2* myocardial relaxation times of 16 ms, consistent with moderate focal iron deposition ➡.*

T2 Mapping in Myocarditis

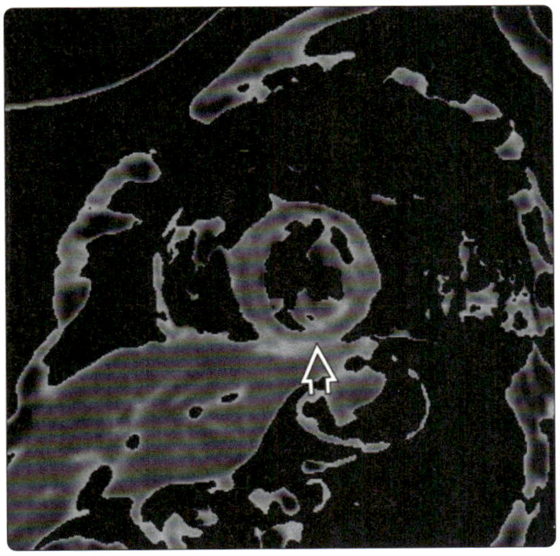

LGE in Myocarditis

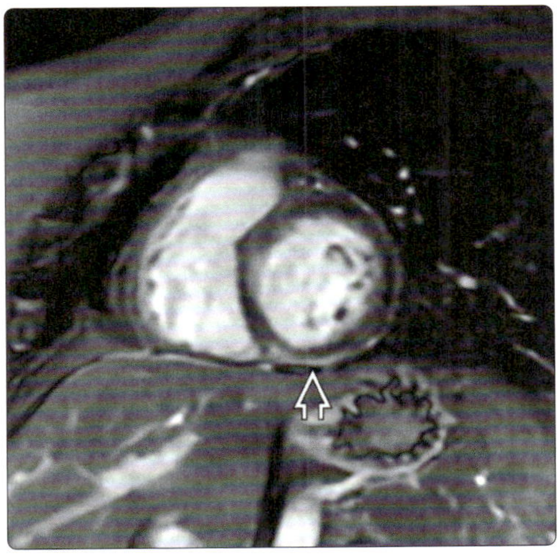

(Left) *T2 map shows elevated T2 values of up to 70 ms in the inferior midleft ventricular segment, consistent with the presence of myocardial edema ➡.* **(Right)** *Corresponding T1-weighted inversion recovery LGE acquisition in the same patient shows subepicardial high signal intensity in the inferior wall, consistent with inflammatory changes ➡.*

Terminology

In cardiac imaging, the term strain is used to describe myocardial shortening and thickening during the cardiac cycle, both of which are fundamental features of myocardial fiber function.

Synonyms

- Speckle-tracking echocardiography (STE)
- Feature tracking (FT) cardiovascular MR (CMR)

Definitions

There are 3 commonly used directional types of strain that are all perpendicular (or '"normal") to each other, which can be measured globally or per myocardial segment.

- Longitudinal strain: Percentage base-to-apex shortening during systole
- Circumferential strain: Percentage circumferential shortening of myocardium in systole in short-axis orientation
- Radial strain: Percentage thickening of myocardium during systole

Cardiac strain is a dimensionless measurement of the deformation that occurs in the myocardium when it contracts.

- End-diastolic length or thickness serves as reference and is compared to end-systolic length or thickness (a.k.a. Lagrangian strain)
- Shear strains are less commonly measured
- Torsion (or "twist") refers to circumferential-longitudinal strain or rotational motion of myocardium caused by clockwise rotation of basal segments and counterclockwise rotation of apical segments
- Strain rate refers to changes in strain over time and may be superior to peak strain because it is less influenced by cardiac load

By convention, shortening, thinning, and counterclockwise rotation are represented with negative values (i.e., < 0), and lengthening, thickening, and clockwise rotation are represented with positive (i.e., > 0) values.

Imaging Protocols

Strain is mostly used to assess the left ventricle (LV) but is increasingly being used to assess right ventricle (RV) and left atrial (LA) function.

Speckle-Tracking Echocardiography

This measures strain from the random, naturally occurring ultrasonographic speckle pattern in the myocardium.

- Most commonly used echocardiographic method to measure strain
- Has superior reproducibility when compared to tissue Doppler echocardiography (TDE), but TDE allows for more accurate measurement of strain rates

Cardiovascular MR

FT is most commonly used method to measure strain from CMR.

- Measures strain from time-averaged cine loops (i.e., acquired over multiple heart beats) using small regions of myocardium

Strain-encoding (SENC) can be used to measure pixel level strain. This is the only advanced method that is US FDA approved.

- Measures strain by tracking parallel moving planes inside and parallel to imaging plane

Clinical Indications

Myocardial Ischemia

- Global or regional circumferential strain can unmask ischemic myocardial segments

Nonischemic Cardiomyopathies

- Strain can be impaired in myocarditis, and in dilated, hypertrophic and arrhythmogenic cardiomyopathy, and has been shown to be independent predictor of outcomes

Cardio-Oncology

- Absolute global longitudinal strain (GLS) drop ≥ 5% or relative drop ≥ 15% compared to baseline is considered indicative of cardiotoxicity

Valvular Heart Disease

- Strain imaging can potentially aid in selecting timing of intervention

Pulmonary Hypertension

- Strain imaging of RV can unmask systolic dysfunction, even in patients with normal RV ejection fraction

Congenital Heart Disease

- Strain imaging has been used for early diagnosis of dysfunction and prediction of adverse outcomes in tetralogy of Fallot, Fontan palliation, transposition of the great arteries, and Ebstein anomaly

Normal Values

Global Longitudinal Strain

- STE mean = -20% (95 CI: -20 to -19%)
- CMR mean for males = -19% (95% CI: -26 to -13%); mean for females = -21% (95 CI: -29 to -14%)

Most commonly used cutoff for normal is more negative than -18%

- Gray zone: -18 to -16%
- Significant myocardial dysfunction: Less negative than -16%

Global Circumferential Strain

- STE mean = -23% (95% CI: -25 to -22%)
- CMR mean = -20% (95% CI: -26 to -14%)

Global Radial Strain

- STE mean = 47% (95% CI: 44-51%)
- Less reproducible with CMR

Left Atrial Strain

Reservoir strain: Difference in peak LA strain and strain at ventricular end-diastole

- STE mean: -42%; reservoir strain less negative than -20 to -23% is abnormally low

Pump strain: Difference between strain values in end-diastole and onset of atrial contraction

- STE mean: -14%; lower limit of normal: Less negative than -6%

Clinical Implications

The principal value of strain imaging lies in its ability to quantify myocardial contraction and to reveal global and segmental functional abnormalities, independent of changes in ejection fraction.

- GLS is more sensitive than ejection fraction to assess systolic dysfunction
- LA strain is strong marker of LV filling pressure

Selected References

1. Smiseth OA et al: Myocardial strain imaging: theory, current practice, and the future. JACC Cardiovasc Imaging. ePub, 2024
2. Rajiah PS et al: Myocardial strain evaluation with cardiovascular MRI: physics, principles, and clinical applications. Radiographics. 42(4):968-90, 2022
3. Kawel-Boehm N et al: Reference ranges ("normal values") for cardiovascular magnetic resonance (CMR) in adults and children: 2020 update. J Cardiovasc Magn Reson. 22(1):87, 2020
4. Pedrizzetti G et al: Principles of cardiovascular magnetic resonance feature tracking and echocardiographic speckle tracking for informed clinical use. J Cardiovasc Magn Reson. 18(1):51, 2016
5. Yingchoncharoen T et al: Normal ranges of left ventricular strain: a meta-analysis. J Am Soc Echocardiogr. 26(2):185-91, 2013
6. Ibrahim el-SH: Myocardial tagging by cardiovascular magnetic resonance: evolution of techniques--pulse sequences, analysis algorithms, and applications. J Cardiovasc Magn Reson. 13(1):36, 2011

STE Strain in Amyloid

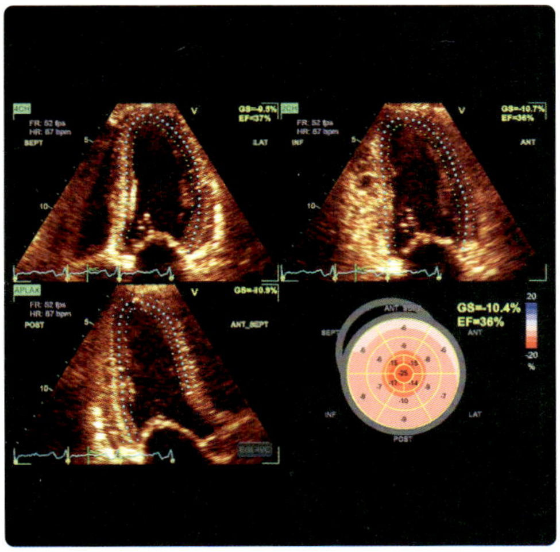

FT-CMR Strain in Amyloid

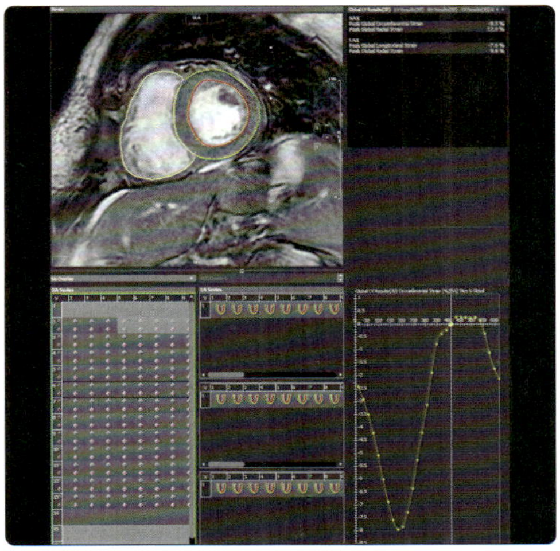

(Left) *This is a 54-year-old male patient with cardiac amyloid with mild to moderately reduced ejection fraction of 36% but severely abnormal longitudinal strains ranging from -10.9 to -9.5%.* **(Right)** *FT-CMR of the same patient shows short-axis global circumferential strain (GCS) of -9.3%, long-axis global longitudinal strain (GLS) of -7.6%, and global radial strain (GRS) of 9.6%.*

CMR SENC in Cardiotoxicity

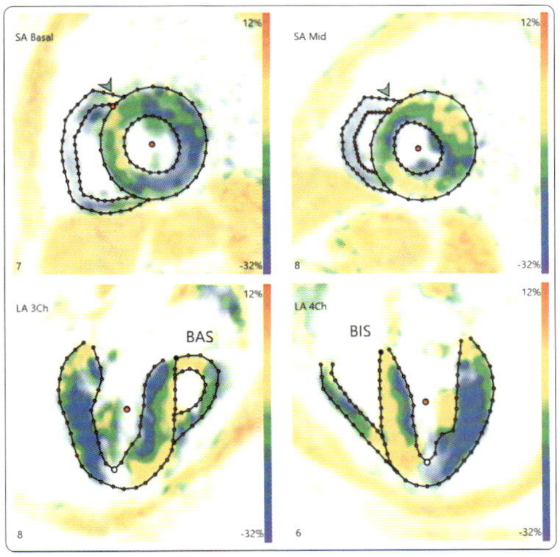

CMR SENC in Early Hypertensive CMP

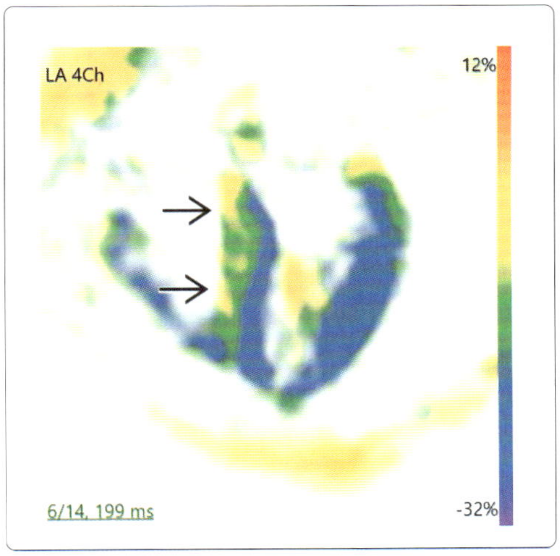

(Left) *This is a 59-year-old female with Hodgkin lymphoma on doxorubicin. Cardiovascular MR (CMR) strain-encoding (SENC) analysis shows a normal left ventricular ejection fraction of 58% with severely abnormal strain (green, yellow, and red areas).* **(Right)** *CMR SENC strain analysis shows a normal left ventricular ejection fraction of 62% but evidence of abnormal septal motion (green and yellow areas) ⇨.*

Nonischemic Dilated Cardiomyopathy

KEY FACTS

TERMINOLOGY

- Left ventricular (LV) dilation with systolic dysfunction ± right ventricular (RV) dilation/dysfunction

IMAGING

- MR is gold standard for ventricular volumes and quantitative function
  - Ventricular dilatation (indexed to body surface area)
  - Midwall septal pattern of LGE can be seen in idiopathic dilated cardiomyopathy (present in ~ 30%)
  - Epicardial or midmyocardial LGE may suggest etiologies, such as sarcoid, myocarditis, Chagas disease
  - Presence of LGE is associated with increased risk of major adverse cardiac events
  - Patterns of LGE may suggest specific etiology
  - Apical LV thrombus can be seen with severe LV dysfunction
- Echocardiography remains initial test in evaluation of suspected cardiomyopathy
  - Gold standard for assessment of valvular heart disease
- Cardiac CTA can exclude obstructive coronary artery disease

CLINICAL ISSUES

- Many patients may be asymptomatic
- Severity of LV dilation/dysfunction and concomitant RV dilation/dysfunction are associated with prognosis
- ~ 25% of patients may have improvement in LV function over time
- Standard guideline-directed medical therapy for heart failure
- Device therapy with implantable cardioverter defibrillator ± biventricular pacing for appropriate patients

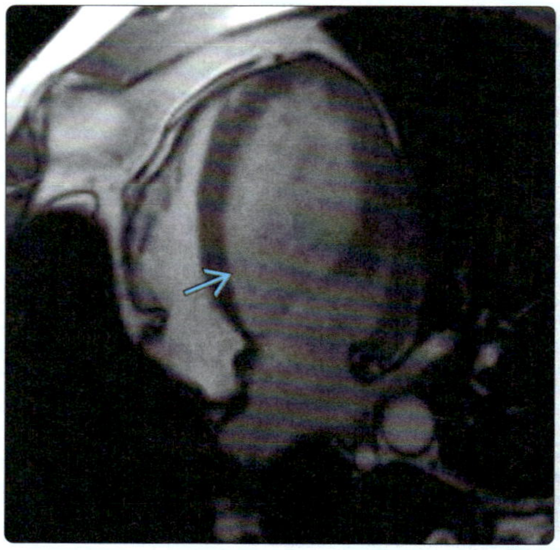

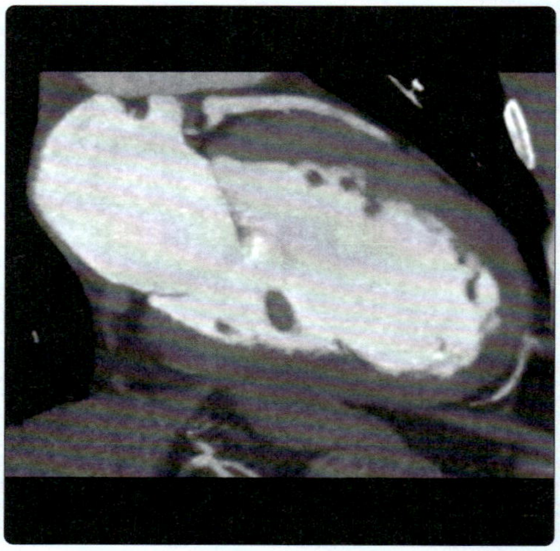

(Left) *Four-chamber SSFP cine MR shows left ventricular (LV) dilatation ➔ and severe systolic dysfunction. Cardiac MR is the gold standard for the assessment of LV volumes and quantitative ventricular function. SSFP images allow for excellent tissue contrast.* **(Right)** *Vertical long-axis (2-chamber) cardiac CT shows LV dilatation with severe systolic dysfunction. Like cardiac MR, CECT provides excellent tissue contrast.*

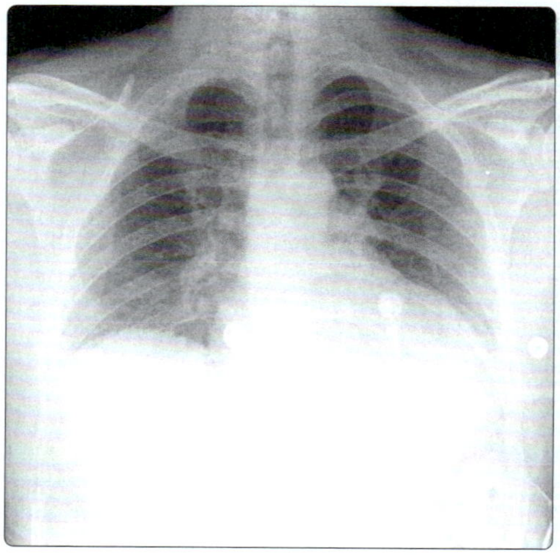

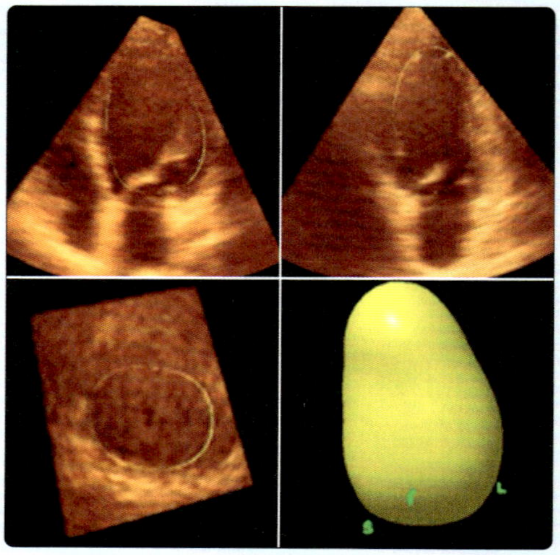

(Left) *AP radiograph shows cardiomegaly, low lung volumes, and prominent pulmonary vasculature. AP technique can magnify cardiac silhouette.* **(Right)** *3D echocardiogram shows LV dilatation and severe systolic dysfunction. 3D echocardiography can improve the accuracy of LV volume and ejection fraction (EF) measurement by avoiding the geometric modeling necessary in 2D techniques. In some cases, definition of the endocardial border can be limited due to low spatial resolution.*

TERMINOLOGY

Abbreviations

- Dilated cardiomyopathy (DCM)

Synonyms

- Idiopathic DCM

Definitions

- Left ventricular (LV) chamber dilation with systolic dysfunction ± right ventricular (RV) dilation/dysfunction
  - LV dilatation is assessed by LV diameter (2D echocardiography) or quantitative LV volumes [cardiac MR (CMR), 3D echo, MUGA]
  - Systolic dysfunction [LV ejection fraction (EF) < 55%]
- Multiple possible etiologies
  - Idiopathic
  - Familial (genetic)
  - Infectious
  - Toxic (e.g., alcohol, cocaine)
  - Metabolic (e.g., hypophosphatemia, hypocalcemia, uremia)
  - Myocarditis
  - Infiltrative disease (e.g., hemochromatosis, sarcoid)
  - Peripartum cardiomyopathy
  - Connective tissue disease
  - Chemotherapy (e.g., doxorubicin)
  - Endocrinopathies (e.g., thyroid dysfunction, pheochromocytoma, Cushing disease)
  - Current definition excludes ischemic, hypertensive, and valvular heart disease

IMAGING

General Features

- Best diagnostic clue
  - Cardiomegaly

Radiographic Findings

- Radiography
  - Cardiomegaly with cardiac silhouette > 50% of thoracic diameter on posteroanterior view
  - Atrial enlargement
  - Findings of decompensated congestive heart failure (pulmonary edema, pleural effusion)

CT Findings

- Cardiac CTA can exclude obstructive coronary artery disease in low to intermediate risk population
- Volume-rendered multiphase datasets can accurately quantify ventricular volumes, mass, and EF
  - Typically done in patients with contraindications for MR

MR Findings

- MR cine
  - Evaluates functional impact of cardiomyopathy
  - Gold standard for ventricular volumes and function
    - Ventricular dilatation (indexed to body surface area)
    - Decreased global or regional function
  - Apical LV thrombus can be seen due to slow flow
- 1st-pass perfusion
  - Stress perfusion can exclude obstructive disease
- LGE
  - Determine nonischemic pattern of LGE
  - Linear midmyocardial LGE of septum (basal and mid) can be seen in idiopathic DCM (present in ~ 30%)
    - Due to interstitial or reparative fibrosis
  - Epicardial or midmyocardial LGE may suggest etiologies, such as sarcoid, myocarditis, Chagas disease
  - Subendocardial pattern seen in 13%
    - Either due to unusual nonischemic fibrosis or silent infarct by coronary embolus or recanalized ruptured plaque
  - No specific enhancement can be seen in 59% of patients
  - Presence of LGE is associated with increased risk of major adverse cardiac events
    - Superior to conventional parameters like EF
  - Guides implantable cardioverter defibrillator (ICD) placement
    - Using LGE, 19% of additional patients get ICD; 11% avoid ICD
- T1 and extracellular volume (ECV) mapping
  - LGE images may be normal despite presence of diffuse fibrosis
  - Increased native T1 and ECV seen in diffuse fibrosis
  - Independent predictor of all-cause mortality and composite heart failure endpoint
- Myocardial strain
  - Can detect subtle abnormalities
  - Global longitudinal strain and long-axis strain are associated with adverse outcome
  - 1% increase in global longitudinal strain increases risk of all-cause mortality regardless of LVEF and LGE

Echocardiographic Findings

- LV dysfunction/dilation ± RV involvement
- Easily accessible and relatively inexpensive

Nuclear Medicine Findings

- PET
  - Can exclude prior infarct or ischemia

Imaging Recommendations

- Best imaging tool
  - MR is most accurate method for assessing LV volumes, mass, and EF
    - Patterns of LGE may suggest specific etiology
    - Presence and extent of LGE has prognostic importance
  - Echocardiography remains initial test in evaluation of suspected cardiomyopathy
    - In some patients, limited acoustic windows may reduce diagnostic accuracy
- Protocol advice
  - Echocardiography is most common initial test in evaluation of suspected cardiomyopathy
  - Cardiac MR and CT should be considered based on patient-specific parameters

DIFFERENTIAL DIAGNOSIS

Restrictive Cardiomyopathy

- Increased resistance to ventricular filling due to abnormal myocardial stiffness

- Biatrial enlargement with normal ventricular size
- Diastolic dysfunction
- Chest radiography findings of congestive heart failure without cardiomegaly

Hypertrophic Cardiomyopathy

- Genetic disease of cardiac sarcomere
- Hypertrophy tends to be asymmetric involving basal interventricular septum, but disease may manifest with atypical patterns of hypertrophy (e.g., midcavity or apical)

Valvular Heart Disease

- Chronic mitral regurgitation and aortic regurgitation can lead to LV dilatation and systolic dysfunction
  - Echocardiography is imaging test of choice for evaluation of valvular heart disease
  - Cardiac MR can be useful in patients with limited or inconclusive echo data; phase-contrast imaging can be used to calculate regurgitant volumes
- Severe aortic stenosis
  - Longstanding severe LV pressure overload can cause LV systolic dysfunction and chamber dilatation

PATHOLOGY

General Features

- Etiology
  - Multiple possible causes
    - Common causes include viral infections as well as genetic mutations
  - In many cases, specific etiology is not identified, though thorough evaluation for reversible causes is warranted
- Genetics
  - Familial DCM is estimated to account for ~ 25% of idiopathic cases
    - Mode of inheritance is usually autosomal dominant, although cases of autosomal recessive, X-linked, and mitochondrial inheritance have been described
  - Inherited syndromes
    - DCM may be important component of inherited disorders, such as neuromuscular disease (i.e., muscular dystrophies)

Staging, Grading, & Classification

- New York Heart Association (NYHA) criteria is most often used to assess functional class of patients with heart failure and is associated with prognosis

Gross Pathologic & Surgical Features

- LV dilation, which may be associated with RV dilation
  - Associated biatrial enlargement may also be seen
- Thrombi, particularly in LV apex, may be seen

Microscopic Features

- Interstitial and perivascular fibrosis
- Variation in myocyte size

CLINICAL ISSUES

Presentation

- Most common signs/symptoms
  - Dyspnea with exertion, impaired exercise capacity, orthopnea, paroxysmal nocturnal dyspnea, and peripheral edema
- Other signs/symptoms
  - Arrhythmia, conduction disturbance, thromboembolic complications

Demographics

- Age
  - Risk for morbidity and mortality with older age
- Sex
  - M > F
- Ethnicity
  - Black populations have almost 3x greater risk for developing DCM, which is not fully attributed to differences in risk factors, such as hypertension, tobacco use, and EtOH consumption
- Epidemiology
  - Prevalence of 36 per 100,000; may be underestimate since patients may have subclinical cardiomyopathy
  - Increased prevalence and worse prognosis in men and Black population
  - 25% of DCM may be genetic in etiology

Natural History & Prognosis

- Patients may be asymptomatic
- In those who develop symptomatic congestive heart failure, annual mortality rate is ~ 10%
- ~ 25% of patients may have improvement in LV function over time
- Severity of LV dilation/dysfunction and concomitant RV dilation/dysfunction are associated with prognosis
- Presence of LGE is associated with worse prognosis
  - Presence of fibrosis and extent of midwall LGE in myocarditis are independently associated with all-cause mortality and are incremental to LVEF and other conventional prognostic factors

Treatment

- Standard medical therapy for heart failure
  - ACE inhibitors, β-blockers, aldosterone receptor blockers, ARB/neprilysin inhibitors, diuretics, digoxin
- Anticoagulation to reduce risk of thromboembolism in patients with atrial fibrillation
- Device therapy with ICD ± biventricular pacing
- Cardiac transplantation

DIAGNOSTIC CHECKLIST

Consider

- Ischemic etiology should be excluded

Image Interpretation Pearls

- CMR provides most detailed tissue characterization
- LGE patterns can help identify specific etiology

SELECTED REFERENCES

1. Li Y et al: Cardiac MRI to predict sudden cardiac death risk in dilated cardiomyopathy. Radiology. 307(3):e222552, 2023
2. Marrow BA et al: Emerging techniques for risk stratification in nonischemic dilated cardiomyopathy: JACC review topic of the week. J Am Coll Cardiol. 75(10):1196-207, 2020

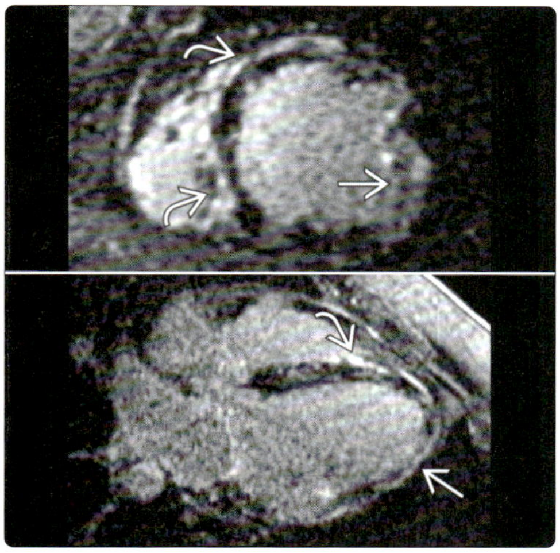

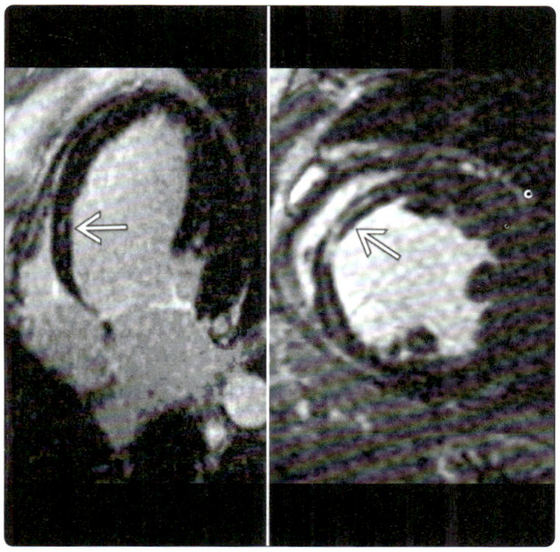

(Left) *Short-axis and 4-chamber LGE MR show extensive epicardial LGE in septal segments* *as well as patchy subendocardial LGE of the lateral segments* *. Right ventricle (RV) endomyocardial biopsy showed nonspecific fibrosis with no evidence of myocarditis or sarcoidosis.* **(Right)** *Combined 4-chamber and short-axis LGE MR show a linear focus of LGE in a midwall distribution involving the midanteroseptum and midinferoseptum* *and dilated LV. This pattern of LGE is typical of a nonischemic dilated cardiomyopathy.*

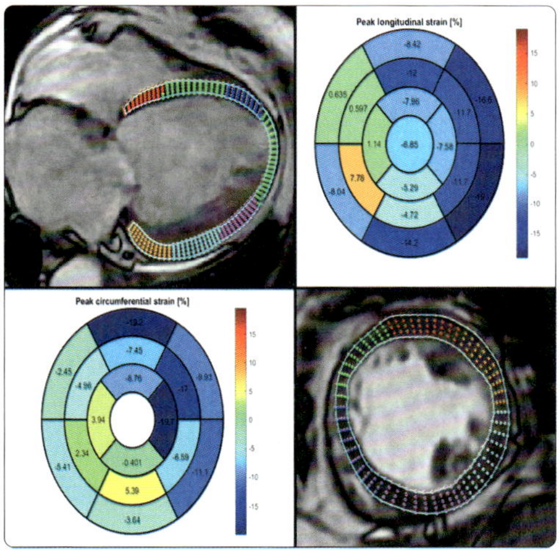

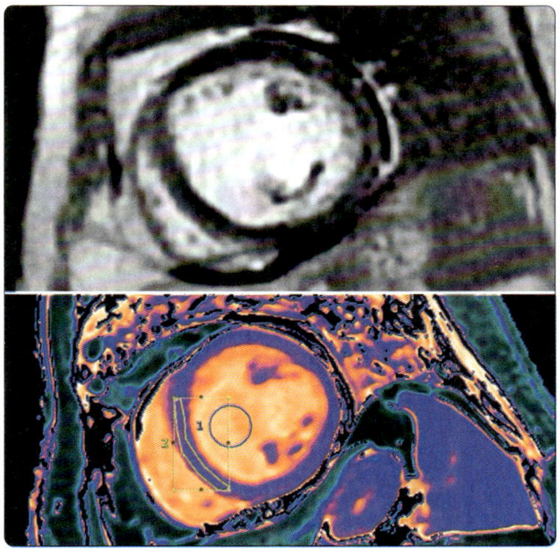

(Left) *Longitudinal (top row) and circumferential (bottom row) MR strain images show impaired global and longitudinal strain (GLS: -7.1%, GCS: -6.4%). The LV is also dilated with decreased systolic function (LVEF: 27%).* **(Right)** *Short-axis LGE MR shows no definite myocardial enhancement, but there are diffusely elevated native T1 values (1,133 ms) and ECV (35%). The overall findings are consistent with nonischemic dilated cardiomyopathy. (Courtesy M. Barbosa, MD.)*

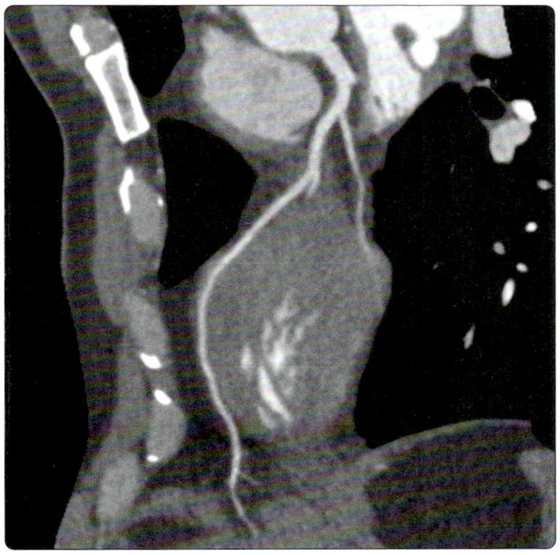

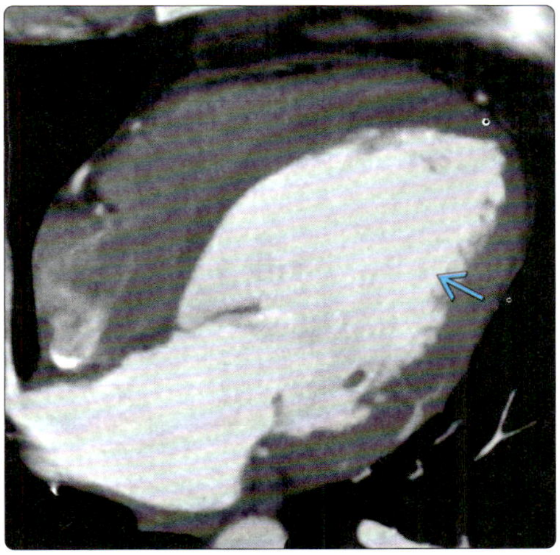

(Left) *Curved MPR coronary CTA of the left main artery and left anterior descending artery shows no evidence of coronary artery disease in a patient presenting with new-onset dilated cardiomyopathy.* **(Right)** *Four-chamber cardiac CT during diastole shows LV dilation* *in the same patient. There is no evidence of wall thinning or calcification to suggest a prior infarct, and there is no evidence of LV thrombus. All these findings point to a nonischemic etiology.*

KEY FACTS

TERMINOLOGY

- Hypertrophic cardiomyopathy (HCM)
  - Hypertrophic obstructive cardiomyopathy or idiopathic hypertrophic subaortic stenosis when left ventricular outflow tract (LVOT) obstruction is present
- Genetic disease affecting proteins of myocardial sarcomere & associated myofilaments

IMAGING

- Left ventricular (LV) wall thickness > 15 mm, but degree of hypertrophy can vary
- Most common location is basal septal hypertrophy with other patterns, including concentric, midcavitary, & apical
- Cardiac CT: Can be used in patients with nondiagnostic echocardiography & contraindication to MR
- Echocardiography: 1st-line modality
- MR: Most useful in assessment of LGE & papillary muscle abnormalities
- LGE can be diffuse or focal; often involves segments with most hypertrophy as well as right ventricular insertion sites

TOP DIFFERENTIAL DIAGNOSES

- Systemic arterial hypertension
- Aortic stenosis
- Athlete's heart
- Infiltrative cardiomyopathy

CLINICAL ISSUES

- High-risk factors on imaging
  - Wall thickness > 30 mm
  - LVOT gradient > 30 mmHg
  - Extensive LGE, > 15 % of myocardial mass
  - LV ejection fraction < 50%
  - Apical aneurysm

(Left) *Short-axis cine MR in end-diastole shows an asymmetric increased anterior septal wall thickness of 23 mm, consistent with hypertrophic cardiomyopathy (HCM) with anteroseptal hypertrophy ➔.* **(Right)** *Short-axis LGE MR in the same patient shows patchy LGE in the basal anteroseptum involving the area of maximal hypertrophy ➔.*

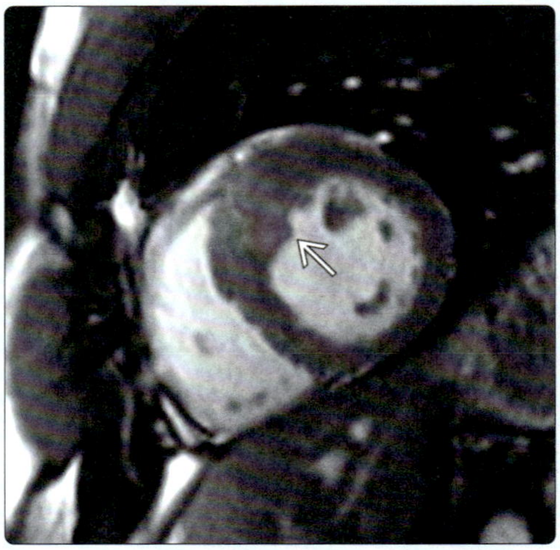

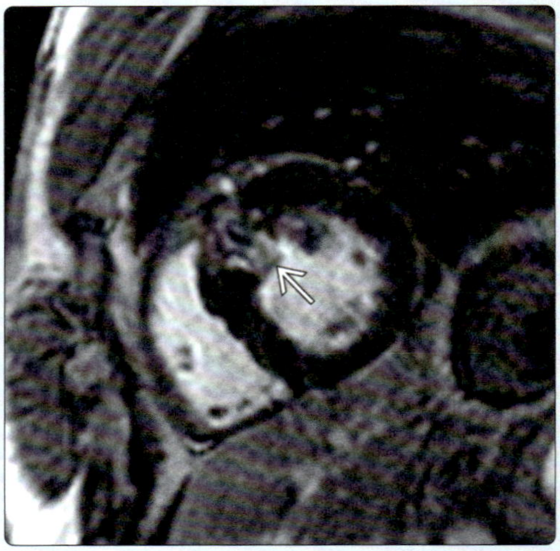

(Left) *Three-chamber cine MR in diastole shows HCM with an asymmetric increased thickness of the basal anteroseptum measuring 20 mm ➔ adjacent to the left ventricular outflow tract. Asymmetric septal hypertrophy is the most common morphologic variant of HCM.* **(Right)** *Vertical long-axis (2-chamber) cine MR in end-diastole shows HCM with focal left ventricular hypertrophy ➔ involving the basal to midanterior wall measuring 22 mm.*

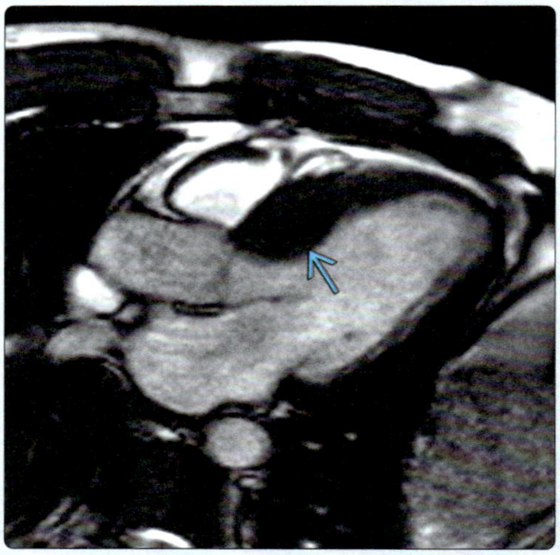

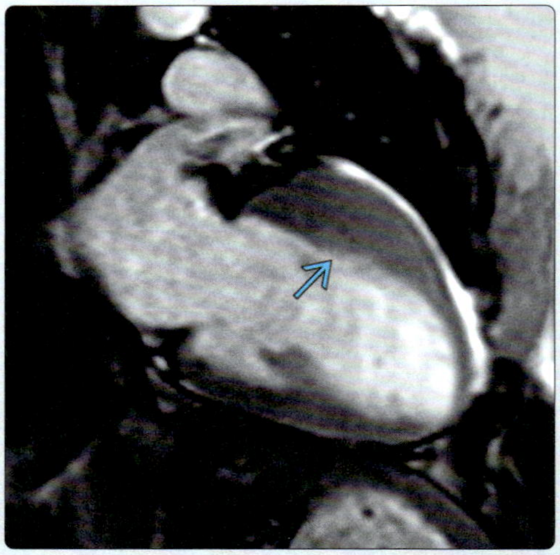

TERMINOLOGY

Abbreviations

- Hypertrophic cardiomyopathy (HCM)

Definitions

- Genetic disease affecting proteins of myocardial sarcomere & associated myofilaments
  - Left ventricular (LV) hypertrophy without secondary cause
    - Hypertrophy can be present in various patterns, such as asymmetric septal (most common), concentric, midcavitary, or apical

IMAGING

General Features

- Best diagnostic clue
  - Myocardial hypertrophy not explained by another disease
    - Most common diagnostic criterion of HCM is LV wall thickness > 15 mm, although HCM can be present with any degree of hypertrophy
- Size
  - LV mass may be ↑
- Morphology
  - Sigmoid: 40-50%; basal septal protuberance; concave septum
    - More mild, isolated basilar septal hypertrophy can be incidental finding in older adult patients
  - Reverse curve: 30-40%; convex septum; high association with abnormal genes
  - Neutral: 10%; straight septum
  - Apical: 10%
  - Mixed pattern
  - Burned out: Dilated cardiomyopathy in end stage
  - Other features: Obstruction; apical aneurysm; right ventricular (RV) involvement

CT Findings

- In patients with nondiagnostic echocardiogram & contraindication to MR

MR Findings

- Accurate quantification of myocardial thickness & LV mass
  - Hypertrophy often > 15 mm; hypertrophied:nonhypertrophied ratio > 1.3
  - Global LV mass accurately measured by drawing endocardial & epicardial contours in end-diastolic SSFP
  - Segmental wall thickness can be quantified: American Heart Association model
- Pattern & extent of LV hypertrophy can be variable
  - Asymmetric: Basal septal; midventricular; apical; lateral wall; mass-like
    - Basal septal: Most common (60% of HCM)
    - Midventricular: Associated with apical aneurysm & thrombus
    - Apical: Thickness > 15 mm; apical:basal thickness ratio > 1.3-1.5; spade-like LV cavity in true apical form
    - Mass-like: Mimics cardiac mass, but myocardial tags deform & normal perfusion
  - Concentric: HCM accounts for 5% of patients with concentric hypertrophy; difficult to distinguish from hypertension
  - RV hypertrophy in 1/3
  - Can also be classified as sigmoid, reverse curve, neutral, apical, mixed, burnt-out
- LV outflow obstruction
  - Seen in up to 30% in MR, in basal septal type
  - Flow acceleration in left ventricular outflow tract (LVOT)
  - Velocity & gradient can be quantified using phase-contrast MR
    - ≥ 50 mmHg is considered obstructive
    - May be present at rest or only with provocation
      - > 50% of patients with minimal gradient at rest develop significant gradient with exercise
    - In midventricular type, gradient is seen in midcavity
      - Gradient > 30 mmHg is associated with bad prognosis & apical aneurysm
- Systolic anterior motion mitral valve
  - Due to venturi effect from high-velocity jet in LVOT
  - Results in posteriorly directed mitral regurgitation
- Perfusion imaging
  - Myocardial ischemia & microvascular dysfunction can be seen: Leading to fibrosis
- LGE due to fibrosis: Seen in up to 80%
  - Midmyocardial enhancement, often hazy
  - Most pronounced in hypertrophied segments
  - Can often be seen at anterior & posterior RV insertion sites (junction of RV & septum)
    - Full-thickness LGE in burnt-out phase
  - LGE is associated with markers of risk of sudden cardiac death (SCD), ventricular arrhythmia, worsening heart failure, implantable cardioverter-defibrillator (ICD) discharge
    - Extensive LGE defined as > 15% of myocardium
- T1 mapping
  - High native T1 & extracellular volume (ECV); may be abnormal even without LGE
  - Values elevated but less so than seen with amyloid
- Functional evaluation
  - ↑ ejection fraction (EF) (hyperdynamic); ↓ or normal cavity size; ↓ end-systolic volume (ESV) size
  - Strain imaging: Measures deformation of myocardial segment from initial length
    - ↓ systolic strains: Circumferential shortening, longitudinal shortening, & wall thickening in hypertrophied segments
      - Due to muscle disorganization
    - ↑ ventricular torsion: Accounts for ↑ EF
    - Myocardial tagging can be used to distinguish HCM from mass
- Complications
  - Burnt-out phase (10%): LV dilation, myocardial thinning, transmural LGE; apical aneurysm
    - Mimics dilated cardiomyopathy
  - Apical aneurysm, thromboembolism
- Mitral/papillary muscle abnormalities
  - Phenotypical variations of HCM

- Narrowing of LVOT caused by papillary muscle abnormalities without significant myocardial hypertrophy
- High-risk factors: Wall thickness > 30 mm; LVOT gradient > 30 mmHg; extensive LGE; LVEF < 50%; apical aneurysm
- Adequacy of treatment evaluation: For myectomy or septal ablation
  - Evaluation of septal reduction; extent of myocardial necrosis; size of LVOT; LVOT velocities
  - Induced infarcts by alcoholic septal ablation: Evaluated using LGE
- Family screening: High EF, delayed relaxation; deep myocardial crypts in basal inferoseptal segment; high native T1 & ECV; mitral valve abnormalities

Imaging Recommendations

- Best imaging tool
  - Echocardiography: 1st-line modality
  - MR: Most useful in assessment of LGE & papillary muscle abnormalities

DIFFERENTIAL DIAGNOSIS

Systemic Arterial Hypertension

- Thickening < 16 mm; EF: Normal or low
- LGE: Absent or minimal; T1/ECV: Lower than HCM
- ↑ LV wall stress; ↓ anteroseptal systolic strain

Athlete's Heart: Endurance Athletes

- Concentric thickening; dilation of LV (< 6.5 cm), left atrial (LA) & RV
- Normal EF & diastolic function; no LGE
- Regression after 3-month deconditioning

Infiltrative Cardiomyopathy

- Concentric LV thickening
  - Fabry disease: LGE in basal inferolateral wall; low native T1 values
  - Hemochromatosis: Low T2*
  - Amyloidosis: Diffuse subendocardial LGE; native T1 amyloid > HCM
  - Danon disease: Midmyocardial LGE; usually spares septum

Ventricular Septal Bulge

- Often asymptomatic finding in older adult patients
- However, isolated septal hypertrophy can be seen in HCM
- Associated findings
  - Focal hypertrophy of basilar septum, often < 15 mm
  - Septum inferior to focal bulge usually < 12 mm thickness
  - In 3-chamber plane, inferolateral wall < 11 mm thickness
  - Anteroseptal angle < 110°
  - Genetic testing usually negative
    - No family history of HCM or SCD
  - Older age at diagnosis (often > 60 years)
  - LVOT obstruction rare
  - LGE uncommon (but also may be absent with HCM)

PATHOLOGY

General Features

- Etiology
  - Mutations in various genes encoding for proteins of sarcomere & associated structural myofilaments
- Genetics
  - Autosomal dominant in most cases with incomplete penetrance & variable expressivity resulting in clinical heterogeneity among patients & family members
    - Genotype-positive/phenotype-negative or subclinical HCM patients require continued surveillance
  - Autosomal recessive, X-linked, & mitochondrial modes of inheritance are less common

Microscopic Features

- Myocyte & myofibrillar disarray with herringbone or pinwheel configuration on microscopy
- Myocyte hypertrophy
- ↑ in both interstitial fibrosis & replacement fibrosis

CLINICAL ISSUES

Presentation

- Most common signs/symptoms
  - Most affected patients are asymptomatic
  - Severe disease → exertional chest pain, dyspnea, syncope, & palpitations
  - Symptoms due to ventricular arrhythmia, LVOT obstruction, myocardial ischemia, diastolic dysfunction, heart failure

Demographics

- Age
  - Can present from infancy to adulthood
- Sex
  - No predominance
- Epidemiology
  - Prevalence is 1 per 500 in general population

Natural History & Prognosis

- Most patients have benign course; significant in certain patients
- SCD
  - Most common cause of young people & young athletes
  - Due to ventricular tachycardia & fibrillation
- Congestive heart failure
  - Diastolic dysfunction is often early finding
  - Systolic dysfunction can develop in small percentage
- Atrial fibrillation

Treatment

- Exercise restrictions to reduce risk of SCD
- Calcium channel or β-blockers improve symptoms of LVOT obstruction
- Septal myomectomy or catheter-based alcohol septal ablation for symptomatic relief in patients with LVOT obstruction & favorable anatomy
- ICD in patients at high risk for SCD, > 15 % LGE

SELECTED REFERENCES

1. Llamas-Esperón GA et al: Hypertrophic cardiomyopathy. Proposal for a new classification. Arch Cardiol Mex. 92(3):377-89, 2022
2. Maron MS et al: How to image hypertrophic cardiomyopathy. Circ Cardiovasc Imaging. 10(7), 2017
3. Baxi AJ et al: Hypertrophic cardiomyopathy from A to Z: genetics, pathophysiology, imaging, and management. Radiographics. 36(2):335-54, 2016

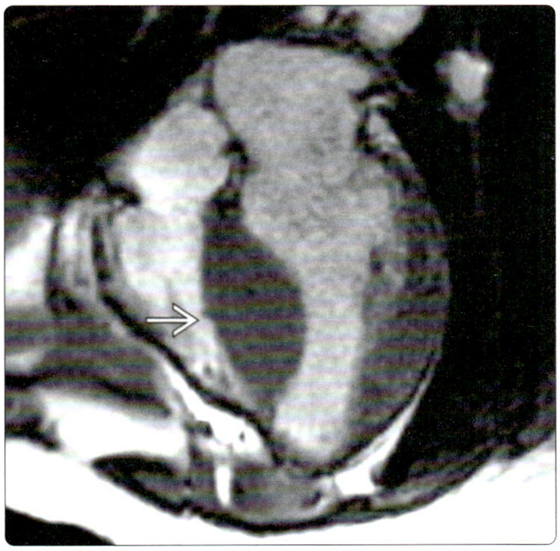

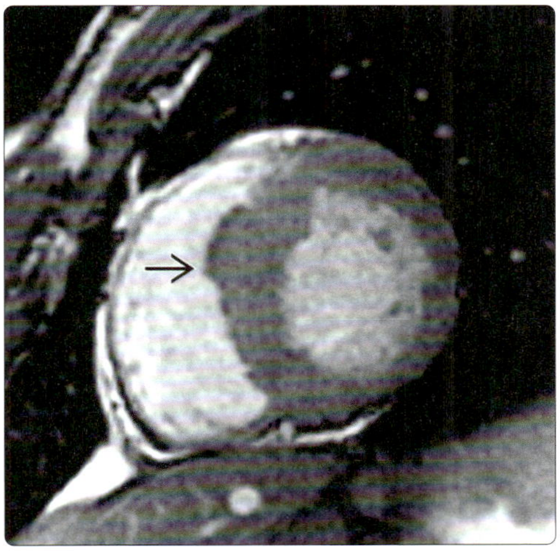

(Left) *Four-chamber SSFP cine MR demonstrates HCM with severe asymmetric septal hypertrophy ➡, consistent with the reverse curve type of HCM. The maximal thickness at midanteroseptum was 29 mm.* **(Right)** *Short-axis cine MR demonstrates HCM with anteroseptal hypertrophy ⇨ measuring 19 mm. The accurate measurement of the degree and extent of septal thickness in end diastole is important in the evaluation for potential treatments, such as alcohol septal ablation and septal myomectomy.*

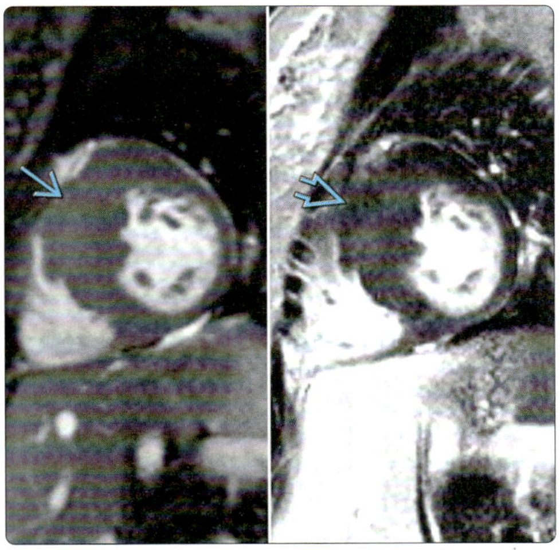

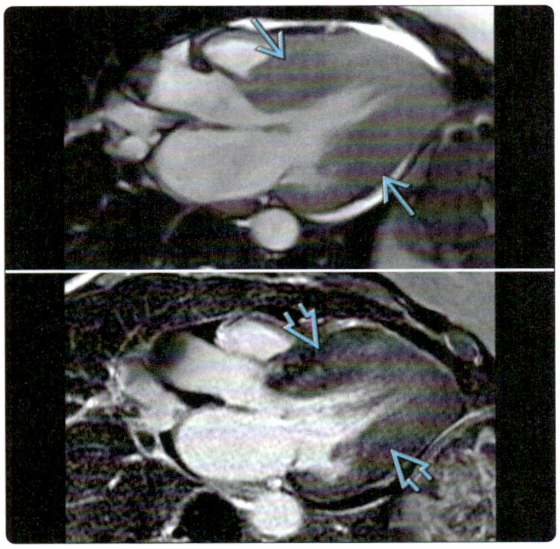

(Left) *Short-axis SSFP MR (left) in a 12-year-old girl shows mass-like thickening of the septum ⇨ at the midcavity level measuring up to 35 mm. LGE MR (right) shows hazy midmyocardial enhancement ⇨, most notably in the hypertrophied septum.* **(Right)** *Three-chamber SSFP MR (top) shows diffuse myocardial hypertrophy ⇨ with most segments measuring > 25 mm. LGE MR (bottom) shows diffuse hazy midmyocardial enhancement ⇨ involving all segments.*

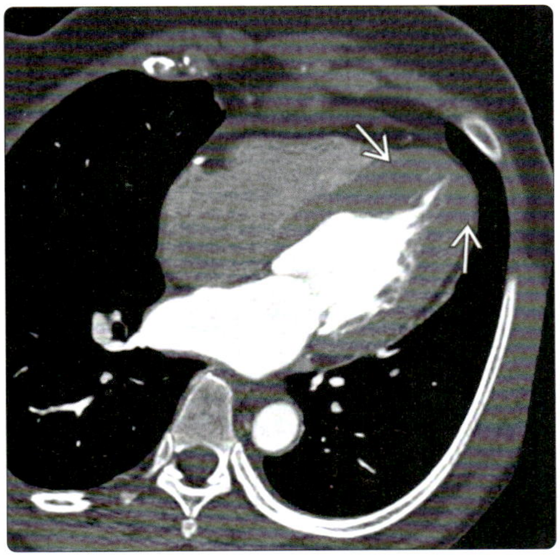

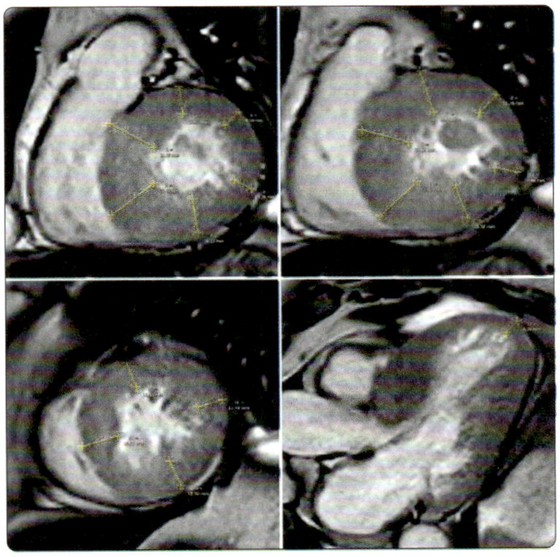

(Left) *Four-chamber cardiac CT in diastole demonstrates the apical variant of HCM ➡ with a spade-like configuration of the left ventricular cavity. The apical myocardium measured 18 mm. Cardiac CT can be considered in patients with a nondiagnostic echocardiogram and contraindications to cardiac MR.* **(Right)** *Short-axis (basal, mid, and apical level) and 3-chamber views in a patient with hypertrophic obstructive cardiomyopathy show the measurements of wall thickness at the end-diastolic phase.*

(Left) *Short-axis cine MR demonstrates HCM with asymmetric anteroseptal left ventricular hypertrophy. The maximal thickness of the septum is 25 mm.* **(Right)** *Short-axis LGE MR demonstrates the foci of LGE ➔ involving the anterior and posterior right ventricular insertion sites, which can be seen in HCM.*

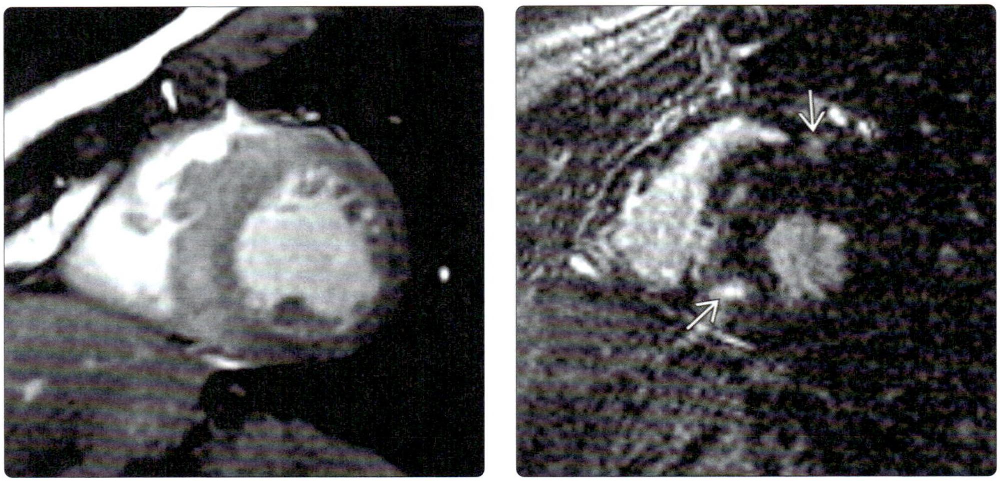

(Left) *Three-chamber cine MR demonstrates left ventricular hypertrophy involving the mid and apical segments of the left ventricle with an associated small apical aneurysm ➔. The left ventricular outflow tract appears largely unobstructed.* **(Right)** *Three-chamber LGE MR in the same patient demonstrates the same small left ventricular aneurysm ➔ at the apex.*

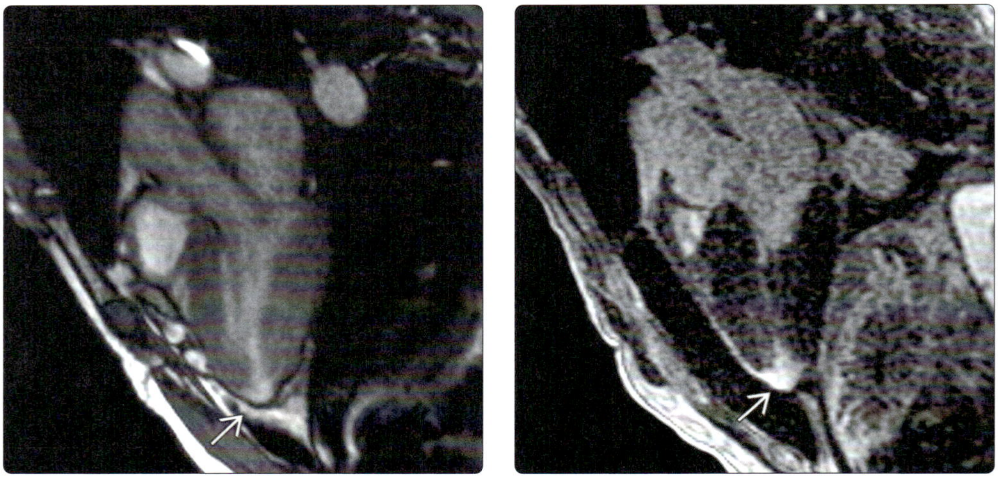

(Left) *Vertical long-axis (2-chamber) cine MR in end diastole demonstrates left ventricular hypertrophy predominantly involving the mid and apical segments of the left ventricle. The maximal thickness was 17 mm.* **(Right)** *Vertical long-axis (2-chamber) LGE MR shows a patchy focus of LGE involving the apical anterior segment ➔, indicating myocardial fibrosis.*

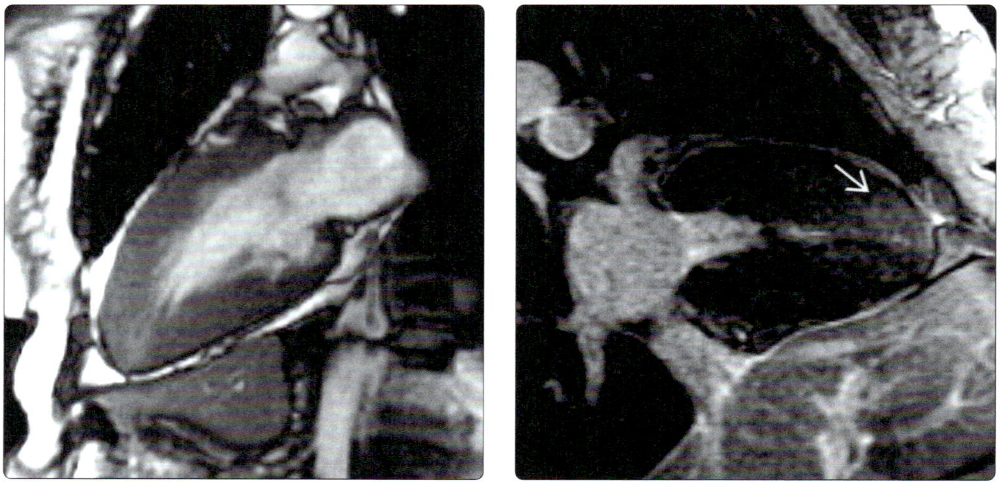

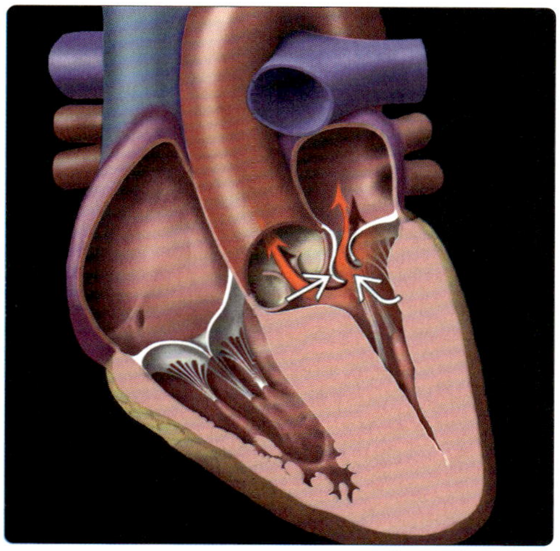

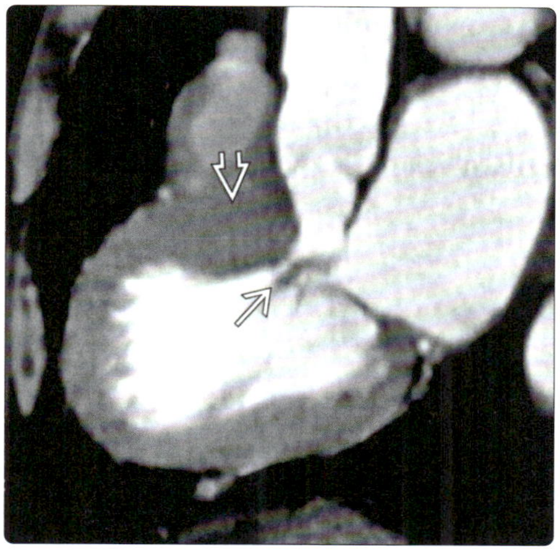

(Left) *Graphic shows concentric HCM with systolic anterior motion (SAM) of the anterior mitral valve leaflet* ➡ *with resulting noncoaptation of the leaflets and mitral valve regurgitation* ➡. **(Right)** *Three-chamber coronary CTA shows hypertrophic obstructive cardiomyopathy with asymmetric septal hypertrophy* ➡ *resulting in narrowing of the left ventricular outflow tract and, thus, flow acceleration, which in turn leads to SAM of the anterior mitral valve leaflet* ➡.

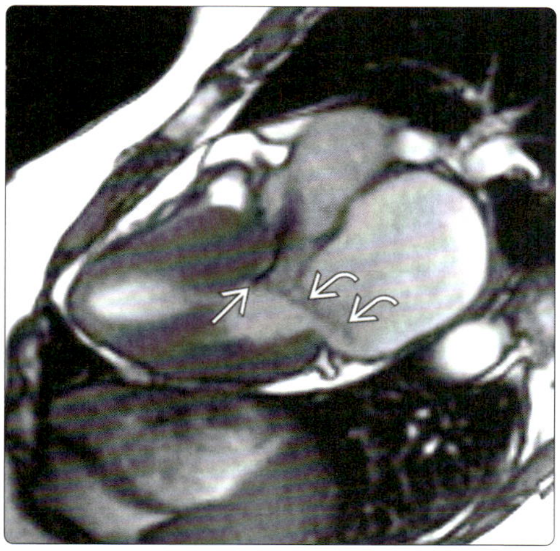

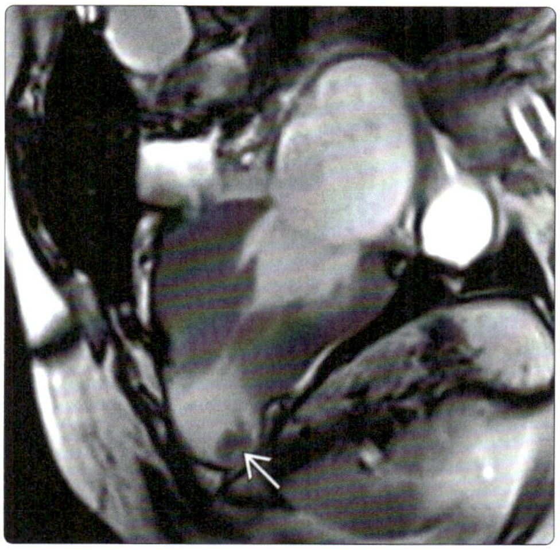

(Left) *Three-chamber cine MR demonstrates HCM with significant asymmetric septal hypertrophy with SAM of the mitral valve resulting in turbulent flow across the left ventricular outflow tract* ➡ *with an associated eccentric, posteriorly directed jet of mitral regurgitation* ➡. **(Right)** *Vertical long-axis (2-chamber) cine MR shows HCM with midventricular hypertrophy associated with an apical aneurysm and left ventricular thrombus* ➡.

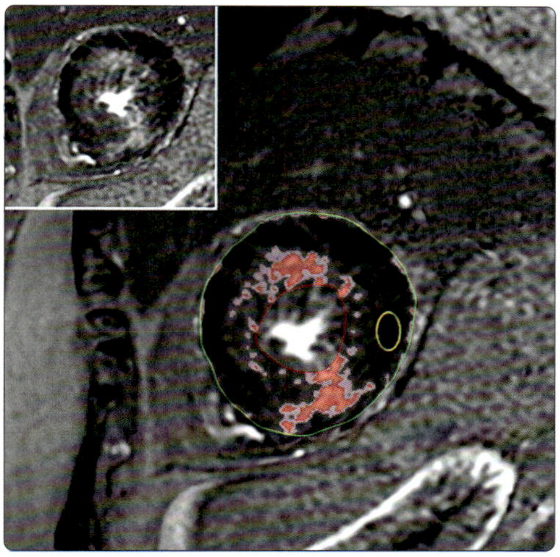

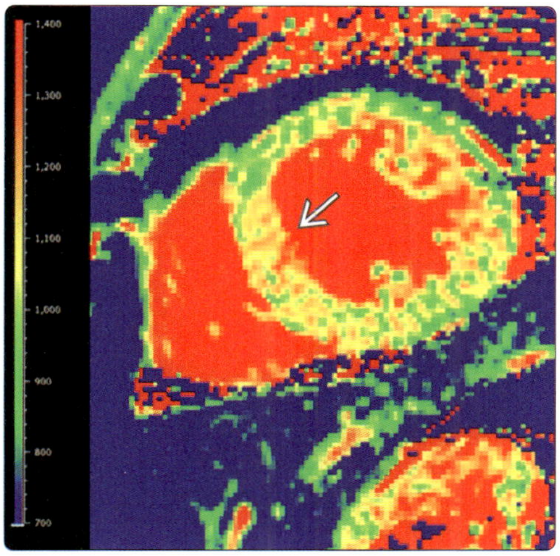

(Left) *Short-axis delayed-enhancement MR in apical HCM shows the quantification of LGE with 16.2% of hyperenhancement (red areas) and 16.4% of intermediate enhancement (purple areas). A region of interest (yellow circle) is placed over normal myocardium. Inset shows patchy midwall LGE mostly in anterior and inferior segments.* **(Right)** *T1 map in a patient with HCM shows mildly elevated native T1 values at septal segments of 1,137 ms due to fibrosis* ➡ *with global T1 value of entire myocardium of 1,047 ms.*

Athlete's Heart

KEY FACTS

TERMINOLOGY

- Athlete's heart encompasses spectrum of structural, functional, and electrical adaptations heart undergoes in response to regular high-intensity exercise
- Can potentially mimic pathologic changes associated with inherited or acquired cardiac disorders

IMAGING

- Left ventricular (LV) and right ventricular (RV) dilatation with increased ventricular mass
- LV wall thickening, usually ≤ 12 mm
- LV ejection fraction (EF) and RVEF may be normal or slightly decreased at rest; EF markedly increases during exercise
- Findings tend to decrease or resolve after cessation of exercise training (physical deconditioning or detraining)
- Standard echocardiography is 1st-line exam for differentiating athlete's heart from pathologic LV hypertrophy (LVH)
- Cardiac MR superior to echocardiography in differentiating athlete's heart from pathologic causes of LVH, such as hypertrophic cardiomyopathy
- Tissue characterization with LGE and T1 mapping further aid to differential diagnosis of hypertrophy

TOP DIFFERENTIAL DIAGNOSES

- Hypertrophic cardiomyopathy
- Dilated cardiomyopathy
- Arrhythmogenic cardiomyopathy

CLINICAL ISSUES

- Patients most often asymptomatic
- May present with palpitations and arrhythmia; most common = atrial fibrillation
- Exercise-induced cardiac remodeling is considered benign entity

(Left) *Short-axis MR cine at end-diastole shows concentric symmetric left ventricular hypertrophy in a 20-year-old male college football player with high ECG voltages who had left ventricular hypertrophy at echo.* **(Right)** *Four-chamber MR at end-diastole in the same patient shows mild left ventricular dilatation.*

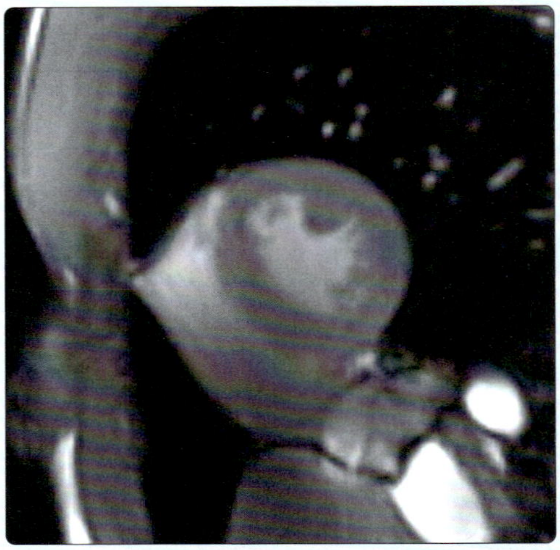

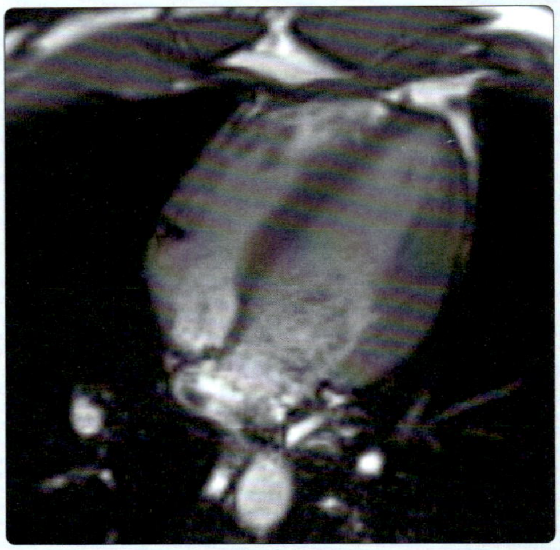

(Left) *Short-axis phase-sensitive inversion recovery (PSIR) LGE in the same patient shows no evidence of myocardial fibrosis or scarring.* **(Right)** *Four-chamber PSIR in the same patient shows no LGE. The patient was asymptomatic. Findings are in keeping with athlete's heart.*

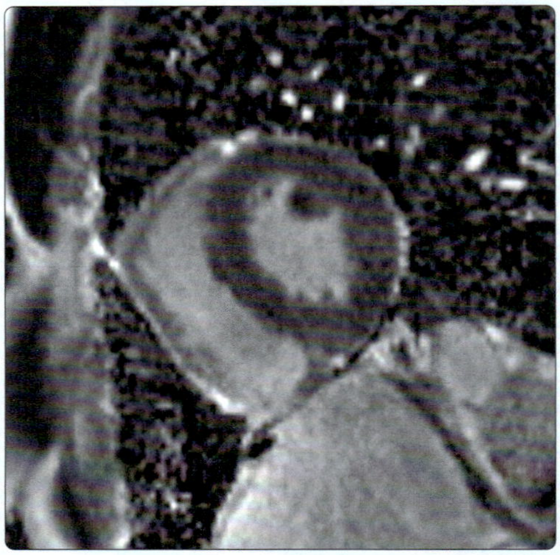

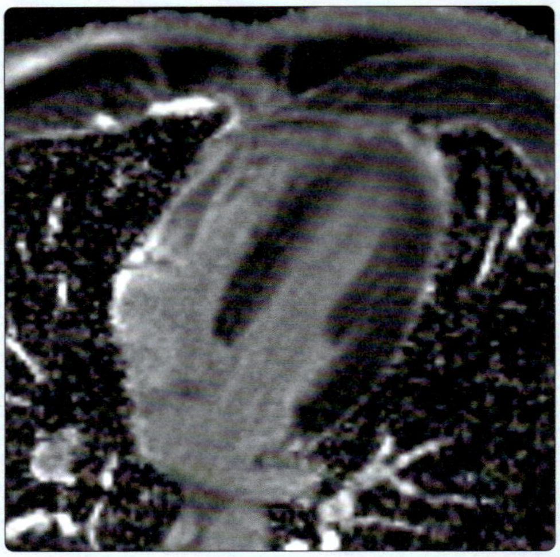

TERMINOLOGY

Synonyms

- Exercise-induced cardiac remodeling (EICR)

Definitions

- Athlete's heart encompasses spectrum of structural, functional, and electrical adaptations heart undergoes in response to regular high-intensity exercise
  - Volumes and pressure loads of exercise induce adaptive increase in cardiac chamber size and wall thickness, which is usually accompanied by lower heart rate at rest
  - Increased contractile function that allows heart to eject larger volumes during exercise
  - It can potentially mimic pathologic changes associated with inherited or acquired cardiac disorders

IMAGING

General Features

- Best diagnostic clue
  - Main findings: Left ventricular (LV) dilatation, LV hypertrophy (LVH) right ventricular (RV) dilatation ± hypertrabeculation
  - LV ejection fraction (EF) and RVEF may be normal or slightly decreased at rest; EF markedly increases during exercise
  - LV dilatation: Usually mild to moderate dilatation; main differential diagnosis is dilated cardiomyopathy
  - LVH: Concentric or eccentric hypertrophy
    - Concentric hypertrophy: More common in strength training; main differential diagnosis is hypertrophic cardiomyopathy (HCM)
    - Eccentric hypertrophy: More common in endurance training
  - LV wall thickening, usually ≤ 12 mm; consider other causes of LVH if thickening is > 12 mm, especially ≥ 15 mm
  - Heart remodeling is most often balanced within right and left cardiac chambers
    - During intense endurance exercise right heart is exposed to disproportional afterload and wall stress
    - RV dilatation: Symmetrical and without regional wall motion abnormalities
      - Most often accompanied by harmonic enlargement of left cardiac chambers
  - Findings tend to decrease or resolve after cessation of exercise training (physical deconditioning or detraining)
    - Physical deconditioning response is heterogeneous, and some patients may show persistent LV dilatation and hypertrophy even years after suspending high-intensity physical activity
  - Acute strenuous activity (high-intensity cycling) has been associated with postrace cardiac troponin I increase, increased T1 relaxation time, and RV dysfunction, including reduced strain
  - When cardiac changes do not decrease or resolve after detraining, consider alternative diagnoses

Imaging Recommendations

- Best imaging tool
  - Echocardiography is often 1st-line exam
  - Cardiac MR (CMR) is used for confirmation of diagnosis and exclusion of differential diagnostic considerations
  - CMR is reference standard

Echocardiography

- Transthoracic echocardiography is 1st-line exam for differentiating athlete's heart from other causes of pathologic LVH
  - LV end-diastolic diameter > 60 mm should raise suspicion of idiopathic dilated cardiomyopathy when LV dilation is out of proportion to athlete's conditioning
  - Maximal end-diastolic septal wall thickness is usually ≤ 12 mm in males and ≤ 9 mm in females
  - Low-normal or decreased LVEF with preserved or augmented stroke volume
  - Pulsed tissue Doppler shows normal or increased myocardial systolic performance at rest
  - Diastolic function is normal or even supranormal (E/A ratio > 2)
- Atrial volumes in athletes up to 60% larger than in nonathletes; may be decreased atrial strain
- Athletes may show slightly decreased global longitudinal strain but increased global circumferential and global radial strains
- Changes may decrease after physical deconditioning, while reverse LV remodeling does not occur in pathologic LVH

Cardiac MR

- Gold standard for assessment of ventricular volumes, LV mass, and global and regional contractile function
  - High interstudy reproducibility of CMR is relevant when assessing individual changes after training cessation
- CMR is superior to echocardiography in differentiating athlete's heart from pathologic causes of LVH, such as HCM
- RV:LV ratio > 1.2 could indicate underlying RV cardiomyopathy
- Tissue characterization with LGE and T1 mapping further aid to differential diagnosis of hypertrophy
  - Studies have shown that LGE can be present in nearly 16% of athlete's, regardless of normal or mildly decreased LVEF
    - Linear nonischemic midwall or subepicardial LGE involving interventricular septum, lateral wall, or RV hinge points
    - LGE is less extensive than in DCM or HCM
  - Extracellular volume (ECV) is lower in athletes than in nonathletes
    - This supports that increased LV mass in athletes occurs due to expansion of cellular compartment while ECV becomes smaller

DIFFERENTIAL DIAGNOSIS

Hypertrophic Cardiomyopathy

- LVH is usually more pronounced (wall thickness ≥ 15 mm) and asymmetrical
- LV cavity tends to be smaller than in athlete's heart
- More severe left atrial enlargement
- Nonischemic LGE of hypertrophic myocardium
- May be accompanied by LV outflow tract obstruction and mitral SAM

Dilated Cardiomyopathy

- LV dilatation tends to be more severe and LVEF is often lower than in athlete's heart
- Myocardial thickness is usually within normal limits or even decreased in advanced cases
- Failure to physiologically increase LVEF during exercise
- Nonischemic septal midwall LGE

Arrhythmogenic Cardiomyopathy

- Physiologic ventricular remodeling and electrical changes may mimic arrhythmogenic cardiomyopathy
- Regional wall motion abnormalities are not feature of athlete's heart
- More severe ventricular dilatation and lower RVEF or LVEF
- Nonischemic LGE of RV or LV

PATHOLOGY

General Features

- Exercise can have profound influence on cardiac size and mass, and this is dependent on type and duration of exercise
  - Intense endurance training has greatest impact on cardiac structure, function, and electrophysiology
  - Cardiac mass and cardiac volumes are ~ 35% and 80% higher in athletes than nonathletes, respectively
- Pathology: Physiologic cardiomyocyte hypertrophy
- Preclinical models have demonstrated association between high-intensity endurance training and myocardial inflammation involving atria and ventricles
- Small patches of interstitial fibrosis have been frequently reported in athletes
  - Unclear if represents underlying cardiomyopathy

CLINICAL ISSUES

Presentation

- Most common signs/symptoms
  - Patients are most often asymptomatic
  - May present with palpitations and arrhythmia
    - Most common is atrial fibrillation
  - Serious ventricular arrhythmias are extremely rare and may be caused by underlying occult cardiomyopathy

Natural History & Prognosis

- EICR is considered benign entity
- Changes tend to decrease or resolve after detraining

DIAGNOSTIC CHECKLIST

Consider

- In cases of increased LV mass and ventricular volumes in patients engaged in recurrent and at least moderate intensity physical activity

Reporting Tips

- Report myocardial mass and maximal myocardial thickness
  - Suggest follow-up after 3 months of suspending physical activity for reassessment of myocardial mass and volumes

SELECTED REFERENCES

1. Claessen G et al: Reduced ejection fraction in elite endurance athletes: clinical and genetic overlap with dilated cardiomyopathy. Circulation. 149(18):1405-15, 2024
2. Ghekiere O et al: Exercise-induced myocardial T1 increase and right ventricular dysfunction in recreational cyclists: a CMR study. Eur J Appl Physiol. 123(10):2107-17, 2023
3. La Gerche A et al: The athlete's heart-challenges and controversies: JACC focus seminar 4/4. J Am Coll Cardiol. 80(14):1346-62, 2022
4. Petek BJ et al: Cardiac effects of detraining in athletes: a narrative review. Ann Phys Rehabil Med. 65(4):101581, 2022
5. Zorzi A et al: Differential diagnosis between athlete's heart and hypertrophic cardiomyopathy: new pieces of the puzzle. Int J Cardiol. 353:77-9, 2022
6. Kübler J et al: Cardiac MRI findings to differentiate athlete's heart from hypertrophic (HCM), arrhythmogenic right ventricular (ARVC) and dilated (DCM) cardiomyopathy. Int J Cardiovasc Imaging. 37(8):2501-15, 2021
7. D'Ascenzi F et al: Female athlete's heart: sex effects on electrical and structural remodeling. Circ Cardiovasc Imaging. 13(12):e011587, 2020
8. Elliott AD et al: Association between physical activity and risk of incident arrhythmias in 402 406 individuals: evidence from the UK Biobank cohort. Eur Heart J. 41(15):1479-86, 2020
9. Millar LM et al: Differentiation between athlete's heart and dilated cardiomyopathy in athletic individuals. Heart. 106(14):1059-65, 2020
10. Trivedi SJ et al: Differing mechanisms of atrial fibrillation in athletes and non-athletes: alterations in atrial structure and function. Eur Heart J Cardiovasc Imaging. 21(12):1374-83, 2020
11. Pelliccia A et al: European Association of Preventive Cardiology (EAPC) and European Association of Cardiovascular Imaging (EACVI) joint position statement: recommendations for the indication and interpretation of cardiovascular imaging in the evaluation of the athlete's heart. Eur Heart J. 39(21):1949-69, 2018
12. Galderisi M et al: The multi-modality cardiac imaging approach to the athlete's heart: an expert consensus of the European Association of Cardiovascular Imaging. Eur Heart J Cardiovasc Imaging. 16(4):353, 2015
13. La Gerche A et al: Exercise-induced right ventricular dysfunction is associated with ventricular arrhythmias in endurance athletes. Eur Heart J. 36(30):1998-2010, 2015
14. Zaidi A et al: Clinical differentiation between physiological remodeling and arrhythmogenic right ventricular cardiomyopathy in athletes with marked electrocardiographic repolarization anomalies. J Am Coll Cardiol. 65(25):2702-11, 2015
15. Spence AL et al: A prospective randomised longitudinal MRI study of left ventricular adaptation to endurance and resistance exercise training in humans. J Physiol. 589(Pt 22):5443-52, 2011
16. Mihl C et al: Cardiac remodelling: concentric versus eccentric hypertrophy in strength and endurance athletes. Neth Heart J. 16(4):129-33, 2008
17. Pelliccia A et al: Remodeling of left ventricular hypertrophy in elite athletes after long-term deconditioning. Circulation. 105(8):944-9, 2002

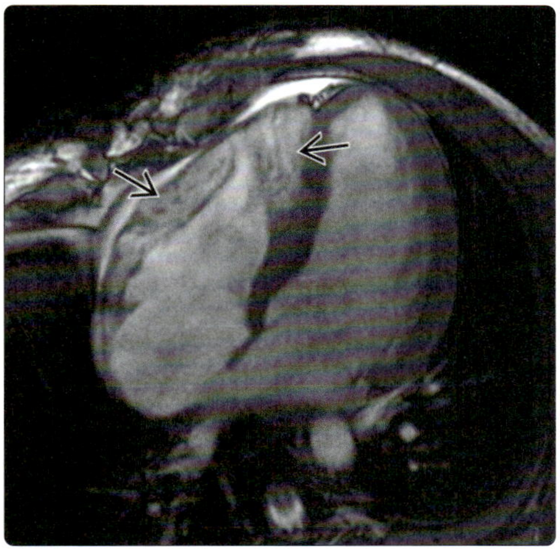

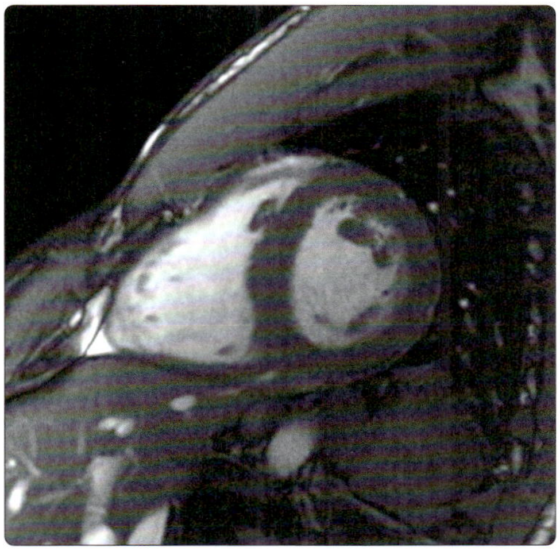

(Left) *SSFP 4-chamber end-diastolic MR cine shows mild biventricular dilatation in a 19-year-old male athlete with occasional palpitations who had a routine health check that revealed tall ECG voltages. There is hypertrabeculation of the right ventricle* ⇒. **(Right)** *Short-axis end-diastolic MR cine in the same patient shows diffuse concentric left ventricular hypertrophy.*

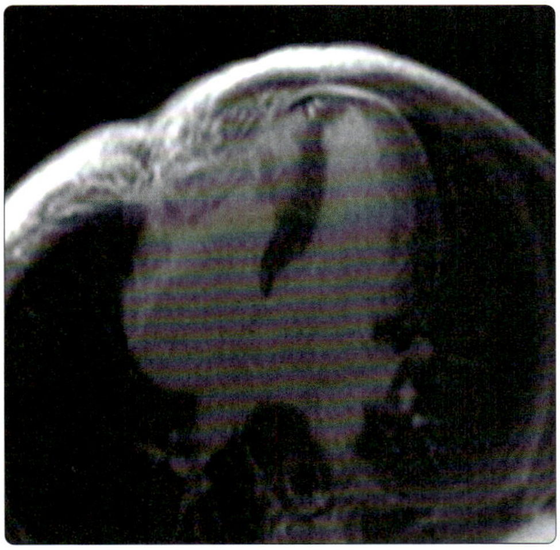

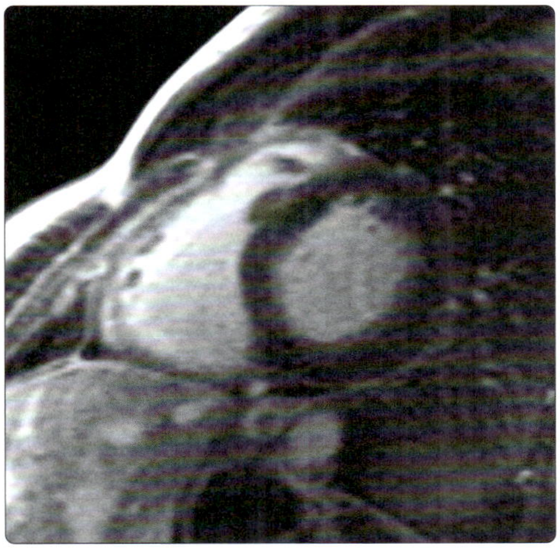

(Left) *LGE PSIR 4-chamber image in the same patient shows no evidence of LGE.* **(Right)** *Short-axis PSIR in the same patient shows no LGE.*

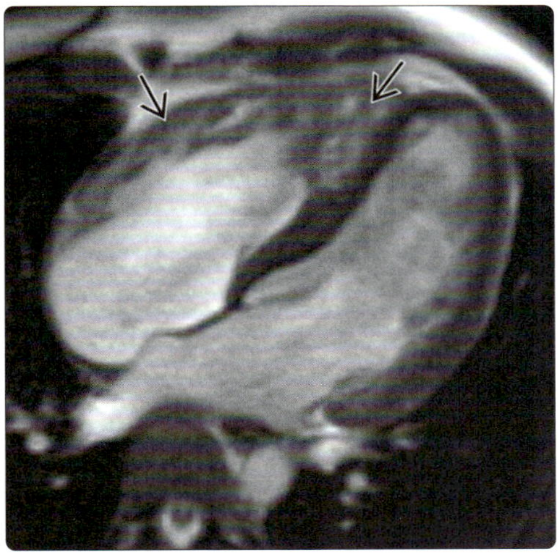

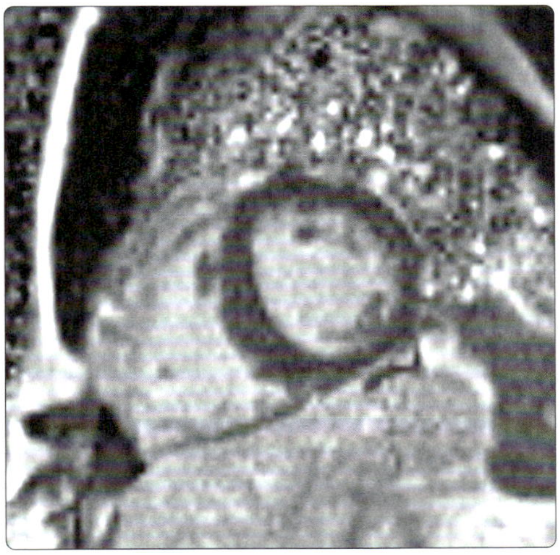

(Left) *A cardiac MR in the same patient was performed 6 months after physical deconditioning (the patient suspended all physical activity). Four-chamber MR cine at end-diastole shows an interval decrease of the left ventricular mass and wall thickness. There is persistent right ventricular hypertrabeculation* ⇒. **(Right)** *Short-axis LGE in the same patient was once again negative. The appearance supports the diagnosis of athlete's heart.*

Sigmoid Septum

KEY FACTS

TERMINOLOGY

- Localized thickening of basal portion of interventricular septum

IMAGING

- Basal septum ≥ 14 mm
  - Basal:midseptum ratio > 1.3
- No evidence of left ventricular hypertrophy (LVH)

TOP DIFFERENTIAL DIAGNOSES

- Sigmoid variant hypertrophic cardiomyopathy
- Hypertensive heart disease

PATHOLOGY

- Basal septal hypertrophy without evidence of cardiomyocyte disarray or scarring

CLINICAL ISSUES

- Considered normal variant that increases in prevalence with age
- Mostly incidental finding with excellent prognosis
- Can be clinically relevant if evidence of left ventricular outflow tract obstruction (LVOTO)
  - Then termed dynamic obstructive basal septal hypertrophy (DOBSH)

DIAGNOSTIC CHECKLIST

- Isolated basal septal hypertrophy without evidence of systolic anterior motion of mitral valve leaflets (SAM) or LVOTO at rest

SCANNING TIPS

- Echocardiography in parasternal long axis
- Cardiac MR cine acquisitions in left 2- and 3-chamber and short-axis views; LGE; 2D &/or 4D flow measurements
- Consider short stack of 3-chamber cine images to assess for LVOTO

(Left) *Sigmoid septum in a 70-year-old man is shown. Parasternal long-axis echocardiogram shows basal septal hypertrophy with otherwise normal thickness of the interventricular septum.* **(Right)** *Corresponding 4-chamber reconstruction of a coronary CTA in the same patient also demonstrates asymmetric thickening of the basal interventricular septum.*

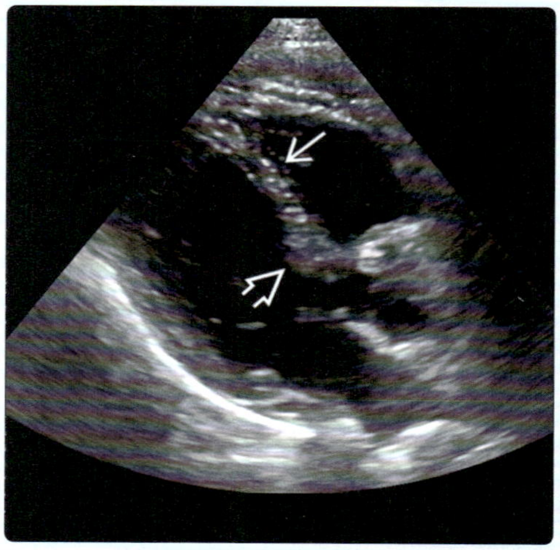

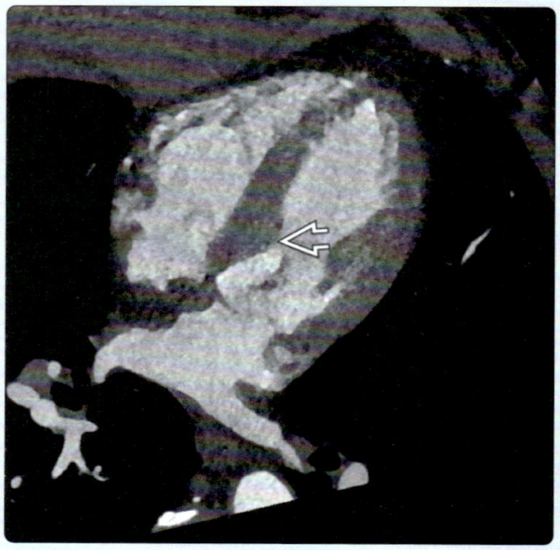

(Left) *Corresponding basal short-axis multiplanar reformation in the same patient shows focal hypertrophy of the anteroseptal segment of up to 18 mm.* **(Right)** *Midventricular short-axis multiplanar reformation shows uniform thickness of the myocardium of 12 mm. The thickness ratio is 18/12 = 1.5 and satisfies the diagnostic criteria for sigmoid septum.*

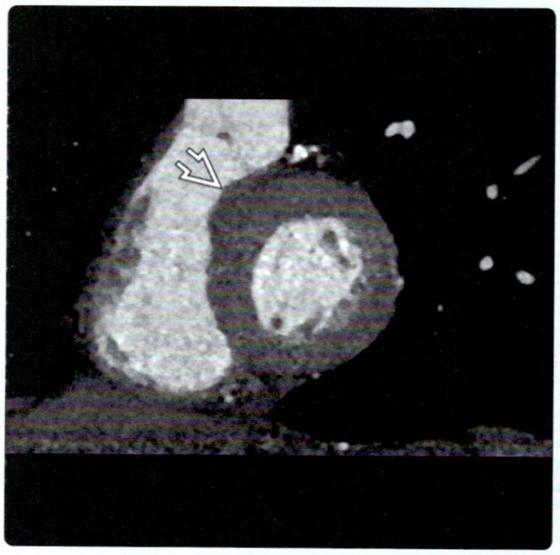

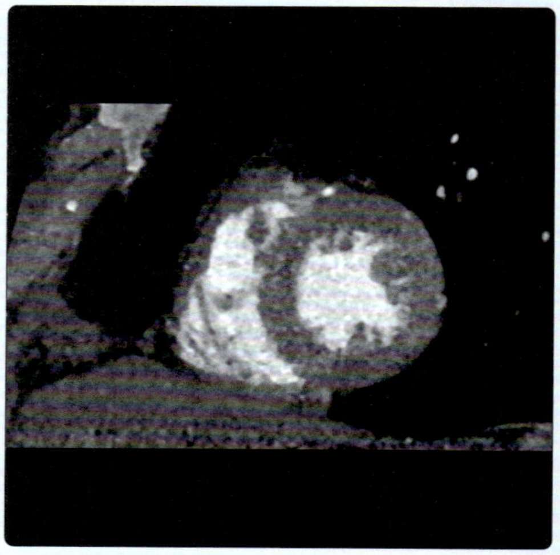

TERMINOLOGY

Synonyms

- Disproportionate ventricular septal hypertrophy
- Disproportionate upper septal thickening
- Localized septal hypertrophy
- Basal ventricular septal hypertrophy
- Ventricular septal bulge (VSB)
- Discrete upper septal thickening
- Upper septal knuckle
- Isolated hypertrophy of basal septum

Definitions

- Localized thickening of basal portion of interventricular septum

IMAGING

General Features

- Best diagnostic clue
  - Isolated basal septal hypertrophy without evidence of systolic anterior motion of mitral valve leaflets (SAM) or left ventricular outflow tract obstruction (LVOTO) at rest
  - Increase in aortic-septal angle
- Location
  - Basal interventricular septum
- Size
  - Basal septum ≥ 14 mm
    - Basal:midseptum ratio > 1.3
- Morphology
  - Thickened myocardium is otherwise normal

Radiographic Findings

- No specific findings; aortic elongation may accompany basal septal hypertrophy (BSH)

CT Findings

- Thickened basal interventricular septum

MR Findings

- Thickened basal interventricular septum
- Dynamic LVOTO in some cases [dynamic obstructive basal septal hypertrophy (DOBSH)]
- No evidence of LGE

Ultrasonographic Findings

- Thickened basal interventricular septum on parasternal long axis
- Dynamic LVOTO in some cases (DOBSH)

Imaging Recommendations

- Best imaging tool
  - Echocardiography (1st-line test); cardiac CT (to assess localized hypertrophy); cardiac MR (to assess LVOTO, scarring, and exclude differentials)
- Protocol advice
  - Echocardiography in parasternal long axis
  - Cardiac MR cine acquisitions in left 2- and 3-chamber and short-axis views; LGE; 2D &/or 4D flow measurements
    - Consider short stack of cine images with center slice in true 3-chamber plane

DIFFERENTIAL DIAGNOSIS

Hypertrophic Cardiomyopathy

- Sigmoidal variant
  - Frequently associated with mitral valve abnormalities and evidence of scarring (LGE)

Hypertensive Heart Disease

- Can manifest as LV hypertrophy (LVH) with different remodeling patterns

PATHOLOGY

General Features

- Basal septal hypertrophy without evidence of cardiomyocyte disarray

Gross Pathologic & Surgical Features

- Basal septal hypertrophy
- Increase in aortic-septal angle

CLINICAL ISSUES

Presentation

- Most common signs/symptoms
  - Mostly discovered as incidental finding
  - Shortness of breath
- Other signs/symptoms
  - May have exertional symptoms compatible with LVOTO

Demographics

- Epidemiology
  - Prevalence increases progressively with increasing age
    - Overall prevalence estimated at 1.5%; can be seen in up to 18% of patients in 8th decade of life

Natural History & Prognosis

- Considered normal variant with excellent prognosis if no evidence of LVOTO

Treatment

- β-blocker treatment can be considered if evidence of LVOTO

DIAGNOSTIC CHECKLIST

Image Interpretation Pearls

- Basal septal thickness ≥ 14 mm without evidence of LVH, SAM, or LVOTO

Reporting Tips

- Clinically relevant if evidence of LVOTO

SELECTED REFERENCES

1. Okada K et al: Optimal left ventricular diameter measurement in subjects with sigmoid septum: comparison with three-dimensional left ventricular volume. J Echocardiogr. 22(1):41-7, 2024
2. Pearson AC: The evolution of basal septal hypertrophy: from benign and age-related normal variant to potentially obstructive and symptomatic cardiomyopathy. Echocardiography. 34(7):1062-72, 2017
3. Turer AT et al: Anatomic and clinical correlates of septal morphology in hypertrophic cardiomyopathy. Eur J Echocardiogr. 12(2):131-9, 2011

KEY FACTS

TERMINOLOGY

- Abnormal diastolic function with normal ventricular cavity size regardless of ventricular wall thickness and systolic function
- Etiologies
  - Noninfiltrative conditions, including idiopathic, familial, hypertrophic cardiomyopathy, scleroderma, and diabetic cardiomyopathy
  - Infiltrative conditions, such as amyloidosis, sarcoidosis, and glycogen storage disease
  - Myocardial diseases, such as hypereosinophilic syndrome, carcinoid, drugs effects, and radiation

IMAGING

- Chest x-ray demonstrates typical appearance of congestive heart failure without significant cardiomegaly
- Echocardiography may show increased left ventricular wall thickness
  - Increased filling pressures or restrictive filling pattern on pulsed wave Doppler of mitral valve
  - Echocardiography alone is often insufficient, particularly when evaluating for specific etiologies
- MR is most comprehensive imaging modality for assessment of cardiomyopathy
  - Patterns of LGE can be diagnostic for specific etiologies of restrictive cardiomyopathy

TOP DIFFERENTIAL DIAGNOSES

- Constrictive pericarditis
- Hypertensive heart disease

DIAGNOSTIC CHECKLIST

- If echocardiogram suggests restrictive cardiomyopathy, consider cardiac MR to evaluate for specific etiologies, which can have implications for treatment

(Left) *Four-chamber echocardiogram shows biventricular thickening, biatrial enlargement, and preserved systolic function, consistent with restrictive cardiomyopathy.* **(Right)** *Pulsed wave spectral Doppler US at the level of mitral anulus in the same patient confirms a restrictive filling pattern with a prominent E wave (increased early atrial diastolic filling) and reduced A wave (late atrial filling from atrial systole). Cardiac MR was performed for further evaluation.*

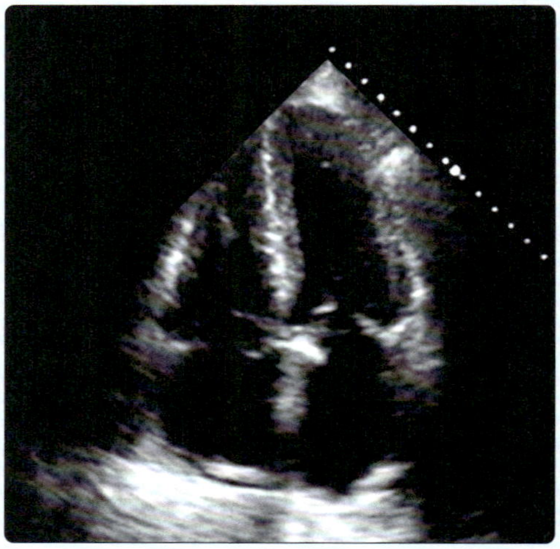

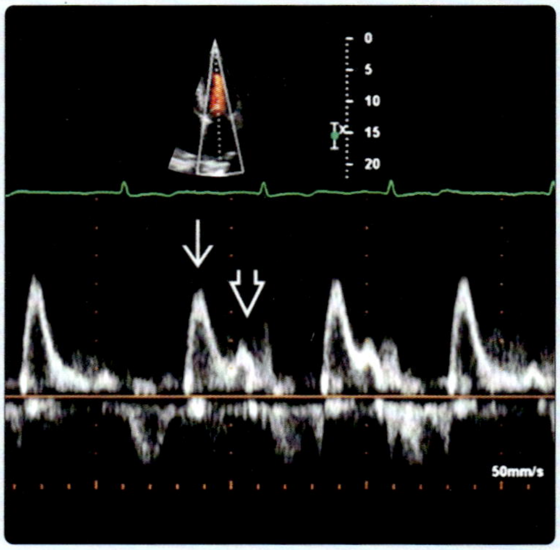

(Left) *Short-axis triple inversion recovery MR in a patient with proven cardiac sarcoidosis shows increased signal intensity at the anterior and septal segments, indicative of edema. Also note the mild thickening of the myocardium in those segments.* **(Right)** *Short-axis delayed enhancement MR in the same patient shows the patchy midwall LGE in the anterior and inferior septal segments, suggestive of myocardial fibrosis.*

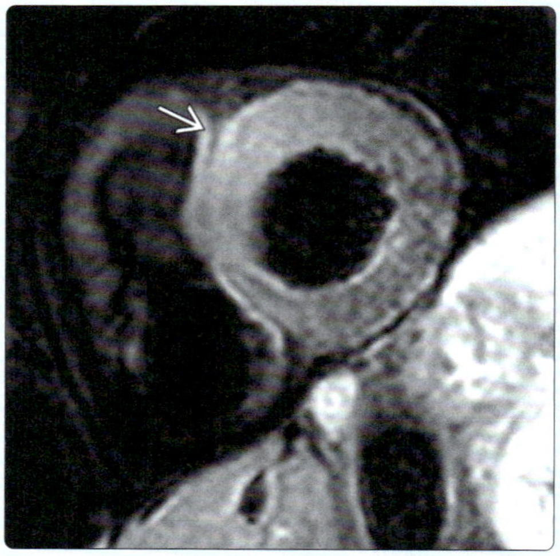

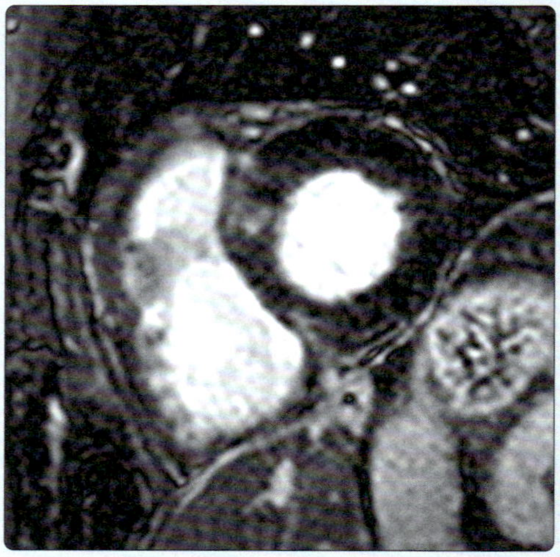

TERMINOLOGY

Definitions

- Abnormal diastolic function regardless of ventricular wall thickness and systolic function
  - Normal ventricular cavity size, atrial dilation
  - Abnormal ventricular compliance that leads to elevated filling pressures
  - Hemodynamics can resemble constrictive pericarditis

IMAGING

General Features

- Best diagnostic clue
  - Congestive heart failure with normal ventricular cavity size
  - Increased filling pressures or restrictive filling pattern on Doppler echocardiography
- Location
  - Left ventricle (LV) &/or right ventricle (RV)
- Size
  - Possible increase in ventricular wall thickness
  - Biatrial enlargement
- Morphology
  - Depending on etiology, can be associated with increased cardiac mass

Radiographic Findings

- Radiography
  - Chest x-ray demonstrates findings of congestive heart failure without significant cardiomegaly
    - Pulmonary venous congestion
    - Pleural effusions
    - May demonstrate biatrial enlargement

CT Findings

- Cardiac CT angiography can accurately depict and quantify ventricular and atrial cavity sizes as well as ventricular wall thickness
  - Useful when evaluating for concomitant coronary artery disease
  - Alternative to MR when it is contraindicated

MR Findings

- Most accurate imaging modality to assess ventricular morphology, function, and tissue characteristics
  - Cine steady-state free precession (SSFP): Small to normal ventricular cavity size with normal systolic function
  - Myocardial wall thickness can provide diagnostic clues
    - Thick: Amyloidosis; lysosomal storage disorders
    - Normal: Iron overload; hypereosinophilic syndromes; radiation heart disease; idiopathic
  - Accurate quantification of ventricular volumes, mass, and function
  - Additional metrics: Time to peak filling; rate of peak filling; early diastolic filling time
  - Patterns of LGE can be diagnostic for specific etiologies
    - Amyloidosis: Diffuse subendocardial with abnormal gadolinium kinetics in blood pool
    - Sarcoidosis: Patchy or diffuse, midmyocardial or subepicardial
    - Hypereosinophilic syndromes: Subendocardial LGE with cavitary thrombus in mid- and apical segments
    - Fabry: Midmyocardial, basal to mid inferolateral
  - T1 and extracellular volume (ECV) mapping: Increased in fibrosis, amyloid; decreased in iron and Fabry diseases
  - T2* imaging: For quantification of myocardial iron: < 20 msec
  - T2W imaging and T2 mapping: For myocardial edema
  - Strain imaging: May show early regional wall motion abnormalities
- Can evaluate for pericardial constriction
  - Pericardial thickening is usually seen (absent in 18%)
  - LGE for evaluation of pericardial inflammation
  - Myocardial adhesions using myocardial tagging
  - Interventricular interdependence using real-time cine imaging of ventricular septum

Echocardiographic Findings

- Echocardiogram
  - Normal LV cavity size and normal systolic function
  - Abnormal diastolic function
    - Mitral inflow Doppler pattern assesses ventricular compliance and filling pressures by comparing early (E) and late (A) diastolic filling
    - Tissue Doppler pattern assesses myocardial motion during early (E') and late (A') diastolic filling
  - Biatrial enlargement

Imaging Recommendations

- Best imaging tool
  - MR is most comprehensive imaging modality for assessment of cardiomyopathy
    - Accurately depicts atrial and ventricular morphology
    - LGE is most sensitive method for identifying scar and fibrosis
    - High sensitivity (88%), specificity (100%), and predictive accuracy (93%) in differentiating restrictive cardiomyopathy from constrictive pericarditis
  - Echocardiography alone is often insufficient, particularly when evaluating for specific etiologies
    - Doppler echo parameters are most reliable noninvasive methods for assessing filling patterns
- Protocol advice
  - SSFP cine images for ventricular morphology and function
  - LGE to assess for myocardial and pericardial patterns of fibrosis or injury may suggest specific etiology

DIFFERENTIAL DIAGNOSIS

Constrictive Pericarditis

- Ventricular interdependence demonstrated in real-time cine imaging of septum
- Pericardial thickening (> 4 mm) may be seen
- Pericardial adhesions via myocardial tagging on MR

Hypertrophic Cardiomyopathy

- Genetic disease with heterogeneous phenotypical expression
- Asymmetric septal thickening is most common type
- Patchy LGE at hypertrophied segments and RV insertion sites

Hypertensive Heart Disease

- Concentric LV hypertrophy in setting of hypertension
- Minimal to no LGE
- Can be associated with elevated filling pressures and diastolic dysfunction

PATHOLOGY

General Features

- Etiology
  - Primary idiopathic restrictive cardiomyopathy is uncommon and has no identifiable cause
  - Familial restrictive cardiomyopathy is also rare entity with autosomal dominant transmission
  - Secondary restrictive cardiomyopathy is most common etiology
    - Noninfiltrative conditions (Interstitial fibrosis/intrinsic myocyte dysfunction)
      - Idiopathic
      - Diabetes
      - Scleroderma
      - Pseudoxanthoma elasticum
    - Infiltrative processes (genetic vs. nongenetic)
      - Amyloidosis
      - Sarcoidosis
      - Gaucher
      - Hurler
    - Storage diseases
      - Iron overload/hemochromatosis
      - Glycogen storage
      - Fabry disease
    - Endomyocardial diseases
      - Hypereosinophilic endomyocardial fibrosis
      - Carcinoid heart disease
      - Radiation-associated myocardial fibrosis
      - Chemotherapy-mediated cardiotoxicity
      - Scleroderma

Staging, Grading, & Classification

- New York Heart Association (NYHA) functional classification of heart failure

Gross Pathologic & Surgical Features

- Increased LV mass and wall thickness
- Biatrial enlargement

Microscopic Features

- 4 different underlying mechanisms
  - Interstitial fibrosis and intrinsic myocardial dysfunction
  - Infiltration of extracellular spaces
  - Accumulation of storage material within cardiomyocytes
  - Endomyocardial fibrosis

CLINICAL ISSUES

Presentation

- Most common signs/symptoms
  - Shortness of breath and exercise intolerance
- Other signs/symptoms
  - Paroxysmal nocturnal dyspnea, orthopnea, edema
  - Fatigue, generalized weakness, cachexia
- Clinical profile
  - Physical exam is consistent with pulmonary and systemic congestion
    - Pulmonary edema
    - Increased central venous pressure (e.g., jugular venous distension, peripheral edema, hepatomegaly, ascites)

Demographics

- Age
  - Increased incidence in older adults but depends on specific etiology
- Sex
  - F > M
- Ethnicity
  - Depends on specific etiology

Natural History & Prognosis

- Historically associated with poor prognosis, but this depends on underlying etiology

Treatment

- Improve symptoms by lowering elevated filling pressures without significantly reducing cardiac output
  - Diuretics and nitrates for preload reduction
  - β-blockers &/or calcium channel blockers may improve diastolic function and reduce afterload in cases of concomitant hypertension
- Medical treatment of underlying systemic disorder
  - Immune-modulating therapy for sarcoidosis
  - Chemotherapy and stem cell transplant for amyloidosis
  - Phlebotomy and chelation therapy for hemochromatosis
- Pacemaker for high-grade atrioventricular block or sick sinus syndrome is associated with atrial fibrillation
- Implantable cardioverter-defibrillator (ICD) for secondary prevention in patients with sustained ventricular arrhythmias
- Cardiac transplantation in medically refractory cases

DIAGNOSTIC CHECKLIST

Image Interpretation Pearls

- Echocardiogram can show increased LV wall thickness and normal cavity size with evidence of increased filling pressures on Doppler
- If echocardiogram suggests restrictive cardiomyopathy, consider cardiac MR to evaluate for specific etiologies, which can have implications for treatment

SELECTED REFERENCES

1. Rapezzi C et al: Restrictive cardiomyopathy: definition and diagnosis. Eur Heart J. 43(45):4679-93, 2022
2. Pereira NL et al: Spectrum of restrictive and infiltrative cardiomyopathies: part 1 of a 2-part series. J Am Coll Cardiol. 71(10):1130-48, 2018
3. Pereira NL et al: Spectrum of restrictive and infiltrative cardiomyopathies: part 2 of a 2-part series. J Am Coll Cardiol. 71(10):1149-66, 2018
4. Garcia MJ: Constrictive pericarditis versus restrictive cardiomyopathy? J Am Coll Cardiol. 67(17):2061-76, 2016
5. Gupta A et al: Cardiac MRI in restrictive cardiomyopathy. Clin Radiol. 67(2):95-105, 2012
6. Quarta G et al: Cardiomyopathies: focus on cardiovascular magnetic resonance. Br J Radiol. 84 Spec No 3:S296-305, 2011
7. Chinnaiyan KM et al: Constrictive pericarditis versus restrictive cardiomyopathy: challenges in diagnosis and management. Cardiol Rev. 12(6):314-20, 2004

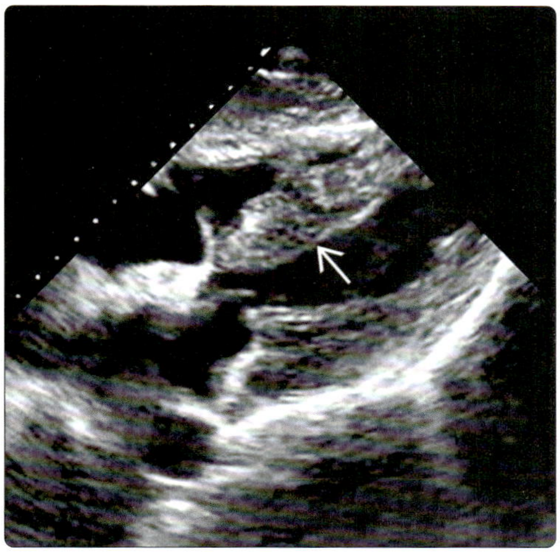

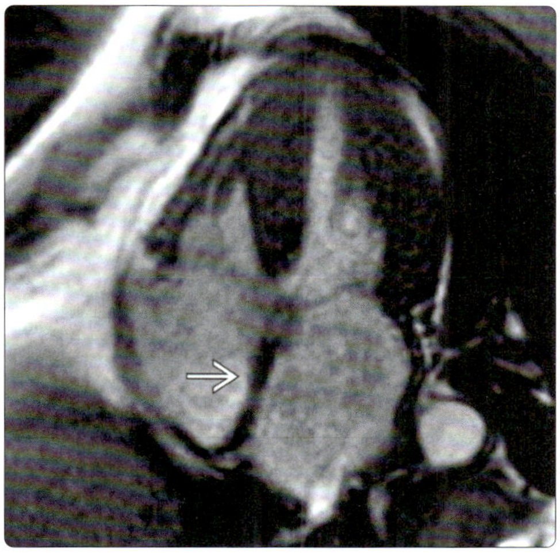

(Left) *Four-chamber echocardiogram shows increased biventricular wall thickness with a speckled pattern ➡ suggestive of amyloidosis, which should be considered in the differential for restrictive cardiomyopathy.* **(Right)** *Four-chamber cine MR in the same patient shows increased biventricular wall thickness and biatrial enlargement, consistent with restrictive cardiomyopathy. Note the increased atrial wall and interatrial septal thickness ➡, which can be seen with amyloidosis.*

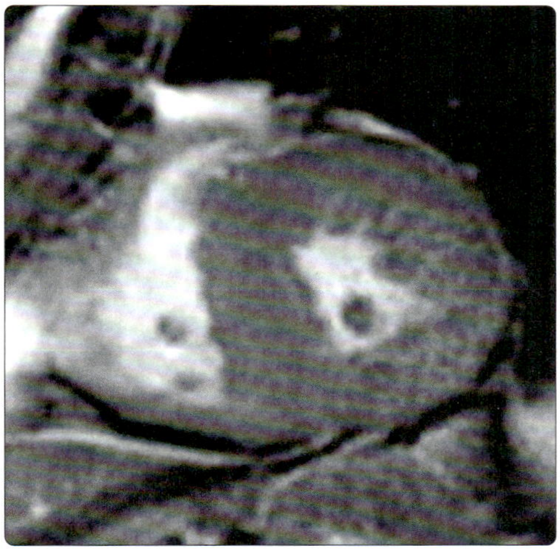

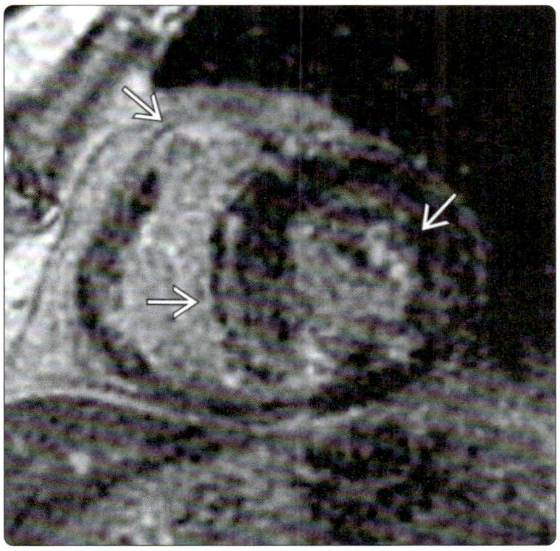

(Left) *Short-axis cine MR shows increased biventricular wall thickness with preserved systolic function.* **(Right)** *Short-axis LGE MR shows a diffuse pattern of LGE involving the septum, inferolateral wall, and anterolateral papillary muscle as well as the free wall of the right ventricle ➡. In the setting of biventricular increase in wall thickness, this extent of LGE is consistent with amyloidosis. In this patient, a right ventricular endomyocardial biopsy confirmed cardiac amyloidosis.*

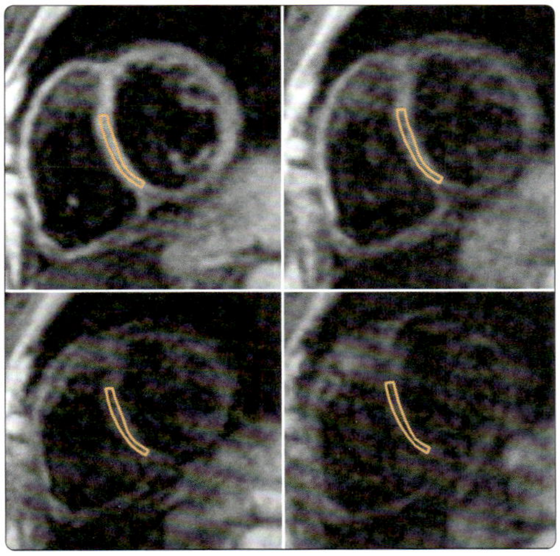

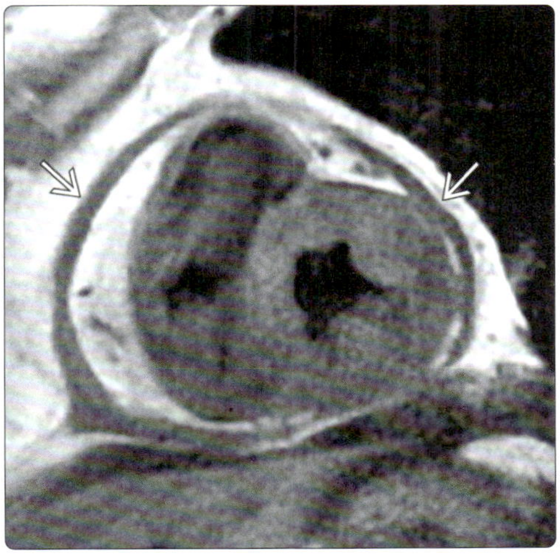

(Left) *Short-axis cardiac MR images in a patient with hemochromatosis show decreased signal of myocardium at different echo times, indicating iron deposition in the myocardium. Overall T2* value of septum was 10 msec, which is lower than normal.* **(Right)** *Short-axis T1 fast spin-echo MR in a patient with constrictive pericarditis shows a significant increase in pericardial thickness ➡, measuring up to 9 mm. Constrictive pericarditis should be considered in the differential for restrictive cardiomyopathy.*

Cardiac Amyloidosis

KEY FACTS

TERMINOLOGY

- Heterogeneous group of diseases characterized by extracellular accumulation of abnormal amyloid fibrillar protein deposits

IMAGING

- Diffuse process that can involve nearly any portion of heart (myocardium, atria, small vessels, conduction system, and valves)
- Concentric thickening of left ventricle and sometimes right ventricle
- Increased echogenicity of myocardium on echocardiogram described as sparkling or granular
- Cardiac MR is best imaging modality to characterize cardiac amyloid and distinguish from other restrictive cardiomyopathies
  - Diffuse pattern of LGE (circumferential, subendocardial, or more diffuse)

TOP DIFFERENTIAL DIAGNOSES

- Hypertrophic cardiomyopathy
- Hypertensive heart disease
- Sarcoidosis
- Glycogen storage diseases

PATHOLOGY

- Types of amyloidosis that affect heart
  - Immunoglobulin light chain (AL) amyloidosis
  - Familial transthyretin-related amyloidosis (ATTR)
  - Senile systemic amyloidosis (wildtype TTR)
  - Secondary amyloidosis (AA)
  - Isolated atrial amyloidosis (atrial natriuretic peptide)

CLINICAL ISSUES

- Prognosis depends on type of amyloid and extent of cardiac and systemic involvement

(Left) *Short-axis cine MR in a 70-year-old woman with progressive congestive heart failure shows concentric increase in left ventricular (LV) wall thickness (maximum of 15 mm) ➔ with a trace pericardial effusion ➩.* **(Right)** *Short-axis LGE MR in the same patient shows a diffuse pattern of late enhancement in a mostly subendocardial and circumferential distribution involving the basal LV ➔ and right ventricle (RV) ➔, typical of cardiac amyloidosis. Endomyocardial biopsy showed light chain (AL) amyloidosis.*

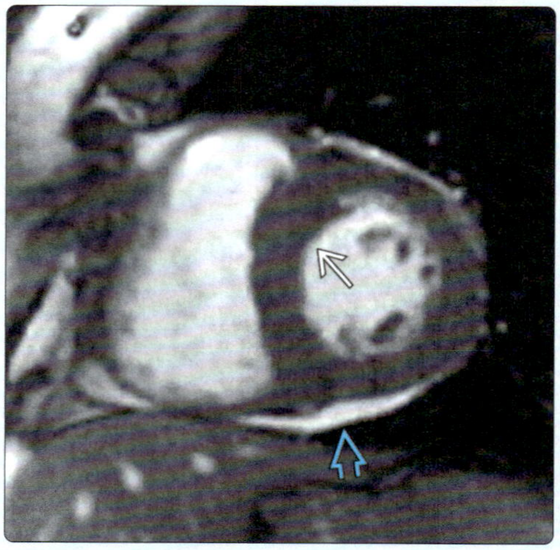

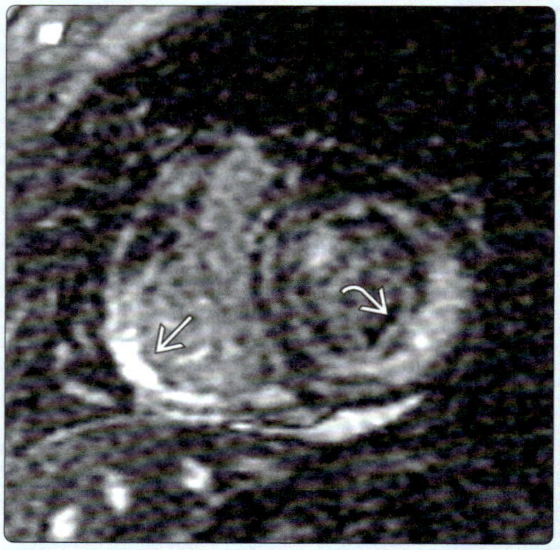

(Left) *Four-chamber cine MR shows a moderate increase in LV wall thickness ➔ with severe biventricular systolic dysfunction [LV ejection fraction (EF) = 31%; RVEF = 28%] with qualitative evidence of significant mitral ➔ and tricuspid regurgitation ➔. Biatrial enlargement is also seen.* **(Right)** *Four-chamber LGE MR shows extensive diffuse LV ➔ and RV ➔ late enhancement. Note that the myocardium is poorly nulled, which is typical of cardiac amyloidosis.*

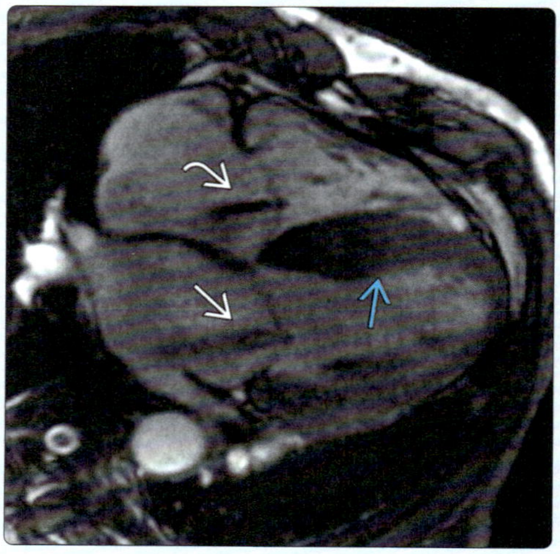

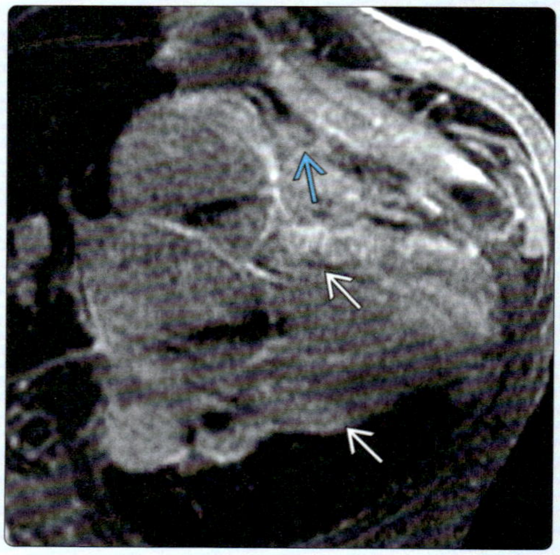

TERMINOLOGY

Definitions

- Heterogeneous group of diseases characterized by extracellular accumulation of abnormal fibrillar amyloid protein deposit
- Cardiac involvement can result in infiltrative cardiomyopathy

IMAGING

General Features

- Best diagnostic clue
  - Restrictive cardiomyopathy in advanced stages
    - Concentric left ventricular (LV) and sometimes right ventricular (RV) wall thickening
    - Circumferential, subendocardial to diffuse LGE
- Location
  - Diffuse process; can involve any portion of heart (myocardium, atria, small vessels, conduction system, and valves)

Echocardiographic Findings

- LV and sometimes RV myocardial thickening
  - Increased echogenicity of myocardium described as speckled, sparkling, or granular
  - Restrictive filling pattern on pulsed-wave Doppler of mitral valve
- Biatrial enlargement and thickening of interatrial septum
- Valvular leaflet thickening

Nuclear Medicine Findings

- Uptake in Tc-99m pyrophosphate scan has 97% sensitivity and 100% specificity in identifying transthyretin-related amyloidosis (ATTR) cardiac amyloidosis

CT Findings

- Cardiac CT can be used to exclude obstructive coronary artery disease in select patients
- Experimental studies can measure extracellular volume (ECV) in CT
- Circumferential late iodine enhancement similar to MR can be seen

MR Findings

- SSFP cine
  - Concentric LV thickening
  - Thickening of RV, atria, and interatrial septum
  - Biatrial enlargement
  - Increased LV mass, normal LV volumes and ejection fraction
- T1 and T2
  - Diffuse low signal
  - Low signal in T2W images implies bad prognosis
- LGE
  - 94% specificity and 80% sensitivity in diagnosis of cardiac amyloidosis
  - Circumferential and typically subendocardial, though can be diffuse
  - Also involves RV, atria, atrial septum
  - Blood pool appears darker due to rapid clearance from blood
    - Acquire LGE earlier than usual (~ 5 minutes after injection)
  - Some studies show poor outcome associated with LGE, whereas others show no or weak correlation
- T1 scout images
  - Altered T1 kinetics with earlier nulling of myocardium before nulling of blood pool
    - Makes it challenging to identify optimal nulling time
  - Poor prognosis if > 50% of myocardium has abnormally short T1
- T1 mapping
  - High native T1, low postcontrast T1, high ECV
  - High T1 is direct marker of cardiac amyloid burden
  - More sensitive for diagnosis of early amyloidosis
  - Elevated native T1 and ECV associated with adverse outcomes, predicts mortality
  - T1 difference between subepicardium and subendocardium > 23 ms predicts mortality
- T2 mapping
  - Low values in amyloidosis
- Distinguishing transthyretin (TTR) from amyloid light chain (AL) amyloidosis is challenging with MR but promising
  - TTR has more LV thickening, more LV mass, more extensive LGE, more RV LGE than AL type
  - Lower T1 values in TTR compared to AL

Imaging Recommendations

- Best imaging tool
  - Cardiac MR is best imaging modality to characterize cardiac amyloidosis and distinguish from other restrictive cardiomyopathies
- Protocol advice
  - LGE
    - Inversion times may be shorter due to diffuse gadolinium retention in areas of infiltration
    - Often have to image earlier after gadolinium administration given abnormal kinetics (~ 5 minutes)
    - Nulling time should be selected after blood pool is nulled

DIFFERENTIAL DIAGNOSIS

Hypertrophic Cardiomyopathy

- Usually asymmetric; concentric pattern challenging to distinguish
- Patchy midmyocardial LGE at hypertrophied areas, RV insertion points

Hypertension

- Concentric LV thickening in documented hypertension
- Diastolic dysfunction; no or minimal LGE

Sarcoidosis

- Infiltrating, noncaseating granulomas
- Nonischemic LGE; edema on T2 MR; mediastinal lymphadenopathy

Glycogen Storage Diseases

- Rare cause of infiltrative cardiomyopathy
- Nonischemic pattern of LGE

PATHOLOGY

General Features

- Etiology
  - Types of amyloidoses that can affect heart
    - Immunoglobulin AL amyloidosis
      - Insoluble monoclonal immunoglobulin light chains or fragments
    - Familial ATTR
      - Deposition of mutant TTR protein
    - Senile systemic amyloidosis (wildtype TTR)
      - Deposition of normal TTR protein
    - Secondary amyloidosis (AA)
      - Deposition of amyloid fibrils derived from serum amyloid A; associated with inflammatory conditions (rheumatoid arthritis, infection)
    - Isolated atrial amyloidosis (atrial natriuretic peptide)
      - Amyloid protein derived from atrial natriuretic peptide
- Genetics
  - Familial TTR-related amyloidosis
    - Autosomal dominant
    - > 70 mutations described in TTR protein
    - 4% of Black population is heterozygous for Val-122-Ile mutation
- Associated abnormalities
  - Systemic involvement is common in AL amyloidosis
    - Hepatic and renal, neurological (carpal tunnel syndrome, neuropathy), macroglossia, dermatological (easy bruising, periorbital purpura)
  - Renal involvement is seen in AA amyloidosis
  - Systemic involvement is typically seen in AL amyloidosis

Staging, Grading, & Classification

- Mayo Clinic staging of AL amyloidosis
  - Lower survival if elevated troponin T and NT-pro-BNP

Gross Pathologic & Surgical Features

- Definitive diagnosis depends on histologic confirmation of amyloid deposition
- Endomyocardial biopsy is gold standard for diagnosis of cardiac involvement

Microscopic Features

- Congo red stain with apple green birefringence under polarized light
- Specific protein types can be identified using immunoelectron microscopy

CLINICAL ISSUES

Presentation

- Most common signs/symptoms
  - Depend on type of amyloid and stage of cardiac involvement
    - Rapidly progressive congestive heart failure in advanced AL amyloidosis
  - Dyspnea is common; angina can be seen in absence of coronary artery disease
  - Arrhythmias, including atrial fibrillation and conduction system disease, leading to bradyarrhythmias
  - Low voltage on electrocardiography
- Other signs/symptoms

Demographics

- Age
  - Variable; depends on type of amyloid
    - Senile amyloidosis is typically > 60 years of age
    - Familial amyloidosis most common > 40 years of age
- Sex
  - Senile amyloidosis is almost exclusively seen in men
  - Isolated atrial amyloidosis is more common in women
- Epidemiology
  - Majority of patients have either AL or TTR amyloidosis

Natural History & Prognosis

- Immunoglobulin AL amyloidosis
  - Poor prognosis with extensive cardiac involvement
  - Progressive disease without definitive treatment of plasma cell disorder
- Familial TTR-related amyloidosis
  - Lower incidence of heart failure and better survival when compared to AL amyloidosis
    - TTR: 3-5 years; AL: < 12 months
- Senile systemic amyloidosis
  - Median survival after onset of symptoms: ~ 8 years
- AA
  - Clinically significant heart failure is rare

Treatment

- Immunoglobulin AL amyloidosis
  - Definitive treatment targeting plasma cell dyscrasia
    - Chemotherapy and autologous stem cell transplant
- Familial TTR-related amyloidosis
  - Definitive treatment involves liver transplant, which can be combined with heart transplant in subset of patients
- AA
  - Treatment of underlying inflammatory condition
- General management of congestive heart failure in cardiac amyloidosis
  - ACE inhibitors can be associated with hypotension, particularly in AL amyloidosis
  - Increased risk of digoxin toxicity secondary to binding of drug to amyloid fibrils
- Senile amyloidosis
  - Clinical trials have shown benefit with stabilizers of amyloid protein (tafamidis and diflunisal)
  - Research involving gene silencing techniques (si-RNA, antisense oligonucleotides)

DIAGNOSTIC CHECKLIST

Consider

- Echocardiogram is most common initial diagnostic test
- Cardiac MR shows excellent diagnostic accuracy
- Technetium pyrophosphate scan identifies TTR type

SELECTED REFERENCES

1. Alwan L et al: Current and evolving multimodality cardiac imaging in managing transthyretin amyloid cardiomyopathy. JACC Cardiovasc Imaging. 17(2):195-211, 2024
2. Oda S et al: Trends in diagnostic imaging of cardiac amyloidosis: emerging knowledge and concepts. Radiographics. 40(4):961-81, 2020

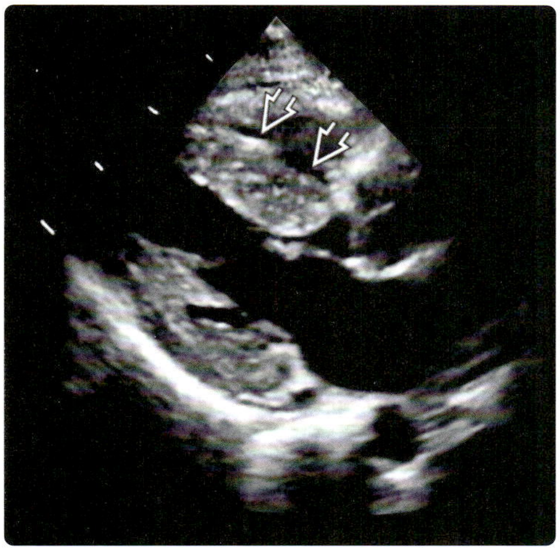

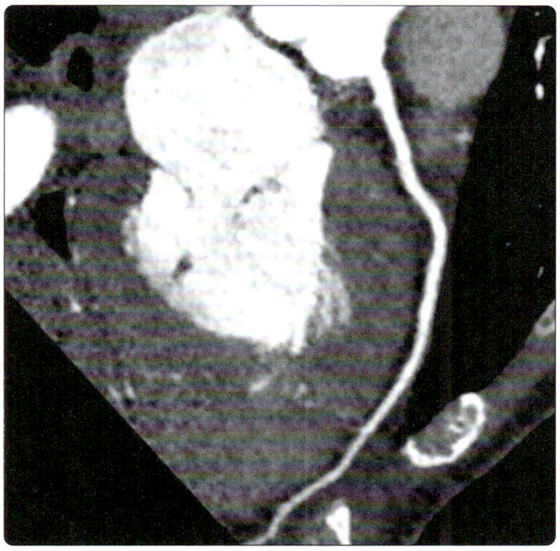

(Left) *Three-chamber echocardiogram shows a concentric increase in LV wall thickness* ➡ *with increased echogenicity of myocardium (speckled appearance), which is suggestive of cardiac amyloidosis.* **(Right)** *Curved MPR CT shows no evidence of left anterior descending artery disease in a patient with typical angina. Remaining coronary arteries were also normal. Subsequent cardiac MR showed diffuse LGE and LV wall thickening, consistent with cardiac amyloidosis. Amyloidosis can be associated with small vessel disease.*

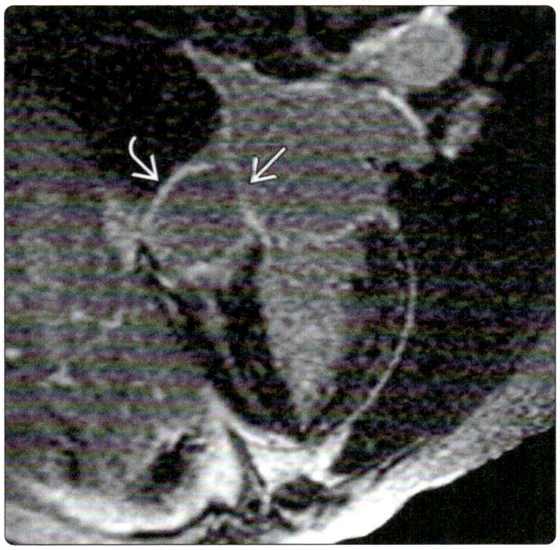

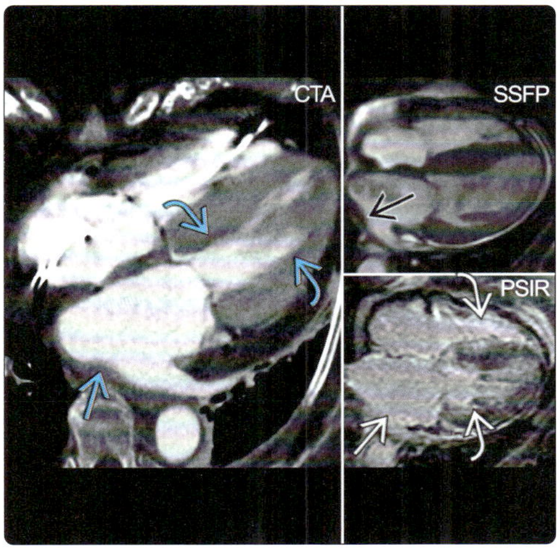

(Left) *Four-chamber LGE MR shows evidence of biatrial late enhancement involving the interatrial septum* ➡ *and superior aspect of the right atrium* ➡*. Small bowel biopsy showed evidence of wildtype TTR, consistent with senile amyloidosis.* **(Right)** *4-chamber CT (left) shows diffuse myocardial hypertrophy with subendocardial hypoperfusion* ➡ *and atrial wall thickening* ➡ *due to amyloid, which correlates with the findings on SSFP MR* ➡*. PSIR image shows subendocardial LGE involving the atria* ➡ *and both ventricles* ➡*.*

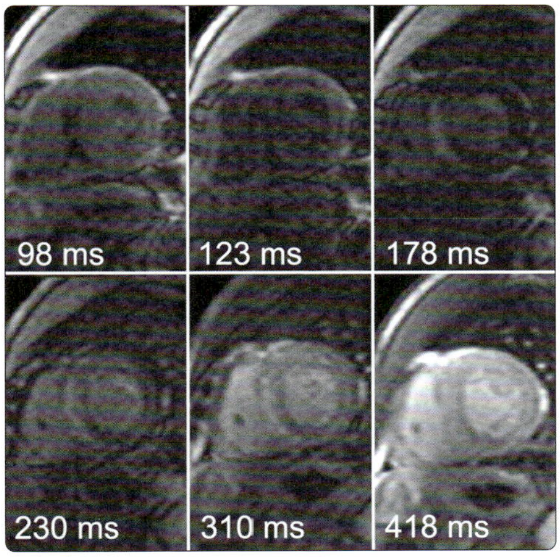

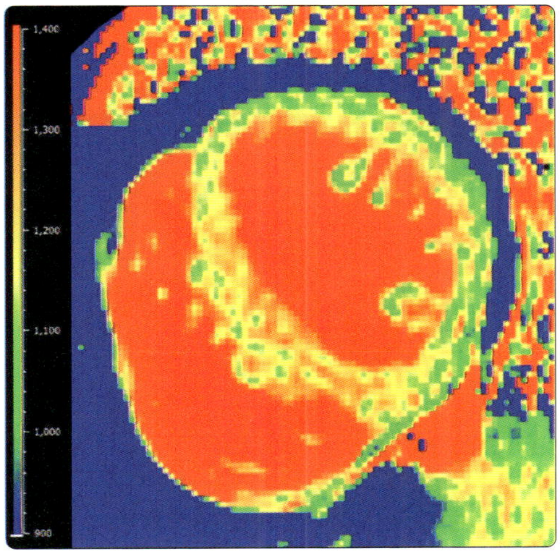

(Left) *Sequential short-axis T1 scout images are shown at different inversion times. Note the early nulling of blood pool (123 ms) and myocardium (178 ms). Amyloidosis might result in abnormal nulling of blood pool and myocardium with abnormal temporal order.* **(Right)** *Color T1 map in a patient with amyloidosis shows elevated native T1 values predominantly in subendocardial areas and septal segments (yellow areas) with a value of 1,215 ms in anteroseptum. The global T1 value of whole myocardium is also elevated (1,145 ms).*

Cardiac Sarcoidosis

KEY FACTS

TERMINOLOGY

- Cardiac sarcoidosis (CS)

IMAGING

- Basilar septum and left ventricular free wall are most common sites of involvement
- Septal involvement likely explains common presentation of complete heart block
- Abnormal enhancement on LGE MR in nonischemic pattern has highest sensitivity/specificity of available noninvasive imaging studies
- Distribution of abnormal LGE MR is most commonly subepicardial or midmyocardial and extends to right ventricular anterior/inferior wall from interventricular septum (hook sign)
- Presence of abnormal LGE has been reported to confer 9x ↑ risk of major adverse cardiac events and 11.5x ↑ risk of sudden death

TOP DIFFERENTIAL DIAGNOSES

- Arrhythmogenic right ventricular dysplasia (ARVD)
  - Ventricular aneurysms, focal wall motion abnormalities, and abnormal LGE MR may be seen in both CS and ARVD
- Myocarditis
  - Overlaps with sarcoid on imaging as CS is form of (granulomatous) myocarditis
- Myocardial infarction
  - Coronary-type LGE MR pattern is seen in ~ 10% of CS cases

CLINICAL ISSUES

- Associated with poorer prognosis compared to sarcoidosis that does not involve heart
- Accounts for 13-25% of deaths from sarcoidosis
- Corticosteroids are mainstay of therapy

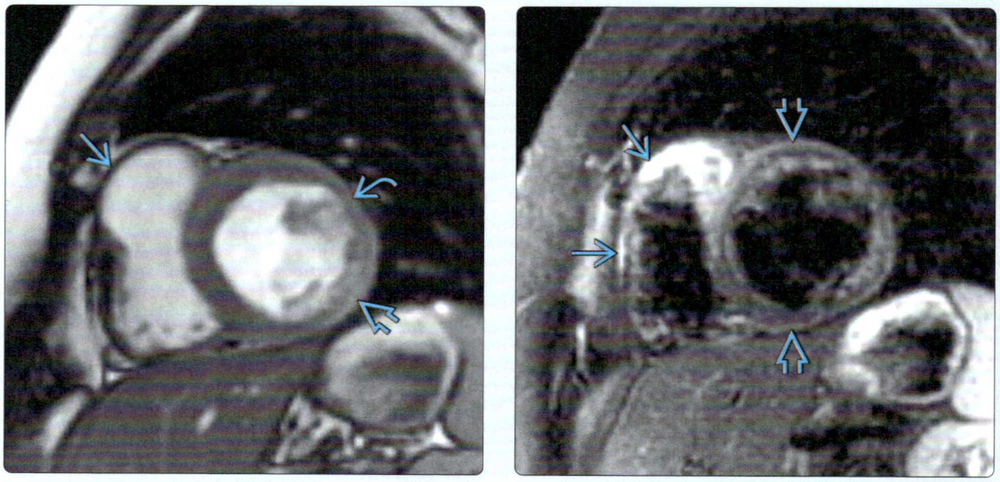

(Left) *Short-taxis SSFP MR during systole in a 51-year-old woman with complete heart block shows areas of thinning of the right ventricular (RV) and left ventricular (LV) myocardium. The RV was dyskinetic in the area of thinning. There is also subtle increased LV subepicardial signal, likely due to edema. The LV ejection fraction was 35%.* **(Right)** *Triple IR MR in the same patient shows diffuse LV subepicardial high signal due to edema. There are multiple areas of edema in the RV.*

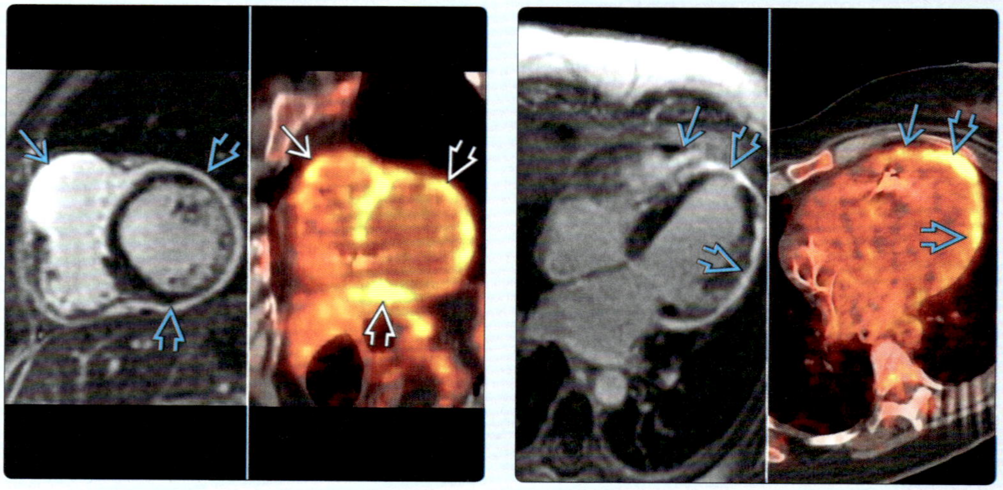

(Left) *Short-axis LGE (left) and FDG PET (right) images in the same patient after defibrillator placement show extensive subepicardial LV and transmural RV MR LGE beautifully correlating with areas of increased LV and RV FDG activity on PET/CT.* **(Right)** *Four-chamber LGE (left) and fused PET/CT (right) images in the same patient again show correlation between the areas of the RV and LV MR LGE and increased FDG activity on PET/CT. Biopsy confirmed sarcoid. (Courtesy S. Kligerman, MD.)*

TERMINOLOGY

Abbreviations

- Cardiac sarcoidosis (CS)

Definitions

- Sarcoidosis: Chronic multisystemic disease of unknown etiology characterized by presence of noncaseating granulomas in affected organs, including lymph nodes and lungs
  - Cardiac involvement occurs in 5% of patients clinically, but much higher percentage (~ 25%) is found at autopsy

IMAGING

General Features

- Best diagnostic clue
  - Cardiac involvement should be suspected in patients with diagnosis of extra CS who present with complete heart block or frequent ventricular arrhythmias
- Location
  - Left ventricular lateral wall and basal septum are most common sites of involvement
    - Septal involvement likely explains common presentation of complete heart block
- Size
  - Granuloma formation may be microscopic or macroscopic
- Morphology
  - Granulomatous infiltration may produce nodules within myocardium
    - As disease progresses, this may evolve into scarring that is seen as thinning of myocardium, resulting in aneurysm formation
    - Occasionally, mild thickening of myocardium is noted, particularly in setting of acute edema/inflammation, and may resemble asymmetric hypertrophy

Imaging Recommendations

- Best imaging tool
  - Cardiac MR
    - Abnormal enhancement on LGE MR images in nonischemic pattern has highest sensitivity/specificity of available noninvasive imaging studies
      - Absence of LGE has high negative predictive value with almost all adverse events occurring in LGE-positive patients
- Protocol advice
  - Cine MR imaging to evaluate overall left ventricular and right ventricular function and look for localized wall motion abnormalities
  - High-resolution LGE MR imaging to detect subtle regions of fibrosis
    - Single-shot techniques may be substituted in arrhythmic patients with slight decrease in sensitivity
    - T2-weighted images and T2 mapping techniques may be useful in detecting edema indicative of active inflammation
  - FDG PET scanning may be useful in patients with pacemakers/defibrillators
    - Also useful for assessing disease activity/response to therapy

Image-Guided Biopsy

- Endomyocardial biopsy is useful when positive, demonstrating noncaseating granulomas consistent with CS
- Very low sensitivity (~ 20%) due to sampling errors, as CS is often patchy and may not involve segments commonly biopsied

Radiographic Findings

- Chest radiographs are helpful in demonstrating common findings of pulmonary involvement, including bilateral hilar and mediastinal adenopathy
  - More advanced cases may show significant interstitial lung disease progressing to honeycombing
- Uncommonly, CS may result in cardiomegaly and signs of heart failure

MR Findings

- T2WI FS
  - High signal intensity indicates presence of myocardial edema due to inflammation in acute phase
  - Hyperintense regions are most often seen in midmyocardium or subepicardium and parallel areas of abnormal LGE
- MR cine
  - Wall motion abnormalities in noncoronary distribution may be seen
  - Occasionally, left ventricular or right ventricular wall aneurysms may be seen secondary to ventricular wall thinning
- LGE enhancement
  - Distribution of abnormal LGE MR is mostly subepicardial or midmyocardial and along right ventricular side of interventricular septum
    - In ~ 10% of cases, LGE MR pattern may be subendocardial, mimicking infarct
  - Abnormal LGE has been reported to confer 9x increased risk of major adverse cardiac events and 11.5x increased risk of sudden death
    - Enhancement of > 20% of left ventricular mass indicates higher risk of death and need for treatment
  - Steroid therapy has been demonstrated to reduce size of hyperenhancement on LGE MR
- Parametric mapping
  - Native T1 and T2 mapping show high values in CS
  - Higher discriminatory accuracy than standard diagnostic criteria
  - T2 mapping may improve detection of active inflammation in CS
  - Native T1 and T2 values decrease after treatment

Nuclear Medicine Findings

- PET/CT
  - May be useful in assessing disease activity in patients with known CS
- Segmental defects are seen on scintigraphy with thallium-201 and FDG PET, which correspond to areas of granulomatous replacement
- Defects decrease on exercise stress thallium imaging, phenomenon known as reverse distribution
  - Helps differentiate from defects secondary to coronary artery disease

- Hybrid PET/MR can simultaneously assess for fibrosis in LGE and disease activity with FDG PET
  - Provide complementary information on disease pathophysiology
  - Strong predictor of major adverse cardiac events
  - Studies have shown it has highest AUC for diagnosis of sarcoid compared to MR and PET/CT

DIFFERENTIAL DIAGNOSIS

Myocarditis

- Inflammatory infiltrate of myocardium with necrosis &/or degeneration of adjacent myocytes, usually viral in origin
- Abnormal enhancement on LGE MR imaging is typically subepicardial in lateral wall but may occur anywhere
- Overlaps with sarcoid on imaging as CS is form of (granulomatous) myocarditis

Arrhythmogenic Cardiomyopathy

- Can involve right ventricle, left ventricle, or both, whereas CS more commonly shows left ventricular or combined dysfunction
- Ventricular aneurysms and focal wall motion abnormalities may be seen in both, as may abnormal LGE MR
- Lymphadenopathy and lung opacities with left ventricular septal involvement are more typical of CS

Acute Myocardial Infarction

- Clinical presentation differs with chest pain, ECG abnormalities, and elevated troponin
- LGE MR shows hyperenhancement in ischemic pattern
  - Subendocardial predominant pattern (with variable transmural extent) conforming to coronary artery territory

PATHOLOGY

General Features

- Etiology
  - Exaggerated immune response to variety of antigens that cause CD4 cell accumulation and release of inflammatory cytokines, leading to granuloma formation
  - Infectious and environmental agents have been implicated as potential antigens
- Genetics
  - Genetic factors may play role

Gross Pathologic & Surgical Features

- Noncaseating epithelioid granulomas are seen
- Granulomas may involve pericardium, myocardium, or endocardium
  - Myocardium is most frequently involved

Microscopic Features

- Microscopic examination reveals T lymphocytes and mononuclear phagocytes, which initially are seen at sites of inflammation
- As disease progresses, there is granuloma formation consisting of aggregated macrophages, epithelioid cells, and giant cells
- Dense band of fibroblasts, collagen, and proteoglycans usually encases aggregate of inflammatory cells

CLINICAL ISSUES

Presentation

- Most common signs/symptoms
  - Majority of patients are asymptomatic
  - Common presentations
    - Conduction abnormalities, most commonly complete heart block
    - Sustained or nonsustained ventricular tachycardia (2nd most common presentation)
- Other signs/symptoms
  - Congestive heart failure may also be seen

Natural History & Prognosis

- Cardiac involvement by sarcoidosis is associated with poorer prognosis compared to sarcoidosis that does not involve heart
- Accounts for 13-25% of deaths from sarcoidosis
- Mortality rate may exceed 40% at 5 years and 55% at 10 years
  - Presence of LGE conveys 11.5x increase in risk of cardiac death

Treatment

- Corticosteroids are mainstay of therapy
- Immunosuppressive therapy in steroid-intolerant patients
- Antiarrhythmic therapy/pacemaker placement depending on electrophysiologic abnormalities

DIAGNOSTIC CHECKLIST

Consider

- CS in patient with known pulmonary sarcoid presenting with complete heart block or frequent ventricular beats

SELECTED REFERENCES

1. Cheng RK et al: Diagnosis and management of cardiac sarcoidosis: a scientific statement from the American Heart Association. Circulation. 149(21):e1197-216, 2024
2. Marschner CA et al: Combined FDG PET/MRI versus standard-of-care imaging in the evaluation of cardiac sarcoidosis. Radiol Cardiothorac Imaging. 5(5):e220292, 2023
3. Cheung E et al: Combined simultaneous FDG-PET/MRI with T1 and T2 mapping as an imaging biomarker for the diagnosis and prognosis of suspected cardiac sarcoidosis. Eur J Hybrid Imaging. 5(1):24, 2021
4. Vita T et al: Complementary value of cardiac magnetic resonance imaging and positron emission tomography/computed tomography in the assessment of cardiac sarcoidosis. Circ Cardiovasc Imaging. 11(1):e007030, 2018
5. Wicks EC et al: Diagnostic accuracy and prognostic value of simultaneous hybrid 18F-fluorodeoxyglucose positron emission tomography/magnetic resonance imaging in cardiac sarcoidosis. Eur Heart J Cardiovasc Imaging. 19(7):757-67, 2018
6. Puntmann VO et al: T1 and T2 mapping in recognition of early cardiac involvement in systemic sarcoidosis. Radiology. 285(1):63-72, 2017
7. Hulten E et al: Cardiac sarcoidosis-state of the art review. Cardiovasc Diagn Ther. 6(1):50-63, 2016
8. Birnie DH et al: HRS expert consensus statement on the diagnosis and management of arrhythmias associated with cardiac sarcoidosis. Heart Rhythm. 11(7):1305-23, 2014

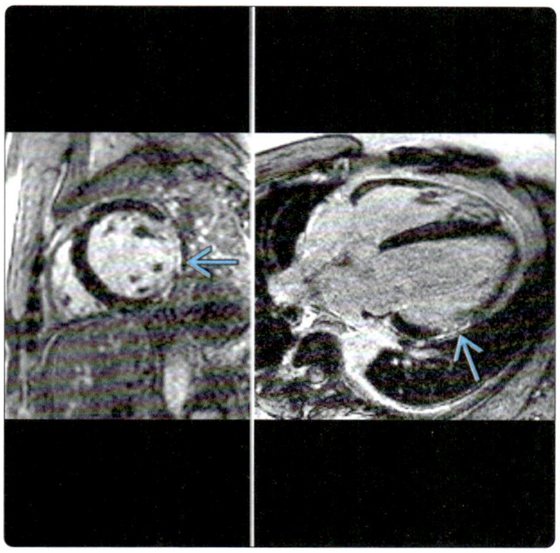

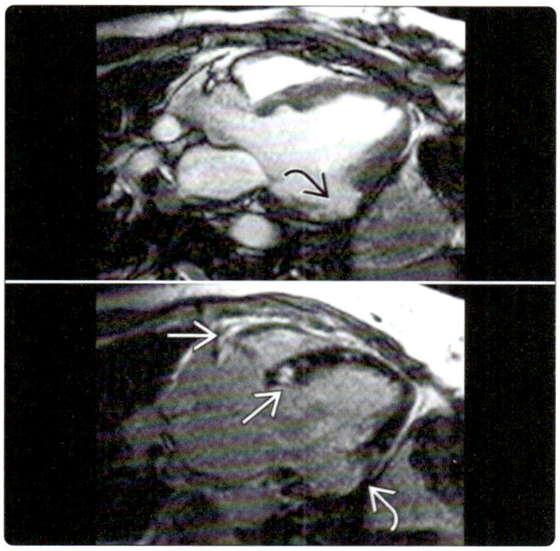

(Left) *Short-axis and 4-chamber LGE MR show transmural enhancement ➔ of the lateral wall with an appearance mimicking myocardial infarction in a patient with cardiac sarcoid (CS) and clean coronaries at catheterization. In ~ 10% of cases, CS may have a subendocardial pattern that simulates coronary artery disease.* **(Right)** *Three-chamber cine (top) and LGE (bottom) MR show a localized aneurysm of the lateral basal wall ↪. Note enhancement of aneurysm wall ↪ and other small foci of enhancement ➔.*

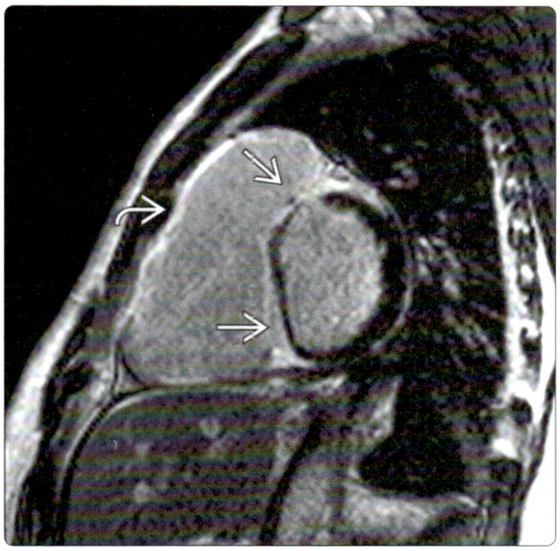

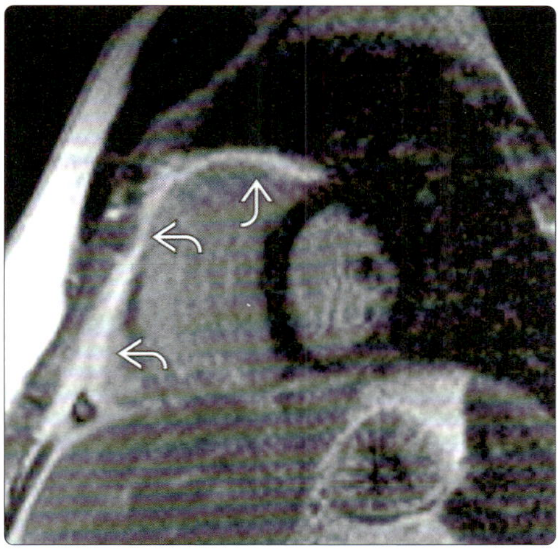

(Left) *Short-axis LGE MR in a patient with proven CS demonstrates enhancement of the septum ➔ and RV free wall ↪. Note also that the RV is dilated.* **(Right)** *Short-axis LGE MR in a patient with arrhythmogenic RV cardiomyopathy demonstrates findings similar to those sometimes seen in CS. Note the dilated RV with abnormal enhancement ↪ of the RV free wall.*

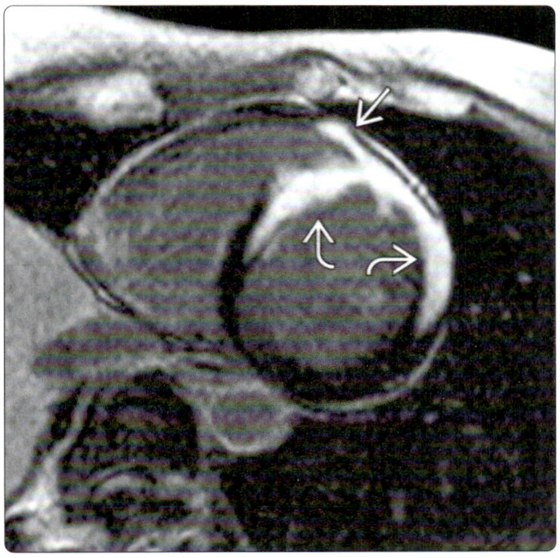

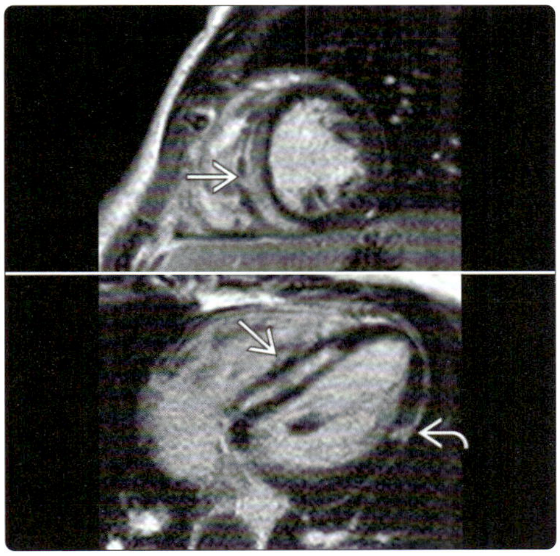

(Left) *Short-axis LGE MR shows extensive enhancement of the anterior and anteroseptal walls ↪. Note the enhancement of the anterior RV wall ➔. This appearance of septal LGE uptake with contiguous extension to the RV has been termed the hook sign.* **(Right)** *Short-axis (top) and 4-chamber (bottom) LGE MR images in a patient with viral myocarditis show septal enhancement ➔, clearly similar to findings in CS. Note also the small focus of enhancement ↪ in the lateral wall.*

Myocarditis

KEY FACTS

TERMINOLOGY

- Inflammatory involvement of myocardium with necrosis &/or degeneration of adjacent myocytes

IMAGING

- New dilated cardiomyopathy in otherwise healthy person shortly after viral syndrome
- 2018 Lake Louis criteria: One T1-based and one T2-based criterion
  - T1-based imaging: Increased native T1, increased ECV or nonischemic LGE
  - T2-based imaging: Increased T2 or regional high T2 signal or high T2 signal intensity ratio

TOP DIFFERENTIAL DIAGNOSES

- Sarcoid cardiomyopathy, ischemic cardiomyopathy
- Nonischemic dilated cardiomyopathy

PATHOLOGY

- Infectious viral etiologies are most frequent

CLINICAL ISSUES

- Variable clinical presentation from subclinical to acute heart failure with hemodynamic compromise

DIAGNOSTIC CHECKLIST

- Cardiac MR study should be performed if patient is symptomatic with clinical suspicion for myocarditis
- MR report should include
  - Ventricular volumes and function
  - Presence or absence of markers of inflammatory activity and injury (T2 ratio, native T2, native T1 and ECV, LGE)
  - Pericardial effusion, thickening or enhancement
- Repeat cardiac MR 1-2 weeks after initial study if no positive criteria are present but onset of symptoms is recent and there is strong suspicion for myocarditis
- Follow-up with MR > 4 weeks after onset of symptoms may have prognostic implications

(Left) *AP radiograph in an 18-year-old man with witnessed cardiac arrest shows normal heart size and extensive pulmonary edema. Troponin T was elevated at 2,707 ng/L.* **(Right)** *4-chamber contrast-enhanced echocardiogram shows that the patient's ejection fraction was 13%. The heart was diffusely hypokinetic. Subsequent coronary CTA showed normal coronaries.*

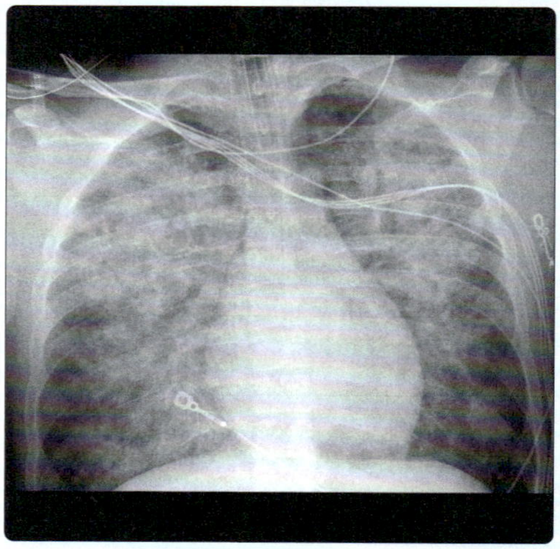

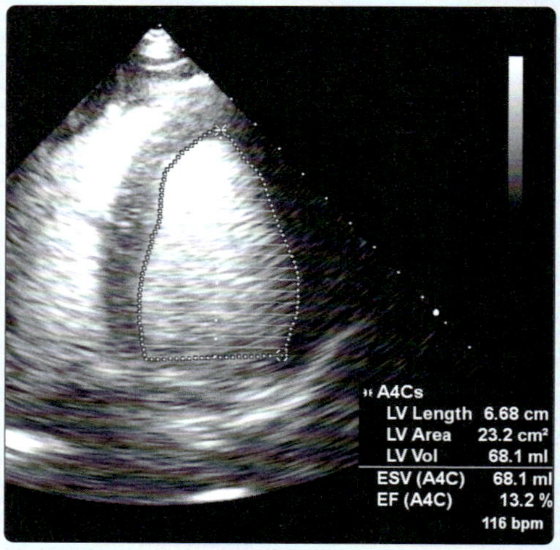

(Left) *SSFP and T2 MR images show subtle increased subepicardial signal. Global myocardial:skeletal muscle ratio was 2.1 on T2 imaging, and T2 mapping was elevated at 60 msec with increased subepicardial signal. Subepicardial hyperperfusion was present.* **(Right)** *Short-axis and 4-chamber 40keV delayed CTA images (left) show subepicardial and midmyocardial enhancement in a young man with elevated troponin and normal coronary arteries. These findings are mirrored on next day cardiac MR.*

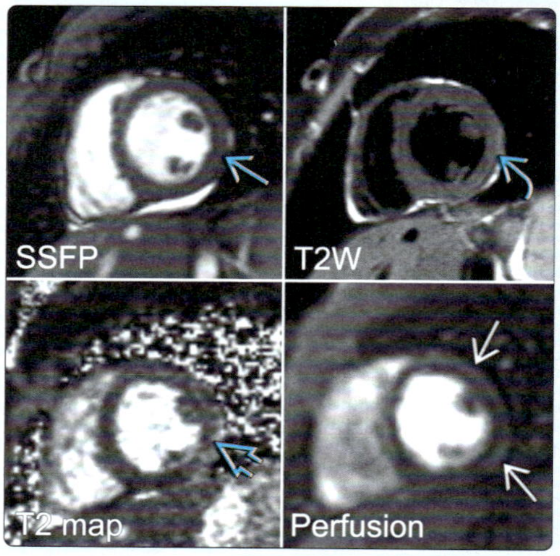

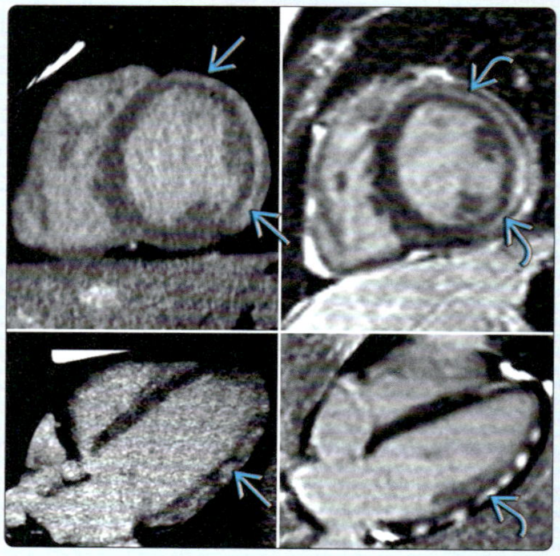

TERMINOLOGY

Definitions

- Inflammatory involvement of myocardium with necrosis &/or degeneration of adjacent myocytes

IMAGING

General Features

- Best diagnostic clue
  - 2018 Lake Louis criteria (LLC): One T1-based and one T2-based criterion
    - T1-based imaging: Increased native T1, increased ECV, or nonischemic LGE
    - T2-based imaging: Increased T2 or regional high T2 signal or high T2 signal intensity ratio
  - New dilated cardiomyopathy in otherwise healthy person shortly after viral syndrome
    - Normal coronary arteries despite enzyme leak and ECG changes

CT Findings

- Cardiac gated CTA
  - Does not have primary role in evaluation of myocarditis
  - Normal coronary arteries help exclude ischemic injury
  - Delayed iodine enhancement can be used
    - Use low monoenergy or iodine map
    - Lower CNR than MR

MR Findings

- T2WI
  - High signal due to inflammation-related edema
  - May be regional or global
  - Global involvement may not be visually appreciated, requiring measurement of left ventricle (LV) signal intensity
    - **T2 signal ratio of LV myocardium to skeletal muscle ≥ 2.0 is consistent with myocarditis**
  - In absence of abnormal LGE, increased T2 is consistent with reversible myocardial injury
  - Pericardial effusion and inflammation may be seen
- T1WI C+
  - Early gadolinium enhancement (EGE) due to myocardial hyperemia and capillary leak
  - Removing EGE from criteria does not significantly reduce diagnostic accuracy
  - **Global relative enhancement (GRE) ratio ≥ 4.0**
    - GRE ratio measures LV myocardial enhancement relative to skeletal muscle enhancement
      - GRE = [(postcontrast LV - precontrast LV)/precontrast LV]/[(postcontrast SM - precontrast SM)/precontrast SM]
    - Normal GRE is < 2.5
- SSFP cine
  - Quantifies LV function, volume, ejection fraction (EF), and end-diastolic LV wall thickness
    - Transient increase in end-diastolic LV wall thickness due to edema
    - May have preserved EF due to increased contractility in surrounding myocardium
    - Excellent for assessing recovery of function
  - ± pericardial effusion, thickening
- LGE
  - **Typical pattern is subepicardial or transmural**
    - May be midwall; patchy focal or multifocal
    - LGE may be extensive in severe cases
    - Subendocardial predominant pattern uncommon but does occur
      - Higher probability of severe lymphocytic myocarditis or giant cell myocarditis
      - Worse clinical features and outcomes
  - LGE in acute myocarditis does not equate to permanent fibrosis
    - In acute phase, LGE can occur with either myocyte injury &/or scarring
    - LGE improves (in 46%) or resolves (in 10%) at 6-month follow-up MR
    - In chronic phase, residual LGE is due to scarring
  - Best independent predictor of sudden cardiac death
    - Large areas of LGE have higher rate of MACE
    - Septal (and midwall) LGE is associated with unfavorable outcome
  - Pericardial LGE may be seen due to pericardial inflammation: Myopericarditis
    - Similarly, pericardial inflammation in pericarditis can lead to adjacent myocardial inflammation: Perimyocarditis
- Parametric mapping
  - Incorporated in updated 2018 LLC
    - Improves diagnostic accuracy over traditional LLC
  - T2 mapping
    - High T2 values are seen due to edema
    - Improved diagnostic accuracy in both acute and chronic phases
  - Native T1 mapping
    - Higher native (i.e., noncontrast) T1 values due to edema, hyperemia, &/or fibrosis
    - Can provide diagnosis of acute myocarditis without intravenous contrast
    - High accuracy (AUC: 0.97) compared to other parameters, including LLC
  - Postcontrast T1 mapping
    - Decreased values due to fibrosis
  - Extracellular volume fraction
    - Requires pre- and postcontrast T1 mapping of myocardium and blood pool, hematocrit
    - Increased ECV in edema and fibrosis
- PET/MR
  - Hybrid technique combining strengths of both techniques

Echocardiographic Findings

- Echocardiogram
  - Normal in less severe cases
  - Demonstrates degree of LV systolic dysfunction
  - Useful in serial monitoring to assess recovery of function
  - May quickly identify other potential causes of new cardiomyopathy (i.e., ischemic or valvular)

Imaging Recommendations

- Best imaging tool
  - Cardiac MR; not only for diagnosis but also for evaluation of progression or resolution of disease

DIFFERENTIAL DIAGNOSIS

Sarcoid Cardiomyopathy

- Can appear identical to myocarditis on MR
- Parenchymal or nodal findings of sarcoid help differentiate
- Clinical scenarios often different
- May require biopsy to differentiate

Ischemic Cardiomyopathy

- Delayed enhancement pattern is subendocardial and confined to coronary territory

Nonischemic Dilated Cardiomyopathy

- Absent or linear midmyocardial LGE
- Some cases secondary to prior myocarditis

Amyloid Cardiomyopathy

- Concentric LV hypertrophy
- Abnormal TI nulling pattern

PATHOLOGY

General Features

- Etiology
  - Often classified as idiopathic
  - Infectious viral etiologies are most frequent
    - Parvovirus B19 is common virus (60-71%)
  - Other causes include autoimmune disorders, toxic/ischemic/mechanical injury, drug related, transplant related
- Endomyocardial biopsy is of limited utility and generally reserved for patients with major clinical manifestations
- Diagnosed by histologic, immunologic, and immunochemical criteria
- Clinicopathologic classification provides prognostic information
- Myocardial damage has 2 main phases
  - Acute phase (first 2 weeks): Myocyte destruction is direct consequence of offending agent
  - Chronic phase: Continuing myocyte destruction is autoimmune in nature

Staging, Grading, & Classification

- WHO Marburg classification (1996)
  - Cell types: Lymphocytic, eosinophilic, neutrophilic, giant cell, granulomatous, or mixed
  - Distribution: Focal (outside vessel lumen), confluent, diffuse, or reparative (in fibrotic areas)
  - Amount: None (grade 0), mild (grade 1), moderate (grade 2), or severe (grade 3)

CLINICAL ISSUES

Presentation

- Most common signs/symptoms
  - Variable clinical presentation from subclinical to acute heart failure with hemodynamic compromise
  - Majority of symptomatic cases with syndrome of heart failure and dilated cardiomyopathy
    - Fatigue and decreased exercise capacity
- Other signs/symptoms
  - ECG changes: ST-segment elevation or T-wave inversion
    - May mimic myocardial ischemia
  - Elevated biomarkers
    - Cardiac biomarkers (CK, CK MB, troponin)
    - Erythrocyte sedimentation rate
  - Cardiogenic shock
  - Sudden cardiac death

Demographics

- Epidemiology
  - Often secondary to infection, either direct viral infection or post viral, immune-mediated reaction
  - True incidence of idiopathic or "viral" myocarditis is unknown
  - Estimated that myocarditis is responsible for
    - 10% of unexplained dilated cardiomyopathy and heart failure
    - 12% of young adults presenting with sudden death

Natural History & Prognosis

- Majority of cases have benign course
- Some patients develop heart failure, serious arrhythmias, disturbances of conduction, or even circulatory collapse
- 2/3 with mild symptoms recover completely
- 1/3 subsequently develop dilated cardiomyopathy

Treatment

- Nonsteroidal antiinflammatory drugs are not effective and may actually enhance myocarditis and increase mortality
- Exercise restriction, electrocardiographic monitoring, anticoagulation, antiarrhythmic drugs in selected patients
- Transplant in cases of cardiogenic shock

DIAGNOSTIC CHECKLIST

Consider

- Cardiac MR should be performed if patient is symptomatic with clinical suspicion for myocarditis (i.e., chest pain, elevated troponin, normal coronary arteries, and suspected viral etiology)

Image Interpretation Pearls

- Updated 2018 LLC: One T1-based and one T2-based criterion
- Repeat cardiac MR 1-2 weeks after initial exam if none of criteria are present but onset of symptoms is recent and there is strong clinical suspicion for myocarditis
- Follow-up with MR > 4 weeks after onset of symptoms may have prognostic implications

SELECTED REFERENCES

1. Li JH et al: Subendocardial involvement as an underrecognized cardiac MRI phenotype in myocarditis. Radiology. 302(1):61-9, 2022
2. Aquaro GD et al: Prognostic value of repeating cardiac magnetic resonance in patients with acute myocarditis. J Am Coll Cardiol. 74(20):2439-48, 2019
3. Ferreira VM et al: Cardiovascular magnetic resonance in nonischemic myocardial inflammation: expert recommendations. J Am Coll Cardiol. 72(24):3158-76, 2018
4. Messroghli DR et al: Clinical recommendations for cardiovascular magnetic resonance mapping of T1, T2, T2* and extracellular volume: a consensus statement by the Society for Cardiovascular Magnetic Resonance (SCMR) endorsed by the European Association for Cardiovascular Imaging (EACVI). J Cardiovasc Magn Reson. 19(1):75, 2017
5. Friedrich MG et al: Cardiovascular magnetic resonance in myocarditis: a JACC White Paper. J Am Coll Cardiol. 53(17):1475-87, 2009

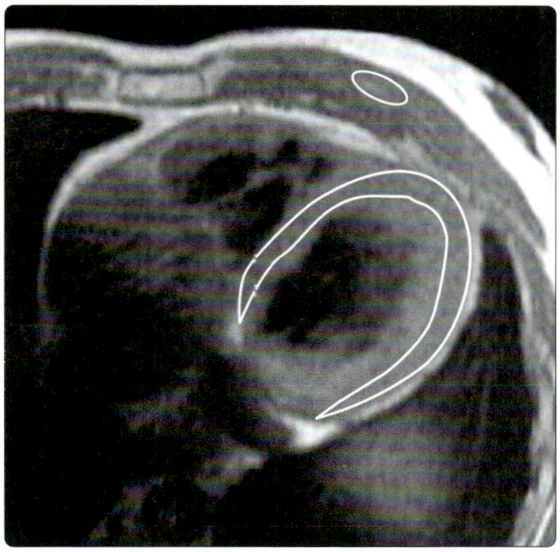
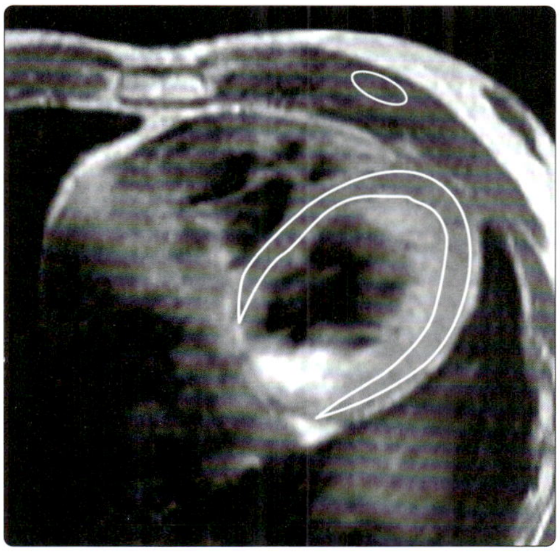

(Left) *Axial T1 MR shows the region of interest (ROI) drawn over the left ventricular myocardium and skeletal muscle.* **(Right)** *Axial T1 C+ MR at the identical slice position with the ROI drawn over identical locations in the left ventricle myocardium and skeletal muscle is used to calculate the global relative enhancement (GRE) ratio (positive GRE is > 4.0). The degree of myocardial relative hyperenhancement is 1 criterion toward the diagnosis of myocarditis.*

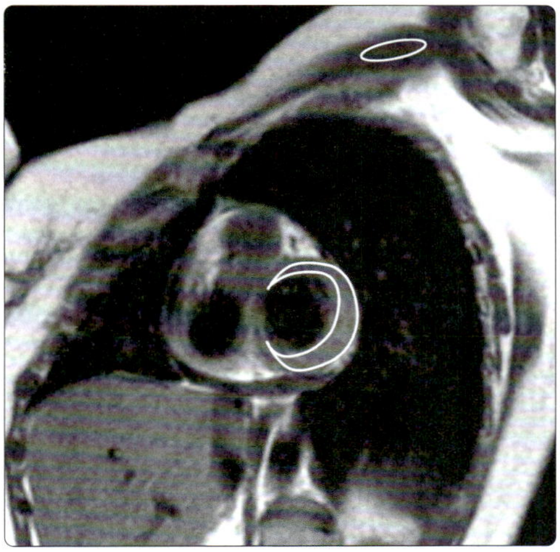
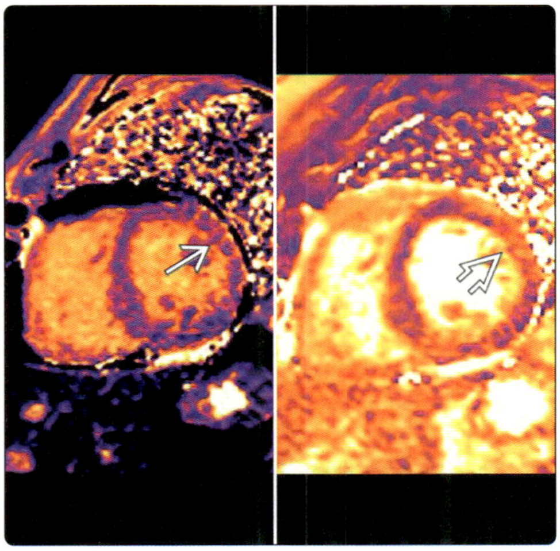

(Left) *Short-axis T2 MR shows the ROI drawn over the left ventricular myocardium and skeletal muscle. The ratio of myocardial T2 signal relative to skeletal muscle signal is 1 criterion toward the diagnosis of myocarditis (abnormal is T2 ratio > 1.9).* **(Right)** *Short-axis T1 color map (left) shows an elevated native T1 value of 1,103 ms in the anterolateral segment in a patient with myopericarditis. T2 color map (right) at the same level shows high T2 value of 61 ms in the same segment due to myocardial edema.*

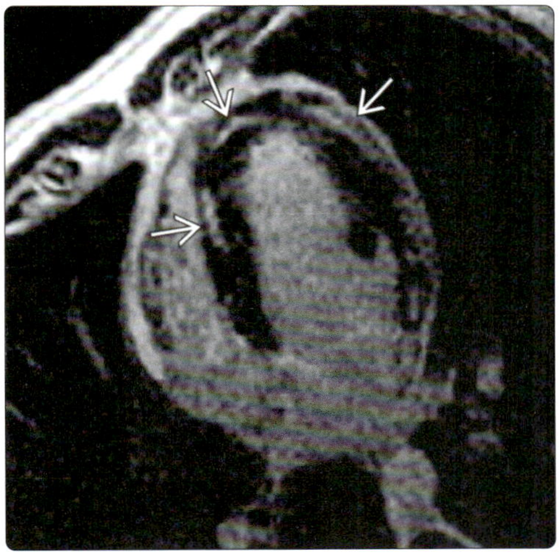
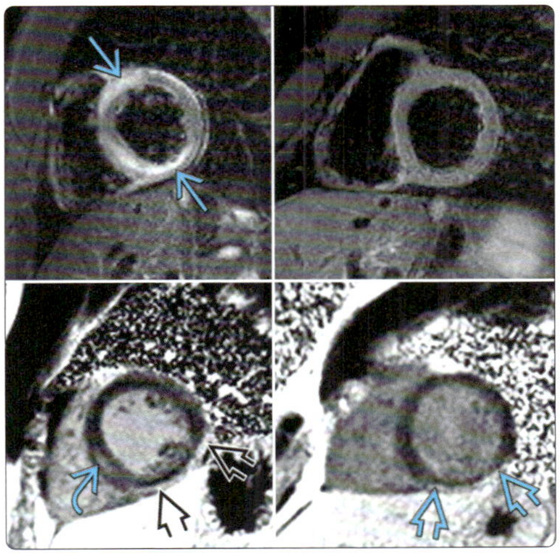

(Left) *LGE MR shows subepicardial LGE in a noncoronary distribution involving multiple regions of the left ventricle.* **(Right)** *STIR images at admission (top left) show extensive myocardial edema, which resolves on the STIR image 6 months later (top right). PSIR image at admission (bottom left) shows midmyocardial and subepicardial LGE. Six months later (bottom right), the midmyocardial LGE has resolved and the subepicardial LGE has improved.*

Post-COVID and Vaccine-Related Myocarditis

KEY FACTS

TERMINOLOGY

- There was early recognition of acute cardiovascular manifestations during course of COVID-19
- Myocarditis and pericarditis cases have been reported after messenger ribonucleic acid (mRNA)-based COVID-19 vaccination with highest risk among adolescent boys and young adult men

IMAGING

- Cardiac MR is noninvasive reference standard for assessment of cardiac chamber size, regional and global ventricular function, and tissue characterization
- Patterns of injury identified at MR after COVID-19 include myocarditis and pericarditis, myocardial ischemia and infarction, and stress-induced cardiomyopathy (rare)
  - Cardiac MR findings are similar to those that are not related to COVID-19
- Myocarditis diagnosis based on revised Lake Louise criteria: Strong evidence of acute myocardial inflammation if at least one T2-based marker of myocardial edema and one T1-based marker of myocardial damage are present
- Acute myocardial infarction pattern: Subendocardial or transmural LGE with corresponding edema (T2 hyperintensity or increased T2 mapping values) and regional wall motion abnormalities

CLINICAL ISSUES

- Minority of patients have persistent cardiac symptoms weeks to months after COVID-19
  - Although they are more common in those with severe COVID-19, symptoms can also persist in previously well individuals with mild COVID-19
- Persistent myocardial inflammation has been linked to chronic cardiovascular symptoms
- COVID-19 vaccine-related myocarditis cases tend to be milder, and imaging abnormalities tend to improve or resolve in 3-6 months

(Left) *Short-axis T2WI with fat saturation (SPAIR) in a 21-year-old man with palpitations and chest pain 1 month after a COVID-19 infection shows basal inferolateral subepicardial hyperintensity ➡, consistent with edema.* **(Right)** *Three-chamber phase-sensitive inversion recovery (PSIR) LGE MR in the same patient shows extensive subepicardial enhancement of the inferolateral wall from basal to apical cavity ➡.*

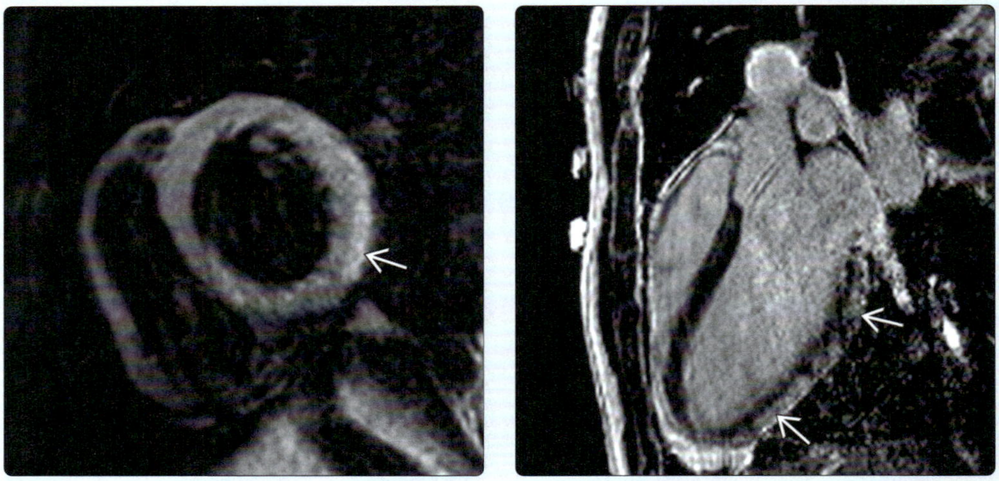

(Left) *Short-axis T1 map obtained at the midcavity in the same patient shows increased native T1 values in the lateral segment ➡ representing myocardial injury/edema.* **(Right)** *Short-axis T2 map obtained at the midcavity in the same patient shows corresponding increased T2 values ➡ in keeping with edema. These findings are consistent with COVID-19 myocarditis.*

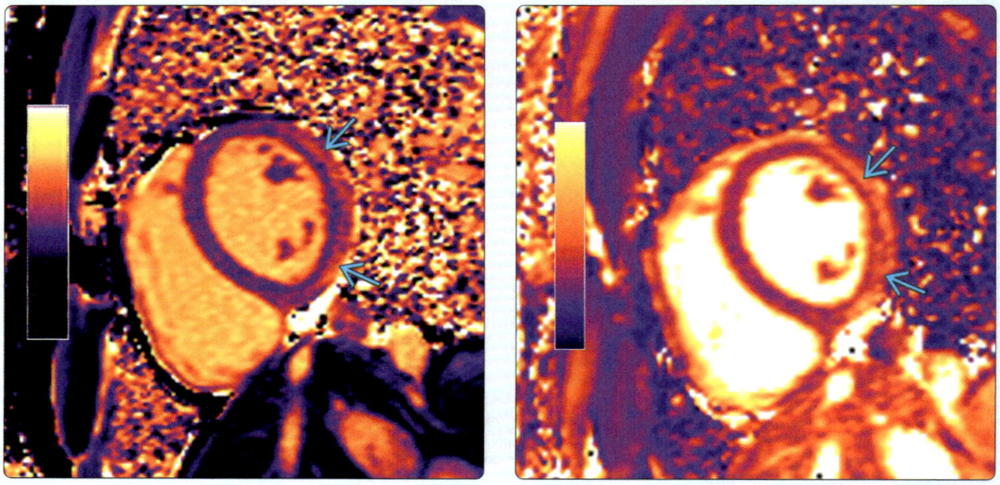

TERMINOLOGY

Background

- Early recognition of acute cardiovascular manifestations related to COVID-19
- Beyond acute phase, some patients have persistent symptoms that last weeks to months after initial infection
  - Has been termed postacute sequelae of SARS-CoV-2 infection (PASC) or "long COVID"
- Most children have mild course of disease during COVID-19
  - Small proportion can develop multisystem inflammatory syndrome that manifests with characteristics similar to those of Kawasaki disease
- Myocarditis and pericarditis cases have been reported after messenger ribonucleic acid (mRNA)-based COVID-19 vaccination
  - Highest risk among adolescent boys and young adult men

Definitions

- American College of Cardiology expert consensus decision pathway on cardiovascular sequelae of COVID-19 in adults proposed standardized terminology to describe cardiovascular sequelae of COVID-19
  - Myocardial injury
    - Elevated troponin level above 99th percentile upper reference limit
  - Myocardial involvement
    - Abnormal myocardium shown at electrocardiography, echocardiography, cardiac MR, &/or histopathologic evaluation; neither symptoms nor elevated troponin level is required
  - Myocarditis
    - Condition defined by presence of cardiac symptoms, elevated troponin level, and abnormal electrocardiographic results, imaging findings, &/or histopathologic findings in absence of flow-limiting coronary artery disease
  - PASC
    - New, returning, or persistent symptoms that are present for 4 or more weeks after SARS-CoV-2 infection

IMAGING

Echocardiography

- Often initial cardiac imaging modality used in evaluation of patients with COVID-19 and suspected cardiovascular involvement
  - Allows for rapid assessment of biventricular function, chamber size, valvular function, myocardial strain, and pericardial abnormalities
- Nonspecific findings
  - Biventricular systolic dysfunction, diastolic dysfunction, impaired left ventricular global longitudinal strain, right ventricular dilatation, and pericardial effusion

Chest CT and Coronary CT Angiography

- Chest CT is frequently performed for evaluation of pulmonary parenchymal changes related to COVID-19, including pneumonia and pulmonary embolism
- Coronary CTA: Less often used to exclude coronary artery disease in setting of chest pain
  - Assessment of coronary artery aneurysms and thrombosis in children with multisystem inflammatory syndrome
  - Late iodine enhancement may be useful if there is contraindication to MR

Cardiac MR

- Noninvasive reference standard for assessment of cardiac chamber size, regional and global ventricular function, and tissue characterization
- Patterns of injury identified at MR after COVID-19
  - Myocarditis and pericarditis
  - Myocardial ischemia and infarction
  - Stress-induced cardiomyopathy (rare)
- Cardiac MR findings are similar to those that are not related to COVID-19
- Myocarditis diagnosis based on revised Lake Louise criteria: Strong evidence of acute myocardial inflammation if at least one T2-based marker of myocardial edema and one T1-based marker of myocardial damage are present
  - T2 markers of edema
    - Regional or global myocardial hyperintensity on T2WI
    - Increased T2 mapping values
  - T1 markers of myocardial damage
    - Increased native T1 mapping values
    - Increased extracellular volume fraction (ECV)
    - Nonischemic LGE
  - Regional or global systolic left ventricular dysfunction and findings of pericarditis are supportive but not required for diagnosis
- LGE, increased native T1 mapping values or increased ECV, and, less frequently, increased native T2 mapping values can persist, especially after cases of severe COVID-19
- Acute myocardial infarction pattern: Subendocardial or transmural LGE with corresponding edema (T2 hyperintensity or increased T2 mapping values) and regional wall motion abnormalities
  - Patients may present embolic infarction pattern (focal and potentially involving multiple territories) after severe COVID-19
- Stress-induced cardiomyopathy: Acute, reversible systolic dysfunction; normal thickening of basal segments with akinesis (ballooning) of mid and apical segments

DIFFERENTIAL DIAGNOSIS

Myocarditis

- Imaging pattern is indistinguishable from other causes of myocarditis, such as other viral myocarditis
- Differential diagnosis is based in presence of history of recent COVID-19 infection or mRNA vaccination

Myocardial Infarction

- Patients with COVID-19 can present with imaging suggestive of embolic myocardial infarction

Kawasaki Disease

- In children with multisystemic inflammatory syndrome
  - Tends to present at older age and with more profound systemic inflammation

CLINICAL ISSUES

Presentation

- Most common signs/symptoms
  - Chest pain and palpitations after COVID-19 infection or mRNA-based COVID-19 vaccination
- Other signs/symptoms
  - Less frequently: Acute heart failure, sudden cardiac death

Demographics

- Myocarditis and myocardial involvement are more common during severe acute COVID-19, although patients with milder disease course can also be affected
- Adolescent and young males aged 12-29 years are at highest risk of mRNA-based COVID-19 vaccine-related myocarditis
  - Risk is 10x higher than females of same age
- Cases tend to be more frequent after 2nd dose; greater than 1st or 3rd and subsequent doses
- When compared to noninfected/nonvaccinated population, relative risk for myocarditis after COVID-19 infection has been estimated to be more than 7x higher than after mRNA-based vaccination

Natural History & Prognosis

- Patients who have recovered from acute COVID-19 are at increased risk of cardiovascular disease for up to 12 months after initial infection
- Minority of patients have persistent cardiac symptoms weeks to months after COVID-19
  - Although they are more common in those with severe COVID-19, symptoms can also persist in previously well individuals with mild COVID-19
- Persistent myocardial inflammation has been linked to chronic cardiovascular symptoms
- COVID-19 vaccine-related myocarditis cases tend to be milder, and cardiac abnormalities (e.g., LGE, increased native T1/ECV, increased T2, T2WI hyperintensity) tend to improve or resolve in 3-6 months

Treatment

- No specific therapy
- Supportive management as per clinical standard of care

Mechanisms of Cardiovascular Injury

- Direct cardiovascular damage by entering endothelial cells and cardiomyocytes via binding to ACE2 receptor
- Indirect cardiovascular damage mediated by systemic inflammation, endothelial dysregulation, and ischemia
- Postacute cardiovascular manifestations are often result of pathophysiologic alterations that occur during acute phase, ongoing inflammation, and endothelial dysfunction
  - Dysregulation of angiotensin-aldosterone axis and autonomous system dysfunction may also contribute to longer term cardiovascular disease
- Potential mechanisms of vaccine-related myocardial injury include
  - Antibody-mediated immunity
  - Molecular mimicry with self antigens
  - Direct cardiotoxicity caused by binding of mRNA vaccine-encoded spike glycoprotein to cardiomyocytes
  - Innate inflammatory response to encoded viral spike glycoprotein

DIAGNOSTIC CHECKLIST

Consider

- Look for increased native T1/ECV, increased T2, T2WI hyperintensity, and LGE in patients with cardiac symptoms after COVID-19 or COVID-19 mRNA-based vaccination

Reporting Tips

- Reasonable to suggest cardiac MR follow-up in 3 to 6 months to assess for interval change and resolution of edema

SELECTED REFERENCES

1. Sánchez Tijmes F et al: Imaging acute and chronic cardiac complications of COVID-19 and after COVID-19 vaccination. Radiographics. 43(9):e230044, 2023
2. Fronza M et al: Myocardial injury pattern at MRI in COVID-19 vaccine-associated myocarditis. Radiology. 304(3):553-62, 2022
3. Hanneman K et al: Combined cardiac fluorodeoxyglucose-positron emission tomography/magnetic resonance imaging assessment of myocardial injury in patients who recently recovered from COVID-19. JAMA Cardiol. 7(3):298-308, 2022
4. Huang S et al: Echocardiography findings in COVID-19 patients admitted to intensive care units: a multi-national observational study (the ECHO-COVID study). Intensive Care Med. 48(6):667-78, 2022
5. Siripanthong B et al: The pathogenesis and long-term consequences of COVID-19 cardiac injury. JACC Basic Transl Sci. 7(3):294-308, 2022
6. Writing Committee et al: 2022 ACC expert consensus decision pathway on cardiovascular sequelae of COVID-19 in adults: myocarditis and other myocardial involvement, post-acute sequelae of SARS-CoV-2 infection, and return to play: a report of the American College of Cardiology Solution Set Oversight Committee. J Am Coll Cardiol. 79(17):1717-56, 2022
7. Xie Y et al: Long-term cardiovascular outcomes of COVID-19. Nat Med. 28(3):583-90, 2022
8. Harrison SL et al: Cardiovascular risk factors, cardiovascular disease, and COVID-19: an umbrella review of systematic reviews. Eur Heart J Qual Care Clin Outcomes. 7(4):330-9, 2021
9. Katsoularis I et al: Risk of acute myocardial infarction and ischaemic stroke following COVID-19 in Sweden: a self-controlled case series and matched cohort study. Lancet. 398(10300):599-607, 2021
10. Huang L et al: Cardiac involvement in patients recovered from COVID-2019 identified using magnetic resonance imaging. JACC Cardiovasc Imaging. 13(11):2330-9, 2020

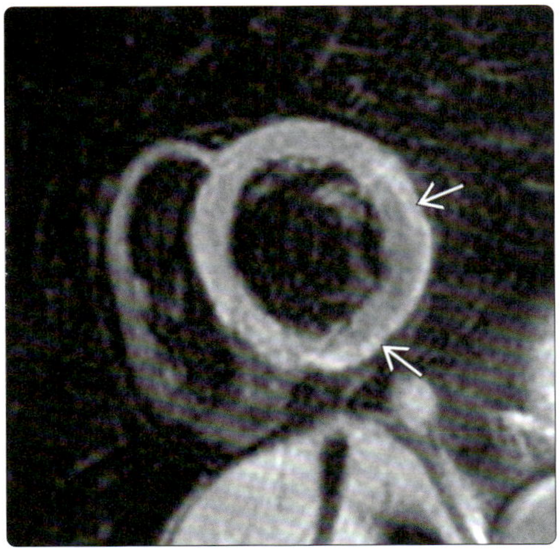

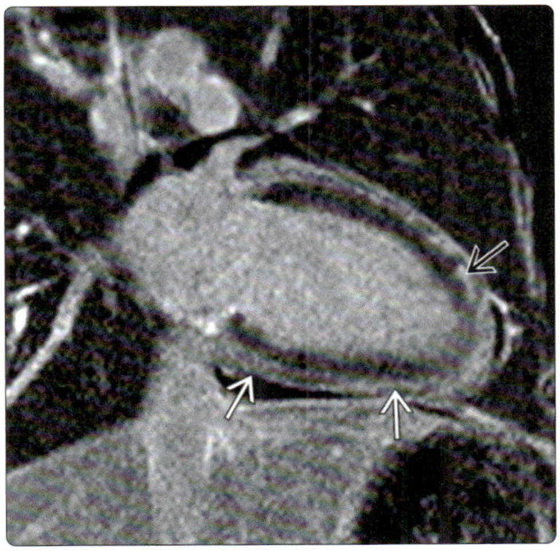

(Left) *Short-axis T2 SPAIR obtained at the midcavity in a 26-year-old man with post messenger ribonucleic acid (mRNA)-based COVID-19 vaccine myocarditis shows subepicardial hyperintensity in the lateral and inferior wall, consistent with edema* →*.* **(Right)** *Two-chamber PSIR in the same patient shows extensive subepicardial LGE involving the apical anterior segment* → *and the inferior wall from base to apex* →*.*

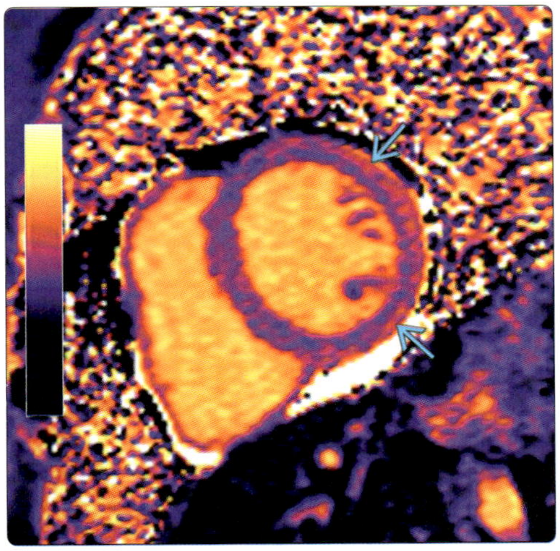

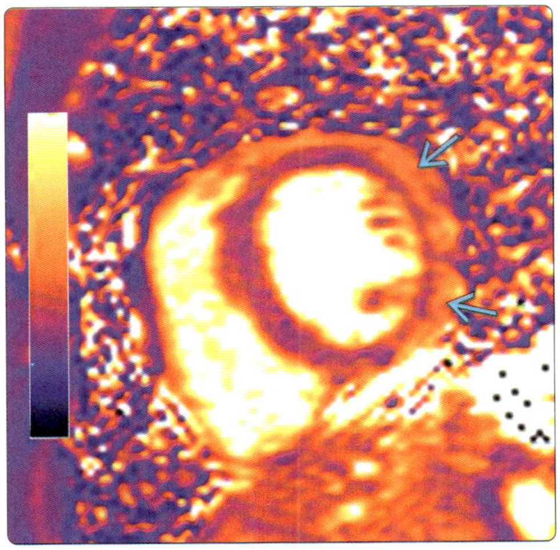

(Left) *Short-axis T1 map obtained at the midcavity in the same patient shows increased native T1 values in the lateral and inferior wall, suggestive of myocardial injury/edema* →*.* **(Right)** *Short-axis T2 map in the same patient shows markedly increased T2 times in the lateral wall* →*, consistent with myocardial edema.*

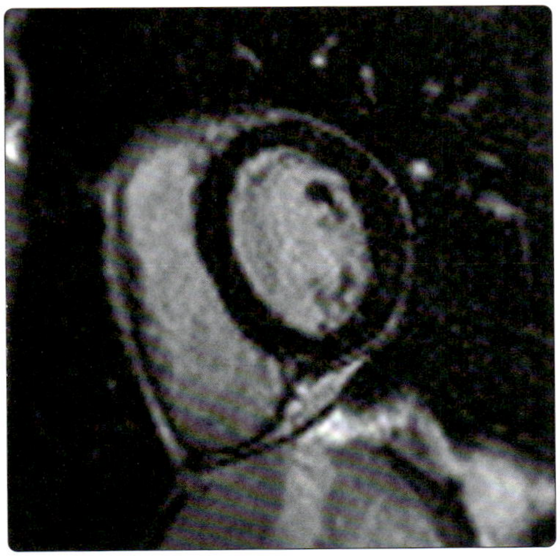

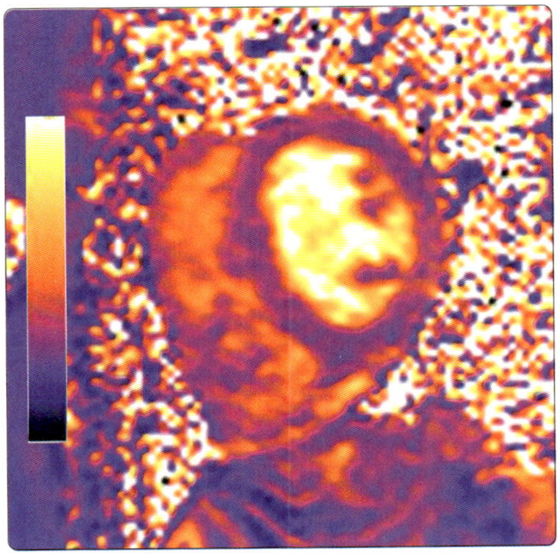

(Left) *Short-axis PSIR follow-up imaging in the same patient after 6 months shows resolved LGE.* **(Right)** *Similarly, short-axis T2 map at the mid-cavity in the same patient shows normalization of the T2 times in the lateral wall, in keeping with resolved myocardial edema. Findings are consistent with resolving myocarditis.*

KEY FACTS

TERMINOLOGY

- Idiopathic disorder characterized by development of subendocardial fibrous and restrictive cardiomyopathy
- This restrictive scarring prevents ventricular filling and causes tethering of papillary muscles, often leading to valvular regurgitation
- Can involve all 4 cardiac chambers, most commonly left ventricle

IMAGING

- Late gadolinium enhancement MR: Best noninvasive tool
  - Late enhancement demonstrates ventricular endocardial fibrosis
  - Can show adjacent typical ventricular layered thrombus
  - Double V sign: Normal myocardium, thickened enhancing endomyocardium, and overlying thrombus with/without calcification
- Echocardiography: 1st-line tool to detect restrictive physiology and obliterative ventricular changes
- Coronary CTA: For exclusion of coronary artery disease and in differentiating chronic thrombus from calcifications

TOP DIFFERENTIAL DIAGNOSES

- Apical thrombus
- Noncompaction of myocardium
- Apical hypertrophic cardiomyopathy

CLINICAL ISSUES

- Primarily disease of young, occurring in children, adolescents, and young adults
- Likely multifactorial aetiology related to dietary, environmental, and infectious factors
- Symptoms or right &/or left heart failure
- Medical therapy includes corticosteroids and immunosuppressive medications
- Surgical endocardectomy with concomitant valve repair/replacement

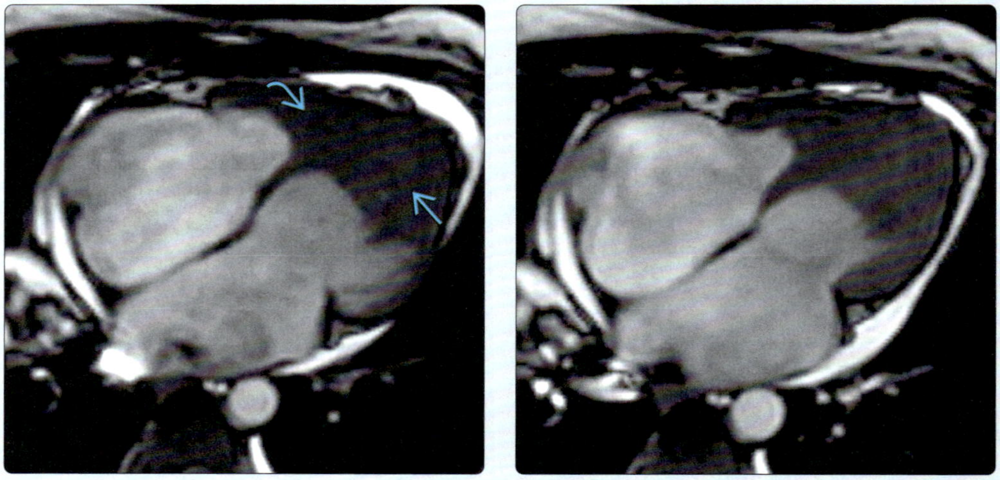

(Left) *Four-chamber SSFP MR during diastole in a patient from India shows isointense signal obliterating the left ventricular (LV) ➡ and right ventricular (RV) ➡ apices and midcavity. The atria are enlarged.* **(Right)** *Systolic SSFP MR shows mild decrease in RV and LV function. However, the large amount of apical soft tissue prevents normal ventricular filling, leading to restriction. In comparison, myocardial stiffening in the amyloid leads to restrictive cardiomyopathy.*

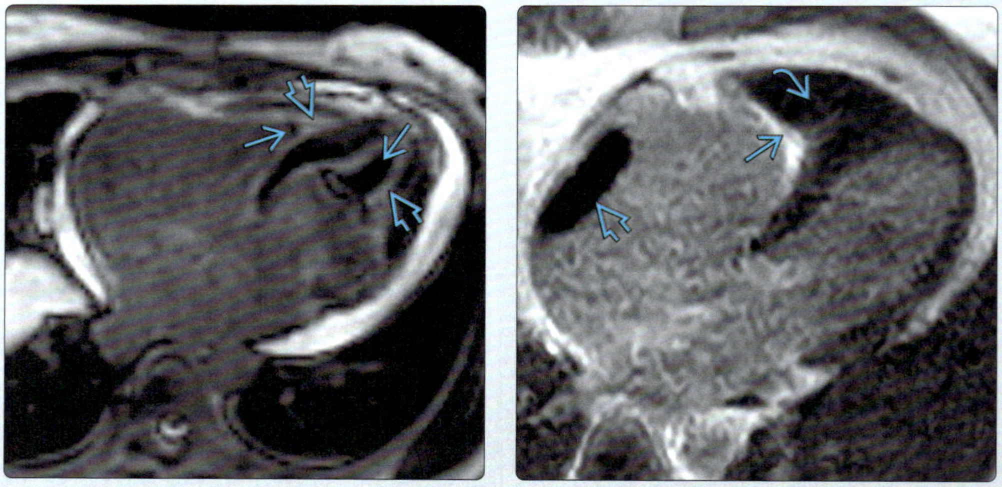

(Left) *LGE MR in the same patient shows low-signal apical thrombus ➡ with subendocardial fibrosis ➡. The scarring and incorporated thrombus decrease LV and RV volumes. This patient was diagnosed with endomyocardial fibrosis (EMF).* **(Right)** *LGE MR in another patient with EMF shows near-complete RV cavity obliteration due to incorporated thrombus ➡ with overlying subendocardial fibrosis ➡. The right atrium is dilated with layering thrombus ➡ due to stasis. (Courtesy R. Kotharih, MD.)*

TERMINOLOGY

Abbreviations

- Endomyocardial fibrosis (EMF)

Synonyms

- Davies disease

Definitions

- Idiopathic disorder characterized by subendocardial fibrosis and restrictive cardiomyopathy
  - This restrictive scarring prevents ventricular filling
  - Tethering of papillary muscles leads to valvular regurgitation
  - Most commonly affects left ventricle

IMAGING

General Features

- Best diagnostic clue
  - Detection of EMF by LGE MR is best noninvasive diagnostic tool
  - May see double V sign at ventricular apex, which is 3-layered appearance consisting of
    - Normal myocardium, thickened enhancing endomyocardium, and overlying thrombus ± calcifications
  - Ventricular apex obliteration by fibrous tissue formation in endomyocardium
  - Atria can be huge, related to severe valvular regurgitation and elevated diastolic ventricular filling pressures
  - Associated signs of right &/or left heart failure: Systemic/pulmonary venous congestion, dilated atria, atrioventricular valve regurgitation
  - Cannot differentiate EMF from Loeffler endocarditis on imaging
- Location
  - 47-50% involve only left ventricle, 14-20% involve only right ventricle, 33-36% involve both ventricles
- Morphology
  - Ventricular volumes are reduced, not dilated
    - Atrial enlargement can be dramatic (secondary to valve regurgitation or restrictive ventricular physiology)

CT Findings

- Not primary imaging modality of choice: Can be used when MR is contraindicated
- Apical obliteration of involved ventricle(s); thrombus may be seen
- Can be useful for differentiating chronic thrombus from calcifications
- Normal or small-sized ventricular cavities; atrial enlargement

Imaging Recommendations

- Best imaging tool
  - Echocardiography: 1st-line tool to detect restrictive physiology and obliterative changes
  - Cardiac MR: Best tool to demonstrate typical EMF pattern and detect mural thrombus
  - Coronary CTA: May be used for exclusion of coronary artery disease and differentiating chronic thrombus from calcifications
- Protocol advice
  - Cardiac MR: Late-enhancement and cine SSFP images are key
    - Subendocardial or endocardial late enhancement indicates inflammatory infiltration (early-stage EMF) or fibrosis (late-stage EMF)
    - Low-signal intracardiac endocardial layering typically represents thrombus
    - Cine SSFP images provide ventricular volumetrics and evaluation of pericardial effusion (common in EMF)

MR Findings

- Cardiac MR
  - Demonstrates typical apical obliteration of involved ventricle(s)
  - Shows small or normal-size ventricle(s) with atrial dilation
  - Detects thrombus and inflammatory/fibrotic changes in endocardial surface on late enhancement
  - May demonstrate fibrosis extending via chordae tendineae to atrioventricular valves where it causes tethering and regurgitation
  - Shows pericardial and pleural effusions, both common in EMF

Echocardiographic Findings

- Apical fibrosis, although apex can be difficult to evaluate
- Thrombi adherent to endocardial surface
- Mitral and tricuspid regurgitation from tethered papillary muscles
- Small or normal-sized ventricle(s) with atrial dilation, often severe
- Restrictive filling pattern by tissue Doppler

Angiographic Findings

- Left and right ventriculography
  - Distortion of chamber morphology by fibrosis and obliteration
  - Variable degrees of mitral and tricuspid regurgitation
  - Hemodynamic findings consistent with restrictive cardiomyopathy
- Invasive coronary angiography typically normal

DIFFERENTIAL DIAGNOSIS

Loeffler Endocarditis

- Cardiac manifestation of hypereosinophilic syndrome
  - Hypereosinophilia variable in EMF
- Indistinguishable on imaging from EMF
- Very similar pathologically to EMF

Apical Thrombus

- Can be attached to areas of prior infarction
- Wall thinning with wall motion abnormalities in myocardial infarction
- Often transmural enhancement restricted to coronary artery territory as well as wall thinning/wall motion abnormalities in myocardial infarction
- Heterogeneous midwall and subepicardial hyperenhancement in nonischemic cardiomyopathies

Left Ventricular Noncompaction

- Characterized by persistent embryonic myocardial morphology
- Noncompacted:compacted myocardium thickness ratio of > 2.3:1.0 is diagnostic
- Noncompaction more frequently affects apex and inferolateral segments of left ventricle
- Late-enhanced sequence is useful in showing absence of endocardial fibrosis and can enhance in noncompacted trabeculae

Apical Hypertrophic Cardiomyopathy

- Thickening of apical myocardium: Ace of spades appearance of cavity
- Late enhancement is useful sequence
  - Late enhancement is located mainly in midwall hypertrophied myocardium, **not** endocardium as in EMF
  - Patchy in distribution, spares endocardial surface

PATHOLOGY

General Features

- Etiology
  - Etiology is not well established; potential causes include
    - Infection
      - Parasites and protozoans (e.g., filariasis, malaria)
    - Inflammation
      - Hypereosinophilic states, EMF similar to late-stage Loeffler endocarditis
    - Nutrition
      - General malnutrition
      - Cassava toxicity, consumed extensively in some tropical African and Latin American countries
    - Drugs
    - Environmental
      - Cerium, rare earth metal found in regional areas of high prevalence

Gross Pathologic & Surgical Features

- Heart size is usually not enlarged, but biatrial enlargement can be seen with valve dysfunction &/or restrictive ventricular physiology
- Ventricular cavities distorted by endocardial thickening and thrombosis of inflow tract and apex of 1 or both ventricles

Microscopic Features

- Endocardial thickening corresponds to endocardial fibrosis
  - Increased number of fibroblasts in endocardium increases local collagen synthesis

CLINICAL ISSUES

Presentation

- Most common signs/symptoms
  - Composed of 2 distinct phases
    - Acute phase with recurrent flare-ups of inflammation
      - Nonspecific symptoms; fever, dyspnea, itching, periorbital edema
      - Pancarditis; pericardial effusion, myocardial edema
    - Chronic phase with hallmark features of restrictive cardiomyopathy
  - Initial manifestation in most patients is right ventricular failure even if there is biventricular involvement
    - Right ventricular involvement
      - Raised jugular venous pulse, hepatomegaly, ascites, peripheral edema
    - Left ventricular involvement
      - Dyspnea, bibasilar crackles, S3
  - At time of diagnosis, most patients are in class III or IV (New York Heart Association)
- Other signs/symptoms
  - Thromboembolic events
    - Secondary to mural thrombi formation along endocardial surfaces

Demographics

- Age
  - Primarily disease of young, occurring in children, adolescents, and young adults
- Sex
  - Women of reproductive age and children are more commonly affected than men
- Epidemiology
  - Tropical EMF
    - 90% of cases in tropical and subtropical regions of Africa, India, and South America
    - EMF is most common type of restrictive cardiomyopathy in tropical countries
    - Likely multifactorial aetiology related to dietary, environmental, and infectious factors
    - Active phase with recurrent flare ups of inflammation leading to chronic phase with restrictive heart failure

Natural History & Prognosis

- Composed of acute and chronic phases
  - In some patients, EMF progresses rapidly to advanced restrictive heart failure and death
  - In remaining patients, often quiescent and asymptomatic for long periods
- Poor overall prognosis: 75% mortality rate at 2 years after onset of symptoms
- Death may be caused by progressive heart failure, secondary to ventricular arrhythmias or PE

Treatment

- Medical
  - Medical treatment for diastolic heart failure
- Surgical
  - Endocardial decortication for classes III and IV
  - Successful surgery has clear benefit on symptoms and seems to favorably affect survival as well
  - Recurrence occurs in 15% of cases postoperatively

SELECTED REFERENCES

1. Rapezzi C et al: Restrictive cardiomyopathy: definition and diagnosis. Eur Heart J. 43(45):4679-93, 2022
2. de Carvalho FP et al: Comprehensive assessment of endomyocardial fibrosis with cardiac MRI: morphology, function, and tissue characterization. Radiographics. 40(2):336-53, 2020
3. Mocumbi AO et al: Endomyocardial fibrosis: an update after 70 years. Curr Cardiol Rep. 21(11):148, 2019
4. Grimaldi A et al: Tropical endomyocardial fibrosis: natural history, challenges, and perspectives. Circulation. 133(24):2503-15, 2016
5. DAVIES JN: Endomyocardial fibrosis in Uganda. Cent Afr J Med. 2(9):323-8, 1956

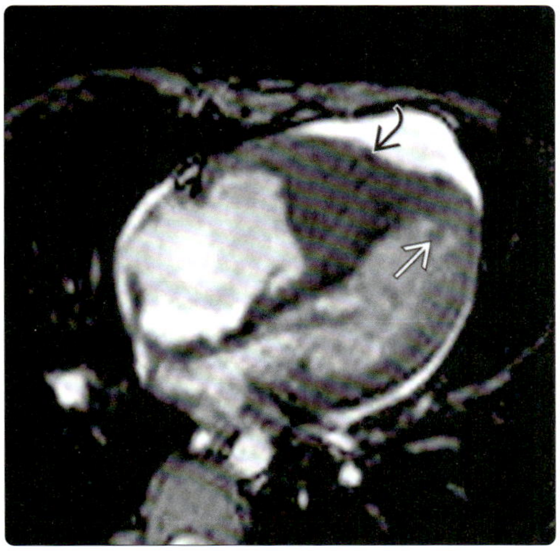

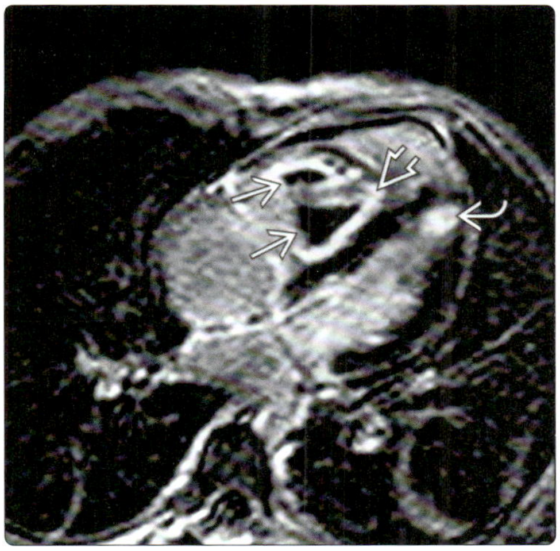

(Left) *Four-chamber view MR cine shows midapical RV obliteration, dilated right atrium/ventricle, and small pericardial effusion. There is also mild LV apical obliteration secondary to thrombus.* **(Right)** *Four-chamber view LGE MR in the same patient shows RV endocavitary thrombus and endomyocardial late enhancement in a patient with eosinophilic leukemia causing Loeffler endocarditis (LE). The LV apex also has focal endocardial late enhancement. MR findings in EMF and LE are identical.*

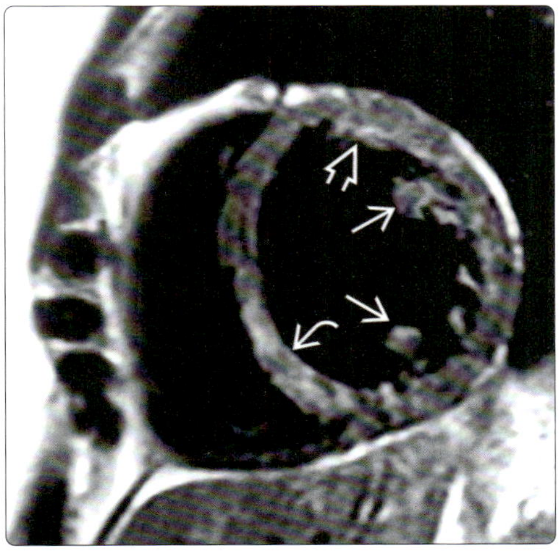

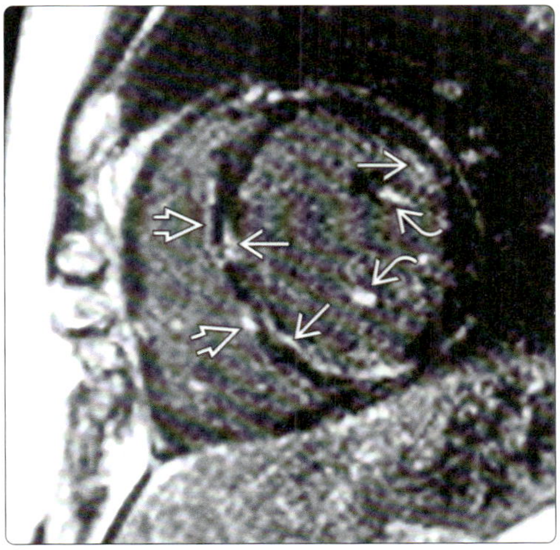

(Left) *Short-axis T2 MR shows high signal in the anterolateral segment, papillary muscles, and inferoseptal segment, consistent with multifocal acute myocardial edema. The patient's peripheral eosinophil count was 27,000 on admission.* **(Right)** *Corresponding short-axis LGE MR in the same patient shows subendocardial LGE in multiple LV segments, endocardial LGE on the RV side of the interventricular septum indicating RV involvement, and papillary muscle LGE.*

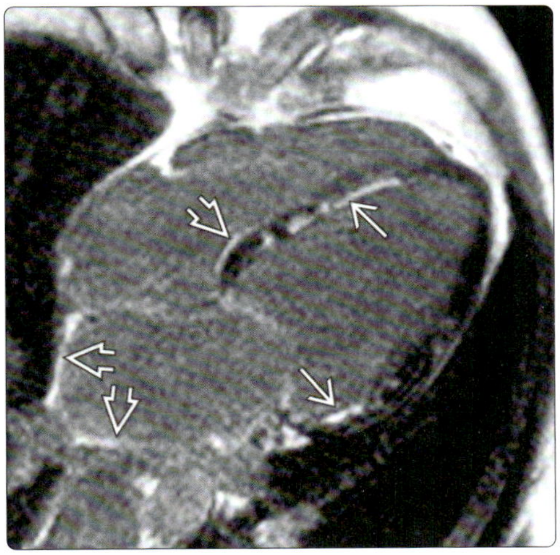

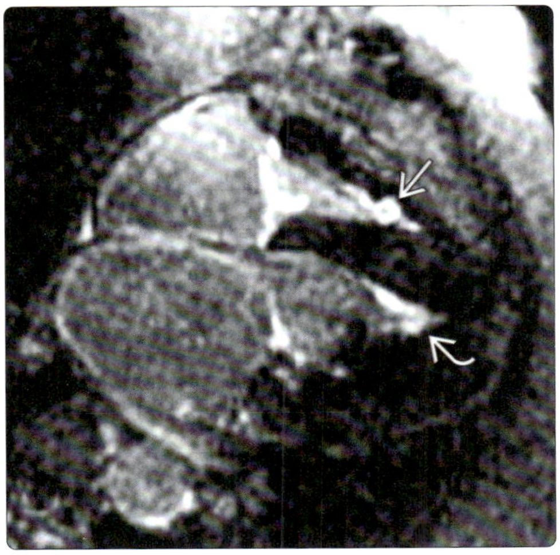

(Left) *Corresponding 4-chamber view in the same patient shows the extent of LV subendocardial LGE and RV endocardial LGE Note biatrial enlargement and enhancement indicative of restrictive physiology and atrial wall fibrosis.* **(Right)** *Four-chamber view LGE MR detects small ventricles with apical obliteration and dilated atria. Note the endomyocardial abnormal delayed enhancement, consistent with fibrosis on both RV and LV with an apical predominance.*

Hypereosinophilic Syndrome

KEY FACTS

TERMINOLOGY

- Unexplained hypereosinophilia (> 1,500/μL) of ≥ 6 months duration associated with organ dysfunction due to eosinophilic infiltration
  - Heart is most commonly involved organ (cardiac involvement in up to 60% of cases)
- Synonyms: Eosinophilic endocarditis, Löffler (or Loeffler) endocarditis

IMAGING

- Cine MR
  - Affected ventricular apices often appear filled with amorphous isointense material that represents thrombus with seemingly apical obliteration
  - Thrombus &/or subsequent intracavitary fibrosis can impair function of chordae tendineae, resulting in valvular regurgitation
  - Restrictive cardiomyopathy can occur secondary to cavity obliteration by thrombus or by fibrosis in later stages of disease
- LGE MR
  - Intense endocardial enhancement is noted involving interface between nonenhancing intracavitary thrombus and nulled myocardium
  - Images with long inversion time (600 ms) are helpful in demonstrating intracavitary thrombi
- Perfusion imaging and early (< 3 minutes) delayed-enhancement MR is often useful to define cleavage plane between thrombus and enhancing, inflamed endocardium

TOP DIFFERENTIAL DIAGNOSES

- Endomyocardial fibrosis
- Apical thrombus
- Apical hypertrophic cardiomyopathy
- Left ventricular noncompaction

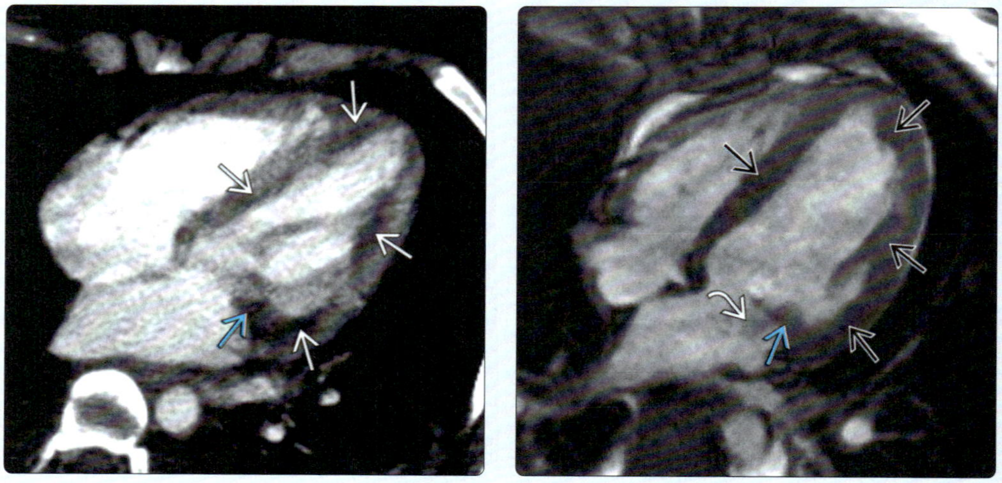

(Left) *Four-chamber reconstruction CT in a 24-year-old woman with rapid clinical decompensation and peripheral eosinophilia of 19,800 cells/μL shows extensive subendocardial hypoenhancement extending posteriorly to involve the mitral valve.* **(Right)** *Four-chamber cine MR in the same patient performed the next day shows areas of irregular thickening of the left ventricular endocardium involving the mitral valve. Mitral regurgitation was present.*

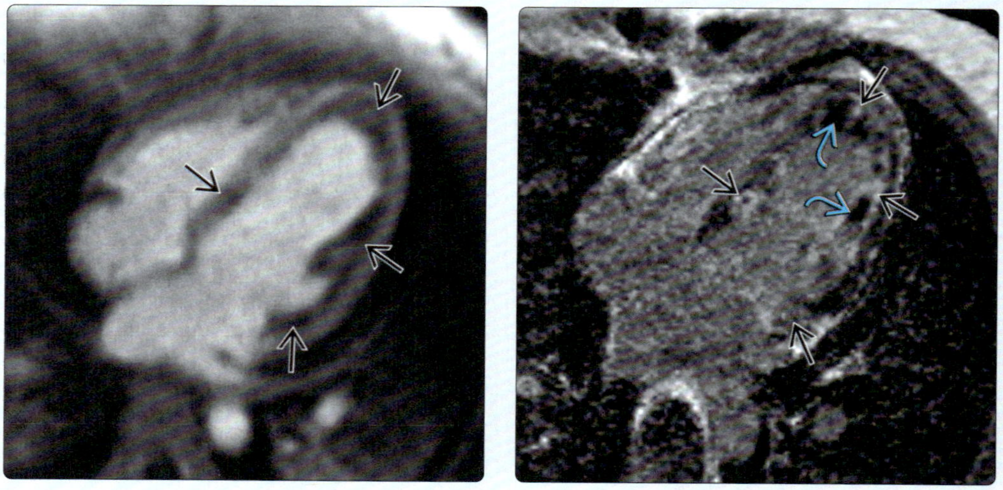

(Left) *First-pass perfusion MR in the same patient shows subendocardial hypoperfusion involving the thickened areas.* **(Right)** *Four-chamber LGE MR in the same patient shows linear subendocardial delayed enhancement in the areas of thickening. Areas of dark signal within the cardiac chamber represent a mix of eosinophilic-laden thrombus and necrotic endocardium. The patient died 5 hours after the examination.*

TERMINOLOGY

Abbreviations

- Hypereosinophilic syndrome (HES)

Synonyms

- Cardiac involvement in HES has many synonyms
  - Loeffler endocarditis
  - Eosinophilic endomyocarditis
  - Nontropical eosinophilic endomyocardial disease

Definitions

- Unexplained hypereosinophilia (> 1,500/μL) of ≥ 6 months duration associated with organ dysfunction due to eosinophilic infiltration
  - Heart is most commonly involved organ (cardiac involvement in up to 60% of cases)

IMAGING

General Features

- Best diagnostic clue
  - Characteristic MR findings are essentially pathognomonic when present
- Location
  - Ventricular endocardium
- Morphology
  - Typically results in arrowhead configuration of 1 or both apices with laminated thrombus layered over inflamed apical ventricular endocardium

Imaging Recommendations

- Best imaging tool
  - Contrast-enhanced MR
    - Gated-cardiac CTA may be substituted in patients unable to undergo MR
  - Echocardiography is often recommended as 1st-line tool but is less sensitive in detecting thrombus
    - Transthoracic echo frequently has technical limitations in evaluation of apices
- Protocol advice
  - Standard cardiac MR exam with SSFP cine imaging plus
    - Perfusion imaging, which can delineate endocardial hypoperfusion and areas of thrombus
    - LGE imaging with inversion time to null myocardium to assess for endocardial fibrosis
    - LGE imaging with longer inversion time (600 ms) to assess for thrombus

MR Findings

- T2WI
  - In acute necrotic stage, subendocardial high signal due to edema can be seen
- MR cine
  - Findings will depend on stage of disease
  - Acute necrotic stage
    - Endocardial thickening, which can be subtle or appear almost mass-like
    - Thrombus often absent or minimal
    - Normal biventricular function
    - Heart may appear relatively normal
  - Thrombotic-necrotic stage
    - Adherent subendocardial thrombus in 1 or both ventricles
    - Ejection fraction still normal
    - Subendocardial injury commonly involves valves, leading to valvular regurgitation
    - Thrombus formation can also impair function of chordae tendinea, leading to valvular regurgitation
  - Late fibrotic stage
    - Apical cavitary obliteration due to fibrosis
    - Reduces ventricular cavity size and causes restrictive cardiomyopathy
      - Often biatrial enlargement, dilation of superior and inferior vena cava, hepatic congestion, etc.
- Delayed enhancement
  - Linear, endocardial-predominant LGE in all stages of disease
    - May be more pronounced in 1 ventricle, but both are pathologically involved
    - Apices more severely involved, especially in later parts of disease process
  - Nonenhancing thrombus, which can be better seen using longer inversion times (600 ms)
  - Triple-layered pattern: Inner dark signal from thrombus; middle layer of enhancement from fibrosis; outer layer of normal myocardium
- 1st-pass perfusion imaging
  - Pronounced subendocardial hypoperfusion
    - In acute stage, may be only abnormal finding on 1st-pass perfusion
  - Nonperfusing ventricular thrombi often present

CT Findings

- Cardiac gated CTA
  - Depending on stage of disease, will demonstrate subendocardial hypoperfusion ± intracavitary thrombus ± findings of restrictive physiology
    - Subendocardial hypoperfusion often evident on both early arterial and portal venous phases
    - Delayed scan may be useful to differentiate thrombus from tumor
    - Retrospectively gated acquisitions may allow evaluation of mitral/tricuspid valve dysfunction

DIFFERENTIAL DIAGNOSIS

Endomyocardial Fibrosis

- One of most common causes of restrictive cardiomyopathy in Africa, Latin America, and Asia
- Imaging appearance similar to cases of Loeffler endocarditis
- Eosinophilia may be present but is absent in up to 70% in acute phase
- LGE may involve subvalvular apparatus

Apical Thrombus

- Often attached to areas of prior infarction

Apical Hypertrophic Cardiomyopathy

- Apical cavity obliteration due to myocardial hypertrophy with thrombus uncommon
- LGE pattern is markedly different with hazy midmyocardial LGE most notably at apex

Left Ventricular Noncompaction

- May have associated thrombi, but these do not obliterate cavity

Other Causes of Restrictive Cardiomyopathy

- Not morphologically similar or confusing but may result in similar physiology

PATHOLOGY

General Features

- Etiology
  - Idiopathic
  - Myeloproliferative variant (10-15% of cases)
    - Seen with eosinophilic myeloid neoplasm
    - Some cases result from *FIP1L1-PDGFRA* gene fusion mutation of tyrosine kinase
    - In > 90% of these cases, patients have complete remission with imatinib, tyrosine kinase inhibitor
  - Lymphocytic variant (15% of cases)
    - Clonal or aberrant T-cell population that produces cytokines causing eosinophilia
  - Overlap HES
    - Eosinophilic disorder limited to single organ with clinically defined eosinophilic syndrome that overlaps in presentation with idiopathic HES
  - Associated HES
    - HES in context of defined disorder such as infection, neoplasm, hypersensitivity reaction, etc.
  - Familial HES
    - Occurrence of HES in > 1 family member, excluding causes of associated HES
- Genetics
  - Most cases are sporadic
    - Familial cases occur but are very rare

Gross Pathologic & Surgical Features

- Eosinophilic infiltration of endocardium leads to subendocardial inflammation and necrosis
  - These changes are most prominent at ventricular apices
- Inflamed endocardium serves as nidus for thrombus formation with subsequent fibrosis
  - This fibrosis often entraps chordae tendineae of mitral &/or tricuspid valves, leading to dysfunction
- Thrombus formation and subsequent endomyocardial fibrosis cause reduction of ventricular cavity volume and marked stiffening of affected ventricle, resulting in restrictive physiology
- Atrial enlargement often occurs as result of valvular dysfunction &/or diminished ventricular compliance

CLINICAL ISSUES

Presentation

- Most common signs/symptoms
  - Dyspnea is most common presenting symptom, followed by chest pain and cough
  - Biventricular congestive heart failure
    - Right heart symptoms often predominate
- Other signs/symptoms
  - Fever, night sweats, weight loss, myalgias, dyspnea, nonproductive cough, and generalized fatigue

Demographics

- Age
  - Patients are typically in 4th or 5th decades at diagnosis, but range is from childhood to late adulthood
- Sex
  - Once thought to have > 80% male predominance, but more recent series suggest only slight male predominance (60%)

Natural History & Prognosis

- 3 stages of disease progression
  - Acute necrotic stage
    - Infiltration of endocardium > myocardium with eosinophils, leading to predominantly endocardial necrosis
  - Thrombotic-necrotic stage
    - Formation of thrombi along damaged endocardium of ventricles and (occasionally) right atrium
  - Late fibrotic stage
    - Endomyocardial fibrosis with entrapment of chordae tendineae, leading to mitral &/or tricuspid regurgitation
    - Restrictive cardiomyopathy due to reduction in cavity size caused by incorporated thrombus
- Cardiac involvement often has poor prognosis with reported 5-year survival rate < 50%

Treatment

- High-dose steroids (> 40 mg/day) are mainstay of therapy for idiopathic and lymphocytic types
- Imatinib is 1st-line therapy for myeloproliferative variant
- Cytotoxic agents/monoclonal antibodies against interleukin 5 often reserved for treatment failures
- Anticoagulation used to treat thrombotic complications
- Conventional heart failure therapy, including diuretics and afterload reduction, may be useful
- Heart transplant is occasionally performed

DIAGNOSTIC CHECKLIST

Consider

- HES in patients with apical cavity obliteration by thrombus along with characteristic circumferential subendocardial delayed enhancement

Image Interpretation Pearls

- Differentiation of HES from apical hypertrophic cardiomyopathy is facilitated by dynamic cine MR and LGE MR imaging

SELECTED REFERENCES

1. Klion AD: Approach to the patient with suspected hypereosinophilic syndrome. Hematology Am Soc Hematol Educ Program. 2022(1):47-54, 2022
2. de Carvalho FP et al: Comprehensive assessment of endomyocardial fibrosis with cardiac MRI: morphology, function, and tissue characterization. Radiographics. 40(2):336-53, 2020
3. Mankad R et al: Hypereosinophilic syndrome: cardiac diagnosis and management. Heart. 102(2):100-6, 2016
4. Perazzolo Marra M et al: Cardiac magnetic resonance features of biopsy-proven endomyocardial diseases. JACC Cardiovasc Imaging. 7(3):309-12, 2014
5. Kleinfeldt T et al: Cardiac manifestation of the hypereosinophilic syndrome: new insights. Clin Res Cardiol. 99(7):419-27, 2010

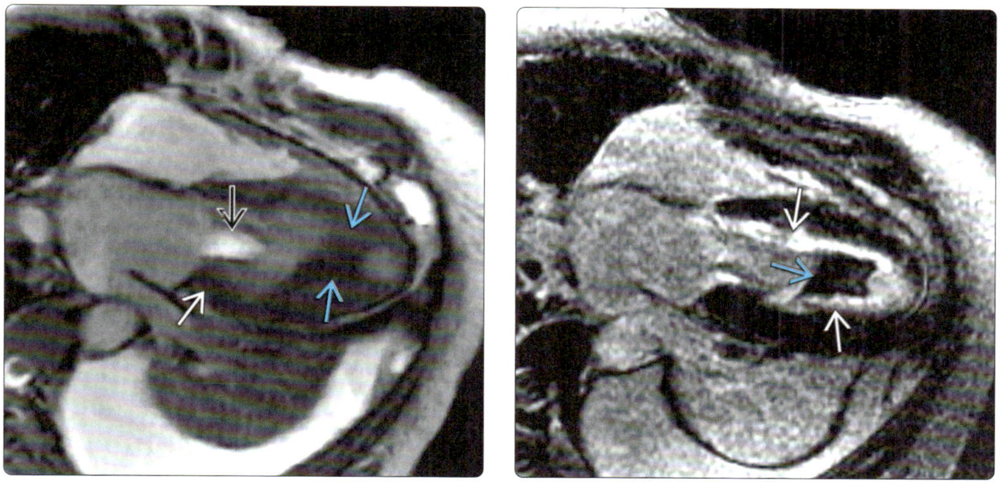

(Left) *Four-chamber SSFP MR shows a large, isointense mass* ➔ *within the left ventricle (LV). There are areas of subendocardial thickening, most notable at the base* ➔. *An early diastolic high-velocity inflow jet is due to a restrictive physiology* ➔, *and the left atrium is enlarged. Mitral regurgitation was present.* **(Right)** *Four-chamber delayed enhancement MR shows diffuse subendocardial enhancement* ➔, *and a large thrombus in the LV* ➔ *spares the apex.*

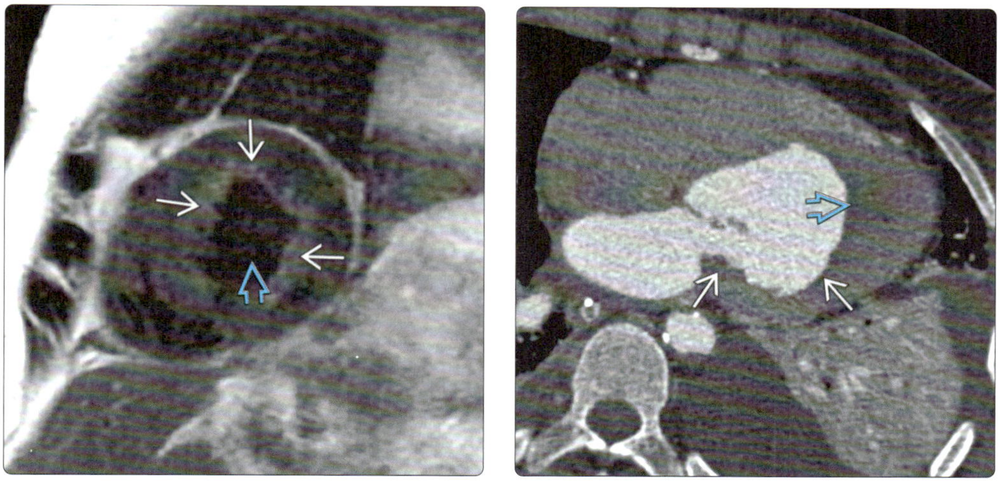

(Left) *Short-axis T2 TSE MR of the LV at the level of the thrombus* ➔ *shows subendocardial high signal* ➔ *due to edema.* **(Right)** *Axial coronary CTA in the same patient performed 11 months later demonstrates increased thrombus* ➔ *and fibrosis obliterating the LV apex, worsening the physiologic restriction. Areas of subendocardial hypoperfusion* ➔ *are also seen. The findings are consistent with late fibrotic stage.*

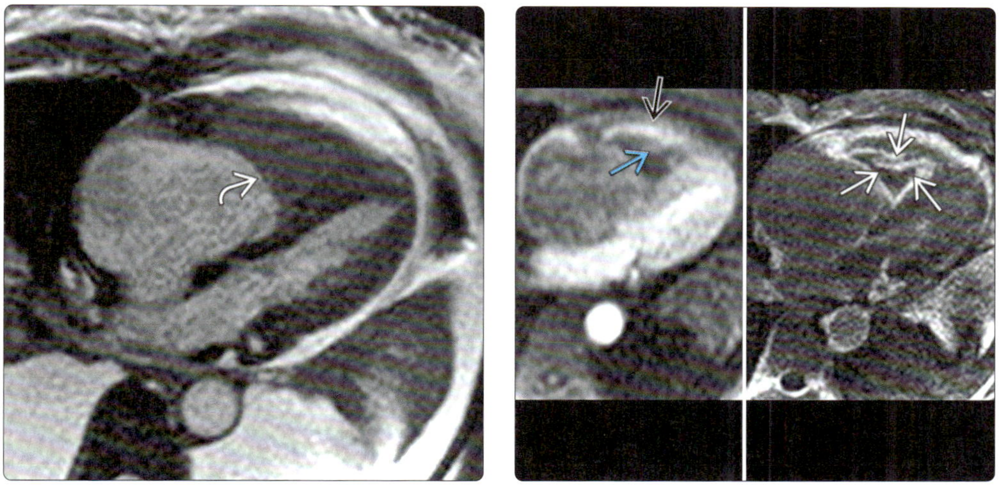

(Left) *Four-chamber cine MR in a patient with Loeffler endocarditis shows thrombus* ➔ *filling much of the right ventricle (RV). The right atrium is markedly dilated.* **(Right)** *Perfusion MR (left) shows RV subendocardial hyperperfusion* ➔ *due to inflammation. The RV thrombus does not enhance* ➔. *LGE MR (right) shows characteristic subendocardial fibrosis* ➔, *which has epithelialized over the thrombus, nearly obliterating the RV cavity and causing restriction.*

KEY FACTS

TERMINOLOGY

- Typically caused by pathogenic desmosomal gene variants, &, less frequently, by variants in nondesmosomal genes
  - Results in apoptosis & early cell death with fibrofatty replacement
  - Predominantly affects right ventricle (RV) with variable left ventricular (LV) involvement
  - Frequently associated with ventricular arrhythmias, including sudden cardiac death, early in disease
  - Marked genotype-phenotype differences are present with *DSP* variants, causing frequent & earlier LV involvement
  - Endurance training accelerates disease progression & may provoke ventricular arrhythmias

IMAGING

- Diagnosis is made using set of major & minor criteria in 6 categories [task force criteria (TFC), 2010]
  - Imaging can supply only 1 major or 1 minor TFC
- Epicardial subtricuspid region & basal RV free wall are most commonly involved
- RV is usually dilated & shows impaired systolic function
- RV aneurysms & microaneurysms are often evident
- RV outflow tract (RVOT) is commonly dilated & poorly contractile
- LV is involved in ≥ 50% of cases & may predominate in some
- Attempts to visualize intramyocardial fat are no longer advised, since they frequently result in misdiagnosis

TOP DIFFERENTIAL DIAGNOSES

- Cardiac sarcoid
- Myocarditis
- RV dilatation in endurance athletes
- RV volume overload
- RV infarction
- Idiopathic RVOT ventricular tachycardia
- Nonarrhythmogenic RV cardiomyopathy fatty infiltration of RV

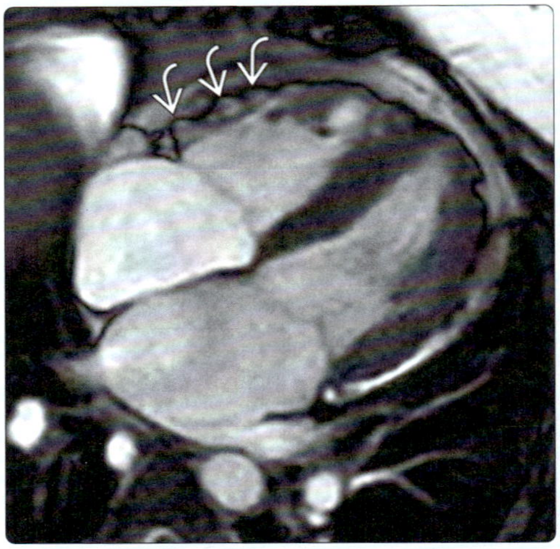

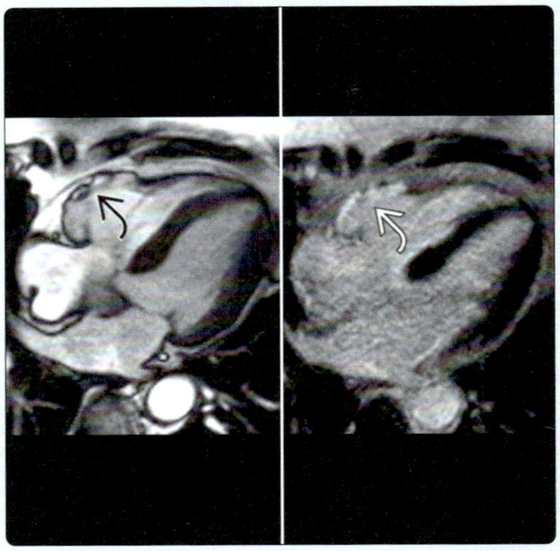

(Left) *Four-chamber SSFP cardiac MR obtained in systole shows several microaneurysms along the right ventricular (RV) free wall in a patient with arrhythmogenic RV cardiomyopathy (ARVC).* **(Right)** *Four-chamber cine SSFP MR (left) in a patient with ARVC shows typical involvement of the subtricuspid region with focal systolic outpouching. LGE MR shows enhancement in this region.*

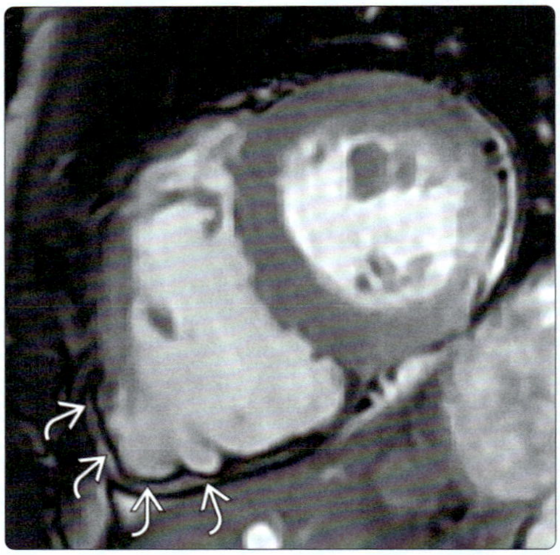

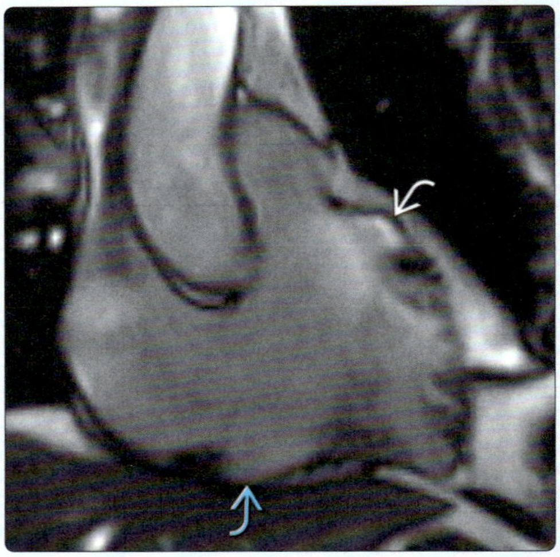

(Left) *Short-axis SSFP cine MR obtained in diastole in an ARVC patient shows dyskinetic bulging of the RV in the region near the junction of the free wall and inferior wall, a common place for ARVC-related abnormalities.* **(Right)** *Systolic RV long-axis SSFP MR from a cardiac MR obtained in a patient with ARVC shows focal dyskinetic regions in the RV outflow tract (OT) just below the pulmonic valve anulus and in the basal RV inferior wall.*

TERMINOLOGY

Abbreviations

- Arrhythmogenic right ventricular cardiomyopathy (ARVC)

Synonyms

- Formerly known as arrhythmogenic right ventricular dysplasia (ARVD)
- Term arrhythmogenic cardiomyopathy (ACM) has been proposed to include both left ventricular (LV) & right ventricular (RV) disease

Definitions

- Distinct entity typically caused by pathogenic variants in desmosomal (i.e., *PKP2*, *DSP*, *DSC2*, *DSG2* & *JUP*) or rarely in nondesmosomal (*TMEM43*) genes
  - Result is apoptosis & early cell death with replacement by fibrofatty tissue
  - Predominantly affects RV with variable LV involvement; is associated with ventricular arrhythmias, including sudden cardiac death (SCD)

IMAGING

General Features

- Best diagnostic clue
  - Diagnosis based on major &/or minor Task Force Criteria (TFC): Combination of functional, structural, electrocardiographic, arrhythmic, pathologic, & family history/genetic information
  - MR abnormalities are important component of TFC but alone are not sufficient to diagnose ARVC
  - Diagnosis is considered definite when 2 major, 1 major & 2 minor, or 4 minor criteria from different categories are present; imaging can only contribute either 1 major or 1 minor or no criterion
- Location
  - RV structural abnormalities are preferentially located in basal to mid RV free wall (particularly subtricuspid region) & basal to mid inferior wall
  - Change in perception of regional structural involvement in ARVC in last decade
    - RV apex abnormalities, previously considered characteristic component of ARVC [triangle of dysplasia: RV outflow tract (OT), RV inflow tract, & apex], now recognized to be less common unless advanced disease
- Size
  - RV is commonly dilated
- Morphology
  - ARVC is regional disease involving some areas of RV free wall & sparing others; extent of RV involvement is variable & may progress over time
    - RV free wall microaneurysms & dyskinetic segments are noted on cine imaging

MR Findings

- Cine SSFP imaging
  - RV is usually dilated with impaired function & regional wall motion abnormalities (RWMA), including akinesia, dyskinesia, & systolic dyssynchrony
  - RV aneurysms & microaneurysms
  - To meet major or minor TFC, MR findings must include both RV RWMA (dyssynchronous RV contraction, dyskinesia, or akinesia) & global RV quantitative abnormality [RV dilation or ↓ RV ejection fraction (RVEF)]
    - Minor: iRVEDV ≥ 100 to < 110 mL/m² (male); ≥ 90 to < 100 mL/m² (female); RVEF > 40% to ≤ 45%
    - Major: iRVEDV ≥ 110 mL/m² (male); ≥ 100 mL/m² (female); RVEF ≤ 40%
- Black blood SE
  - May detect RV or LV intramyocardial fat (caution: Presence of fat is not part of TFC due to high interobserver variability & potential to result in misdiagnosis)
- LGE
  - May demonstrate LGE of RV wall, representing fibrosis in 2/3 of cases, but, similar to fat, is not part of TFC
    - RV LGE can be difficult to visualize on standard 2D images due to thinness of RV wall
  - LV involvement may manifest as LGE, often involving subepicardial mid to apical inferior & lateral walls ± concomitant WMA
    - Septal LGE is unusual in typical ARVC

Echocardiographic Findings

- Echocardiogram
  - Hypokinetic & dilated RV with ↓ RVEF
  - To meet major or minor TFC, echo findings must include both regional RV RWMA (regional RV akinesia, dyskinesia, or aneurysm) & RV quantitative abnormality: Either RVOT dilation [by parasternal long axis (PLAX) or parasternal short axis (PSAX) views] or reduced RV fractional area change (FAC)
    - Minor: PLAX RVOT ≥ 29 to < 32 mm [corrected for body size PLAX/body surface area (BSA) ≥ 16 to < 19 mm/m^2] or PSAX RVOT ≥ 32 to < 36 mm (corrected for body size PLAX/BSA ≥ 18 to < 21mm/m^2) or FAC > 33% to ≤ 40%
    - Major: PLAX RVOT ≥ 32 mm (corrected for body size PLAX/BSA ≥ 19 mm/m^2) or PSAX RVOT ≥ 36 mm (corrected for body size PLAX/BSA ≥ 21 mm/m^2) or FAC ≤ 33%

Imaging Recommendations

- Best imaging tool
  - MR is preferred for RV RWMA evaluation, volumes & function, & tissue characterization
- Protocol advice
  - Cine MR of entire RV is essential
    - Standard long- & short-axis planes recommended with full ventricular coverage
    - Consider adding dedicated long axis RVOT views & stack of axial or 4-chamber planes

DIFFERENTIAL DIAGNOSIS

Cardiac Sarcoidosis

- May mimic ARVC with dilated, poorly functioning RV with biventricular LGE
- Commonly has extensive LV LGE, particularly septal, & manifests with prolonged PR interval, advanced atrioventricular block, prolonged QRS duration, & positive (18) F-FDG PET scan

Myocarditis

- Isolated RV involvement is uncommon; subepicardial LV LGE in basal inferolateral wall is most common pattern

Right Ventricular Dilatation in Endurance Athletes

- Marathon runners & other endurance athletes often develop RV dilation; RV function is usually preserved

Right Ventricular Volume Overload

- Pretricuspid left-to-right shunts
  - Has normal or hyperdynamic RV function
  - Shunt seen: Atrial septal defect, partial anomalous pulmonary venous return, unroofed coronary sinus
- Repaired tetralogy of Fallot
  - Often has significant pulmonic regurgitation with RV volume overload & systolic dysfunction

Right Ventricular Infarction

- Usually associated with inferior wall LV infarct (right coronary artery territory)
- Not commonly associated with localized aneurysm formation

Pitfalls

- RV free wall tether: Pericardial connective tissue joining anterior RV free wall to posterior sternum, mistaken as dyskinesia
- Apicolateral bulge: Seen in 79% as wall motion abnormality in RV at site of insertion of moderator band
- Butterfly apex: Prominent RV apex confused for aneurysm, but isolated apical aneurysm is unusual; normal systolic & diastolic motion
- Pulmonary valve sinuses: Systolic bulge due to filling with blood mimics dyskinesia; located above pulmonary valve anulus

PATHOLOGY

General Features

- Etiology
  - Pathogenic variants in genes coding for desmosomal proteins lead to early apoptosis, likely hastened by "wear & tear," which is exacerbated by endurance exercise
- Genetics
  - Predominantly autosomal dominant inheritance with variable penetrance
    - 5 desmosomal genes (*PKP2, DSP, DSG2, DSC2,* & *JUP*) & *TMEM43* have been implicated in ARVC
  - Family history may provide TFC if 1st-degree relative with proven (major) or suspected (minor) ARVC

Gross Pathologic & Surgical Features

- RV wall thinning & aneurysms

Microscopic Features

- Biopsy findings demonstrating myocyte loss with fibrous replacement may provide TFC

CLINICAL ISSUES

Presentation

- Most common signs/symptoms
  - Early ("concealed") phase: Patients are often asymptomatic but may be at risk of arrhythmic SCD
  - Overt ("electric") phase: Patients present with symptomatic ventricular arrhythmias & RV morphofunctional abnormalities, detectable with imaging
- Clinical profile
  - Should be considered in athletes of any age as cause of syncope or cardiovascular collapse
  - Can lead to isolated RV or biventricular heart failure
- Diagnosis
  - Made on basis of TFC, representing combination of functional, structural, electrocardiographic, arrhythmic, pathologic, & family history/genetic information

Demographics

- Age
  - More clinically apparent in 2nd-4th decades of life
- Sex
  - M:F = 3:1 in younger age groups; M = F in later-onset cases
- Epidemiology
  - Estimated incidence: 1 in 2,000 to 1 in 5,000

Natural History & Prognosis

- Annual mortality rate: ~ 0.08-3.6%
- Disease expression significantly differs across genotypes

Treatment

- Avoid endurance training
- Pharmacotherapy: Antiarrhythmic agents, β-blockers, & heart failure drug therapy, as appropriate
- Implantable cardioverter defibrillator (ICD)
  - Indicated for secondary prevention in patients with history of ventricular tachycardia (VT) or cardiac arrest
  - ARVC risk calculator can help guide primary prevention ICD decisions; in patients with *DSP* variant, DSP Risk Score should be considered
- Catheter ablation of VT may be useful in patients with recurrent ICD therapies
- Heart transplant, predominantly for advanced heart failure or untreatable arrhythmias

DIAGNOSTIC CHECKLIST

Image Interpretation Pearls

- Qualitative RV RWMA & quantitative global volumetric &/or functional abnormalities are key imaging components to meet ARVC structural criteria (TFC)
- Neither myocardial fat nor LGE are components of ARVC diagnostic criteria (TFC); rather, they should be seen as adjunct information that may help with differential diagnosis
- Normal variants of RV wall motion are common sources of diagnostic error with CMR interpretation

SELECTED REFERENCES

1. Sampognaro JR et al: Diagnostic pitfalls in patients referred for arrhythmogenic right ventricular cardiomyopathy. Heart Rhythm. 20(12):1720-6, 2023
2. Malik N et al: Multimodality imaging in arrhythmogenic right ventricular cardiomyopathy. Circ Cardiovasc Imaging. 15(2):e013725, 2022
3. Zghaib T et al: Left ventricular fibro-fatty replacement in arrhythmogenic right ventricular dysplasia/cardiomyopathy: prevalence, patterns, and association with arrhythmias. J Cardiovasc Magn Reson. 23(1):58, 2021

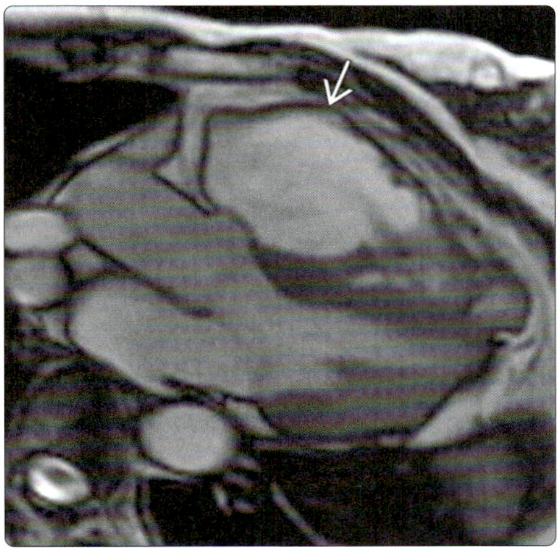

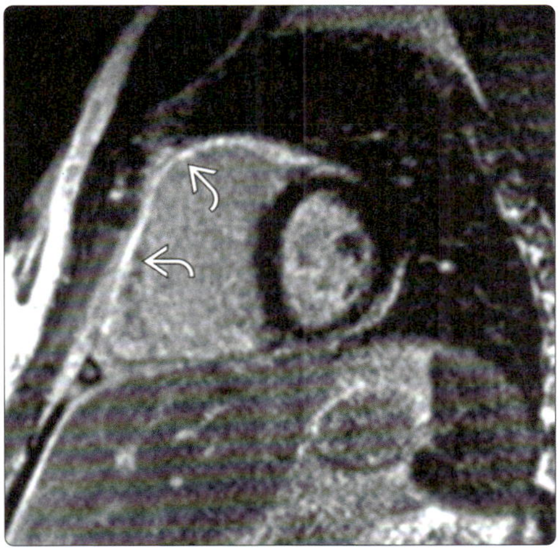

(Left) *RVOT plane SSFP image from a cardiac MR obtained in a patient with advanced ARVC shows a dilated RVOT ➔ that was dyskinetic on cine evaluation.* **(Right)** *Short-axis LGE MR in a patient with ARVC shows diffuse enhancement of the RV ➔, which may be difficult to identify due to thinness of the RV wall. Presence of LGE is not included in the task force criteria (TFC) for diagnosis of ARVC.*

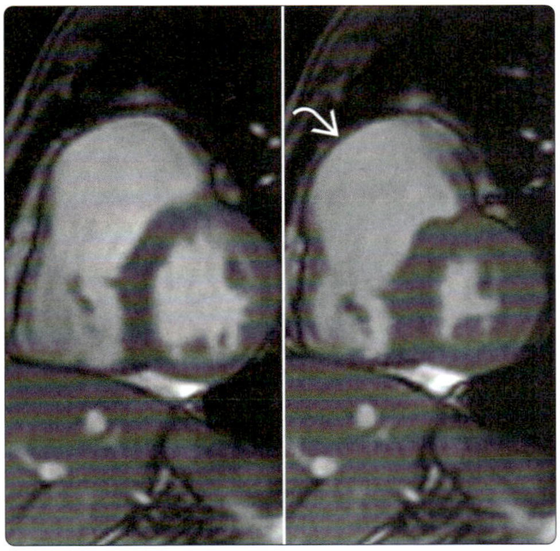

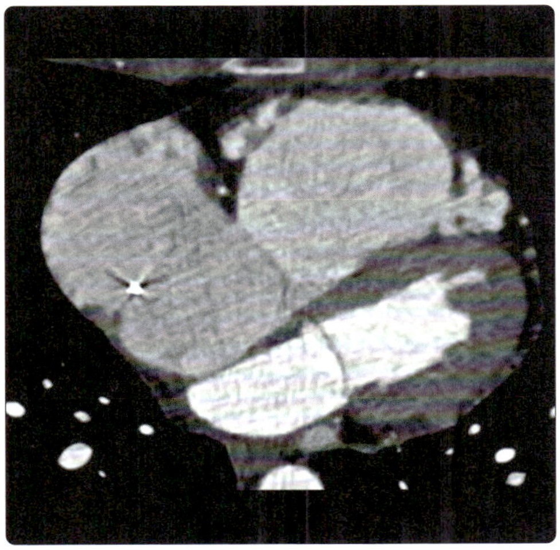

(Left) *Sagittal cine SSFP bright-blood MR through the RVOT in diastole (left) & systole (right) in an adolescent boy with ARVC shows ↑ dilation of the RVOT during systole ➔.* **(Right)** *Axial cardiac CT obtained prior to ablation for ventricular tachycardia shows a dilated RV and partially visualized implantable cardioverter defibrillator (ICD) leading into the right atrium in a patient with severe ARVC.*

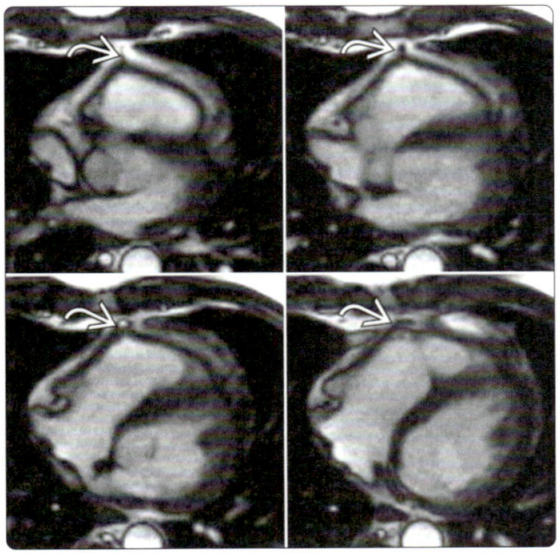

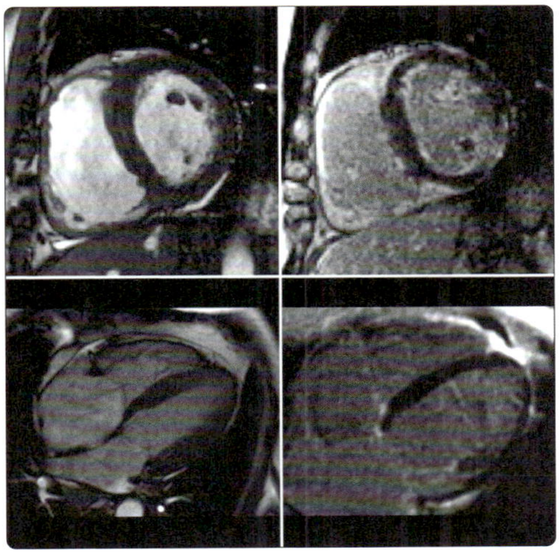

(Left) *Axial cine MR images in a normal patient shows a triangular outpouching from the anterior RVOT, known as tethering ➔, which is best seen on axial images of the superior RV free wall and RVOT region. This finding is a potential pitfall in evaluation of RV wall motion that can be mistaken for pathology.* **(Right)** *Short-axis MR cine (top left) & LGE (top right) images & 4-chamber cine (bottom left) & LGE images (bottom right) are shown in a patient with sarcoid. Note the extensive RV enhancement.*

Arrhythmogenic Cardiomyopathy

KEY FACTS

TERMINOLOGY

- Arrhythmogenic cardiomyopathy (ACM) most often refers to patients with inherited arrhythmogenic myocardial disease
  - Subgroups of patients with exclusively or predominantly left ventricle (LV), right ventricle (RV), or biventricular involvement
    - LV-predominant disease commonly caused by pathogenic variants in *DSP*, *FLNC*, *DES*, and *PLN* genes
    - RV-predominant disease, often caused by *PKP2* pathogenic variants, is further discussed in another document regarding arrhythmogenic right ventricular cardiomyopathy (ARVC)
- Ventricular arrhythmias, including sudden cardiac death, may be early in disease and predate structural disease

IMAGING

- Most affected patients with LV involvement demonstrate subepicardial or transmural LGE
- Both RV and LV might be dilated or normal
- Regional LV wall motion abnormalities (WMA) might be observed at sites of LGE and beyond
- Genotype-based diagnostic schemes currently in development by international expert group
- Acute myocardial injury flares mimicking myocarditis can be seen in some patients

TOP DIFFERENTIAL DIAGNOSES

- Dilated cardiomyopathy
- ARVC
- Myocarditis
- Cardiac sarcoid
- Postinfarction myocardial scar

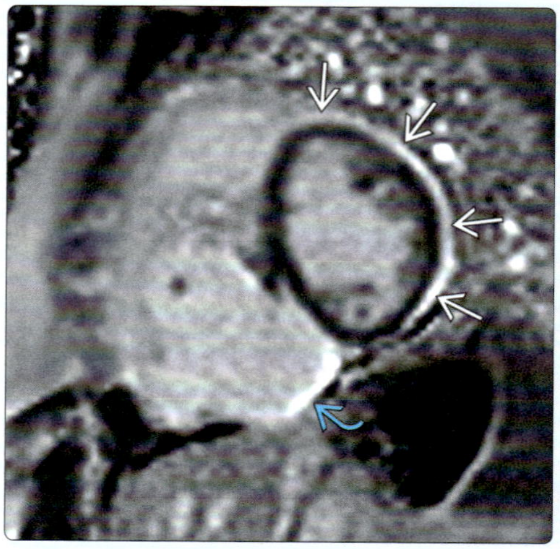
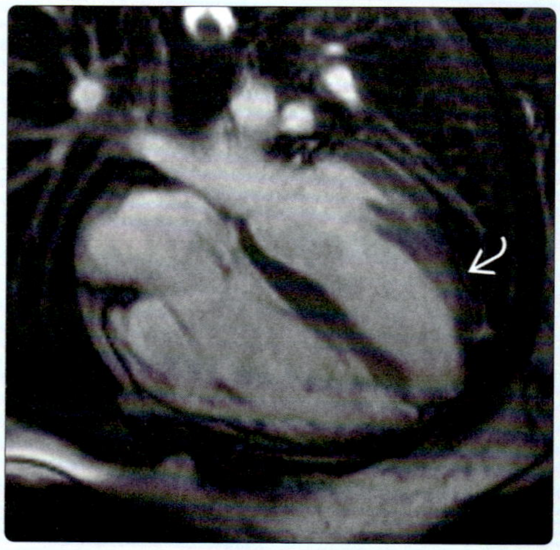

(Left) *Short-axis LGE MR in a 42-year-old arrhythmogenic cardiomyopathy (ACM) patient with a pathogenic desmoglein-2 (DSG2) variant shows a dilated right ventricle (RV) with inferior wall enhancement and a ring-like pattern of subepicardial enhancement in the left ventricle (LV).* **(Right)** *Four-chamber SSFP MR in the same patient shows a dilated RV and subepicardial fat infiltration along the lateral wall of the LV, identified by the dark out-of-phase signal at the interface of fat and myocardium.*

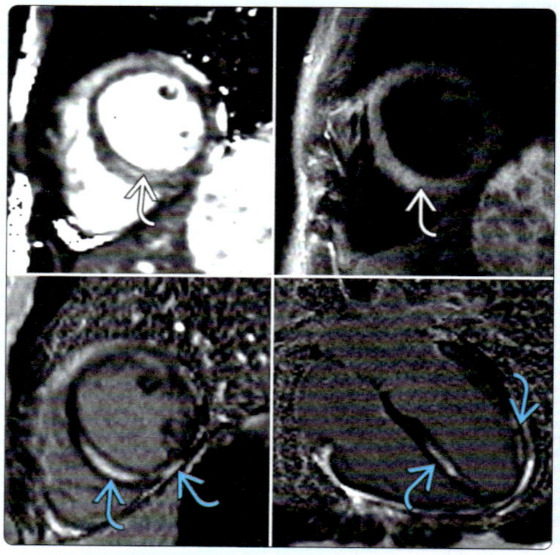
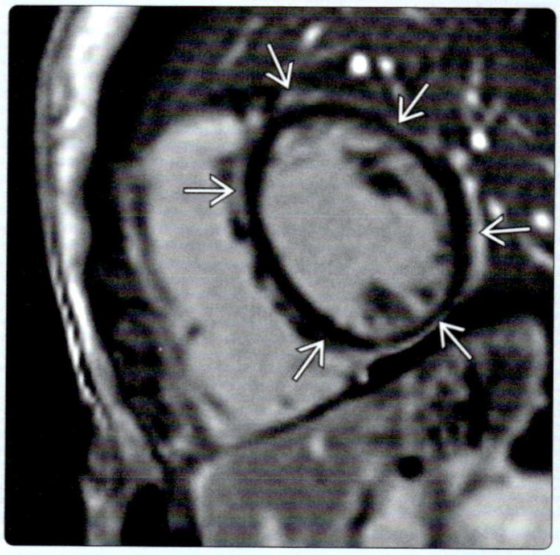

(Left) *Cardiac MR in a patient with a PPA2 mitochondrial cardiomyopathy during a myocardial injury flare mimicking acute myocarditis with chest pain and elevated troponins shows inferoseptal edema on T2 maps and T2 dark blood images and a nonischemic pattern of septal, inferior wall, and lateral wall enhancement.* **(Right)** *Short-axis LGE MR in a patient with DSP cardiomyopathy shows a typical pattern of dilated LV and ring-like subepicardial enhancement involving the LV.*

TERMINOLOGY

Abbreviations

- Arrhythmogenic cardiomyopathy (ACM)

Synonyms

- ACM has been proposed as umbrella term to include left ventricle (LV)-predominant, right ventricle (RV)-predominant, biventricular forms of disease
- Arrhythmogenic left ventricular cardiomyopathy (ALVC)
- Left-dominant ACM
- Biventricular ACM

Definitions

- Focus here is on familial causes of ACM that are LV predominant (ALVC) or biventricular; RV-predominant form (ARVC) is discussed in another document
- Variable definitions of ACM exist
    - In broadest definition, term ACM includes any patient with arrhythmic heart disease, including genetic, acquired, infectious, and inflammatory causes
    - More narrow scope, commonly used in literature and clinical practice, focuses on only inherited arrhythmic myocardial diseases with subtypes defined by pattern of myocardial involvement (RV, LV, or biventricular) &/or underlying pathogenic genetic abnormality
- Underlying genotypes appear to lead to distinct natural courses with large phenotypic overlap
    - Different genetic forms of disease likely exhibit different pathogenetic mechanisms
    - Per definition, predominantly affects LV or both ventricles and is associated with ventricular arrhythmias, including sudden cardiac death
    - Key features often include circumferential fibrous/fibrofatty band between middle and subepicardial 1/3 of myocardium, corresponding to ring-like LGE distribution at cardiac MR

IMAGING

General Features

- Best diagnostic clue
    - Diagnosis may begin with arrhythmia or myocardial dysfunction in probands that lead to genetic testing
    - Family members may be detected by genetic screening
    - Genotype-based diagnostic schemes currently in development by international expert group
- Location
    - LV, RV, and biventricular forms of disease are seen
    - Atrial enlargement also commonly seen in late stages of disease
- Size
    - LV commonly normal in size but might be dilated in late stages of disease
- Morphology
    - Some patients may have electrical abnormalities with normal myocardial structure on imaging
    - Structural disease often manifests as myocardial contractile dysfunction, ventricular dilation, &/or LGE

Radiographic Findings

- Chest radiography findings are usually normal and rarely show LV or biventricular dilatation

CT Findings

- Dilated LV with reduced systolic function (requires multiphase gated image acquisition)

MR Findings

- Global ventricular dilation, reduced function, regional wall motion abnormalities (WMA) may be seen
- Extent of LV LGE is variable in presence, extent, and location
    - LGE absent in many patients
    - Midwall septal LGE is common finding, similar to other types of nonischemic cardiomyopathy, corresponding to fibrous/fibrofatty band between middle and subepicardial 1/3 of myocardium
    - Ring-like LGE involving septum and subepicardial regions circumferentially in LV is common in some genotypes, particularly *DSP*
    - Some patients may present with acute myocardial injury episodes that are indistinguishable from myocarditis, featuring nonischemic LGE and myocardial edema on T2WI

Diagnosis

- In spectrum of ACM, ARVC diagnosis is made using set of major and minor criteria in 6 categories [task force criteria (TFC)], 2010); however, 2010 TFC lack criteria for diagnosis of ALVC and biventricular forms of ACM
- 2020 International Criteria (Padua criteria) have been proposed, which expand upon 2010 TFC to include criteria for RV- and LV-predominant forms of disease; however, further validation may be needed prior to widespread adoption in clinical practice and treatment guidelines
    - MR findings of LV structural and functional abnormalities are included
    - LV LGE (subepicardial or midwall) involving ≥ 1 segment of LV free wall, septum, or both meets 1 major criterion
- Genotype-specific diagnostic criteria with appropriate staging and management recommendations are currently in development

Imaging Recommendations

- Best imaging tool
    - Cardiac MR for evaluation of LV (&/or RV) LGE, global function, and regional WMA
- Protocol advice
    - Axial SSFP cine stacks can be helpful for identification of RV WMA when evaluating for RV involvement

DIFFERENTIAL DIAGNOSIS

Cardiac Sarcoidosis

- Multifocal LV LGE, often with septal involvement
- Atrioventricular block common, whereas only observed in certain forms of ACM/ALVC (e.g., *DES* cardiomyopathy)
- Ring-like enhancement typical for ACM/ALVC and rare in cardiac sarcoidosis
- Endocardial involvement may be seen in cardiac sarcoid but less commonly in ACM/ALV

Arrhythmogenic Right Ventricular Cardiomyopathy

- Predominantly affects RV, but LV involvement common, particularly at advanced stages of disease
- Most consider ARVC subtype of ACM
- 2 most common forms are *PKP2*-mediated and genotype-elusive forms
- Commonly associated with exercise-associated disease progression, including ventricular arrhythmias

Myocarditis

- Typically associated with chest pain, troponin elevation, and fever
- Can be secondary to variety of causes, including infection, autoimmune diseases, and drug toxicity
- May be part of phenotype of *DSP* cardiomyopathy; as part of *DSP* disease spectrum, increased myocarditis episodes seem to be associated with disease progression, and may predispose to higher ventricular arrhythmia burden, particularly if left untreated
- May manifest with subepicardial or midmyocardial LGE, particularly in basal posterolateral wall
- Posterolateral basal LGE (e.g., in *FLNC* and *PLN* cardiomyopathy) or ring-like LGE (e.g., in *FLNC* and *DES* cardiomyopathy) can also be seen in familial arrhythmogenic cardiomyopathies, overlapping with myocarditis patterns

Dilated Cardiomyopathy

- Has major phenotypic overlap with ACM/ALVC
- Mostly genotype-elusive or in ~ 30% caused by genes that do not lead to regional typical LGE formation (e.g., *TTN* or *BAG3*)
- LV systolic dysfunction is predominantly global rather than regional WMA associated with regional LGE
- Distinguished from ALVC/ACM with proportional association of ventricular arrhythmia risk with reduced LV ejection fraction (LVEF), rather than increased risk irrespective of LVEF, as seen in ALVC/ACM

PATHOLOGY

General Features

- Regional LV scarring ± associated LV dilation
- Subepicardial, midmyocardial, or transmural localization of scar, which may include 1 or more segments
- Ring-like scarring is characteristic with some genetic forms

Staging, Grading, & Classification

- Staging guidelines are under development at time of authoring

Gross Pathologic & Surgical Features

- Ventricular fibrosis in nonischemic pattern matching locations of LGE on cardiac MR
- Fibrofatty myocardial replacement may also be seen

CLINICAL ISSUES

Presentation

- Most common signs/symptoms
  - Ventricular arrhythmias might be initial manifestation
  - Some genetic forms, e.g., *DSP* cardiomyopathy, may present with myocardial inflammation episodes mimicking myocarditis; these episodes are also called "hot phase" of disease
  - Ring-like LGE is often associated with low QRS voltages and negative T waves in inferior &/or lateral ECG leads
- Other signs/symptoms
  - Some patients may have heart failure, but it is often observed in advanced stages of disease

Demographics

- Females and males are affected; data on demographics for different genetic forms are limited
- Female patients with *DSP* cardiomyopathy have higher risk for ventricular arrhythmias
- Male patients with *DES* variants have higher risk for ventricular arrhythmias and heart failure events
- Male patients with RBM20 variants have higher risk for end-stage heart failure, but risk of arrhythmias is similar among male and female patients

Natural History & Prognosis

- Variable natural history and prognosis depending on underlying genotype
- Patients with myocardial injury flares likely have higher risk of later arrhythmic events
- LV involvement is shown to be associated with higher incidence of heart failure, heart transplantation, and hot phases

Treatment

- Current approach relies on cardiac MR characterization and genetic testing
- While official guidelines are in development, higher MR LGE burden in *FLNC*, *DES*, RBM20, *DSP*, and *PLN* genotypes is usually viewed as high-risk marker for ventricular arrhythmias
- DSP risk calculator can estimate ventricular arrhythmia risk in primary preventive *DSP* cardiomyopathy patients

SELECTED REFERENCES

1. Bariani R et al: Phenotypic expression and clinical outcomes in patients with arrhythmogenic cardiomyopathies. J Am Coll Cardiol. 83(8):797-807, 2024
2. Carrick RT et al: A novel tool for arrhythmic risk stratification in desmoplakin gene variant carriers. Eur Heart J. 45(32):2968-79, 2024
3. Asatryan B et al: Inflammation and immune response in arrhythmogenic cardiomyopathy: state-of-the-art review. Circulation. 144(20):1646-55, 2021
4. Bariani R et al: 'Hot phase' clinical presentation in arrhythmogenic cardiomyopathy. Europace. 23(6):907-17, 2021
5. Corrado D et al: Diagnosis of arrhythmogenic cardiomyopathy: the Padua criteria. Int J Cardiol. 319:106-14, 2020
6. Segura-Rodríguez D et al: Myocardial fibrosis in arrhythmogenic cardiomyopathy: a genotype-phenotype correlation study. Eur Heart J Cardiovasc Imaging. 21(4):378-86, 2020
7. Smith ED et al: Desmoplakin cardiomyopathy, a fibrotic and inflammatory form of cardiomyopathy distinct from typical dilated or arrhythmogenic right ventricular cardiomyopathy. Circulation. 141(23):1872-84, 2020

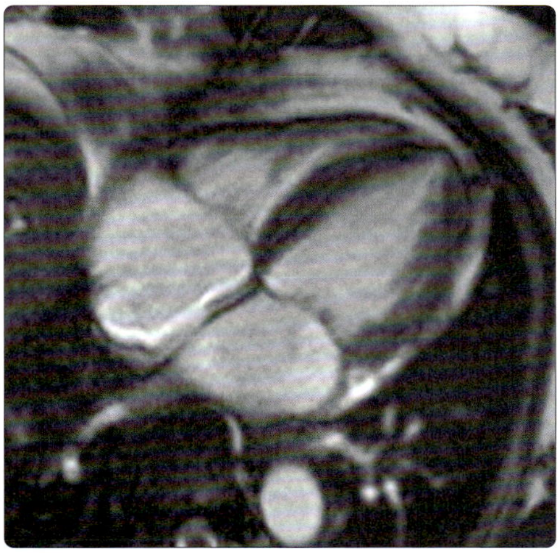

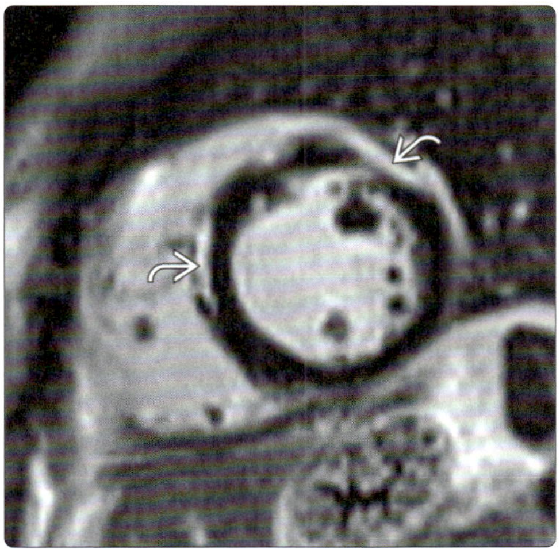

(Left) *Four-chamber cine SSFP MR in the same patient with a familial DSP variant and mild LV structural disease shows normal LV and RV size. On cine images, RV ejection fraction (EF) and LVEF were 55% and 57%, respectively.* **(Right)** *Short-axis LGE MR in a 70-year-old woman with a familial DSP variant, history of premature ventricular contractions, nonsustained ventricular tachycardia, and mild remodeling of the LV shows a nonischemic pattern of enhancement ➔ in the midseptum and anterolateral walls.*

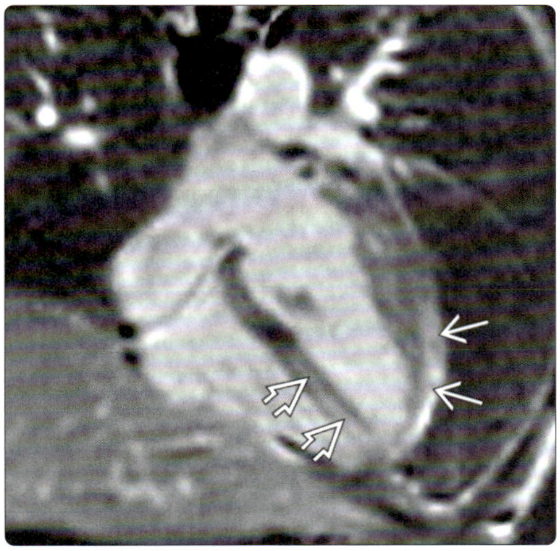

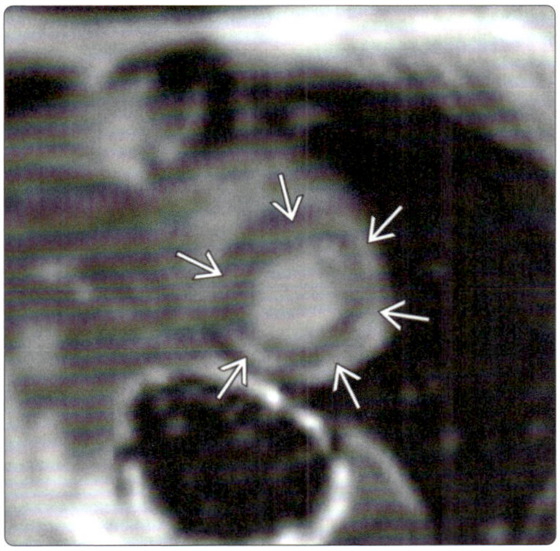

(Left) *Four-chamber LGE MR in a patient with ACM and pathogenic PLN variant shows subepicardial enhancement in the mid to apical lateral wall ➔ and midwall enhancement in the septum ➔. LV and RV were normal in size with mildly reduced LV function (LVEF was 43%).* **(Right)** *Short-axis LGE MR in the same patient with a pathogenic PLN variant shows ring-like enhancement of the apical LV ➔.*

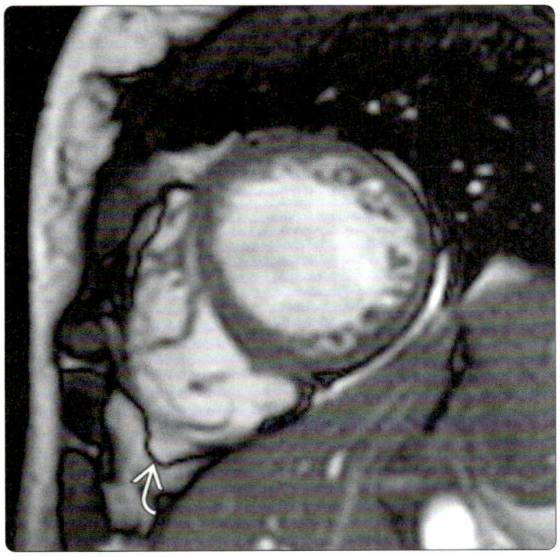

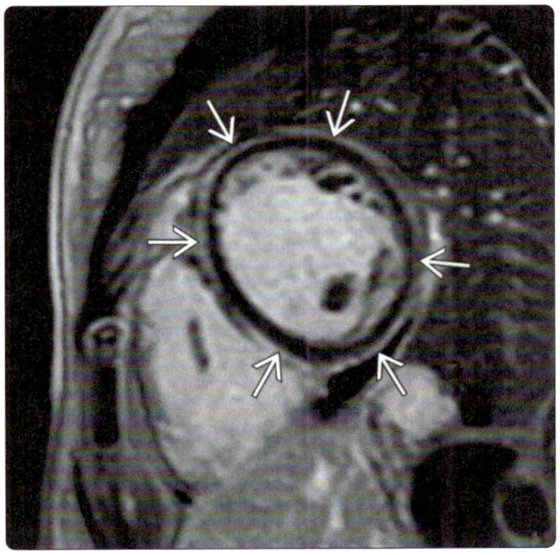

(Left) *Short-axis SSFP cine from cardiac MR in a 22-year-old patient with ACM and both PKP2 and DSP variants shows biventricular disease with RV dyskinesia at the junction of the inferior wall and anterior wall ➔ and a dilated LV.* **(Right)** *Short-axis LGE MR in the same patient with ACM and both PKP2 and DSP variants shows extensive ring-like LGE in the LV ➔.*

Noncompaction Cardiomyopathy

KEY FACTS

TERMINOLOGY

- Excessive left ventricular (LV) trabeculations preferred descriptor rather than LV noncompaction (LVNC)
- Cardiomyopathy with excessive LV trabeculations and deep intertrabecular recesses
- Was thought to be due to arrest of normal embryologic process of myocardial compaction
- Current evidence suggests differential growth of trabeculated and compacted layers

IMAGING

- Predominantly involves midventricle to apex of LV
- Echocardiographic findings/criteria
  - End-systolic ratio of noncompacted:compacted layers > 2:1 on short-axis imaging
  - Predominant location of pathology: Midlateral, midinferior, and apex of LV
  - Color Doppler evidence of deep perfused intertrabecular recesses
  - Coexisting cardiac abnormalities are absent (isolated LVNC)
- MR findings
  - > 2.3:1.0 ratio of noncompacted:compacted myocardium at end-diastole on cine MR
  - LGE MR may demonstrate subendocardial hyperenhancement corresponding to myocardial fibrosis

TOP DIFFERENTIAL DIAGNOSES

- Apical hypertrophic cardiomyopathy
- Dilated cardiomyopathy
- LV thrombus
- Endocardial fibroelastosis
- Healthy individuals

DIAGNOSTIC CHECKLIST

- Important to evaluate for complicating/confounding thrombus

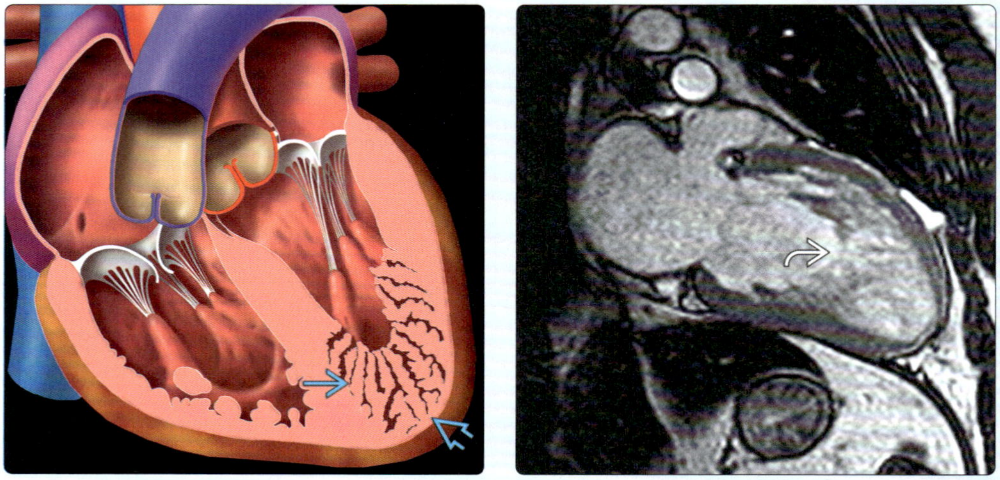

(Left) *Graphic shows extensive trabeculations within the left ventricle (LV) and thinning of the underlying compact myocardium. There is predominant involvement of the left ventricular apex with sparing of the basal segments.* **(Right)** *Vertical long-axis (2-chamber) SSFP cine MR shows extensive hypertrabeculation at the apex, which results in a 2-layered appearance of the myocardium.*

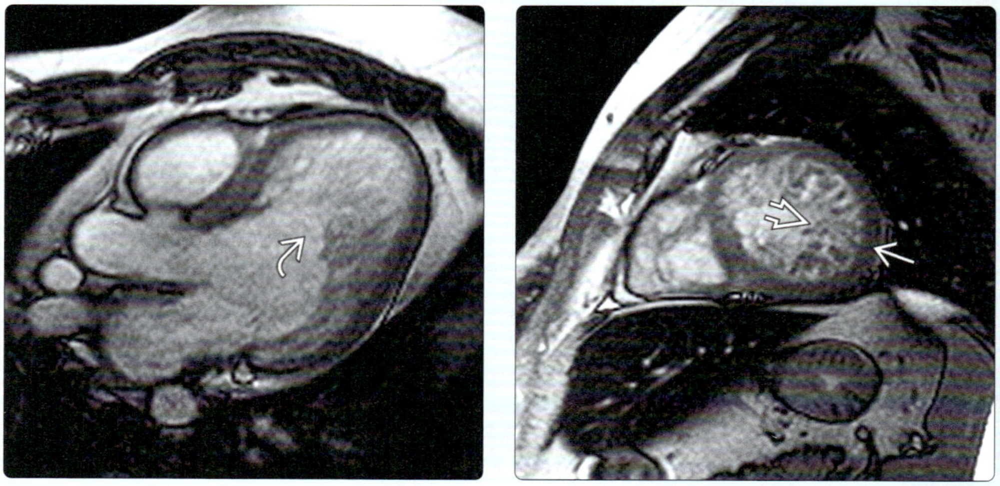

(Left) *Three-chamber SSFP cine MR in the same patient demonstrates the excessive trabeculations at the LV apex. In many cases, there is predominant involvement of the lateral and inferior walls, beginning at the midventricular level and extending to the apex.* **(Right)** *Short-axis SSFP cine MR in the same patient demonstrates the diagnostic finding of a > 2.3 ratio of the thickness of the trabeculated to the nontrabeculated myocardium. Note that diastolic-phase images are used for measurement in MR.*

TERMINOLOGY

Synonyms

- Excessive trabeculation of left ventricle has recently emerged as more accurate term because trabeculated myocardium does not actually coalesce to form compact myocardial wall
- Isolated noncompaction of ventricular myocardium
- Left ventricular (LV) hypertrabeculation

Definitions

- Excessive LV trabeculations and deep intertrabecular recesses
  - American Heart Association classifies LV noncompaction (LVNC) as genetic cardiomyopathy; however, European Society of Cardiology defines as nonclassified entity
    - Recent publications describe spectrum of primary and secondary causes; recommend term excessive trabeculations rather than LVNC

IMAGING

General Features

- Best diagnostic clue
  - Excessive LV trabeculation with delaminated appearance of myocardium into 2 layers
- Location
  - Predominantly involves midventricle to apex of LV
    - Lateral and inferior walls show greatest involvement

Imaging Recommendations

- Best imaging tool
  - Echocardiography is 1st-line imaging modality
  - Cardiac MR plays increasingly important role
  - No diagnostic (imaging or genetic) gold standard to make diagnosis of LVNC
- Protocol advice
  - MR studies should include LGE imaging to evaluate for fibrosis/scarring; consider LGE with long inversion time (~ 600 ms) to exclude thrombus
- **Echocardiographic findings/criteria**
  - End-systolic ratio of noncompacted:compacted layers > 2:1 on short-axis echo
  - Predominant location of pathology: Midlateral, midinferior, and apex of LV
  - Color Doppler evidence of deep perfused intertrabecular recesses
  - Coexisting cardiac abnormalities are absent (isolated LVNC)

MR Findings

- Ratio of noncompacted:compacted myocardium at end-diastole > 2.3
  - Measured in short-axis view for basal and midsegments; long-axis view for apical segments
  - Supplemental information in borderline cases
    - Trabecular mass > 15 g/m^2
    - Trabecular/LV mass > 20-25%
    - Trabeculations (> 2.0) of basal segments (inferior, inferolateral, anterolateral)
    - One segment with ratio > 3.0
  - Best diagnostic performance when multiple criteria are used
    - None of criteria are diagnostic for pathology in isolation; increased trabeculations identified in proportion of normal volunteers
- Subendocardial perfusion defects may be seen on 1st-pass perfusion imaging
- LGE may be in trabeculations or compact myocardium

CT Findings

- Findings on gated CTA are similar to those on cine MR

DIFFERENTIAL DIAGNOSIS

Dilated Cardiomyopathy

- Normal apical trabeculations may be spread apart and appear more prominent
- Use of multiple criteria may help

Apical Hypertrophic Cardiomyopathy

- Characterized by abnormal apical thickening that can mimic prominent trabeculations
- Often complicated by aneurysm formation

Endocardial Fibroelastosis

- Triple-layered pattern in LGE with inner thrombus (dark), middle layer of fibrosis (LGE), and outer layer of normal myocardium (dark)

Excessive Trabeculations in Adults

- Prominent LV trabeculations fulfilling LVNC criteria seen in 25.7- 43.0% of healthy, asymptomatic individuals
  - Not associated with increase in volumes or decrease in function over 10 years of follow-up
- May be seen as response to increased preload (in athletes and pregnancy)
- Interpret prominent trabeculations in context of clinical features

Excessive Trabeculations in Children

- Can be associated with occult neuromuscular disease or genetic/metabolic diseases

PATHOLOGY

General Features

- Etiology
  - Thought to be arrest of trabecular remodeling, which normally occurs during 8-12 weeks of fetal life
    - Current evidence does not support compaction from noncompacted myocardium or its arrest
    - Differential growth of trabeculated and compacted layers determines eventual amount of trabeculations
- Genetics
  - Both familial and sporadic forms of noncompaction have been described
  - Familial recurrence varies widely: 18-50%
    - Autosomal dominant inheritance is more common than X-linked
      - Genetic heterogeneity is common with lack of specific genotype-phenotype association
      - Sarcomere protein gene mutations are common and shared with hypertrophic and dilated cardiomyopathies

- Mutations definitively associated with noncompaction: *ACTC1, DES, DSP, MIB1, MYBPC3, MYH7, NONO, RYR2, TTN, TPM1*
- Many pediatric cases show X-linked patterns of inheritance associated with mutation of *TAFAZZIN* gene
  - Results in wide spectrum of severe X-linked cardiomyopathic phenotypes, including Barth syndrome
  - *TAFAZZIN* mutation is not found in adult cases
- Associated abnormalities
  - Intraventricular thrombus formation due to slow blood movement within heavily trabeculated regions of LV
    - Uncommon if ejection fraction > 35%
  - Ventricular and supraventricular arrhythmias
  - Biventricular noncompaction can occur with variable involvement of right ventricular (RV)
    - RV involvement has been reported in up to 50% of patients in some series
  - Congenital cardiac anomalies (not isolated LVNC)
    - Obstruction of RV or LV outflow tract
    - Complex cyanotic congenital heart disease
  - Subendocardial fibroelastosis

Gross Pathologic & Surgical Features

- Excessive trabeculation of LV that predominantly involves apex and midventricle
  - May also involve RV to lesser degree
- Areas of subendocardial ischemia in severe noncompaction

Microscopic Features

- Interstitial fibrosis of endomyocardium is commonly seen

CLINICAL ISSUES

Presentation

- Most common signs/symptoms
  - Clinical manifestations are highly variable depending on severity of LV involvement and underlying cause
    - Individuals with mild forms of LVNC may remain asymptomatic
  - Congestive heart failure
    - Both systolic and diastolic ventricular dysfunction have been described
    - Restrictive hemodynamics by cardiac catheterization may be present
  - Cardiac arrhythmias
    - Atrial fibrillation has been reported in up to 35% of individuals
    - Ventricular tachyarrhythmias have been reported in up to 50% of individuals
    - Paroxysmal supraventricular tachycardia and complete heart block have also been reported
    - Nonspecific resting ECG abnormalities have been frequently described (> 80%)
  - Thromboembolic events
    - Development of thrombi within prominent ventricular trabeculations due to sluggish blood flow
    - Incidence: 4-40%
    - Cerebrovascular accidents, transient ischemic attacks, pulmonary embolism, and mesenteric infarction have been described in patients with LVNC
    - Atrial fibrillation and impaired systolic function have likewise been implicated in development of systemic emboli

Demographics

- Age
  - Can be present at birth or develop in adulthood
- Sex
  - Slight male predominance
- Epidemiology
  - Median age at diagnosis: 7 years
  - 0.014% prevalence for all patients referred for ECG

Natural History & Prognosis

- Variable prognosis and outcome depending on underlying etiology
- Prognostic value of excessive trabeculations in adults has not been shown to be independent of other myocardial disease

Treatment

- Incidental excessive trabeculations in adults with otherwise normal myocardium and function; management not based on trabeculations but on other cardiovascular symptoms/abnormalities
- Adults with diagnosis of hypertrophic cardiomyopathy or dilated cardiomyopathy + excessive trabeculations; guideline-based management specific for those diseases
  - No evidence of altered prognosis based on extent of trabeculations
  - Standard heart failure therapy (afterload reduction, angiotensin-receptor blockers, etc.) as needed
  - Cardioverter-defibrillator implantation
  - Anticoagulation for prevention of systemic embolism
  - Orthotopic heart transplant
- Children with incidental excessive trabeculations
  - Evaluate for occult neuromuscular, genetic, or metabolic diseases
  - Metabolic cocktail for underlying mitochondrial myopathies

DIAGNOSTIC CHECKLIST

Image Interpretation Pearls

- Noncompacted:compacted ratio of > 2.3:1.0 on diastolic short-axis cine MR in several segments

Reporting Tips

- Excessive trabeculations should be interpreted along with clinical context

SELECTED REFERENCES

1. Pittorru R et al: Left ventricular non-compaction: evolving concepts. J Clin Med. 13(19), 2024
2. Petersen SE et al: Excessive trabeculation of the left ventricle: JACC: cardiovascular imaging expert panel paper. JACC Cardiovasc Imaging. 16(3):408-25, 2023
3. Rojanasopondist P et al: Genetic basis of left ventricular noncompaction. Circ Genom Precis Med. 15(3):e003517, 2022
4. Aung N et al: Prognostic Significance of left ventricular noncompaction: systematic review and meta-analysis of observational studies. Circ Cardiovasc Imaging. 13(1):e009712, 2020
5. Zemrak F et al: The relationship of left ventricular trabeculation to ventricular function and structure over a 9.5-year follow-up: the MESA study. J Am Coll Cardiol. 64(19):1971-80, 2014

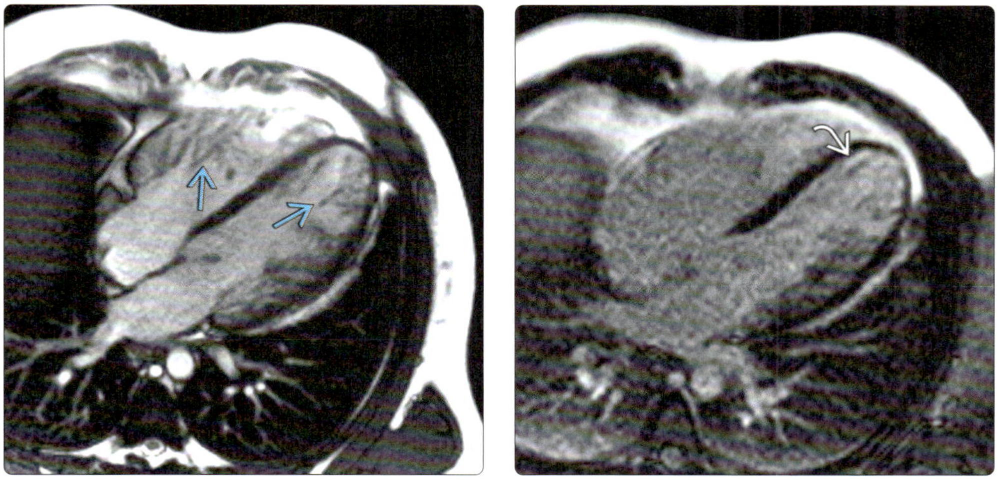

(Left) *Four-chamber cine MR shows involvement of both ventricles. Although the subject of some disagreement due to a lack of clear diagnostic criteria, right ventricular involvement is suspected in up to 40% of patients.* **(Right)** *Four-chamber LGE MR in the same patient shows subendocardial enhancement, consistent with fibrosis at the apex. This finding of abnormal enhancement is directly correlated with ventricular function impairment.*

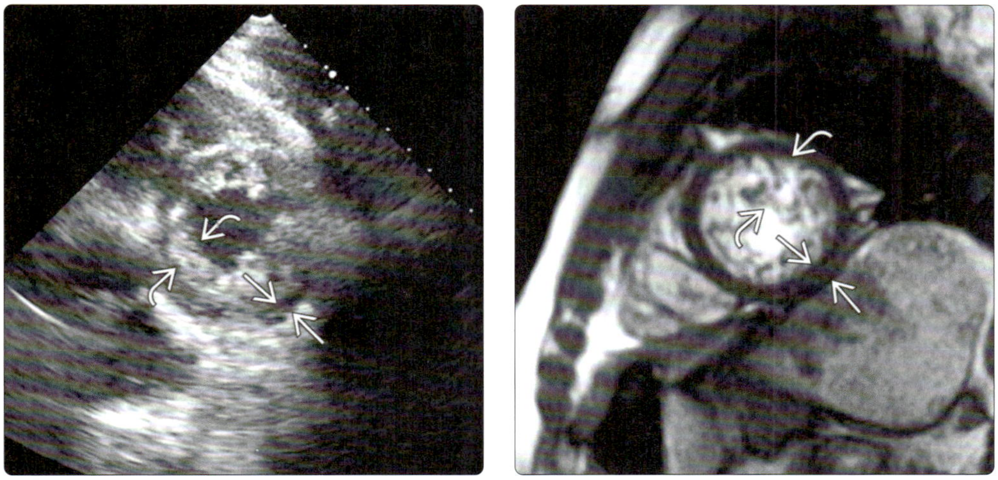

(Left) *Short-axis echocardiogram in the same patient obtained at the apex during systole reveals an abnormal noncompacted :compacted myocardial ratio (> 2:1). Note that echocardiographic diagnosis is made using end-systolic images.* **(Right)** *Short-axis cine MR in the same patient demonstrates an abnormal ratio (> 2.3) of noncompacted :compacted myocardium in diastole. Note the image clarity, making diagnosis of the abnormality relatively straightforward.*

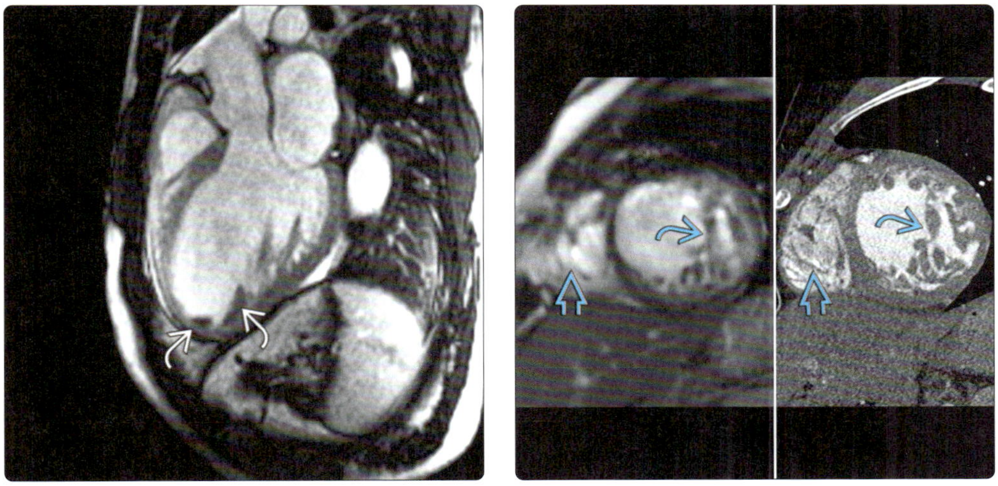

(Left) *Postcontrast MR cine demonstrates thrombi at the LV apex. Thrombi may be difficult to recognize, as they are isointense to the myocardium on precontrast cine images and isoechoic on echocardiography. They may be mistaken for trabeculations.* **(Right)** *Short axis SSFP MR (left) and CT (right) images in a 12-year-old show pronounced biventricular noncompaction with an increase in LV and right ventricle trabeculations. LV ejection fraction was 22%.*

KEY FACTS

TERMINOLOGY

- Chagas heart disease, American trypanosomiasis

IMAGING

- 60-80% of infected patients do not progress to clinical abnormalities
- Chagas cardiomyopathy is most common clinical manifestation
- Echocardiography, cine MR, and gated CTA (advanced clinical phase) show global biventricular dysfunction with segmental akinesis and aneurysms, usually involving left ventricular apex and inferolateral walls
- Left ventricular wall thinning is also noted, particularly involving apex
  - Results in apical aneurysm (vortex lesion), characteristic feature of Chagas heart disease
- Extent of myocardial fibrosis shown on LGE MR correlates with global and regional function assessments and may reveal subclinical Chagas heart disease
- Prevalence of fibrosis on LGE MR images varies with disease severity
  - Typically affects apex and inferolateral regions of left ventricle
  - Indeterminate/asymptomatic phase: 20% positive on LGE MR
  - Symptomatic cardiomyopathy patients: 85% positive on LGE MR
  - Cardiomyopathy patients with ventricular tachycardia: 100% positive on LGE MR

TOP DIFFERENTIAL DIAGNOSES

- Myocarditis
- Ischemic cardiomyopathy
- Apical hypertrophic cardiomyopathy
- Takotsubo cardiomyopathy
- Congenital aneurysm

(Left) *Posteroanterior radiograph shows global cardiomegaly and clear lungs in a patient with chronic Chagas cardiomyopathy. There is no evidence of pulmonary edema or pleural effusion. Chagas disease is a common cause of heart failure in countries where it is endemic.* **(Right)** *Long-axis vertical 2-chamber LGE MR demonstrates abnormal enhancement ➔ of the apex, a finding indicative of myocardial fibrosis in a patient with Chagas cardiomyopathy.*

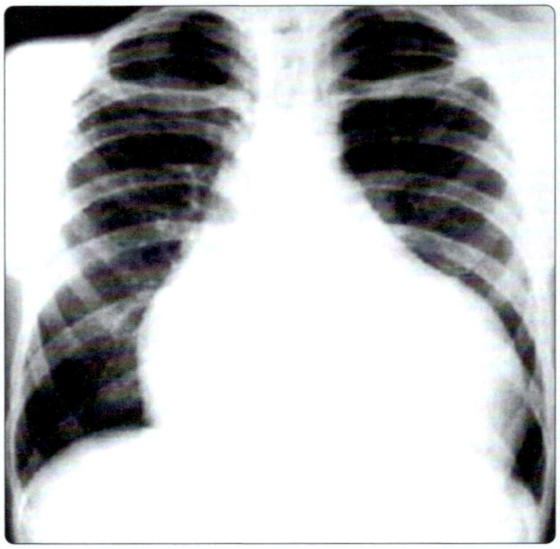

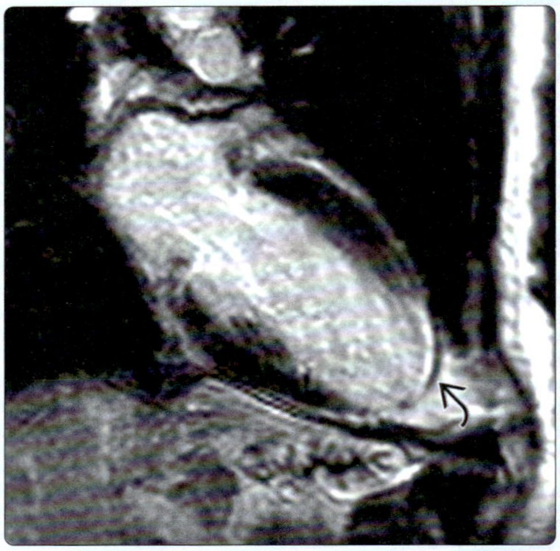

(Left) *Three-chamber LGE MR in a patient with Chagas disease shows abnormal enhancement of the apex ➔ and the inferolateral wall at the basal level ➔. These are the areas of the heart most commonly involved by Chagas cardiomyopathy.* **(Right)** *Long-axis gross pathology specimen shows a typical vortex aneurysm ➔ at the left ventricular apex, a finding characteristic of Chagas cardiomyopathy.*

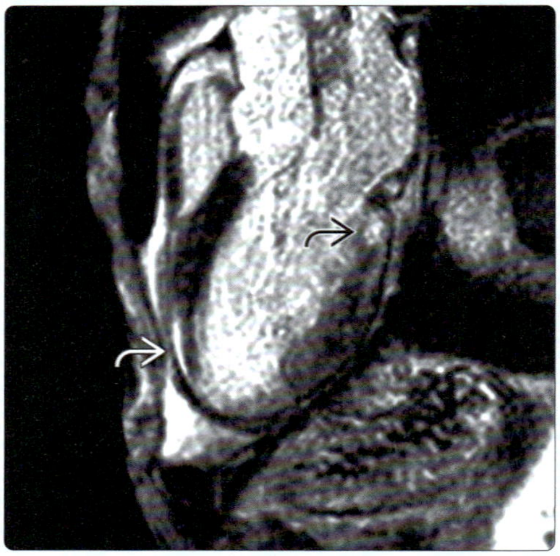

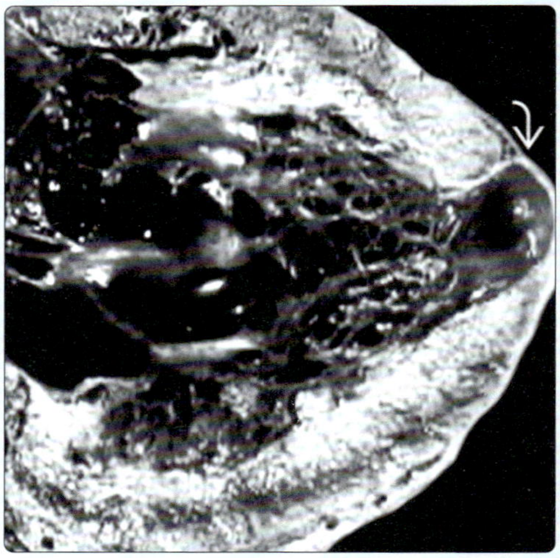

TERMINOLOGY

Synonyms

- Chagas heart disease, American trypanosomiasis

Definitions

- Infection by protozoan parasite *Trypanosoma cruzi* transmitted through feces of infected bloodsucking insects in endemic areas of Latin America

IMAGING

General Features

- Best diagnostic clue
  - Myocardial fibrosis on LGE MR typically affecting apex and inferolateral region of left ventricle (LV) in heart failure patient from endemic region
  - Thinning of LV wall, particularly involving apex, resulting in apical aneurysm (vortex lesion) is characteristic feature of Chagas heart disease
- Location
  - Apex and inferolateral segment of LV
- Morphology
  - 60-80% of infected patients do not progress to clinical abnormalities
    - Termed indeterminate chronic stage
      - Most will have preserved LV morphology and function, but 15-20% may show abnormalities on LGE and T2 MR
  - Progressive chronic disease is seen in 20-40% of cases
    - Most common clinical manifestation: Chagas cardiomyopathy (dilated cardiomyopathy with global cardiac enlargement)

Imaging Recommendations

- Best imaging tool
  - LGE MR demonstrates predominantly midwall and subepicardial hyperenhancement in nonischemic pattern
  - Echocardiography, cine MR, and gated CTA (advanced clinical phase) show global biventricular dysfunction with segmental akinesis and aneurysms, usually involving LV apex and inferolateral walls
- Protocol advice
  - LGE MR provides diagnostic and prognostic information
  - Good correlation observed between LGE and both increased T2 myocardial signal intensity and T1 early gadolinium enhancement

Radiographic Findings

- Global cardiomegaly, pulmonary vascular congestion, pulmonary edema

Echocardiographic Findings

- 1st-line tool for morphologic and functional evaluation
- Increased LV volumes
- Segmental or global wall motion abnormalities
- Apical aneurysm and intracavitary thrombus

MR Findings

- T2WI
  - Defines segments involved by myocardial edema
- MR cine
  - Demonstrates location, extent, and severity of global and regional systolic dysfunction
    - Dysfunction often most severe in apex and lateral wall
- Early gadolinium enhancement
  - Detects myocardial signal intensity gain after gadolinium injection compared to skeletal muscles
- LGE
  - Extent of myocardial fibrosis on LGE MR correlates with global and regional function assessments and may reveal subclinical Chagas heart disease
    - Prevalence of fibrosis varies with disease severity
      - Indeterminate/asymptomatic phase: 20% positive on LGE MR
      - Symptomatic patients with cardiomyopathy: 85% positive on LGE MR
      - Cardiomyopathy patients with ventricular tachycardia: 100% positive on LGE MR
  - Fibrosis is seen as abnormal enhancement on LGE MR
    - Usually nonischemic pattern (midmyocardial and subepicardial location in multiple coronary artery distributions)
    - Subendocardial or transmural enhancement mimicking coronary artery disease (CAD) may be seen in small percentage of cases
    - LGE is adverse prognostic determinant
      - Correlates with clinical severity and inversely with LV ejection fraction and regional wall motion
      - LGE in > 2 segments predicts development of ventricular tachycardia

CT Findings

- Gated coronary CTA is occasionally useful in excluding significant CAD in selected Chagas patients with atypical chest pain

Angiographic Findings

- Typical LV apical aneurysm (vortex lesion)
- Normal epicardial coronary arteries

DIFFERENTIAL DIAGNOSIS

Viral Myocarditis

- Serologic tests for *Trypanosoma cruzi* are negative
- Geographic history does not include endemic regions
- Imaging in viral myocarditis often occurs in acute phase and frequently shows T2 signal abnormalities (edema) and early gadolinium enhancement

Ischemic Cardiomyopathy

- May also result in apical aneurysm
- LGE MR findings follow ischemic pattern (beginning in subendocardium and extending toward epicardium) in coronary artery distribution
- Subendocardial involvement is hallmark for ischemic lesions

Apical Hypertrophic Cardiomyopathy

- Often complicated by formation of apical aneurysm, which usually shows delayed enhancement
- LV function is preserved

Takotsubo Cardiomyopathy

- Form of nonischemic cardiomyopathy in which there is sudden temporary dysfunction of myocardium

- Dysfunction manifests as apical dilatation or "ballooning"
- Usually triggered by severe emotional stress

Congenital Aneurysm

- Imaging pattern may be indistinguishable from that of Chagas disease, showing fibrotic apical aneurysms
  - LGE MR is abnormal in 70%
- Serologic tests for *Trypanosoma cruzi* are negative
- Geographic history does not include endemic regions

PATHOLOGY

General Features

- Etiology
  - Caused by flagellate protozoa *Trypanosoma cruzi*
  - Insect vectors of Chagas disease belong to Hemiptera order, Reduviidae family, and Triatominae subfamily ("kissing bugs")
- Associated abnormalities
  - Megaesophagus and megacolon

Gross Pathologic & Surgical Features

- Cardiomegaly with ventricular wall thinning/aneurysm formation

Microscopic Features

- Intracellular parasite multiplication → rupture of infected cells → inflammatory response → fibrosis
- Cellular lesions mainly affect myocytes (causing myocytolysis) and nervous cells (leading to autonomic denervation)
- Arteriolar dilatation with organized thrombi and severe diffuse fibrosis in watershed myocardial regions (LV apex and basal inferior LV wall)

CLINICAL ISSUES

Presentation

- Most common signs/symptoms
  - Typically, arrhythmias, cardiac failure, thromboembolic phenomena, or sudden death
  - Atypical chest pain without evidence of coronary artery disease (15-20% of patients)
  - Chagas heart disease is most frequent and serious manifestation of symptomatic chronic disease

Demographics

- Age
  - Symptomatic acute phases mainly occur in newborns or young children
  - Chronic Chagas cardiomyopathy is generally detected in 3rd-5th decades of life
- Sex
  - Chronic cardiomyopathy occurs earlier and is more severe in males than in females
- Epidemiology
  - In USA, according to estimates, 300,000 immigrants from Latin America are infected with *Trypanosoma cruzi*
  - Internationally, estimated 8 million people are infected in Latin America
    - 30,000 new cases per year

Natural History & Prognosis

- Acute phase (1 week after initial infection)
  - Usually asymptomatic
  - Cardiac involvement in 90%
    - Myocarditis or pericardial effusion
    - Spontaneous resolution in > 90% of patients
  - Mortality in < 5% of cases
    - Death results from acute myocarditis &/or meningoencephalitis
- Chronic phase
  - Indeterminate form: No symptoms; normal ECG; normal radiologic study of heart, esophagus, and colon
    - 60-80% of patients in indeterminate phase remain asymptomatic and never develop chronic lesions
  - Clinical forms: Cardiac, digestive, and mixed
    - In endemic areas, Chagas heart disease is most common cause of cardiomyopathy and leading cause of cardiovascular death of patients aged 30-50 years (12,500 deaths annually)
    - Seen 10-30 years after infection at rate of 2-3% per year
  - Independent prognostic factors in chronic Chagas disease
    - Cardiomegaly with impaired LV function (New York Heart Association class III/IV)
    - Nonsustained ventricular tachycardia

Treatment

- Acute phase: Always requires treatment with benznidazole; cures 100% of children < 2 years old and 60-70% of acutely infected older patients
- Chronic cardiac phase
  - Diuretics, digitalis, angiotensin-converting enzyme inhibitors, and other standard heart failure therapies
  - Class III antiarrhythmic drugs (sotalol and amiodarone)
  - Anticoagulant treatment is justified in patients at risk for thromboembolic complications
  - Heart transplant

DIAGNOSTIC CHECKLIST

Consider

- Chagas disease in patients from endemic areas who present with new-onset heart failure

Image Interpretation Pearls

- Look for apical aneurysm and abnormal enhancement on LGE MR

SELECTED REFERENCES

1. Gómez-Ochoa SA et al: Myocardial fibrosis by magnetic resonance and outcomes in chagas disease: a systematic review and meta-analysis. JACC Cardiovasc Imaging. 17(5):552-5, 2024
2. Veluswami K et al: Unraveling the missing pieces: exploring the gaps in understanding Chagas cardiomyopathy. Cureus. 16(8):e66955, 2024
3. Uellendahl M et al: Cardiac magnetic resonance-verified myocardial fibrosis in Chagas disease: clinical correlates and risk stratification. Arq Bras Cardiol. 107(5):460-6, 2016
4. Regueiro A et al: Myocardial involvement in Chagas disease: insights from cardiac magnetic resonance. Int J Cardiol. 165(1):107-12, 2013
5. Rochitte CE et al: Myocardial delayed enhancement by magnetic resonance imaging in patients with Chagas' disease: a marker of disease severity. J Am Coll Cardiol. 46(8):1553-8, 2005

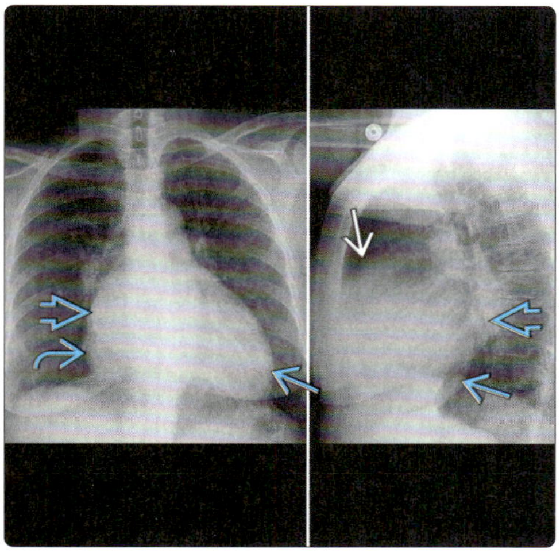

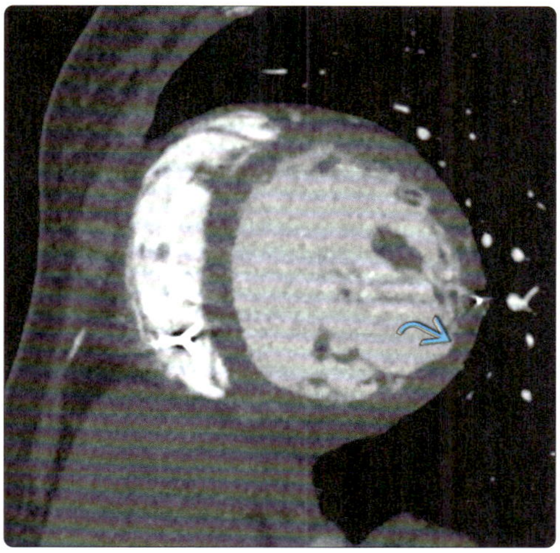

(Left) *PA (left) and lateral (right) CXR in a 57-year-old Brazilian woman shows left atrial and left ventricular (LV) enlargement > right atrium and right ventricle (RV) enlargement. Patient's T. cruzi IgG antibody was elevated from prior infection.* **(Right)** *CECT shows marked LV dilation (EDV = 178 ml/m2) and more mild RV dilation (EDV = 101 ml/m2). LV and RV ejection fractions were 32% and 28%, respectively. Note thinning of the inferolateral segment. Coronaries were normal on CT and catheterization.*

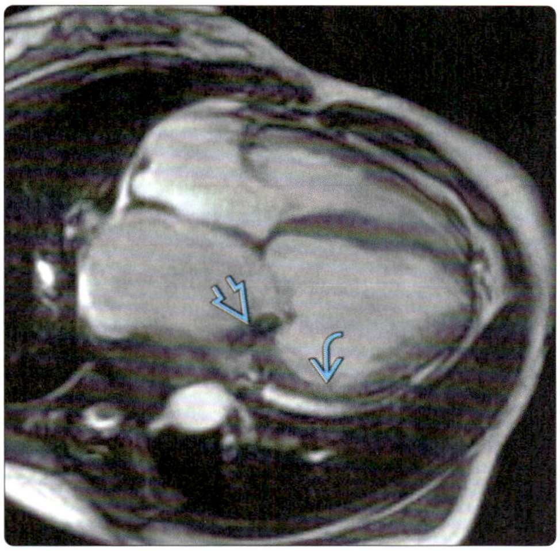

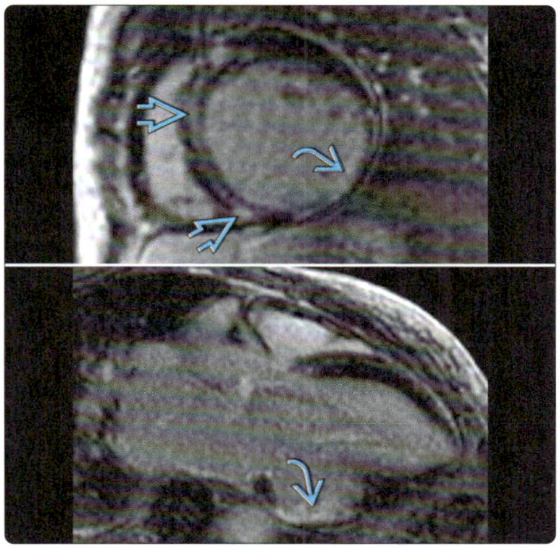

(Left) *Four-chamber SSFP MR during systole in the same patient as above shows severe left heart enlargement with severe mitral regurgitation. The right heart is more mildly enlarged. Thinning of the inferolateral wall is present.* **(Right)** *Short-axis (top) and modified 3-chamber (bottom) LGE images show near transmural inferolateral LGE with numerous additional areas of nodular and linear midmyocardial LGE elsewhere. Inferolateral LGE is common in Chagas cardiomyopathy. (Courtesy S. Kligerman, MD.)*

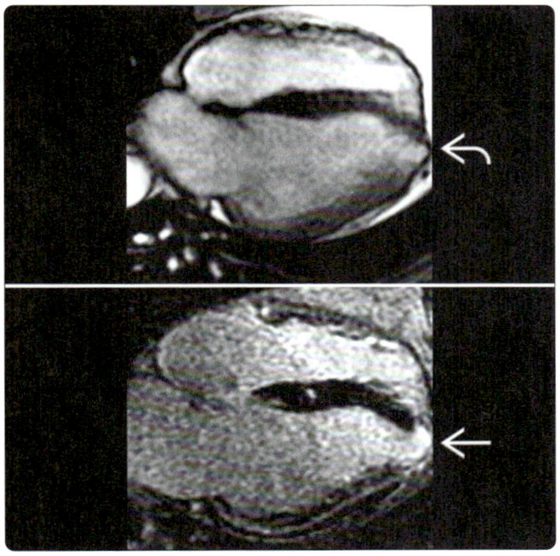

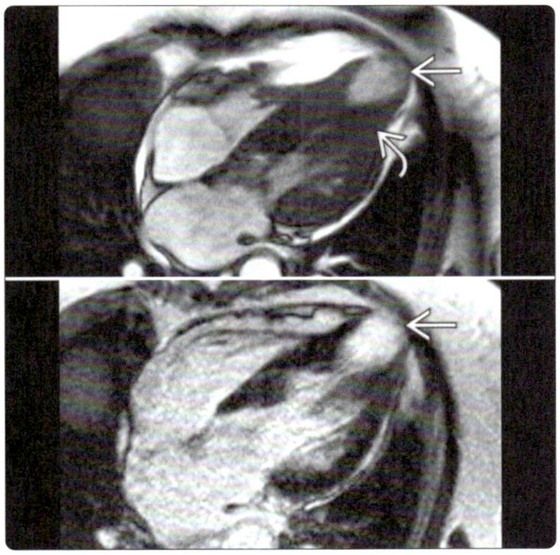

(Left) *Four-chamber cine (top) and LGE (bottom) MR images of a Chagas aneurysm show systolic outpouching on the cine image and enhancement of the apex on the LGE MR.* **(Right)** *Four-chamber cine (top) and LGE (bottom) MR images in a patient with apical hypertrophic cardiomyopathy show an apical aneurysm. Note there are hypertrophic changes in the adjacent segments that produce cavity obliteration in the systolic cine image (top), a finding not seen in Chagas aneurysms.*

Iron Overload Syndromes

KEY FACTS

TERMINOLOGY

- Iron overload syndromes
- Primary form: Hemochromatosis
  - Autosomal recessive genetic disorder resulting in abnormal uptake of dietary iron
- Secondary form: a.k.a. transfusional siderosis, secondary hemochromatosis, or transfusional iron overload
  - Results from transfusion therapy of hereditary anemias characterized by ineffective erythropoiesis and hemolysis
  - Thalassemia major and intermedia are most common worldwide

IMAGING

- Low signal intensity of heart &/or liver on T2 MR should suggest diagnosis of iron overload
- Excess iron levels can be displayed qualitatively on T2 or T2* MR by hypointense signal changes in affected organs
- T2* MR can be used to quantify myocardial iron levels

TOP DIFFERENTIAL DIAGNOSES

- Hemochromatosis
  - Normal appearance of spleen and bone marrow suggests hemochromatosis
- Transfusional iron overload
  - Abnormal amounts of iron accumulate first in reticuloendothelial system of liver, spleen, and bone marrow
  - Pancreas is initially spared but may be involved once reticuloendothelial system capacity is exceeded
  - Cardiac imaging findings are indistinguishable from those of hemochromatosis

CLINICAL ISSUES

- Congestive heart failure in setting of significant cardiac involvement
- Transfusional iron overload is treated by chelation therapy using deferoxamine (intravenous or subcutaneous) often coupled with deferiprone orally

(Left) *Vertical long-axis (2-chamber) cine SSFP MR in a patient with iron overload cardiomyopathy demonstrates abnormally low signal intensity in both the myocardium → and the liver →. The left ventricle is dilated, a finding commonly seen as the disease progresses.* **(Right)** *Axial NECT shows diffusely increased attenuation throughout the myocardium →, consistent with extensive myocardial iron deposition. The left ventricular cavity is dilated →, indicative of systolic dysfunction.*

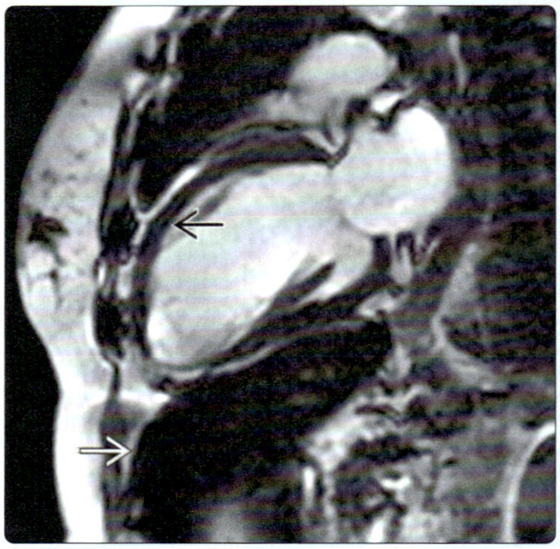

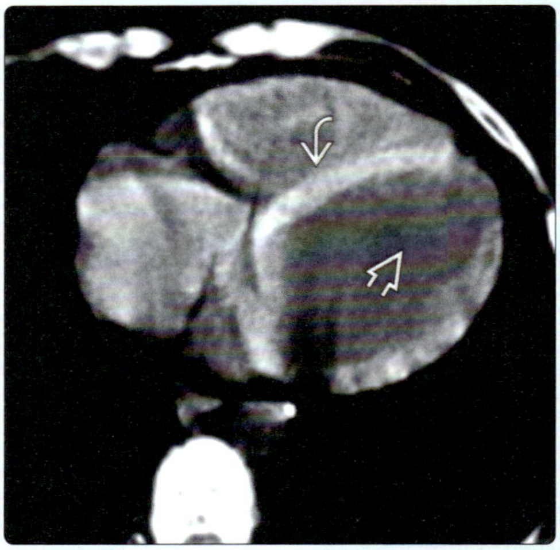

(Left) *SSFP cine MR shows a dark, amorphous artifact in the right ventricle →, consistent with the banding artifact often seen on SSFP. This artifact is accentuated by the field inhomogeneity induced by the extensive iron present in the patient's tissues due to iron overload.* **(Right)** *Short-axis cine MR images in the same patient using SSFP (left) and GRE (right) sequences illustrate the extensive banding artifact present on SSFP →, which can often be circumvented by using GRE cine images.*

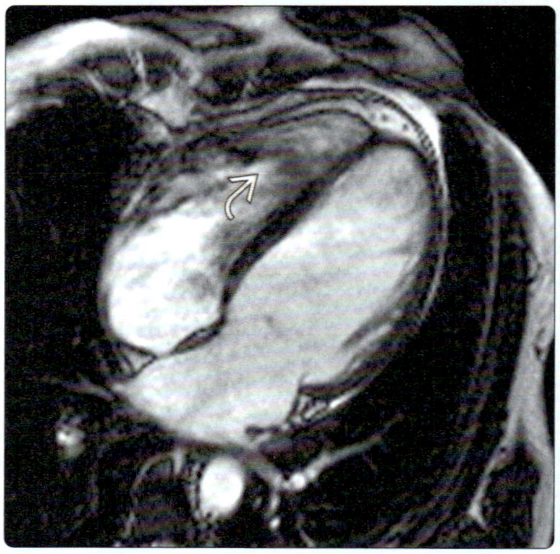

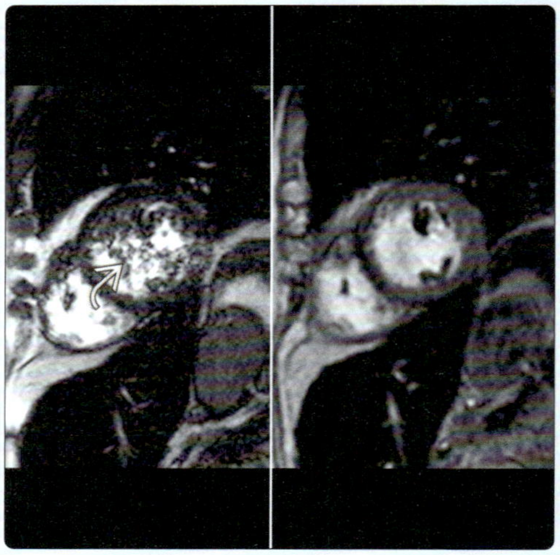

TERMINOLOGY

Abbreviations

- Iron overload syndromes (IOSs)

Definitions

- Primary form: Hemochromatosis
  - Autosomal recessive genetic disorder resulting in abnormal uptake of dietary iron
  - Progressive increase in total body iron stores with abnormal multiorgan parenchymal iron deposition
    - Not in reticuloendothelial system
  - Liver is primary site of abnormal iron deposition (leading to cirrhosis), although abnormal iron deposition can also occur in heart (resulting in cardiomyopathy), pancreas (causing diabetes), or pituitary gland (resulting in hypogonadism)
    - Cirrhosis and hepatocellular carcinoma are greatly increased in frequency along with heart failure in untreated cases
- Secondary form: a.k.a. transfusional siderosis, secondary hemochromatosis, or transfusional iron overload
  - Results from transfusion therapy used in treatment of hereditary anem as characterized by ineffective erythropoiesis and hemolysis
    - Thalassemia major and intermedia are most common worldwide
      - Commonly require 1-2 transfusions/month beginning in early infancy
      - 1 unit of packed cells contains 200-250 mg of iron (normal dietary uptake = 1-2 mg/d)
      - Cardiac involvement is most common cause of death with 50% of patients dying before age 35
  - Excessive iron is initially localized to reticuloendothelial system, but when storage is overwhelmed, iron is deposited in multiple tissues in pattern similar to hemochromatosis
    - Liver, spleen, and bone marrow are initially involved
    - Pancreas is initially spared but may become involved later as iron overload progresses

IMAGING

General Features

- Best diagnostic clue
  - Low signal intensity of heart &/or liver on T2 MR should suggest diagnosis of iron overload
  - Excess iron levels can be displayed qualitatively on MR by hypointense signal changes in affected organs on T2 or T2* images
- Location
  - Diffuse involvement of myocardium is characteristic, but inhomogeneous involvement occasionally occurs
  - Initially begins in epicardium, then extends to myocardium and endocardium
- Morphology
  - Although initially there may be restrictive phenotype, progressive cardiac iron loading results in dilated cardiomyopathy phenotype associated with systolic dysfunction

Imaging Recommendations

- Best imaging tool
  - T2* MR at 1.5T can be used to quantify myocardial iron levels; lower T2* is associated with higher iron levels
- Protocol advice
  - Breath-hold T2* GRE MR with varying echo times (TEs) or T2* maps can be obtained to estimate cardiac iron load
  - Standard short- and long-axis cine MR series should be obtained for evaluation of cardiac function

CT Findings

- NECT
  - Global hyperdensity of myocardium &/or liver may be noted
- Dual-energy CT
  - Attenuation values of septal muscle correlated with T2* MR values

MR Findings

- T2* GRE
  - Can be done in single breath-hold using GRE sequence with multiple TEs
  - Signal dropout with progressively longer TE is greatly accelerated in patients with cardiac iron deposition
  - Iron deposition results in local field inhomogeneities that result in T2* shortening
    - Degree of T2* shortening is closely correlated with degree of iron deposition
    - Signal intensity measurements are typically obtained on short-axis midventricular images using region of interest positioned in septum
    - Quantification best validated at 1.5T
    - Postprocessing with dedicated software facilitates calculation of myocardial T2* values from plot of signal intensity relative to changing TE
      - T2* value < 10 ms indicates severe iron loading (in one study, ~ 89% of thalassemia patients with new-onset failure had T2* < 10 ms)
      - T2* value of 10-20 ms indicates mild to moderate iron loading
      - T2* value > 20 ms is in normal range (normal mean: ~ 40 ms)
  - Efficacy of iron reduction treatment is also best assessed in this way
    - Since 1999, improved survival in patients with thalassemia major in UK likely due to early detection of cardiac iron overload using T2*
- MR cine
  - Hyperdynamic contractility in unaffected anemic patients
    - Apparently normal function is abnormal in these patients and may be early marker of cardiac involvement
- SSFP cine MR may show reduced signal of myocardium, since this sequence is relatively T2 weighted
- Significant iron loading may be present before function becomes abnormal
  - However, once functional abnormalities develop, rapid progression to severe failure, arrhythmia, or death occurs
- T1 mapping
  - Low T1 values are seen in iron deposition

- Good correlation between T1 and T2*
- T1 may detect missed iron in 1 out of 3 subjects with normal T2*
- Complementary to T2*

Ultrasonographic Findings

- Echocardiography may show restrictive physiology in initial stages and systolic dysfunction in later stages
  - Not recommended as screening tool (insensitive)

DIFFERENTIAL DIAGNOSIS

Hemochromatosis

- Both primary and secondary forms of IOS produce dark liver on MR
  - However, there is poor correlation between hepatic and cardiac iron loading in either disorder
- Normal appearance of spleen and bone marrow
- Pancreas and pituitary involvement is seen early

Transfusional Iron Overload

- Abnormal amounts of iron accumulate first in reticuloendothelial system of liver, spleen, and bone marrow
- Pancreas is initially spared but may be involved once reticuloendothelial system capacity is exceeded
- Cardiac imaging findings are indistinguishable from those of hemochromatosis

PATHOLOGY

General Features

- Etiology
  - Excess unbound iron deposited in myocardium is highly cardiotoxic
    - Mitochondrial respiratory chain function is impaired, resulting in inadequate ATP production and eventual heart failure
- Genetics
  - Hemochromatosis is autosomal recessive genetic disorder characterized by excessive uptake of dietary iron
    - 80% of cases are due to mutation in *HFE* gene, most commonly p.C282Y mutation
      - Mutation leads to inadequate production of hepcidin, protein that negatively modulates uptake of dietary iron
      - No excretory pathway in humans to eliminate excess iron, and thus iron build-up ensues
      - Patients homozygous for gene show low penetrance for clinical disease with probably < 3% developing significant disease
  - β-thalassemia is most common worldwide hereditary anemia, resulting in transfusional iron overload
    - Homozygous patients will develop severe anemia early in life and require transfusions to survive
    - Iron loading predominantly results from transfusions but may also reflect downregulation of hepcidin production related to ineffective erythropoiesis
      - This results in excessive dietary uptake of iron
- Associated abnormalities
  - Hemochromatosis
    - Excessive liver deposition with development of cirrhosis, portal hypertension, and hepatocellular carcinoma
    - Excessive pancreatic iron deposition can result in type 1 diabetes mellitus
    - Abnormal deposition in skin causes bronze skin color
    - Pituitary hypogonadism
  - Transfusional iron overload/thalassemia
    - Severe anemia may be present if transfusion is inadequate
    - Frontal bossing (protuberance of frontal bones) may develop due to bone marrow expansion

CLINICAL ISSUES

Presentation

- Most common signs/symptoms
  - Congestive heart failure in setting of significant cardiac involvement

Demographics

- Age
  - Hemochromatosis
    - Often presents in 4th and 5th decades; M > F
  - Transfusional siderosis
    - Cardiac involvement usually by early adulthood
- Epidemiology
  - *HFE*-related primary form occurs predominantly in White populations of Northern European descent
    - Prevalence of p.C282Y gene homozygosity is 1:200 in this population

Natural History & Prognosis

- Once iron-related cardiac impairment has developed, natural history is that of inexorable progression to heart failure and death

Treatment

- Transfusional iron overload is treated by chelation therapy using deferoxamine (intravenous or subcutaneous) often coupled with deferiprone orally
- Hemochromatosis is treated by weekly phlebotomy until iron levels return to normal range, and then bimonthly

DIAGNOSTIC CHECKLIST

Consider

- IOSs when low cardiac or hepatic signal intensity noted on T2W MR

SELECTED REFERENCES

1. Meloni A et al: Myocardial iron overload by cardiovascular magnetic resonance native segmental T1 mapping: a sensitive approach that correlates with cardiac complications. J Cardiovasc Magn Reson. 23(1):70, 2021
2. Torlasco C et al: Role of T1 mapping as a complementary tool to T2* for non-invasive cardiac iron overload assessment. PLoS One. 13(2):e0192890, 2018
3. Carpenter JP et al: On T2* magnetic resonance and cardiac iron. Circulation. 123(14):1519-28, 2011
4. Kirk P et al: Cardiac T2* magnetic resonance for prediction of cardiac complications in thalassemia major. Circulation. 120(20):1961-8, 2009
5. Modell B et al: Improved survival of thalassaemia major in the UK and relation to T2* cardiovascular magnetic resonance. J Cardiovasc Magn Reson. 10:42, 2008

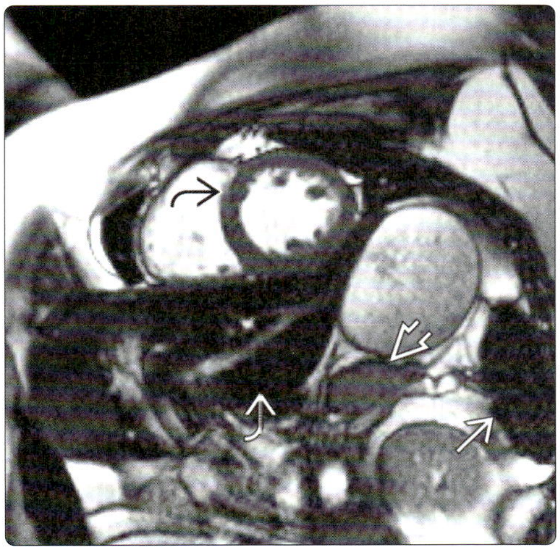

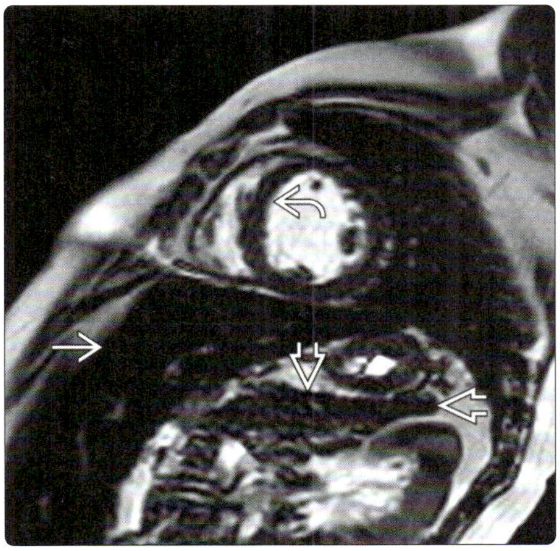

(Left) *Short-axis cine MR of a mild transfusional ion overload syndrome (IOS) shows normal myocardial signal* ➩ *but very dark liver* ➩ *and spleen* ➩ *signals, as they are part of the reticuloendothelial system. Note that the pancreas is normal in signal intensity* ➩, *as expected early in transfusional IOS.* **(Right)** *Short-axis SSFP cine MR of a severe transfusional IOS shows low pancreatic signal* ➩ *as well as cardiac* ➩ *and hepatic* ➩ *involvement.*

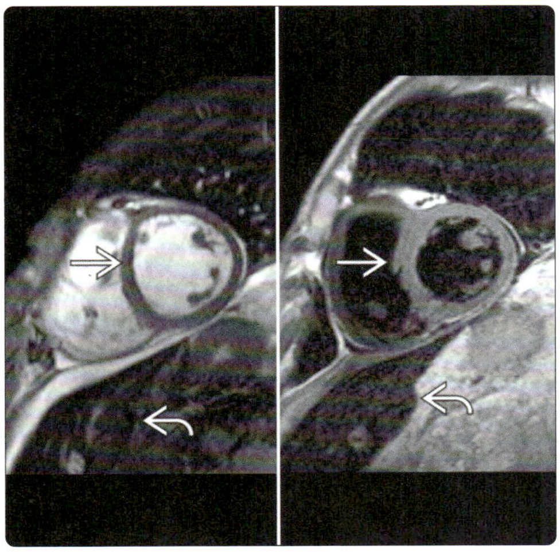

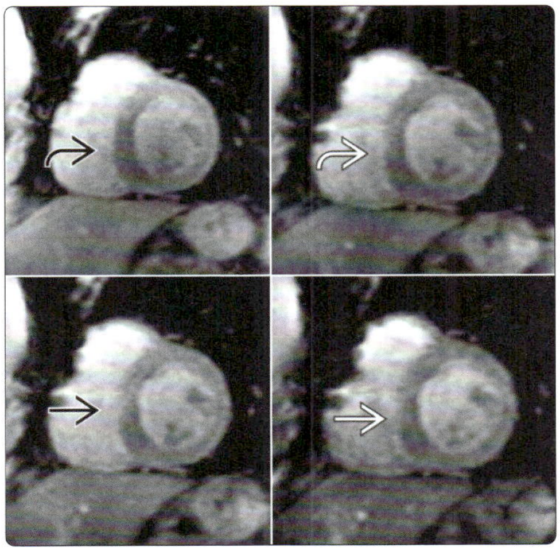

(Left) *Short-axis cine MR (left) and T2 FSE MR (right) of a hemochromatosis patient show hepatic iron overload (low hepatic signal* ➩*) but normal cardiac signal intensity* ➩. *There can be significant discrepancy in the degree of iron loading between the liver and the heart.* **(Right)** *Short-axis GRE MR with varying echo times (TE) (4* ➩, *7* ➩, *10* ➩, *and 15* ➩ *ms) were obtained at a single slice location and show no signal dropout with increasing TE that would indicate abnormal iron deposition.*

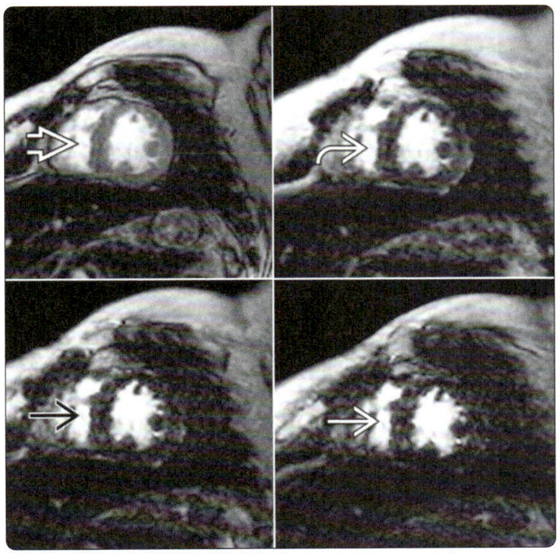

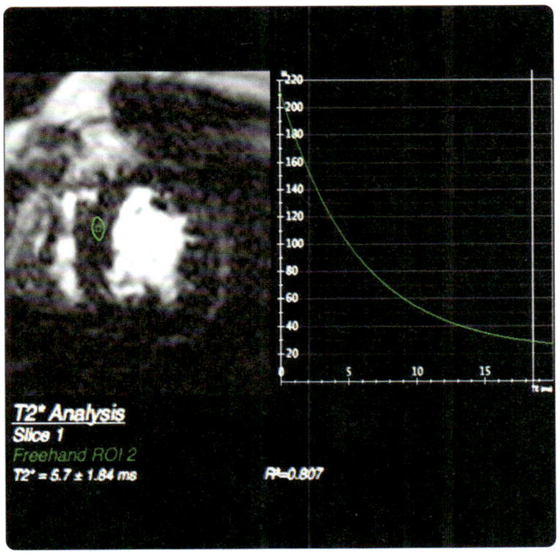

(Left) *Short-axis GRE MR with varying TE (2.4* ➩, *5.4* ➩, *8.3* ➩, *and 11.3* ➩ *ms) were obtained at a single slice location and show extensive signal dropout at increasing TE, which indicates abnormal iron deposition.* **(Right)** *Software analysis of the signal intensity of a selected region of the septum relative to the varying TE allows calculation of the T2* value of the myocardium. The T2* value of 5.7 ms, which is consistent with severe iron loading in a patient with thalassemia, is shown.*

Takotsubo Cardiomyopathy

KEY FACTS

TERMINOLOGY

- Reversible left ventricular (LV) systolic dysfunction in absence of significant coronary artery stenosis
- a.k.a. stress cardiomyopathy or apical ballooning syndrome
- Classically described following periods of severe emotional or physical stress

IMAGING

- Initial imaging test is usually echocardiogram or left ventriculogram during cardiac catheterization
- Cardiac MR is best modality to distinguish from other causes of LV dysfunction, such as myocarditis or ischemic injury
  - Increased T2 signal (edema), T1, and extracellular volume (ECV) in areas of hypokinesis
  - Areas of hypokinesis/akinesis recover on follow-up imaging
  - Apical, midventricular, and basal hypokinesis seen in up to 80%, 40%, and 4%, respectively
- LGE MR
  - Typically characterized by absence of significant LGE
  - ~ 9% can have minimal or subtle LGE, particularly when lower signal intensity threshold is used

CLINICAL ISSUES

- Initial presentation can closely resemble that of acute myocardial infarction or acute coronary syndrome
- In hospital, mortality range is 0-8%
- Most patients typically recover LV function within 4 weeks
- Most common complication is heart failure ± pulmonary edema

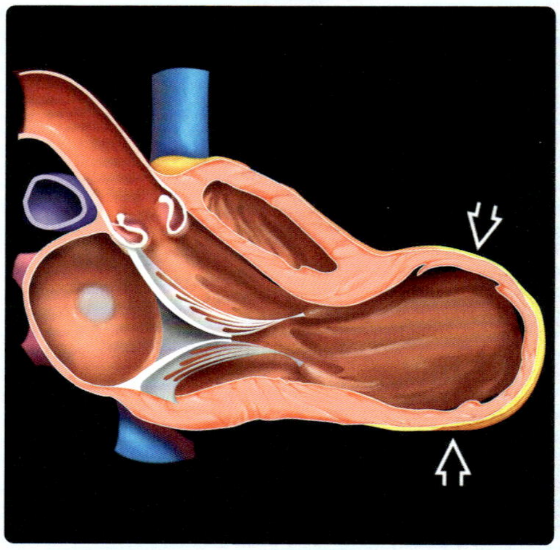

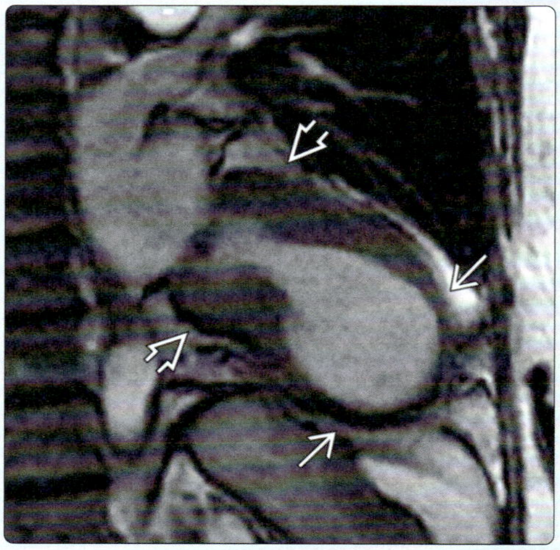

(Left) *Three-chamber graphic shows the most common type of stress cardiomyopathy with severe hypokinesis and thinning of all apical segments ➙, resulting in apical ballooning. This results in a left ventricular (LV) shape resembling the Japanese octopus trap (takotsubo), which gives the entity its name.* **(Right)** *Vertical long-axis (2-chamber) cine MR in systole shows a typical pattern of stress cardiomyopathy with akinesis of the mid to apical LV ➙ and normal contraction of the basal LV ➙.*

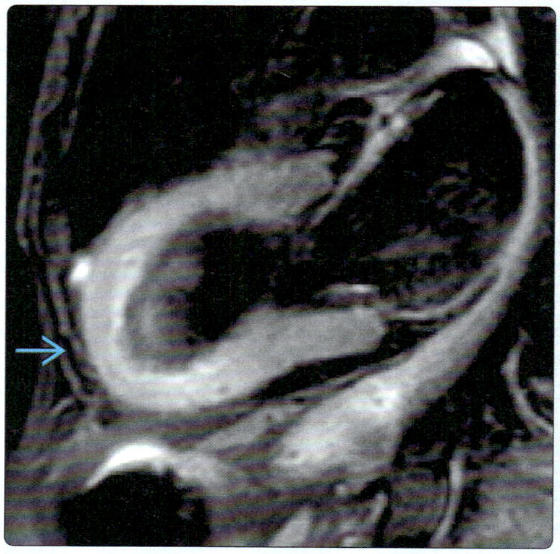

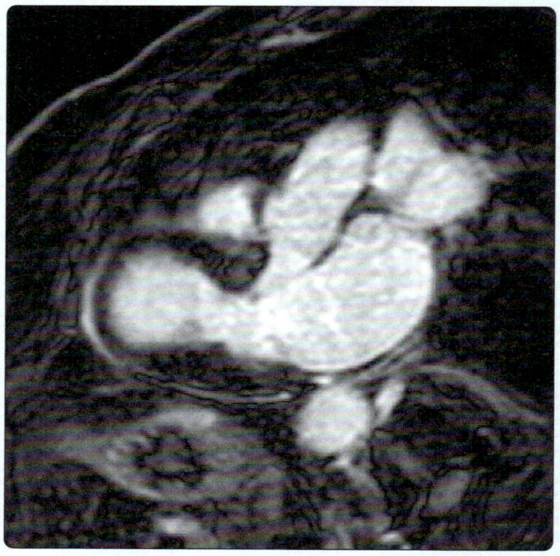

(Left) *Two-chamber T2 MR in a patient with Takotsubo cardiomyopathy shows the presence of myocardial edema in the apical segment, which is seen as high signal in the myocardium →.* **(Right)** *Delayed-enhancement MR shows no focal LGE of the myocardium in a patient with Takotsubo cardiomyopathy. Low-intensity LGE may be seen in up to 9% of the patients with Takotsubo cardiomyopathy.*

TERMINOLOGY

Synonyms

- Stress-induced cardiomyopathy
- Apical ballooning syndrome

Definitions

- Reversible dysfunction of left ventricle (LV) in absence of significant coronary artery stenosis
  - Classically described following periods of severe emotional or physical stress
    - In recent prospective multicenter study, stressful trigger was identified in ~ 70% of patients
  - Often accompanied by acute chest pain, ischemic ST segment abnormalities, and elevation of cardiac biomarkers

IMAGING

General Features

- Best diagnostic clue
  - Regional wall motion abnormalities in setting of recent emotional or physical stress
  - In its most common variant, LV during systole resembles Japanese octopus pot, which has narrow mouth and large round base
    - Tako = octopus; tsubo = pot
  - Wall motion abnormalities often extend beyond single coronary artery territory
- Location
  - Most common variant features distinct apical ballooning with hypokinesis of mid to apical LV with preserved or hyperdynamic function at base
  - Other patterns of LV dysfunction include biventricular, midventricular, and basal ("reverse")

Imaging Recommendations

- Best imaging tool
  - Initial imaging test often echocardiography or left ventriculogram during cardiac catheterization with normal or nonobstructive coronary arteries
  - Cardiac MR is best imaging modality to distinguish from other causes of LV dysfunction, such as myocarditis or ischemic injury

Nuclear Medicine Findings

- Myocardial perfusion defects can be seen and may be related to microvascular dysfunction
  - Can be difficult to exclude ischemic heart disease on basis of nuclear myocardial perfusion

CT Findings

- Cardiac gated CTA
  - Absence of obstructive epicardial coronary artery disease (CAD)
  - Functional assessment on multiphase reconstructions can show patterns of wall motion abnormalities consistent with stress-induced cardiomyopathy
    - CT used in patients with contraindications to MR

MR Findings

- T2WI FS
  - Increased T2 signal (edema) in areas of hypokinesis
    - Edema is diffuse, may extend beyond wall motion abnormalities, and resolves in few weeks
      - Acute myocardial infarction: Focal edema; can take up to 3 months to resolve
- MR cine
  - Areas of hypokinesis/akinesis can occur in various patterns
    - Apical ballooning ("classic") in 60-80%
    - Midventricular hypokinesis in 20-40%
    - Basal hypokinesis ("reverse") in 1-4%
    - Focal hypokinesis < 1%
    - Right ventricle involvement in 13.4%
      - Associated with higher mortality, in-hospital death, thromboembolic events, stroke, cardiogenic shock, use of assist device, pulmonary edema, and malignant arrhythmias
  - Improvement in function at 3-4 months MR is confirmatory
    - Recovery may take up to 12 months in small minority (5%)
    - Recurrence in 5-11%; may have different pattern
  - LV thrombus is relatively uncommon finding
  - Pericardial effusion is seen in ~ 40% of patients
- LGE
  - Typically absent
  - Recent studies have shown LGE in up to 40%
    - Some studies showed no correlation between LGE and adverse outcome, while other studies showed higher risk of cardiogenic shock and longer time for recovery
    - Low-intensity LGE usually resolves; persistent LGE with wall motion abnormalities indicates infarction
- Parametric mapping
  - Increased T2 values due to myocardial edema
  - Increased T1 values with comparable accuracy to T2 MR
  - Extracellular volume (ECV) may be increased in affected myocardium
- Wall motion and ejection fraction usually recover on follow-up imaging, but native T1 and ECV values may not return to normal

Echocardiographic Findings

- Regional wall motion abnormalities
- Can be limited by acoustic windows
- Does not allow myocardial tissue characterization

Angiographic Findings

- Absence of significant CAD
  - 10% can have incidental CAD with > 75% stenosis: Carefully evaluate if CAD causes wall motion abnormality
  - Takotsubo not necessarily excluded in presence of CAD
- Left ventriculogram shows typical regional wall motion abnormalities
- Rarely, multivessel epicardial spasm is evident, which may be spontaneous or induced by ergonovine or acetylcholine infusion

Image-Guided Biopsy

- Endocardial biopsy shows nonspecific findings without evidence of myocardial necrosis

DIFFERENTIAL DIAGNOSIS

Acute Myocardial Infarction

- Given presentation of chest pain, ischemic ECG changes, and regional wall motion abnormalities, CAD should always be excluded
  - Anatomic assessment with coronary angiography or cardiac CT
- Ischemic pattern of LGE on cardiac MR
  - Subendocardial or transmural LGE in distribution of coronary artery
  - Edema can be seen larger than extent of LGE

Acute Myocarditis

- Subepicardial or midmyocardial pattern of LGE
- Increase in T2 signal and increased early global relative enhancement can be seen in both stress cardiomyopathy and myocarditis

Coronary Vasospasm

- Prinzmetal angina
- Due to focal coronary artery vasospasm
- May be associated with acute myocardial infarction, serious ventricular arrhythmias, and sudden death

PATHOLOGY

General Features

- Etiology
  - Precipitated by emotional or physical stress in most patients
  - Precise pathophysiology is not well established
    - Increased sympathetic activity with catecholamine release has been suggested as central mechanism
      - Switching β-2 adrenoreceptor coupling from positively inotropic Gs-cAMP pathway to negative inotropic GI signaling pathway
    - Brain-heart axis is potential mechanism
      - Recent fMRI study showed hypoconnectivity of central brain regions associated with autonomic functions and regulation of limbic system in patients with this cardiomyopathy
    - Microvascular dysfunction
    - Coronary vasospasm driven by α-adrenergic receptors
    - Inflammation

Microscopic Features

- Endomyocardial biopsy shows disorganized contractile proteins, increased collagen-1, and no evidence of cell necrosis

CLINICAL ISSUES

Presentation

- Most common signs/symptoms
  - Initial presentation can closely resemble that of acute myocardial infarction or acute coronary syndrome
    - Chest pain and dyspnea
    - Spectrum of ECG changes, including ST elevation, ST depression, T-wave inversion
  - Mild elevation of cardiac biomarkers (troponin I or T, CK-MB)
    - Degree of elevation of biomarkers often does not correlate with extent of ventricular dysfunction
  - Congestive heart failure
    - Elevated jugular venous pressure on exam
    - Pulmonary edema
    - Hypotension
- Other signs/symptoms
  - Patients may have more serious presentations, such as cardiogenic shock or ventricular fibrillation

Demographics

- Epidemiology
  - May account for 2% of patients presenting with acute coronary syndrome
  - Majority of cases are in postmenopausal females
  - M:F = 1:6

Natural History & Prognosis

- Mortality range in hospitals: 0-8%
  - Most patients recover LV function within 4 weeks
  - Recurrence occurs in ~ 10% of patients
- Most common complication is heart failure ± pulmonary edema
  - May have increased risk of thrombus formation in akinetic apex
  - Tachy- and bradyarrhythmias
  - Transient LV outflow tract obstruction has been described
- Recent studies suggest that there can be persistent abnormalities in myocardial deformation, energetics despite normalization of LV ejection fraction

Treatment

- Supportive care with standard heart failure medications [β-blockers, angiotensin-converting enzyme (ACE) inhibitor, diuretics]
  - Optimal duration of therapy is unclear
- Intraaortic balloon counterpulsation in cases of refractory shock
- Anticoagulation in cases of apical thrombus formation

DIAGNOSTIC CHECKLIST

Consider

- Echocardiogram &/or LV ventriculogram are often 1st imaging tests
- Cardiac MR can help distinguish between other causes of cardiomyopathy and allows for additional myocardial tissue characterization

Image Interpretation Pearls

- On cardiac MR, both myocarditis and stress cardiomyopathy can present with myocardial edema and increased early global relative enhancement

SELECTED REFERENCES

1. Citro R et al: Negative prognostic impact of biventricular ballooning in Takotsubo syndrome: when two is not better than one. Chest. 160(4):1179-80, 2021
2. Priya S et al: Review of multi-modality imaging update and diagnostic work up of Takotsubo cardiomyopathy. Clin Imaging. 80:334-47, 2021
3. Ojha V et al: Advanced cardiac magnetic resonance imaging in takotsubo cardiomyopathy. Br J Radiol. 93(1115):20200514, 2020

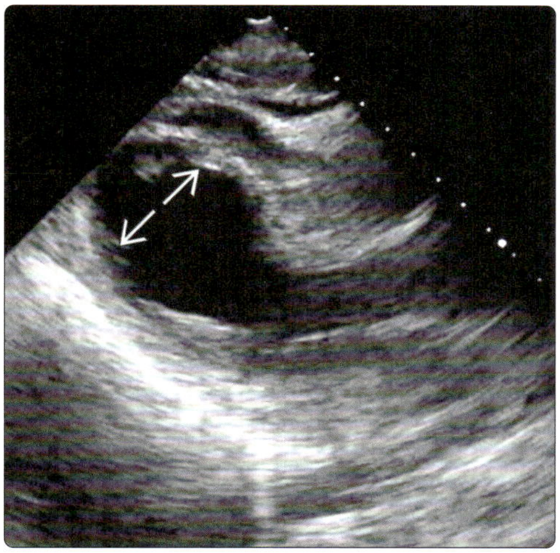

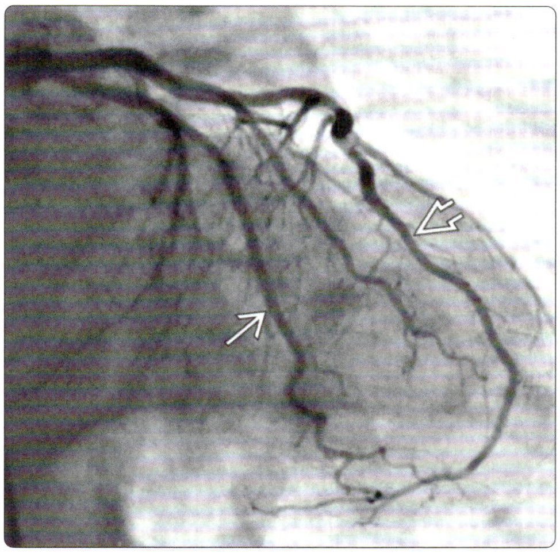

(Left) *Three-chamber echocardiogram shows hypokinesis of the mid to apical LV → in an older adult woman presenting with chest pain and anterior ST elevations shortly after learning of the death of a loved one.* **(Right)** *Coronary angiography in the same patient shows absence of significant obstructive coronary artery disease of the left circumflex (LCx) → and left anterior descending (LAD) coronary → arteries. The right coronary artery (RCA) (not shown) was also normal.*

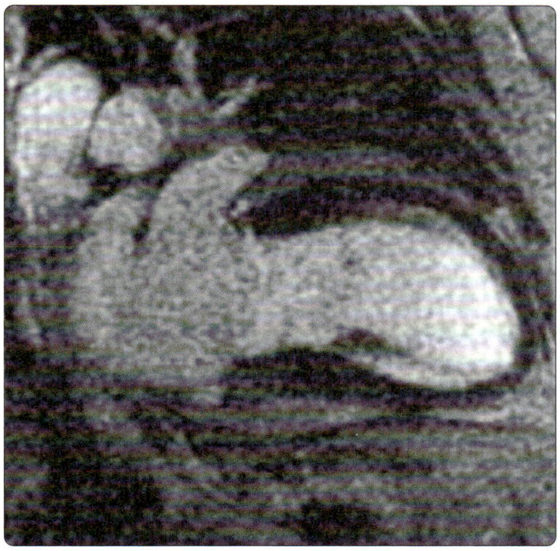

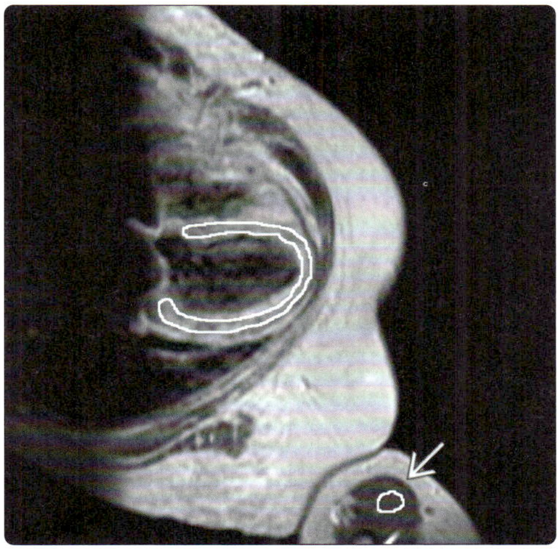

(Left) *Vertical long-axis (2-chamber) LGE MR of the LV shows no focal areas of abnormal late enhancement, which is typical in stress-induced cardiomyopathy.* **(Right)** *Axial T1WI spin-echo sequence after administration of gadolinium is shown. The early global relative enhancement ratio is calculated by comparing pre- and postcontrast signal intensity in the myocardium normalized to the skeletal muscle →. In this case of stress cardiomyopathy, the ratio was abnormal at 9.*

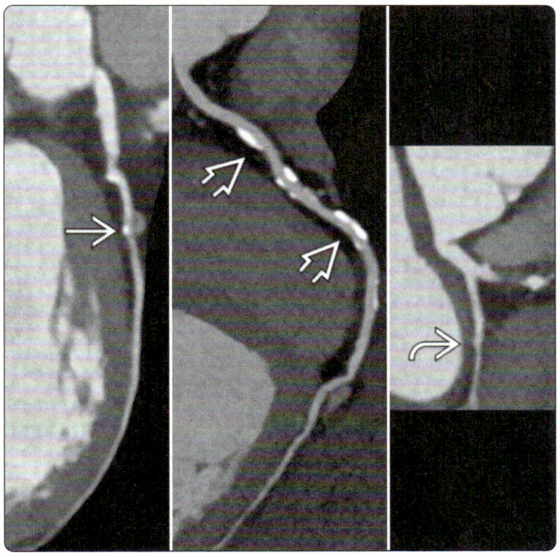

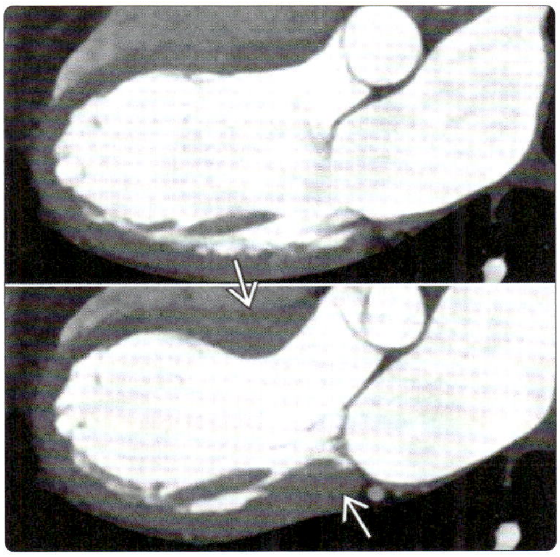

(Left) *Retrospective EKG gated coronary CTA was performed in a female patient who presented with acute chest pain without significant troponin elevation. Curved MPR of the LAD →, RCA →, and LCx → demonstrates scattered calcified plaques but no obstructive disease.* **(Right)** *Composite 3-chamber CT views (top-diastole; bottom-systole) in the same patient show akinesia of the apical and midsegments with preserved contractility of the basal segments → during systole, consistent with Takotsubo cardiomyopathy.*

Muscular Dystrophy

KEY FACTS

TERMINOLOGY

- Inherited muscle diseases with progressive weakness and wasting of skeletal muscles of varying distribution and severity
- Heart is involved in several muscular dystrophies, sometimes even without significant skeletal muscle involvement

IMAGING

- Cardiac MR is best imaging tool for early identification of cardiac involvement
  - Subepicardial LGE pattern is seen, often prior to onset of left ventricular systolic dysfunction
  - Regional wall motion abnormalities are also seen in early stages
  - ↑ native T1; ↓ postcontrast T1; ↑ extracellular volume in early stages
  - Excessive trabeculations and hypertrophy may be associated
  - Accurately quantifies ventricular volumes and function
- Cardiac MR is useful in screening family members with carrier genes
- Cardiac CT is utilized only in patients with contraindications for MR
- Cardiac CT is performed with retrospective ECG gating and triphasic contrast injection to quantify biventricular volumes and functions

TOP DIFFERENTIAL DIAGNOSES

- Myocarditis; sarcoidosis
- Chagas disease; Fabry disease
- Ischemic cardiomyopathy
- Nonischemic dilated cardiomyopathy

CLINICAL ISSUES

- Early initiation of standard heart failure treatment delays onset and progression of LV systolic dysfunction

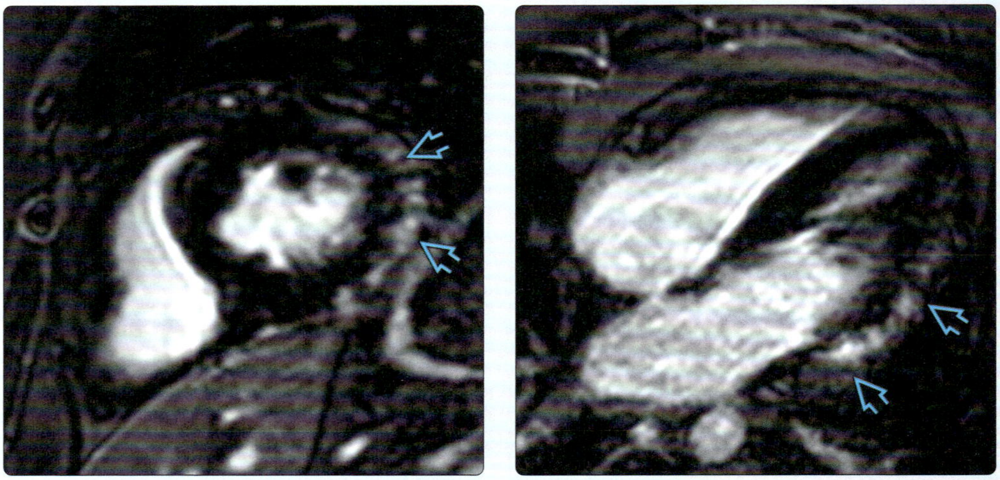

(Left) *Short-axis LGE cardiac MR in a 20-year-old man with Duchenne muscular dystrophy and restrictive lung disease demonstrates a subepicardial pattern of LGE in the lateral wall, indicative of fibrosis.* **(Right)** *Four-chamber LGE MR in the same patient shows the subepicardial pattern of LGE in the anterolateral wall, indicative of fibrosis. The degree of LGE in Duchenne patients correlates with degree of left ventricular (LV) dysfunction.*

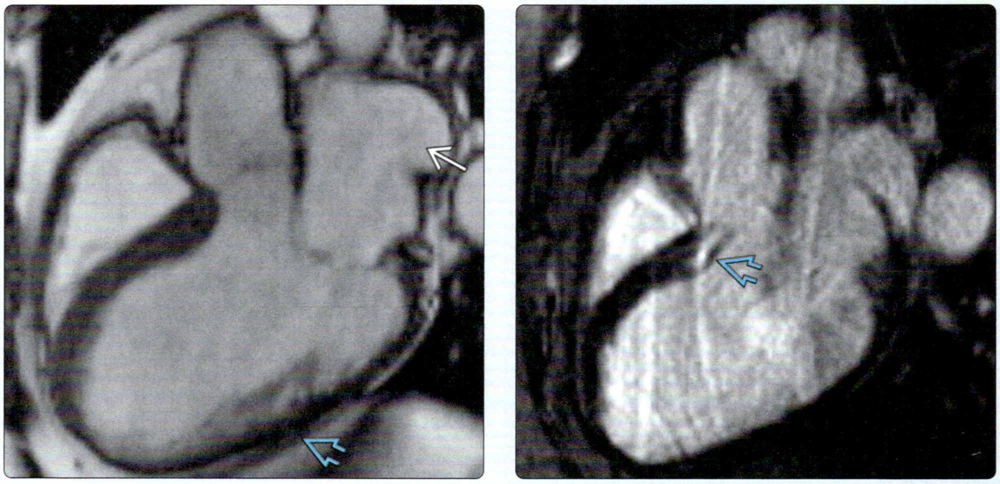

(Left) *Three-chamber cine SSFP cine MR in a 66-year-old man with Becker muscular dystrophy shows marked dilation of the LV and mild dilation of left atrium. Severely depressed LV systolic function (LV ejection fraction: 25 %) was detected.* **(Right)** *Three-chamber LGE MR in the same patient demonstrates a focal midmyocardial LGE in the basal anteroseptal segment, indicative of fibrosis.*

TERMINOLOGY

Abbreviations

- Muscular dystrophy (MD)

Definitions

- Inherited muscle diseases with progressive weakness and wasting of skeletal muscles of varying distribution and severity
  - Genetic mutation of proteins involved in muscular structure and contraction
  - Heart is involved in several muscular dystrophies
    - May be predominant manifestation
    - Due to shared proteins of cardiac and skeletal muscles

IMAGING

General Features

- Role of imaging
  - Early diagnosis of cardiac involvement
    - Early initiation of treatment to halt progression to heart failure and adverse remodeling

CT Findings

- Not primary imaging modality of choice
  - Utilized only when MR is contraindicated
    - Mainly due to indwelling pacemakers/implantable cardioverter defibrillators (ICDs)
- Quantification of ventricular volumes and function
  - Requires retrospective ECG gating
  - Triphasic contrast bolus to opacify entire heart
  - Comparable to MR
- Qualitative evaluation
  - Ventricle dilation or hypertrophy
  - Global or regional dysfunction
  - Excessive trabeculations may be seen
- Delayed iodine enhancement
  - Subepicardial or midmyocardial enhancement
  - Inferior quality compared to MR due to lower CNR
- Skeletal muscle atrophy and fatty replacement also shown

MR Findings

- Ideal imaging modality in identifying early cardiac involvement
  - Findings can be seen even with normal echocardiography
  - Can be used to screen family members
- Black-blood imaging for morphology
  - Dilation of ventricles; hypertrophy in some
  - Myocardial fat infiltration may be seen
  - Lipomatous hypertrophy of atrial septum
  - Atrophic changes in the skeletal muscles
- Cine SSFP
  - Morphologic changes as above
    - Excessive trabeculations in Duchenne MD (DMD), myotonic dystrophy (DM)
      - □ Ratio of trabeculated to compacted myocardium in end diastole > 2.3
  - Functional changes: Global systolic dysfunction
    - Accurate quantification of ventricular volumes and function; useful in monitoring response to therapy
- Strain imaging
  - Regional wall motion abnormalities are seen earlier than onset of global systolic dysfunction
    - Used to diagnose occult cardiac dysfunction
    - Potential for evaluating response to therapy
  - DMD: Lower global and circumferential strain
    - Localized to basal inferolateral wall or diffusely to basal lateral, inferior wall, and septum
    - Precedes systolic dysfunction and LGE
    - May predict LGE-positive segments
    - Captures left ventricular (LV) function decline better than ejection fraction (EF)
  - Emery-Dreifuss MD (EDMD): ↓ systolic circumferential strain, inferior segment
- LGE
  - DMD and Becker MD (BMD)
    - Subepicardial LGE; inferolateral wall
      - □ Mechanical stress on structurally abnormal myocardium
    - More sensitive than echo/LV systolic dysfunction
    - Similar findings in gene-carrying family members
    - Degree of LGE correlates with degree of dysfunction
      - □ Transmural pattern of fibrosis is independent predictor of adverse events, even with preserved LVEF (> 45%)
      - □ Correlation between LGE, LVEF, and genotype
    - Septal midmyocardial and regional transmural patterns in advanced cases
  - EDMD: Early fibrosis not seen prior to systolic dysfunction
  - Limb-Girdle MD (LGMD)
    - Lamin A/C cardiomyopathy
      - □ Fibrosis seen before systolic dysfunction and LV dilatation
      - □ Midmyocardial; basal ventricular septum
      - □ Lateral wall subepicardial pattern also seen
    - LGMD2I (*FKRP* gene mutation) and LGMD2c
      - □ Early midmyocardial scarring can be seen
      - □ ↓ EF, ↑ LV volumes/mass
  - Myotonic muscular dystrophy (DM)
    - LGE seen in up to 13% of patients
      - □ Mild midwall fibrosis of septum may be seen
      - □ Dilation, hypertrophy, reduced LV mass, noncompaction, systolic dysfunction more common
      - □ Some LGE may be due to fat infiltration in epimyocardial region; impaired right ventricle contractility
  - X-linked dilated cardiomyopathy
    - Subepicardial or midmyocardial pattern
      - □ With LV dilation and systolic dysfunction
- Parametric mapping
  - ↑ native T1; ↓ postcontrast T1; ↑ extracellular volume (ECV)
    - Due to diffuse fibrosis
    - Has been shown in DMD and BMD
    - More sensitive than LGE
    - Identifies early involvement of myocardium
    - DMD: Native T1 predicts disease severity better than ECV; higher ECV predictive of lower LV EF

Imaging Recommendations

- Best imaging tool
  - Cardiac MR for early identification of cardiac involvement
    - Myocardial fibrosis and quantification of volumes and function
  - Cardiac CT is utilized when MR is contraindicated
- Protocol advice
  - Cardiac MR should include cine, LGE, and parametric mapping
  - Cardiac CT is performed with retrospective ECG gating and triphasic contrast injection

DIFFERENTIAL DIAGNOSIS

Nonischemic Dilated Cardiomyopathy

- May show linear or patchy midmyocardial LGE
- No skeletal muscle abnormalities

Myocarditis

- Global and regional wall motion abnormalities may be seen
- Acute: High T2 signal, T2 values, and native T1 values; early (EGE) and LGE
  - Subepicardial or midmyocardial; lateral wall or septum
- Chronic: Wall thinning; wall motion abnormality; LGE; no T2 signal or EGE

Sarcoidosis

- Usually chronic presentation with heart block
- Wall motion abnormalities; thinning in chronic; LV dilation
- Subepicardial or midmyocardial LGE; rarely subendocardial or transmural

Chagas Disease

- Caused by *Trypanosoma cruzi* infection
- Myocardial edema, wall motion abnormalities, aneurysm, thrombi, fibrosis
- LGE: Heterogeneous; subepicardial (1/4), subendocardial (1/4), or transmural

Fabry Disease

- Glycogen storage disease: Deficiency of alpha-galactosidase
- Subepicardial/midmyocardial LGE; basal inferolateral wall
- Myocardial thickening is present
- Native T1 mapping shows low values due to fat; high values can be seen when fibrosis develops

Ischemic Cardiomyopathy

- LGE always involves subendocardium with variable transmurality
- Matching wall motion abnormalities in coronary vascular distribution

PATHOLOGY

Molecular Basis

- DMD and BMD: X-linked; mutations in dystrophin
  - Dystrophin stabilizes cell membrane of myocytes
- EDMD: X-linked recessive; rarely autosomal recessive
  - Nuclear envelopathies: Mutations in genes encoding emerin and lamin A/C
- LGMD: Mutations in sarcoglycan subunits; usually AR; rarely AD
- DM: Mutations in DMPK or zinc finger proteins; AD; DM1 and DM2
- Facioscapulohumeral MD: AD

CLINICAL ISSUES

Presentation

- Most common signs/symptoms
  - Heart failure, heart block, arrhythmias, sudden death

Natural History & Prognosis

- DMD: Most common and severe form in children
  - Delayed cardiac presentation due to inactivity
  - All have cardiac involvement in 3rd decade
- BMD: Later- and slower-onset skeletal myopathy
  - 70 % have cardiac involvement
  - Manifestation is worse than DMD due to physical activity
- EDMD: Heart commonly involved; presents in 3rd decade or earlier
  - Starts in atria → → AV node → → ventricles
  - Sudden cardiac death (SCD) may be presenting feature
    - Commonly have pacemaker implanted
- LGMD: Heterogeneous presentation; some are similar to EDMD2
  - Weakness of proximal muscles
  - Dilated cardiomyopathy; conduction disorder; SCD
- DM: Conduction defects and sudden death common
  - LV dilation and hypertrophy (20%); LV systolic dysfunction (14%)
  - Clinical heart failure less common
- X-linked dilated cardiomyopathy
  - Nonischemic dilated cardiomyopathy
- Facioscapulohumeral MD
  - Hypertrophy, conduction defects, arrhythmia

Treatment

- Early initiation of heart failure treatment to delay onset and progression of LV systolic dysfunction
  - ACE inhibitors; β blockers
- Reverse remodeling in patients with X-linked dystrophinopathy

DIAGNOSTIC CHECKLIST

Consider

- MR for early diagnosis and screening of family members

Image Interpretation Pearls

- History and features of MD
- Subepicardial pattern of LGE in MR

SELECTED REFERENCES

1. Petersen SE et al: Excessive trabeculation of the left ventricle: JACC: cardiovascular imaging expert panel paper. JACC Cardiovasc Imaging. 16(3):408-25, 2023
2. Marty B et al: Comprehensive evaluation of structural and functional myocardial impairments in Becker muscular dystrophy using quantitative cardiac magnetic resonance imaging. Eur Heart J Cardiovasc Imaging. 20(8):906-15, 2018
3. Olivieri LJ et al: Native T1 values identify myocardial changes and stratify disease severity in patients with Duchenne muscular dystrophy. J Cardiovasc Magn Reson. 18(1):72, 2016
4. Otto RK et al: Cardiac MRI in muscular dystrophy: an overview and future directions. Phys Med Rehabil Clin N Am. 23(1):123-32, xi-xii, 2012

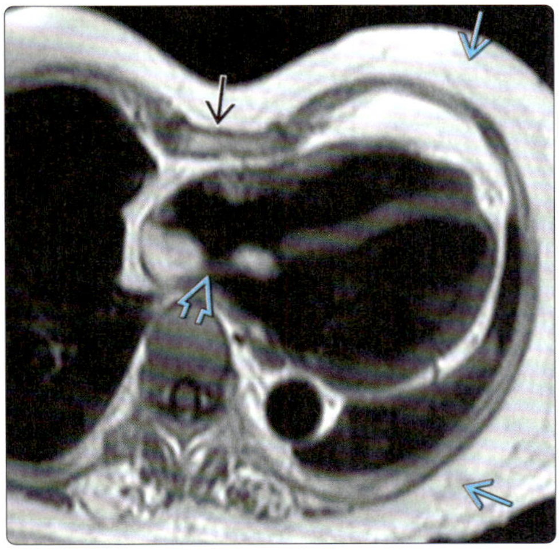
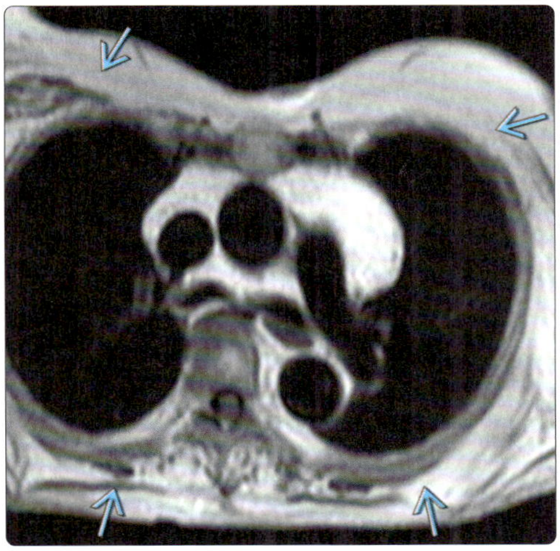

(Left) *Axial black-blood MR in a 74-year-old man with history of facioscapulohumeral muscular dystrophy shows fatty atrophy of the skeletal muscles. There is also lipomatous hypertrophy of the interatrial septum, sparing the fossa ovalis. Note the pectus excavatum with Haller index of 6.2.* **(Right)** *Axial black-blood MR in the same patient at a higher level shows fatty atrophy of the paraspinal/erector spinae, latissimus dorsi, rotator cuff, serratus anterior, and pectoralis major/minor muscles.*

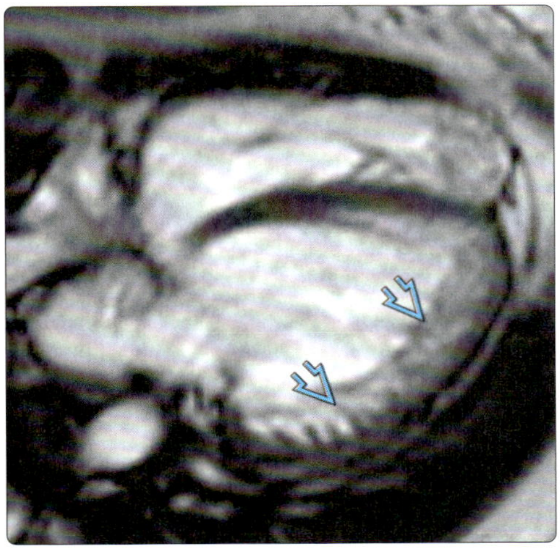
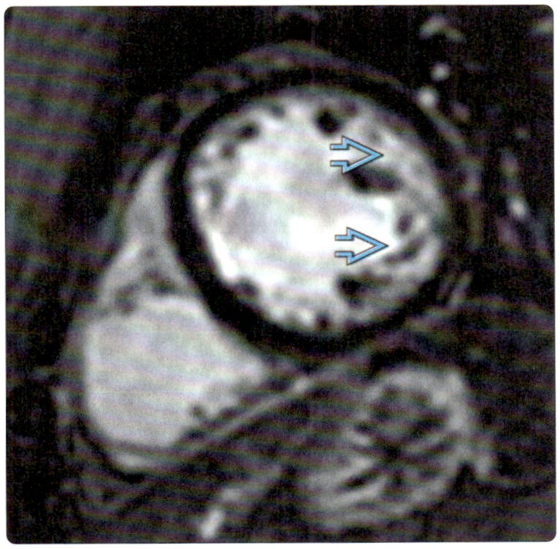

(Left) *Four-chamber SSFP cine MR obtained in diastole in a 41-year-old woman with Duchenne muscular dystrophy shows excessive trabeculations of the lateral and apical segments of the LV with a ratio of trabeculated:nontrabeculated myocardium > 2.3.* **(Right)** *Short-axis LGE MR in the same patient shows excessive trabeculations in the lateral wall. There is no abnormal LGE.*

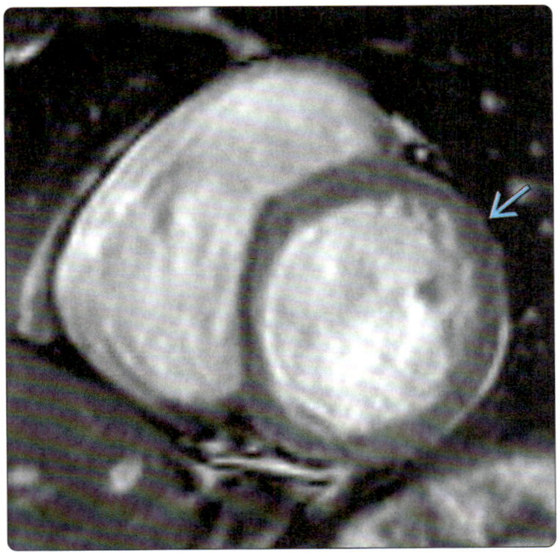
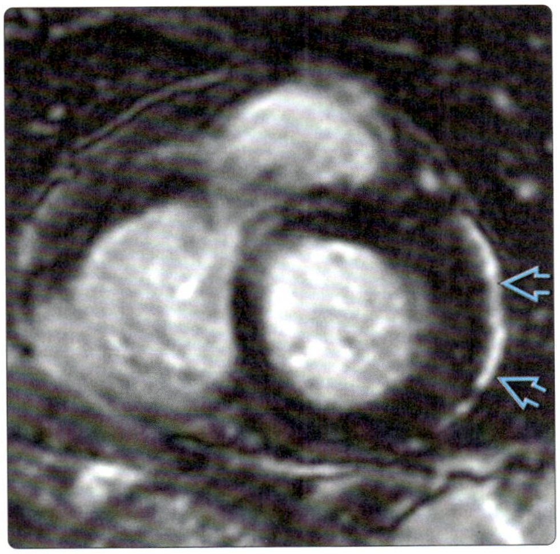

(Left) *Short-axis SSFP cardiac cine MR in a 29-year-old man with type 1 myotonic dystrophy demonstrates focal myocardial thinning of the anterolateral segment of the mid LV wall.* **(Right)** *Short-axis LGE MR in the same patient at a higher level shows focal subepicardial LGE in the basal lateral wall of the LV, consistent with fibrosis.*

KEY FACTS

TERMINOLOGY

- X-linked multisystem lysosomal storage disorder caused by mutations in *GLA* gene
- Impaired breakdown and accumulation of globotriaosylceramide (Gb3) and related glycosphingolipids in lysosomes of different tissues, including heart, blood vessels, kidneys, and CNS

IMAGING

- Concentric left ventricular hypertrophy
- Right ventricular hypertrophy in 30% to 40% of patients
- Nonischemic midmyocardial LGE in basal to midinferolateral wall
- Diffusely decreased native T1 relaxation times due to intracellular glycosphingolipid accumulation

TOP DIFFERENTIAL DIAGNOSES

- Hypertrophic cardiomyopathy
- Cardiac amyloidosis
- Athlete's heart
- Hypertensive heart disease

CLINICAL ISSUES

- Left ventricular hypertrophy, dysrhythmias, diastolic and systolic dysfunction, sudden cardiac death
- More frequent in males (X-linked)
- 2-4% of patients with unexplained left ventricular hypertrophy
- Treatment
    - Enzyme replacement therapy or pharmacologic chaperone therapy

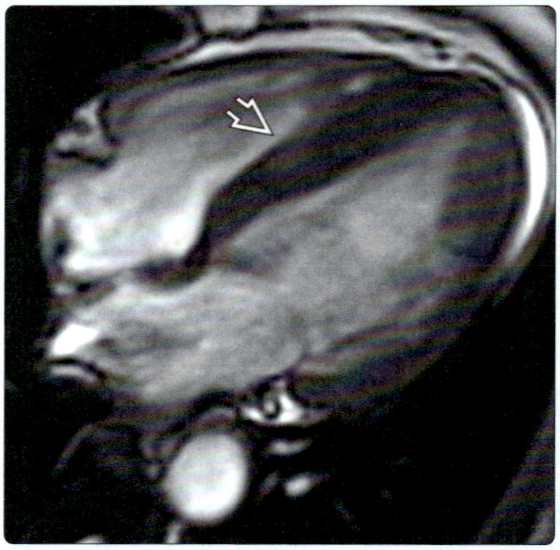
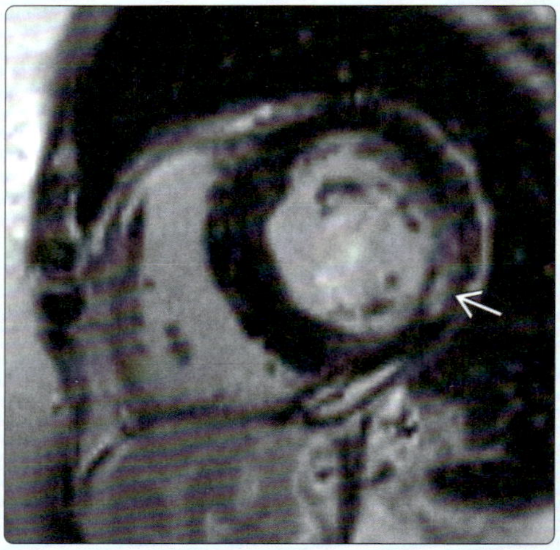

(Left) *Four-chamber SSFP MR in a 66-year-old woman with known Fabry disease shows slightly asymmetric hypertrophy that predominates in the interventricular septum* ➨. **(Right)** *Short-axis LGE (PSIR) MR shows nonischemic, patchy midmyocardial LGE involving the basal inferolateral wall* ➨.

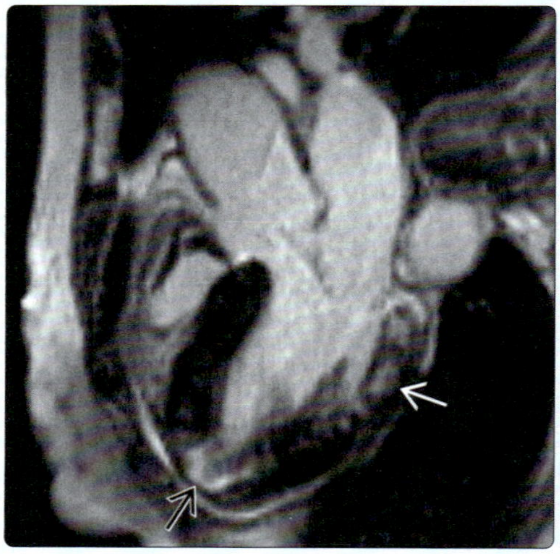
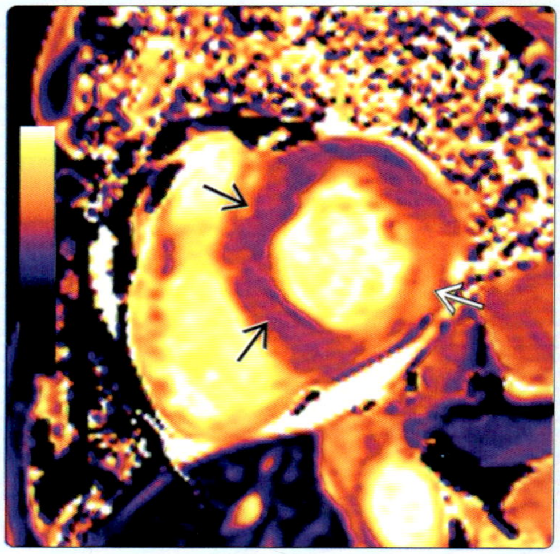

(Left) *Three-chamber LGE (PSIR) MR shows patchy, nonischemic midmyocardial enhancement of inferolateral segment* ➨ *and apex* ➨. **(Right)** *T1 map with modified Look-Locker inversion recovery (MOLLI) technique in a short-axis slice at the basal cavity shows diffusely decreased native T1 times of the hypertrophic myocardium* ➨ *(1134 ms at 3T, measured at the interventricular septum; lower limit of normal 1153 ms). T1 times are increased in the inferolateral segment at the site of LGE* ➨*, consistent with fibrosis.*

TERMINOLOGY

Synonyms

- Anderson-Fabry disease

Definitions

- X-linked lysosomal storage disorder caused by mutations in *GLA* gene
  - Deficiency or dysfunction of enzyme alpha-galactosidase A (α-Gal A)
  - Impaired breakdown and accumulation of globotriaosylceramide (Gb3) and related glycosphingolipids in lysosomes of different tissues
    - Including heart, blood vessels, kidneys, and CNS
  - Gb3 storage disrupts cellular processes and triggers inflammation and fibrosis

IMAGING

General Features

- Best diagnostic clue
  - Concentric left ventricular (LV) wall thickening with decreased native T1 relaxation times
- Location
  - Basal to mid inferolateral midwall LGE

CT Findings

- CECT
  - Concentric myocardial thickening of left ventricle

MR Findings

- Cine MR
  - Concentric LV wall thickening: Most common pattern
  - Less frequently, asymmetric septal hypertrophy, LVOT obstruction, midcavitary obstruction, or apical hypertrophy
  - Right ventricular (RV) hypertrophy in 30-40% of patients
  - Thinning of basal inferolateral wall once fibrosis has developed
  - Decreased LV ejection fraction: Typically late finding in end-stage disease
  - Valvular disease: Valve thickening and regurgitation
  - Mild aortic root dilatation
- Strain
  - Decreased global longitudinal strain and abnormal segmental longitudinal strain in basal inferolateral wall
- LGE
  - Nonischemic pattern of enhancement
  - Midwall LGE in basal to midinferolateral wall: Most common
  - Less frequently, midwall LGE of apical segments
  - LGE may develop before LV hypertrophy, particularly in women
- T1 mapping
  - Diffusely decreased native T1 relaxation times due to glycosphingolipid accumulation
  - T1 mapping is useful to differentiate Fabry cardiomyopathy from other hypertrophic phenotypes, such as hypertrophic cardiomyopathy and amyloidosis
  - Decreased native T1 times in up to 59% of patients with Fabry disease and no LV hypertrophy
    - Identification of patients with early cardiac involvement and predicts progression
  - T1 times can pseudonormalize or even be elevated in later stages of disease due to inflammation and fibrosis
  - Normal native T1 does not exclude underlying diagnosis of Fabry cardiomyopathy
  - Extracellular volume (ECV) is frequently normal during early stages of disease
  - ECV may be elevated due to chronic inflammation
- Edema imaging and T2 mapping
  - Mildly increased T2 mapping values and T2 hyperintensity corresponding to areas of LGE
  - Reflects mild chronic inflammation
- 3 stages of cardiac involvement have been proposed based on native T1 times, wall thickness, and LGE
  - Storage stage
    - Normal or decreased native T1 times
    - No wall thickening
    - No LGE
  - Inflammation and myocyte hypertrophy phase
    - Decreased native T1 times
    - Nonischemic LGE
    - ± LV hypertrophy
  - Fibrosis and impairment phase
    - Pseudonormalization or elevation of native T1
    - Extensive LGE
    - ± LV hypertrophy

Ultrasonographic Findings

- Nonspecific findings
  - LV hypertrophy
  - Thickened papillary muscles
  - Impaired global longitudinal strain and segmental longitudinal strain in inferolateral wall
  - Diastolic dysfunction
    - Impaired tissue Doppler velocities
    - Higher E/e ratios
    - Shortened isovolumic relaxation time
  - Tricuspid and mitral insufficiency; valvular leaflets thickening
  - Binary sign (i.e., hyperechogenic endocardium and hypoechogenic midwall) is no longer considered specific for Fabry disease

Imaging Recommendations

- Best imaging tool
  - Cardiac MR, including LGE and native T1 mapping
- Protocol advice
  - Key sequences: Multiplanar cine, native T1 mapping, multiplanar LGE

DIFFERENTIAL DIAGNOSIS

Hypertrophic Cardiomyopathy

- Hypertrophy more frequently asymmetric
- Amorphous or patchy LGE at septum
- Usually increased native T1

Cardiac Amyloidosis

- Altered T1 nulling pattern
- Diffuse subendocardial or transmural LGE
- Significantly increased native T1 and ECV

Athlete's Heart

- Normal native T1 times and normal/decreased ECV
- Usually no LGE
  - Nonspecific midmyocardial LGE may be seen, typically at RV insertion points

Hydroxychloroquine Cardiotoxicity

- Presents with severe hypertrophy and LGE that can progress rapidly
- Typical treatment history with decades of antimalarial therapy

Hypertensive Heart Disease/Aortic Stenosis

- Normal or increased native T1 times
- No or minimal LGE

PATHOLOGY

General Features

- Accumulation of Gb3 in cardiomyocytes, endothelial cells of intramyocardial vessels or endocardium, valvular fibroblasts, and conduction tissue
- Activation of hypertrophic signaling and inflammatory pathways leading to myocyte hypertrophy, dysfunction, and fibrosis
- Involvement of intramural vessels can induce myocardial ischemia
- Presence of fibrosis and involvement of conduction tissue can prompt conduction disturbances and ventricular arrhythmias

CLINICAL ISSUES

Presentation

- Most common signs/symptoms
  - LV hypertrophy, dysrhythmias, diastolic and systolic dysfunction, sudden cardiac death
  - Chest pain, myocardial infarction with nonobstructed coronary arteries (MINOCA), atrioventricular valvular disease
- Other signs/symptoms
  - When multisystemic involvement is present
    - Neurologic: Small vessel ischemia, thromboembolic ischemic strokes secondary to cardiac involvement, basilar artery dolichoectasia
    - Renal: Proteinuria, end-stage renal failure, renal cysts
    - Pulmonary: Chronic obstructive airways disease
- 2 main clinical phenotypes: Classic and late onset
  - Classic: Severely decreased or absent α-Gal A activity
    - Early onset (pediatric age) with multisystemic involvement
  - Late onset: Residual α-Gal A activity
    - Predominant involvement of single organ during adulthood, usually heart

Demographics

- X-lined disease often more severe in males
  - Classic phenotype: 1 in 35,000-50,000 newborns
  - Late onset: 1 in 1,200-3,000 newborns
- In females, X-chromosome random inactivation results in mosaicism and heterogeneous manifestations: From asymptomatic or mild phenotypes manifesting later in life to severe presentations resembling classic phenotype
- 2-4% of patients with unexplained LV hypertrophy
- 0.5-1% of all patients with suspected hypertrophic cardiomyopathy

Treatment

- Enzyme replacement therapy
- Pharmacologic chaperone therapy
  - For certain cases with residual α-Gal A activity

DIAGNOSTIC CHECKLIST

Reporting Tips

- Attention to: LV and RV thickening, presence and extension of LGE, presence of myocardial edema, measurement of focal T1 times
- If patient is being followed in same center, standardized measurements of T1 relaxation times can be provided in report to assess for change

SELECTED REFERENCES

1. Pieroni M et al: Anderson-Fabry disease management: role of the cardiologist. Eur Heart J. 45(16):1395-409, 2024
2. Averbuch T et al: Anderson-Fabry disease cardiomyopathy: an update on epidemiology, diagnostic approach, management and monitoring strategies. Front Cardiovasc Med. 10:1152568, 2023
3. Gagnon LR et al: Review of hydroxychloroquine cardiotoxicity: lessons from the COVID-19 pandemic. Curr Heart Fail Rep. 19(6):458-66, 2022
4. Pieroni M et al: Cardiac involvement in Fabry disease: JACC review topic of the week. J Am Coll Cardiol. 77(7):922-36, 2021
5. Augusto JB et al: Myocardial edema, myocyte injury, and disease severity in Fabry disease. Circ Cardiovasc Imaging. 13(3):e010171, 2020
6. Camporeale A et al: Predictors of clinical evolution in prehypertrophic Fabry disease. Circ Cardiovasc Imaging. 12(4):e008424, 2019
7. Tower-Rader A et al: Multimodality imaging assessment of Fabry disease. Circ Cardiovasc Imaging. 12(11):e009013, 2019
8. Karur GR et al: Use of myocardial T1 mapping at 3.0 T to differentiate Anderson-Fabry disease from hypertrophic cardiomyopathy. Radiology. 288(2):398-406, 2018
9. Walter TC et al: Segment-by-segment assessment of left ventricular myocardial affection in Anderson-Fabry disease by non-enhanced T1-mapping. Acta Radiol. 58(8):914-21, 2017
10. Thompson RB et al: T_1 mapping with cardiovascular MRI is highly sensitive for Fabry disease independent of hypertrophy and sex. Circ Cardiovasc Imaging. 6(5):637-45, 2013

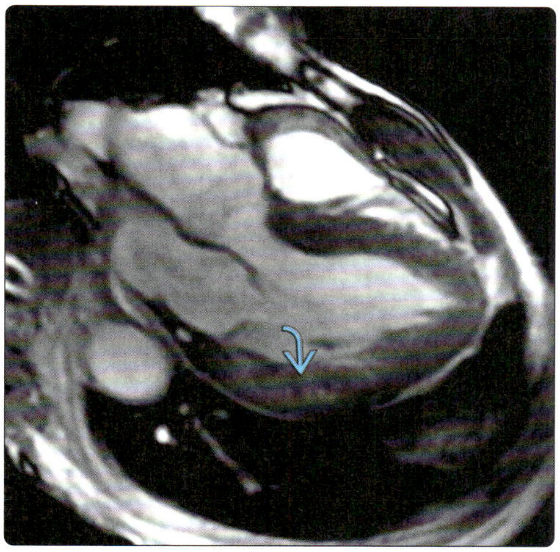

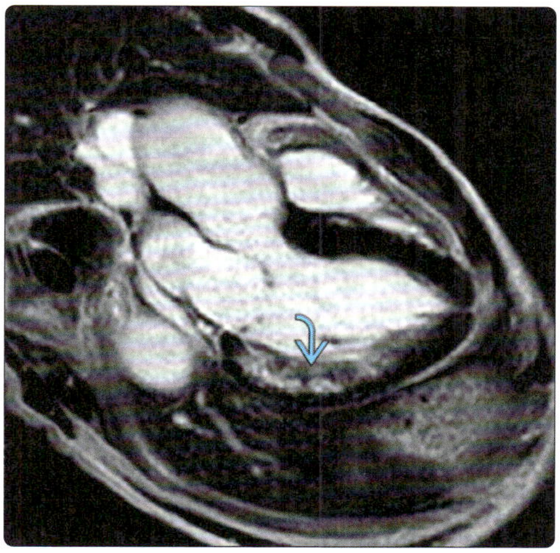

(Left) *Four-chamber SSFP MR obtained after administration of contrast shows diffuse myocardial hypertrophy. Areas of midmyocardial enhancement can be seen in the inferolateral segments* ➚ *at the base and midcavity level.* **(Right)** *Three-chamber PSIR MR in the same patient shows the pronounced LGE isolated to the inferolateral segments* ➚.

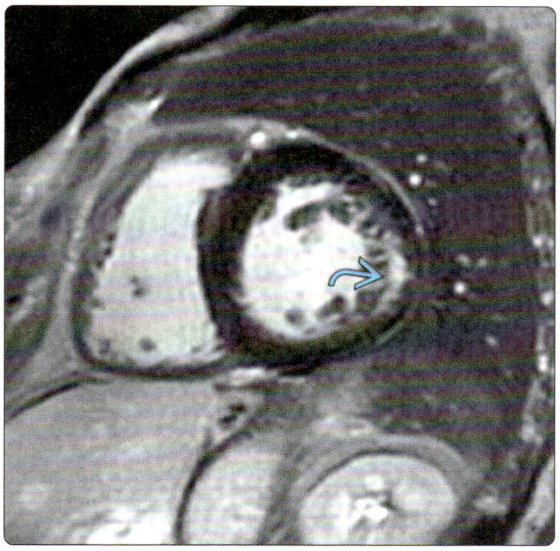

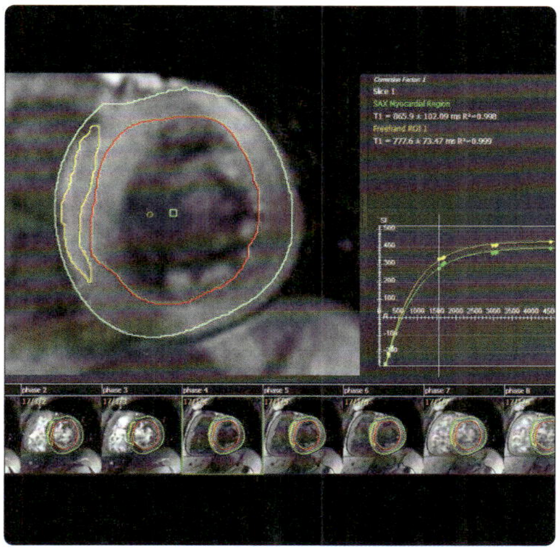

(Left) *Short-axis PSIR MR in the same patient shows that the LGE is isolated to the inferolateral segments* ➚. **(Right)** *Native T1 mapping shows dramatic decrease in the native T1 values at the base, which are 866 msec due to myocardial sphingolipid accumulation (lower limit of normal on this 3T scanner is 1115 msec). This decrease is even more pronounced in the septal segments, which have a native T1 value of 778 msec as they exclude the region of fibrosis in the inferolateral segment. (Courtesy S. Kligerman, MD.)*

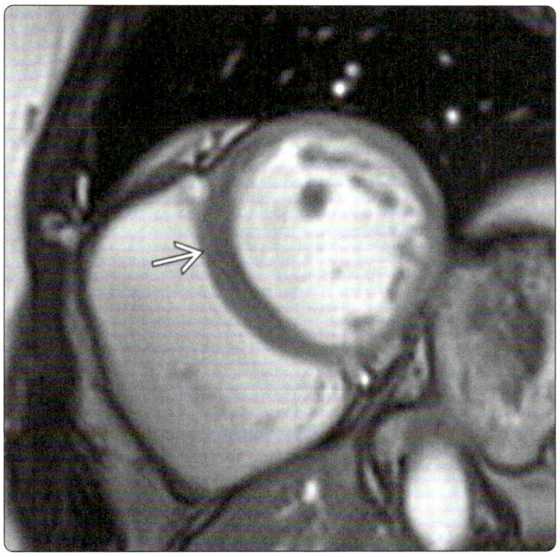

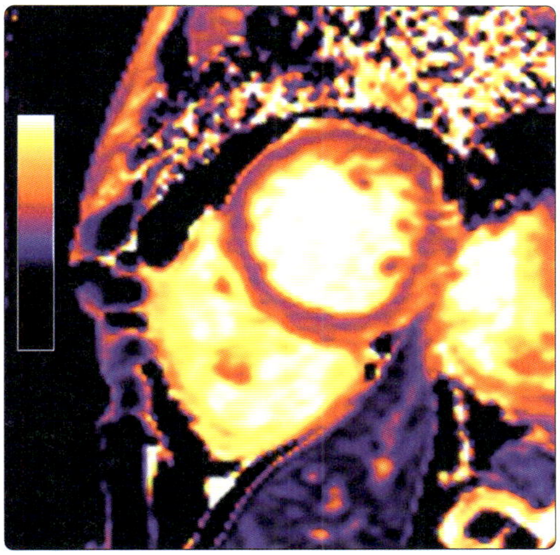

(Left) *Short-axis SSFP MR at diastole in a 45-year-old woman with known Fabry disease and atypical presentation without significant left ventricular hypertrophy shows only mild asymmetric thickening of the interventricular septum (up to 11 mm* ➡*).* **(Right)** *T1 map (MOLLI) in the same patient with a short-axis slice at the midcavity shows diffusely decreased native T1 times (1142 ms at 3T measured at the interventricular septum; lower limit of normal 1153 ms).*

Mechanical Circulatory Assist Devices

KEY FACTS

TERMINOLOGY

- Mechanical pump device used to augment cardiac output for failing ventricle

IMAGING ANATOMY

- Implantable devices typically consist of
  - Inflow cannula, implanted pump device, outflow cannula
- Percutaneous devices have no implanted component and are temporary by design
- Indicators of normal left ventricular assist device function include
  - Neutral interventricular septum; aortic valve closed throughout cardiac cycle

ANATOMY-BASED IMAGING ISSUES

- Field of view should include from aortic arch to abdomen
- Use retrospectively ECG-gated CT with contrast
  - Dacron conduits are not visible radiographically
  - Orientation of inflow cannula in left ventricle is important; ideally, no contact with ventricular walls
- MR is contraindicated

PATHOLOGY-BASED IMAGING ISSUES

- Aortic stenosis occurs in 88% of patients with left ventricular assist device
- Right heart failure occurs in 20-30% of cases

CLINICAL IMPLICATIONS

- Bridge to cardiac transplant
- "Destination" therapy
- Bridge to myocardial recovery

POST-PROCEDURE COMPLICATIONS

- Infection
- Device failure
- Postoperative bleeding

(Left) *PA chest radiograph in a patient with a HeartMate 3 (HM3) left ventricular assist device (LVAD) shows the inflow cannula, proximal outflow cannula, and driveline are radiographically visible. Note that the remainder of the outflow cannula connecting the device to the ascending aorta is not typically visible radiographically.* **(Right)** *Double oblique MIP in the same patient shows the course and patency of the LVAD outflow cannula. This portion is not typically visible radiographically.*

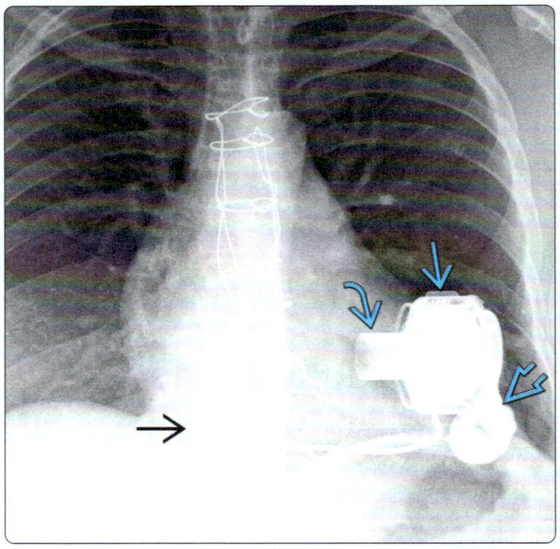

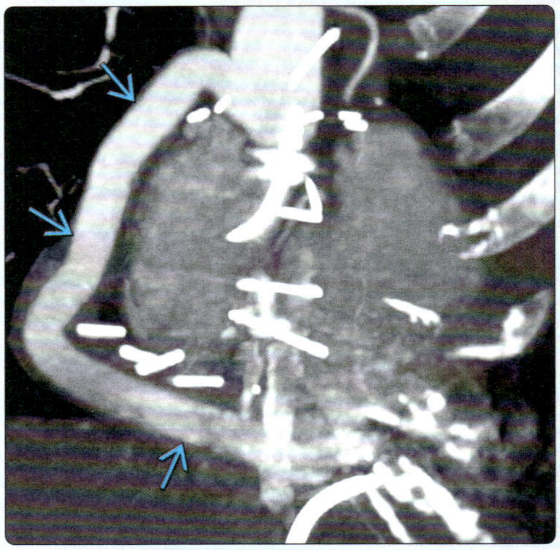

(Left) *Anteroposterior chest radiograph shows a HeartMate II LVAD. The outflow cannula is not radiopaque at its insertion into the ascending aorta. The inflow cannula is at the left apex.* **(Right)** *Graphic shows a HeartMate II (HMII) LVAD. The inflow cannula is in the left ventricular (LV) apex, and the outflow cannula inserts into the ascending aorta. The pump device is smaller in this model, although an external power source (not shown) is still required.*

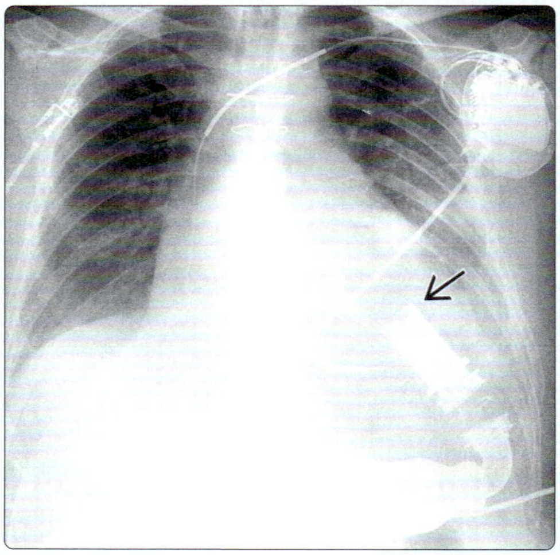

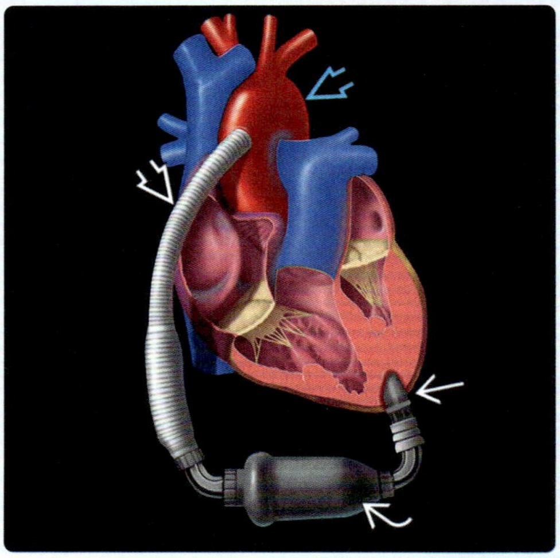

TERMINOLOGY

Definitions

- Mechanical pump device used to augment cardiac output for failing ventricle
  - Left ventricular assist device (LVAD)
    - Diverts oxygenated blood from left heart into aorta, bypassing left ventricular function
  - Right ventricular assist device (RVAD)
    - Diverts blood from right ventricle to pulmonary artery, bypassing right ventricular function
- FDA approval of first LVAD as bridge to transplant was in 1994
  - Heartmate II, III, and HeartWare Ventricular Assist Device (HVAD) are only commercially FDA-approved adult ventricular assist device (VAD) options in North America
  - SynCardia total artificial heart (TAH) is only FDA-approved device in its class
- Impella
  - Transfers oxygenated blood via catheter tip in left ventricle to outlet in ascending aorta by axial flow

IMAGING ANATOMY

General Anatomic Considerations

- Device components are variable
  - Implantable devices are typically composed of
    - Inflow cannula, implanted pump device, and outflow cannula
  - Percutaneous devices have no implanted component and are temporary by design
    - May access left atrium by transseptal puncture via femoral vein; blood is returned via femoral artery cannula (TandemHeart)
    - May access left ventricle by crossing aortic valve via femoral artery or subclavian artery (Impella)
      - Distal tip coiled ideally 3-4 cm across aortic valve and too deep into left ventricle
  - Helium-inflated balloon of intraaortic balloon pump (IABP) inflates during diastole to improve coronary and cerebral blood flow
- Cannula position
  - Inflow cannula at left ventricular apex aligned posteriorly without contacting ventricular wall or angulation
  - Outflow cannula may insert into ascending aorta (2nd or 3rd generation) or ascending/descending aorta (Jarvik 2000 LVAD)
    - May be displaced from retrosternal position to protect cannula in case of repeat sternotomy
    - Coronary grafts may be connected to outflow cannula; hence, chest CT needed before explanation
- Indicators of normal LVAD function
  - Neutral interventricular septum; aortic valve closed throughout cardiac cycle
  - Minimal aortic regurgitation; significant reduction in mitral regurgitation from preop

PATHOLOGY-BASED IMAGING ISSUES

Key Concepts

- Aortic stenosis occurs in 88% of patients with LVAD
- Aortic insufficiency worsens over time with LVAD use
- Right heart failure occurs in 20-30% of cases
  - Increases morbidity and mortality from LVAD
    - Hepatic congestion and bleeding
    - Decreased left ventricular filling
  - Myocardial disease or increased pulmonary vascular resistance
- VAD results in 81% and 70% survival at 1 year and 2 years, respectively

CLINICAL IMPLICATIONS

Clinical Importance

- More effective treatment for end-stage heart failure than medical therapy

Indications

- Bridge to cardiac transplant
  - Effective hemodynamic support
- "Destination" therapy
  - For permanent use in patients not eligible for transplant
- Bridge to myocardial recovery
  - Severe refractory cardiogenic shock

Contraindications

- Impella contraindicated in mechanical aortic valve, aortic valve stenosis, moderate to severe aortic insufficiency

Best Procedure Approach

- Preperitoneal pocket is preferred placement site
- Impella can be implanted via femoral artery or subclavian artery approach

Imaging Findings

- **Radiography**
  - Can visualize radiopaque structures; typically pump component; Dacron conduits are not visible
  - Percutaneous devices are typically placed via femoral vessels
  - Bend relief disconnection; snap ring is out of plane &/or lucency between snap ring and underlying graft
  - TAH: 2 radiolucent pneumatic chambers and 4 mechanical prosthetic valves over cardiac silhouette
- **Echocardiography**
  - Intraoperative and perioperative assessment
  - Evaluation of hemodynamics, valvular and myocardial recovery, left ventricular thrombus after VAD placement
  - Septal deviation to left may indicate right heart failure
  - Transthoracic echocardiogram limited by metal artifact shadowing, smaller acoustic window; transesophageal echocardiogram limited for inflow and outflow limbs of VAD
- **CT**
  - Can visualize conduits as well as more radiodense components; evaluates inflow and outflow cannula
  - Thrombus assessment within LV, inflow or outflow cannula
    - CT limited for device pump thrombosis; echocardiogram well suited
  - Evaluates valvular disease, thickening of leaflets, and valve area for functional analysis
  - Gas or fluid collections around device may indicate infection

- Neointimal hyperplasia; low attenuation between outflow graft and outer Gore-Tex graft of HeartMate II LVAD implant
  - Mimics thrombus

Imaging Protocols

- Retrospectively ECG-gated contrast-enhanced cardiac CT
  - Additional standard nongated CECT of abdomen
  - Include entire subcutaneous course of driveline for infection assessment
  - Unenhanced CT sufficient for mediastinal or retroperitoneal hematoma evaluation
- MR is contraindicated

Imaging Pitfalls

- Portions of outflow cannula may not be visible radiographically
- Impella curled tip should be within left ventricle; outflow portion should be in ascending aorta
- IABP radiopaque tip ideally within center of aortic arch or ~ 2 cm above carina
- TandemHeart tip should be within left atrium; outflow portion should be in femoral arteries
- Neointimal hyperplasia can mimic graft thrombus

EQUIPMENT

Types

- Extracorporeal nonpulsatile
- Extracorporeal pulsatile
- Implantable pulsatile
- TAH

Components

- Pump: Surgically implanted in abdomen
- Inflow conduit: Conducts blood from left ventricular apex to pump
- Outflow conduit: Conducts blood from pump to ascending or descending aorta or main pulmonary artery
- Internal valves: Ensures unidirectional flow
- External power source
- External controller: System function settings, system status

Devices

- 1st-generation pulsatile pumps simulate cardiac cycle
  - HeartMate XVE Implantable; Thoratec VAD; Novacor Implantable
- 2nd-generation nonpulsatile continuous flow pumps
  - HeartMate II and Jarvik 2000 (commonly available); INCOR; DeBakey VAD
- 3rd-generation continuous centrifugal flow pump
  - HeartWare and HeartMate III
  - LVAD or biventricular support
  - Compared to 2nd generation, better event-free survival, less pump thrombosis, stroke, or bleeding
- Percutaneous ventricular assist device (pVAD): Impella, TandemHeart
- TAH; preferred in massive myocardial damage and failed cardiac transplant
  - SynCardia TAH most commonly used

POST PROCEDURE

Expected Outcome

- Typically bridge to cardiac transplant or myocardial recovery
- Reverse remodeling while on LVAD has been described

Complications

- Infection
  - Driveline site infection is most common LVAD-associated infection
- Device failure
  - Low-flow rates
    - Cannula obstruction due to hypertrophic ventricular wall, right heart failure, thrombus, reverse left ventricular remodeling
    - Tamponade, hypovolemia
  - Pump thrombosis can involve inflow and outflow cannula or pump housing
  - Tearing at cannula attachment site; bend relief disconnection, kinking of outflow grafts, driveline fracture
- Postoperative bleeding
  - Hemopericardium, mediastinal hemorrhage, tamponade
  - Focal accumulations of blood around inflow or outflow cannulas may be expected postoperative finding
  - Hemolysis due to thrombosis, malpositioned cannulas, bend relief disconnection, and postoperative complications
- Cardiac complications
  - Aortic stenosis or insufficiency, arrhythmia from cannula contact with ventricle wall
  - Development of right ventricular failure can occur due to increased preload from increased left ventricular outflow
- Thromboembolism
  - Pulmonary, cerebral, other end organs
- Pleural complications
  - Pneumothorax, hemothorax
- Abdominal
  - Hemoperitoneum, bowel obstruction, abscess, gastrointestinal bleeding with continuous-flow devices
- Explantation complications
  - Tear of cannula or graft, diaphragmatic defects, left ventricular pseudoaneurysm and thrombus
- Complications of Syncardia TAH
  - Left superior pulmonary vein and inferior vena cava compression, device malfunction due to air leak
- IABP complications
  - Limb ischemia, vascular perforation or dissection, hematoma

SELECTED REFERENCES

1. Scott A et al: Preoperative computed tomography assessment of risk of right ventricle failure after left ventricular assist device placement. ASAIO J. 69(1):69-75, 2023
2. Cole SP et al: Imaging for temporary mechanical circulatory support devices. J Cardiothorac Vasc Anesth. 36(7):2114-31, 2022
3. Dilsizian V et al: Best practices for imaging cardiac device-related infections and endocarditis: A JACC: Cardiovascular Imaging Expert Panel Statement. JACC Cardiovasc Imaging. 15(5):891-911, 2022
4. Kligerman S et al: Imaging of cardiac support devices. Radiol Clin North Am. 58(1):151-65, 2020

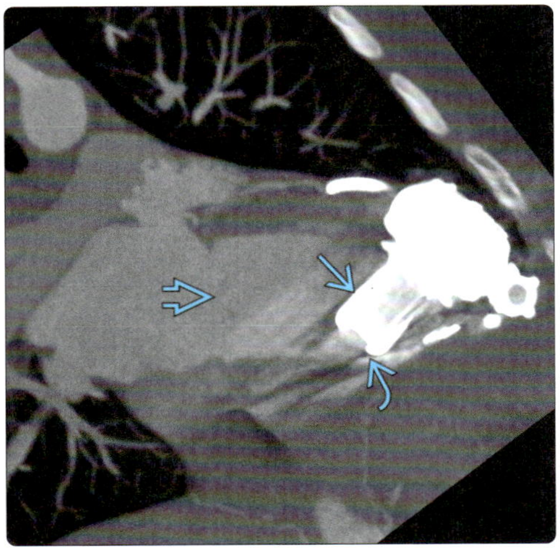

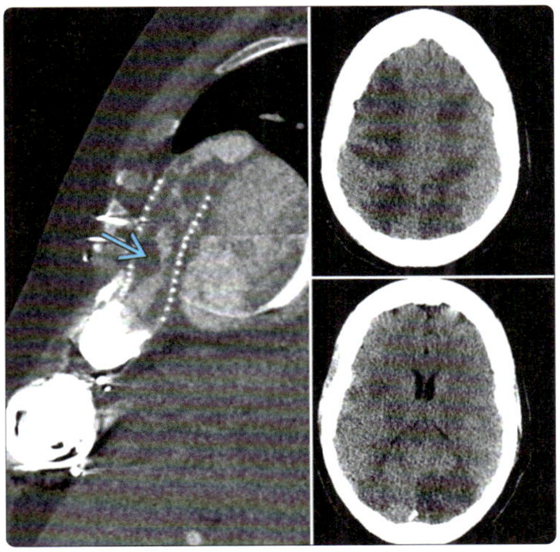

(Left) *Sagittal oblique CT in a patient with a HHM3 LVAD and low-flow shows the inflow cannula oriented inferoseptally and abutting the inferior LV septum . The inflow cannula should be oriented along the axis of the LV toward the mitral valve .* **(Right)** *Sagittal oblique CECT of the outflow cannula of a HMII LVAD (left) shows large volume thrombus . Head CT performed 1 day later (right) shows extensive bilateral infarcts, which are likely due to a combination or emboli and hypoperfusion.*

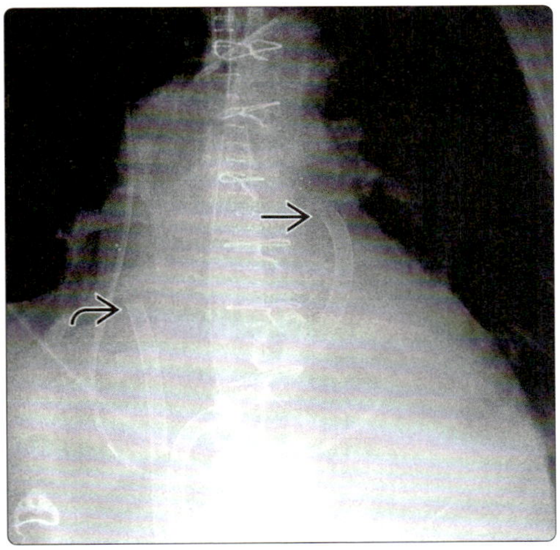

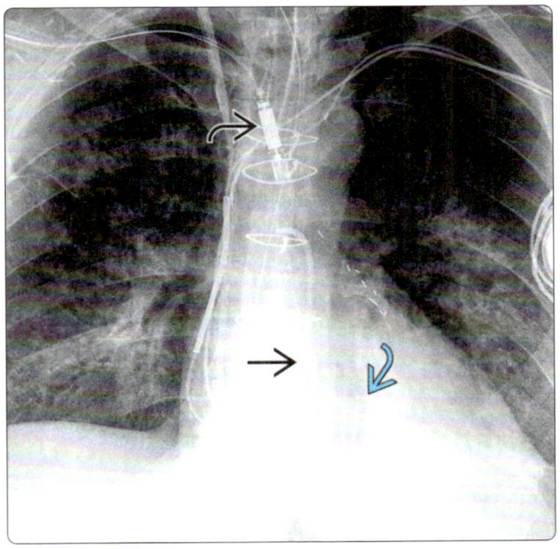

(Left) *AP chest radiograph shows a right ventricular assist device with its inflow cannula in the right atrium and its outflow cannula in the right ventricular outflow tract . The pump device is external to the patient, placed via the femoral vein.* **(Right)** *Percutaneous LVAD (Impella) is shown. The pigtail is just beyond aortic valve, not reaching the LV apex. The inlet area is located proximal to the pigtail in the mid LV, and the outlet area is in the ascending aorta.*

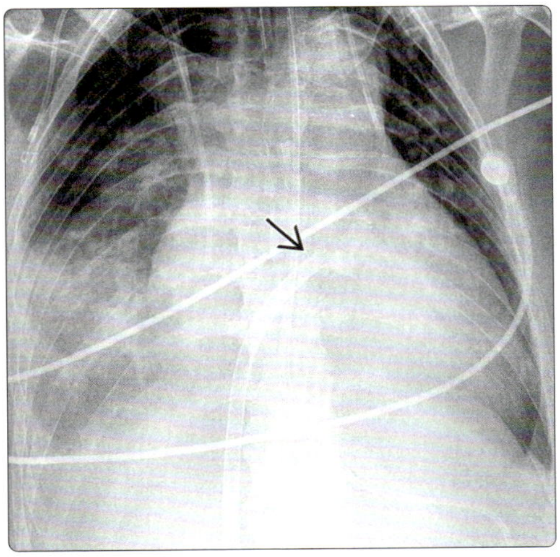

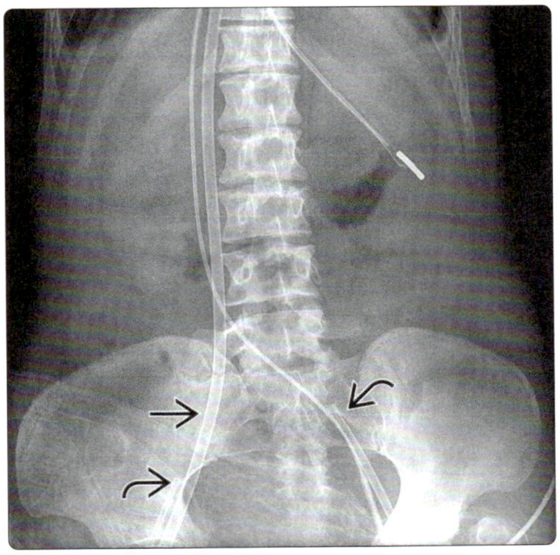

(Left) *AP chest radiograph shows a TandemHeart LVAD placed via the right femoral vein. The inflow cannula of the device accesses the left atrium via a transseptal puncture.* **(Right)** *AP abdominal radiograph in the same patient shows the inflow cannula placed via the right femoral vein. The pump is external to the patient, and the outflow cannula is placed in the femoral artery for retrograde perfusion of the aorta and systemic circulation.*

Heart Transplant

KEY FACTS

TERMINOLOGY

- Most frequent form: Orthotopic cardiac allograft transplantation
- Operative technique: Biatrial anastomosis, bicaval anastomosis
- Acute cellular rejection
  - T-cell-mediated inflammatory response leading to myocardial edema and myocyte damage
  - Occurs with decreasing frequency with increasing time interval since transplantation
  - Usually detected by endomyocardial biopsy in asymptomatic stage
- Coronary transplant vasculopathy
  - Diffuse intimal thickening of coronary vessels with potential luminal narrowing and obstruction, ischemia, and graft failure
- Transplant coronary atherosclerosis
  - Follows normal pattern of coronary artery disease

IMAGING

- Assessment of left ventricular function
  - Echocardiography, MR
- Assessment of cardiac allograft vasculopathy and transplant coronary atherosclerosis
  - Ischemia imaging by stress echocardiography, myocardial perfusion imaging, and MR
  - Invasive angiography + intravascular ultrasound; coronary CTA
- Assessment of acute rejection
  - Endomyocardial biopsy; gallium-67 scintigraphy
  - Impaired diastolic function: Echocardiography, MR
  - Imaging of edema by MR

CLINICAL ISSUES

- Acute rejection occurs most frequently in 1st year
- Graft vasculopathy has increasing prevalence in following years, ~ 50% after 10 years

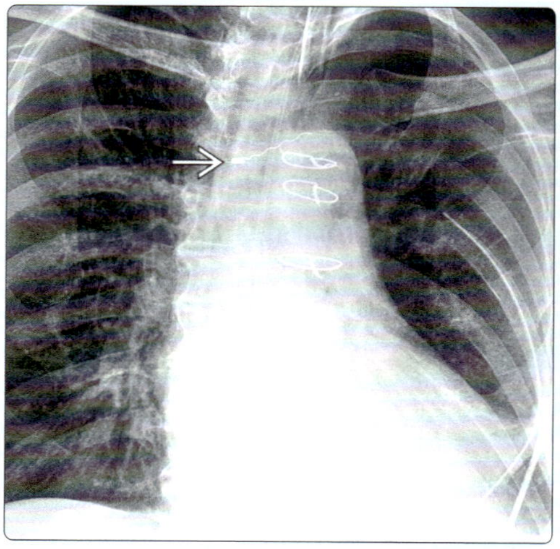
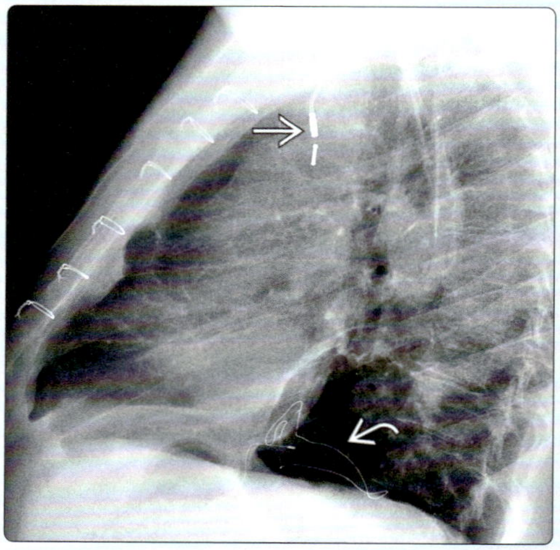

(Left) *Anteroposterior chest radiograph in a patient after a heart transplant shows retained portions of a cardiac pacing wire ➔ in the left brachiocephalic vein and sternotomy wires, which may be clues to the history of orthotopic heart transplant when that clinical information is unavailable.* **(Right)** *Lateral chest radiograph status post heart transplantation shows retained cardiac pacing wire fragments ➔ and left ventricular epicardial pacing wires ➔.*

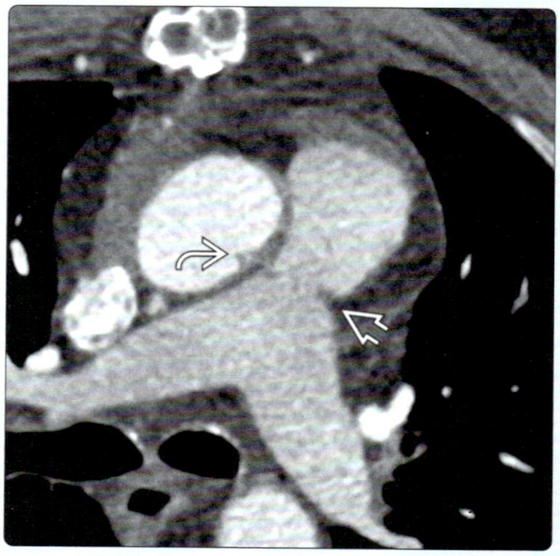
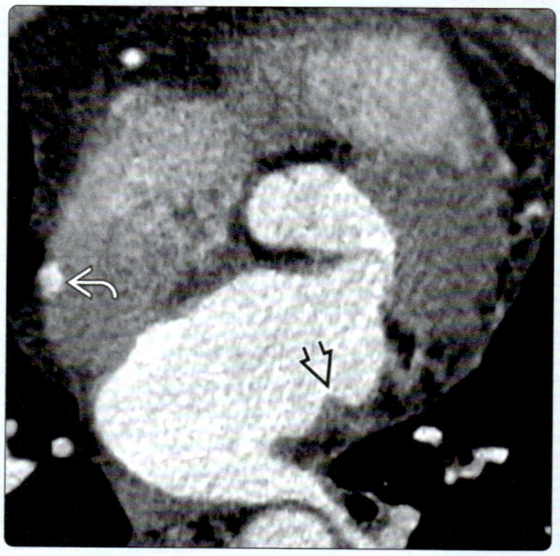

(Left) *Axial CECT status post median sternotomy shows suture material and indentations at the aortic ➔ and pulmonary arterial ➔ anastomoses that are present in all commonly performed orthotopic heart transplantations.* **(Right)** *Axial CECT in a patient status post orthotopic heart transplantation shows suture material at the right atrial wall ➔, atrial waist due to anastomosis at the left atrium ➔, and characteristic biatrial elongation.*

TERMINOLOGY

Definitions

- Most frequent form: Orthotopic cardiac allograft transplantation
  - Replacement of patient's heart with human donor's organ
  - Bicaval technique now considered preferable
    - Recipient's right atrium removed with excised heart
    - Donor's right atrium preserved
    - Anastomosis at superior and inferior vena cava, left atrium, aorta, and pulmonary artery
  - Biatrial technique still performed
    - Anastomosis at right and left atria, aorta, and pulmonary artery
    - Associated with higher rates of
      - Early and late tricuspid regurgitation
      - Early need for permanent pacemaker placement
- Other forms of transplantation
  - Heterotopic cardiac allograft transplantation
    - Infrequently performed
  - Cardiac xenograft transplantation
    - Very rare
- Common complications of cardiac transplantation
  - Acute cellular rejection
  - Cardiac allograft vasculopathy (CAV)

IMAGING

General Features

- Most common procedure: Orthotopic cardiac allograft transplantation
  - Bicaval anastomosis: Anastomosis of
    - Superior and inferior vena cava
    - Left atrium, aorta, and pulmonary artery
  - Biatrial anastomosis (a.k.a. Shumway technique): Anastomosis of
    - Right and left atrium
    - Aorta and pulmonary artery
  - Total transplantation (a.k.a. Banner technique): Anastomosis of
    - Vena cava superior and inferior, aorta, pulmonary artery and veins
- Common complications of cardiac transplantation
  - Early postoperative complications (< 30 days)
    - Pneumonia, pulmonary interstitial/alveolar edema, pneumothorax and pneumomediastinum, pleural effusion, sternal dehiscence
  - Intermediate postoperative complications (1-12 months)
    - Allograft failure and rejection
    - CAV
  - Late posttransplant complications (> 12 months)
    - Coronary atherosclerosis
      - May have been transplanted with heart
      - May develop in accelerated form after transplant
    - Malignancies: Lung cancer, lymphoma

Imaging Recommendations

- Best imaging tool
  - Echocardiography
    - Used for assessing left and right ventricular function
  - Cardiac MR
    - Best modality to identify transplant rejection and left and right ventricular failure
  - Invasive coronary angiography, intravascular ultrasound, and coronary CTA
    - Used for identifying coronary atherosclerosis and CAV
  - MR and gallium-67 scintigraphy
    - May identify transplant rejection
  - Endomyocardial biopsy (EMB)
    - Frequently performed for rejection monitoring
- Protocol advice
  - Monitoring allograft systolic function important in suspected or known rejection
  - LGE imaging and T2WI should be included in cardiovascular MR protocol
  - Renal insufficiency is common in transplant patients
    - Iodinated contrast and gadolinium should be used judiciously and with precautions
  - Heart rate control may be challenging when performing coronary CTA

Echocardiographic Findings

- Used to assess left ventricular systolic and diastolic functions
  - Left ventricular diastolic dysfunction can be early sign of acute cellular rejection
- Wall motion abnormalities in stress echocardiography can indicate presence of hemodynamically relevant coronary atherosclerosis or coronary allograft vasculopathy

Angiographic Findings

- Invasive coronary angiography
  - Often performed in serial fashion (annually) to monitor for coronary atherosclerosis and CAV
    - Focal stenosis suggests coronary atherosclerosis
    - Diffuse narrowing suggests CAV
    - Both can be present without detectable narrowing
  - Intracoronary ultrasound may be used to identify coronary artery affection not identified by angiography
    - Concentric intimal thickening in case of transplant vasculopathy
    - Eccentric lesions in case of transplant atherosclerosis

Radiographic Findings

- Double right atrial contours (overlap of donor and recipient right atria in orthotopic transplant)
- Residual cardiac pacer wire fragments in thoracic veins

CT Findings

- Atrial waist due to anastomosis of right and left donors and recipient atria
- Coronary calcium
  - May occur in both CAV or coronary atherosclerosis
- Coronary CTA
  - May be difficult to perform posttransplantation when heart rate is high and difficult to control
  - Diffuse plaque involving both proximal and distal parts of vessel with distal pruning in CAV
  - Localized eccentric plaque and stenosis (especially in proximal part) in case of coronary artery disease

MR Findings

- Best method to quantify left and right ventricular function
- Allows assessment of entire myocardium compared to EMB
- Detection of transplant vasculopathy
  - Several techniques have been suggested
    - Stress myocardial perfusion MR
    - LGE of coronary artery wall
    - Subendocardial delayed enhancement suggestive of silent myocardial infarction (MI)
- Detection of acute rejection
  - Abnormal T2 prolongation is strong predictor of rejection when clinically suspected
  - High negative predictive value of T2 relaxation times
  - Quantitative T2 mapping can improve T2 detection
  - Can be used to monitor treatment response
    - Elevated T2 values in patients with acute rejection was found to be normalized within 2 months after treatment
  - T1 mapping could be useful in diagnosis of acute rejection (≥ grade 2) and tracking recovery after treatment
    - Sensitivity 93%, specificity 79%, and negative predictive value 99%

DIFFERENTIAL DIAGNOSIS

Left Ventricular Dysfunction Following Heart Transplantation

- Consequence of allograft rejection
- Consequence of ischemia
  - Coronary atherosclerosis
  - CAV
- Consequence of recipient disease reaffecting transplanted heart (infrequent)
  - Amyloid, sarcoid, hemochromatosis, giant cell myocarditis

Coronary Arterial Narrowing or Occlusion Following Heart Transplantation

- Often lack of symptoms due to denervation of transplanted heart
- Manifests as shortness of breath or reduced left ventricular function
- Sequel of transplant vasculopathy
  - Coronary vessel wall thickening and luminal narrowing with diffuse pattern and concentric morphology
- Sequel of coronary artery disease
  - Focal occurrence and eccentric morphology

PATHOLOGY

General Features

- Etiology
  - Disease processes that require transplantation
    - Nonischemic cardiomyopathy: 50%
    - Ischemic cardiomyopathy: 40%
    - Valvular heart disease: 3%
    - Adult congenital heart disease: 2%

CLINICAL ISSUES

Demographics

- Epidemiology
  - Over 5,000 cardiac transplants are performed worldwide annually
    - 2,000-3,000 in USA each year
  - Prevalence of CAV
    - 8% within 1st year
    - 32% within first 5 years
    - 50% within first 10 years

Natural History & Prognosis

- EMB may be used for surveillance or diagnosis of rejection
- 1-year survival of heart transplant recipients: 90%
- 5-year survival rate: ~ 70%
- Graft half-life: ~ 10 years
- Causes of death
  - In 1st year after surgery
    - Graft failure and infectious disease are leading causes of death
    - Infectious disease accounts for almost 33% of deaths
    - Acute rejection accounts for 12% of deaths
  - Beyond 1st year
    - Transplant vasculopathy
    - Malignancies
      - Lung cancer is most common
      - Lymphoproliferative disorders and skin cancer are also common
      - Incidence of any malignancy is 35% by 10 years

Treatment

- Retransplantation is required in 2% of cases
- Posttransplant immunosuppression often includes
  - Calcineurin inhibitors (ciclosporin, tacrolimus, etc.)
  - mTOR inhibitors (sirolimus, everolimus, etc.)
  - Antimetabolites (mycophenolate, azathioprine) and steroids (prednisone)

DIAGNOSTIC CHECKLIST

Consider

- Orthotopic transplantation shows elongated left atrium due to anastomosis of donor's heart with recipient's atria
- 2 atrial appendages may be present
- Impaired left ventricular function may be due to
  - Rejection
  - Ischemia
  - Suboptimal donor heart
  - Recipient disease (re)affecting transplanted heart
- Malignancies occur at increased rates in transplant patients

SELECTED REFERENCES

1. Kamel MA et al: Cardiac allograft vasculopathy: challenges and advances in invasive and non-invasive diagnostic modalities. J Cardiovasc Dev Dis. 11(3), 2024
2. Randhawa MK et al: Role of radiology in assessment of postoperative complications of heart transplantation. Radiol Clin North Am. 62(3):453-71, 2024
3. Ortega-Legaspi JM et al: Diagnosis and management of cardiac allograft vasculopathy. Heart. 108(8):586-92, 2022

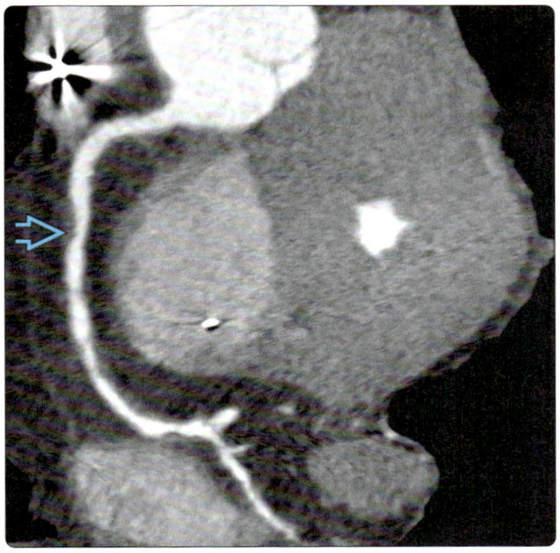

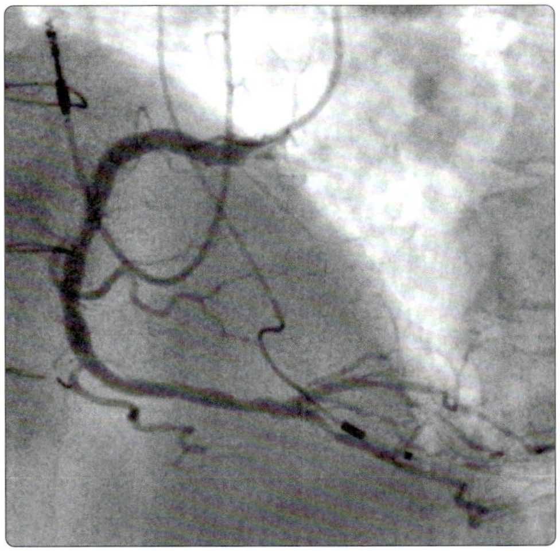

(Left) *Double oblique reformat from an ECG-gated CTA in a patient status post orthotopic heart transplantation shows diffuse luminal narrowing of the right coronary artery secondary to a noncalcified plaque ⇨. CTA may be difficult to perform in transplant patients with high heart rates.* **(Right)** *Angiography of the right coronary artery in the same patient shows diffuse luminal narrowing and irregularity. Angiography may be used as a surveillance technique for coronary allograft vasculopathy.*

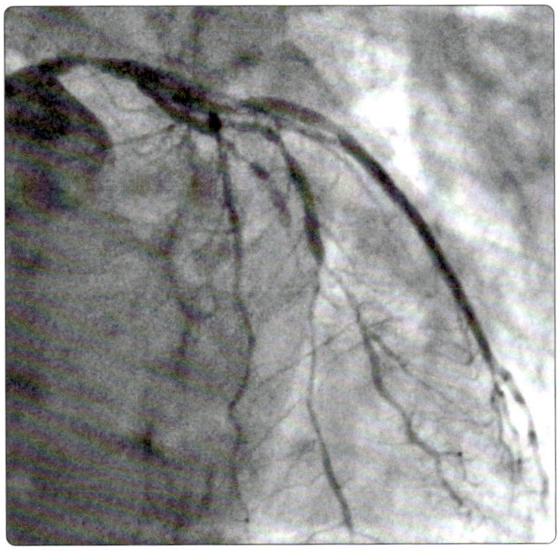

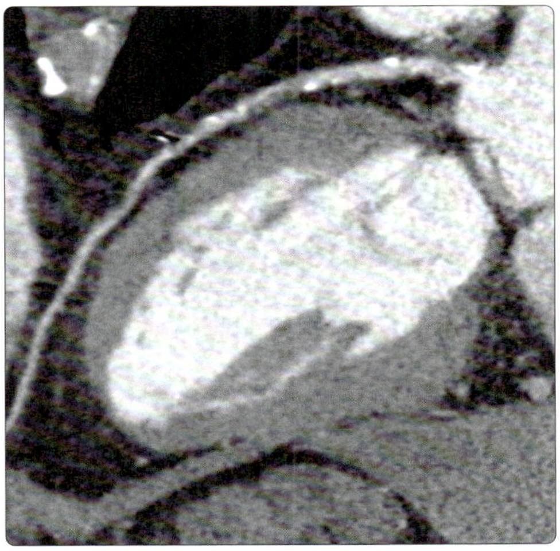

(Left) *Angiography of the left anterior descending (LAD) artery shows diffuse luminal narrowing of the coronary arteries, consistent with cardiac allograft vasculopathy. Plaque in this disease tends to be concentric and diffuse.* **(Right)** *Curved MPR coronary CTA shows moderate amount of calcified and noncalcified plaques in the LAD coronary artery leading to at least moderate stenosis in a patient 3 years after heart transplant.*

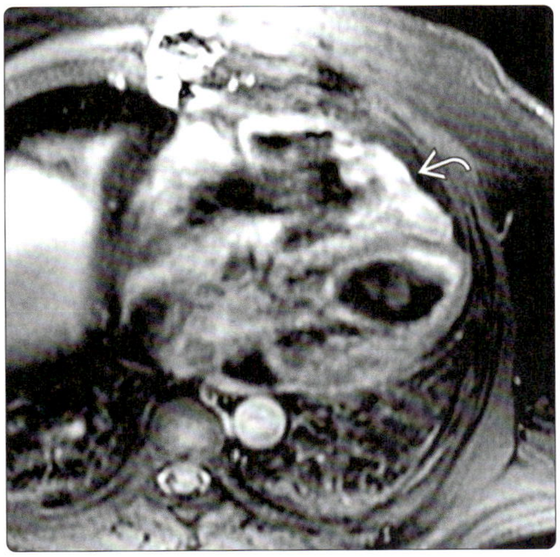

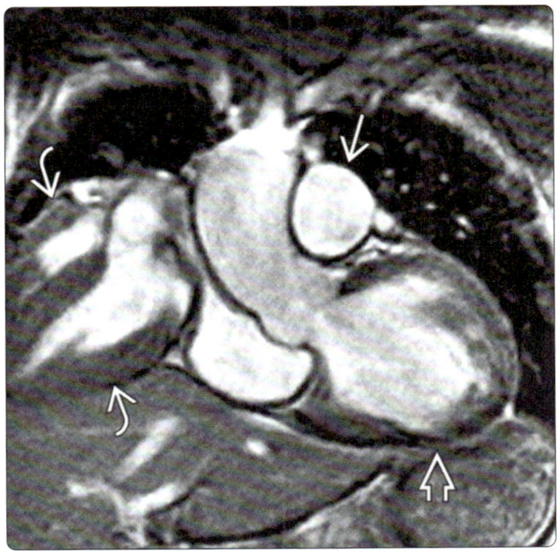

(Left) *Four-chamber T2WI FS cardiac MR shows diffuse hyperintensity of the right ventricular free wall ➩, suspicious for mural edema and transplant rejection. Abnormal T2 prolongation is a strong predictor of rejection when clinically suspected.* **(Right)** *Coronal SSFP cardiac MR shows a heterotopic heart transplant ➩. The native pulmonary artery ➡ and left ventricle ⇨ are enlarged. This transplant is rarely performed and is used in patients with severe pulmonary arterial hypertension or a small donor heart.*

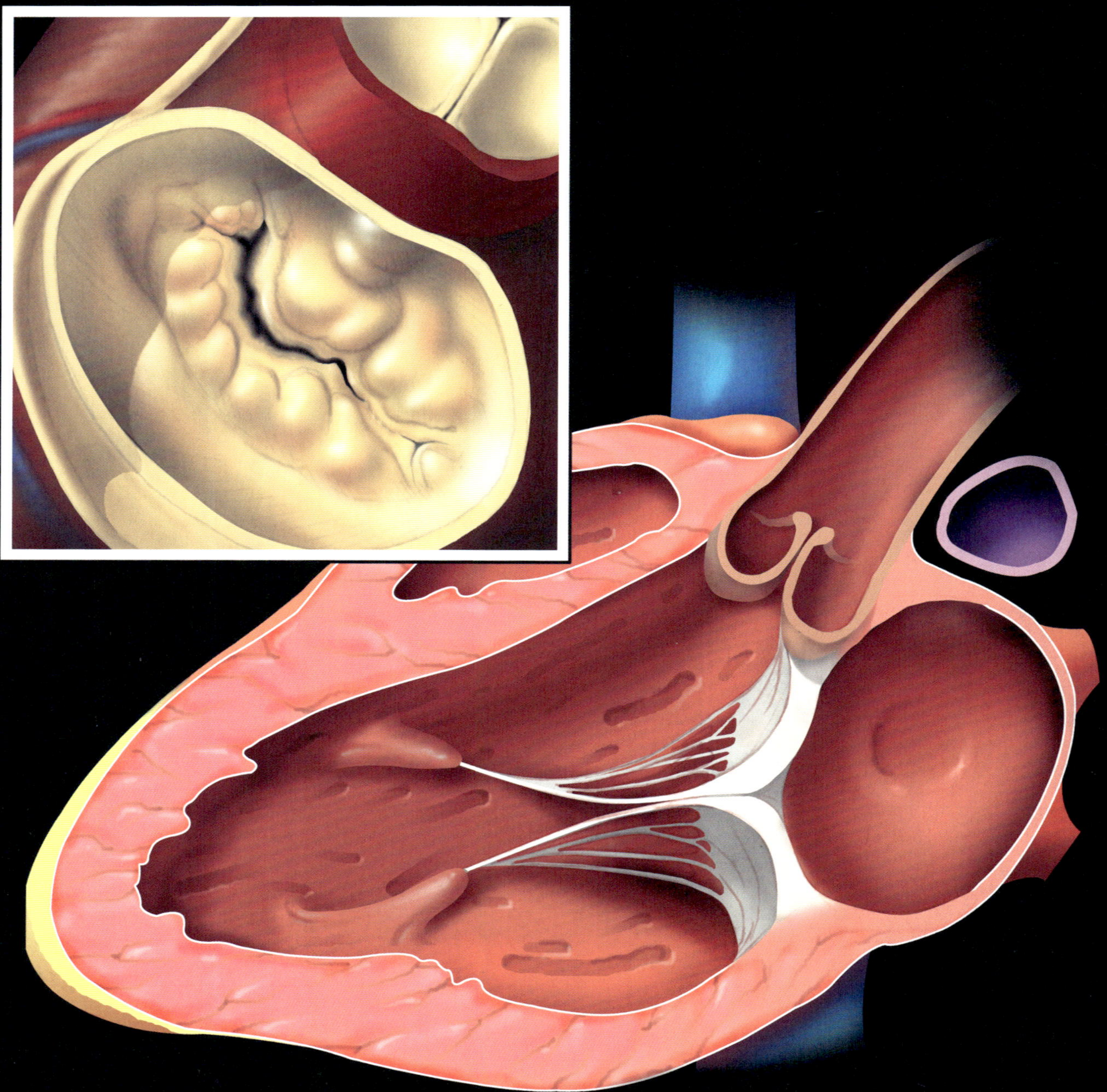

SECTION 4

Valvular

Introduction

Valvular heart disease is very common and surgical repair of valve disease comprises ~ 10-20% of all cardiac surgical procedures. Echocardiography is the initial modality used to evaluate patients with suspected valvular dysfunction.

Echocardiography (echo) is widely available and portable, has excellent temporal resolution, and is relatively cost-effective. Valvular assessment during echo can be limited due to patient body habitus, anatomic location of certain valves, and interoperator variability.

CT and MR imaging are used to characterize valvular dysfunction in select patients. MR can evaluate valvular anatomy, quantify valvular regurgitation, and measure velocities and gradients across valves. MR is beneficial, as it can also quantify ventricular mass and function, which aids the surgeon in appropriately timing valve replacement surgery. CT is used for preprocedural evaluation before the transcatheter valvular replacement. This chapter describes the role of CT and MR in the evaluation of valvular disease.

Anatomy and Physiology

There are 2 atrioventricular (tricuspid and mitral) and 2 semilunar (pulmonic and aortic) valves. The pulmonic and aortic valves each have 3 cusps and open during systole when ventricular pressure exceeds the pressure in the pulmonary trunk or aorta, respectively. The tricuspid and mitral valves open during ventricular diastole. An important identifying feature of the morphologic right ventricle is that the tricuspid and pulmonic valves are separated from each other by a muscular ridge of tissue called the crista supraventricularis or conus, whereas the mitral and aortic valves are in fibrous continuity, a defining feature of the left ventricle.

The main function of the cardiac valves is to allow unidirectional blood flow through the cardiac chambers while maintaining a low-pressure gradient. Generally, valve regurgitation causes chamber dilatation, such as left atrial and left ventricular dilation in mitral regurgitation. Valve stenosis causes ventricular hypertrophy, such as left ventricular hypertrophy with aortic stenosis, and atrial dilation, such as left atrial dilation in the setting of mitral stenosis.

Role of MR

Steady-state free precession (SSFP) MR with ECG gating is the primary sequence used for the evaluation of cardiac valve morphology and for measuring the orifice area. Images are acquired in multiple orthogonal planes to the valve of interest in addition to the standard cardiac views (e.g., 4 chamber, paraseptal long axis, and 3 chamber). Valvular stenosis and regurgitation cause turbulent blood flow, leading to spin dephasing and signal voids (black jets). A black jet originating from the valve directed forward into the receiving chamber or vessel indicates valvular stenosis, whereas a jet directed retrograde from the valve indicates valvular regurgitation. Unlike echocardiography, MR cannot use the size and magnitude of the dephasing jet to quantify the degree of valve stenosis or regurgitation; these should be used simply as markers to diagnose the abnormality.

MR is widely considered the noninvasive reference standard for determining myocardial mass, ventricular volumes, and ventricular function. Ventricular function and volumes are calculated after tracing the ventricular cavity contour at end-systole and end-diastole, usually on short-axis images. These measurements are summed to yield end-systolic and end-diastolic volumes, which are then used to calculate ventricular stroke volume and ejection fraction. The myocardial mass is calculated by tracing the endocardial and epicardial borders at end-diastole and summing the measurements. The calculated volumes and myocardial mass are corrected for the patient's body surface area and then compared to a standard table of reference normals. Calculated ventricular function and volumes are used by the surgeon and cardiologist to assess the effect of the valvular abnormality on the heart and may influence the timing of surgery.

Several **direct** and **indirect** methods are available for **quantifying** the degree of **valve regurgitation** or **stenosis**. **Direct quantification** of the degree of valve regurgitation or stenosis can be performed with velocity-encoded cine (VEC) phase-contrast (PC) techniques. Traditional PC sequences used for flow quantification are acquired through-plane during a single breath hold. However, given the complexity of flow dynamics, the localization of a single through-plane PC sequence may not be truly perpendicular to the plane of flow or may be remote from the region of peak velocity, leading to inaccuracies in measurement. However, creation of in-plane PC sequences allows for the acquisition of a time-resolved cine sequence for all 3 planes at the same time using respiratory and cardiac gating. While this sequence, termed 4D-flow, often takes around 10 minutes to complete, through-plane measurements can be obtained anywhere in the 3-dimension slab.

Direct measurement of the maximal valve opening area or the size of the regurgitation orifice (so-called valve planimetry) can be performed with SSFP imaging in a plane parallel to the valve of interest. **Indirect quantification** of valve regurgitation can be performed by comparing ventricular stroke volumes. Under normal circumstances, the right and left ventricular stroke volumes are equal. In the presence of a single regurgitant valve, the stroke volume increases on the abnormal side, and the difference between the stroke volumes of the 2 ventricles is equal to the regurgitant volume. Importantly, this method is inaccurate when there are cardiac shunts or when more than 1 valve is abnormal.

Role of CT

Excluding preoperative assessment prior to transcatheter valvular replacement, ECG-gated CT is a 2nd-line modality in evaluating patients with suspected valvular disease due to its use of ionizing radiation and intravenous contrast. CT is used in select patients, such as those who have contraindications to MR (e.g., claustrophobia or MR-incompatible pacemaker) or those with nondiagnostic or limited echocardiography due to body habitus or emphysema. One advantage of CT is that it can assess the burden of coronary artery disease prior to valve replacement surgery. For assessing postoperative complications, CT is often the study of choice due to its excellent spatial resolution and speed of acquisition.

Compared to MR, CT has a superior spatial resolution, which is now as low as 0.2 mm. While the temporal resolution is down to 66 m/sec with certain scanners, CT has a lower temporal resolution when compared with both echocardiography and MR. Ideally, valve evaluation is conducted on a 64-slice (or higher) CT scanner with most studies being acquired in < 6 sec. The voltage, pitch, and tube current vary depending on the patient's weight and heart rate. Patients with a low body mass index can have excellent image quality with reduced tube voltages of 70-100 kV, which also allows for reduced contrast dose. While 140 kV can be used in select patients with extremely large body habitus, it should be avoided in nearly all instances. However, with newer photon-counting CT technology, 140 kV is often recommended for improved spectral separation. Computer software that allows automated adjustment of many parameters is now available. Image reconstruction parameters vary depending on preferences, but submillimeter isotropic images should be used for evaluation.

Imaging obtained during the entire cardiac cycle (low-pitch helical acquisition or long z-axis axial acquisition) is usually used for valve assessment to visualize leaflet mobility and coaptation. Tube current modulation, limited field of view, and iterative reconstruction are helpful in reducing the radiation dose.

The degree of aortic valve calcification positively correlates with the aortic stenosis severity. The amount of calcification can be quantified using the Agatston method. Measurement of maximal valve area (valve planimetry) has shown excellent correlation in predicting the severity of aortic stenosis when compared with direct measurement by transesophageal echocardiography or indirect measurement using the continuity equation in transthoracic echocardiography.

Transcatheter Valve Replacement

The use of CT for preprocedural evaluation in transcatheter valve replacement has significantly increased in recent years due to the expansion of transcatheter approaches for valves other than the aortic valve. Currently, transcatheter procedures for mitral, tricuspid, and pulmonary valve replacements are performed, all of which require CT evaluation prior to the procedure.

Transcatheter aortic valve replacement (TAVR) can be performed via transfemoral/subclavian, transapical, transaortic, or carotid access. Preprocedural CTA is used to assess aortic and anulus size, aortic calcification pattern, degree of aortic valve calcification, distance of the coronary arteries to the aortic anulus, recommended fluoroscopic projection angle, and peripheral access suitability. Additionally, CTA of the chest, abdomen, and pelvis is performed to evaluate for peripheral access suitability (e.g., minimal iliac and subclavian artery luminal diameter; minimal common femoral artery diameter; and the presence of dissection, vascular tortuosity, and circumferential vascular calcification).

Valve-in-valve procedures have evolved as an important treatment strategy in patients with degenerating prosthetic valves. In these patients, it is important to measure the internal diameter of the failed valve prior to the procedure. Furthermore, CT and MR may also be used in patients who are undergoing percutaneous repair of other valvular disorders, such as the MitraClip device in patients with mitral regurgitation, or transcatheter pulmonic valve replacement in patients with pulmonic regurgitation. CT plays an important role in detecting complications after transcatheter valve replacement, such as paravalvular leak, aortic dissection, and complications at the access site, such as pseudoaneurysm or hematoma.

Special Cases

Valvular Masses

Most valvular masses are vegetations related to endocarditis, which is common in intravenous drug users and patients with prosthetic valves. Echocardiography is the primary modality used to diagnose vegetations. Gated CT can often visualize even small submillimeter vegetations and can accurately delineate a perivalvular abscess and important extracardiac findings (e.g., septic emboli). Soft tissue contrast of MR can help differentiate a valvular mass from a vegetation in addition to assessing valvular injury do to endocarditis.

Papillary fibroelastoma (PF) is the most common primary cardiac neoplasm. It is rare and typically affects left-sided valves (aortic > mitral). Patients are generally asymptomatic but may present with symptoms/signs of peripheral thromboembolism (e.g., stroke or limb ischemia). Unlike a vegetation, a PF does lead to valvular destruction. Most PF are < 1 cm in size and may have low or high T2 signal on MR. They may be difficult to visualize on CT or MR due to their small size. Larger tumors enhance following administration of a gadolinium chelate contrast agent. Myxoma, sarcoma, hemangioma, or metastatic tumors rarely involve cardiac valves.

Valvular Prostheses

Valve replacement surgery is most commonly performed on the aortic and mitral valves. There are 2 types of artificial valves: Bioprosthetic (tissue) and mechanical. Tissue valves have a shorter lifespan compared to artificial valves but do not require lifelong anticoagulation. Annuloplasty with a ring device is most commonly used in the setting of tricuspid or mitral regurgitation.

While MR can be used, echocardiography and CT are the primary tools used in assessing postsurgical complications (e.g., endocarditis, perivalvular abscess, dehiscence, obstruction, perivalvular leak, or pseudoaneurysm) related to valvular prostheses.

Important Considerations for Reporting

Valvular anatomy and morphology
- Number of leaflets
- Morphology of leaflets: Prolapse, rupture, calcification, thickening, or fusion
- Presence of perivalvular aneurysm, abscess, etc.
- Cross-sectional valvular area

Valvular function
- Stenosis or regurgitation
- Valve opening and closing pattern

Valvular effect on cardiac function
- Ventricular ejection fractions and end-diastolic volumes
- Diastolic filling
- Regional and global ventricular wall motion
- Myocardial mass

Associations that may influence surgical approach
- Myocardial viability (MR)
- Obstructive coronary artery disease (CT)
- Thrombus; aortic coarctation

Selected References

1. Zoghbi WA et al: Guidelines for the evaluation of prosthetic valve function with cardiovascular imaging: a report from the American Society of Echocardiography developed in collaboration with the Society for Cardiovascular Magnetic Resonance and the Society of Cardiovascular Computed Tomography. J Am Soc Echocardiogr. 37(1):2-63, 2024
2. Reid A et al: Multimodality imaging in valvular heart disease: how to use state-of-the-art technology in daily practice. Eur Heart J. 42(19):1912-25, 2021

Anatomy of Cardiac Skeleton

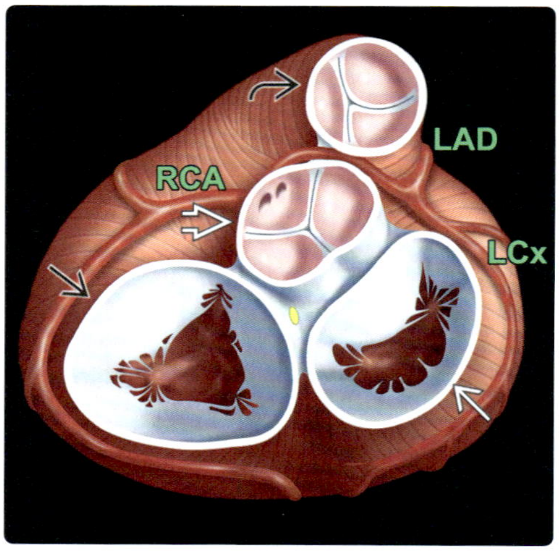

Normal Trileaflet Aortic Valve

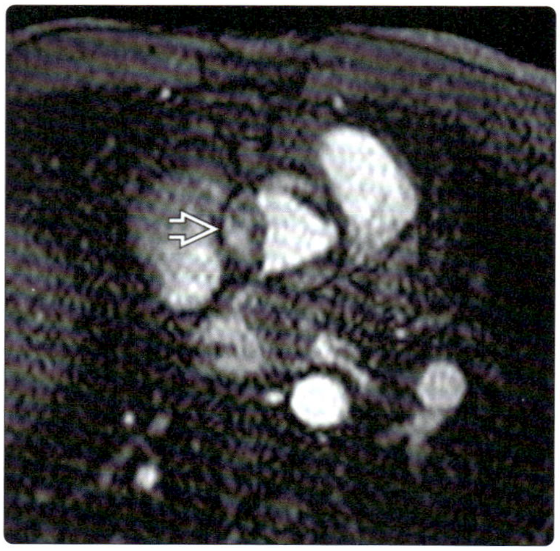

(Left) *Graphic demonstrates the anatomy of the cardiac skeleton between the atria and ventricles. The cardiac skeleton consists of thick, fibrous connective tissue and provides support for the valve orifices. Note that the mitral ➡ and aortic ➡ valves are in fibrous continuity, whereas the tricuspid ➡ and pulmonic ➡ valves are separated by a muscular infundibulum. Also note the anomalous left main coronary artery.* **(Right)** *Axial steady-state free precession (SSFP) MR shows a normal trileaflet aortic valve ➡ during ventricular systole.*

Tricuspid Leaflets and Mitral Valves

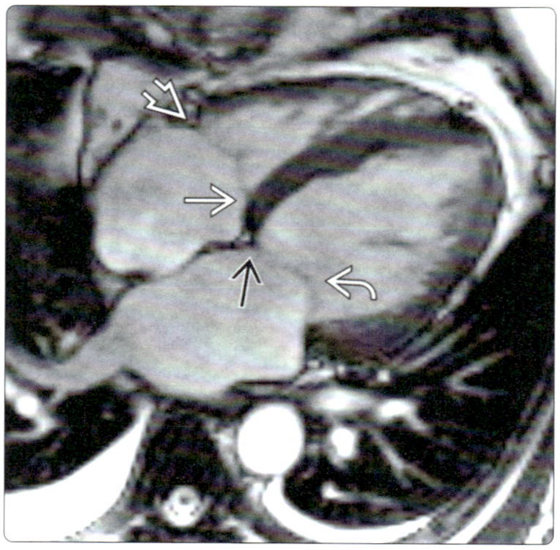

Normal Thin Leaflets

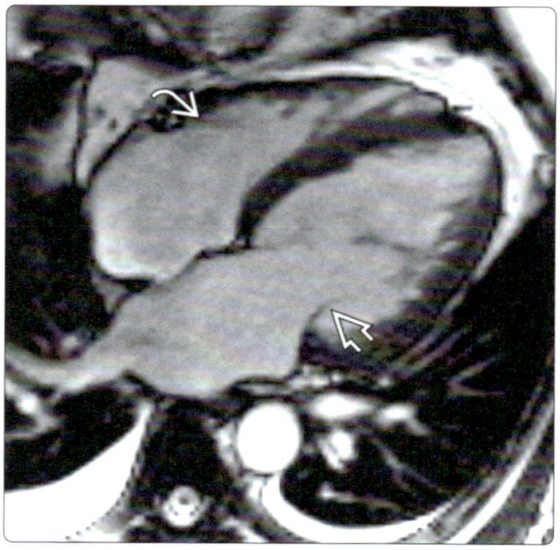

(Left) *Four-chamber SSFP MR shows normal thin leaflets of the tricuspid ➡ and mitral ➡ valves, which are closed during ventricular systole. The hinge point of the septal tricuspid valve leaflet ➡ is normally more apical than the septal mitral valve leaflet ➡ hinge point.* **(Right)** *Four-chamber SSFP MR in the same patient shows normal thin leaflets of the tricuspid ➡ and mitral ➡ valves, which are open during ventricular diastole.*

Closed Pulmonic Valve

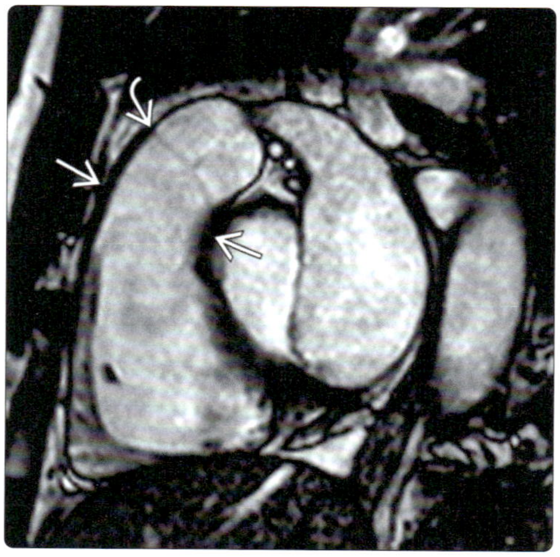

Aortic and Mitral Valves

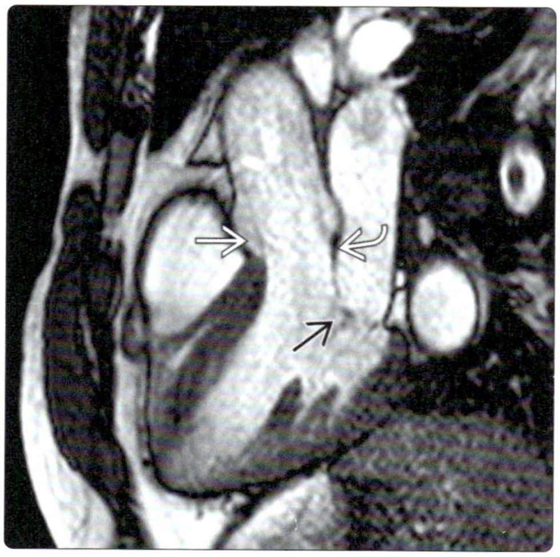

(Left) *Right ventricular outflow tract (RVOT) SSFP MR shows a normal, thin, closed pulmonic valve ➡ situated on top of the RVOT ➡, which connects it to the body of the right ventricle and separates it from the tricuspid valve.* **(Right)** *Left ventricular outflow tract (LVOT) SSFP MR shows that the aortic valve ➡ is open and the mitral valve ➡ is closed during ventricular systole. Note that the aortic and mitral valves are directly adjacent to each other (so-called fibrous continuity). Also note intravalvular fibrosa ➡.*

Right Ventricle and Right-Sided Cardiac Valves

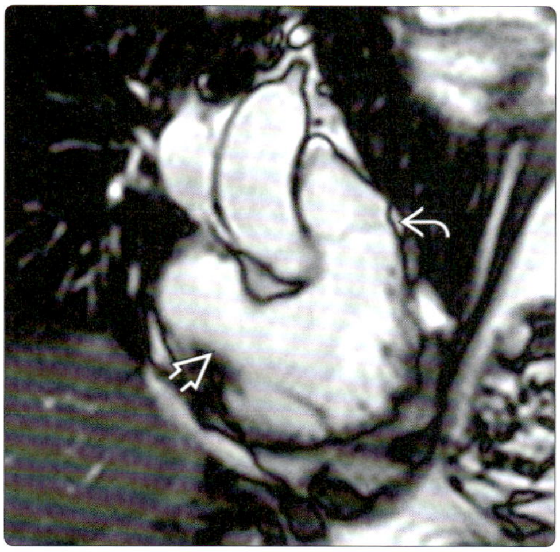

Aortic Regurgitation

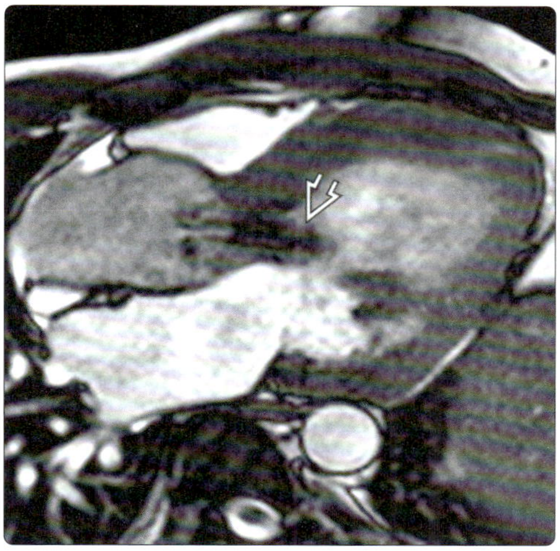

(Left) *RVOT long-axis SSFP MR shows the normal anatomy of the right ventricle and right-sided cardiac valves. Note that the pulmonic valve ➡ is separated from the tricuspid valve ➡ by a muscular infundibulum known as the crista supraventricularis.* **(Right)** *LVOT SSFP MR shows a black jet ➡ originating from the aortic valve directed posteriorly into the left ventricle during ventricular diastole, indicating aortic regurgitation.*

Black Jet

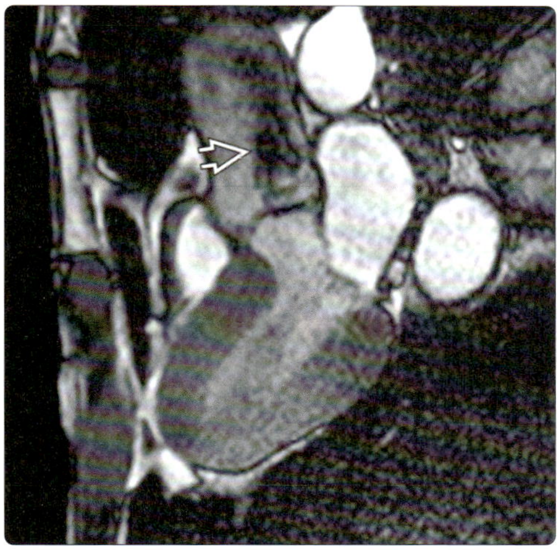

Regurgitant Jet

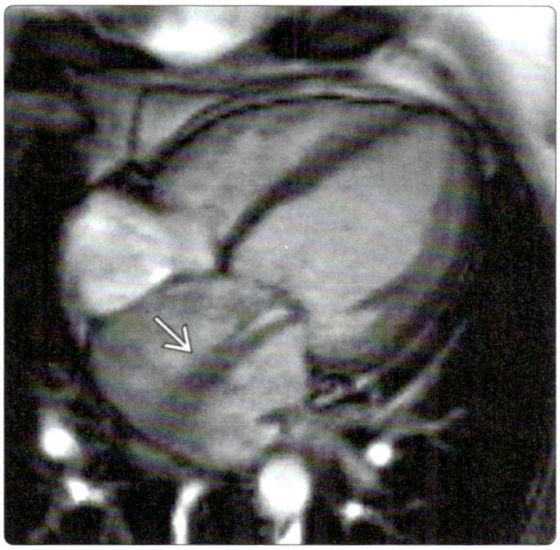

(Left) *LVOT systolic SSFP MR shows a black jet ➡ originating from the aortic valve directed into the ascending aorta, which indicates aortic stenosis. Importantly, the size and magnitude of the jet cannot be used to quantify the degree of stenosis or regurgitation on MR, as it varies depending on the echo time used in acquisition.* **(Right)** *Four-chamber SSFP MR during systole shows a regurgitant jet ➡ extending retrograde from the mitral valve to the posterior wall of the left atrium.*

Bicuspid Aortic Valve

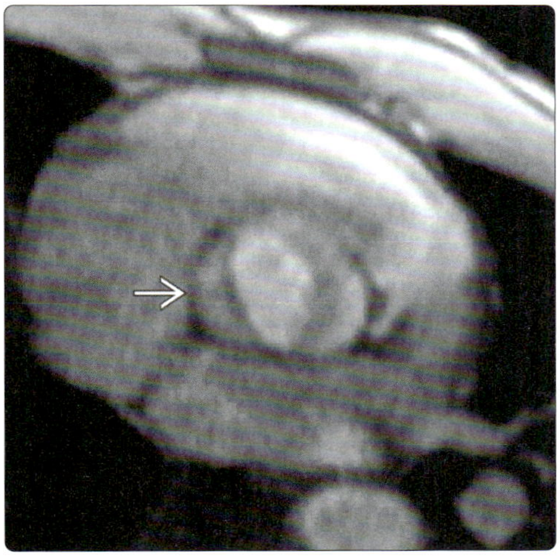

Phase Image

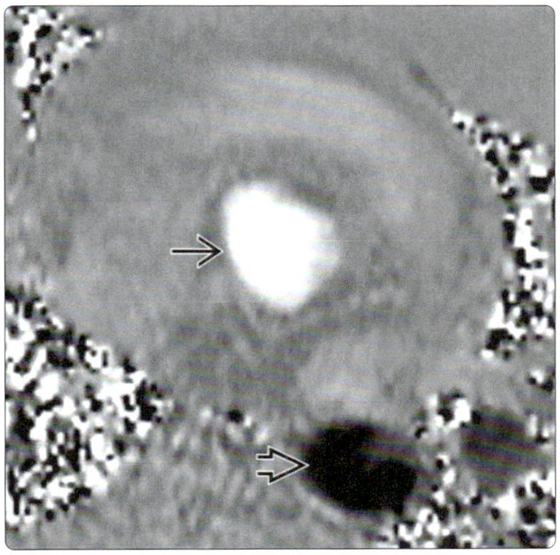

(Left) *Magnitude image from a velocity-encoded cine (VEC) MR sequence obtained during systole shows a fish mouth appearance of the aortic valve, consistent with a bicuspid aortic valve ➡.* **(Right)** *In this phase image from a VEC MR sequence in the same patient, direction is encoded into the signal so that blood flowing toward the head is encoded as bright signal ➡ and blood flowing toward the feet, as in the descending aorta ➡, is encoded as dark signal.*

(Left) *Magnitude image from a VEC MR sequence obtained during diastole shows incomplete coaptation of the aortic valve ➔ leading to aortic regurgitation.* **(Right)** *Corresponding phase image shows aortic regurgitation ➔. In the magnitude image, blood flowing both in and out of plane is designated as bright signal, whereas the phase image encodes the direction of blood flow, confirming retrograde regurgitant flow. VEC MR is useful in quantitating the degree of regurgitation or valve stenosis.*

Magnitude Image

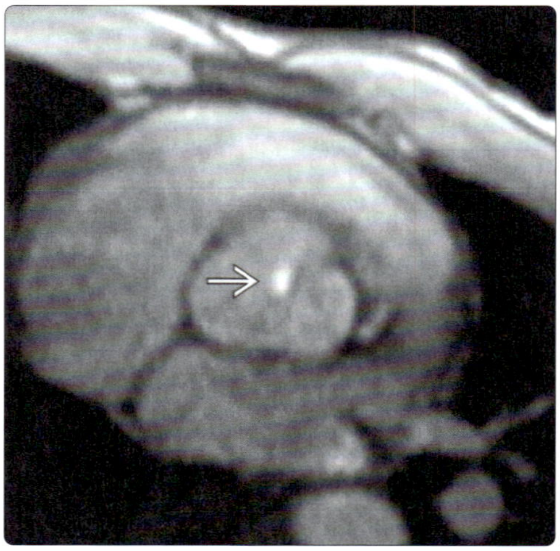

Aortic Regurgitation

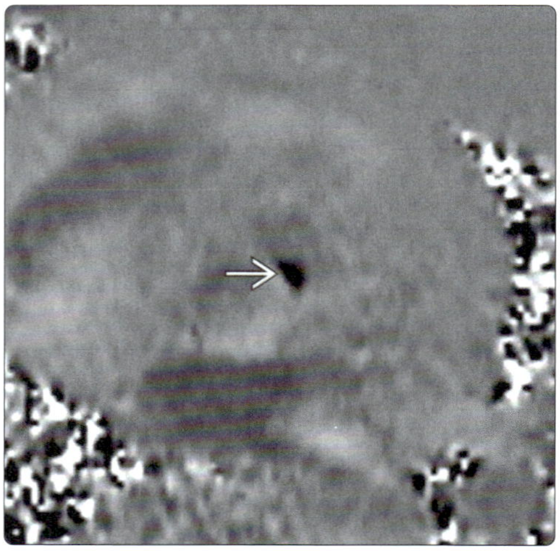

(Left) *Four-chamber (left) and short-axis (right) CT images show marked thickening of the tricuspid valve ➔ due to endocarditis in an intravenous drug user.* **(Right)** *Four-chamber view SSFP MR shows a well-seated mitral valve prosthesis ➔. There is a round, low-signal nodule ➔ attached to the ventricular side of the prosthesis, which represents a thrombus.*

Endocarditis of Tricuspid Valve

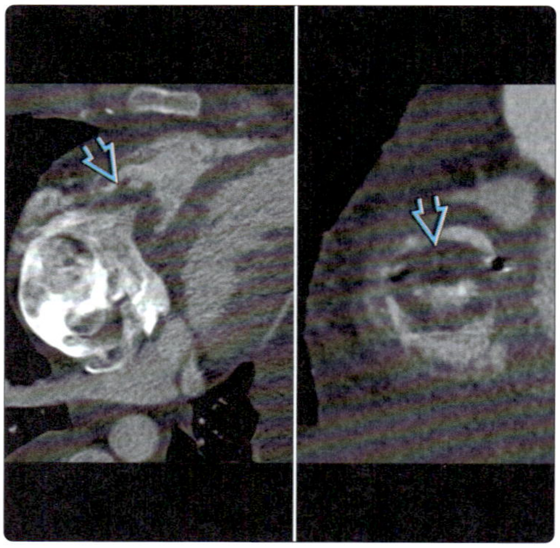

Mitral Valve Prosthesis

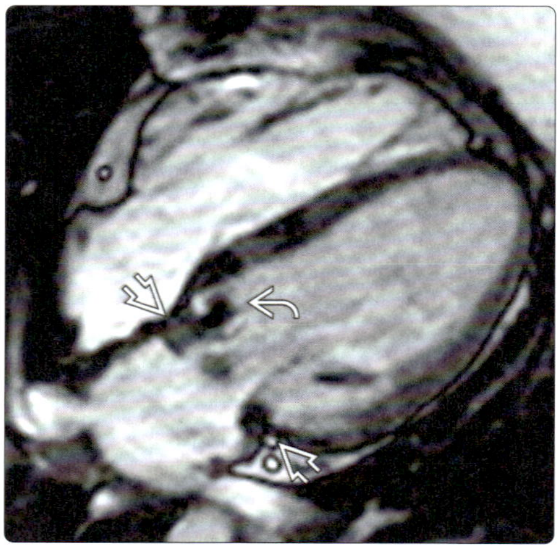

(Left) *Axial oblique gated cardiac CTA shows a small, 3-mm soft tissue nodule ➔ arising from the aortic valve ➔ due to a fibroelastoma.* **(Right)** *CT shows a large hypoattenuation mass on the pulmonary valve ➔ and a smaller hypoattenuation mass on the tricuspid valve ➔. The patient was asymptomatic with a normal WBC count, making endocarditis unlikely. Synchronous papillary fibroelastomas, which are very rare, were confirmed pathologically.*

Papillary Fibroelastoma

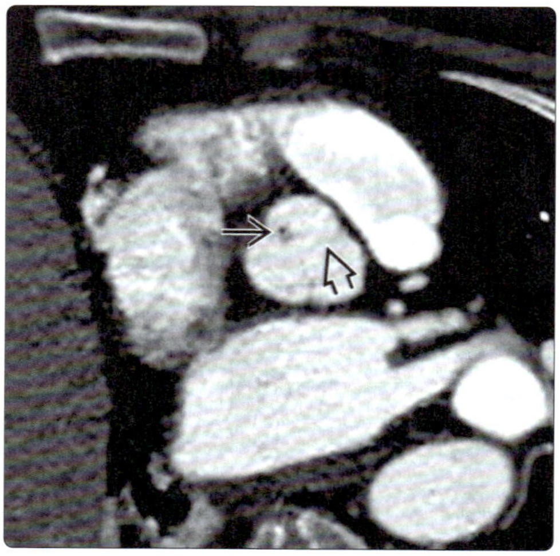

Multiple Papillary Fibroelastomas

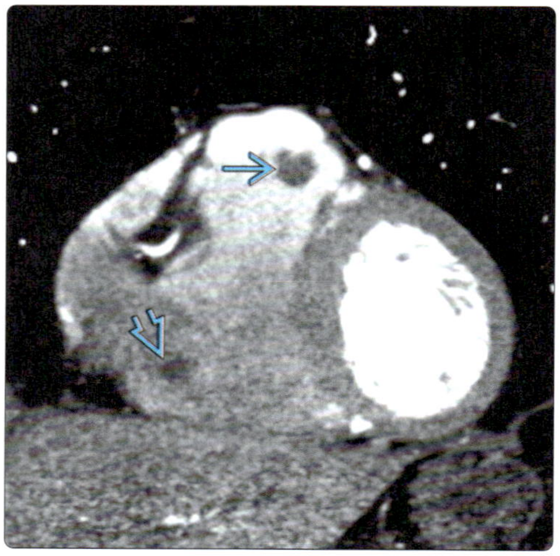

Calcified Aortic Valve

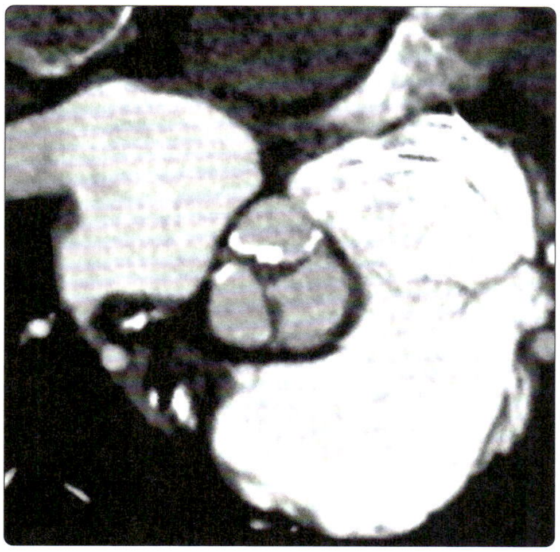

Severe Stenosis

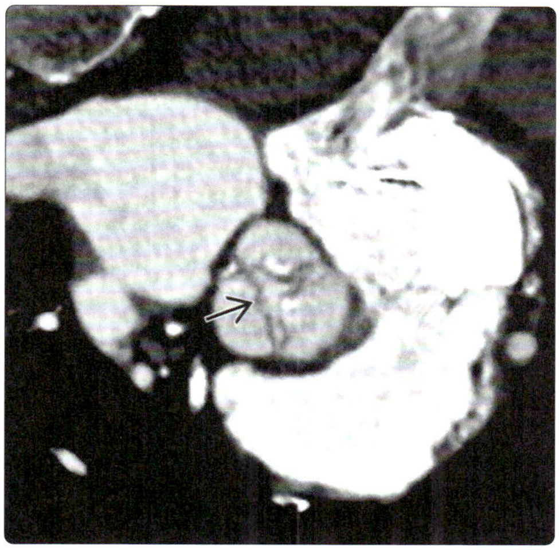

(Left) *Aortic valve short-axis cardiac CT during diastole shows a heavily calcified aortic valve with thickening of all 3 leaflets. Without systolic images, bicuspid or unicuspid valve cannot be excluded, as leaflets may be fused.* **(Right)** *Aortic valve short-axis CT obtained at midsystole in the same patient shows a markedly reduced opening area ⇒ of the aortic valve, indicating severe stenosis. The valve is confirmed to be tricuspid, although partial peripheral fusion of some cusps has occurred.*

Systolic Orifice Area of Valve

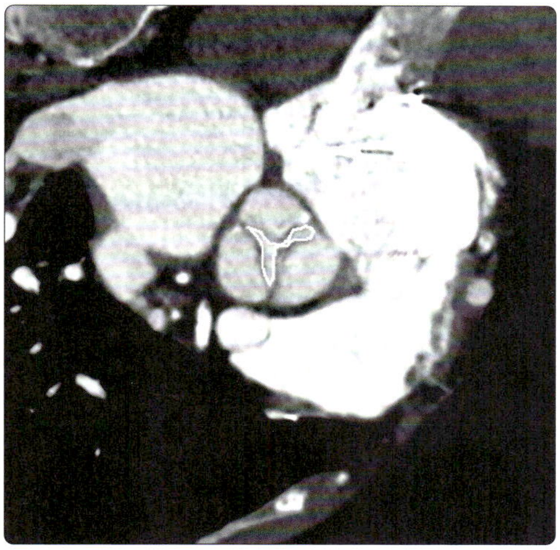

Aortic Leaflet Calcification in Severe Stenosis

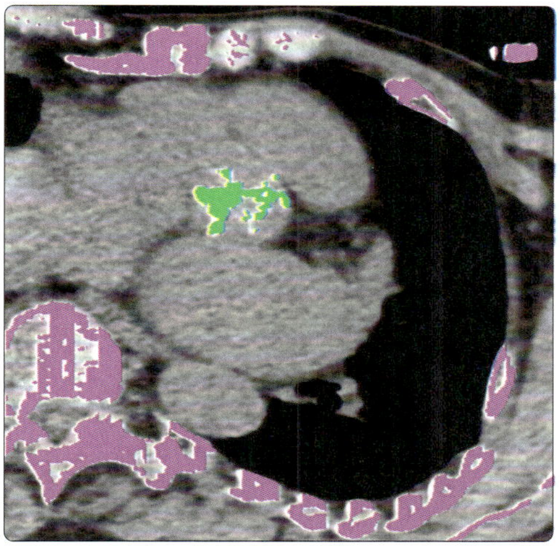

(Left) *Short-axis CT obtained at midsystole in the same patient has a region of interest tracing the systolic orifice area of the valve that is 0.78 cm² (valve planimetry). A normal opening area is > 2 cm². A stenosis is considered severe if it is < 1 cm². Opening areas < 0.7 cm² are often classified as critical stenoses.* **(Right)** *Axial oblique view from a noncontrast-gated cardiac CT shows extensive aortic leaflet calcification in severe stenosis. Aortic valve calcium is highlighted in green and calcium score is calculated as 2,263.*

Anulus Plane

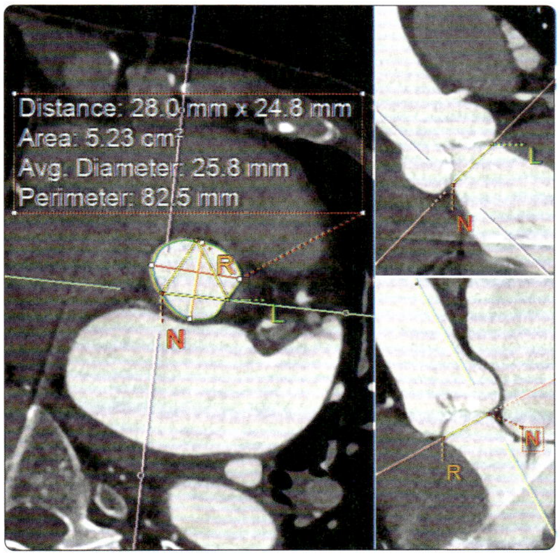

Cardiac CT Angiogram

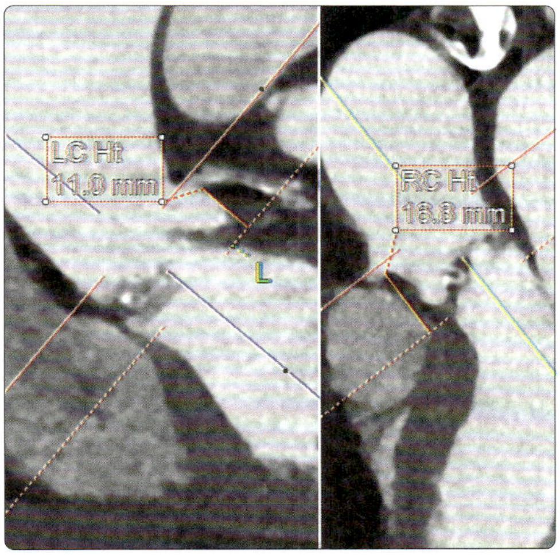

(Left) *Cardiac CTA is utilized in pre-TAVR evaluations to size the anulus plane, which determines the appropriate valve size for the procedure. Short-axis and long-axis images in the same patient show the anulus plane, which was created by marking hinge points below each cusp.* **(Right)** *Cardiac CTA is helpful for assessment of potential coronary occlusion during TAVR. Coronary height, the distance between the inferior aspect of the coronary artery and annulus plane, is an important surrogate of potential coronary occlusion.*

KEY FACTS

TERMINOLOGY

- Raphe represents visible fusion point between 2 underdeveloped coronary cusps
- Bicuspid aortic valve (BAV) is most common congenital cardiovascular malformation, affecting 1-2% of population

IMAGING

- BAV has 2 cusps of generally unequal size
- Usually, ridge or raphe lies across 1 cusp

TOP DIFFERENTIAL DIAGNOSES

- Other valve anomalies
- Aortic stenosis

PATHOLOGY

- Associations
  - Congenital left-sided obstructive lesions
  - Aortic dilation, aneurysms, & dissection
  - Ventricular septal defect & coronary artery anomalies
- BAV classification
  - Sievers classification is based on number of raphes (type 0, 1, & 2); orientation of leaflet & valvular function (regurgitation or stenosis) also included
  - New recommended nomenclature (3 types): Fused BAV > 2-sinus BAV > partial-fusion BAV

CLINICAL ISSUES

- Symptoms result from development of either valvular stenosis or regurgitation
- BAV is predisposed to infective endocarditis
- Serial assessment of aortic valve to evaluate chamber dimensions & valvular & ventricular functions
- Aortic valve replacement indicated for severe valve dysfunction, symptomatic patients, or abnormal left ventricular dimensions & function

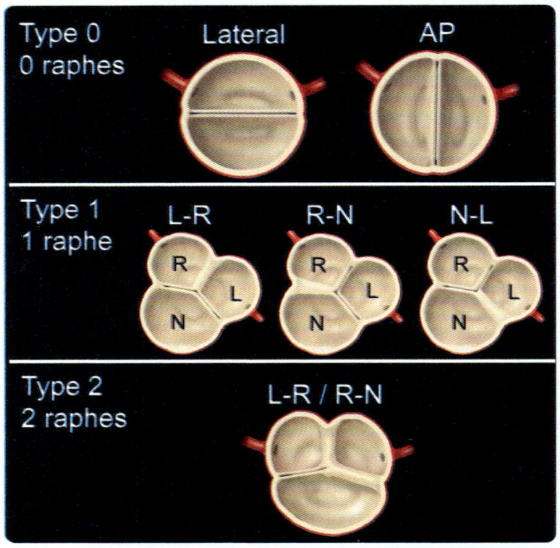

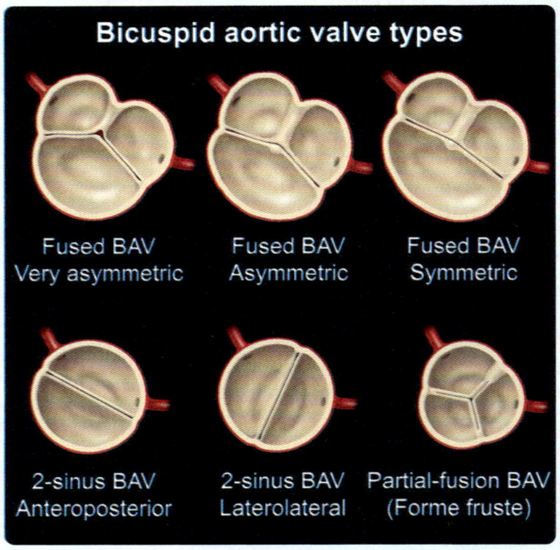

(Left) *Graphic depicts Sievers classification of bicuspid aortic valves (BAVs). Based on the number of raphes, BAV is classified into 3 groups: Type 0 (top), type 1 (middle), & type 2 (bottom). Different phenotypes of type 0 and type 1 are also present.* **(Right)** *Updated recent classification of BAV is shown. Three main groups are present: Fused BAV, 2-sinus BAV, & partial-fusion BAV. Fused BAV is further grouped based on the symmetry of the leaflets (top). 2-sinus BAV is divided in 2, depending on the orientation of leaflets (bottom).*

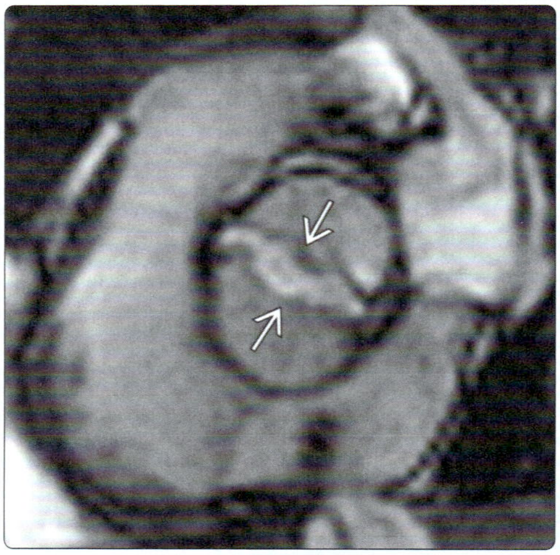

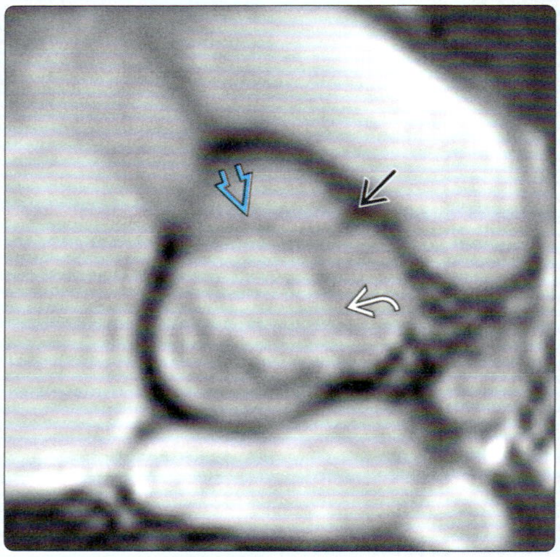

(Left) *Short-axis cine image from a cardiac MR during end-systole shows a morphologic BAV with 2 leaflets ➔ with AP orientation. Note that there is no raphe. This is classified as Sievers type 0 or 2-sinus BAV. Note incomplete opening of the valve, indicating mild aortic stenosis.* **(Right)** *Short-axis cine true FISP MR through the aortic valve during systole demonstrates fusion of the right ⇨ and left ➔ aortic valve leaflets with raphe ⇨, resulting in a fish mouth appearance. It is classified as Sievers type 1 or fused BAV.*

TERMINOLOGY

Abbreviations

- Bicuspid aortic valve (BAV)

Definitions

- Raphe represents visible fusion point between 2 underdeveloped coronary cusps
- Commissure represents opening between aortic valve cusps (leaflets)

IMAGING

General Features

- Best diagnostic clue
  - Dilated aortic root with systolic doming & diastolic prolapse of 2 aortic cusps
  - Eccentric closure plane in systole
- Size
  - BAV has 2 cusps of generally unequal size
    - Ridge or raphe often seen across larger cusp
- Morphology
  - Thickened leaflets with either AP or horizontal (right-left) orientation

Imaging Recommendations

- Best imaging tool
  - Echocardiography, MR
    - Serial follow-up for BAV & aortic root &/or ascending aorta diameter ≥ 4.0 cm at interval dependent of aortic size & growth rate

Radiographic Findings

- Characteristic calcification along valve commissures & anulus
- Frequently, prominent calcified ridge along raphe
- Cardiomegaly, if BAV is accompanied by significant aortic regurgitation
- Ascending aortic enlargement
  - May have poststenotic ascending aortic aneurysm due to stenotic jet
  - Ascending aorta may also enlarge due to aortopathy associated with BAV, which is unrelated to valve stenosis

CT Findings

- NECT
  - Allows quantification of aortic valve calcium (Agatston score)
    - Severity of valve calcium correlates with peak & mean aortic valve gradients in cases of stenosis
- Cardiac gated CTA
  - Accurately detects number of valve leaflets, valve motion, & valve calcium on cine CT
  - Classic fish mouth shape of open valve in systole
  - Raphe in middle of 1 fused cusp often mimics trileaflet aortic valve in diastole
  - Quantifies degree of aortic valve stenosis using planimetry for measuring systolic valve opening area
  - Semiquantitatively grades aortic valve regurgitation by planimetry of anatomic regurgitant orifice in diastole
  - Allows for evaluation of associated aortic pathology (e.g., dilation, aneurysm, dissection)

MR Findings

- SSFP cine
  - Detects antegrade spin-dephasing flow void artifact in cases of valve stenosis or retrograde flow void jet across regurgitant orifice
  - Quantifies left ventricular volume & function, which helps monitor therapy or time surgical intervention
- Double IR FSE
  - Accurate morphologic characterization of valve cusps, presence of raphe & valve orientation (AP or right-left)
  - Black-blood assessment of thoracic aorta
- Velocity-encoded cine phase-contrast MR
  - Provides peak systolic flow velocities, from which pressure gradient across valve can be calculated using modified Bernoulli equation
  - Provides regurgitant volume & regurgitant fraction in cases of aortic regurgitation
  - 4D flow MR provides new insights on aortic flow patterns in different phenotypes
    - Right-left type: Anterior flow distribution, higher axial wall shear stress (WSS) at aortic root, dilation at root & ascending aorta along convexity
    - Right-noncoronary type: Posterior outflow jet at sinotubular junction that shifts to anterior/right anterior in mid- & distal ascending segment; higher circumferential WSS in mid- & distal ascending aorta; dilation of arch & ascending aorta; sparing root
- MR angiography
  - For evaluation of thoracic aorta & aneurysm
  - Associated anomalies, such as coarctation

Echocardiographic Findings

- BAV shows doming configuration in long-axis view when it opens during systole

DIFFERENTIAL DIAGNOSIS

Other Valve Anomalies

- Unicuspid aortic valve, quadricuspid aortic valve (QAV)

Aortic Stenosis

- Senile calcified aortic stenosis, subaortic stenosis, supravalvular stenosis

PATHOLOGY

General Features

- Etiology
  - Embryologic abnormality in conotruncal channel
  - Congenital: There are 2 functional cusps caused by fusion during embryology (raphe present) or de novo development of 2 cusps (raphe absent)
  - Acquired BAVs are secondary to inflammatory processes (e.g., rheumatic fever) or calcification of normal trileaflet aortic valve resulting in fusion of 2 cusps
- Genetics
  - Abnormal & inadequate production of microfibrillar proteins, such as fibrillin-1
  - Abnormal endothelial nitric oxide synthase also implicated
  - Associated with familial clustering suggesting autosomal dominant inheritance with reduced penetrance

- Incidence as high as 10-17% in 1st-degree relatives
- Echocardiography is recommended screening tool for offspring & 1st-degree relatives of patients

- Associated abnormalities
  - Associated with congenital left-sided obstructive lesions
    - Coarctation of aorta, supravalvular stenosis (Williams syndrome), interrupted aortic arch
  - BAV is associated with aortic dilation, aneurysms, & dissection
    - Aortic aneurysm may be due to poststenotic dilation
    - Aortic root may also have inherent abnormal connective tissue with cystic medial necrosis similar to disorders, such as Marfan syndrome
    - Even after valve replacement for BAV, there is risk of subsequent aortic dissection
  - Other associated congenital syndromes
    - Patent ductus arteriosus
    - Familial aortic dissection
    - Turner syndrome (30% of patients have BAV)
  - Ventricular septal defect, sinus of Valsalva aneurysm, & coronary artery anomalies

Staging, Grading, & Classification

- Classification on 3 anatomic characteristics that influence prognosis & treatment
  - Sievers classification: Main category is based on number of raphes: 0 (type 0), 1 (type 1), or 2 (type 2)
    - Subcategory based on positioning of leaflets in type 0 (AP vs. lateral) & raphes in type 1 (L-R, R-N, N-L)
    - Functional status of valve: Quantifies opening & closing (stenosis or regurgitation)
  - Recent classification endorsed by multiple societies: 3 BAV types
    - Fused BAV (most common): 3 aortic sinuses with 2 cusps & 2 commissures; raphe usually present
      - R-L (70-80%) > R-N (20-30%) > L-N (3-6%)
    - 2-sinus BAV (2nd common): 2 aortic sinuses with 2 cusps & 2 commissures; no raphe
      - Lateral orientation of leaflets (most common); AP orientation
    - Partial-fusion BAV: 3 aortic sinuses with 3 cusps & 3 commissures; small, partial raphe (< 50% of 1 commissure)

Gross Pathologic & Surgical Features

- With aging, valve is predisposed to sclerosis & calcification

CLINICAL ISSUES

Presentation

- Most common signs/symptoms
  - Generally asymptomatic
    - Frequent incidental finding on echocardiography
  - Symptoms result from development of either valvular stenosis or regurgitation
- Other signs/symptoms
  - BAV is predisposed to infective endocarditis
    - Lifetime risk of developing infective endocarditis on BAV is 10-30%
  - Symptoms may also develop secondary to associated aortopathies (i.e., aortic dilation & dissection)

Demographics

- Age
  - BAV may be identified in patients of any age
- Sex
  - M:F > 3:1
- Epidemiology
  - BAV is most common congenital cardiovascular malformation, present in 1-2% of population
    - Since BAV may be silent through adulthood, incidence is likely underestimated
    - Incidence is not affected by geography or race

Natural History & Prognosis

- Aortic valve stenosis is most frequent complication
  - BAVs are present in majority of patients presenting with aortic stenosis at age 15-65
  - BAV in which right & noncoronary cusps are fused is more frequently associated with changes of stenosis or insufficiency in pediatric population
    - This arrangement is more commonly associated with myxomatous mitral valve & ascending aortic dilation
  - BAV in which right & left cusps are fused is less commonly associated with stenosis or insufficiency in children
    - This arrangement is much more commonly associated with coarctation of aorta & with functionally normal valve
- Overall prognosis of BAV is good

Treatment

- Serial assessment of aortic valve to evaluate valvular function, chamber dimensions, & ventricular function
- Modify coronary artery disease risk factors since their presence may accelerate BAV sclerosis & calcification
  - Treatment of hypercholesterolemia with statin if present
- Balloon aortic valvuloplasty is treatment of choice in pediatric cases
  - Valve repair or replacement becomes necessary later in childhood or adolescence
  - Ross procedure (pulmonary autograft) is considered in younger patients as alternative to prosthetic valve replacement
- Aortic valve replacement is indicated for severe valve dysfunction, symptomatic patients, or abnormal left ventricular dimensions & function
  - Transcatheter aortic valve replacement has been studied in patients with high risk for open surgery
- Aortic valve repair may be performed in cases of severe isolated aortic regurgitation
- Aortic replacement is recommended in cases of BAV with
  - Aortic dilation > 5.5 cm (class I), or
  - Aortic diameter 5.0-5.5 cm + additional risk factor for dissection (family history of dissection, aortic growth > 0.5 cm per year, aortic coarctation; class 2a), or
  - Aortic diameter ≥ 4.5 cm with indication for surgical aortic valve replacement (SAVR) (class 2a)

SELECTED REFERENCES

1. Michelena HI et al: International consensus statement on nomenclature and classification of the congenital bicuspid aortic valve and its aortopathy, for clinical, surgical, interventional and research purposes. Radiol Cardiothorac Imaging. 3(4):e200496, 2021

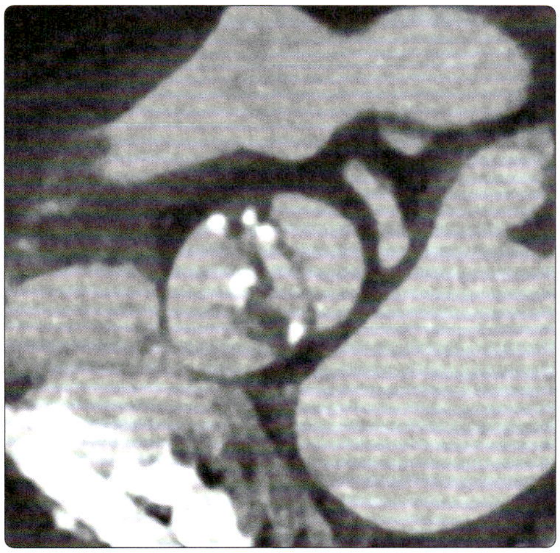

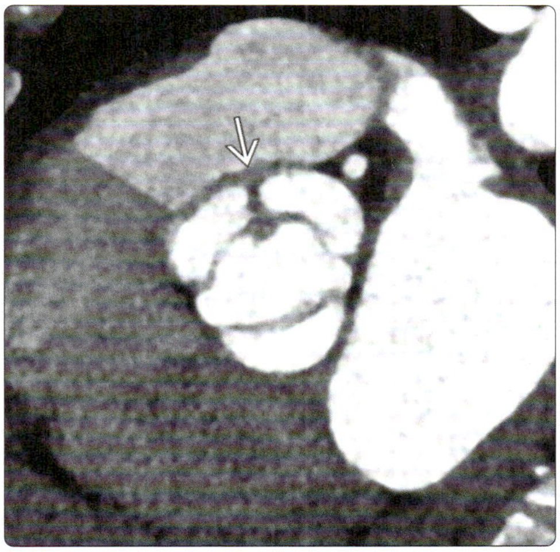

(Left) *Short-axis image of aortic valve shows BAV without raphe can be classified as Sievers type 0 or 2-sinus BAV. Note the thickening and calcification of the leaflets associated with severe aortic stenosis.* **(Right)** *Short-axis image of the aortic valve shows a BAV with the fusion of left and right coronary cusps, which can be classified as Sievers type 1 (L-R) or fused BAV (asymmetric). Note the large opening area of the valve during systole, indicating absence of aortic stenosis.*

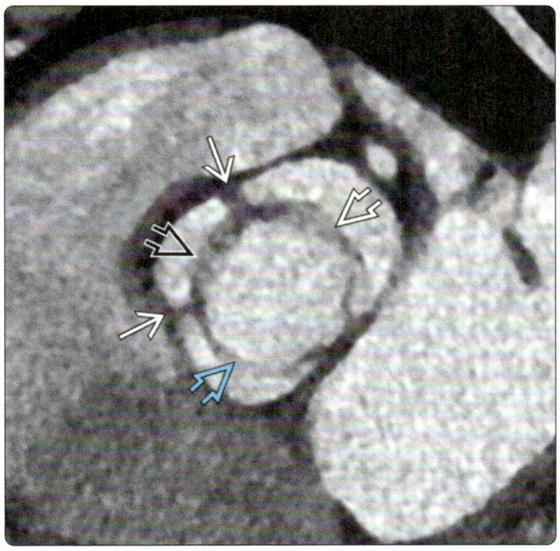

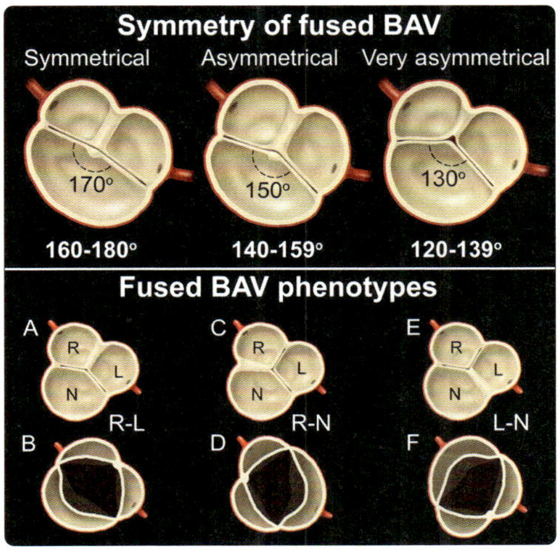

(Left) *Short-axis image of the aortic valve during systole shows fusion of left -right and right-noncoronary leaflets with 2 raphes, consistent with Sievers type 2 BAV, which is classified as fused BAV based on recent suggested nomenclature.* **(Right)** *Graphic of the phenotypes of fused BAV based on the location of fusion and symmetry of the leaflets is shown.*

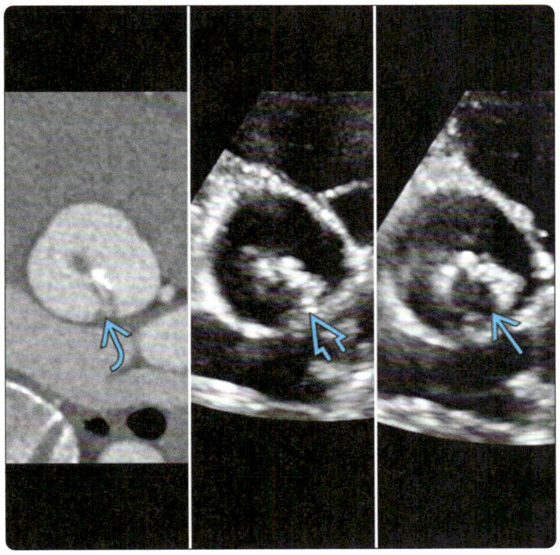

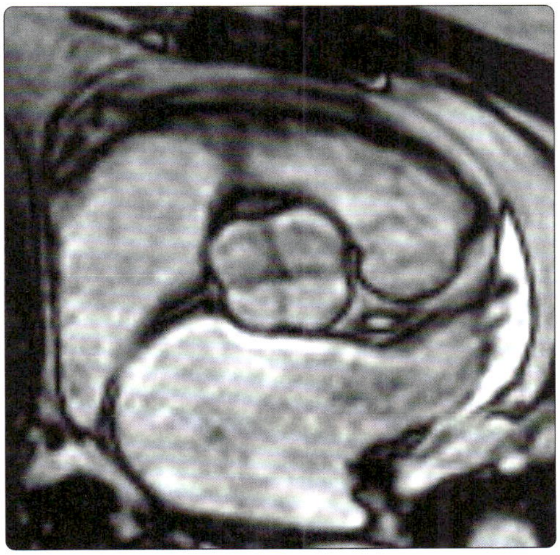

(Left) *Diastolic CT (left) shows a thickened and calcified unicuspid aortic valve (UAV) with one commissural attachment. The UAV is regurgitant and stenotic. Echocardiogram images during diastole (center) and systole (right) show the stenotic UAV, which affects 0.2% of people.* **(Right)** *SSFP MR during diastole in an asymptomatic older man shows a quadricuspid aortic valve (QAV), which very rare. It is often an incidental finding or associated with aortic regurgitation. (Courtesy S. Kligerman, MD.)*

(Left) *Oblique SSFP MR shows a BAV ➔ can be classified as Sievers type 0 or 2-sinus BAV. Note that RV = right ventricle.* **(Right)** *Oblique axial phase-contrast MR in the same patient demonstrates a technique for measuring peak velocity across the stenotic valve. A region of interest (blue outline) is drawn just superior to the aortic valve at peak systole to determine the maximal blood velocity. The maximum velocity is used to determine the pressure gradient across the valve through the modified Bernoulli equation ($\Delta P = 4v^2$).*

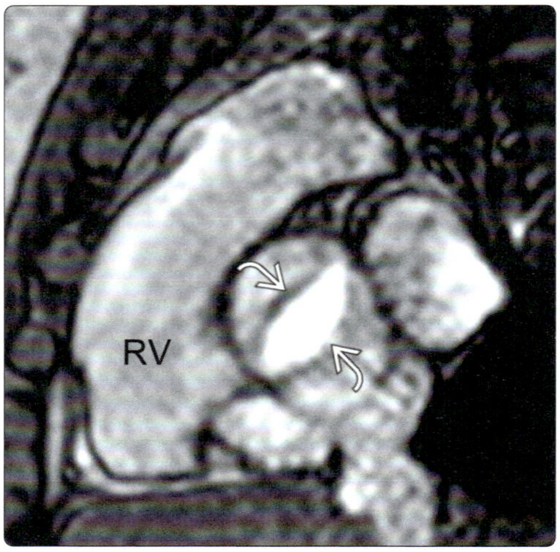

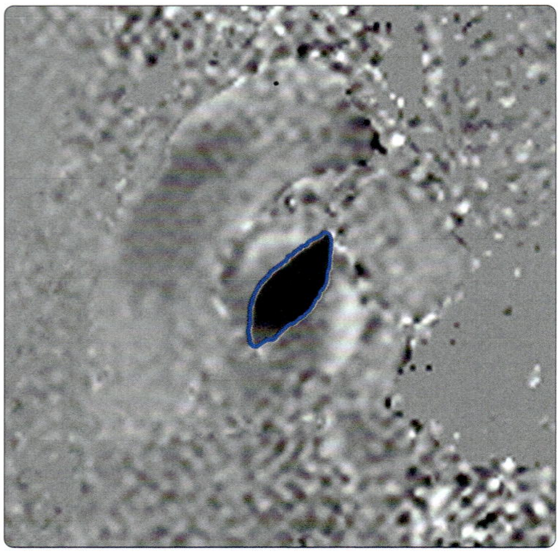

(Left) *Short-axis coronary CTA at the valve level in diastole shows a congenital bicuspid valve with 2 cusps. Note the small piece of calcium ➔. There is no malcoaptation to suggest aortic regurgitation.* **(Right)** *Short-axis coronary CTA at the valve level in systole in the same patient shows reduced opening area ➔, indicating significant aortic stenosis.*

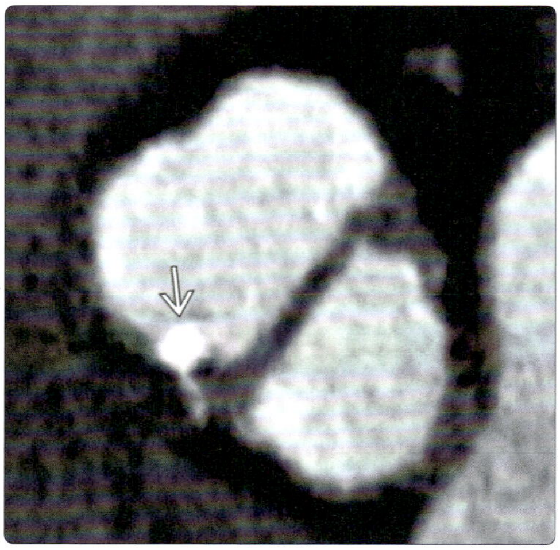

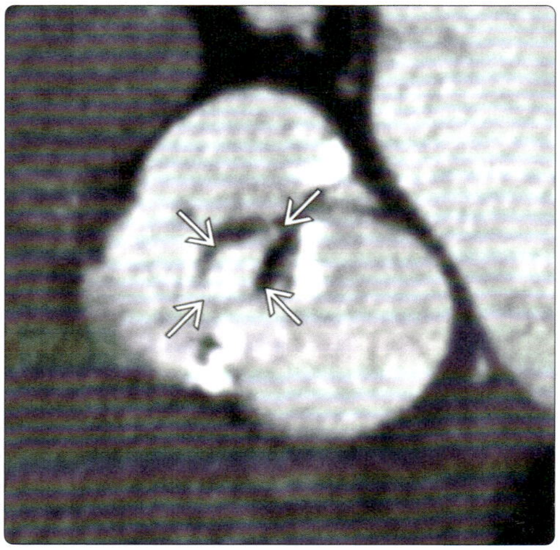

(Left) *LVOT SSFP MR in a 25-year-old man shows a spin-dephasing flow void artifact ➔, indicating flow acceleration due to aortic stenosis. Note the concentric left ventricular (LV) hypertrophy. Note that LA = left atrium.* **(Right)** *Oblique axial SSFP MR in the same patient shows restricted right-left leaflet opening ➔ and a BAV. Valve planimetry measures the total valve opening area and is a useful adjunct to phase-contrast MR in determining stenosis severity.*

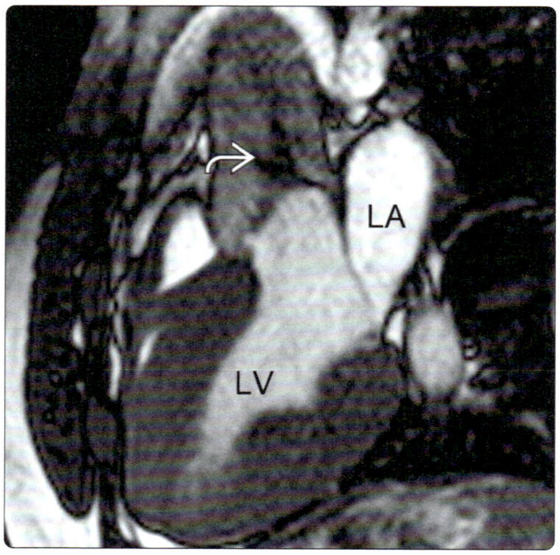

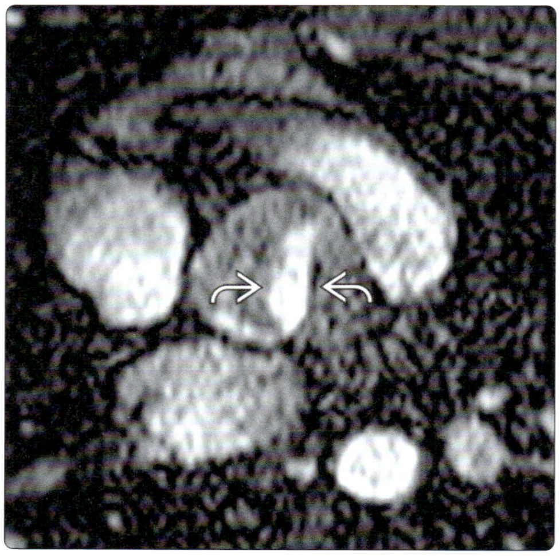

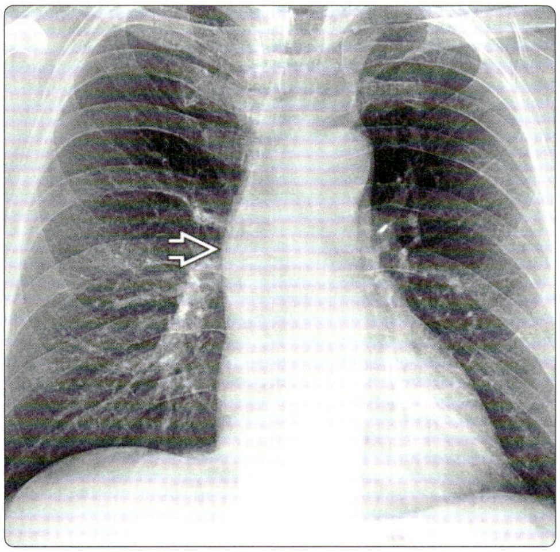

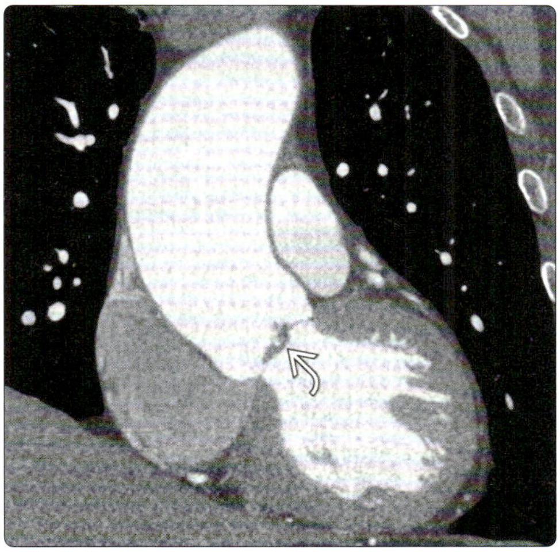

(Left) *Frontal radiograph in a 64-year-old man shows a convex ascending aortic segment, suggesting ascending aortic enlargement. This finding is often seen in aortic valve stenosis, although it is nonspecific.* **(Right)** *Oblique coronal cardiac CT in the same patient confirms ascending aortic aneurysm. Note the thickened aortic valve leaflet, which is suggestive of aortic stenosis.*

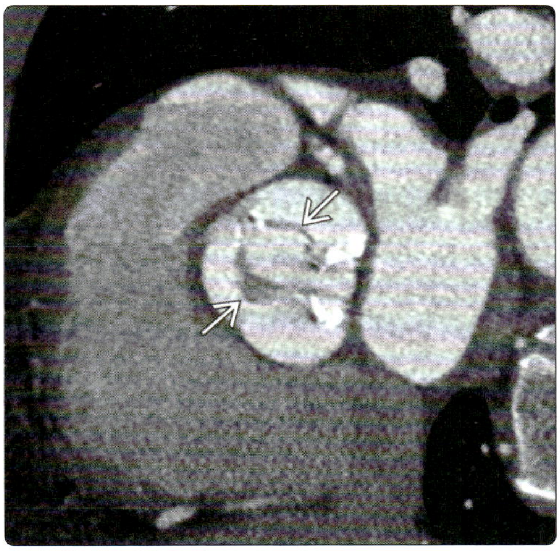

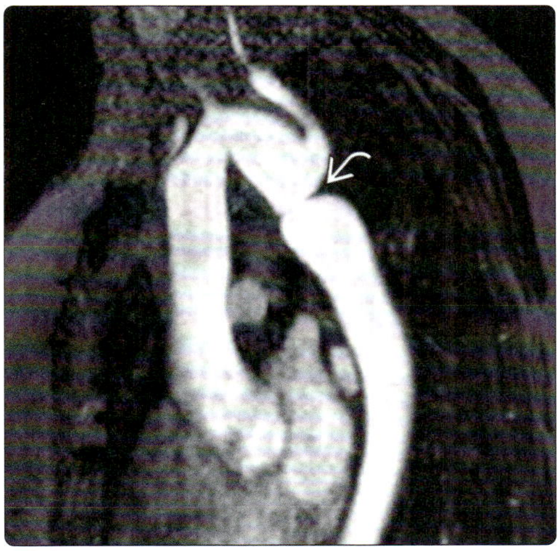

(Left) *Double oblique axial cardiac CT in systole in the same patient shows restricted AP aortic valve opening and calcification with thickening of bileaflet valve cusps. The valve configuration has been termed a fish mouth appearance.* **(Right)** *Oblique sagittal MRA in a patient with a congenital BAV shows aortic coarctation. Aortic coarctation and pseudocoarctation are often associated with BAV.*

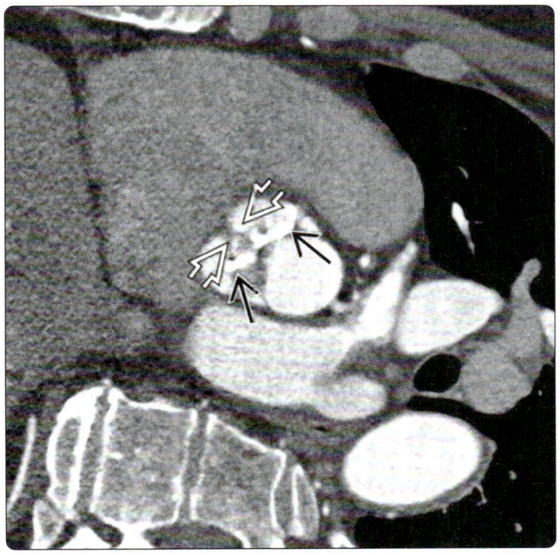

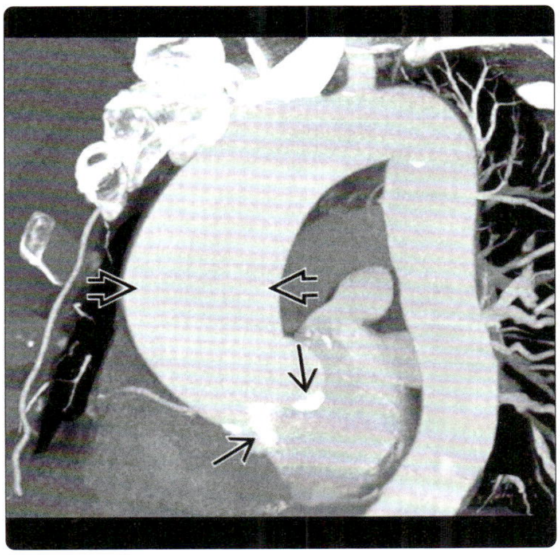

(Left) *Sagittal reformat CT transverse to the aorta below the level of the sinuses of Valsalva shows a fused raphe between the right and noncoronary cusps. There are associated valvular calcifications.* **(Right)** *Sagittal MIP reformat CT shows the heavily calcified aortic valve and aneurysmal ascending aorta.*

Aortic Stenosis

KEY FACTS

TERMINOLOGY

- Narrowing of aortic outflow tract, which causes flow obstruction
  - Valvular (most common); subvalvular (rare); supravalvular (extremely rare)

IMAGING

- Doppler echocardiogram: High transvalvular velocity systolic jet and high-pressure gradient
  - Except: Low-flow, low-gradient aortic stenosis (AS)
- CT, MR, transesophageal echocardiogram: Narrowing of aortic valve orifice (area < 1.5 cm^2)

TOP DIFFERENTIAL DIAGNOSES

- Degenerative calcified AS
- Rheumatic heart disease
- Bicuspid aortic valve
- Subvalvular AS

CLINICAL ISSUES

- Asymptomatic over long period; symptoms late (syncope, dyspnea, heart failure)
- Left ventricular function is important parameter to predict outcome
- Dominant cause: Bicuspid valve (< 70 years) or degenerative calcified stenosis (> 70 years)
- Aortic valve replacement is only effective treatment (surgical or transcatheter route)

DIAGNOSTIC CHECKLIST

- Echocardiography: ↑ transvalvular pressure gradient and velocity (standard tool)
- Cardiac CT: Calcific stenosis; planimetric sizing of aortic valve orifice area
- MR: Comprehensive evaluation of valve, aorta, and myocardium

(Left) *Severe aortic valve Ca^{++} of all 3 cusps is the hallmark for aortic stenosis (AS). 3D VRT shows the aortic valve, right ventricular pacemaker →, triangular narrowing or orifice area, right coronary cusp →, left coronary cusp →, and noncoronary cusp → with irregular Ca^{++}.* **(Right)** *Three-chamber cardiac CT in a patient with subvalvular AS shows a thin membrane → causing left ventricular outflow tract obstruction.*

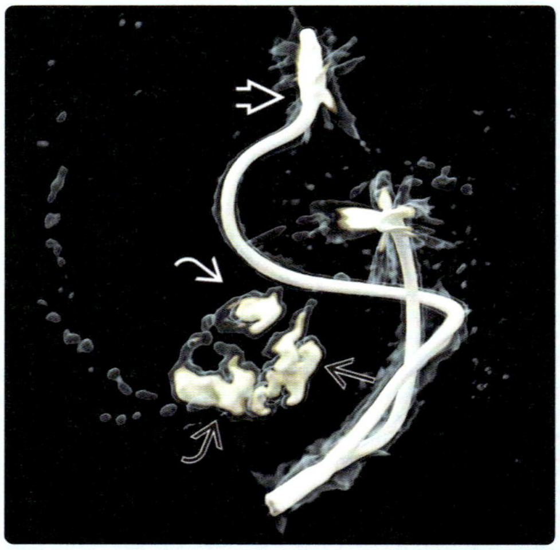

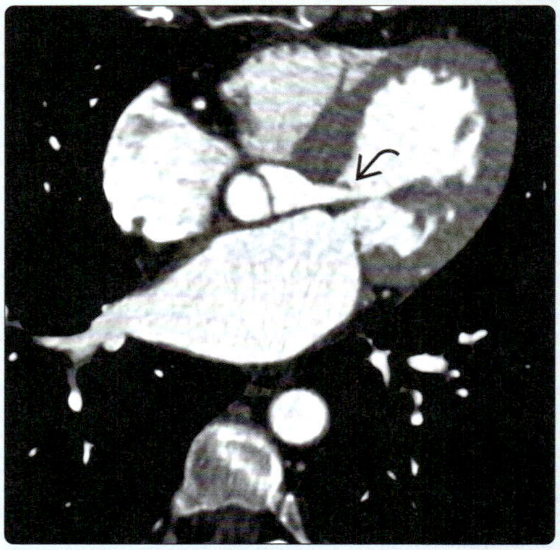

(Left) *Double-oblique cardiac CT in the aortic valve plane shows a bicuspid valve with a calcified raphe → between the right and left coronary cusps. Note the decreased systolic aortic valve orifice area →.* **(Right)** *Axial oblique cardiac CT shows a tricuspid valve that is severely calcified → and has fibrous thickening of leaflets, indicating the degenerative or rheumatic nature of the disease.*

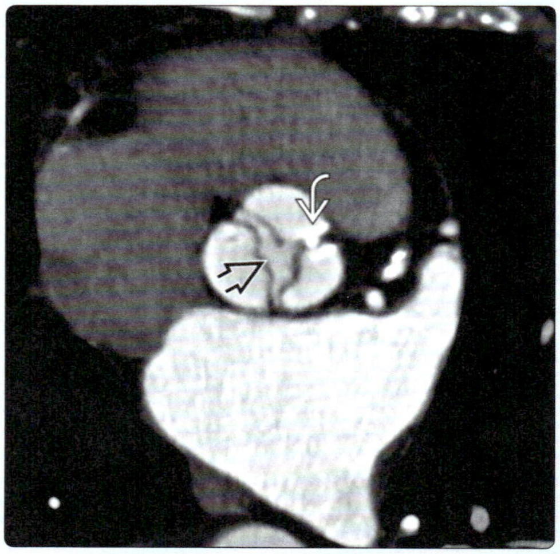

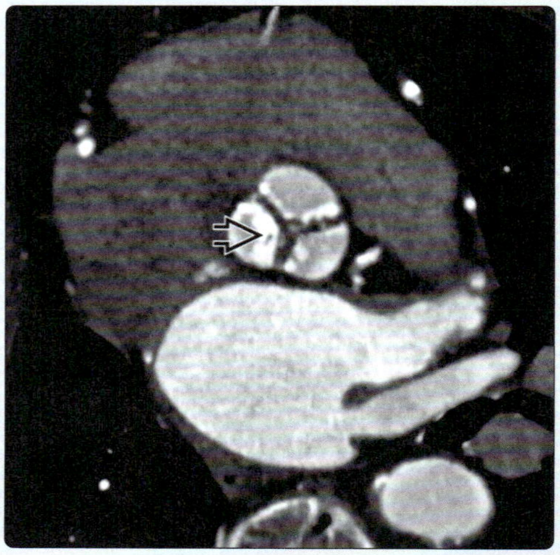

TERMINOLOGY

Abbreviations

- Aortic stenosis (AS)

Definitions

- AS is valve narrowing, which restricts flow of blood from left ventricle (LV) into aorta

IMAGING

General Features

- Best diagnostic clue
  - Echocardiography is cornerstone of AS diagnosis
  - High-velocity systolic blood jet ejected into ascending aorta with ↑ transvalvular pressure gradient and velocity
- Morphology
  - Thickening, fusion, &/or calcification of aortic valve (AV) apparatus
- Concentric LV hypertrophy (LVH) (> 12-mm myocardium thickness)

CT Findings

- NECT
  - Calcium score of AV for prediction of severe AS
    - Highly likely = > 3,000 in males and > 1,600 in females; likely = > 2,000 in males and > 1,200 in females; unlikely = < 1,600 in males and < 800 in females
  - Larger AV calcification associated with ↑ risk for development of heart failure
- Cardiac gated CTA
  - Thickening and calcification of AV leaflets
  - Preplanning for transcatheter AV replacement (TAVR) and post-TAVR evaluation
  - CT myocardial strain in AS assesses degree of LV dysfunction and compensatory changes by quantifying myocardial deformation
    - CT strain predicts both reverse myocardial remodeling and survival in patients undergoing transcatheter AV implantation (TAVI)
  - Identify patients with transthyretin amyloid cardiomyopathy (up to 15% of patients with severe AS)
    - Using pre- and postcontrast imaging, late-enhanced CT can provide measurement of myocardial extracellular volume (ECV) to diagnose cardiac amyloid
    - Photon-counting CT can provide ECV measurement without need for noncontrast scan
- 4D CT
  - Recommended standard in work-up prior to AVR/implantation for AS
  - Quantify morphologic and functional properties of LV myocardial contractility and strain
  - CT offers advantage of direct planimetry to measure AV orifice area (AVA), though thresholds for AS are not defined
    - Hybrid method using CT for LV outflow tract (LVOT) and echocardiography for velocities (AVA hybrid) sets higher threshold of < 1.2 cm^2 for severe AS

MR Findings

- Typically used in patients with suboptimal echocardiography or borderline severity on echo
- Cine SSFP
  - Restricted systolic opening of AV; thickening and low signal of valves from calcification
  - Effective orifice area can be calculated similar to echo using LVOT area and stroke volume
  - Accurate assessment of LV volumes, mass, and ejection fraction (EF); MR is gold standard
- Phase-contrast MR
  - Peak velocity and pressure gradient can be quantified
    - Image slice placed perpendicular (through plane) to jet
    - Lower values than echo due to lower temporal resolution
  - 4D flow MR
    - Entire jet is visualized and can better localize region of peak velocity
    - Different systolic flow patterns in bicuspid valve and its subtypes
      - Right-handed helical and anterior flow in type 1 left-handed helical and posterior with type 2
      - Transvalvular pressure gradient measurement throughout cardiac cycle
- T1 mapping
  - High native T1 in severe symptomatic AS
  - Native T1 and ECV can be used to track LV mass regression post AVR
  - ECV fraction is independent predictor of mortality
- LGE
  - Detects areas of myocardial fibrosis in severe AS: Associated with ↑ all-cause mortality
  - Identify patients with coexisting amyloid cardiomyopathy
- TAVR evaluation: Valve measurements can be performed in MR in those with contraindications to CT

Echocardiographic Findings

- Echocardiogram
  - Transthoracic echocardiography (TTE)
    - Calcified, thickened valve leaflets
    - LV systolic impairment, LVH, and eventual LV dilatation; relative apical sparing (RASP)
    - Visualization of AV morphology
      - Bicuspid vs. tricuspid vs. other
    - Planimetry of anatomic AVA
      - 1.5-2 cm^2 = mild AS; 1-1.5 cm^2 = moderate AS; < 1cm^2 = severe AS
  - Transesophageal echocardiography (TEE)
    - Better visualization of AV
  - Color and pulsed Doppler
    - Indicate severity of stenosis (if normal LV function)
      - Mean transvalvular gradient: < 20, 20-40, > 40 mmHg with mild, moderate, and severe AS, respectively
      - Peak transvalvular velocity: 2.5-3, 3-4, > 4 m/sec with mild, moderate, and severe AS, respectively
      - Dimensionless index (< 0.25)
    - Calculation of AVA by continuity equation [velocity time integral (VTI)]

- Dobutamine exercise stress echocardiography in asymptomatic moderate to severe AS can provoke symptoms to aid patient risk stratification

Nuclear Medicine Findings

- **Positron emission tomography**
  - PET/CT 18F-fluorodeoxyglucose (FDG) for valvular metabolic activity
    - Used to measure inflammation in valves of patients with AS
    - Correlates with macrophage burden
  - 18F-sodium fluoride (NaF) for calcification activity
    - 18F-NaF binds to sites of newly developing microcalcifications
    - Predicts disease progression with respect to CT calcium scoring, echocardiography, and adverse events

Imaging Recommendations

- Best imaging tool
  - Echocardiography is 1st-line imaging for evaluation of AS
  - ECG-gated CTA for preoperative TAVR assessment

DIFFERENTIAL DIAGNOSIS

Supravalvular Conditions

- Supravalvular AS
- Aortic coarctation
- Ascending aortic aneurysm or dilatation
- Supravalvular membrane
- Aortic dissection involving root

Subvalvular Conditions

- Hypertrophic cardiomyopathy
- Subaortic membrane
- Congenital LVOT obstruction

PATHOLOGY

General Features

- Etiology
  - Degenerative/calcifying disease
  - Rheumatic (less common)

Staging, Grading, & Classification

- 3 grades by echocardiography
  - Mild (grade I): AVA > 1.5 cm^2; mean transvalvular pressure gradient < 20 mmHg; peak velocity 2.5-2.9 m/sec
  - Moderate (grade II): AVA = 1.0-1.5 cm^2; mean transvalvular pressure gradient = 20-40 mmHg; peak velocity 3-3.9 m/sec
  - Severe (grade III): AVA < 1 cm^2 (or AVA indexed to body surface area < 0.6 cm/m^2); mean transvalvular pressure gradient > 40 mmHg; peak velocity > 4 m/sec
- Special subtype: Low flow, low gradient
  - Paradoxical (normal LVEF; mean transvalvular pressure gradient < 40 mmHg)
  - Classic (reduced LVEF < 40%; mean gradient < 40 mmHg)

Gross Pathologic & Surgical Features

- Stenotic cusps with nodular calcium deposits on leaflets

CLINICAL ISSUES

Presentation

- Most common signs/symptoms
  - Syncope, angina, dyspnea, arrhythmia, ↑ risk sudden cardiac death, and heart failure
- Clinical profile
  - Asymptomatic over long period ("mystery killer"); symptoms develop late

Demographics

- Age
  - Estimates of incidence rates of severe AS vary from 4-7% in individuals > 65 years

Natural History & Prognosis

- Bicuspid valve is dominant cause for patients < 70 years old; calcific degenerative for patients > 70 years old
- ↑ sudden cardiac death, especially in symptomatic patients

Treatment

- Surgical AVR recommended in symptomatic patients with severe, high-gradient AS
  - Coronary artery bypass grafting if needed for concomitant obstructive coronary artery disease
- Transcatheter AVR recommended in older patients (> 75 years of age) or high surgical risk
- Mortality rate
  - ~ 4% for AVR; ~ 7% with accompanying coronary artery bypass grafting; ~ 10% with repair of another valve
- AVR 10-year survival rate: ~ 85%

DIAGNOSTIC CHECKLIST

Consider

- Calcific AS is predominant
  - ~ 100% of patients exhibit valve calcium
- LV function is important parameter to predict outcome

SELECTED REFERENCES

1. Bernhard B et al: Myocardial analysis from routine 4D cardiac-CT to predict reverse remodeling and clinical outcomes after transcatheter aortic valve implantation. Eur J Radiol. 175:111425, 2024
2. Abecasis J et al: Prevalence and significance of relative apical sparing in aortic stenosis: insights from an echo and cardiovascular magnetic resonance study of patients referred for surgical aortic valve replacement. Eur Heart J Cardiovasc Imaging. 24(8):1033-42, 2023
3. Aquino GJ et al: Myocardial characterization with extracellular volume mapping with a first-generation photon-counting detector CT with MRI reference. Radiology. 307(2):e222030, 2023
4. Bernhard B et al: Routine 4D cardiac CT to identify concomitant transthyretin amyloid cardiomyopathy in older adults with severe aortic stenosis. Radiology. 309(3):e230425, 2023
5. Vahanian A et al: 2021 ESC/EACTS guidelines for the management of valvular heart disease. Eur Heart J. 43(7):561-632, 2022
6. Fukui M et al: Baseline global longitudinal strain by computed tomography is associated with post transcatheter aortic valve replacement outcomes. J Cardiovasc Comput Tomogr. 14(3):233-9, 2020
7. Pawade T et al: Why and how to measure aortic valve calcification in patients with aortic stenosis. JACC Cardiovasc Imaging. 12(9):1835-48, 2019

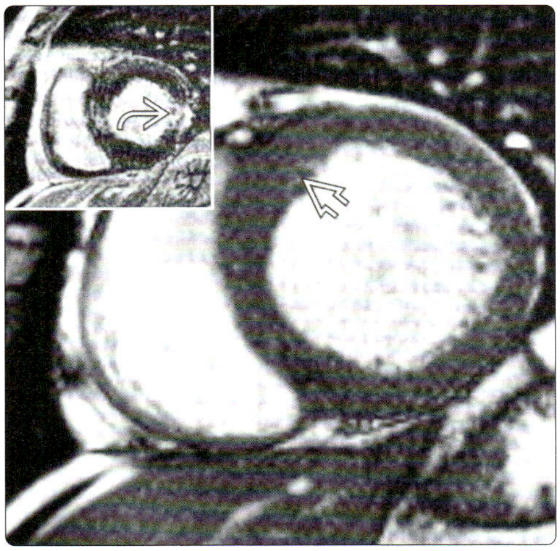

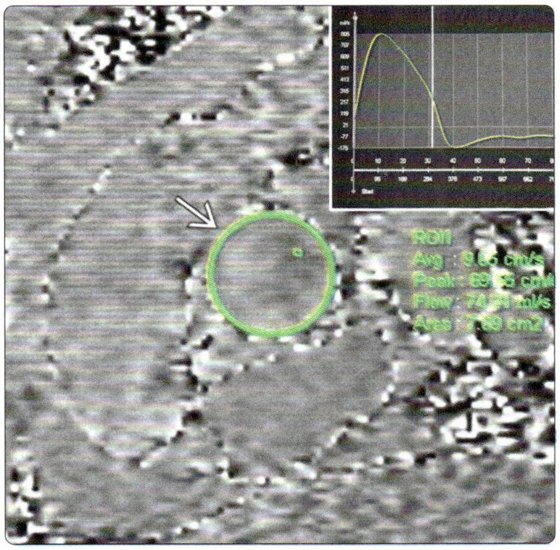

(Left) *Cine image shows asymmetric left ventricular hypertrophy, frequently seen in severe AS. Inset shows LGE, consistent with myocardial fibrosis (8.2% of patients with severe AS).* **(Right)** *Phase-contrast flow across the ascending aorta provides peak velocity through the entire cardiac cycle (inset). Bernoulli equation (peak pressure = 4 x peak velocity squared) provides peak pressure.*

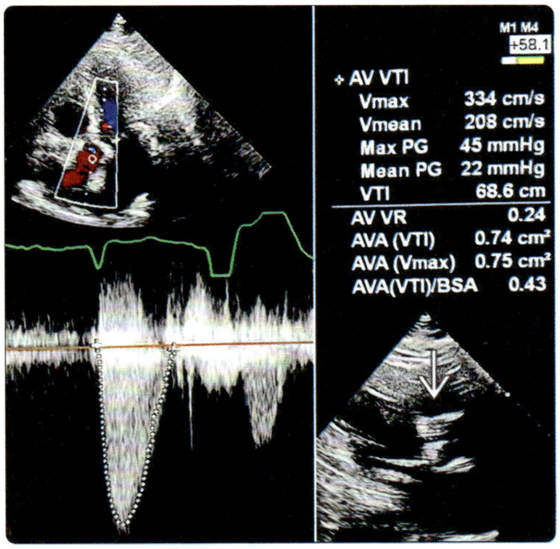

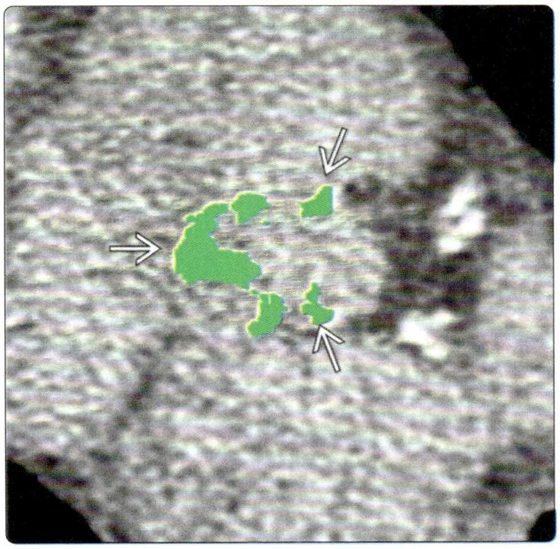

(Left) *Doppler velocities of flow at aortic valve show moderate AS (mean transvalvular pressure gradient: 22 mmHg, peak velocity: 3.3 m/sec). Note the severely calcified, stenotic aortic valve leaflets (inset).* **(Right)** *However, severe aortic valve calcification is noted on noncontrast CT. The calcium score of the aortic valve is > 2,000. Based on multimodality assessment of the aortic valve, this patient went on to aortic valve replacement.*

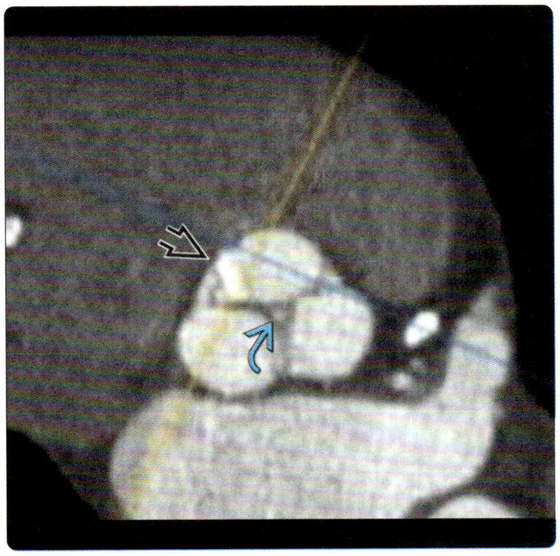

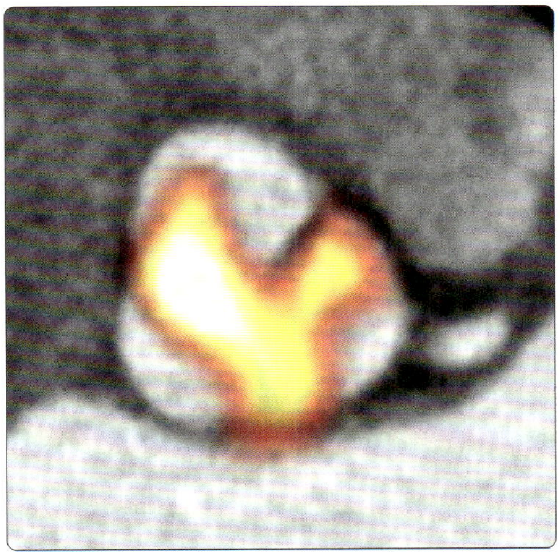

(Left) *Image shows a minimally calcified aortic valve. Additionally, there is lack of coaptation of the leaflets during diastole consistent with aortic regurgitation, which is likely mild.* **(Right)** *However, coregistered PET using 18F-fluoride shows striking AV uptake, consistent with aortic leaflet inflammation.*

KEY FACTS

TERMINOLOGY

- Incomplete closure of cusps during diastole leading to retrograde blood flow into left ventricle

IMAGING

- Best diagnostic tool: Echocardiography (Doppler regurgitant jet)
- MR and CT are alternative modalities
- Axial imaging is useful addition in cases of discordant echocardiography and clinical findings

TOP DIFFERENTIAL DIAGNOSES

- Aortic root disease
- Rheumatic or degenerative/calcific heart disease
- Infective endocarditis
- Trauma
- Bicuspid valve

CLINICAL ISSUES

- Acute aortic regurgitation (AR): Immediate signs of severe left heart failure due to volume overload
- Chronic AR: Progressive signs of left heart failure

DIAGNOSTIC CHECKLIST

- Consider different etiologies of acute and chronic AR
- Acute and chronic AR can be distinguished by size of left atrium and left ventricle (radiograph)
- Acute: Normal size of left atrium (but often pulmonary edema and severe clinical symptoms)
- Chronic: Enlarged left atrium and left ventricle (symptoms late)
- Echocardiography: Doppler regurgitation jet, jet length/width, pressure half-time method
- CT: Incomplete closure of leaflets and aortic root dimensions
- MR: Regurgitant flow, fraction, and left ventricular volume

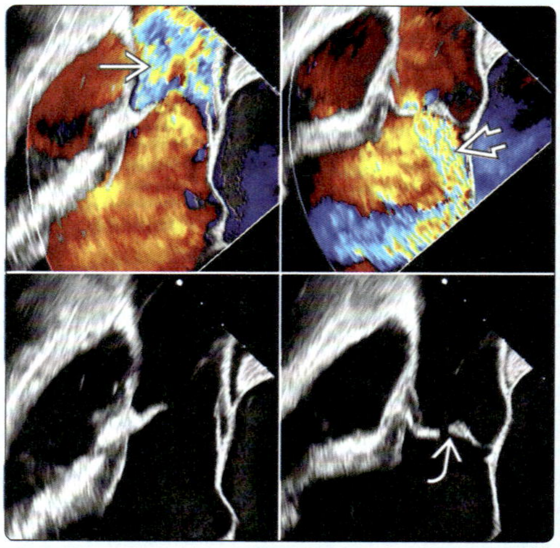

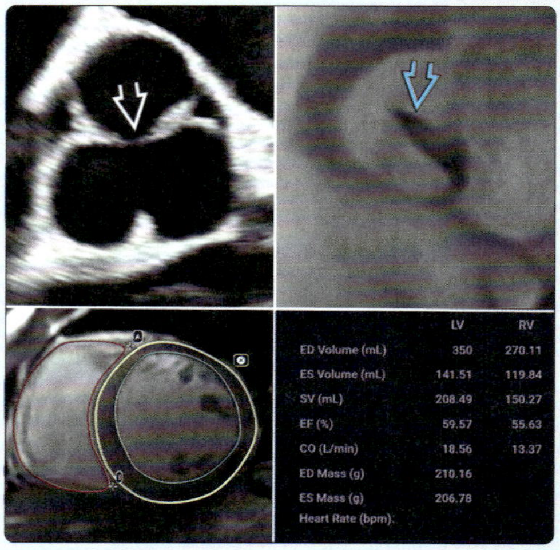

(Left) *Echocardiogram images show anterograde flow in the ascending aorta (AA) during systole (➡, top left). At end-diastole (ED), there is a large eccentric aortic regurgitation (AR) jet (➡, top right) with lack of coaptation of the aortic valve (AV) (➡, bottom right).* **(Right)** *Echocardiogram shows a bicuspid AV ➡, and SSFP MR just inferior to the AV shows the eccentric AR jet ➡. The left ventricle (LV) is dilated (bottom) with an ED volume of 153 ml/m2. AR volume via differences in stroke volumes (SV) is 58.2 ml. Valves were otherwise normal.*

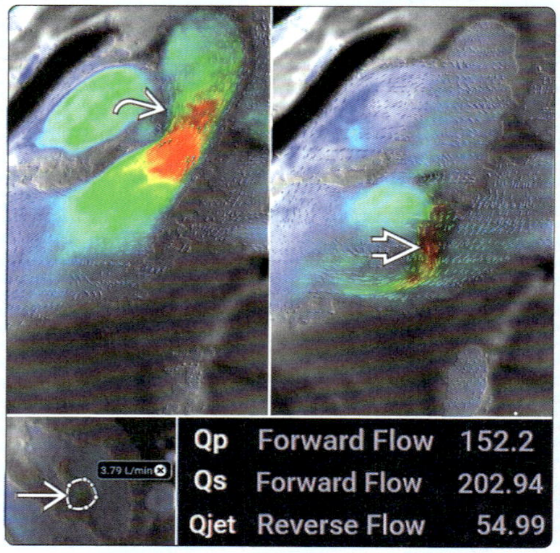

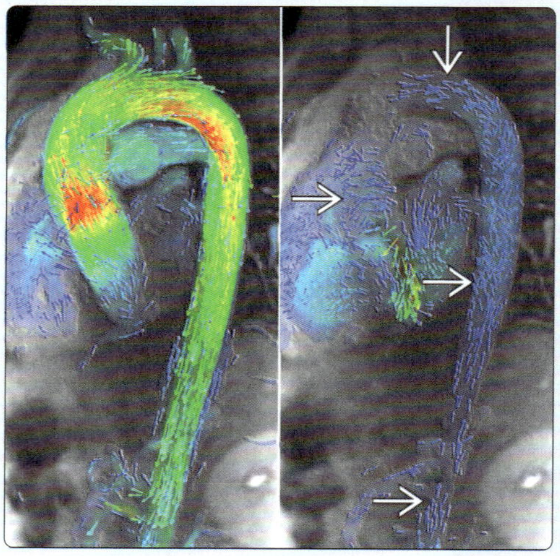

(Left) *During systole, there is anterograde aortic flow (➡, left) with a large diastolic eccentric AR jet (➡, right). AA flow (Qs) = 203 mL and PA flow (Qp) is 152 mL. Direct AR jet measurement (➡, bottom left) shows reverse volume of 55 mL, similar to Qs-Qp of 53 mL. AR is moderate at 26%.* **(Right)** *4D flow during systole (left) shows normal aortic flow with anterograde vector arrows. Holodiastolic flow reversal in the abdominal and thoracic aorta with retrograde vector arrows (right, ➡) signifies severe AR. (Courtesy S. Kligerman, MD.)*

TERMINOLOGY

Abbreviations

- Aortic regurgitation (AR)

Synonyms

- Aortic insufficiency

Definitions

- Incomplete closure of cusps during diastole leading to retrograde blood flow into left ventricle (LV)

IMAGING

General Features

- Best diagnostic clue
  - Retrograde blood flow into LV
- Acute AR
  - No LV dilatation
  - Pulmonary edema due to volume overload
- Chronic AR
  - Eccentric LV hypertrophy and dilatation
  - Dilatation of ascending aorta and aortic root is common
  - Valve calcification is uncommon in pure AR

CT Findings

- CTA
  - Aortic root ± ascending aortic dilation frequent
  - Measurement of aortic anulus, maximal sinus of Valsalva diameter, sinotubular junction diameters
  - Evaluation of sinotubular junction effacement
- Cardiac gated CTA
  - Incomplete coaptation of cusps during diastole results in regurgitant orifice ("central valvular leakage" area)
  - Detects moderate and severe AR; can miss mild AR
  - Cusp: Thickening, calcification, or vegetations; dilated LV at late stage

MR Findings

- Incomplete coaptation of leaflets with retrograde diastolic jet through valve into LV
- Diastolic flow void (jet) area in LV on flow-sensitive sequences provides rough estimation of severity
- Planimetry of effective regurgitant orifice correlates with regurgitant volume (RV) and regurgitant fraction (RF)
- Ventricle dilatation in severe chronic AR
  - MR is gold standard for functional assessment, ventricular volumes, and myocardial mass
- 2D or 4D phase-contrast MR: Highly accurate and reproducible quantification of AR
  - Direct quantification of RV and RF by acquisition perpendicular to ascending aorta
  - Flow curves are generated and allow calculation of stroke volume, cardiac output, RV and RF (RV/stroke volume)
- Severity of AR
  - Variable measurements
    - Mild: < 20%
    - Moderate: 20-40%
    - Severe: > 40%
    - **Or**
    - Mild: ≤ 15%
    - Moderate: 16-25%
    - Moderate severe 26-45%
    - Severe > 45 %
  - AR volume measured by MR is lower than echo in native valves and higher than echo following transcatheter aortic valve replacement (TAVR)
  - Holodiastolic flow reversal in descending aorta indicates severe AR and is strongest additional parameter after echocardiography for evaluating severity of AR
- Determining timing of surgery
  - AR > 33% has 85% sensitivity, 92% specificity for identifying patients who will progress to surgery
  - Severe LV dilation [LV end-diastolic volume (LVEDV) > 246 mL)]
  - Quantification of regurgitation has better association with events than LV indices
  - MR superior to echo in predicting which patients require surgery for chronic AR
    - RV > 50 mL: 50% underwent surgery with 0% for < 50 mL
- Pre- and post-TAVR evaluation alternative to CT
- Contrast-enhanced MR is useful for quantification of degree of myocardial fibrosis in patients with chronic AR
  - Patients with high degrees of myocardial fibrosis have demonstrated suboptimal outcomes post aortic valve replacement
  - Contrast-enhanced MR can help to stratify patients being considered for aortic valve replacement
- LV tracing of endocardial and epicardial borders on 2-chamber views provides reproducible measures of LV volumes, mass, and ejection fraction
  - Postprocessing software can derive myocardial strain measurements to quantify the degree of LV dysfunction

Echocardiographic Findings

- Echocardiogram
  - Acute AR
    - Reduced opening motion and premature closure of valve
    - Delayed opening of mitral valve
    - Minimal dilatation of LV cavity with normal function
  - Chronic AR
    - Marked dilatation of LV cavity with decreased function
- M-mode
  - High-frequency flutter of anterior mitral valve leaflet is indirect sign
- Color Doppler
  - Most sensitive method for assessment of AR: Vena contracta (proximal jet height)
  - Central or eccentric retrograde jet
- Continuous-wave Doppler
  - Measurement of regurgitant jet velocity and calculation of pressure half-time (PHT) is defined as time taken for initial maximal pressure gradient across AV to fall by 50% during diastole
- LV morphology
  - Serial monitoring of LV size and function are useful indicators for timing of surgery

DIFFERENTIAL DIAGNOSIS

Aortic Root Disease

- Dilatation of aortic root (most common cause of pure AR) ± ascending aortic aneurysm
  - Etiologies: Degenerative/atherosclerotic, cystic medial necrosis, Marfan syndrome, aortitis
- Dissection

Rheumatic or Degenerative/Calcific Heart Disease

- Thickened &/or calcified leaflets prevent closure during diastole
- Associated with AS and mitral valve disease

Infective Endocarditis

- Vegetations that prevent coaptation of cusps
- Perforation of cusp

Trauma

- Rupture of sinus of Valsalva
- Loss of commissural support producing prolapse

Bicuspid Valve

- Thickening of leaflets produces incomplete closure &/or prolapse

PATHOLOGY

General Features

- Etiology
  - Secondary to diseases of aortic valve leaflets &/or wall of aortic root
- Valve leaflets
  - Thickening, shortening, and retraction of 1 or more leaflets
  - Perforation of valve leaflet or vegetation that prevents coaptation of leaflets
- Ascending aorta
  - Dilatation secondary to degeneration, dissection, hypertension, and infection

Staging, Grading, & Classification

- 3 grades by Doppler echocardiography
  - Grade I: Mild
    - Vena contracta < 3 mm [or < 25% of LV outflow tract (LVOT)]
    - PHT > 500 ms
    - RV < 30 mls
  - Grade II: Moderate
    - Vena contracta = 3-6 mm (or 25-65% of LVOT)
    - PHT = 200-500 ms
    - RV 30-59 mls
  - Grade III: Severe
    - Vena contracta > 6 mm (or > 65% of LVOT)
    - PHT < 200 ms
    - RV ≥ 60 mls

CLINICAL ISSUES

Presentation

- Most common signs/symptoms
  - Chronic AR is asymptomatic over long period until signs of heart failure develop
- Other signs/symptoms
  - Decrescendo diastolic murmur
- Acute AR
  - Immediate signs of severe left heart failure due to volume overload
  - Infectious endocarditis can cause acute AR
- Chronic AR
  - Progressive signs of left heart failure

Demographics

- Age
  - Variable age manifestation dependent on etiology
  - Prevalence: 4.9% [Framingham Heart Study (FHS)]
  - Increasing prevalence with age: 8.5% female, 13% male at 54 years of age (FHS)

Natural History & Prognosis

- Without surgery, patients with symptomatic AR live ~ 2-4 years
- LV function is important parameter to define clinical management and optimal time point of surgery
- If heart failure NYHA III-IV: High mortality with 25% annually

Treatment

- Medical management
  - Vasodilators, calcium channel blockers, arrhythmia control, antibiotic therapy in cases of infective endocarditis
- Surgical management
  - Decision for operative management is based on clinical symptoms, AR severity, and degree of LV remodeling

DIAGNOSTIC CHECKLIST

Consider

- Acute AR and chronic AR can be distinguished by size of left atrium and LV (radiograph)
  - Acute AR: Normal left atrial size (but often pulmonary edema and severe clinical symptoms)
  - Chronic AR: Enlarged left atrium and LV (symptoms late)
- Echocardiography is primary imaging modality
- ECG gated cardiac CT
  - Detect moderate and severe AR (usually incidentally on coronary artery study)
  - Evaluate etiology (aortic aneurysm, dissection, etc.)
- Cardiac MR to define best timing of surgery (RV and LV volume measurements)

Image Interpretation Pearls

- Radiograph: Enlarged ascending aorta and LV
- Echocardiography: Vena contracta, PHT method
- CT: Incomplete diastolic coaptation of cusps
- Cardiac MR: RF, ventricular volumes

SELECTED REFERENCES

1. Ranard LS et al: Imaging methods for evaluation of chronic aortic regurgitation in adults: JACC state-of-the-art review. J Am Coll Cardiol. 82(20):1953-66, 2023
2. Vahanian A et al: 2021 ESC/EACTS guidelines for the management of valvular heart disease. Eur Heart J. 43(7):561-632, 2022
3. Kammerlander AA et al: Diagnostic and prognostic utility of cardiac magnetic resonance imaging in aortic regurgitation. JACC Cardiovasc Imaging. 12(8 Pt 1):1474-83, 2019

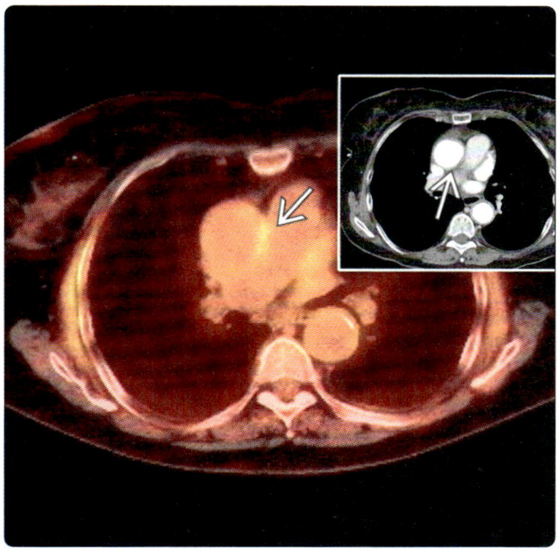

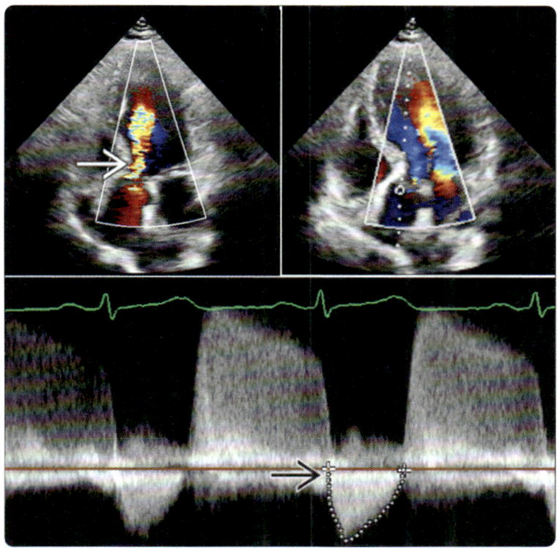

(Left) *Axial FDG PET/CT shows increased uptake in the aortic root wall* ➔ *in a patient with severe AR on a background of biopsy-proven giant cell arteritis. Inset shows aortitis with arterial wall thickening on enhanced CT.* **(Right)** *Color Doppler echocardiogram in the same patient shows a large retrograde pulse jet* ➔ *into the LV. Doppler waveform demonstrates reversal of flow across the aortic valve* ⇨*.*

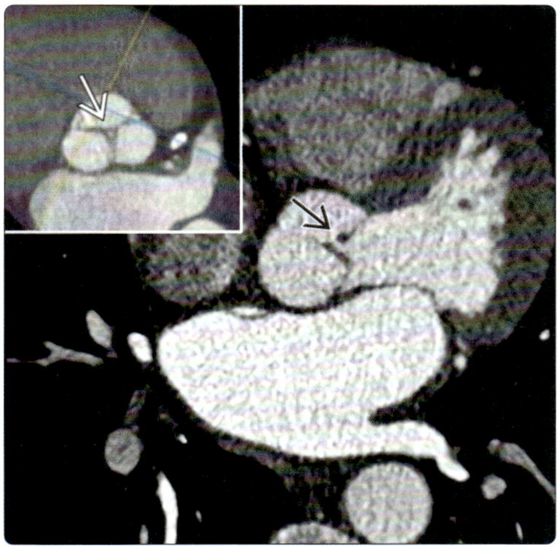

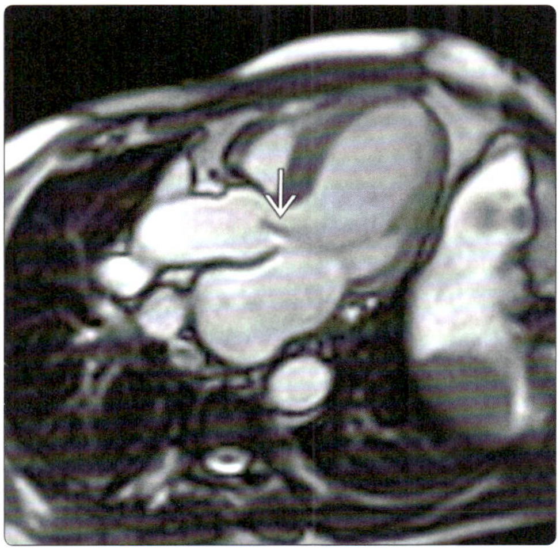

(Left) *Axial oblique CT demonstrates failure of aortic valve coaptation* ⇨ *in diastole. Inset shows true transvalvular view demonstrating a regurgitant orifice* ➔ *during ventricular diastole.* **(Right)** *Three-chamber MR shows a flow void secondary to a high-flow regurgitant jet into the aortic valve* ➔*. The size of the flow void can indicate regurgitant severity. (Image is a corollary of the Austin Flint murmur.)*

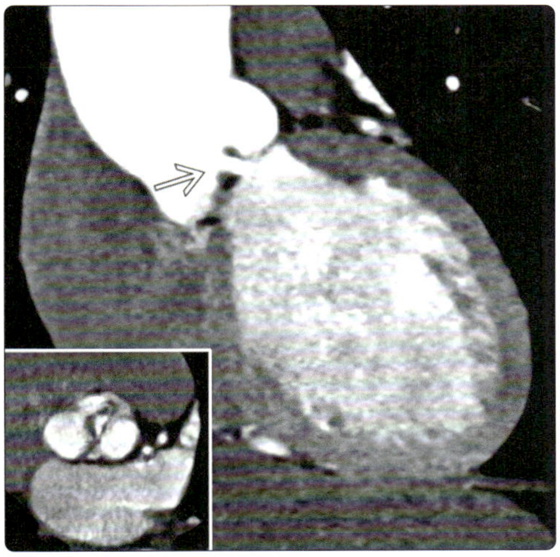

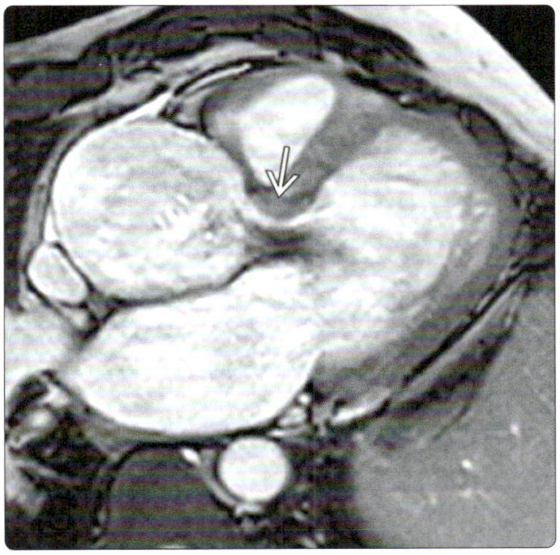

(Left) *Left sagittal oblique diastolic cardiac CT shows incomplete coaptation of aortic cusps* ➔*, which results in regurgitant orifice, leading to severe aortic insufficiency. Axial oblique inset (orthogonal to regurgitant jet) shows a bicuspid valve with fusion of the right and noncoronary cusps.* **(Right)** *Three-chamber SSFP cine MR in diastole shows a dephasing regurgitant jet* ➔ *in the LV outflow tract with a regurgitant fraction of 59%, consistent with severe regurgitation. Also note severe dilation of the aortic root measuring 6.4 cm.*

Mitral Stenosis

KEY FACTS

TERMINOLOGY

- Obstruction to left ventricular blood inflow at level of mitral valve (MV)

IMAGING

- Acceleration of flow at MV level during left ventricular diastole
- Narrowed orifice, often related to commissural &/or chordal fusion
- Left atrial (LA) dilatation

TOP DIFFERENTIAL DIAGNOSES

- Mitral annular calcification
- Obstruction from tumor (myxoma) or atrial thrombus
- Cor triatriatum or other LA obstruction

PATHOLOGY

- Rheumatic heart disease most common
- Degenerative; congenital

CLINICAL ISSUES

- Symptoms appear 20-40 years after acute rheumatic fever in developed countries
- Medical therapy to reduce afterload and treat arrhythmias
- Frequent atrial fibrillation and associated LA thrombus
- Anticoagulation is necessary to avoid risk of stroke
- Dilatation of left atrium, ↑ LA pressures, and eventual right heart failure
- Mild MV stenosis may 1st present with symptoms during exercise; symptoms at rest develop if MV orifice area < 1.5 cm^2

DIAGNOSTIC CHECKLIST

- Transthoracic echocardiography is primary imaging modality: ↑ transvalvular pressure gradient
- ECG gated cardiac CT and cardiac MR useful to clarify etiology of nonprimary valvular mitral stenosis, demonstrate commissural and chordal fusions (4D volume renderings), quantify mitral stenosis severity

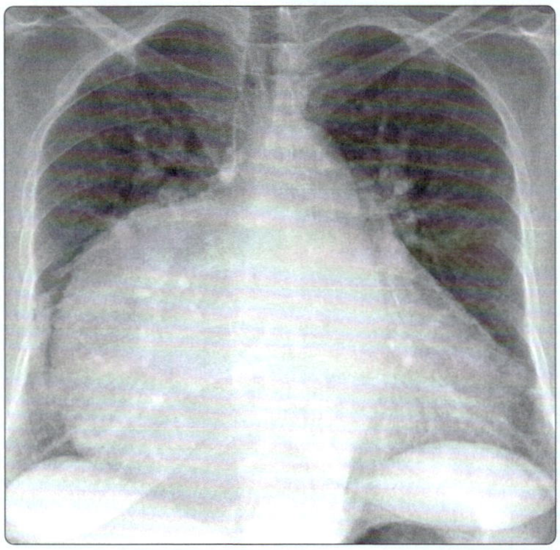

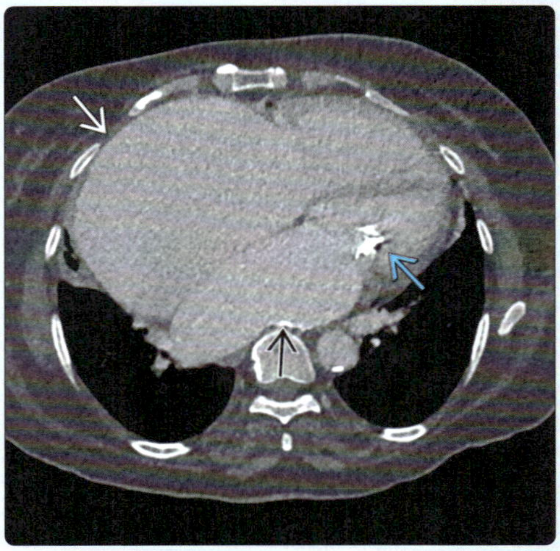

(Left) *PA chest radiograph shows gross cardiomegaly with splaying of the bronchi as a result of left and right atrial enlargement due to severe mitral valve stenosis with secondary pulmonary venous hypertension.* **(Right)** *Axial nongated contrast-enhanced CT of the chest in the same patient demonstrates heavily calcified mitral valve leaflets → and dilated left atrium with patchy calcification along the wall →. Note the grossly dilated right atrium → secondary to pulmonary venous hypertension from severe mitral valve stenosis.*

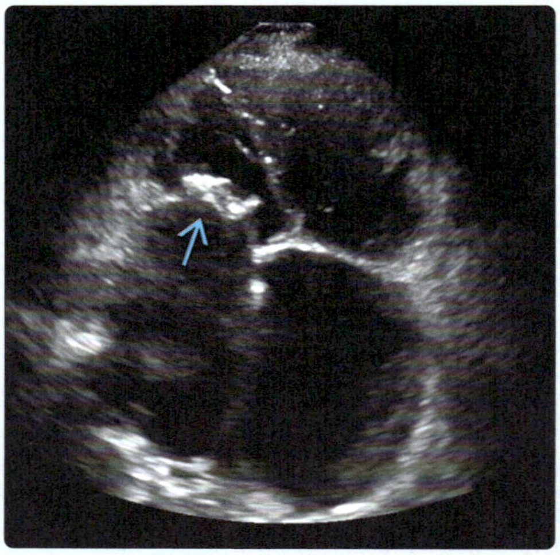

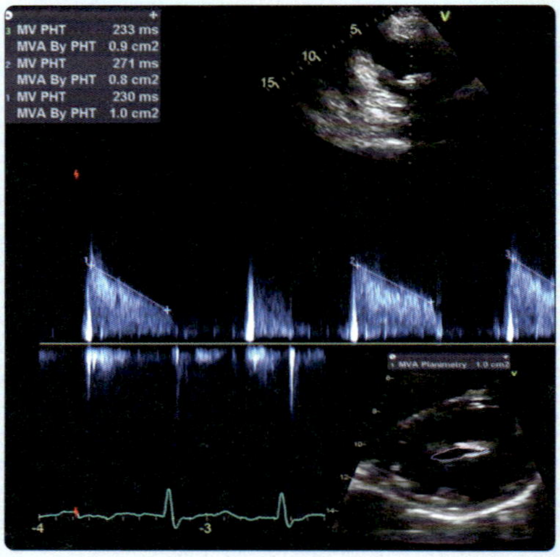

(Left) *Four-chamber echocardiogram in the same patient demonstrates thickened mitral valve leaflets → and a dilated left atrium. The right atrium is grossly dilated as a result of secondary pulmonary venous hypertension.* **(Right)** *Echocardiogram in the same patient demonstrates a pressure half-time measurement between 230-271 ms. Lower right image shows direct planimetry of the mitral valve area measuring 1 cm^2. The findings are consistent with severe mitral valve stenosis.*

TERMINOLOGY

Abbreviations

- Mitral stenosis (MS)

Definitions

- Obstruction to left ventricular blood inflow at level of mitral valve (MV)

IMAGING

General Features

- Best diagnostic clue
  - Acceleration of flow at MV level during left ventricular diastole
- Morphology
  - Thickened &/or calcific leaflets, often with commissural fusion
  - Chordal thickening &/or fusion
  - Left atrial dilatation

Radiographic Findings

- Chest radiography
  - Left atrial enlargement, possible left atrial calcification if longstanding
    - Right retrocardiac double density
    - Enlargement of left atrial appendage (LAA) created extra "mogul" inferior to pulmonary artery (PA)
    - Splaying of carina
    - Left atrium (LA) extending posteriorly toward spine on lateral view
  - Pulmonary venous hypertension (PVH)
  - PA, right ventricle, and right atrium enlargement due to group 2 pulmonary hypertension

CT Findings

- NECT
  - Calcification of MV, mitral anulus, &/or chordae tendinea
- Cardiac gated CT
  - "Doming" of anterior leaflet during diastolic opening and immobility of posterior leaflet (4D cine imaging)
  - Narrowing of MV orifice
  - Thickening &/or calcification of valve leaflets, fusion of chordae tendinea
  - LA enlargement and left atrial thrombi (hypodense, nonenhancing mass) frequent
- NECT and CECT
  - 8% prevalence of MV calcification by 60 years, ~ 1/2 of which will have evidence of MS

MR Findings

- Thickened mitral leaflets
- Fixed mitral leaflets with restricted opening
- Distinctive features of rheumatic MS
  - Hockey stick appearance of anterior leaflet in 2- or 4-chamber views: Bowing of thickened and fibrotic anterior leaflet
  - Fish mouth appearance in short-axis image due to commissural fusion, valve calcification, or both
- MVA can be measured on cine SSFP MR in image perpendicular to direction of flow in valve
- Diastolic flow dephasing (jet) entering left ventricle
- Phase contrast can be used to calculate peak systolic velocity and gradients
- Secondary signs: LA enlargement; main PA enlargement; right ventricle enlargement
- Nonvalvular disease, such as cardiac tumor or ball-valve thrombus, can be seen

Echocardiographic Findings

- Echocardiogram
  - Transthoracic echocardiography
    - Fusion of leaflets with poor leaflet separation in diastole
    - LA enlargement
    - "Doming" of anterior MV leaflet
  - Transesophageal echocardiography
    - 4D images demonstrate commissural fusion and reduced orifice area
    - Better visualizes left atrial/appendage thrombus
- Color Doppler
  - Increased transmitral pressure gradient as estimated by modified Bernoulli equation
  - MVA (by either continuity equation or pressure half-time method)
    - Pressure half-time method may be inaccurate in setting of left ventricular diastolic dysfunction
  - High-velocity flow jet in left ventricle

Imaging Recommendations

- Best imaging tool
  - ECG
    - Transthoracic as baseline examination
    - Transesophageal to clarify etiology, before surgery, and to rule out left atrial or LAA thrombi
- Protocol advice
  - ECG gated cardiac CT
    - Multiphase image reconstruction with multiplanar reformations (MPR): 2-chamber, 3-chamber, 4-chamber, and short-axis views
    - 4D cine imaging

DIFFERENTIAL DIAGNOSIS

Mitral Annular Calcification

- Calcification of mitral anulus is common, especially in older patients
- Does not typically involve valve leaflets
- However, in severe cases, may encroach on base of leaflets and limit leaflet excursion
- Extends from mitral anulus toward base of leaflets, compared to rheumatic disease, which begins at commissures and tips of leaflets

Mitral Valve Obstruction Not Secondary to Valvular Stenosis

- Atrial myxoma obstructing valve orifice (e.g., by diastolic prolapse)
- Ball-valve thrombus in LA
- Valve itself is normal

Left Atrial Obstruction Remote From Mitral Valve

- Cor triatriatum

PATHOLOGY

General Features

- Etiology
  - Rheumatic heart disease (> 95%)
  - Degenerative
  - Congenital
  - Infective endocarditis
  - Mucopolysaccharidoses, including Hunter-Hurler, Whipple, and Fabry diseases
  - Malignant carcinoid syndrome
- Associated abnormalities
  - Pulmonary hypertension, elevated right-sided pressures, and tricuspid regurgitation
- Rheumatic heart disease
  - Thickening → fusion → calcification of mitral leaflets, mitral anulus, and proximal chordae tendineae

Staging, Grading, & Classification

- Clinically significant MS is defined by MVA ≤ 1.5 cm^2
- Graded
  - At risk: Mild valve "doming" during diastole; normal transmitral flow velocity; no hemodynamic consequences; no symptoms
  - Progressive: Commissural fusion, valve "doming" during diastole and MVA > 1.5 cm^2; increased transmitral flow velocities, diastolic pressure half time < 150 ms; LA increased, normal PA pressure; no symptoms
  - Asymptomatic severe: Commissural fusion, valve "doming" during diastole and MVA ≤ 1.5 cm^2; diastolic pressure half time ≥ 150 ms; increased LA size, PA systolic pressure > 50 mmHg; no symptoms
  - Symptomatic severe: Commissural fusion, valve "doming" during diastole and MVA ≤ 1.5 cm^2; diastolic pressure half time ≥ 150 ms; increased LA size, PA systolic pressure > 50 mmHg; decreased exercise tolerance, exertional dyspnea

Gross Pathologic & Surgical Features

- Thickening and fusion of MV apparatus
  - Commissure thickening in 30%; cusps thickening in 15%
  - Chordae in 10%; combination of lesions in 45%
- MV apparatus has funnel-shaped appearance related to commissural and chordal fusion
- Thickened, adherent leaflets inhibit valve function
- Calcium deposits in leaflets and occasional in anulus

CLINICAL ISSUES

Presentation

- Most common signs/symptoms
  - Dyspnea
- Mild mitral valve stenosis may 1st present with symptoms during exercise
- Exertional dyspnea frequently with cough and wheezing
- Stress-induced pulmonary edema (pregnancy)
- ↑ LA pressures causing PH
- Chest pain simulating coronary artery disease in 15%
- Frequent atrial fibrillation results in increased risk of thrombus
  - LA thrombi
    - Up to 30% in severe MS and atrial fibrillation

Demographics

- Age
  - Mean age at clinical presentation: 50-70 years
- Sex
  - F:M = 2:1
- Epidemiology
  - Prevalence: 1.6% of females and 0.4% of males

Natural History & Prognosis

- Symptoms appear 20-40 years after acute rheumatic fever in developed countries
- Severe disability (New York Heart Association class II) 5-10 years after initial symptoms
- 10-year survival rate without surgery is 50-60% if asymptomatic at time of diagnosis
  - 10-year survival rate without surgery is < 15% if presenting with severe clinical symptoms
- Mortality caused by progressive pulmonary and systemic congestion (60-70%) or pulmonary embolism (10%)

Treatment

- Medical therapy to reduce afterload and treat arrhythmias (most common atrial fibrillation)
- Percutaneous balloon mitral valvuloplasty with mortality rate of 1-2% and 70-80% of patients are free of recurrent symptoms at 10 years
- Surgical valvotomy with mortality rate of 1-3% and 5-year survival rate > 90%
- MV replacement with mortality rate of 3-8%

DIAGNOSTIC CHECKLIST

Consider

- Transthoracic echocardiography is primary imaging modality (increased transvalvular pressure gradient)
- Transesophageal echocardiography (TEE) is standard to rule out LAA thrombi in atrial fibrillation
  - 3D TEE useful to identify commissural fusion
- ECG gated cardiac CT and cardiac MR useful
  - Clarify etiology of nonprimary valvular MS (obstruction by myxoma, thrombus, etc.)
  - 4D volume renderings demonstrate commissural and chordal fusions
  - Planimetry comparable to other measures of MS severity

Image Interpretation Pearls

- "Doming" of valve during diastole with hockey stick appearance of anterior MV leaflet
- Irregularly thickened leaflets with narrowing of orifice area typical for rheumatic disease

SELECTED REFERENCES

1. Otto CM et al: 2020 ACC/AHA guideline for the management of patients with valvular heart disease: a report of the American College of Cardiology/American Heart Association Joint Committee on Clinical Practice Guidelines. Circulation. 143(5):e72-227, 2021
2. Al-Sabeq B et al: Imaging in mitral stenosis. Curr Opin Cardiol. 35(5):445-53, 2020
3. Al-Taweel A et al: Degenerative mitral valve stenosis: diagnosis and management. Echocardiography. 36(10):1901-9, 2019
4. Wunderlich NC et al: Rheumatic mitral valve stenosis: diagnosis and treatment options. Curr Cardiol Rep. 21(3):14, 2019

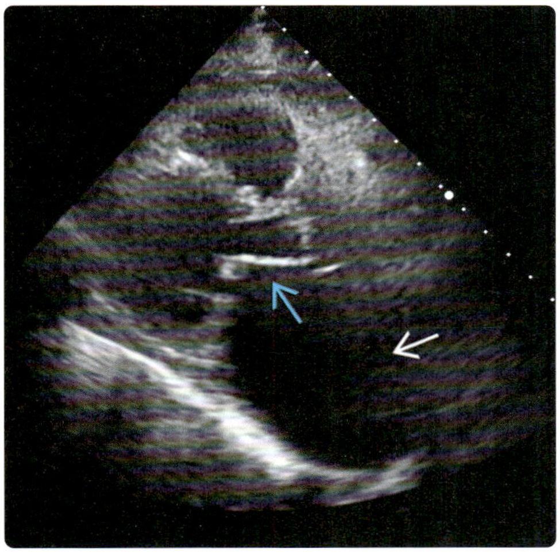

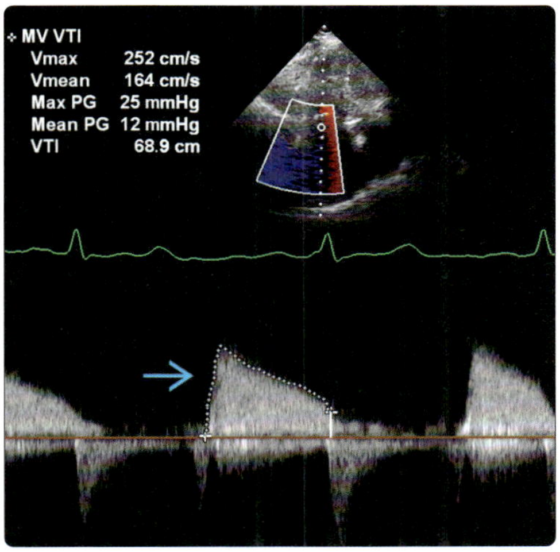

(Left) *Transthoracic echocardiogram in the same patient shows mildly thickened mitral valve leaflets with a hockey stick-like appearance of the anterior leaflet* ➡ *in keeping with the patient's known history of rheumatic heart disease. Note the dilated left atrium* ➡ *secondary to mitral stenosis.* **(Right)** *Doppler echocardiogram in the same patient shows an elevated transmitral gradient (12 mmHG) in keeping with severe mitral stenosis. This is calculated by tracing the transmitral diastolic flow* ➡*.*

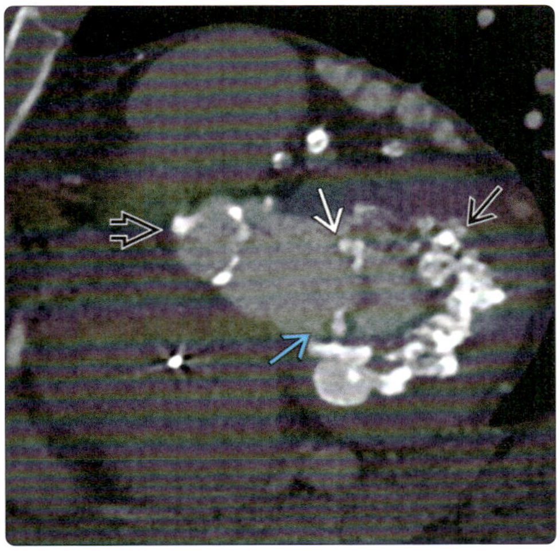

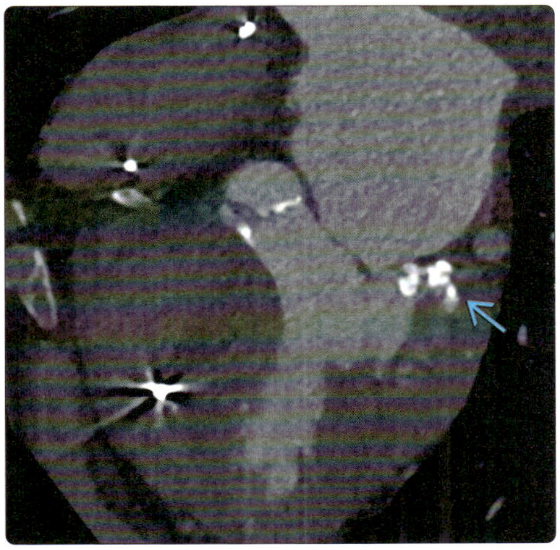

(Left) *Short-axis oblique 2D MPR view at the level of the mitral anulus demonstrates severe mitral annular calcification* ➡ *with calcification extending along the anterior* ➡ *and posterior* ➡ *mitral valve leaflets. Aortic valve calcification* ➡ *is also seen.* **(Right)** *Four-chamber contrast-enhanced CT shows mitral annular calcification with calcification* ➡ *extending along the posterior mitral valve leaflet.*

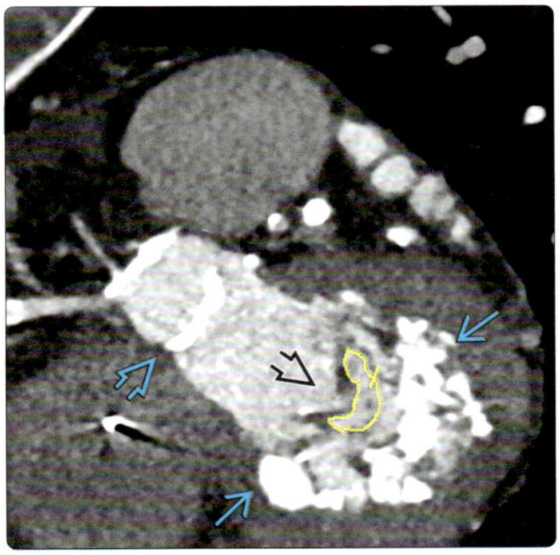

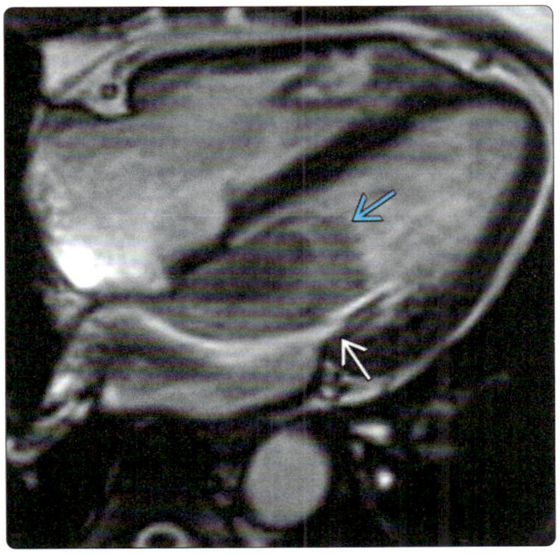

(Left) *Short-axis MPR on contrast-enhanced CT in the same patient demonstrates a mitral annular calcification* ➡ *with calcification extending along the mitral valve leaflets, resulting in a a narrow mitral valve area* ➡*. Aortic valve calcification* ➡ *is again seen.* **(Right)** *Four-chamber MR SSFP cine demonstrates a heterogeneous mobile mass arising from the interatrial septum in keeping with an atrial myxoma* ➡*. The mass extends into the left atrial outflow tract, resulting in a functional mitral stenosis* ➡*.*

Mitral Valve Prolapse

KEY FACTS

TERMINOLOGY

- Mitral valve prolapse (MVP): Systolic extension of mitral valve leaflets > 2 mm into left atrium (LA)
  - "Billowing" leaflet: Part/all of leaflet bows posteriorly into LA > 2 mm beyond mitral annular plane
  - "Flail" leaflet: Chordal rupture to portion of leaflet allows retrograde extension of free edge of leaflet into LA
- Myxomatous mitral valve disease: Inflammatory and infiltrative disease of mitral valve that involves excess collagen and proteoglycan deposition in valve tissue
  - Results in edematous leaflet thickening, elongation, redundancy, and dysfunction

IMAGING

- May relate to problem with mitral valve or subvalvular apparatus (chordae tendineae and papillary muscles)
- Important to localize abnormality based on Carpentier classification
  - Anterior leaflet divided into 3 segments: A1, A2, A3
  - Posterior leaflet divided into 3 scallops: P1, P2, P3
- Echocardiography (ECG)
  - Transesophageal echo is gold standard for accurate characterization by Carpentier classification
- Cardiac MR
  - Able to accurately assess degree of MVP and quantify degree of mitral regurgitation if present
  - Late gadolinium enhancement in papillary muscles/myocardium is associated with ↑ risk of sustained ventricular tachycardia, sudden cardiac death and syncope

TOP DIFFERENTIAL DIAGNOSES

- Myxomatous mitral valve disease
- Hereditary connective tissue disease
- Infectious endocarditis
- Rheumatic disease
- Trauma

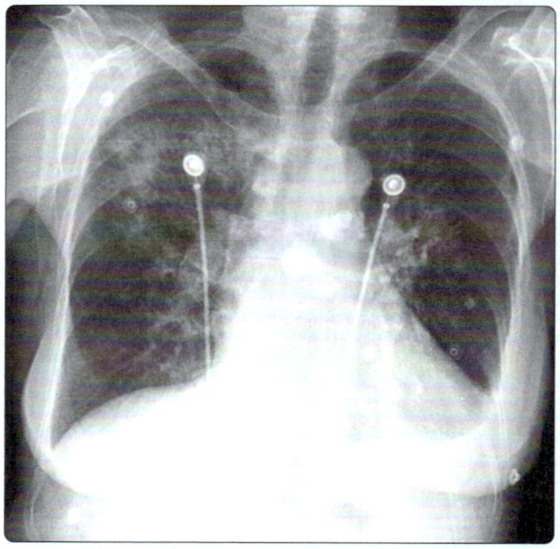
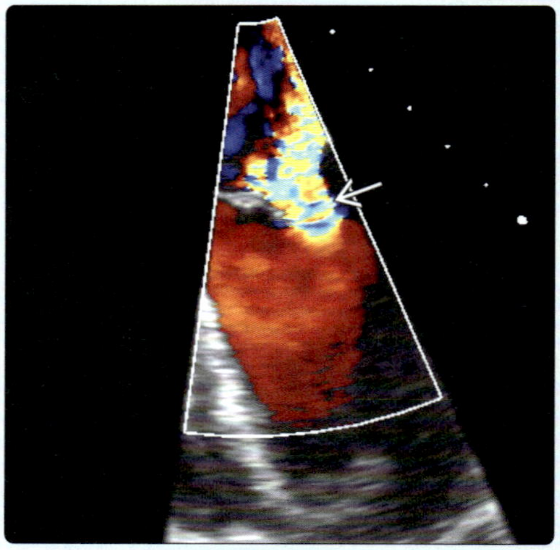

(Left) *AP radiograph in a 71-year-old woman with severe dyspnea shows asymmetric consolidation and ground-glass opacity in the right mid- and upper lung. The patient was afebrile, and her WBC count was normal.* **(Right)** *Image from a transesophageal echocardiogram obtained during systole shows severe mitral regurgitation (MR). Echocardiogram showed rupture of the chordae tendineae attached to the posterior leaflet (PL) of the mitral valve (MV).*

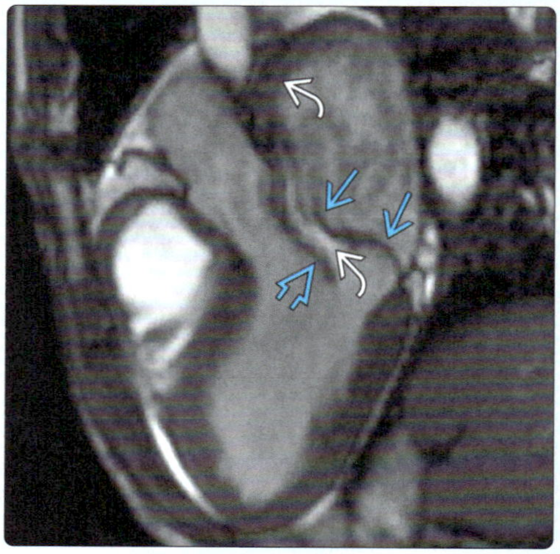
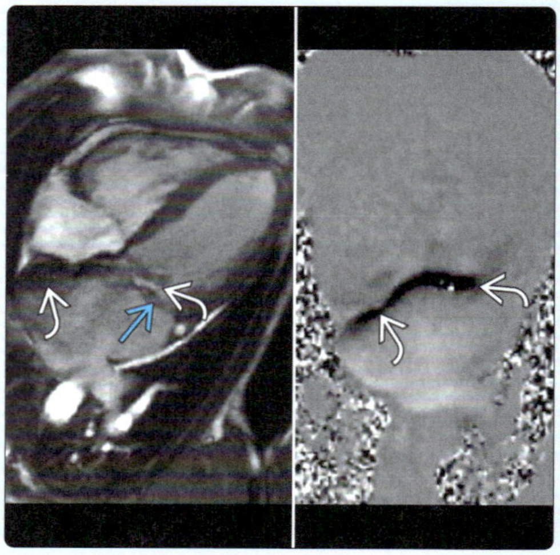

(Left) *Three-chamber SSFP MR shows a flail PL of the MV, which prolapses into the left atrium with a large MR jet directed superiorly and to the right. Both the PL and normally positioned anterior leaflet are thickened and elongated, likely related to myxomatous degeneration.* **(Right)** *SSFP (left) and in-plane phase-contrast MR images (right) show the flail PL and large MR jet. The direction of the jet toward right-sided pulmonary veins causes the asymmetric pulmonary edema on CXR. (Courtesy S. Kligerman, MD.)*

TERMINOLOGY

Abbreviations

- Mitral valve prolapse (MVP)

Definitions

- MVP: Systolic extension of mitral valve leaflets > 2 mm into left atrium (LA)
  - 2 main forms
    - "Billowing" leaflet: Entire leaflet or portion of leaflet bows posteriorly into LA > 2 mm beyond mitral annular plane; tips of leaflets remain in left ventricle (LV)
    - "Flail" leaflet: Chordal or papillary muscle rupture to portion of leaflet allows retrograde extension of free edge of leaflet into LA
- Mitral regurgitation: Systolic retrograde flow of blood from LV into LA
- Myxomatous mitral valve disease: Inflammatory and infiltrative disease of mitral valve
  - Involves excess collagen and proteoglycan deposition in valve tissue
  - Results in edematous leaflet thickening, elongation, redundancy, and dysfunction
  - Most common cause of mitral prolapse and regurgitation requiring surgery in Western world
  - Synonyms: Barlow syndrome or floppy valve disease

IMAGING

General Features

- Best diagnostic clue
  - Systolic extension of mitral valve leaflets into LA > 2 mm
  - If chordal rupture is present and free edge prolapses significantly into LA, "flail" portion of leaflet is present
- Location
  - May relate to problem with mitral valve or subvalvular apparatus (i.e., chordae tendineae or papillary muscles)
  - Important to localize abnormality based on Carpentier classification
    - Anterior leaflet divided into 3 segments: A1, A2, and A3
    - Posterior leaflet divided into 3 scallops: P1, P2, and P3
- Morphology
  - With myxomatous mitral valve disease, there is diffuse thickening of mitral valve leaflets, which become elongated and redundant and eventually prolapse

Radiographic Findings

- Chest radiography
  - May show LV and LA dilatation if mitral prolapse is associated with significant mitral regurgitation
  - In acute MR due to chordal or papillary muscle rupture, can see asymmetric edema in right upper lobe due to direction or regurgitant jet toward right superior pulmonary vein

CT Findings

- NECT
  - May show LA and LV dilatation if mitral prolapse is associated with significant mitral regurgitation
- CECT
  - With myxomatous mitral valve disease, diffuse thickening of mitral valve leaflets may be evident even on nongated CT examinations
- Cardiac gated CTA
  - Thickened mitral valve leaflets with systolic "bowing" > 2 mm into LA beyond mitral annular plane during systole
  - Incomplete closure of leaflets during ventricular systole if insufficiency

Echocardiographic Findings

- Echocardiogram
  - 2D echocardiography (ECG)
    - Thickening (3-5 mm) of 1 or both valve leaflets
    - Symmetrical bowing of valve leaflets > 2 mm behind plane of anulus
    - Asymmetrical buckling of free edge of 1 or both leaflets into LA when chordae have ruptured ("flail" leaflet)
    - Mitral annular disjunction is frequently seen in association with MVP (31-68%)
  - Transesophageal ECG
    - Detailed anatomy of mitral valve and chordae
- Color Doppler
  - Eccentric systolic high-velocity flow jet of mitral regurgitation

Angiographic Findings

- Conventional
  - Buckling of mitral valve
  - Scalloped valve edges reflecting redundant valve tissue
  - Retrograde systolic flow jet if mitral regurgitation

MR Findings

- MR cine
  - Same criteria used in ECG: Symmetrical bowing of valve leaflets > 2 mm behind plane of anulus
    - Thickening of leaflets may be seen
    - 100% sensitivity in detection of MVP syndrome compared to ECG
  - Coexistent mitral regurgitation as eccentric retrograde systolic flow jet
  - Accurate in measuring mitral valve anulus, necessary for repair or valve implantation
- Phase-contrast MR
  - Detect and quantify mitral regurgitation: Direct or indirect
  - Plane needs to be perpendicular to mitral valve regurgitant orifice
- Tissue characterization
  - LGE in papillary muscles and wall of LV
  - Could be due to fibrosis or proteoglycan deposition
  - LGE in papillary muscles and myocardium is associated with ↑ risk of adverse outcomes, e.g., sustained ventricular tachycardia, sudden cardiac death, and syncope

Imaging Recommendations

- Best imaging tool
  - Transesophageal ECG
- Protocol advice
  - ECG

- Transthoracic ECG may demonstrate findings and can recognize associated regurgitation
- Transesophageal ECG is gold standard for accurately localizing problem by Carpentier classification scheme and determining repairability
  - ECG-gated cardiac CT
    - Useful 2nd-line imaging modality
    - Retrospective gating and multiphase reconstructions necessary to allow dynamic assessment
    - 4D cine imaging; multiplanar reformations (MPRs) (3-chamber, 2-chamber, and 4-chamber views)
- Cardiac MR
  - Cine SSFP images in 3-chamber view (allows adequate evaluation for A2/P2 prolapse only)
    - Additional planes may be required to evaluate A1/P1 and A3/P3 portions of valve
      - Due to saddle shape of valve, stack of 3-chamber images spanning entire mitral valve is required
  - Postcontrast imaging is important to assess for myocardial fibrosis

DIFFERENTIAL DIAGNOSIS

Myxomatous Mitral Valve Disease

- a.k.a. Barlow syndrome, floppy valve disease, and MVP syndrome
- Most common cause of MVP worldwide

Hereditary Connective Tissue Disease

- Marfan syndrome, Ehlers-Danlos syndrome, osteogenesis imperfecta

Infectious Endocarditis

- Prolapse of perforated leaflets, free leaflet margins, or vegetations (mimicking leaflet prolapse)

Rheumatic Disease; Trauma

- Diseased subvalvular apparatus (e.g., ruptured chordae) mostly leading to "flail" leaflet

PATHOLOGY

General Features

- Etiology
  - Primary (familial or nonfamilial) or secondary
  - Condition may be inherited, especially in association with connective tissue disorders, such as Marfan syndrome
  - Flail leaflet
    - Papillary muscle rupture due to infarct involving patent ductus arteriosus (PDA), endocarditis, trauma, iatrogenic
    - Chordae tendineae rupture due to myxomatous degeneration, endocarditis, rheumatic heart disease

Gross Pathologic & Surgical Features

- Edematous, thickened, elongated, and redundant mitral valve leaflets in myxomatous mitral valve disease
- If advanced disease is present, chordal thinning and rupture may be present (results in "flail" portion of leaflet)

Microscopic Features

- Myxomatous mitral valve disease
  - Inflammatory cell and fibroblast infiltration of leaflets
  - Disarray of collagen/elastin and excess deposition of proteoglycans

CLINICAL ISSUES

Presentation

- Most common signs/symptoms
  - Most patients are asymptomatic (60%) or experience syncope, palpitations, or atypical chest pain
  - Atrial fibrillation due to progressive LA enlargement
  - Symptoms of heart failure develop in presence of concomitant chronic mitral regurgitation
  - Irregular heartbeat or palpitations, especially while lying on left side
  - May be associated with numerous symptoms of dysautonomia, including anxiety, panic attacks, headaches, fatigue, depression
- Other signs/symptoms
  - Systolic "click" ± murmur
- Clinical profile
  - Strong hereditary component for MVP
  - Present in 90% of Marfan syndrome cases or if 1st-degree relative is affected
  - Sudden cardiac death < 2% (most likely ventricular tachyarrhythmia), more frequent in familial form
  - Fibrin emboli and ↑ risk of cerebrovascular accidents in patients < 45 years of age

Demographics

- Age
  - Manifestation usually between 20-40 years
- Sex
  - F:M = 2:1
- Epidemiology
  - Most prevalent cardiac valvular abnormalities affecting 2-5% of population

Natural History & Prognosis

- Spectrum ranges from normal life to severe mitral regurgitation requiring surgery
- At risk for development of endocarditis, arrhythmias, and spontaneous rupture of chordae

Treatment

- Most patients with MVP require no specific precautions

DIAGNOSTIC CHECKLIST

Consider

- ECG is primary imaging modality

Image Interpretation Pearls

- Localization to A1, A2, and A3 or P1, P2, and P3 aids in surgical planning

SELECTED REFERENCES

1. Malagoli A et al: Arrhythmic mitral valve prolapse: a practical approach for asymptomatic patients. Eur Heart J Cardiovasc Imaging. 25(3):293-301, 2024
2. Figliozzi S et al: Myocardial fibrosis at cardiac MRI helps predict adverse clinical outcome in patients with mitral valve prolapse. Radiology. 306(1):112-21, 2023
3. Adabifirouzjaei F et al: Mitral valve prolapse-the role of cardiac imaging modalities. Struct Heart. 6(2):100024, 2022

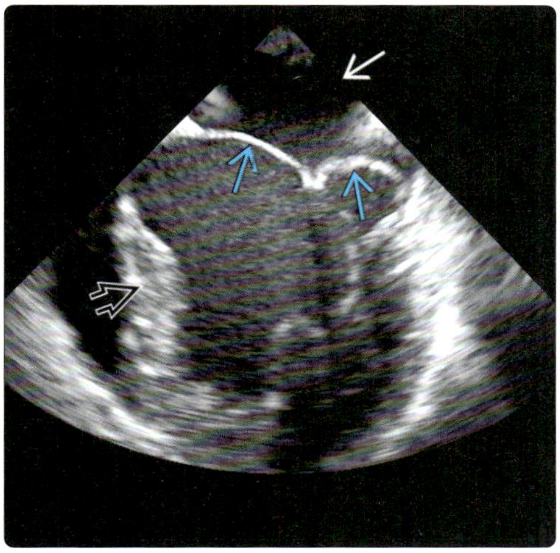

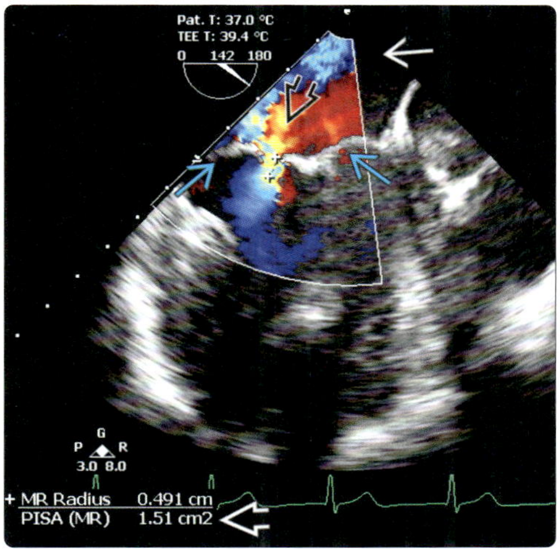

(Left) *Transesophageal echocardiogram shows billowing of the anterior and posterior MV leaflets into the partially visualized left atrium. The left ventricle is annotated to help with orientation.* **(Right)** *Transesophageal color Doppler echocardiogram in the same patient demonstrates prolapse of the anterior and posterior MV leaflets with a large, eccentric regurgitant jet into the left atrium. A proximal isovelocity surface area (PISA) of > 1 cm² suggests severe MR.*

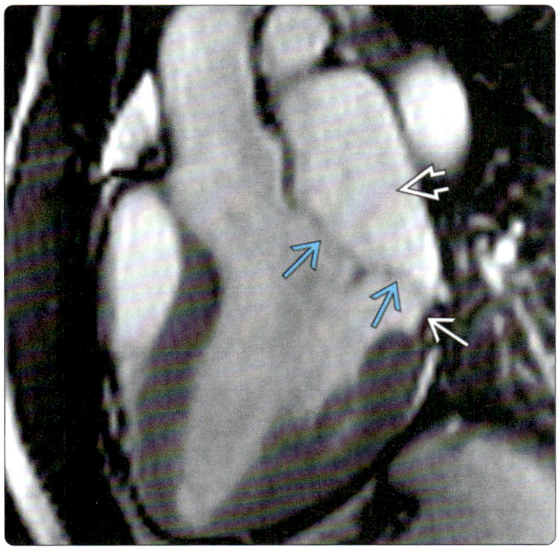

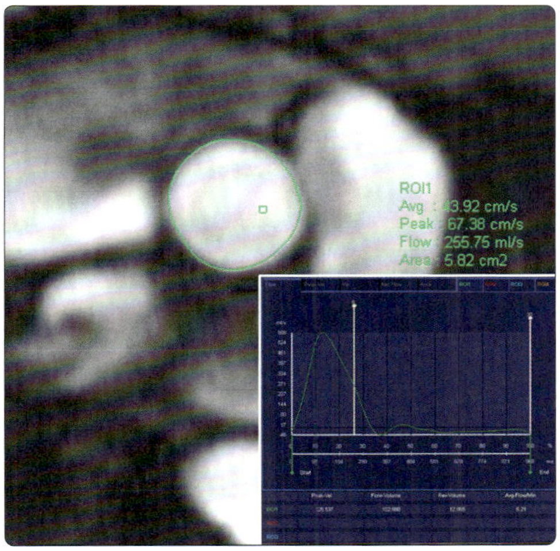

(Left) *Three-chamber SSFP MR in the same patient shows "billowing" of the anterior and posterior mitral leaflets into the left atrium. Mitral annular disjunction is present in this case.* **(Right)** *MR can measure aortic forward flow using phase-contrast flow sequences. The inset shows blood flow across the ascending aorta during a cardiac cycle. The aortic forward flow can be subtracted from left ventricular stroke volume to give the mitral regurgitant fraction (assuming no other valvular disease).*

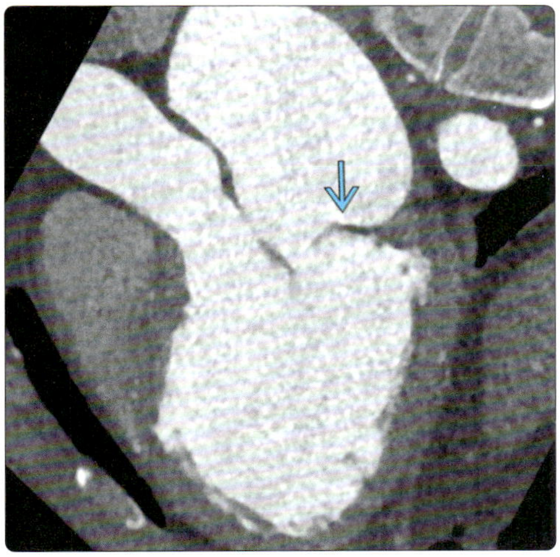

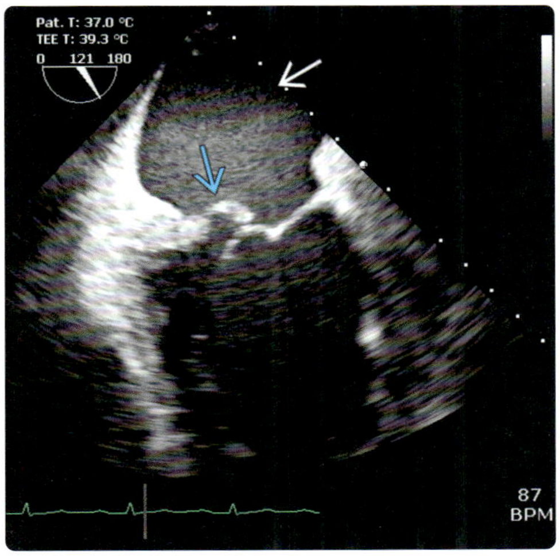

(Left) *Three-chamber MPR contrast-enhanced CT demonstrates "billowing" of the PL posterior to the mitral anulus plane.* **(Right)** *Two-chamber transesophageal echocardiogram in the same patient demonstrates prolapse of the P2 segment of the posterior MV leaflet and dilated left atrium.*

KEY FACTS

TERMINOLOGY

- Mitral regurgitation (MR)
- Incomplete closure of mitral valve during systole resulting in retrograde blood flow into left atrium (LA)

IMAGING

- Retrograde flow from left ventricle (LV) into LA during systole
- Acute MR: Usually normal heart size, often with asymmetric pulmonary edema (most severe in right upper lobe)
- Chronic MR: Dilated LA and LV; pulmonary artery and right heart dilatation late in disease
- Echocardiography is most commonly utilized for diagnosis and surveillance imaging
- Key imaging biomarkers of risk have been identified in primary MR: reduced left ventricular ejection fraction, impaired strain, and LV fibrosis

TOP DIFFERENTIAL DIAGNOSES

- Degenerative mitral valve disease (60-70%)
- Ischemic MR (20%)
- Infective endocarditis (2-5%)
- Rheumatic heart disease (2-5%)

PATHOLOGY

- Classified based on causes (ischemic vs. nonischemic) and mechanisms (functional vs. organic)
- Graded by echocardiography based on size of vena contracta, regurgitant volume, regurgitant fraction, and effective regurgitant orifice area

DIAGNOSTIC CHECKLIST

- Regardless of imaging modality used, try to differentiate between ischemic and nonischemic etiologies as well as functional vs. organic causes of MR, as this may significantly affect management

(Left) *Echocardiogram shows at least moderate mitral regurgitation with the regurgitant jet reaching the back wall* → *of the left atrium. Note dilation of the left atrium* ⇒*, commonly seen in chronic mitral regurgitation.* **(Right)** *Corresponding cardiac 4-chamber SSFP MR in the same patient shows the mitral regurgitant jet into the left atrium* ⇒.

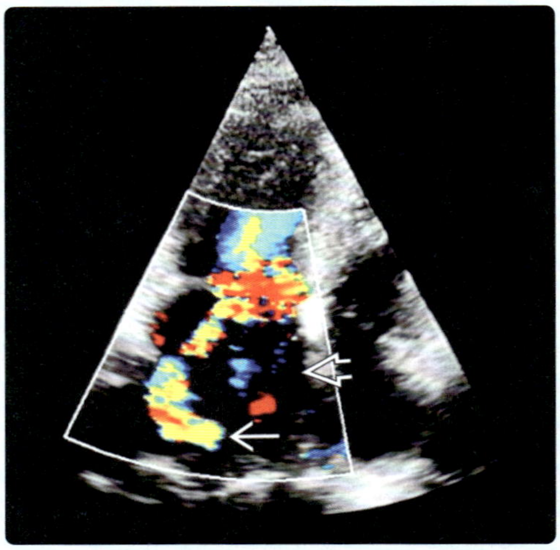

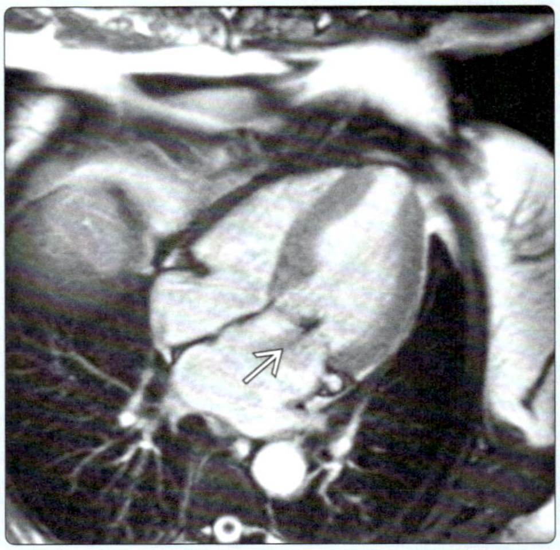

(Left) *Phase-contrast sequence across the ascending aorta above the valve cusp tips* → *allows measurement of aortic forward flow (inset). Subtracting left ventricular (LV) stroke volume yields the mitral regurgitant volume.* **(Right)** *A more indirect method is to subtract the LV stroke volume from the right ventricular stroke volume, which yields the mitral regurgitant volume.*

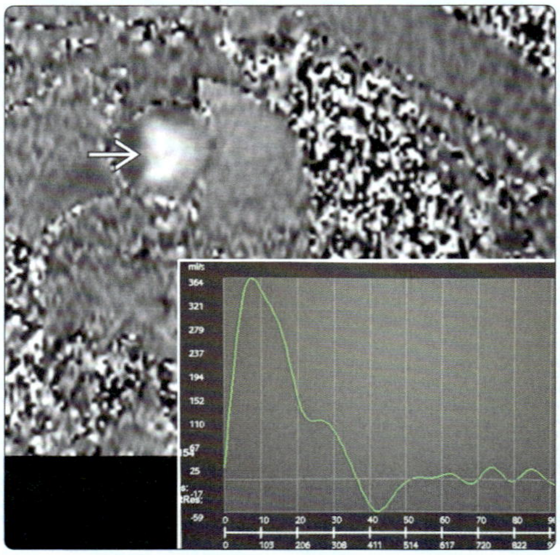

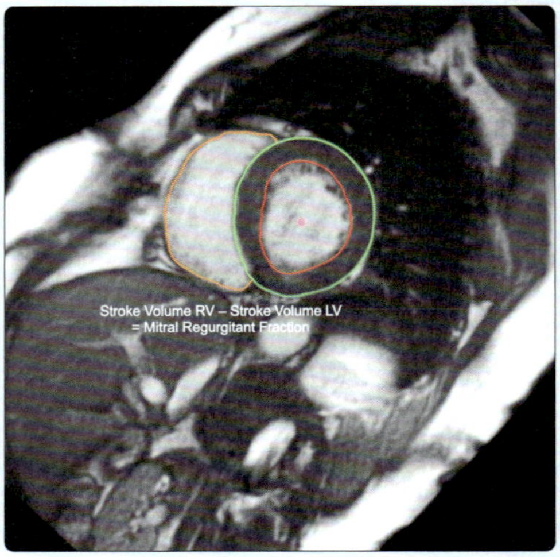

TERMINOLOGY

Abbreviations

- Mitral regurgitation (MR)

Definitions

- Incomplete closure of mitral valve (MV) during systole resulting in retrograde blood flow into left atrium (LA)
  - Classified as primary (degenerative) MR or secondary (functional) MR
    - Primary MR is characterized by leaflet prolapse or flail, leading to loss of leaflet tip/edge coaptation
    - Secondary MR is consequence of left ventricular or left atrial remodeling and dysfunction, leading to coaptation loss due to leaflet tethering, preventing adequate leaflet tip/edge approximation

IMAGING

General Features

- Best diagnostic clue
  - Retrograde flow through MV into LA during systole

CT Findings

- Cardiac gated CTA
  - Multiphase studies show similar morphologic findings as echocardiography and MR
    - Limited by lack of ability to assess flow
    - Volumetric assessment of LA (at end-systole) is useful in predicting risk of atrial fibrillation (AFib)
  - Can quantify left ventricular volume and function with similar accuracy as MR imaging

MR Findings

- Systolic flow dephasing (jet) into LA
- Gold standard for functional assessment; left ventricular ejection fraction (LVEF), volumes, and mass
  - LA and LV dilatation is common in chronic MR
- Phase contrast may be used to quantitate severity
  - Direct method for isolated MR = LV stroke volume (LVSV) - aortic forward flow
    - Indirect method for isolated MR = LVSV - right ventricle stroke volume (RVSV)
  - MR in patients with aortic regurgitation (AR) = LVSV - (AR volume + forward aortic flow)
  - MR in patients with ASD = LVSV - aortic forward flow
  - MR in patients with tricuspid regurgitation (TR)
    - TR = RVSV: Forward stroke volume
  - MR in restrictive VSD and unidirectional left-right-right shunt
    - LVSV - PA forward flow
  - MR may also be measured directly using short-axis phase-contrast (PC) sequence at level of mitral inflow
    - Through plane and in-plane motion of mitral anulus is challenge for conventional 2D PC cine
    - Improved accuracy with 4D flow enables retrospective valve tracking
- MR more accurate than echocardiography for MR severity using postsurgical remodeling as reference standard
  - Higher degree of MR associated with greater degree of remodeling
  - No correlation between PISA-derived regurgitant volume (RVol), and postsurgical remodeling
- MR typically performed in patients with severe MR in echocardiography for greater diagnostic certainty and deciding surgery
- MR best predictor of which patients will develop symptoms or have indication for surgery
- LGE
  - In primary MR, LGE of papillary muscles is associated with complex ventricular arrhythmias
- 4D flow
  - Advantages include single acquisition, single sequence, and retrospective analysis that allow valve tracking to account for motion throughout cardiac cycle
- Predictors of worse outcome in asymptomatic patients
  - Dilated LV; borderline reduced LVEF; dilated LA; progressive dilatation of LV and worsening of LVEF

Echocardiographic Findings

- Doppler echocardiography
  - Combined evaluation with color, pulsed-wave, and continuous-wave Doppler is utilized
- Quantitative 2D echocardiography
  - Useful for estimation of LV and LA volumes
  - Problems include inconsistency between measures and noncircular, eccentric, and nonholosystolic jets
- 3D echocardiography
  - Evaluation of annular size and localization of MV dysfunction in setting of prolapse/flail leaflets

Imaging Recommendations

- Best imaging tool
  - Echocardiography is most commonly utilized for diagnosis and surveillance imaging

DIFFERENTIAL DIAGNOSIS

Degenerative Mitral Valve Disease (60-70%)

- Myxomatous degeneration (a.k.a. Barlow syndrome)
  - Elongated, redundant, and thickened leaflets secondary to mucopolysaccharide deposition
  - Often results in MV prolapse (MVP) or flail leaflet
- Primary flail leaflets
  - Usually result of ruptured chordae
  - Posterior leaflet involved in 70% of cases

Ischemic Mitral Regurgitation (20%)

- Ventricular remodeling results in functional MR
  - Left ventricular remodeling and dilatation → apical displacement of papillary muscles → traction on MV via chordae → incomplete coaptation (despite normal MV leaflets)
  - Malcoaptation from annular flattening and dilatation
- Papillary muscle rupture: Rare but can cause severe acute MR

Infective Endocarditis (2-5%)

- Perforation of leaflets
- Vegetations may prevent complete leaflet coaptation

Rheumatic Heart Disease (2-5%)

- Thick (and often calcified), stiff leaflets and chordae, often with chordal and commissural fusion

PATHOLOGY

General Features

- Genetics
  - Some genetic causes: Familial MVP, Marfan syndrome, and other connective tissue diseases

Staging, Grading, & Classification

- Graded by echo based on size of vena contracta (VC), RVol, regurgitant fraction (RF), and effective regurgitant orifice (ERO) area
  - Mild: VC 1-3 mm, RVol < 30 mL, RF < 30%, ERO < 0.2 cm^2
  - Moderate: VC 4-6 mm, RVol 30-59 mL, RF 30-49%, ERO 0.2-0.39 cm^2
  - Severe: VC ≥ 7 mm, RVol ≥ 60 mL, RF ≥ 50%, ERO ≥ 0.4 cm^2
    - Severity is graded more stringently in individuals with ischemic MR
      - Severe disease at lower threshold
    - Severe ischemic MR: RVol > 45 mL, RF > 40%, ERO > 0.3 cm^2
- Recommended MR grading
  - Primary (based on RF): Mild < 20%, moderate 20-39%, severe 40-50%, very severe > 50%
  - Secondary (based on RV): Mild < 30 mL, moderate 30-60 mL, severe ≥ 60 mL

CLINICAL ISSUES

Presentation

- Most common signs/symptoms
  - Acute MR (uncommon)
    - Almost always severe symptoms
    - LA is normal in size with increase in pressure leading to pulmonary edema
    - Reduced forward output (shock) may develop due to LV volume overload
  - Chronic MR (most common)
    - May be asymptomatic until late in course of disease
    - Risk of morbidity and mortality depends not only on severity of disease but also on underlying causes and mechanisms
    - In general, with severe chronic MR, > 90% of patients either die or require surgery within 10 years
- Other signs/symptoms
  - AFib
    - Common consequence of chronic MR
    - Associated with increased LA volumes

Demographics

- Age
  - Typically older individuals in industrialized nations
  - Younger patients in countries with endemic rheumatic fever
- Epidemiology
  - Moderate to severe MR is most common valve disease in USA

Treatment

- Medical management: Varies according to mechanism of disease (organic or functional)
  - Organic disease
    - Medical management otherwise has shown little efficacy in management of chronic organic MR
      - Notable exception is anticoagulation in setting of AFib related to chronic MR
  - Functional disease
    - Medical therapy is similar to typical heart failure regimens and is typically based on long-acting β-blocker (e.g., carvedilol) and ACE-inhibition
- Surgical management
  - Only approach shown to provide sustained relief of symptoms of heart failure
  - May involve valve repair (usually preferred) or valve replacement, ± annuloplasty
    - MV repair
      - May involve valvular, subvalvular, &/or annular procedures to restore leaflet coaptation
    - MV replacement
      - Bioprosthetic: Less durable but does not require anticoagulation; typically utilized in older individuals (> 65 years)
      - Mechanical: More durable but requires chronic anticoagulation; typically used in younger individuals
      - Choice is also influenced by patient preference and ability to maintain anticoagulation
      - Either approach must aim to preserve integrity and function of mitral subvalvular apparatus
- Transcatheter management
  - Transcatheter edge-to-edge repair is of benefit to patients with severely symptomatic primary MR who are at high or prohibitive risk for surgery as well as to select subset of patients with secondary MR who remain severely symptomatic despite guideline-directed management and therapy for heart failure
  - MATTERHORN trial: In patients with heart failure and secondary MR who were at high surgical risk, transcatheter edge-to-edge repair was noninferior to surgical MV repair or replacement

DIAGNOSTIC CHECKLIST

Image Interpretation Pearls

- Grading is typically based on echocardiography
- MR imaging protocol includes contiguous LVOT cines perpendicular to MV commissures and cines through commissures
- Regardless of imaging modality used, try to differentiate between ischemic and nonischemic etiologies as well as functional vs. organic causes of MR, as this may significantly affect management

SELECTED REFERENCES

1. Baldus S et al: Transcatheter repair versus mitral-valve surgery for secondary mitral regurgitation. N Engl J Med. 391(19):1787-98, 2024
2. Otto CM et al: 2020 ACC/AHA guideline for the management of patients with valvular heart disease: executive summary: a report of the American College of Cardiology/American Heart Association joint committee on clinical practice guidelines. Circulation. 143(5):e35-71, 2021
3. Reid A et al: Multimodality imaging in valvular heart disease: how to use state-of-the-art technology in daily practice. Eur Heart J. 42(19):1912-25, 2021
4. Garg P et al: Assessment of mitral valve regurgitation by cardiovascular magnetic resonance imaging. Nat Rev Cardiol. 17(5):298-312, 2020

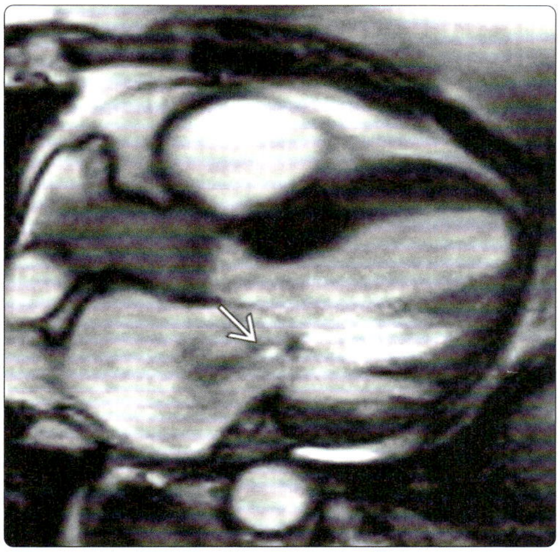

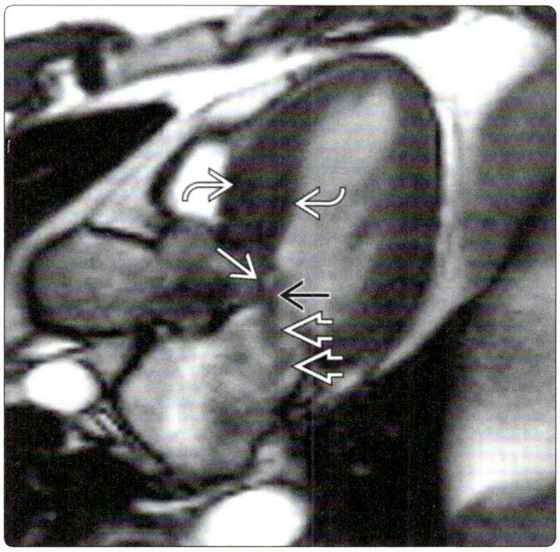

(Left) *Three-chamber SSFP cine MR in early systole shows LV dilatation and a centrally oriented jet ➔. The tethering of valve leaflets to the dilated LV wall resulted in failure of coaptation (functional mitral regurgitation).* **(Right)** *Three-chamber SSFP cine MR in a patient with septal hypertrophy ➔ shows an eccentric mitral regurgitation jet ➔ posteriorly into the left atrium related to systolic anterior motion of anterior mitral valve leaflet ⇨. Note presence of systolic jet in the LV outflow tract ➔ below the aortic valve.*

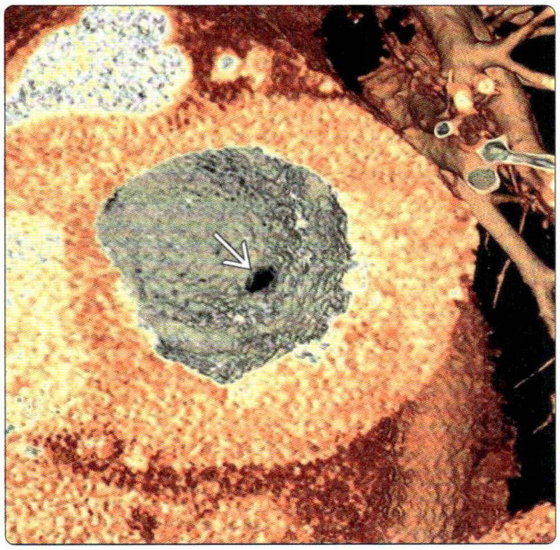

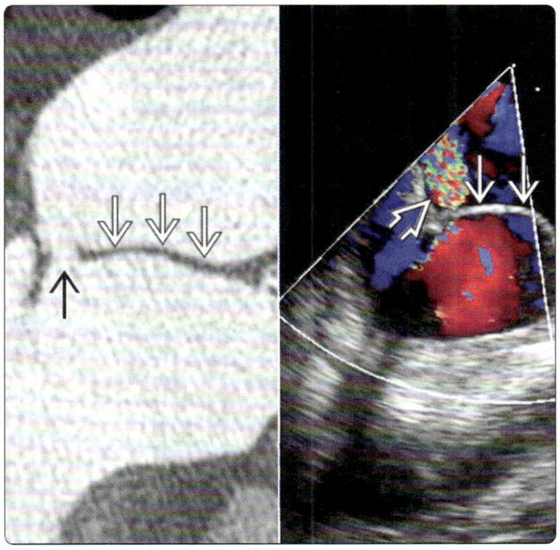

(Left) *Thick-slab short-axis volume-rendered cardiac gated CTA at the level of the mitral valve in systole (valve closed) demonstrates an 8-mm perforation ➔ in the anterior leaflet.* **(Right)** *MPR from the same examination (left) and intraoperative transesophageal echocardiogram (right) oriented through the anterior leaflet of the mitral valve ➔ show discontinuity at the site of perforation ⇨ on the MPR and eccentric mitral regurgitation into the left atrium on the echo ➔.*

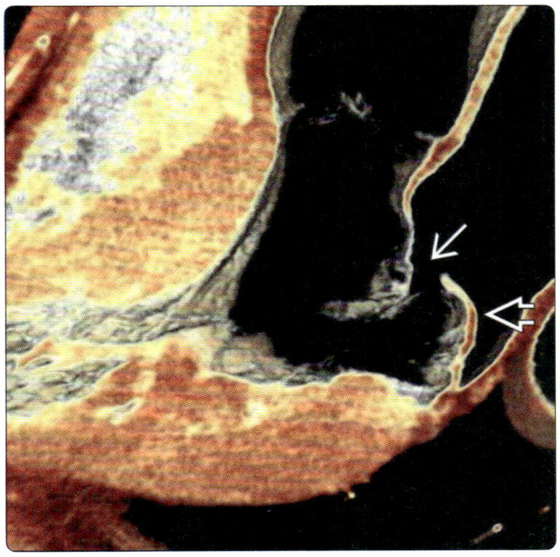

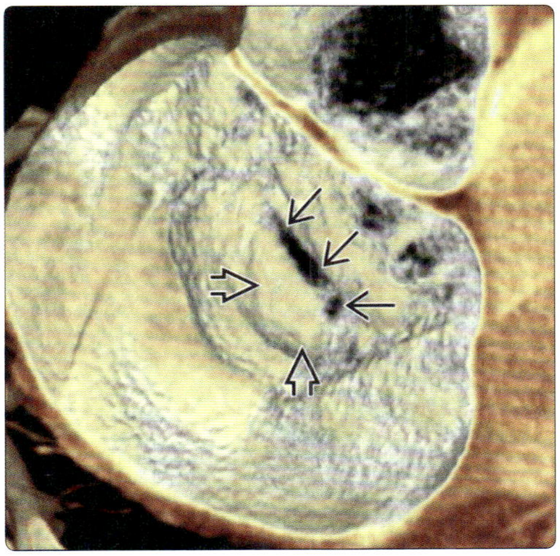

(Left) *Thin-slab volume-rendered 3-chamber cardiac gated CTA during systole demonstrates a flail P2 scallop ➔ of the posterior leaflet of the mitral valve, resulting in a large area of incomplete coaptation ➔.* **(Right)** *Thick-slab short-axis volume-rendered CTA during systole (same patient), looking at the mitral orifice from the left atrial perspective, also demonstrates the flail P2 scallop ⇨ and the resultant region of incomplete coaptation ⇨.*

KEY FACTS

IMAGING

- J-, C-, U-, or O-shaped mitral annular calcification (MAC) on radiography or reconstructed CT
- "Eggshell" or rim-calcified mass in same location containing lower density material (toothpaste-like necrotized calcium)
- NECT usually sufficient for diagnosis
- Cardiac CTA may be useful for presurgical planning to assess myocardial involvement, distinguish whether leaflets are calcified or not, and distinguish caseous calcification from tumor
- Hyperechogenic, dense calcification with acoustic shadowing
- Echodense mass with echolucent center (liquefaction necrosis)
- May mimic neoplasm on echocardiography
- Calcium usually dark on all MR pulse sequences
    - Helpful for differential diagnosis of caseous calcification vs. neoplasm

TOP DIFFERENTIAL DIAGNOSES

- MAC may be pitfall on calcium scoring CT as MAC can mimic atherosclerotic calcification in left circumflex coronary artery

PATHOLOGY

- In patients with end-stage renal disease, *ENPP1* genotype associated with higher severity of systemic arterial calcification
- Not usually associated with mitral valve stenosis or regurgitation
- If extensive calcification, myocardium may be involved
- Caseous calcification: Toothpaste-like, white material = liquefaction necrosis

(Left) *Left ventricular (LV) long-axis SSFP MR shows a mass ➡ wedged into inferior left atrioventricular (AV) groove, slightly hypointense to myocardium. Note the very thin, hypointense rim. Caseous MAC may be difficult to differentiate from neoplasm or aneurysm on MR and echocardiography. (Courtesy W. Eicher, MD.)* **(Right)** *LV long-axis T1 C+ MR (same patient) shows no enhancement of AV groove mass ➡. Note the thin, hypointense rim corresponding to calcification on CT. (Courtesy W. Eicher, MD.)*

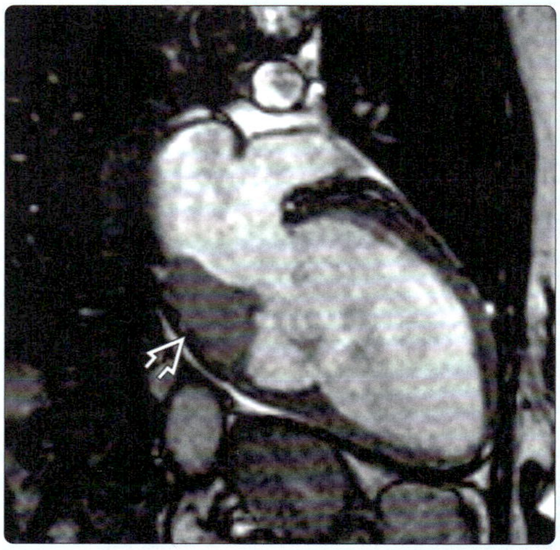

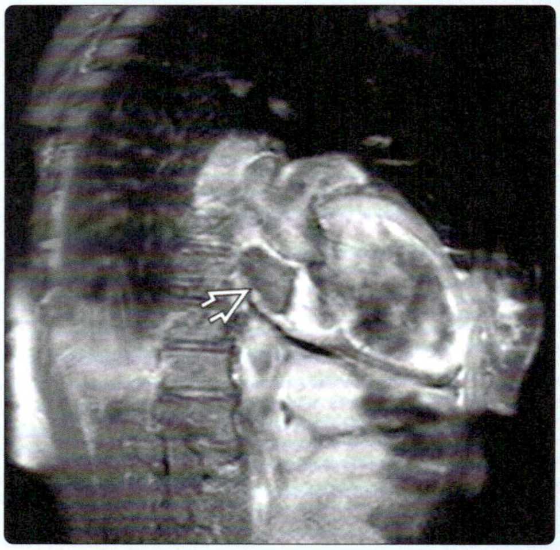

(Left) *LV long-axis cardiac CT (same patient) shows a hyperdense (compared to myocardium) lesion in the left atrioventricular groove with rim or "eggshell" calcification ⇨, which is characteristic of caseous MAC. (Courtesy W. Eicher, MD.)* **(Right)** *Axial nonenhanced cardiac gated CT (same patient) shows that the content of the rim-calcified lesion is also of high-density material ➡, consistent with liquified caseous mitral annular calcification. (Courtesy W. Eicher, MD.)*

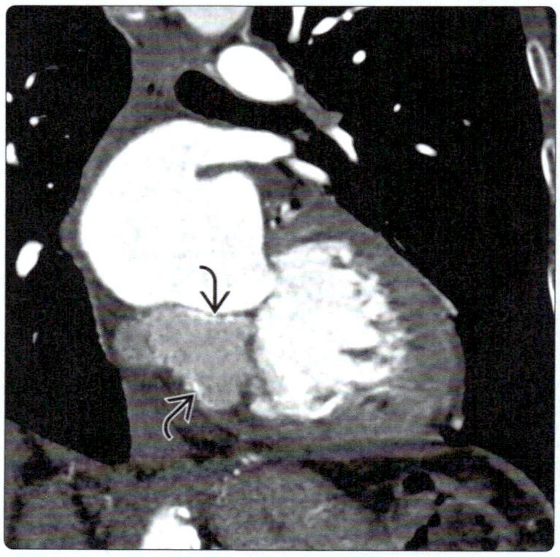

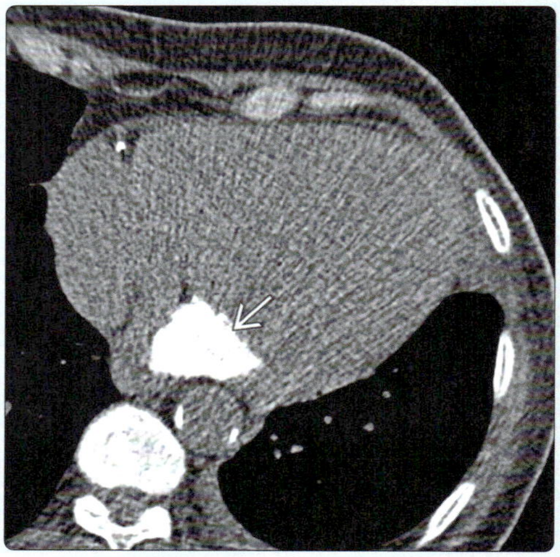

TERMINOLOGY

Abbreviations

- Mitral annular calcification (MAC)

Synonyms

- Annular mitral valve calcification

Definitions

- Chronic degenerative calcification of fibrous mitral valve anulus
- May develop caseous necrosis

IMAGING

General Features

- Best diagnostic clue
  - J-, C-, U-, or O-shaped MAC
  - "Eggshell" or rim-calcified mass in same location containing lower density material (toothpaste-like necrotized calcium)
- Location
  - Posterior base (early stage) and full anulus (late stage)
- Morphology
  - Dense calcification
    - Rare variant: Caseous calcification (due to liquefaction necrosis)

Imaging Recommendations

- Best imaging tool
  - Radiograph (lateral views)
  - Computed tomography
  - Echocardiography
- Protocol advice
  - CT
    - NECT usually sufficient for diagnosis
    - Contrast-enhanced cardiac ECG gated CT may demonstrate relationship to surrounding structures (e.g., left circumflex coronary artery)
    - Cardiac CT may be useful for presurgical planning to assess myocardial involvement, distinguish whether leaflets are calcified or not, and distinguish caseous calcification from tumor
  - Transthoracic echocardiography
    - B-mode, M-mode, and Doppler

Radiographic Findings

- Incomplete calcification of posterior anulus (forming J-, C-, or U-shaped MAC)
- Entire anulus calcified (O-shaped) in late cases
  - Best seen on lateral projections

CT Findings

- NECT
  - Dense calcification within unenhanced cardiac tissue along expected location of posterior or entire anulus
  - Sparing of mitral valve leaflets
  - May protrude into lumen
  - May involve papillary muscles when severe

Echocardiographic Findings

- Echocardiogram
  - Hyperechogenic, dense calcification with acoustic shadowing
  - Caseous MAC uncommon variant
    - Echogenic mass with echolucent center (liquefaction necrosis)
    - May mimic neoplasm on echocardiography
- M-mode
  - Measurement of anulus thickness as predictor for stroke and cardiovascular disease
- Color Doppler
  - Concomitant regurgitation or stenosis (rare)

MR Findings

- Calcium usually dark on all pulse sequences
  - In expected location of mitral anulus
- Helpful for differential diagnosis of caseous calcification vs. neoplasm
  - No contrast enhancement

DIFFERENTIAL DIAGNOSIS

Mitral Stenosis

- Thickening and calcification involving valve leaflets
- MAC involves anulus and rarely only valve itself
- When severe, MAC causes mitral stenosis or regurgitation, primarily due to mechanical obstruction of valvular function

End-Stage Renal Disease

- Extraosseous calcification develops due to secondary hyperparathyroidism
- Frequently combined with systemic vascular calcification (tunica media)

Atherosclerosis

- MAC linked with aortic atheroma and coronary artery disease
- MAC may be pitfall on calcium-scoring CT as MAC can mimic atherosclerotic calcification in left circumflex coronary artery

Multivalvular Calcific Disease

- MAC associated with aortic valve calcification, and aortic stenosis may develop

Caseous Mitral Annular Calcification

- Rim-calcified mass containing liquified calcium, which appears toothpaste-like on surgery or pathology (a.k.a. toothpaste tumor) or cheese-like (hence "caseous")

PATHOLOGY

General Features

- Etiology
  - End-stage renal disease
    - Secondary hyperparathyroidism and alterations in calcium metabolism leading to extraosseous calcium deposits
  - Atherosclerosis
    - Association with cardiovascular disease, such as stroke, coronary artery disease, and aortic atheroma
    - May be later state of atherosclerosis
  - Multivalvular calcification: Association with MAC
  - Tuberculosis

- Genetics
  - Genetics may play role
    - In patients with end-stage renal disease, *ENPP1* genotype associated with higher severity of systemic arterial calcification
- Associated abnormalities
  - Not usually associated with mitral valve stenosis or regurgitation

Gross Pathologic & Surgical Features

- Calcification of fibrous base of mitral anulus
- Fibroelastic deficiency
- If extensive calcification, myocardium may be involved
  - Prevalence: 12% of surgical specimens
- Caseous calcification: Toothpaste-like, white material

Microscopic Features

- Calcium deposits
- Liquefaction necrosis (in case of caseous calcification)

CLINICAL ISSUES

Presentation

- Most common signs/symptoms
  - Usually asymptomatic
  - Sometimes mass effect if extensive calcium deposits; if atrioventricular node affected, atrioventricular block may develop
- Other signs/symptoms
  - Rarely signs of coexistent mitral insufficiency or stenosis
  - Caseous MAC may cause systemic embolization
  - Despite presence of MAC, mitral valve repair has favorable results

Demographics

- Age
  - Increased incidence with age
    - > 35% of older adult population
- Sex
  - More common in females
- Epidemiology
  - Prevalence in Framingham Heart Study population: 14%
  - Prevalence in end-stage renal disease: ~ 40%

Natural History & Prognosis

- Slow progression over time
- Increased risk of stroke
  - Dependent of MAC thickness measured by echocardiography
  - 1 mm increase → 10% increased risk
  - MAC is independent predictor of incident ischemic stroke in treated hypertensive patients with left ventricular hypertrophy
- 3x increased mortality in patients with chronic kidney disease
- Predisposing factor for infective endocarditis
  - Bacterial endocarditis found in 19% of surgical specimens
- Marker for severe coronary artery disease in patients < 65 years of age
- Higher prevalence of coronary artery disease and aortic atheroma
- Association with incidental atrial fibrillation
  - Progression of MAC detected by CT associated with increased risk of atrial fibrillation
- Caseous necrosis rare sequela of MAC
  - May cause embolic strokes

Treatment

- Nonspecific if asymptomatic (e.g., calcium metabolism regulation in end-stage renal disease)
- Surgery considered if symptoms due to mass effect or systemic embolization
  - 5-year survival after surgery: 76%
  - Caseous MAC more frequently surgically resected due to higher prevalence of systemic embolization

DIAGNOSTIC CHECKLIST

Consider

- MAC is benign degenerative disease
- Most frequently incidental finding on chest x-ray or CT
  - Particularly in patients with end-stage renal disease or systemic atherosclerosis
- Caseous calcification rare variant that may mimic tumor
  - CT and MR can differentiate

Image Interpretation Pearls

- Posterior anulus base calcification (J-, C-, or U-shaped) and full anulus (O-shaped) at late stage
- Best seen on lateral radiograph projections and CT

SELECTED REFERENCES

1. Stankowski K et al: Multimodality imaging of caseous mitral annular calcification complicated by possible systemic embolizations. Int J Cardiovasc Imaging. ePub, 2024
2. Bitar ZI et al: Caseous calcification of the mitral annulus: mimicking a cardiac mass. Eur J Case Rep Intern Med. 10(9):004000, 2023
3. Mergen V et al: Cardiac virtual noncontrast images for calcium quantification with photon-counting detector CT. Radiol Cardiothorac Imaging. 5(3):e220307, 2023
4. Mayr A et al: The spectrum of caseous mitral annulus calcifications. JACC Case Rep. 3(1):104-8, 2021
5. O'Neal WT et al: Mitral annular calcification progression and the risk of atrial fibrillation: results from MESA. Eur Heart J Cardiovasc Imaging. 19(3):279-84, 2018
6. Dingli P et al: Caseous mitral annular calcification mimicking a lung tumor on chest X-ray. J Family Med Prim Care. 6(2):442-4, 2017
7. Chan V et al: Impact of mitral annular calcification on early and late outcomes following mitral valve repair of myxomatous degeneration. Interact Cardiovasc Thorac Surg. 17(1):120-5, 2013
8. Higgins J et al: Cardiac computed tomography facilitates operative planning in patients with mitral calcification. Ann Thorac Surg. 95(1):e9-11, 2013
9. Okada Y: Surgical management of mitral annular calcification. Gen Thorac Cardiovasc Surg. 61(11):619-25, 2013
10. Eller P et al: Impact of ENPP1 genotype on arterial calcification in patients with end-stage renal failure. Nephrol Dial Transplant. 23(1):321-7, 2008
11. d'Alessandro C et al: Mitral annulus calcification: determinants of repair feasibility, early and late surgical outcome. Eur J Cardiothorac Surg. 32(4):596-603, 2007
12. Lubarsky L et al: Images in cardiovascular medicine. Caseous calcification of the mitral annulus by 64-detector-row computed tomographic coronary angiography: a rare intracardiac mass. Circulation. 116(5):e114-5, 2007
13. Poh KK et al: Prominent posterior mitral annular calcification causing embolic stroke and mimicking left atrial fibroma. Eur Heart J. 28(18):2216, 2007
14. Sharma R et al: Mitral annular calcification predicts mortality and coronary artery disease in end stage renal disease. Atherosclerosis. 191(2):348-54, 2007
15. Cury RC et al: Epidemiology and association of vascular and valvular calcium quantified by multidetector computed tomography in elderly asymptomatic subjects. Am J Cardiol. 94(3):348-51, 2004

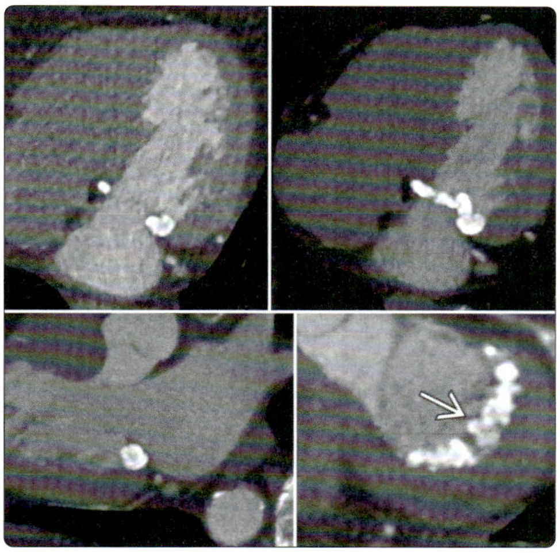

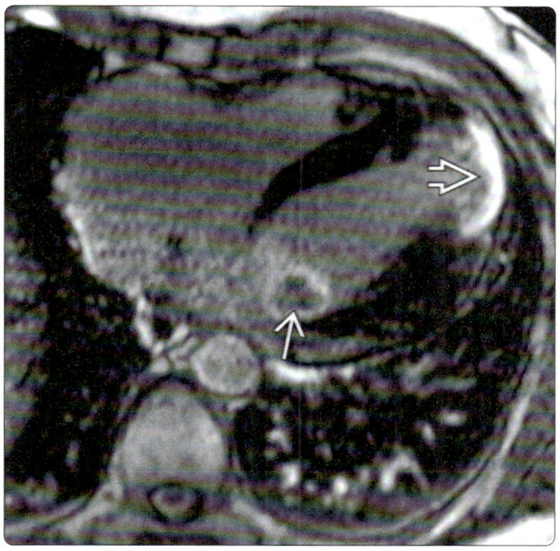

(Left) *Cardiac CT in 4-chamber, 3-chamber, and mitral valve short-axis views shows the typical appearance of MAC. Note the reversed C shape* ➡ *on the short-axis view and the predominantly inferior and lateral AV groove involvement.* **(Right)** *LGE MR in a patient with a remote transmural apical myocardial infarction shows a rounded lesion with low internal signal* ➡ *in the AV groove near the mitral anulus and a slightly enhancing rim* ➡*, corresponding to MAC seen on CT (not shown).*

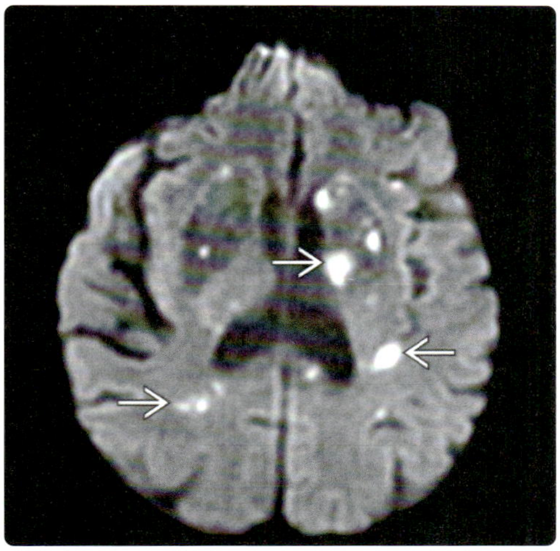

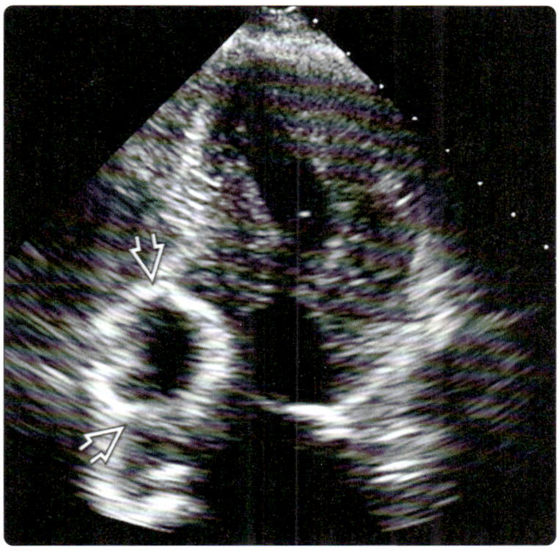

(Left) *Axial DWI MR demonstrates multiple bilateral, hyperintense-signal foci* ➡*, consistent with multiple small embolic infarcts.* **(Right)** *Apical 2-chamber transthoracic echocardiogram in the same patient shows an echolucent mass with a hyperechoic rim* ➡ *at the posterior mitral anulus. Clinically, the etiology was uncertain, and MR and CT were subsequently performed for characterization.*

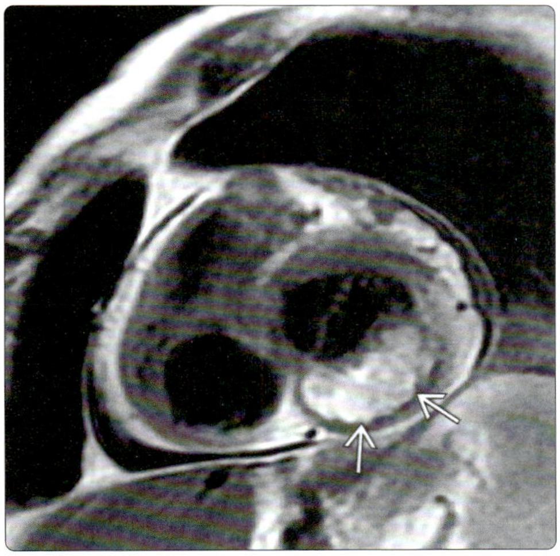

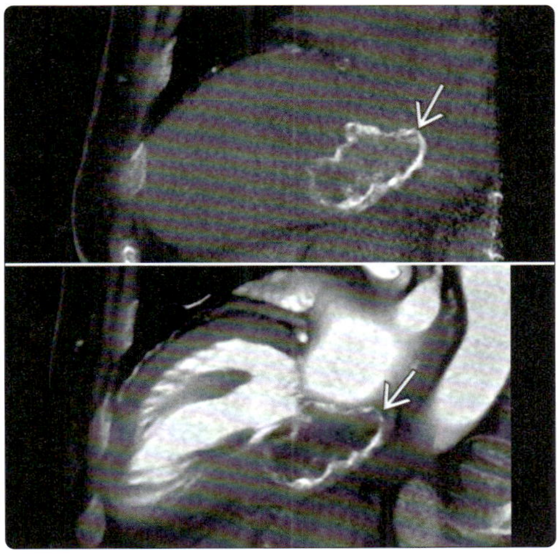

(Left) *Short-axis T2 FSE MR in the same patient shows a high-signal mass lesion* ➡ *in the left AV groove along the posterior mitral anulus.* **(Right)** *Paraseptal long-axis NECT and volume-rendered thick-slab enhanced cardiac CT in the same patient demonstrate a rim-calcified mass* ➡ *containing lower density material, indicating caseous MAC, likely with some content embolization leading to the cerebral infarct.*

(Left) *Portable chest radiograph shows coarse, C-shaped calcification projected over the expected location of the mitral valve, seen to the left of the midline* ➡. **(Right)** *Lateral chest radiograph shows coarse, C-shaped calcification projected over the expected location of the mitral valve* ➡.

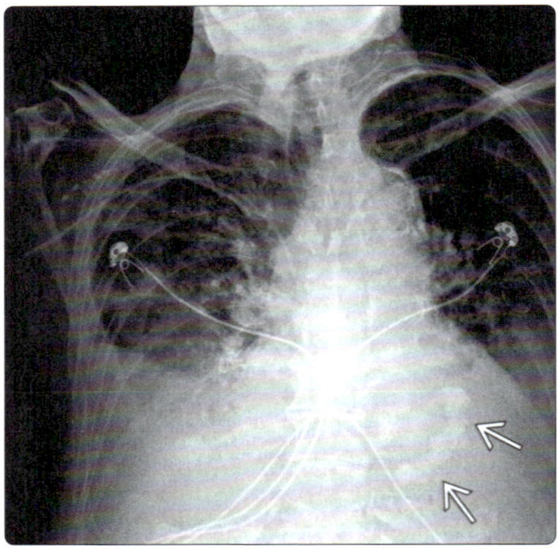

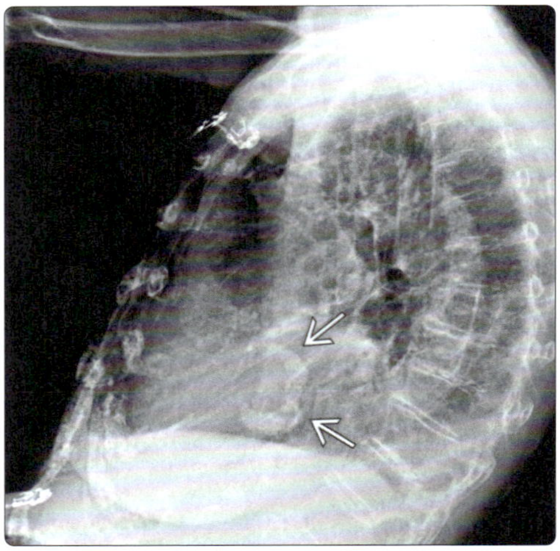

(Left) *Three-chamber cardiac CT angiogram demonstrates the typical CT appearance of caseous mitral valve annular calcification* ↷*, featuring a central region with lower attenuation compared to the calcified shell* ➡. **(Right)** *Coronal MIP cardiac CT shows nodular, coarse C-shaped calcification at the mitral anulus* ➡.

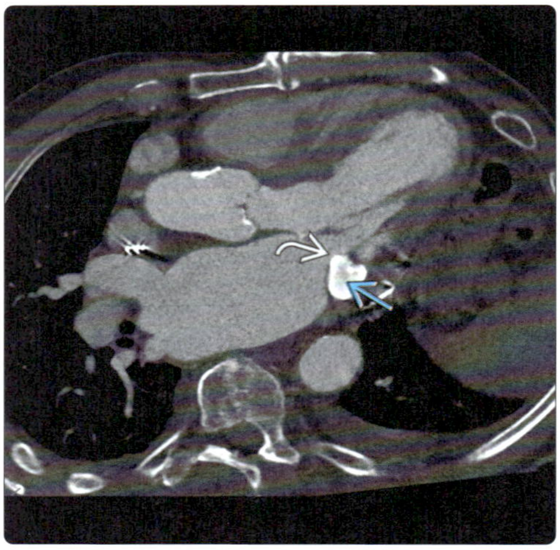

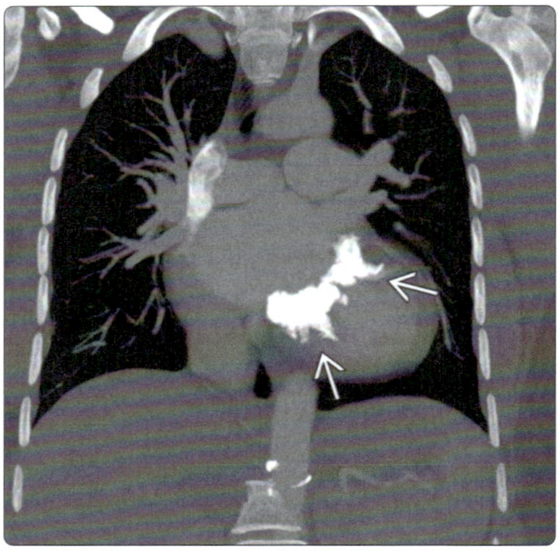

(Left) *Multidetector computed tomography (MDCT) shows the anatomic delineation of the mitral anulus* ➡ *in a patient with MAC* ↷*, which is crucial for identifying the feasibility of transcatheter mitral valve replacement (TMVR).* **(Right)** *Volume-rendered 3D reconstruction shows the placement of a virtual transcatheter mitral valve replacement in a patient with MAC* ➡ *to predict the neo-left ventricular outflow tract* ➡.

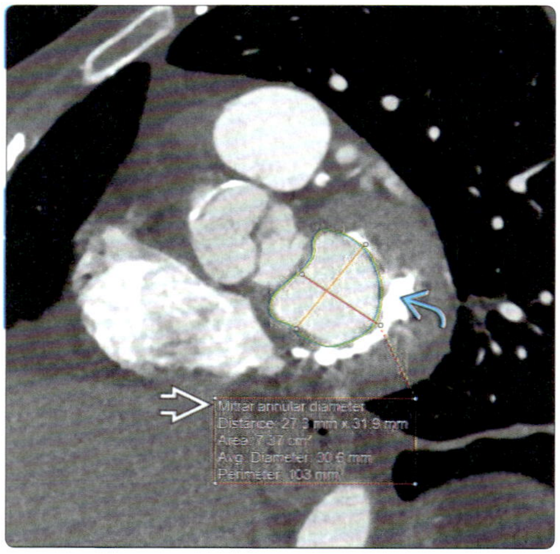

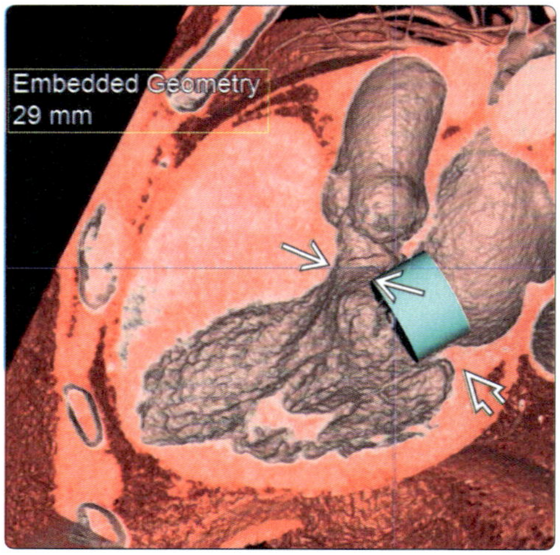

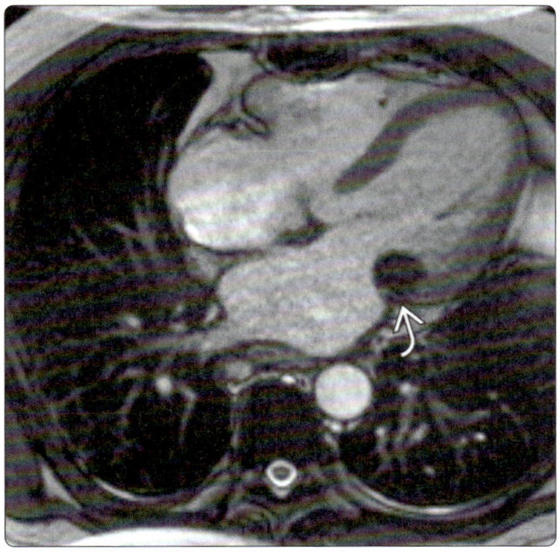

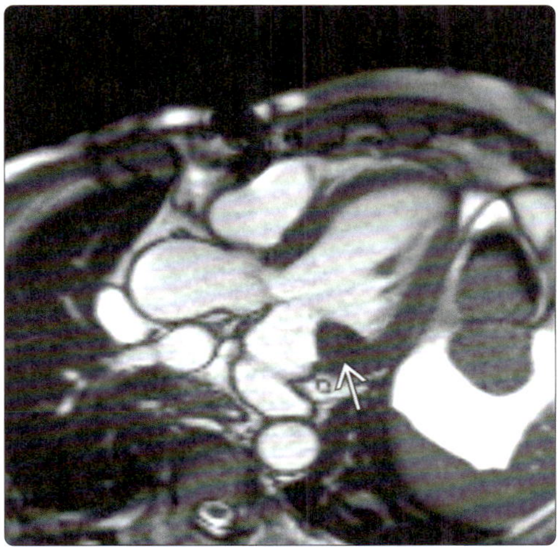

(Left) *Three-chamber SSFP MR shows a low signal intensity noncontracting, immobile, nodular bulge near the hinge point of the posterior mitral leaflet ⮫.* **(Right)** *Four-chamber SSFP MR shows a nodular bulge at the posterior mitral anulus ➡, which is hypointense compared to myocardium.*

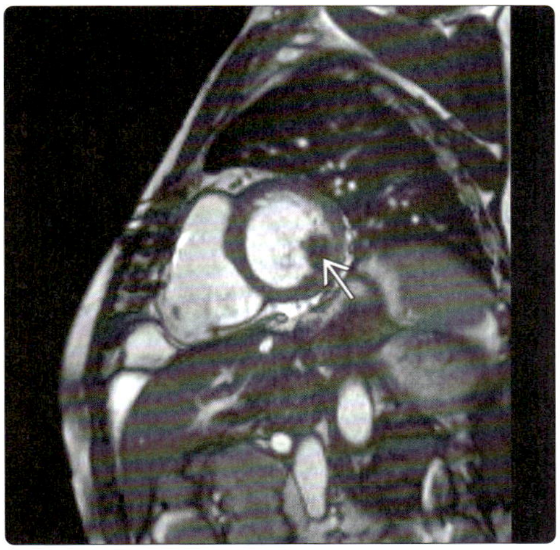

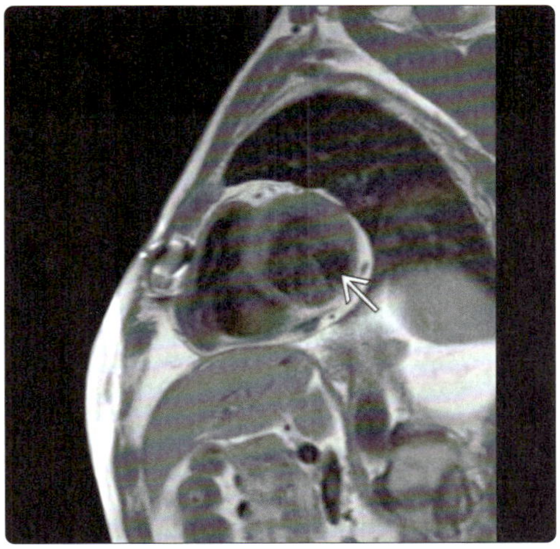

(Left) *Short-axis SSFP MR shows a noncontracting, immobile, nodular mass ➡ adjacent to the posterior lateral mitral anulus.* **(Right)** *Short-axis double inversion recovery MR in the same patient shows persistence of hypointensity of the nodular mass at the posterior mitral anulus ➡.*

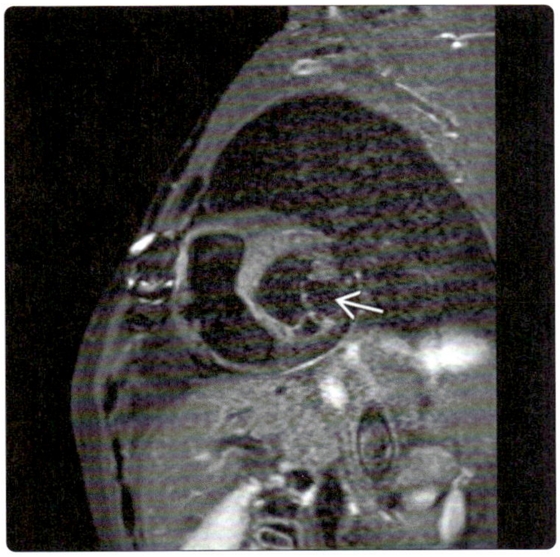

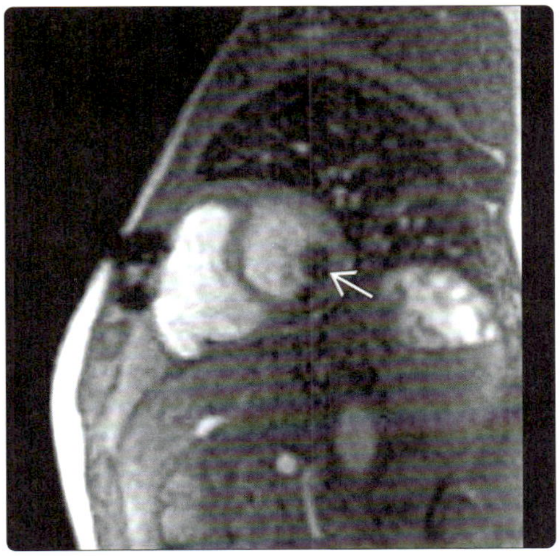

(Left) *Short-axis triple inversion recovery MR confirms a non-fat-containing, multilobulated, hypointense mass at the posterior mitral anulus ➡.* **(Right)** *Short-axis early perfusion MR postgadolinium administration shows absence of 1st-pass enhancement of the low-signal mass adjacent to the mitral anulus. Characteristics of caseous necrosis include a hypointense appearance on all pulse sequences ➡, the typical location, and shape, and absence of enhancement.*

KEY FACTS

TERMINOLOGY

- Structural abnormality of mitral valve apparatus characterized by significant (> 5 mm) atrial displacement of mitral valve anulus from basal left ventricular myocardium

IMAGING

- Detachment (≥ 5 mm) of left inferolateral myocardial wall from posterolateral portion of mitral anulus; best measured in systole
- Echocardiography is 1st-line imaging modality
- MR provides comprehensive characterization of mitral annular disjunction (MAD) and risk stratification
  - Cine MR images perpendicular to mitral anulus, 5 mm thickness, no gap, temporal resolution of ≤ 45 milliseconds
  - Atrial displacement of mitral anulus hinge point from basal left ventricular myocardium
    - MAD distance is measured parallel to disjunction from hinge point in left atrium to top of basal left ventricular myocardium
  - More common in anterior and inferior anulus
  - Involves 30-240° of mitral anulus circumference
  - Mitral valve prolapse (MVP) is usually associated
  - LGE can be seen in basal inferolateral wall and posteromedial papillary muscle; associated with arrhythmia

TOP DIFFERENTIAL DIAGNOSES

- Pseudo-MAD
- Mitral anulus pseudoaneurysm

CLINICAL ISSUES

- Up to 98% prevalence of MAD in surgical series of MVP patients with severe mitral regurgitation
- Association between MAD and ventricular arrhythmia is recognized

(Left) *Four-chamber color Doppler echocardiogram shows severe mitral regurgitation in a patient with known mitral valve prolapse (MVP).* **(Right)** *Corresponding echocardiogram in the same patient confirms mitral annular disjunction (MAD) ➔ of the posterior mitral leaflet > 5 mm.*

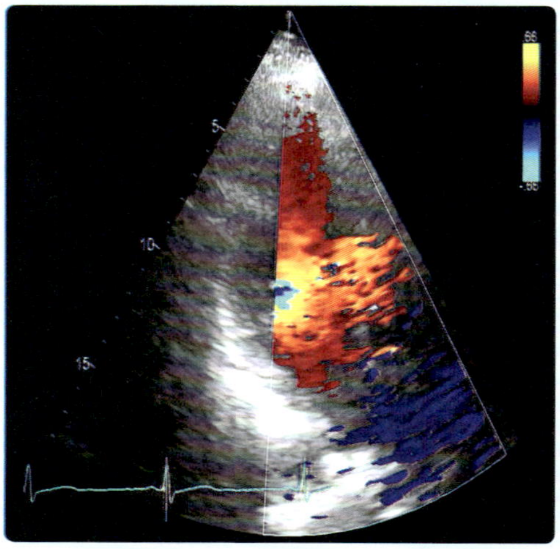

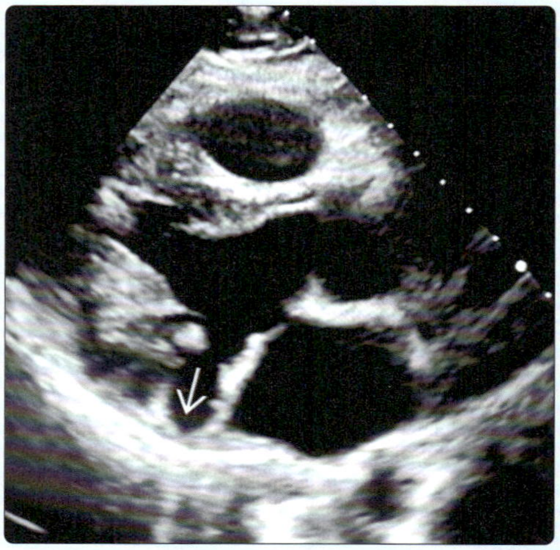

(Left) *Tissue Doppler echocardiogram shows a high-velocity midsystolic spike of the mitral valve anulus ➔, which resembles a German military helmet with a spike.* **(Right)** *Three-chamber reconstructed cardiac CT shows 6-mm MAD with separation of the mitral anulus from the left ventricular basal myocardium ⇨. Note also MVP ⇨.*

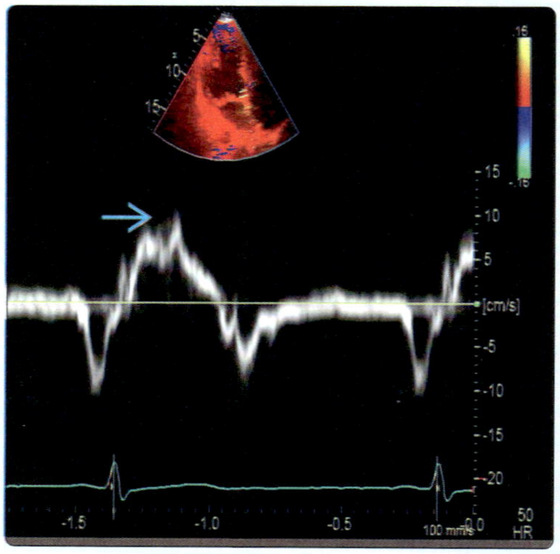

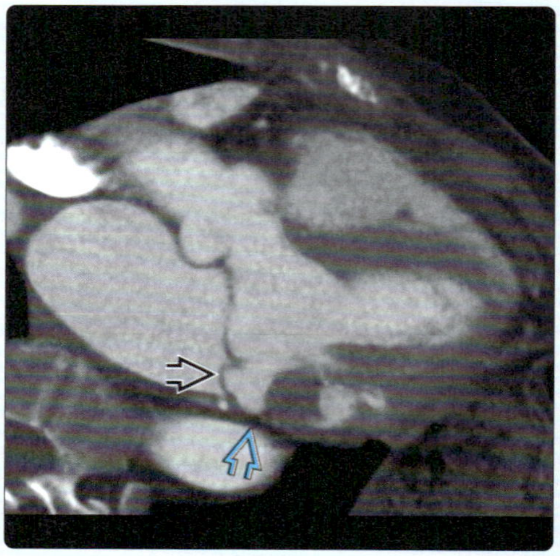

TERMINOLOGY

Abbreviations

- Mitral annular disjunction (MAD)

Definitions

- Structural abnormality of mitral valve apparatus characterized by significant (> 5 mm) atrial displacement of mitral valve anulus from basal left ventricular myocardium

IMAGING

General Features

- Best diagnostic clue
  - Detachment (≥ 5 mm) of left inferolateral myocardial wall from posterolateral portion of mitral anulus; best measured in systole
    - Some authors use > 2 mm of detachment distance as threshold
- Location
  - Posterolateral anulus is frequently implicated
  - Left ventricle (LV) anterior wall (28%), inferior wall (26%), posterolateral wall (9%)
- Size
  - Detachment (≥ 5 mm); this can be > 10 mm in severe cases
  - Various cutoffs have been described, starting from 1 mm
- Morphology
  - Increased distance between posterior mitral leaflet insertion and left ventricular myocardium of ≥ 5 mm

CT Findings

- MAD is evaluated in long-axis 2-chamber, 3-chamber, and 4-chamber reconstructions
- MAD measured in 3-chamber reconstruction in systole phase
- ≥ 5 mm considered significant
  - MAD associated with female sex, smaller anulus size, and posterior leaflet length
- Mitral valve prolapse (MVP) often associated
- May see hypertrophy isolated to inferior and inferolateral segments at base near mitral anulus

MR Findings

- Cine: Atrial displacement of mitral anulus hinge point from basal left ventricular myocardium
  - Displacement reported from 1-15 mm
  - ≥ 5 mm considered significant
  - Involves 30-240° of mitral anulus circumference
    - Evaluated in short-axis images
  - More common in anterior and inferior anulus
    - Inferolateral location is associated with MVP and cardiac arrhythmia
- MAD distance is measured parallel to disjunction from hinge point in left atrium (LA) to top of basal left ventricular myocardium
  - Evaluate long-axis cine images throughout cardiac cycle
  - Measure in 3-chamber view in systole
- MVP is usually associated
  - Single/bileaflet prolapse ≥ 2 mm beyond annular plane in long axis into LA
  - Classic MVP = > 5-mm prolapse
  - Distance from top of prolapsed leaflet during peak systole to mitral anulus plane
- May see isolated myocardial hypertrophy in inferior and inferolateral segments at base near mitral anulus
  - Mechanism of left ventricular basal hypertrophy in MAD is unknown
  - Potentially related to changes in myocardial energetics in response to repetitive traction by MAD &/or MVP
- Delayed enhancement
  - Can be seen in basal left ventricular wall, including inferior and lateral wall and papillary muscles
  - Associated with arrhythmia
  - Higher MAD distance in patients with LGE
- Strain imaging
  - Lower radial and circumferential strain in basal inferolateral segments

Ultrasonographic Findings

- Significant (≥ 5-mm) atrial displacement of mitral annular hinge point from left ventricular myocardium
  - > 2 mm is minimum displacement that can be detected using echocardiography
  - Diagnosis is straightforward when displacement ≥ 6 mm
  - Measured in parasternal long axis at end of systole
- Often associated with MVP where 1 or both of mitral valve leaflets billow into LV during systole
- Can be associated with thinning or elongation of posterior mitral valve leaflet
- Rarely can be associated with focal left ventricular myocardial thinning or outpouching at site of disjunction
- Transesophageal echocardiogram: Required for young patients with MVP, mitral regurgitation, and arrhythmias
  - Better performance than transthoracic echocardiogram
  - Measured in 4-chamber midesophageal view at 0° during systole
  - 3D transesophageal echocardiogram provides more quantitative information
- Tissue Doppler: Pickelhaube sign (German helmet with spike)
  - High-velocity, midsystolic spike of mitral valve anulus, > 16 cm/sec

Imaging Recommendations

- Best imaging tool
  - Echocardiography is 1st-line imaging modality
  - MR provides comprehensive characterization of MAD and risk stratification
- Protocol advice
  - Cine MR images perpendicular to mitral anulus, 5 mm thickness, no gap, temporal resolution of ≤ 45 milliseconds

DIFFERENTIAL DIAGNOSIS

Pseudomitral Annular Disjunction

- Prolapsing mitral leaflet folds during systole and juxtaposes along LA wall, mimicking hinge point
  - Hinge point is still attached to top of basal left ventricular myocardium, distinguishing it from MAD
- Evaluate cine images throughout cardiac cycle to determine if anulus hinge point is displaced to LA wall

Mitral Anulus Pseudoaneurysm

- Complication of mitral valve surgery, infective endocarditis, myocardial infarction
- Focal outpouching from mitral anulus
- Correlate with clinical and surgical history

PATHOLOGY

General Features

- Separation of mitral valve anulus from left ventricular myocardium results in excessive annular motion
- Outward curling of posterior anulus increases anulus diameter during systole, myocardial stretch, poor coaptation, and myxomatous degeneration of leaflets
- Abnormal tugging on submitral apparatus → papillary muscle hypertrophy, myocardial hypertrophy, and fibrosis
  - This serves as arrhythmogenic substrate
- MVP and myxomatous valve also seen

Staging, Grading, & Classification

- Classification system by Carmo, P et al
  - Type I: Excessive annular mobility with absence of visualized separation between anulus and basal left ventricular myocardium
  - Type II: Anulus-ventricular separation (i.e., disjunction) of < 5 mm
  - Type III: Disjunction > 5 mm

Gross Pathologic & Surgical Features

- High prevalence of MAD in myxomatous mitral valve
- Myxomatous mitral valve and left ventricular fibrosis at level of papillary muscle and inferobasal wall
- Left ventricular fibrosis is associated with mechanical injury of myocardium as consequence of continuous traction of prolapsing leaflets and elongation of chordae tendinea
- Positive correlation between severity of MAD and number of diseased mitral valve scallops supports association between MAD and severity of MVP
- Increased risk of failure of surgical mitral valve repair if MAD not recognized

CLINICAL ISSUES

Presentation

- Most common signs/symptoms
  - Symptoms and clinical findings overlap with that of MVP
  - Symptomatic dysrhythmias, presyncope, palpitations, dyspnea, chest pain
- Other signs/symptoms
  - Can be isolated imaging finding
  - Can present with sudden cardiac death, midsystolic auscultatory click of MVP, displaced apical impulse with associated left ventricular dilation, systolic murmur of mitral regurgitation
  - ECG: Biphasic or inverted T waves, ST-depression, QT prolongation, right bundle branch block, polymorphic ventricular tachycardia, QRS-T wave discordance in inferior leads, paroxysmal ventricular contractions
  - Electroanatomic mapping: Low-voltage fractionated complexes in hypertrophied left ventricular basal myocardium

Demographics

- MAD has been reported in up to 16-92% of patients with MVP
  - Recent studies report 30% prevalence in MVP
- 7.2-8.7% prevalence in general population
- F > M

Natural History & Prognosis

- Up to 98% prevalence of MAD in surgical series of MVP patients with severe mitral regurgitation
- Association between MAD and ventricular arrhythmia is recognized
  - In patients with greater MAD and presence of LGE
  - Abnormal annular motion and leaflet traction leads to myocardial stress, valve degeneration, and myocardial stretch of posterobasal LV and papillary muscles

Treatment

- β-blockers may be theoretically beneficial, but there are no randomized studies available in arrhythmic MVP patients
- Implantable cardioverter-defibrillators may have role in MVP with high arrhythmic burden to reduce risk of out-of-hospital cardiac arrest
- Targeted catheter ablation may have role in MVP with high arrhythmic burden
- Surgical repair may have role in management of patients with MVP with high arrhythmic burden

DIAGNOSTIC CHECKLIST

Consider

- MVP

Image Interpretation Pearls

- Hinge point of mitral anulus should be defined
- MAD distance is measured parallel to disjunction in 3-chamber systolic image
- Frequently associated with MVP
- LGE at basal inferolateral wall and posterior papillary muscle can be seen

Reporting Tips

- Report: MAD distance, presence of MVP, height of prolapsing leaflet, single/bileaflet prolapse, flail leaflets, paradoxical outward curling of anulus, basal left ventricular hypertrophy, LGE of myocardium &/or papillary muscles, and extracellular volume

SELECTED REFERENCES

1. Alfares FA et al: Mitral annular disjunction: an under-recognized entity in pediatrics. JACC Case Rep. 29(9):102297, 2024
2. Compagnucci P et al: Arrhythmic mitral valve prolapse and sports activity: pathophysiology, risk stratification, and sports eligibility assessment. J Clin Med. 13(5), 2024
3. Troger F et al: Mitral annular disjunction in out-of-hospital cardiac arrest patients-a retrospective cardiac MRI study. Clin Res Cardiol. 113(5):770-80, 2024
4. Van der Bijl P et al: Mitral annular disjunction in the context of mitral valve prolapse: identifying the at-risk patient. JACC Cardiovasc Imaging. 17(10):1229-45, 2024
5. Gulati A et al: Mitral annular disjunction: review of an increasingly recognized mitral valve entity. Radiol Cardiothorac Imaging. 5(6):e230131, 2023

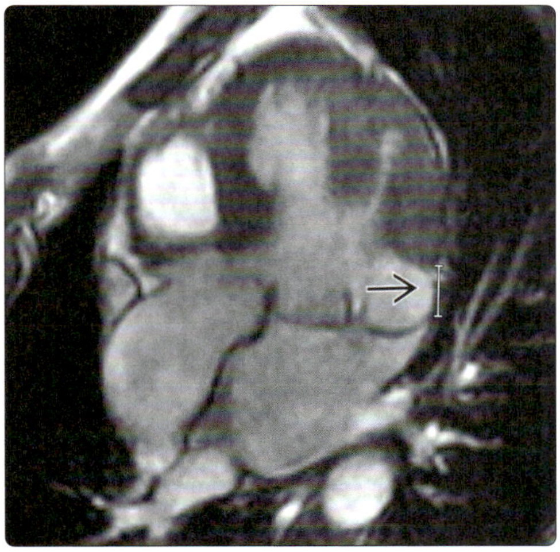

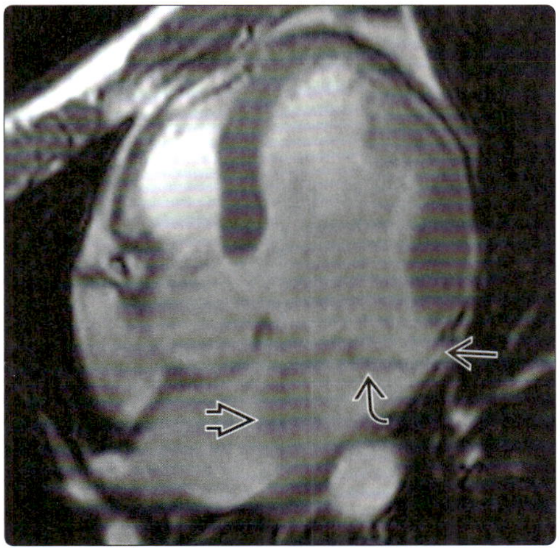

(Left) *Three-chamber cine SSFP MR shows separation of the mitral anulus hinge point from the left ventricular basal myocardium towards the left atrium by 14 mm, consistent with MAD.* **(Right)** *Three-chamber cine MR shows MAD measuring 6 mm, MVP, and moderate mitral regurgitation.*

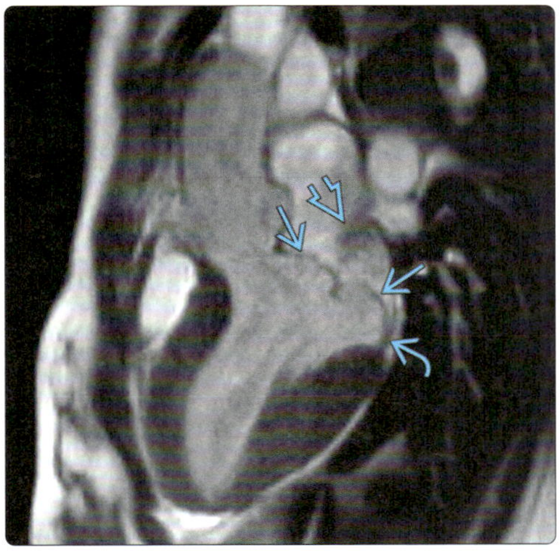

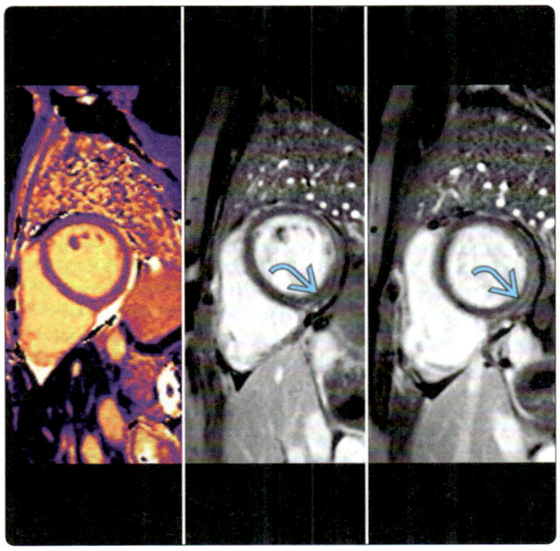

(Left) *Three-chamber MR in a 20-year-old with Ehlers-Danlos syndrome and palpitations shows bileaflet MVP, moderate mitral regurgitation, and MAD measuring 8 mm.* **(Right)** *Precontrast T1 tissue mapping at 3T (left) shows borderline elevated native T1 values of 1,180 msec. Short-axis delayed-enhancement sequences at the base show thin, linear, midmyocardial delayed enhancement isolated to the inferior and inferolateral segments at the base near the mitral anulus. (Courtesy S. Kligerman, MD.)*

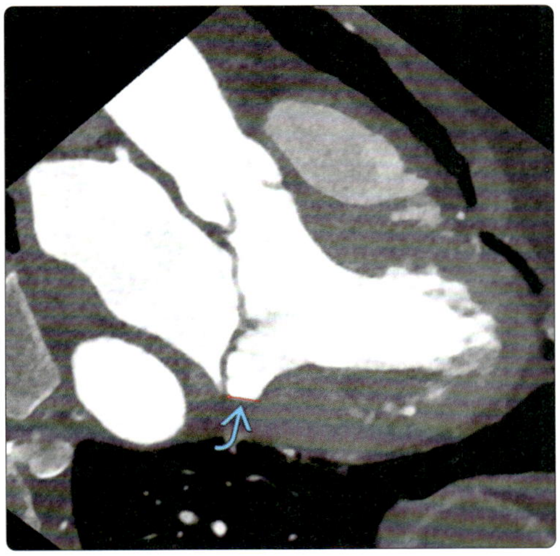

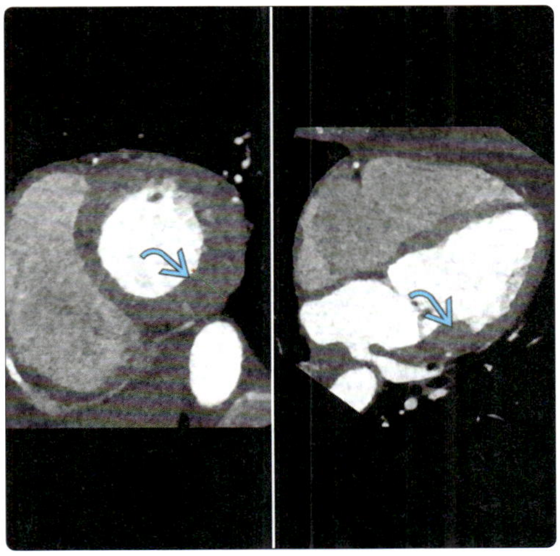

(Left) *Three-chamber cardiac CTA during end-systole in a 51-year-old woman with an arrhythmia shows prolapse of the posterior leaflet of the mitral valve and 7 mm of MAD.* **(Right)** *CECT in the same patient at end-diastole shows there is conspicuous thickening isolated to the inferior and inferolateral segments at the base, measuring up to 17 mm. The exact cause of this hypertrophy is unknown. (Courtesy S. Kligerman, MD.)*

KEY FACTS

TERMINOLOGY

- Tricuspid stenosis (TS)
- Reduced valve area (< 1 cm^2 = severe TS)

IMAGING

- Echocardiography is best modality to diagnose
  - Thickened and distorted with limited leaflet mobility
  - Decreased separation of leaflet tips and diastolic doming of valve
  - High transvalvular pressure gradient on Doppler (2-mmHg pressure gradient is considered abnormal)
  - Frequently associated tricuspid regurgitation
  - Right atrial (RA) enlargement
  - Dilated inferior vena cava
- CT
  - Calcified and thickened tricuspid valve (TV) leaflets with dilated right atrium
  - Limited diastolic leaflet motion
  - Hepatic venous congestion with dilated venae cavae
- MR
  - Diastolic flow void jet from TV into right ventricle
  - Limited diastolic leaflet motion
  - RA enlargement

TOP DIFFERENTIAL DIAGNOSES

- Rheumatic heart disease
- Obstruction of TV
  - RA tumor, such as myxoma, or vegetation obstructing valve orifice
- Congenital TS
- Complication of other disease
  - Carcinoid syndrome, medications (methysergide, ergotamine, fenfluramine ± phentermine), eosinophilic endomyocardial fibrosis, endomyocardial fibroelastosis, lupus

(Left) *Composite image shows thickening of the pulmonic and tricuspid valve leaflets with associated valve stenosis due to carcinoid heart syndrome. Fibrous endocardial plaques develop on the tricuspid and pulmonic valves due to tumor metabolites being secreted directly into the hepatic veins in patients with liver metastases.* **(Right)** *Axial CECT of the liver in the same patient shows numerous contrast-enhancing masses, representing carcinoid metastases.*

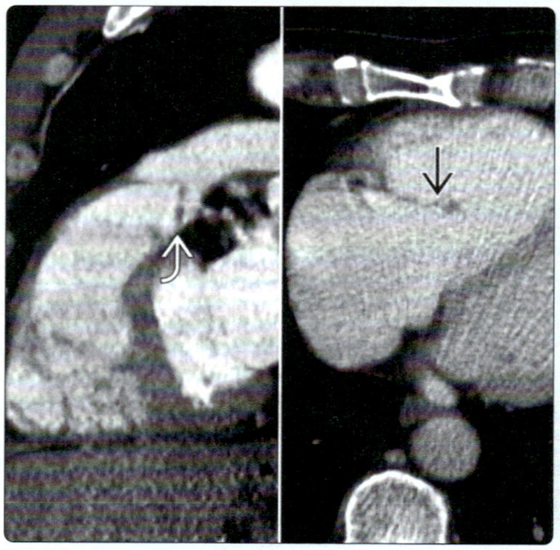

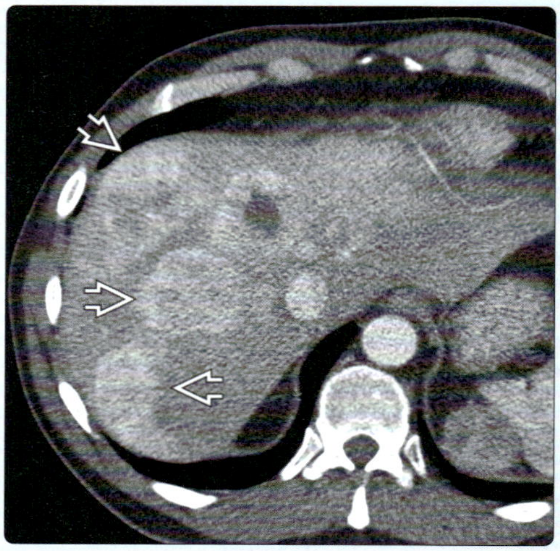

(Left) *Patient with rheumatic heart disease s/p mitral and aortic valve replacement is shown. Four-chamber view shows increased diastolic velocity across the tricuspid valve with mean Doppler gradient 5 mmHg at an HR of 55, compatible with tricuspid stenosis.* **(Right)** *Corresponding diastolic 4-chamber cardiac CT shows thickened tricuspid valve leaflets with decreased opening compatible with tricuspid stenosis. This is a patient with rheumatic heart disease after mitral and aortic valve replacement.*

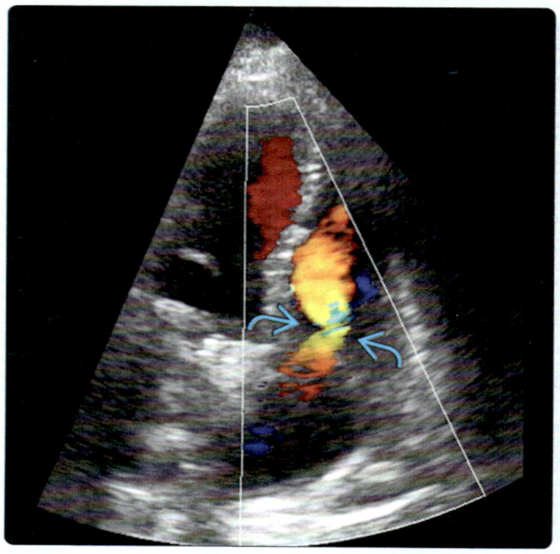

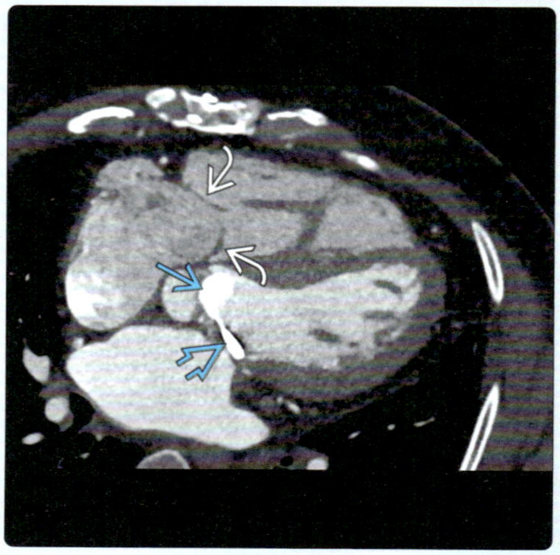

TERMINOLOGY

Abbreviations

- Tricuspid stenosis (TS)

Definitions

- Reduced valve area (< 1 cm^2 = severe TS); normal = 4 cm^2

IMAGING

General Features

- Best diagnostic clue
  - Mean Doppler gradient ≥ 5 mmHg across valve considered significant TS
- Morphology
  - Thickened and diastolic, domed tricuspid leaflets
  - Right atrial (RA) enlargement; dilated inferior vena cava (IVC)

Radiographic Findings

- Radiography
  - Marked RA enlargement
  - Dilation of superior vena cava and azygos vein
  - Pulmonary arteries appear normal unless associated mitral valve disease

CT Findings

- CECT
  - Thickened tricuspid valve (TV) leaflets; dilated RA (area > 20 cm^2)
  - Narrow TV anulus
  - Hepatic venous congestion with dilated venae cavae

MR Findings

- Thickened TV leaflets
- Restricted diastolic opening
- Diastolic flow jet from TV into right ventricle
- RA enlargement

Echocardiographic Findings

- Echocardiogram
  - 2D echocardiography
    - Fused leaflets, diastolic doming, RA and IVC enlargement
    - Normal right ventricular function
- Color Doppler
  - Diastolic high-velocity turbulent flow across valve
  - High transvalvular pressure gradient on Doppler (2-mmHg pressure gradient is considered abnormal)

DIFFERENTIAL DIAGNOSIS

Rheumatic Heart Disease

- Most common cause of TS
- Nearly always associated with mitral stenosis
  - 3% of rheumatic TS is isolated
- 50% associated with functional TS

Obstruction of Tricuspid Valve

- RA tumor, such as myxoma, or vegetation obstructing valve orifice
- Extracardiac neoplasm ("tumor thrombus")
- Pacemaker lead-induced stenosis

Congenital Tricuspid Stenosis

- Rare; associated with right ventricular hypoplasia, pulmonic stenosis/atresia, atrial septum defects, ventricular septum defects, patent ductus arteriosus

Complication of Other Disease

- Carcinoid syndrome, medications (methysergide, ergotamine, fenfluramine ± phentermine), eosinophilic endomyocardial fibrosis, endomyocardial fibroelastosis, lupus

PATHOLOGY

General Features

- Etiology
  - Very uncommon isolated valvular abnormality
  - Rheumatic heart disease is most common cause
    - Usually presents in combination with tricuspid regurgitation (TR) and left heart valvular disease
  - Carcinoid syndrome is 2nd most common cause
    - Tumor products secreted directly into hepatic veins cause deposition of fibrous endocardial plaques on tricuspid and pulmonic valves
  - Tumors resulting in TV obstruction (functional TS)
  - Other causes (uncommon): Infective endocarditis, nonbacterial thrombotic endocarditis, hypereosinophilic syndrome, iatrogenic and congenital (atresia-stenosis)

CLINICAL ISSUES

Presentation

- Most common signs/symptoms
  - Commonly coexisting TR or left valvular disease masks clinical symptoms of TS
  - TS symptoms relate to systemic venous congestion (typically out of proportion to dyspnea in absence of left valvular disease)
    - Fatigue, exertional syncope, abdominal discomfort (hepatomegaly and ascites) and peripheral edema related to low cardiac output
    - Fluttering sensation in neck due to giant A waves and slow descent in jugular venous pulse
- Other signs/symptoms: Opening snap of TV
  - Lungs are clear unless concomitant mitral valve disease
- Progressive fatigue and anorexia
- Effort intolerance

Natural History & Prognosis

- Symptoms develop over extended period
- Most patients have coexisting mitral valvular disease

DIAGNOSTIC CHECKLIST

Consider

- Rheumatic fever in setting of multivalvular disease

SELECTED REFERENCES

1. Otto CM et al: 2020 ACC/AHA guideline for the management of patients with valvular heart disease: a report of the American College of Cardiology/American Heart Association Joint Committee on Clinical Practice Guidelines. Circulation. 143(5):e72-227, 2021
2. Golamari R et al: Tricuspid stenosis. StatPearls, 2018
3. Shah S et al: Multimodal imaging of the tricuspid valve: normal appearance and pathological entities. Insights Imaging. 7(5):649-67, 2016

KEY FACTS

IMAGING

- CT
  - Dilated inferior vena cava and hepatic veins with systolic reflux of contrast
- MR
  - 4-chamber views and paraseptal long-axis SSFP views are most helpful for diagnosis
  - Systolic spin-dephasing flow void (jet) directed from tricuspid valve into right atrium during systole
- 2D echocardiography
  - Right ventricle (RV) volume overload pattern: Right atrial enlargement, RV enlargement, diastolic ventricular septal flattening, and dilated inferior vena cava and hepatic veins
  - Size of regurgitant jet orifice at valve and in right atrium is utilized to assess severity and grade regurgitation
  - Most widely used modality for diagnosis

TOP DIFFERENTIAL DIAGNOSES

- Primary tricuspid regurgitation
  - Rheumatic heart disease
  - Ebstein anomaly
  - Carcinoid syndrome
  - Infectious endocarditis
  - Trauma, atrial tumors, pacemaker leads
- Secondary tricuspid regurgitation
  - Most common cause of tricuspid regurgitation
  - Right heart failure of any etiology (most commonly resulting from left heart failure)

CLINICAL ISSUES

- Trace to mild tricuspid regurgitation is common and detected by echocardiography in > 70% of patients
- Considered physiologic when jet does not extend > 1 cm into atrium

(Left) *Frontal radiograph shows right atrial, left atrial, and appendage enlargement in a patient with rheumatic heart disease.* **(Right)** *Axial CECT in the same patient shows right atrial enlargement from severe tricuspid regurgitation. The left atrium is dilated and partially calcified from longstanding mitral stenosis. Leaflet calcification is associated with rheumatic mitral stenosis.*

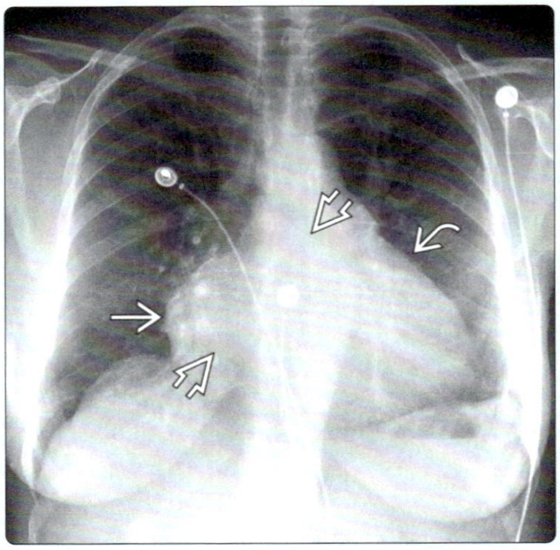

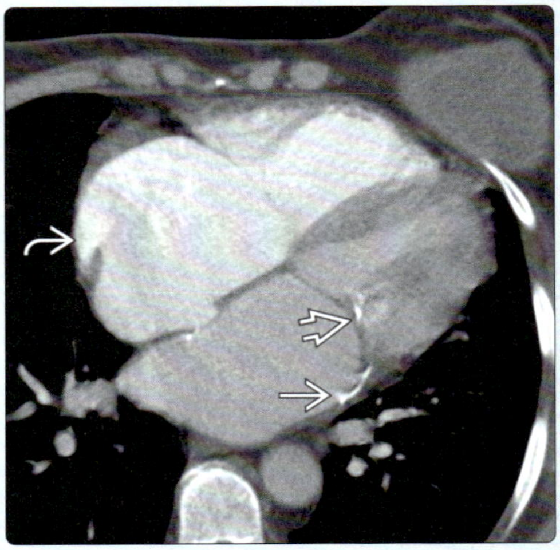

(Left) *Four-chamber SSFP MR shows regurgitant flow across the tricuspid valve (TV) into the right atrium during systole. The right atrium and right ventricle are dilated, and bilateral pleural effusions are also noted.* **(Right)** *Short-axis velocity-encoded phase-contrast cine MR in the same patient shows the regurgitant jet. It is difficult to accurately quantify tricuspid regurgitation by phase-contrast MR due to excursion of the valve plane during the cardiac cycle.*

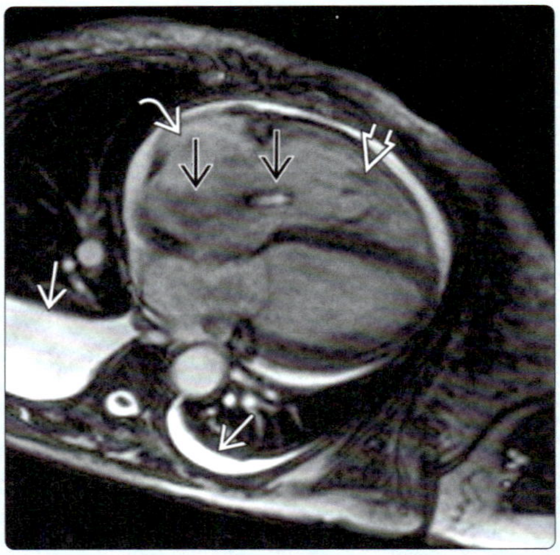

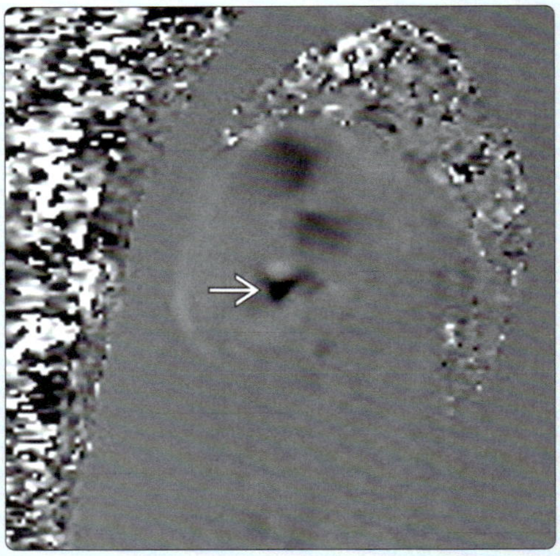

TERMINOLOGY

Abbreviations

- Tricuspid regurgitation (TR)

IMAGING

Radiographic Findings

- Radiography
  - Cardiomegaly with enlarged right atrium and right ventricle (RV)
  - Distention of azygos vein and superior vena cava
  - Filling of retrosternal clear space on lateral view from RV enlargement

CT Findings

- Cardiac gated CTA
  - Tricuspid valve (TV) can be visualized with appropriate contrast injection protocol
    - Triphasic contrast injection results in good opacification of right heart and may allow morphologic assessment of TV
      - Contrast bolus at high flow rate, followed by contrast-saline mixture, followed by saline
  - Retrospective ECG gating allows for functional assessment of RV, including RV volumes and RV ejection fraction (EF)
  - Retrospective gating also assesses leaflet motion, areas of malcoaptation, and commissure to commissure gap distances, which may assist in transcatheter repair
  - TV annular dimensions and relationship of anulus with right coronary artery and RV
  - Diastolic ventricular septal flattening and shift toward left ventricle due to volume overload
  - Dilated right atrium, RV, TV anulus, and systemic veins
  - Incomplete closure of TV in ventricular systole and regurgitant orifice; may be seen better with delayed CT

MR Findings

- Cine SSFP 4-chamber, RV long-axis and short-axis views are most useful
- Systolic spin-dephasing flow void (jet) directed from TV into right atrium during systole
  - In short-axis plane, jet area and normalized signal intensity can quantify severity of TR
    - With severe TR, jet in short-axis plane is larger and has lower signal intensity (jet size varies with sequence type)
    - Effective regurgitant orifice area can also be measured for quantifying TR
- Dilation of right atrium, RV, and tricuspid anulus
  - Assessment of right atrial volume is generally performed qualitatively rather than quantitatively
- Dilation of superior vena cava, inferior vena cava, hepatic and azygos veins ± systolic flow reversal
- Diastolic ventricular septal flattening toward left ventricle
- Calculation of low RVEF is helpful in predicting poor outcomes in patients with isolated, severe TR undergoing surgical repair
  - MR recommended for evaluation of RV volumes and function in severe TR, especially with suboptimal echocardiograms
  - Predicts all cause and cardiac mortality, especially in surgeries for functional TR
- Phase-contrast MR assesses forward pulmonic flow, which can be subtracted from RV stroke volume to quantify TR
  - Direct quantification of TR in short axis is difficult and requires complex software for tracking tricuspid anulus throughout cardiac cycle
  - 4D flow allows quantification of TR without dedicated plane or planning
  - Regurgitant fraction (RF) ≥ 40% is considered hemodynamically significant
- Tricuspid leaflet morphology can be assessed with breath-hold or navigator-gated sequences with data throughout cardiac cycle
  - Tricuspid anulus can be measured for surgical planning
- Using ventricular volumes and stroke volume from cine images and phase-contrast images can calculate TR (volume and RF)
  - In absence of pulmonary regurgitation
    - TR volume = RV stroke volume - pulmonary net volume
  - In presence of pulmonary regurgitation
    - TR volume = RV stroke volume - (pulmonary net volume + pulmonary regurgitant volume)
- RF = regurgitant volume/stroke volume x 100%

Ultrasonographic Findings

- Grayscale ultrasound
  - 2D echocardiography
    - RV volume overload pattern: Right atrial enlargement, RV enlargement, diastolic ventricular septal flattening, and dilated inferior vena cava and hepatic veins
  - 3D echocardiography
    - More accurate than 2D echocardiography to determine RV size and function
- Color Doppler
  - Systolic high-velocity flow jet in right atrium
  - Size of regurgitant jet orifice at valve and in right atrium is one of many methods utilized to assess severity and grade regurgitation
    - Vena contracta width of 7 mm or greater (severe TR)
  - Systolic flow reversal in inferior vena cava or hepatic veins

Imaging Recommendations

- Best imaging tool
  - Echocardiography
- Protocol advice
  - Triphasic contrast injection or delayed-phase CT imaging (60 seconds) may be helpful in providing homogeneous right chamber contrast opacification
  - Conventional MR gradient-echo (longer echo time) images demonstrate regurgitant jet better than SSFP pulse sequences

DIFFERENTIAL DIAGNOSIS

Primary Tricuspid Regurgitation

- Endocardial cushion defects
- Rheumatic heart disease
  - Thickening of valve leaflets &/or chordae tendineae
- Ebstein anomaly

- Downward displaced septal and posterior leaflets lead to "atrialized" RV
- Excessive motion and delayed closure of valve causes TR
- Carcinoid syndrome
  - Stiffened and immobile leaflets
  - Tumor metabolites from liver metastases are secreted directly into hepatic veins, causing fibrous endocardial plaque to deposit on right-sided valves
- Infectious endocarditis
  - Vegetations on valve leaflets
  - Predominantly in IV drug users
- Trauma, atrial tumors, pacemaker leads

Secondary Tricuspid Regurgitation

- Most common cause of TR
- Related to RV dilation resulting in improper coaptation of valve leaflets
  - Right heart failure of any etiology (most commonly resulting from left heart failure)
  - RV hypertension secondary to pulmonic stenosis
  - Primary pulmonary hypertension and mitral valve disease
  - RV systolic pressure gradients > 55 mmHg produce functional TR
  - Endomyocardial fibrosis

PATHOLOGY

General Features

- Etiology
  - Any disease that causes abnormalities in TV apparatus (anulus, leaflets, chordae, and papillary muscles) can cause TR
  - Primary causes: Pacemaker leads, injury to valve (trauma, endocarditis, carcinoid syndrome, rheumatic valve disease), congenital anomaly (Ebstein anomaly), ischemic disease (papillary muscle rupture), and myxomatous degeneration
  - Secondary causes: Dilation of RV and right atrium resulting in dilation of TV anulus &/or tethering of TV leaflets
  - Posttransplantation
    - Moderate to severe TR in 15-20% of heart transplant recipients
    - May be avoided if modified inferior vena caval anastomosis is performed
  - Severe TR is occasionally idiopathic
    - Proposed mechanism: Annular dilatation due to aging, atrial fibrillation, or other causes
- Associated abnormalities
  - Underlying cause of TR
    - Left ventricular failure; chronic lung disease; LV inflow obstruction
  - Secondary findings of systemic venous hypertension
    - Hepatic congestion with resultant cirrhosis
- Deformation and retraction of valve cusps in primary diseases
- Myxomatous degeneration
- Valve leaflets
  - Rheumatic heart disease
    - Thickening; shortening and retraction of 1 or more leaflets; shortening of chordae
  - Infectious endocarditis
    - Shortening and retraction of 1 or more leaflets; shortening of chordae
  - Traumatic destruction of leaflet
  - Carcinoid syndrome
    - Fibrous plaques deposit on right-sided leaflets
    - Occurs in setting of hepatic metastases
- Chordae tendineae
  - Thickening and retraction due to rheumatic fever

CLINICAL ISSUES

Presentation

- Most common signs/symptoms
  - Wide spectrum; depends on severity and chronicity of regurgitation
    - In absence of pulmonary hypertension, trace to mild TR is common, well tolerated, and usually asymptomatic
- Other signs/symptoms
  - Pulsations in neck from prominent V waves in jugular venous pulse
- Fatigue, exhaustion, and right heart failure
- Hepatomegaly, ascites, and peripheral edema

Demographics

- Epidemiology
  - Trace to mild TR is common and detected by echocardiography in > 70% of patients
  - Considered physiologic when jet extends ≤ 1 cm into atrium
  - Severe TR present in > 1.6 million patients in USA
  - 20-30% of patients with severe left-sided heart disease have at least moderate TR

Treatment

- Medical therapy includes preload and afterload reduction in setting of severe TR and RV failure
- Surgical therapy is more common with primary TR
- Secondary (functional) TR is often treated surgically if another indication for cardiac surgery is also present
  - e.g., mitral valve surgery, aortic valve surgery, or coronary artery bypass graft
- Annuloplasty is most common procedure
  - Usually performed at time of left-sided valve surgery
  - 30-40% of patients have residual TR
  - < 5% require valve replacement in 5 years
- Valve replacement surgery when annuloplasty is not feasible or has failed
  - 5-year survival rate post surgery: ~ 70%
  - 10-year survival rate post surgery: ~ 40%
- Transcatheter repair/replacement of TR will likely be increasingly used for treatment

SELECTED REFERENCES

1. Rajiah PS et al: Utility of CT and MRI in tricuspid valve interventions. Radiographics. 43(7):e220153, 2023
2. Otto CM et al: 2020 ACC/AHA guideline for the management of patients with valvular heart disease: a report of the American College of Cardiology/American Heart Association joint committee on clinical practice guidelines. Circulation. 143(5):e72-227, 2021

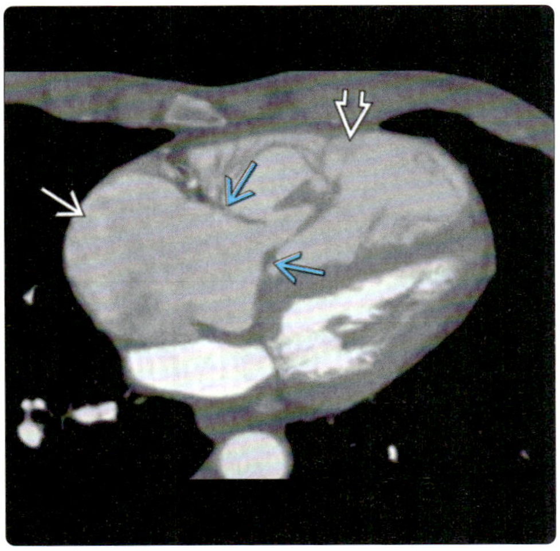

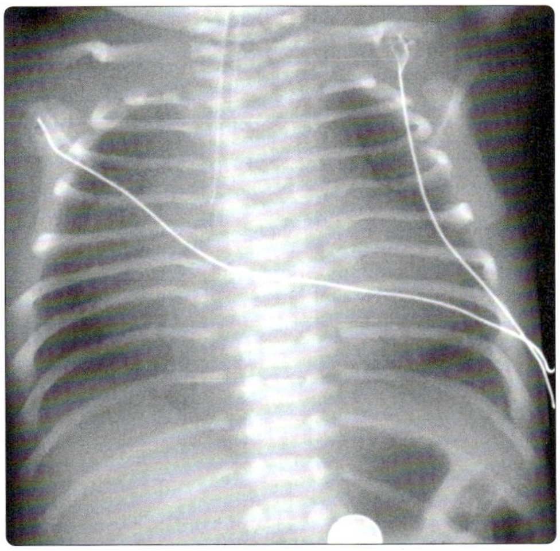

(Left) *End-diastolic 4-chamber MinIP shows a dilated right atrium and right ventricle with thickened, noncoapting TV leaflets in a patient with carcinoid syndrome.* **(Right)** *Frontal radiograph in a newborn shows massive cardiac enlargement from right atrial enlargement associated with Ebstein anomaly. There is decreased pulmonary vasculature, which is a typical finding with this disorder. The endotracheal tube intubates the right main bronchus.*

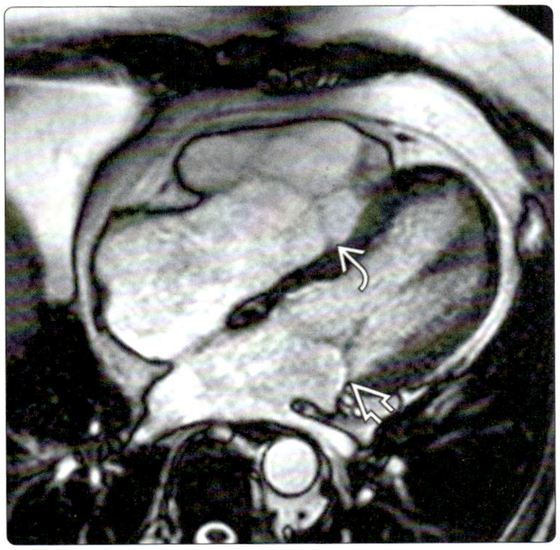

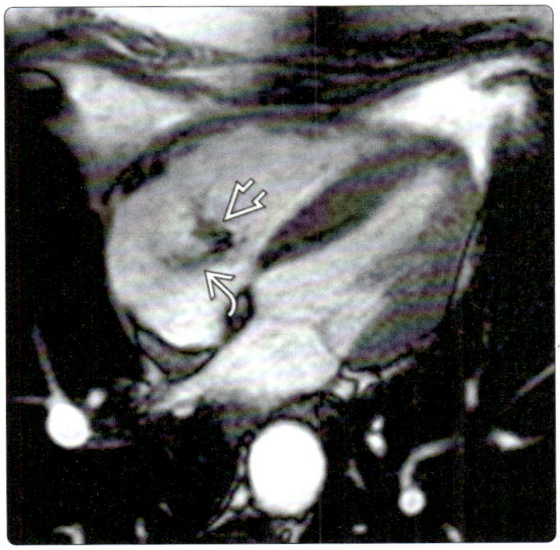

(Left) *Four-chamber SSFP MR shows marked right atrial dilation from tricuspid regurgitation associated with Ebstein anomaly. Note "atrialization" of the right ventricle from apical displacement of the TV leaflets relative to the mitral valve.* **(Right)** *Four-chamber SSFP MR shows a dephasing flow jet directed from the TV into the right atrium, indicating tricuspid regurgitation. There is an associated valve vegetation from endocarditis.*

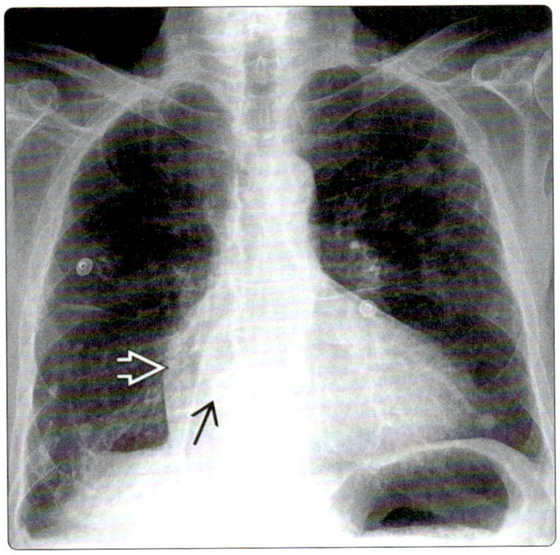

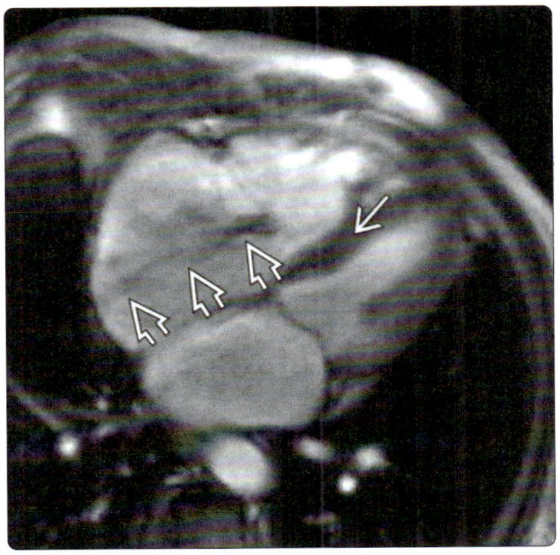

(Left) *Frontal radiograph shows mild left atrial dilation and a markedly enlarged right atrium. The apparent left ventricular dilation is a result of right heart enlargement causing clockwise rotation of the cardiac chambers.* **(Right)** *Four-chamber MR in the same patient shows a dephasing jet extending toward the posterior right atrial wall, suggestive of moderate to severe tricuspid regurgitation. There is flattening of the interventricular septum indicating volume overload.*

KEY FACTS

TERMINOLOGY

- Carcinoid tumor secretion of vasoactive substances causing clinical syndrome of flushing, diarrhea, and bronchospasm

IMAGING

- Echocardiography
  - Thickened, retracted, highly reflective tricuspid &/or pulmonary valve leaflets
- MR
  - Enlarged right atrium
  - Thickening of tricuspid and pulmonary valve leaflets
  - Quantification of tricuspid/pulmonic regurgitation
- F18 FDG, although FDG uptake is limited due to low proliferative activity
- PET/CT with 68Ga-labeled somatostatin receptor agonists, such as DOTATOC, DOTATATE, and DOTANOC
- Radiolabeled octreotide (Octreoscan) is less sensitive with less spatial resolution

TOP DIFFERENTIAL DIAGNOSES

- Rheumatic heart disease
- Other causes of tricuspid or pulmonary valve disease

CLINICAL ISSUES

- Cardiac involvement in 50% of carcinoid syndrome cases
  - May be only presentation
- Progressive signs of right heart failure
- Symptoms are partially controlled with somatostatin analogues, serotonin antagonists, and α-adrenergic blockers
- Systemic chemotherapy reduces tumor burden
- Selective hepatic artery chemotherapy or embolization is used for liver disease
- Valve replacement for severe disease
- Bioprosthetic valve replacement is undertaken for severely diseased valves with close monitoring required for potential bioprosthetic valve thrombosis

(Left) *Four-chamber (left) and coronal oblique (right) images from a routine CT chest in a patient with metastatic carcinoid tumor show thickening of the tricuspid (TV) and pulmonic (PV) valve leaflets. The right atrium (RA) is dilated, and the right ventricle is hypertrophied. The left heart is normal. Note hepatic metastasis.* **(Right)** *Two-chamber images during systole (top) show fixed, thickened TV leaflets with severe tricuspid regurgitation. Octreotide scan (bottom left) shows numerous hepatic metastases.*

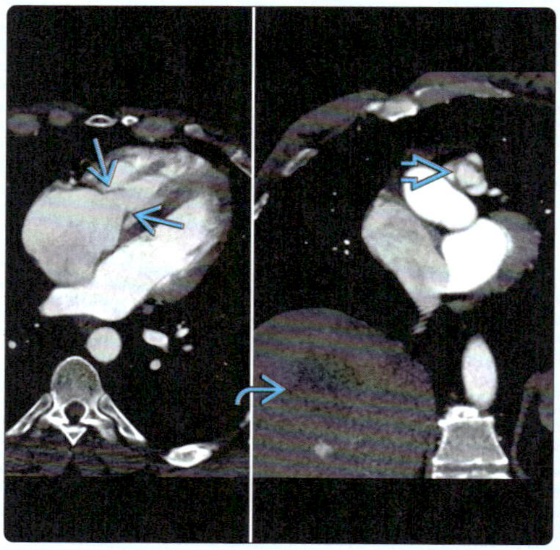

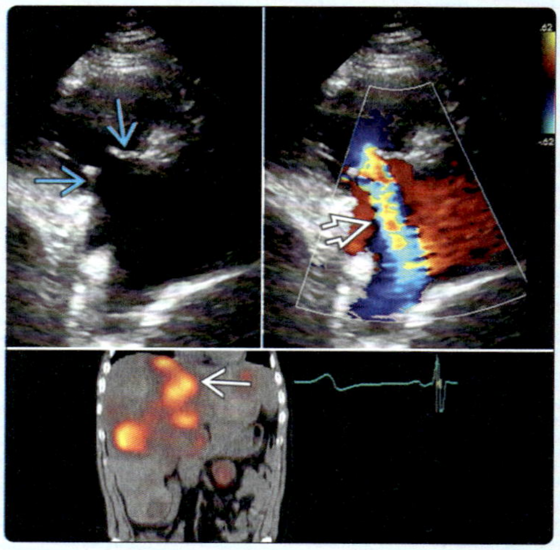

(Left) *Four-chamber MR during diastole (left) in the same patient shows the fixed and thickened TV leaflets. Right ventricular outflow tract (RVOT) during systole (right) shows a high-velocity jet across the very thickened PV. A portion of the tricuspid regurgitant jet can be seen. The aortic valve is normal.* **(Right)** *PA (left) and lateral (right) radiographs a few weeks later in the same patient show prosthetic valves in the pulmonic and tricuspid positions.*

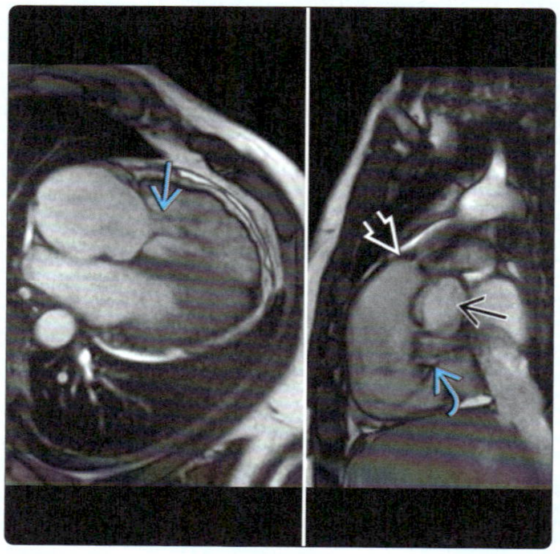

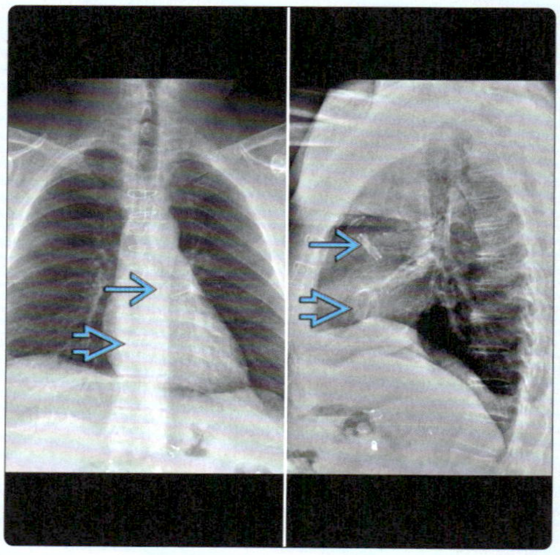

TERMINOLOGY

Definitions

- Secretion of vasoactive substances by carcinoid tumor causing clinical syndrome of flushing (90%), diarrhea (70%), and bronchospasm (10%)
  - Develops from neuroendocrine cells of enterochromaffin cell origin in submucosa
    - Most have midgut origin (ileocecal region/appendix)
    - Origin can also be from lung
      - Due to common origin of foregut and respiratory diverticulum during 4th week of fetal development
    - Origin cannot be found in 18% of patients
  - Clinical symptoms occur when secretory products are directly released into systemic circulation or when hepatic metabolism is overwhelmed
    - Cells secrete vasoactive substances
      - Serotonin [5-hydroxytryptamine (5-HT)] production is most prominent, especially in midgut tumors
      - Bradykinins, tachykinins, histamine, substance P, and ACTH also reported
    - Tumor products activate mitogenic pathways on exposed endocardial surfaces inducing valvular fibrosis
    - Tricuspid and pulmonary valves are involved on upstream side where vasoactive substance levels are highest
    - 2nd most common cause of tricuspid stenosis
      - Concomitant regurgitation is always present
    - Left heart can be involved in pulmonary carcinoid or patent foramen ovale but is less likely due to pulmonary deactivation of vasoactive substances

IMAGING

General Features

- Best diagnostic clue
  - Echocardiography shows thickened, retracted, highly reflective tricuspid &/or pulmonary valve leaflets
- Location
  - Tricuspid and pulmonary valves are most commonly involved; tricuspid regurgitation (TR) is most common abnormality
  - Left heart involvement is seen in 7% of patients with bronchial carcinoids or right-to-left intracardiac shunts
- Thickened leaflets similar to rheumatic involvement
- Flow abnormalities related to degree of valve involvement

CT Findings

- CTA
  - Thickened, retracted tricuspid and pulmonic valves
    - Fixed, nonmobile leaflets
  - Enlarged right atrium and ventricle
  - Pulmonary nodules in primary pulmonary disease
  - ↓ pulmonary vascularity in presence of severe pulmonary stenosis

MR Findings

- Cine SSFP sequence shows tricuspid and pulmonary regurgitation and stenosis
  - Tricuspid leaflets may be shortened, thickened, and retracted and show incomplete coaptation
- Cine SSFP: Quantification of ventricular function and volumes
- Phase-contrast MR: Quantification of tricuspid and pulmonary stenosis/regurgitation
- Delayed enhancement of valve leaflets due to fibrosis

Echocardiographic Findings

- Echocardiogram
  - Color Doppler is used to semiquantitatively identify jets
  - Continuous wave (CW) spectral Doppler is used to measure peak transvalvular velocities and pressure half time (inversely proportional to valve area)
    - Tricuspid valve: Regurgitation (97%), stenosis (59%)
      - Tricuspid leaflets may be shortened, thickened, retracted and show incomplete coaptation
      - Leaflets and papillary muscles may appear highly reflective
      - CW Doppler shows characteristic dagger-shaped profile with early peak pressure and rapid decline due to rapid equalization of right atrial and ventricular pressures
    - Pulmonic valve: Regurgitation (50%), stenosis (25%); pulmonic valve leaflets characteristically stay open in fixed position

Nuclear Medicine Findings

- PET
  - F18 FDG, although FDG uptake is limited due to low proliferative activity
  - 68Ga-labeled somatostatin receptor agonists, such as DOTATOC, DOTATATE, and DOTANOC PET/CT, rapidly becoming noninvasive gold standard staging test
  - Ga68-DOTATOC PET/CT demonstrated to be > 97% sensitive and 92% specific for identification of metastatic neuroendocrine neoplasms; DOTATATE PET most common method for detection of cardiac neuroendocrine tumor metastases
  - Somatostatin receptor scintigraphy can distinguish patients who will qualify for and benefit from somatostatin antagonist and peptide treatment
- SPECT
  - Radiolabeled octreotide using either conventional scintigraphy or SPECT imaging: Inferior resolution and less sensitive than PET
- Valvular carcinoid syndrome due to valvular fibrosis and not tumor infiltration → no uptake on PET or SPECT imaging

Imaging Recommendations

- Best imaging tool
  - Transthoracic echocardiography (TEE) is gold standard with cardiac MR or CTA being useful adjunctive tools

DIFFERENTIAL DIAGNOSIS

Rheumatic Heart Disease

- More commonly affects left-sided heart valves; most commonly affects mitral valve

Endocarditis

- Injury to valve often with vegetation &/or perforation; valve thickening and fibrotic in carcinoid syndrome

Endomyocardial Fibrosis

- Can lead to encasement of valve that is similar to carcinoid syndrome
- More extensive involvement of endocardial surfaces, often with thrombus formation

Ebstein Anomaly

- Displacement of septal and posterior leaflets toward apex; large atrialized portion of right ventricle

Fenfluramine and Phentermine Usage

- Associated with group 1 pulmonary hypertension
- Involves both left- and right-sided valves
- Medications banned by FDA

PATHOLOGY

General Features

- Genetics
  - Most carcinoid tumors are sporadic
  - Foregut carcinoids are associated with type 1 multiple endocrine neoplasia in ~ 10% of cases and also (rarely) with type 2 multiple endocrine neoplasia or type 1 neurofibromatosis
- Macroscopically, valves appear thickened and may be partly fused
  - Extensive diffuse infiltration from valves to myocardium may cause restrictive cardiomyopathy

Gross Pathologic & Surgical Features

- Coaptation of nodular thickened valve leaflets impaired by fibrous plaque coating leaflets and papillary muscles

Microscopic Features

- Fibrous plaques are composed of smooth muscle cells mixed with mucopolysaccharide and collagen
- Fibrous plaques may be mediated by serotonin 1B receptor subtype, which induces fibroblast proliferation on in vitro stimulation

CLINICAL ISSUES

Presentation

- Most common signs/symptoms
  - Cutaneous flushing (90%), diarrhea (70%), and bronchospasm (10%)
- Other signs/symptoms
  - Cardiac involvement in 50% of carcinoid syndrome cases but may be only presentation
    - Progressive signs of right heart failure
- N-terminal (NT)-prohormone BNP (NT-proBNP) useful screening serum biomarkers
  - Both have diagnostic and prognostic significance for cardiac involvement
- Measurement of either 24-hr urine 5-HIAA or plasma 5-HIAA mandatory for diagnosis and follow-up

Natural History & Prognosis

- 50% of patients with carcinoid tumor will develop carcinoid syndrome
- 50% of patients with carcinoid syndrome will develop cardiac involvement
- Mean life expectancy with carcinoid heart disease: 1.6 years; without carcinoid heart disease: 4.6 years

Treatment

- Medical
  - Therapy for right heart failure (includes ACE inhibitors)
  - Partial symptom control of and antiproliferative effects via serotonin antagonists, α-adrenergic blockers
    - Somatostatin analogues are mainstay therapy
  - Systemic chemotherapy to reduce tumor burden
  - Neuroendocrine tumors peptide receptor radionuclide therapy (PRRT)
- Monitoring/surveillance: If cardiac involvement suspected, NT-proBNP levels and TTE recommended; if no cardiac signs or symptoms, periodic NT-proBNP screening recommended
  - Levels > 260 ng/mL warrant further evaluation with TTE
- 2017 expert consensus document recommends ongoing follow-up with NT-proBNP levels if TTE findings are unremarkable, with surveillance TTE every 6 months for mild heart failure, and every 3 months for moderate or greater heart failure
- Interventional
  - Selective hepatic artery chemotherapy or embolization for liver disease burden
  - Balloon angioplasty for valvular stenosis
  - Radiofrequency ablation for liver tumor debulking
  - Selective internal radiation therapy with yttrium-90
- Surgical
  - If small, may be resectable; becoming increasingly used as has been proven to have better outcomes
  - Valve replacement in severe TR (high on-table mortality)
  - Transcatheter pulmonic/tricuspid valve replacement has been described for severe valvular disease patients who are not operative candidates
    - Absence of rigid anulus for pulmonary and tricuspid valves risks dislodgement
  - Bioprosthetic valve replacement is undertaken for severely diseased valves, with close monitoring required for potential bioprosthetic valve thrombosis
    - Transcatheter valve-in-valve implantation may be useful in patients with bioprosthetic degeneration
      - Rigid frame of conventional bioprosthesis provides scaffold secure seating
  - Tricuspid edge-to-edge repair (TEER) generally not considered for significant TR as severe retracted and fixed tricuspid leaflets limits ability to deploy clips
- Multidisciplinary approach becoming more emphasized to deal with systemic and cardiac disease

SELECTED REFERENCES

1. Namkoong J et al: A systematic review and meta-analysis of the diagnosis and surgical management of carcinoid heart disease. Front Cardiovasc Med. 11:1353612, 2024
2. Das S et al: Carcinoid heart disease management: a multi-disciplinary collaboration. Oncologist. 28(7):575-83, 2023
3. Wang Y et al: Gastroenteropancreatic neuroendocrine tumor metastasis to the heart: evaluation of imaging manifestations. Curr Probl Diagn Radiol. 52(5):340-5, 2023
4. Grozinsky-Glasberg S et al: European Neuroendocrine Tumor Society (ENETS) 2022 guidance paper for carcinoid syndrome and carcinoid heart disease. J Neuroendocrinol. 34(7):e13146, 2022
5. Pellikka PA et al: Carcinoid heart disease. Clinical and echocardiographic spectrum in 74 patients. Circulation. 87(4):1188-96, 1993

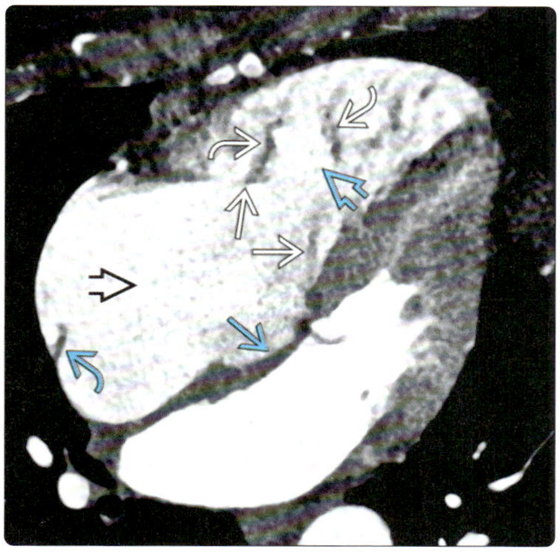

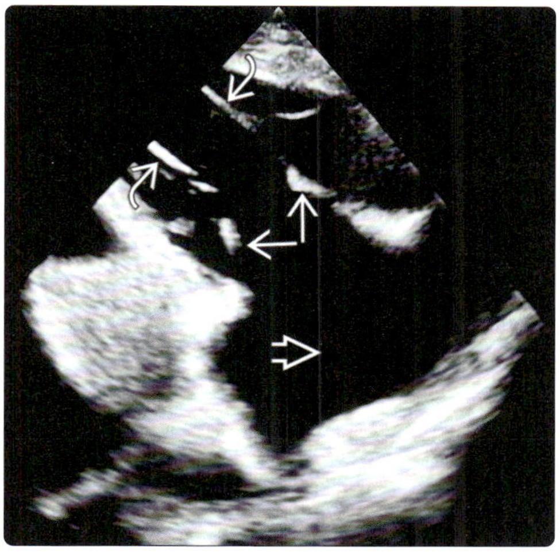

(Left) *Cardiac CT during systole shows thickened and fixed tricuspid leaflets with thickened RV trabeculae and a severely dilated RA and right ventricle . Increased RA pressures causes bowing of the interatrial septum to the left. Normal crista terminalis are noted.* **(Right)** *Two-chamber echocardiogram shows very thickened tricuspid leaflets fixed open in systole and a severely dilated RA secondary to torrential tricuspid regurgitation. Note also the very thickened RV trabeculae .*

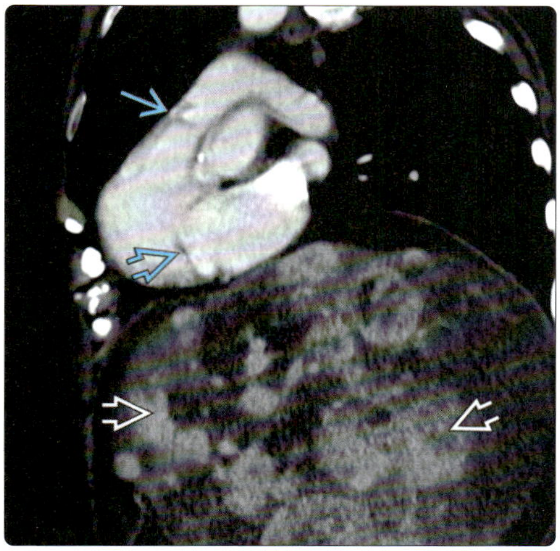

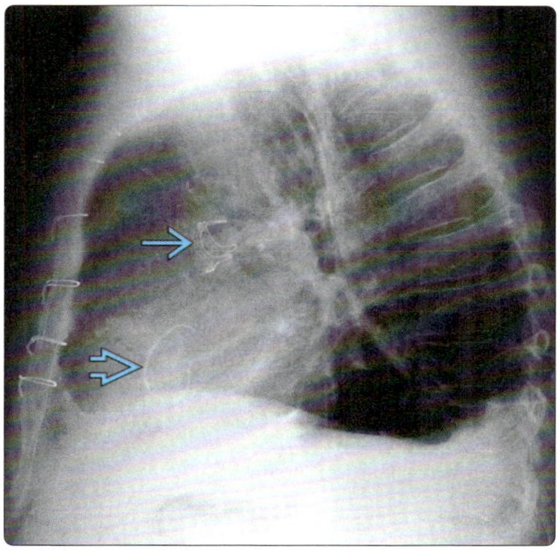

(Left) *Nongated chest CT in a patient with metastatic neuroendocrine cancer with liver metastases shows a dilated right heart with thickening of both the PV and TV due to carcinoid valve disease.* **(Right)** *Lateral radiograph 2 weeks later in the same patient shows findings of tricuspid annuloplasty and a bioprosthetic PV .*

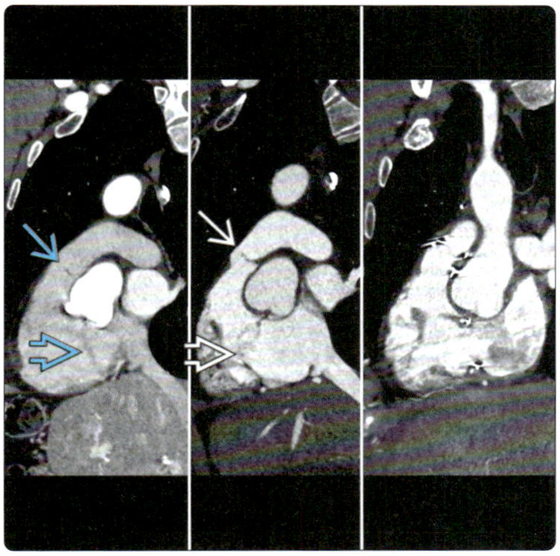

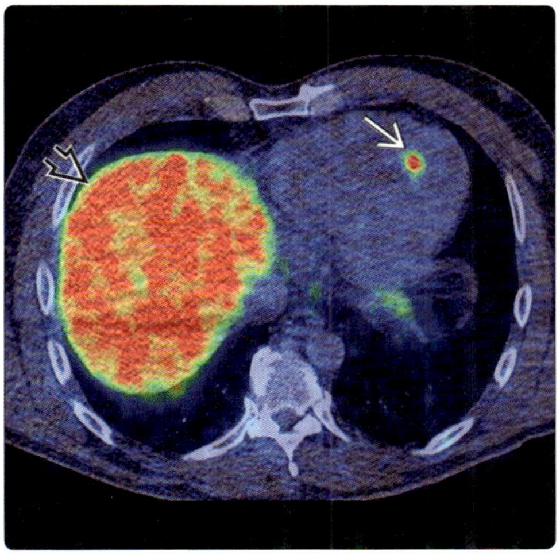

(Left) *RVOT CECT in 2021 (left) in a patient with a metastatic neuroendocrine tumor shows mild thickening of both the PV and TV . Repeat CT 1 year later (middle) shows worsening PV and TV thickening. The patient underwent replacement of both valves a few weeks later (right).* **(Right)** *Axial fused 68Ga-DOTATATE PET/CT shows a focal cardiac metastasis in the apical interventricular septum along with extensive hepatic metastatic disease .*

KEY FACTS

TERMINOLOGY

- Pulmonary stenosis (PS)
- Lesion resulting in obstruction of right ventricular outflow tract (RVOT)

IMAGING

- Radiography: Enlargement of pulmonary trunk and left pulmonary artery (LPA)
- CT
  - Poststenotic dilation of pulmonary trunk and LPA
  - Thickened, immobile valve leaflets
  - Small valve area and anulus
  - Pericardial calcification involving aorta and pulmonary trunk may rarely produce acquired PS
- MR: Determination of presence and extent of PS
  - Doming or windsock appearance of pulmonic valve
  - Narrowing of valve orifice

TOP DIFFERENTIAL DIAGNOSES

- Hypoplasia of right PA (RPA)
- Pulmonary embolism of RPA
- Proximal interruption of RPA

PATHOLOGY

- Majority of cases are congenital in etiology
- Acquired: Carcinoid syndrome, rheumatic heart disease, and infective endocarditis
- Severity of PS is determined by peak velocity of peak pressure gradient across valve

CLINICAL ISSUES

- Treatment
  - Trivial and mild PS: Observation and endocarditis prophylaxis prior to surgical procedures
  - Moderate and severe PS: Balloon valvuloplasty or surgical valvotomy

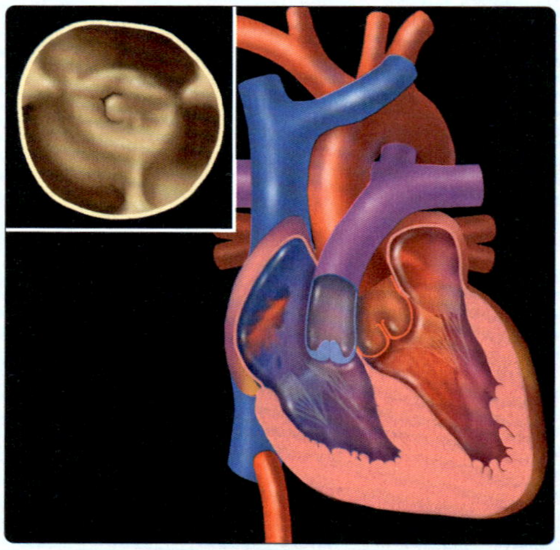

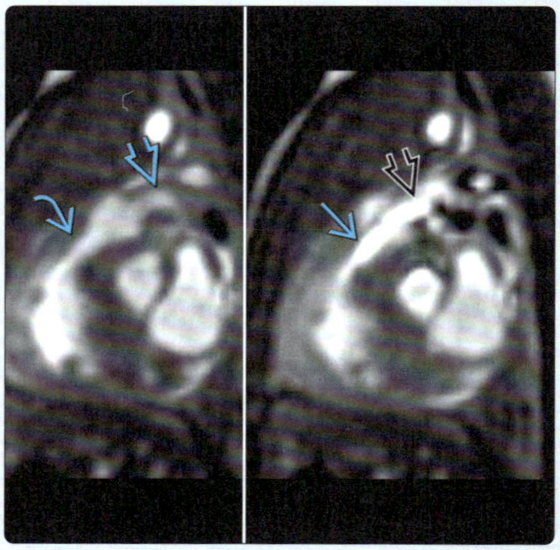

(Left) *Graphic shows morphologic features of pulmonary stenosis (PS) characterized by diffuse thickening of the pulmonary valve (PV) leaflets and fusion near the commissures, which results in narrowing of the valve orifice (insert).* **(Right)** *Images in a newborn with Williams syndrome show severe right ventricular outflow tract (RVOT) narrowing and hypoplasia of the main pulmonary artery (PA), best seen on diastole (left). On systole (right), there is subvalvular and supravalvular stenoses.*

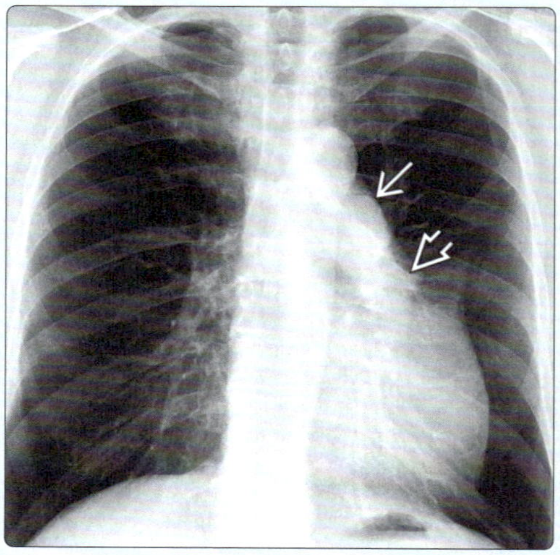

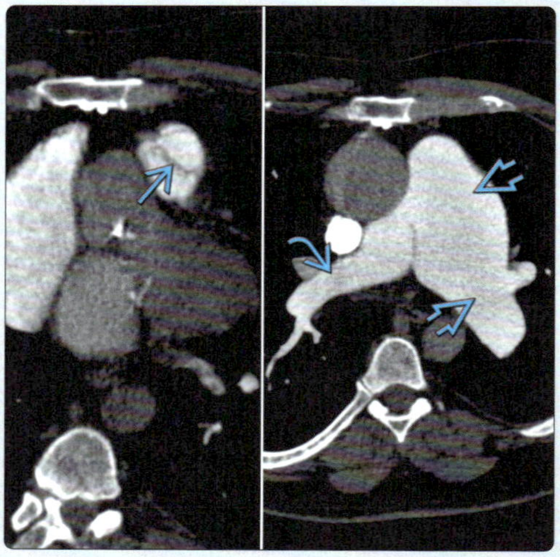

(Left) *Frontal chest radiograph in a patient with congenital PS demonstrates poststenotic dilatation of the pulmonary trunk and left PA (LPA), which are characteristically enlarged in PS.* **(Right)** *CTA in the same patient shows a thickened bicuspid PV. The main artery and PA are dilated, and the right PA is normal in size. Severe PS was confirmed on MR.*

TERMINOLOGY

Abbreviations

- Pulmonary (pulmonic) stenosis (PS)

Synonyms

- Pulmonary (pulmonic) valvular stenosis

Definitions

- Lesion resulting in obstruction of pulmonary valve and poststenotic dilatation of pulmonary trunk and left pulmonary artery (PA)

IMAGING

General Features

- Best diagnostic clue
  - Enlargement of pulmonary trunk and left PA (LPA)
- Location
  - Valvular (90%), subvalvular, supravalvular

Radiographic Findings

- Radiography
  - **Enlargement of pulmonary trunk**
    - Convexity along left mediastinal border inferior to aortic arch
  - Enlargement of LPA may be present
  - Right ventricular (RV) enlargement

CT Findings

- CECT
  - Dilatation of pulmonary trunk and LPA
  - RV enlargement
  - Focal pericardial calcification involving aorta and pulmonary trunk reported as unusual cause of acquired PS
- Cardiac gated CTA
  - Thickened valve leaflets
  - Small pulmonary valve area and anulus
  - Restricted systolic opening of leaflets
  - Hypoplasia of supravalvular pulmonary trunk may be present

MR Findings

- MR cine
  - Morphologic abnormalities of pulmonary valve
    - Thickening ± fusion of valve leaflets
    - Narrowing of valve orifice (planimetry to measure)
    - Restricted systolic opening of valve
      - Doming or windsock appearance of valve
  - High-velocity stenotic jet produces dark signal through valve
  - Enlargement of pulmonary trunk and LPA
  - RV hypertrophy, dilation, and dysfunction quantified
  - Supravalvular: Narrowing of PA sinotubular junction above valve
  - Subvalvular: RV hypertrophy and narrowing
  - Associated congenital anomalies
- Phase-contrast imaging
  - Visualization of stenotic jet through valve into PA
  - Quantification of PS: Velocity and pressure gradient
- MR angiography
  - Enlargement of pulmonary trunk and LPA

Echocardiographic Findings

- Echocardiogram
  - Thickening of valve leaflets
  - Restricted systolic motion and reduced mobility of valve leaflets
  - Doming or windsock appearance of pulmonic valve
  - Poststenotic dilatation of PA
- Color Doppler
  - Systolic high-velocity flow jet in pulmonary outflow tract

Angiographic Findings

- Conventional
  - Patients with severe PS usually undergo cardiac catheterization for confirmatory pressure assessment
    - Concomitant balloon valvuloplasty may be performed
  - Useful in evaluating morphology of pulmonary outflow tract, PAs, and RV

DIFFERENTIAL DIAGNOSIS

Congenital Hypoplasia of Right Pulmonary Artery

- Small right PA (RPA) on CT and MR
- Small right main bronchus
- Rudimentary right lung is present

Massive Embolism of Right Pulmonary Artery

- On radiograph, asymmetrical large main PA and LPA
  - Oligemia of right lung
- CT and MR: Pulmonary embolism is demonstrated

Proximal Interruption of Right Pulmonary Artery

- Failed development of proximal right main PA
- On radiograph, small right hilum and lung
- Absence of RPA on CT and MR
- Collateral systemic and bronchial arteries seen on right

Aberrant Left Pulmonary Artery (Pulmonary Sling)

- Congenital anomaly in which LPA originates from RPA
- Forms "sling" around trachea, passing between trachea and esophagus
- Associated anomalies of tracheobronchial tree and cardiovascular system

Pulmonary Hypertension

- Dilation of main PA, RPA, and LPA (not asymmetric)
  - Main PA > 29 mm or > size of ascending aorta at same level on CT or MR
- Etiologies classified into 5 groups in WHO classification

Idiopathic Dilation of Pulmonary Trunk

- Congenital dilatation of pulmonary trunk ± involvement of RPA and LPA
- Diagnosed only after excluding pulmonary hypertension
  - Normal pressures in PA and RV

PATHOLOGY

General Features

- Etiology
  - Congenital
    - Most common etiology of PS

- Isolated in 80% of cases
- Additional forms of congenital heart disease present in 20% of cases
  - Tetralogy of Fallot (TOF), complete atrioventricular (AV) canal, double-outlet RV, univentricular heart
- Acquired
  - Carcinoid syndrome
    - Most common cause of acquired PS
    - Associated with tricuspid valvular disease
  - Rheumatic heart disease
    - Stenosis is rare even if valve is affected
    - Mitral and aortic valve are affected
  - Masses
    - Extrinsic: Narrowing RV outflow tract (RVOT)
    - Intrinsic: Thrombus, vegetation
  - Following surgeries
- Subvalvular stenosis
  - Congenital ventricular septal defect (VSD) with associated RVOT obstruction; levo-transposition of great arteries (L-TGA)
  - Iatrogenic (surgeries/interventions), hypertrophic cardiomyopathy, infiltrative diseases, compression by tumor or vascular structure
- Supravalvular stenosis
  - At pulmonary trunk or more distally; may be membrane
  - Can be seen with PA hypoplasia

- Genetics
  - Considered to be multifactorial in origin
  - Familial forms have been described
  - May be associated with genetic disorders
    - Valvular PS
      - Noonan syndrome: Markedly dysplastic valve, leaflet thickening, little commissural fusion
    - Supravalvular PS
      - Congenital rubella syndrome
      - Williams syndrome
- Associated abnormalities
  - Atrial septal defect
  - VSD
  - Patent foramen ovale
  - TOF

Staging, Grading, & Classification

- **Severity classification by velocity**
  - Mild PS: Peak velocity < 3 m/sec
  - Moderate PS: Peak velocity 3-4 m/sec
  - Severe PS: Peak velocity > 4 m/sec
- **Severity classification by peak gradient**
  - Mild PS: < 36 mmHg
  - Moderate PS: 36-64 mmHg
  - Severe PS: > 64 mmHg

Gross Pathologic & Surgical Features

- Thickening of valve leaflets
  - Calcification may be present
- Partial fusion of commissures
- Valve is typically dome-shaped or conical in configuration
- Narrowing of central orifice
- Congenital: Trileaflet/unicuspid/bicuspid/dysplastic

Microscopic Features

- Thickening of valve leaflets
- Dysplastic valves may be composed of myxomatous tissue
  - Present in 10-15% of patients with valvular PS

CLINICAL ISSUES

Presentation

- Most common signs/symptoms
  - Presentation depends on severity of symptoms
    - Mild PS
      - Typically asymptomatic
    - Moderate or severe PS
      - Signs and symptoms of systemic venous congestion
      - Mimics congestive heart failure
- Other signs/symptoms
  - Cyanosis in setting of concomitant patent foramen ovale or atrial septal defect

Demographics

- Age
  - Age at presentation depends on severity of obstruction
- Sex
  - M:F = 1:1
- Epidemiology
  - Represents 10% of all congenital cardiac defects
  - 8-12% of all congenital cardiac defects in children
    - Isolated PS with intact ventricular septum is 2nd most common defect

Natural History & Prognosis

- Severity of stenosis determines morbidity and mortality
  - Mild to moderate PS
    - Usually well tolerated
  - Severe PS
    - Decreased cardiac output, RV hypertrophy, congestive heart failure, and cyanosis may develop

Treatment

- Trivial and mild PS
  - Observation
- Moderate and severe PS
  - Balloon valvuloplasty or surgical valvotomy
    - Mild pulmonic regurgitation and RV dilatation may develop following valvuloplasty

DIAGNOSTIC CHECKLIST

Consider

- Pulmonic stenosis in patients with pulmonary trunk and LPA enlargement

SELECTED REFERENCES

1. Correction to: 2020 ACC/AHA guideline for the management of patients with valvular heart disease: a report of the American College of Cardiology/American Heart Association Joint Committee on Clinical Practice Guidelines. Circulation. 148(20):e185, 2023
2. Marchini F et al: Pulmonary valve stenosis: from diagnosis to current management techniques and future prospects. Vasc Health Risk Manag. 19:379-90, 2023

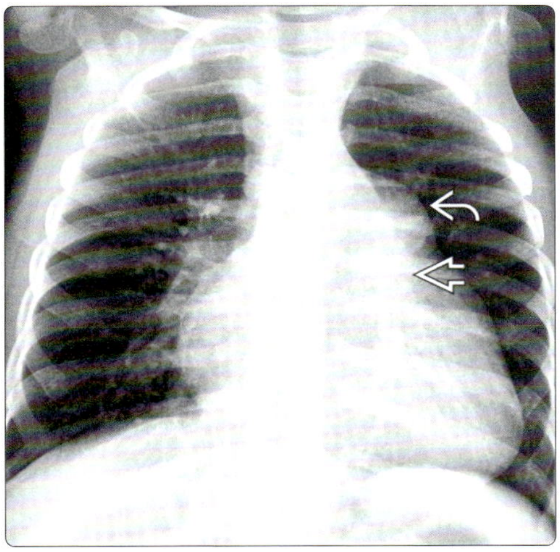

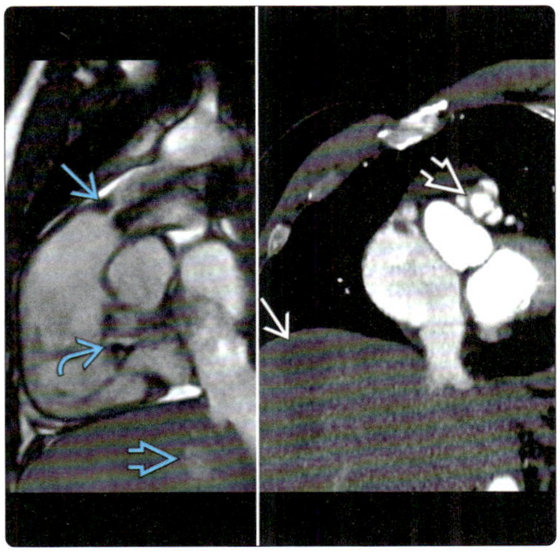

(Left) *Frontal chest radiograph in a patient with congenital PS demonstrates enlargement of the pulmonary trunk and LPA. PA enlargement is the most common radiographic appearance of PS.* **(Right)** *RVOT SSFP MR left) in a patient with a metastatic carcinoid tumor shows severe PS with thickening of the PV. There is also severe tricuspid regurgitation. Coronal oblique CT shows the thickened pulmonary valve. Liver metastases are seen on both MR and CT.*

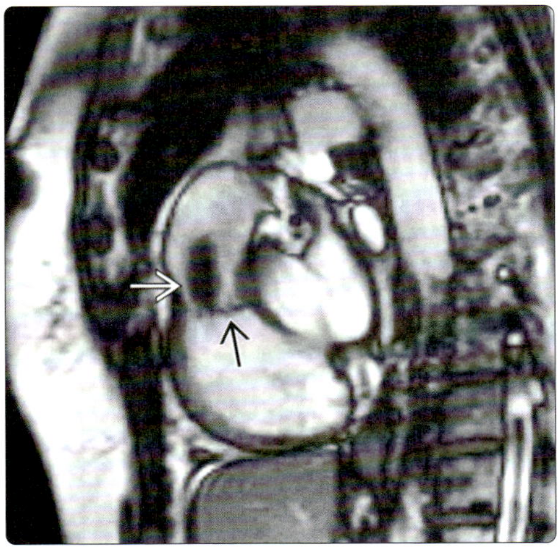

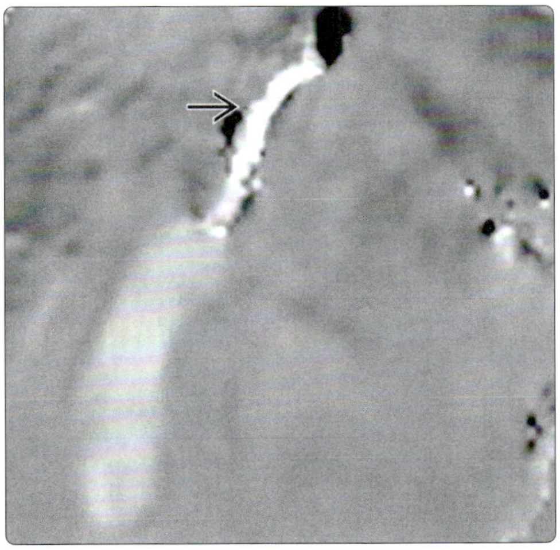

(Left) *Oblique sagittal RVOT SSFP cardiac MR shows a jet of signal dephasing arising from the pulmonic valve, consistent with severe PS. Thickening of the PV leaflets is also noted. Patients with moderate or severe PS are typically treated with balloon valvuloplasty or surgical valvulotomy.* **(Right)** *Corresponding RVOT phase-contrast velocity map shows slit-like, turbulent flow through the PV, indicative of severe stenosis.*

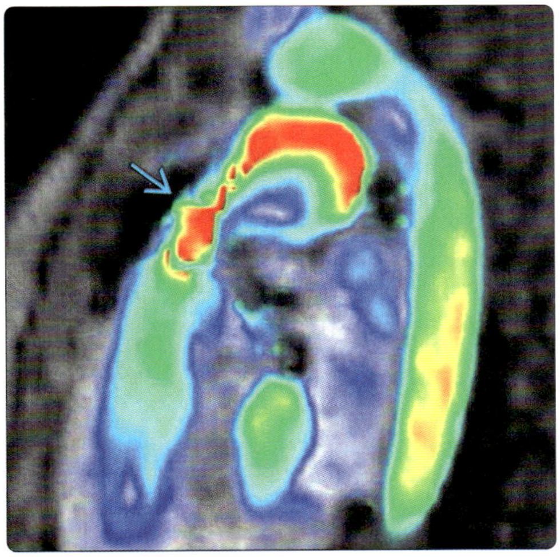

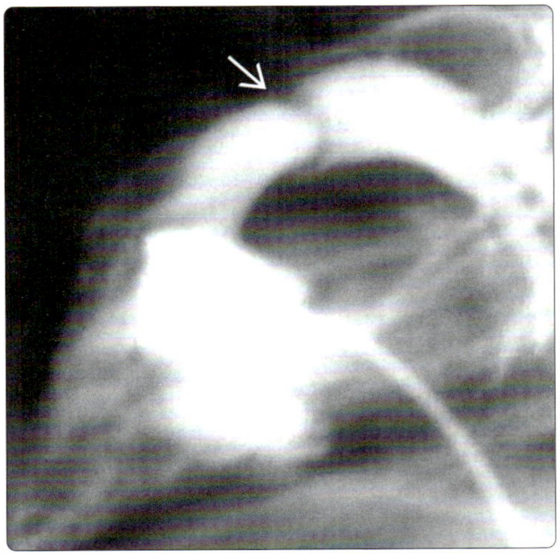

(Left) *Sagittal oblique 4D flow phase-contrast MR in a patient with PS shows high-velocity flow acceleration through the PV.* **(Right)** *Catheter angiography in the right ventricle shows an area of circumferential, high-grade stenosis of the PV with mild poststenotic dilatation of the main PA.*

Pulmonary Regurgitation

KEY FACTS

TERMINOLOGY

- Reversed flow from pulmonary artery (PA) through incompetent or absent pulmonary valve into right ventricle (RV) in diastole

IMAGING

- Diastolic flow jet entering RV from main PA as visualized on cardiac MR or echocardiography
- Trace pulmonary regurgitation (PR) is seen in up to 75% of normal patients and is of no clinical consequence
- Patients with clinically significant PR most often have history of prior intervention on pulmonary anulus/pulmonary valve for relief of obstruction in cases of tetralogy of Fallot (TOF) or congenital valvular pulmonic stenosis
- Chest radiographs in cases of significant PR show dilated PA with normal pulmonary blood flow

TOP DIFFERENTIAL DIAGNOSES

- Surgical/procedural complication
    - Postoperative TOF patients with prior pulmonary valve resection
    - Balloon valvuloplasty for congenital pulmonary valve stenosis
- Atrial septal defect
- Pulmonary hypertension

CLINICAL ISSUES

- Patients known to have lesions predisposing to PR (prior TOF or pulmonic stenosis repair) should have surveillance imaging to detect and quantify

DIAGNOSTIC CHECKLIST

- Consider PR when chest x-ray shows prominent PA and enlarged RV without shunt vascularity
- Although severity of PR may be estimated with echocardiography, quantification best performed with MR

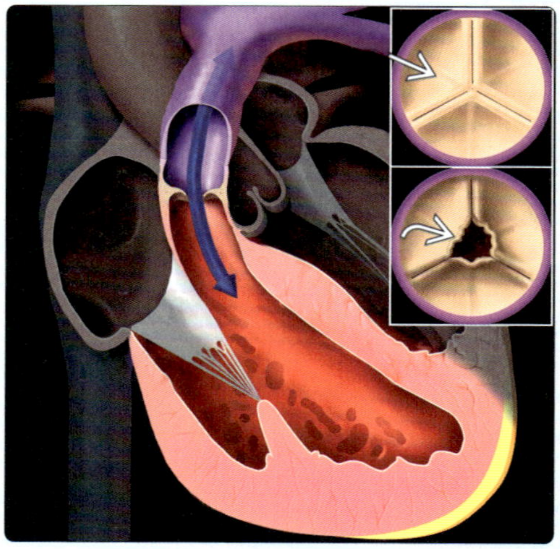

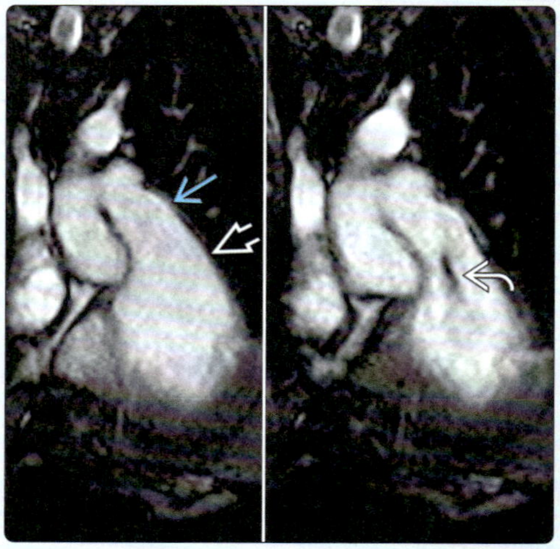

(Left) *Graphic shows direction of pulmonary regurgitation (PR) jet (blue arrow). Insets show normal diastolic appearance of the pulmonary valve and diastolic failure of coaptation in a trileaflet pulmonary valve leading to PR.* **(Right)** *SSFP cine MR shows enlarged right ventricle (RV) and pulmonary artery (PA) in systole (L) and diastole (R). Note regurgitant jet of PR seen in diastole emanating from abnormal pulmonary valve in this patient post balloon valvuloplasty for congenital pulmonary stenosis.*

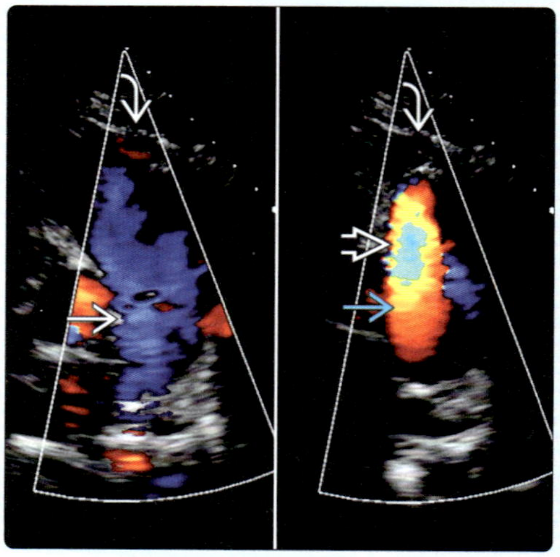

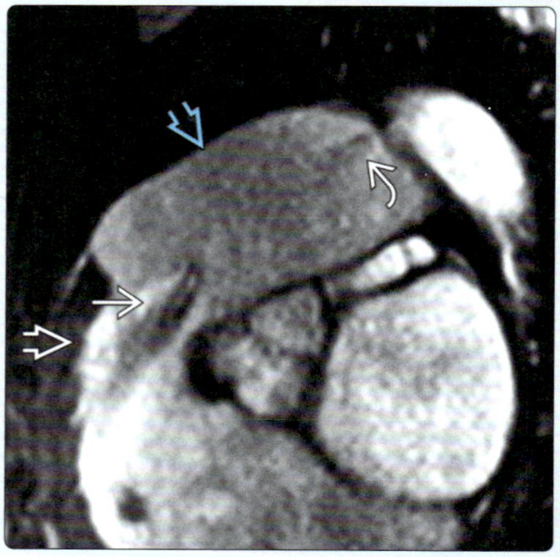

(Left) *Color Doppler echocardiogram of the RV and RV outflow tract (RVOT) shows forward systolic flow (blue jet) extending from the RV into the PA with reversal in diastole (red jet). Note the aliasing in the regurgitant diastolic jet due to the high velocity. The RV apex is noted.* **(Right)** *Short-axis cine MR of an RVOT shows a jet of PR extending into the RV from a dilated PA in a patient with a patent ductus arteriosus (PDA) and pulmonary hypertension. Note the flow jet from PDA to PA.*

TERMINOLOGY

Abbreviations

- Pulmonary regurgitation (PR)

Synonyms

- Pulmonary insufficiency (PI)

Definitions

- Reversed flow from pulmonary artery (PA) through incompetent or absent pulmonary valve into right ventricle (RV) during diastole

IMAGING

General Features

- Best diagnostic clue
  - Diastolic flow jet entering RV from main PA as visualized on cardiac MR or echocardiography
    - Significant PR is most often seen in patients postoperative tetralogy of Fallot (TOF) repair or post balloon valvuloplasty for valvular pulmonic stenosis
- Location
  - Jet of PR begins at level of pulmonary valve (when present) and extends into RV cavity
- Morphology
  - Significant PR leads to enlargement of RV and main PA
  - Diastolic flow through pulmonary valve into RV

Radiographic Findings

- Radiography
  - Dilated PA with normal pulmonary blood flow pattern
  - RV enlargement secondary to volume overload in moderate to severe cases

MR Findings

- Cine steady-state free precession (SSFP) or gradient-echo (GRE) images show retrograde diastolic flow jet into RV
  - In cases of free PR (e.g., postoperative TOF patients post patch annuloplasty) bulk to-and-fro flow may be observed rather than flow jet
  - Regurgitant orifice may be seen during diastole if residual valve tissue present
- Cine MR imaging represents gold standard methodology for accurate assessment of RV size and function
  - RV size and function are key determinants of whether valve repair/replacement is necessary
- Through plane velocity-encoded phase-contrast flow or 4D flow can measure regurgitant volume and fraction
  - Residual or coexisting pulmonic stenosis gradients can be assessed simultaneously
  - Significant pulmonary regurgitant fraction (PRF) by MR: Mild: < 20%; moderate: 20-40%; severe: > 40%
- MRA
  - Enlargement of main PA and RV
    - Asymmetric enlargement of left PA may indicate preceding or coexisting pulmonic stenosis

Echocardiographic Findings

- Echocardiogram
  - Trace PR is seen in up to 75% of normal patients and is of no clinical consequence
  - PV often difficult to visualize on echocardiogram
- Color Doppler
  - Diastolic flow jet into RV emanating from valve, best seen on parasternal long-axis view
  - Severity estimated by diameter of regurgitant jet at its origin just below valve
    - Severe regurgitant jets reach 1-2 cm into RV and last through 75% of diastole

CT Findings

- CTA
  - May show dilatation of main PA and RV if significant PR present
    - Cross-sectional view of valve may show regurgitation orifice in diastole due to incomplete coaptation
  - In cases where MR not feasible, gated CT may provide useful substitute method for measuring RV size and function
    - CT may overestimate RV end-diastolic volume (RVEDV) and underestimate pulmonary regurgitant fraction (PRF) vs. MR

Angiographic Findings

- Right heart catheterization rarely necessary but can demonstrate regurgitant flow and enlargement of PA and RV
  - "Ventricularization" of PA pressure indicates severe PR with equalization of diastolic RV and PA pressures

Imaging Recommendations

- Best imaging tool
  - Cardiac MR is most accurate means to serially follow RV function and volumes in order to guide timely intervention

DIFFERENTIAL DIAGNOSIS

Surgical/Procedural Complication

- Postoperative TOF patients who have undergone RV outflow tract (RVOT) enlargement surgery &/or valve resection
  - Older patients with patch annuloplasty repairs often have free PR with no discernible valve tissue
- Balloon valvuloplasty for congenital pulmonary valve stenosis
  - Significant PR most common significant complication; seen in up to 35% of cases

Congenital Heart Diseases

- Atrial septal defect
  - Produces RV enlargement, but no abnormal diastolic flow is seen through RVOT on MR or echocardiography
  - Usually has shunt vascularity that is not present in PR
- Primary pulmonary valve abnormalities
  - Congenital absence of pulmonary valve often presents in neonates with cyanosis, massive enlargement of hilar PAs, and free PR

Pulmonary Hypertension

- Usually shows more rapid tapering (pruning) of branch vessels as they extend peripherally from hilar regions
- PR often seen as associated condition but is usually mild, pulmonary valve is normal and rarely alters management of underlying disorder

Other Diseases

- Carcinoid syndrome, infective endocarditis, Marfan syndrome, iatrogenic (i.e., PA catheter) rheumatic heart disease

PATHOLOGY

General Features

- Etiology
  - Acquired causes are most common
    - Pulmonary valvotomy often part of TOF repair and balloon valvuloplasty for PS
    - Pulmonary hypertension
    - Endocarditis, carcinoid heart disease less common
- Genetics
  - Variable, depending on etiology

Staging, Grading, & Classification

- Severity can be measured with cardiac MR and estimated with echocardiography
  - Velocity-encoded phase-contrast MR can directly measure forward flow, regurgitant flow, and regurgitant fraction
  - Grading of PR by regurgitant fraction: Mild PR: < 20%; moderate PR: 20-40%; severe: > 40%
  - Echocardiography with color Doppler can estimate severity by measuring size of regurgitant jet, its density and width, and deceleration rate

Gross Pathologic & Surgical Features

- Incompetence of pulmonary valve
  - Due to valve resection or disruption in treatment of TOF or valvuloplasty patients
  - Due to annular dilatation in severe pulmonary hypertension

CLINICAL ISSUES

Presentation

- Most common signs/symptoms
  - Mild PR: Usually none
  - Longstanding or severe PR may result in right heart failure and dyspnea on exertion
- Clinical profile
  - PR often seen in postoperative TOF or pulmonary stenosis (PS) patients
    - Symptoms of RV volume overload may be clinically inapparent until significant RV failure is present
      - Decision regarding timing of pulmonary valve replacement increasingly performed using MR data

Demographics

- Age
  - Varies with underlying lesion
    - If severe, congenital PR may be noted shortly after birth; if due to treatment of underlying congenital lesion, such as PS, it will be apparent after treatment (balloon valvuloplasty); often not clinically apparent for years after initial intervention
- Epidemiology
  - Usually benign condition when mild
    - Patients known to have lesions predisposing them to PR (prior TOF or PS repair) should have surveillance imaging to evaluate

Natural History & Prognosis

- Most often mild and clinically insignificant, requiring no treatment
  - Most often seen secondary to pulmonary hypertension and occurring in otherwise normal valve
- More significant degrees of regurgitation usually associated with underlying abnormality
  - Most often represents significant complication of prior repaired congenital heart disease (e.g., post valvuloplasty for PS, post RVOT enlargement as part of repair of TOF)

Treatment

- While mild PR is often well tolerated, PR associated with repaired TOF or PS is often severe and may require valve replacement
  - Valve replacement undertaken when progressive deleterious impact on RV function is demonstrated
    - In asymptomatic patients with severe PR, indications for PV replacement include 2 or more of following: RVEDV > 150 mL/m² or z-score > 4; RV end-systolic volume (RVESV) > 80 mL/m²; RV ejection fraction (RVEF) < 47%; LVEF < 55%; residual RVOT obstruction; residual shunt
    - As patients may not have symptoms until RV failure supervenes, close follow-up of at-risk patients with MR is suggested
  - Valve treatment options consist of anulus repair or prosthetic valve replacement
    - Increasingly, transcatheter valve replacement techniques are being utilized
- In patients with secondary pulmonary valve regurgitation, prognosis is related to underlying etiology (i.e., pulmonary arterial hypertension or chronic left-sided inflow obstruction); treatment is directed to primary disorder

DIAGNOSTIC CHECKLIST

Reporting Tips

- MR is current reference standard for evaluating PR and RV performance (volumes and function)
  - RVEDV and RVESV analysis using MR is essential for timing of valve replacement

SELECTED REFERENCES

1. Stefanescu Schmidt AC et al: Transcatheter pulmonary valve replacement with balloon-expandable valves: utilization and procedural outcomes from the IMPACT registry. JACC Cardiovasc Interv. 17(2):231-44, 2024
2. Almeida-Pinto R et al: Pulmonary valve replacement: a new paradigm with tissue engineering. Curr Probl Cardiol. 48(8):101212, 2023
3. Bokma JP et al: Improved outcomes after pulmonary valve replacement in repaired tetralogy Of Fallot. J Am Coll Cardiol. 81(21):2075-85, 2023
4. Laflamme E et al: Outcome and right ventricle remodelling after valve replacement for pulmonic stenosis. Heart. 108(16):1290-5, 2022
5. Rommel JJ et al: Causes and hemodynamic findings in chronic severe pulmonary regurgitation. Catheter Cardiovasc Interv. 92(3):E197-203, 2018
6. Alvarez-Fuente et al: Timing of pulmonary valve replacement: how much can the right ventricle dilate before it loses its remodeling potential? Pediatric Cardiology. 37(3): 601-5, 2016
7. Rajiah P et al: CT and MRI of pulmonary valvular abnormalities. Clin Radiol. 69(6):630-8, 2014

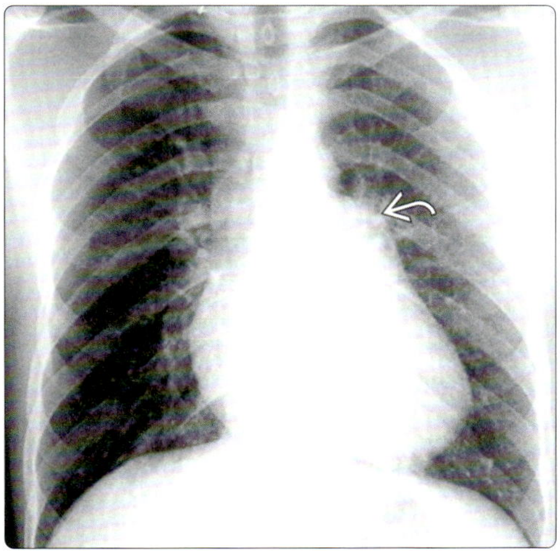

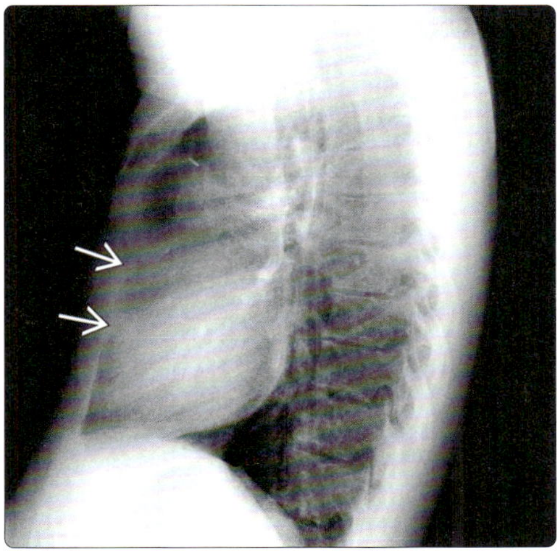

(Left) *Frontal chest radiograph shows a prominent main PA* ➔ *with normal hilar PAs and normal pulmonary blood flow in a patient with severe PR from prior TOF repair. Note that no shunt vascularity is present.* **(Right)** *Lateral chest radiograph shows RV enlargement* ➔ *in the same patient. Note that no left ventricular enlargement is seen and that the hilar PAs are normal in size.*

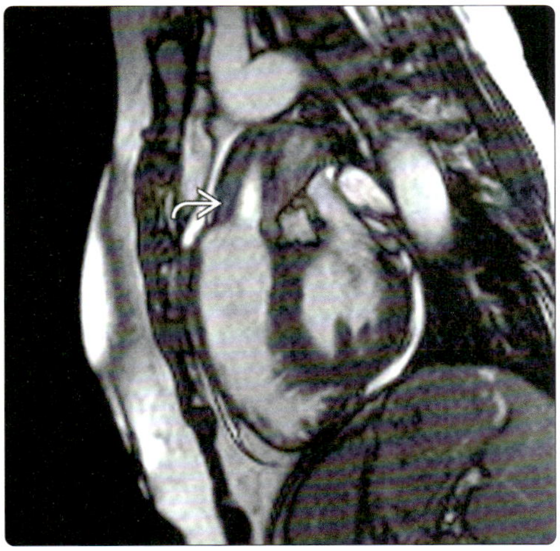

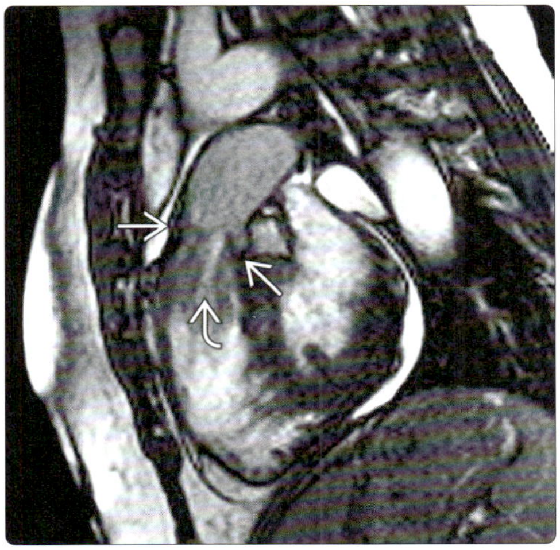

(Left) *RVOT SSFP cine MR through the pulmonic valve and RVOT shows a prominent systolic flow jet* ➔ *in this patient with carcinoid valve disease. Note the positions of the thickened pulmonic valve leaflets.* **(Right)** *RVOT cine MR in diastole through the pulmonic valve shows diastolic flow jet of PR* ➔ *in the same patient. Note the immobility of the abnormally thickened pulmonic valve leaflets* ➔*, which show little change in position when compared to the systolic images.*

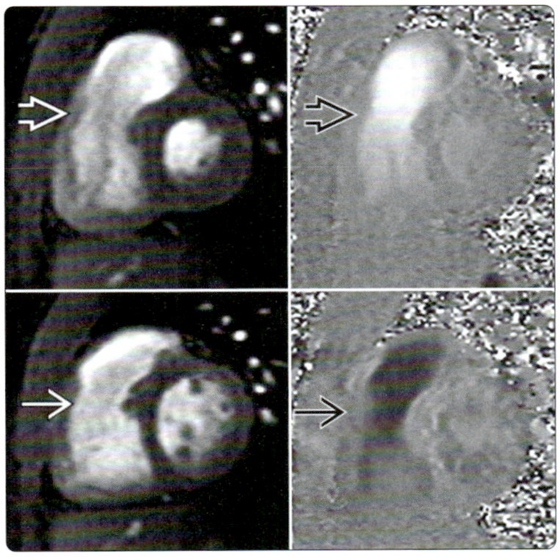

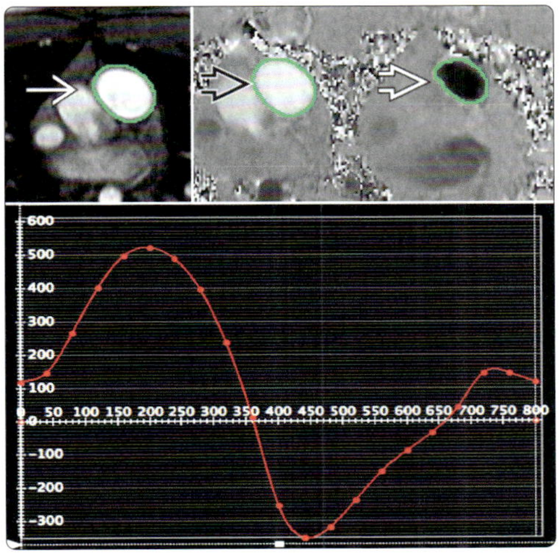

(Left) *Short-axis cine MR (systole* ➔ *and diastole* ➔*) and in-plane matched flow images (systole* ➔ *and diastole* ➔*) show free PR and no discernible valve tissue in this postoperative TOF patient.* **(Right)** *Transverse cine MR* ➔ *and velocity-encoded through-plane flow studies (systole* ➔ *and diastole* ➔*) show severe PR in this patient. Using the flow-velocity data, forward and regurgitant flow can be calculated and rendered graphically and the regurgitant fraction calculated (33%).*

KEY FACTS

IMAGING

- CT: Provides anatomic information of valves, functional quantification and mapping for procedure planning
- MR: Visualization and quantification of valvular function; accurate and reproducible quantification of ventricular volumes and function

TOP DIFFERENTIAL DIAGNOSES

- **Rheumatic heart disease**
  - Most frequent cause of multivalvular disease
  - Most common combination is mitral stenosis with aortic stenosis or aortic regurgitation
  - Classic radiographic findings: Double density of left atrial enlargement, pulmonary venous hypertension, and enlarged pulmonary arteries
- **Degenerative calcification**
  - Frequently occurs in mitral regurgitation and aortic stenosis
  - Most common cause of multivalvular disease in developed countries, which is likely from aging population
  - Primary single-valve lesions often cause secondary dysfunction in upstream valve
- **Infective endocarditis**
  - Extension of infection through mitral-aortic intervalvular fibrosa may cause mitral regurgitation and aortic regurgitation
- **Marfan syndrome**
  - Mitral valve prolapse is most common primary valve abnormality
  - Most patients develop annuloaortic ectasia, which leads to incomplete leaflet coaptation and aortic regurgitation
- **Carcinoid syndrome**
  - Tumor metabolites from liver metastases cause right-sided valve dysfunction

(Left) *Frontal radiograph shows a double-density sign ➔ and left atrial appendage dilation ➔ from marked left atrial enlargement due to mitral stenosis. Note a 2nd convex bulge ➔ from associated right atrial enlargement due to tricuspid regurgitation in rheumatic heart disease.* **(Right)** *Lateral radiograph in the same patient shows posterior displacement of the left lower lobe bronchus ➔ from massive left atrial dilation. Diminished retrosternal clear space is due to right heart enlargement.*

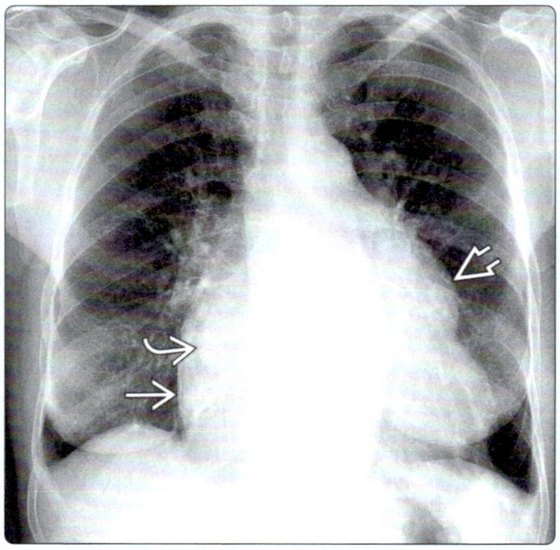

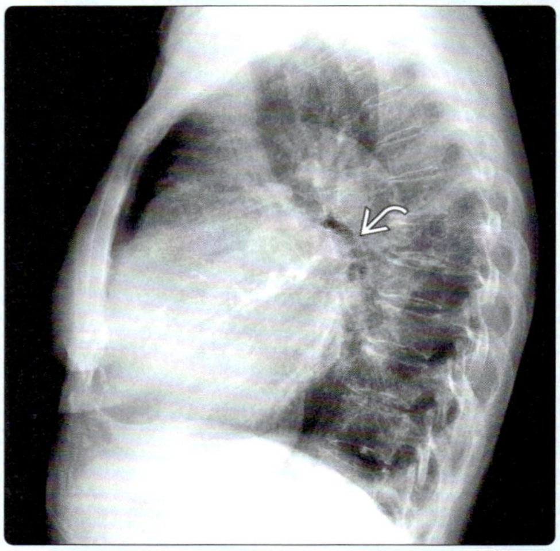

(Left) *Axial CECT in the same patient shows enlargement of the left atrium with left atrial wall calcification ➔ from longstanding mitral stenosis due to rheumatic heart disease. The right border ➔ of the left atrium is responsible for the double-density sign seen on the frontal radiograph.* **(Right)** *Frontal radiograph in the same patient after treatment shows a single-chamber pacemaker lead ➔ in the right ventricle, mechanical mitral valve replacement ➔, and tricuspid annuloplasty ring ➔.*

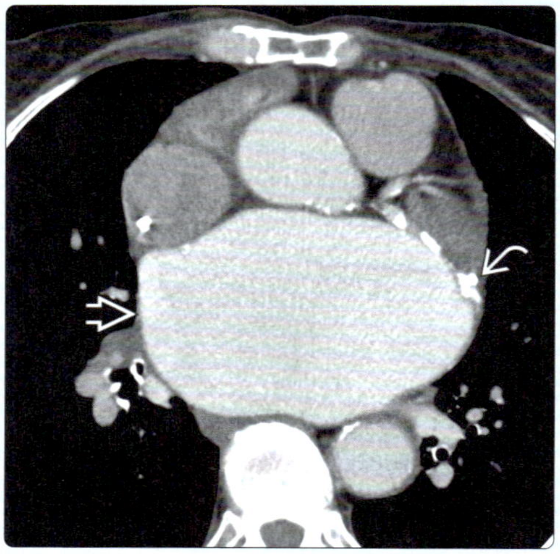

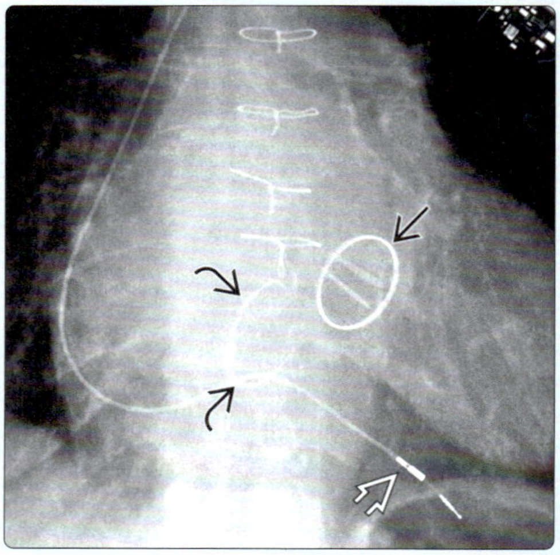

IMAGING

Imaging Recommendations

- MR: Visualization and quantification of valvular function; accurate and reproducible quantification of ventricular volumes and function
  - Aortic stenosis (AS) = peak velocity to calculate peak systolic gradient on phase-contrast images using modified Bernoulli equation (peak gradient = 4 x peak velocity squared)
  - Aortic insufficiency = systolic forward volume - diastolic backward volume on phase-contrast images
  - Mitral regurgitation (MR) = left ventricular stroke volume - aortic phase contrast
    - If aortic insufficiency = left ventricular stroke volume - (aortic insufficiency + aortic forward volume)
  - Pulmonic stenosis = peak velocity to calculate peak systolic gradient on phase-contrast images using modified Bernoulli equation (peak gradient = 4 x peak velocity squared)
  - Pulmonary regurgitation = forward volume - backward volume on phase-contrast images
  - Tricuspid regurgitation (TR) = right ventricular stroke volume - pulmonary phase contrast
  - If pulmonary insufficiency = right ventricular stroke volume - (pulmonary insufficiency + pulmonary forward volume)
- CT: Provides anatomic information of valves; functional quantification when echocardiography is suboptimal or MR contraindicated and is used for intervention planning
- 1st-line imaging tool is echocardiography

DIFFERENTIAL DIAGNOSIS

Rheumatic Heart Disease

- Complication of group A streptococcal pharyngitis
- Most frequent cause of multivalvular disease; incidence declining over past 5 decades in developed countries
- Most common combination is mitral stenosis (MS) with AS or aortic regurgitation (AR)
- Classic radiographic findings include double density of left atrial enlargement, pulmonary venous hypertension (i.e., cephalization), and enlarged pulmonary arteries from pulmonary hypertension
- Calcification of mitral valve leaflets (**not just anulus**) or left atrial wall may be seen in MS

Degenerative Calcification

- Most common cause of multivalvular disease in developed countries (aging population)
- Frequently results in MR and AS
- Primary single-valve lesions often cause secondary dysfunction in upstream valve
  - Pulmonic stenosis can lead to functional TR from elevated right ventricular end-diastolic pressure
  - Mitral and aortic valve disease can lead to functional TR from pulmonary hypertension and right heart failure
  - Aortic valve disease can lead to functional MR from elevated left ventricular end-diastolic pressure

Infective Endocarditis

- Extension of infection through mitral-aortic intervalvular fibrosa may cause MR and AR

Hypertrophic Cardiomyopathy

- Asymmetric septal hypertrophy and systolic anterior motion of mitral valve cause sub-AS and MR

Marfan Syndrome

- Mitral valve prolapse is most common primary valve abnormality, leads to MR
- Most patients (60-80%) develop annuloaortic ectasia (tulip-bulb appearance of ascending aorta with effacement of sinuses of Valsalva extending to sinotubular junction)
- Annuloaortic ectasia leads to incomplete leaflet coaptation and AR
- Patients with Ehlers-Danlos syndrome can have similar valve abnormalities

Carcinoid Syndrome

- Tumor metabolites from liver metastases are secreted directly into hepatic veins, causing fibrous endocardial plaque to deposit on right-sided valves (combined tricuspid and pulmonic valve disease)
- Left-sided valves may be affected in patients with atrial septal defect or patent foramen ovale

Radiation-Induced Valvular Disease

- Most common in patients treated with mantle radiation therapy for Hodgkin lymphoma
- Left-sided ≥ right-sided valves

CLINICAL ISSUES

Demographics

- 20% of patients with native valve disease have multivalvular involvement
- Mean age: 64 years; 84% men

Natural History & Prognosis

- Combined aortic and mitral valve disease
  - Rheumatic valvular disease
    - Left ventricle is small, stiff, and hypertrophied in cases of AS and MS
    - Severe MS is usually accompanied by mild AR
    - Combination of MS and severe AR is uncommon
  - AS and MR can produce severe pulmonary congestion
- Combined tricuspid and left-sided valve disease
  - Functional TR occurs in most patients with significant MR due to elevated pulmonary arterial pressures and right ventricular dysfunction
- Significant triple-valve disease is rare and usually is result of rheumatic heart disease

SELECTED REFERENCES

1. Otto CM et al: 2020 ACC/AHA guideline for the management of patients with valvular heart disease: a report of the American College of Cardiology/American Heart Association Joint Committee on clinical practice guidelines. Circulation. 143(5):e72-227, 2021
2. Unger P et al: Pathophysiology and management of multivalvular disease. Nat Rev Cardiol. 13(7):429-40, 2016

(Left) *Composite image in a patient with rheumatic-induced aortic and mitral stenoses shows marked calcification and thickening of the aortic ➔ and mitral valve ➔ leaflets. The left atrium is dilated, measuring > 4 cm (AP dimension).* **(Right)** *Frontal radiograph shows a single-chamber pacemaker lead in the right ventricle and a double-density sign ➔ of left atrial enlargement. The carinal angle ➔ measures > 90° and is a late indirect sign of left atrial enlargement.*

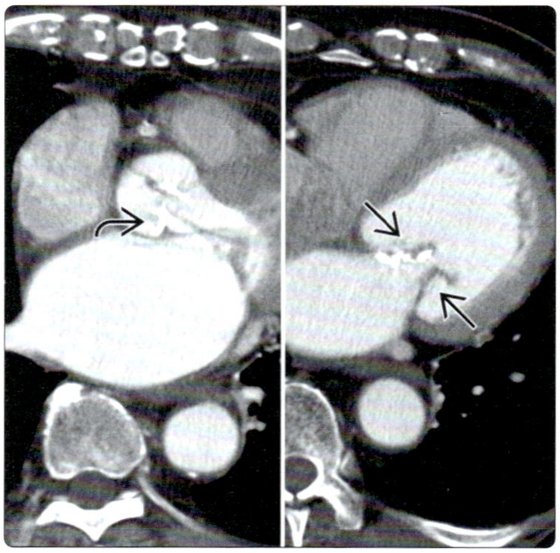

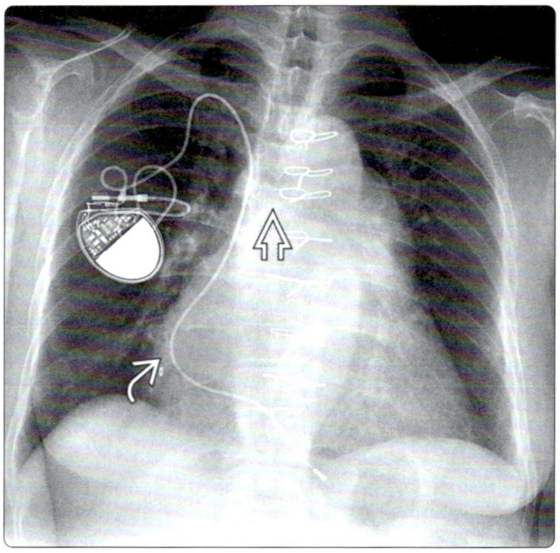

(Left) *Left ventricular outflow tract SSFP MR during ventricular systole shows spin-dephasing jets of aortic stenosis ➔ and mitral regurgitation ➔ in this patient with rheumatic heart disease. Patients with mitral stenosis often have concomitant mitral regurgitation.* **(Right)** *Axial CECT in the same patient after treatment shows mechanical mitral ➔ and aortic ➔ prosthetic valves. The mitral and aortic valves are the most commonly affected valves in rheumatic heart disease.*

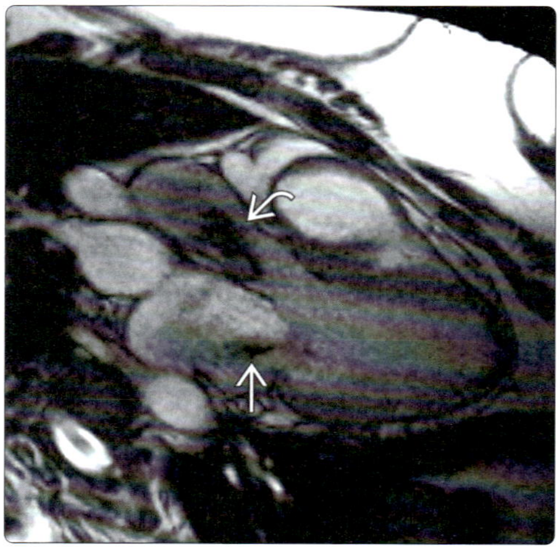

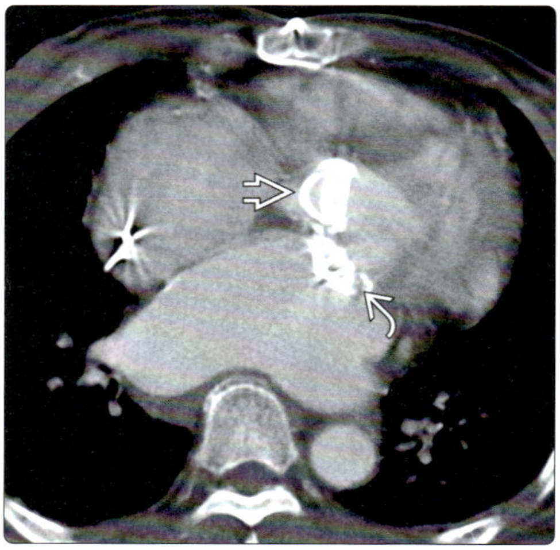

(Left) *Frontal radiograph shows mechanical aortic ➔ and mitral ➔ ball in cage valves and a tricuspid valve annuloplasty ring ➔. Rheumatic heart disease is the most frequent cause of multivalvular disease, although its incidence has been declining.* **(Right)** *Short-axis SSFP MR shows thickening of the mitral valve leaflets ➔ in a patient with rheumatic mitral stenosis. Rheumatic heart disease most commonly affects the mitral and aortic valves, leading to mitral stenosis and aortic stenosis/regurgitation.*

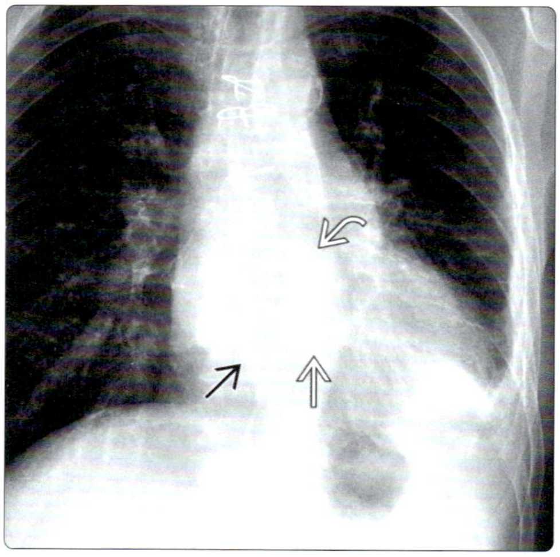

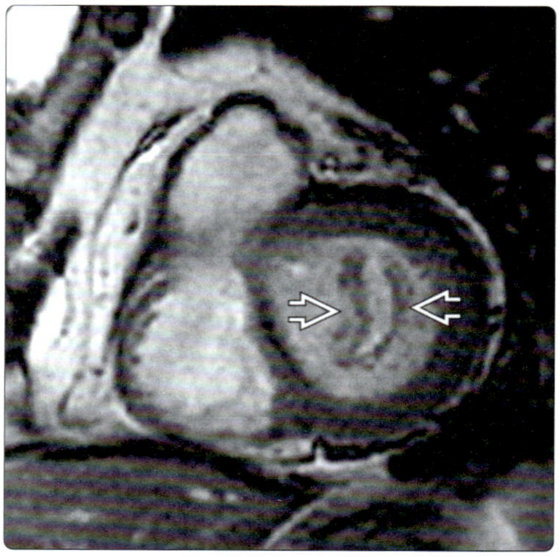

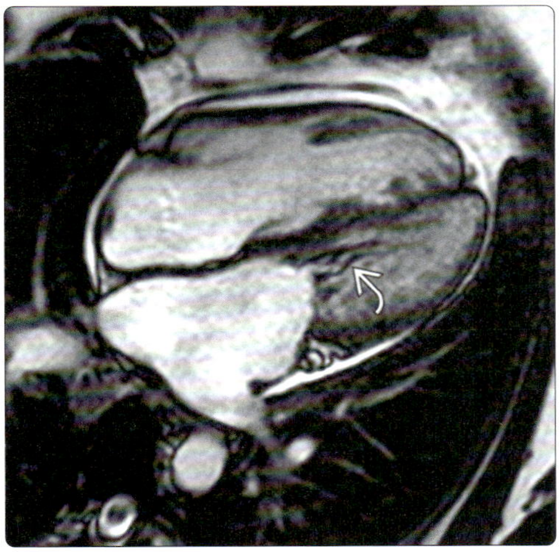

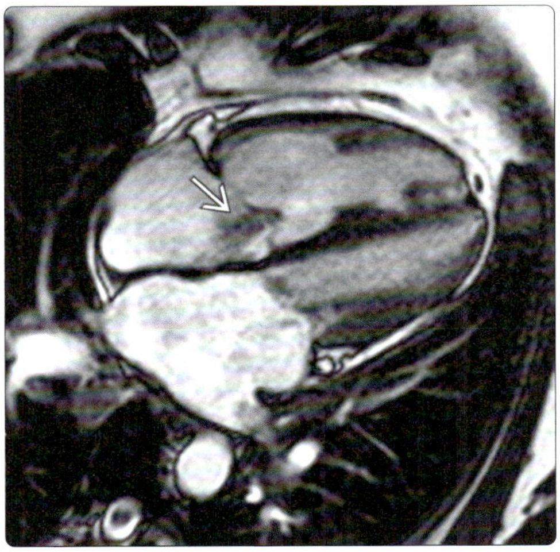

(Left) *Four-chamber SSFP MR in diastole shows restricted mitral valve opening, leaflet thickening, and a spin-dephasing flow jet into the left ventricle, indicating mitral stenosis.* **(Right)** *Four-chamber SSFP MR in the same patient now in systole shows a spin-dephasing regurgitant flow jet into the right atrium, indicating tricuspid insufficiency. Mitral valve disease often leads to functional tricuspid regurgitation from pulmonary hypertension and right heart failure.*

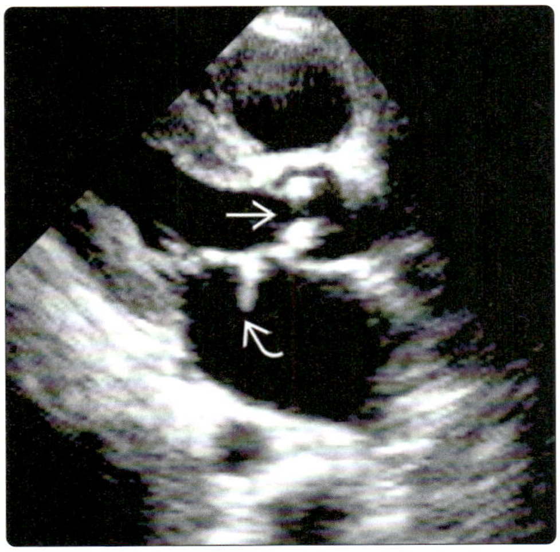

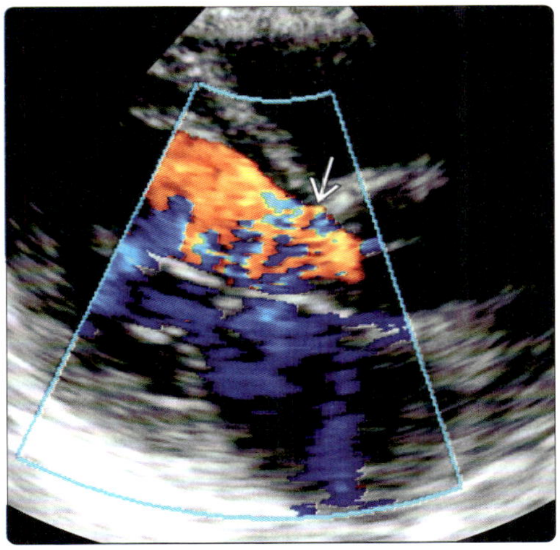

(Left) *Transthoracic echocardiogram parasternal long-axis view in systole shows mitral and aortic valve nodular thickening, consistent with vegetations in a patient with endocarditis.* **(Right)** *Transthoracic echocardiogram parasternal view with color Doppler in diastole in the same patient shows severe aortic regurgitation. Echocardiography is the best imaging tool to evaluate valvular disease.*

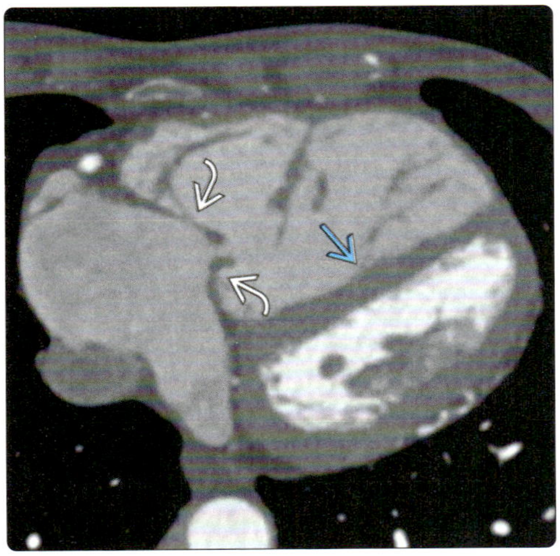

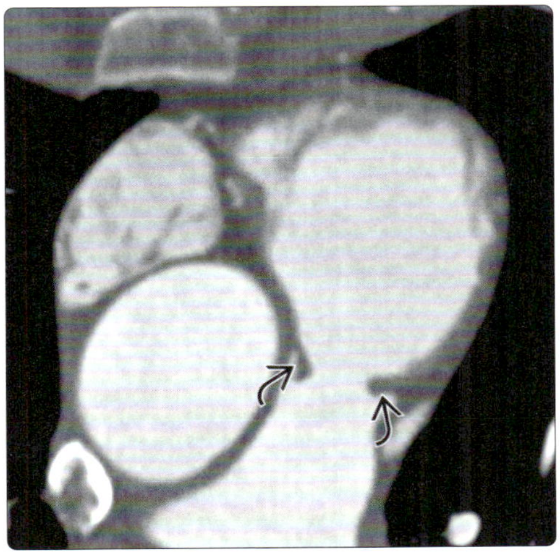

(Left) *Four-chamber CECT during diastole in a patient with carcinoid syndrome shows thickened tricuspid valve leaflets with a limited opening, compatible with tricuspid stenosis. Also note dilation of the right chambers and flattening of the interventricular septum.* **(Right)** *CECT during diastole in a patient with carcinoid syndrome shows thickened and shortened pulmonic valve leaflets, compatible with free pulmonic regurgitation.*

Infective Endocarditis

KEY FACTS

TERMINOLOGY

- Infection of endocardium, prosthetic cardiac valves, or cardiac implantable electronic devices (CIEDs)

IMAGING

- Heart valves are most commonly involved; cardiac chambers less frequently
- Prosthetic valves and CIEDs can be affected
- Transesophageal echocardiography (TEE)/ECG-gated cardiac CT angiogram are best diagnostic tools
- Cardiac CT can show typical lesions; useful for valvular lesion characterization (soft tissue mass vs. calcification), paravalvular involvement, and prosthetic valve infection; less sensitive than TEE for vegetations

CLINICAL ISSUES

- Predisposing factors: Prosthesis, implantable cardioverter-defibrillator, pacemakers, intravenous drug abuse, immunodeficiency
- Septic emboli and hematogenous seeding to remote sites are frequent (often neurologic symptoms)
- Diagnosis is based on clinical and imaging findings according to modified Duke criteria (major and minor)

DIAGNOSTIC CHECKLIST

- Vegetations: Hypodense, irregular, or round-shaped masses of few mm up to > 1 cm; may be mobile
- Perivalvular abscess: Fluid accumulation
- Perivalvular pseudoaneurysm: Contrast agent-filled cavity, typically arising from aortic or mitral anulus plane
- Leaflet perforation
- Fistula: Communication between cardiac chambers &/or aortic root
- Prosthetic valves: Paravalvular leak, dysfunction
- Valvular regurgitation (&/or stenosis) may occur

(Left) *Thickened prosthetic valve leaflets and a linear vegetation arising from 1 of the bioprosthetic leaflets in a patient with a bioprosthetic aortic valve replacement is shown.* **(Right)** *CT confirmed thickened bioprosthetic aortic valve leaflets with subvalvular vegetations corresponding to the transesophageal echocardiography (TEE), consistent with infective endocarditis (IE).*

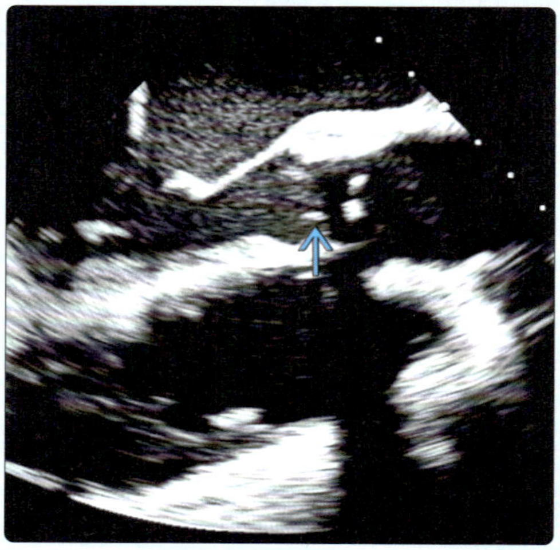

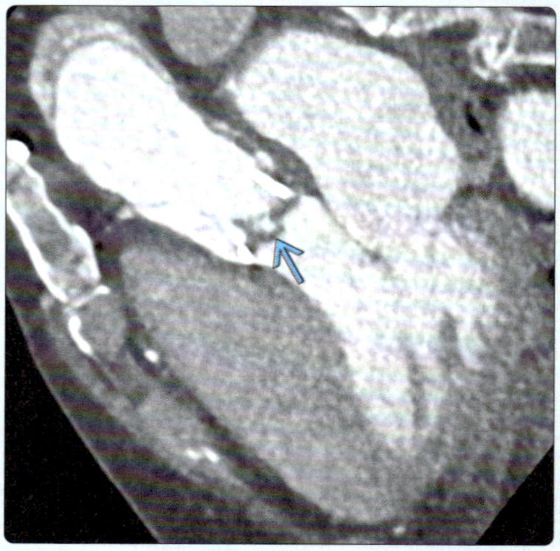

(Left) *Additional CT findings to the TEE included a low-density collection in the paravalvular tissues adjacent to the bioprosthetic valve with extension into the fibrous anulus.* **(Right)** *The infection extended into the mitral annulus and onto the anterior leaflet of the mitral valve where there is a vegetation evident.*

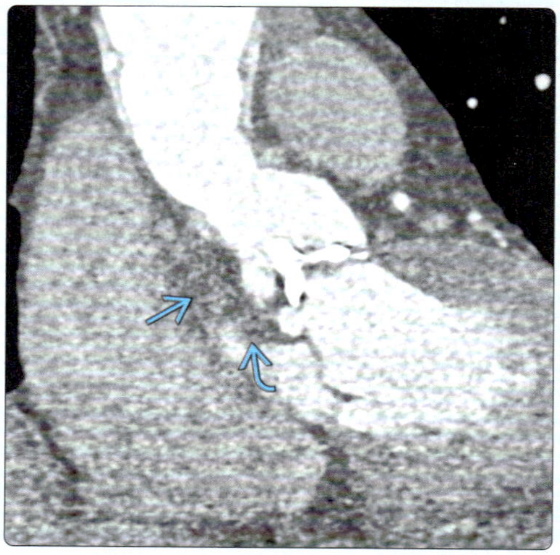

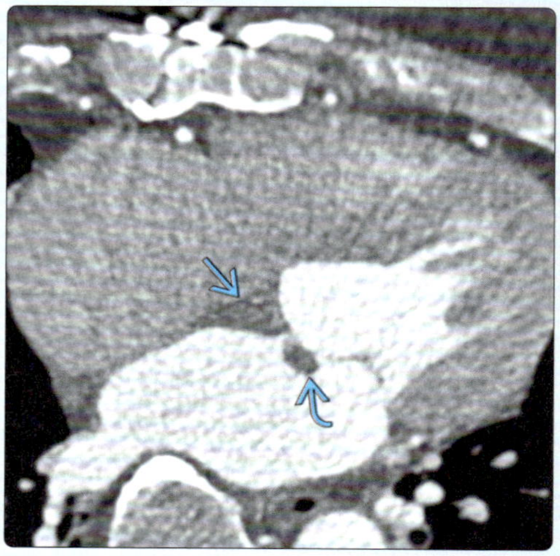

TERMINOLOGY

Abbreviations

- Infective endocarditis (IE)

Definitions

- Infection of endocardium, prosthetic cardiac valves, or cardiac implantable electronic devices (CIEDs)

IMAGING

General Features

- Location
  - Endocardial surfaces of heart
    - Valves are most commonly involved
    - Cardiac chambers are less frequently involved
  - Prosthetic valves, CIEDs
- Specific findings
  - Vegetation: Irregular mass adherent to endocardium/device
    - Can be mobile, can cause regurgitation/stenosis
  - Leaflet perforation: Tiny defect in leaflet
  - Leaflet pseudoaneurysm: Saccular outpouching
  - Perivalvular abscess: Cavity with purulent material without luminal communication
  - Perivalvular pseudoaneurysm: Cavity with luminal communication
  - Perivalvular fistula: Connection between 2 cavities through aberrant tract
  - Prosthetic valve dehiscence: Destruction of prosthetic valve sewing ring: Inadequate sealing, paravalvular leak (PVL)

CT Findings

- Cardiac gated CTA
  - Vegetations
    - Focal, irregular mass(es) or thickening, low to intermediate signal
    - Mobile, prolapses into chambers
    - Usually on lower pressure side
    - Prosthetic valves: Valve leaflet or sewing ring, usually on ventricular side of aortic valve
  - Perivalvular abscess and pseudoaneurysm
    - Erosion through myocardium, annuli, or aortic root
    - Fluid and fat stranding surrounding pseudoaneurysm
    - May fill with contrast and fistulize with surrounding structures
    - May involve coronary arteries
  - As good as TEE for abscess, fistula, valve destruction; less sensitive for vegetations
  - Leaflet perforations
    - Challenging to detect; at edge/tip of leaflet
  - Leaflet pseudoaneurysm
    - Saccular outpouching of leaflet; loss of homogeneous curvature
  - Perivalvular abscess
    - Earliest finding: Increased attenuation of fat around aortic root (1-30 HU)
    - Soft tissue stranding
    - Low-attenuation (20-50 HU) or heterogeneous collection adjacent to valve
    - Rim enhancement is rarely seen: In delayed phase
  - Perivalvular pseudoaneurysm
    - Contrast-filled outpouching (200-400 HU) from valve/chamber
    - Saccular/fusiform, narrow neck, variable size
    - Changes size with cardiac cycle
  - Fistula
    - Associated more with prosthetic valves
    - Aberrant tract connects 2 cavities, beyond valve
    - Aortocavitary: Right sinus → right ventricle (RV); NC sinus → RV; left sinus → left ventricle (LV)
    - Gerbode defect: LV → right atrium (RA)
  - Prosthetic valve dehiscence
    - More common in mechanical valves
    - Malalignment of prosthesis
    - Rocking motion of valve > 15° compared to annular motion
    - Defect between prosthesis and anulus: Connects 2 associated chambers (PVL)
  - Evaluation of coronary arteries before surgery-anatomic relationship to abscess and exclusion of significant coronary stenosis

MR Findings

- Not commonly used for assessment of endocarditis
  - Prosthetic valves produce artifacts
- Can assess flow in pseudoaneurysm and through fistula
- Can quantify valvular regurgitation/stenosis

Echocardiographic Findings

- Echocardiogram
  - 2D transthoracic echocardiography (TTE)
    - 1st-line imaging modality
    - More sensitive than CT for small vegetations and leaflet perforations
  - TEE
    - More sensitive than TTE
    - Detailed anatomy of vegetation; mobility
    - Paravalvular abscess, pseudoaneurysm, fistula

Nuclear Medicine Findings

- PET/CT
  - Abnormal metabolic activity in native or prosthetic valve
  - Prosthetic endocarditis
    - If TEE or CTA are inconclusive
    - Evaluate extracardiac components of CIED (pocket infection)
  - Embolic complications of IE (abscess)

Imaging Recommendations

- Best imaging tool
  - TEE more sensitive for vegetations
  - Cardiac CTA: Superior evaluation of perivalvular structures + coronary artery evaluation prior to surgery
    - Avoids risk of embolization with invasive angiography
  - PET/CT for prosthetic valve IE or CIED
- Protocol advice
  - Cardiac CT
    - Contrast bolus adjusted to valve evaluated
    - Retrospective ECG gating without tube-current modulation: For comprehensive evaluation

- Delayed phase (> 70 seconds): For perivalvular abscess

DIFFERENTIAL DIAGNOSIS

Papillary Fibroelastoma

- No constitutional symptoms
- Native valves; > left side; on high-pressure side
- Highly mobile; attached by stalk to valve

Nonbacterial Thrombotic Endocarditis

- No signs of infection; associated with neoplasms, autoimmune diseases
- Native valves; > left side; on high-pressure side
- < 1 cm; irregular; broad based; valve destruction less common

Thrombus

- Acute onset; subtherapeutic anticoagulation; any time after surgery
- Prosthetic valves; tricuspid > mitral > aortic; on high-pressure side
- Large; irregular; low attenuation

Hypoattenuated Leaflet Thickening

- Subclinical thrombus in bioprosthetic valve leaflets
- Thick leaflets; may have reduced leaflet motion

Pannus

- Subacute or chronic onset, > 1 year after surgery
- Prosthetic valve; mitral > aortic; on low-pressure side
- Disk plane; centripetal growth under valve ring; higher attenuation; calcification may be seen

PATHOLOGY

General Features

- Etiology
  - Bacterial infection (common)
    - *Staphylococcus aureus* and *Streptococcus* (80%) or *Enterococcus faecalis* (10%)
    - HACEK group (*Haemophilus*, *Actinobacillus*, *Cardiobacterium*, *Eikenella*, *Kingella*) may cause large vegetations > 1 cm
  - Fungal infection
    - *Candida*, *Aspergillus* (especially in prosthetic valves or compromised immune system)

Staging, Grading, & Classification

- Modified Duke criteria
  - Major criteria
    - Positive echocardiography &/or ECG-gated cardiac CT angiogram &/or FDG PET/CT
      - Specific valvular lesions or new onset of regurgitation or abnormal metabolic activity
    - Positive blood culture with typical microorganism
  - Minor criteria
    - Fever (> 38 °C)
    - Immunologic phenomena (Osler nodes, positive rheumatoid factor, etc.)
    - Vascular phenomena (major arterial emboli, intercerebral hemorrhage, septic pulmonary embolism, etc.)
    - Predisposing cardiac condition (e.g., valvular disease, pacemaker, prosthesis, etc.) or intravenous drug abuses
- Diagnosis
  - Definite
    - 2 major or 1 major and 3 minor criteria
    - Pathology or bacteriology of specific valvular lesions
  - Possible
    - 1 major and 1 minor or 3 minor criteria
  - Rejected
    - Alternative firm diagnosis

CLINICAL ISSUES

Presentation

- Fever, anorexia, weight loss, and changing heart murmur; signs of heart failure (dyspnea), petechiae
- Septic emboli with associated complaints, e.g., neurologic symptoms (most common)
- Diagnosis based on clinical and imaging findings according to modified Duke criteria (major and minor)

Demographics

- Epidemiology
  - Predisposing factors
    - Degenerative or rheumatic valve disease
    - Prosthetic valves, pacemakers, defibrillators
    - Intravenous drug users
    - Immunodeficiency

Natural History & Prognosis

- 50-75% with prior conditions, including mitral valve prolapse, rheumatic, congenital, degenerative valve disease, or prosthetic valves
- IE of prosthetic valve frequently extends to cause abscesses, fistulas, and valve dehiscence resulting in paravalvular regurgitation
- Septic emboli and hematogenous seeding to remote sites are frequent (mostly neurologic symptoms)
- Severe disease with high mortality up to 40%
  - Mortality increases if perivalvular involvement

Treatment

- Long-term intravenous antibiotic therapy based on microbial profile
- Indications for surgery
  - Congestive heart failure due to valvular dysfunction
  - Antimicrobial therapy failure
  - Unstable prosthesis
  - Perivalvular invasion
  - Fungal or other highly resistant organisms

SELECTED REFERENCES

1. Baddour LM et al: Update on cardiovascular implantable electronic device infections and their prevention, diagnosis, and management: a scientific statement from the American Heart Association: endorsed by the International Society for Cardiovascular Infectious Diseases. Circulation. 149(2):e201-16, 2024
2. Broncano J et al: Multimodality imaging of infective endocarditis. Radiographics. 44(3):e230031, 2024
3. Fowler VG et al: The 2023 Duke-International Society for Cardiovascular Infectious Diseases criteria for infective endocarditis: updating the modified Duke criteria. Clin Infect Dis. 77(4):518-26, 2023

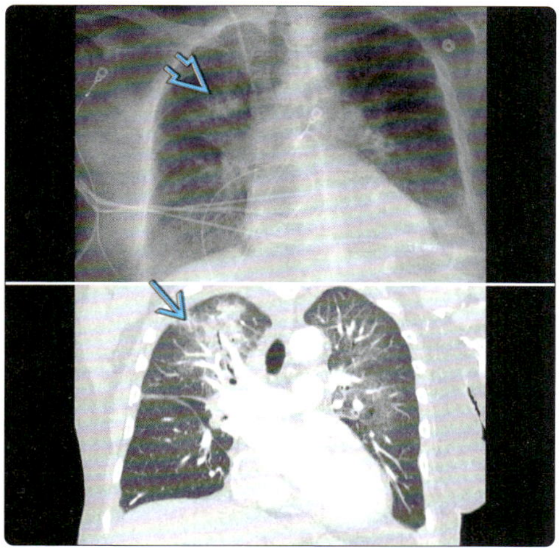

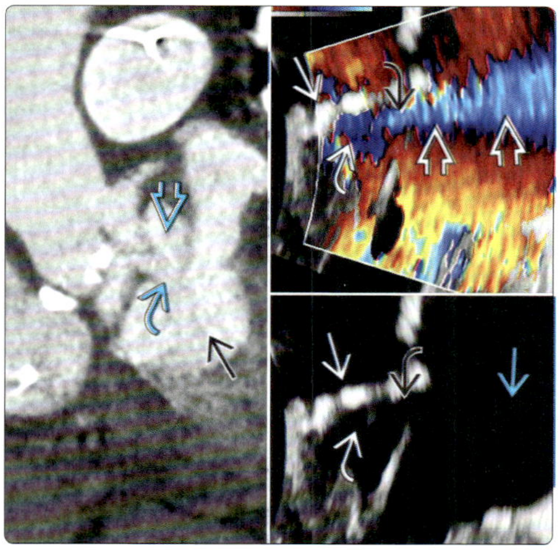

(Left) *AP CXR (top) in a man with sepsis shows asymmetric pulmonary edema, which is most severe in the right upper lobe* ➡. *This finding* ➡ *is mirrored on CTA (bottom).* **(Right)** *CTA (left) shows a subvalvular pseudoaneurysm* ➡ *eroded through the roof of and fistulized* ➡ *with the left atrium (LA)* ➡ *due to IE. Echocardiogram (right) shows a high-velocity jet* ➡ *through the fistula* ➡ *from the LVOT* ➡ *to LA* ➡. *The jet was directed toward the right superior pulmonary vein causing asymmetric edema. Note calcified aortic valve* ➡.

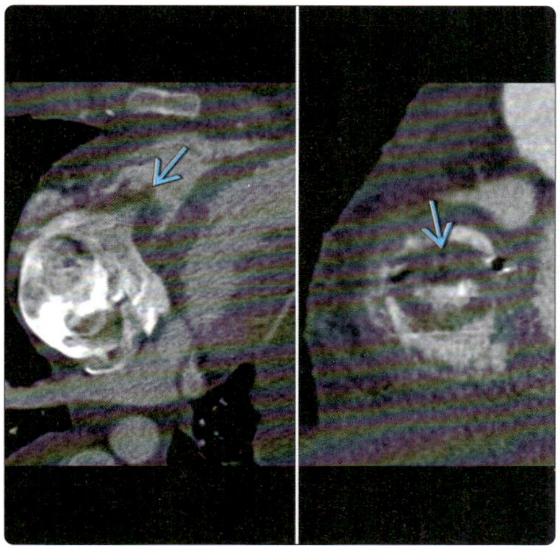

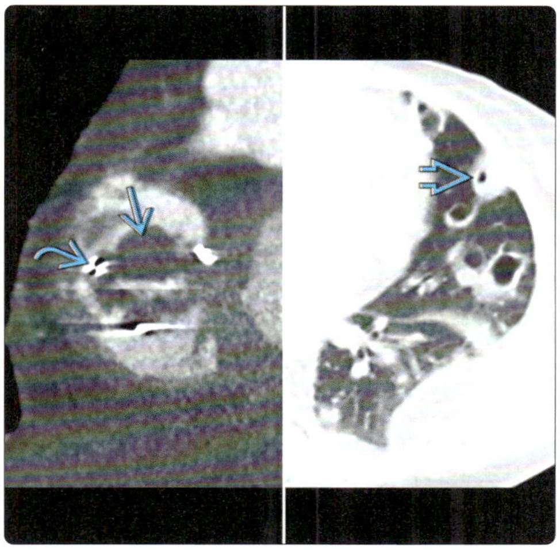

(Left) *Four-chamber (left) and short-axis (right) images from a gated CTA in a 28-year-old IV drug user shows confluent soft tissue along the tricuspid valve (TV) leaflets* ➡. *The right atrium is enlarged due to severe tricuspid regurgitation seen on echocardiogram. Patient underwent TV replacement.* **(Right)** *The patient returns to the ED 7 months later with repeat TV endocarditis (left)* ➡ *of the bioprosthetic valve* ➡. *Numerous bilateral septic emboli* ➡ *are present (right).*

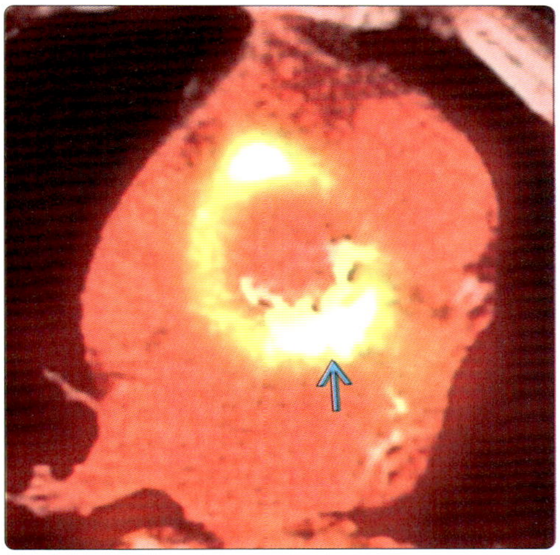

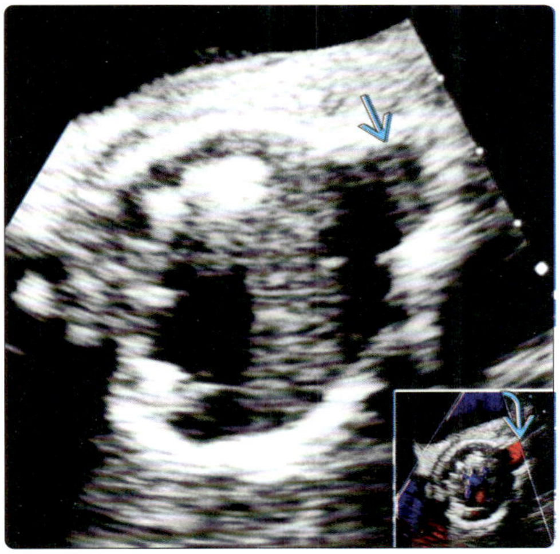

(Left) *A patient with prior transarterial aortic valve implantation (TAVI) is shown. FDG PET/CT demonstrates intense uptake along the TAVI* ➡ *wall, consistent with prosthetic valve endocarditis.* **(Right)** *Echocardiogram in the same patient shows an out pouching into the paravalvular aortic anulus* ➡ *external to TAVI with internal flow (see color Doppler inlay* ➡*).*

KEY FACTS

TERMINOLOGY

- Condition characterized by cardiac valve damage secondary to previous rheumatic fever
  - Rheumatic fever is complication of group A β-hemolytic streptococcal pharyngitis (strep throat) in children and adolescents
  - Rheumatic valve disease may first become apparent years or decades after initial infection
- May include valvular stenosis, regurgitation, left ventricular and left atrial enlargement, pericarditis, and heart failure
- Most commonly affects mitral valve (MV) followed by aortic and tricuspid valve

IMAGING

- Dilated left atrial appendage and left atrium
  - Right-sided double-density sign on frontal radiograph due to appearance of enlarged left atrium
- Calcification of anterior and posterior leaflets of MV (**not** mitral annular calcification)
- Thickening and incomplete opening of MV leaflets
- Stress echocardiography is utilized if there is discordance between findings at rest and clinical findings with exercise
- Phase-contrast MR technique is used to quantify peak velocity of stenotic jet and amount of mitral regurgitation

TOP DIFFERENTIAL DIAGNOSES

- Other reasons for left atrial inflow obstruction
- Secondary mitral regurgitation
- Carcinoid with septal defect, congenital disease
- Medications
- Mucopolysaccharidoses, autoimmune disease

PATHOLOGY

- Immune-mediated reaction to *Streptococcus* bacterium
- MV may demonstrate fish mouth or button hole configuration

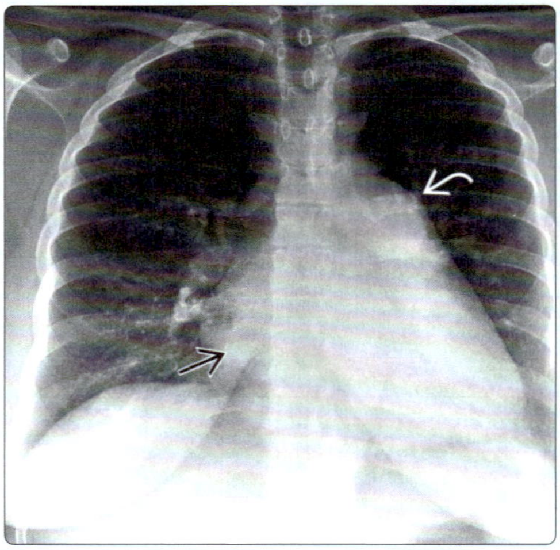

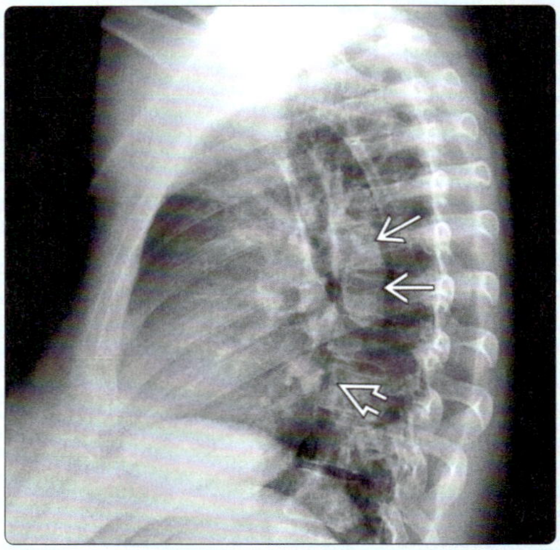

(Left) *PA radiograph shows right retrocardiac double density →, indicating left atrial enlargement, and convex pulmonary trunk segment → due to pulmonary hypertension (secondary to chronic pulmonary venous hypertension).* **(Right)** *Lateral radiograph demonstrates an enlarged left main pulmonary artery → as it arches over the posteriorly displaced left main stem bronchus and enlarged left atrium →. The constellation of these findings is characteristic for rheumatic mitral valve disease.*

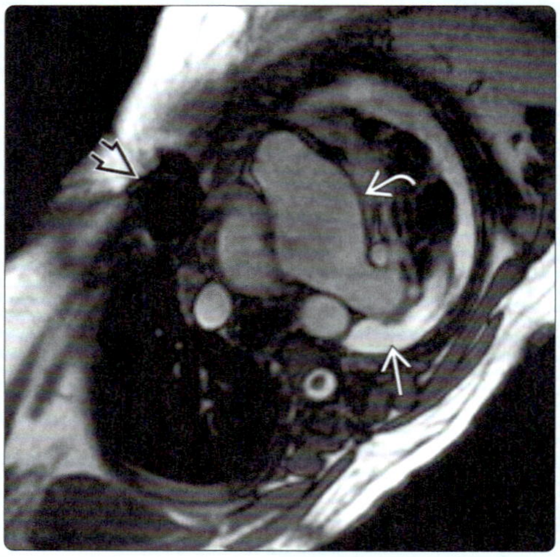

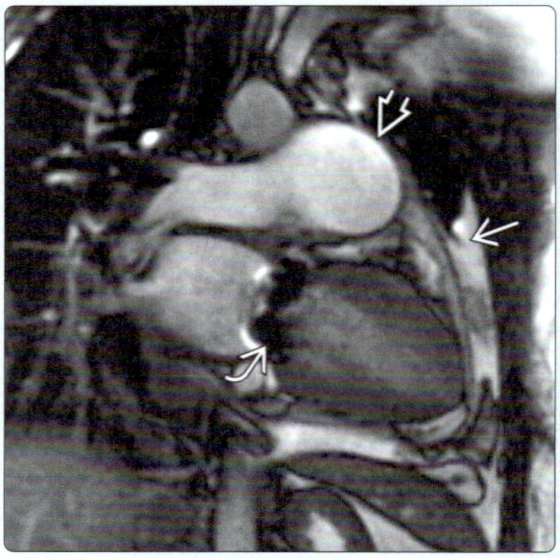

(Left) *Oblique SSFP MR at the level of the pulmonary trunk → in a patient with rheumatic mitral valve stenosis demonstrates markedly enlarged central pulmonary arteries due to longstanding pulmonary hypertension. Note the artifact from sternotomy wires → and left pleural effusion →.* **(Right)** *Long-axis SSFP MR in the same patient demonstrates an artifact from prosthetic mitral valve replacement →, mild left atrial enlargement, and marked pulmonary arterial enlargement →. Note the pleural effusion →.*

TERMINOLOGY

Definitions

- Condition characterized by cardiac valve damage secondary to previous rheumatic fever
  - Rheumatic fever is complication of group A β-hemolytic streptococcal pharyngitis (strep throat) in children and adolescents
  - Rheumatic valve disease may first become apparent years or decades after initial infection
- May include valvular stenosis, regurgitation, left ventricular and left atrial enlargement, pericarditis, and heart failure
- Most commonly affects mitral valve (MV), followed by aortic and tricuspid valve
  - Mitral regurgitation (MR) > mitral stenosis (MS) > aortic regurgitation (AR) > aortic stenosis

IMAGING

Radiographic Findings

- Dilated left atrial appendage and left atrium
  - Right-sided double-density sign on frontal radiograph due to appearance of enlarged left atrium
  - Posterior displacement and slight elevation of left mainstem bronchus
- Calcification of left atrial wall
- Normal:slightly enlarged cardiothoracic ratio
- Calcification of MV leaflets
- Interstitial pulmonary edema &/or pulmonary venous redistribution

CT Findings

- NECT
  - Enlarged left atrium
  - Calcification of anterior and posterior leaflets of MV (**not** mitral annular calcification)
  - May show calcified left atrial wall
    - Rarely, extensive calcifications may result in porcelain heart appearance
- Cardiac gated CTA
  - Thickening and incomplete opening of MV leaflets in diastole
    - Essential to perform multiphase imaging and reconstruction
    - Allows for MV planimetry, although not commonly employed clinically
  - Allows assessment of additional valvular involvement
    - Aortic valve > tricuspid valve
  - May demonstrate left atrial appendage thrombus
  - Helpful for preoperative assessment

MR Findings

- MR cine
  - Cine SSFP images demonstrate valvular regurgitation &/or stenosis
    - MV: Dephasing (dark) retrograde jet in systole indicates insufficiency; antegrade jet in diastole indicates stenosis
    - Aortic valve: Retrograde jet in diastole indicates insufficiency; antegrade jet in systole indicates stenosis
  - May demonstrate diastolic "doming" of MV, indicating stenosis
  - Quantification of valvular abnormality
    - Stenosis: Using planimetry technique, anatomic valve area is measured by planimetry in diastole for MS
      - Requires thin, contiguous slices
      - MV area is overestimated in MR by 8% compared to transthoracic echocardiogram (TTE) but comparable to transesophageal echocardiogram (TEE)
    - Regurgitation: Measurement of effective regurgitant orifice area
      - Regurgitant jet area can be measured but variable and dependent on pulse sequence parameters
  - Evaluates entire MV apparatus
    - May reveal thickening or retraction of chordae tendineae
  - Secondary changes on heart can be evaluated and quantified; ventricular volumes and function
  - Enlarged left atrium ± left atrial appendage thrombus
    - Accuracy of MR for detection of left atrial appendage thrombus is limited
  - Pericardial thickening and effusion may be seen
- Phase-contrast technique to quantify peak velocity of stenotic jet and amount of MR
  - Stenosis can be quantified on either through-plane images perpendicular to MV jet or in-plane images parallel to jet
    - Peak velocity and pressure gradient quantified
  - Regurgitation is usually quantified indirectly as (stroke volume of left ventricle-forward flow in aorta)/stroke volume of left ventricle x 100%
    - Direct measurement of regurgitation is challenging due to valve excursion in systole; requires advanced software for valve tracking
- LGE
  - Abnormal LGE may be seen in left atrial wall
  - LGE is useful for diagnosis of thrombus; thrombus has dark signal at long inversion times of 600 ms
  - Pericardial enhancement may be seen due to inflammation
  - Myocarditis may be seen in acute phase, progressing to dilated cardiomyopathy
  - Presence of myocardial fibrosis detected by LGE is associated with poorer prognosis after MV surgery

Echocardiographic Findings

- Modality of choice for initial evaluation and for assessment of disease progression
- Doppler echocardiography is used to calculate pressure half-time valve area and transvalvular gradient
- Color Doppler can show both MS and MR
- 3D echocardiography is emerging modality that allows for accurate planimetry of valve area
- Stress echocardiography is utilized if there is discordance between findings at rest and clinical findings with exercise
- **2023 World Heart Federation** guideline introduced new echocardiography findings for diagnosis of rheumatic heart disease (RHD)
  - Screening: To detect suspected cases in patients ≤ 20 years of age; if positive, confirmatory echo is needed

- Confirmatory: To confirm diagnosis by experts
  - Exclude other common causes of mild valvular disease [(MVP) bicuspid aortic valve] before diagnosing RHD
- RHD is classified into 4 stages based on risk of progression (A: Minimal RHD; B: Mild RHD; C-D: Advanced RHD); borderline, definite, or latent RHD terms are no longer recommended

DIFFERENTIAL DIAGNOSIS

Other Reasons for Left Atrial Inflow Obstruction

- Decreased left ventricular compliance
  - Restrictive cardiomyopathy
  - Endomyocardial fibrosis
  - Dilated cardiomyopathy
- Chronic aortic stenosis
- Myxoma or other masses

Secondary Mitral Regurgitation

- Myocardial infarction

Carcinoid

- Presence of patent foramen ovale may result in predominantly left-sided valve involvement

PATHOLOGY

General Features

- Etiology
  - Pathogenesis is believed to be immune-mediated reaction to *Streptococcus* bacterium
    - 0.3 % of children with group A β-hemolytic streptococcus develop acute rheumatic fever
      - Pancarditis with valvular insufficiency, heart failure, and sudden death may be present
- End result of what is believed to be autoimmune reaction to group A *Streptococcus* leading to fibrinoid degeneration, which results in verrucous appearance of lesions on valve

Gross Pathologic & Surgical Features

- MV may demonstrate fish mouth or button hole configuration
- Pericardium and epicardium are thickened and may demonstrate fibrinous exudates
  - Pericardial adhesions may be present; however, unlike in other settings, in this setting, adhesions do not result in pericardial constriction

Microscopic Features

- Presence of Aschoff nodules that are characterized by monocyte-/macrophage-appearing cells and loss of normal adjacent myocardial muscle with fibrous tissue replacement

CLINICAL ISSUES

Presentation

- Other signs/symptoms
  - Systemic venous hypertension due to chronic severe MS and elevated pulmonary vascular resistance and right heart failure
    - Hepatomegaly
    - Edema
    - Ascites
  - Disease may worsen in pregnant patients or may initially present during pregnancy because of increased cardiac output and heart rate
  - Typical murmur of MS is diastolic rumble at apex
  - Atrial fibrillation
- Clinical profile
  - Dyspnea, orthopnea, paroxysmal nocturnal dyspnea
  - Fatigue due to low cardiac output
  - Chest pain due to right ventricular ischemia/failure in severe pulmonary hypertension
  - Syncope
  - Hemoptysis
  - Ortner syndrome (hoarseness due to left atrium compressing left recurrent laryngeal nerve)

Treatment

- Can prevent its development by giving antibiotics when strep throat is detected
- Control and treat elevated pulmonary venous pressure and heart failure
- Asymptomatic patients with
  - Severe MS should undergo close clinical follow-up and yearly echocardiogram
  - Moderate MS should undergo echocardiogram every 1-2 years
  - Mild MS should undergo echocardiogram every 3-5 years
- Symptomatic patients with moderate to severe MS &/or pulmonary hypertension undergo intervention
  - MV replacement
  - Percutaneous mitral balloon valvuloplasty may be used in acute settings or prophylactic treatment for women of childbearing age
- MV annuloplasty has been proposed in patients with MR
  - Does not reduce mortality

DIAGNOSTIC CHECKLIST

Image Interpretation Pearls

- Convex left atrial appendage segment, right double density, and pulmonary venous redistribution are classic findings of rheumatic MV disease in radiograph
  - Convex pulmonary artery segment and large central pulmonary arteries may develop due to back pressure in chronic rheumatic MV disease

SELECTED REFERENCES

1. Rwebembera J et al: 2023 World Heart Federation guidelines for the echocardiographic diagnosis of rheumatic heart disease. Nat Rev Cardiol. 21(4):250-63, 2024
2. Williamson J et al: Echocardiographic screening for rheumatic heart disease: a brief history and implications for the future. Heart Lung Circ. 33(7):943-50, 2024
3. Seitler S et al: Cardiac imaging in rheumatic heart disease and future developments. Eur Heart J Open. 3(2):oeac060, 2023
4. Writing Committee Members et al: 2020 ACC/AHA guideline for the management of patients with valvular heart disease: a report of the American College of Cardiology/American Heart Association Joint Committee on Clinical Practice Guidelines. J Thorac Cardiovasc Surg. 162(2):e183-353, 2021
5. Mutnuru PC et al: Cardiac MR imaging in the evaluation of rheumatic valvular heart diseases. J Clin Diagn Res. 10(3):TC06-9, 2016

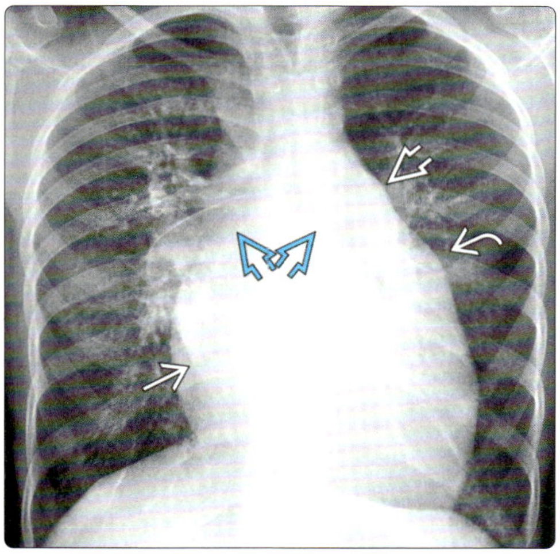

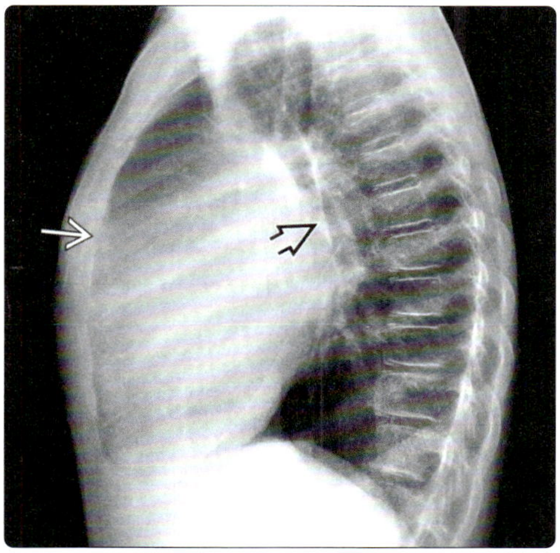

(Left) *PA radiograph shows cardiomegaly with retrocardiac double density ➡, carinal splaying ⇨, and convex left atrial appendage segment ➡ due to left atrial enlargement from rheumatic heart disease. Note the convex pulmonary artery segment ➡ due to secondary pulmonary hypertension.* **(Right)** *Lateral radiograph shows retrosternal clear space filling ➡, indicating right heart enlargement secondary to pulmonary hypertension. Posterior displacement of the left mainstem bronchus ⇨ indicates enlarged left atrial.*

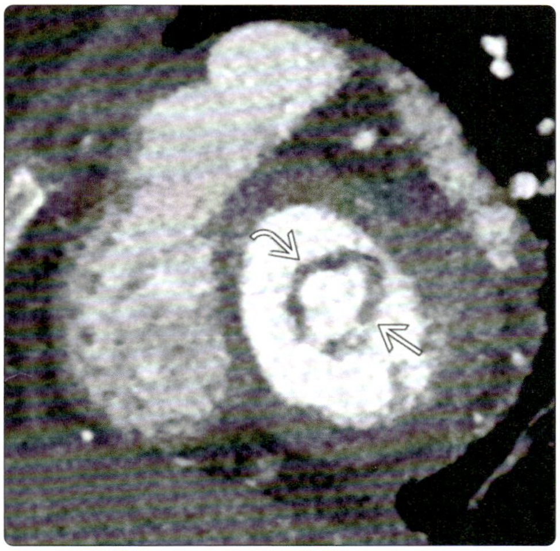

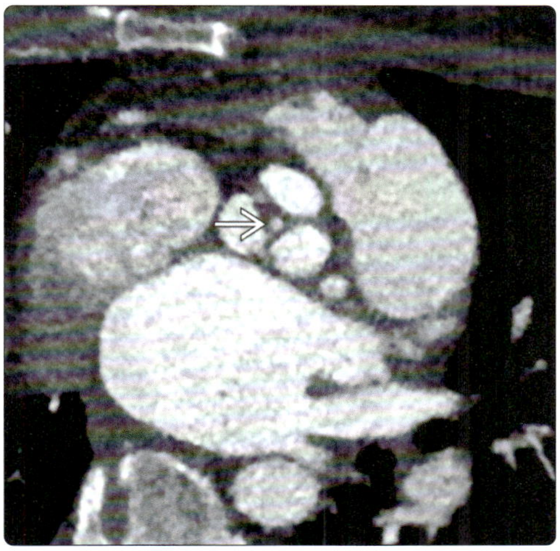

(Left) *Short-axis cardiac CT reconstruction in the mitral valve plane shows thickened anterior ➡ and posterior ➡ mitral leaflets with an incomplete diastolic opening, resulting in a fish mouth appearance in a patient with untreated rheumatic heart disease.* **(Right)** *Short-axis cardiac CT of the aortic valve in the same patient shows thickened cusps and incomplete diastolic closure with central malcoaptation, resulting in a moderate-sized regurgitant orifice ➡.*

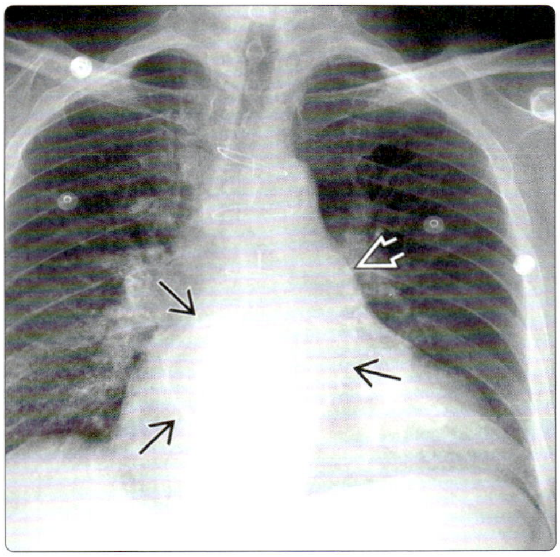

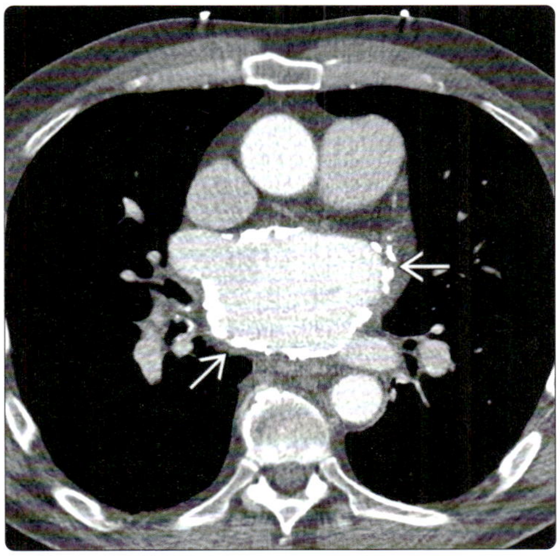

(Left) *PA radiograph shows cardiomegaly with diffuse calcification ⇨ of the left atrial wall. A mechanical mitral valve prosthesis and sternotomy wires are present. Note the convex pulmonary artery segment ➡ and enlarged central pulmonary arteries, indicating pulmonary hypertension secondary to longstanding pulmonary venous hypertension.* **(Right)** *Axial cardiac CT shows left atrial enlargement and confirms diffuse wall calcification ➡.*

Radiation Valvular Disease

KEY FACTS

TERMINOLOGY

- Cardiac valvular damage secondary to previous radiation, characterized by fibrosis and calcification
- Usually secondary to mediastinal irradiation
- Apparent 10-20 years after radiation

IMAGING

- Echocardiography is 1st-line imaging test
- MR is used when echocardiography is suboptimal
  - Thick aortic leaflet, mitral leaflet, aortomitral curtain
  - Stenosis: Restricted opening; forward dephasing jet
  - Regurgitation: Incomplete leaflet coaptation; retrograde jet
  - Planimetry: Valve opening area for stenosis; regurgitant orifice for regurgitation
- CTA is used when percutaneous procedure is considered
  - Thick and calcified aortic and mitral valve leaflets and aortomitral curtain

TOP DIFFERENTIAL DIAGNOSES

- Rheumatic valvular disease
- Chronic uremia/hemodialysis
- Drug-induced valvulopathies

PATHOLOGY

- Valve involvement is early indicator of late heart damage
- Valves are commonly involved by radiation (up to 81% of autopsy in dose > 35 Gy)

CLINICAL ISSUES

- Conventional reparative techniques are limited
- Valve replacement is preferable with aortomitral reconstruction
- Symptoms 1-2 decades after radiation exposure

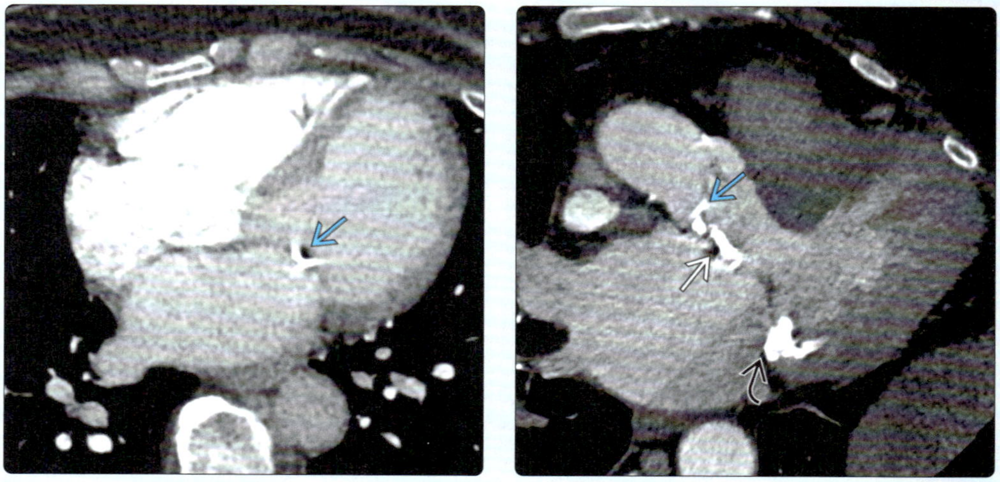

(Left) *Axial contrast-enhanced CT in a patient with a history of mediastinal radiation shows a thickened and calcified anterior mitral leaflet →, consistent with mitral stenosis. Restricted diastolic opening was also seen (not shown here).* **(Right)** *Three-chamber reconstructed CTA in a patient with a history of mediastinal radiation shows calcification in the aortic valve leaflet →, which is extending along the aortomitral curtain ➡ into the anterior mitral leaflet. There is also posterior mitral annular calcification ↷.*

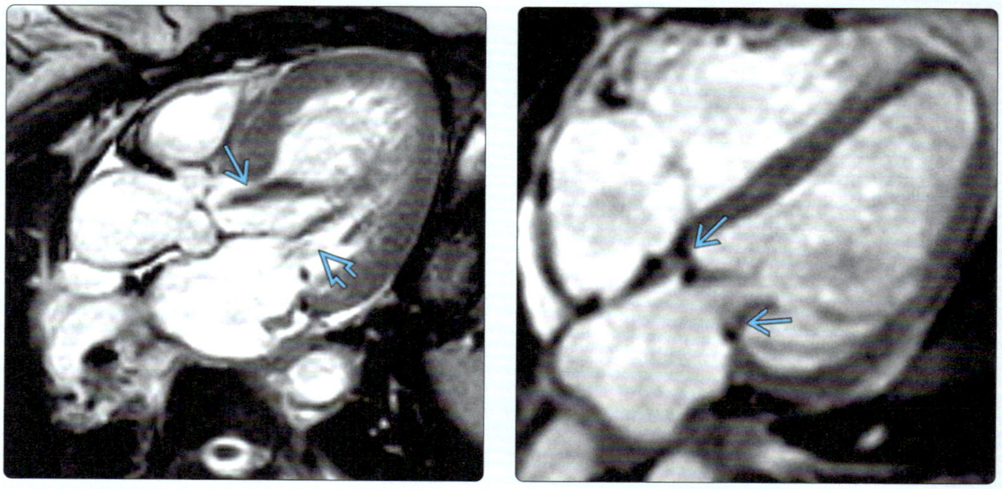

(Left) *Three-chamber cine SSFP MR in diastole in a patient with radiation valve disease shows multivalvular involvement. There is a jet of aortic regurgitation → and restricted opening of the mitral valve ⇒, indicative of mitral stenosis.* **(Right)** *Four-chamber cine SSFP MR shows thick mitral leaflets →, consistent with mitral stenosis in a patient who had radiation therapy for lymphoma. Left-sided heart valves are more frequently affected due to higher pressures.*

TERMINOLOGY

Definitions

- Cardiac valvular damage secondary to previous radiation, characterized by fibrosis and calcification
  - Usually secondary to mediastinal irradiation
  - Manifests 10-20 years after radiation
- Regurgitation followed by stenosis
- Affects aortic/mitral valves more due to higher pressures

IMAGING

General Features

- Best diagnostic clue
  - Thick, calcified aortic/mitral valve leaflets & aortomitral curtain

CT Findings

- Cardiac gated CTA
  - Thick and calcified valve leaflets and aortomitral curtain
  - Dynamic evaluation with retrospective ECG gating
    - Stenosis-restricted opening
    - Regurgitation: Incomplete coaptation
  - Quantification
    - Planimetry: Valve opening area for stenosis; regurgitant orifice for regurgitation
    - Ventricular dilation, hypertrophy, systolic dysfunction
  - Associated findings
    - Coronary artery, pericardial, vascular disease
    - Extracardiac: Lung fibrosis, focal vertebral changes

MR Findings

- Cine SSFP
  - Thick aortic and mitral valves and fibrosa
  - Stenosis: Restricted opening; forward dephasing jet
  - Regurgitation: Incomplete leaflet coaptation; retrograde jet
  - Quantification
    - Planimetry for valves
    - Ventricular dilation, hypertrophy, and dysfunction
- Phase contrast: Quantification of stenosis, regurgitation

Imaging Recommendations

- Best imaging tool
  - Echocardiography is 1st-line imaging test
  - MR is used when echocardiography is suboptimal
  - CTA is used when percutaneous procedures are considered

DIFFERENTIAL DIAGNOSIS

Rheumatic Valvular Disease

- Mitral (regurgitation > stenosis) > aortic (regurgitation > stenosis)
- Commissural fusion and mitral leaflet tip involvement is present, unlike radiation

Chronic Renal Disease

- Premature valve disease due to secondary hyperparathyroidism, hypertension, hypercholesterolemia
- Structural deterioration of aortic and mitral valves with fibrosis, calcification, valve dysfunction

Drug-Induced Valvulopathies

- Ergots, methysergide, fenfluramine, phentermine
- Mitral and aortic valve thickening; mitral leaflet tethering

PATHOLOGY

General Features

- Risk factors for radiation cardiotoxicity
  - High radiation dose (> 30 Gy) or dose fraction (> 2 Gy/day)
  - Tumor close to heart; large field size
  - Old unguided imaging techniques; cobalt source
  - Young age at exposure; long duration after exposure
  - Associated chemotherapy and cardiovascular risk factors
- Valves are commonly involved by radiation
  - Up to 81% of autopsies in dose > 35 Gy
  - Valve involvement is early indicator of late heart damage
- Associated abnormalities
  - Vascular: Coronary artery disease; microvascular dysfunction; myocardial infarction; porcelain aorta; arteritis
  - Myocardial: Cardiomyopathy; fibrosis; diastolic dysfunction; systolic dysfunction
  - Pericardial: Acute pericarditis; chronic pericarditis; effusion; tamponade; constriction; effusive-constriction
  - Conduction: Complete heart block; sick sinus syndrome; prolonged QT; sudden cardiac death

Staging, Grading, & Classification

- Early finding: Valve retraction results in regurgitation
- Late finding: Valve thickening, calcification, stenosis

Gross Pathologic & Surgical Features

- Damage to surrounding myocardial endothelium
- Cusp/leaflet fibrosis, retraction, calcification of valve
  - Involvement of adjacent structures: Valve anulus; subvalvular apparatus; aortomitral curtain

CLINICAL ISSUES

Presentation

- Most common signs/symptoms
  - Majority of patients (71%) have no symptoms
  - Minority have moderate or severe dysfunction
  - Symptoms 1-2 decades after radiation exposure

Natural History & Prognosis

- Asymptomatic disease: Mean of 11.5 years after irradiation
- Symptomatic: Mean of 16.5 years after irradiation

Treatment

- Valve replacement is preferable
- TAVR in severe disease with comorbidities

SELECTED REFERENCES

1. Belzile-Dugas E et al: Radiation-induced aortic stenosis: an update on treatment modalities. JACC Adv. 2(1):100163, 2023
2. Lee C et al: Valvular Heart disease associated with radiation therapy: a contemporary review. Struct Heart. 7(2):100104, 2023
3. Desai MY et al: Radiation-associated cardiac disease: a practical approach to diagnosis and management. JACC Cardiovasc Imaging. 11(8):1132-49, 2018

Valvular Prosthesis

KEY FACTS

IMAGING

- Ball-in-cage valves
  - **Hufnagel valve** (1952): 1st caged ball valve, implanted in descending aorta
  - **Starr-Edwards** (1965): Initial models used stellite alloy cage; later bare metal cage and Silastic rubber ball
- Tilting disc valves
  - **Björk-Shiley** flat (1969) and convexoconcave (1975) disc valves
  - **Medtronic-Hall** (previously Hall-Kaster) tilting disc valve (1977)
- Bileaflet valves
  - **St. Jude Medical** (1977): 1st all-carbon (Pyrolite) valve
  - **On-X** (1996): Pure carbon structure, lower INR target
- Tissue valves (bioprosthesis)
  - **Carpentier-Edwards** porcine xenograft: Pressure-fixed, glutaraldehyde-preserved, and wire-mounted porcine or pericardial valve
  - **Mitroflow** bovine pericardial valve: Single piece of glutaraldehyde-preserved bovine pericardium sewn onto nonradiopaque polymer stent
- Catheter-delivered valves
  - May be delivered via transfemoral or transapical approach
  - Cardiac and vascular CT used for procedure planning (femoral access feasibility, valve sizing)
  - Initially, transcatheter approach was used for aortic valves; today, it can also be employed for mitral, tricuspid, and pulmonary valve replacements
- Sutureless valves
  - Rapid deployment valves, shorter operational time
  - **3F Enable** (Medtronic), **Perceval S** (Sorin), **Intuity Elite** (Edwards Lifescience)

(Left) *PA (inset = lateral) radiograph demonstrates a bileaflet tilting disc mitral valve replacement, which had a paravalvular leak between the mitral anulus and the prosthetic valve ring repaired by transcatheter placement of 2 Amplatzer occluder devices. Note that the devices have 2 dense radiopaque ends.* **(Right)** *Average-weighted (inset = volume-rendered) CT MPR in mitral plane shows the calcified mitral annulus and 2 occluder devices across the paravalvular regurgitant orifice.*

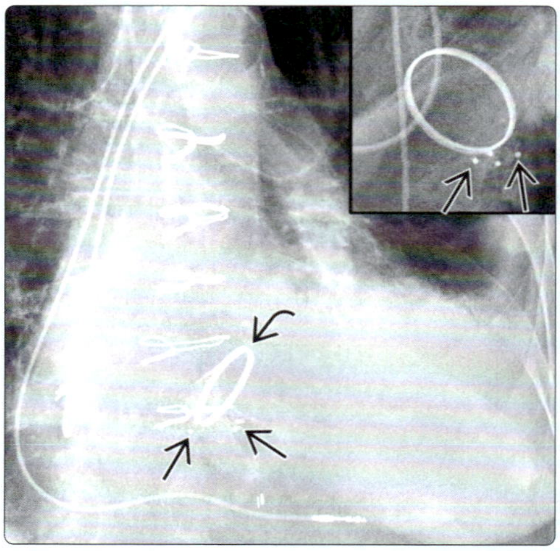

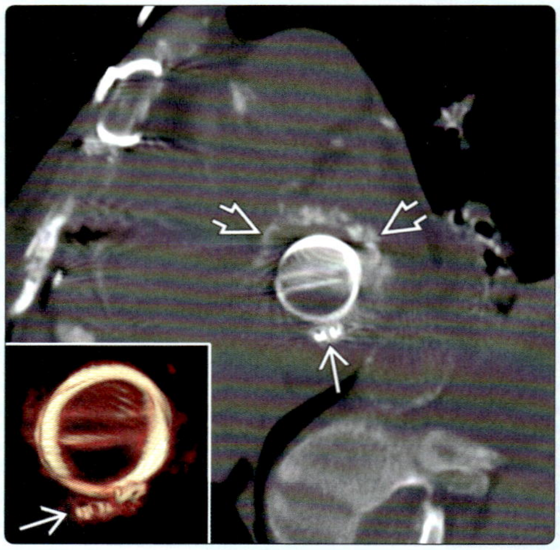

(Left) *Oblique combined volume-rendered and left ventricular long-axis multiplanar reconstruction cardiac CT shows Starr-Edwards valves normally seated in aortic and mitral valve positions. Note that the radiopaque-caged ball is visible in the mitral valve in the open position.* **(Right)** *Volume-rendered multiplanar reconstructed cardiac CT in systole demonstrates Starr-Edwards valves in the aortic and mitral valve positions. The ball now occludes the prosthetic valve anulus (closed position).*

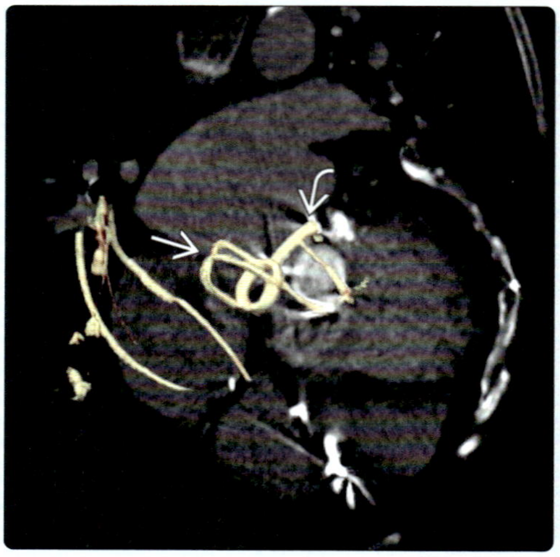

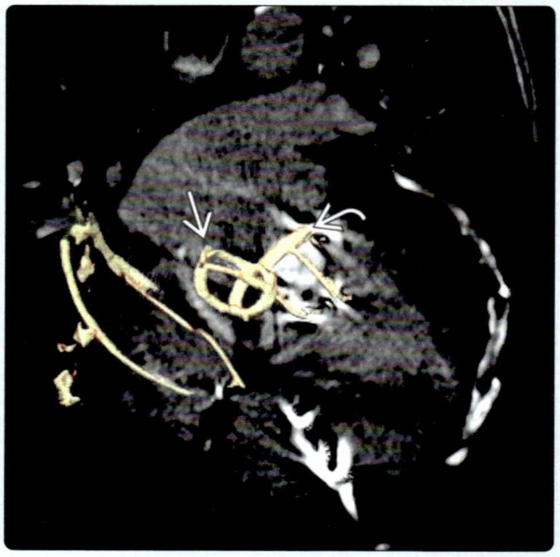

IMAGING

General Features

- Location
  - Most common in aortic position, followed by mitral, tricuspid, and pulmonic
- **Ball-in-cage valves**
  - Hufnagel valve
    - 1st caged ball valve (1952)
  - Harken-Soroff valve
    - 1st in situ ball-in-cage aortic valve (1960)
  - Starr-Edwards valve [1960 (mitral) - 2007]
    - Initial models used stellite alloy cage; later changed to bare metal cage, Silastic rubber ball
- **Nontilting disc valves**
  - Kay-Shiley: Flat disc; widely used mitral valve replacement
  - Beall-Surgitool: Flat disc (initially Teflon, later Pyrolite)
  - Cooley-Cutter: Biconical silicone rubber disc later replaced with Pyrolite disc, full-flow orifice
- **Tilting disc valves**
  - Björk-Shiley flat (1969-1987) and convexoconcave (1975) disc valves
    - Convexoconcave disc was developed to improve flow across valve, but new design led to strut fractures in 2% of cases and required prophylactic valve replacements
      - Consequently, convexoconcave and even complication-free flat disc valve production was terminated in 1986
  - Lillehei-Kaster tilting disc valve (1970-1987)
    - 2 side prongs hold valve in place
    - Omniscience (1978) and Omnicarbon (1984) valves are newer models and are still in production
  - Medtronic-Hall (previously Hall-Kaster) tilting disc valve (1977-2009)
    - Titanium housing with Pyrolite disc
    - Strut traverses hole in disc
    - Widespread use; for aortic and mitral valves
- **Bileaflet valves**
  - St. Jude Medical (1977)
    - 1st all-carbon (Pyrolite) valve
  - Carbomedics (1986)
    - Housing can be rotated within sewing ring
    - Pyrolite housing and Pyrolite discs
    - 1st totally supraannular mechanical valve
  - On-X (1996)
    - Pure carbon structure
    - Lower INR target of 1.5-2.0
    - Reduction in bleeding, clot formation, and stroke
  - Open pivot valves
    - Low level of hemolysis and thromboembolic events
    - For aortic and mitral valve replacement
    - Multiple different vendors (Medtronic, Abbott, ATS, etc.) currently offer open pivot valve systems
- Mechanical valves have longer durability with low structural valve deterioration (SVD) rate but more thromboembolic complications than tissue valves
- Lifelong anticoagulation is necessary
- **Tissue valves (bioprosthesis)**
  - Ionescu-Shiley bovine pericardial valve (1971)
    - 3 leaflets sutured to titanium frame covered with Dacron
    - Aortic, mitral, and tricuspid
    - Develops significant leaflet calcification, especially in patients < 70 years old
  - Carpentier-Edwards Perimount valve (1981)
    - Pressure-fixed, glutaraldehyde-preserved, and wire-mounted porcine or pericardial valve
    - Aortic valve replacement
    - > 20 years of follow-up data shows excellent durability
  - Hancock porcine xenograft (1982)
    - Glutaraldehyde-preserved porcine valve mounted on Dacron-covered polypropylene strut
    - Currently, 2nd-generation (Hancock II and Hancock II Ultra) valves are available for aortic mitral valve replacement
  - Mitroflow aortic valve (1982, Europe; 2007, USA)
    - Single piece of glutaraldehyde-preserved bovine pericardium sewn onto nonradiopaque polymer stent
    - Radiopaque silicone sewing ring is visible on radiographs and CT
    - 4th-generation valves are available
    - SVD is secondary to leaflet calcification and stiffening
  - Pulmonary autograft (Ross procedure)
    - Substituting patient's aortic valve with patient's pulmonary valve
    - Might be used in young patients when anticoagulation is contraindicated or undesirable
    - Allows growth of valve in children
  - Edwards RESILIA aortic valve (2018)
    - Leaflet tissue is designed to resist calcium build-up
    - No SVD or paravalvular leak after 5 year follow-up; however, impact of RESILIA tissue on long-term durability is not clear at this point
  - Medtronic Avalus (2017) and Avalus Ultra (2024)
    - Enables future valve-in-valve replacements
    - Radiopaque coil enhances visibility under fluoroscopy
- 3 months of anticoagulation are required for tissue valves until sewing ring becomes endothelialized
  - Higher risk of SVD requiring reoperation
- No anticoagulation is required thereafter
- **Catheter-delivered valves**
  - Initially, transcatheter approach was used for aortic valves; today, it can also be employed for mitral, tricuspid, and pulmonary valve replacements
  - Transfemoral approach is preferred
    - Other approaches: Transapical, transaortic, transsubclavian, transcarotid, caval-aortic
  - Cardiac and vascular CT used for procedure planning
    - Aortoiliac system is analyzed for access feasibility
    - Identification of valvular anatomy and anulus plane
    - Measurements for sizing and implantation feasibility
    - Evaluation of possible contraindications or situations requiring different approaches
      - Low coronary heights (aorta), small neo-left ventricular outflow tract (mitral), close relationship to left main (pulmonary) or right coronary artery (tricuspid)
  - Edwards SAPIEN 3 transcatheter heart valve system

- Bovine pericardium leaflets sewn onto balloon-expandable stainless steel frame
- 99% deployment accuracy, 90% survival at 5 years
- Can be used for valve-in-valve procedure

- Medtronic CoreValve Evolut
  - Porcine pericardium sewn onto nitinol alloy stent (nickel titanium)
- Boston scientific ACURATE neo2
  - Aortic valve system with open frame and supraannular leaflets
- Abbot Portico transcatheter aortic heart valve
  - Porcine pericardium sealing cuff
- Medtronic Melody transcatheter pulmonary valve
  - Bovine jugular vein valve sutured within platinum-iridium frame
- Medtronic Harmony transcatheter pulmonary valve
  - Especially for larger right ventricular outflow tract (RVOT)
  - Porcine pericardial tissue valve sewn in self-expanding nitinol frame with polyester cloth covering
- Edwards Alterra Adaptive Prestent
  - Used in conjunction with Edwards SAPIEN 3 valve system in pulmonary position
  - Allows deployment of SAPIEN valve in larger conduits or native RVOT
- Edwards EVOQUE tricuspid valve system
  - 1st transcatheter tricuspid valve system
  - Self-expanding nitinol frame, bovine pericardial tissue similar to SAPIEN and Perimount valves
  - 9 ventricular anchors provide secure positioning

- **Sutureless valves**
  - Rapid deployment aortic valves
  - No extensive placement or tying of sutures
  - Shorter operational time (cross-clamp and CPB duration)
  - Facilitates minimally invasive valve surgery
    - 3F Enable (Medtronic): Equine pericardium mounted on self-expanding nitinol frame, 1 guiding suture
    - Perceval S (Sorin): Double sheet design, no sutures
    - Intuity Elite (Edwards Lifescience): Balloon expandable, implanted by catheter delivery system, 3 guiding sutures

Imaging Recommendations

- Best imaging tool
  - Transthoracic ECG (TEE): 1st-line imaging for evaluation of valve function and status of left ventricle
    - TEE: Preferred for mitral and tricuspid valves
  - EKG-gated CT and cardiac MR for evaluation of leaflet function and etiology of prosthetic valve dysfunction
    - Provides information about paravalvular and surrounding structure
    - MR better in bioprosthetic valves (artifacts limit evaluation of mechanical valves)

DIFFERENTIAL DIAGNOSIS

Aortic Calcifications

- Can mimic aortic valve replacement on nongated CT

Annuloplasty Ring

- Usually open ring on radiography or CT

CLINICAL ISSUES

Presentation

- Indications for mechanical valves
  - Age: < 50 years
    - Longer expected life: Better durability of mechanical valves is preferred; lifetime anticoagulation is necessary
    - Bioprosthetic valves have higher risk of SVD in younger patients (15-year risk; 30% for age 40 years, 50% for age 20 years)
  - Anticoagulation is required for other reasons
  - Patient preference (avoid risk of reoperation)
  - Compliant patient for monitoring
  - Small aortic root (may preclude valve-in-valve procedure)
  - High risk of reintervention (e.g., porcelain aorta, prior radiation therapy)
- Indications for bioprosthetic valves
  - Age: > 70 years
    - Shorter life expectancy &/or multiple comorbidities: Lower risk from thromboembolism
    - Lower risk of SVD in older adult patients (15-year risk; < 10% for age > 70 years)
  - Contraindication or high risk for anticoagulation
  - Patient preference (avoid anticoagulation and valve sounds)
  - Limited access to medical care or noncompliant patient
  - Access to surgical centers with low operative mortality rate
  - Possible pregnancy
- Choice of type of prosthetic valve should be shared decision-making process

Natural History & Prognosis

- Bleeding or thrombotic complications account for 50% of complications of tissue valves and 75% of complications of mechanical valves
- Risk of thromboembolic events is higher with mechanical valves than tissue valves; higher with mitral than aortic valves; higher in early (< 3 months) vs. late postoperative phase
- Mechanical prostheses usually cause subclinical mild chronic hemolysis (50-95%)
- Valve thrombosis occurs in 0.1% per year in aortic position and in 0.35% per year in mitral position
- Prosthetic valve endocarditis (PVE) occurs in 1.4-3.1% at 1 year and in 3.2-5.7% at 5 years (cumulative)
  - 0.5-3.1% incidence rate during 1st year after transcatheter aortic valve implantation (TAVI)
- PVE agents
  - Most common; coagulase negative staphylococci, *Staphylococcus aureus*, and streptococci

SELECTED REFERENCES

1. Rajiah PS et al: Utility of CT and MRI in tricuspid valve interventions. Radiographics. 43(7):e220153, 2023
2. Singh SK et al: Polymeric prosthetic heart valves: a review of current technologies and future directions. Front Cardiovasc Med. 10:1137827, 2023
3. Canan A et al: Pre- and postprocedure imaging of transcatheter pulmonary valve implantation. Radiographics. 42(4):991-1011, 2022
4. Bartus K et al: Final 5-year outcomes following aortic valve replacement with a RESILIA™ tissue bioprosthesis. Eur J Cardiothorac Surg. 59(2):434-41, 2021

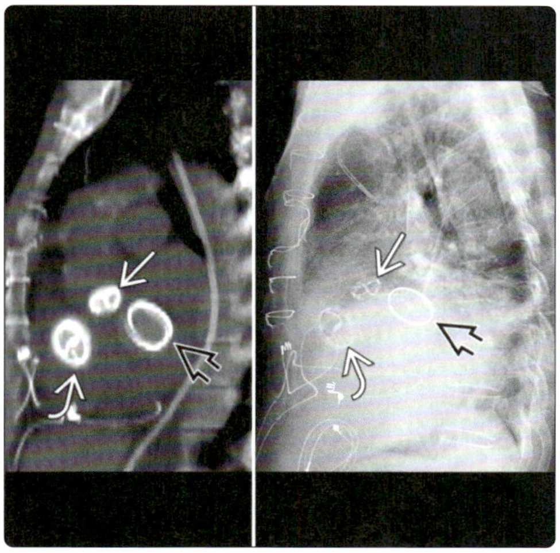

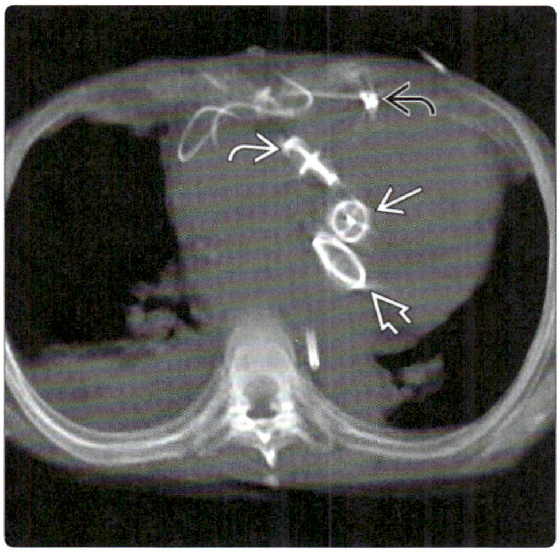

(Left) *Lateral radiograph and thick MPR CT in a patient with rheumatic heart disease show Medtronic-Hall valves in aortic and tricuspid positions and St. Jude-type valve in the mitral position. Note the single curved strut in the Medtronic-Hall valves traversing through a central disc opening.* **(Right)** *Axial thick MPR NECT shows Medtronic-Hall valves in aortic and tricuspid positions and St. Jude-type valve in the mitral position. Note also the epicardial screw-in lead.*

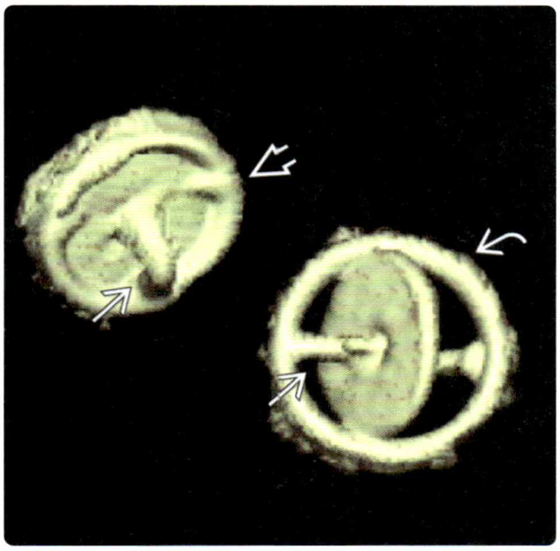

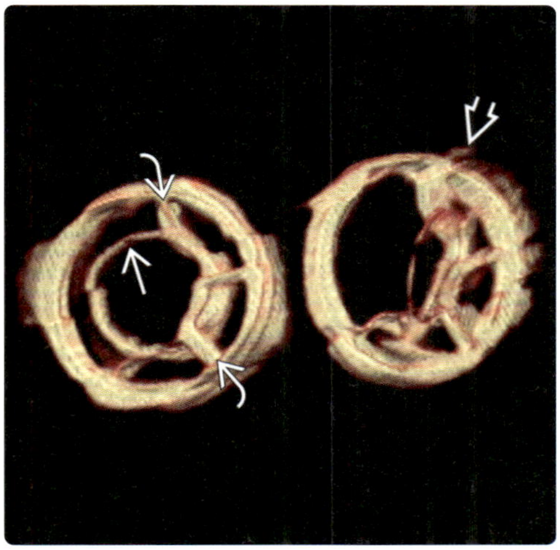

(Left) *Oblique coronary CTA volume rendering in diastole shows normal closed aortic and open mitral Medtronic-Hall tilting disc valve replacements. Note that a single strut traverses the central disc opening.* **(Right)** *Oblique coronary CTA volume rendering in systole shows normal open aortic and closed mitral Björk-Shiley tilting disc valve prostheses. The disc has a radiopaque ring but is otherwise radiolucent. Note that 2 struts keep the disc in place.*

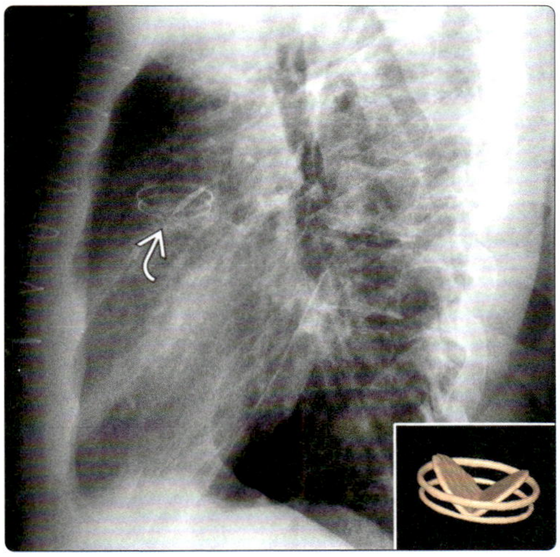

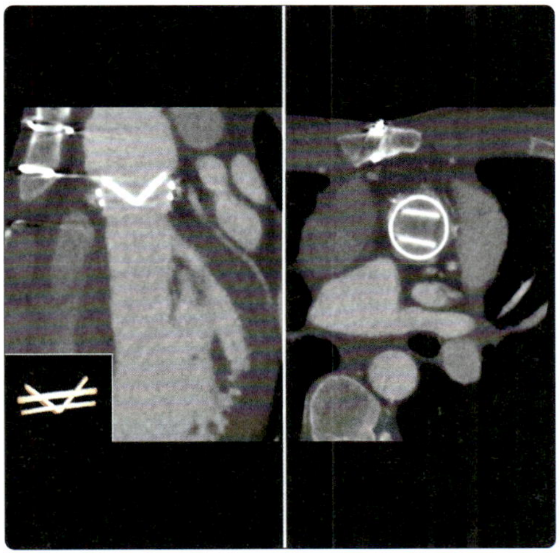

(Left) *Lateral radiograph (inset = volume rendered) demonstrates On-X bileaflet mechanical valve in the aortic position.* **(Right)** *Two-chamber (inset + volume-rendered) cardiac CT in the same patient shows the normal appearance of a well-seated bileaflet prosthetic valve. Aortic valve axial short-axis view demonstrates normal opening of the leaflets during systole.*

(Left) *Oblique volume-rendered cardiac CT shows St. Jude mechanical prosthetic valves in the aortic and mitral valve positions. This diastolic reconstruction shows the open position of the mitral valve and the closed position of the aortic valve.* **(Right)** *Three-chamber cardiac CT combined volume-rendered and MPR reconstruction in the same patient show a large subvalvular defect with contrast extending into the perivalvular area, consistent with endocarditic pseudoaneurysm .*

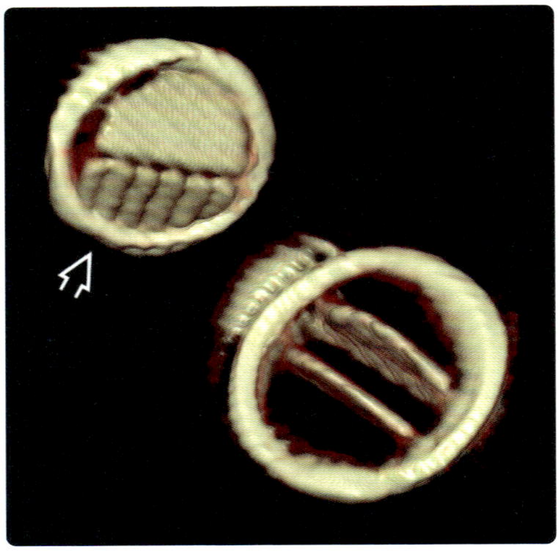

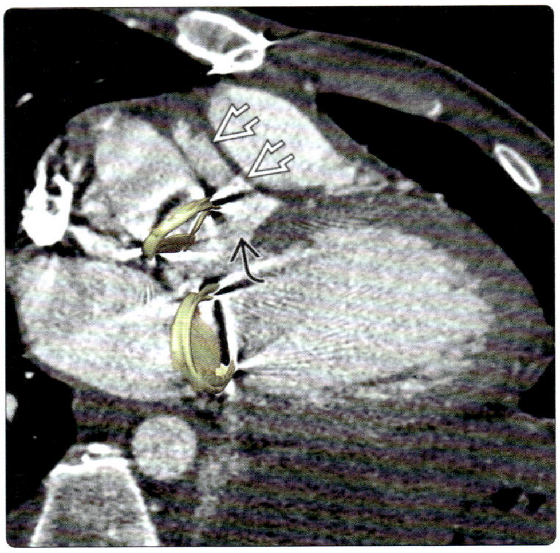

(Left) *Fluoroscopy with CT is a road map to determine the optimal fluoroscopic plane for transcatheter aortic valve replacement (TAVR) and coronary ostia location. A stented valve during deployment is centered around anulus markers (red dots); note coronary markers and TEE probe .* **(Right)** *AP radiograph shows well-seated TAVR with stented Edwards SAPIEN valve in aortic position. Note 2 valves (retracted and fully deployed) in the descending aorta due to malposition during partial deployment.*

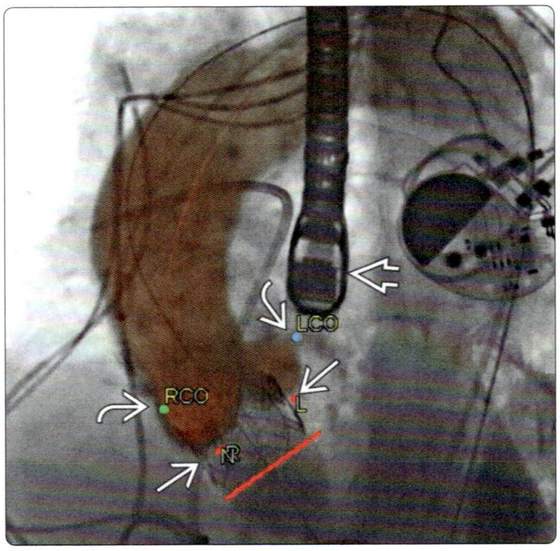

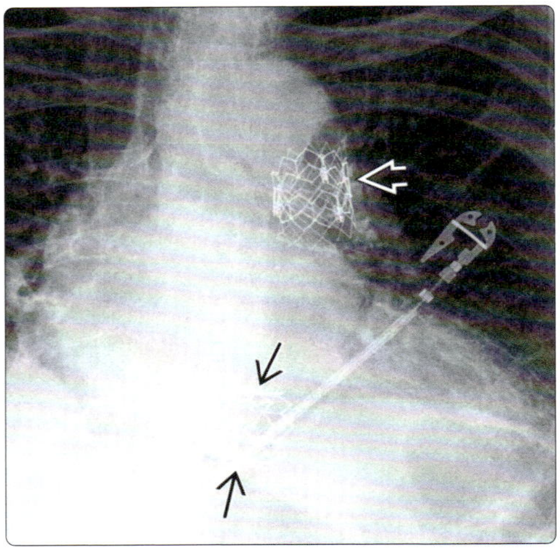

(Left) *PA radiograph shows the normal appearance of TAVR with the Medtronic core valve in the aortic position. Three-chamber cardiac view CT MIP also shows calcification of the native aortic leaflets around the stent.* **(Right)** *Short-axis cardiac CT demonstrates a well-seated aortic valve and normal closing and opening of the bioprosthetic leaflets at the diastole and systole, retrospectively.*

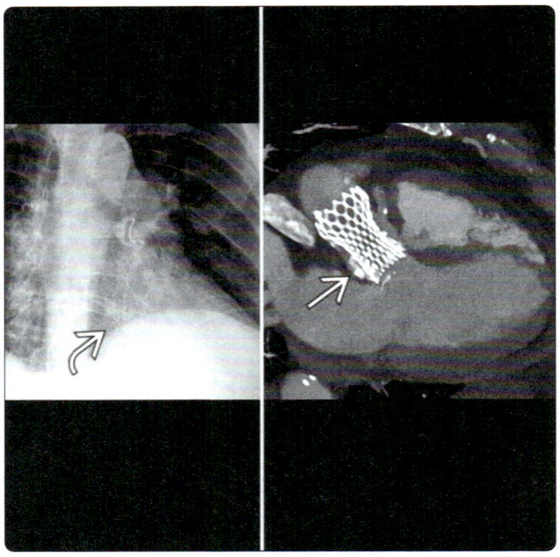

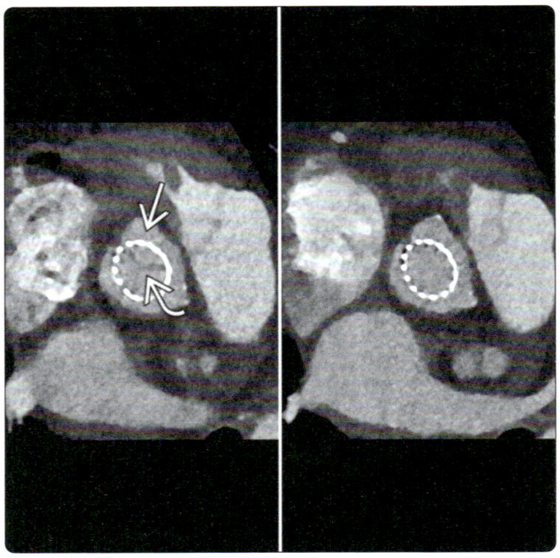

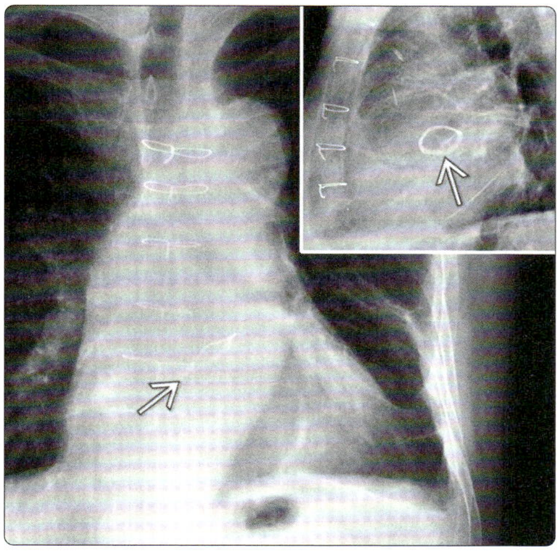

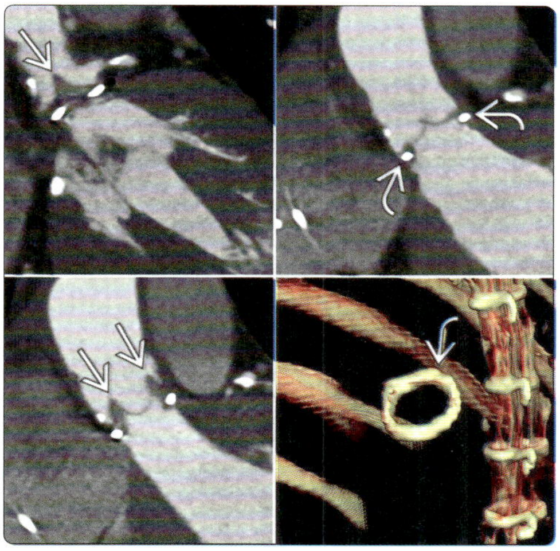

(Left) *PA and lateral (inset) radiographs show the normal appearance of Mitroflow bioprosthetic aortic valve replacement. Note the characteristic appearance of the radiopaque silicone sewing ring . The stent that holds the pericardial leaflets in place is radiolucent and not seen (unlike Carpentier-Edwards valve).* **(Right)** *Aortic root long-axis and volume-rendered cardiac CT in the same patient show the 3 low-attenuation struts that hold up the pericardium. Note the radiopaque sewing ring .*

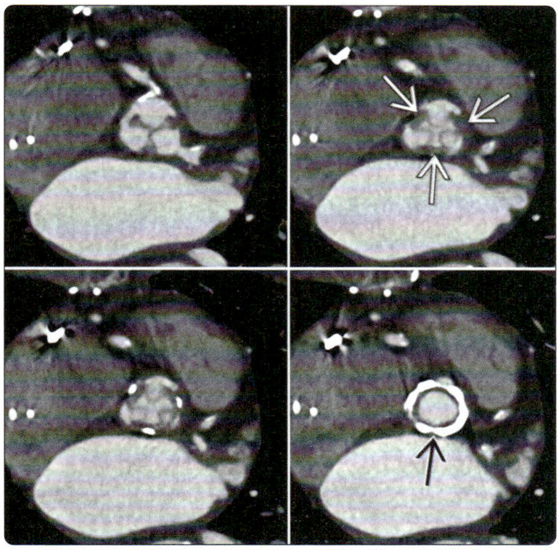

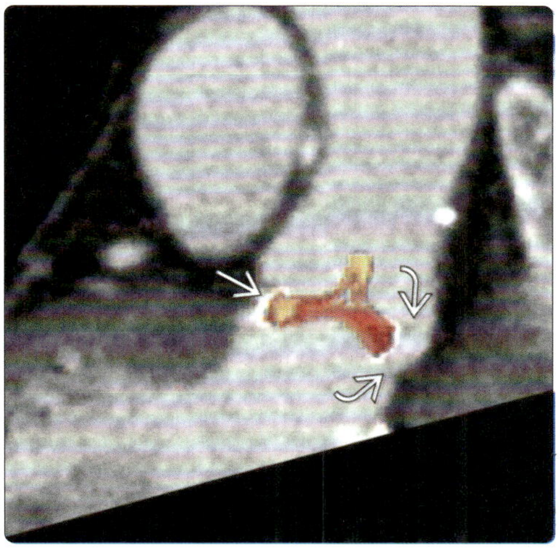

(Left) *Aortic valve short-axis cardiac CT from the level of valve coaptation (top left) down to the anulus shows the normal appearance of the Mitroflow valve. Note radiolucent stents inside the circumferential pericardium, allowing for leaflet-like function of the pericardium.* **(Right)** *Aortic root long-axis MPR/VRT cardiac CT shows the normal connection of Carpentier-Edwards bioprosthesis to aortic anulus on one side but dehiscence with paravalvular regurgitant orifice on the other side .*

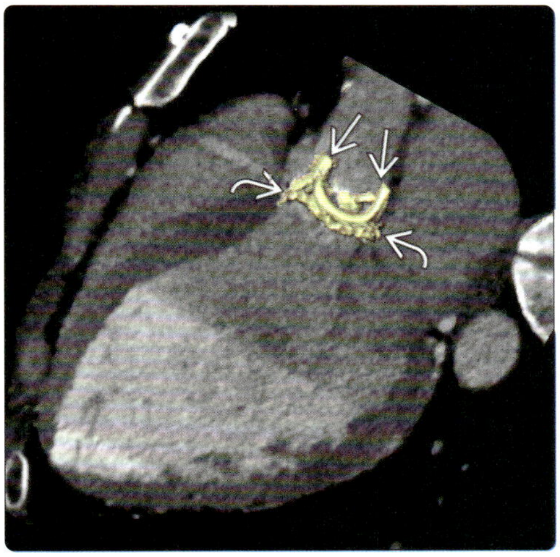

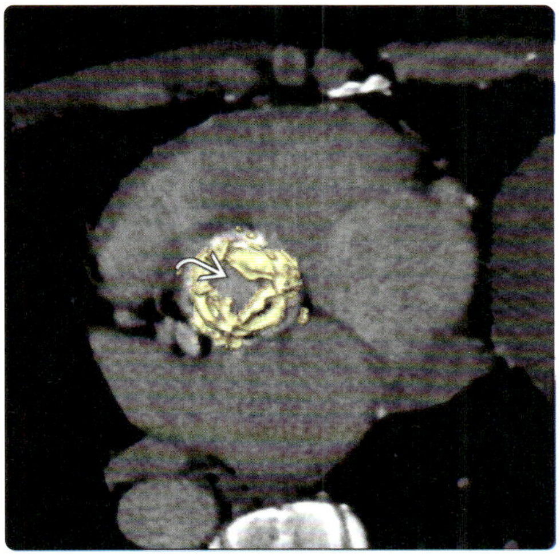

(Left) *Three-chamber cardiac CT shows well-seated Carpentier-Edwards bioprosthetic aortic valve replacement. The metallic struts are visible , and the valve sewing ring extends all the way to the aortic anulus without a gap to suggest paravalvular leak.* **(Right)** *Aortic valve short-axis cardiac CT shows the normally seated Carpentier-Edwards aortic valve in systole. Note that the leaflets are densely calcified, and the systolic opening orifice is reduced, consistent with stenosis.*

Prosthetic Valve Complications

KEY FACTS

IMAGING

- General imaging findings
  - Structural valve deterioration: Broken or disrupted metallic leaflets (metallic valve); degeneration and calcification of leaflets (bioprosthetic valve)
  - Pannus/thrombus (rather mechanic)
  - Infective endocarditis (vegetations, abscess, cusp perforation): May or may not cause dysfunction
  - Paravalvular leak
  - Dehiscence (rocking valve motion > 15° in any 1 plane)
  - Perivalvular abscess and pseudoaneurysm may be seen
  - Regurgitation (more common) or stenosis (less common)
  - Frozen disc: Causes severe regurgitation
  - Hypoattenuated leaflet thickening (HALT) (bioprosthetic valves) ± restricted leaflet motion
- Transthoracic echocardiography is 1st-line imaging
  - Transesophageal echocardiography is better to clarify etiology, especially for mitral valve prosthesis
- Cardiac CT is adjuvant imaging technique that permits
  - Visualization of calcification, HALT and degenerative changes of bioprosthesis
  - Evaluation of etiology of valve dysfunction
  - Identification of pannus formation, presence of thrombus
  - Assessment of leaflet motions
- Fluoroscopy is gold standard for suspected frozen leaflet evaluation

CLINICAL ISSUES

- Chronic: Gradual onset of congestive heart failure symptoms (dyspnea, fatigue, pulmonary edema)
- Acute: Acute heart failure symptoms
  - Most common etiology is infective endocarditis
- Severe clinical symptoms if prosthetic valve dysfunction is caused by acute infective endocarditis
- Sepsis, thromboembolic events (stroke)
- Systemic emboli if right-sided valve dysfunction

(Left) *Oblique fluoroscopy in systole and diastole shows aortic St. Jude-type bileaflet tilting disc with a frozen leaflet ➔ and a normally functioning leaflet ↷. Frozen disc in closed position causes stenosis, and open position results in regurgitation. Note mitral valve replacement ⇨.* **(Right)** *Volume-rendering technique (VRT) cardiac CT shows mitral and aortic bileaflet tilting disc prostheses. Note the frozen leaflet ➔ and a normally functioning leaflet ↷.*

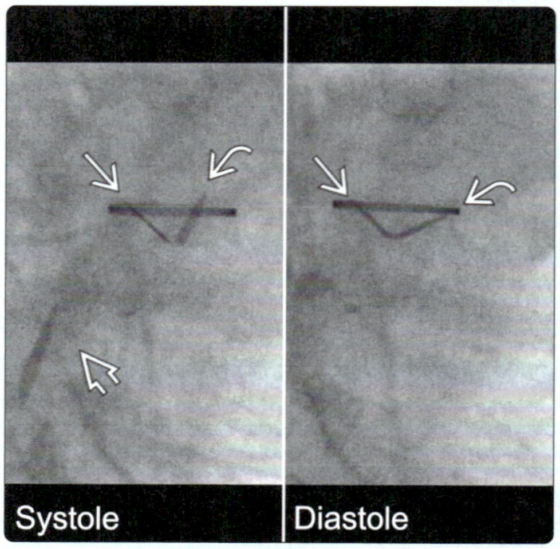

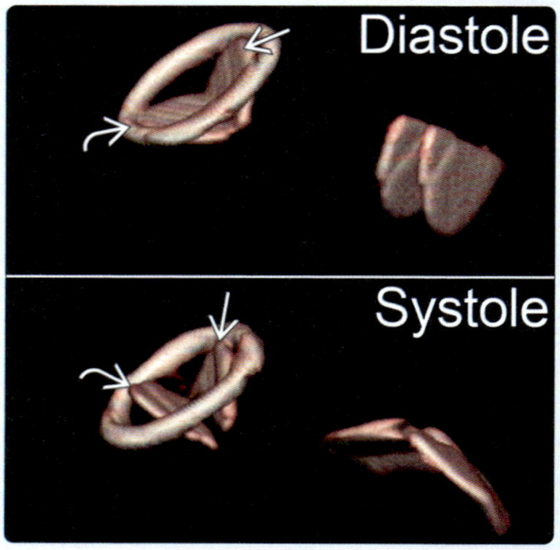

(Left) *Oblique cardiac CT shows a bileaflet tilting disc valve in aortic position with contrast extravasating from left ventricular outflow tract (LVOT) into perivalvular tissue ➔, consistent with pseudoaneurysm due to endocarditis. No paravalvular connection between LVOT and aortic lumen was seen.* **(Right)** *Aortic valve short-axis cardiac CT in combined multiplanar reformation and VRT view shows a prosthetic valve nearly circumferentially surrounded by large contrast collection, consistent with a pseudoaneurysm ➔.*

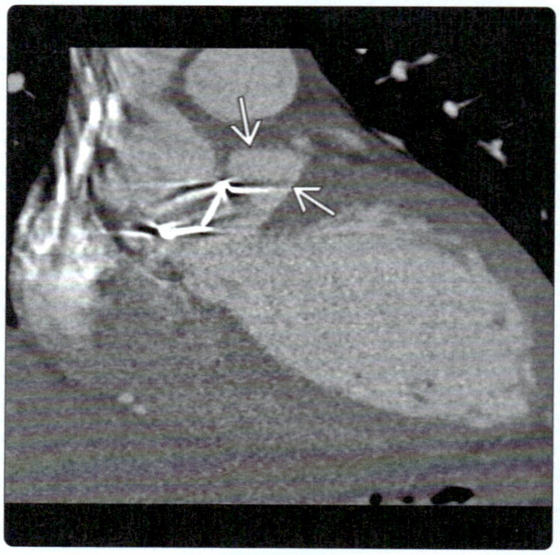

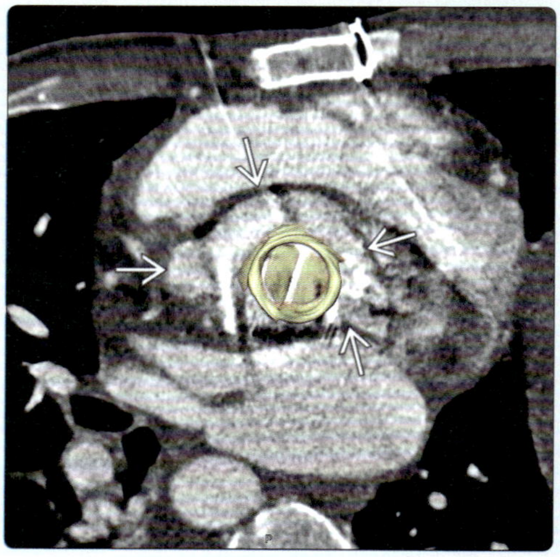

TERMINOLOGY

Synonyms

- Prosthetic valve dysfunction (PVD)

IMAGING

General Features

- **Structural valve deterioration/dysfunction (SVD)**
  - Any change in valve function resulting from intrinsic abnormality
  - Leads to stenosis or regurgitation (more common)
  - Mostly seen in bioprosthetic valves; risk ↑ over time, especially after 7-8 years
  - Mitral valve (MV) > atrioventricular (AV); due to higher mechanical stress on leaflets
  - **Mechanical valves**: Very rare, observed > 3 or 4 decades after surgery
    - Strut fracture, occluder fracture or escape, broken or disrupted metallic leaflets, loss of leaflet mobility, ball (Starr-Edwards) or disc dislodgement, sewing cuff separation from housing
  - **Bioprosthetic valves**: More aggressive in younger patients
    - Most common cause: Degeneration of valve due to calcification (best evaluated on CT)
    - Other causes: Tearing of cuff, disruption of annular housing or sewing ring
- **Prosthetic valve obstruction (PVO)**
  - Thrombus, pannus, or combination of both; differentiation is crucial
  - Thrombus most common cause of obstruction of mechanical valves
    - History of inadequate anticoagulation
    - Occurs at any time after surgery; most common in 1st year; above or below prosthesis
    - Tricuspid valve (TV) >> MV = AV (~ 20% of TV replacements)
    - Irregularly shaped mass attached to leaflet
    - Lower density on CT than pannus (< 145 HU)
      - Sensitivity of 87.5% and specificity of 95.5%
  - Pannus seen in both mechanical and prosthetic valves
    - Usually 12 months after surgery
    - Below prosthesis; MV > AV
    - Circular mass extending from sewing ring
    - Calcification may present
    - Higher density on CT than thrombus (> 145 HU)
- **Hypoattenuated leaflet thickening (HALT)**
  - Hallmark of subclinical leaflet thrombosis
  - Restricted leaflet motion (RLM) may be associated
  - Hypoattenuation affecting motion (HAM) = HALT with significant RLM (> 50%)
  - Start from base (area of leaflet attachment) and extend to varying degrees to edges of leaflets
  - 1st described in transcatheter aortic valve replacement, but has been reported after surgical bioprosthetic valve replacement and with sutureless valves
  - Asymptomatic patients with absence of any ↑ in velocities or pressure gradient on echocardiography
  - Best seen on cardiac gated CT
  - ↑ risk of systemic thromboembolism
  - Complete resolution or regression of both leaflet thickening and RLM with anticoagulation
- **Dehiscence**
  - Suture line breakdown leading to separation of prosthetic valve from anulus
  - Rocking valve motion > 15° in any plane
  - Endocarditis (most common), aneurysm of ascending aorta, severe calcification of native valve
  - Manifests as paravalvular leak
- **Paravalvular leak**
  - Abnormal blood flow through channel between prosthesis and anulus
  - 2-10% in prosthetic aortic valves, 7-17% in prosthetic MVs
  - Endocarditis-induced dehiscence (most common), dehisced sutures or improper implantation of valve
  - Similar risk in mechanical and bioprosthetic valves
  - Minor; well tolerated, asymptomatic, mild hemolytic anemia
  - < 1% clinically significant heart failure or severe anemia
- **Pseudoaneurysm**
  - 7-25% of patients with composite grafts
- **Valvular regurgitation or stenosis**
  - Mostly seen in bioprosthesis due to degeneration
- **Frozen disc**
  - Severe regurgitation or stenosis, depending on position
- **Embolism**
  - Often associated with mechanical valves due to inadequate anticoagulation
- **Bleeding**
  - Mechanical valves, mostly due to anticoagulation therapy
- **Hemolysis**
  - 50-95% of patients with mechanical valves have subclinical mild hemolysis; severe hemolytic anemia occurs due to paravalvular leak, infection, or obstruction
- **Endocarditis**
  - 1st year: Equal frequency at aortic and mitral position and on mechanical and bioprosthetic valves
  - 18 months: Bioprosthetic valves have greater risk
  - May present with vegetations, aortic wall thickening > 5 mm, perivalvular abscess, and pseudoaneurysm
  - Mechanical valves: Often starts at sewing cuff or from thrombi near sewing ring; leads to paravalvular leak, ring abscess, extension of infection into adjacent tissue
  - Bioprosthetic valves: Limited to cusps and rarely includes sewing cuff or leads to periprosthetic abscess

CT Findings

- Cardiac gated CTA
  - Useful for establishing specific etiology of PVD, complementary to echocardiography
  - Useful for mechanical prosthesis if echocardiography is limited by massive metal artifacts
  - 4D dynamic cine imaging for
    - Valve function; dynamic leaflet motion, opening and closing angles
    - Dehiscence; gap between aortic anulus and opposing margin of valve allows continuous column of contrast from left ventricular outflow tract (LVOT) into aortic root

- Paravalvular leak; contrast-filled structure adjacent to valve area continuous with LVOT and aorta
- Pseudoaneurysm; outpouching of contrast
- Presence, extent, differentiation of thrombus from pannus
- Vegetation; irregular, low-attenuation mobile masses adherent to leaflet or sewing ring
- Perivalvular abscess; perivalvular fluid collection with surrounding soft tissue inflammation and fat stranding; can have peripheral rim enhancement on delayed phase
- Coexistent valvular regurgitation or stenosis
- Evaluation of HALT and RLM

- Coronary CT angiography
  - Exclusion of coronary artery disease (CAD) (stenosis > 50%) before surgery
  - Evaluation of occlusion of coronary ostium due to misplacement of valve after surgery
- Multienergy CT (spectral, photon-counting)
  - Virtual noncontrast can be used to identify calcification and sutures without additional acquisition
  - Iodine-only images and monoenergetic images can enhance visualization of prosthetic valve
  - Additional filters can be used, such as metal reduction filter to reduce artifacts
- Protocol advice: Retrospective ECG gating for data in multiple cardiac phases without tube modulation
  - Noncontrast CT or virtual nonenhanced DECT: Differentiate sutures from pseudoaneurysm/leak, identify valvular calcification
  - Delayed phase can be used in cases of suspected pseudoaneurysm or abscess

MR Findings

- May quantify stenosis or regurgitation for specific valve
- Better evaluation of bioprosthetic valves than metallic
- Metallic components may cause artifacts (signal void)

Echocardiographic Findings

- Echocardiogram
  - Transthoracic echocardiography 1st-line imaging modality to evaluate prosthetic valve function
  - Transesophageal better than transthoracic to clarify etiology of PVD, particularly of MV prosthesis
- Color Doppler
  - De novo regurgitation (more common) or stenosis (rare)
    - Mechanical prosthesis: Mild regurgitation is normal; each type has specific retrograde flow pattern [except Starr-Edwards (no regurgitation)]
    - Bioprosthesis: No regurgitation but may develop if chronic-degenerative dysfunction
  - Paravalvular leakage: Eccentric Doppler jet, typically with half moon or sickle shape
  - Thrombus or pannus: Eccentric inflow pattern because leaflet motion is impaired (thrombus = lower echogenicity; pannus = higher echogenicity)

Angiographic Findings

- Mechanical valve: Rocking of dehiscing prosthesis, strut separation
- Paravalvular leakage, regurgitation, and stenosis
- Exclusion of CAD before redo surgery
  - Invasive catheter manipulation is associated with high risk of embolization if mobile vegetations/thrombus

Nuclear Medicine Findings

- F-18 FDG PET/CT has been used for diagnosing prosthetic valve endocarditis
  - Abnormal ↑ in FDG uptake has positive predictive value of 85% and negative predictive value of 67%

Fluoroscopic Findings

- Gold standard for suspected frozen leaflet evaluation

CLINICAL ISSUES

Presentation

- Most common signs/symptoms
  - Dependent on whether acute or chronic dysfunction
    - Chronic: Gradual onset of congestive heart failure symptoms (dyspnea, fatigue, pulmonary edema)
    - Acute: Acute heart failure symptoms
      - Most common etiology is infective endocarditis
- Clinical profile
  - Severe clinical symptoms if PVD is caused by acute infective endocarditis
    - Sepsis, thromboembolic events (stroke, rarely myocardial infarction)
    - Systemic emboli (e.g., pulmonary) if right-sided PVD

Demographics

- Epidemiology
  - Bioprosthesis
    - Preferred in older adults (> 70 years); Ross procedure in children and adolescents
    - Limited long-term durability: 30% SVD after 10 years due to degeneration beginning in 4th-5th postop year
    - Advantage: No long-term anticoagulation necessary
  - Metallic prosthesis: Excellent long-term durability, low risk of SVD

Natural History & Prognosis

- Failure of mechanical valve apparatus is rare; consider thrombosis or pannus as well as dehiscence
- Failure of bioprosthesis is more common with > 25% in 10 years resulting in higher rate of reoperation
- ↑ risk of infective endocarditis with bioprostheses

Treatment

- Medical therapy for vegetations, endocarditis, HALT
- Surgery is indicated for severe dysfunction, dehiscence, severe thromboembolism, or severe recurrent bleeding
- Transcatheter valve-in-valve; high and extreme-risk patients with bioprosthetic aortic valve in absence of endocarditis

SELECTED REFERENCES

1. Carlson S et al: Multimodality imaging for prosthetic valves evaluation: current understanding and future directions. Prog Cardiovasc Dis. 72:66-77, 2022
2. Verma M et al: Imaging spectrum of valvular and paravalvular complications of prosthetic heart valve at CT angiography. Radiol Cardiothorac Imaging. 3(4):e210159, 2021
3. Rajiah P et al: Multimodality imaging of complications of cardiac valve surgeries. Radiographics. 39(4):932-56, 2019
4. Rashid HN et al: Subclinical leaflet thrombosis in transcatheter aortic valve replacement detected by multidetector computed tomography - a review of current evidence. Circ J. 82(7):1735-42, 2018

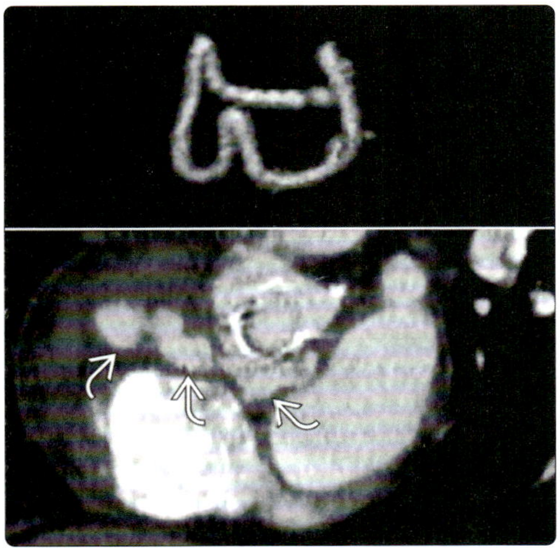

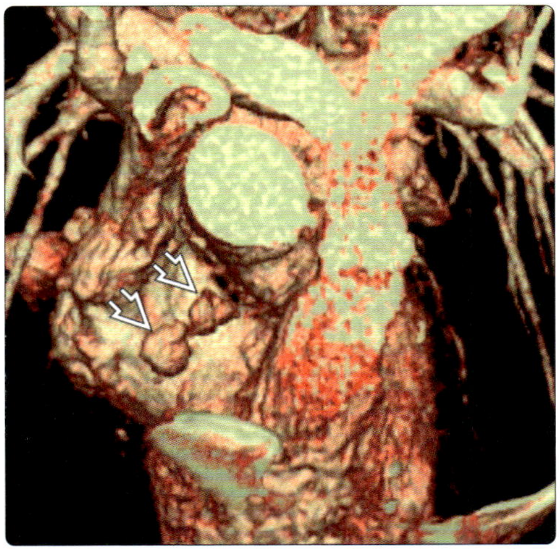

(Left) *Oblique CTA shows an aortic Carpentier-Edwards porcine tissue valve (inset shows volume rendering of valve frame). Three discrete extraluminal contrast cavities ➔ with surrounding fat stranding indicate prosthetic valve endocarditis with paravalvular abscess.* **(Right)** *Oblique coronary CTA volume rendering in the same patient shows 2 of the abscess cavities filled with contrast ➔.*

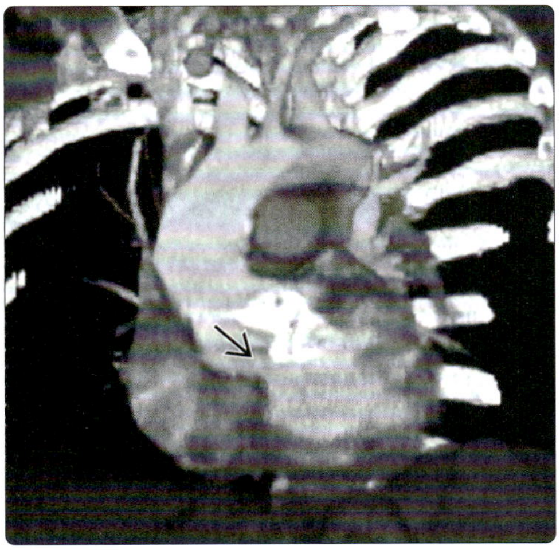

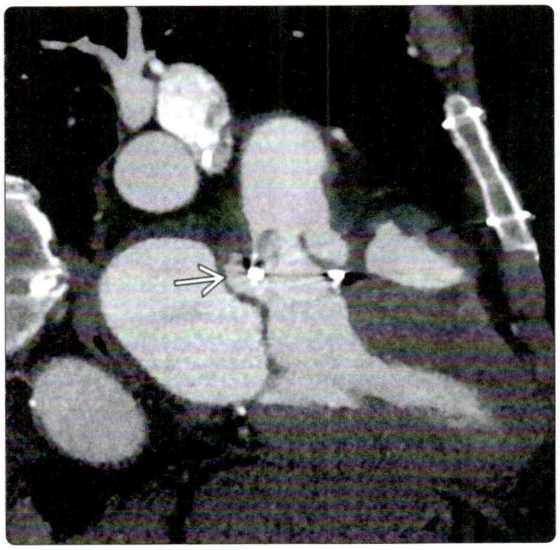

(Left) *Coronal oblique nongated CECT volume rendering in a patient with a prosthetic valve and endocarditis shows a tilting disc valve not fully extending to the aortic anulus, indicating dehiscence. Note the paraprosthetic regurgitant orifice ➔.* **(Right)** *Three-chamber cardiac CT in endocarditis shows bioprosthetic aortic valve replacement and contrast collection extending from the LVOT posteriorly ➔, representing a pseudoaneurysm.*

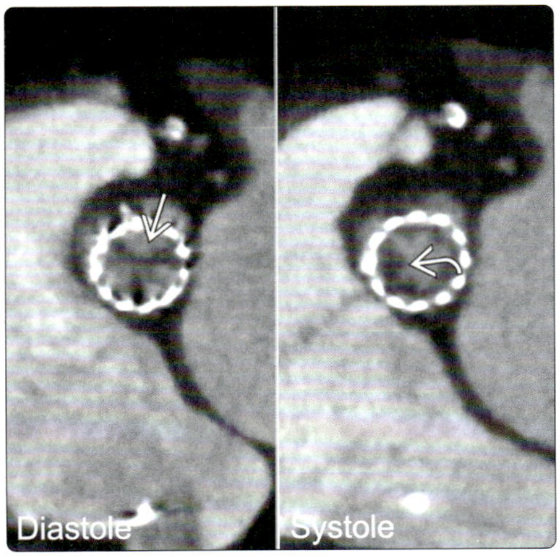

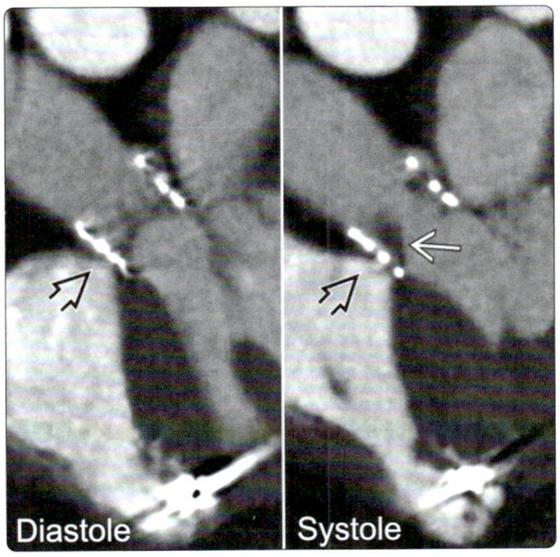

(Left) *Aortic valve short-axis cardiac CT shows normal closing of the bioprosthetic valve leaflets in diastole with mild hypoattenuated leaflet thickening (HALT) ➔ of all 3 leaflets. At systole, there is mild (< 50%) restricted motion of the posterior leaflet ➔.* **(Right)** *Aortic root long-axis cardiac CT demonstrates restricted leaflet motion ➔ of the posterior leaflet (< 50%) with HALT during systole. Note the normal closure of the leaflet during diastole and a well-seated Edwards-SAPIEN prosthetic valve ➔ in place.*

Left Ventricular Apical Aortic Conduit

KEY FACTS

IMAGING

- **Definition**: Extraanatomic valved graft connecting left ventricular apex to descending thoracic aorta
- Typically used in patients with severe aortic stenosis and porcelain aorta or other condition precluding median sternotomy (e.g., retrosternal coronary grafts)
- Rarely, complex congenital left ventricular outflow tract anomalies ± hypoplastic ascending aorta and arch
- **CT**
  - Gated CT best delineates graft course, implantation angle, proximal and distal anastomoses, and potential complications
  - Signs of infection include stranding, fluid collection with rim enhancement, and gas formation tracking to skin (fistula)
- **MRA**
  - Demonstrates morphologic and functional imaging of heart, conduit, and aorta
  - Phase-contrast MR may be used to quantify ventricular outflow fraction through valved conduit
- **Echocardiography**
  - May not visualize entire conduit, but presence of Doppler gradients across native left ventricular outflow tract indirectly suggests graft obstruction

PATHOLOGY

- Performed in presence of conditions precluding median sternotomy or aortic disease (porcelain aorta) or congenital disease precluding in situ valve replacement

CLINICAL ISSUES

- Avoid need to redo sternotomy
- Transcatheter aortic valve replacement in native valve position or conduit valve has been described to treat late apicoaortic conduit stenosis

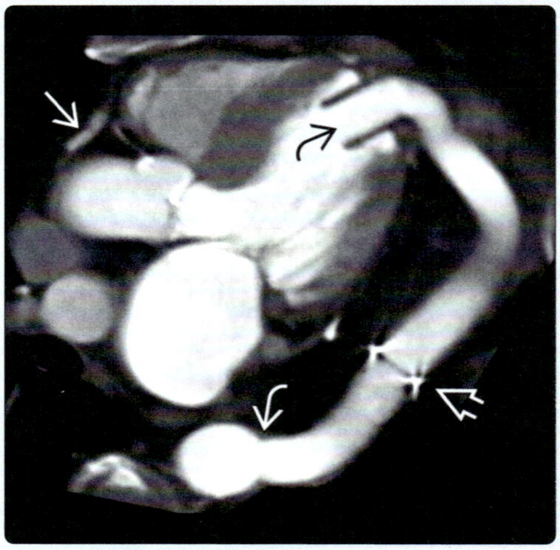

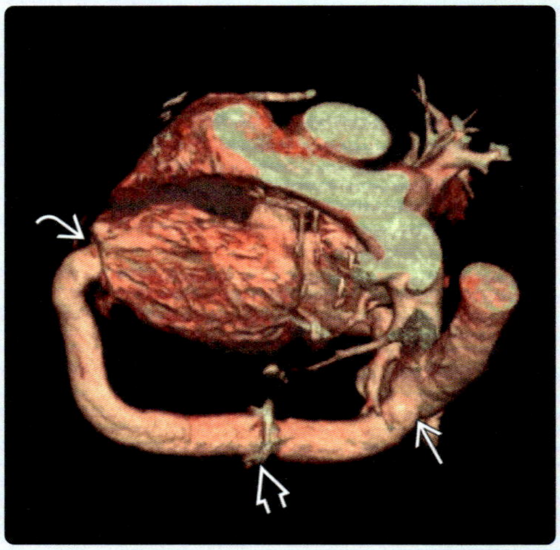

(Left) *Oblique cardiac CT shows an apicoaortic conduit in a patient with aortic stenosis, prior coronary artery bypass grafting (CABG) , and increased risk for redoing of sternotomy. Note the slightly oblique but unobstructed inflow cannula ostium , prosthetic valve with the conduit, and distal anastomosis to the descending thoracic aorta .* **(Right)** *Oblique cardiac CT VRT shows apicoaortic conduit exiting the left ventricular (LV) apex , prosthetic valve , and distal anastomosis with the descending aorta .*

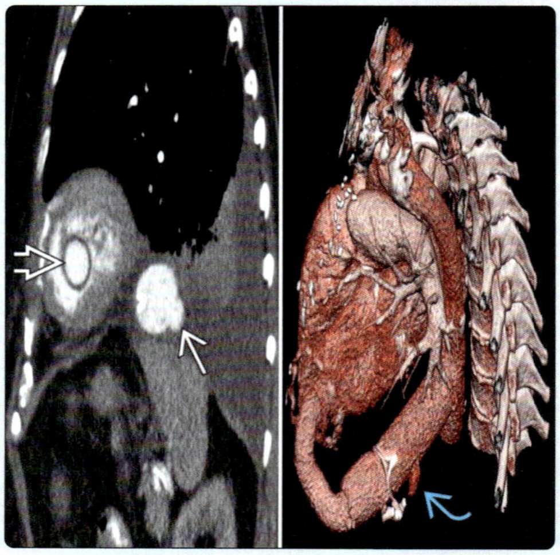

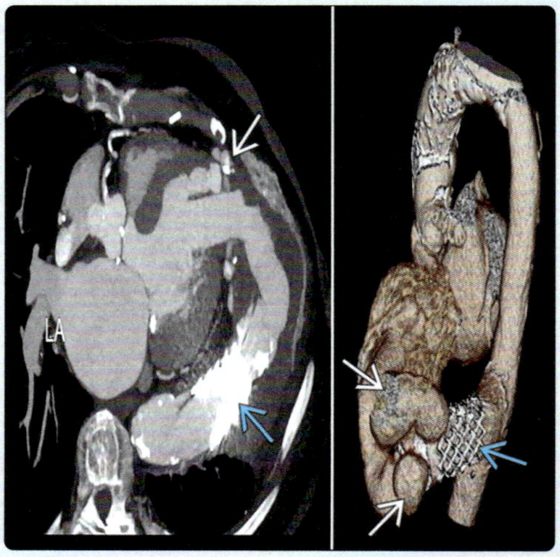

(Left) *Oblique CECT VRT shows a Carpentier-Edwards bioprosthetic valve with a small outpouching of contrast distal to the valve , corresponding to a cannulation site. Sagittal CECT reveals the inflow cannula in the LV and a small contrast leak beyond the conduit lumen .* **(Right)** *Oblique three-chamber cardiac CT and VRT show an LV conduit with stenting and multiple pseudoaneurysms near the apex in a patient with bicuspid aortic valve stenosis and prior CABG.*

TERMINOLOGY

Synonyms

- Apical aortic conduit; apicoaortic conduit
- Apicoaortic bypass

Definitions

- Extraanatomic valved graft connecting left ventricular apex to descending thoracic aorta

IMAGING

General Features

- Best diagnostic clue
  - Graft connected proximally to apex of left ventricle and distally to descending thoracic aorta or (rarely) to great vessels

Imaging Recommendations

- Best imaging tool
  - ECG-gated CT: Best delineates graft course, implantation angle, proximal and distal anastomoses, and potential complications
  - MR: Demonstrates graft course and may provide flow information
  - Echocardiography: May not visualize entire conduit, but presence of Doppler gradients across native left ventricular outflow tract indirectly suggests graft obstruction

Radiographic Findings

- Radiography
  - Complete metallic ring (conduit valve) or stented bioprosthetic valve can be seen in midportion of graft
    - May be visible lateral to apex on frontal radiograph and projected over inferior middle mediastinum on lateral views

CT Findings

- Ring of suture cuff can be seen as high-attenuation material surrounding inflow canula at apex and mimic pseudoaneurysms
- Signs of infection include stranding, fluid collection with rim enhancement, and gas formation tracking to skin (fistula)
  - May demonstrate pseudoaneurysms at anastomotic sites

MR Findings

- Morphologic and functional imaging of heart, conduit, and descending aorta
- Phase-contrast MR may be used to quantify ventricular outflow fraction through valved conduit

DIFFERENTIAL DIAGNOSIS

Ventricular Assist Device

- Apical left ventricular inflow cannula anastomosis with distal insertion into pump, not aorta
- 2nd tube graft from pump to (usually) ascending aorta (outflow cannula)

In Situ Valve Replacement

- May demonstrate complete metallic ring on radiograph; however, location will correspond to that of replaced valve

Coarctation Repair With Extraanatomic Bypass

- Tube graft from ascending aorta to descending aorta
- Not valved conduit

PATHOLOGY

General Features

- Performed in presence of conditions precluding median sternotomy or aortic disease (porcelain aorta) or congenital disease precluding in situ valve replacement
- Requires left thoracotomy approach

CLINICAL ISSUES

Demographics

- Age
  - Utilized in 2 distinctly different populations
    - 2-week- to 19-year-old patients
    - Older adult (~ 70 years) high-risk patients
- Sex
  - M = F (for congenital indications)
- Indications
  - Most common: Severe aortic stenosis in setting of porcelain aorta &/or patent coronary bypass graft precluding median sternotomy
  - Multiple previous sternotomies
  - Prior sternal wound infection
  - Multiple failed aortic valve replacements
  - Rarely: Complex congenital left ventricular outflow tract anomalies ± hypoplastic ascending aorta and arch

Natural History & Prognosis

- Longest known survival of functioning conduit graft is > 24 years

Treatment

- Transcatheter aortic valve replacement in native valve position or conduit valve has been described to treat late apicoaortic conduit stenosis

DIAGNOSTIC CHECKLIST

Consider

- Extend range of gated CT from arch/great vessels to below diaphragm (distal anastomosis location varies)

Image Interpretation Pearls

- Evaluate angle of apical graft with respect to ventricular septum as this may be flow limiting

SELECTED REFERENCES

1. Perlman GY et al: First transcatheter valve-in-valve implantation in an apicoaortic conduit. Catheter Cardiovasc Interv. 91(7):E86-9, 2018
2. Jneid H et al: Transcatheter aortic valve replacement as a treatment for late apicoaortic conduit obstruction in a patient with severe aortic stenosis. Circulation. 127(11):e491-4, 2013
3. Domoto S et al: Apicoaortic bypass for a patient with structural valve deterioration of a 19 mm bioprosthetic valve. Interact Cardiovasc Thorac Surg. 14(1):105-7, 2012
4. Filsoufi F et al: Apicoaortic conduit. Semin Thorac Cardiovasc Surg. 24(3):202-5, 2012
5. Nance JW et al: Apicoaortic conduits: indications, complications, and imaging techniques. J Thorac Imaging. 27(3):141-7, 2012
6. Elmistekawy E et al: Apico-aortic conduit for severe aortic stenosis: technique, applications, and systematic review. J Saudi Heart Assoc. 22(4):187-94, 2010

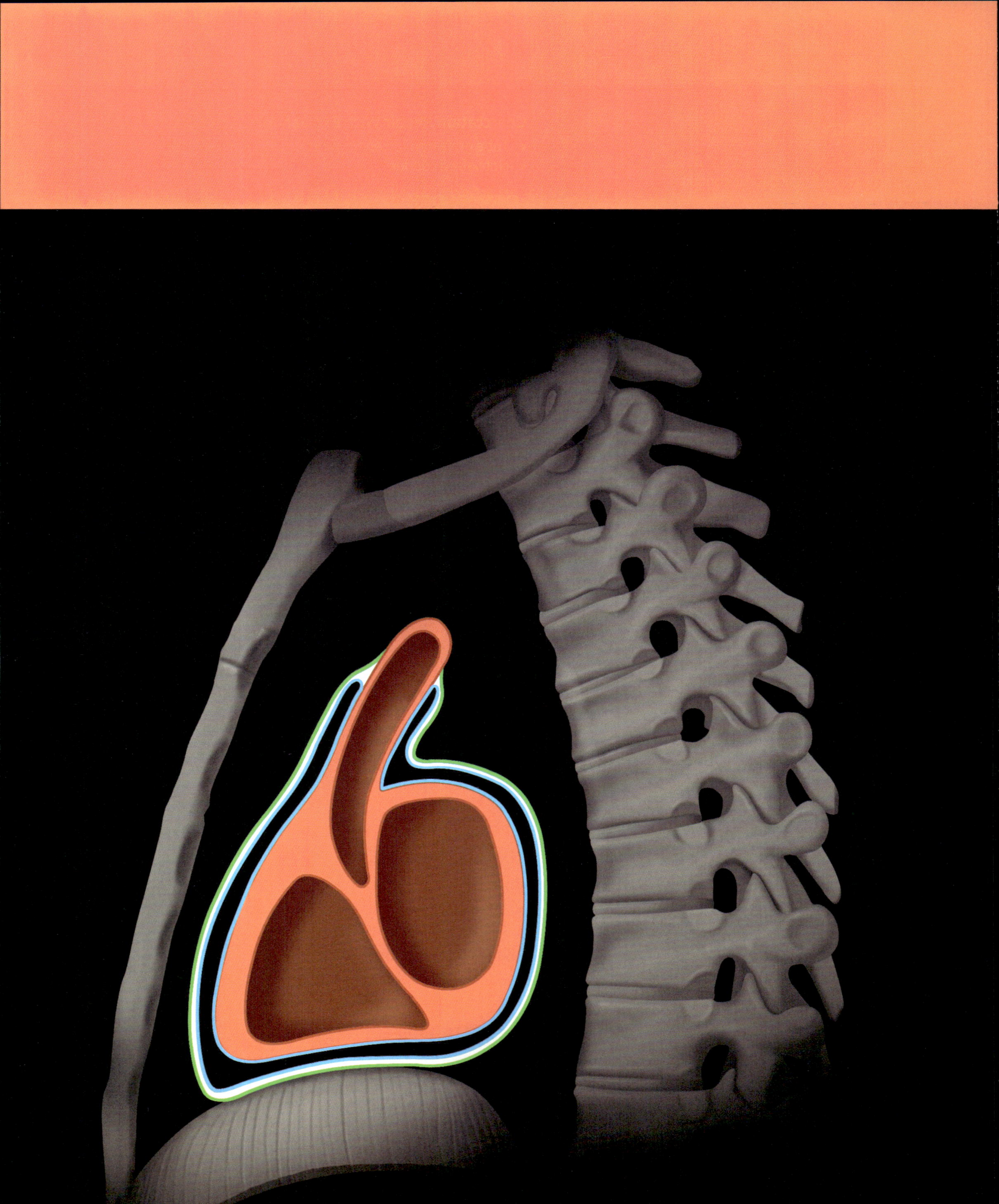

SECTION 5

Pericardial

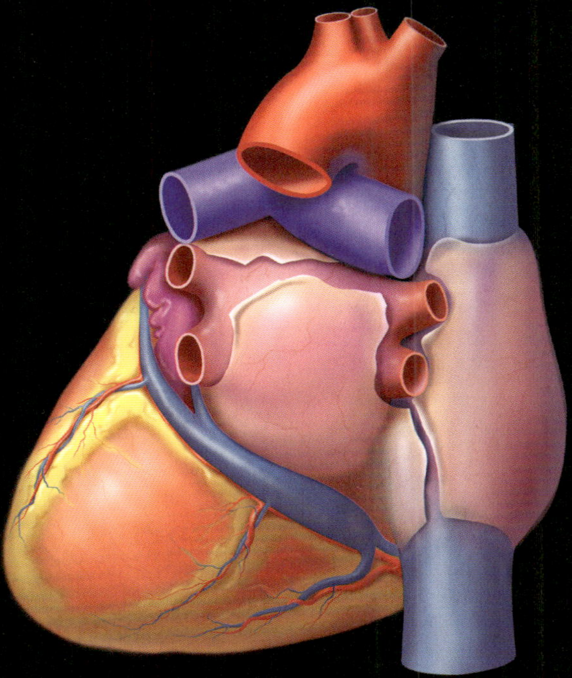

Introduction

A spectrum of lesions varying from inflammatory to neoplastic etiologies can involve the pericardium and alter cardiac function. The clinical presentation ranges from nonspecific to unequivocal physical and physiologic findings. Noninvasive imaging techniques, such as echocardiography, CT, and cardiac MR (CMR), play an important role in resolving the diagnostic dilemma in patients with suspected pericardial disease.

Imaging Test Selection

Echocardiography is the 1st-line imaging modality in the evaluation of pericardial pathologies. CT and CMR enjoy a number of advantages, especially in cases of loculated or hemorrhagic effusion, constrictive pericarditis, and pericardial masses. CT and CMR not only provide excellent delineation of the pericardial anatomy but can also aid in the characterization of different pericardial lesions. Although certain pericardial abnormalities can be identified on chest radiography, this modality plays a limited role. Cardiac catheterization can provide invasive hemodynamics in challenging cases of pericardial constriction.

Pericardial Effusion and Cardiac Tamponade

Common causes of pericardial effusion include heart failure, infection (viral, bacterial, and tuberculosis), neoplasia, injury (from trauma, myocardial infarction, and aortic dissection), and radiation therapy. Detection of pericardial effusion may also occur in asymptomatic patients who are imaged for other reasons.

Large pericardial effusion can be seen on chest radiographs as an enlarged cardiac silhouette (water bottle configuration) and the absence of pulmonary edema. Echocardiography is the modality of choice with simple pericardial effusion appearing as an anechoic space within the pericardial cavity. Further investigation with CT and CMR is indicated when loculated or hemorrhagic effusion or pericardial thickening is suspected or when findings on echocardiography are inconclusive. Because of the wide field of view, CT and CMR can easily identify loculated effusions, especially those in anterior locations.

CT attenuation measurement can facilitate initial characterization of pericardial fluid. On CT, simple pericardial effusion (transudate) has density similar to water attenuation (< 10 HU). Attenuation greater than water suggests hemopericardium, purulent exudates, malignancy, or effusion associated with hypothyroidism. Chylopericardium, which is rare, may resemble transudate effusion.

Acute hemopericardium has higher density (range: 60-80 HU), whereas subacute hematomas may resemble exudative effusion and, sometimes, can be difficult to distinguish from transudative effusion. On MR, nonhemorrhagic fluid appears as low signal on T1-weighted images and has high signal intensity on T2-weighted and cine steady-state free procession (SSFP) images. Conversely, hemorrhagic effusion is characterized by high signal intensity on T1-weighted images and low intensity on T2-weighted and cine images. Subacute and chronic hematomas are usually heterogeneous with both high- and low-signal regions on T1-weighted images. When pericardial effusion is secondary to a malignancy, an irregularly thickened pericardium or pericardial nodularity may be observed. Pericardial thickening and enhancement is seen in pericardial inflammation. Small amounts of pericardial fluid can be misinterpreted on CT because their appearance is similar to pericardial thickening. MR can distinguish low signal of normal parietal pericardium from high signal intensity of small effusion on T2-weighted and cine images.

Acute accumulation of pericardial fluid may result in an effusion under tension or cardiac tamponade. Tamponade occurs when cardiac chambers are compressed to the point of compromising systemic venous return to the right heart chamber. Transthoracic echocardiography (TTE) is the imaging modality of choice to assess cardiac tamponade. However, the size of effusion does not always reflect the hemodynamic significance of pericardial effusion. Typical echocardiographic findings include late diastolic collapse of the right atrium and early diastolic collapse of the right ventricle. Persistence of right atrial collapse for > 1/3 of the cardiac cycle is highly sensitive and specific for tamponade. Left atrial collapse, which can also occur in tamponade, is very specific but not sensitive for tamponade. Other findings include respiratory variation in mitral and tricuspid inflow, ventricular interdependence, plethora of inferior vena cava, and prominence of diastolic reversals in hepatic veins by pulsed Doppler. CT and CMR are useful when TTE is inconclusive due to larger body habitus or in postoperative setting, and more detailed quantification of pericardial effusion is necessary, especially when loculated.

Pericarditis

Pericarditis refers to inflammation of the pericardium in response to a host of conditions and may or may not be associated with pericardial effusion. Pericarditis may occur as an isolated abnormality or manifestation of an underlying abnormality. Pericarditis can present with or without constriction of the heart.

Nonconstrictive Pericarditis

Nonconstrictive pericarditis can be further classified as acute or chronic. Pericarditis may occur as an isolated abnormality or as a manifestation of an underlying abnormality. The underlying cause may be infection (usually viral-like coxsackievirus B, echovirus, or tuberculosis), inflammatory (such as systemic lupus erythematosus, rheumatoid arthritis, and uremia), HIV, or radiation. The diagnosis of pericarditis is usually suspected clinically and supported by ECG and serum enzymes. Complementary diagnostic modalities can be used when nonimaging diagnostic tools are inconclusive and for detection of complications related to pericarditis.

The chest radiograph is often normal, although it should be considered to exclude other pulmonary or mediastinal pathologies. TTE is often the initial imaging modality of choice. TTE is recommended to exclude cardiac tamponade, guide diagnostic or therapeutic pericardiocentesis, and when there are features of constrictive physiology. In the proper clinical setting, smooth pericardial thickening (≥ 4 mm) with enhancement on cardiac CT and CMR is suggestive of acute pericarditis. With increasing duration of pericardial inflammation, the smooth pericardium may eventually become irregular. When associated with pericardial effusion, CT attenuation and MR signal characteristics will vary depending on transudative or exudative effusion. One of the important drawbacks of CT is the inability to differentiate small pericardial effusions from pericardial thickening. On CMR, the signal intensity of the pericardium may vary depending on the extent of inflammatory or granulation tissue in acute pericarditis and fibrous tissue or calcification in chronic pericarditis.

Imaging Modalities in Evaluation of Pericardial Disease

Echocardiography	Cardiac CT	Cardiac MR
Advantages		
1st-line imaging modality for initial diagnosis and follow-up of pericardial disease	Superior anatomic details; 3D postprocessing and cine capabilities; not operator dependent	Better contrast resolution and superior tissue characterization; direct multiplanar and cine imaging; less operator dependent
Low cost, safe, widely available, and does not use ionizing radiation; quickly performed, especially as bedside test in hemodynamically unstable patients	Visualization of entire heart and pericardium, easy detection of pericardial calcification; detection and characterization of extracardiac findings that may explain presenting symptom(s); best test to evaluate associated or causative lung findings, such as edema or cancer	Visualization of entire heart and pericardium; morphologic and functional information; detection and characterization of extracardiac findings
Limitations		
Operator dependent with limited acoustic window and narrow field of view; technical difficulties in postcardiac surgery and with patients who are obese or have chronic obstructive pulmonary disease; limited tissue characterization	Relatively higher cost, ionizing radiation, and occasional need for iodinated contrast; challenges in patients with tachycardia and irregular heartbeat; no capability for direct flow velocity quantification	More cost and time consuming; contraindicated in patients with some metallic devices and in patients with glomerular filtration rate < 30 mL/min; detection of calcification can be challenging

As on CT, postcontrast enhancement can be seen on CMR. The use of delayed enhancement and CMR is proposed to be a more sensitive method for identifying pericardial inflammation. In general, CT and CMR are used in cases of therapeutic difficulties and complications from acute pericarditis, such as failure to respond to treatment in the recurrent setting, to monitor disease activity and treatment response, or in chronic pericarditis with constrictive features. Cross-sectional imaging may also be considered when linked to specific conditions, such as neoplastic disorders, and involvement from an adjacent anatomic structure, such as empyema.

Constrictive Pericarditis

Constrictive pericarditis represents the end stage of an inflammatory process. In resource-rich countries, the most frequent causes are cardiac surgery and radiation therapy, as opposed to infection, and mostly tuberculosis in resource-limited countries. Constrictive pericarditis can clinically mimic restrictive cardiomyopathy, hepatic disease, and congestive heart failure. Clinically, it is difficult to differentiate between constrictive pericarditis and restrictive cardiomyopathy, but correct distinction between them is very important since only constrictive pericarditis can benefit from surgical pericardial stripping, and restrictive cardiomyopathy would not improve.

On chest radiograph, pericardial calcifications are strongly suggestive of constrictive pericarditis. However, calcifications are seen in only 20-40% of constrictive cases.

Echocardiography is usually the initial diagnostic imaging modality. An important reason to use echocardiography early in the diagnostic process is to rule out other more common causes of right-sided heart failure. Precise assessment of pericardial thickening may be difficult, but diastolic septal motion (septal bounce), a respiratory shift in the position of the interventricular septum, inferior vena cava plethora, and the presence of myocardial tethering are classic 2D features associated with pericardial constriction (none of them particularly sensitive or specific, however). Respiration-correlated Doppler techniques are particularly useful in the diagnosis of constrictive pericarditis. In restrictive cardiomyopathy, the mitral inflow velocity rarely shows respiratory variation, and hepatic vein systolic flow reversals are more prominent with inspiration.

Up to 20% of patients with constrictive pericarditis lack the typical respiratory changes in the presence of mixed constrictive-restrictive disease &/or markedly elevated left atrial pressure.

In equivocal situations after echocardiography, additional testing is greatly supported by the excellent anatomic depiction of the pericardium at CT and MR imaging. CT findings are centered on the demonstration of thickened (≥ 4 mm) or calcified pericardium with other signs of constriction, including distorted ventricles (conical, tubular, or bullet-shaped), sigmoid-shaped interventricular septum, large atria, coronary sinus, and inferior vena cava.

On CMR, changes similar to those on CT are appreciated. Unlike CT, calcification may not be very well visualized on CMR. Spin-echo sequences are useful to detect thickened pericardium, whereas limited pericardial thickening and pericardial effusions are better seen on cine sequences sensitive to pericardial fluid. Pericardial thickening may be limited to the right side of the heart or even to a smaller area, such as the atrioventricular groove. Neither pericardial thickening nor calcification are diagnostic of constrictive pericarditis, unless the patient also has symptoms of physiologic constriction.

Diastolic flattening of the septum and abrupt cessation of diastolic filling in cine images are features suggestive of constriction. Real-time MR imaging of the ventricular septum in the short-axis plane is highly accurate in diagnosing pericardial constriction. Exaggerated ventricular interdependence seen as exaggerated diastolic septal bowing/flattening toward the left ventricle in inspiration is indicative of constriction. Myocardial tagging, which uses a grid-like pattern, can assist in evaluating adherence and immobility of the pericardial-myocardial interface. However, the presence or absence of pericardial adhesions neither diagnoses nor excludes constrictive pericarditis.

Effusive Constrictive Pericarditis

Effusive constrictive pericarditis is a relatively uncommon pericardial syndrome characterized by elements of pericardial effusion/tamponade and features of constrictive pericarditis. In patients with effusive constrictive pericarditis, hemodynamics related to pericardial construction typically persist even after the pericardial fluid has been removed. Noninvasive imaging demonstrates key imaging findings of pericardial effusion, thickened pericardium, and hemodynamic evidence of constrictive physiology, which can be readily demonstrated by TTE, cardiac CT, or CMR.

Transient constrictive pericarditis can be seen in acute/subacute period of pericarditis. This may show features of constriction along with pericardial inflammation. These patients may benefit from medications and may not necessarily need pericardial stripping procedure.

Pericardial Masses

Pericardial masses are often detected initially on chest radiograph or TTE. CT and CMR are useful for further characterization of these masses. CT attenuation or MR signal intensity, contrast enhancement characteristics, and the presence or absence of blood flow on cine MR images can help differentiate pericardial masses. CT and MR imaging also provide a road map for cases that are considered suitable for surgical resection. Extension into or from the mediastinum and lungs can be readily assessed with CT and CMR.

Pericardial Cysts

Pericardial cysts are considered congenital in origin and often detected incidentally. On chest radiograph, they often present as radiopacity similar to water/soft tissue in the right cardiophrenic angle. On TTE, these appear as an echolucent lesion. However, smaller cysts and those outside the vicinity of a cardiac chamber may not be detected. It is important that they are not misinterpreted as pleural effusion. Contrast echocardiography may be used to exclude an anomalous systemic vein that may present in that location.

On cross-sectional imaging, pericardial cysts demonstrate smooth, thin walls and appear inseparable from the heart border. When connection with the pericardial cavity is maintained, it is known as a pericardial diverticulum and is often indistinguishable from a cyst. On CT, the attenuation is similar to that of water, and pericardial cysts do not enhance after contrast material administration. On MR imaging, they are nonenhancing and typically have low or intermediate signal intensity on T1-weighted images and homogeneous high intensity on T2-weighted images. Occasionally, highly proteinaceous content can be seen giving high signal intensity on T1-weighted images. Pericardial cysts may be at an unusual location and, occasionally, can be indistinguishable from thymic or bronchogenic cysts.

Pericardial Tumors

Primary pericardial tumors are rare, and most neoplastic pericardial diseases are related to metastases from extracardiac malignancies. Sometimes, the pericardium may be involved by a primary cardiac neoplasm of benign or malignant etiology. Benign pericardial tumors include lipoma, fibroma, teratoma, and hemangioma. Malignant tumors include mesothelioma and sarcomas. Lung, breast, and esophageal cancers and melanoma, lymphoma, and leukemia are common extracardiac malignancies that may involve the pericardium.

Chest radiograph plays no significant role. The use of TTE may be limited to detection and follow-up of pericardial effusion. Pericardial thickening/nodularity related to metastasis may be appreciated. Cardiac CT and CMR, in addition to characterization of pericardial tumor and effusion, also demonstrate local tumor extension.

Lipoma typically has low attenuation consistent with fat on CT images and high signal intensity on T1-weighted spin-echo images. Presence of fat &/or calcium in a pericardial mass on CT or MR suggests teratoma. Fibroma, although difficult to characterize on CT, demonstrates characteristically low signal intensity on T2-weighted images and is nonenhancing or shows heterogeneous enhancement because of poor vascularization.

Sarcomas typically present as large, heterogeneous, enhancing masses, often with foci of necrosis, and are frequently associated with pericardial effusion/hemopericardium. Primary malignant mesothelioma of the pericardium may manifest as pericardial effusion accompanied by pericardial nodules or plaques.

Congenital Absence of Pericardium

Most defects involving the pericardium are congenital but can be iatrogenic in nature or occur secondary to trauma. The partial form of congenitally absent pericardium is more common and occurs along the left side of the heart. It can also occur on the right side or at the diaphragmatic surface, although infrequently. On chest radiographs, leftward displacement of the heart and aortic knob, flattened left cardiac silhouette, long prominent pulmonary artery, radiolucency between the aortic knob and the main pulmonary artery, and a radiolucent band between the left hemidiaphragm and the base of the heart have been described. Exaggerated cardiac motion (especially along the posterior wall of the left ventricle), the false appearance of an enlarged right ventricular cavity due to shifting of axis, compressed atria, and altered apical imaging window toward the axilla can be appreciated on TTE. The findings on CT and MR imaging rely on the lack of visualization of the pericardium and on other signs, including displacement of the cardiac axis to the left side and posteriorly, prominent atrial appendage, and separation of the aorta and main pulmonary artery due to lung tissue interposition.

Patients with pericardial defects may also have 1 or more associated congenital abnormalities, such as patent ductus arteriosus, mitral valve stenosis, atrial septal defect, or tetralogy of Fallot, which are also detectable on CT or CMR. The partial absence of the pericardium is usually associated with an increased, but rare, risk of herniation and strangulation of the left atrial appendage. Surgical closure or enlargement of the defect is sometimes necessary to alleviate herniation.

Selected References

1. Wang TKM et al: Cardiac magnetic resonance imaging techniques and applications for pericardial diseases. Circ Cardiovasc Imaging. 15(7):e014283, 2022
2. Kligerman S: Imaging of pericardial disease. Radiol Clin North Am. 57(1):179-99, 2019
3. Rajiah P et al: MRI of the pericardium. Radiographics. 39(7):1921-2, 2019
4. Alajaji W et al: Noninvasive multimodality imaging for the diagnosis of constrictive pericarditis. Circ Cardiovasc Imaging. 11(11):e007878, 2018

Pericardial Effusion

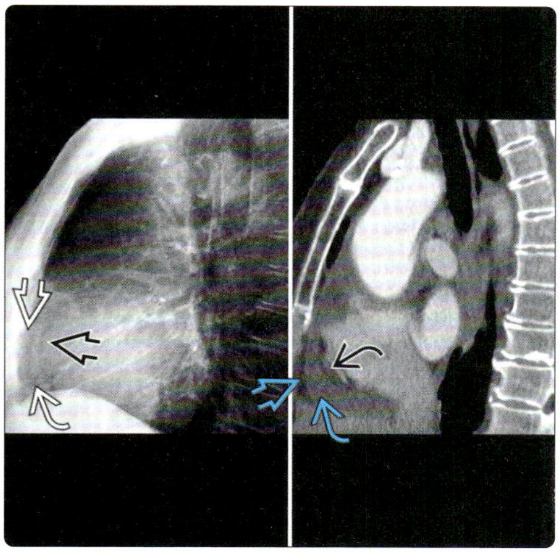

Pericardial Effusion

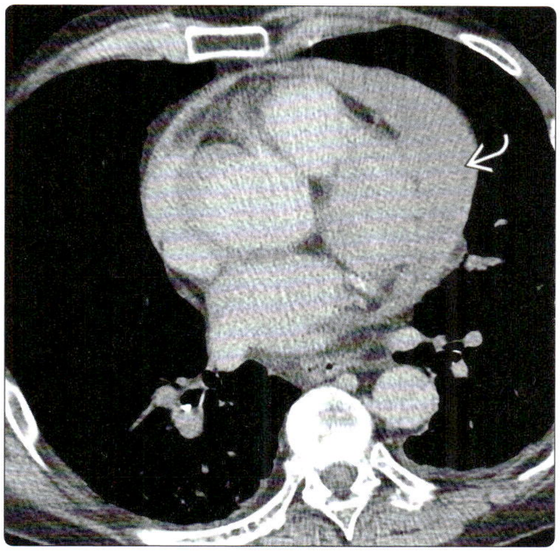

(Left) *Lateral chest radiograph shows opacity corresponding to a pericardial effusion ➡, which separates the retrosternal fat stripe ➡ (dark line parallel to the sternum, anterior to the effusion) and the epicardial fat stripe ➡ (dark line behind the effusion), the Oreo cookie sign. Sagittal CECT shows a pericardial effusion ➡ separating the retrosternal fat stripe ➡ and the epicardial fat stripe ➡.* **(Right)** *Axial CECT shows high-density pericardial fluid ➡, consistent with hemopericardium.*

Pericardial Effusion, Physiology

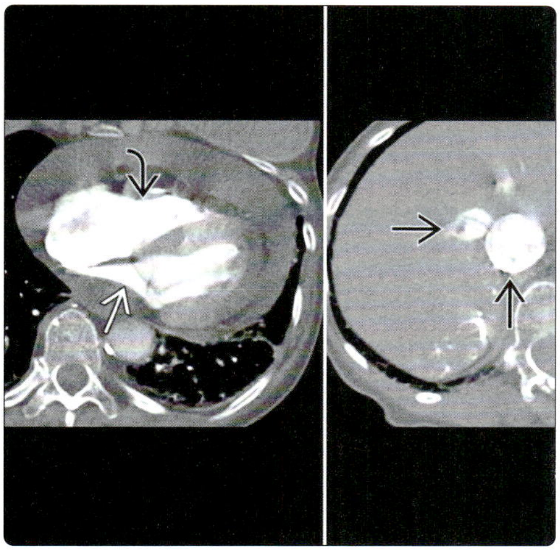

Pericardial Effusion, Physiology

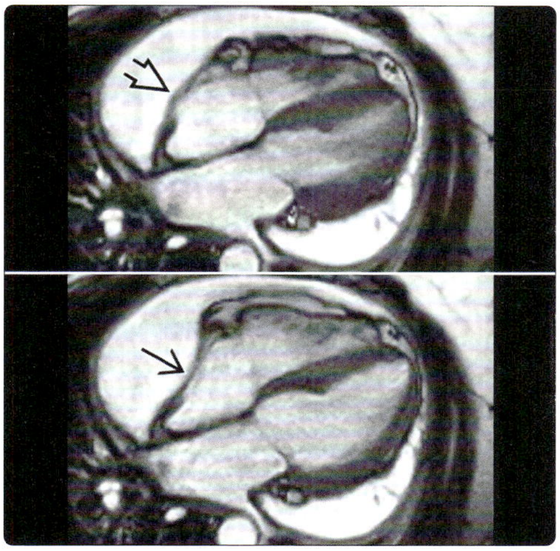

(Left) *Axial CTA shows large pericardial effusion with collapse of the right ventricle and some inversion of the anterior surface of the heart ➡. Also seen are an attenuated left atrium ➡ and reflux of contrast into the inferior vena cava and hepatic veins ➡, consistent with tamponade physiology.* **(Right)** *Four-chamber SSFP MRs show large pericardial effusion resulting in compression of the right atrial wall during early diastole ➡, consistent with cardiac tamponade. Note the normal configuration during systole ➡.*

Pericardial Calcification

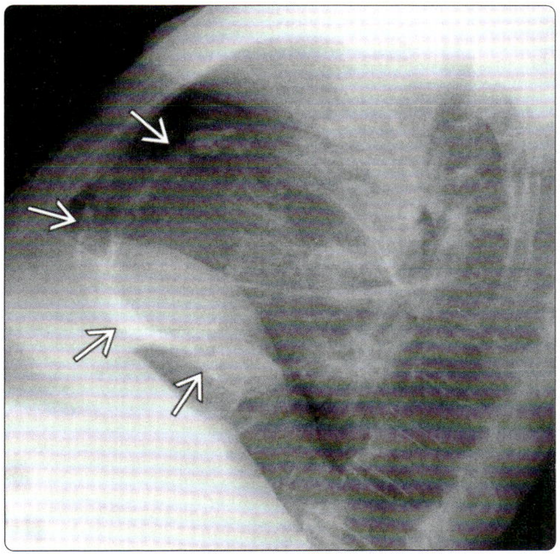

Pericardial Calcification

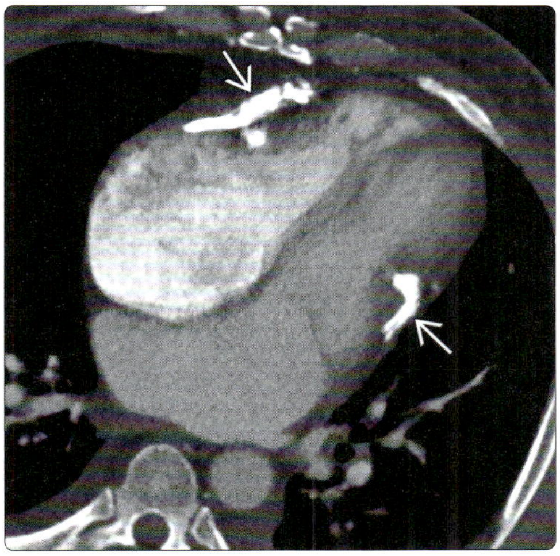

(Left) *Lateral chest radiograph shows extensive curvilinear calcification ➡ surrounding the heart shadow, consistent with pericardial calcification.* **(Right)** *Axial CT in the same patient shows extensive nodular pericardial calcification ➡, which compresses both ventricles and results in tubular, narrowed, and a deformed appearance of ventricles. Biatrial dilation is also present. Findings are commonly associated with constrictive pericarditis.*

(Left) *Short-axis DIR MR shows circumferential thickening of the pericardium with complex small pericardial effusion. Note that both parietal ➡ and visceral ➡ layers are significantly thickened. Normal pericardial thickness should be < 2 mm.* **(Right)** *Short-axis SSFP MR in the same patient shows circumferential pericardial thickening and small pericardial effusion. Note the heterogeneous appearance of the pericardial fluid with low-intensity areas demonstrating the complex nature of the fluid.*

Pericardial Thickening

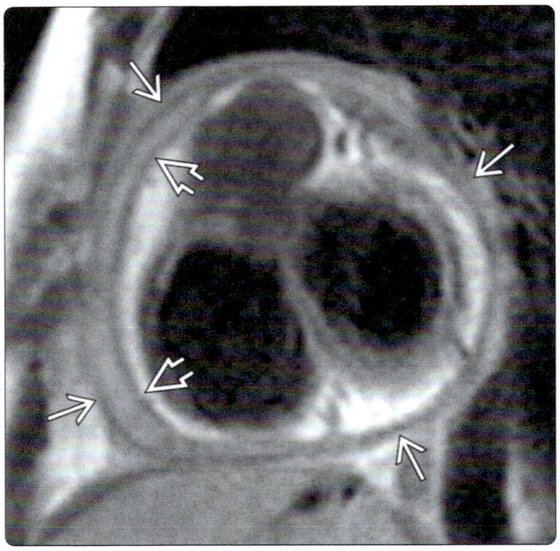

Pericardial Thickening

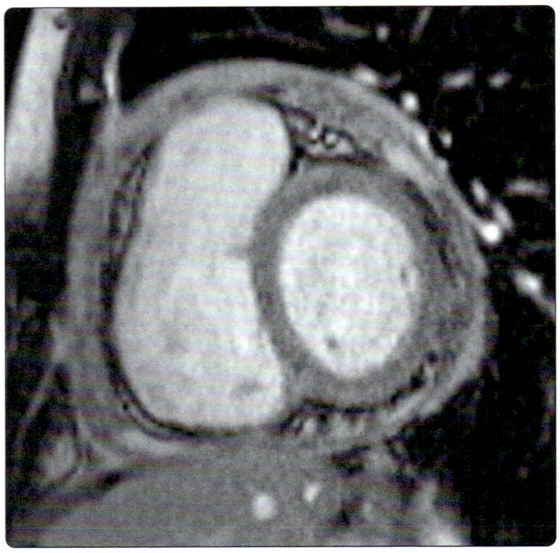

(Left) *Short-axis real-time cine images in the same patient show interventricular septal flattening during inspiration ➡ compared to the normal appearance of the septum during expiration ➡, demonstrating ventricular interdependence, a sign of constrictive physiology.* **(Right)** *Postcontrast MR shows diffuse circumferential enhancement of the pericardium ➡ in the same patient, indicating ongoing pericardial inflammation. The patient was diagnosed with acute inflammatory constrictive pericarditis.*

Ventricular Interdependence

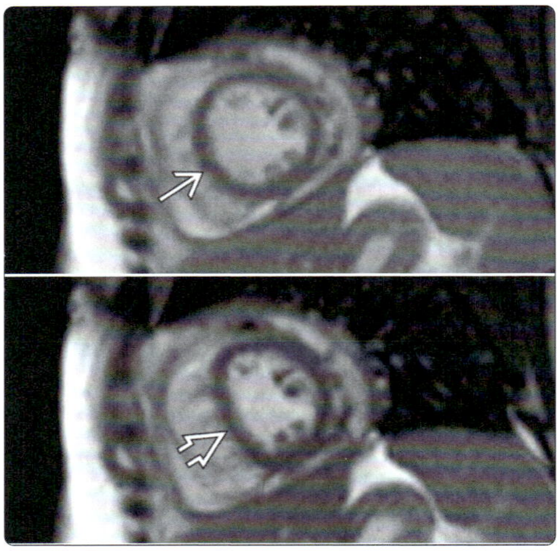

Pericardial LGE

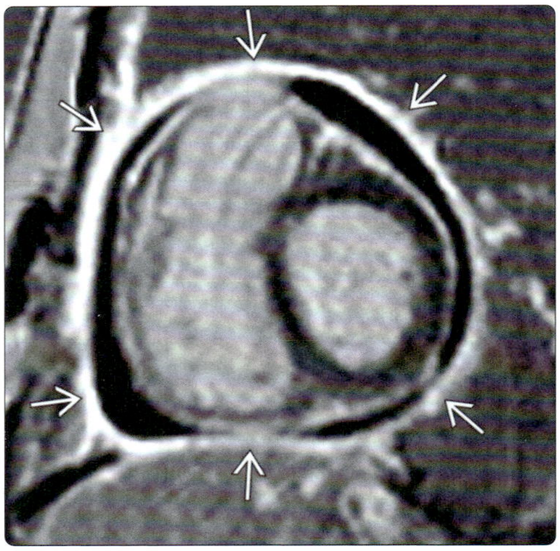

(Left) *Axial T2 fast spin-echo MR shows a bilobed right pericardial mass with homogeneous high signal intensity ➡ and a thin, smooth single septation.* **(Right)** *Axial T1 C+ FS MR in the same patient obtained at a similar level shows no enhancement of the mass ➡ and dark intrinsic signal similar to cerebrospinal fluid, which is indicative of a simple pericardial cyst.*

Pericardial Cyst

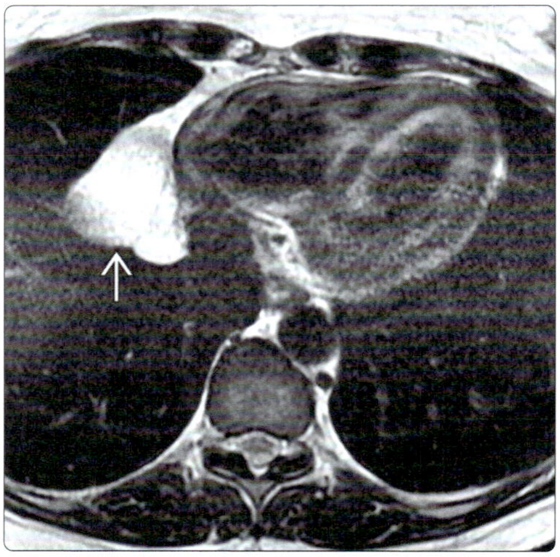

Pericardial Cyst

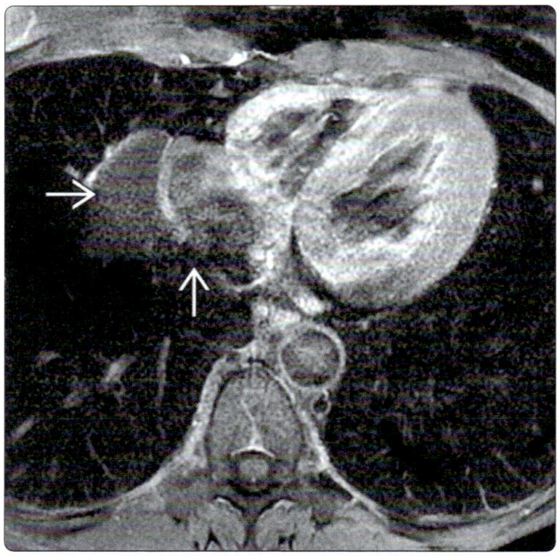

Pericardial Metastatic Disease

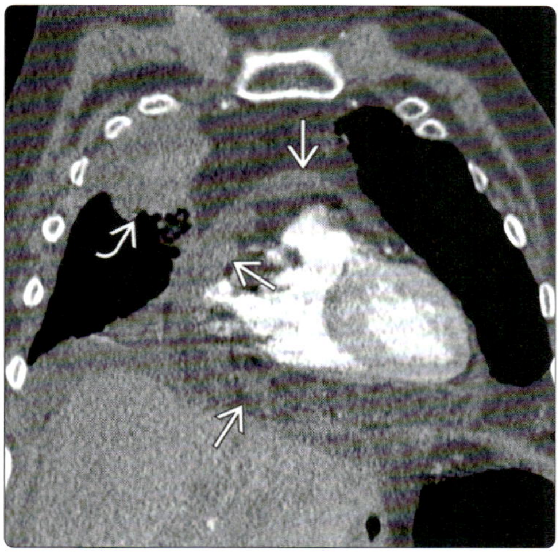

Primary Pericardial Lymphoma

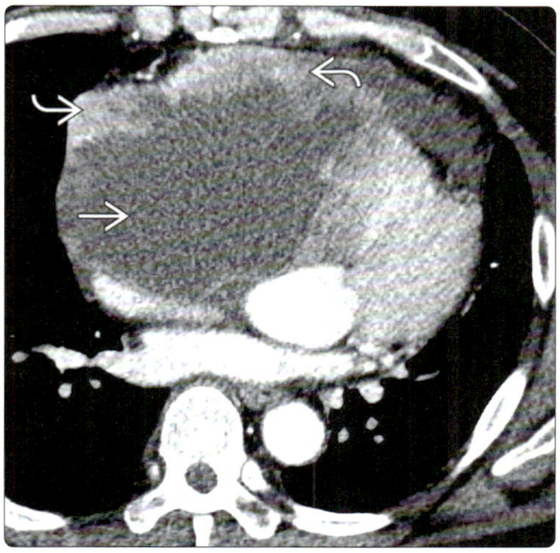

(Left) *Coronal CT shows nodular thickening and enhancement of the pericardium ➡ in a patient with right lung cancer ➡, consistent with pericardial metastatic disease.* **(Right)** *Axial CT shows a heterogeneous, irregular, lobulated, heterogeneously enhancing, large soft tissue mass involving the atrioventricular groove ➡ and pericardium ➡ in setting of lymphoma. Given lymphoma elsewhere, this is secondary cardiac involvement. Primary pericardial lymphoma can rarely occur.*

Primary Pericardial Sarcoma

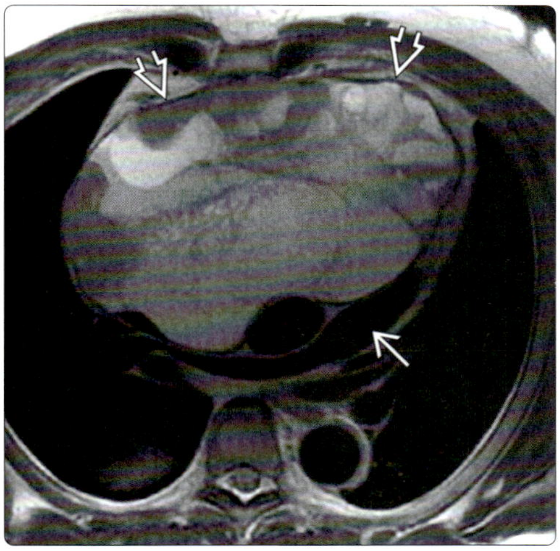

Primary Pericardial Sarcoma

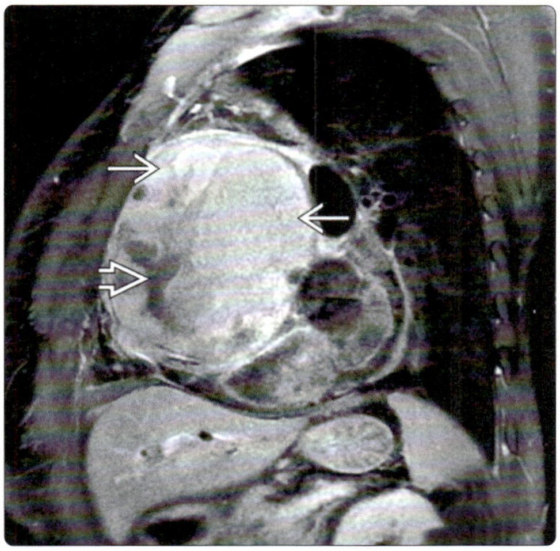

(Left) *Axial T2 FS MR shows a large, complex, heterogeneous-signal mass ➡ centered within the space between the heart ➡ and the overlying pericardial layers.* **(Right)** *Sagittal T1 C+ MR in the same patient shows a mass centered anterior to the right ventricle and great vessels with mass effect displacing the chambers posteriorly. Heterogeneous enhancement ➡ with nonenhancing areas is suggestive of necrosis ➡ in this case of primary pericardial sarcoma.*

Partial Absence of Pericardium

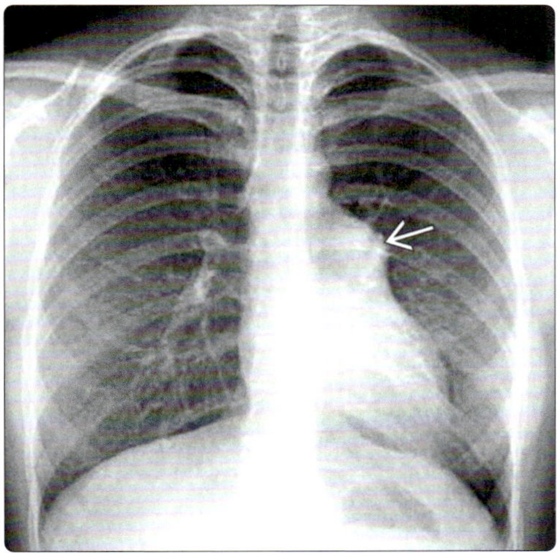

Partial Absence of Pericardium

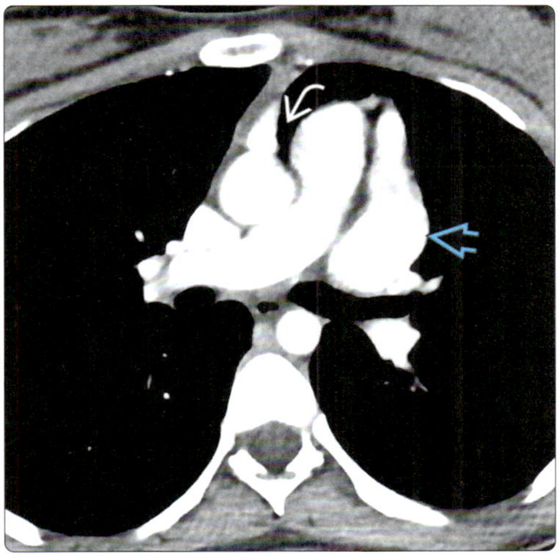

(Left) *Frontal radiograph demonstrates prominent convex deformity of the left atrial appendage ➡ secondary to partial absence of the pericardium.* **(Right)** *Axial CECT in the same patient shows interposition of lung tissue between the aorta and the main segment of the pulmonary artery ➡, indicating the absence of the pericardium in this area. Note the prominence of the atrial appendage ➡.*

TERMINOLOGY

Synonyms

- Parietal pericardium = fibrous pericardium [plus its inner layer (serous pericardium)] = often simply referred to as pericardium
- Visceral pericardium = serous pericardium = epicardium

Definitions

- Pericardium: Double-layered sac of serous and fibrous membranes connected to mediastinum, sternum, and diaphragm (outer layer), which envelops cardiac surfaces and proximal great vessels and venae cavae (inner layers)
- Sac contains small physiologic amount of fluid (15-50 mL) that enables nearly friction-free motion of heart within mediastinum
- Outer layer composed of fibrous pericardium and parietal portion of serous pericardium
  - Resulting layer up to 2 mm thick; often simply referred to as pericardium
  - Opposing visceral serous pericardium that covers heart; often referred to as epicardium
- Serous layer of pericardium formed by single layer of mesothelial cells

IMAGING ANATOMY

Overview

- Epicardium covers heart and epicardial fat layer within which coronary arteries and cardiac veins run; epicardium gives heart glistening appearance when pericardial sac is opened during surgery
- At pericardial reflections, serous pericardium folds upon itself and continues as parietal serous pericardium, which is fused with fibrous pericardium; these 2 layers form parietal pericardium or simply pericardium (as opposed to epicardium)
- Pericardial reflections form potential spaces called sinuses, which have several extensions known as pericardial recesses

GROSS ANATOMY

Fibrous Pericardium

- Outer layer of parietal pericardium, composed of several interwoven layers of collagen fibers with few interspersed elastic fibrils; this leaves only limited capacity to stretch
  - Consequently, rapidly accumulating effusions may lead to cardiac compression and tamponade physiology, even if only moderate in size, whereas slowly accumulating effusions may become quite large but not lead to tamponade
  - Inner aspect of fibrous pericardium lined with thin layer of serous pericardium

Serous Pericardium

- Lines both heart and epicardial fat (epicardium) as well as fibrous pericardium; consists of single layer of mesothelial cells

Pericardial Attachments

- Fibrous pericardium interweaves with great vessel adventitia and is anchored to central tendon of diaphragm inferiorly and to sternum anteriorly via sternopericardial ligament
- Epicardium is in direct continuity with cardiac fat layer (epicardial fat); pericardium surrounded by fat anteriorly (pericardial fat) and posteriorly
  - Pericardial fat pad = accumulations of pericardial fat near left ventricular apex and cardiophrenic angles; may mimic masses on radiographs but readily identified as benign fat on CT or MR

Pericardial Sinuses

- Reflection of pericardium posterior to atria forms oblique sinus, which is cul-de-sac that extends to carina; pericardial reflection posterior to aorta and pulmonary trunk and cranial to left atrium forms transverse sinus
- Sinuses connect with several recesses formed by pericardial reflections along junction of right atrium and superior vena cava (post caval recess) and along pulmonary vein ostia (right and left pulmonary venous recesses)
  - Inferior aortic recess lies between ascending aorta and right atrium and extends to transverse sinus
  - Superior pericardial recess covers posterior right proximal 3 cm of aortic root and right pulmonary artery and extends to transverse sinus
- Sinuses and recesses: Potential spaces that become visible when filled with fluid
  - Small amounts of physiologic fluid in sinuses may mimic adenopathy or mediastinal masses on CT
  - Pericardial fluid in superior pericardial recess may mimic aortic dissection or intramural hematoma on CT

Pericardiophrenic Bundle

- Space between mediastinal portion of parietal pleura and parietal pericardium contains nerve and vascular bundle running in craniocaudal direction
  - Bundle contains phrenic nerves and pericardiophrenic artery and veins
  - Traverses mediastinum and extends to both right and left diaphragm
  - Surgical injury to this bundle may result in diaphragmatic paralysis or elevation

ANATOMY IMAGING ISSUES

Imaging Recommendations

- Normal pericardial thickness on CT is 2 mm; abnormally thick pericardium > 3 mm may be associated with constriction, although not diagnostic
  - Of note, normal-thickness pericardium does not exclude constriction
- CT best test to identify pericardial calcifications
- MR best test to identify pericardial adhesions; achieved by applying tag lines orthogonal to pericardium on cine imaging

Imaging Pitfalls

- Pockets of fluid within pericardial recesses and sinuses can be mistaken for mediastinal adenopathy or masses

ANTERIOR VIEW OF PERICARDIAL SAC IN SITU AND WITH ANTERIOR PARIETAL PERICARDIUM REMOVED

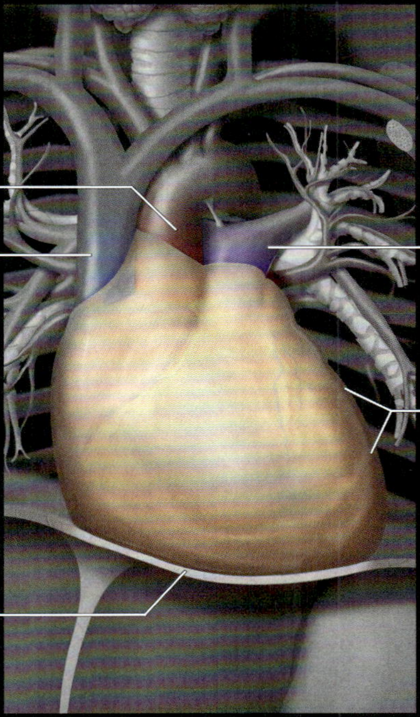

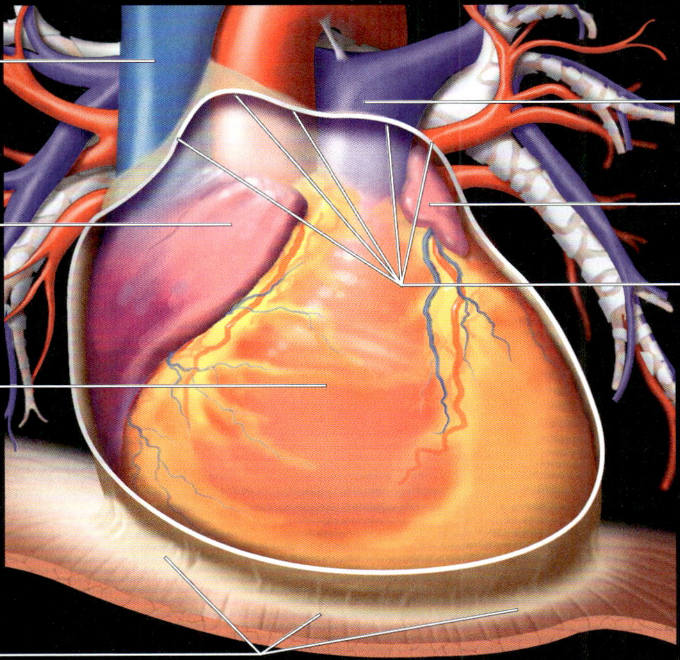

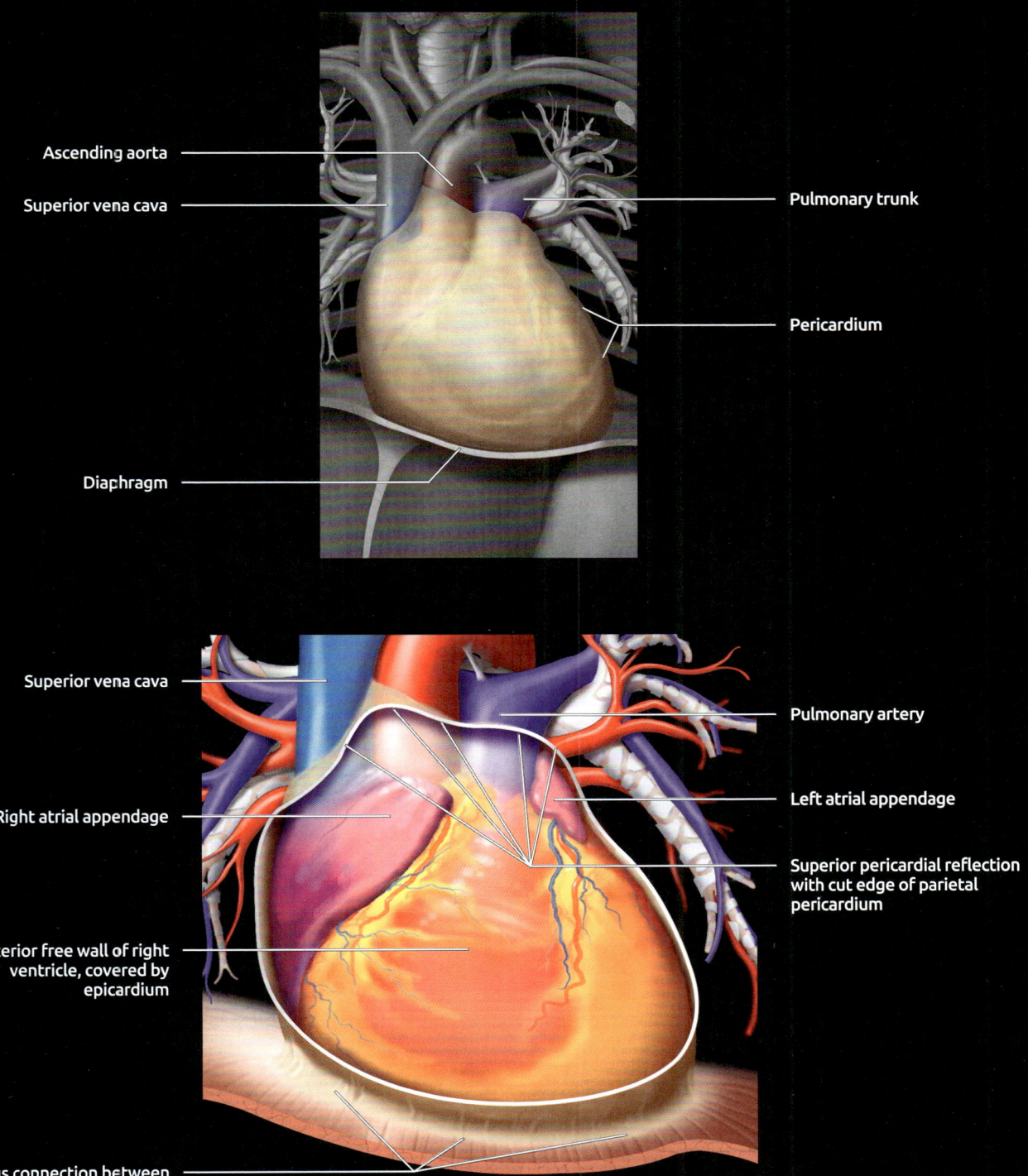

(Top) *The pericardium is a sac-like membrane that surrounds the heart and the origins of the great vessels. It has a conical shape with the apex of the cone oriented inferiorly and to the left. The pericardium normally contains 15-50 mL of serous fluid that provides lubrication of its apposing serous surfaces during cardiac motion. Although the heart can move relatively freely and change its morphology within the pericardial cavity, the pericardium poses some restrictions on cardiac motion and pericardial fluid volume.* **(Bottom)** *Anterior view shows the heart and pericardium with portions of the anterior parietal pericardium removed to allow viewing of the heart and its glistening visceral pericardium. Note that the pericardial reflections are ~ 3 cm above the origins of the aorta and pulmonary arteries. Note coronary arteries, cardiac veins, and epicardial fat "shining through" the glistening epicardium, a.k.a. visceral pericardium or epicardium.*

VISCERAL PERICARDIUM, POSTERIOR VIEW, PARIETAL PERICARDIUM WITH HEART REMOVED

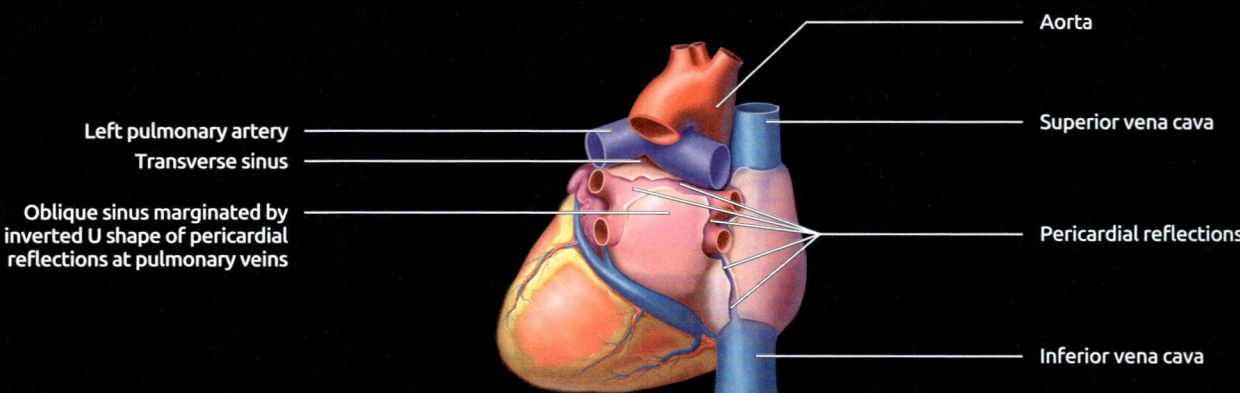

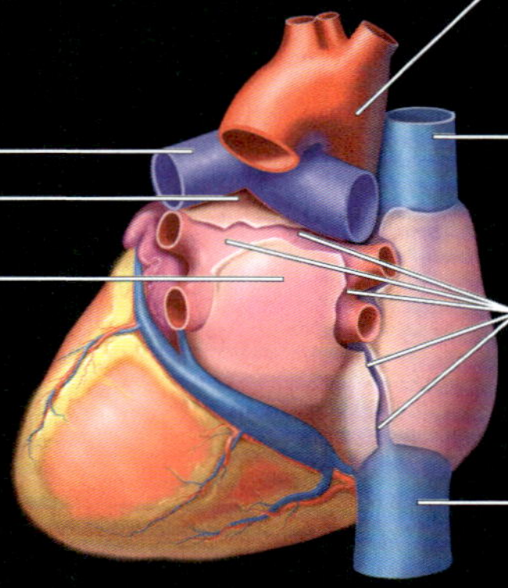

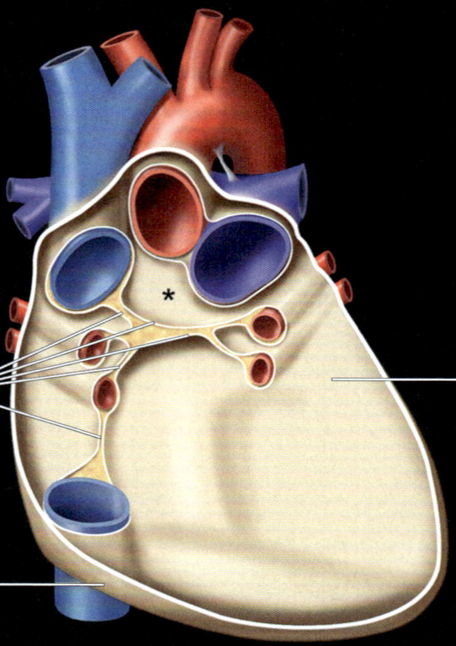

(Top) *Posterior graphic of the heart after removal of the parietal pericardium shows cut edges of the pericardial reflections at the pulmonary veins and venae cavae. Most of the heart is covered by the serous visceral pericardium. The space above the left atrial roof and below the pulmonary artery and posterior to the aortic root is termed the transverse sinus. After opening the pericardium, the surgeon may put a finger or instrument through this space, and, occasionally, a bypass graft is routed through it.* **(Bottom)** *Anterior view shows the posterior portions of the parietal pericardium and its reflections with the heart removed (view from inside the pericardial space). Asterisk denotes transverse sinus.*

CROSS-SECTIONAL APPEARANCE OF PERICARDIUM

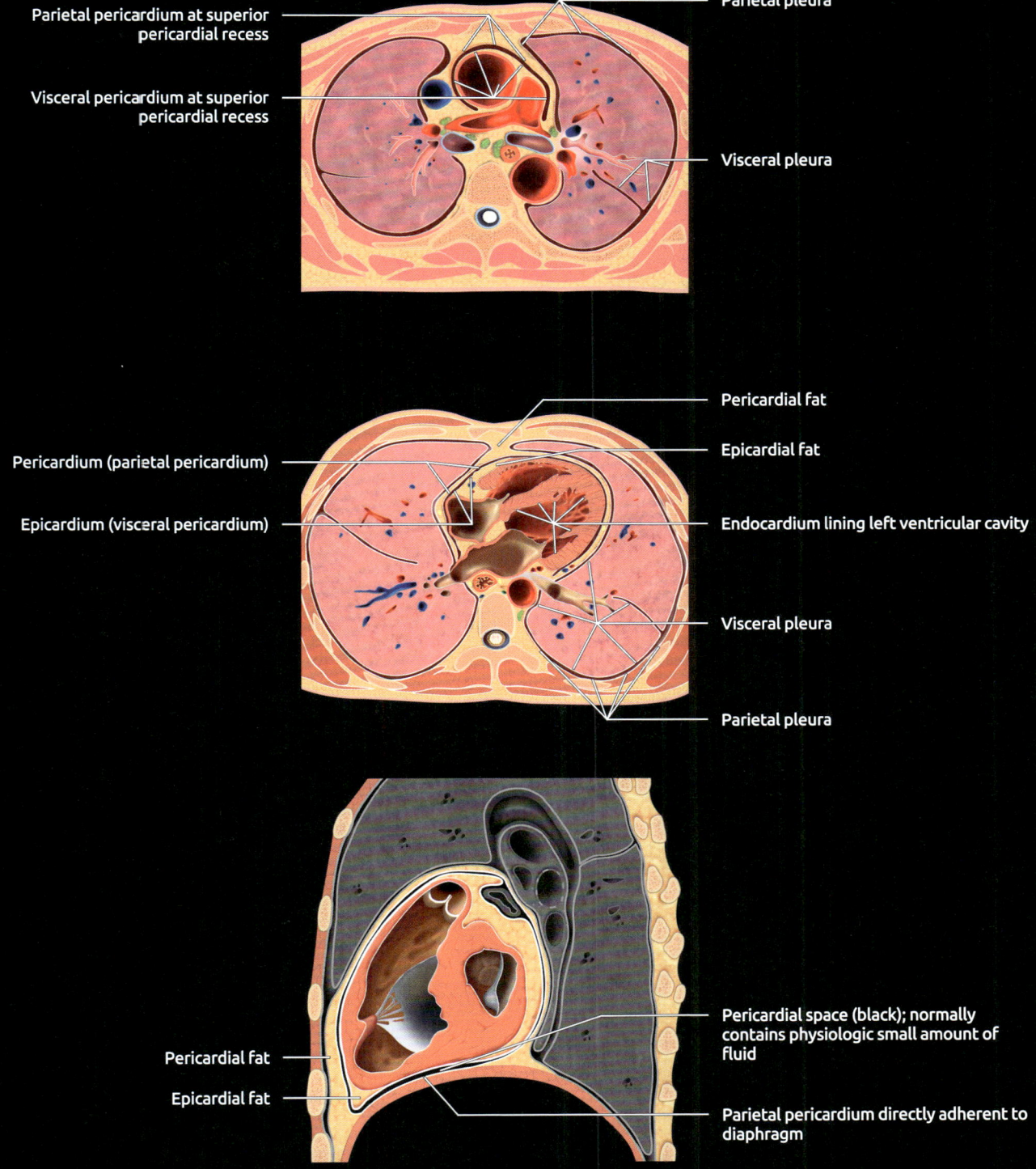

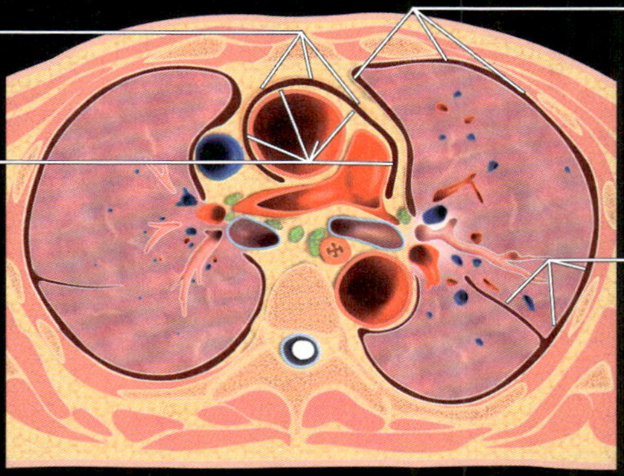

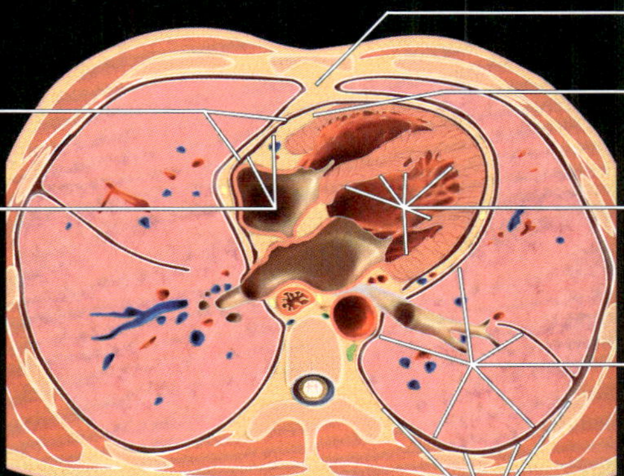

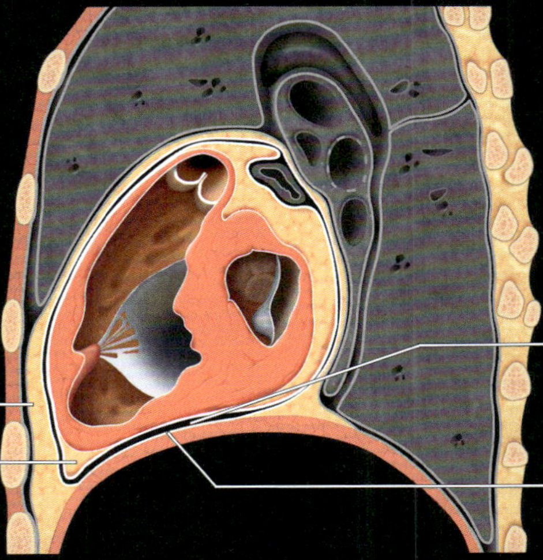

(Top) *Graphic shows an axial section at the level of the pulmonary artery bifurcation. The superior aortic recess is illustrated, which extends ~ 3 cm above the aortic root.* **(Middle)** *Graphic shows an axial section at the level of the fossa ovalis. The pericardium covers nearly all surfaces of the heart. The parietal pericardium is directly attached to the parietal pleural laterally. The phrenic nerve, artery, and vein run in a craniocaudal direction within the space between the pleura and pericardium.* **(Bottom)** *Graphic shows a sagittal section through the heart at the level of the right ventricular outflow tract. The pericardium separates the pericardial or mediastinal fat from the epicardial fat. The coronary arteries are embedded in the epicardial fat and are therefore a.k.a. the epicardial arteries.*

PERICARDIAL ANATOMY ON AXIAL MDCT

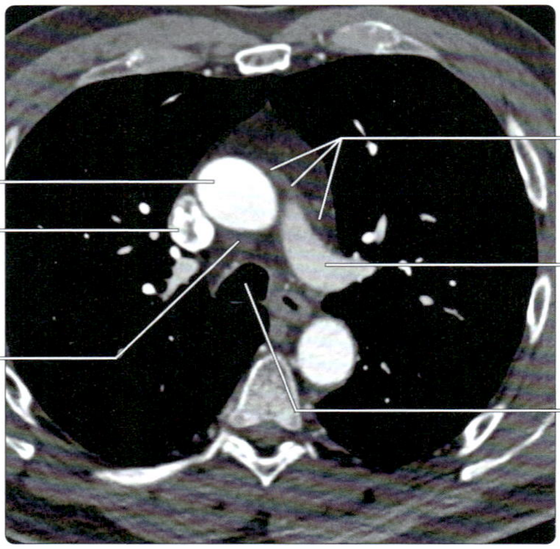

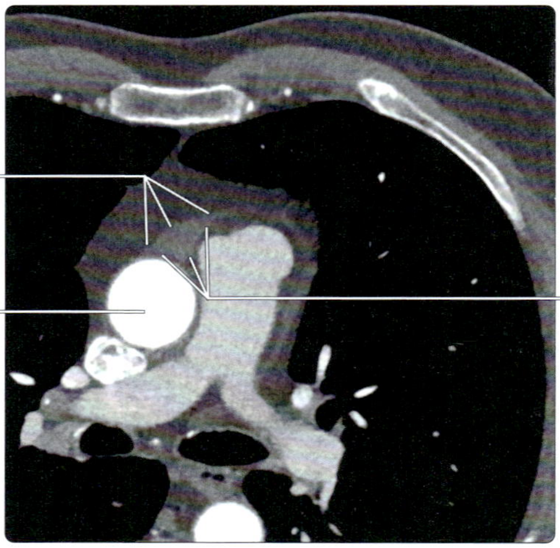

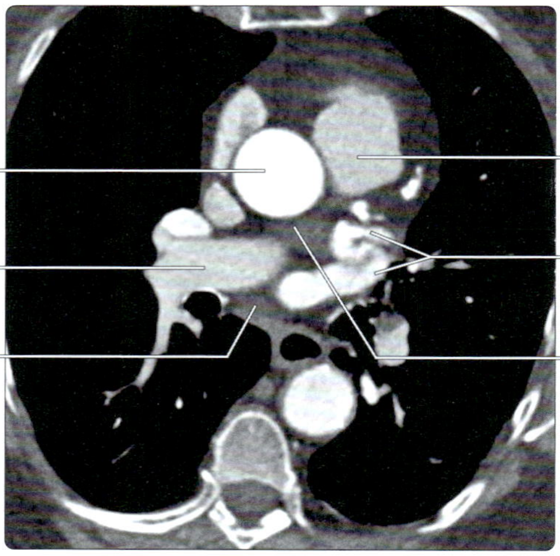

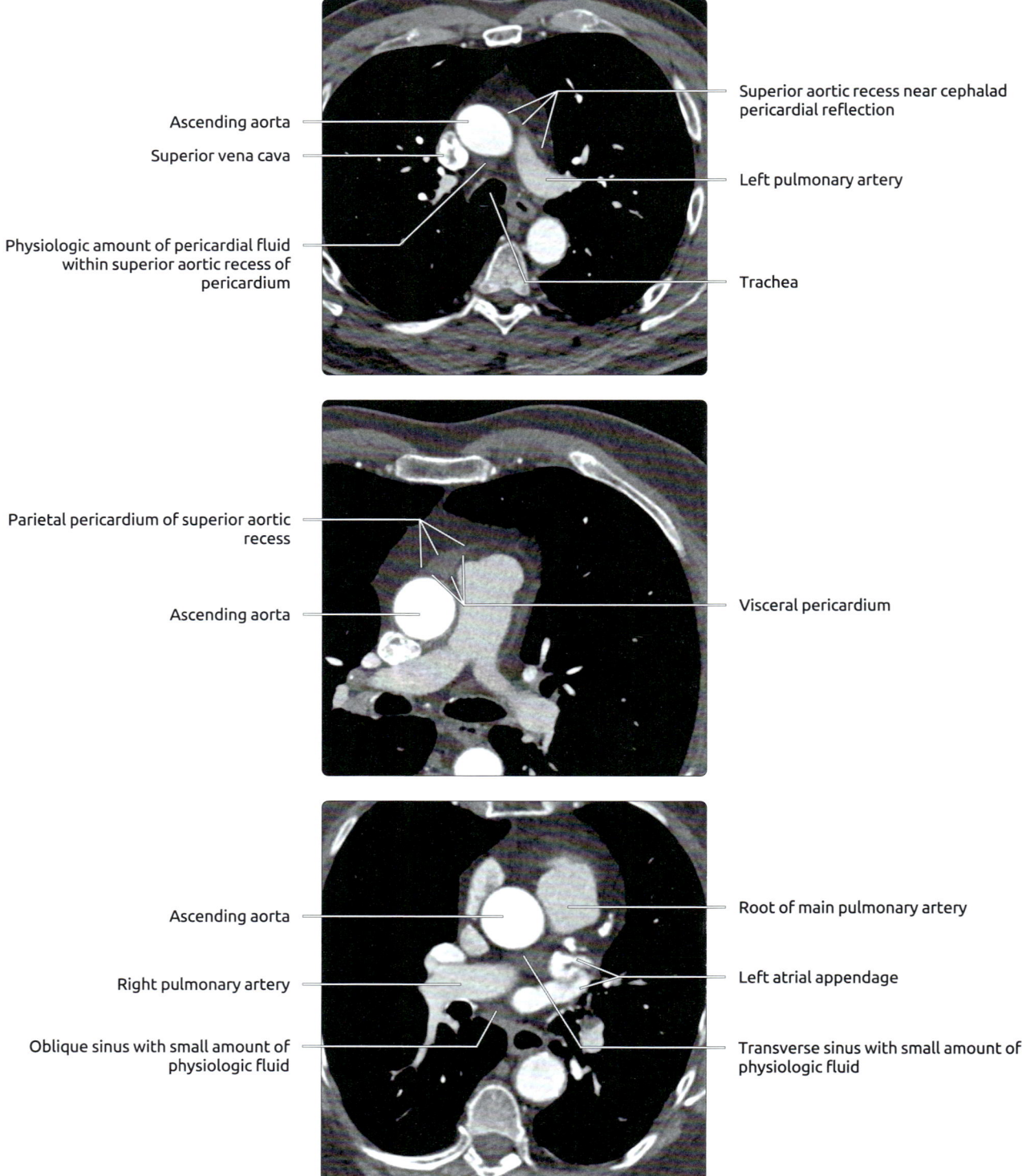

(Top) *Axial contrast-enhanced cardiac CT at the level of the trachea just above the carina shows the most cephalad extent of the pericardium, the superior aortic recess. Small amounts of fluid in this recess may mimic pathology, such as adenopathy, masses, and aortic dissection.* **(Middle)** *Axial contrast-enhanced cardiac CT at the level of the pulmonary trunk shows a small amount of fluid separating the epicardium from the parietal pericardium between the ascending aorta and pulmonary artery.* **(Bottom)** *Axial contrast-enhanced cardiac CT at the level of the left atrial appendage shows a small fluid collection posterior to the aorta and pulmonic valve. This fluid is within the transverse sinus, which is a potential space that can be used to route a bypass graft through.*

PERICARDIAL ANATOMY ON AXIAL MDCT

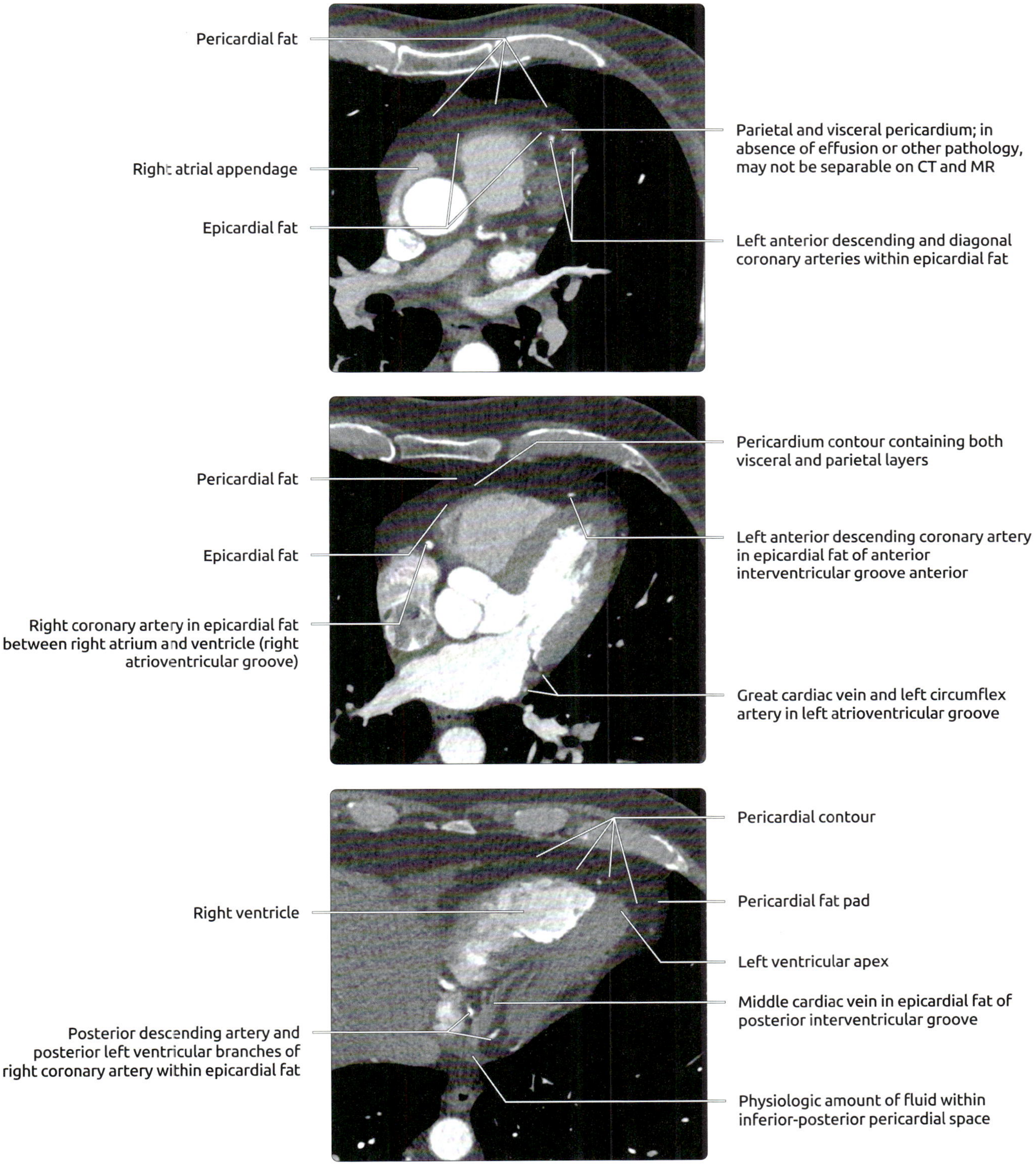

(Top) *Axial contrast-enhanced cardiac CT at the level of the left superior pulmonary vein shows the left anterior descending coronary artery and diagonal branch within the epicardial fat off the anterior interventricular groove, just posterior to the pericardial contour.* **(Middle)** *Axial contrast-enhanced cardiac CT at the level of the left ventricular outflow tract shows thin contour of pericardium separating the pericardial fat and the epicardial fat. Both the right atrioventricular groove (or sulcus) and the anterior interventricular groove are shown.* **(Bottom)** *Axial contrast-enhanced cardiac CT at the level of the middle cardiac vein shows the epicardial fat of the posterior interventricular groove.*

PERICARDIAL ANATOMY ON BLACK-BLOOD MR

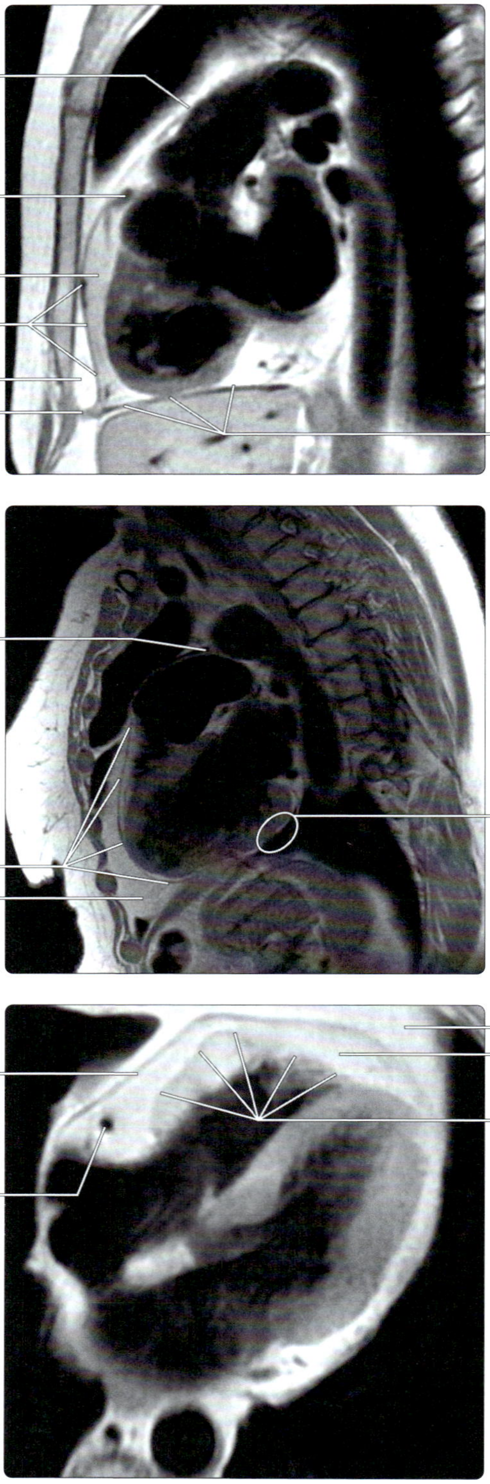

(Top) *Sagittal FSE black-blood MR shows the pericardial contour separating the pericardial fat (anterior, between sternum and pericardium) from the epicardial fat (between pericardium and myocardium/great vessels). In the absence of effusions or other pathology, both MR and CT cannot resolve the epicardium and pericardium as separate structures, and these therefore appear as 1 curvilinear line.* **(Middle)** *Left ventricular long-axis FSE MR shows pericardium as a curvilinear line surrounding the heart. The visibility of the pericardium depends on the location and is best along the anterior cardiac surface (epicardial and pericardial fat on either side). Often, the pericardium is not visualized along the posterolateral and inferior walls of the left ventricle because of a paucity of pericardial fat at these locations.* **(Bottom)** *Four-chamber FSE MR shows pericardium anteriorly and poorly or nonvisible pericardium laterally. This is due to absence of mediastinal or pericardial fat between lung (black) and pericardium.*

PERICARDIAL ANATOMY ON WHITE-BLOOD CINE & LGE IMAGING

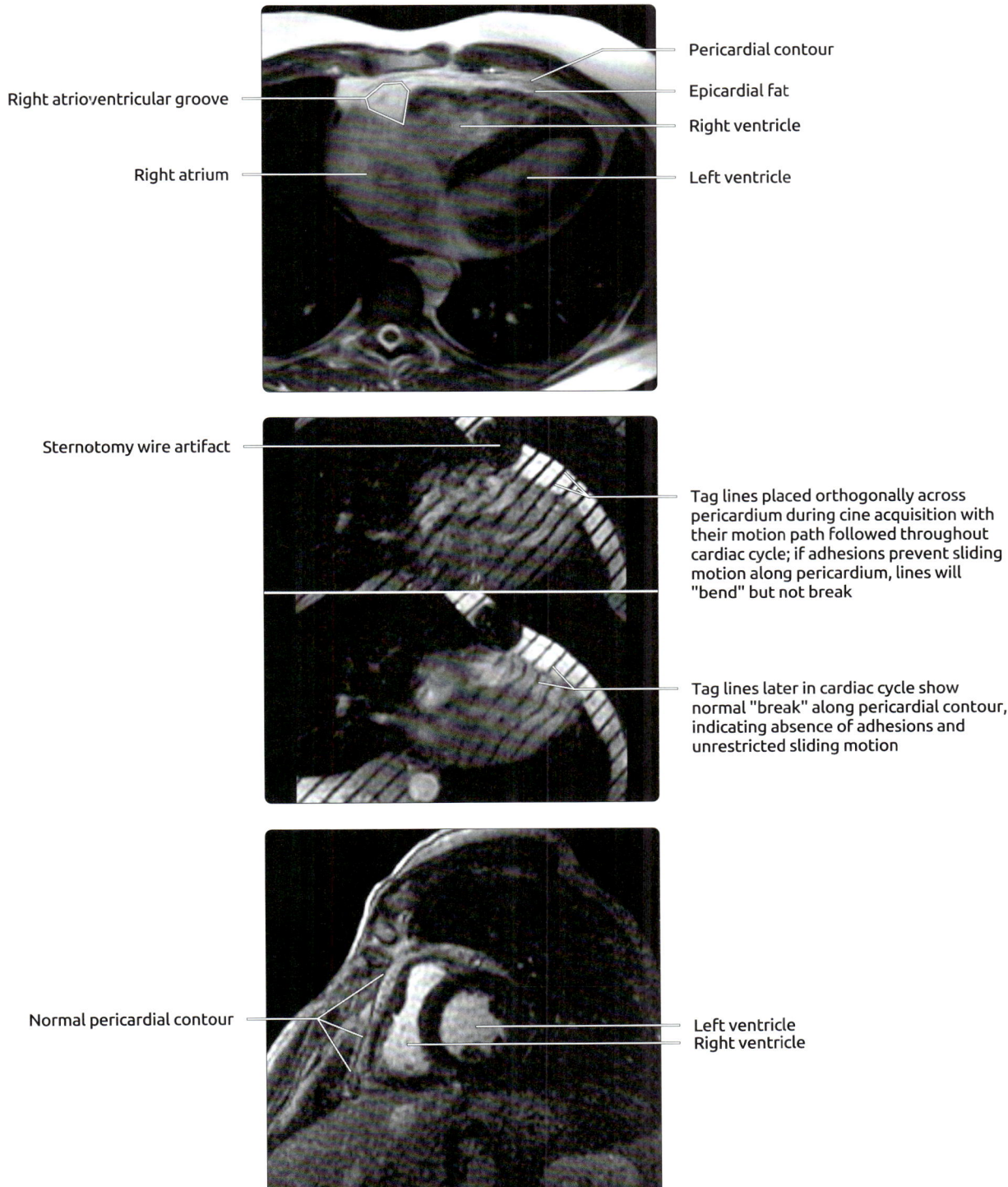

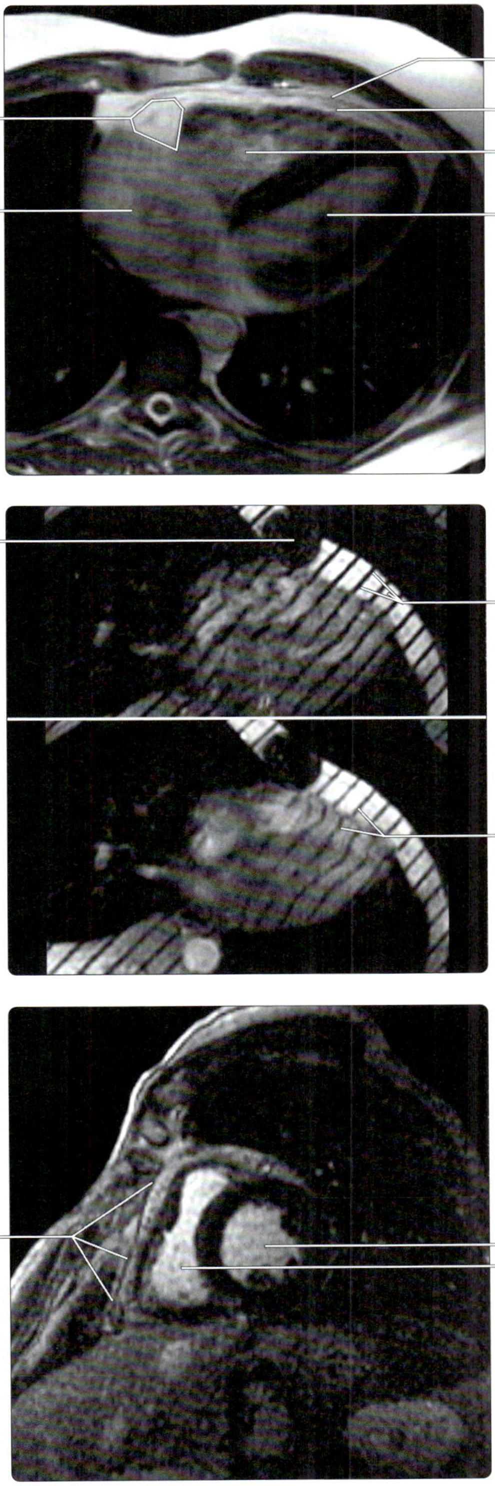

(Top) *Axial SSFP white-blood cine MR shows pericardium anteriorly as a curved line separating anterior pericardial fat from epicardial fat.* **(Middle)** *Tagged gradient-echo cine MR images in different phases of the cardiac cycle show tag lines when they were recently deposited (top) and later in the cardiac cycle (bottom). If normal motion occurs, the tag lines move with the tissue in which they were deposited and appear to fracture or break the location where they traverse the pericardium, as shown here.* **(Bottom)** *LGE MR in left ventricular short axis shows normal black pericardium. The inversion time was optimized for nulling of left ventricular myocardial signal. Inflamed or infected pericardium enhances and will appear white.*

Acute Pericarditis: Infectious

KEY FACTS

TERMINOLOGY

- Pericarditis due to infectious agent

IMAGING

- Radiography
  - Signs of pericardial effusion
- CT
  - Thickening best seen on portal venous phase of contrast
  - Best characterizes calcification or gas
  - May see septations or loculations
- MR
  - Evaluates pericardial thickening/effusion
  - Evaluates signs of tamponade/constriction
  - STIR imaging may detect pericardial inflammation
  - Tagged cine T1-weighted GRE may demonstrate tethering of pericardium

TOP DIFFERENTIAL DIAGNOSES

- Iatrogenic pericarditis
  - Pericardiotomy, radiation therapy
- Inflammatory pericarditis
  - Rheumatoid arthritis, systemic lupus erythematosus
- Metabolic disorders
  - Renal failure
- Neoplastic disease

CLINICAL ISSUES

- Pleuritic chest pain
- Fever, tachycardia, dyspnea

DIAGNOSTIC CHECKLIST

- Look for signs of tamponade and constriction
- Pericardial calcifications may suggest chronic/remote infectious pericarditis
- Enhancing pericardium separated by complex fluid

(Left) *Anteroposterior chest radiograph in a patient with acute pericarditis and chest pain shows enlargement of the cardiac silhouette with globular water bottle morphology, typical for a large pericardial effusion.* **(Right)** *Axial CECT in a patient with acute pericarditis shows thickening and enhancement of both the visceral and the parietal pericardial layers separated by pericardial effusion. Viral disease is the most common cause of infectious pericarditis.*

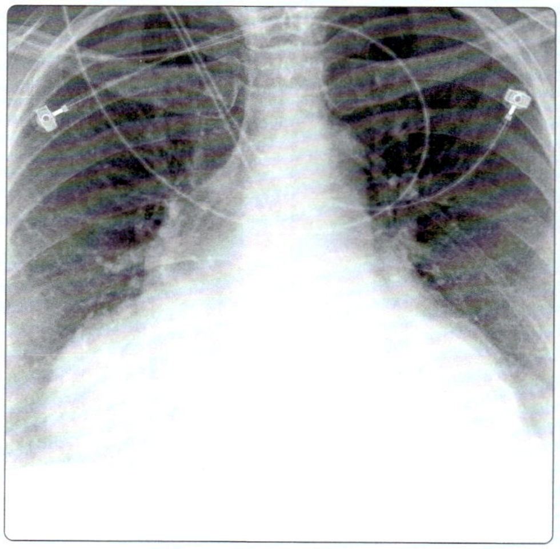

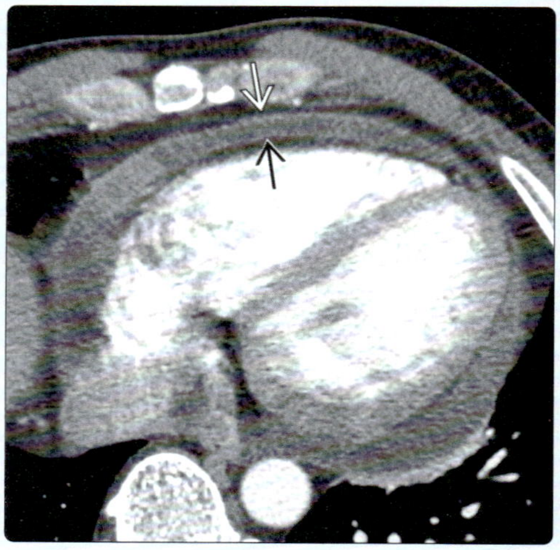

(Left) *Lateral radiograph in a patient with acute pericarditis shows opacity separating the relatively lucent epicardial and anterior mediastinal fat, the Oreo cookie sign. The lateral chest radiograph is more sensitive for pericardial fluid and calcification than is the frontal radiograph.* **(Right)** *Sagittal CECT in the same patient shows the small, circumferential pericardial effusion. CT allows direct evaluation of the entire pericardium and associated thoracic disease.*

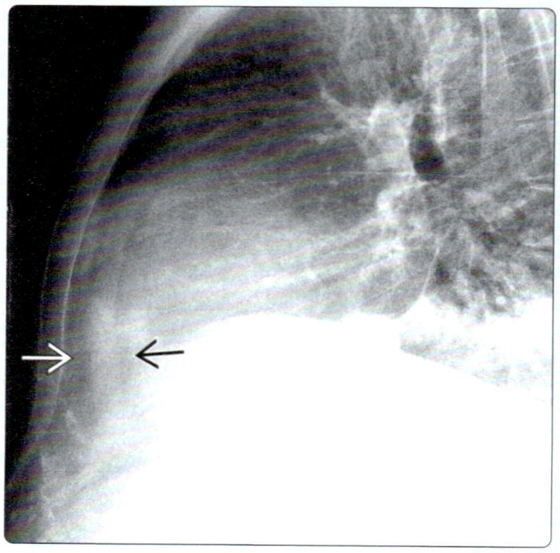

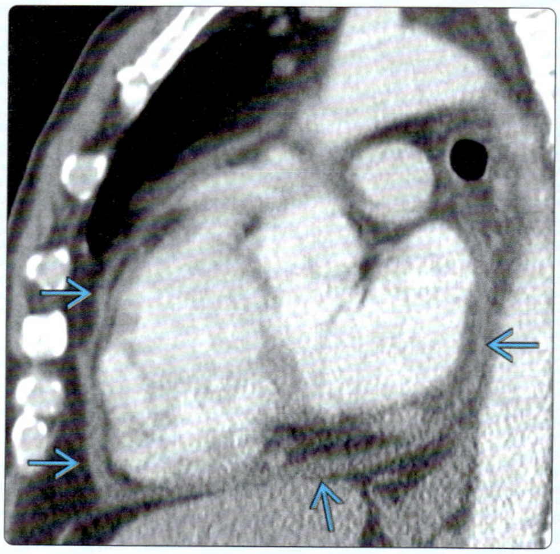

TERMINOLOGY

Definitions

- Acute inflammation of pericardium

IMAGING

General Features

- Best diagnostic clue
  - Typical imaging characteristics of pericardial effusion
  - Thickened and enhancing pericardium
- Location
  - Pericardium
- Size
  - Varying size of pericardial fluid or purulent material
- Morphology
  - Loculations with enhancing septation may be present

Radiographic Findings

- Radiography
  - Radiographs may appear normal until pericardial fluid exceeds 250 mL
  - Pericardial effusion: Water bottle-shaped; Oreo cookie sign
    - Posteroanterior chest radiograph
      - Enlargement of cardiac silhouette
      - Flask- or water bottle-shaped cardiac silhouette
    - Lateral radiograph
      - Sandwich or Oreo cookie sign: Separation of lower density retrosternal pericardial fat from cardiac epicardial fat by higher density effusion
  - Rapid increase in size of cardiac silhouette over short period of time may be related to pericardial effusion

CT Findings

- NECT
  - Varying degree of pericardial fluid
  - Best characterizes calcification
  - Pericardial thickening difficult to assess without contrast
  - High-attenuation pericardial fluid (> 30 HU) may suggest purulent effusion, hemorrhage, neoplastic pericarditis
  - Can be difficult to differentiate simple pericardial effusion from pericarditis without contrast
    - Inflammatory stranding in adjacent mediastinal fat
    - Mediastinal inflammation and associated abscess
- CECT
  - Varying degree of pericardial fluid
  - Pericardial enhancement
    - Best seen during portal venous phase
    - May be absent in arterial phase of contrast
  - Septations within pericardial fluid or loculated fluid
  - Rarely, gas bubbles from gas-producing organism or prior instrumentation
  - May demonstrate features of tamponade
    - Mass effect on right heart or coronary sinus
    - Straightening or bowing of interventricular septum
    - Signs of elevated right heart pressure

MR Findings

- T1WI
  - Pericardial thickening
    - May see areas of low signal due to calcification in acute-on-chronic pericarditis
  - Variable signal pericardial fluid
    - May be intermediate to high signal due to high protein and cell content
  - Adjacent fat stranding
- T2WI
  - High signal may not be seen as in simple effusion
    - Lower T2 signal may be seen due to high protein and cell content
  - Loculations and septations best seen on T2W and SSFP imaging
- T1WI C+
  - Enhancing pericardium and septations
  - Streaky enhancement of adjacent fat, especially in chronic cases
- SSFP cine
  - Usually bright signal pericardial fluid with varying degrees of internal signal
  - Evaluates signs of tamponade physiology
  - Evaluates signs of elevated right heart pressure
  - Real-time cine imaging of septum for ventricular interdependence
- Black blood SE
  - Evaluates pericardial thickening
  - STIR: Pericardial inflammation/edema or masses
- Tagged cine T1-weighted GRE
  - May demonstrate tethering of pericardium
- LGE
  - Pericardial enhancement indicates inflammation
  - Enhancement of adjacent fat
  - Enhancement of myocardium &/or epicardium indicates associated myocarditis &/or epicarditis

Echocardiographic Findings

- Echocardiogram
  - Often 1st imaging modality employed
  - Effusions of varied size ± septations
  - Tamponade in extreme cases
  - May be limited by acoustic windows
    - Difficult to image entire pericardium

Imaging Recommendations

- Best imaging tool
  - Echocardiogram
  - MR for detailed characterization and functional evaluation
  - CT for anatomic assessment and to help delineate underlying cause

DIFFERENTIAL DIAGNOSIS

Idiopathic Pericarditis

- 26-86% of acute pericarditis
- May be due to undiagnosed viral infection

Iatrogenic Pericarditis

- Radiation therapy: High incidence when > 4,000 rad
- May develop post pericardiotomy in 10-40% of cardiac operations

Inflammatory Pericarditis

- Rheumatoid arthritis, systemic lupus erythematosus, scleroderma, rheumatic fever, sarcoidosis

Metabolic Disorders

- Renal failure
  - Dialysis decreases incidence
- Hypothyroidism

Cardiovascular Disorders

- Myocardial infarction (MI)
  - Pericarditis complicates 5-8% of acute MIs
  - Dressler syndrome now rare
- Proximal extension of ascending aortic dissection and rupture into pericardium

Neoplastic Disease

- Hematogenous metastasis or direct extension
- Effusion usually large, out of proportion to tumor size; often hemorrhagic
- May demonstrate enhancing pericardial nodules and noncardiac metastatic foci

Drug Reaction

- Penicillin, procainamide, hydralazine, isoniazid, methysergide, phenytoin, anticoagulants

Trauma

- Penetrating trauma, esophageal rupture

Intrapericardial Teratoma

- Seen in young children
- Large, heterogeneous, multiloculated cystic mass arising from near junction of aortic root and right atrium

Pericardial Cyst

- Usually grows outward from parietal pericardium with no mass effect on heart
- Nonenhancing

PATHOLOGY

General Features

- Etiology
  - Viral agent most common cause of acute pericarditis
    - Coxsackievirus B, adenovirus, influenza
    - HIV
    - Hepatitis A and B
  - Pyogenic (bacterial) pericarditis uncommon
    - Most often *Staphylococcus*, *Streptococcus*, or gram-negative species
  - Tuberculous pericarditis
    - Suspected when insidious onset in high-risk groups
    - 1-2% of patients with pulmonary disease
    - May exist without obvious pulmonary involvement
    - Increasing incidence in resource-limited countries with high prevalence of HIV
  - Other uncommon infectious causes
    - Fungal, parasitic (*Echinococcus*), chlamydia
    - Amebic liver abscess can erode into pericardium; amebiasis may spread hematogenously as well
  - Extension of myocardial abscess related to infectious endocarditis or mediastinal abscess
  - Secondary to esophageal or lung cancer invasion and subsequent infection
- Acute pericarditis may be serous, fibrinous, sanguineous, hemorrhagic, or purulent

Gross Pathologic & Surgical Features

- Exudative effusion with protein and cellular debris
  - Specific gravity > 1,020 g/L
  - Bread and butter appearance on gross pathology
- Caseation requires exclusion of tuberculous pericarditis

CLINICAL ISSUES

Presentation

- Most common signs/symptoms
  - Pleuritic chest pain
    - Aggravated by thoracic motion
    - Relieved by upright position, leaning forward
  - Fever, tachycardia, dyspnea
  - Pericardial friction rub
- Other signs/symptoms
  - Kussmaul sign: Paradoxical rise in jugular vein pressure with jugular vein distention
  - Pulsus paradoxus: > 10-mmHg drop in systolic blood pressure and cardiac output

Natural History & Prognosis

- Most resolve with appropriate therapy and cessation of inciting factor
- Purulent pericarditis almost always fatal if untreated
  - Mortality rate in treated patients: 40%
- May progress to chronic effusive pericarditis

Treatment

- Colchicine, NSAIDs, and, potentially, corticosteroids
- Antimicrobial agents in bacterial pericarditis
- Pericardiocentesis for relief of tamponade
- Surgical debridement in advanced cases

DIAGNOSTIC CHECKLIST

Consider

- Pericardial fluid evaluation
  - Cell count + differential, stains, and culture for aerobic and anaerobic bacteria, acid-fast and fungal agents
  - Viral cultures and viral nucleic acid detection assays
  - Cytology to exclude neoplasm

Image Interpretation Pearls

- Thickened and enhancing pericardium separated by complex fluid with loculations/strands
- Pericardial calcifications may suggest chronic/remote infectious pericarditis
- Look for signs of tamponade and constriction

SELECTED REFERENCES

1. Conte E et al: The contemporary role of cardiac computed tomography and cardiac magnetic resonance imaging in the diagnosis and management of pericardial diseases. Can J Cardiol. 39(8):1111-20, 2023
2. Kligerman S: Imaging of pericardial disease. Radiol Clin North Am. 57(1):179-99, 2019

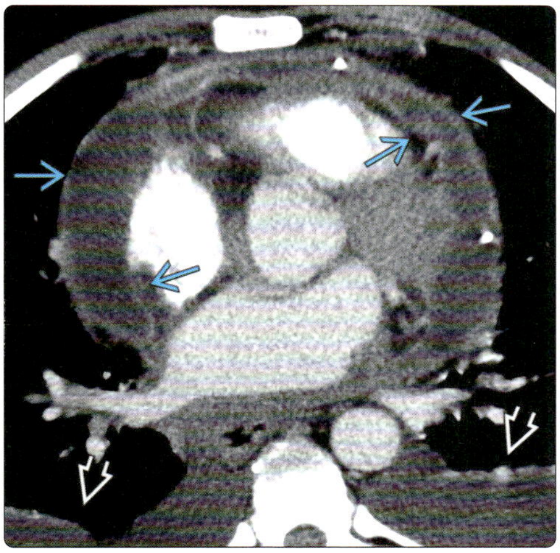

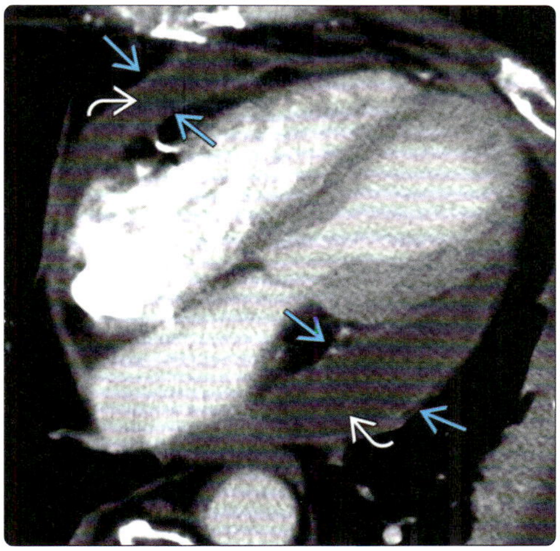

(Left) *Axial CECT in a patient with HIV and tuberculous pericarditis shows diffuse thickening and enhancement of the pericardial layers* → *and pericardial and bilateral pleural effusions* ➡*. A pericardial drain is in place. Tuberculous pericarditis may occur without pulmonary symptoms, particularly in patients with HIV.* **(Right)** *Axial CECT in a patient with pericarditis* → *and pericardial effusion* ➡ *after partial pericardiectomy shows tubular morphology of the ventricles, as seen in tamponade physiology.*

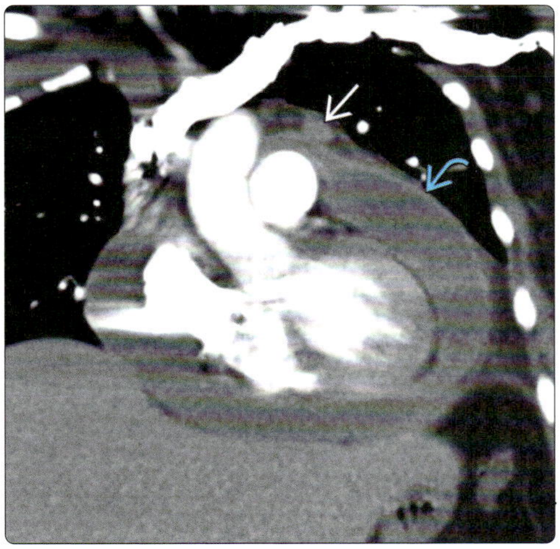

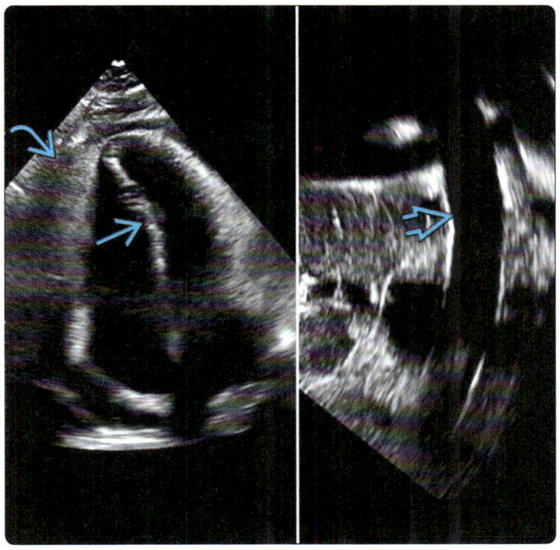

(Left) *Ten-mm average image from a CTPA in a 38-year-old woman shows a large circumferential pericardial effusion with thickening and enhancement* →*. Scattered prominent lymph nodes* ➡ *are present.* **(Right)** *Echo images in the same patient show the larger pericardial effusion (left,* →*) with inversion of the septum to the left* → *with associated diastolic septal bounce. Image through the inferior vena cava (IVC) (*⇨*, right) shows little respiratory variation in the IVC size, suggestive of tamponade.*

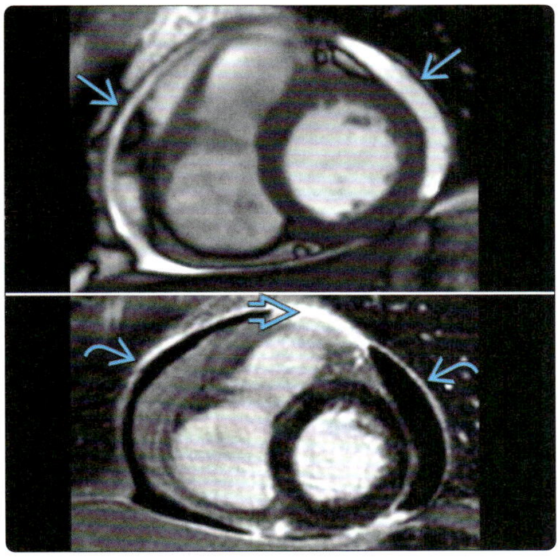

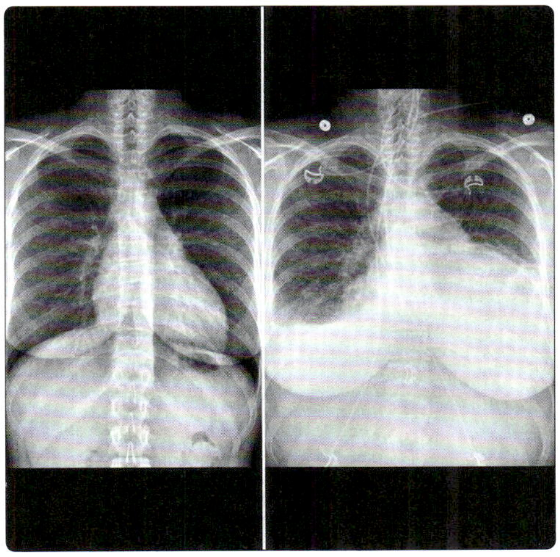

(Left) *Short-axis cine (top) and PSIR delayed enhancement (bottom) images in a patient with viral pericarditis show moderate circumferential pericardial effusion with pericardial thickening* → *and enhancement* →*. Focal pericardial adhesions* ⇨ *are present.* **(Right)** *PA radiograph (left) in a 38-year-old woman is normal. AP radiograph performed 10 days later (left) shows bilateral effusions, pulmonary edema, and marked enlargement of the cardiac silhouette due to a pericardial effusion from viral pericarditis.*

KEY FACTS

TERMINOLOGY

- Pericarditis not secondary to infection
  - Uremic pericarditis in chronic kidney disease (CKD)
  - Pericarditis in rheumatic disease
  - Pericarditis in postcardiac injury syndrome
  - Posttraumatic pericarditis
  - Drug-induced pericarditis

IMAGING

- Radiography
  - Pericardial effusion: Flask- or bottle-shaped silhouette on AP image
  - Pericardial effusion: Fat pad or Oreo cookie sign on lateral image
- CT/MR
  - Effusion with pericardial thickening and enhancement
    - Best seen on portal venous phase on CT
    - Seen on both T1W postcontrast and LGE imaging
- Tamponade or constrictive physiology may be present
  - Inversion of septum toward left
  - Septal bounce on retrospective ECG-gated cardiac CT or MR
  - Compression of atria or free wall of right ventricle
  - Dilation of superior and inferior vena cava
- Associated CT findings that can point toward underlying cause
  - Dialysis catheter in chronic renal disease
  - Coexistent pleuritis in patients with lupus
  - Findings of subacute myocardial infarction or recent sternotomy in postcardiac injury syndrome
  - Linear paramediastinal opacity from radiation
  - Findings of trauma or malignancy

TOP DIFFERENTIAL DIAGNOSES

- Infectious pericarditis
- Hemopericardium
- Volume overload
- Primary pericardial malignancy

(Left) *Axial NECT from 2006 in a patient with chronic renal failure (CRF) and poor compliance with dialysis shows a small pericardial effusion ➡. The patient had chest pain, leukocytosis, and elevated blood urea nitrogen (BUN) levels. A diagnosis of uremic pericarditis was made, and the patient's symptoms resolved after dialysis.* **(Right)** *In 2008, the same patient presented with similar symptoms and abnormal lab values after missing dialysis. A small effusion ➡ is present. Symptoms resolved after dialysis.*

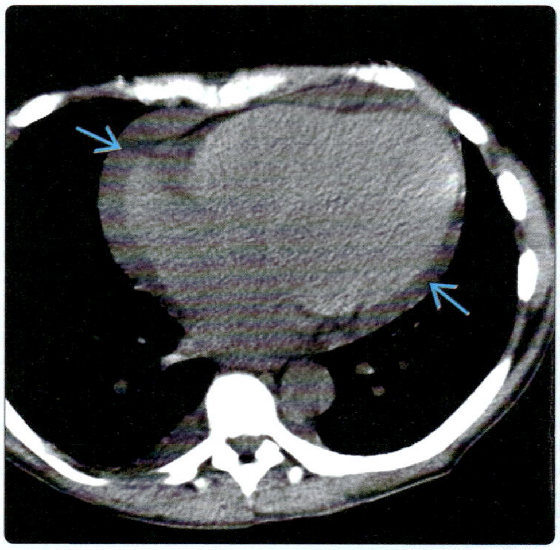

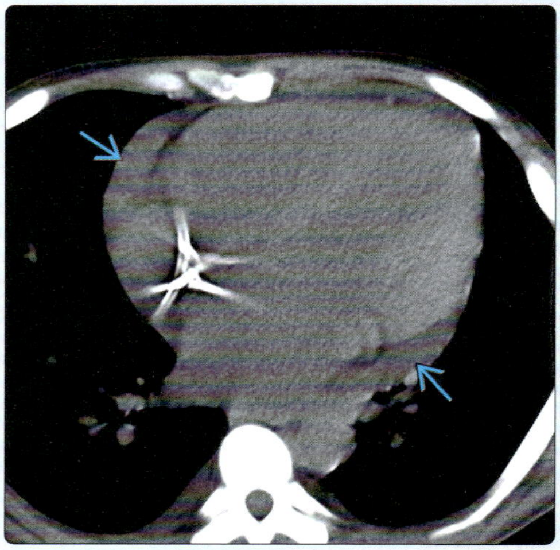

(Left) *Axial CECT from 2010 in the same patient shows circumferential, rind-like pericardial thickening ➡. Between 2006-2010, the patient was admitted for multiple episodes of uremic pericarditis.* **(Right)** *Axial CECT from 2012 shows rind-like pericardial thickening ➡ and a small area of pericardial calcification ➡. The ventricles have a more conical shape due to the stiffness of the pericardium. Eight months later, the patient underwent pericardiectomy for treatment of constrictive pericarditis.*

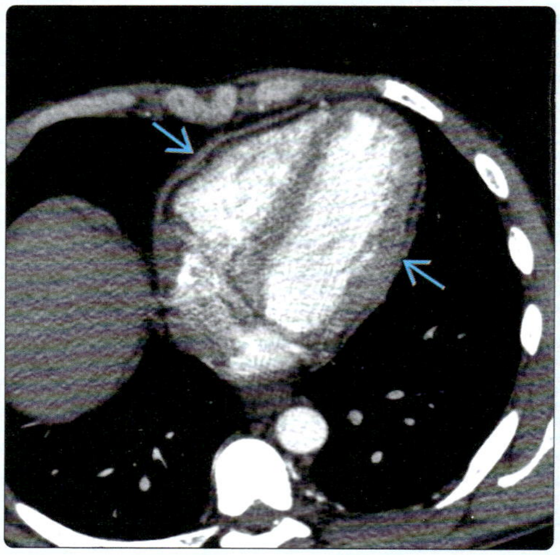

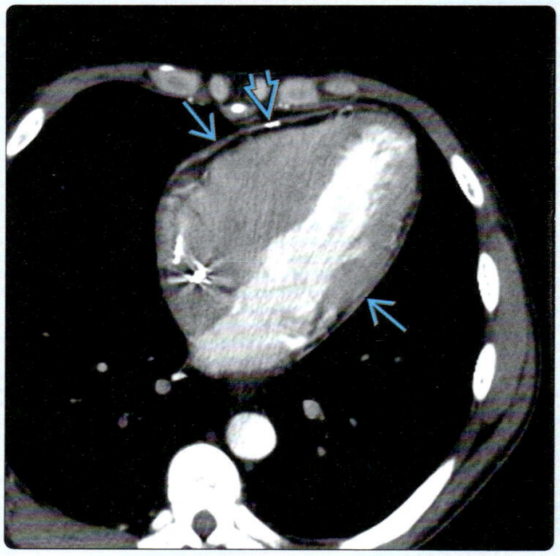

TERMINOLOGY

Definitions

- Pericarditis not secondary to infection

Associated Syndromes

- Uremic pericarditis in chronic kidney disease (CKD)
- Pericarditis in rheumatic disease
  - Autoimmune diseases
    - Most notably lupus and rheumatoid arthritis
  - Vasculitis
  - Infiltrative diseases (sarcoid and IgG4-related disease)
  - Autoinflammatory diseases
- Pericarditis in postcardiac injury syndrome
  - Post-myocardial infarction (MI) pericarditis
    - Early post-MI pericarditis
      - Occurs within 5 days of MI
    - Late post-MI pericarditis (Dressler syndrome)
      - Occurs 2-8 weeks after MI
  - Postpericardiotomy syndrome
    - Occurs days to weeks after cardiac surgery
- Posttraumatic pericarditis
  - Blunt or penetrating trauma
  - Iatrogenic: Cardiac procedures, radiation
- Drug-induced pericarditis
- Pericarditis due to malignancy

IMAGING

General Features

- Best diagnostic clue
  - Pericardial thickening and effusion
  - Pericardial enhancement

Radiographic Findings

- Radiography
  - Pericardial effusion
    - Flask- or bottle-shaped silhouette on frontal
    - Fat pad or Oreo cookie sign on lateral
  - Small pericardial effusions or thickening not well evaluated on radiography

CT Findings

- Pericardial effusion
  - May be increased in attenuation (> 20 HU) due to proteinaceous/hemorrhagic fluid
- Enhancement of pericardial lining may be present
  - Best seen on portal venous phase of imaging
- Pericardial thickening
- Tamponade or constrictive physiology may be present
  - Need to look for secondary signs on CT
- Look for associated CT findings that can point toward underlying cause
  - Dialysis catheter in chronic renal disease
  - Coexistent pleuritis in patients with lupus
  - Myocardial hypoperfusion in postcardiac injury syndrome
  - Linear paramediastinal ground glass from radiation
  - Findings of trauma or malignancy

MR Findings

- Pericardial thickening and effusion; may be loculated
- Pericardial enhancement due to inflammation
  - Seen on both T1W postcontrast and LGE imaging
- Features of pericardial constriction or tamponade can occur
- Look for findings that can point toward underlying cause

Echocardiographic Findings

- Echocardiogram
  - Effusion: Persistent echo-free space between parietal and visceral pericardium throughout cardiac cycle
    - May show fibrinous strands
  - Thickening of pericardium
  - Findings of tamponade or pericardial constriction

DIFFERENTIAL DIAGNOSIS

Infectious Pericarditis

- Viral, bacterial, or granulomatous

Hemopericardium

- Cases of trauma or aortic dissection

Volume Overload

- Will produce transudative pericardial effusion

Primary Pericardial Malignancy

- Can mimic pericarditis in early stages

PATHOLOGY

Gross Pathologic & Surgical Features

- Thickened, highly vascular pericardium, adhesions, serous or hemorrhagic pericardial effusion

CLINICAL ISSUES

Presentation

- Most common signs/symptoms
  - Pericarditis (sharp retrosternal pain aggravated by lying down and relieved by sitting up; friction rub)
  - Pericardial effusion (dyspnea if sizable)
  - Pericardial tamponade (tachycardia, hypotension, inspiratory jugular venous distention, paradoxical pulse)
  - Pericardial constriction in late disease

Natural History & Prognosis

- Quite variable
- Commonly resolves with treatment and cessation of inciting factors
- Can lead to constrictive pericarditis in some cases

Treatment

- Reduce inflammation with NSAIDs, etc.
- Treat underlying cause
- Pericardiocentesis if persistent or progressive effusion
- Pericardial window in rare cases

SELECTED REFERENCES

1. Kawano Y et al: Evaluation and management of pericarditis in rheumatic diseases. J Cardiovasc Pharmacol. 83(6):491-502, 2023
2. Verma BR et al: Multimodality imaging in patients with post-cardiac injury syndrome. Heart. 106(9):639-46, 2020
3. European Society of Cardiology: Post-cardiac injury syndrome: aetiology, diagnosis, and treatment. Published October 31, 2017. Accessed April 10, 2024. https://www.escardio.org/Journals/E-Journal-of-Cardiology-Practice/Volume-15/Post-cardiac-injury-syndrome-aetiology-diagnosis-and-treatment

(Left) *Five-mm short-axis minIP 1 week after discharge for left circumflex (LCx) territory myocardial infarction shows hypoattenuation of the inferolateral wall ➔ due to LCx infarct. A moderate-sized pericardial effusion ➔ with associated pericardial enhancement ➔ due to pericarditis, secondary to postcardiac injury syndrome, is present.* **(Right)** *Four-chamber reconstruction shows thinning and hypoattenuation of the lateral basal wall ➔ and pericardial effusion with associated enhancement ➔.*

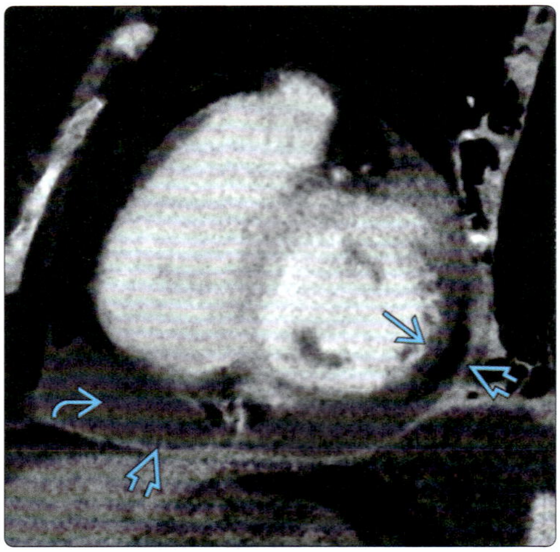

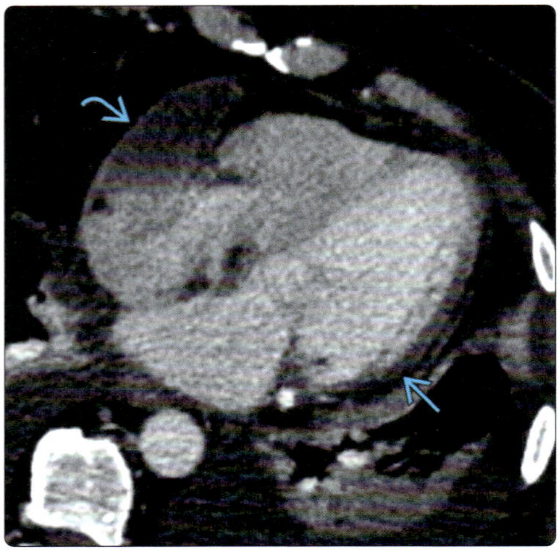

(Left) *PA radiograph in a 31-year-old woman with lupus presenting to the emergency department with dyspnea and chest pain shows globular enlargement of the cardiac silhouette. Moderate pleural effusions are present.* **(Right)** *Axial image from a CTPE study shows a large, circumferential pericardial effusion with enhancement of the pericardium ➔ and associated mass effect on the right atrium ➔, raising the possibility of tamponade. Moderate loculated pleural effusions are also present.*

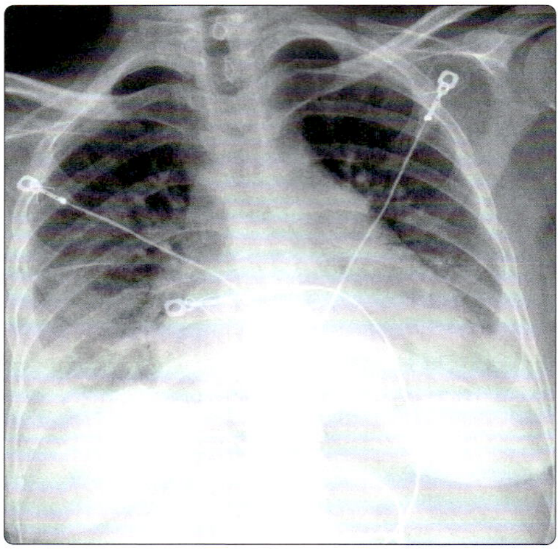

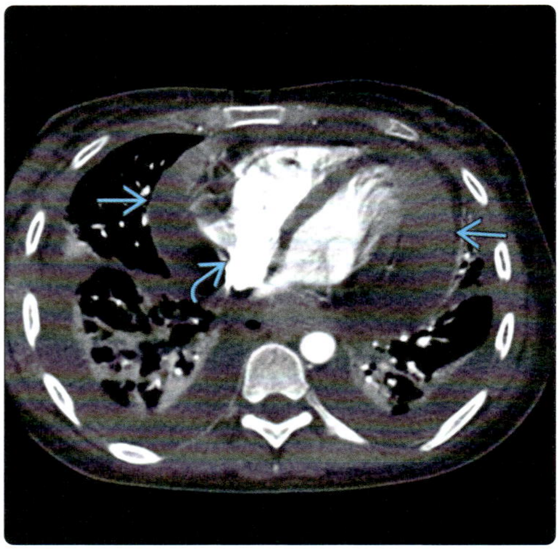

(Left) *Four-chamber echocardiogram a few hours later in the same patient shows the large, hypoechoic pericardial effusion ➔ measuring over 28 mm in maximum diameter. Right atrial collapse ➔ during systole is seen. Additional findings of cardiac tamponade were also present. The pericardium was also thickened, which is not well seen on this image.* **(Right)** *PA radiograph in the same patient shows that, due to tamponade, a pericardial drain ➔ was placed.*

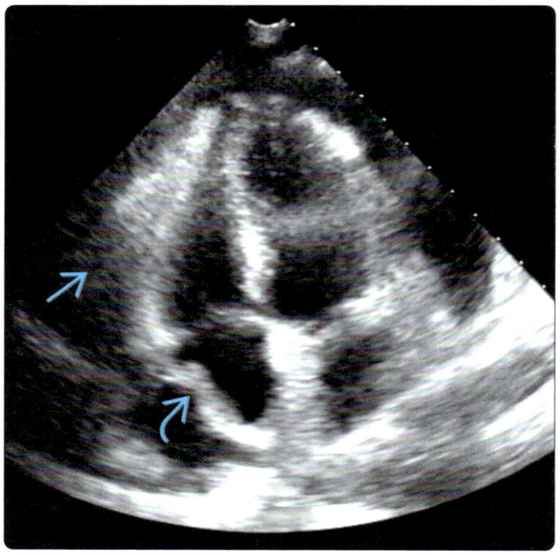

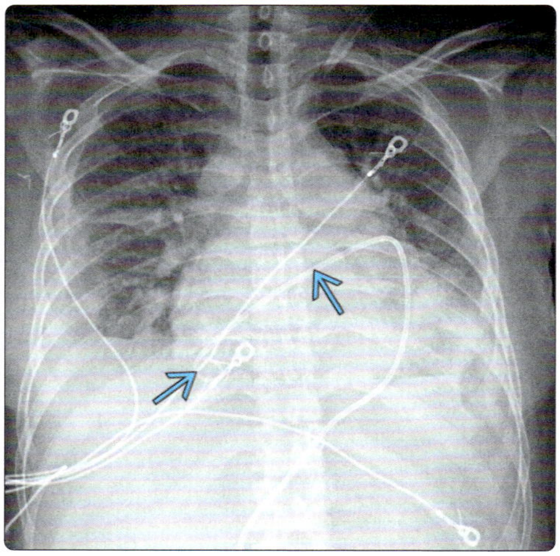

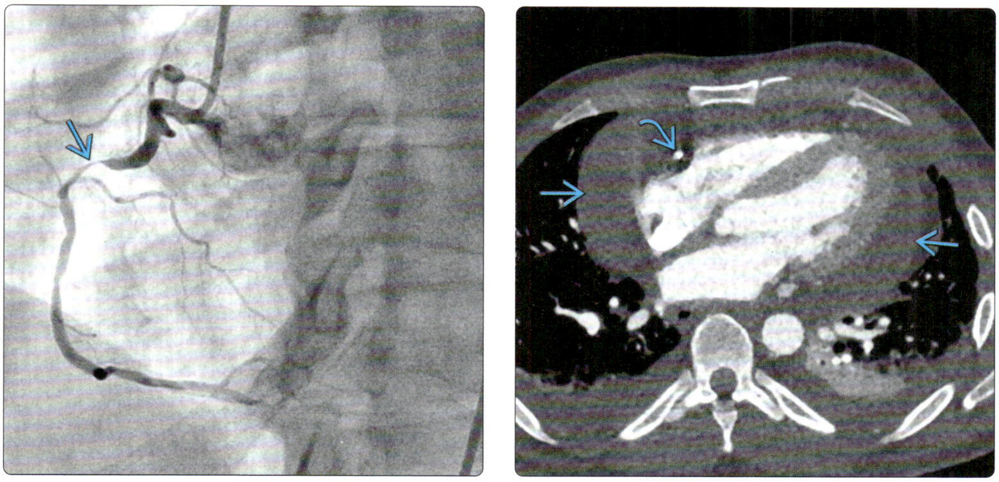

(Left) *Coronary angiogram in a 55-year-old man presenting to the emergency department with severe chest pain and elevated troponin shows a severe stenosis → in the proximal right coronary artery (RCA). The patient underwent RCA stent placement.* **(Right)** *CT angiogram in the same patient, who developed worsening shortness of breath 3 days after the procedure, shows a large circumferential pericardial effusion with mild pericardial enhancement →. Note RCA stent →. Findings are suggestive of early post-myocardial infarct pericarditis.*

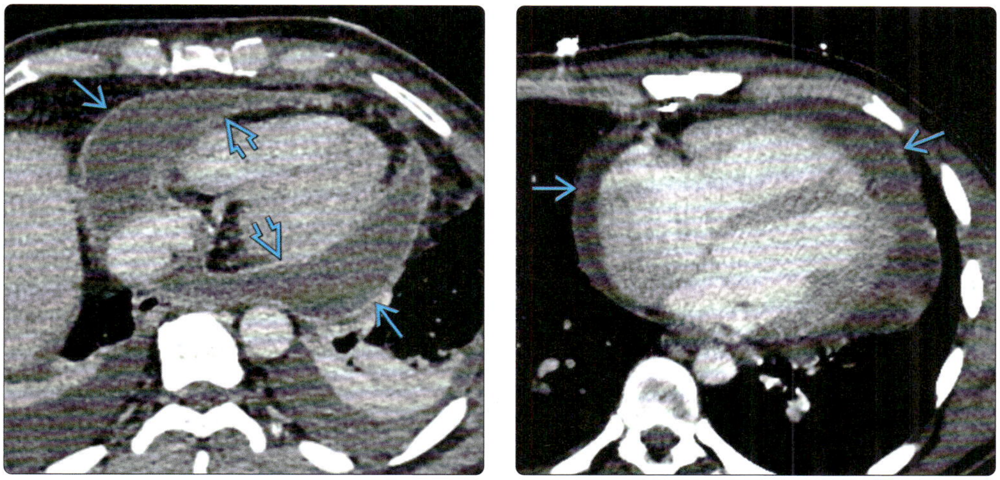

(Left) *Portal venous phase axial image in the same patient performed immediately after the CT angiogram better illustrates visceral → and parietal → pericardial enhancement.* **(Right)** *Chest CT obtained 3 days after sternotomy for pulmonary thromboendarterectomy in a 43-year-old man shows a lobulated pericardial effusion with pericardial enhancement →. Findings are consistent with postpericardiotomy syndrome, which can occur days to weeks after cardiac surgery.*

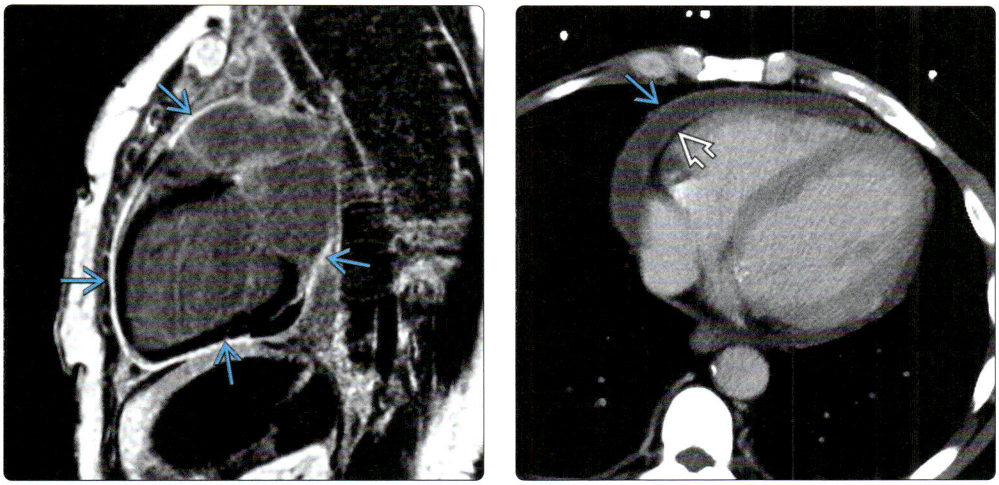

(Left) *Two-chamber MR in a woman with lupus-related dilated cardiomyopathy shows a dilated left ventricle and circumferential pericardial delayed enhancement → due to numerous recurrent episodes of pericarditis.* **(Right)** *Portal venous-phase CECT in a patient with renal failure shows enhancement of the parietal → and visceral → pericardium. A diagnosis of uremic pericarditis was made based on history, clinical exam, and laboratory tests. The patient's symptoms resolved after dialysis.*

Chronic Inflammatory Pericarditis

KEY FACTS

TERMINOLOGY

- No strict definition of chronic inflammatory pericarditis, although some criteria have been suggested
  - Acute pericarditis: Acute inflammation of pericardium that resolves in majority of patients
  - Incessant pericarditis: Inflammation of pericardium that persists for 4-6 weeks after acute episode
  - Chronic pericarditis: Inflammation of pericardium lasting > 3 months; often associated with pericardial fibrosis
    - Chronic pericarditis is not synonymous with constrictive pericarditis
  - Recurrent pericarditis: Relapse of pericarditis with ~ 4-6 weeks between previous and current episode
    - Recurrent pericarditis not associated with development of constrictive pericarditis

IMAGING

- CT is best imaging modality to detect calcification
- MR is best tool to assess for acute, incessant, recurrent, and chronic pericarditis, as it can assess anatomy, physiology, inflammation, and fibrosis
- Pericardial thickness > 4 mm is considered abnormal on CT and MR
- As pericardial inflammation progresses from acute to chronic stages, pericardial thickness often decreases as inflammation resolves and fibrosis progresses
- Large pericardial effusions are uncommon, as fibrosis of pericardial space limits accumulation of fluid
- Presence and extent of postcontrast enhancement will vary depending on degree of inflammation and fibrosis

TOP DIFFERENTIAL DIAGNOSES

- Constrictive pericarditis
- Neoplastic pericarditis
- Myocarditis

(Left) *Chest CT in a 53-year-old woman with chest pain in early January shows a small pericardial effusion ➙ with mild haziness in the pericardial fat ➙ suggestive of inflammation. Based on history, laboratory values, physical examination, and imaging findings, a diagnosis of acute pericarditis was made. The patient was treated with NSAIDs.* **(Right)** *Four-chamber CECT in the same patient at the end of January shows resolution of the pericardial effusions. The pericardium ➙ is minimally thickened in a few areas.*

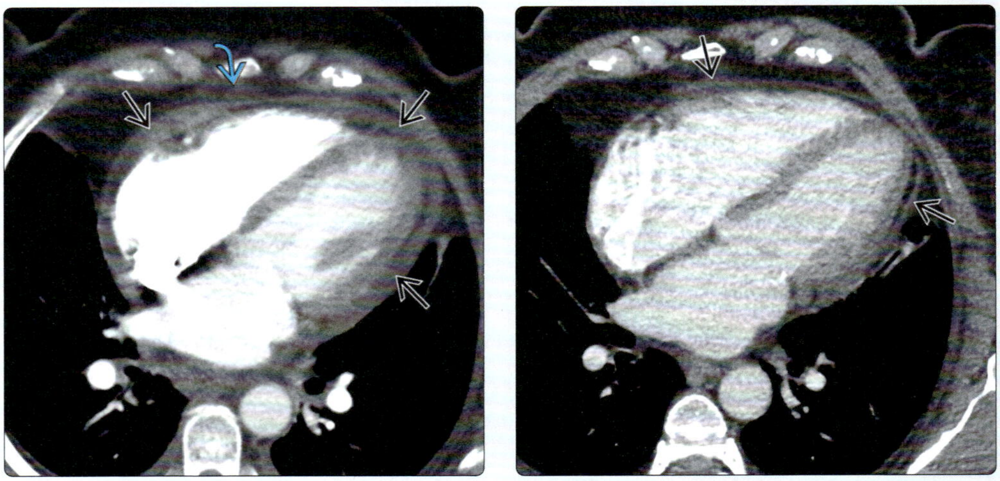

(Left) *Four-chamber CECT in same patient in mid-February shows recurrent pericardial effusion ➙ with pericardial enhancement ➙, consistent with recurrent pericarditis.* **(Right)** *Four-chamber CECT in the same patient in early April again shows resolution of pericardial effusion. In many areas, pericardium ➙ is thickened. Although echo and MR showed no evidence of constriction, patient underwent partial pericardial resection due to continued chest pain. Pathology showed dense pericardial adhesions and fibrosis.*

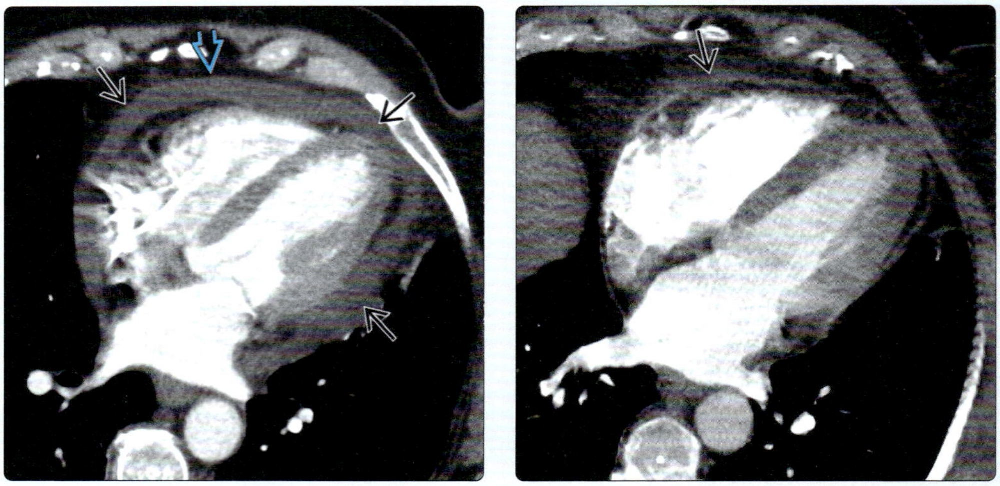

TERMINOLOGY

Synonyms

- Chronic pericarditis
- Chronic sclerosing pericarditis
- Chronic fibrosing pericarditis

Definitions

- No strict definition of chronic pericarditis, although some criteria have been suggested
  - Acute pericarditis: Acute inflammation of pericardium that resolves in majority of patients
  - Incessant pericarditis: Inflammation of pericardium that persists for 4-6 weeks
  - Chronic pericarditis: Inflammation of pericardium lasting > 3 months; often associated with pericardial fibrosis
  - Recurrent pericarditis: Relapse of pericarditis with ~ 4-6 weeks between previous and current episode
- Chronic pericarditis is not synonymous with constrictive pericarditis
  - While many patients have pericardial fibrosis, not all patients with pericardial fibrosis have physiologic constriction
  - However, nearly all patients with pericardial constriction do have pericardial fibrosis

IMAGING

General Features

- Best diagnostic clue
  - Thickening of pericardium
  - Effusion, if present, is often small
    - Large effusions in setting of chronic pericarditis are not common due to developing fibrosis, which can limit fluid accumulation
  - Calcification may be present
- Location
  - Pericardium
- Size
  - Normal pericardial thickness is ~ 2 cm or less on CT and MR
  - Pericardial thickness > 4 mm is considered abnormal on CT and MR
    - Important to remember that up to 20% of patients with pericardial constriction have normal pericardial thickness
    - As pericardial inflammation progresses from acute to chronic stages, pericardial thickness often decreases as inflammation resolves and fibrosis progresses
    - In most instances, pericardial thickening is not subtle

Radiographic Findings

- Given that pericardial effusions are often small, radiography in patients with chronic pericarditis is often normal unless calcification is visible

CT Findings

- Thickening of pericardium ± calcification
  - Best imaging tool to detect calcification
- Large pericardial effusions are uncommon, as fibrosis of pericardial space limits accumulation of fluid
- May be difficult to differentiate mild pericardial thickening from small pericardial effusion in some patients
  - Portal venous phase of contrast may better differentiate pericardial thickening and enhancement from fluid

MR Findings

- T1WI
  - Thickening of pericardium ± calcification
  - Imaging findings vary depending on degree of pericardial inflammation and fibrosis
  - Pericardium will often appear intermediate signal to myocardium on T1 MR
  - Low-signal pericardial effusion, if present, is often small in size
- T2WI
  - In cases of incessant and recurrent pericarditis, pericardial inflammation can be seen as high signal on T2 MR
  - When pericardium is predominantly replaced by fibrous tissue in longstanding chronic fibrous pericarditis, signal intensity on T2W sequences is often low
- T1WI C+
  - Presence and extent of postcontrast enhancement will vary depending on degree of inflammation and fibrosis
    - Acute and subacute inflammation leads to neovascularity, which increases contrast enhancement on 1st-pass perfusion and T1WI C+
    - Degree of enhancement may be decreased or even absent in cases of diffuse fibrous and calcific pericarditis as vascularity of pericardium is decreased
  - In cases of incessant or recurrent pericarditis, postcontrast imaging will show pericardial enhancement
  - As fibrosis increases, degree of immediate postcontrast enhancement may decrease
- SSFP cine
  - Pericardial thickening often appears as intermediate to low signal intensity
  - Thickening of visceral and pleural pericardium may be separated by small pericardial effusion, or 2 layers may be adherent
  - Real-time cine sequences of ventricular septum during inspiration and expiration are performed to demonstrate ventricular interdependence, feature of pericardial constriction
- Delayed enhancement
  - Similar to 1st-pass perfusion imaging and T1WI C+, presence and extent of delayed enhancement will vary depending on degree of inflammation and fibrosis
  - In cases of incessant and recurrent pericarditis, neovascularity will lead to delayed enhancement
    - Enhancing visceral and parietal pericardium may be separated by small pericardial effusion
    - In other areas, layers may be fused due to fibrosis
    - Assess adjacent subepicardial layer of myocardium for inflammation due to perimyocarditis
  - Fibrous pericarditis may also show delayed enhancement
- 1st-pass perfusion imaging
  - In cases of incessant or recurrent pericarditis, 1st-pass perfusion imaging may show rapid signal increase in pericardium due to inflammation
  - In cases of fibrous thickening often seen with chronic pericarditis, 1st-pass perfusion imaging may be normal

- Gradient-echo tagging sequence
  - Allows for evaluation of pericardial adhesions
  - Does not diagnose constrictive pericarditis

Imaging Recommendations

- Best imaging tool
  - MR is best tool to assess for acute, incessant, recurrent, and chronic pericarditis, as it can assess anatomy, physiology, inflammation, and fibrosis
    - CT is better for assessing calcification
- Protocol advice
  - Similar protocol advice for evaluation of acute or constrictive pericarditis
    - Cine SSFP sequences in standard cardiac planes
    - T1 and T2 sequences
    - 1st-pass perfusion
    - Postcontrast T1W sequence in same plane as T1W precontrast sequence
    - Delayed enhancement imaging
    - Real-time cine sequences of ventricular septum during inspiration and expiration
    - Gradient-echo tagging

DIFFERENTIAL DIAGNOSIS

Constrictive Pericarditis

- Patients with constrictive pericarditis will have chronic pericarditis and pericardial fibrosis
  - However, not all patients with chronic or recurrent pericarditis will have physiologic constriction
- Constriction can be seen transiently during acute pericarditis or associated with effusion (effusive constrictive pericarditis)

Neoplastic Pericarditis

- In patient with malignancy, development of pericardial effusion or pericardial thickening must raise concern for malignant pericardial disease
- In some instances, there are enhancing nodules or masses in or adjacent to pericardium that can help differentiate between them
- Pericardiocentesis or pericardial biopsy may be necessary to differentiate

Myocarditis

- Myocarditis can cause adjacent inflammation of adjacent pericardium (myopericarditis), and patients can present with similar symptoms as patients with pericarditis
  - Similarly, patients with pericarditis can present with adjacent myocardial inflammation (perimyocarditis)
    - While differentiation between 2 may be difficult in acute phase, recurrent or chronic cases of myocarditis are even less common
      - In perimyocarditis, degree of pericardial inflammation usually exceeds degree of myocardial inflammation and vice versa

PATHOLOGY

Staging, Grading, & Classification

- Acute pericarditis
  - Acute pericardial inflammation with mesothelial cell necrosis, inflammatory cells, neovascularity, and fibrin deposition
- Fibrinous pericarditis
  - Subacute and chronic inflammation of pericardium with fibrin deposition on pericardial surface, reactive mesothelial cells, chronic inflammation, and granulation tissue
- Chronic fibrosing pericarditis
  - Fibrotic thickening of pericardium with collagen deposition, mesothelial cell hyperplasia, and calcification

Gross Pathologic & Surgical Features

- Fibrinous pericarditis: Bread and butter appearance
- Chronic fibrosing pericarditis: Shaggy, leather-like pericardium

CLINICAL ISSUES

Presentation

- Most common signs/symptoms
  - Incessant pericarditis: Continued pain after acute episode
  - Recurrent pericarditis: Symptoms often less severe or absent with subsequent episodes of pericardial inflammation
  - Fibrous pericarditis without inflammation: Often asymptomatic in absence of constriction

Natural History & Prognosis

- Recurrent pericarditis: Good prognosis; no documented cases of development of constrictive pericarditis

Treatment

- Determine and treat underlying abnormality if present
- Various medications, such as aspirin, NSAIDs, colchicine, corticosteroids
- IVIG, anakinra, and azathioprine may be considered in noninfectious, corticosteroid-dependent, recurrent pericarditis not responsive to colchicine

SELECTED REFERENCES

1. Jost JS et al: Prevalence of pericardial effusion in autosomal dominant polycystic kidney disease. Clin Kidney J. 16(11):2041-7, 2023
2. Kligerman S: Imaging of pericardial disease. Radiol Clin North Am. 57(1):179-99, 2019
3. Xu B et al: Imaging of the pericardium: a multimodality cardiovascular imaging update. Cardiol Clin. 35(4):491-503, 2017
4. Cremer PC et al: Complicated pericarditis: understanding risk factors and pathophysiology to inform imaging and treatment. J Am Coll Cardiol. 68(21):2311-28, 2016
5. Aquaro GD et al: Role of tissue characterization by cardiac magnetic resonance in the diagnosis of constrictive pericarditis. Int J Cardiovasc Imaging. 31(5):1021-31, 2015
6. Cosyns B et al: European Association of Cardiovascular Imaging (EACVI) position patimodper: mulality imaging in pericardial disease. Eur Heart J Cardiovasc Imaging. 16(1):12-31, 2015
7. Bogaert J et al: Pericardial disease: value of CT and MR imaging. Radiology. 267(2):340-56, 2013
8. Klein AL et al: American Society of Echocardiography clinical recommendations for multimodality cardiovascular imaging of patients with pericardial disease: endorsed by the Society for Cardiovascular Magnetic Resonance and Society of Cardiovascular Computed Tomography. J Am Soc Echocardiogr. 26(9):965-1012.e15, 2013
9. Zurick AO et al: Pericardial delayed hyperenhancement with CMR imaging in patients with constrictive pericarditis undergoing surgical pericardiectomy: a case series with histopathological correlation. JACC Cardiovasc Imaging. 4(11):1180-91, 2011

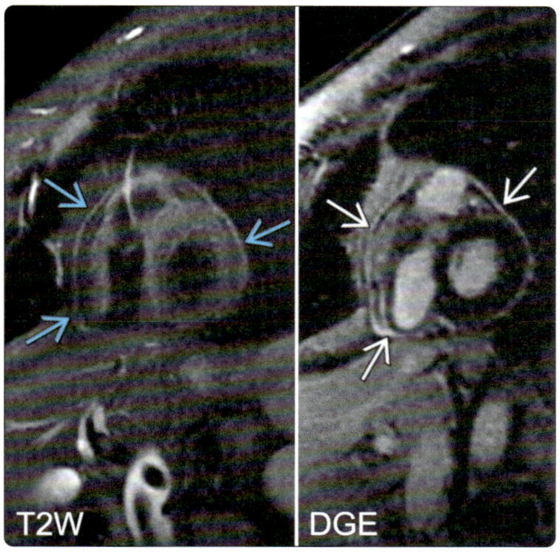

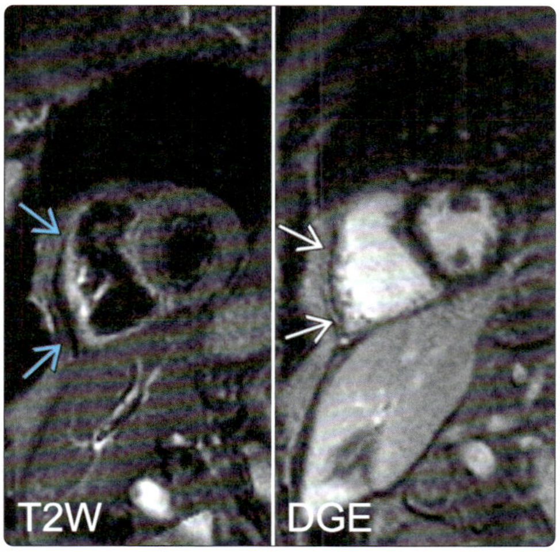

(Left) *Short-axis T2 triple IR (left) and LGE (right) cardiac MR images in the same patient at the end of February show pericardial edema* → *and enhancement* ➡. *The LGE may be secondary to acute pericardial inflammation or fibrosis.* **(Right)** *Short-axis T2 triple IR (left) and LGE (right) cardiac MR in the same patient (obtained in May) show resolution of pericardial edema* → *and mild linear LGE* ➡ *due to fibrosis.*

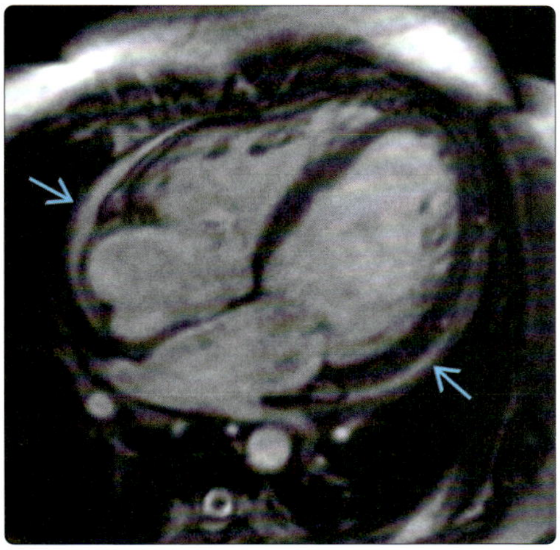

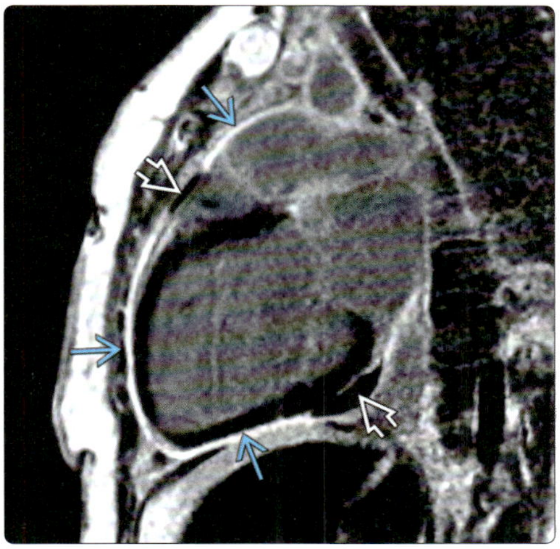

(Left) *Four-chamber SSFP cine MR in a 31-year-old woman with systemic lupus erythematosus and recurrent episodes of pericarditis and pleuritis shows a dilated left ventricle due to a nonischemic dilated cardiomyopathy. There is also mild thickening of the parietal pericardium* →. **(Right)** *Two-chamber LGE cardiac MR in the same patient shows the diffuse pericardial LGE* → *with a small effusion* ➡.

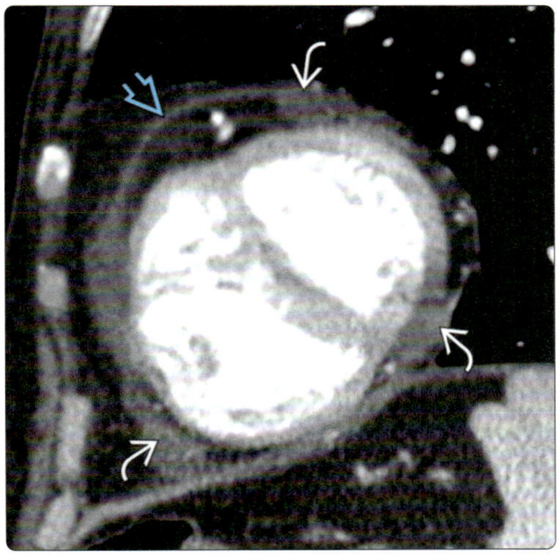

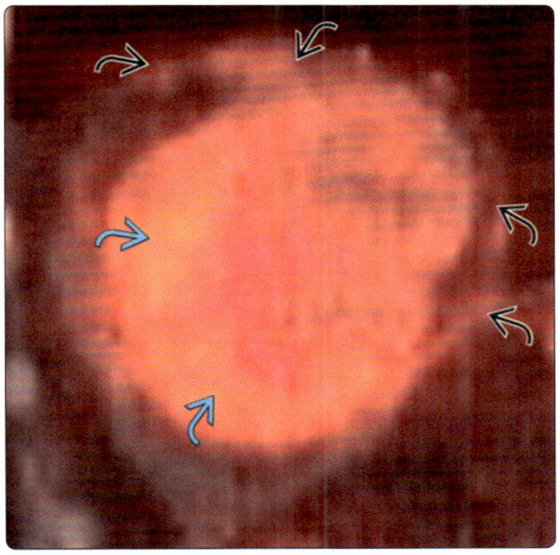

(Left) *Short-axis CECT in a 50-year-old woman with lupus, pulmonary hypertension (PHTN), and chest pain shows right ventricular hypertrophy and a combination of pericardial fluid* ➡ *and mild thickening* ⇨. *The pericardial fluid collections appear somewhat nodular, as much of the pericardium is scarred.* **(Right)** *Fused FDG PET shows intense right ventricle uptake due to PHTN* ⇨. *There is also mild pericardial inflammation* ⇨. *Subsequent heart and lung transplant showed diffuse pericardial fibrosis.*

Constrictive Pericarditis

KEY FACTS

TERMINOLOGY

- Noncompliant pericardium leading to impaired ventricular diastolic filling and reduced cardiac output

IMAGING

- Echocardiography and MR are best modalities to make diagnosis
- MR: High sensitivity for distinguishing constrictive pericarditis from restrictive cardiomyopathy
  - Early diastolic septal bounce, which is accentuated during early inspiration on free-breathing cine MR
  - Thickening and enhancement of pericardium
- CT: Evaluate findings associated with constrictive pericarditis
  - Pericardial thickening and calcification
    - Thickened pericardium does not make diagnosis of constrictive pericarditis
    - Some patients with constrictive pericarditis have normal-thickness pericardium

TOP DIFFERENTIAL DIAGNOSES

- Restrictive cardiomyopathy
- Cardiac tamponade
- Pericarditis without constriction

PATHOLOGY

- Causes include postmyocardial infarction, post radiation, postsurgical, post infectious, posttraumatic, and idiopathic
- In developed countries, most common etiologies are idiopathic (presumed viral) and post CABG

CLINICAL ISSUES

- Symptoms of right heart failure
- Surgical stripping of pericardium
- Medical treatment is difficult and does not affect natural progression or prognosis of disease

DIAGNOSTIC CHECKLIST

- Pericardial thickening, pericardial enhancement, and presence of calcifications

(Left) *Lateral radiograph in a patient with a history of tuberculous pericarditis shows extensive pericardial calcification →.* **(Right)** *Five-mm thick CT pulmonary angiogram in the same patient shows the extensive pericardial calcification →. There is compression and deformity of the free wall of the right ventricle ↷. CT is the imaging modality of choice for the detection of the pericardial calcification.*

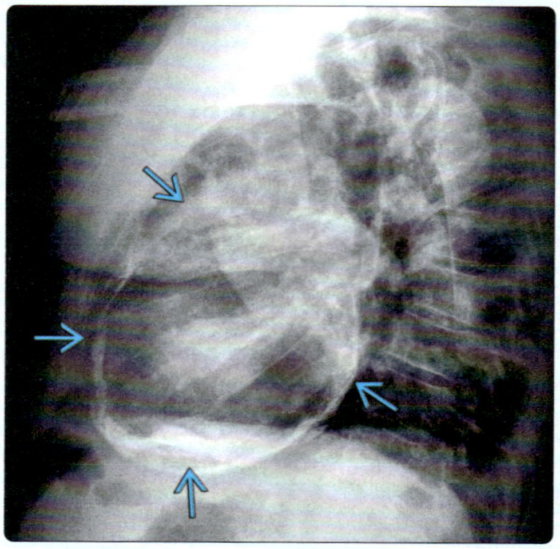

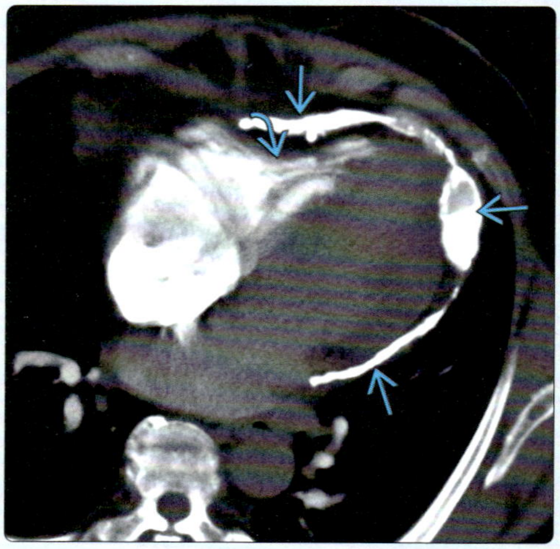

(Left) *Short-axis T2 MR shows circumferential low signal due to pericardial calcification → that is better seen on CT.* **(Right)** *Real-time cine MR obtained during early inspiration shows inversion of the septum ⇨, which had a normal configuration on expiration (not shown here). This variation of septal morphology on MR confirms exaggerated ventricular interdependence and a constrictive physiology. There is associated biatrial enlargement.*

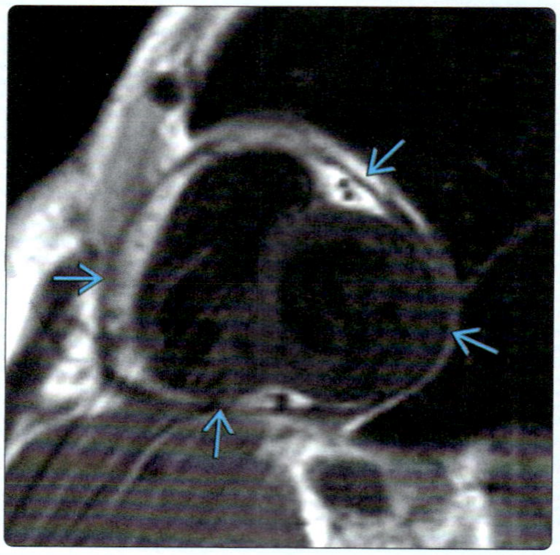

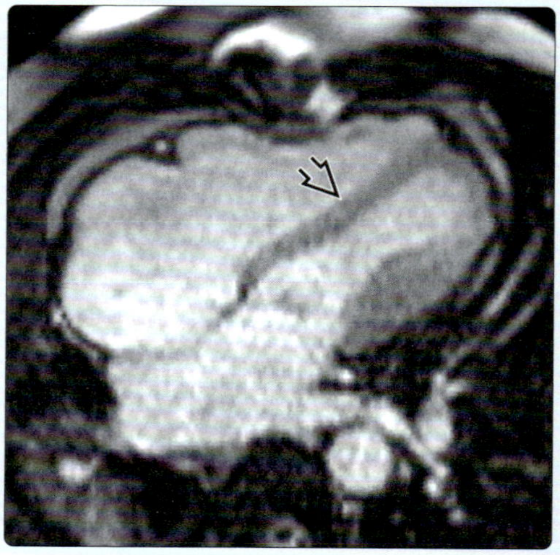

TERMINOLOGY

Definitions

- Noncompliant pericardium due to pericardial scarring leading to impaired ventricular diastolic filling and reduced cardiac output

IMAGING

General Features

- Best diagnostic clue
  - Ventricular interdependence makes diagnosis on both echocardiogram and MR
    - Real-time cine imaging is best MR sequence to diagnose ventricular interdependence
  - Other findings associated with diagnosis
    - Pericardial thickening
      - Thickening > 4 mm commonly seen but does not denote constriction
    - Pericardial calcifications
      - Commonly associated with constrictive pericarditis, but physiologic constriction can occur without calcifications and vice-versa
    - Hepatic venous congestion, enlargement of atria, dilated superior vena cava/inferior vena cava (SVC/IVC) and hepatic veins, ascites, pleural effusions
- Location
  - Pericardium
- Morphology
  - Thickening and calcification of pericardium is common
    - May be absent in 20% of patients
  - Tubular or conical-shaped heart
  - Biatrial enlargement with dilation of SVC and IVC

Radiographic Findings

- Radiography
  - Pericardial calcification
  - Biatrial enlargement and pleural effusion in absence of pulmonary edema
  - Often normal

CT Findings

- NECT
  - Pericardial findings in constrictive pericarditis
    - Pericardial calcification
      - CT best at identifying calcification
      - Calcification associated with, but not diagnostic of, constrictive pericarditis
    - Pericardial thickening
      - Thickening defined as > 4 mm
      - Pericardium often severely thickening and calcified in constrictive pericarditis
      - Pericardium may appear normal on CT and patient can still have constrictive pericarditis (in 18%)
  - Nonspecific findings associated with ↑ atrial pressures
    - Hepatic congestion, dilated hepatic veins, dilated SVC and IVC, biatrial enlargement, ascites, pleural effusions
- CECT
  - Similar findings to NECT
  - Pericardial enhancement can help delineate between pericardial thickening and effusion
  - Conical-shaped ventricles with biatrial enlargement
- Cardiac gated CTA
  - Improved assessment of pericardium and heart due to ECG gating
  - Diastolic septal bounce can be seen on retrospectively gated CTA

MR Findings

- T1WI
  - Thick pericardium (> 4 mm)
  - Calcification has low signal
  - Fibrous tissue has low to intermediate signal
- T2WI
  - Calcification has low signal
  - Fibrous thickening has low to intermediate signal
  - Pericardial effusion often absent or very small due to fibrosed pericardial space
- STIR
  - Pericardial thickening
  - Occasional high signal due to pericardial inflammation
- SSFP cine
  - Real-time cine MR sequence
    - Best sequence to assess for ventricular interdependence in constrictive pericarditis
    - Inspiration in normal patients causes minimal septal excursion to left
    - Inspiration in constrictive pericarditis causes marked septal flattening, which is most conspicuous during early inspiration and resolves on expiration
      - ↑ in right ventricular (RV) pressures during early inspiration as RV cannot normally distend as it is encased by stiff pericardium
    - Respiratory variation absent in restrictive cardiomyopathy and cor pulmonale
  - Gated cine SSFP
    - Pericardial thickening = intermediate signal
    - Cardiac chambers may have conical appearance
    - Atrial dilation
    - Classic diastolic septal bounce and abrupt cessation of diastolic filling
  - Pericardial tagging
    - Tagging diagnoses pericardial adhesions, not constrictive pericarditis
- Delayed enhancement
  - Useful in identifying pericardial inflammation
    - May represent transient or reversible, inflammatory constriction
    - May benefit from antiinflammatory therapy
    - Patients with inflammation at baseline have higher clinical improvement
- Phase-contrast MR
  - Can be used to assess mitral and tricuspid valve inflow and E/A waves
- Variants of pericardial constriction
  - Focal constriction
    - Strategically located focal thickening: Atrioventricular (AV) groove, basal ventricles
  - Constriction with normal thickness
    - Seen in 18% due to noncompliant pericardium

- Effusive constrictive pericarditis
  - Tamponade physiology due to tense pericardial effusion and constrictive physiology due to stiff, noncompliant pericardium
  - Seen in < 7% of patients with tamponade
  - Features of constriction persist after removal or resolution of pericardial fluid
- Inflammatory constriction
  - Seen in resolution phase of acute pericarditis due to noncompliant pericardium
  - Transient; subsides in few months
- Occult constriction
  - Manifests only on rapid fluid challenge

Echocardiographic Findings

- Primary diagnostic tool
  - Inspiratory septal shift to left and expiratory shift to right
  - Change in mitral and tricuspid inflow during respiration
    - Inspiration: ↓ mitral inflow (E) and ↑ tricuspid inflow
    - Reverse during expiration
  - ↓ hepatic vein diastolic forward flow with end-diastolic flow reversal
  - Minimal changes in SVC flow during respiration
  - Ventricular septal bounce
  - Anulus reversus: Tissue Doppler (e') shows medial mitral annular velocities > lateral velocities
    - Due to tethering of pericardial to lateral anulus
  - Anulus paradoxus: Normal to slightly ↓ E/e' velocity in constrictive pericarditis despite ↑ filling pressure
    - ↓ e' in restrictive cardiomyopathy, thus ↑ E/e'
- Suboptimal in demonstration of pericardial thickening

Imaging Recommendations

- Best imaging tool
  - Echocardiography is primary tool but has limitations
  - MR is ideal as it can assess anatomy and physiology
    - Can also distinguish between constrictive pericarditis and restrictive cardiomyopathy
    - Identifies constriction associated with inflammation, which benefits from antiinflammatory therapy
  - CT is best tool to identify pericardial anatomy and calcification
  - Cardiac catheter for physiology (right and left heart catheter)
- Protocol advice
  - Imperative to perform real-time cine MR in short-axis or 4-chamber planes during deep inspiration and expiration to assess for respiratory variation in septal morphology

DIFFERENTIAL DIAGNOSIS

Pericarditis Without Constriction

- Pericardial thickening, effusion, and enhancement; less effusion and enhancement in chronic phases
- No physiologic changes of constriction

Restrictive Cardiomyopathy

- Numerous causes, including amyloid, sarcoid, Loeffler endocarditis, endomyocardial fibrosis, chemotherapy, radiation, hemochromatosis, and Fabry disease
- LGE MR is extremely helpful in detecting LGE within myocardium related to restrictive cardiomyopathy
- No ventricular interdependence in real-time cine MR

Pericardial Tamponade

- Collapse of RV free wall in early diastole and right atrial free wall in late diastole and early systole
- Compression of cardiac chambers; dilated IVC, SVC

Right Heart Failure

- Other causes of right heart failure, such as pulmonary hypertension, shunts, RV dysplasia, RV infarction can have similar clinical picture
- MR can exclude other causes of right heart failure

PATHOLOGY

General Features

- Etiology
  - Caused by idiopathic, infectious, iatrogenic, and traumatic processes
    - In developed countries, most common etiologies are idiopathic (presumed viral) and post coronary artery bypass graft surgery (CABG)
    - In developing world, infectious etiologies (tuberculosis has highest total incidence)

Gross Pathologic & Surgical Features

- > 50% of cases with pericardial calcification will have constrictive pericarditis

CLINICAL ISSUES

Presentation

- Most common signs/symptoms
  - Symptoms of right heart failure: Dyspnea, orthopnea
  - Symptoms are often vague with insidious onset
  - Kussmaul sign: ↑ jugular venous pressure during inspiration

Treatment

- Surgical stripping of pericardium
  - Entire pericardium is difficult to remove
- Pericardial constriction may recur despite treatment
- Transient or reversible constriction: Responds to antiinflammatory therapy (NSAIDs, steroids, colchicine)

DIAGNOSTIC CHECKLIST

Consider

- Assessing both morphologic (pericardial thickness, pericardial enhancement) and physiologic parameters (septal bounce, ventricular interdependence)

SELECTED REFERENCES

1. Gillombardo CB et al: Constrictive pericarditis in the new millennium. J Cardiol. 83(4):219-27, 2024
2. Conte E et al: The contemporary role of cardiac computed tomography and cardiac magnetic resonance imaging in the diagnosis and management of pericardial diseases. Can J Cardiol. 39(8):1111-20, 2023
3. De Paula Morales KR et al: Multimodality imaging for investigating constrictive pericarditis. Eur Heart J Cardiovasc Imaging. 25(1):e64, 2023
4. Lloyd JW et al: Multimodality imaging in differentiating constrictive pericarditis from restrictive cardiomyopathy: a comprehensive overview for clinicians and imagers. J Am Soc Echocardiogr. 36(12):1254-65, 2023

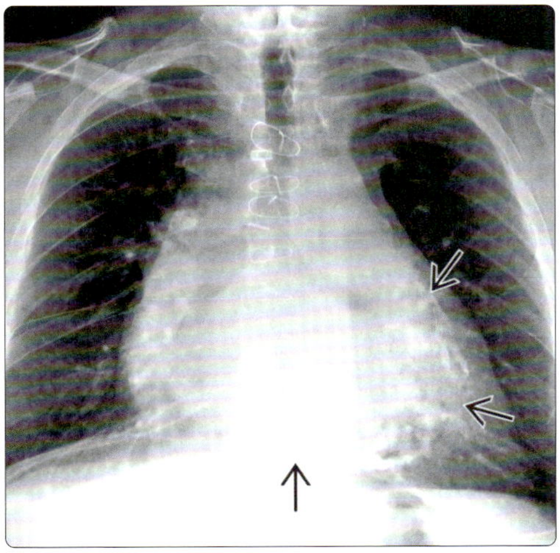

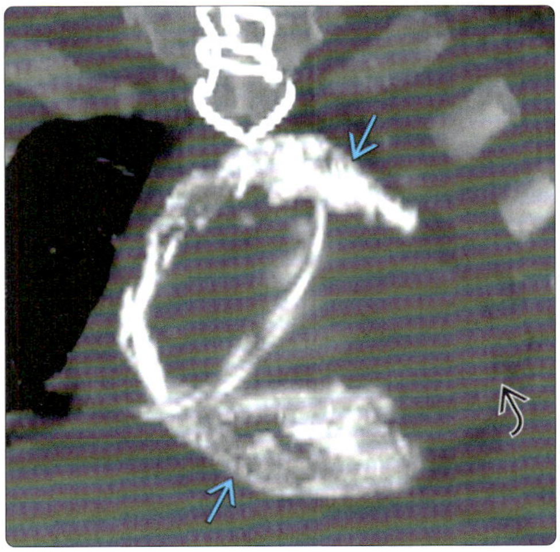

(Left) *PA radiograph in a patient status post cardiac surgery shows cardiomegaly with multiple areas of pericardial calcification →, most pronounced overlying the ventricles.* **(Right)** *MIP coronal reformatted cardiac CT shows extensive pericardial calcification → centered about the ventricles and at the atrioventricular groove. Portions of the pericardium appear normal →. A thickened and calcified pericardium does not necessarily make the diagnosis of constrictive pericarditis.*

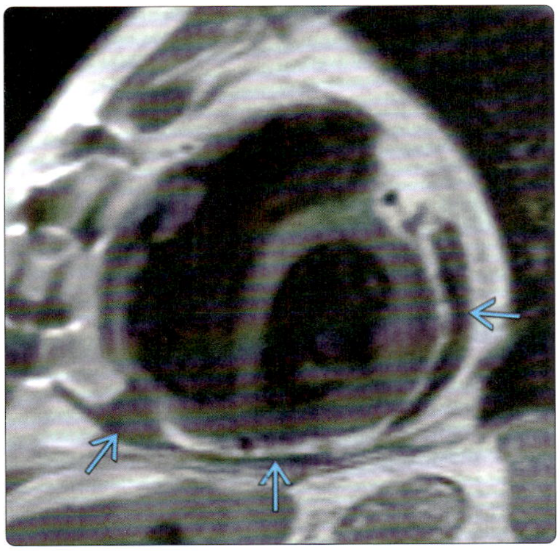

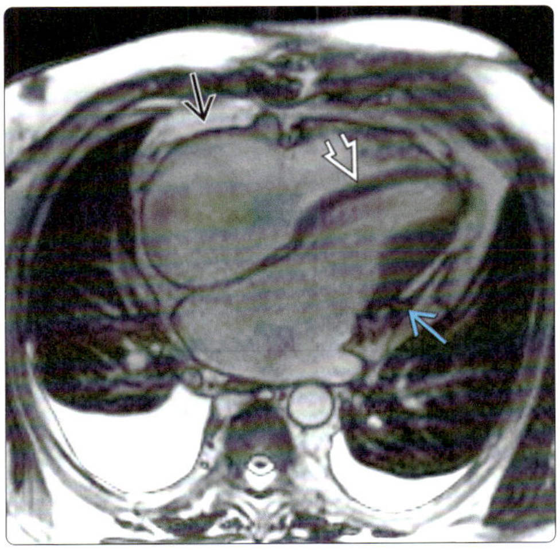

(Left) *Short-axis T1 MR cardiac MR in the same patient performed at the same level shows low signal along the pericardium → corresponding to areas of pericardial calcification seen on CT. The pericardium was > 1 cm in thickness in multiple areas.* **(Right)** *Four-chamber cine MR shows biatrial enlargement with pleural effusions. There is a thickened pericardium → but no pericardial effusion. The pericardium appears normal over the atria →. An early diastolic septal bounce → is present.*

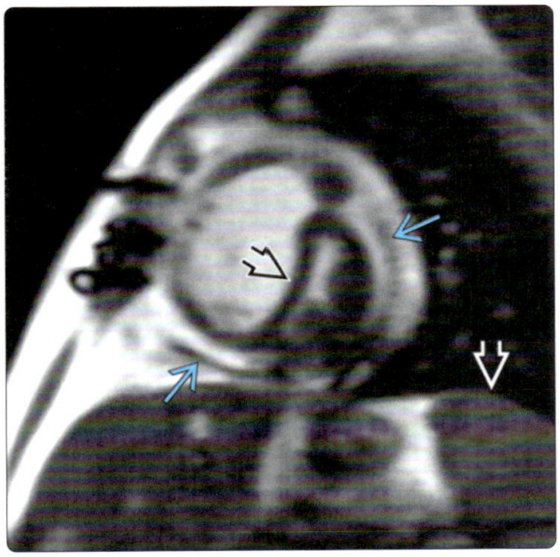

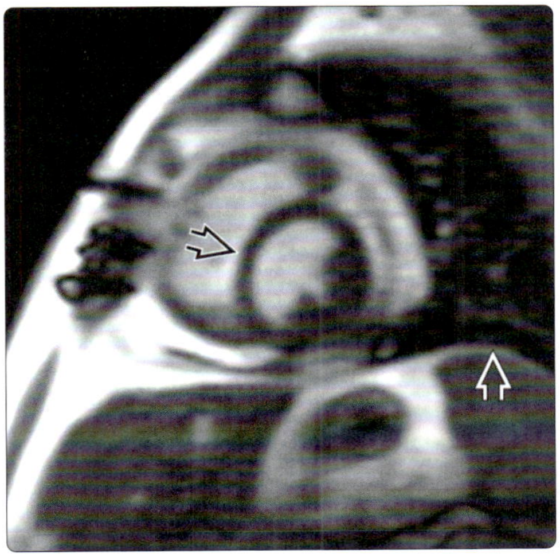

(Left) *Short-axis real-time cine MR shows inferior movement of the diaphragm → during early inspiration with pronounced septal inversion →. Pericardial thickening → is again seen.* **(Right)** *Short-axis real-time cine MR shows superior movement of the diaphragm → during expiration and a normal appearance to the septum →. This confirms exaggerated ventricular interdependence and the diagnosis of constrictive pericarditis.*

Pericardial Cyst

KEY FACTS

IMAGING

- Smoothly marginated, rounded mass
- Unilocular in 80-90%, multilocular in 10-20%
- Most commonly adjacent to right cardiophrenic (CP) angle
  - Right CP angle in 75%
  - 2nd most common location left CP angle
  - May occur anywhere in mediastinum around heart
- Round mass at CP angle on radiographs
  - Sharp, smooth contours
  - Partly spherical with incomplete borders
- Typically fluid attenuation on CT
  - Can be higher attenuation due to proteinaceous fluid
- Typically water signal intensity on MR
  - T1: Homogeneous low or intermediate signal intensity
  - T2: Homogeneous high signal intensity
  - Signal can vary depending on proteinaceous fluid
- No internal enhancement
- Limited imaging protocol required
  - MR
    - Axial and coronal T1, T1 C+, and T2
  - CT
    - Axial CECT

TOP DIFFERENTIAL DIAGNOSES

- Pericardial diverticulum

PATHOLOGY

- Benign cyst of mediastinum

CLINICAL ISSUES

- Generally incidental imaging finding requiring no treatment
- No literature to support percutaneous drainage

DIAGNOSTIC CHECKLIST

- T2-hyperintense, T1-hypointense mass without septations in right costophrenic angle diagnostic of pericardial cyst

(Left) *Posteroanterior radiograph demonstrates a rounded mass at the left cardiophrenic angle ➡, which is smoothly marginated and contiguous with the left heart border.* **(Right)** *Lateral radiograph confirms the position of the mass near the left ventricular apex. It appears smoothly marginated within the left cardiophrenic angle ➡ and contiguous with the left heart border. No calcification or fluid/lipid levels are present.*

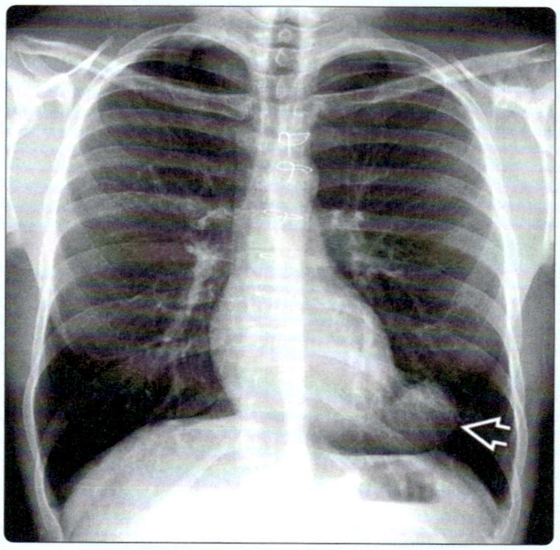

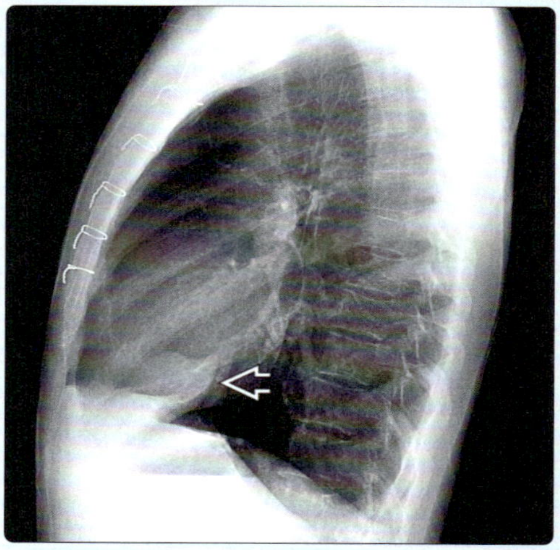

(Left) *Coronal CECT demonstrates a rounded mass that abuts the lateral left ventricle ➡. This is a homogeneous, fluid-attenuation, thin-walled mass with no enhancement. Note a clean fat plane separating the mass from the left ventricle, representing normal epicardial fat.* **(Right)** *Axial CECT shows a rounded, fluid-attenuation, nonenhancing, thin-walled mass ➡ contiguous with the pericardium but separated from the myocardium by epicardial fat. These findings are diagnostic for a pericardial cyst.*

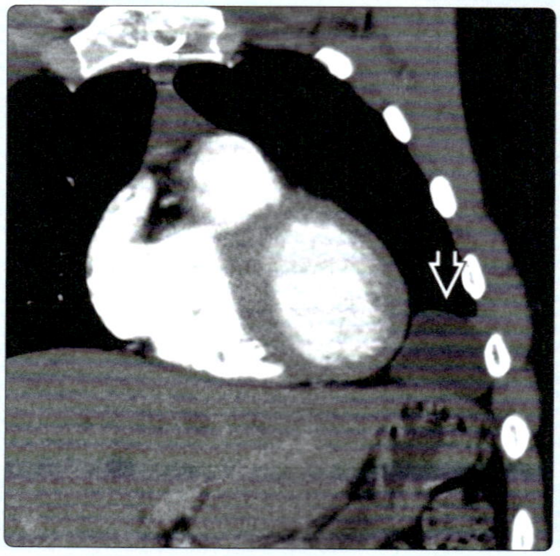

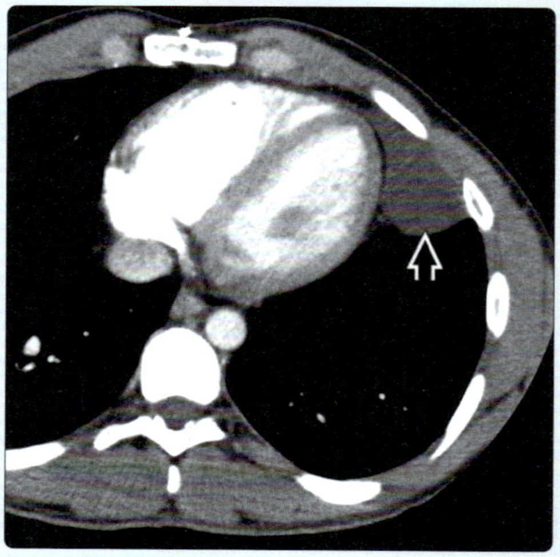

TERMINOLOGY

Definitions

- Fluid-containing mass arising from pericardium, abuts heart
- Embryologic defect in coelomic cavity development or sequela of pericarditis

IMAGING

General Features

- Best diagnostic clue
  - Smoothly marginated, rounded mass adjacent to heart at cardiophrenic (CP) angles
  - Most commonly right anterior CP angle
  - Often water attenuation on CT
    - Can have higher attenuation due to proteinaceous fluid
  - Often follows water signal intensity on MR
    - Signal can vary depending on proteinaceous fluid in cyst
  - Unilocular in 80-90%, multilocular in 10-20%
- Location
  - CP angle
    - Right: 75%, left: 10-40%
- Size
  - 2-30 cm in diameter
- Morphology
  - Smoothly marginated
  - Rounded, teardrop-shaped
  - May change shape with cardiac cycle (mass volume does not change)
  - May prolapse into pleural fissures

Radiographic Findings

- Radiography
  - Rounded mass at right or left CP angle
    - Sharp, smooth contours
    - Partly spherical with incomplete borders (silhouetted by heart)
  - May rarely occur in mediastinum distant from CP angle
    - In these cases, difficult to distinguish pericardial cyst from bronchogenic or thymic cyst
  - May change shape with body positioning, respiration, or cardiac cycle

CT Findings

- NECT
  - Smoothly marginated
  - Wall imperceptible or thin
  - Noncalcified
  - Water attenuation (< 10 HU); usually, no septations
    - Can have higher attenuation due to proteinaceous fluid
- CECT
  - No internal septations or enhancement
  - No wall enhancement

MR Findings

- T1WI
  - Uniform low or intermediate signal intensity
  - Occasionally, high signal intensity due to proteinaceous fluid
- T2WI
  - Homogeneous high signal (follows water signal)
    - Rarely intermediate or low signal due to proteinaceous fluid
- DWI
  - Homogeneous high signal on diffusion-weighted images
  - ADC map: Homogeneous high signal with high ADC values
- T1WI C+
  - No internal septations or enhancement, although may be bilobed
  - No rim enhancement
- MR findings diagnostic, generally requiring no further intervention
- Phase-contrast imaging may detect slow internal flow

Echocardiographic Findings

- Anechoic space between epicardium and parietal pericardium

Imaging Recommendations

- Best imaging tool
  - Echocardiography or MR
- Protocol advice
  - Limited protocol suffices
    - Axial and coronal T1 and T1 C+ MR
    - Axial and coronal T2 MR
    - Coronal imaging helpful to demonstrate relationship to heart and pericardium
- Echocardiography
  - Anechoic in appearance
  - Distinguishes solid from cystic masses
  - Defines relationships with cardiac chambers
- CT and MR useful to
  - Examine entire pericardium
  - Distinguish myocardial from pericardial disease
  - Further characterize pericardial masses

DIFFERENTIAL DIAGNOSIS

Loculated Pleural Effusion

- Fluid density at CT
- May show other loculations or free effusion
- Enhancing septations may be present
- History is pertinent
  - Loculated effusion more common postoperatively

Pericardial Diverticulum

- Focal outpouching of pericardial sac; communicates directly with pericardial cavity
- May be different stage in same developmental process as pericardial cyst; may be acquired following pericarditis and effusion
- Similar imaging features as pericardial cyst
- Changes in size or shape with body position or respiration due to fluid draining back into pericardial cavity

Bronchogenic Cyst

- Imaging characteristics identical to pericardial cyst
- Most commonly in middle mediastinum around carina

- When infected or containing secretions, may appear as solid tumor or may have air-fluid level

Esophageal Duplication Cyst

- Imaging characteristics identical to pericardial cyst
- Adjacent to esophagus
- Can get infected

Thymic Cysts

- Imaging characteristics identical to pericardial cyst
- Usually in anterior mediastinum

Hematoma

- MR particularly useful
  - Acutely demonstrates homogeneous high signal intensity on T1 and T2
  - Subacutely shows heterogeneous signal intensity and areas of high signal intensity on T1 and T2
  - Chronically may show dark peripheral rim and low signal intensity areas that may represent calcification, fibrosis, or hemosiderin deposition on T1
  - High signal intensity areas on T1 or T2 may correspond to hemorrhagic fluid
  - No enhancement on T1 C+

Pericardial Fat Pad

- Echo-free space may be seen by echocardiography
  - May be difficult to distinguish from pericardial fluid
- Distinguishing feature: Fat density on CT

Enlarged Pericardial Lymph Nodes

- Mantle radiation therapy: Cardiac blockers used to protect heart; area may be undertreated
  - Fat pad sign: Enlarging recurrent nodes from lymphoma in undertreated pericardial lymph nodes
  - Appearance or enlargement of fat pad heralds development of adenopathy
  - Nodes may be irradiated since field was blocked initially

Pericardial Metastases

- Lung and breast cancers are most common
- Effusion and irregularly thickened pericardium or pericardial mass
- Enhancement common on CT or MR
- Most have low signal intensity on T1 and high signal intensity on T2 MR

Neurofibroma

- May cause CP angle mass
- Generally solid but may have cystic components
- Enhancement internally on CT or MR

Hydatid Cyst

- Cystic mass with well-defined edges
- Internal trabeculations correspond to daughter membranes
- May be pericardial or intramyocardial
- May appear as solid mass if cyst replaced by necrotic matter
  - Contains membrane residues and granulomatous foreign body inflammatory reaction

Pancreatic Pseudocyst

- History is pertinent
- May show peripancreatic inflammatory changes and fluid collections
- Usually extends through esophageal hiatus

PATHOLOGY

General Features

- Etiology
  - Anomalous outpouching of parietal pericardium
  - Occurs by 4th week of gestation
  - Occurs as coalescing spaces form intraembryonic body cavity
- Benign cyst of mediastinum

Gross Pathologic & Surgical Features

- Invariably connected to pericardium
- Only few show visible communication with pericardial sac

Microscopic Features

- Fibrous tissue lined by single layer of bland mesothelium
- Differentiate from bronchogenic cyst and esophageal duplication cyst by cell lining
  - Absence of bronchial or gastrointestinal epithelium, respectively

CLINICAL ISSUES

Presentation

- Most common signs/symptoms
  - Usually asymptomatic, incidental finding
  - Prevalence: 1 in 100,000
- Other signs/symptoms
  - If symptomatic, presents with chest pain, dyspnea, and cough
    - Symptoms secondary to large size and mass effect
  - Pericardial tamponade may rarely occur

Demographics

- Age
  - 30-50 years

Treatment

- Generally, incidental imaging finding requiring no treatment
- Surgery if symptomatic due to mass effect

DIAGNOSTIC CHECKLIST

Consider

- CT often diagnostic
- MR considered imaging gold standard

Image Interpretation Pearls

- T2-hyperintense, T1-hypointense mass without septations in right CP angle diagnostic of pericardial cyst

SELECTED REFERENCES

1. Meredith A et al: Pericardial cyst. StatPearls, 2024
2. Rajiah P et al: MRI of the pericardium. Radiographics. 39(7):1921-2, 2019
3. Tower-Rader A et al: Pericardial masses, cysts and diverticula: a comprehensive review using multimodality imaging. Prog Cardiovasc Dis. 59(4):389-97, 2017

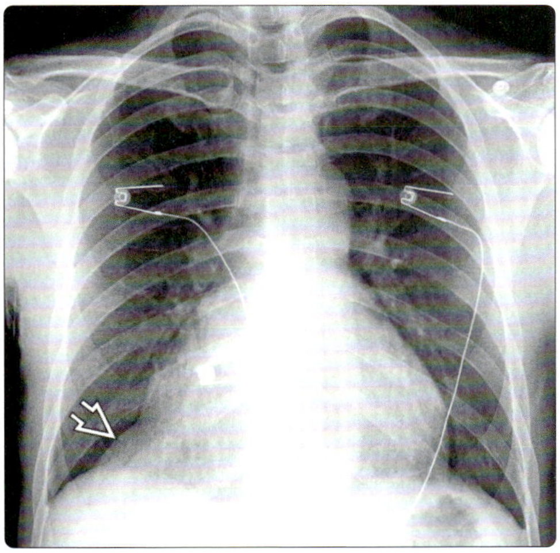

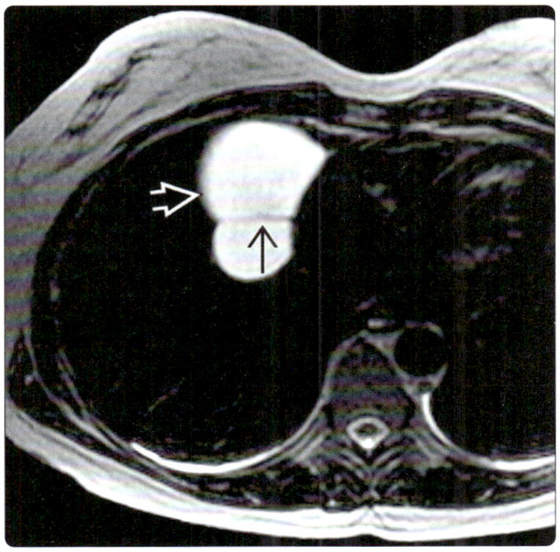

(Left) *Anteroposterior radiograph demonstrates a rounded mass in the right cardiophrenic angle contiguous with the right heart border* ➡. **(Right)** *Axial T2 MR shows a lobulated mediastinal mass at the right cardiophrenic angle, which shows homogeneously high T2 signal intensity* ➡. *The bilobed nature gives the appearance of a single thin, smooth septation* →. *The mass broadly adheres to the pericardium. The appearance and location are characteristic for a pericardial cyst.*

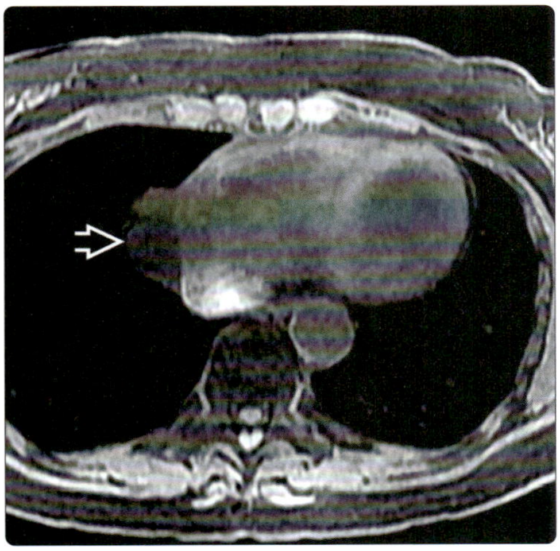

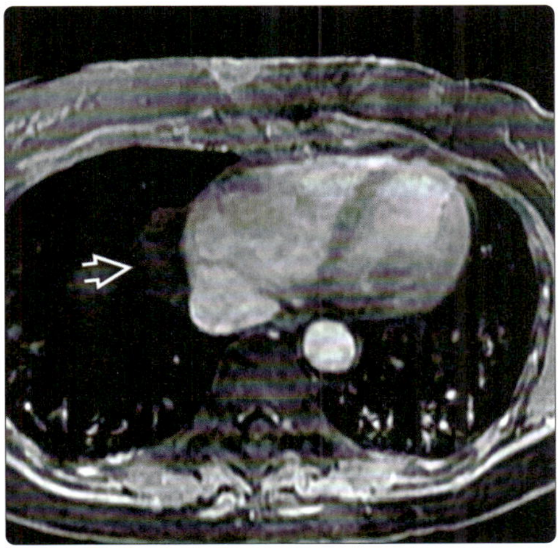

(Left) *Axial T1 MR demonstrates a lobulated mass* ➡ *at the right costophrenic angle with homogeneously low signal. No signs of invasion exist, and broad adherence to the pericardium is present.* **(Right)** *Axial T1 C+ MR demonstrates absence of enhancement of the mass or its walls* ➡, *compatible with a pericardial cyst.*

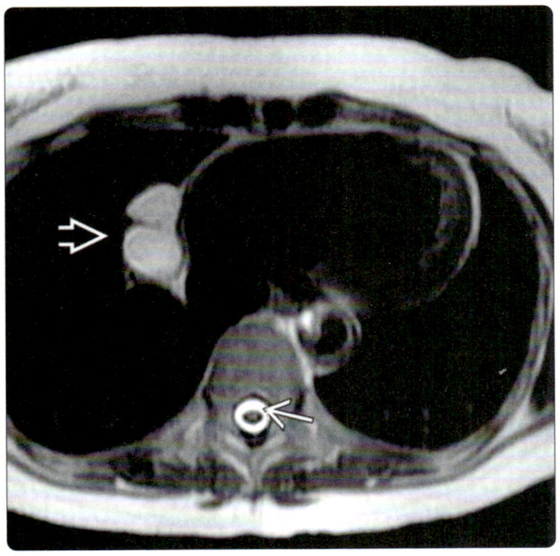

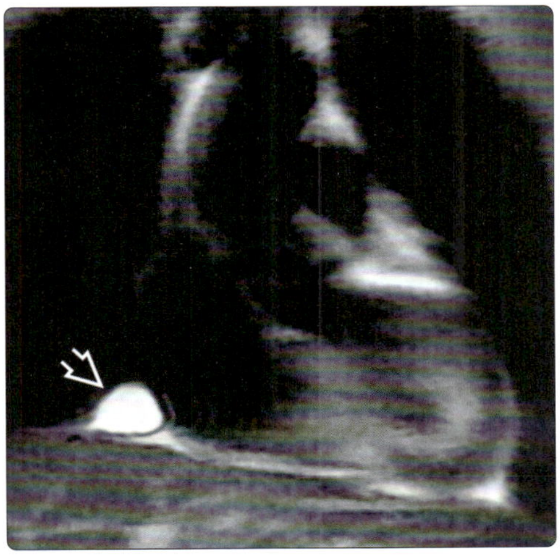

(Left) *Axial T2 FSE MR in the same patient demonstrates homogeneous high signal, consistent with fluid* ➡. *Note that the signal intensity of the cyst is similar to that of cerebrospinal fluid* → *(allowing for general variation of signal strength within the image), which can be used as an internal reference for fluid signal intensity.* **(Right)** *Coronal T2 FSE MR in the same patient localizes the lesion to the right cardiophrenic angle* ➡.

KEY FACTS

TERMINOLOGY

- Congenital absence of pericardium; may be partial or complete right, complete left, or complete

IMAGING

- Radiography
  - Lung interposition between pulmonary trunk and aortic arch
  - Lung interposition between left hemidiaphragm and base of heart
  - Conspicuous left atrial appendage
  - Leftward shift of cardiac silhouette
- CT: Leftward shift and rotation of heart
  - Absence of visible pericardium in affected region
- MR: Absence of hypointense pericardial line
  - Excessive mobility of myocardium
  - Large difference in heart volume between end-systole and end-diastole in affected patients

TOP DIFFERENTIAL DIAGNOSES

- Postsurgical changes (lobectomy, pneumonectomy)
- **Radiographic findings** can mimic other entities, such as
  - Pericardial cyst
  - Pericardial effusion
  - Loculated pleural effusion
  - Left ventricular aneurysm

PATHOLOGY

- Interruption of vascular supply to developing pericardium during embryogenesis

CLINICAL ISSUES

- Most complete defects are clinically insignificant
- Foramen-type defects (subtype of partial pericardial absence defects) may be lethal
- Treatment
  - Surgical closure or enlargement of pericardial defect

(Left) *PA chest radiograph in a patient with partial absence of the pericardium shows the cardiac silhouette shifted to the left ("Snoopy's nose") and the lung interposed between the aortic arch ➔ and pulmonary trunk ➔.* **(Right)** *Axial CECT in a patient with total pericardial absence demonstrates leftward and clockwise rotation of the heart. Note the absence of visible pericardium. Also note the unusual position of the left ventricle ➔ with the apex pointing posteriorly.*

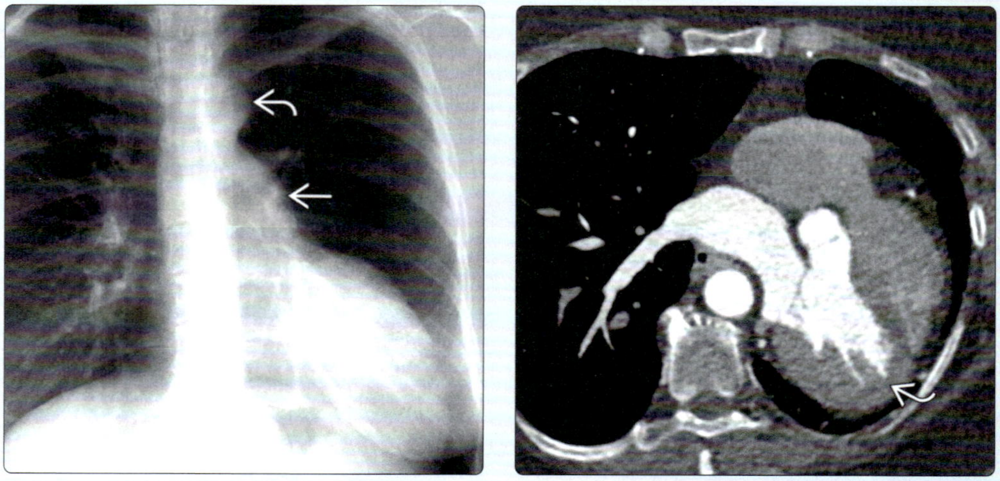

(Left) *Axial CECT in a patient with congenital absence of the left pericardium shows leftward rotation of the heart and great vessels. Normally, the ascending aorta and pulmonic trunk are intrapericardial, but the lung may be interposed ➔ due to pericardial absence.* **(Right)** *Axial CECT in the same patient demonstrates leftward rotation and shift of the heart resulting in the right and left ventricles broadly abutting the left lateral chest wall. Note that the right pericardium ➔ is visible, but the left pericardium is absent.*

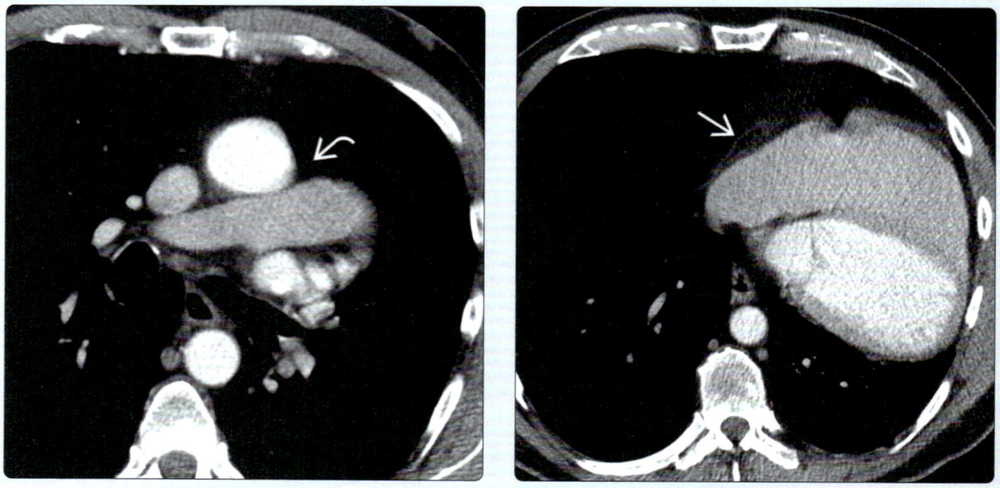

TERMINOLOGY

Definitions

- Congenital absence of pericardium; may be partial or complete right, complete left, or complete

IMAGING

General Features

- Best diagnostic clue
  - Absence of visible pericardium + shift of heart
- Location
  - Partial defects usually occur along lateral left ventricular wall but may occur anywhere

Radiographic Findings

- Radiography
  - **Lung interposition between pulmonary trunk and aortic arch**
  - Lung interposed between left hemidiaphragm and base of heart
  - **Snoopy sign** in complete absence of pericardium
    - Leftward shift and rounding of cardiac silhouette ("Snoopy's nose")
      - May also be seen in partial absence of left pericardium
      - May not be present in younger patients with complete absence
    - Convex prominent left atrial appendage ("Snoopy's ear")
      - Common in partial absence of left pericardium

CT Findings

- NECT
  - **Lung interposition between pulmonary trunk and ascending aorta**
  - Leftward shift and levorotation of heart
  - Absence of visible pericardium in affected region(s)
    - Even in normal persons, intact pericardium may not be seen over left atrial appendage and left ventricle

MR Findings

- Absence of hypointense pericardial line
- Excessive myocardial mobility, especially at apex
- Large difference between end-systolic and end-diastolic volumes

DIFFERENTIAL DIAGNOSIS

Postsurgical Changes

- Segmentectomy, lobectomy, or pneumonectomy
- Surgical material and volume loss on side of surgery
- Heart and mediastinum may shift into postsurgical side
- Compensatory overinflation of other side

Atelectasis/Collapse

- Volume loss resulting in displacement of diaphragm, fissures, hili, or mediastinum
- Sharply defined opacity obscuring vessels without air bronchogram

Radiographic Findings

- Can mimic other entities, such as
  - Pericardial cyst
  - Pericardial effusion
  - Loculated pleural effusion
  - Left ventricular aneurysm

PATHOLOGY

General Features

- Etiology
  - Interruption of vascular supply to developing pericardium during embryogenesis

Staging, Grading, & Classification

- 2/3 are isolated cases
- 1/3 are associated with other congenital abnormalities
  - Cardiac: Bicuspid aortic valve, septal defects, tetralogy of Fallot, mitral valve stenosis, persistent ductus arteriosus
  - Extracardiac: Pectus excavatum deformity, pulmonary sequestration, diaphragmatic hernias

CLINICAL ISSUES

Presentation

- Most common signs/symptoms
  - Complete absence: Usually asymptomatic
  - Partial absence: Nonexertional paroxysmal chest pain, tachycardia, palpitations, death
    - Symptoms due to herniation of parts of myocardium, while other parts remain fixed

Demographics

- Sex: 70% male patients
- Prevalence: 0.002-0.004%

Natural History & Prognosis

- Most complete defects are clinically insignificant
- Subtype of partial absence may be lethal
  - Foramen-type defects may cause herniation of left atrial appendage or left ventricle that results in strangulation of myocardium

Treatment

- Surgical
  - Closure of pericardial defect
  - Enlargement of pericardial defect to prevent strangulation of heart

DIAGNOSTIC CHECKLIST

Consider

- Absence of pericardium when there is lung interposition between pulmonary trunk and aortic arch, particularly if associated with left shift of heart

SELECTED REFERENCES

1. Newman B: Congenital absence of the pericardium: pearls and pitfalls. Semin Ultrasound CT MR. 43(1):47-50, 2022
2. Rajiah P et al: MRI of the pericardium. Radiographics. 39(7):1921-2, 2019
3. Lopez D et al: Congenital absence of the pericardium. Prog Cardiovasc Dis. 59(4):398-406, 2017
4. Shah AB et al: Congenital defects of the pericardium: a review. Eur Heart J Cardiovasc Imaging. 16(8):821-7, 2015
5. Alpert JB et al: Imaging the post-thoracotomy patient: anatomic changes and postoperative complications. Radiol Clin North Am. 52(1):85-103, 2014

Pericardial Effusion

KEY FACTS

TERMINOLOGY

- ↑ fluid in pericardial space

IMAGING

- Radiography
  - Frontal: Water bottle sign; globular enlargement of cardiopericardial silhouette
  - Lateral: Fat pad sign; pericardial fluid outlined by surrounding fat
- CT
  - Water-attenuation fluid: Often transudative
  - High-attenuation fluid: Hemorrhage, purulent fluid, malignancy
  - Associated pericardial thickening and calcification
  - Cardiac chambers: Constriction and tamponade
- MR: Assessment of complicated effusion
  - 93% accuracy for constrictive pericarditis
- Echocardiography: Imaging modality of choice

TOP DIFFERENTIAL DIAGNOSES

- Pericardial cyst
- Pericardial malignancy
- Dilated cardiomyopathy

CLINICAL ISSUES

- Signs/symptoms
  - May be asymptomatic
  - Chest pain, friction rub
  - Cardiac tamponade: Rate of fluid accumulation is more significant than volume or composition
- Treatment
  - Small effusions may not require treatment
  - ↑ hemodialysis in chronic renal failure
  - Antiinflammatory agents for acute idiopathic/viral pericarditis
  - Percutaneous or surgical drainage
  - Emergent management of tamponade

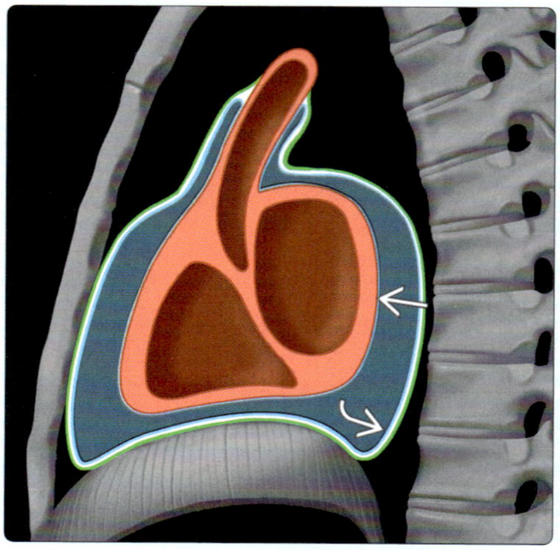

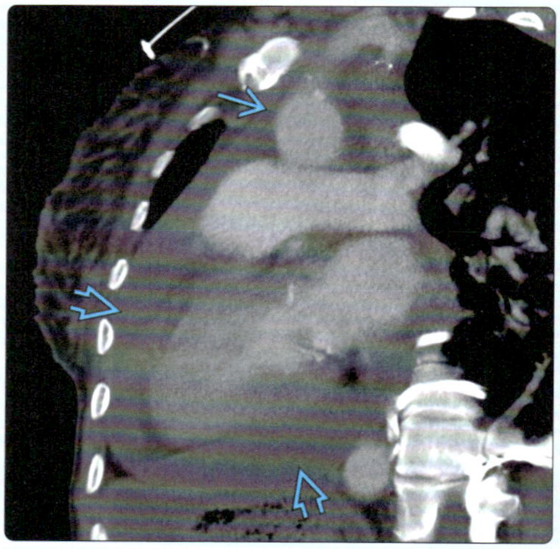

(Left) *Graphic shows features of pericardial effusion. Pericardial fluid is located in the potential space between the serous layers of the parietal pericardium* ➔ *and visceral pericardium (epicardium)* ➔. **(Right)** *Two-chamber CECT using a 10-mm-thick projection in a woman with renal failure shows a large pericardial effusion* ➔. *Note the superior extent of the parietal pericardium* ➔ *where it attaches to the aortic arch.*

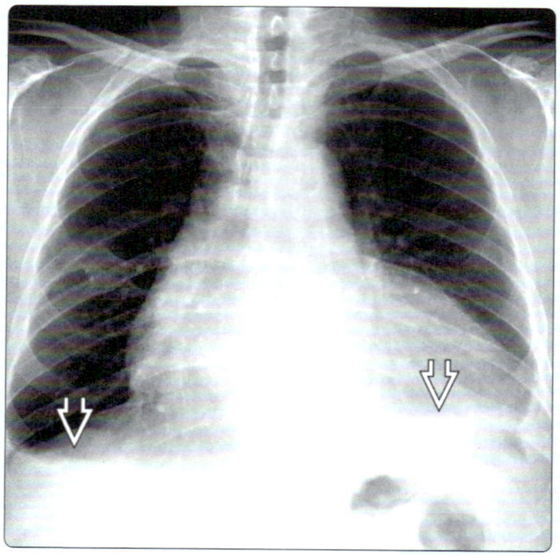

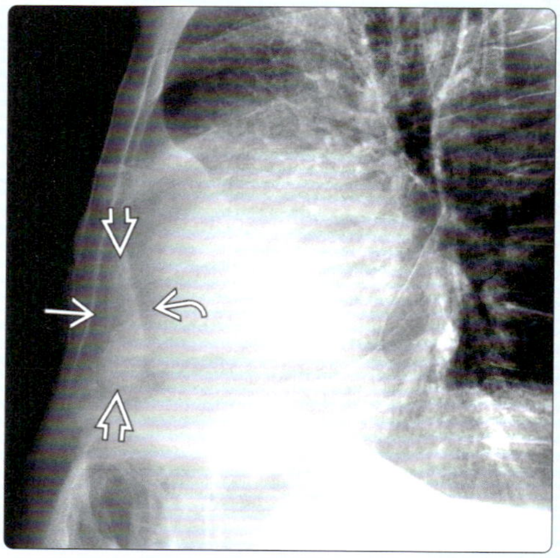

(Left) *PA chest radiograph in a patient with congestive heart failure demonstrates enlargement of the cardiac silhouette and bilateral pleural effusions* ➔. **(Right)** *Lateral chest radiograph in the same patient shows a pericardial effusion manifesting as the fat pad sign. A water-attenuation stripe* ➔ *between the retrosternal mediastinal fat (a.k.a. pericardial fat)* ➔ *and the subepicardial fat* ➔ *represents a pericardial effusion.*

TERMINOLOGY

Definitions

- Abnormal ↑ of fluid within pericardial sac

IMAGING

General Features

- Best diagnostic clue
  - Radiography: Fat pad sign on lateral radiograph
  - CT and MR: Fluid in pericardial space
- Location
  - CT and MR
    - Common to see small amount of fluid in pericardial space
      - This is often seen along inferior and posterior aspect of heart
    - As fluid volume ↑, effusion begins to extend anteriorly
    - In moderate to large effusions, pericardial fluid can circumferentially surround heart
- Anatomic considerations
  - 2 apposed pericardial layers with intervening potential (pericardial) space
  - Normally contains 15-50 mL of fluid
- Normal pericardium in CT and MR
  - No distinction between serous and fibrous pericardial layers is possible
  - Frequent visualization of small amount of physiologic fluid and fluid-filled pericardial sinuses and recesses
  - Can be difficult to distinguish between small amount of pericardial fluid and mild thickening of pericardium

Radiographic Findings

- Frontal chest radiograph
  - Moderately large (> 250-mL) pericardial effusion
    - Water bottle sign
      - Globular symmetric enlargement of cardiopericardial silhouette
      - Normal superior mediastinum
  - Rapid enlargement of cardiac silhouette on serial radiography commonly associated with pericardial effusion
- Lateral chest radiograph
  - Fat pad sign, a.k.a. Oreo cookie sign, sandwich sign, or bun sign
    - > 2-mm water density stripe between retrosternal and subepicardial fat

CT Findings

- NECT
  - Water-attenuation pericardial fluid
    - Heart failure, renal failure, malignancy
  - High-attenuation (> 20-HU) pericardial fluid
    - Hemorrhage, purulent effusion, malignancy
    - Hemopericardium: Attenuation is initially high but ↓ over time
  - High sensitivity for detection of pericardial calcification
- CECT
  - Assessment for thickening, nodules, masses
  - Enhancement of serous pericardium and pericardial thickening from inflammation
    - Enhancement best seen on portal venous phase of imaging
    - Can occasionally see inflammation of mediastinal fat
  - Assessment of cardiac chambers
    - Signs of constriction: Tubular ventricles, flattened/sigmoid interventricular septum
  - Signs of cardiac tamponade
    - Flattening of anterior surface of heart and right cardiac chambers
    - Angulation or bowing of interventricular septum
    - Enlarged vena cava
    - Periportal edema
    - Compression of coronary sinus

MR Findings

- General
  - Uncomplicated effusion
    - T1WI: Hypointense; T2WI: Hyperintense; PSIR: Dark
  - Complicated effusion: Septations, debris
  - Hemorrhagic effusion
    - T1WI: Hyperintense; T2WI: Hypointense
    - Hemopericardium
      - Acute phase: Homogeneous hyperintensity
      - Subacute phase (1-4 weeks): Heterogeneous signal, foci of hyperintensity on T1WI and T2WI
      - Chronic phase (> 4 weeks): Hypointense foci (calcification, fibrosis), dark peripheral rim
      - No contrast enhancement
  - Assessment of pericardium and cardiac chambers
    - MR: 93% accuracy for differentiation between constrictive pericarditis (pericardial thickening of > 4 mm) and restrictive cardiomyopathy

Echocardiographic Findings

- High sensitivity for pericardial fluid
  - Echo-free space between pericardial layers
  - ↓ parietal pericardial motion
- Assessment of constrictive pericarditis
- Assessment of suspected tamponade
  - Mass effect
    - Diastolic compression/collapse of right heart chambers
    - Abnormal cardiac filling
    - Compression of pulmonary trunk and thoracic inferior vena cava
  - Abnormal motion
    - Lack of inspiratory collapse of dilated inferior vena cava
    - Cardiac swing within pericardium
    - Doppler flow velocity paradoxus: Respiratory variation in Doppler velocities
    - Paradoxical motion of interventricular septum

Imaging Recommendations

- Best imaging tool
  - Echocardiography: Modality of choice for initial pericardial imaging

- CT and MR: Evaluation of complications of pericardial effusion; hemorrhage; loculation; calcification; constriction

DIFFERENTIAL DIAGNOSIS

Pericardial Cyst

- Focal, water-attenuation cyst abutting pericardium
- May mimic loculated pericardial effusion

Pericardial Thickening

- Can be difficult to differentiate small amount of pericardial fluid from thickening
- Areas of calcification or ↑ attenuation of pericardium more suggestive of chronic thickening

Dilated Cardiomyopathy

- May mimic pericardial effusion on radiograph

Fluid in Pericardial Recesses

- Several pericardial recesses and sinuses
- Small physiologic amount of fluid in these structures is normal

PATHOLOGY

General Features

- Etiology
  - Obstruction of lymphatic or venous drainage
  - Left ventricular failure: Most common causes of pericardial effusion
  - Myocardial infarction
  - Uremic effusion: 50% of patients with chronic renal failure
  - Infection
    - Acute pericarditis: 90% idiopathic or viral
    - Tuberculosis
      - Most common cause of constrictive pericarditis in developing world
      - Tamponade, frequent complication
    - Endocarditis, sepsis
  - Postcardiac surgery: Typical spontaneous resolution
    - Up to 6% may become clinically significant; cardiac tamponade
  - Autoimmune disease
    - Rheumatoid arthritis: Effusion in 2-10%
    - Systemic lupus erythematosus (SLE): Up to 50% with symptomatic effusion
    - Systemic sclerosis: Up to 70% with small effusion
  - Neoplasia
  - Thermal injury
  - Blunt/penetrating trauma
  - Hypoalbuminemia, myxedema
  - Drug reaction, radiation, trauma
  - Effusive constrictive pericarditis
    - Constrictive physiology ± associated pericardial effusion or tamponade
    - Persistent elevated right chamber pressures after pericardial fluid drainage

Pathophysiology

- Pericardial effusion: Rate of fluid accumulation
  - Gradual ↑ in pericardial fluid: May accommodate > 1 L without tamponade
  - Rapid ↑ in pericardial fluid: Cardiac tamponade, impaired cardiac filling
- Cardiac tamponade
  - ↓ intracardiac volume; ↑ diastolic filling pressures
  - ↑ intrapericardial pressure with cardiac compression
- Rate of fluid accumulation is more significant than fluid volume or composition

CLINICAL ISSUES

Presentation

- Most common signs/symptoms
  - Depends on cause of effusion and rapidity of development
  - May be asymptomatic
  - Dyspnea, which is worse when lying down
  - Pericardial friction rub in acute pericarditis
- Other signs/symptoms
  - Pericardial tamponade
    - Anxiety, dyspnea, chest pain, jugular vein distention
    - Tachycardia, hypotension
    - Paradoxical pulse: > 10-mmHg drop in systolic arterial pressure during inspiration
    - Beck triad
      - Muffled heart sounds
      - Hypotension
      - Jugular vein distention

Treatment

- Most effusions are treated by treating underlying cause; i.e., diuresis in setting of congestive heart failure
- ↑ hemodialysis; renal failure-related effusion
- ↑ effusion or effusion > 250 mL
  - Consider pericardiocentesis (image guided)
    - 93% success rate
  - Surgical drainage
    - Preferred for hemopericardium and purulent effusion
    - Pericardial window, subxiphoid pericardiotomy
    - Pericardiectomy
    - Balloon pericardiotomy in recurrent tamponade
      - Emergent management of tamponade
- Antiinflammatory agents for acute idiopathic/viral pericarditis

DIAGNOSTIC CHECKLIST

Image Interpretation Pearls

- Recognition of normal fluid-filled pericardial recesses, which may mimic lymph nodes and congenital cysts

SELECTED REFERENCES

1. Wang TKM et al: Cardiac magnetic resonance imaging techniques and applications for pericardial diseases. Circ Cardiovasc Imaging. 15(7):e014283, 2022
2. Chetrit M et al: Imaging-guided therapies for pericardial diseases. JACC Cardiovasc Imaging. 13(6):1422-37, 2020
3. Kligerman S: Imaging of pericardial disease. Radiol Clin North Am. 57(1):179-99, 2019
4. Cummings KW et al: Imaging of pericardial diseases. Semin Ultrasound CT MR. 37(3):238-54, 2016
5. Bogaert J et al: Pericardial disease: value of CT and MR imaging. Radiology. 267(2):340-56, 2013

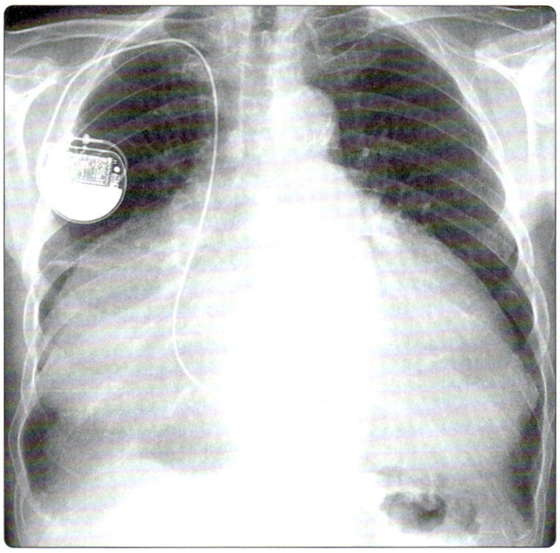

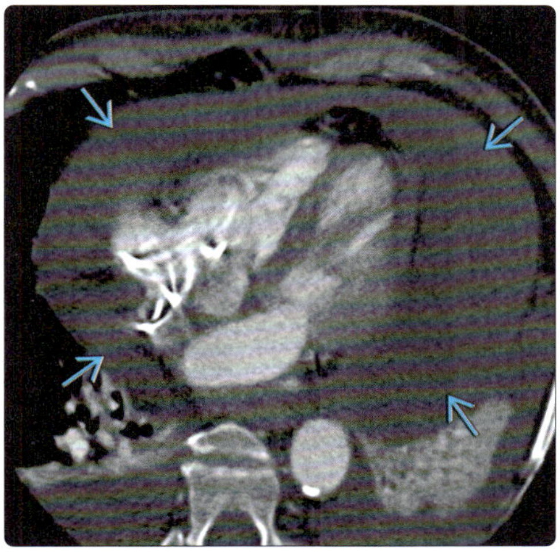

(Left) *PA chest radiograph shows a large pericardial effusion manifesting with the water bottle sign, characterized by globular enlargement of the cardiopericardial silhouette and a normal superior mediastinum. Pericardial fluid may slowly accumulate and attain a large volume without producing cardiac tamponade.* **(Right)** *Axial CT in the same patient shows the massive circumferential transudative pericardial effusion* [→]. *Despite the large size, there was no tamponade on ECG.*

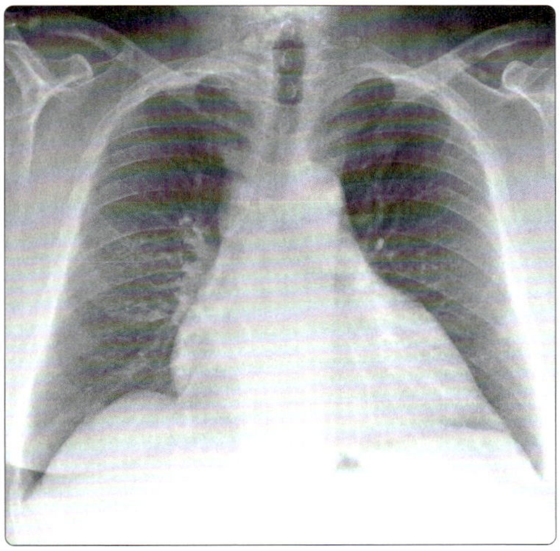

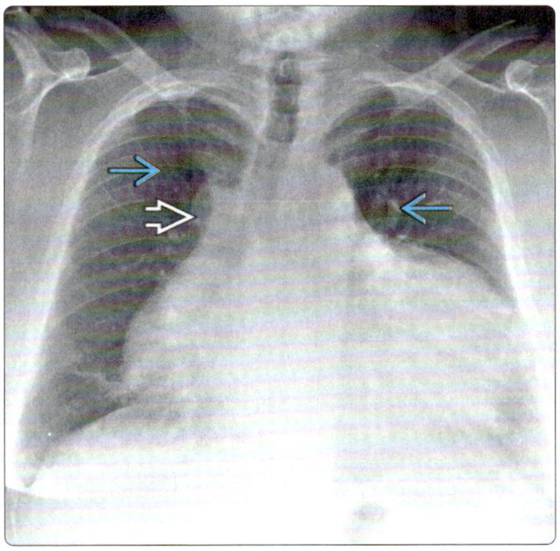

(Left) *PA radiograph in a 66-year-old man with renal failure shows only a mildly enlarged cardiac silhouette.* **(Right)** *PA radiograph obtained 2 weeks later due to worsening dyspnea shows an globular cardiac silhouette. In addition, the pulmonary vasculature* [→] *and azygous vein* [⇨] *are more distended. Given this cardiac configuration and rapid increase in size, a larger pericardial effusion was suggested. Rate of fluid accumulation is more significant in developing clinical symptoms.*

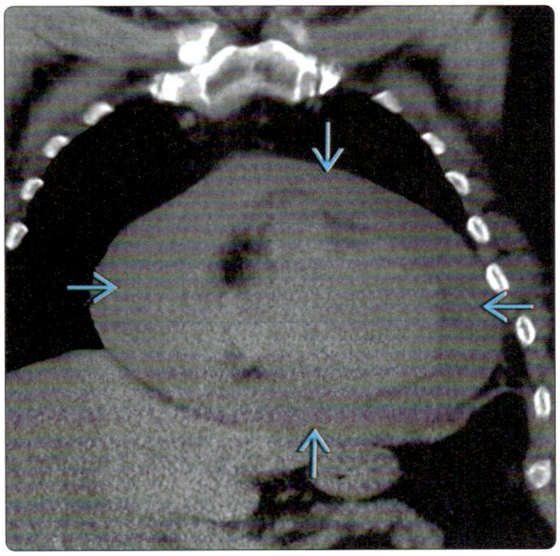

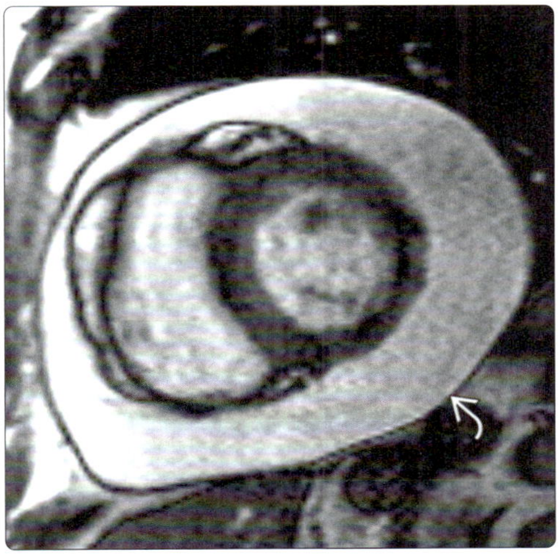

(Left) *Coronal NECT in the same patient shows the large circumferential pericardial effusion* [→]. *Although there was concern for tamponade given the rapid accumulation, there was no evidence of this on echocardiogram.* **(Right)** *Short-axis SSFP cine MR in a patient with a large pericardial effusion shows circumferential, high-signal pericardial fluid. The combined parietal serous and fibrous pericardial layers are within a thin, low-signal, linear structure* [↗] *surrounding the fluid, which is accentuated by a chemical shift artifact.*

(Left) *Axial CECT in a 31-year-old woman with lupus shows a moderate-sized pericardial effusion with enhancement of the visceral* → *and parietal* → *pericardium due to inflammation. There are also moderate, bilateral pleural effusions, which are partially loculated.* **(Right)** *Four-chamber chest CT in a patient with acute TB pericarditis shows a loculated pericardial effusion with enhancement of the visceral* → *and parietal* → *pericardium. Exudate material that was PCR positive for TB was present in the pericardial fluid.*

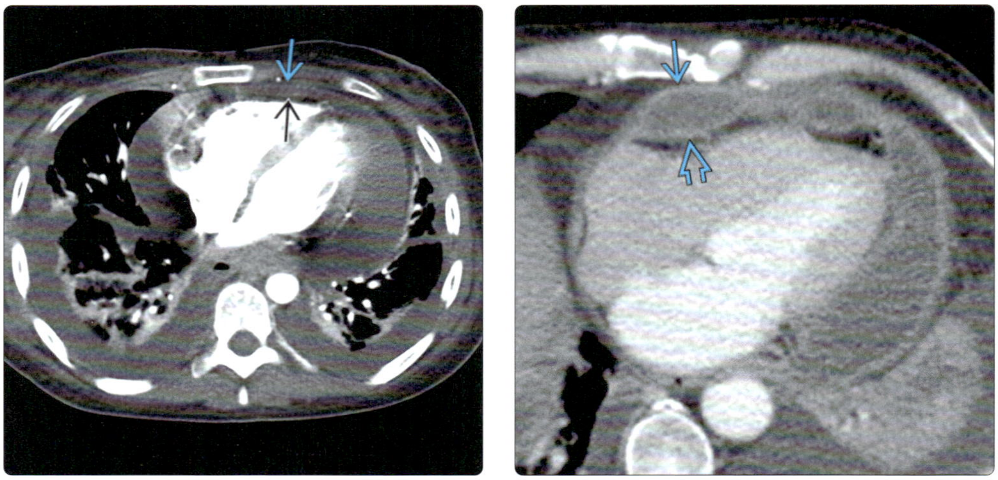

(Left) *Axial CECT in a patient with TB pericarditis shows a water-attenuation pericardial effusion, enhancement of the serous pericardium* →*, infiltration of the adjacent mediastinal fat, right paraesophageal lymphadenopathy* →*, and bilateral pleural effusions.* **(Right)** *Axial CECT in a patient with infectious pericarditis shows a large pericardial effusion and pericardial thickening and enhancement* →*. Note the bilateral pleural effusions, which are larger on the left than on the right.*

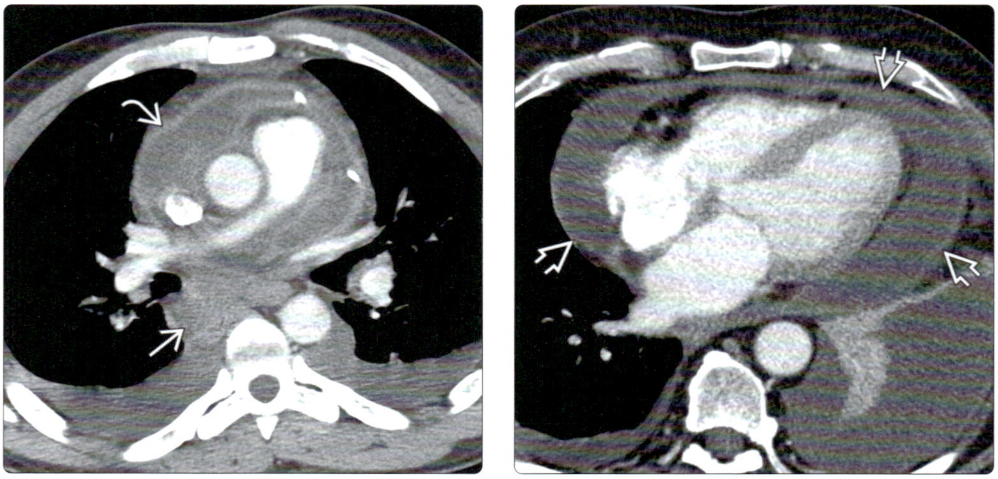

(Left) *Axial chest CT in a 51-year-old man with chronic renal failure shows a small to moderate pericardial effusion* →*. Although there is linear enhancement of the parietal pericardium* →*, it is relatively subtle during the systemic arterial phase.* **(Right)** *Axial CECT during the portal venous phase in the same patient demonstrates enhancement of both the parietal* → *and visceral* → *pericardium that are more conspicuous than during the systemic arterial phase. A diagnosis of uremic pericarditis was made.*

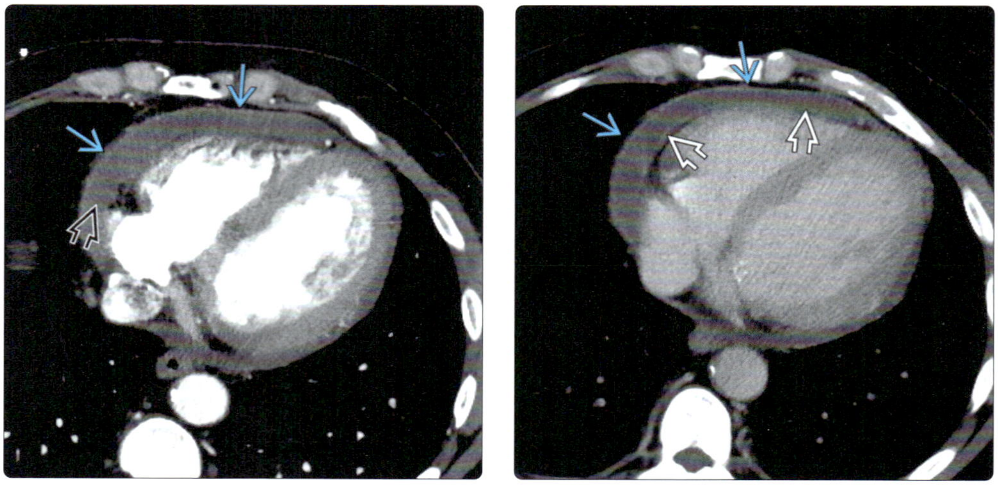

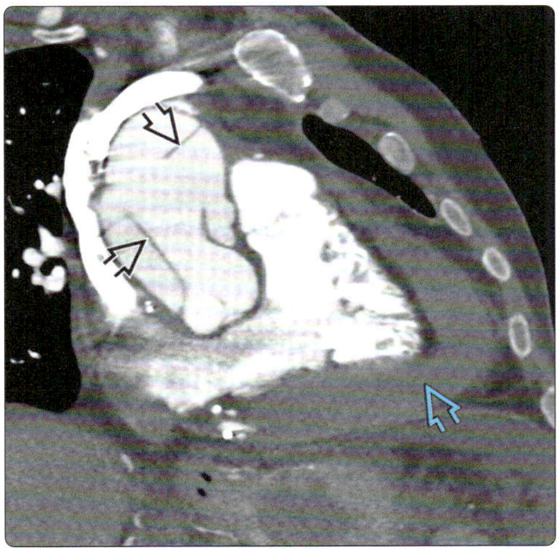

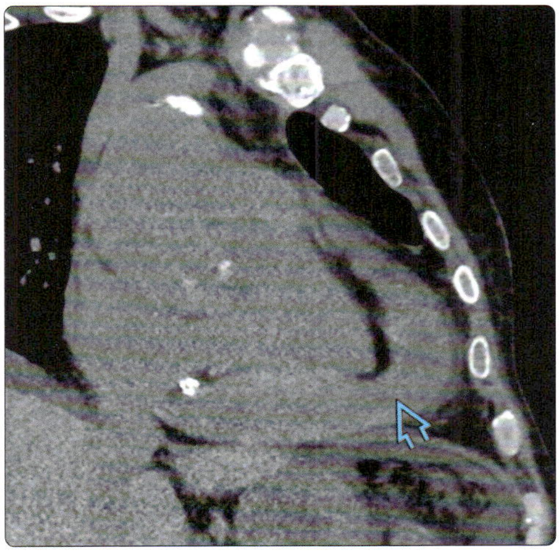

(Left) *Right ventricular outflow tract (RVOT) ECG-gated cardiac CTA in a 63-year-old man demonstrates a type A dissection of aorta and pericardial effusion surrounding the ventricles.* **(Right)** *RVOT NECT in the same patient demonstrates high attenuation in the pericardial space due to accumulation of blood, which is consisted with hemopericardium. NECT is better in identification of high-attenuation pericardial fluid.*

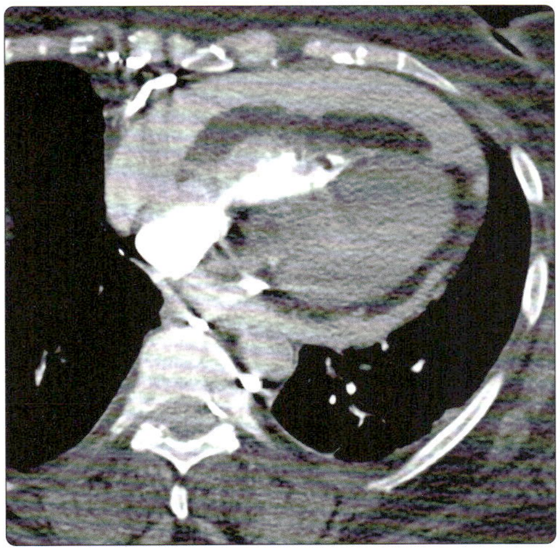

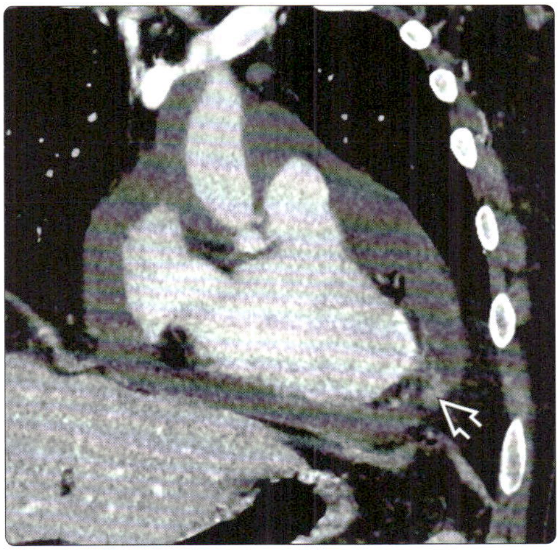

(Left) *Axial CECT in a patient with pericardial tamponade after traumatic catheter placement shows high-attenuation pericardial fluid due to extravasated contrast and blood from superior vena cava laceration and mass effect on the right ventricle. Tamponade was confirmed on ECG.* **(Right)** *RVOT CECT in a patient with a pericardial effusion shows a subtle, enhancing nodule. Pericardiocentesis revealed a bloody effusion with malignant cells. A primary pericardial angiosarcoma was proven on biopsy.*

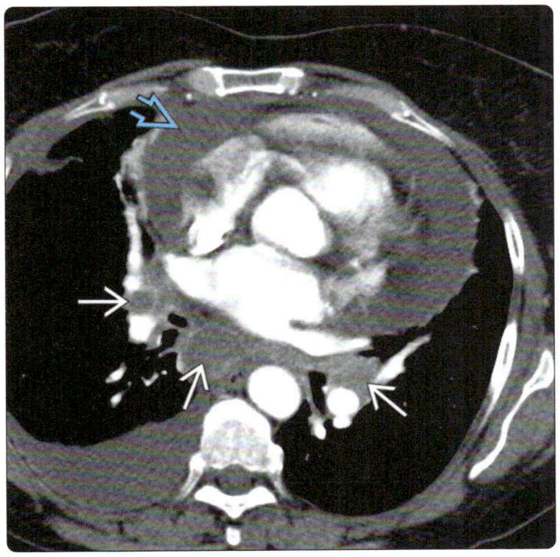

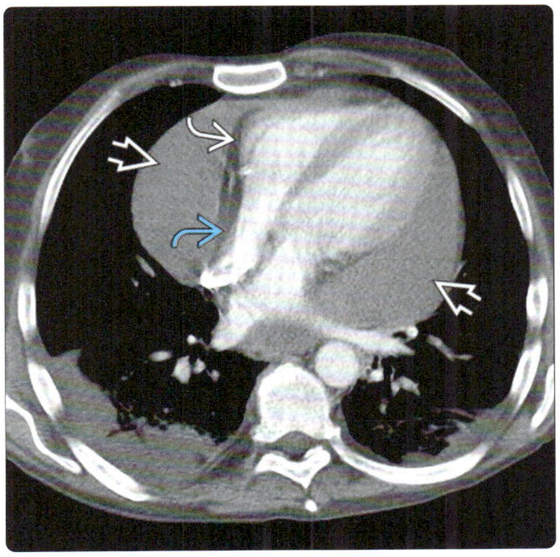

(Left) *Axial oblique CECT in a 58-year-old woman with lung cancer shows a moderate-sized pericardial effusion and nodal metastases. Although there were no enhancing nodules, malignant cells were seen on pericardiocentesis.* **(Right)** *Axial CECT in a patient with lung cancer shows a large pericardial effusion compressing the right atrium and ventricle, highly suggestive of cardiac tamponade, which was proven on ECG. Draining of the effusion showed malignant cells.*

KEY FACTS

TERMINOLOGY

- Compression of heart chambers by pericardial fluid, gas, or solid tissue with hemodynamic sequelae
  - Pressure-volume curve of space between visceral and parietal layers depends on rate of accumulation

IMAGING

- Serial chest radiographs: Rapid increase in cardiac silhouette
- Echocardiography: Primary tool for diagnosis of tamponade
  - Tamponade physiology in setting of > 50 mL of fluid
  - Diastolic collapse of right atrium is earliest sign, followed by persistence in systole
- MR: Functional images may demonstrate collapse of right atrium and ventricle and enlarged systemic veins
  - Not commonly used in tamponade due to acute nature
- CT: Moderate to large pericardial effusion with
  - Contrast reflux within inferior vena cava, azygos vein and hepatic veins
    - Contrast refluxing into azygous vein is suggestive of tamponade in setting of pericardial effusion
  - Collapse of right atrial or right ventricular free wall
  - Septal flattening
  - Echocardiogram of cardiac catheterization should be performed to confirm or exclude diagnosis

CLINICAL ISSUES

- Spectrum of severity, ranging from asymptomatic to complete cardiovascular collapse
- Acute tamponade
  - Tachycardia and pulsus paradoxus (exaggerated inspiratory drop of systolic blood pressure > 10 mmHg)
  - Treat with pericardiocentesis
- Subacute or chronic tamponade
  - Signs of right heart failure predominate
  - Hepatomegaly, ascites, peripheral edema

(Left) *CTPA in a 38-year-old woman shows a large circumferential pericardial effusion with pericardial enhancement ⇨. There is question of mild collapse of the free wall of the right ventricle (RV) ⇨, concerning for tamponade. The superior vena cava (SVC) and inferior vena cava (IVC) were also dilated.* **(Right)** *Four-chamber CECT shows partial collapse of the right atrium ⇨, which is concerning for tamponade.*

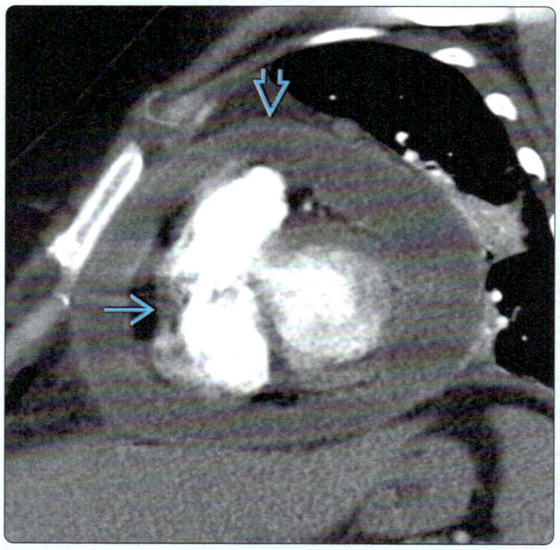

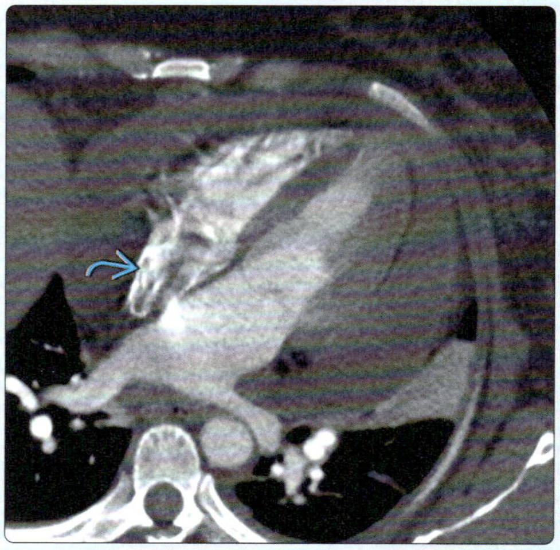

(Left) *In the same patient, echocardiogram (left) during early diastole shows RV free wall collapse ⇨. During inhalation, a late diastolic image (right) shows the normal configuration of the RV free wall, but flattening and inversion of the septum ⇨, also due to tamponade. A large pericardial effusion ⇨ is seen.* **(Right)** *Globular cardiac silhouette, azygous vein distention, and mild edema is seen just after pericardial drain placement ⇨ in the emergency department. The cause of the acute pericarditis was unknown.*

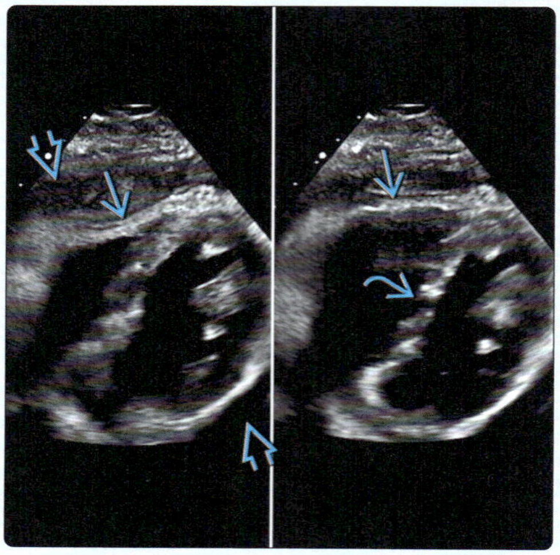

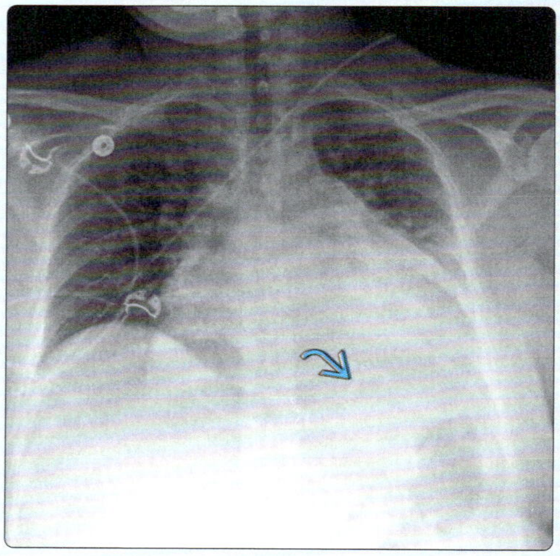

TERMINOLOGY

Definitions

- Compression of heart chambers by pericardial fluid, gas, or solid tissue with hemodynamic sequelae
  - Potential space separates visceral and parietal serosal layers and normally contains up to 50 mL of serous fluid (plasma ultrafiltrate)
    - Pressure-volume curve behavior of this finite space depends on rate of accumulation
    - Impairment of diastolic filling of ventricles leads to reduction in cardiac output; if untreated, will lead to cardiac arrest

IMAGING

General Features

- Best diagnostic clue
  - Collapse of right-sided cardiac chambers on echocardiogram, CT, or MR
- Location
  - Pericardial space between visceral (inner) and parietal (outer) pericardial layers
    - Earliest pericardial fluid collects adjacent to posterolateral left ventricular or inferolateral right ventricle walls
    - Moderate-sized collections of fluid (100-500 mL) then tend to accumulate adjacent to anterior free wall of right ventricle (> 5 mm)

Radiographic Findings

- Rapid increase in size of cardiac silhouette on serial chest radiographs
- Findings of large pericardial effusion
  - Globular shape of heart, Oreo cookie sign on lateral radiograph, etc.
- Pulmonary edema and pleural effusions may be present
- Chest radiograph may be normal

Fluoroscopic Findings

- Often right heart catheterization is performed under fluoroscopy
  - Right atrial (RA) pressures are elevated, and systole is followed by large X descent, but diastolic equalization of pressures leads to diminished Y descent
  - If intraatrial pressures fail to decrease as fluid is drained, effusive-constrictive pericarditis should be considered

CT Findings

- Dilated inferior vena cava (IVC) and superior vena cava (SVC)
  - Distension of jugular veins can also be present
- Contrast reflux within IVC, azygos vein, and hepatic veins
  - Contrast refluxing into azygous vein implies significant hemodynamic disturbance and with acute pericardial effusion suggests tamponade
- Partial collapse of right ventricular (RV) free wall or RA may be seen during nongated studies
- Flattening or inversion of interventricular septum
- Compression of coronary sinus
- Pericardial effusion, often large
  - Attenuation of fluid can help delineate underlying etiology
- Pericardial enhancement often present
- Tension pneumopericardium
  - Air filling pericardial space leading to compression of heart
    - Common causes include trauma, recent surgery, positive pressure ventilation, fistulous connective between pericardium and gas-containing space, such as to tracheobronchial tree, pleural, peritoneum, or GI tract

MR Findings

- Delayed enhancement
  - Can be used to detect grade and severity of ongoing pericardial inflammation
- Simple, transudative effusions have low signal on T1 images and high signal on T2 FSE and SSFP images
- Complex effusions, such as exudative and hemorrhagic fluid, have high signal on T1 and intermediate signal on T2 spin-echo images
  - Hemorrhagic effusions can evolve into chronic hematoma with low signal intensity and dark foci signifying hemosiderin deposition surrounded by dark peripheral rim
- On SSFP cine sequences
  - RA and ventricular collapse; early phase during diastole
  - Dilated systemic veins (IVC and SVC) and hepatic veins
  - Heart may appear to be "swinging" in pericardial space
  - Flattening or inversion of interventricular septum
- With use of double-inversion recovery in FSE sequences, signal depends on presence of flow within collection
  - Free-flowing collections, such as transudates, have no signal
  - Complex collections without flow have intermediate to high signal

Echocardiographic Findings

- Hypoechoic band between pericardial layers
- Size of effusion does not indicate its hemodynamic significance
- In large effusions, heart may "swing" within pericardial fluid on beat-to-beat basis correlating with electrical alternans
- Earliest sign is diastolic collapse of right atrium, followed by persistent collapse in systole
  - Duration of right atrium collapse > 1/3 of ventricular systole is highly specific for cardiac tamponade
- Early diastolic RV free wall collapse
- Paradoxical motion of septum
- > 35% respiratory difference in transmitral inflow velocities and tricuspid inflow of > 80% correlated best with tamponade physiology in comparison hemodynamic studies
- Plethoric IVC with no respirophasic change; most sensitive, not specific
- Hepatic vein diastolic flow reversal on expiration
- Small collections may be visible only during ventricular systole; effusions > 25-50 mL are seen as echo-free space throughout cardiac cycle

Imaging Recommendations

- Best imaging tool
  - Echocardiography showing tamponade physiology in setting of > 50 mL fluid

DIFFERENTIAL DIAGNOSIS

Constrictive Pericarditis

- Due to noncompliance of pericardium rather than rapid accumulation of fluid
  - Is chronic process, whereas tamponade is more acute
- Can be similar physiologically
- Pericardial often thickened &/or calcified in constrictive pericarditis
- Pericardial effusion often small in constrictive pericarditis

Effusive-Constrictive Pericarditis

- Presence of tense pericardial effusion in setting of pericardial constriction
- Persistence of elevated RA pressure after removal of pericardial fluid
- Primarily diagnosed with echocardiogram and cardiac catheterization

Pericardial Effusion Without Tamponade

- Pericardial effusions are common
- If pericardial effusion is slowly accumulating, pericardium can slowly stretch and accommodate large volume of fluid without tamponade
- While there may be signs suggesting tamponade on CT, echocardiogram should be used for physiologic assessment

PATHOLOGY

General Features

- Etiology
  - Infectious
    - Viral causes: Commonly adeno- or coxsackievirus
    - Bacterial: Tuberculosis
  - Hemorrhage
    - Aortic dissection or aortic aneurysm rupture into pericardial space
    - Traumatic or iatrogenic (ablation of arrhythmias, pacemaker implantation)
  - Acute myocardial infarction
  - Renal failure
  - Neoplasm
    - Lung (most commonly), breast, or lymphoma

CLINICAL ISSUES

Presentation

- Most common signs/symptoms
  - Spectrum of severity, ranging from asymptomatic to complete cardiovascular collapse
  - In acute tamponade, features include
    - Tachycardia (most sensitive sign)
    - Pulsus paradoxus
      - Exaggerated inspiratory drop of systolic blood pressure > 10 mmHg
      - Driven by reciprocal changes in left and right heart filling and output
      - Most specific sign
    - Diastolic filling is reduced as intrapericardial pressure rises
    - Reduced preload may lead to shock
    - Beck triad: Hypotension, jugular vein distension, muffled heart sounds
  - In subacute or chronic tamponade, signs of right heart failure predominate
    - Hepatomegaly, ascites, peripheral edema
    - Compression of left recurrent laryngeal nerve by may lead to hoarseness (Ortner syndrome)
- Other signs/symptoms
  - ECG: Classic ECG pattern of widespread ST segment elevation and PR depression seen in < 60% of patients

Treatment

- Interventional
  - Pericardiocentesis for acute tamponade
    - Beware: Hemopericardium may be due to aortic dissection, and pericardiocentesis may be catastrophic
  - Echocardiographic guidance reduces major complications from 20% to < 1.5%
  - Extrapleural subxiphoid approach recommended
  - Drainage should continue until aspirated volume is < 25 mL/day
- Surgical
  - Recurrent effusions may be treated by repeat pericardiocentesis, surgical creation of pericardial window (creating communication with pleural space)
  - Video-assisted thoracoscopic pericardiectomy is alternative to open thoracotomy
  - Surgical pericardiectomy in patients for whom medical therapy and repeated pericardiocentesis unsuccessful
- Intrapericardial thrombin: Has been used successfully as "bailout strategy" by promoting hemostasis and acting as sealing agent
- Mechanical ventilation with positive airway pressure should be avoided in tamponade

SELECTED REFERENCES

1. Hoit BD: Pericardial effusion and cardiac tamponade pathophysiology and new approaches to treatment. Curr Cardiol Rep. 25(9):1003-14, 2023
2. Saeed S et al: Natural course of electrocardiogram changes and the value of multimodality imaging in acute pericarditis. Cardiology. 148(3):219-27, 2023
3. Chetrit M et al: Imaging-guided therapies for pericardial diseases. JACC Cardiovasc Imaging. 13(6):1422-37, 2020
4. Chiabrando JG et al: Management of acute and recurrent pericarditis: JACC state-of-the-art review. J Am Coll Cardiol. 75(1):76-92, 2020
5. Imazio M et al: Cardiac tamponade: an educational review. Eur Heart J Acute Cardiovasc Care. 10(1):102–9, 2020
6. Tuck BC et al: Clinical update in pericardial diseases. J Cardiothorac Vasc Anesth. 33(1):184-99, 2018
7. Appleton C et al: Cardiac tamponade. Cardiol Clin. 35(4):525-37, 2017
8. Azarbal A et al: Pericardial effusion. Cardiol Clin. 35(4):515-24, 2017
9. Xu B et al: Imaging of the pericardium: a multimodality cardiovascular imaging update. Cardiol Clin. 35(4):491-503, 2017
10. Adler Y et al: 2015 ESC guidelines for the diagnosis and management of pericardial diseases: the Task Force for the Diagnosis and Management of Pericardial Diseases of the European Society of Cardiology (ESC)Endorsed by: the European Association for Cardio-Thoracic Surgery (EACTS). Eur Heart J. 36(42):2921-64, 2015
11. Dawson D et al: Contemporary imaging of the pericardium. JACC Cardiovasc Imaging. 4(6):680-4, 2011. Erratum in: JACC Cardiovasc Imaging. 4(7):819, 2011

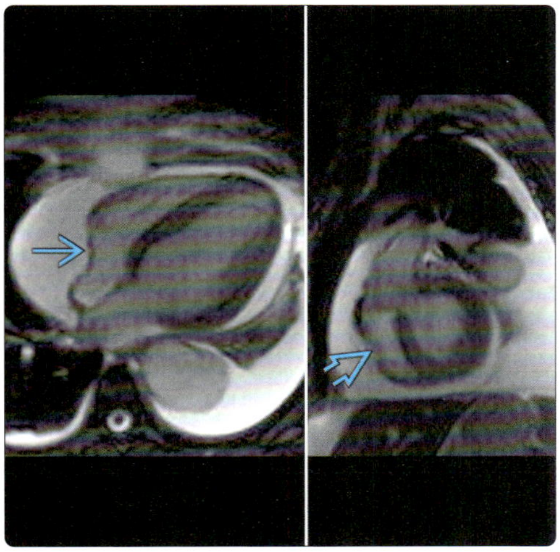

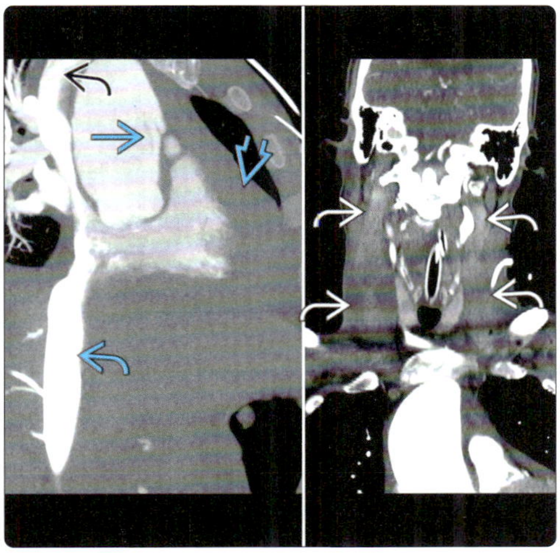

(Left) *SSFP MR images obtained during early diastole show collapse and inversion of the right atrial (left) and RV free wall (right) in a young patient with lupus and pericardial tamponade.* **(Right)** *MIP image (left) in a patient with a type A dissection and tamponade from hemopericardium shows IVC and SVC distention with extensive IVC reflux. Coronal MPR (right) shows marked jugular venous distention .*

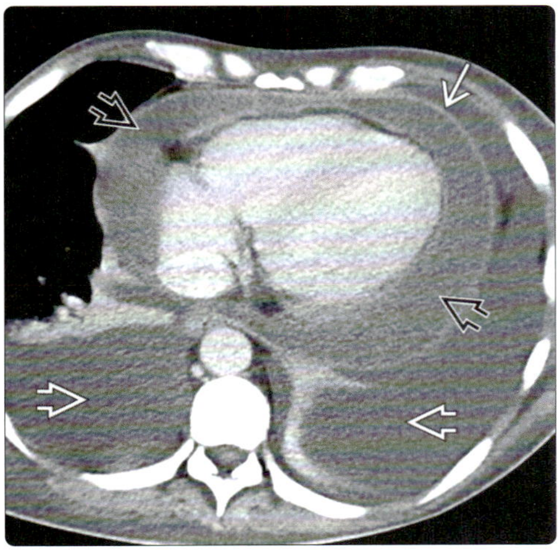

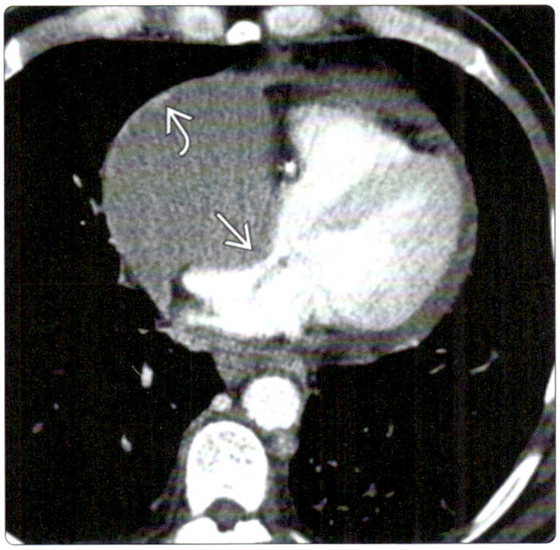

(Left) *Axial CTA shows a large pericardial effusion and enhancing pericardium , features consistent with acute pericarditis. Also note the large bilateral pleural effusions . The patient required a pericardial drain due to tamponade physiology.* **(Right)** *This 64-year-old patient presented obtunded with large pericardial effusion causing severe compression on the right atrial free wall . Note subtle pericardial nodules , consistent with metastases from an unsuspected primary lung cancer.*

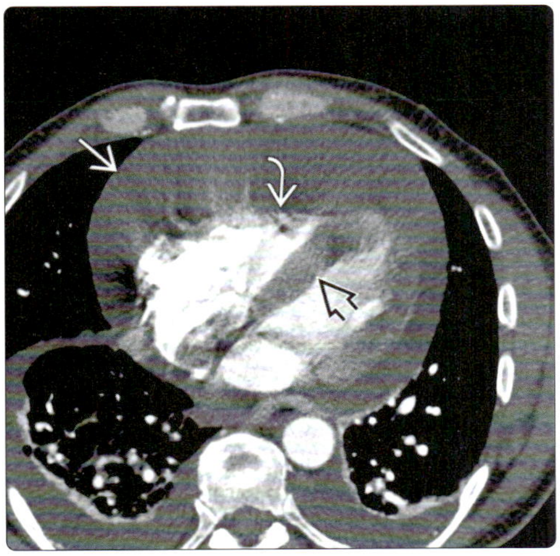

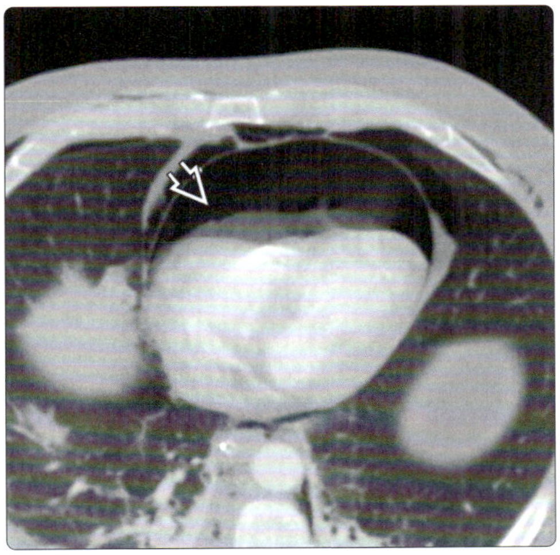

(Left) *Axial CT in a patient with gastric cancer shows pericardial effusion , compression of the RV free wall , and straightening of the interventricular septum . These findings are consistent with tamponade physiology. RV compression is not sensitive but a specific sign of tamponade.* **(Right)** *Axial CECT in a patient in a recent high-speed motor vehicle collision shows tension pneumopericardium with compression of the heart in the pericardial space leading to tamponade.*

KEY FACTS

TERMINOLOGY

- Primary benign tumor arising from pericardium

IMAGING

- Focal masses of variable size, which exert mass effect on surrounding structures without signs of invasion
  - Can envelop and compress normal cardiac structures
  - Plexiform neurofibroma (PNF) and paraganglioma can be locally invasive
- Lipoma
  - Encapsulated mass with homogeneous fat attenuation
- Lymphangioma
  - Cystic mass, usually large, arising from pericardium
  - Can be difficult to differentiate from pericardial cyst
- Hemangioma
  - Soft tissue mass that characteristically shows slow, progressive enhancement with contrast
  - During early pulmonary or systemic arterial phases, enhancement may be absent
  - Associated with hemopericardium in some cases
- PNF
  - Homogeneous soft tissue mass with contrast enhancement
  - Associated with neurofibromatosis type 1 (NF1) and multiple neurofibromas
  - Can be locally invasive
- Paraganglioma
  - Most are either mediastinal or cardiac in origin
  - Avidly enhancing
  - Numerous small feeding vessels supply tumor
  - Can be locally invasive

CLINICAL ISSUES

- Most are incidental findings and have good prognosis
  - Most require no treatment
- Some may need to be resection due to large size and compression
  - Complete surgical resection recommended

(Left) *Axial CT shows a moderate-sized mass with homogeneous fat attenuation ⇨ with the pericardium, consistent with a lipoma. The mass is located between the visceral ⇨ and parietal ⇨ layers of the pericardium.* **(Right)** *Axial chest CT in a woman with an incidentally discovered mass on breast MR shows a homogeneous 12 x 7 cm fluid attenuation mass along the pericardium, which has the appearance of a pericardial cyst ⇨.*

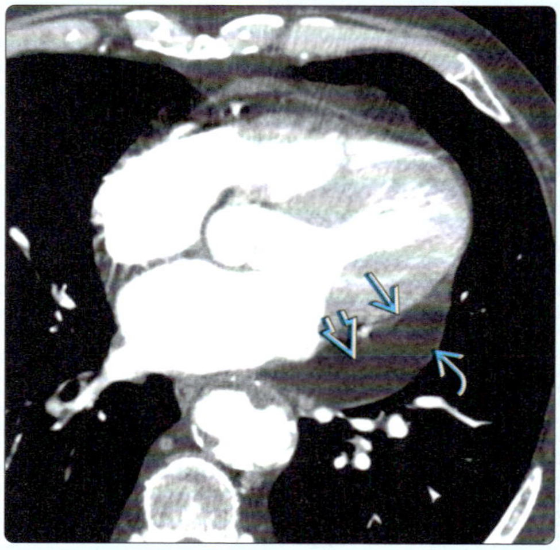

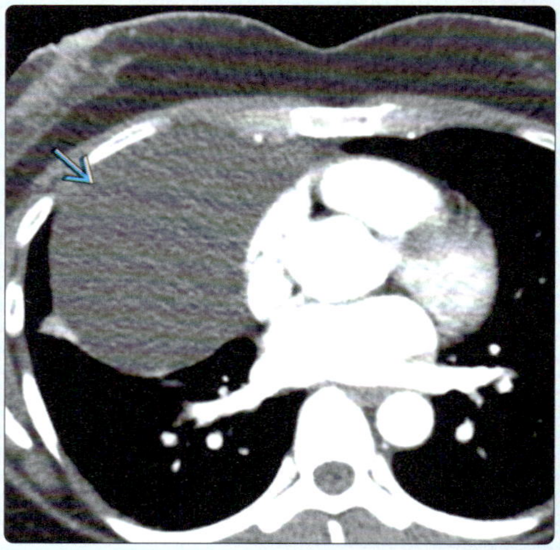

(Left) *T2 MR from the outside breast MR shows scattered flow voids ⇨ in the hyperintense mass. Scattered septations ⇨ are also present. Findings would not be typical for a pericardial or mediastinal cyst.* **(Right)** *T1 C+ MR from the breast MR shows numerous areas of linear and nodular enhancement ⇨ within the mass, which is predominantly hypointense. The MR findings are suggestive of a lymphangioma, which was confirmed on resection.*

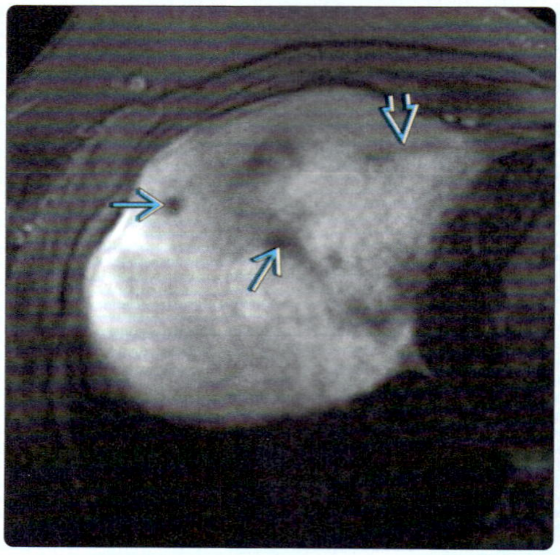

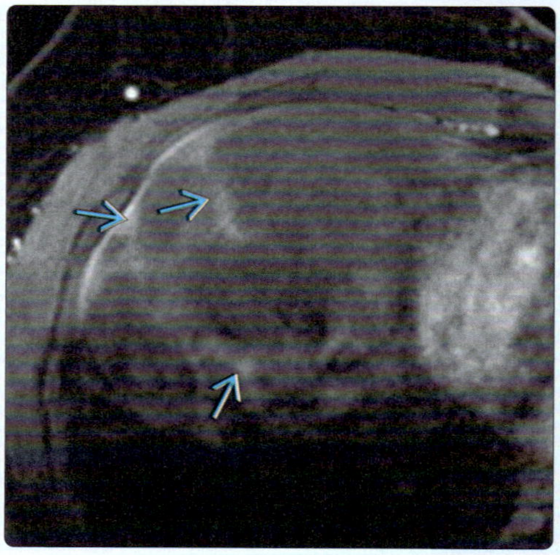

TERMINOLOGY

Definitions

- Primary benign tumor arising from pericardium
- Lipoma
- Lymphangioma
- Hemangioma
- Plexiform neurofibroma (PNF)
- Paraganglioma
  - Often included in lists of pericardial tumors, although it does not arise from pericardium proper

IMAGING

General Features

- Best diagnostic clue
  - Benign mass centered within pericardium without evidence of disease outside pericardium
- Location
  - Pericardium
- Size
  - Tend to be solitary, well-defined masses of variable size
  - Can occasionally be multiple
    - Multiple PNF in neurofibromatosis type 1 (NF1)
    - Multiple paragangliomas associated with certain genetic mutations (*SDHA*, *SDHAF2*, *SDHB*, *SDHC*, and *SDHD*)
- Morphology
  - Focal masses of variable size, which exert mass effect on surrounding structures without signs of invasion
    - Can envelop and compress normal cardiac structures
    - PNF and paraganglioma can be locally invasive

Radiographic Findings

- Often undetectable unless quite large

CT Findings

- Lipoma
  - Encapsulated mass with homogeneous fat attenuation within pericardium
- Lymphangioma
  - Cystic mass, usually large, arising from pericardium
  - Can be difficult to differentiate from pericardial cyst
  - Septations may be visible in some cases
- Hemangioma
  - Soft tissue attenuation mass that characteristically shows slow, progressive enhancement with contrast
  - During early pulmonary or systemic arterial phases, enhancement may be absent
    - Can be difficult to differentiate from cyst
    - Septations may be present
  - Associated with hemopericardium in some cases
- PNF
  - Homogeneous soft tissue attenuation mass
  - Enhancement after contrast typical
- Paraganglioma
  - Usually mediastinal or cardiac origin; not technically arising from pericardium but may appear pericardial on imaging
    - Paragangliomas that arise along roof of left atrium (LA)
      - Cardiac in origin, as they arise from paraganglia in LA wall
    - Paragangliomas in aorticopulmonary (AP) window
      - Arise from AP window paraganglia in epicardial space
  - Avidly enhancing masses, often with interspersed areas of hypoattenuation
    - Numerous small feeding vessels supplying tumor are often present
  - Few calcifications may be present
- PNF and paraganglioma can be locally invasive

MR Findings

- MR findings are variable, depending on tumor type
- Lipoma
  - Follow fat signal on all sequences
- Lymphangioma
  - Septated cystic mass with flow voids
  - SSFP and T2W imaging: Hyperintense to myocardium
  - T1W: Hypointense to myocardium
  - Perfusion: None or very mild
  - T1W+: Septations and rim enhance
- Hemangioma
  - SSFP and T2W: Hyperintense to myocardium
  - T1W: Isointense to myocardium
  - Perfusion: None or mild
  - T1W+: Progressive enhancement
- PNF
  - SSFP: Isointense to hyperintense to myocardium
  - T2W: Hyperintense to myocardium
  - T1W: Isointense to myocardium
  - Perfusion: Mild perfusion
  - T1W+: Diffuse postcontrast enhancement
- Paraganglioma
  - SSFP: Hyperintense to myocardium
  - T2W: Very intense signal
  - T1W: Isointense to myocardium
  - Perfusion: Avid perfusion
  - T1W: Avid postcontrast enhancement

Echocardiographic Findings

- Most tumors will be echogenic on echocardiogram
- Associated with variable degree of hypoechoic pericardial fluid

Nuclear Medicine Findings

- PET
  - Often show no abnormal uptake on FDG PET
    - Paraganglioma will show uptake on both FDG PET and Ga-68 DOTATATE PET
- MIBG scintigraphy
  - For paraganglioma imaging

Imaging Recommendations

- Best imaging tool
  - While CT is excellent tool to assess for tumor, subtle tumor can be missed even after administration of IV contrast
    - In general, portal venous phase of imaging will be better to assess for tumor than arterial phase of imaging

- MR is preferred tool to assess for pericardial tumor
- Protocol advice
  - ECG-gated CT
    - Consider arterial, portal venous phase, and delayed imaging for certain masses
  - Same protocol for other cardiac and pericardial masses

DIFFERENTIAL DIAGNOSIS

Pericardial Metastases

- Much more common
- Usually disseminated nodularity through pericardium
- Invasive features

Lipomatous Hypertrophy of Interatrial Septum

- In typical location with dumbbell morphology and sparing of fossa ovalis
- Lipoma is encapsulated tumor

Pericardial Cyst

- Can mimic pericardial lymphangioma on CT
- MR would show typical septations and flow voids

Erdheim-Chester Disease and IgG4 Disease

- Infiltrative soft tissue primarily in epicardial fat
  - Rarely solid mass in pericardium
- Avid 1st-pass perfusion, pronounced enhancement on T1W imaging, and very intense uptake on LGE imaging
- Often findings outside pericardium
  - Erdheim-Chester disease (ECD) often with characteristic imaging findings in perirenal fat

Pericardial Hematoma

- Can present as heterogenous-signal pericardial mass
- Often associated with trauma, surgery, or anticoagulation

High-Flow Vascular Malformation

- Can mimic paraganglioma
  - Numerous large feeding vessels and less well defined
- Pronounced early arterial enhancement unlike hemangioma

Unifocal Castleman Disease

- Avidly enhancing mass that can mimic paraganglioma
- Hard to differentiate based on CT or MR alone
- MIBG imaging can help differentiate

PATHOLOGY

General Features

- Histologically identical to extrapericardial counterparts
- Lipoma
  - Encapsulated masses composed mainly of mature fat with surrounding thin layer of fibrous tissue
  - Tends to be less well-defined than lipomas elsewhere
- Lymphangioma
  - Embryologic remnants of sequestered lymphatics that do not connect to efferent channels
  - Multiloculated cystic mass
  - Composed of aggregates of lymphatic channels containing serous &/or proteinaceous fluid
  - Devoid of erythrocytes, unlike hemangioma
- Hemangioma
  - 3 subtypes
    - Capillary: Smaller capillary-like vessels
    - Cavernous: Multiple thin-walled, dilated vessels
    - Arteriovenous: Thick-walled dysplastic arteries, venous-like vessels, and capillaries
  - Pericardial hemangiomas usually cavernous subtype, although they can be mixed
    - Irregular, cavernous spaces lined by single layer of endothelial cells set in loose fibrous stroma; some of endothelial cells can be lined by smooth muscle
    - Spaces are filled with blood, unlike lymphangioma
- PNF
  - Similar to neurofibroma seen elsewhere in body
    - Benign peripheral nerve sheath tumor that arises from Schwann cells
    - Irregularly thickened, distorted, and tortuous configurations in form of plexus
    - Can be locally invasive
  - Associated with NF1
- Paraganglioma
  - Do not typically arise from pericardium proper
    - Paragangliomas along roof of LA arise from paraganglia cells in LA wall
    - Intrapericardial paragangliomas in AP window arise from paraganglia tissue in that region
  - Can be quite large, measuring up to 15 cm
  - Hemorrhage is often visible on gross examination due to vascularity of tumor
  - Can be locally invasive and, occasionally, malignant

CLINICAL ISSUES

Presentation

- Most common signs/symptoms
  - Most benign tumors are incidental findings
  - Can cause symptoms due to local compression
  - Hemangioma can cause hemopericardium and tamponade

Natural History & Prognosis

- Most are incidental findings and have good prognosis
- Some may need to be resection due to large size and compression
- PNF and paraganglioma can be locally invasive

Treatment

- Most benign tumors do not require any treatment
- Complete surgical resection is recommended in cases causing symptomatic compression
  - Tumors can recur if incomplete resection

SELECTED REFERENCES

1. Pichler Sekulic S et al: Pericardial lymphangioma: a rare benign albeit variably symptomatic tumefactive lesion. Cardiovasc Pathol. 57:107402, 2022
2. Jacob D et al: Benign pericardial hemangioma-a rare cause of cardiac tamponade. Indian J Radiol Imaging. 31(3):754-7, 2021
3. Burke A et al: The 2015 WHO classification of tumors of the heart and pericardium. J Thorac Oncol. 11(4):441-52, 2016
4. Restrepo CS et al: Primary pericardial tumors. Radiographics. 33(6):1613-30, 2013

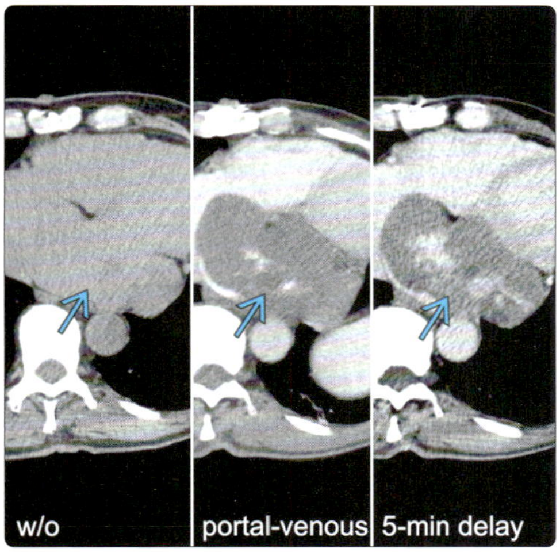

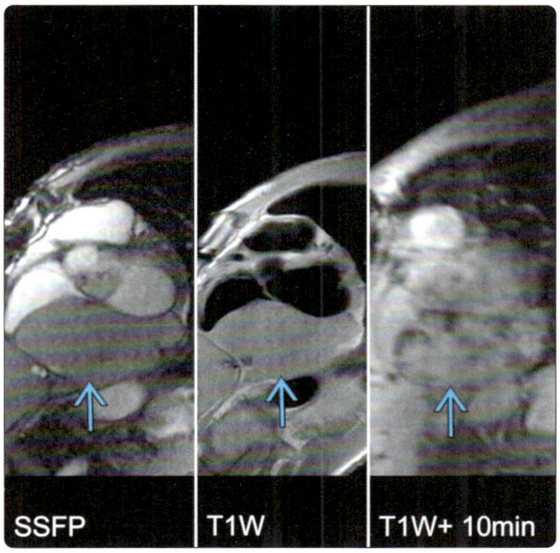

(Left) *CT images in a 63-year-old man show a 11.5 x 6 cm mass along the inferior aspect of the pericardium ⇒. Without contrast (left), the mass is inconspicuous. After contrast, it shows progressive nodular enhancement.* **(Right)** *SSFP (left), T1 double IR (center), and VIBE postcontrast (right) images show the mass ⇒, which is hyperintense and isointense to myocardium on SSFP and T1 images, respectively, and shows diffuse enhancement 10 minutes post contrast. A pericardial hemangioma was confirmed on resection.*

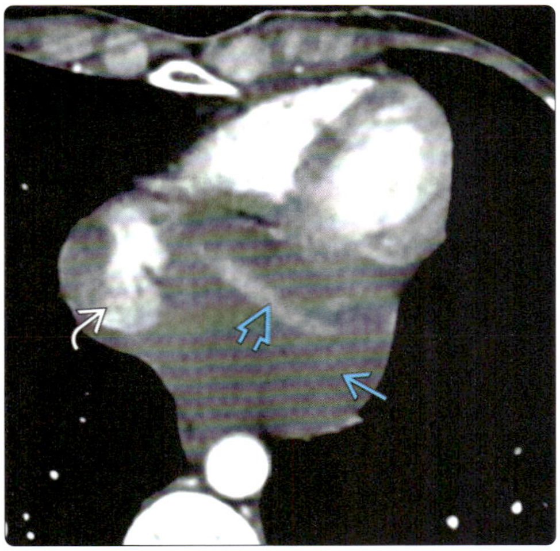

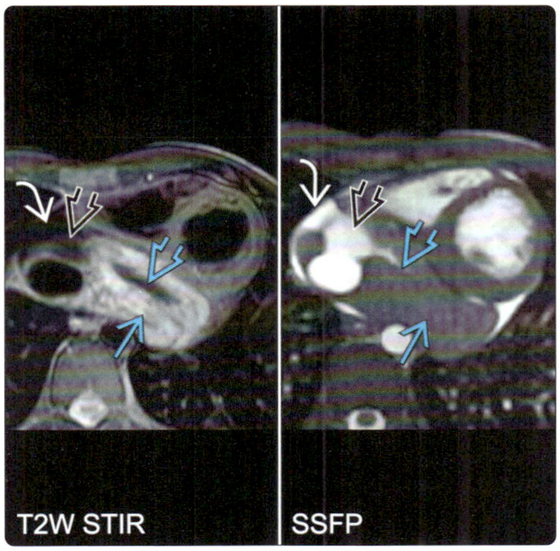

(Left) *Axial CT in a 21-year-old with neurofibromatosis type 1 (NF1) shows a biopsy-proved intrapericardial plexiform neurofibroma (PNF) ⇒ encasing the coronary sinus ⇒ and portions of the inferior vena cava ⇒.* **(Right)** *On STIR (right) and SSFP (left) sequences, the PNF ⇒ is hyperintense and iso- to slightly hyperintense to the myocardium, respectively. The mass envelops the coronary sinus ⇒, which is extrinsically compressed but drains freely into the right atrium ⇒. An associated small pericardial effusion ⇒ is present.*

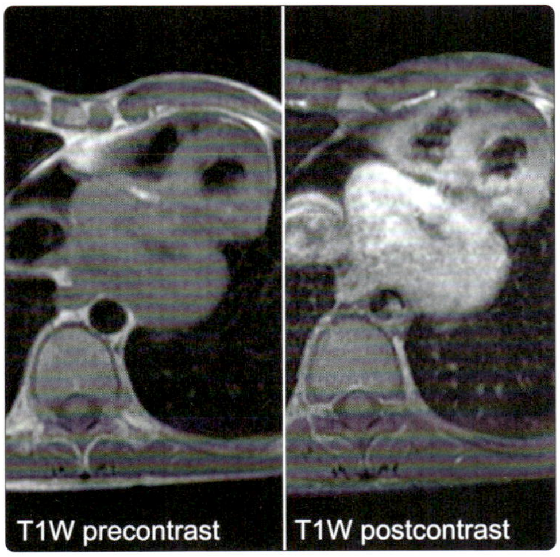

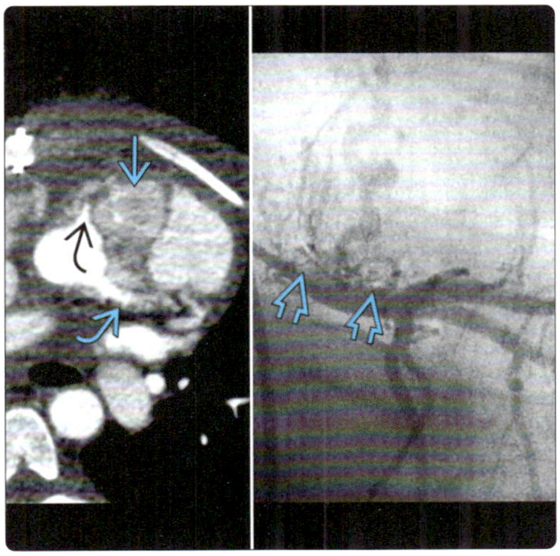

(Left) *T1 MR without (left) and with (right) contrast shows the PNF is isointense to the myocardium precontrast and has diffuse enhancement post contrast.* **(Right)** *CTA (left) shows an avidly enhancing AP window paraganglioma ⇒, which encases the right coronary artery ⇒ and abuts the left main, which has a shaggy appearance ⇒ due to small vessels feeding the mass, as seen on angiogram (right) ⇒. Although often classified as a pericardial tumor, it does not arise from the pericardium but from paraganglia cells near the aortic root.*

Pericardial Germ Cell Tumors

KEY FACTS

TERMINOLOGY

- Benign teratoma or malignant germ cell tumor (GCT) arising from pericardium

IMAGING

- Malignant GCT and benign pericardial teratoma appear similar on imaging
- Large cystic and soft tissue mass in young child arising from pericardial reflection near junction between right aspect of aortic root and right atrial appendage
- Will commonly compress right atrium
- Typically extends superiorly along right aspect of ascending aorta
- Tumor is often quite heterogeneous with areas of soft tissue interspersed with areas of cystic change and necrosis
- Soft tissue components avidly enhance
- Associated with moderate to large pericardial effusion

PATHOLOGY

- All pericardial tumors are histologically identical to their extrapericardial counterparts
- Most cases of malignant GCT are yolk sac tumors
    - Associated with elevated α-fetoprotein

CLINICAL ISSUES

- Symptoms associated with compression of cardiac structures or tamponade physiology
- Teratoma
    - Infants can be diagnosed in utero during screening ultrasound
- Malignant GCT
    - Often diagnosed in early childhood
- Treatment is surgical resection, either prenatal or postnatal
    - Survival not as good with malignant GCT

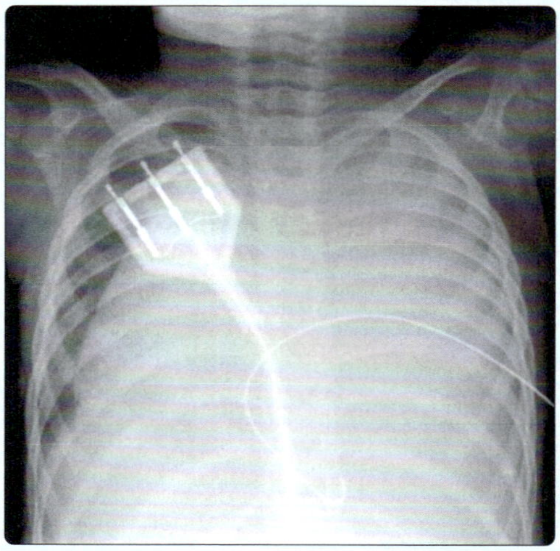

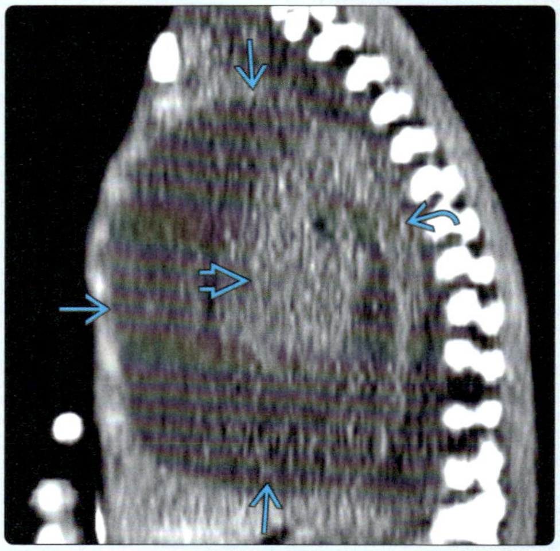

(Left) *AP radiograph in a 21-month-old girl shows massive enlargement of the cardiac silhouette, which fills nearly the entire chest.* **(Right)** *Sagittal NECT shows the heart ➡ floating in a massive pericardial effusion ➡. The aorta ➡ can be seen posteriorly.*

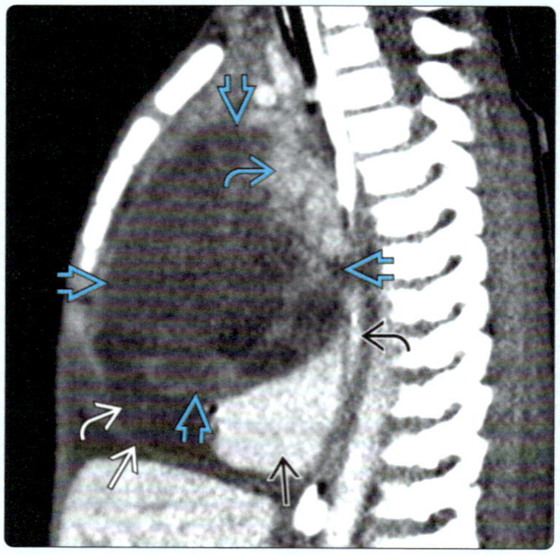

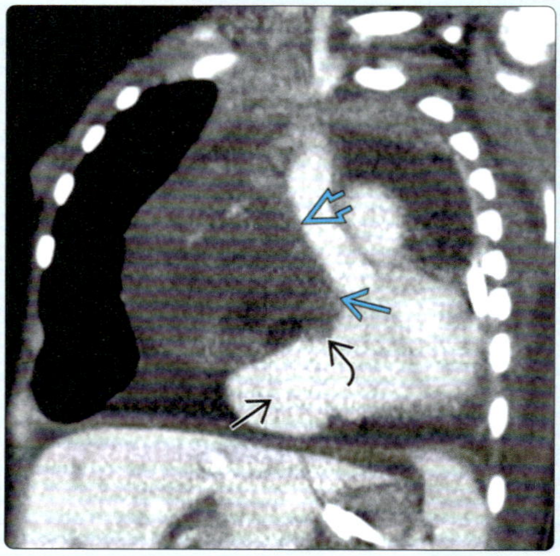

(Left) *Contrast-enhanced CT in the same patient after pericardiocentesis shows a moderate pericardial effusion ➡ with enhancement ➡. A large, heterogeneous pericardial mass ➡ with fluid, enhancing septations, and enhancing soft tissue ➡ is seen. The right atrium (RA) ➡ and left atrium (LA) ➡ are compressed.* **(Right)** *The mass arises from the right aspect of the aortic root ➡ and extends superiorly along the ascending aorta ➡. It sits on top of and compresses the RA ➡ with an area ➡ concerning for invasion.*

TERMINOLOGY

Definitions

- Germ cell tumor (GCT) arising from pericardium

IMAGING

General Features

- Best diagnostic clue
  - Large cystic and soft tissue mass in young child arising from pericardial reflection near junction between right aspect of aortic root and right atrial appendage
- Location
  - Pericardium
- Size
  - Large, solitary mass, which can measure > 10 cm
- Morphology
  - Large tumor with variable degrees of soft tissue, lipid, cystic change, and necrosis
  - Usually associated with moderate to large pericardial effusion

Radiographic Findings

- Large mass deforming cardiothymic silhouette

CT Findings

- Large, solitary mass seen in young children, commonly arising from pericardial reflection near junction between right aspect of aortic root and right atrial appendage
- Commonly compresses right atrium
- Typically extends superiorly along right aspect of ascending aorta
- Tumor is quite heterogeneous with areas of soft tissue interspersed with areas of cystic change and necrosis
  - Fat attenuation often present in teratoma
- Soft tissue components enhance avidly
- Associated pericardial effusion may be large
- Malignant GCT and benign pericardial teratoma appear similar on CT

MR Findings

- Large mass compressing right atrium and displacing aorta
- Characteristic signal appearance of mass, which demonstrates variable degree of cystic change and necrosis
  - T1W: Isointense to hyperintense to muscle; often numerous areas of low signal due to necrosis; areas of bright signal may be due to hemorrhage
  - T2W and SSFP: Hyperintense to skeletal muscle with numerous areas of bright fluid signal in areas of necrosis and cystic change
  - Perfusion: Variable 1st-pass perfusion often with areas of pronounced enhancement
  - T1W+: Avid areas of enhancement involving soft tissue components; areas of necrosis and cystic change will not enhance
  - LGE: Areas of uptake in solid portions of mass
- Associated pericardial effusion, usually large
- Imaging appearance similar between teratoma and malignant GCT

Echocardiographic Findings

- Large, heterogeneous mass
- Associated with hypoechoic pericardial effusion

DIFFERENTIAL DIAGNOSIS

Pericardial Metastases

- Uncommon in young child without history of malignancy
- Unlikely for metastases to be very large single mass

Primary Pericardial Hemangioma

- Rare tumor with intermediate T1 and high T2 signal
- Nodular, intense, peripheral early enhancement with progressive filling on delayed acquisitions

Cardiac Fibroma

- Can present as large mass in young child
- However, fibroma arises from myocardium
- Imaging characteristics are different from GCT
  - Fibroma is solid mass with dramatic diffuse LGE on MR

PATHOLOGY

General Features

- Histologically identical to GCTs elsewhere
- Malignant GCT
  - Most cases are yolk sac tumors
    - Associated with elevated α-fetoprotein
  - Attach to ascending aorta near aortic root
  - Multilocular cystic tumor with areas of necrosis
- Teratoma
  - Gross specimens appear similar to malignant GCT
  - Most consist of endodermal, mesodermal, and neuroectodermal tissue in varying proportions

CLINICAL ISSUES

Presentation

- Most common signs/symptoms
  - Symptoms associated with compression of cardiac structures or tamponade physiology
  - May present with intrauterine fetal demise
  - Can be diagnosed in utero during screening ultrasound
    - Associated hydrops fetalis and pericardial effusion

Demographics

- Malignant GCT
  - Most commonly reported in young children < 3 years of age
  - Most common in females
- Benign teratoma
  - More commonly diagnosed during prenatal ultrasound
  - Gestation age of presentation: 21-34 weeks

Treatment

- Surgical resection, either prenatal or postnatal
- Adjuvant chemotherapy &/or radiation for malignant GCT

SELECTED REFERENCES

1. Medina Perez M et al: Cardiac and pericardial neoplasms in children: radiologic-pathologic correlation. Radiographics. 43(9):e230010, 2023
2. Burke A et al: The 2015 WHO classification of tumors of the heart and pericardium. J Thorac Oncol. 11(4):441-52, 2016
3. Rychik J et al: Fetal intrapericardial teratoma: natural history and management including successful in utero surgery. Am J Obstet Gynecol. 215(6):780.e1-7, 2016

(Left) *Sagittal SSFP cardiac MR in the same patient shows the heterogeneous pericardial mass surrounding the ascending aorta and severely compressing both the RA and LA. The large pericardial effusion has increased in size since the recent CT.* **(Right)** *The large, heterogeneous mass shows areas of high signal, which may be due to cystic change &/or necrosis. It appears to be arising from the right aspect of the aortic root. The LA is severely compressed.*

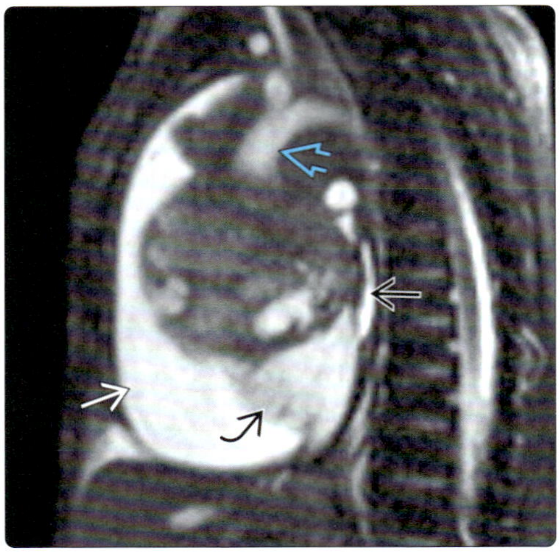

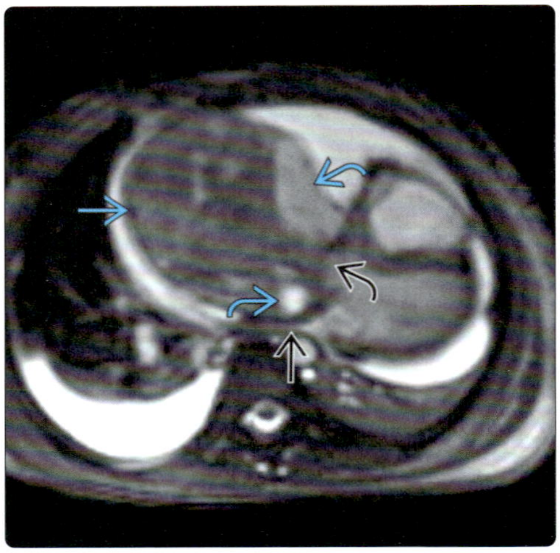

(Left) *T2 MR in the same patient shows the heterogeneous, relatively high-signal mass with variable degrees of soft tissue and hyperintense fluid signal.* **(Right)** *On T1 MR, the mass is heterogeneous with the soft tissue component being isointense to hyperintense to muscle. Multiple areas of high signal are present, likely due to areas of hemorrhage &/or proteinaceous fluid.*

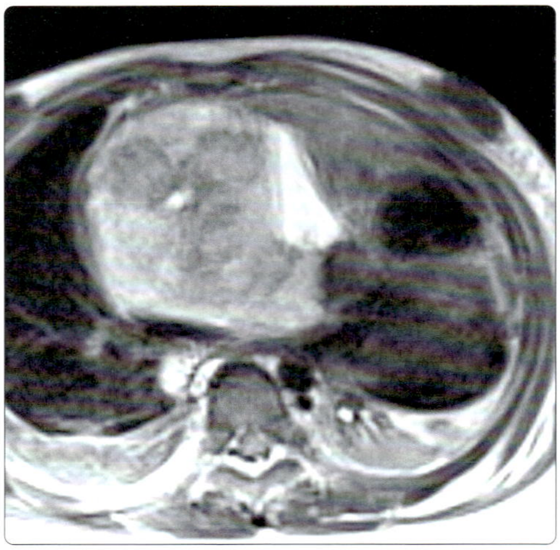

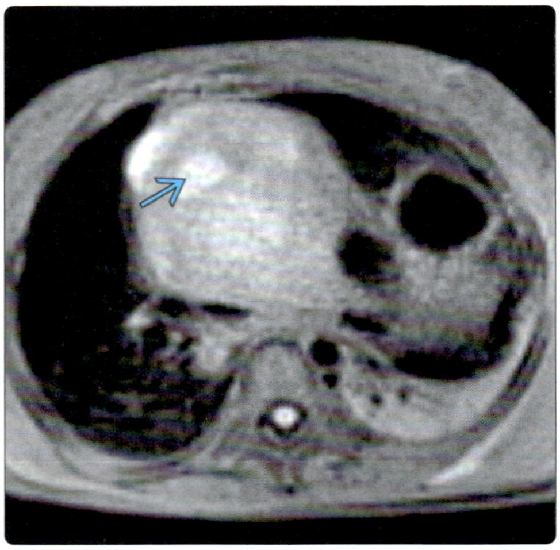

(Left) *After administration of contrast, there are numerous areas of avid enhancement throughout the mass.* **(Right)** *Gross pathologic specimen shows the soft tissue mass with multiple cystic areas, areas of hemorrhage, and areas of necrosis. Pathologic diagnosis confirmed an intrapericardial malignant germ cell tumor with yolk sac differentiation.*

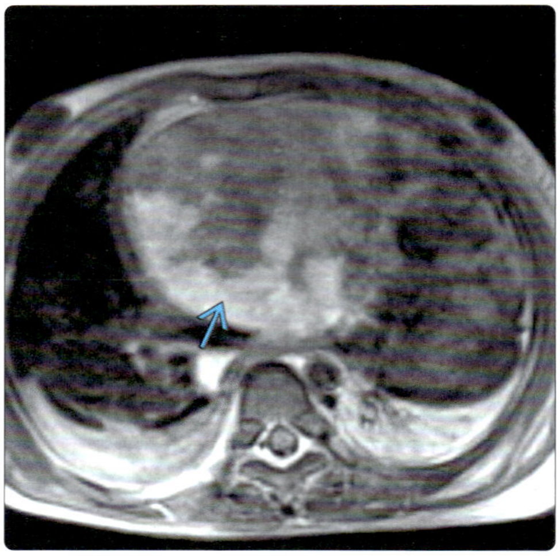

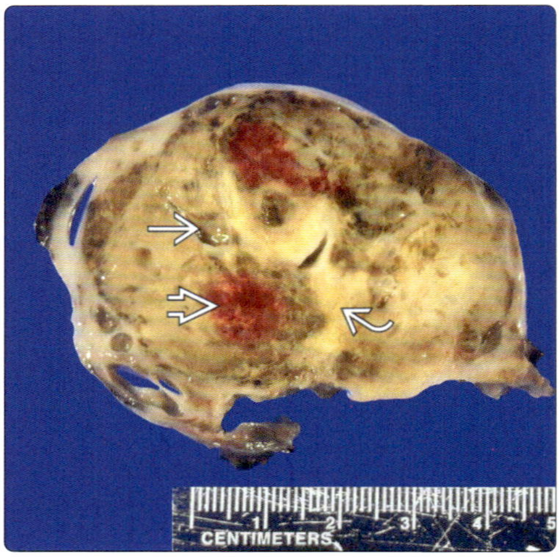

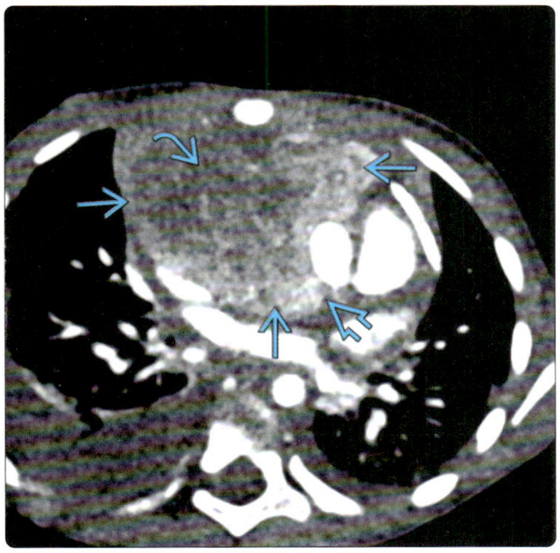

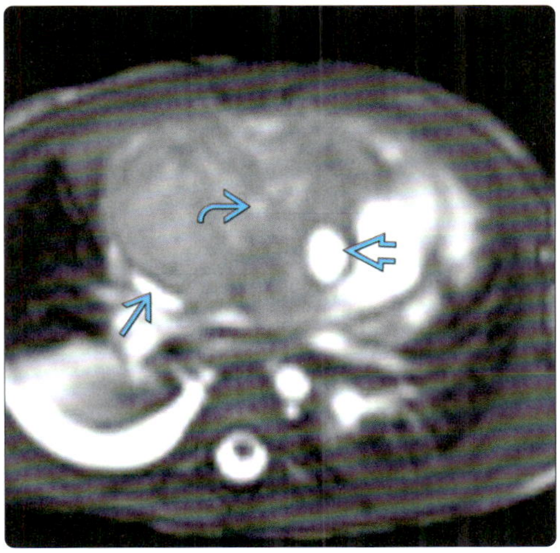

(Left) *CT in a 28-month-old girl who presented with a large pericardial effusion shows a 7 x 7 cm intrapericardial mass with intermixed areas of enhancement and fluid attenuation. The mass extends and appears to arise near the right side of the aortic root.* **(Right)** *On SSFP MR, the mass is primarily hyperintense to skeletal muscle, compresses the superior vena cava, and envelops the ascending aorta. Focal hyperintensity within the mass likely represents areas of cystic change &/or necrosis.*

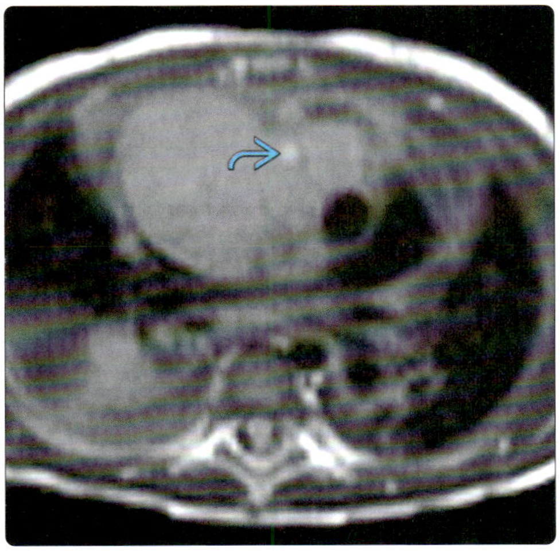

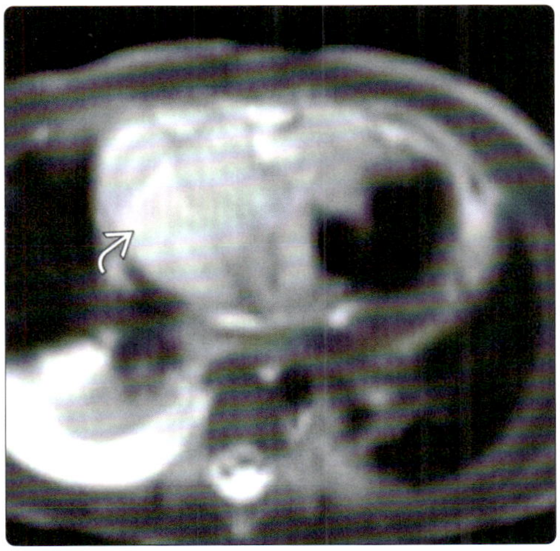

(Left) *Axial precontrast T1 MR in the same patient shows the mass is hyperintense to skeletal muscle. A small focus of hyperintensity within the mass likely represents focal hemorrhage.* **(Right)** *T2 HASTE MR shows heterogeneous stroma and T2 hyperintensity of the large mass. Also present is right pleural effusion and adjacent relaxation atelectasis.*

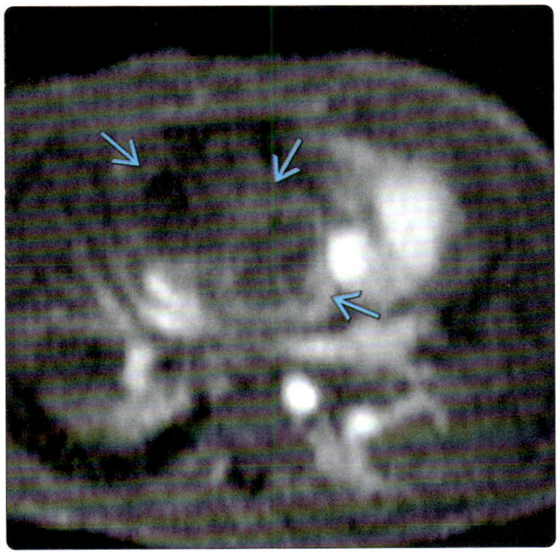

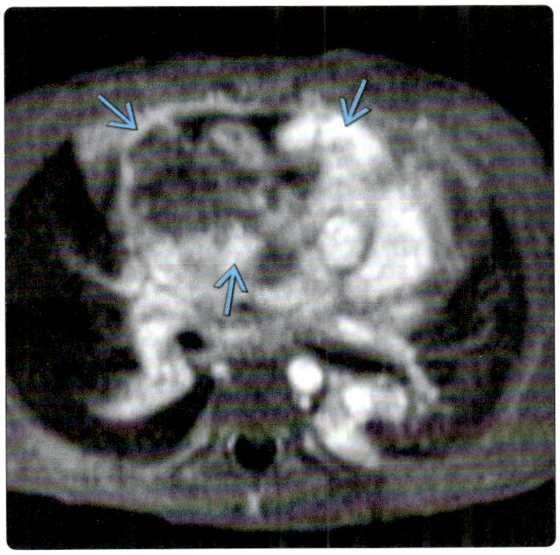

(Left) *First-pass perfusion imaging in the same patient shows rapid contrast enhancement of portions of the mass.* **(Right)** *T1 postcontrast MR shows extensive areas of enhancement within the mass. Nonenhancing portions of the mass are secondary to areas of cystic change &/or necrosis. The patient underwent a total resection of the mass, which was found to be a malignant mixed germ cell tumor with a predominant yolk sac component.*

Pericardial Lymphoma

KEY FACTS

TERMINOLOGY

- Primary lymphoma arising from pericardium

IMAGING

- 2 main morphologies
  - Disseminated form with numerous confluent nodules and masses throughout pericardium
    - Associated with variably sized pericardial effusion
    - Soft tissue invasion into epicardial and pericardial fat is common
  - Primary effusion lymphoma (PEL)
    - Rare form of lymphoma secondary to HHV-8 infection, commonly seen in patients with HIV or who are immunocompromised for other reasons
    - Can present as large, isolated pericardial effusion with some degree of pericardial thickening
    - Masses are absent
    - Requires pathologic analysis of pericardial fluid to make diagnosis
    - Assess for multicentric Castleman disease, which is also HHV-8 related

TOP DIFFERENTIAL DIAGNOSES

- Pericardial metastases
- Infiltrative disease of epicardial fat can mimic malignant pericardial tumors
- Pericarditis
- Pericardial mesothelioma

PATHOLOGY

- Disseminated form
  - Most commonly diffuse large B-cell lymphoma
  - Other subtypes (T-cell lymphoma, small lymphocytic lymphoma, Burkitt lymphoma) less common
- PEL
  - Rare aggressive B-cell lymphoma that can involve pleural, pericardium, &/or peritoneum

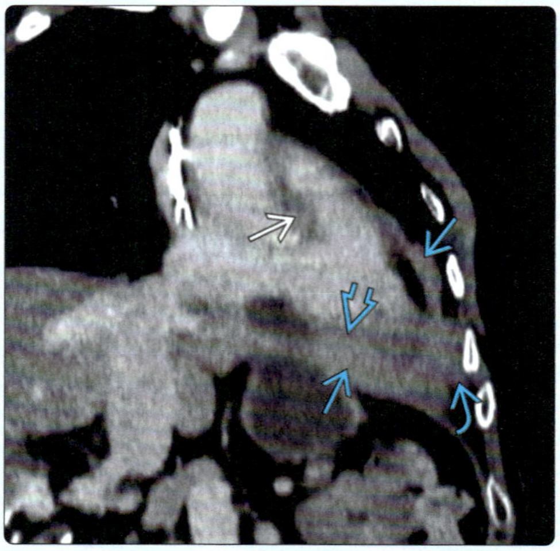

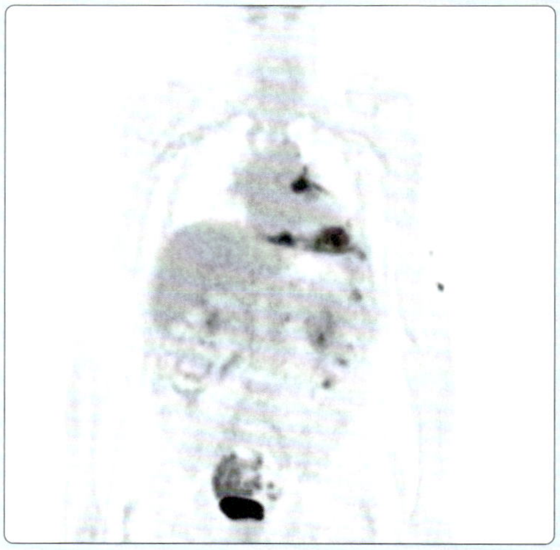

(Left) *Right 3-chamber reconstruction from a chest CT shows confluent soft tissues masses within the pericardium, some of which is invading into the epicardial and pericardial fat. Tumor is also in the superior pericardial recess.* **(Right)** *40-mm MIP image from a PET/CT shows multiple areas of uptake in the pericardium and epicardial fat. No tumor was seen elsewhere. Pericardial biopsy showed diffuse large B-cell lymphoma.*

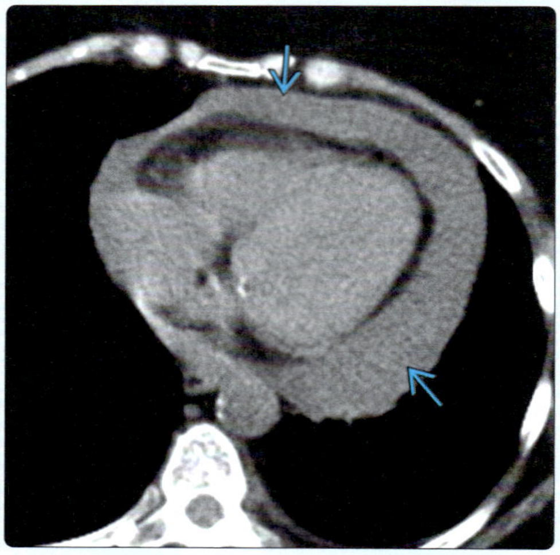

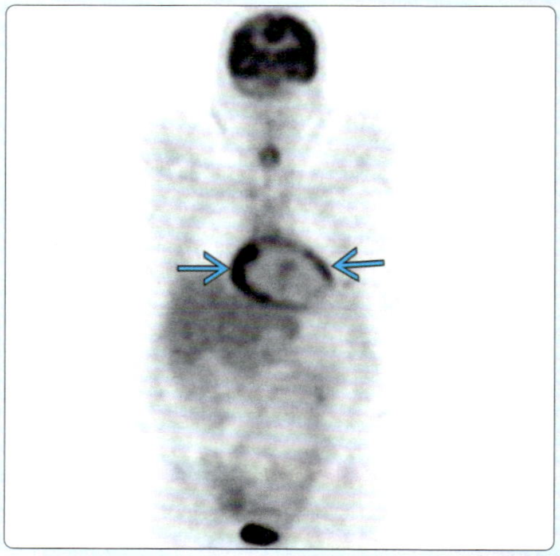

(Left) *CT in a 60-year-old woman with history of poorly controlled HIV infection shows a moderate-sized pericardial effusion. Patient was treated for pericarditis without improvement. Fluid evaluation showed a high-grade B-cell lymphoma. Subsequent work-up of lymphomatous cells showed HHV-8 and EBV infections. The patient was diagnosed with primary effusion lymphoma (PEL).* **(Right)** *Coronal image from a PET in a patient with PEL shows diffuse pericardial uptake without disease elsewhere.*

TERMINOLOGY

Definitions

- Primary lymphoma arising from pericardium

IMAGING

General Features

- Best diagnostic clue
  - Complex pericardial effusions with nodules; often associated with infiltration of epicardial fat
  - Recurrent pericardial effusion in immunocompromised patient, often with HIV
- Location
  - Pericardium
- 2 subtypes
  - Disseminated form
    - Numerous confluent pericardial nodules
    - May invade into pericardial and epicardial fat
      - Can envelop coronary arteries
      - Most notably in right atrioventricular groove
    - Associated with variably sized pericardial effusion
  - Primary effusion lymphoma (PEL)
    - Isolated pericardial effusion with some degree of pericardial thickening
    - Masses are absent
    - Requires pathologic analysis of pericardial fluid to make diagnosis

Radiographic Findings

- Globular enlargement of cardiac silhouette due to pericardial effusion

CT Findings

- Disseminated form
  - Nodules in pericardium with variably sized effusion
    - Tumor invading epicardial fat
- PEL
  - Moderate to large pericardial effusion
    - Variable thickening and enhancement
    - Masses absent

MR Findings

- Pericardial lymphoma
  - Areas of nodularity or pericardial thickening with variably sized pericardial effusion
    - Tumor infiltrating into epicardial space
  - Signal characteristics of masses
    - SSFP and T1W: Isointense to hypointense to muscle
    - T2W: Isointense to hyperintense to skeletal muscle
    - Perfusion: Mild, if present, but often absent
    - T1W+: Variable enhancement but often less than other tumors
  - PEL
    - No cases with MR reported in literature

Nuclear Medicine Findings

- PET
  - Uptake in pericardium and masses in disseminated form
  - Pericardial uptake in PEL

DIFFERENTIAL DIAGNOSIS

Pericardial Metastases

- Secondary lymphomatous involvement of pericardial or other metastases much more common

Infiltrative Diseases of Epicardial Fat

- Erdheim-Chester disease (ECD) and IgG4 disease
  - Avid 1st-pass perfusion and enhancement on T1W+ and LGE imaging
    - Atypical for lymphoma
  - ECD often with characteristic findings in perirenal fat

Pericarditis

- Can mimic lymphoma, but clinical symptoms different

Pericardial Mesothelioma or Sarcoma

- Can have similar appearance
- Usually more avid enhancement

PATHOLOGY

General Features

- All pericardial tumors are histologically identical to their extrapericardial counterparts
- Most commonly diffuse large B-cell lymphoma
  - Other subtypes (T-cell lymphoma, small lymphocytic lymphoma, Burkitt lymphoma) less common
- PEL
  - Rare aggressive B-cell lymphoma
  - Associated with HHV-8 and EBV coinfection
  - Can involve pleural, pericardium, &/or peritoneum

CLINICAL ISSUES

Presentation

- Most common signs/symptoms
  - Symptoms associated with pericardial constriction or cardiac tamponade

Demographics

- Variable age based on subtype
- PEL
  - Seen in immunocompromised patients, often with HIV
    - Mean age in HIV-PEL: 45 years

Natural History & Prognosis

- Treatment depends on extent and type of lymphoma
- Lymphoma
  - Given rarity of this disease, survival is unclear
- PEL
  - No standardized therapy
  - Worse prognosis
    - Concurrent untreated HIV
    - Involvement of pericardium
    - Single vs. multiple cavity involvement
    - Coexistent multicentric Castleman disease

SELECTED REFERENCES

1. Gathers DA et al: Primary effusion lymphoma: a clinicopathologic perspective. Cancers (Basel). 14(3), 2022
2. Kim Y et al: Current concepts in primary effusion lymphoma and other effusion-based lymphomas. Korean J Pathol. 48(2):81-90, 2014

Pericardial Sarcoma

KEY FACTS

TERMINOLOGY

- Primary sarcoma arising from pericardium

IMAGING

- 2 main morphologies
  - Solitary or dominant mass
    - More common in sarcoma
    - Pathology often shows pericardial tumor dissemination even in absence of visible disease
  - Disseminated form with numerous confluent nodules and masses throughout pericardium
    - More common in mesothelioma and lymphoma but also seen with sarcoma
- Pericardial effusion, which can be quite large
  - Assess for pericardial constriction or tamponade
  - In early disease, can be difficult to differentiate from pericarditis
- Masses will enhance with contrast administration

TOP DIFFERENTIAL DIAGNOSES

- Pericardial metastases
- Pericardial mesothelioma
- Pericardial lymphoma
- Pericarditis

PATHOLOGY

- Multiple subtypes of pericardial sarcoma
  - Synovial sarcoma
    - Most commonly reported in literature
  - Undifferentiated sarcoma
  - Angiosarcoma
  - Less common subtypes: Leiomyosarcoma, spindle cell sarcoma, fibrosarcoma, and others

CLINICAL ISSUES

- Very poor prognosis
- Surgery can be attempted in cases of isolated tumor without disseminated disease but uncommon

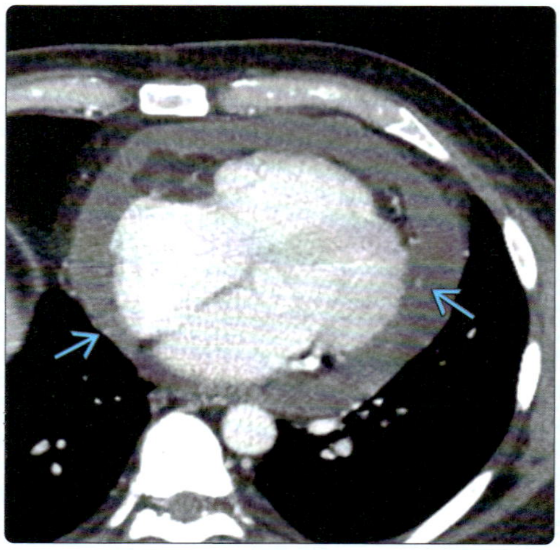

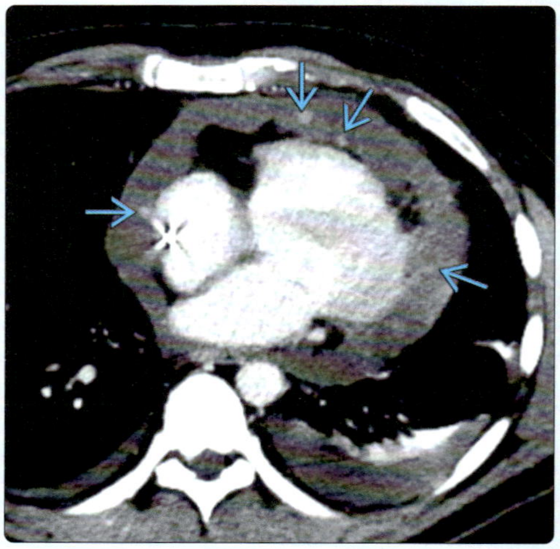

(Left) *Axial CT in a 50-year-old man with dyspnea shows a circumferential enhancing pericardial effusion with a lobulated contour. Scattered, very subtle foci of nodular hyperattenuation → are present. The findings were initially thought to represent pericarditis.* **(Right)** *Axial CECT in the same patient 8 weeks later shows increased size and conspicuity of enhancing pericardial nodules →. Biopsy showed angiosarcoma, and a diagnosis of primary pericardial angiosarcoma was made given isolated pericardial disease.*

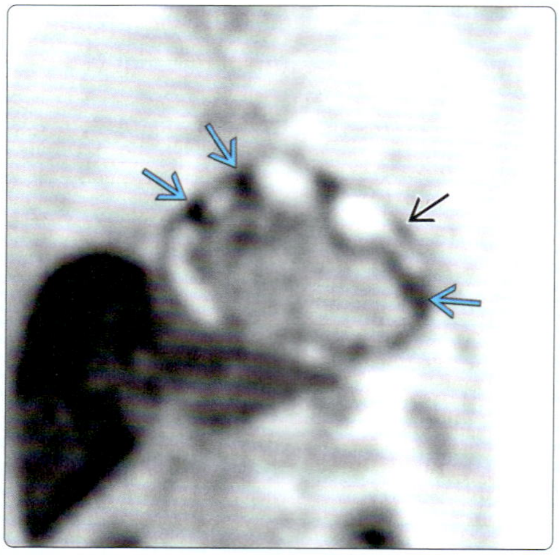

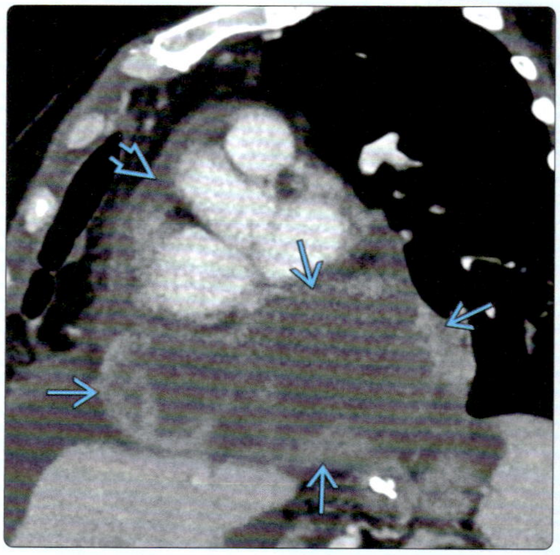

(Left) *Coronal PET/CT in the same patient 1 week later shows mild circumferential pericardial uptake → with areas of more pronounced nodular uptake →. No abnormal uptake is seen outside pericardium.* **(Right)** *Short-axis CECT in a 59-year-old man shows a 17 x 9 cm mass along the inferior aspect of the pericardium → with multiple areas of rim, nodular, and septation enhancement. A small pericardial effusion ⇒ is present with associated pericardial enhancement. Biopsy showed an undifferentiated sarcoma.*

TERMINOLOGY

Definitions

- Primary sarcoma arising from pericardium

IMAGING ANATOMY

General Features

- Best diagnostic clue
  - Dominant pericardial mass often with smaller pericardial tumor deposits with associated pericardial effusion
  - No evidence of disease outside pericardium
- Location
  - Pericardium
- Size
  - Variable depending on morphology
    - Solitary or dominant mass can be quite large (> 20 cm)
    - Disseminated form with numerous confluent soft tissues masses of variable size throughout pericardium
- Morphology
  - Solitary or dominant mass
    - More common
  - Disseminated form with numerous confluent nodules and masses throughout pericardium
    - Less common
  - Pericardial effusions occur with both morphologies and may be predominant finding

Radiographic Findings

- Can present with "water bottle" heart due to large pericardial effusion
- In cases with dominant or solitary pericardial mass, more focal distortion of cardiomediastinal silhouette

CT Findings

- Sarcomas are more likely to present with dominant or solitary pericardial mass compared to pericardial mesothelioma or lymphoma
  - Tumor can often be found throughout pericardium remote from dominant mass on surgery/pathology, even in absence of visible disease on imaging
- Can present as infiltrating nodules and masses throughout pericardium
  - In some cases, degree of nodularity is very mild, and tumor could be imperceptible, even with intravenous contrast
- Masses will enhance with contrast administration
  - Enhancement may best be seen on portal venous phase
- Often associated with moderate to large pericardial effusion
  - Pericardium will often be thickened and loculated
  - In early disease, may mimic pericarditis
  - Can lead to pericardial constriction or tamponade

MR Findings

- Pericardial sarcoma
  - Masses tend to follow signal characteristics of sarcomas seen elsewhere
  - Signal characteristics of masses compared to myocardium
    - SSFP: Isointense to mildly hyperintense; often heterogeneous
    - T1W: Isointense to mildly hyperintense; often heterogeneous
    - T2W: Hyperintense; often heterogeneous
    - Perfusion: Present
    - T1W+: Enhancement of tumor and pericardium; areas of necrosis will not enhance
      - Angiosarcoma will enhance to greater degree than other sarcomas
      - Synovial cell sarcomas will enhance to lesser degree than other sarcomas
      - However, this is not reliable method to differentiate
    - LGE: Heterogeneous enhancement
  - More likely than mesothelioma to invade myocardium
  - Even in dominant mass morphology, MR may localize additional areas of tumor deposit in pericardium
- Pericardial effusion is nearly always present
  - Effusion will appear complex and loculated
  - Diffuse pericardial enhancement even remote to areas of visible tumor
  - Pathology often shows disseminated tumor in pericardium, even in cases with only single enhancing lesion on imaging

Echocardiographic Findings

- Tumors are echogenic
- Associated with variable degree of hypoechoic pericardial fluid
- Pericardial thickening and nodularity often present

Nuclear Medicine Findings

- PET
  - Avid uptake on FDG PET

Imaging Recommendations

- Best imaging tool
  - MR
- Protocol advice
  - ECG-gated CT
  - Scan entire chest to assess for extrapericardial involvement
    - Portal venous phase better than arterial phase
      - Obtain noncontrast, arterial, and portal venous phases
      - Although radiation dose will be high with 3 phases, aggressive nature of these malignancies make this less of concern
  - MR
  - SSFP imaging through heart and pericardium
    - Entire axial or 4-chamber stack SSFP through heart and pericardium
    - Consider SA stack through ventricle and atria
    - Additional planes as needed to assess for myocardial invasion
  - T1W imaging ± fat saturation
    - Axial or 4-chamber stack through heart and pericardium
    - Additional planes as needed
    - Consider 3D T1W sequence (VIBE, LAVA, etc.)
  - T2W imaging ± fat saturation

- Axial or 4-chamber stack through heart and pericardium
- Additional planes as needed
- 1st-pass perfusion through mass
- T1W postcontrast in same planes as T1W precontrast imaging
  - 3D T1W sequence (VIBE, LAVA, etc.)
- LGE not essential but can be performed
  - Consider TI for myocardial inversion and longer TI of 600 ms
- Consider sequences to assess for constrictive pericarditis
  - Real-time free-breathing short-axis cine images with deep inspiration and expiration for ventricular interdependence, tagged cines for pericardial adhesions

DIFFERENTIAL DIAGNOSIS

Pericardial Metastases

- Much more common that primary pericardial tumors

Pericardial Mesothelioma

- Difficult to differentiate on imaging alone
- More likely to show disseminated tumor encasing heart

Pericardial Lymphoma

- Often associated with epicardial and myocardial infiltration

Infiltrative Disease of Epicardial Fat Mimicking Malignant Pericardial Tumors

- Erdheim-Chester disease (ECD) and IgG4 disease
  - Both often show diffuse infiltration of epicardial fat
  - ECD may show characteristic soft tissue infiltration of perirenal fat (hairy kidney sign), periaortic adventitial fat (coated aorta), and other systemic manifestations

Pericarditis or Abscess

- Viral, bacterial, or tuberculous pericarditis or abscess can present with pronounced pericardial thickening, loculations, and soft tissue attenuation/signal foci within pericardium
- Clinical symptoms are quite different between populations

Pericardial Hematoma

- Can present as variable signal mass in pericardium with heterogeneous pericardial fluid signal/attenuation, especially if chronic
- Often associated with trauma, surgery, or anticoagulation

PATHOLOGY

General Features

- Histologically identical to their extrapericardial counterparts
- Sarcoma
  - Various subtypes
    - Synovial sarcoma
      - Derived from primitive mesenchymal cells that differentiate into neoplastic cells that are similar to synovial tissue
      - 95% of cases involve t(X;18) translocation
      - Composed of spindle cells, epithelial cells, or both
      - Subtypes based on proportion, distribution, and differentiation of epithelial and spindle cells
    - Angiosarcoma
    - Undifferentiated sarcoma
      - Subtypes include high-grade pleomorphic sarcoma, pleomorphic sarcoma with giant cells, and pleomorphic sarcoma with predominant inflammation
    - Less common subtypes (leiomyosarcoma, spindle cell sarcoma, fibrosarcoma, rhabdomyosarcoma, liposarcoma)
  - Molecular and genetic testing should be performed on tissue to assess for certain genetic mutations that might be more amenable to specific therapies

CLINICAL ISSUES

Presentation

- Most common signs/symptoms
  - Symptoms associated with pericardial constriction or cardiac tamponade
    - Chest pain that gets worse with deep breathing, lying flat, or cough
    - Shortness of breath
    - Tachycardia

Demographics

- Variables ages
  - Synovial cell sarcoma tends to be younger patients in their 30s and more common in men

Natural History and Prognosis

- Very poor prognosis

Treatment

- Surgical resection can be attempted if tumor localized, which is rare
- Various forms of chemotherapy and radiation can be attempted but usually of limited success

DIAGNOSTIC CHECKLIST

Consider

- Consider pericardial sarcoma infiltrative masses or single dominant mass centered within pericardium without disease outside of pericardium

SELECTED REFERENCES

1. Jin H et al: Multimodal imaging features of primary pericardial synovial sarcoma: a case report. Front Oncol. 13:1181778, 2023
2. Medina Perez M et al: Cardiac and pericardial neoplasms in children: radiologic-pathologic correlation. Radiographics. 43(9):e230010, 2023
3. Luo Y et al: Case report: a young man with giant pericardial synovial sarcoma. Front Cardiovasc Med. 9:829328, 2022
4. Duran-Moreno J et al: Pericardial synovial sarcoma: case report, literature review and pooled analysis. In Vivo. 33(5):1531-8, 2019
5. Burke A et al: The 2015 WHO classification of tumors of the heart and pericardium. J Thorac Oncol. 11(4):441-52, 2016
6. Restrepo CS et al: Primary pericardial tumors. Radiographics. 33(6):1613-30, 2013
7. Cheng Y et al: Pericardial synovial sarcoma, a potential for misdiagnosis: clinicopathologic and molecular cytogenetic analysis of three cases with literature review. Am J Clin Pathol. 137(1):142-9, 2012

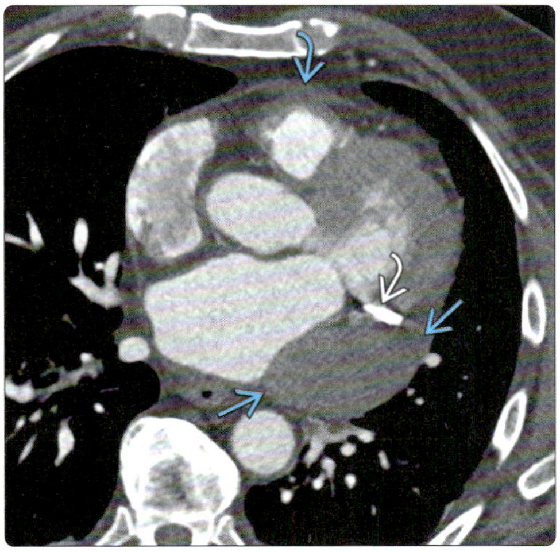

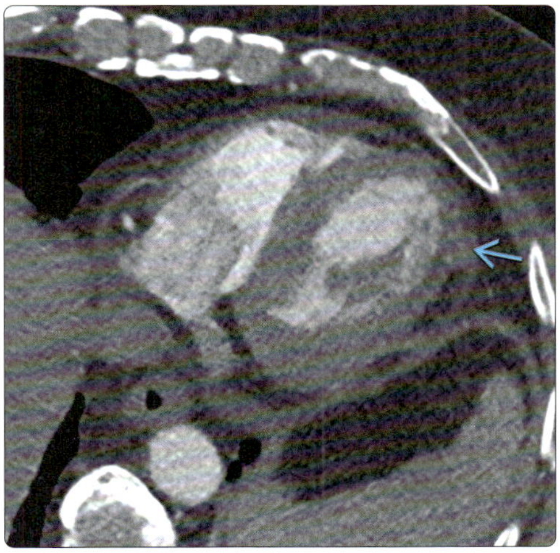

(Left) *Axial CT performed in a 55-year-old man with a stent placement for an LCx infarct shows a 5.8-cm pericardial mass with mass effect on the adjacent left atrium. There is only a small amount of pericardial fluid. This was the only mass initially perceived.* **(Right)** *Closer evaluation of an axial CECT in the same patient shows shows a 2nd, smaller, 1-cm nodule centered on the epicardial fat likely with myocardial invasion inferior and anterior to the dominant mass.*

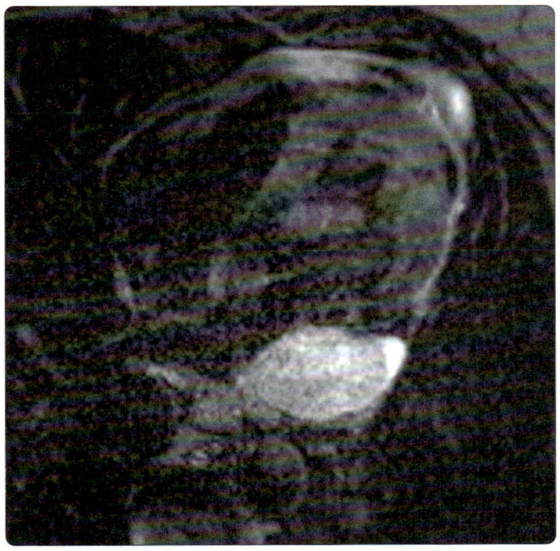

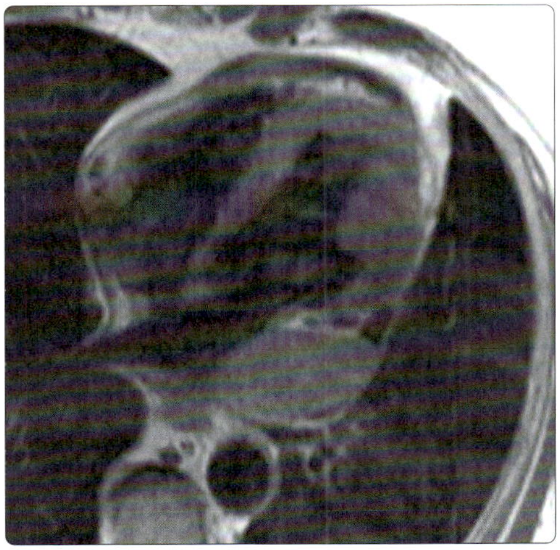

(Left) *Four-chamber T2 STIR MR in the same patient shows hyperintense signal of the dominant mass.* **(Right)** *Four-chamber T1 MR in the same patient shows that the mass is slightly heterogeneous but is primarily isointense to hyperintense to the nearby myocardium.*

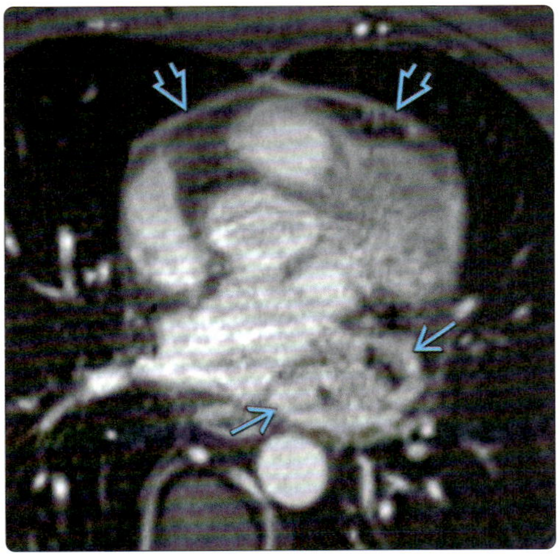

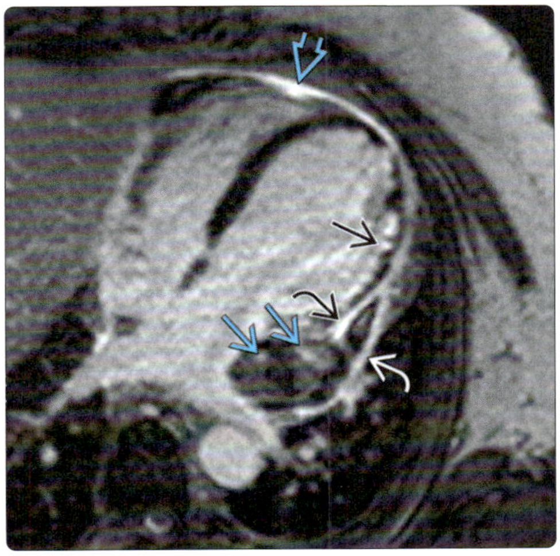

(Left) *Four-chamber T1 C+ MR postcontrast shows avid enhancement of the mass. Note diffuse pericardial enhancement.* **(Right)** *Inversion recovery MR shows foci of LGE in the mass, which splits visceral and parietal pericardium. There is diffuse pericardial enhancement. Subendocardial LGE is from a prior LCx infarct. Biopsy showed a high-grade synovial sarcoma composed primarily of spindle cells. More inferior lesion (not shown) had similar imaging characteristics.*

Pericardial Mesothelioma

KEY FACTS

TERMINOLOGY

- Primary mesothelioma arising from pericardium
- Although very rare, it is most common primary malignancy of pericardium

IMAGING ANATOMY

- 2 main morphologies
  - Disseminated form with numerous confluent nodules and masses throughout pericardium
    - Most common
  - Solitary or dominant mass
    - Less common
    - Pathology often shows tumor disseminated in pericardium, although there may be no visible tumor remote from dominant mass on imaging
- Pericardial effusion, which can be quite large, seen with both morphologies
  - In early disease, it can be difficult to differentiate mesothelioma from acute or chronic pericarditis
- Patients often present with findings of pericardial construction due to tumor encasing heart

TOP DIFFERENTIAL DIAGNOSES

- Pericardial metastases
  - Much more common
- Primary pericardial sarcoma
  - Can mimic mesothelioma
  - More likely to present with solitary or dominant mass
- Primary pericardial lymphoma
  - Very rare
  - Most often associated with lymphomatous infiltration of epicardial fat &/or myocardium

CLINICAL ISSUES

- Rapidly progressive tumor
- Very poor prognosis with median survival of 6 months

(Left) *Axial CECT shows circumferential soft tissue attenuation throughout the pericardium →. This leads to a narrowing of the ventricles and leftward inversion of the interventricular septum →, suggestive of pericardial constriction, which was confirmed on echocardiogram.* **(Right)** *Short-axis reconstruction from the chest CT shows the circumferential soft tissue →, which is seen invading into the epicardial fat in sone regions →.*

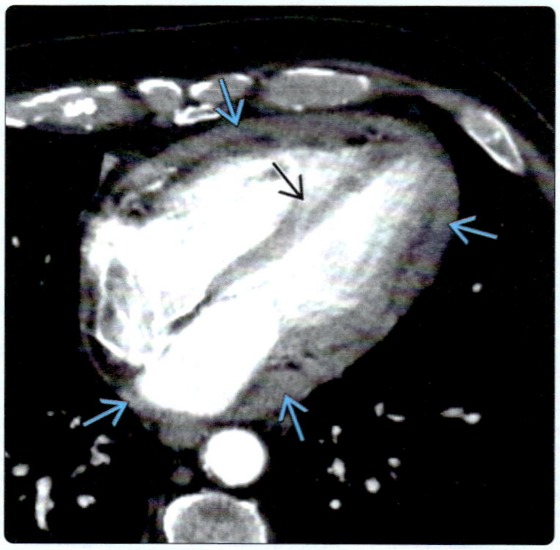

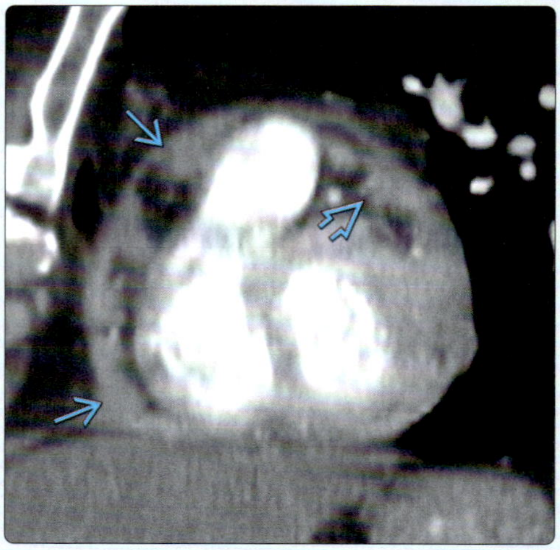

(Left) *Axial FDG PET/CT shows intense circumferential pericardial thickening and uptake. The exam was otherwise normal. Pericardial biopsy showed pericardial mesothelioma.* **(Right)** *Axial image from a calcium score CT performed < 12 months before presentation shows no perceptible abnormality.*

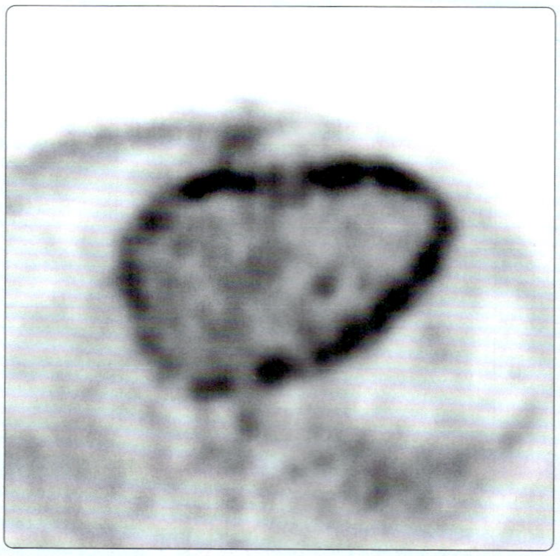

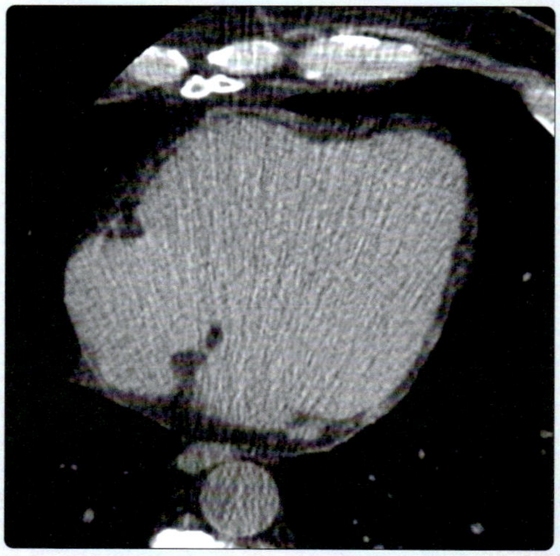

TERMINOLOGY

Synonyms

- Primary pericardial mesothelioma (PPM)

Definitions

- Mesothelioma arising from pericardium

IMAGING ANATOMY

General Features

- Best diagnostic clue
  - Most commonly disseminated and infiltrative masses centered within pericardium without evidence of disease outside pericardium
- Location
  - Pericardium
- Size
  - Variable depending on morphology
    - In cases of large solitary mass, which is less common, tumor can measure > 20 cm
- Morphology
  - Disseminated form with numerous confluent nodules and masses throughout pericardium
    - Most common presentation
      - Soft tissue lesions may invade into epicardial fat or pericardial fat
      - Myocardial invasion can occur but rare with mesothelioma
  - Solitary or dominant mass
    - Less common with pericardial mesothelioma
      - More common with pericardial sarcoma
    - MR may be able to elucidate additional pericardial lesions compared to CT
    - Pathology often shows tumor disseminated in pericardium, although there may be no visible tumor remote from dominant mass
  - Pericardial effusion, which can be quite large, seen with both morphologies
    - Effusion often loculated with pericardial thickening and septations
    - In early disease, pericardial nodularity may be subtle
    - Often initially misdiagnosed as pericarditis or even simple pericardial effusion

Radiographic Findings

- Disseminated form
  - Globular enlargement of cardiac silhouette commonly associated with large pericardial effusion
  - May have calcification or ossification, which may be visible on radiograph
- Solitary mass
  - Visible on radiograph if mass large enough to alter cardiomediastinal silhouette or if associated with moderate to large pericardial effusion
  - Masses can show calcification or ossification, which may be visible on radiograph

CT Findings

- Disseminated form
  - Numerous confluent soft tissue masses infiltrating throughout pericardium and encasing heart with associated complex pericardial effusion
    - Heart becomes encased by tumor
    - Can lead to pericardial constriction
      - Flattening or leftward bowing of interventricular septum
      - Dilation of superior and inferior vena cava
      - Septal bounce if retrospective ECG gating performed
  - Associated complex pericardial effusion that may be large
    - Pericardium will have lumpy, bumpy appearance
      - During early phases of disease, can be difficult to differentiate from acute or chronic pericarditis
      - Patients often misdiagnosed as having pericarditis
    - Pericardium often shows multiple septations or loculations
      - In early disease, can mimic simple pericardial effusion
  - Tumor and pericardium will enhance after administration of contrast
    - Enhancement or masses and pericardium better seen on portal venous phase on contrast
  - Calcification can occur
  - Tumor will often infiltrate into pericardial recesses, especially superior pericardial recess
    - Myocardial invasion is rare
- Dominant mass form
  - Variable degree of enhancement and necrosis in dominant mass, which can be quite large
    - Need to evaluate pericardium for additional smaller lesions that may be subtle
  - Even in cases where only single mass is visible on CT, tumor often found throughout pericardium on pathology
  - Associated pericardial effusion and pericardial enhancement
    - Pericardial enhancement may be diffuse, suggesting pericardial tumor infiltration remote to dominant mass
    - Can lead to pericardial constriction
- Metastatic disease to regional lymph nodes, lung, and pleural can occur

MR Findings

- Disseminated form
  - Infiltrating tumor throughout pericardial space with associated pericardial thickening and effusion
  - Tumor masses
    - SSFP: Heterogeneous but often isointense to hyperintense to muscle
    - T1W: Heterogeneous but often isointense to mildly hyperintense muscle
    - T2W: Heterogeneous but typically hyperintense to skeletal muscle
    - Perfusion: Variable but mild to moderate 1st-pass perfusion
    - T1W+: Enhancement of solid tumors and pericardial thickening/septations

- LGE: Diffuse enhancement of pericardium and tumor; dominant mass(es) may show areas of necrosis
  - Pericardium and pericardial septations often follow signal characteristics of masses with thickening and avid enhancement
  - Variable amount of pericardial fluid, which follows fluid signal on all sequences
- Dominant mass form
  - Signal characteristics of masses
    - SSFP: Isointense to mildly hyperintense to muscle; often heterogeneous
    - T1W: Isointense to mildly hyperintense; often heterogeneous
    - T2W: Hyperintense to skeletal muscle; often heterogeneous
    - Perfusion: Variable but usually present
    - T1W+: Enhancement of tumor and pericardium; areas of necrosis will not enhance
    - LGE: Diffuse enhancement of pericardium and tumor; dominant mass(es) may show areas of necrosis
  - Pericardium may show diffuse enhancement
- Metastatic disease to regional lymph nodes, lung, and pleural can occur

Echocardiographic Findings

- Tumor will be echogenic on echocardiogram
- Associated with variable degree of hypoechoic pericardial fluid
- Pericardial thickening and nodularity often present

Nuclear Medicine Findings

- Tumor(s) show avid uptake on FDG PET
- Often diffuse pericardial uptake

Imaging Recommendations

- Best imaging tool
  - MR is preferred modality
  - While CT is also good, subtle tumor can be missed even after administration of IV contrast
    - In general, portal venous phase of imaging will be better to assess for tumor than arterial phase of imaging
  - PET/CT has better accuracy for staging compared to CT
- Protocol advice
  - CT
    - ECG gated
    - Should scan entire chest to assess for disease outside pericardium
    - Portal venous phase better than arterial phase
      - Ideally will obtain noncontrast, arterial, and portal venous phases
      - Although radiation dose will be high with 3 phases, aggressive nature of these malignancies make this less of concern
    - Should scan entire chest to assess for disease outside pericardium
  - MR
    - ECG gated
    - SSFP imaging through heart and pericardium
      - Entire axial or 4-chamber stack SSFP through heart and pericardium
      - Consider short-axis stack through ventricle and atria
      - Additional planes as needed
    - T1W imaging ± fat saturation
      - Axial or 4-chamber stack through heart and pericardium
      - Additional planes as needed
      - Consider 3D T1W sequence (VIBE, LAVA, etc.)
    - T2W imaging ± fat saturation
      - Axial or 4-chamber stack through heart and pericardium
      - Additional planes as needed
    - 1st-pass perfusion through mass
    - T1W postcontrast in same planes as T1W precontrast imaging
      - 3D T1W sequence (VIBE, LAVA, etc.)
    - LGE not essential but can be performed
      - Consider inversion time (TI) for myocardial inversion and longer TI of 600 msec
    - Consider sequences to assess for constrictive pericarditis
      - Real-time free-breathing cine images with deep inspiration and expiration

CLINICAL IMPLICATIONS

- Although exceptionally rare, mesothelioma is most common primary pericardial malignancy

DIFFERENTIAL DIAGNOSIS

Pericardial Metastases

- Much more common that primary tumors
- Findings suggestive of pericardial malignancy should evoke work-up to assess for primary tumor outside pericardium

Primary Pericardial Sarcoma

- Less common than pericardial mesothelioma
  - However, can have identical imaging appearance
- More commonly presents with solitary or dominant pericardial mass compared to mesothelioma

Primary Pericardial Lymphoma

- Rare for lymphoma to just involve pericardium
- Usually associated with infiltration of epicardial fat &/or myocardium

Infiltrative Disease of Epicardial Fat Can Mimic Malignant Pericardial Tumors

- Erdheim-Chester disease (ECD) and IgG4-related disease can mimic mesothelioma
  - Both will show avid 1st-pass perfusion and pronounced enhancement on T1W+ and LGE imaging
  - ECD often with characteristic imaging findings in perirenal fat
  - These are primarily epicardial processes and not pericardial

Pericarditis or Abscess

- Bacterial or tuberculous pericarditis or abscess can present with pronounced pericardial thickening, loculations, and soft tissue attenuation/signal foci within pericardium

- However, clinical symptoms are quite different between populations

Benign Pericardial Tumors (e.g., Hemangioma or Neurofibroma)

- In some instances, can mimic mesothelioma in case of solitary mass
  - However, these tumors are noninvasive
    - Displace or envelop structures without evidence of invasion
- Pericardial neurofibroma associated with neurofibromatosis type 1
- Hemangioma associated with hemopericardium

Pericardial Hematoma

- Can present as variable signal mass in pericardium with heterogeneous pericardial fluid signal/attenuation, especially if chronic
- Often associated with trauma, surgery, or anticoagulation

PATHOLOGY

General Features

- Most common primary pericardial malignancy
- Pericardium, like pleura, is lined by mesothelial cells
  - Microscopic findings are identical to pleural mesothelioma
  - Most cases are epithelioid with biphasic and sarcomatoid being less common; can be difficult to differentiate from pleural mesothelioma if there is focal mass invading both pleural and pericardium
- Tumor grows along visceral and parietal surfaces of pericardium, eventually encasing heart
- Cardiac invasion is uncommon but can occur

Staging, Grading, & Classification

- Similar to pleural mesothelioma, there are 3 subtypes
  - Epithelioid
    - Most common subtype in PPM
  - Sarcomatoid
  - Biphasic
- Metastatic disease to lymph nodes, pleura, and lung can occur

CLINICAL ISSUES

Presentation

- Most common signs/symptoms
  - Symptoms associated with pericardial constriction or cardiac tamponade
    - Chest pain that worsens with deep breathing, lying flat, or cough
    - Shortness of breath
    - Tachycardia
    - Palpitations
    - Lower extremity edema

Demographics

- Can occur at any age from 20 months to 85 years
- Mean age: 57 years
  - Younger age than pleural mesothelioma
- Association with asbestos exposure not as well documented
  - Italian cohort showed occupation exposure to asbestos was significantly associated with risk of disease
    - Odds ratio: 3.68

Natural History & Prognosis

- Very poor prognosis with median survival of 6 months

Treatment

- Surgical resection can be attempted if tumor is resectable
  - However, unresectable in majority of cases
- Chemotherapy with platinum agent can improve median survival to 13 months

DIAGNOSTIC CHECKLIST

Consider

- Primary malignant pericardial tumor in presence of infiltrative masses or single dominant mass centered within pericardium without evidence of disease outside pericardium

Image Interpretation Pearls

- Mesothelioma is most common primary pericardial malignancy
- However, metastatic disease is much more common
- Even in cases where there appears to be single dominant lesion, disease is often present in other regions of pericardium pathologically

SELECTED REFERENCES

1. Roset-Altadill A et al: Epicardial space: comprehensive anatomy and spectrum of disease. Radiographics. 44(4):e230160, 2024
2. Arrossi AV: Pericardial mesotheliomas. Adv Anat Pathol. 30(4):253-8, 2023
3. Bonde A et al: Mesotheliomas and benign mesothelial tumors: update on pathologic and imaging findings. Radiographics. 43(3):e220128, 2023
4. Brydges H et al: Primary pericardial mesothelioma: a population-based propensity score-matched analysis. Semin Thorac Cardiovasc Surg. 34(3):1113-9, 2022
5. Marinaccio A et al: Association between asbestos exposure and pericardial and tunica vaginalis testis malignant mesothelioma: a case-control study and epidemiological remarks. Scand J Work Environ Health. 46(6):609-17, 2020
6. McGehee E et al: Treatment and outcomes of primary pericardial mesothelioma: a contemporary review of 103 published cases. Clin Lung Cancer. 20(2):e152-7, 2019
7. Burke A et al: The 2015 WHO Classification of Tumors of the Heart and Pericardium. J Thorac Oncol. 11(4):441-52, 2016

(Left) *PA radiograph in a 22-year-old man who presented to the emergency department with shortness of breath shows globular enlargement of the cardiac silhouette.* **(Right)** *Coronal CT from a CT pulmonary angiogram shows multiple areas of fluid and soft tissue filling the pericardium. The remainder of the chest CT was normal. Subsequent neck, abdominal, and pelvic CT were normal. The findings were concerning for a pericardial tumor, so the patient was referred for cardiac MR.*

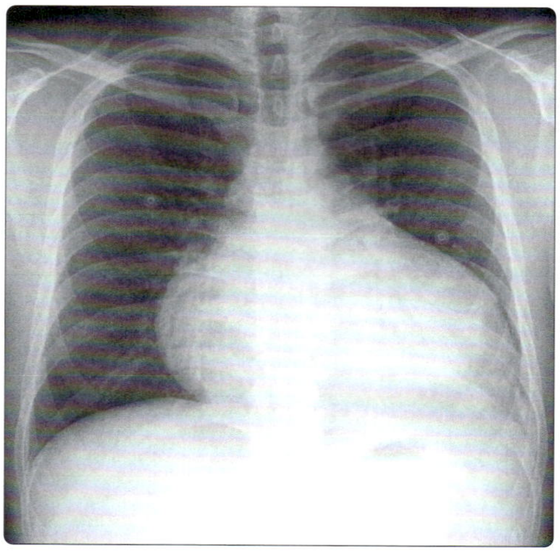

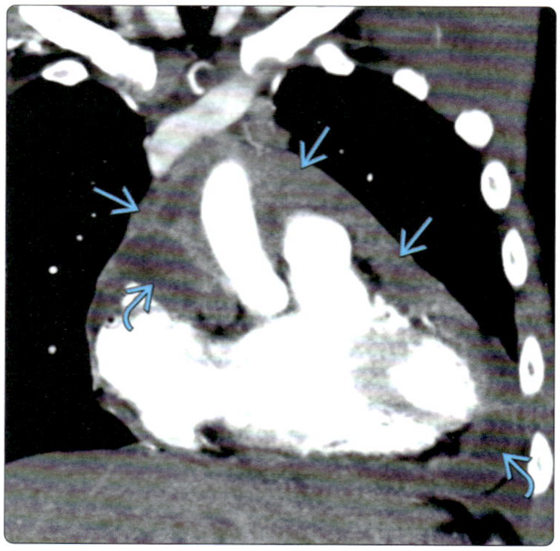

(Left) *Axial SSFP MR from a cine sequence shows hypointense soft tissue filling the much of the pericardial space with extension into the superior pericardial recess. Scattered areas of fluid are also present. Findings of pericardial constriction were also present.* **(Right)** *Axial T1 without contrast MR shows soft tissue filling the majority of the pericardial space with extension into the superior pericardial recess. Scattered areas of fluid are also present.*

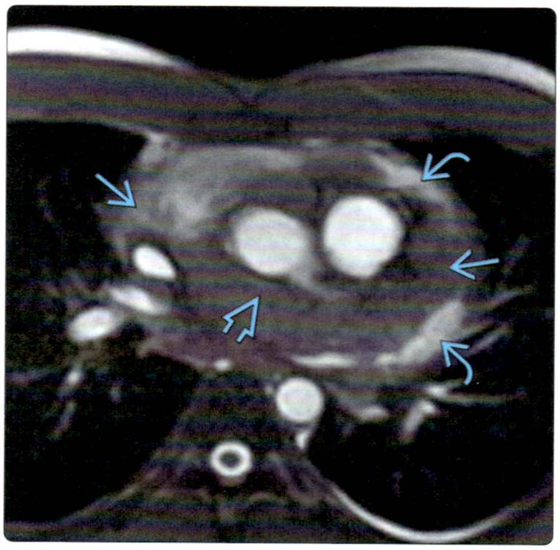

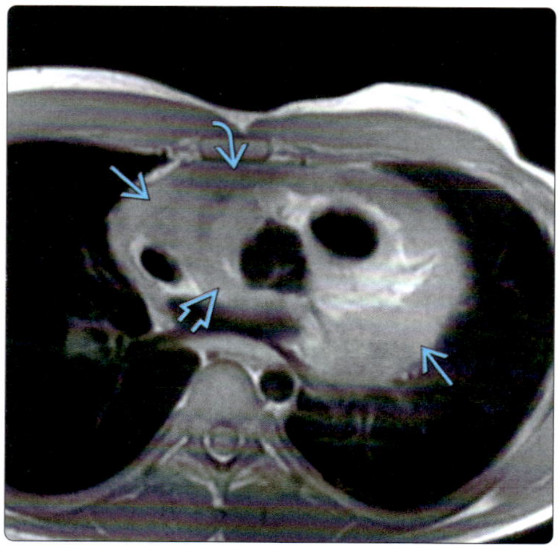

(Left) *Axial T1 postcontrast VIBE image shows avid enhancement of the pericardial soft tissue. While pericardial metastases are most common, a primary tumor, such as a pericardial mesothelioma, was considered given the absence of findings outside the pericardium.* **(Right)** *Coronal PET/CT shows intense uptake throughout the pericardium. There was no evidence of disease elsewhere. Pericardial mesothelioma was confirmed on biopsy. The patient died < 5 months after presentation.*

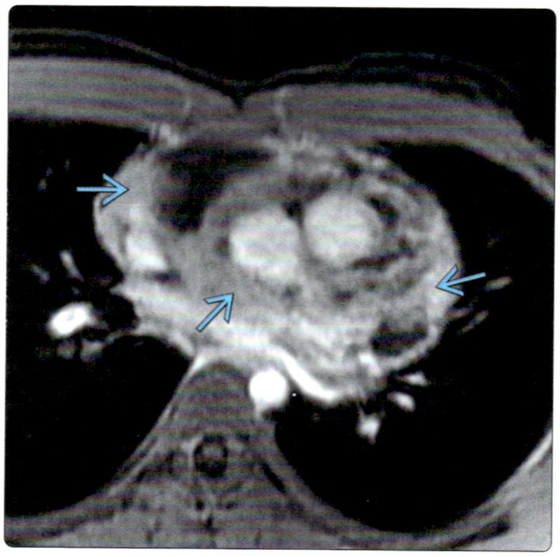

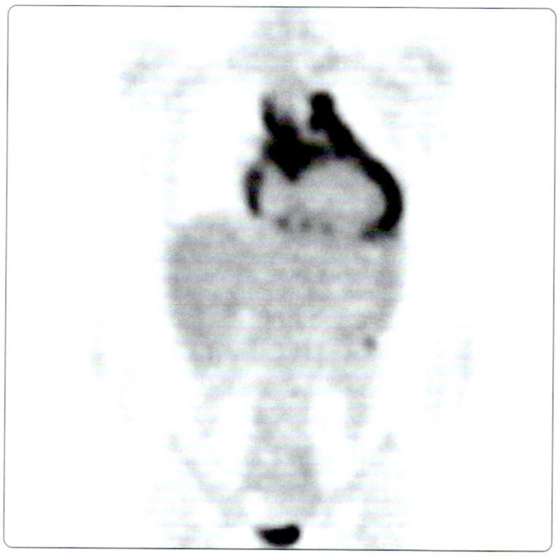

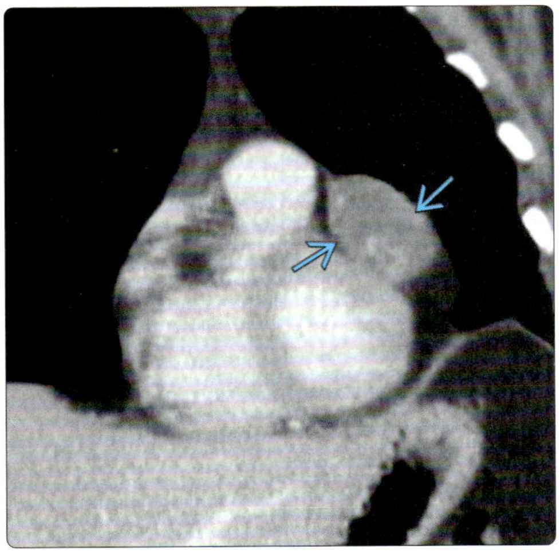

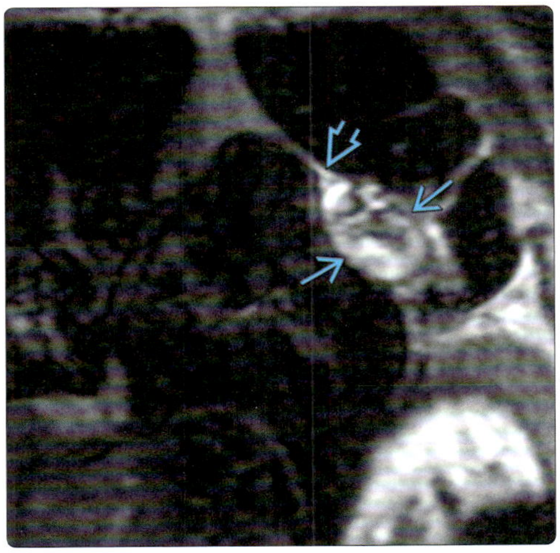

(Left) *Coronal CT shows a 5.2 x 3.7 cm focal mass arising from the pericardium. Areas of increased attenuation were thought to be due to enhancement, although this could not be confirmed without noncontrast imaging.* **(Right)** *Coronal T2 FS MR in the same patient shows the mass as being predominantly hyperintense with central hypoattenuation. The mass appears to split the pericardium, which best seen more superiorly.*

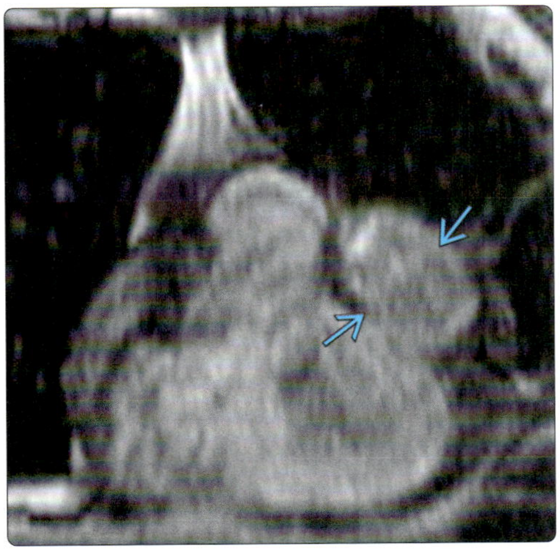

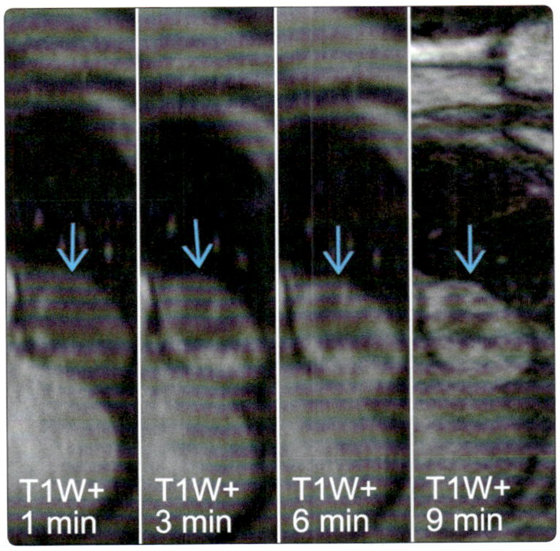

(Left) *Coronal T1 3D VIBE sequence precontrast in the same patient shows the mass is heterogeneous but predominantly hypointense to myocardium with foci of signal that is isointense and hyperintense to myocardium.* **(Right)** *T1 3D VIBE imaging after contrast administration shows progressive peripheral nodular enhancement of the same mass, thought to be a pericardial hemangioma based on enhancement pattern. Complete excision of the mass revealed epithelioid mesothelioma. There was no recurrence 3 years later.*

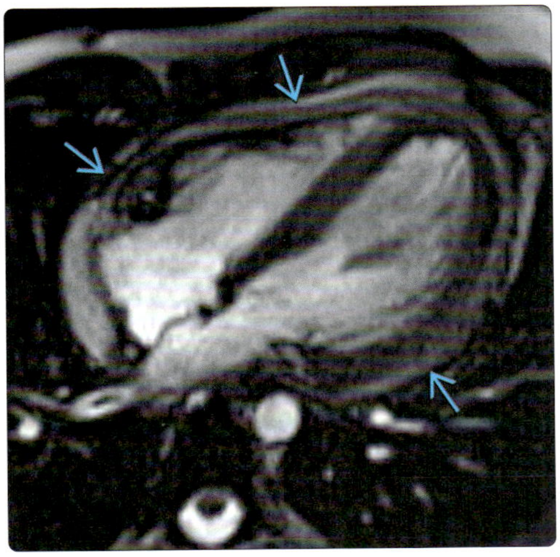

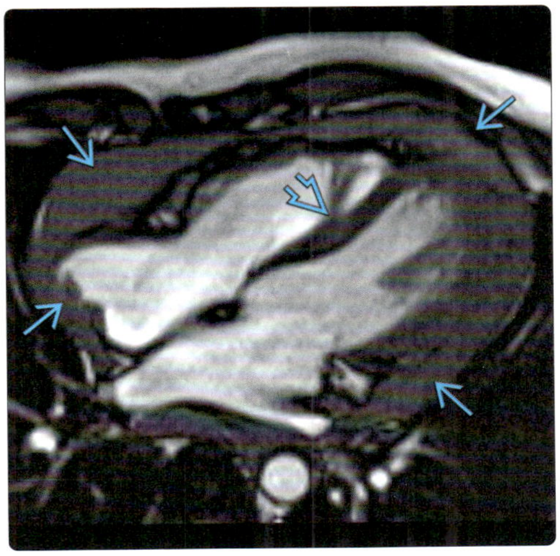

(Left) *SSFP MR in a young man who presented with shortness of breath shows circumferential pericardial thickening without mass. The patient was thought to have chronic pericarditis. There was no evidence of pericardial constriction.* **(Right)** *MR < 10 months later shows complete encasement of the heart by a confluent pericardial mass diagnosed as an epithelioid mesothelioma on biopsy. There is leftward inversion of the interventricular septum due to constriction. (Courtesy N. Choh, MD.)*

Pericardial Metastases

KEY FACTS

TERMINOLOGY

- Metastases (mets) to pericardium occurs via
  - Direct extension
  - Lymphatic spread
  - Hematogenous spread
- Primary pericardial tumors 100-1,000x less common than metastatic disease

IMAGING

- **Radiography**
  - Findings related to pericardial effusion
  - Associated signs of malignancy
- **CT**
  - Pericardial effusion often heterogeneous
  - Pericardial enhancement and nodularity
  - Pericardial soft tissue masses and nodules
  - Additional signs of malignancy
- **MR**
  - Heterogeneous signal pericardial fluid and thickening
  - Enhancing soft tissue nodules in pericardium
  - Pericardial enhancement
  - Assess for constriction or tamponade

TOP DIFFERENTIAL DIAGNOSES

- Primary pericardial tumors
- Benign pericardial effusion
- Pericarditis
- Erdheim-Chester disease

PATHOLOGY

- Most common primary sites
  - Lung, breast, lymphoma, upper GI

CLINICAL ISSUES

- Very poor prognosis

DIAGNOSTIC CHECKLIST

- New pericardial effusion in patient with known malignancy should always raise concern for mets

(Left) *Staging axial CT in a patient with a history of melanoma shows numerous complex pericardial effusions with a mixture of fluid and soft tissue masses ➡. Masses are in the oblique sinus ➡, transverse sinus ➡, and superior pericardial recess ➡. Although a similar appearance can be seen with a pericardial mesothelioma, metastases are much more common.* **(Right)** *Three-chamber CECT reconstruction shows circumferential malignant pericardial effusion with multiple enhancing masses ➡.*

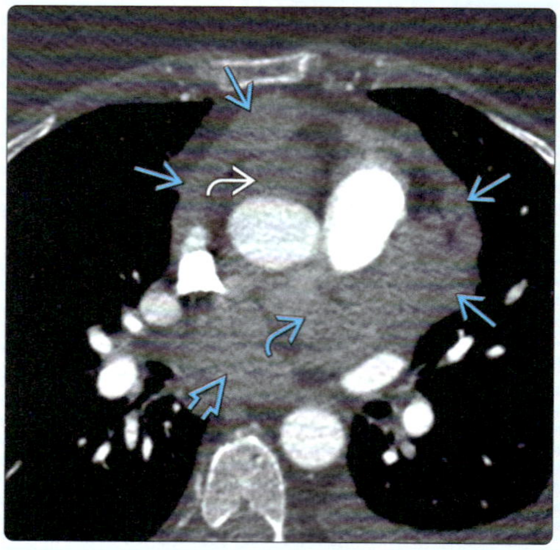

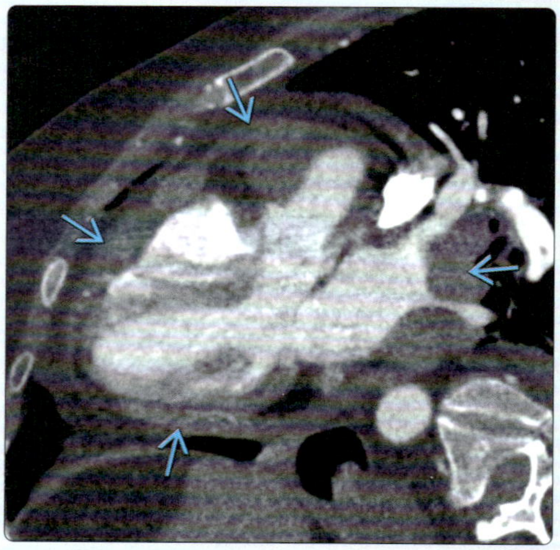

(Left) *Parasternal long-axis echocardiogram in the same patient shows the left ventricle ➡, left atrium ➡, aorta ➡, and right ventricular outflow tract ➡ corresponding to the 3-chamber CT reconstruction. A complex pericardial effusion is present with numerous areas of echogenicity ➡ due to metastatic melanoma.* **(Right)** *Axial T1 C+ MR images in a 62-year-old woman shows a large, fungating forearm melanoma ➡. Brain metastases ➡ are present.*

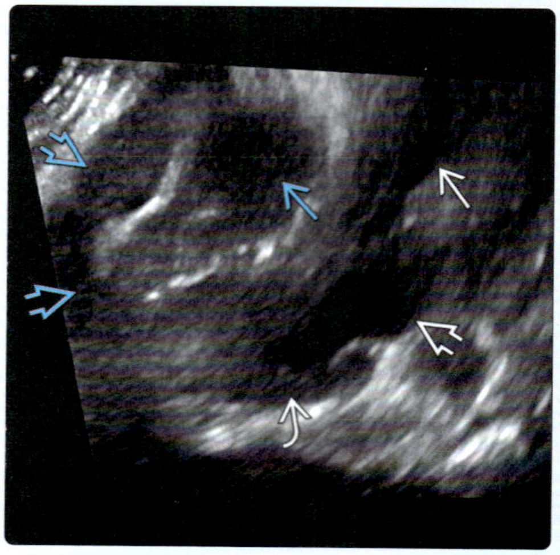

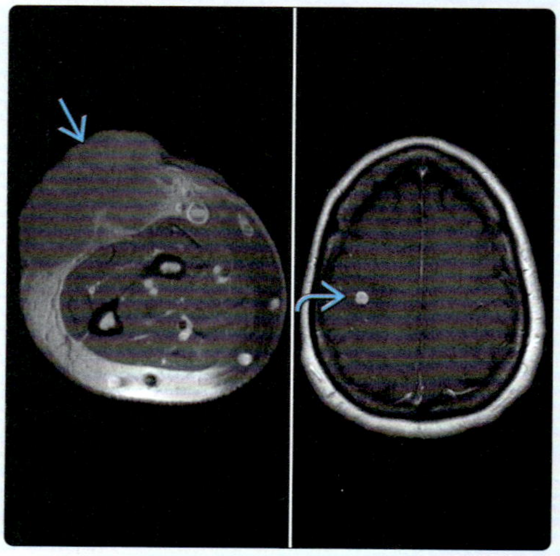

TERMINOLOGY

Definitions

- Metastases (mets) to pericardium occurs via
  - **Lymphatic spread**
    - Visceral pericardium contains most of pericardial lymphatics
    - Lymphatic channels come together near aortic root
  - **Direct extension**
    - Lung cancer
    - Lymphoma
  - **Hematogenous spread**
    - Uncommon with pericardial mets
- Primary pericardial tumors 100-1,000x less common than metastatic disease

IMAGING

General Features

- Best diagnostic clue
  - New pericardial effusion or nodules in patient with known malignancy should always raise concern for mets
  - Other extracardiac thoracic mets
- Location
  - Pericardium
- Morphology
  - Pericardial effusion
    - Nodules and masses
    - Loculated fluid collections
    - Heterogeneous attenuation fluid
    - Nodular enhancement of pericardium
  - Pericardial nodules and masses
    - Seen in pericardium proper and pericardial recesses

Radiographic Findings

- Radiography
  - Initial abnormality detected may be lung or mediastinal mass
  - Typical findings of pericardial effusion
    - May simulate cardiomegaly (if quantity of fluid exceeds 250 mL)
    - "Water bottle" heart, if large
    - Oreo cookie sign on lateral radiography
  - Associated signs of malignancy
    - Mediastinal lymphadenopathy in 80%
    - Pleural effusions in 50%
    - Osseous mets

CT Findings

- NECT
  - Pericardial effusion
    - Can be difficult to differentiate from simple pericardial effusion
    - Lobulated contours
    - Heterogeneous fluid attenuation
  - Soft tissue masses in pericardium or recesses
    - Often displacing normal anatomic structures
    - Infiltration into epicardial or pericardial fat
  - Associated signs of malignancy
    - Lung or bone mets, lymphadenopathy, pleural effusion, etc.
- CECT
  - Pericardial effusion
    - ± thickening/enhancement
    - ± pericardial nodules/masses
    - Best seen on portal venous phase
      - □ May better demonstrate solid and cystic components
      - □ May demonstrate associated myocardial involvement
  - Soft tissue masses in pericardium, often displacing normal anatomic structures
  - Associated lymphadenopathy

MR Findings

- T1WI
  - Low-signal pericardial effusion
    - May be heterogeneous due to blood products
  - Hypointense to isointense pericardial nodules and masses
  - Thickening of pericardium
- T2WI
  - High-signal pericardial effusion
    - May be heterogeneous
  - Hyperintense pericardial nodules and masses
  - Thickening of pericardium
- T1WI C+
  - Most mets enhance
  - Pericardial enhancement
- Better assessment of extent of disease than with CT
- Can assess for constrictive pericarditis or tamponade

Echocardiographic Findings

- Procedure of choice for initial evaluation of suspected pericardial effusion
  - Moderate effusion: Echo-free space 10-20 mm
  - Severe effusion: Echo-free space > 20 mm
- Echogenic material in pericardium
  - May represent tumor or blood products

Imaging Recommendations

- Best imaging tool
  - Echocardiography for initial evaluation
  - Portal venous-phase CT
  - Cardiac gated MR for further evaluation

DIFFERENTIAL DIAGNOSIS

Primary Pericardial Tumors

- **100-1,000x less common than pericardial mets**
- Can appear identical to mets
- Evidence of disease elsewhere in mets

Benign Pericardial Effusion

- Can be difficult to differentiate from mets in absence of soft tissue deposits
  - May require pericardiocentesis for diagnosis
- Numerous causes of pericardial effusions in patients with cancer
  - Radiation therapy
    - Estimated rate of 10%
      - □ As high as 50% in some cancer

- Most common with radiation field to heart and mediastinum
  - Lymphoma, breast, lung, esophageal
- More common in older patients with preexisting cardiovascular disease
- Increases toxicity of certain cancer drugs
- Chemotherapy and immune checkpoint inhibitors (ICI)
  - 4x increased incidence of pericarditis and pericardial effusion with ICIs
  - May be related to undetected pericardial mets
- Lymphatic obstruction from enlarged mediastinal lymph nodes

Pericarditis

- May mimic mets
- Cancer patients often immunocompromised
  - Can increase risk of infectious pericarditis
- Radiation and drug therapy also cause pericarditis

Erdheim-Chester Disease

- Soft tissue infiltration of epicardial fat
- Pericardial and pleural involvement can occur
- Classic perirenal findings

PATHOLOGY

General Features

- Etiology
  - Mets to pericardium more common than mets to epicardium or myocardium
  - Direct extension of tumor
  - Lymphatic spread
  - Primary sites
    - Lung (most common)
      - Adenocarcinoma most common
      - 1/3 of patients with lung cancer have pericardial mets at autopsy
    - Breast (2nd most common)
      - In women, breast and lung account for > 90% of pericardial mets
      - 1/4 of patients with metastatic breast cancer have malignant pericardial effusion at autopsy
    - Lymphoma
    - Upper GI
    - Gynecologic
- **Malignant pericardial disease overwhelmingly secondary to mets**
  - Primary tumors very rare

Gross Pathologic & Surgical Features

- Hemorrhagic and fibrinous exudates
- Various-sized nodules
- Diffuse pericardial thickening can occur
  - Mimics pericardial mesothelioma

Microscopic Features

- False-negative rate of cytology < 20%
- Hemorrhagic exudates
- Epithelial tumors grow along pericardial surface or tumor in lymphatics
- Immunohistochemistry differentiates tumor from reactive mesothelial cells

CLINICAL ISSUES

Presentation

- Most common signs/symptoms
  - Asymptomatic (50%)
  - Findings of tamponade or constrictive pericarditis
    - Hypotension and tachycardia
    - Chest pain, cough, peripheral edema
    - Dyspnea out of proportion to radiographic abnormality
  - Arrhythmia common
- Other signs/symptoms
  - Signs of cardiac tamponade
    - Kussmaul sign: Increased distention of jugular veins with inspiration
    - Friedreich sign: Rapid diastolic descent of venous pulse
    - Pulsus paradoxus: Decrease of > 10 mmHg in diastolic pressure on inspiration

Demographics

- Age
  - Determined by incidence of primary malignancy
- Sex
  - Equal distribution

Natural History & Prognosis

- Very poor prognosis
- > 80% die within 5 years of detection
- Cardiac tamponade from fluid accumulation in pericardial sac
  - Decreased cardiac output, progressive decrease in cardiac diastolic filling
  - Rapid accumulation poorly tolerated
  - Recurrent pericardial effusion in 50%
- Constrictive pericarditis from encasement of heart
- Newer immunotherapy can worsen survival in some tumors

Treatment

- Treatment of cardiac tamponade from malignant pericardial effusion
  - Pericardiocentesis or pericardial window: Primary treatment choice with catheter drainage
  - Pericardial sclerosis or pericardiectomy
  - Radiation therapy
- Surgical resection uncommon

DIAGNOSTIC CHECKLIST

Image Interpretation Pearls

- Malignant pericardial effusion is often 1st sign of cardiac or pericardial metastatic disease

SELECTED REFERENCES

1. Mori S et al: Pericardial effusion in oncological patients: current knowledge and principles of management. Cardiooncology. 10(1):8, 2024
2. Gong J et al: Pericardial disease in patients treated with immune checkpoint inhibitors. J Immunother Cancer. 9(6), 2021
3. Karpathiou G et al: Pericardial and pleural metastases: clinical, histologic, and molecular differences. Ann Thorac Surg. 106(3):872-9, 2018

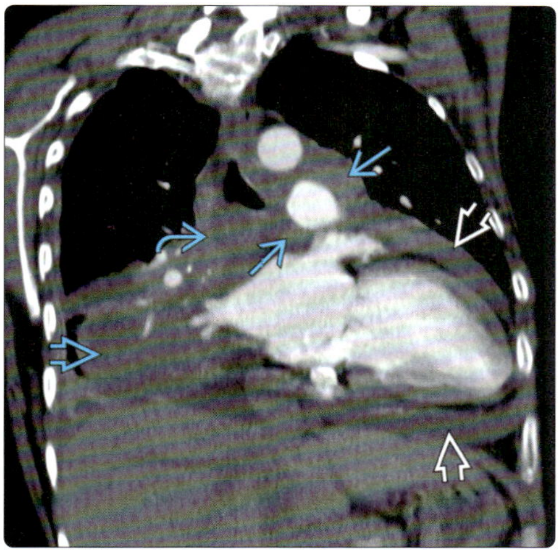

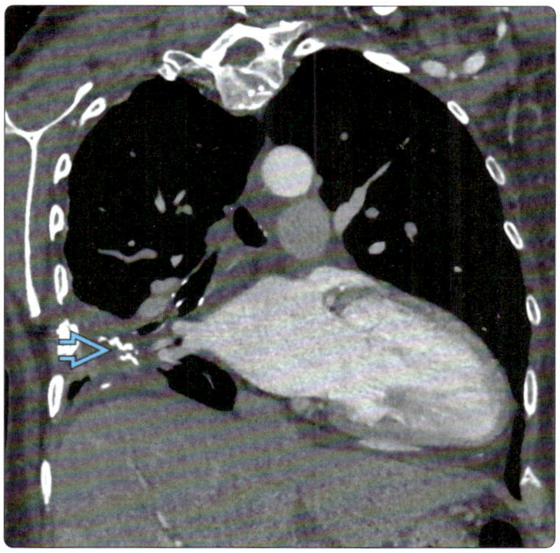

(Left) *CT in a 58-year-old woman shows a large right lower lobe necrotic mass and mediastinal lymphadenopathy. There is a pericardial effusion, and soft tissue surrounds pulmonary artery. Biopsy revealed a lung adenocarcinoma with EGFR mutation. Pericardiocentesis confirmed metastases. Patient was started on targeted immunotherapy.* **(Right)** *Coronal oblique CECT (same patient) in 2023 shows treated right lower lobe cancer and resolution of malignant nodal and pericardial disease.*

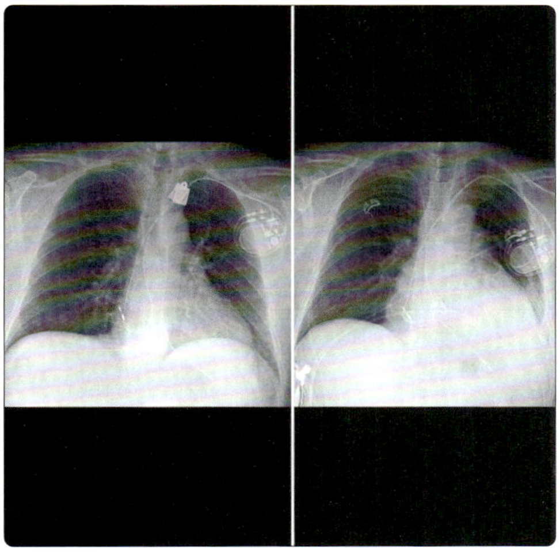

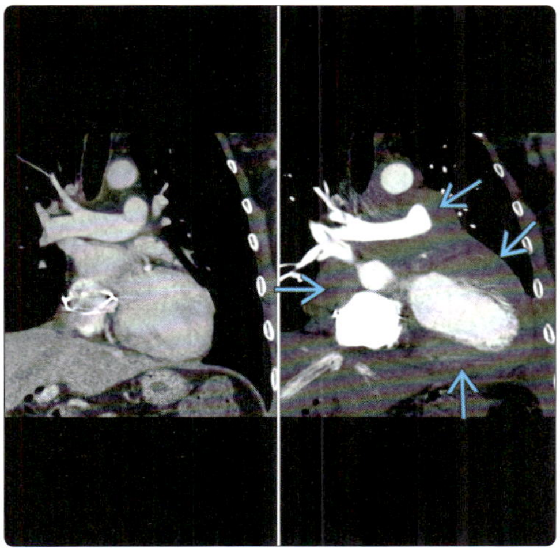

(Left) *AP radiograph in a 37-year-old man with T-cell lymphoma shows a normal radiograph (left). Two months later, the patient developed dyspnea. Radiograph (right) shows enlargement of cardiac silhouette with a moderate left effusion and left basilar atelectasis. The pulmonary vasculature is normal.* **(Right)** *At the time of the normal chest x-ray, CT shows a normal heart and pericardium (left). Two months later (right), there is diffuse soft tissue infiltration of epicardial fat and the pericardium, concerning for lymphoma.*

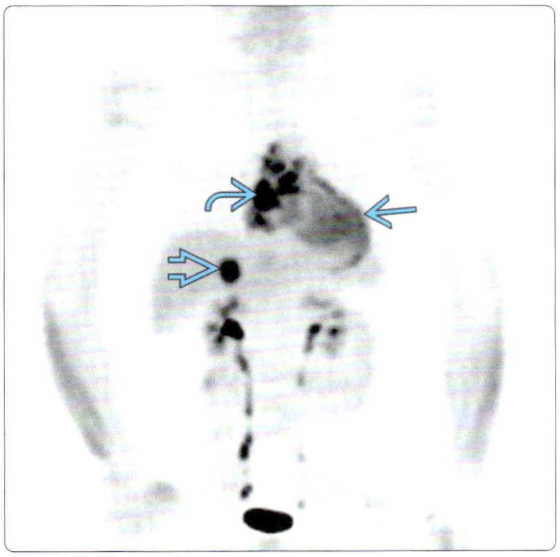

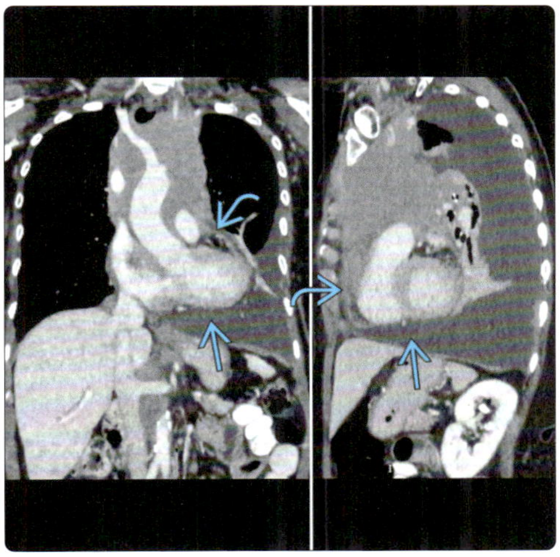

(Left) *AP PET image in the same patient shows areas of uptake in both the pericardium and epicardial fat. A liver mass is also present. Pericardiocentesis confirmed metastatic T-cell lymphoma.* **(Right)** *Coronal (left) and sagittal (right) CT images in a patient with large B-cell lymphoma show a large anterior mediastinal mass directly invading through the pericardium with pericardial thickening and nodularity. Pericardial enhancement is seen inferiorly.*

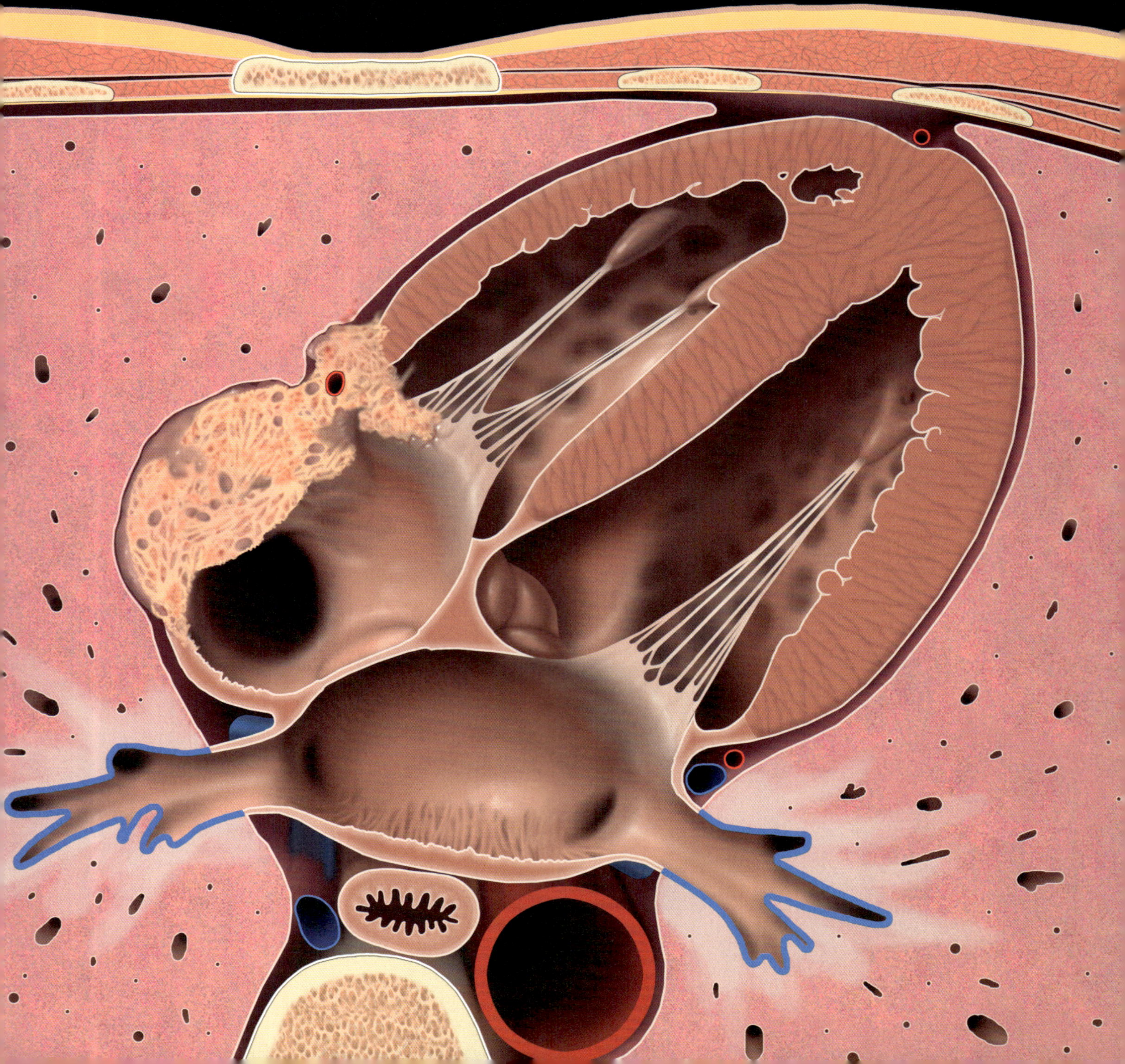

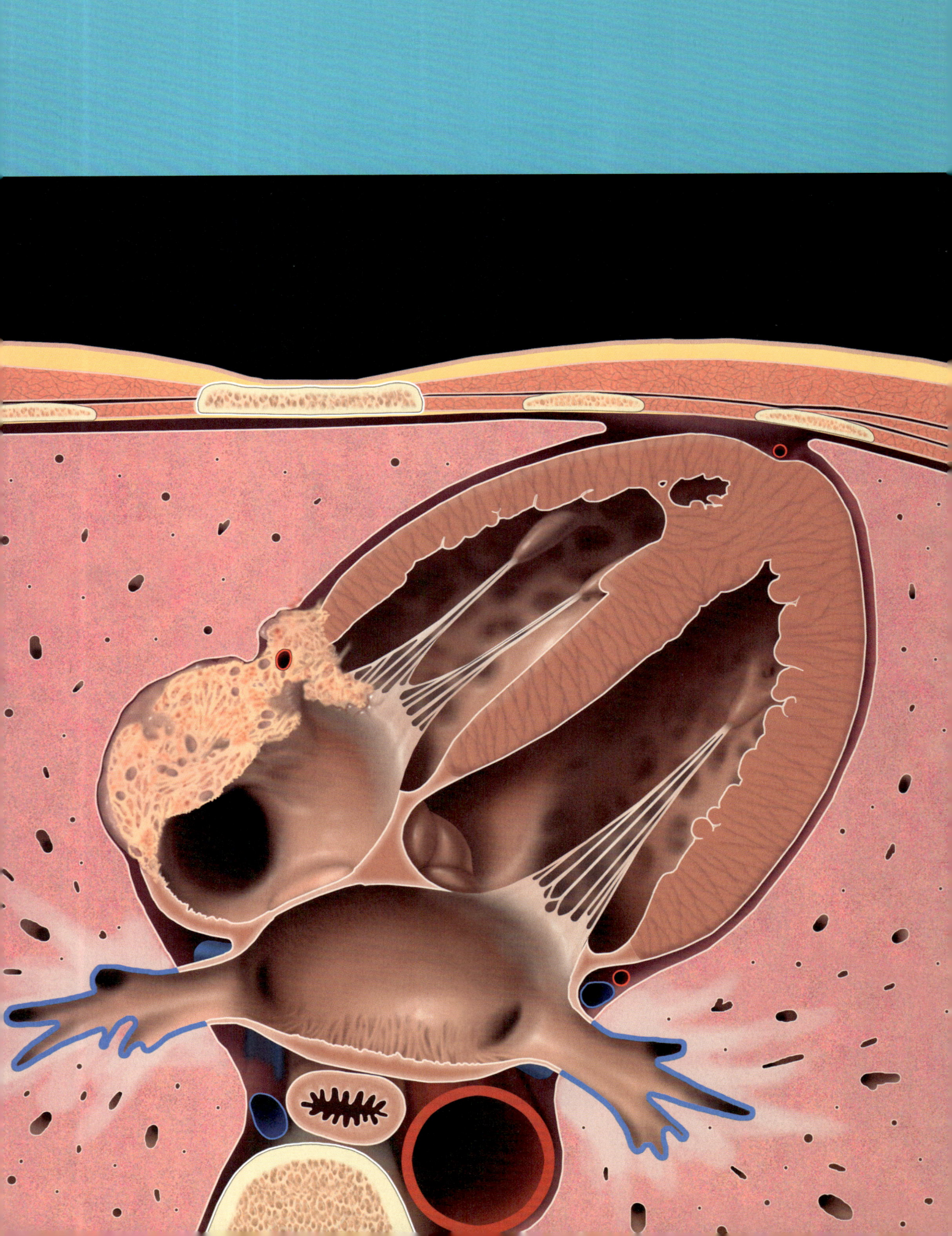

Introduction

Evaluation of a known or suspected cardiac neoplasm has become an increasingly common source of referrals for further cross-sectional imaging, particularly using cardiac MR. This chapter discusses the imaging modalities available for the evaluation of cardiac masses and their respective advantages and disadvantages. It also briefly considers the anatomic and imaging characteristics of various types of masses, most of which are covered in detail in dedicated chapters. Finally, the chapter proposes a systematic imaging approach to the evaluation of known or suspected cardiac neoplasms that aims to narrow the set of differential diagnostic considerations with a high degree of confidence.

Imaging Considerations

The goals of imaging a cardiac mass should be to make the proper diagnosis, assess its anatomic relationship to other cardiovascular structures to help determine resectability, and to assess treatment response in the appropriate setting. To make the proper diagnosis, one should localize the lesion to a specific chamber and determine whether the lesion is intracavitary, intramural, or epicardial/pericardial in location, which will greatly narrow the differential diagnosis. Then, one should determine the composition of the lesion (i.e., cystic vs. solid, heterogeneous vs. homogeneous, fat vs. calcium containing), evaluate the lesion margins (well defined vs. infiltrating), determine the tumor vascularity with perfusion imaging, evaluate the enhancement pattern on postcontrast imaging, and assess for hemodynamic effect.

While echocardiography is widely available and readily performed, it has significant limitations in characterizing solid masses owing to its poor soft tissue contrast. Also, in many patients, lack of acoustic windows limits visualization of cardiac structures. Cardiac CT has unrestricted imaging windows, and its soft tissue contrast resolution is superior to that of echocardiography but inferior to that of MR. Its temporal resolution is inferior to that of echocardiography or MR, and it requires ionizing radiation. CT is superior to MR and echo for identification of calcification and for feeding arteries of vascular lesions. However, for small, highly mobile lesions, echocardiography may be the test of choice due to high temporal resolution.

MR provides the most comprehensive assessment of cardiac masses, including soft tissue characterization as well as 1st-pass perfusion, postcontrast enhancement, and late gadolinium enhancement (LGE) of the mass with a single administration of contrast. MR cine imaging can simultaneously visualize the lesion borders and evaluate its impact on cardiac function. The most significant advantage of MR is that of improved soft tissue contrast. The pattern of early and delayed enhancement demonstrated by a given lesion can also frequently provide important information leading to the correct diagnosis. For example, thrombus (which is the most common cardiac mass) has LGE properties that allow conclusive differentiation from a normal myocardium as well as most neoplasms. On the other hand, a cardiac fibroma typically shows little to no perfusion or early enhancement on T1W imaging but shows intense uptake on LGE. Additionally, emerging T1 and T2 mapping sequences can provide additional parameters for lesion characterization.

CT protocols are dependent on the chamber of interest and may include noncontrast, arterial, and delayed acquisitions. The excellent spatial resolution of CT allows for detailed anatomic characterization of the mass in relation to vital cardiac structures. Multiphasic datasets can be acquired to determine the behavior of the mass throughout the cardiac cycle, which can aid in the diagnosis.

An additional modality that can be helpful in evaluation of cardiac masses is positron emission tomography (PET) utilizing F-18 fluorodeoxyglucose (FDG). This is typically used in combination with low-dose CT for anatomic location and attenuation correction and more recently in combination with MR (PET/MR). Due to variable physiologic myocardial uptake of F-18 FDG, the assessment of cardiac masses may require special patient preparation (diet). PET/CT can also help assess for metastatic disease or to determine the effectiveness of treatment.

Suggested MR Protocol

MR may also be requested to evaluate for cardiac/pericardiac infiltration from masses adjacent to the heart. In this scenario, lesion characterization is less important. Cine SSFP, T1 images with fat saturation (to demonstrate the fat plane), and early as well as delayed contrast-enhanced sequences at the location of the mass are necessary.

Intracavitary Lesions

Myxomas make up ~ 50% of all primary benign cardiac neoplasms. Myxomas are located in the left atrium in ~ 75-80% of cases and are usually attached to the fossa ovalis. The location of myxomas within the right atrium tends to be a little more heterogeneous. **Precontrast SSFP cine images often demonstrate higher signal intensity than the myocardium, owing to the high T2 signal of the myxoid matrix present. This fact is helpful in differentiating these lesions from thrombi, which are isointense to the myocardium precontrast.** Similarly, myxomas tend to be bright on T2W sequences. First-pass perfusion of myxomas is variable but usually mild. T1W postcontrast imaging usually does show scattered areas of enhancement in the mass. Myxomas usually demonstrate heterogeneous enhancement on delayed enhancement images with a short inversion time. The fibrous stalk of the myxoma, if it can be visualized, shows homogeneous intense LGE. On long inversion time images, the gelatinous component of the lesion may be quite dark, mimicking the appearance of a thrombus.

Thrombus is the most common cardiac "mass," although it is not a neoplasm. Thrombi are often seen in the left atrium in patients with atrial fibrillation or in the left ventricular apex in patients with apical infarct. First-pass perfusion, postcontrast T1W enhancement, and LGE should be absent. In some instances of chronic thrombus, enhancement along the edge of the thrombus can occur due to fibrous tissue deposition. Although they may have low signal on long inversion time LGE imaging like some myxomas, **thrombi are isointense to the myocardium on noncontrast SSFP cine imaging.**

Metastases can extend into the cardiac chambers via the inferior vena cava from renal or hepatic carcinomas or via the pulmonary veins from lung carcinomas. Of the intracavitary entities, usually only metastatic lesions show intense enhancement on LGE imaging.

Valvular Lesions

Papillary fibroelastoma (PF) is recognized as the most common primary cardiac tumor by the 2021 revised WHO classification system. They are small (≤ 1-cm) excrescences found on any endocardial surface but are most commonly seen on valve surfaces (90%). Although PFs can embolize, it is often discovered incidentally on an echocardiogram performed for another indication. On MR, PFs often show homogeneous LGE. Due to their small size, PFs can be difficult to localize on MR and may be better visualized on multiphase cardiac CTA.

Vegetations are best thought of as infected thrombi attached to valves. While their signal characteristics mimic those of thrombi, associated valvular destruction with regurgitation and embolization are common. Septic emboli in the lung help confirm the diagnosis in right-sided vegetations.

Intramural Lesions, Malignant

Metastatic disease is reported to be ~ 40x more common than primary cardiac neoplasia in pathologic series. Cardiac metastases almost always occur in the setting of advanced, known malignancy. Metastatic lesions may be well defined or infiltrative with poorly defined margins. Most are bright on T2W imaging and demonstrate 1st-pass perfusion and conspicuous postcontrast enhancement. Heterogeneous enhancement on LGE is common. Pericardial effusions are frequently associated.

Primary cardiac sarcomas are rare, and they can mimic lymphoma or metastatic disease. Angiosarcomas make up ~ 50% of sarcomas and are usually right atrial in origin. They are highly invasive and usually invade into the epicardial fat, especially in the region of the right atrioventricular groove where it commonly envelops the right coronary artery (RCA). Right ventricle and pericardial invasion are also common. Angiosarcomas are very hyperintense on T2W imaging and show intense 1st-pass perfusion and postcontrast T1W enhancement. Other sarcomas have a left atrial predominance and include undifferentiated pleomorphic sarcoma, leiomyosarcomas, osteosarcoma, fibrosarcomas, synovial sarcoma, and rhabdomyosarcoma. They are often very aggressive, commonly obstruct pulmonary veins, and invade along and through the atrial wall. Enhancement is more variable.

Primary cardiac lymphoma are a rare B-cell tumors with an infiltrating, aggressive appearance. They tend to involve the right heart and can encase the RCA. However, compared to angiosarcomas, they do not enhance as avidly on 1st-pass perfusion and T1W postcontrast imaging. Additionally, they are often not as hyperintense to the myocardium on T2W imaging as an angiosarcoma.

Intramural Lesions, Benign

Lipomatous hypertrophy of the interatrial septum is not a neoplasm but refers to infiltration of the interatrial septum by unencapsulated adipocytes. It spares the fossa ovalis, resulting in the classic dumbbell appearance.

Lipomas are rare, benign tumors that are true neoplasms composed of fat with a surrounding capsule. They may arise along the epicardium or in an intramural location. They show characteristic fat suppression on MR.

Paragangliomas are typically well-encapsulated lesions seen in patients with symptoms of catecholamine excess. They are very vascular lesions and tend to occur in the atria, along the atrioventricular sulcus, and at the roots of the great vessels. They are light bulb bright on T2 images with a salt and pepper appearance due to the presence of flow voids. They demonstrate intense 1st-pass perfusion and T1W postcontrast enhancement.

Intramural Lesions in Pediatric Patients

Rhabdomyoma is the most common cardiac neoplasm in children and is most often seen in children with tuberous sclerosis. The lesions are often multiple and typically involve the ventricular free walls and interventricular septum. Their signal intensity is similar to a normal myocardium on cine and LGE imaging, meaning that **they null (or go dark) similar to a normal myocardium**.

Fibroma is the 2nd most common childhood neoplasm. It is a solitary mass of fibroblasts and collagen that typically involves the ventricular free walls and interventricular septum. In older children and adults, fibromas may be dark on T2 imaging, a characteristic finding. **On LGE imaging, they show intense enhancement (bright signal), differentiating them from rhabdomyomas.**

Epicardial/Pericardial Lesions

Metastatic lesions involve the pericardium more frequently than the myocardium. They often result in nodular regions of pericardial thickening and are usually associated with pericardial effusions or hemopericardium.

Pericardial cysts, although not neoplasms, may sometimes cause mass effect requiring differentiation from more serious lesions. Their internal signal is homogeneous. While they often follow typical fluid signal, they may be T1W hyperintense and T2W hypointense with proteinaceous fluid.

Hemangiomas and **lymphangiomas** are both tumors of endothelial cells and contain either blood (hemangiomas) or lymph (lymphangiomas). Both are bright on T2 images, but only hemangiomas demonstrate increased vascularity on perfusion imaging.

Tumor Mimics/Pseudomasses

Occasionally, cardiac and paracardiac structures may have a confusing echocardiographic appearance and simulate a mass. In most instances, normal cardiac structures may mimic a true cardiac lesion. For instance, a prominent Chiari network or eustachian ridge can be mistaken for a right atrial mass. These anatomic structures can be well evaluated on cardiac MR or ECG-gated CTA.

Differential Diagnosis

The diagnostic path starts with localizing the epicenter of the lesion as being intracavitary, intramural, or epicardial. Defining the lesion as sharply marginated or infiltrating is helpful in the analysis of intramural and epicardial lesions. Perfusion and LGE sequences will indicate the vascularity of the lesion and help to narrow the differential diagnosis. For example, an intracavitary mass with well-defined borders arising in the left atrium attached to the fossa ovalis will likely be a myxoma. On the other hand, a bulky infiltrating lesion arising in the wall of the left atrium and demonstrating vigorous enhancement will likely be a primary sarcoma (or a metastatic lesion) even if it protrudes into the left ventricular cavity.

Selected References

1. Lorca MC et al: Radiologic-pathologic correlation of cardiac tumors: updated 2021 WHO tumor classification. Radiographics. 44(6):e230126, 2024
2. Beroukhim RS et al: Accuracy of cardiac magnetic resonance imaging in diagnosing pediatric cardiac masses: a multicenter study. JACC Cardiovasc Imaging. 15(8):1391-405, 2022

Comparison of Imaging Modalities for Evaluating Cardiac Neoplasms

Echocardiography	Cardiac CT	Cardiac MR
Advantages		
Availability, portability, and relatively rapid image acquisition; good spatial resolution and excellent temporal resolution	Highest spatial resolution for anatomic assessment; less operator dependent; fair soft tissue contrast; calcium delineation	Superior soft tissue contrast and tissue characterization; assessment of function; perfusion imaging without radiation
Disadvantages		
Need adequate acoustic window; ↓ soft tissue contrast resolution compared with CT or MR	Relatively poor temporal resolution; ionizing radiation; iodinated contrast	Not universally available; need skilled technologist

Suggested MR Imaging Protocol

Sequences	Imaging Planes	Coverage	Imaging Information Obtained
Single-shot SSFP and HASTE/FSE	Axial/sagittal/coronal stack	Entire thorax	Overview of cardiac/mediastinal structures; lesion localization
Cine SSFP	Short- and long-axis stack	Heart base to apex	Lesion visualization; cardiac function
T1W and T2W FSE/fat suppression	Short and long axis	Tailored to lesion	Lesion tissue characterization
Perfusion imaging	Short and long axis	Tailored to lesion	Lesion vascularity
T1W post contrast	Short and long axis	Tailored to lesion	Enhancement characteristics
LGE images with time inversion to null myocardium	Short- and long-axis stack	Tailored to lesion	Enhancement characteristics
LGE images with long time inversion (~ 600 ms)	Short- and long-axis stack	Tailored to lesion	Thrombus detection
Parametric mapping (T1 and T2)	Short or long axis	Tailored to lesion	Lesion tissue characterization

Cardiac Masses by Location

Location	Lesion	Typical Imaging Features	Differentiating MR Features
Intracavitary	Thrombus	Any chamber; variable shape	Isointense to myocardium on cine SSFP; nulls at inversion time ~ 600 ms
	Myxoma	85% left atrial (fossa ovalis); 10-12% right or biatrial	Hyperintense to myocardium on SSFP; stalk enhances
	Metastasis	Solitary or multiple; mass effect	Transvenous extension; heterogeneous enhancement
Valvular	Papillary fibroelastoma	Small-stalked mass arising along valve or endocardium	Usually low signal on cine and T1 images
	Vegetations	Perivalvular or attached to thickened, abnormal valve	May have concomitant embolic disease
Intramural, malignant	Metastasis	Multiple infiltrative lesions in patients with malignancy	Heterogeneous enhancement
	Primary sarcoma	Solitary bulky, infiltrative mass; right atrial angiosarcoma most common (50%)	Heterogeneous enhancement
	Lymphoma	Typically large, infiltrative mass; right ventricle involvement common	Variable enhancement, often < metastases
Intramural, benign	Lipomatous hamartoma of interatrial septum	Fatty signal in interatrial septum with barbell shape	Fat suppression
	Lipoma	Intramural or epicardial; rarely protrudes into cavity	Fat suppression
	Paraganglioma	Well-defined lesion in patient with catecholamine excess	Light bulb bright on T2 images; hypervascular
Intramural, in children	Rhabdomyoma	Commonly multiple; associated with tuberous sclerosis	Isointense to myocardium on all sequences
	Fibroma	Large intracavitary ventricular mass	Bright on LGE imaging (may have dark core)
Epicardial /pericardial	Metastasis	Pericardial involvement > myocardial	Effusions common, may result in symptoms
	Cyst	Well defined, nonenhancing; contiguous with pericardium	Homogeneous signal with no enhancement
	Hemangioma	Multicystic; epicardial, pericardial, intramural or cavitary	High T1 and T2 signal; hypervascular
	Lymphangioma	Multicystic lesion; intramural, epicardial, or pericardial	Low T1 signal, high T2 signal; hypovascular

MR of Cardiac Left Ventricular Thrombus

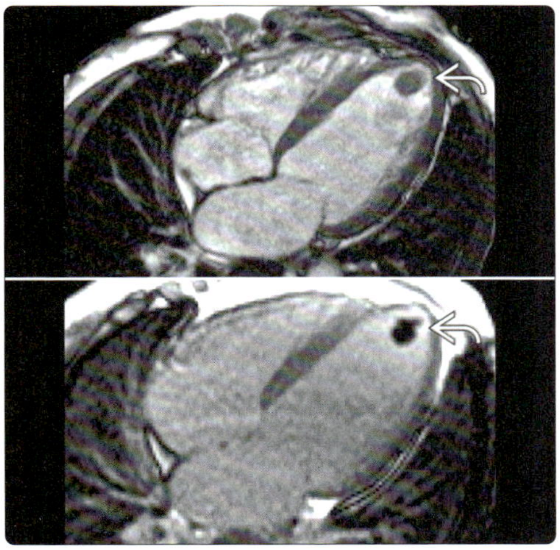

Cardiac MR of Left Atrial Thrombus

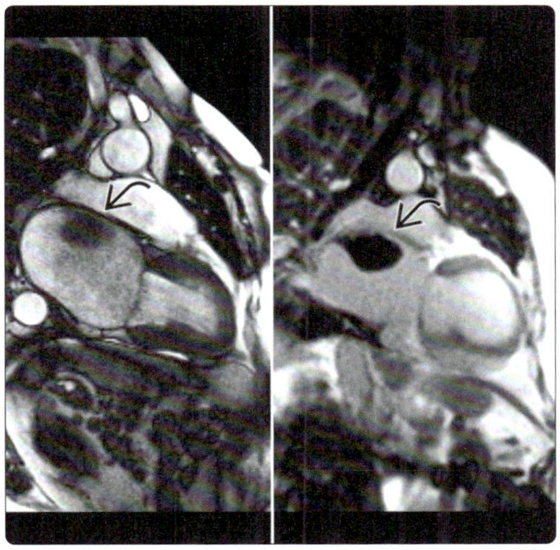

(Left) *Four-chamber SSFP cine MR (top) and late gadolinium enhancement (LGE) MR obtained with an inversion time of 600 ms (bottom) show an apical thrombus ➪. Note that the thrombus is isointense to myocardium on the cine image, which is different from the appearance of myxomas.* **(Right)** *Vertical long-axis (2-chamber) SSFP cine MR (left) and LGE MR (right) in a patient with atrial fibrillation show a left atrial thrombus ➪. Note that the thrombus is isointense to the myocardium on SSFP cine imaging.*

SSFP of Left Atrial Myxoma

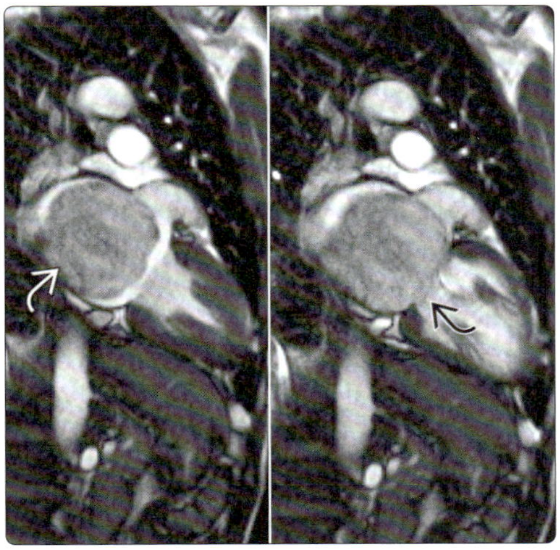

Cardiac MR of Right Atrial Myxoma

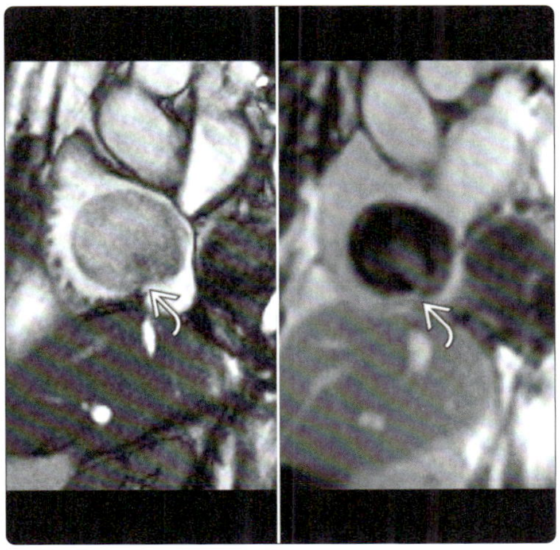

(Left) *Two-chamber SSFP cine MR in systole (left) and diastole (right) show a left atrial (LA) myxoma ➪, which is conspicuously hyperintense to myocardium. The myxoma nearly obstructs the mitral valve in diastole ➪.* **(Right)** *SSFP cine (left) and 600 ms inversion time LGE (right) images show a right atrial myxoma attached inferiorly via a short stalk ➪, which enhances on LGE. The rest of the mass shows little enhancement, which can mimic thrombus. The bright signal on SSFP imaging would not be seen with thrombus.*

MR of Papillary Fibroelastoma

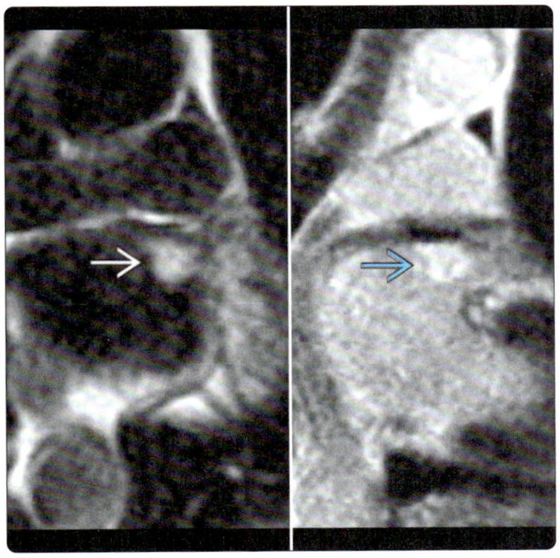

MR of Renal Cell Carcinoma Metastases

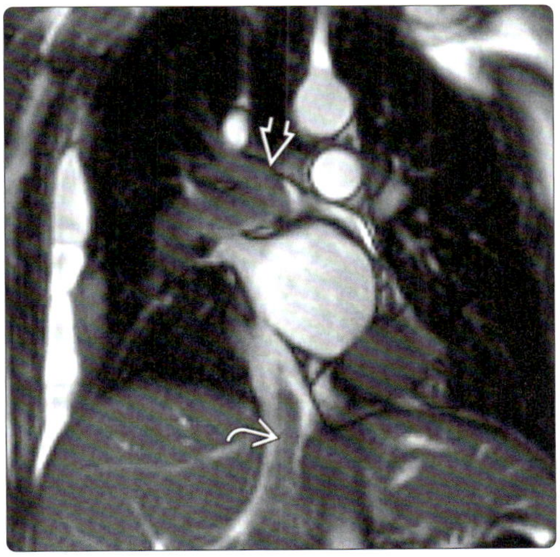

(Left) *T2 (left) and LGE (right) images show an atypical papillary fibroelastoma in the left atrium ➡. Note the lesion demonstrates LGE ➡ on imaging delayed to 20 minutes.* **(Right)** *Coronal oblique SSFP cine MR in a patient with renal cell carcinoma shows tumor extending through the inferior vena cava ➪ into the right atrium. There is also a tumor embolism to the right pulmonary artery ➡.*

(**Left**) *Four-chamber cine MR in diastole (top) and systole (bottom) show large vegetations of the tricuspid valve ➔ that are associated with significant valvular dysfunction ➔.* (**Right**) *Four-chamber SSFP cine MR (top) and LGE MR (bottom) show a metastasis from colon carcinoma producing an intracavitary lesion of the right ventricular apex ➔. Note the high signal of the lesion ➔ on LGE imaging. Of the intracavitary lesions, metastases tend to show the greatest enhancement.*

SSFP of Tricuspid Valve Vegetations

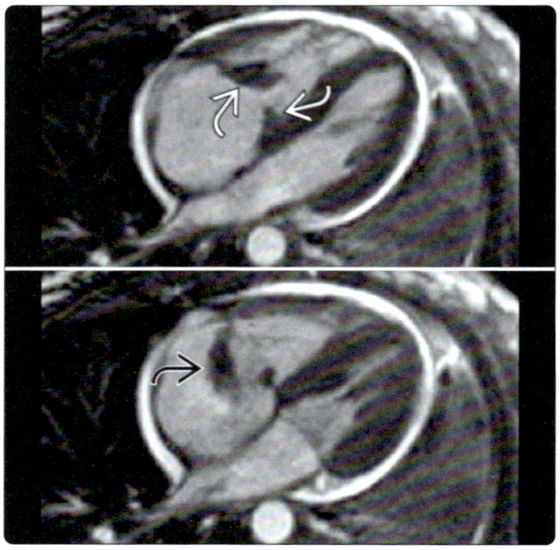

MR of Cardiac Metastases

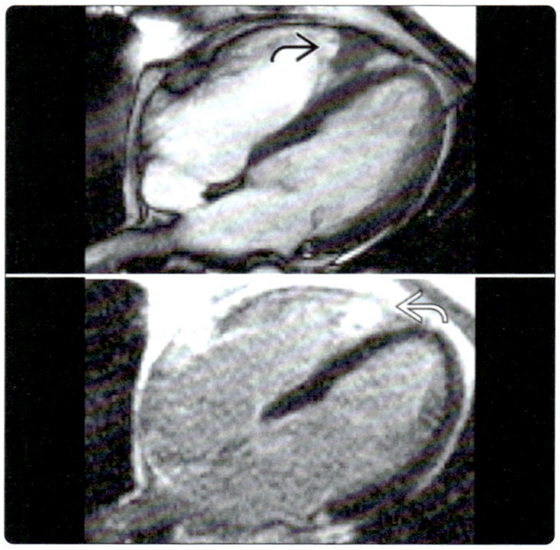

(**Left**) *Short-axis SSFP cine MR (left) and T1 FSE MR (right) show rhabdomyomas of the anterior and inferior left ventricular walls ➔. The lesions have signal intensity similar to that of normal myocardium on all sequences.* (**Right**) *Short-axis SSFP cine MR (top left), LGE MR (top right), 3-chamber SSFP cine MR (bottom left), and LGE MR (bottom right) of a fibroma of the right ventricular outflow tract (RVOT) show that the lesion is sharply demarcated from normal myocardium ➔ and has intense delayed enhancement ➔.*

Cardiac MR of Rhabdomyomas

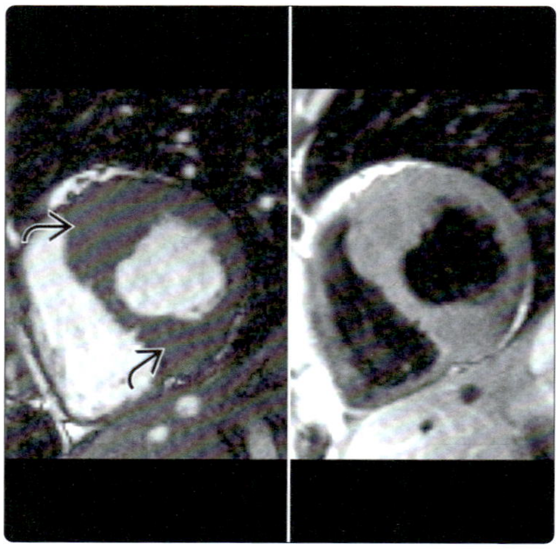

MR of Cardiac Fibroma

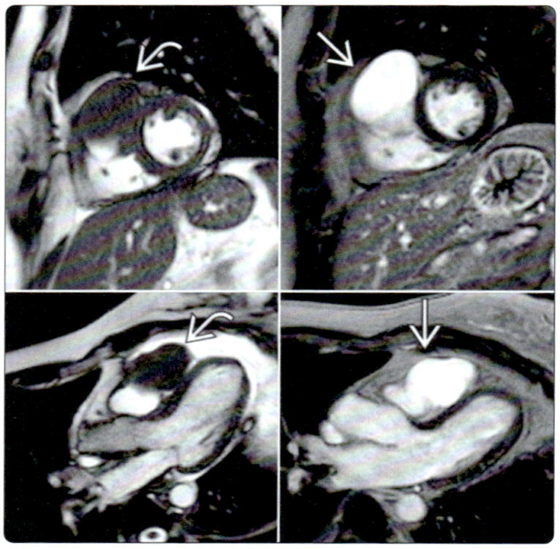

(**Left**) *Cardiac paraganglioma ➔ is known to show a characteristic MR appearance: Isointense on T1, bright on T2 with associated flow voids, and intense 1st-pass perfusion with extensive uptake on LGE imaging.* (**Right**) *Four-chamber cine MR of an angiosarcoma shows the characteristic right atrial location. Note the infiltration of the right atrial wall ➔ by this aggressive lesion and the pedunculated intracavitary components ➔.*

MR of Paraganglioma

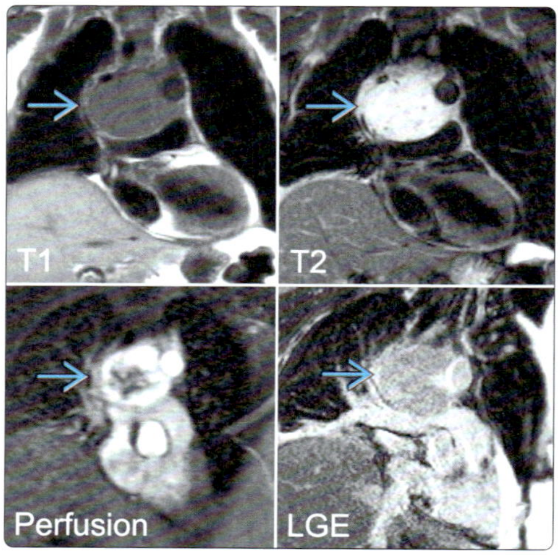

MR of Right Atrial Angiosarcoma

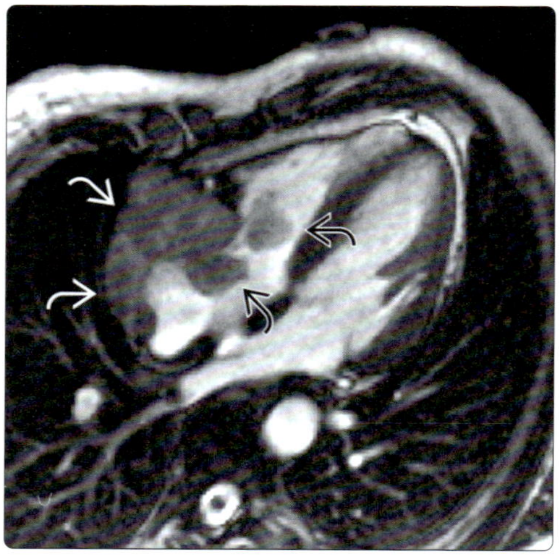

Primary Left Atrial Osteosarcoma

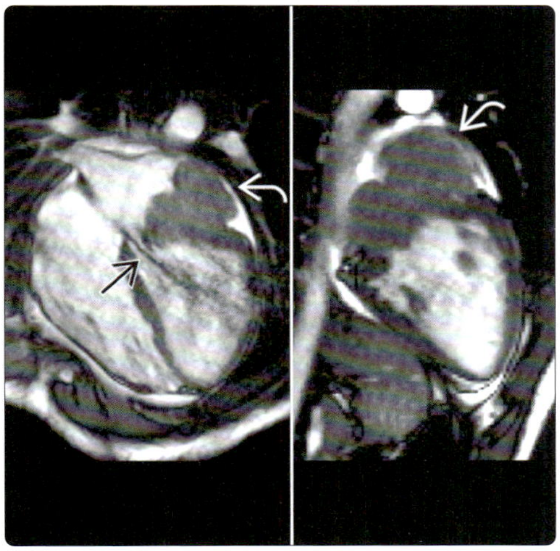

SSFP of Cardiac Lymphoma

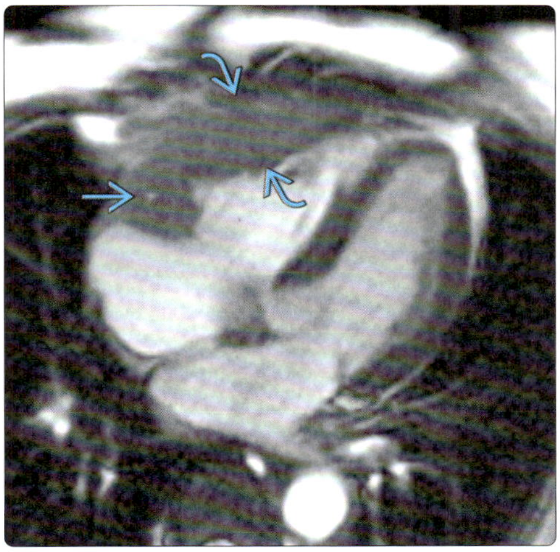

(Left) *Four- (left) and 2-chamber SSFP cine MR (right) of a bulky, infiltrating LA mass due to an osteosarcoma show the importance of lesion margins and MR appearance in differentiating benign and malignant lesions. Note the nearly total obstruction of the mitral valve is clearly seen, as is the turbulent flow produced.* **(Right)** *Four-chamber SSFP cine MR shows primary cardiac lymphoma infiltrating the right ventricular free wall. Lymphoma often encases the right coronary artery, as seen here.*

Hyperintense T1W Signal in Metastatic Melanoma

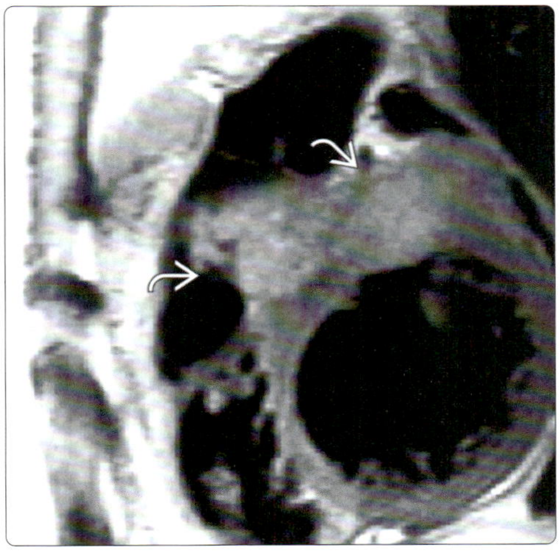

MR of Cardiac Metastases From Lung Cancer

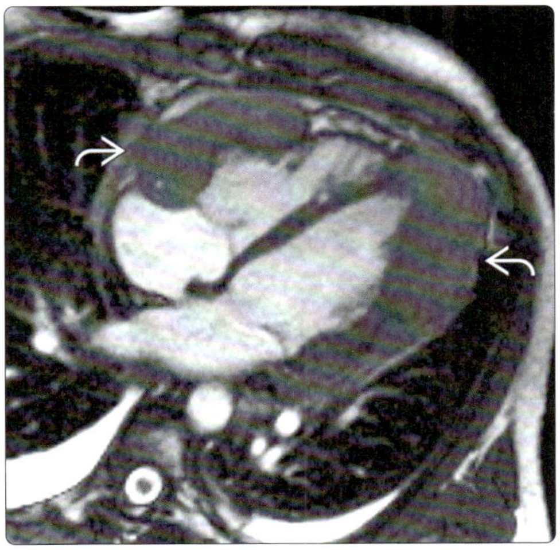

(Left) *RVOT T1 FSE MR demonstrates high signal intensity lesions infiltrating the RVOT in a patient with metastatic melanoma. The high signal on precontrast T1 (likely due to melanin) is highly suggestive of this diagnosis.* **(Right)** *Horizontal long-axis (4-chamber) cine MR shows 2 infiltrating lesions of the myocardium in a patient with lung carcinoma. Metastatic lesions are often multiple and show poor definition of margins, as seen in this case.*

MR in Renal Cell Carcinoma Metastases

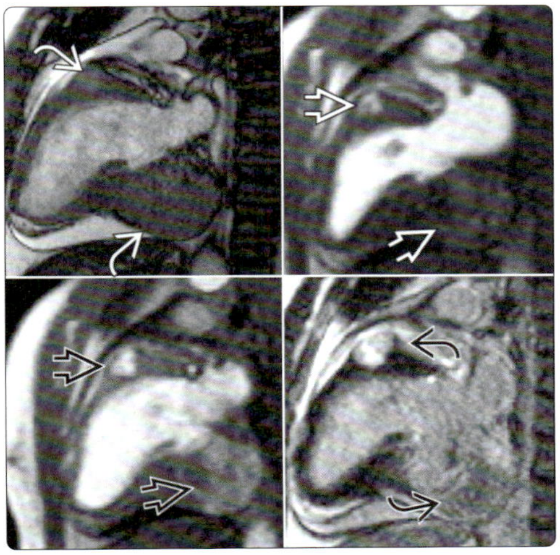

Cardiac MR of Pseudomasses

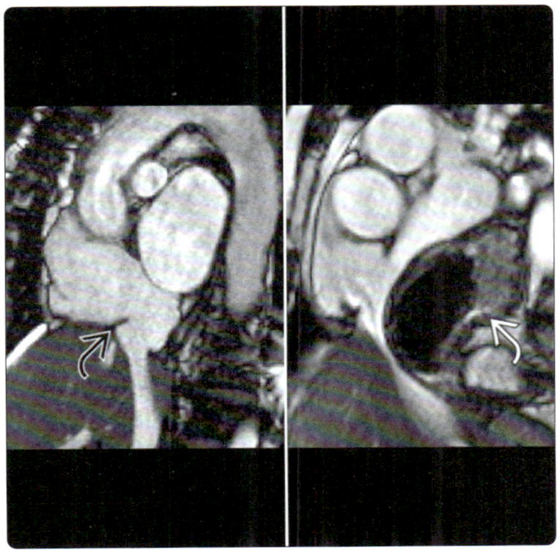

(Left) *Vertical long-axis (2-chamber) cine MR, perfusion early and late arterial phases, and LGE MR of hypervascular renal cell carcinoma metastases in the anterior and inferior left ventricular walls show that the lesions enhance on perfusion and LGE.* **(Right)** *Short-axis SSFP cine MR of a prominent eustachian valve (left) and a large hiatal hernia (right) illustrate the fact that various structures can mimic a cardiac mass.*

Tumor Mimics

KEY FACTS

TERMINOLOGY

- Pseudomasses: Entities that appear as masses on initial imaging (usually echo) but often are either normal structures or clinically insignificant variant lesions; usually resolved with cross-sectional imaging (CT or MR)
- Pseudomasses (including thrombi) make up ~ 1/3 of cases referred to MR for "cardiac mass"

IMAGING

- **Crista terminalis**: Normal structure denoting site of embryologic fusion of primitive right atrium (RA) with sinus venosus
  - Usually recognized on cine MR as part of RA wall
  - Often best appreciated on 4-chamber or axial view
- **Eustachian valve**: Variably prominent but normal ridge of tissue at junction of inferior vena cava (IVC) with RA
  - Recognized by characteristic location at junction of IVC with RA
- **Lipomatous hypertrophy of interatrial septum**: Infiltration of interatrial septum by fatty hyperplasia
  - Recognized by characteristic fat signal and specific location
  - Typically spares fossa ovalis
- **Thrombus**: Not actually mimic, but true mass, yet not neoplasm
  - Often adheres to sites of prior ventricular infarction
  - Uniformly low in signal on delayed enhancement MR images with long inversion time (600 ms)
- **Mitral annular calcification** (particularly tumefactive variant)
  - CT: Calcific density in characteristic location
  - MR: Low signal on all sequences
- **Less common mimics**: Sinus of Valsalva aneurysms, aneurysms of membranous septum adjacent to ventricular septal defects

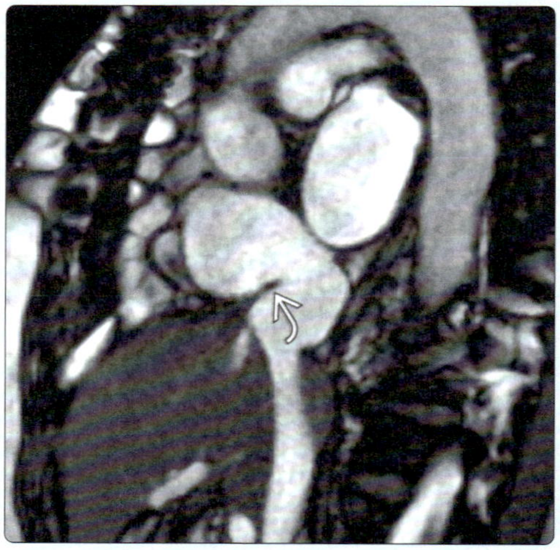

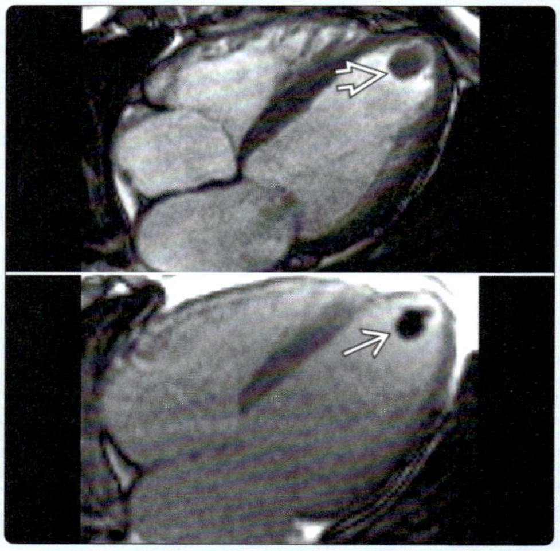

(Left) *Short-axis cine SSFP MR shows a prominent eustachian valve at the right atrium (RA)-inferior vena cava (IVC) junction, which may have a mass-like appearance on echocardiography.* **(Right)** *Four-chamber SSFP cine MR (top) and LGE MR with a long inversion time (TI) of 600 ms (bottom) show a thrombus in the left ventricle (LV) apex. Note that the thrombus is isointense to myocardium on cine MR and dark on LGE MR. Patient has an apical myocardial infarction, which was better seen on LGE MR images with a standard TI.*

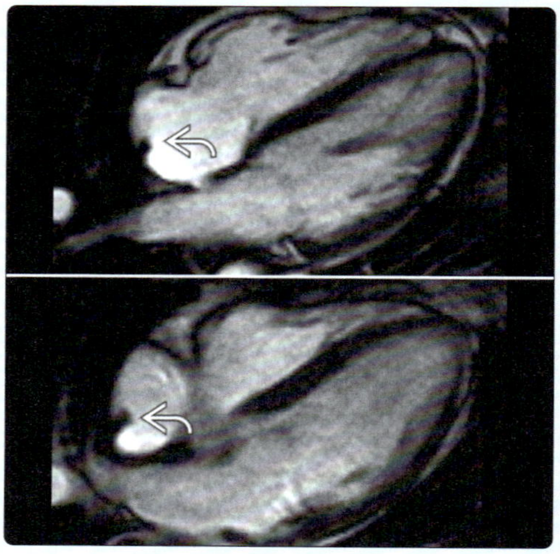

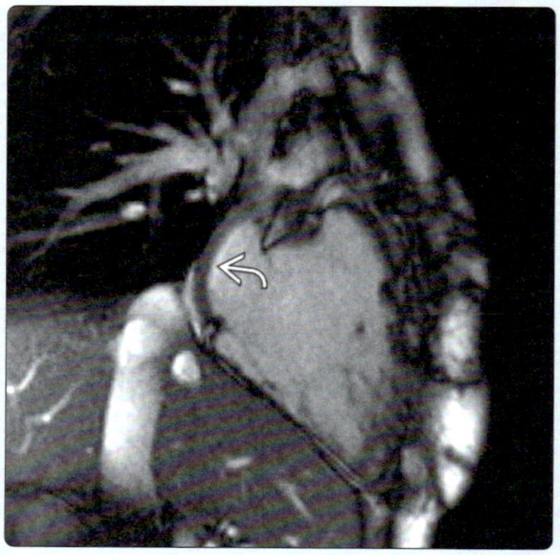

(Left) *Two sequential 4-chamber SSFP cine MR images show a prominent crista terminalis along the RA margin. Note its polypoid appearance and characteristic location at the intersection of the right atrial appendage with the superior vena cava (SVC)-RA junction. Also, it is isointense to the myocardium on these cine images and on all sequences obtained.* **(Right)** *Vertical long-axis (2-chamber) cine MR in the plane of the crista terminalis in the same patient shows its vertical extent and characteristic location.*

TERMINOLOGY

Synonyms

- Pseudomasses

Definitions

- Entities that appear as masses on initial imaging (usually echo) but often are either normal structures or clinically insignificant variant lesions; usually resolved with cross-sectional imaging (CT or MR)
  - **Normal cardiac variants**
    - **Crista terminalis**
      - Normal fibromuscular ridge indenting right atrium (RA)
      - Demarcates site of fusion of embryologic primitive RA with sinus venosus
    - **Eustachian valve**
      - Variably prominent ridge of tissue at junction of inferior vena cava (IVC) with RA
      - Directs blood flow toward foramen ovale in fetal life
      - When prominent, can be mistaken for mass on echo
    - Other congenital remnants of valve of sinus venosus in RA
      - **Thebesian valve**: At junction of coronary sinus with RA
      - **Chiari network**: Net-like structure thought to be variant of eustachian valve but much more mobile
    - **Taenia sagittalis**
      - Most prominent pectinate muscle in RA
      - Remnant of septum spurium
    - **Coumadin (warfarin) ridge**
      - Band-like structure in left atrium (LA) between left superior pulmonary vein and left atrial appendage (LAA)
      - Described as Q-tip sign on transesophageal echocardiography (TEE)
      - Mistaken for thrombus or mass in echocardiography
  - **Intracardiac benign abnormalities**
    - **Lipomatous hypertrophy of interatrial septum (LHIAS)**
      - Unencapsulated hyperplasia of normal fat cells often contiguous with epicardial fat
      - Fat infiltrates interatrial septum and expands it to diameter > 2 cm but spares fossa ovalis, creating dumbbell shape
      - May be hot on FDG PET due to composition of brown fat, which is FDG avid
    - **Mitral annular calcification (MAC)**
      - Calcification of fibrous anulus of mitral valve usually occurs as degenerative change
      - Occurs earlier and is more extensive in renal failure
      - May appear mass-like in some cases, especially if caseous MAC
    - **Sinus of Valsalva aneurysm**
      - Abnormal enlargement of single sinus, usually right (~ 80%)
      - Usually congenital in origin, less commonly due to endocarditis
    - **Membranous septal aneurysm** associated with ventricular septal defect (VSD)
      - Redundant septal tissue arising adjacent to membranous VSD that may appear mass-like
      - May partially occlude VSD
    - **Valvular vegetation**
      - Associated with endocarditis
      - Can erode into valve, leading to regurgitation
  - **Extracardiac lesions**: Less common causes of confusion on imaging
    - Hiatal hernia
    - Large amount of mediastinal or pericardial fat
  - **Thrombus**
    - Actually mass, not pseudomass, but not neoplasm
  - Pseudomasses and thrombi make up ~ 1/3 of cases referred to MR for "cardiac mass"

IMAGING

General Features

- Best diagnostic clue
  - Some of these lesions are incidentally detected in otherwise normal individuals
    - Often, CT or MR imaging requested because of confusing echocardiographic findings

MR Findings

- Crista terminalis usually recognized on cine MR images as being part of RA wall
  - Often best appreciated on 4-chamber or axial view
  - Cine imaging in oblique sagittal plane helpful to demonstrate its vertical orientation along margin of RA
  - Has same signal characteristics as RA wall on all sequences
- Eustachian valve has characteristic location at junction of IVC with RA
  - Best seen on sagittal cine images through RA-IVC junction
  - Signal characteristics same as myocardium
- LHIAS recognized by characteristic fat signal and sparing of fossa ovalis
  - Bright on T1 and T2 with signal dropout on fat-suppressed images
  - Does not enhance with contrast
  - Fat may occasionally extend superiorly along RA wall
- Thrombus
  - Recognized by characteristic intracavitary location
    - Found in LA or atrial appendage in cases of atrial fibrillation or atrial stasis from restrictive cardiomyopathy, particularly amyloid
    - Found in left ventricle (LV) adjacent to infarcts/aneurysms
    - May be seen in RA secondary to central lines
  - May be mobile with adherent stalk (mimicking myxomas)
  - Isointense to myocardium on cine SSFP imaging
    - Differentiates from myxomas, which are higher in signal intensity than myocardium on cine SSFP
  - No contrast uptake on perfusion MR or postcontrast imaging
    - Chronic thrombus can show mild peripheral enhancement

- Typically, low signal on LGE MR with long inversion time (600 ms)
- MAC
  - Low in signal on all imaging sequences
  - Does not enhance
  - Caseous necrosis variant may have high signal on T1 sequences
  - Often predominantly involves posterior leaflet, but entire anulus is involved in more severe cases
- Vegetation
  - Often erodes through valve, leading to regurgitation
  - LGE extends into tissue around vegetation
  - Right-sided vegetations associated with septic emboli
  - Often extends across valve plane
- Miscellaneous/uncommon lesions
  - Sinus of Valsalva aneurysm
    - May contain signal, and, hence, appear solid on black-blood MR due to slow flow
    - May protrude into right ventricle (RV)/RV outflow tract (RVOT)
    - Occasionally complicated by rupture, usually into RV (90%) or RA, resulting in left-to-right shunt
  - Membranous septal aneurysm associated with VSD
    - Often demonstrates mobility on cine MR
    - May have windsock appearance with flow jet visible on cine MR
    - May prolapse through membranous VSD into RV/RVOT
  - Hiatal hernia easily recognized on MR
    - Often indents posterior wall of LA
  - Coumadin ridge
    - Nodular, pedunculated, or linear structure between left superior pulmonary vein and LAA
    - Signal and enhancement, similar to that of LA

CT Findings

- Findings often similar to MR findings, but soft tissue contrast is inferior
  - Crista terminalis and eustachian valve location and morphology as per MR
  - LHIAS recognized by fat attenuation and sparing of fossa ovalis, leading to dumbbell morphology
  - MAC
    - Calcific density easily visualized on CT
      - Rarely undergoes caseous necrosis and may then have lower central density with calcific rim
  - Vegetations
    - In setting of infective endocarditis
    - May see septic emboli in right-sided disease
  - Miscellaneous/uncommon lesions
    - Hiatal hernia easily recognized on CT ± oral contrast
    - Mediastinal or pericardial fat or fluid easily resolved with CT
    - Sinus of Valsalva aneurysm detectable on echocardiography-gated CT

Imaging Recommendations

- Best imaging tool
  - MR or CT usually resolve diagnosis; MR often preferred due to superior soft tissue contrast resolution

DIFFERENTIAL DIAGNOSIS

Varies With Lesion Type

- Crista terminalis may mimic true mass in RA wall, such as angiosarcoma or metastasis
  - Recognized as part of wall, at characteristic location, with no invasive features
- Vegetation may mimic papillary fibroelastoma (PF)
  - PF not usually associated with valvular destruction
  - Diffuse LGE in PF but no LGE in surrounding tissue
  - PF on downstream side of valve
- Eustachian valve may mimic thrombus or IVC extension of intraabdominal tumor, such as renal, adrenal, or hepatocellular carcinoma
  - Recognized as part of RA-IVC junction and not true intraluminal mass
- LHIAS may mimic true neoplasm of fat cells (lipoma)
  - Recognized by characteristic location and sparing of fossa ovalis
- Thrombus may mimic intracavitary masses, such as myxoma
  - T2W: Myxomas usually hyperintense due to gelatinous composition, thrombus low signal
  - LGE MR: Thrombi become darker with longer inversion time (600 ms); myxomas will often have enhancing stalk
- MAC
  - True nature usually evident on CT or MR

CLINICAL ISSUES

Presentation

- Most common signs/symptoms
  - Usually none; patients present for MR or CT imaging to resolve confusing echocardiographic studies
  - Thrombi usually in setting of atrial fibrillation, cardiomyopathy, or postmyocardial infarction

DIAGNOSTIC CHECKLIST

Consider

- Referrals from echocardiography for RA mass may represent pseudomass
- Comprehensive imaging with MR is usually best technique to determine true nature of cardiac mass

Image Interpretation Pearls

- Cine MR imaging useful to localize mass as intramural, epicardial, or intracavitary, significantly narrowing differential diagnoses
- MR perfusion imaging helpful to determine contrast uptake/vascularity of suspected cardiac mass
- LGE MR often useful in tissue characterization of true cardiac masses and in excluding pseudomasses

SELECTED REFERENCES

1. Lorca MC et al: Radiologic-pathologic correlation of cardiac tumors: updated 2021 WHO tumor classification. Radiographics. 44(6):e230126, 2024
2. Shenoy C et al: Cardiovascular magnetic resonance imaging in suspected cardiac tumour: a multicentre outcomes study. Eur Heart J. 43(1):71-80, 2021
3. Tyebally S et al: Cardiac tumors: JACC cardiooncology state-of-the-art review. JACC CardioOncol. 2(2):293-311, 2020

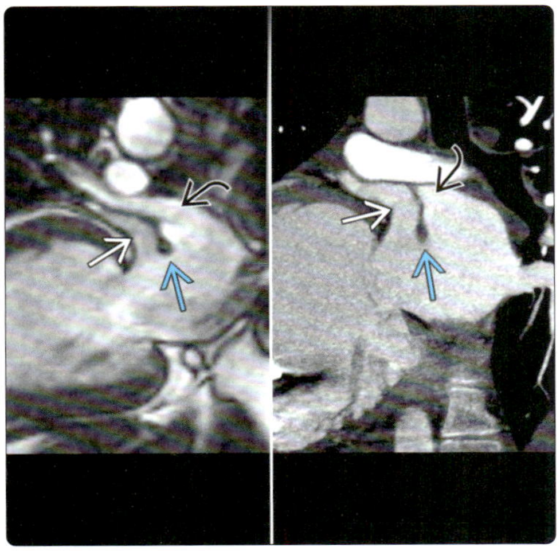

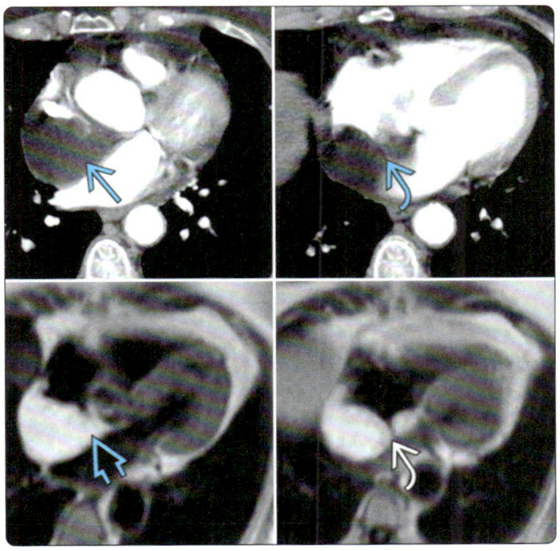

(Left) *Two-chamber cine MR (left) and CTA (right) images demonstrate a "coumadin ridge" seen as a soft tissue structure interposed between the left atrial appendage and the left upper lobe pulmonary vein.* **(Right)** *Axial CT images (top) show a fatty lesion in the interatrial septum, which inferiorly spares the fossa ovalis (FO). T1W MR images (bottom) show the homogeneously bright fatty lesion, which spares the FO. Findings are diagnostic of lipomatous hypertrophy of the interatrial septum.*

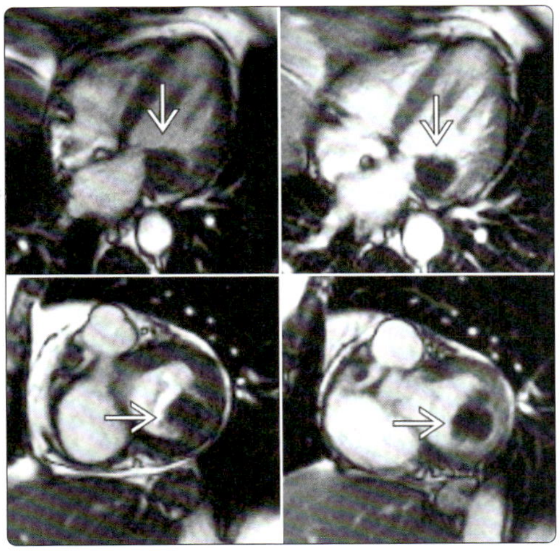

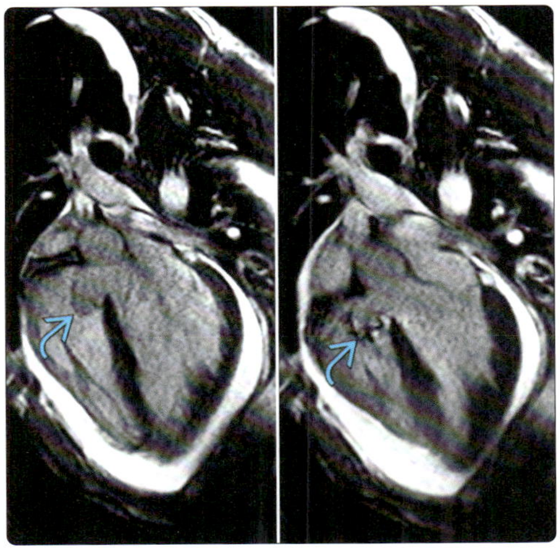

(Left) *Four-chamber (top) and short-axis (bottom) cine MR images show bulky posterior mitral annular calcification. Precontrast images (left) and postcontrast images (right) show no enhancement and uniform low signal.* **(Right)** *Modified 4-chamber SSFP cine MR shows aneurysm of membranous ventricular septum prolapsing from LV to right ventricle (RV) through the associated membranous ventricular septal defect (VSD). Turbulent transseptal flow results in perilesional flow artifacts noted in the systolic image (right).*

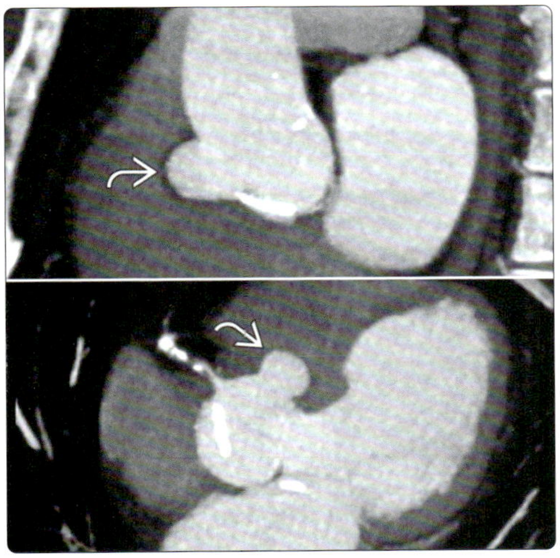

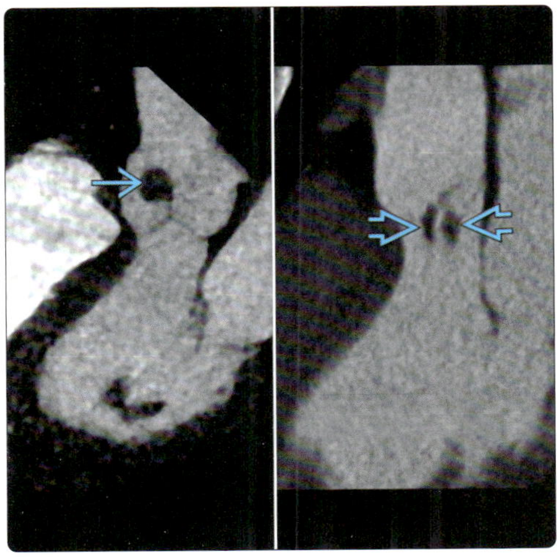

(Left) *Oblique sagittal (top) and axial (bottom) CT images show a right sinus of Valsalva (SOV) aneurysm, which is the most common location for a congenital SOV aneurysm. These can occasionally mimic a mass.* **(Right)** *Papillary fibroelastoma (left) is most commonly on the downstream side of a cardiac valve, is rounded, and does not injure the valve. A vegetation (right) is more commonly irregular in shape, straddles the valve, erodes through the valve causing regurgitation.*

Lipomatous Hypertrophy, Interatrial Septum

KEY FACTS

TERMINOLOGY

- Lipomatous hypertrophy of interatrial septum
- Massive fatty deposits
- Lipomatous hamartoma

IMAGING

- Characteristic dumbbell-shaped lesion sparing fossa ovalis
- Typically, area with greatest fatty deposition will be superior to fossa ovalis
- Characteristic bright T1 signal with signal loss on fat-suppressed sequences
- FDG-PET scan shows focal increased uptake
- Echogenic lesion within interatrial septum

TOP DIFFERENTIAL DIAGNOSES

- Lipoma
- Liposarcoma
- Teratoma
- Myocardial infarction
- Arrhythmogenic right ventricular dysplasia

PATHOLOGY

- No capsule present
- Proliferation of fat cells rather than hypertrophy
- Mature adipose tissue with cells resembling brown fat
- Associated with large amount of epicardial fat and increased body mass index

CLINICAL ISSUES

- Most commonly asymptomatic
- Rare reports of association with supraventricular arrhythmias and sudden death
- May present as obstructive right atrial mass and exertional dyspnea
- Prevalence increases with age

(Left) *Noncontrast cardiac CT shows a fat-density mass in the interatrial septum* ➔*, respecting the fossa ovalis* →*.* **(Right)** *Fused axial images in the same patient show FDG-avid uptake within the fatty mass* ➔ *due to the high metabolic activity of brown fat.*

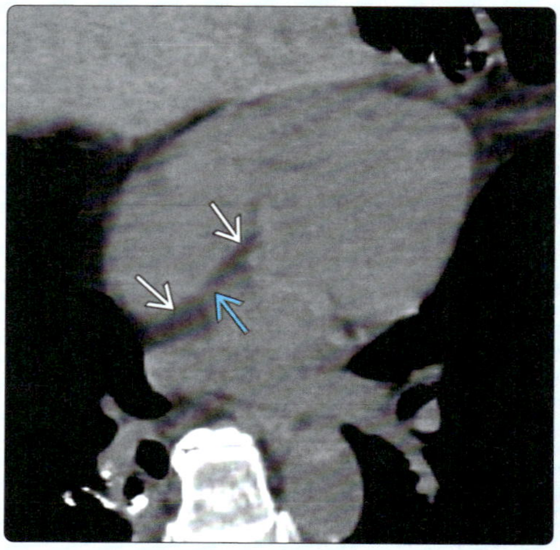

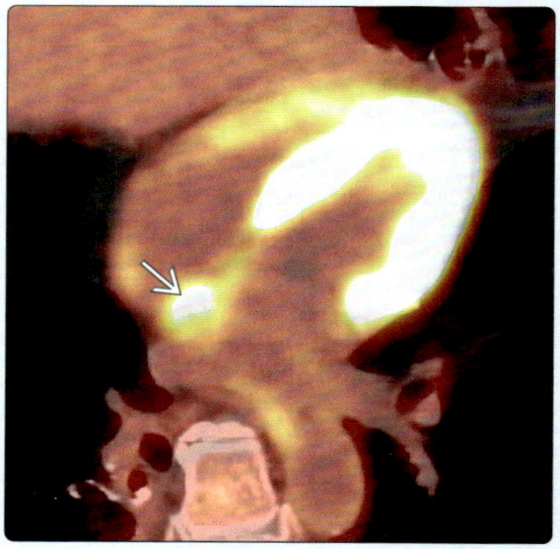

(Left) *Coronal FDG PET performed for oncologic reasons in the same patient demonstrates focal increased uptake within the region of the atria* →*, corresponding to hypermetabolic brown fat activity within the lipomatous hypertrophy of interatrial septum (LHIS).* **(Right)** *Four-chamber SSFP cine MR shows a fatty mass in the interatrial septum* →*, sparing the fossa ovalis.*

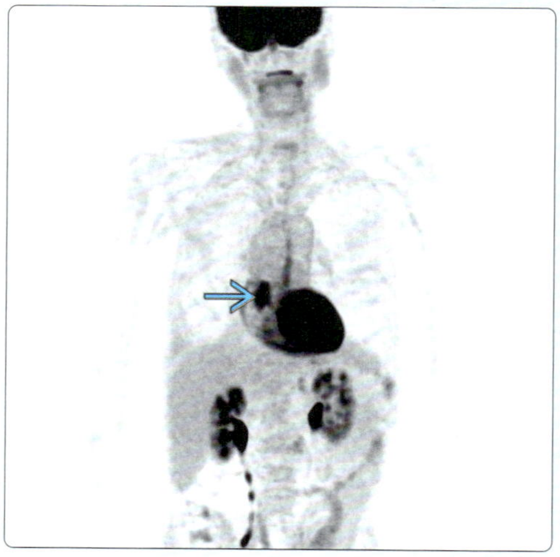

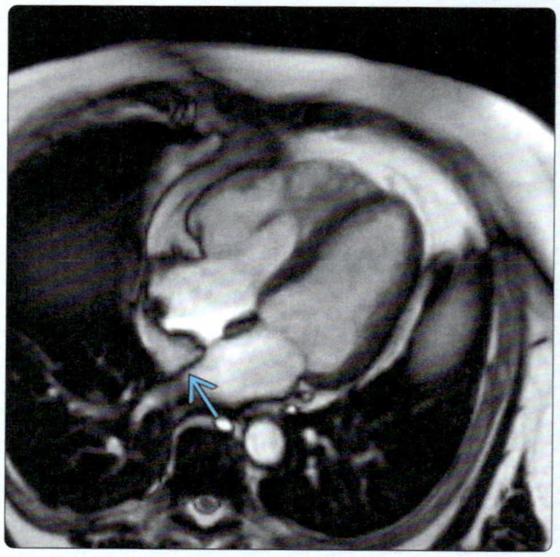

TERMINOLOGY

Abbreviations

- Lipomatous hypertrophy of interatrial septum (LHIS or LHIAS)

Synonyms

- Lipomatous hypertrophy of atrial septum
- Lipomatous hamartoma
- Lipomatous hyperplasia
- Massive fatty deposits

Definitions

- Nonencapsulated, nonneoplastic deposition of excessive amounts of fat within interatrial septum
  - First described in 1964 by JT Prior
- Not true neoplasm

IMAGING

General Features

- Best diagnostic clue
  - Characteristically dumbbell-shaped fatty lesion in atrial septum sparing fossa ovalis
    - Typical appearance is not always present
- Location
  - Within septum secundum
    - Spares fossa ovalis
- Size
  - Typically, 11-28 mm in diameter; can be larger
    - Cutoff values vary by definition
      - Range: ~ 10-15 mm
  - Normal septum is up to 6 mm thick
    - Septum at fossa ovalis is ~ 1 mm thick
  - Amount of fatty deposit increases with age
- Morphology
  - Characteristically, area of greatest amount of fatty deposition will be superior to fossa ovalis
  - 80% demonstrate dumbbell shape or hourglass shape

Imaging Recommendations

- Best imaging tool
  - Incidental finding that usually does not require imaging unless one imaging modality is equivocal, and exclusion of mass is required
    - MR: Black-blood double inversion and triple inversion recovery (IR) FSE sequences
- Protocol advice
  - FSE sequences without fat saturation (hyperintense on double IR) followed by fat saturation (hypointense on triple IR)

Radiographic Findings

- Radiography
  - Chest radiograph does not detect this abnormality

CT Findings

- NECT
  - Low-attenuation (fat) material within otherwise water-density heart in region of atrial septum
  - May also demonstrate increased mediastinal and epicardial fat
- CTA
  - Dumbbell-shaped, fat-density lesion in atrial septum that spares fossa ovalis
  - May be contiguous with epicardial fat
  - Usually incidental diagnosis
  - Multiplanar reconstructions may be helpful to determine caval obstruction

MR Findings

- Double IR FSE
  - Bright signal in T1-weighted sequence
- Triple IR FSE
  - Signal drop in same position in T1-weighted sequence with fat saturation
- Atrial septal location with sparing of fossa ovalis
- Dumbbell shape

Nuclear Medicine Findings

- PET
  - FDG PET shows focal increased FDG uptake
    - Due to metabolically active brown fat
  - Standardized uptake value (SUV) of LHIS ~ 1.6-6.1x > SUV of adjacent blood pool
  - Positive correlation of SUV and thickness of LHIS on CT
  - Image fusion with CT will confirm location during staging and may avoid pitfall of diagnosing metastatic disease

Echocardiographic Findings

- Echogenic lesion within interatrial septum
- Typically echo-dense globular shape with sparing of fossa ovalis
- Often incidental diagnosis that requires no further follow-up
  - Occasionally, findings are equivocal, and further testing (such as MR) may be necessary to exclude cardiac mass

DIFFERENTIAL DIAGNOSIS

Lipoma

- Primary cardiac lipomas are rare
- True lipoma has fibrous capsule whereas lipomatous hypertrophy does not
- Does not have brown fat cells
- Multiple fat deposits or lipomas may be seen in setting of tuberous sclerosis

Liposarcoma

- Rare
- Usually large, filling entire cavity
- Signs of malignancy (e.g., invasion of neighboring structures, mass effect, metastasis)

Teratoma

- Rare
- Demonstrates mass effect
- Not dumbbell-shaped
- May demonstrate fat or lipid collection but also various other tissues (e.g., soft tissue, hair, teeth, bone)

Myocardial Infarction

- Linear fat is within myocardium but not within atrial septum

Arrhythmogenic Right Ventricular Dysplasia

- Fat is typically within right ventricular myocardium
    - Occasionally within left ventricular myocardium
    - Virtually never within atrial septum

Myxoma

- Most common primary cardiac neoplasm
- May be adjacent to fossa ovalis but is usually connected to septum via stalk and is mobile
- Does not have features of fat on either CT or MR

Other Benign Tumors

- Rhabdomyoma
- Fibroma
- Mesothelioma
- Typically no fat-density/signal characteristics

Thrombus

- May adhere to atrial wall
- Will not follow characteristics of fat on either CT or MR

Metastatic Disease

- Usually no fat-density/signal characteristics
- Other cardiac or extracardiac metastatic deposits

PATHOLOGY

General Features

- Etiology
    - Hyperplasia rather than hypertrophy of local fat cells
    - Fat infiltration between myocardial fibers
- Associated abnormalities
    - Associated with large amount of epicardial fat and increased body mass index

Gross Pathologic & Surgical Features

- If resected, will show features characteristic of mass-like fat deposits
    - Constrained by normal structures
- No capsule present

Microscopic Features

- Proliferation of fat cells rather than hypertrophy
- Mature adipose tissue with cells resembling brown fat
- Vacuolated cytoplasm and centrally placed nuclei
- Myocytes are distributed within lesion

CLINICAL ISSUES

Presentation

- Most common signs/symptoms
    - Most commonly asymptomatic
- Other signs/symptoms
    - Rare reports of association with supraventricular arrhythmias and sudden death
    - Syncope
    - May present as obstructive right atrial mass and exertional dyspnea
        - Obstruction of superior vena cava

Demographics

- Age
    - Prevalence increases with age
- Sex
    - No predilection
- Reported prevalence: 1-8%
    - Prevalence of 2.2% on recent prospective CT study
- More common in obese persons

Natural History & Prognosis

- Usually asymptomatic
- Rarely may cause obstructive symptoms that necessitate resection

Treatment

- Usually no treatment is necessary
- Rarely resection of obstructive variants
- May necessitate change in type of transcatheter closure device used for closing concomitant patent foramen ovale or atrial septal defect
    - Amplatzer devices are stiff, and some cannot bridge thickness > 6-7 mm

DIAGNOSTIC CHECKLIST

Consider

- Add fat-saturated T1WI (triple IR FSE) to regular T1WI (double IR FSE) for differentiating from cardiac masses, such as melanoma

Image Interpretation Pearls

- Fat-density material (CT) or signal intensity identical to nearby epicardial fat on all MR pulse sequences in atrial septal location with sparing of fossa ovalis is diagnostic of LHIS

SELECTED REFERENCES

1. Șoşdean R et al: Importance of multimodality cardiac imaging in the diagnosis of lipomatous hypertrophy of the interatrial septum-a view beyond standard situations. Life (Basel). 14(4), 2024
2. Coulier B et al: Lipomatous hypertrophy of interatrial septum causing hot spot on 18FDG PET/CT. Diagn Interv Imaging. 100(3):197-8, 2019
3. Rocha RV et al: Adipose tumors of the heart. J Card Surg. 33(8):432-7, 2018
4. Motwani M et al: MR imaging of cardiac tumors and masses: a review of methods and clinical applications. Radiology. 268(1):26-43, 2013
5. Lee SH et al: Visceral obesity of the heart: extensive lipomatous hypertrophy of interatrial septum. J Cardiovasc Ultrasound. 20(3):161-2, 2012
6. Rigatelli G et al: Anatomo-functional characterization of interatrial septum for catheter-based interventions. Am J Cardiovasc Dis. 1(3):227-35, 2011
7. Pugliatti P et al: Lipomatous hypertrophy of the interatrial septum. Int J Cardiol. 130(2):294-5, 2008
8. Tugcu A et al: Lipomatous hypertrophy of the interatrial septum presenting as an obstructive right atrial mass in a patient with exertional dyspnea. J Am Soc Echocardiogr. 20(11):1319.e3-5, 2007
9. Fan CM et al: Lipomatous hypertrophy of the interatrial septum: increased uptake on FDG PET. AJR Am J Roentgenol. 184(1):339-42, 2005
10. Kuester LB et al: Lipomatous hypertrophy of the interatrial septum: prevalence and features on fusion 18F fluorodeoxyglucose positron emission tomography/CT. Chest. 128(6):3888-93, 2005
11. Heyer CM et al: Lipomatous hypertrophy of the interatrial septum: a prospective study of incidence, imaging findings, and clinical symptoms. Chest. 124(6):2068-73, 2003
12. Iacovoni A et al: [Lipomatous hypertrophy of the interatrial septum: its assessment with TEE, CT and MRI.] G Ital Cardiol. 28(11):1273-7, 1998
13. Meaney JF et al: CT appearance of lipomatous hypertrophy of the interatrial septum. AJR Am J Roentgenol. 168(4):1081-4, 1997
14. Burke AP et al: Lipomatous hypertrophy of the atrial septum presenting as a right atrial mass. Am J Surg Pathol. 20(6):678-85, 1996
15. Shirani J et al: Clinical, electrocardiographic and morphologic features of massive fatty deposits ("lipomatous hypertrophy") in the atrial septum. J Am Coll Cardiol. 22(1):226-38, 1993

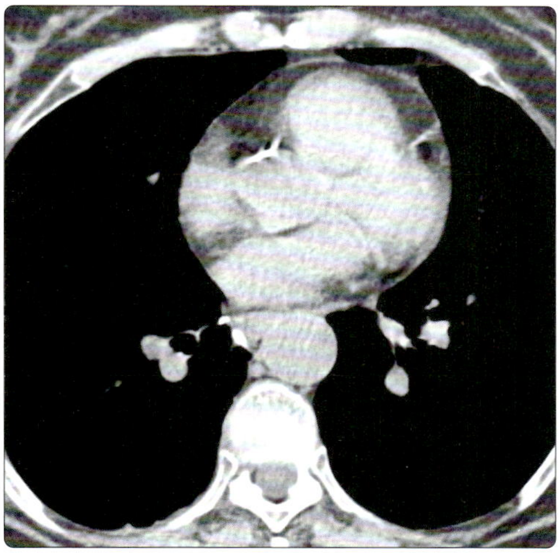

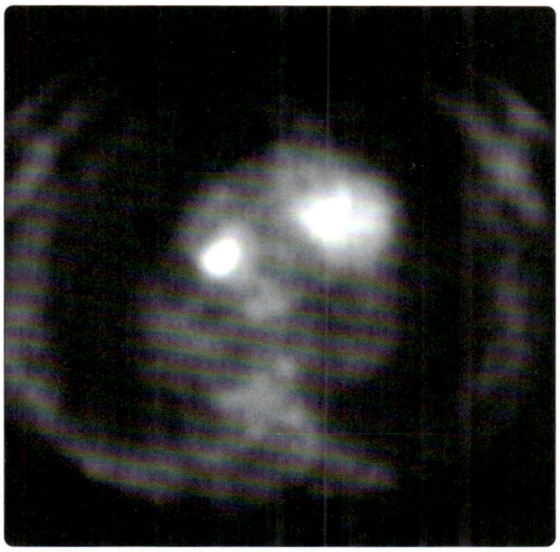

(Left) *Axial MDCT without contrast demonstrates a low-attenuation lesion within the superior aspect of the atrial septum, measuring ~ 15 mm in thickness. Hounsfield units are lower than for blood pool (negative numbers), and attenuation is similar to that of epicardial fat.* **(Right)** *Axial FDG PET in the same patient demonstrates abnormal hypermetabolic activity within the lesions, which is characteristic for lipomatous hypertrophy of the atrial septum. This phenomenon is due to the presence of brown fat.*

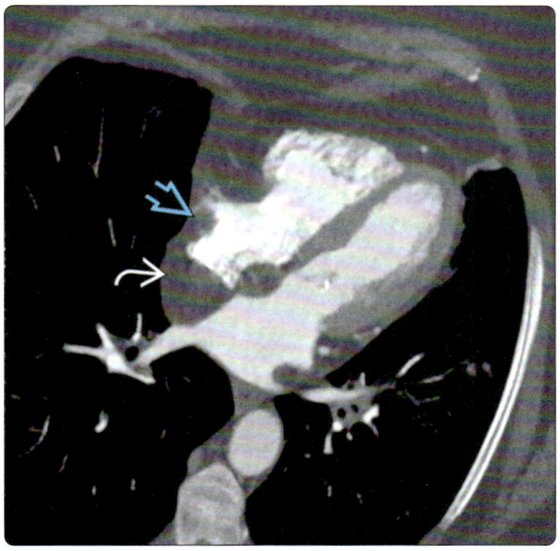

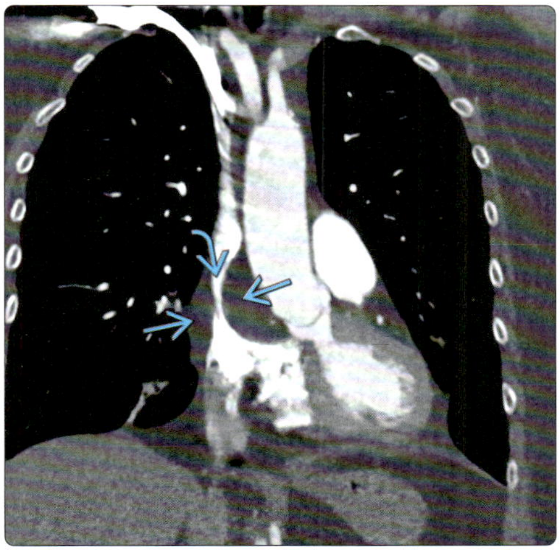

(Left) *Four-chamber cardiac CT shows a fat-density, dumbbell-shaped mass in the interatrial septum extending to the right atrial free wall* ➔*. Note also lipomatous hypertrophy of the crista terminalis* ⇨*.* **(Right)** *Coronal cardiac CT in the same patient shows the fatty mass* → *from the lipomatous hypertrophy of the interatrial septum extending cephalad to the cavoatrial junction and causing narrowing the superior vena cava (SVC)* ⇨*.*

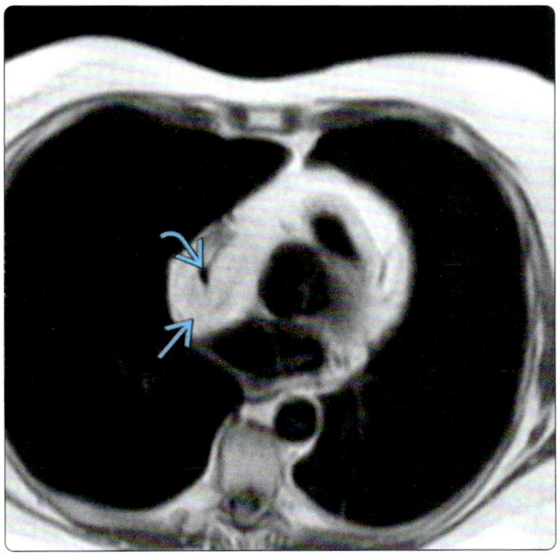

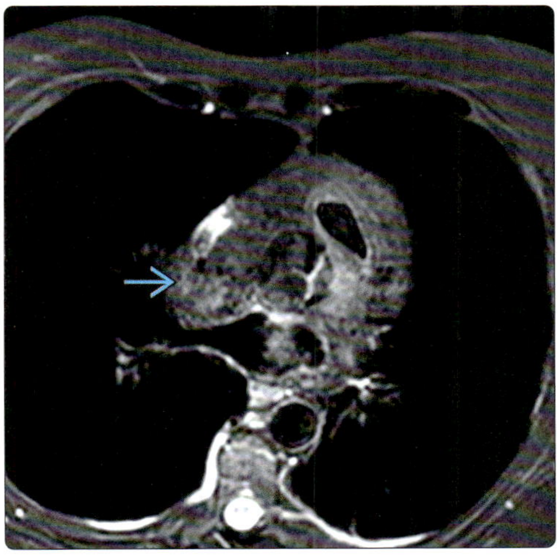

(Left) *Double inversion recovery sequence (black-blood MR) shows the hyperintense mass* → *(similar signal intensity to the subcutaneous fat) in the LHIS, extending to the superior cavoatrial junction and causing narrowing of the SVC* ⇨*.* **(Right)** *Triple inversion recovery sequence (cardiac STIR MR) in the same patient shows suppression of the signal intensity of the mass (hypointense), which is characteristic of a fatty mass* →*.*

Cardiac Thrombus

KEY FACTS

TERMINOLOGY

- Clot within cardiac chamber typically resulting from flow disturbance or akinetic or dyskinetic wall due to prior infarct/aneurysm or cardiomyopathy

IMAGING

- Intraluminal filling defect
- Nonenhancing mural rim of tissue lining infarction
- Underlying infarct may be evident from myocardial thinning, linear myocardial calcification, linear subendocardial fatty metaplasia, aneurysm, or wall motion abnormality
- Left ventricular mural thrombus in 40-60% of patients with anterior myocardial infarction if no anticoagulant therapy
- Thrombus is usually 35-50 HU, whereas remote normal myocardium is 80-100 HU
- Left atrium thrombus is common in atrial fibrillation and mitral stenosis
- May demonstrate calcification if old thrombus
- LGE technique is highly sensitive for detecting intracardiac thrombus
- If thrombus is suspected, long inversion time (TI = 600 ms at 1.5T and 875 ms at 3T) has been shown to be most decisive
- Cardiac MR is best imaging technique
- Chronic vascularized thrombus may show some enhancement

PATHOLOGY

- Thrombus is most frequent intracardiac mass
- Central layers: Fibroblasts, macrophages
  - May be organized
- Superficial layers: Fibrin, platelets, and red blood cells

CLINICAL ISSUES

- Left chambers: Stroke, systemic emboli
- Right chambers: Pulmonary emboli

(Left) *Three-chamber LGE MR shows a large anteroapical left anterior descending territory transmural left ventricle (LV) infarct ⇨ with aneurysm formation and a broadly attached signal void mass ➡ within the lumen, consistent with LV thrombus.* **(Right)** *Short-axis LGE MR in the same patient shows the transmural abnormal LGE ⇨ and thinning of the myocardium, which indicate remote infarct. Nonenhancing, broadly attached thrombus ➡ along the anterior septum is present. Matching dyskinesia was evident on cine images.*

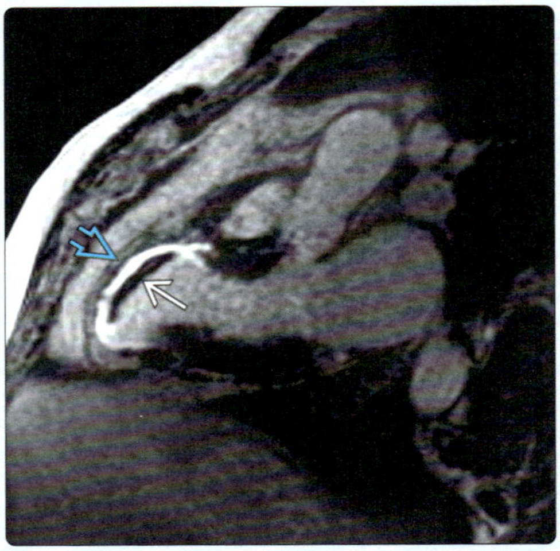

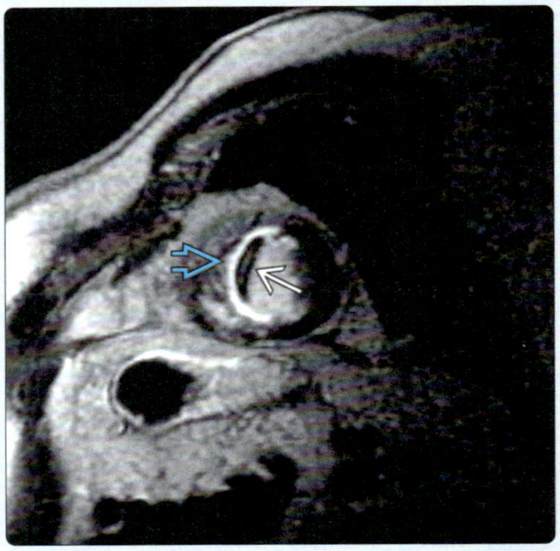

(Left) *Axial 4-chamber CECT shows enlargement and apical low-attenuation LV filling defect, consistent with LV thrombus ➡ in nonischemic cardiomyopathy. Note normal papillary muscle ⮥ and normal-thickness LV wall without fatty metaplasia or calcification.* **(Right)** *Axial CECT in a patient with cardiomyopathy shows a well-circumscribed, low-attenuation filling defect within dilated right atrial appendage ➡. Note small right and moderate left pleural effusions and left basilar atelectasis.*

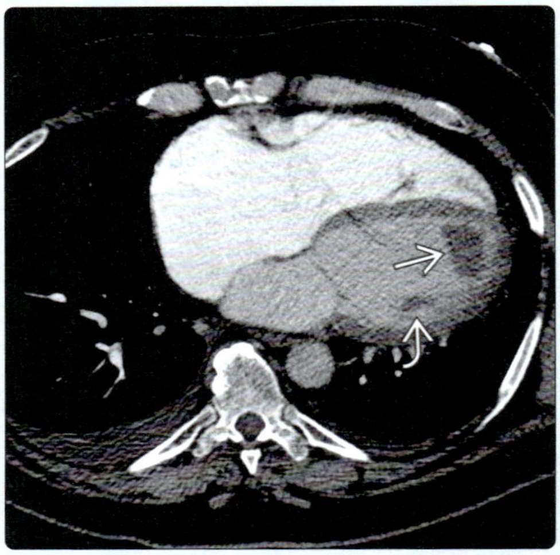

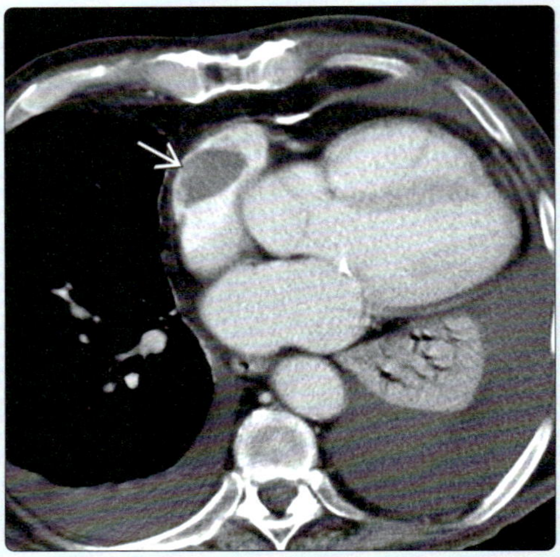

TERMINOLOGY

Definitions

- Clot formation within cardiac chamber, typically from flow disturbance or akinetic or dyskinetic wall due to prior infarct/aneurysm or cardiomyopathy; abnormal endothelium may contribute

IMAGING

General Features

- Best diagnostic clue
  - Intraluminal filling defect
    - In setting of infarct or dilated hypokinetic myopathic ventricle or atrium
  - Nonenhancing mural rim of tissue lining infarction
- Location
  - Left ventricle (LV) mural thrombus in 40-60% of patients with anterior myocardial infarction if no anticoagulant therapy
  - Left atrium (LA) thrombus often in setting of atrial fibrillation and mitral stenosis
  - May occur in any chamber
- Morphology
  - Broad-based lining of akinetic wall if due to LV infarct/aneurysm
  - May be ovoid or lobular intraluminal mass or filling defect
    - May be pedunculated with connection to wall
    - Could be mobile

CT Findings

- NECT
  - May demonstrate calcification if old thrombus
- CECT
  - Filling defect and underlying signs of LV infarction
  - Mural thrombus may mimic wall of normal thickness
    - Look for signs of infarction (calcium or fatty metaplasia)
    - Thrombus appears slightly lower in attenuation compared to remote normal myocardium
      - Thrombus 35-50 HU; remote: 80-100 HU
- Cardiac gated CTA
  - May demonstrate mobility of pedunculated thrombi
  - Wall motion abnormality in underlying myocardium
  - Underlying chronic infarction, aneurysm, or pseudoaneurysm may be seen
    - Laminated mural thrombus may be subtle finding
- Dual-energy CT
  - Absence of significant iodine uptake in cardiac soft tissue mass is consistent with thrombus
    - < 1.7 mg/mL has high specificity and sensitivity in rapid kVp-switching technology

MR Findings

- T1WI
  - Iso- or hypointense relative to myocardium (old thrombus)
  - Hyperintense in subacute thrombus due to methemoglobin
- T2WI
  - Iso- or hypointense relative to myocardium (old thrombus)
  - Hypointense in subacute thrombus due to methemoglobin
- T2WI FS
  - Iso- or hypointense relative to myocardium (old thrombus)
- SSFP cine
  - Iso- or hypointense relative to myocardium (old thrombus)
  - Underlying wall motion abnormality can be evaluated
  - Valvular lesions can be evaluated
- Dynamic 1st-pass perfusion
  - No enhancement
- LGE
  - No contrast enhancement
    - Long inversion time (TI = 600 ms); has been shown to be most decisive
      - Chronic vascularized thrombus may show some enhancement
  - LGE may be seen in adjacent myocardium due to infarct
    - Subendocardial or transmural
- Parametric mapping techniques
  - Intermediate values in native T1 mapping
- General
  - Typically, thrombus has homogeneous signal
    - Heterogeneous signal with calcification
    - Occasionally thrombus may be layered on underlying neoplasm, resulting in heterogeneous signal and enhancement
  - Reduces in size after anticoagulation

Echocardiographic Findings

- Echocardiogram
  - 1st-line technique for ventricular thrombus
    - 70-80% sensitive; 90-95% specific
  - Ventricular thrombi are usually anterior and apical
  - May be laminar and adherent to wall or pedunculated and mobile echogenic masses in areas of hypokinesis
  - Criteria for increased risk of embolization
    - Increased mobility, protrusion into ventricular chamber
    - Visualization in multiple views
    - Contiguous zones of akinesis and hyperkinesis
  - Experimental use of antifibrinogen-labeled echogenic immunoliposomes for thrombus-specific enhancement of echogenicity

Angiographic Findings

- Conventional
  - Filling defect may be free floating (atrial thrombus ball)
  - May be negative if thrombus is broadly adherent to wall
    - Only hint may be presence of wall motion abnormality on ventriculography

Imaging Recommendations

- Best imaging tool
  - Cardiac MR

Image-Guided Biopsy

- Biopsy performed to differentiate neoplasm from benign thrombus may be false-negative for neoplasm if mass is covered with reactive thrombus

DIFFERENTIAL DIAGNOSIS

Neoplasms

- Benign or malignant lesions
- Malignant lesion: Invades atrial or ventricular wall; involves multiple chambers; irregular margins; pericardial effusion may be present
- Typically show contrast enhancement

Pseudothrombus Due to Mixing Artifacts

- Seen as filling defect, typically in LA appendage
- Higher attenuation than thrombus, > 80 HU
- Attenuation in LA appendage/ascending aorta > 0.25
- Delayed-phase CT: Artifact disappears, whereas thrombus remains
- Dual-energy CT: Iodine > 1.74 mg/mL

Normal Anatomic Structures

- Crista terminalis, tenia sagittalis, coumadin ridge, Eustachian valve, papillary muscles, moderator band, etc., may be confused with thrombus
- Normal structures show same signal and contrast enhancement as normal myocardium

Valve Vegetations

- Sick patient
- Irregular mass attached to valve
- May show contrast enhancement

PATHOLOGY

General Features

- Etiology
  - Right atrium thrombus
    - Low cardiac output state
    - Atrial fibrillation
    - Central catheters or pacemaker wires, transvenous ablation procedures
    - Embolic thrombus from deep venous thrombosis or extension of tumor-thrombus from kidney, liver, or adrenal glands
    - Rheumatic tricuspid stenosis, heart surgery, cardiomyopathy, or extension of tumor-thrombus from kidney, liver, or adrenal glands
    - Heart surgery
    - Cardiomyopathy
  - Right ventricle thrombus
    - Rare; same as right atrium thrombus
  - LA thrombus
    - Atrial fibrillation is most common
    - Mitral stenosis
    - LA appendage is most common site
  - LV thrombus
    - Myocardial infarction, LV aneurysm
    - Sequela of nonischemic cardiomyopathy
    - Sequela of chemotherapy or toxins (e.g., carbon monoxide)
    - Paraneoplastic syndrome
- Most frequent intracardiac mass

Gross Pathologic & Surgical Features

- Freshly thrombosed blood at surface
- May have organized thrombus in deep layers

Microscopic Features

- May be layered and adherent to myocardium
- Central layers: May be organized
  - Fibroblasts
  - Macrophages
- Superficial layers: Fibrin, platelets, and red blood cells

CLINICAL ISSUES

Presentation

- Symptoms of underlying condition
  - Most frequently myocardial infarction
    - Ventricular aneurysm
  - Cardiomyopathy
- May be asymptomatic until complication occurs
- Left chambers: Stroke, peripheral emboli
  - 10% of mural LV thrombi result in systemic emboli
- Right chambers: Pulmonary emboli

Demographics

- Age
  - Parallels myocardial infarction as most common underlying cause

Natural History & Prognosis

- Mural thrombus formation within 48-72 hours postmyocardial infarction carries poor prognosis from associated complications
- Found in 30-40% of anterior myocardial infarction but in < 5% of inferior myocardial infarction

Treatment

- Anticoagulation for 3-6 months with warfarin
  - Observational studies suggest some benefit in prevention of thromboembolism
- Aspirin may prevent further platelet deposition
- Percutaneous LA appendage transcatheter occlusion in high-risk patients with atrial fibrillation to prevent stroke

DIAGNOSTIC CHECKLIST

Consider

- If presumed thrombus does not resolve with anticoagulation, consider differential diagnoses

Protocol Advice

- Perform LGE at long TI (600 ms) to diagnose thrombus

SELECTED REFERENCES

1. Jenista ER et al: Revisiting how we perform late gadolinium enhancement CMR: insights gleaned over 25 years of clinical practice. J Cardiovasc Magn Reson. 25(1):18, 2023
2. Chaosuwannakit N et al: Left ventricular thrombi: insights from cardiac magnetic resonance imaging. Tomography. 7(2):180-8, 2021
3. Pazos-López P et al: Value of CMR for the differential diagnosis of cardiac masses. JACC Cardiovasc Imaging. 7(9):896-905, 2014

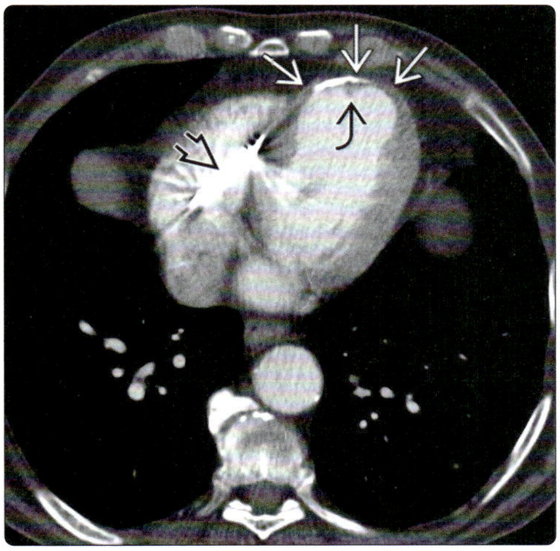

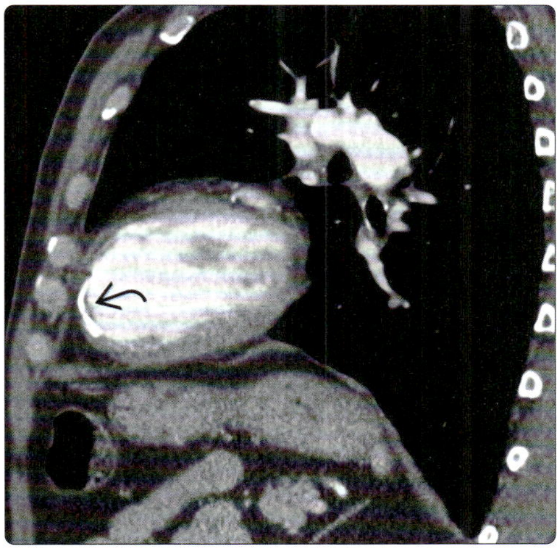

(Left) *Axial CECT shows an artifact from an implantable cardioverter-defibrillator in the right ventricle and thinning of the LV apical wall, linear calcification, and a small soft tissue density just inside the calcification, typical of remote myocardial infarction with luminal thrombus formation.* **(Right)** *Sagittal CECT in the same patient shows wall thinning and calcification with a suggestion of an LV aneurysm. Note the thin, low-density rim lining the infarct, which indicates a thrombus.*

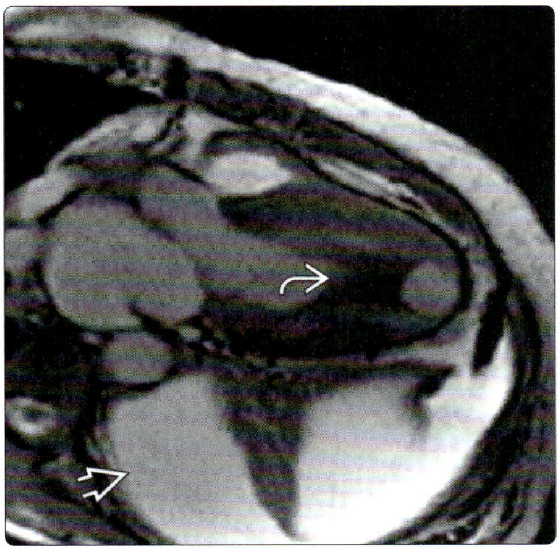

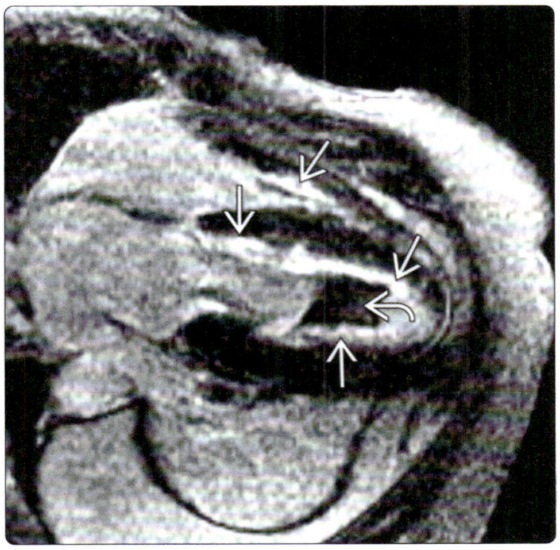

(Left) *Three-chamber SSFP cine MR shows a low-signal thrombus adherent to the mid anteroseptal and inferolateral walls, which correspond to different coronary territories. Note the large left pleural effusion.* **(Right)** *Four-chamber LGE MR in the same patient shows diffuse left and right ventricular subendocardial delayed hyperenhancement spanning all coronary territories and a nonenhancing ventricular thrombus in a patient with Loeffler endocarditis.*

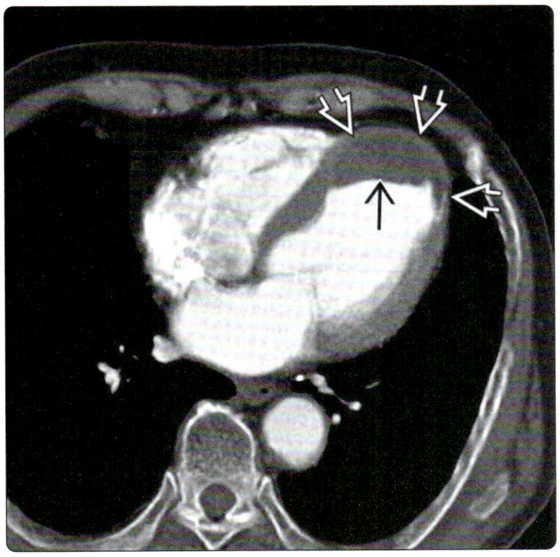

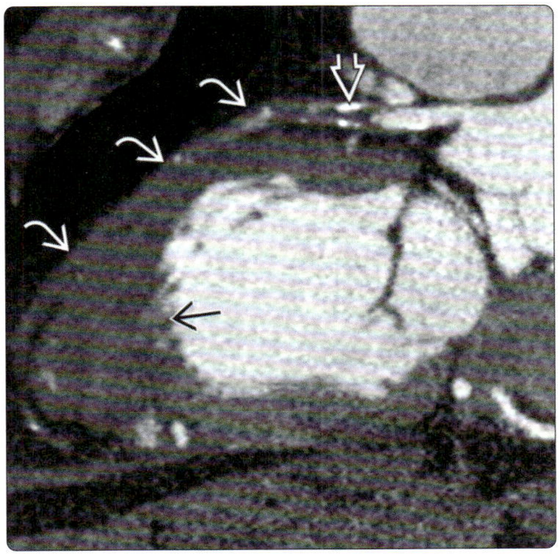

(Left) *Axial CECT shows a thinned rim of apical myocardium with an aneurysm that is difficult to separate from the thrombus, which is of only slightly lower attenuation.* **(Right)** *Oblique cardiac CT 5 hours after onset of chest pain shows complete nonfilling of the LAD coronary artery due to acute proximal plaque rupture or occlusion. Note apical LV filling defect.*

(Left) *LGE 2-chamber view shows transmural enhancement and thinning in the apical segments ➲, indicating old infarct. Myocardial nulling ➲ is seen at TI of 265 ms, and a 1.5-cm nonenhancing mass in the apex ➔ appears dark on PSIR imaging.* **(Right)** *The same patient with TI of 600 ms shows infarction ➲, normal myocardium ➲, and thrombus ➔. Thrombi persistently appear black against gray or bright normal and infarcted structures. Best diagnostic clue: Persistent darkness on high TI LGE acquisition.*

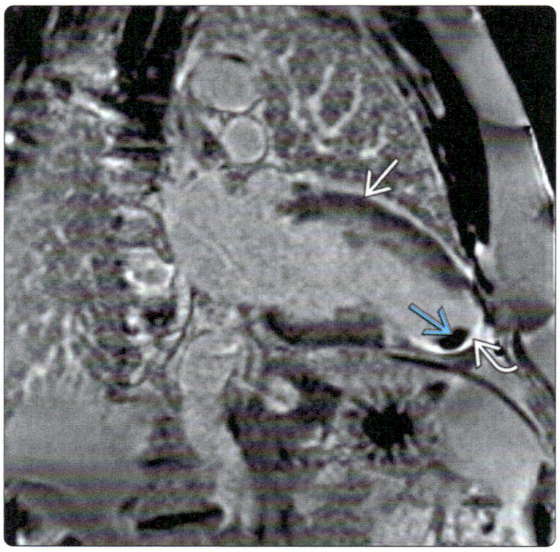

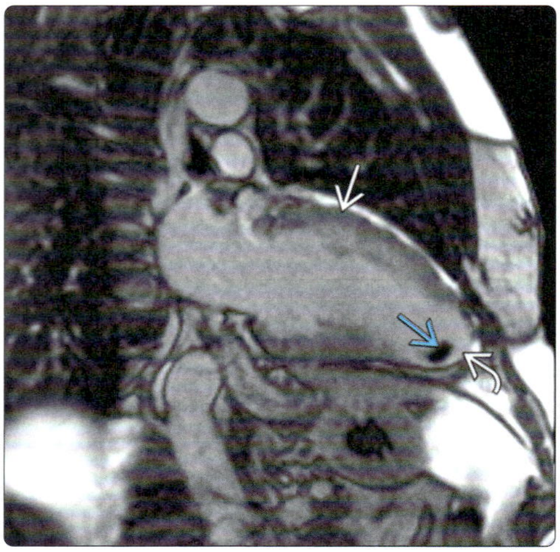

(Left) *Cardiac CECT for transcatheter aortic valve replacement (TAVR) assessment reveals a large filling defect with hypodensity in the left atrial appendage ➲.* **(Right)** *The same patient with a subsequent flash scan of the entire aorta, typically performed immediately after the cardiac exam, shows complete opacification of the left atrial appendage, consistent with mixing artifact ➲. This highlights the importance of delayed-phase imaging in distinguishing between mixing artifact and thrombus.*

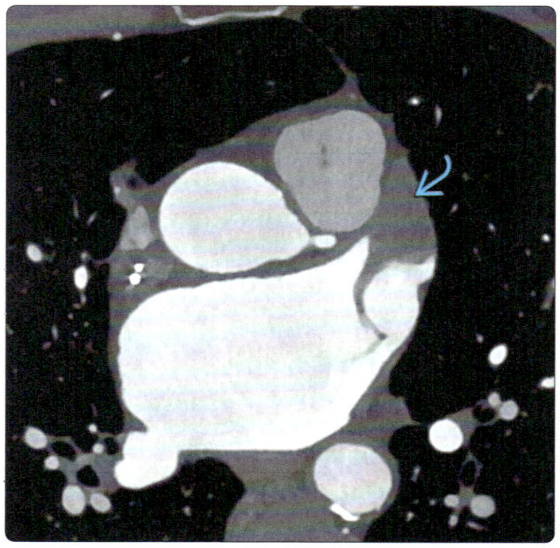

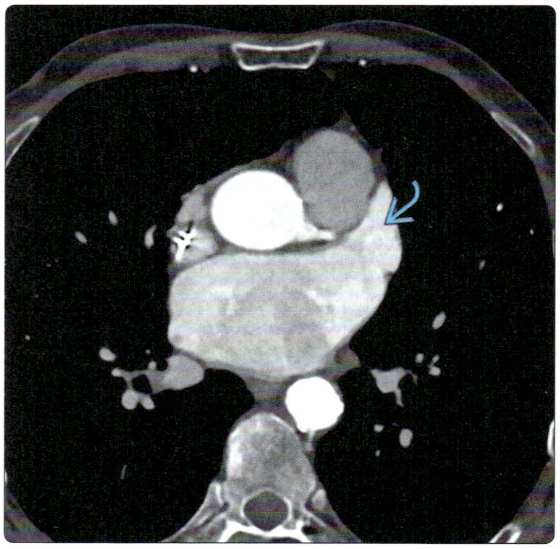

(Left) *Chest CECT shows a hypodense, ovoid area in the apical left ventricle ➲, which could represent a slow mixing of contrast due to the early pulmonary arterial phase, although thrombus cannot be excluded based on this image.* **(Right)** *Subsequent abdomen CTA with a later contrast phase demonstrates optimal filling ➲ of the apical LV, confirming the absence of a thrombus.*

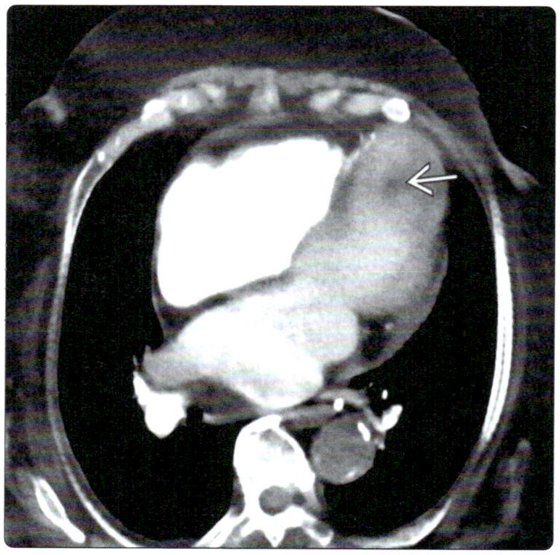

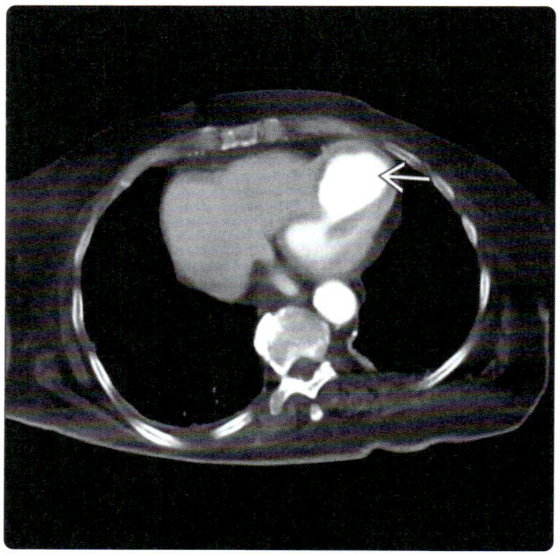

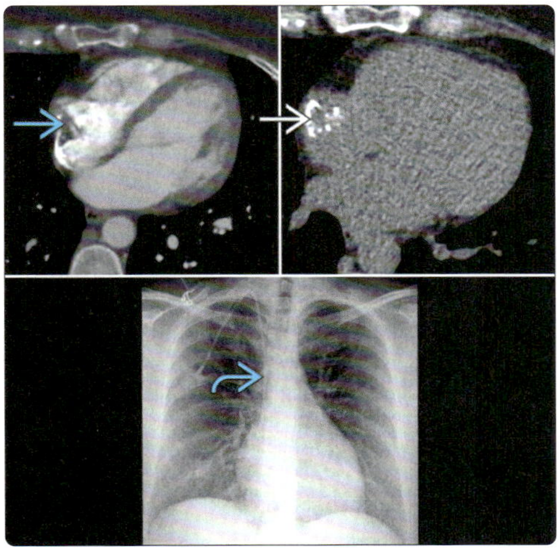

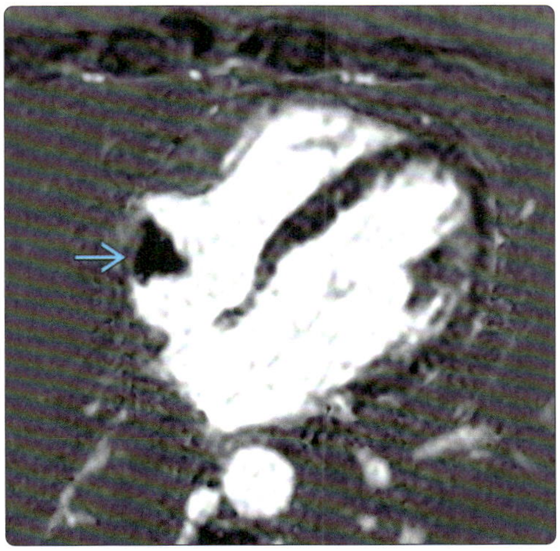

(Left) *Chest x-ray, NECT, and CECT of the chest reveal a mediport catheter with associated calcified mass in the right atrium, appearing relatively hypodense on the CECT.* **(Right)** *Four-chamber LGE MR in the same patient shows a nonenhancing mass attached to the right ventricle free wall, with no early perfusion and appearing dark on long TI (not shown), consistent with an RA thrombus associated with a central catheter.*

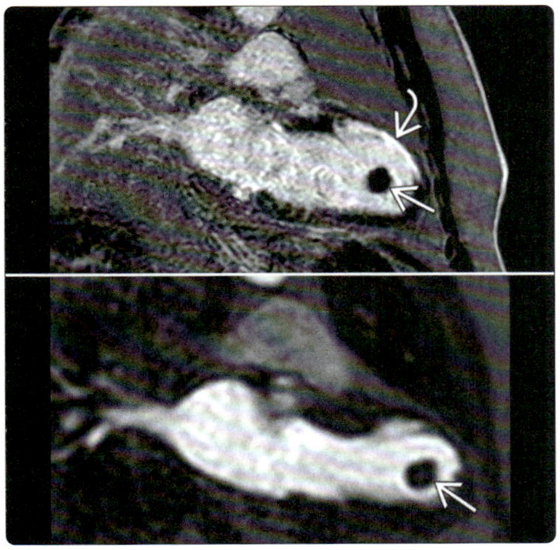

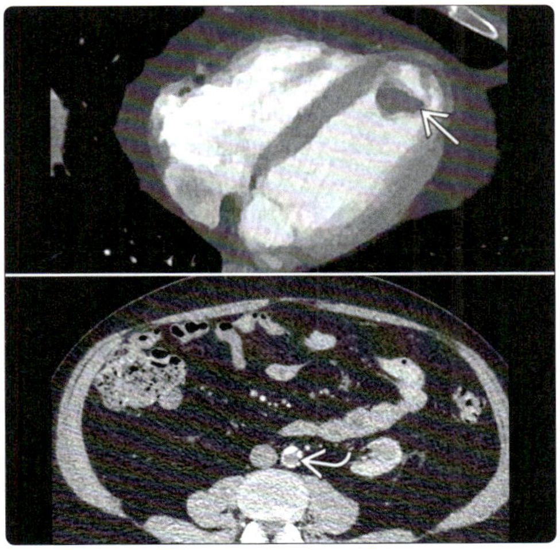

(Left) *Early perfusion and late gadolinium images reveal a nonenhancing cardiac thrombus in the mid to apical left ventricle, with subendocardial to transmural enhancement in the anterior LV wall. The thrombus was mobile on cine images (not shown) and was attached to the wall by fine trabeculations.* **(Right)** *The patient later presented with acute lower limb ischemia due to thrombus in lower aorta. The cardiac thrombus was highly mobile on cardiac MR, posing a significant risk of dislodgement.*

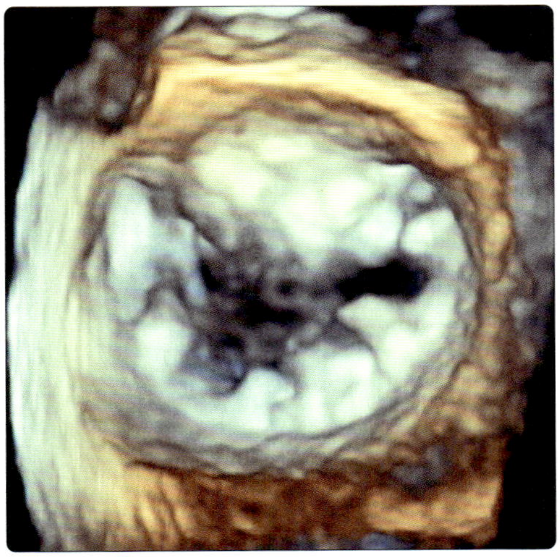

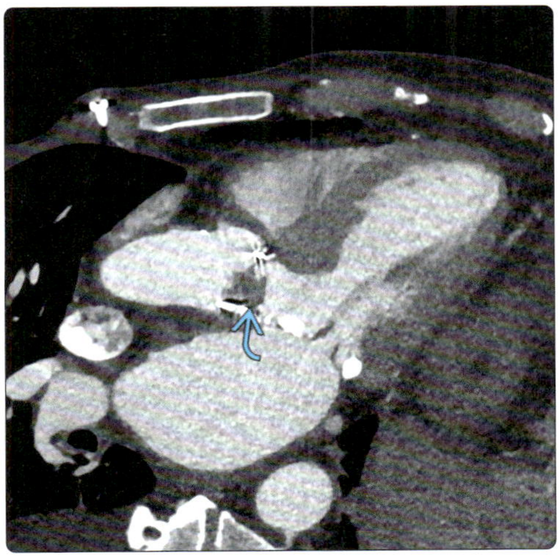

(Left) *3D echocardiography of the aortic valve in end-systole reveals severe thickening of the leaflets, indicating significant aortic stenosis.* **(Right)** *Three-chamber cardiac CT reveals a lobulated hypodensity beneath the aortic bioprosthetic valve in an afebrile patient, noncompliant with blood thinners. The hypodensity, typically facing the LV outflow tract, is suggestive of a thrombus.*

Cystic Tumor of Atrioventricular Node

KEY FACTS

TERMINOLOGY

- Benign congenital mass located in triangle of Koch along atrial septum near atrioventricular (AV) node

IMAGING

- 2-mm to 3-cm rounded cystic lesion along interatrial septum in region of AV node
- Internal characteristics will vary based on fluid composition
  - Variable homogeneous attenuation on CT ranging from hypodense to hyperdense
  - T1WI, T2WI, and SSFP will range from homogeneously low signal to high signal
- Delayed enhancement sequences most commonly show no LGE
- Homogeneous anechoic to hyperechoic mass in expected location in echo
- Can be associated with other midline defects in 10% of cases

TOP DIFFERENTIAL DIAGNOSES

- Lipomatous hypertrophy of interatrial septum
- Lipoma
- Atrial myxoma
- Metastasis

PATHOLOGY

- Endodermal congenital abnormality rather than true tumor
- Composed of cysts, ducts, and solid nests of cells
- Multicystic mass in region of AV node

CLINICAL ISSUES

- Given its location near AV node, can lead to arrhythmia (complete heart block or partial AV block)
  - Most common tumor to cause sudden cardiac death
- More common in women (3:1)
- Surgical excision is preferred treatment

(Left) *Four-chamber chest CECT reconstruction in a 63-year-old woman with hepatic cirrhosis who presented to the ED after experiencing a life-threatening arrhythmia shows a hypoattenuation mass in the anterior aspect of the interatrial septum in the expected location of the atrioventricular (AV) node. The mass has an attenuation of 21 HU.* **(Right)** *Four-chamber echocardiogram (left) and SSFP cardiac MR (right) in the same patient shows that the mass is anechoic on echo and homogeneously high signal on SSFP.*

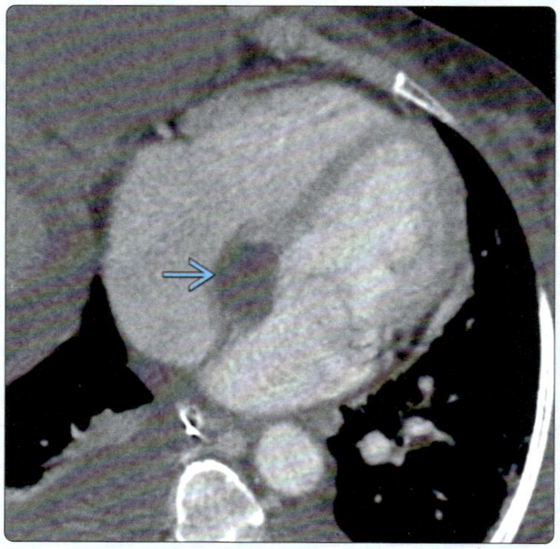

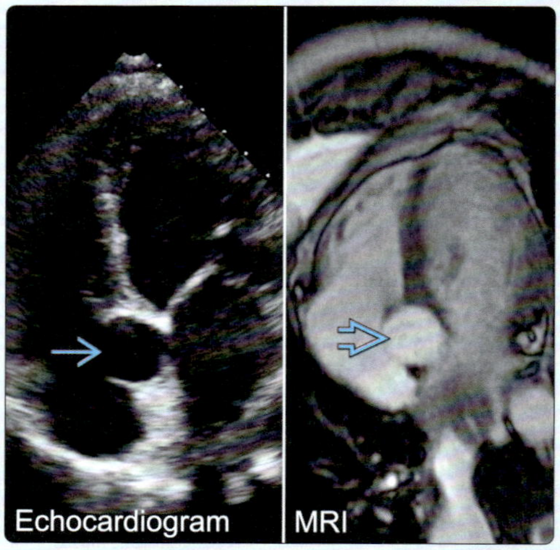

(Left) *T1W TSE (left), T2W TSE (center), and T2 STIR (right) images through the mass in the same patient show relatively homogeneous low signal and high signal on the T1W and T2W sequences, respectively.* **(Right)** *MR perfusion in the same patient shows no evidence of 1st-pass enhancement in the mass. There is no evidence of LGE on magnitude imaging with a TI of 300 msec or 600 msec. Lower signal on the longer 600-msec TI sequence suggests the mass is composed of material with a long T1 relaxation, such as fluid.*

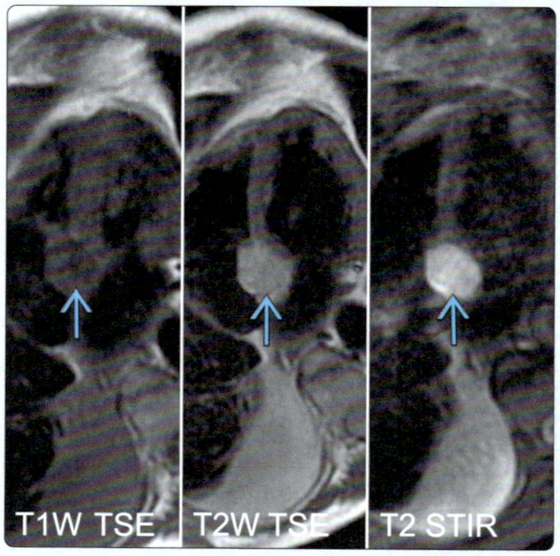

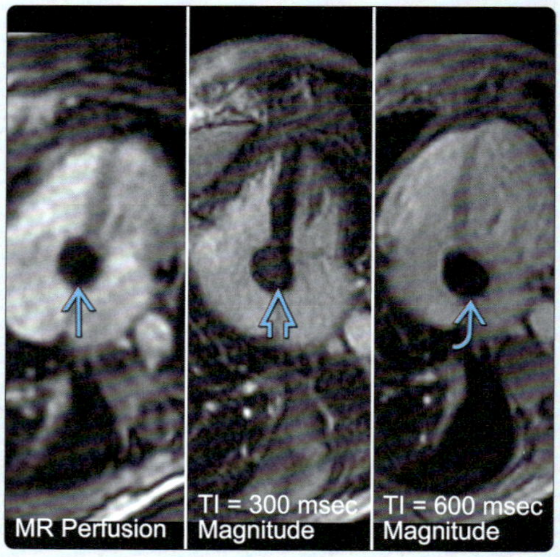

TERMINOLOGY

Abbreviations

- Cystic tumor of atrioventricular node (CTAVN)

Synonyms

- Mesothelioma of atrioventricular (AV) node
  - Older, incorrect term as it does not have mesothelial origin

Definitions

- Benign congenital mass located in triangle of Koch along atrial septum near AV node

IMAGING

General Features

- Best diagnostic clue
  - Cystic lesion along interatrial septum in region of AV node
- Location
  - Interatrial septum near expected location of AV node
  - Often within triangle of Koch
    - Located in paraseptal endocardium of right atrium
    - Borders
      - Anterior: Septal leaflet of tricuspid valve
      - Posterior: Tendon of Todaro (fibrous extension from eustachian ridge)
      - Inferior: Ostium of coronary sinus
      - These structures form triangle with superior point being central fibrous body of heart
      - AV node located just inferior to central fibrous body within superior aspect of Koch triangle
    - Important landmark for electrophysiology procedures given location of AV node
- Size
  - 2 mm to 3 cm
- Morphology
  - Benign, round, cystic lesion localized to region of AV node

Radiographic Findings

- Not visible on radiography

CT Findings

- Round, cystic lesion along anterior aspect of interatrial septum localized to region of AV node
- Variable homogeneous attenuation ranging from hypodense to hyperdense
- Variable enhancement reported in literature
  - No enhancement to homogeneous internal enhancement
- Can be associated with other midline defects in 10% of cases
  - Complex congenital heart disease, septal defects, thyroglossal duct cyst, omphalocele, etc.

MR Findings

- Round lesion along interatrial septum localized to region of AV node
- Internal characteristics will vary depending on internal fluid composition
  - T1WI: Range from homogeneously low signal to high signal
  - T2WI: Range from homogeneous high signal to low signal
  - SSFP: Usually homogeneous high signal but can be isointense to hypointense
- Perfusion ranges from no perfusion to slow internal perfusion
- T1WI postcontrast findings varied based on case reports
  - No enhancement
  - Enhancement of rim of cyst
  - Diffuse homogeneous enhancement
- Delayed enhancement sequences most commonly show no LGE
  - Some case reports mention diffuse enhancement on LGE
  - Internal signal characteristics can be variable depending on internal fluid composition, inversion time (TI), and whether magnitude or phase-sensitive inversion recovery sequences are used
- Can be associated with other midline defects in 10% of cases
  - Complex congenital heart disease, septal defects, thyroglossal duct cyst, omphalocele, etc.

Echocardiographic Findings

- Homogeneous, anechoic to hyperechoic mass in interatrial septum near expected location of AV node

Imaging Recommendations

- Best imaging tool
  - Cardiac MR
  - Cardiac CT can help localize lesion
- Protocol advice
  - MR with standard cardiac mass protocol
    - Cine SSFP imaging through standard planes as well as through mass in multiple planes
    - T1W, T1W + fat saturation, T2W, and T2W + fat-saturation images through mass
    - 1st-pass perfusion through mass
      - Consider running perfusion for at least 60 sec to assess for slow internal perfusion
    - T1W postcontrast imaging through mass
    - LGE through myocardium and mass
      - Recommend using TI for standard myocardial nulling as well as long TI near 600 msec
      - Consider performing TI scout through mass

DIFFERENTIAL DIAGNOSIS

Lipomatous Hypertrophy of Interatrial Septum

- Fat attenuation on CT and all MR sequences
- Conspicuously spares fossa ovalis, which may lead to dumbbell shape

Lipoma

- Septal lipomas are rare, especially in this specific location
- Fat attenuation on CT and all MR sequences

Atrial Myxoma

- Atrial mass usually localized to region of fossa ovalis when in left atrium with more variable locations in right atrium

- Myxoma is not centered within atrial septum in region of AV node
  - However, in some instances, it can be difficult to localize cystic tumor of AV node to atrial septum due to its thinness
- Myxoma unlikely to have typical cystic appearance on MR
  - Reports of myxoma mimicking cyst are primarily based on case reports with echocardiographic imaging

Metastasis

- Rare for isolated metastases to atrial septum in this specific location
- Not expected to be homogeneous in attenuation and signal on CT and MR sequences, respectively

PATHOLOGY

General Features

- Rare choristomatous lesions composed of ectopic glands of endodermal origin
  - Endodermal congenital abnormality rather than true tumor
  - Arises from foregut endodermal rests
- Originates during embryogenesis of heart
  - AV nodal region is area of embryonic fusion where these ectopic glands can become trapped
- Associated with midline defects in 10% of cases

Gross Pathologic & Surgical Features

- Multicystic mass in region of AV node

Microscopic Features

- Composed of cysts, ducts, and solid nests of cells
  - Benign cysts lined by flattened cuboidal or squamous epithelium

CLINICAL ISSUES

Presentation

- Most common signs/symptoms
  - Given its location to AV node, can lead to arrhythmia (complete heart block or partial AV block)
    - Smallest tumor known to cause sudden cardiac death
- Other signs/symptoms
  - Can be asymptomatic or incidental finding on autopsy

Demographics

- Age
  - Congenital lesion that can be seen from birth, with oldest reported age of 89 years
- Sex
  - More common in women (3:1)

Natural History & Prognosis

- Benign congenital lesion
- Can be incidental finding that is asymptomatic
- May cause heart block, other arrhythmia, and sudden cardiac death
  - Ventricular tachycardia and ventricular fibrillation may be fatal, even in presence of pacemaker
- No longitudinal studies available to assess for changes in size and imaging characteristics

Treatment

- Surgical excision is preferred treatment
- Pacemaker does not prevent sudden cardiac death

DIAGNOSTIC CHECKLIST

Consider

- Consider cystic tumor of AV node when simple-appearing cystic lesion is seen in region of AV node on echocardiogram, CT, or MR

Image Interpretation Pearls

- Diagnosis is based on presence of cystic lesion in characteristic location
- Variable attenuation and signal characteristics on CT and MR, respectively, but lesion is characteristically homogeneous without aggressive features

SELECTED REFERENCES

1. Inserra MC et al: MR imaging of primary benign cardiac tumors in the pediatric population. Heliyon. 9(9):e19932, 2023
2. Maleszewski JJ et al: The 2021 WHO classification of tumors of the heart. J Thorac Oncol. 17(4):510-8, 2022
3. Ojha V et al: Cystic tumor of the atrioventricular node in a patient with intermittent complete heart block. BMJ Case Rep. 14(6):e244442, 2021
4. Cohle SD: Cystic tumour of the atrioventricular node: case report and literature review. Forensic Sci Res. 4(3):287-9, 2019
5. Fiset S et al: Multimodality imaging of a rare atrioventricular nodal tumor. Circ Cardiovasc Imaging. 11(10):e008159, 2018
6. Klimek-Piotrowska W et al: Geometry of Koch's triangle. Europace. 19(3):452-7, 2017
7. Luc JGY et al: Cystic tumor of the atrioventricular node: a review of the literature. J Thorac Dis. 9(9):3313-8, 2017
8. Saremi F et al: Fibrous skeleton of the heart: anatomic overview and evaluation of pathologic conditions with CT and MR imaging. Radiographics. 37(5):1330-51, 2017
9. Burke A et al: The 2015 WHO classification of tumors of the heart and pericardium. J Thorac Oncol. 11(4):441-52, 2016
10. Cavanaugh J et al: Sudden cardiac death due to arrhythmogenic right ventricular cardiomyopathy and cystic tumor of the AV node. Forensic Sci Med Pathol. 9(3):407-12, 2013

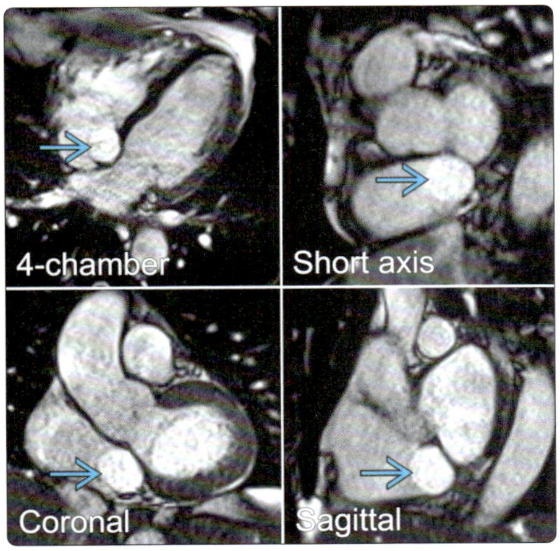

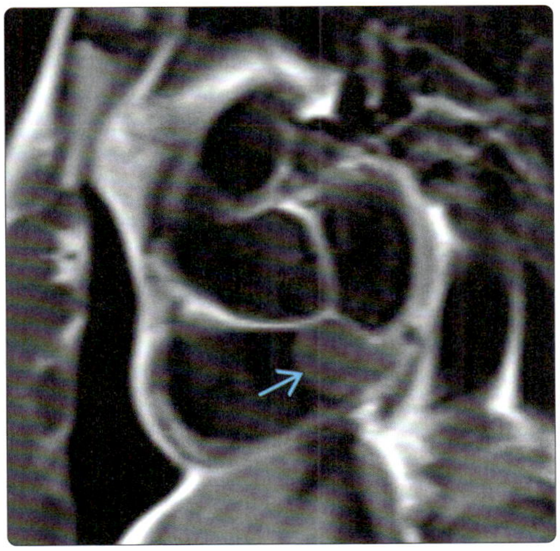

(Left) *Four-chamber short-axis, coronal, and sagittal images from cine SSFP sequences in a 49-year-old man with history of arrhythmia with a septal mass seen on echocardiogram demonstrates a homogeneously hyperintense 2.9 x 2.1 cm mass in the interatrial septum near the expected location of the AV node* →. **(Right)** *Short-axis T1W FSE in the same patient shows the mass is isointense to skeletal muscle* →.

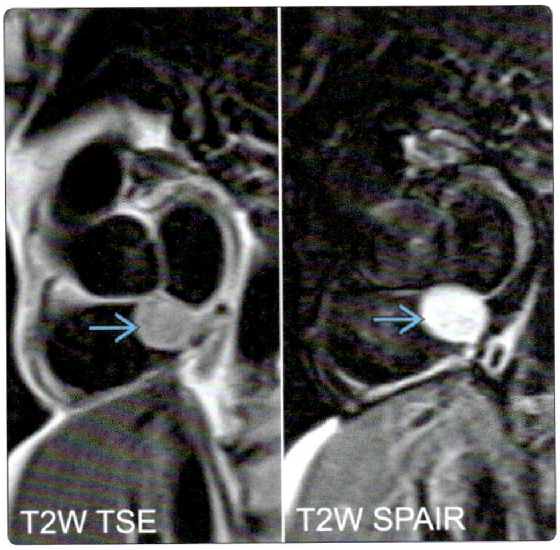

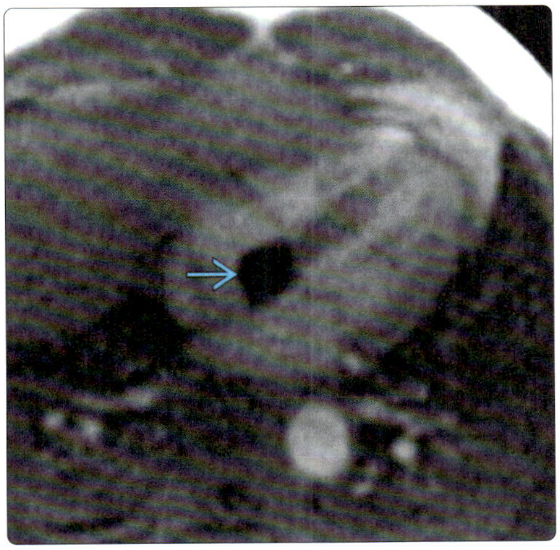

(Left) *Short-axis T2W TSE MR (left) and T2W SPAIR with fat saturation (right) in the same patient shows the hyperintense mass in the interatrial septum in the expected location of the AV node* →. **(Right)** *First-pass MR perfusion in the same patient shows no evidence of enhancement in the mass* →.

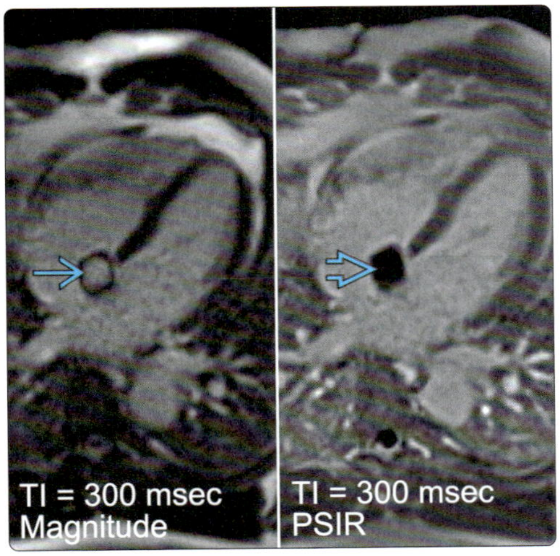

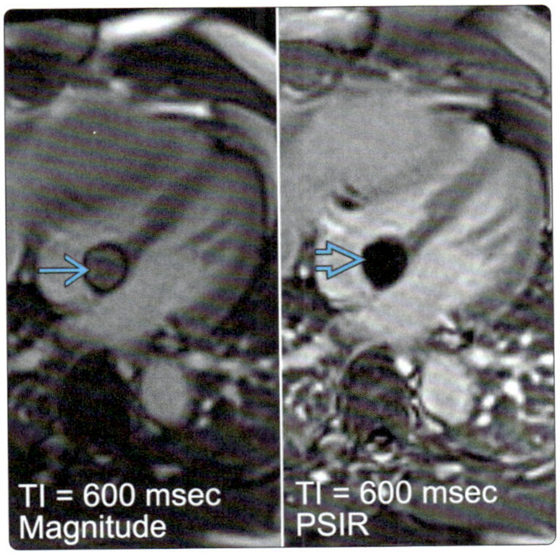

(Left) *LGE images in the same patient with a TI of 300 msec shows the mass as having bright internal signal* → *on the magnitude image but dark internal signal* ⇒ *on the PSIR image, indicative of the cystic nature of the mass. There was no evidence of LGE.* **(Right)** *Even with a prolonged TI of 600 msec, the mass still demonstrates relatively high internal signal* → *on the magnitude image and dark internal signal* ⇒ *on the PSIR image, further supporting the cystic nature of the mass. There was no evidence of LGE.*

Intracardiac Blood Cysts

KEY FACTS

TERMINOLOGY

- Intracardiac blood cysts (IBCs)
- May also be referred to as hematic cysts

IMAGING

- Most commonly found around atrioventricular valves, though they can appear in any chamber of heart
- Typically anechoic on ultrasound with thin, echogenic covering; agitated saline studies may be useful to evaluate blood flow around suspected cyst
- EKG-gated contrast CT typically reveals homogeneous mass with areas of calcification and without contrast uptake; cyst may change its size during follow-up
- IBCs typically T1 hypointense or hyperintense and T2 hyperintense; this may be used to distinguish IBCs from hydatid cysts, which are isointense on both T1 and T2

TOP DIFFERENTIAL DIAGNOSES

- Other cardiac masses, e.g., myxoma, cardiac hydatid cyst, endocardial hematic cyst, etc.

CLINICAL ISSUES

- Commonly asymptomatic, incidental finding during chest imaging; depending on size and location of cyst, may cause valvular dysfunction or outflow obstruction, which can present with new murmurs or dyspnea
- IBCs may also cause systemic embolization, possibly resulting in stroke or sudden death

DIAGNOSTIC CHECKLIST

- Assess cardiac function via echocardiogram and cardiac MR, if possible
- Closely monitor if operative removal is deferred

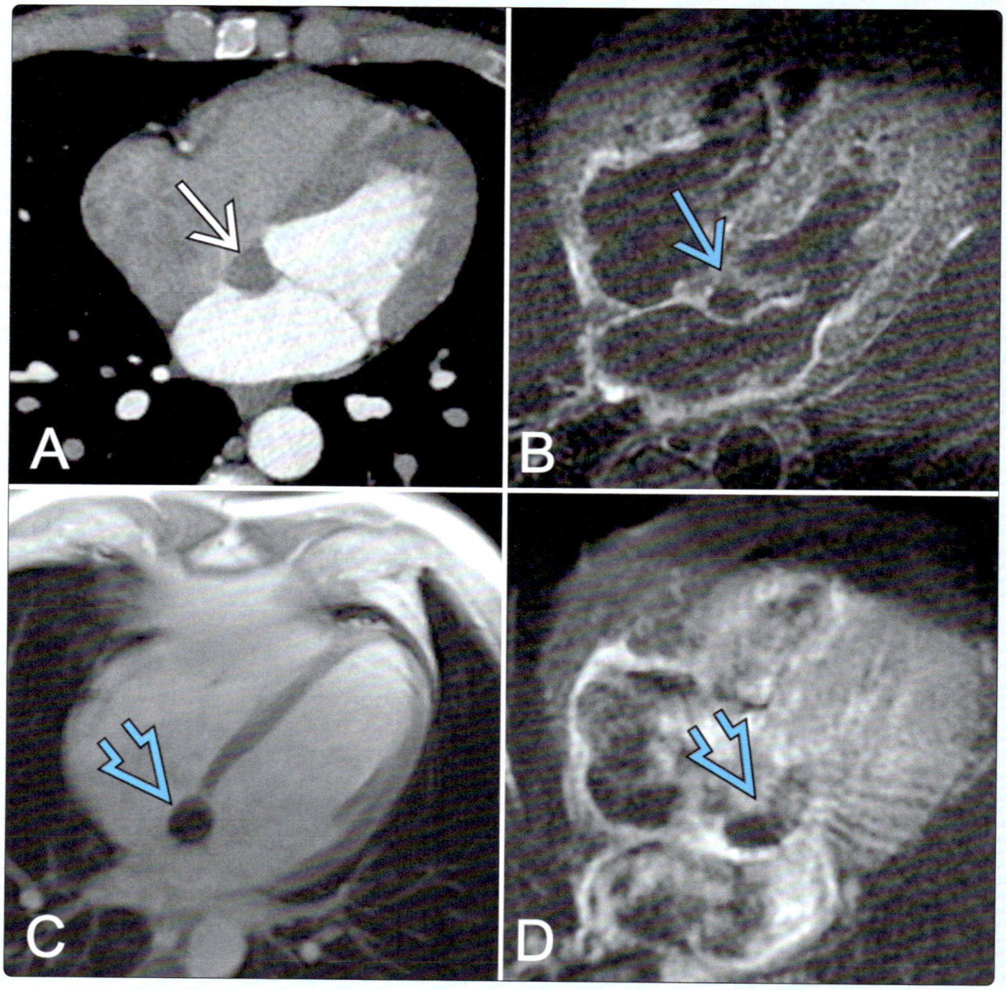

Axial postcontrast CT (A) shows a relatively isointense mass ➡ at the level of the mitral valve without contrast uptake. Axial LGE MR (C) in the same patient shows the cyst ⇨ is hypointense on T1-weighted imaging. T2- (B) and T1-weighted (D) MR images in a different patient show an intracardiac cyst ⇨ that appears hypointense on both sequences.

TERMINOLOGY

Abbreviations

- Intracardiac blood cysts (IBCs)

Synonyms

- Hematic cysts

IMAGING

CT Findings

- EKG-gated contrast CT typically reveals homogeneous mass with areas of calcification and without contrast uptake
- Cyst may change its size during follow-up

MR Findings

- IBCs are typically T1 hypointense or hyperintense and T2 hyperintense; this may be used to distinguish IBCs from hydatid cysts, which are isointense on both T1 and T2
- IBCs do not take up gadolinium contrast as they are not vascularized

Ultrasonographic Findings

- Typically anechoic on ultrasound with thin, echogenic covering; agitated saline studies may be useful to evaluate blood flow around suspected cyst

DIFFERENTIAL DIAGNOSIS

Cardiac Myxoma

- Presentation may be variable depending on location and size
  - Dyspnea or embolic event if left-sided (left atrium most common)
  - Symptoms of right-sided heart failure
  - May show constitutional symptoms, such as fatigue and weight loss
- Typically display heterogeneous attenuation on CT

Infective Endocarditis

- Clinical presentation: Constitutional signs, such as fever and weight loss, Roth spots, Janeway lesions
- CT may show vegetation, valve destruction, or filling defects
- Endocardial tissue inflammation may be evident on cardiac MR
- Vegetation/abscess may be contrast enhancing in cardiac MR

PATHOLOGY

General Features

- Etiology
  - Most commonly found along closure lines of atrioventricular valves
  - IBCs more frequently found on left side of heart in children; in adults, most common site is mitral valve
  - Pathogenesis of IBCs unclear; speculated they may arise from blood retained in crevices during valve formation; also been suggested that retained Chiari network may be predisposing factor in adult IBCs
  - Could be secondary to cardiovascular surgery, trauma, or inflammatory process

Gross Pathologic & Surgical Features

- Cystic masses most commonly found around atrioventricular valves, though they can appear in any chamber of heart

Microscopic Features

- IBCs demonstrate collagenous, fibrinoid casing and commonly contain calcified interior contents; inner wall of cyst is commonly demarcated by thin layer of typical endothelium

CLINICAL ISSUES

Presentation

- Most common signs/symptoms
  - Commonly asymptomatic, incidental finding during chest imaging; depending on size and location of cyst, may cause valvular dysfunction or outflow obstruction, which can present with new murmurs or dyspnea
  - IBCs may also cause systemic embolization, possibly resulting in stroke or sudden death

Demographics

- Rare and represent only 1.5% of all primary cardiac masses
- No sex preference
- Most commonly in infants, primarily at mitral valve

Natural History & Prognosis

- Infantile IBCs most common and typically spontaneously regress (in most cases, before 6 months)

Treatment

- No consensus guidelines for management of IBCs
- Infantile cysts most commonly regress spontaneously within few months
- Management of IBCs is primarily surgical
  - Urgency of surgery is dictated by symptomatic burden
    - Neonatal cases typically handled with watchful waiting if no symptoms are present; in adult cases of asymptomatic IBCs, removal is generally still recommended to reduce likelihood of embolization or future valvular dysfunction

DIAGNOSTIC CHECKLIST

Consider

- Assess cardiac function via echocardiogram and cardiac MR, if possible
- Closely monitor if operative removal is deferred

SELECTED REFERENCES

1. Baltodano-Arellano R et al: Case report and literature review: cardiac hematic cyst. Front Cardiovasc Med. 11:1417074, 2024
2. Clusa NM et al: Right atrium blood cyst: minimally invasive surgical approach. JTCVS Tech. 16:128-31, 2022
3. Li M et al: Clinical and echocardiographic characteristics of cardiac blood cysts. J Cardiol. 80(3):261-7, 2022
4. Beale RA et al: Mitral valve blood cyst diagnosed with the use of multimodality imaging. CASE (Phila). 5(3):173-6, 2021
5. Bortolotti U et al: Blood cysts of the cardiac valves in adults: review and analysis of published cases. J Card Surg. 36(12):4690-8, 2021
6. Karagözlü S et al: Giant intracardiac blood cyst of the mitral valve in a pediatric patient: a case report. Echocardiography. 37(6):922-5, 2020

Atrial Myxoma

KEY FACTS

IMAGING

- Myxomas are most common of all primary cardiac neoplasms
- Intracavitary mass originating from interatrial septum near fossa ovalis
- 60-75% in left atrium; followed by right atrium
- CT
  - Typically low-attenuation intracavitary mass
  - Calcification in ~ 50% of right atrial myxomas
- MR
  - Heterogeneous mass, heterogeneous enhancement
  - May change position during cardiac cycle
  - May exhibit stalk; may prolapse through or obstruct atrioventricular valve
  - Cine SSFP to evaluate mobility, valvular obstruction, and flow acceleration
- Echocardiography is generally initial imaging modality
- MR is optimal imaging modality for evaluation of myxoma

TOP DIFFERENTIAL DIAGNOSES

- Intracardiac thrombus
- Cardiac metastasis
- Cardiac lipoma
- Primary malignant cardiac tumor

CLINICAL ISSUES

- ~ 60% of affected patients are female
- Classic triad: Symptoms of valvular obstruction + embolic events + constitutional symptoms
- Treated with surgical resection; 3-year survival > 95%
- May recur after removal in 5% of cases

DIAGNOSTIC CHECKLIST

- Consider cardiac myxoma in patients with well-defined, noninvasive atrial mass
- Stalk-like connection to interatrial septum may be evident on cross-sectional imaging
- Risk of systemic embolization if left atrial myxoma

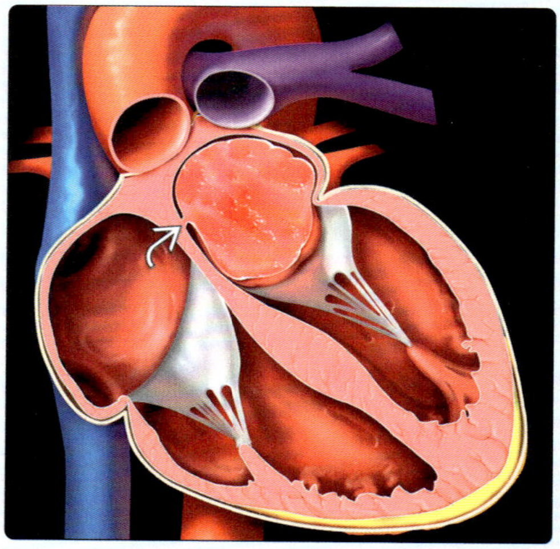

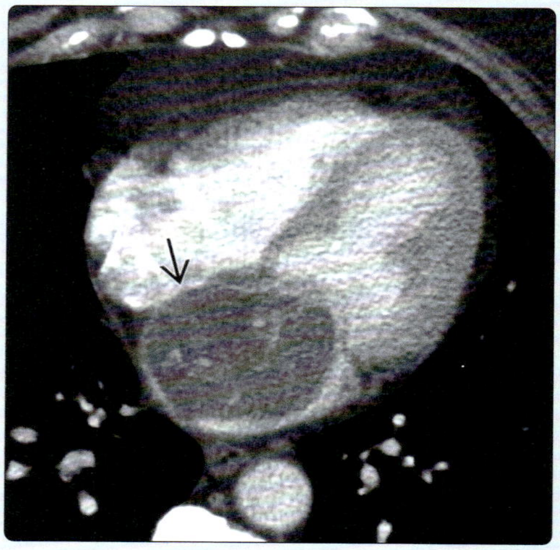

(Left) *Graphic shows the typical morphologic features of cardiac myxoma with a thin, short stalk ➔ connecting the heterogeneous left atrial mass to the interatrial septum. Large lesions may obstruct the mitral valve during systole (ball-valve mechanism).* **(Right)** *Axial CECT in a patient with a left atrial myxoma shows a heterogeneous left atrial mass with smooth borders, internal vascularity, and characteristic attachment to the interatrial septum ➔ near the fossa ovalis.*

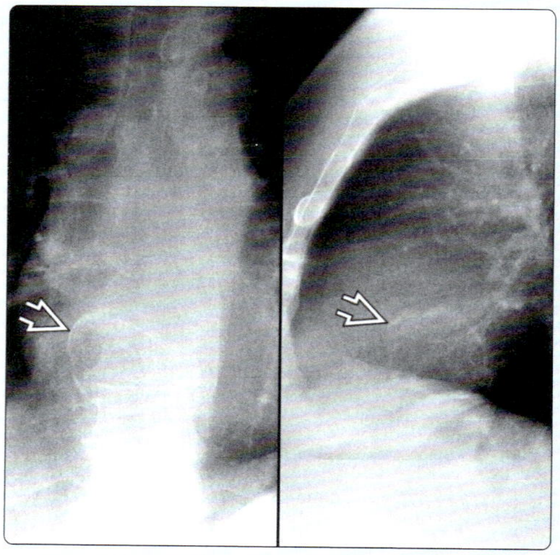

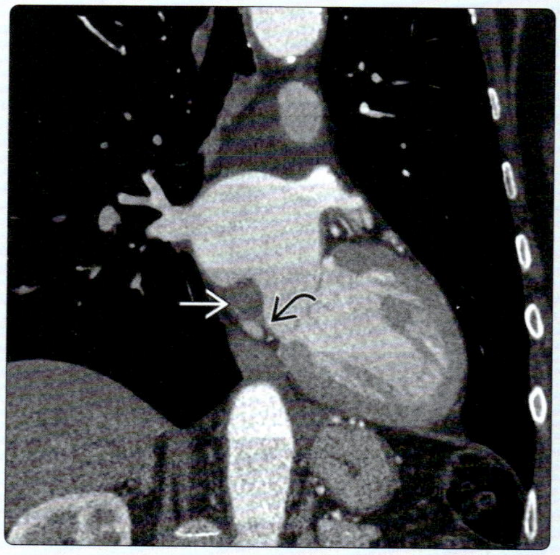

(Left) *PA (left) and lateral (right) chest radiographs show an ovoid right atrial myxoma with peripheral curvilinear calcification ➔. The right atrium is the 2nd most common location, and right atrial myxomas are more likely to exhibit calcification (~ 50%) than left atrial myxomas.* **(Right)** *Vertical long-axis (2-chamber view) cardiac CT shows a round mass ➔ in the left atrium. Note that the mass has a long pedicle ➔.*

TERMINOLOGY

Definitions

- Most common primary cardiac neoplasm (45%)

IMAGING

General Features

- Location
  - ~ **60-75% in left atrium**, followed by right atrium
    - Usually attached to left side of atrial septum
  - Rare sites: Ventricle, valve, inferior vena cava, pulmonary artery/vein
- Size
  - 1- to 15-cm diameter (mean = 5.8 cm at pathology)
- Morphology
  - Usually solitary; may be multiple in familial forms
  - Ovoid/round lesion with lobular or smooth contours
  - Connected via 1 or multiple stalks

Radiographic Findings

- Left atrial myxomas rarely calcify, but 50% of right atrial myxomas calcify
- Findings may mimic atrioventricular valve stenosis

CT Findings

- NECT
  - Low-attenuation intracavitary mass
    - Occasionally cystic; may be occult on NECT
    - May change position during cardiac cycle
  - **Calcification in ~ 50% of right atrial myxomas**, rare in left atrial myxomas
- CECT
  - May exhibit heterogeneous, low-grade enhancement

MR Findings

- **Majority are heterogeneous on MR**
  - Iso- or hypointense on T1WI
  - Usually hyperintense on T2WI
- **Cine SSFP images**: **Evaluation of mobility**, **valve obstruction**, flow acceleration, stalk visualization
  - Mass generally hypointense to blood pool
- 1st-pass perfusion often absent
- **Heterogeneous, low-grade LGE**
- Parametric mapping: High native T1, high T2 values, and extracellular volume have been reported

Echocardiographic Findings

- Tumor typically hyperechoic
- Assessment of tumor mobility and cardiac physiology

Nuclear Medicine Findings

- May be mildly FDG avid
- If very FDG avid, consider alternative malignancy

DIFFERENTIAL DIAGNOSIS

Intracardiac Thrombus

- Common; usually in posterolateral atrium or appendage
- Associated with atrial fibrillation and mitral valve disease
- Acute thrombus does not enhance; chronic thrombus may have slight peripheral enhancement
- No prolapse through mitral valve
- Both thrombus and myxoma can be mobile

Cardiac Metastasis

- More often multiple and enhancing
- Often associated with pericardial effusion, lymphadenopathy, or other metastases

Primary Malignant Cardiac Tumor

- Most often angiosarcoma
- May exhibit pericardial effusion, lung metastases

Papillary Fibroelastoma

- Most common tumor of valvular epithelium
- Usually solitary and ≤ 1 cm

PATHOLOGY

General Features

- Genetics
  - **90% sporadic**; 10% in setting of Carney complex: Autosomal dominant syndrome of multiple endocrine neoplasia, pigmented skin and mucosal lesions, cardiac + extracardiac mucinous neoplasms (53% have cardiac myxomas, often relapsing)

Gross Pathologic & Surgical Features

- Usually soft, gelatinous or friable, frond-like tumor
- 80% of cases exhibit hemorrhage, thrombus, or hemosiderin

CLINICAL ISSUES

Presentation

- Most common signs/symptoms
  - Symptoms of valvular obstruction (40%)
  - Peripheral embolization (stroke, myocardial infarction)
  - Constitutional (30%): Fatigue, weight loss, fever
  - Arrhythmias or other electrocardiographic changes
  - May be associated with auscultation abnormalities
    - Mimics mitral valve disease
    - Tumor plop in ~ 15% of cases

Demographics

- Age
  - **Mean age at presentation: 50 years**
  - Range: 1 month to 81 years
- Sex
  - ~ **60%** of affected patients are **female**

Natural History & Prognosis

- Very slow growth, **3-year survival rate > 95%**

Treatment

- Surgical resection, traditionally via sternotomy
- May recur after removal in 5% of cases
- Newer, minimally invasive techniques promising

SELECTED REFERENCES

1. Griborio-Guzman AG et al: Cardiac myxomas: clinical presentation, diagnosis and management. Heart. 108(11):827-33, 2022
2. Young PM et al: Computed tomography imaging of cardiac masses. Radiol Clin North Am. 57(1):75-84, 2019
3. Hoey ET et al: MRI assessment of cardiac tumours: part 1, multiparametric imaging protocols and spectrum of appearances of histologically benign lesions. Quant Imaging Med Surg. 4(6):478-88, 2014

(Left) *Four-chamber SSFP MR shows a round right atrial mass ➡ closely apposed to the interatrial septum.* **(Right)** *Four-chamber T2 MR in the same patient shows a uniform high T2 signal ➡ within the mass, indicating high water content. Myxoma is the most common primary benign cardiac tumor and is distinguished from thrombus by enhancement with gadolinium and increased or heterogeneously high T2 signal, as seen in this case.*

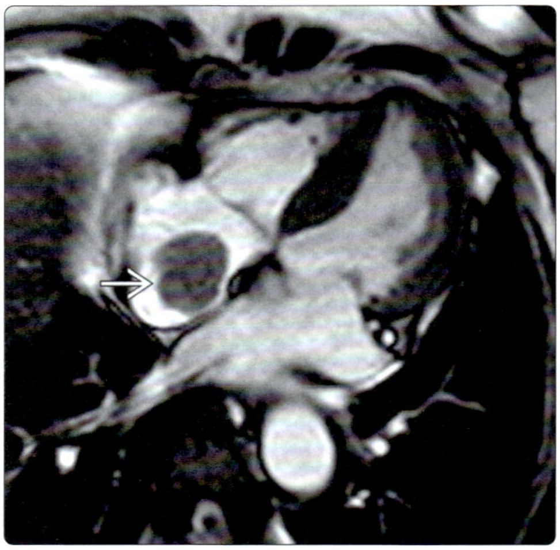

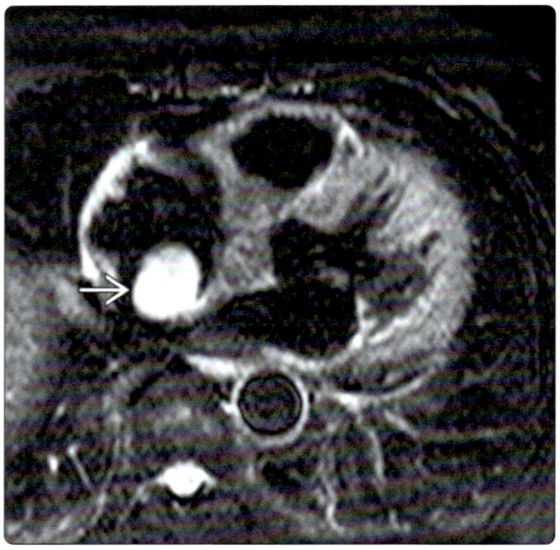

(Left) *Four-chamber 1st-pass perfusion image demonstrates a lobulated mass in the right atrium ➡ with no significant perfusion enhancement. Myxomas usually show no early perfusion enhancement.* **(Right)** *Four-chamber cine SSFP MR in systole (top) and diastole (bottom) shows a large left atrial myxoma attached to the interatrial septum that prolapses through and obstructs the mitral valve ➡ during diastole, an uncommon but characteristic and distinguishing feature from thrombus.*

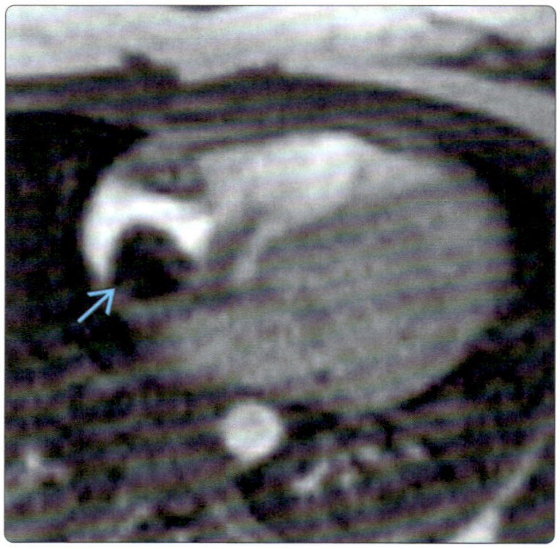

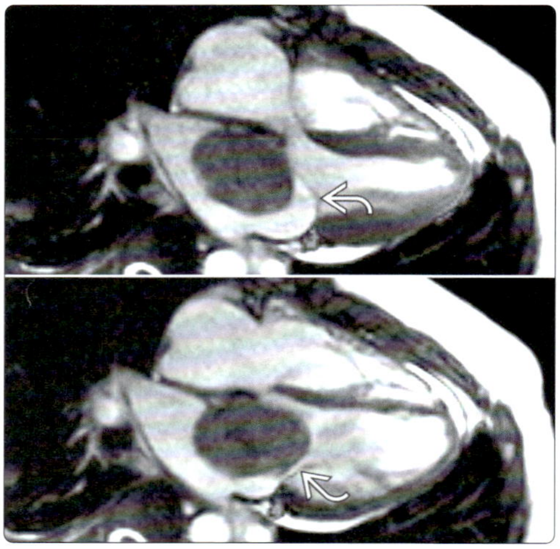

(Left) *Coronal oblique cardiac CT shows high-density contrast ➡ in the superior vena cava outlining a mass ➡ within the right atrium.* **(Right)** *Oblique axial cardiac CT in the same patient shows the oval-shaped mass ➡ with punctate calcifications adjacent to the interatrial septum. The right atrium is the 2nd most common location for intracardiac myxoma. Calcification can be seen in ~ 50% of right atrial myxomas.*

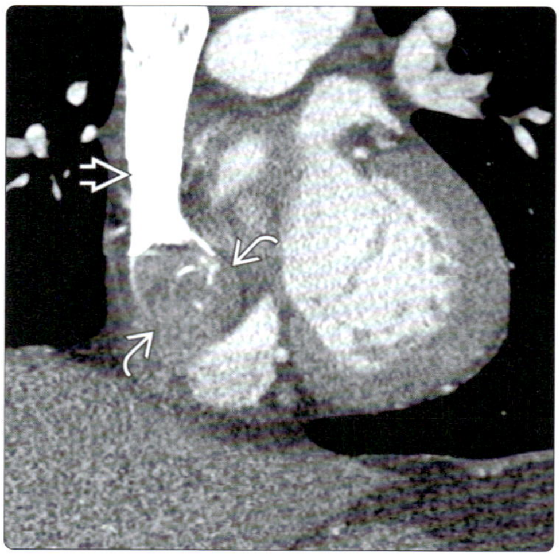

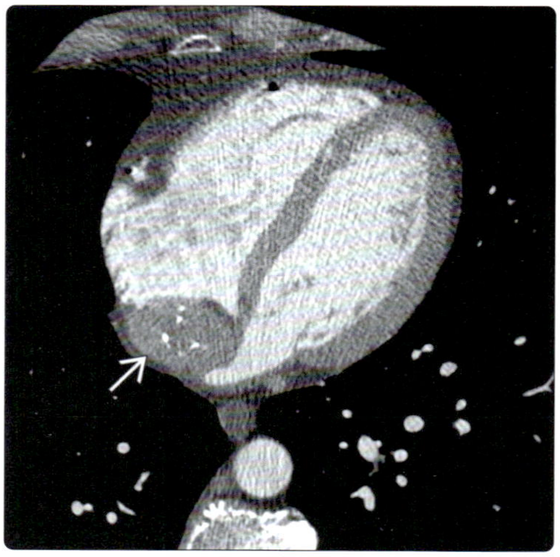

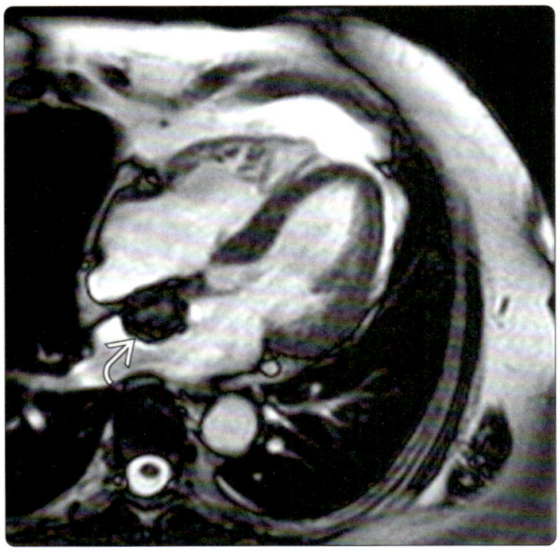

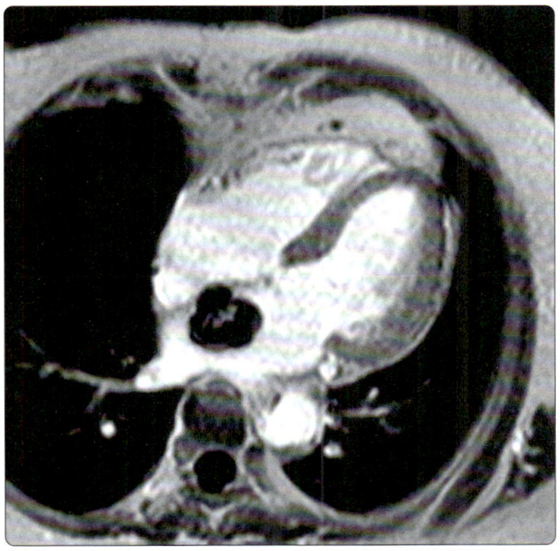

(Left) *Four-chamber SSFP MR shows a round, low signal intensity left atrial mass ⮫ located immediately adjacent to the interatrial septum.* **(Right)** *Four-chamber LGE MR in the same patient shows mostly low signal in the mass, indicating no enhancement. Despite the absence of enhancement in the mass, the characteristic location makes atrial myxoma the most likely diagnosis in this case.*

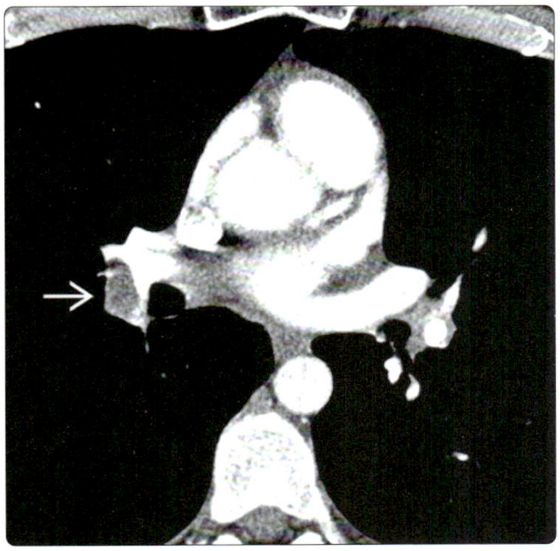

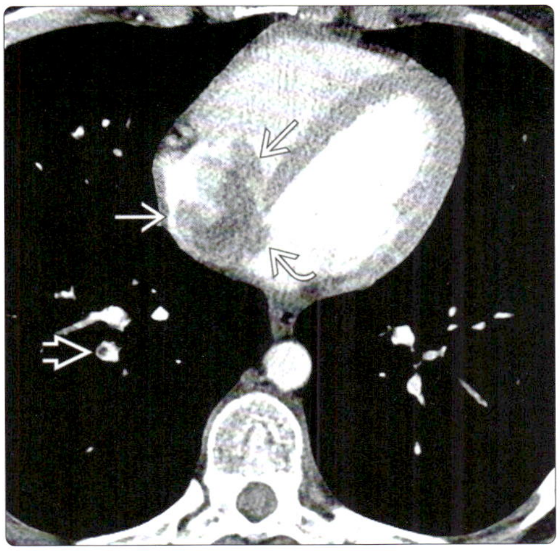

(Left) *Axial CECT shows multiple pulmonary tumor emboli ➔ in a patient with a right atrial myxoma.* **(Right)** *Axial CECT in the same patient shows a lobulated, frond-like right atrial mass ➔ arising from the interatrial septum ⮫, which was an atrial myxoma. Note the pulmonary artery filling defects, consistent with tumor emboli ⇨. The embolic event is a component of the classic triad of atrial myxoma. Villous myxomas are more likely to develop embolic complications.*

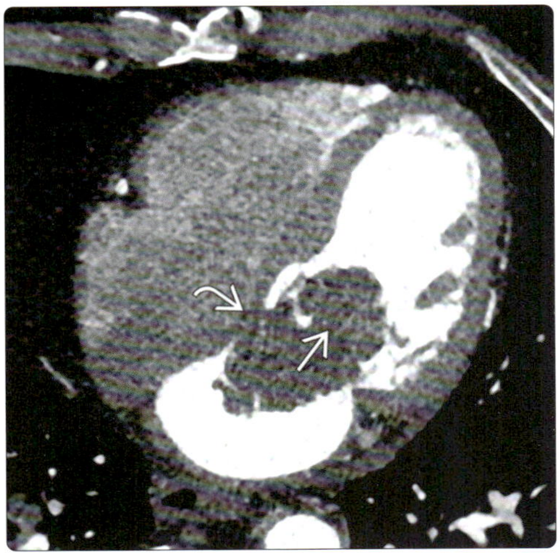

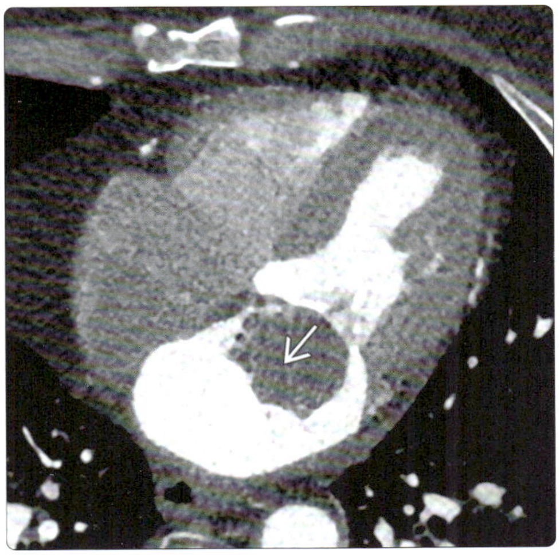

(Left) *Four-chamber cardiac CTA in end-diastole shows a large left atrial myxoma attached to the interatrial septum ⮫, prolapsing through ➔ and obstructing the mitral valve during diastole, a distinguishing feature from thrombus.* **(Right)** *Four-chamber cardiac CTA in end-systole shows a large left atrial myxoma retracted back into the left atrium during systole ➔.*

Papillary Fibroelastoma

KEY FACTS

TERMINOLOGY

- Benign endocardial papilloma that predominantly affects cardiac valves

IMAGING

- Pedunculated, valvular/paravalvular mass
- 2nd most common benign primary cardiac neoplasm
- Most arise from heart valves; aortic valve is commonest
- Typically on aortic side of aortic valve; atrial side of mitral valve
- Round, oval, or irregular in shape
  - Connected via thin stalk
  - Arises from body of valves, away from free edge

TOP DIFFERENTIAL DIAGNOSES

- Thrombus
  - May be indistinguishable from fibroelastoma
- Vegetations
  - Often at leaflet tips
  - Mostly associated with leaflet destruction
- Atrial myxoma
  - Typically arises from interatrial septum

PATHOLOGY

- Gelatinous mass with characteristic sea anemone appearance; produced by multiple narrow branching papillary fronds

CLINICAL ISSUES

- Patients are generally asymptomatic
- Patients may become symptomatic if tumor fragments or thrombus on surface of tumors result in embolic event
- Transient ischemic attacks or stroke from cerebrovascular occlusion
- Myocardial infarction or sudden cardiac death from coronary artery occlusion
- Treatment: Simple surgical excision with possible leaflet repair or valve replacement

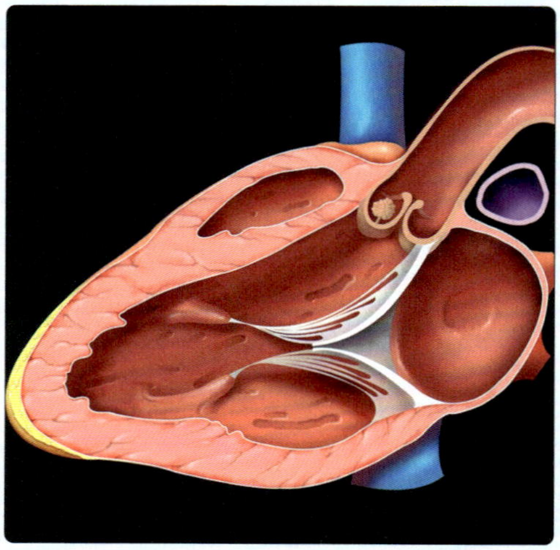
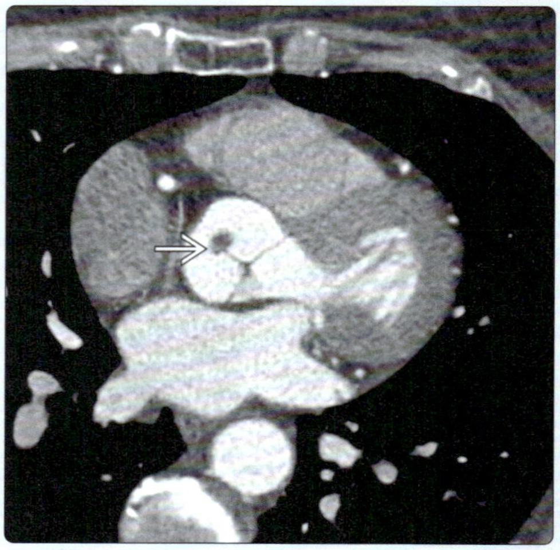

(Left) *Three-chamber graphic shows a small mass with a thin stalk and multiple frond-like projections arising from the aortic side of the aortic valve. Note the normal thickening of the cusps at the central coaptation site (nodules of Arantius).* **(Right)** *Axial cardiac CT shows a small, rounded mass ➡ with a microlobulated surface arising from the aortic side of the aortic valve. It is connected via a thin stalk to the right coronary cusp. These findings are characteristic for papillary fibroelastoma.*

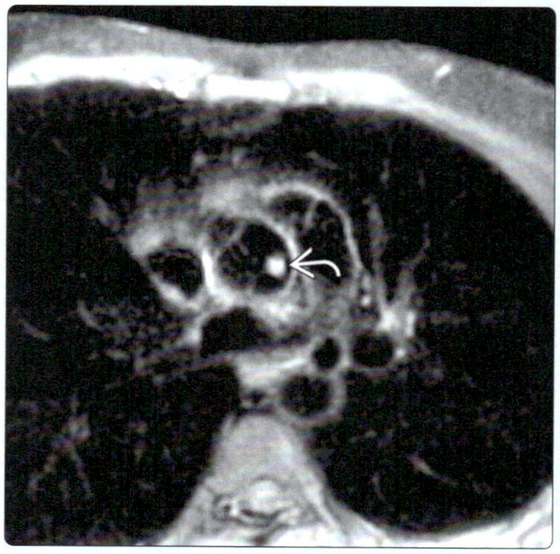
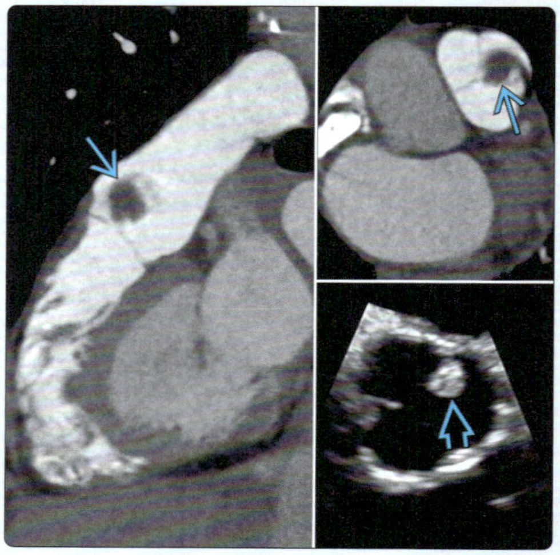

(Left) *Aortic root short-axis FS FSE MR demonstrates a small, rounded mass ➡ arising from the left coronary cusp. Note that the mass is not near the center of the valve.* **(Right)** *CT right ventricular outflow tract (RVOT) and axial images show a lobulated, hypodense mass at the pulmonary artery surface of the pulmonary valve ➡. Corresponding hyperechoic mass ➡ of the pulmonary valve is seen on echocardiography.*

TERMINOLOGY

Definitions

- Benign endocardial papilloma that predominantly affects cardiac valves

IMAGING

General Features

- Best diagnostic clue
  - Pedunculated, valvular/paravalvular mass
- Location
  - Tends to arise from heart valves in 90% of cases
    - Aortic valve (29%), mitral valve (25%), pulmonary valve (13%), tricuspic valve (17%)
  - Typically on aortic side of aortic valve and on atrial side of mitral valve
  - ~ 16% of tumors may arise from nonvalvular surfaces
- Size
  - Range: 2-28 mm (median: 8 mm); 99% of all tumors measure < 20 mm
- Morphology
  - Round, oval, or irregular in shape
  - Speckled appearance or "stippling" around tumor perimeter has also been described

MR Findings

- Attached by stalk to valve; away from free edge or on endocardial surface of affected chamber
- Hypointense, mobile mass in SSFP images
- T2-weighted images: Intermediate signal intensity similar to myocardium due to high fibrous content
- May lead to turbulence in blood flow; perilesional flow artifact
- Delayed enhancement may be seen

Imaging Recommendations

- Best imaging tool
  - Echocardiography has been primary imaging modality in years past, although MR is rapidly becoming gold standard for evaluation of cardiac masses
- Protocol advice
  - Lesions are best detected on bright-blood SSFP sequences on MR due to their inherent low signal; tumors tend to be obscured by blood pool on conventional spin-echo black-blood images

DIFFERENTIAL DIAGNOSIS

Thrombus

- May be indistinguishable from fibroelastoma
- Results in higher incidence of valvular dysfunction

Atrial Myxoma

- Typically arises from interatrial septum
- Generally larger than fibroelastoma
- Calcification, hemorrhage, or necrosis common

Vegetation

- Often at leaflet tips; not typically attached with stalk
- May be mobile
- Destruction of valve leaflets, associated regurgitation
- Clinical features of fever, murmurs, emboli, small vessel vasculitis

Aortic Valve Rheumatoid Nodules

- Complication of rheumatoid arthritis
- Nodules represent granulomas

Nodules of Arantius

- Normal structure at coaptation center of aortic cusps
- May rarely hypertrophy and mimic vegetations or masses

PATHOLOGY

General Features

- Associated abnormalities
  - Rheumatic valvulitis, valvular fibrosis, &/or calcification
  - Hypertropic cardiomyopathy
  - Aortic aneurysm
  - Congenital heart disease

Gross Pathologic & Surgical Features

- Gelatinous mass with characteristic sea anemone appearance; produced by branching papillary fronds
  - Fronds are best seen by immersing tumor in water

CLINICAL ISSUES

Presentation

- Most common signs/symptoms
  - Patients are generally asymptomatic
    - Most lesions are incidentally discovered at autopsy or while undergoing coronary surgery, echocardiography, or cardiac catheterization
- Other signs/symptoms
  - May become symptomatic if tumor fragments or thrombus on surface of tumors result in embolic event
    - Transient ischemic attack or stroke from cerebrovascular occlusion
    - Dyspnea from pulmonary emboli
    - Myocardial infarction or sudden cardiac death from coronary artery occlusion

Demographics

- Epidemiology
  - 2nd most common benign primary cardiac neoplasm
  - Accounts for ~ 75% of all cardiac valvular tumors
- Age: Mean: 60 years

Natural History & Prognosis

- Patients are generally asymptomatic with little incidence of valvular dysfunction; in setting of thromboembolic events, lesions can be surgically excised with virtually no reported recurrence

Treatment

- Simple surgical excision with possible leaflet repair or valve replacement

SELECTED REFERENCES

1. Lorca MC et al: Radiologic-pathologic correlation of cardiac tumors: updated 2021 WHO tumor classification. Radiographics. 44(6):e230126, 2024
2. Val-Bernal JF et al: Cardiac papillary fibroelastoma: retrospective clinicopathologic study of 17 tumors with resection at a single institution and literature review. Pathol Res Pract. 209(4):208-14, 2013

Cardiac Lipoma

KEY FACTS

TERMINOLOGY

- Benign encapsulated cardiac mass composed of mature adipocytes

IMAGING

- Best diagnostic clue
  - Fat attenuation cardiac lesion on CT (negative HU)
  - Follows fat signal intensity on all MR pulse sequences
  - No enhancement or invasion
- Common locations
  - Left ventricle and right atrium most commonly affected chambers
- Distribution
  - Subendocardial (50%) > subepicardial (25%) > intramyocardial (25%)
- May protrude into chamber lumen when subendocardial
- May grow within pericardial space when subepicardial

TOP DIFFERENTIAL DIAGNOSES

- Lipomatous hypertrophy of interatrial septum
- Cardiac or pericardial teratoma
- Liposarcoma
- Thrombus
- Atrial myxoma
- Other benign and malignant tumors

CLINICAL ISSUES

- Usually asymptomatic
- May cause arrhythmias
- Subepicardial tumors may cause compression symptoms
- Intraluminal subendocardial tumors may cause location-specific symptoms, such as valve obstruction or syncope
- Treatment
  - No treatment necessary if asymptomatic; imaging follow-up to assess growth
  - Surgical resection if symptomatic

(Left) *Short-axis cardiac CT in a patient with decreased ventricular function and palpitations shows a large fat attenuation left ventricular filling defect ➡ adherent to left ventricular lateral wall.* **(Right)** *Four-chamber cardiac CT in the same patient shows broad attachment of the fat attenuation mass to the left ventricular wall and papillary muscles. The mass was resected surgically due to symptoms and was confirmed to be a lipoma. (Courtesy B. Ghoshhajra, MD.)*

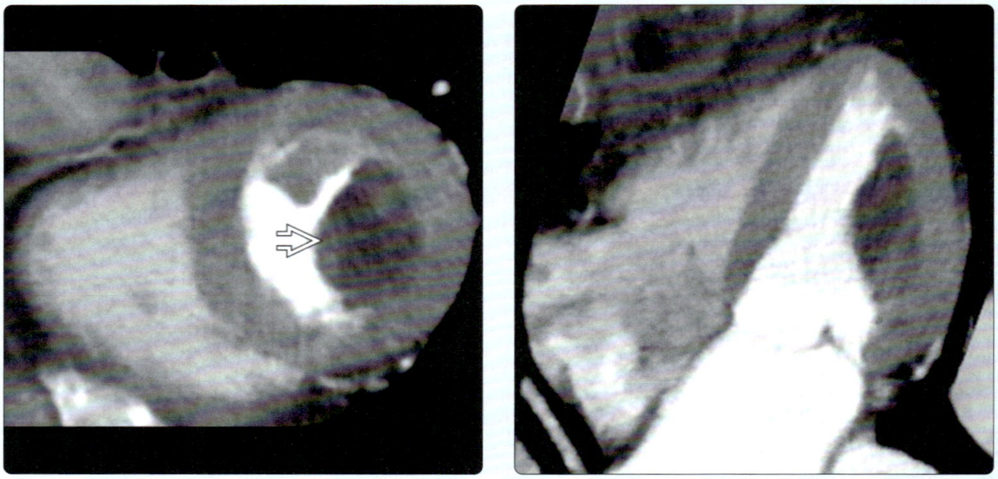

(Left) *Short-axis T1 FSE MR in the same patient shows a left ventricular mass with high signal intensity ➡, similar to adjacent subepicardial fat ↪.* **(Right)** *LVOT view from a retrospectively gated cardiac CT shows a low-attenuation mass ➡ in the anteroseptal wall of the left ventricle. The lesion's attenuation is similar to subcutaneous fat ↪ and became more rounded during systole. This suggests that the lesion is composed of tissue that is softer than the surrounding myocardium, such as fat.*

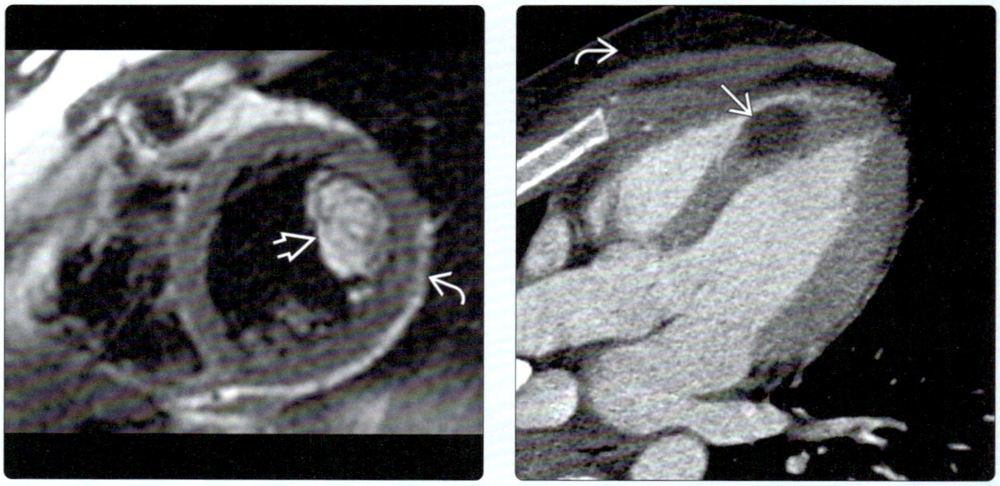

TERMINOLOGY

Definitions

- Benign encapsulated cardiac mass composed of mature adipocytes

IMAGING

General Features

- Best diagnostic clue
  - Fat attenuation (negative HU) lesion on CT
  - Follows fat signal intensity on all MR pulse sequences
- Location
  - Location
    - Left ventricle and right atrium most commonly affected chambers
  - Distribution
    - Subendocardial (50%)
    - Subepicardial (25%)
    - Intramyocardial (25%)
  - May protrude into chamber lumen when subendocardial
  - May grow within pericardial space when subepicardial
  - Rarely arises from cardiac valves
  - Rarely, multiple cardiac lipomas
    - Multiple myocardial fatty foci (MFF) deposition described in tuberous sclerosis
- Size
  - Variable, ranging from few mm to > 15 cm
  - Often large at diagnosis
  - Slow growing
- Morphology
  - Sessile or polypoid encapsulated mass with sharp demarcation

Radiographic Findings

- Radiography
  - Chest radiography
    - **Usually normal**
    - ± signs of valve obstruction distal to lipoma if intracavitary
    - May manifest as mass causing mediastinal contour abnormality
    - ± calcifications
    - ± nonspecific cardiomegaly

CT Findings

- NECT
  - Fat attenuation lesion (< -50 HU) within otherwise water or soft tissue density cardiac chambers/myocardium
  - Dilatation of obstructed chambers/vasculature
- CECT
  - Fat attenuation mass usually predominantly intraluminal or subepicardial
    - Filling defect on CECT
  - May originate within left ventricular myocardium
  - No enhancement ± thin, nonenhancing septation
  - No signs of local invasion
  - Encasement of coronary artery may occur
  - Useful for preoperative planning and determining resectability

MR Findings

- T1WI
  - Homogeneous high signal intensity mass; capsule has low signal intensity or is inapparent
  - May exhibit few thin septations
  - Fat saturation images demonstrate signal dropout
- T2WI
  - Follows fat signal; homogeneous
- PD/intermediate
  - Follows fat signal
- T1WI C+
  - No significant enhancement
- MRA
  - Filling defect in cardiac chambers

Echocardiographic Findings

- Echocardiogram
  - Sensitive tool to demonstrate lesion extent and effect on cardiac function
  - Echogenic intraluminal spherical or polypoid mass
  - Usually broad-based attachment, not very mobile
  - Transesophageal echocardiography helpful in guiding transvenous biopsy in equivocal cases

Angiographic Findings

- Nonspecific filling defect in cardiac chamber

Nuclear Medicine Findings

- PET
  - Usually no uptake

Imaging Recommendations

- Best imaging tool
  - MR or CT usually diagnostic
- Protocol advice
  - T1WI with fat saturation: Characterizes fat content, capsule, and nonfatty components
    - Solid nonfatty components suggest alternative diagnosis (e.g., teratoma, liposarcoma)

DIFFERENTIAL DIAGNOSIS

Lipomatous Hypertrophy of Interatrial Septum

- Not true neoplasm
- No capsule; differentiating feature from lipoma
- May contain brown fat; may be FDG avid on PET
- Dumbbell appearance of atrial septum due to sparing of fossa ovalis

Cardiac or Pericardial Teratoma

- Rare, usually manifests in infancy
- ± large amount of fat
- May have mature tissues from all 3 germ cell layers
- ± cardiac compression or pericardial effusion

Liposarcoma

- Very rare; soft tissue ± fat components
- May invade neighboring structures
- May produce obstructive symptoms
- 4 pathologic types: Well differentiated, myxoid, round cell, pleomorphic

Thrombus

- Common locations
  - Left atrial appendage
  - Left ventricular apex following infarct
- Does not follow signal characteristics of mediastinal fat on all sequences

Atrial Myxoma

- Most common benign primary tumor
- Typically arises in left atrium
- Hypointense on T1 MR
- Close association with interatrial septum

Cardiac Sarcoma

- Angiosarcoma is most common primary cardiac malignancy
- Restricted to heart and pericardium
- Hypodense mass involving cardiac wall &/or chambers on CT
  - Infiltration/invasion of pericardium, myocardium, mediastinum
- MR
  - Heterogeneous isointensity on T1
  - Heterogeneous high signal intensity on T2
  - Heterogeneous enhancement

Cardiac and Pericardial Metastases

- Most common: Lung, breast, melanoma, lymphoma
- Pericardial effusion is typical
- Associated with lung and osseous metastases, pleural effusion, and lymphadenopathy
- MR
  - Most exhibit low signal intensity on T1
    - Melanoma and hemorrhagic metastases may exhibit high signal intensity
  - High signal intensity on T2
  - Most enhance

PATHOLOGY

General Features

- Usually solitary subendocardial, myocardial, or subepicardial homogeneous circumscribed tumor
- True cardiac lipomas are rare
  - 2nd most common **benign primary** cardiac **neoplasm**
    - Most common **mass** is thrombus
    - Most common **neoplasm** (primary or secondary) is metastasis
    - Most common benign primary neoplasm is myxoma
    - Most common malignant primary cardiac neoplasm is angiosarcoma

Gross Pathologic & Surgical Features

- Spheric, sessile, or polypoid mass of homogeneous yellow fat
- Usually 1-15 cm; may be as massive as 4,000 g
  - Subepicardial tumor often grows to large size
  - Subendocardial tumor is usually small with broad attachment

Microscopic Features

- True lipomas are encapsulated and contain neoplastic mature adipocytes
- Lipoma does not contain brown fetal fat cells like lipomatous hypertrophy of interatrial septum
- May have entrapped myocytes at interface of tumor with myocardium but not distributed within tumor

CLINICAL ISSUES

Presentation

- Most common signs/symptoms
  - Symptoms depend on location and size of mass
    - Majority asymptomatic
    - May cause arrhythmias
    - Subepicardial tumors may cause compression symptoms
    - Intraluminal subendocardial tumors may cause location-specific symptoms, such as valve obstruction or syncope
- Other signs/symptoms
  - Rare reports of sudden cardiac death

Demographics

- Epidemiology
  - All ages; equal sex distribution
  - More common in overweight patients

Natural History & Prognosis

- Frequently incidentally found on autopsy
- Progressive obstructive or compressive symptoms may require surgery
- Generally good outcome
- Rarely recurs following surgery

Treatment

- No treatment necessary if asymptomatic; follow-up imaging to assess growth
- Surgical resection if symptomatic

DIAGNOSTIC CHECKLIST

Consider

- T1 MR with fat saturation to document fat content

Image Interpretation Pearls

- If soft tissue component, consider liposarcoma or teratoma as alternate diagnosis

SELECTED REFERENCES

1. Kadoya Y et al: Noninvasive diagnosis of a massive cardiac lipoma with multimodality imaging. J Nucl Cardiol. 33:101815, 2024
2. Roset-Altadill A et al: Epicardial space: comprehensive anatomy and spectrum of disease. Radiographics. 44(4):e230160, 2024
3. Shu S et al: The value of multimodality imaging in diagnosis and treatment of cardiac lipoma. BMC Med Imaging. 21(1):71, 2021
4. Rocha RV et al: Adipose tumors of the heart. J Card Surg. 33(8):432-37, 2018
5. Díaz Angulo C et al: Imaging findings in cardiac masses (part I): study protocol and benign tumors. Radiologia. 57(6):480-8, 2015
6. Girrbach F et al: Epicardial lipoma–a rare differential diagnosis in cardiovascular medicine. Eur J Cardiothorac Surg. 41(3):699-701, 2012
7. Adriaensen ME et al: Mature fat cells in the myocardium of patients with tuberous sclerosis complex. J Clin Pathol. 64(3):244-5, 2011
8. Adriaensen ME et al: Fatty foci in the myocardium in patients with tuberous sclerosis complex: common finding at CT. Radiology. 253(2):359-63, 2009
9. Gaerte SC et al: Fat-containing lesions of the chest. Radiographics. 22 Spec No:S61-78, 2002
10. Vander Salm TJ: Unusual primary tumors of the heart. Semin Thorac Cardiovasc Surg. 12(2):89-100, 2000

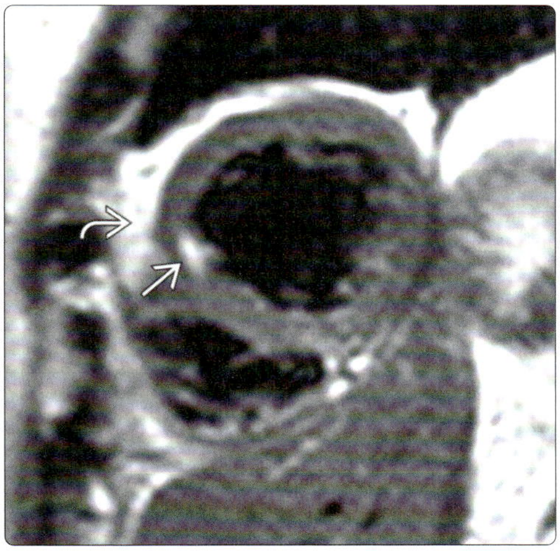

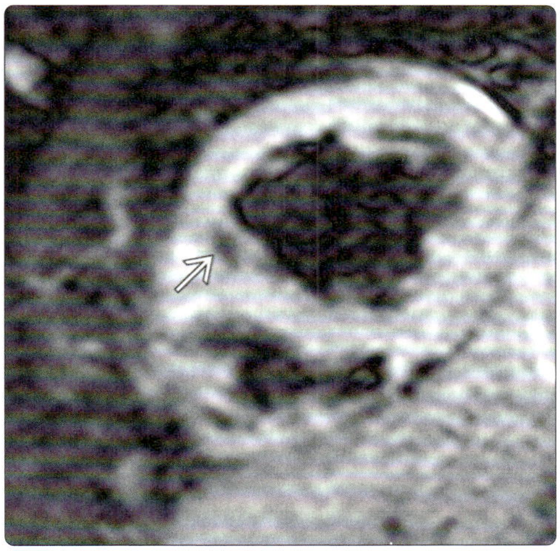

(Left) *Short-axis T1 MR shows a small, high signal intensity ovoid lesion ➔ in the myocardium of the upper interventricular septum, similar in signal intensity to nearby subepicardial fat ➔.* **(Right)** *Short-axis T1 FS MR in the same patient shows complete signal loss ➔ in the ovoid lesion. This confirms the presence of fat and is consistent with an intramyocardial lipoma.*

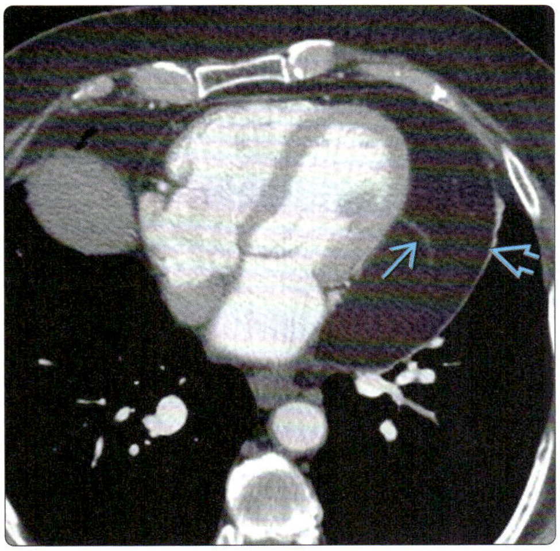

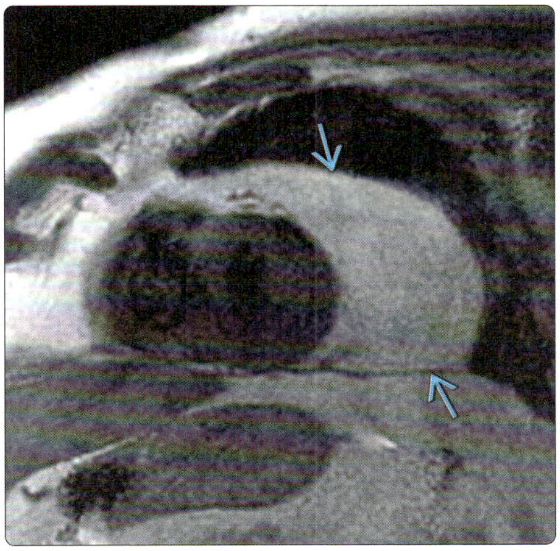

(Left) *Axial CECT shows a large, fat-containing subepicardial mass ➔, consistent with lipoma. Note the small, linear soft tissue strand ➔ within the lipoma, a common ancillary finding.* **(Right)** *Short-axis T1 MR in the same patient shows a hyperintense subepicardial mass ➔ with signal intensity that matches the intraabdominal and chest wall fat, consistent with lipoma. Growth into the pericardial space was confirmed at surgery. (Courtesy B. Carter, MD.)*

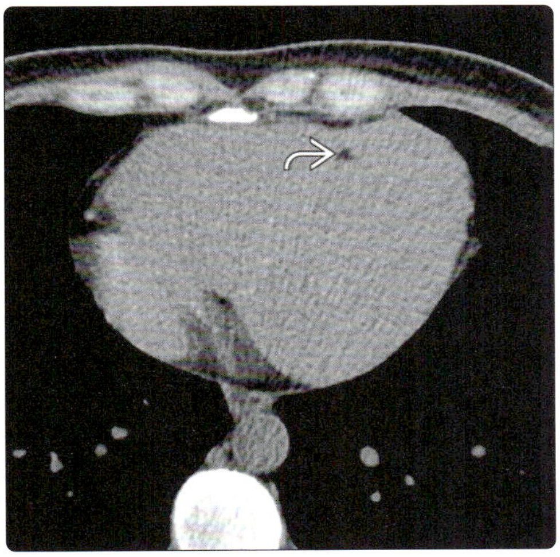

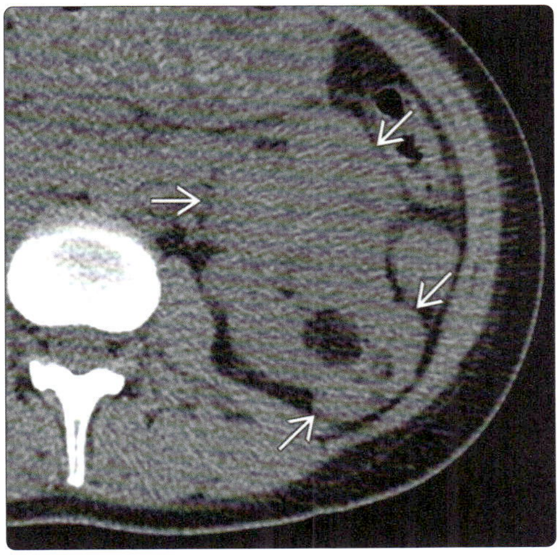

(Left) *Axial NECT shows a well-defined, fat attenuation lesion ➔ within the interventricular septum.* **(Right)** *Axial NECT in the same patient shows multiple lobulated masses ➔ arising from the anterior and posterior left kidney. The masses contain macroscopic fat and are diagnostic of angiomyolipomas. The presence of multiple angiomyolipomas as well as fat-containing intramyocardial lesions are most commonly associated with tuberous sclerosis.*

KEY FACTS

TERMINOLOGY

- Benign tumor composed of vascular endothelial cells

IMAGING

- Hypervascular mass without aggressive features
- ~ 70% intramural, 15% endocardial/intracavitary, and 15% epicardial/pericardial
- Can occur in any chamber or wall
- MR provides most comprehensive assessment
  - Isointense and hyperintense to myocardium on T1W and T2W imaging, respectively
  - Variable perfusion with mild to extensive enhancement
  - Progressive enhancement over time with typically extensive LGE
- Isoattenuating on CT with progressive contrast enhancement

TOP DIFFERENTIAL DIAGNOSES

- Location dependent
  - Intracavitary: Myxoma; metastases
  - Intramural: Metastases; rhabdomyoma
  - Epicardial: Metastases; paraganglioma; lymphangioma

CLINICAL ISSUES

- Rare tumors estimated to make up 2.8% of all primary cardiac masses
- Surgery usually recommended if diagnosis is uncertain or if lesion is symptomatic
- Treatment is surgical excision
  - Sometimes, complete surgical excision is not possible due to intramural location, but recurrence is uncommon
- Many are asymptomatic, incidental findings detected on imaging for unrelated finding, such as murmur
- When symptomatic, dyspnea on exertion and arrhythmias are most common manifestations
- Rarely may be seen in Kasabach-Merritt syndrome with recurrent thrombocytopenia and coagulopathy associated with multiple systemic hemangiomas

(Left) *Axial NECT (top left) shows an isoattenuating epicardial soft tissue mass ➡ with progressive central enhancement ➡ 1 minute (top right) and 3 minutes (bottom left) post contrast. Echo (bottom right) shows a heterogeneous mass ➡, which is inseparable from left ventricle (LV) ➡.* **(Right)** *In the same patient, the mass ➡ is mildly, moderately hyperintense to myocardium on SSFP MR ➡, and T2W and is isointense to myocardium on T1W imaging ➡ with mild immediate postcontrast enhancement ➡.*

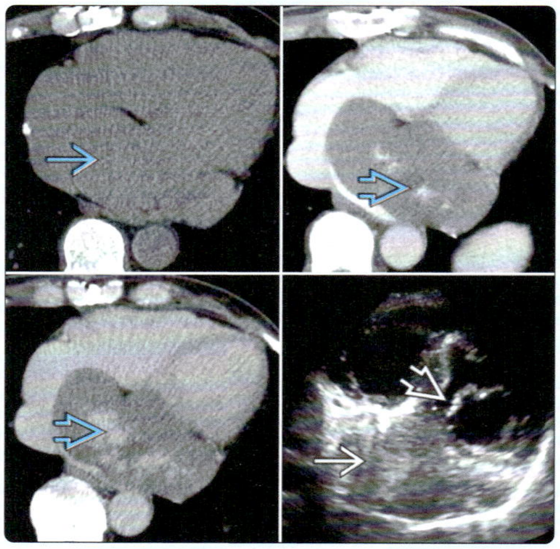

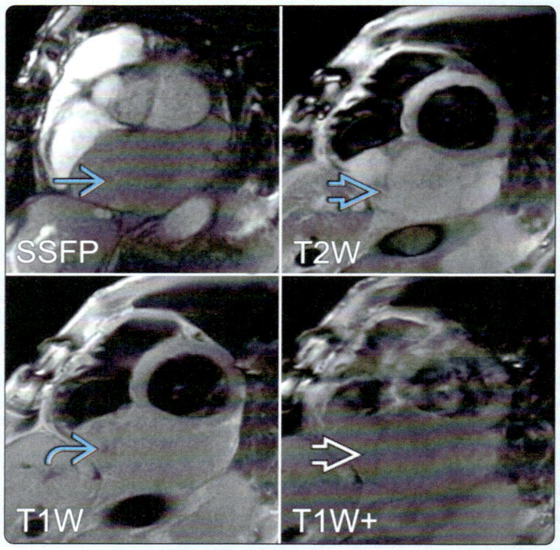

(Left) *LAVA images in the same patient (top row) show progressive contrast enhancement ➡ of the mass. LGE (bottom left) shows diffuse enhancement ➡ commonly seen in hemangiomas. PET/CT shows mild FDG uptake ➡ in the mass (SUVmax = 2.8). Biopsy confirmed a hemangioma.* **(Right)** *Axial (top row) and short-axis (bottom row) T2 MR (left column) and SSFP cine MR (right column) show an epicardial hemangioma ➡. Note that the lesion has sharply defined margins and internal septations.*

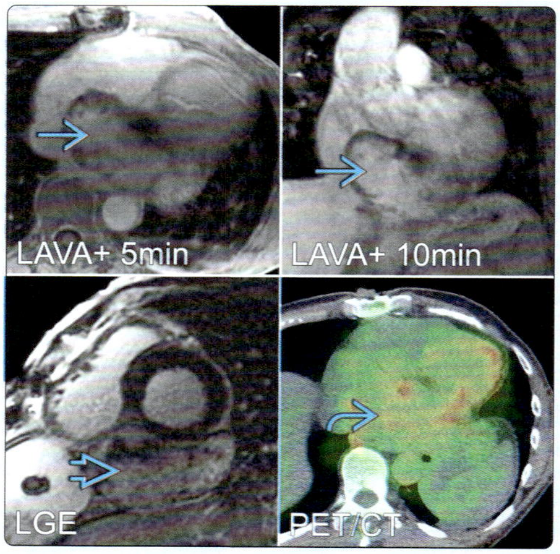

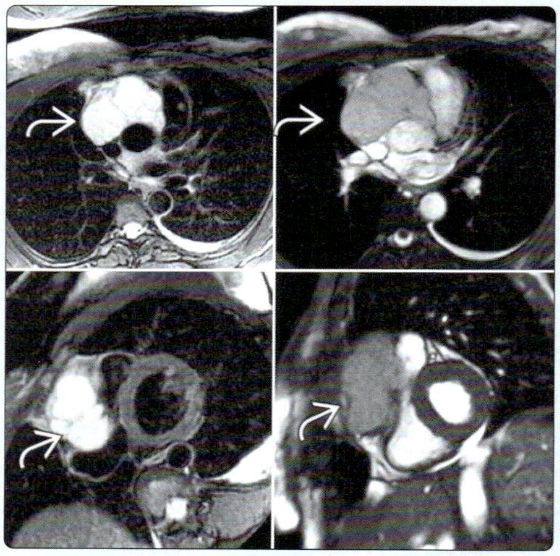

TERMINOLOGY

Synonyms

- Angioma

Definitions

- Benign tumor composed of vascular endothelial cells

IMAGING

General Features

- Best diagnostic clue
  - Hypervascular mass without aggressive features
- Location
  - ~ 70% intramural, 15% endocardial/intracavitary, and 15% epicardial/pericardial
  - Can occur in any chamber or wall
    - Atria slightly more common than ventricles in childhood; right atrium > left atrium
    - Ventricles or interventricular septum slightly more common in adult series
- Size
  - Variable, ranging from small (~ 5- to 10-mm) polypoid intracavitary lesion to large intramural or epicardial mass (> 10 cm)
    - Most 2-6 cm in size
- Morphology
  - When intracavitary, may be rounded or polypoid in appearance with short stalk, similar to myxoma
  - When mural or epicardial, often amorphous and may mold to adjacent structures

Radiographic Findings

- Radiography
  - May show enlargement of cardiac silhouette when large

CT Findings

- NECT
  - Homogeneous mass that may be intramural or epicardial
    - May not be visible without contrast
- CECT
  - Progressive enhancement post contrast
    - Small endocavitary lesions may require careful contrast bolus timing to be best demonstrated
  - Septations, if present, may enhance

MR Findings

- T1WI
  - Isointense to mildly hyperintense
- T2WI
  - Hyperintense; septations may be present
- STIR
  - Hyperintense; septations may be present
- T1WI C+
  - Progressive enhancement over time
  - In some instances, central scar may lead to diminished uptake relative to periphery
- 1st-pass perfusion imaging
  - Quite variable
  - Enhancement on perfusion imaging may be heterogeneous &/or late
- LGE
  - Heterogeneous with conspicuous areas of intense LGE

Echocardiographic Findings

- Heterogeneous but commonly hyperechoic

Nuclear Medicine Findings

- PET
  - Only few case reports with PET/CT
  - FDG uptake ranges from none to mild

Imaging Recommendations

- Best imaging tool
  - Multisequence multiplanar MR provides most comprehensive assessment
- Protocol advice
  - 1st-pass perfusion imaging very helpful in demonstrating hypervascular nature of mass, limiting differential
  - Cine MR important to assess borders of lesion to determine degree of infiltration and likelihood of complete resection

DIFFERENTIAL DIAGNOSIS

Depends on Location

- Intracavitary lesions
  - Myxoma
    - Usually has attachment to fossa ovalis, which is uncommon with hemangioma
    - 1st-pass perfusion MR usually shows minimal enhancement or enhancement of stalk only
- Intramural lesions
  - Childhood
    - Rhabdomyoma
      - ◻ Most often seen in patients with tuberous sclerosis
      - ◻ Isointense to myocardium on all sequences, particularly LGE MR and 1st-pass perfusion MR
    - Fibroma
      - ◻ Usually hypointense on T2 MR, not markedly hyperintense, as is hemangioma
      - ◻ Does not enhance on 1st-pass perfusion MR
      - ◻ Enhancement in LGE MR: May have dark center, particularly if imaged early, similar to hemangioma
  - Adulthood
    - Metastases
      - ◻ 20-40x more common than primary tumors
      - ◻ Most often have infiltrating, poorly marginated appearance
      - ◻ Enhancement on LGE MR heterogeneous, similar to hemangioma
      - ◻ Hypervascular metastases (renal cell, melanoma, etc.) may have prominent 1st-pass perfusion uptake
      - ◻ Usually seen in patients with advanced known malignancy
      - ◻ Typically more aggressive in appearance than hemangioma with higher incidence of pericardial effusion
    - Cardiac angiosarcoma
      - ◻ Ill-defined tumor often centered in right atrioventricular groove
      - ◻ Very hypervascular on 1st-pass perfusion MR

- Heterogeneous uptake on LGE MR, similar to hemangioma
- Very aggressive tumor with cardiac invasion and pericardial dissemination

- Epicardial
  - Childhood
    - Teratomas
      - Complex multiloculated cystic tumors
      - Usually arise from aortic root near roof of right atrium
    - Lymphatic malformation
      - Tumors of dilated lymphatic channels that do not communicate with lymphatic tree
      - Minimal or no contrast uptake; low in signal on T1 images
    - Neurofibroma
      - Rare location in neurofibromatosis type 1 (NF1)
      - Does not show progressive enhancement
  - Adulthood
    - Metastases
      - Most common cause of epicardial/pericardial neoplastic disease
      - Pericardial effusions extremely common and may be cause of clinical presentation
    - Paraganglioma
      - Hyperintense with salt and pepper appearance on T2W imaging
      - Typical locations with cardiac lesions usually on roof of left atrium
      - Much less frequently intracavitary
      - Marked 1st-pass perfusion and T1W+, usually greater than hemangioma
      - Heterogeneous on LGE MR, similar to hemangioma
      - May present with symptoms of catecholamine excess

PATHOLOGY

General Features

- Associated abnormalities
  - Rarely, hemangiomas of GI tract

Gross Pathologic & Surgical Features

- May be clearly demarcated, lobular tumor or have infiltrating margins, resulting in difficulty in resection

Microscopic Features

- May be cavernous, capillary, or arteriovenous in type; mixed cavernous/capillary types in 20% of cases
- Cavernous type is most common (50%) and similar to cavernous hemangiomas elsewhere
  - Usually intramural in location
- Capillary types 2nd most common (23%) and composed of lobules of endothelial cells
  - Often endocardial (50%) and project intraluminally
  - May mimic myxoma
- Arteriovenous malformation (AVM)-type lesions have areas of dysplastic, thickened arterial and venous structures similar to AVMs elsewhere
  - Most often intramural in location

CLINICAL ISSUES

Presentation

- Most common signs/symptoms
  - Many are asymptomatic, incidental findings detected on imaging for unrelated finding, such as murmur
  - When symptomatic, dyspnea on exertion/shortness of breath and arrhythmias are most common manifestations
  - Rarely may be seen in Kasabach-Merritt syndrome with recurrent thrombocytopenia and coagulopathy associated with multiple systemic hemangiomas
- Other signs/symptoms
  - Uncommonly, pericardial effusions or congestive heart failure may develop
    - Rarely, may present with syncope or sudden death

Demographics

- Age
  - All ages reported, from infancy to old age, with median age of 43 years
- Sex
  - Slight male predominance in most reported series
- Epidemiology
  - Rare tumors estimated to make up 2.8% of all primary cardiac masses
    - Usually sporadic, uncommonly seen as part of hemangiomatosis syndrome

Natural History & Prognosis

- Most remain asymptomatic, and spontaneous regression has been occasionally reported

Treatment

- Surgery usually recommended if diagnosis is uncertain or if lesion is symptomatic

DIAGNOSTIC CHECKLIST

Consider

- Hemangioma should be in differential diagnosis for hypervascular intramural lesions lacking other aggressive features
  - Particularly in patients without known malignancy

Image Interpretation Pearls

- Variable perfusion with progressive enhancement
  - Note that some large hemangiomas may show delayed or absent filling of center of lesion

SELECTED REFERENCES

1. Beroukhim RS et al: Accuracy of cardiac magnetic resonance imaging in diagnosing pediatric cardiac masses: a multicenter study. JACC Cardiovasc Imaging. 15(8):1391-405, 2022
2. Li W et al: Cardiac hemangioma: a comprehensive analysis of 200 cases. Ann Thorac Surg. 99(6):2246-52, 2015
3. Beroukhim RS et al: Characterization of cardiac tumors in children by cardiovascular magnetic resonance imaging: a multicenter experience. J Am Coll Cardiol. 58(10):1044-54, 2011
4. Burke A et al: Tumors of the Heart and Great Vessels. Armed Forces Institute of Pathology, 1996
5. Burke A et al: Hemangiomas of the heart. A clinicopathologic study of ten cases. Am J Cardiovasc Pathol. 3(4):283-90, 1990

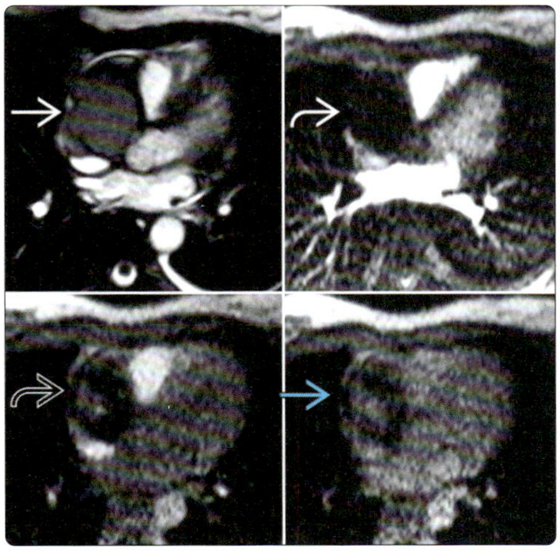

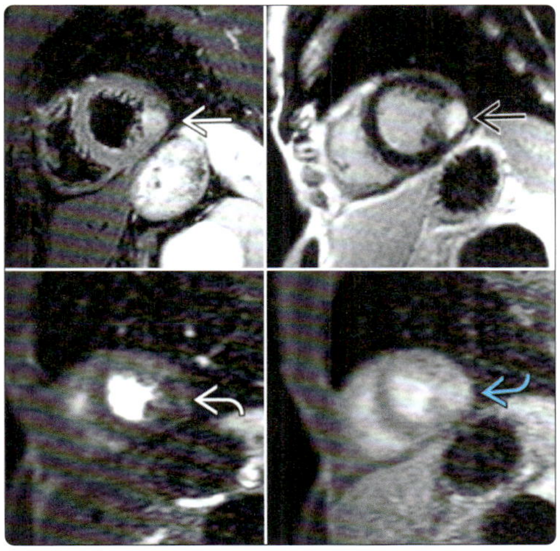

(Left) *Axial cine MR shows an epicardial hemangioma ➡ as a sharply marginated lesion. Perfusion images obtained in the early ➡, middle ➡, and late phase ➡ of IV contrast administration show slow, progressive enhancement of the lesion.* **(Right)** *Short-axis view of an intramural hemangioma of the LV shows the usual hyperintense T2 signal ➡. LGE MR ➡ shows enhancement, while the early ➡ and late ➡ perfusion images show progressive enhancement.*

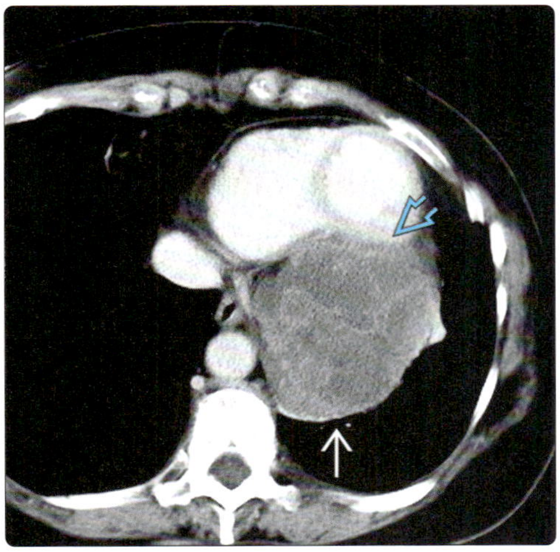

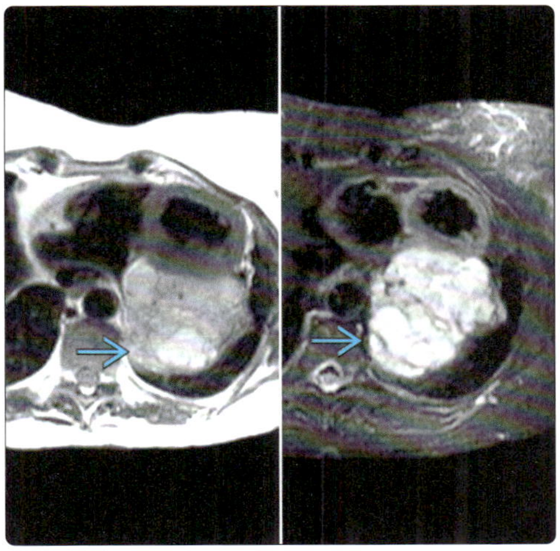

(Left) *Axial CECT shows a large epicardial hemangioma ➡ with enhancing internal septations. The mass is inseparable from the LV ➡.* **(Right)** *Axial T2 (left) and STIR (right) MR images in the same patient show the hemangioma ➡ arising along the posterior margin of the LV. Note the internal septations evident on both.*

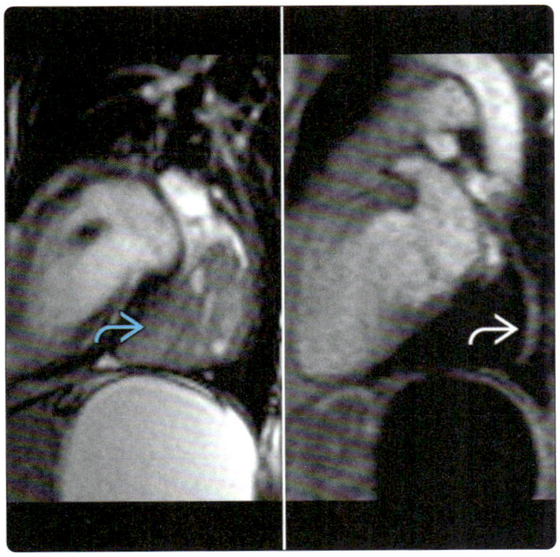

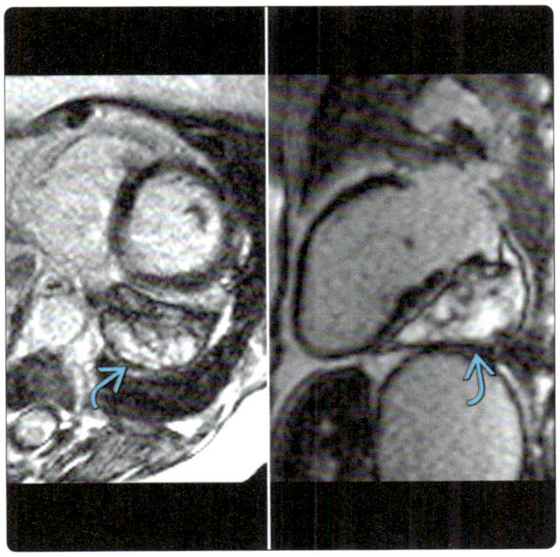

(Left) *Sagittal SSFP MR (left) shows a complex epicardial mass along the posterior cardiac margin ➡ with cystic and solid components. Perfusion image (right) shows peripheral rim enhancement ➡. The center filled in much later. Many large, cavernous hemangiomas will show this pattern of peripheral early enhancement with delayed or absent central enhancement due to a central scar.* **(Right)** *Short-axis LGE (left) and 2-chamber (right) MR images show characteristic heterogeneous enhancement of an LV hemangioma ➡.*

KEY FACTS

TERMINOLOGY

- Tumors that arise from cardiac autonomic paraganglia and are commonly located in atria (L > R) along atrioventricular (AV) grooves, near roots of aorta and pulmonary artery
- 90% benign; ~ 1/3 hormonally active

IMAGING

- **Radiograph**
  - Mediastinal mass that splays carina or causes left atrial enlargement
- **CT**
  - Hypervascular, insinuating mass in characteristic location
- **MR**
  - T1 iso- to mildly hypointense, T2 hyperintense, diffusion restricting, avidly enhancing mass

TOP DIFFERENTIAL DIAGNOSES

- Metastatic disease
- Angiosarcoma
- Hemangioma

CLINICAL ISSUES

- Often are incidental findings and asymptomatic
  - Many patients present with symptoms from catecholamine production in functional tumors, such as hypertension, headache, or flushing
- **Treatment**
  - Surgical resection; catecholamine blockade may be helpful

DIAGNOSTIC CHECKLIST

- Consider screening entire chest for additional lesions
  - High-resolution images with 3D anatomic modeling may help surgeon to visualize and plan approach
- Describe any large feeding vessels, involvement of coronary arteries or other structures
  - Try to visualize defect that would be left if tumor were cut out and describe location and size

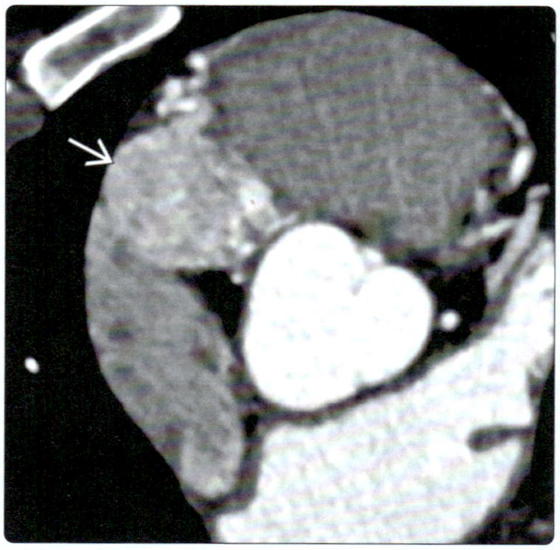

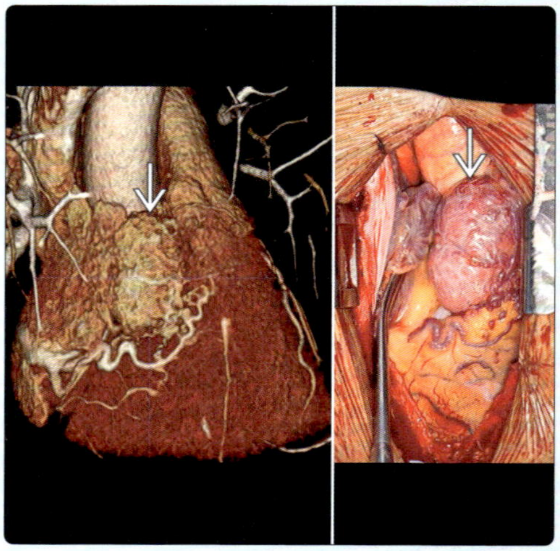

(Left) *Axial CECT demonstrates an enhancing, hypervascular, infiltrative but well-defined mass ➡ in the right atrioventricular (AV) groove. This was a paraganglioma on pathology.* **(Right)** *Oblique volume-rendered CT is shown with correlative operative findings. This paraganglioma ➡ was well depicted preoperatively, as was its blood supply from an enlarged acute marginal artery. The blood supply of cardiac paragangliomas is usually from coronary arteries, especially from the right coronary artery.*

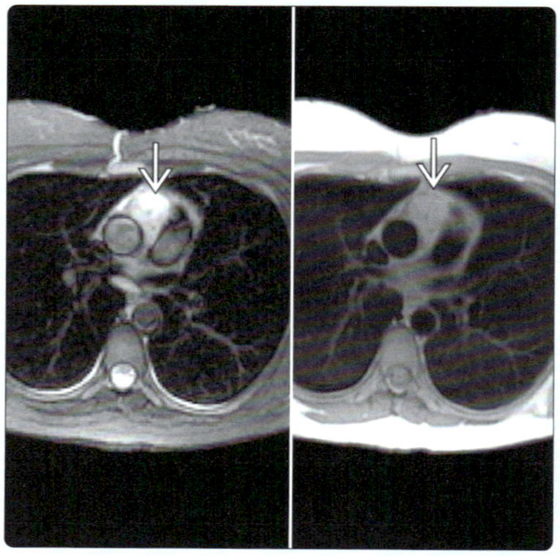

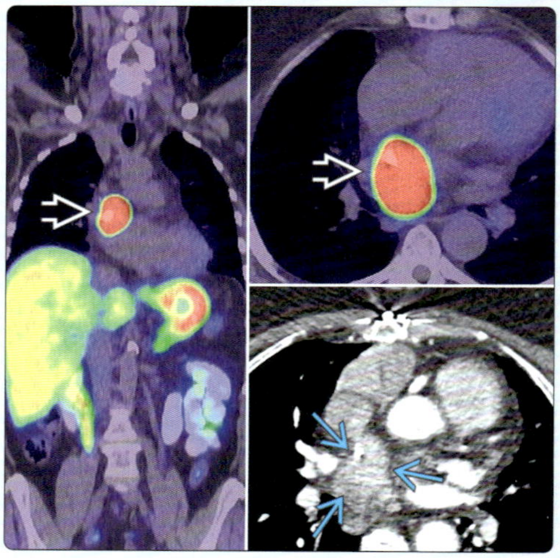

(Left) *Cardiac MR demonstrates a T2-hyperintense (left) and T1-isointense (right) mass ➡ wedged between the root of the aorta and the main pulmonary artery is a paraganglioma. There also was avid enhancement (not shown).* **(Right)** *Ga-68 DOTATATE scan and CT show avid uptake in a mass on the superior left atrium ➡. The cardiac CT reveals a vascular mass ➡ in the same region. Paragangliomas, targeted by DOTATATE, express high levels of somatostatin receptors.*

TERMINOLOGY

Synonyms

- Pheochromocytoma, cardiac neuroendocrine tumor

Definitions

- Tumors that arise from cardiac autonomic paraganglia
- 90% benign; ~ 1/3 hormonally active

IMAGING

General Features

- Best diagnostic clue
  - Invasive but well-defined hypervascular mass associated with atria &/or atrioventricular (AV) grooves
- Location
  - Posterior wall of left atrium or left atrial roof along AV grooves; interatrial septum; along coronary arteries; roots of aorta and pulmonary artery
    - More often project into pericardial space than atrial cavity
- Size
  - Any
- Morphology
  - Insinuating, hypervascular, relatively well defined

CT Findings

- Hypervascular, insinuating mass in characteristic location
- May have central hypodensity due to necrosis
- No fat or calcification

MR Findings

- T1 iso- to mildly hypointense; high signal due to hemorrhage; flow voids may be seen
- Light bulb sign: Intensely high signal in T2 spin-echo images
- Intense contrast enhancement; may contain areas of necrosis

Nuclear Medicine Findings

- Somatostatin receptor analogue nuclear studies can localize and stage these neoplasms
- In-111 octreotide or Ga-68 DOTA-PET: Highly specific
- I-131/I-123 MIBG scan: High false-negative rate
- F-18 FDG PET is specific for primary tumor and metastasis

Imaging Recommendations

- Best imaging tool
  - CT or MR can show intensely enhancing mass
- Protocol advice
  - Cover entire chest to look for additional lesions along sympathetic chains

DIFFERENTIAL DIAGNOSIS

Hemangioma

- Benign vascular neoplasm; more common in ventricles
- High T2 signal, heterogeneous enhancement

Angiosarcoma

- Malignant tumor with infiltrative features
- More common in right atrium

Metastases

- Nodular lesions or masses or pericardial effusion

PATHOLOGY

General Features

- Genetics
  - Usually sporadic
  - 1/4-1/3 are familial
- Groups of epithelioid cells arranged in organoid fashion with nests, cords, and trabeculae

Gross Pathologic & Surgical Features

- Encapsulated or infiltrative; tumors have to be "cut" out rather than "shelled" out
- Highly vascular tumors at risk of blood loss
- Highly vascular stroma with chief cells and sustentacular cells

CLINICAL ISSUES

Presentation

- Most common signs/symptoms
  - Often are incidental findings and asymptomatic
  - Symptoms from catecholamine production, such as hypertension, headache, or flushing
- Other signs/symptoms
  - Palpitations, syncope

Demographics

- Usually ~ 3rd and 4th decades of life

Natural History & Prognosis

- Complete resection can be curative
- There is risk of developing additional tumors in patients with specific genetic mutations, such as *SDHB*
- Up to 20% of patients also have associated synchronous paragangliomas in other locations
- There are reports of metastatic spread

Treatment

- Surgical resection; catecholamine blockade may be helpful

DIAGNOSTIC CHECKLIST

Consider

- High-resolution images with 3D anatomic modeling may help surgeon to visualize and plan approach

Image Interpretation Pearls

- Hypervascular, insinuating, but well-defined mass involving atria &/or AV grooves

Reporting Tips

- Describe any large feeding vessels, involvement of coronary arteries or other structures
- Try to visualize defect that would be left if tumor were cut out and describe location and size

SELECTED REFERENCES

1. Punzo B et al: Advanced imaging of cardiac paraganglioma: a systematic review. Int J Cardiol Heart Vasc. 53:101437, 2024
2. Carvalho JG et al: Multimodality imaging of cardiac paragangliomas. Radiol Cardiothorac Imaging. 5(4):e230049, 2023

KEY FACTS

TERMINOLOGY

- Hamartoma of developing cardiac myocytes
- Most common primary benign cardiac tumor in pediatric patients, highly associated with tuberous sclerosis
- 50% of solitary tumors and 100% of multiple tumors are associated with tuberous sclerosis

IMAGING

- Almost always arise in ventricular myocardium; may prolapse into ventricular cavity
- Echocardiography: 1st-line test; echogenic mass
- CT: Isoattenuating to adjacent myocardium with minimal or no differential contrast enhancement
- May also see fatty intramyocardial lesions in tuberous sclerosis
- MR: Homogeneous and well-circumscribed masses
    - T1: Isointense; T2: Slightly hyperintense; perfusion: Hypointense; delayed enhancement: Isointense
- Echocardiography and MR: Complementary imaging modalities
- Echocardiography: Better for small (< 5-mm) or completely intramural lesions
- MR: Better for intracavitary lesions and extracardiac extension

TOP DIFFERENTIAL DIAGNOSES

- Fibroma; myxoma; myocardial fatty foci in tuberous sclerosis; thrombus

CLINICAL ISSUES

- Almost all will spontaneously regress as child ages and can be managed conservatively
    - Frequently associated with tuberous sclerosis
- Most will be followed to document regression, usually with echocardiography but occasionally with MR if better seen by that modality

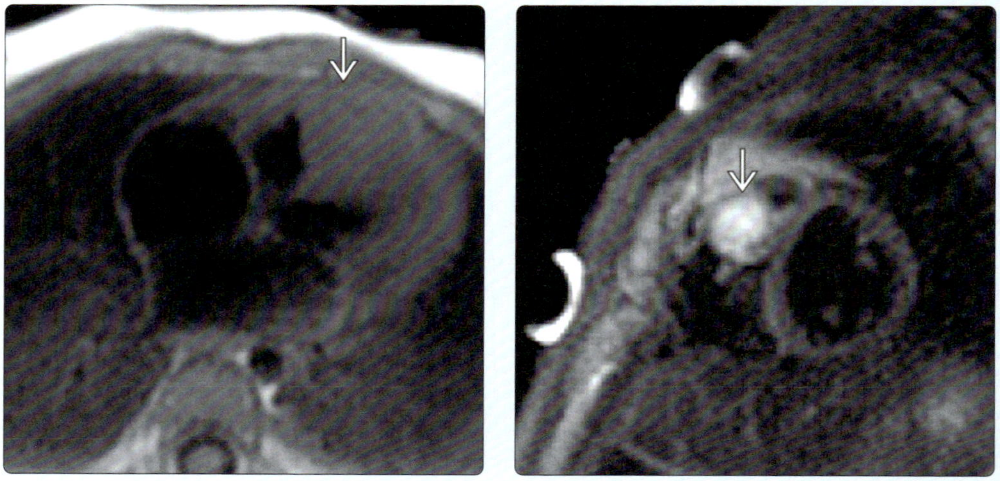

(Left) *Axial T1-weighted MR through the heart shows a large, well-defined right ventricular (RV) mass ➔, which is isointense to the myocardium.* **(Right)** *Short-axis T2-weighted MR in the same patient shows a well-circumscribed, hyperintense mass in the right ventricle ➔. MR is better than echocardiography for the identification of the intracavitary mass and extracardiac extension of the mass.*

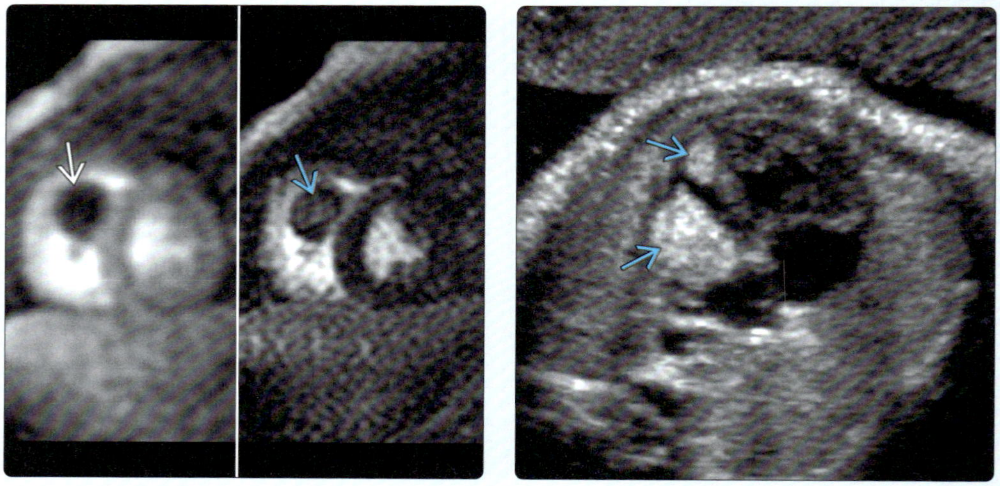

(Left) *MR perfusion (left) and LGE (right) images in the same patient demonstrate no significant perfusion ➔ or delayed enhancement ➙ in the mass. Rhabdomyomas are the most common primary benign cardiac tumor in pediatric patients.* **(Right)** *Prenatal US shows 2 echogenic RV masses ➙ due to rhabdomyomas. The patient was diagnosed with tuberous sclerosis after birth. (Courtesy S. Kligerman, MD.)*

TERMINOLOGY

Synonyms

- Cardiac hamartoma

Definitions

- Hamartoma of developing cardiac myocytes
  - Most common primary benign cardiac tumor in pediatric patients, highly associated with tuberous sclerosis

IMAGING

General Features

- Best diagnostic clue
  - Pediatric myocardial tumor with homogeneous signal (more common in patients with tuberous sclerosis)
- Location
  - Usually attached to myocardium
  - Intramyocardial or intracavitary; can result in flow obstruction
- Morphology
  - Generally well circumscribed
  - Solitary or multiple
    - 50% of solitary tumors and 100% of multiple tumors are associated with tuberous sclerosis
  - Homogeneous; may have fatty degeneration

CT Findings

- Isoattenuating to adjacent myocardium with minimal or no differential contrast enhancement
- Ventricular wall or intracavitary
- May demonstrate fatty degeneration
- Fatty lesions and pseudolesions may be associated in tuberous sclerosis
  - Ventricular septum, free wall of left ventricle/right ventricle (LV/RV), papillary muscles

MR Findings

- Well-circumscribed and homogeneous masses
- Almost always arise in ventricular myocardium; may prolapse into ventricular cavity
- T1: Isointense to myocardium; T2: Mildly hyperintense
- Perfusion: Hypointense to myocardium
- Delayed enhancement: Isointense to myocardium
- MR is better than echocardiography for intracavitary lesions and for determining extracardiac extension
- Myocardial fatty foci (MFF) in tuberous sclerosis
  - High T1 and T2 with fat saturation; chemical shift in SSFP

Echocardiographic Findings

- Homogeneous, echogenic, intramyocardial, or intracavitary mass(es)

Imaging Recommendations

- Best imaging tool
  - Echocardiography and MR: Complementary imaging modalities
  - Echocardiography: Better for small (< 5-mm) or completely intramural lesions
  - MR: Better for intracavitary lesions and extracardiac extension

DIFFERENTIAL DIAGNOSIS

Fibroma

- Solitary, well-defined, intramyocardial tumor
- Septum or free wall; may have calcification; large size
- Heterogeneous; T1: Isointense with hypointense core; delayed enhancement with central hypointense core

Myxoma

- More common in left atrium, attached to fossa ovalis
- Lobulated with heterogeneous signal
- Typically hyperintense in T2 images

Myocardial Fatty Foci in Tuberous Sclerosis

- Also common in patients with tuberous sclerosis
- Follow fat signal on MR and attenuation on CT

PATHOLOGY

Staging, Grading, & Classification

- Rhabdomyomas are seen in 50% of tuberous sclerosis

Gross Pathologic & Surgical Features

- Usually characterized by nodules of rounded myocytes with large vacuoles and strands of glycogen-rich cytoplasm

CLINICAL ISSUES

Presentation

- Most common signs/symptoms
  - Typically asymptomatic, incidental imaging finding
  - May present with obstruction of ventricular outflow or inflow (former more common); arrhythmia; heart failure
- Other signs/symptoms
  - Fetal tumors: May have stillbirth or hydrops fetalis

Demographics

- Usually discovered in fetal imaging or infants or small children
- Very rare in patients > 6 years of age

Natural History & Prognosis

- Partial or complete spontaneous regression in fetal life or before 6 years of age
- Worse prognosis: Large tumor size (> 2 cm); arrhythmia; hydrops

Treatment

- Surgical resection in patients with complications: Outflow obstruction or arrhythmia
  - Good prognosis after excision

DIAGNOSTIC CHECKLIST

Consider

- Looking for other signs of tuberous sclerosis

SELECTED REFERENCES

1. Morin CE et al: Imaging of pediatric cardiac tumors: a COG Diagnostic Imaging Committee/SPR Oncology Committee white paper. Pediatr Blood Cancer. 70 Suppl 4:e29955, 2023
2. Parato VM et al: Imaging of cardiac masses: an updated overview. J Cardiovasc Echogr. 32(2):65-75, 2022
3. Uysal SP et al: Tuberous sclerosis: a review of the past, present, and future. Turk J Med Sci. 50(SI-2):1665-76, 2020

Fibroma

KEY FACTS

TERMINOLOGY

- Fibrous hamartoma
- Benign congenital cardiac neoplasm composed of fibroblasts and abundant collagen

IMAGING

- Solitary myocardial mass most evident as area of altered contraction on cine imaging
- Most commonly arises in left ventricular free wall, interventricular septum, or right ventricular free wall
- Most often solid, well-defined mass
  - Less commonly has infiltrative appearance
- Calcifications seen in 15-20% on CT
- Isointense ventricular wall mass that does not show contraction on cine MR imaging
- Hypointense on T2WI in adults, particularly centrally
  - T2 hypointensity is very uncommon in any other cardiac tumor and strongly suggests fibroma when seen
- Late gadolinium enhancement (LGE) MR shows intense hyperenhancement
- MR perfusion imaging can help differentiate from aggressive lesions, as fibromas do not show enhancement on 1st-pass perfusion imaging

TOP DIFFERENTIAL DIAGNOSES

- Rhabdomyoma
- Hypertrophic cardiomyopathy
- Metastases
- Hemangioma
- Rhabdomyosarcoma

CLINICAL ISSUES

- 80% children; 20% adolescents and adults
- Surgical excision is treatment of choice
- Recurrence is uncommon even after incomplete resection
- Arrhythmias are common mode of presentation

(Left) *Axial graphic shows a large mass compressing both ventricles. Note its intramural location within the right ventricular (RV) free wall and solitary nature. These findings are typical of fibroma.* **(Right)** *Short-axis SSFP cine MR images in diastole (left) and systole (right) show a fibroma as a noncontractile mass ➡ arising in the anterior RV wall.*

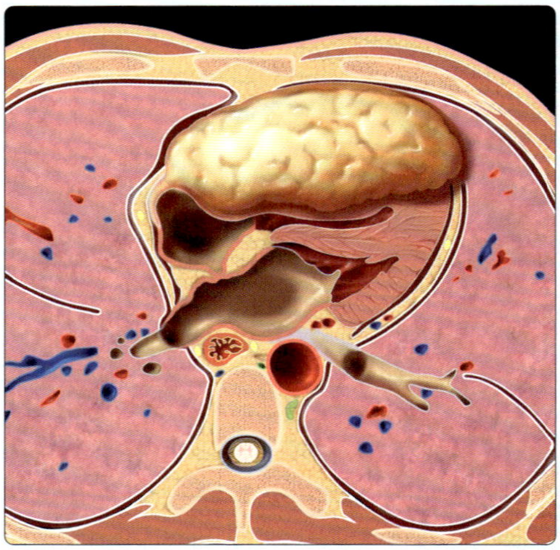

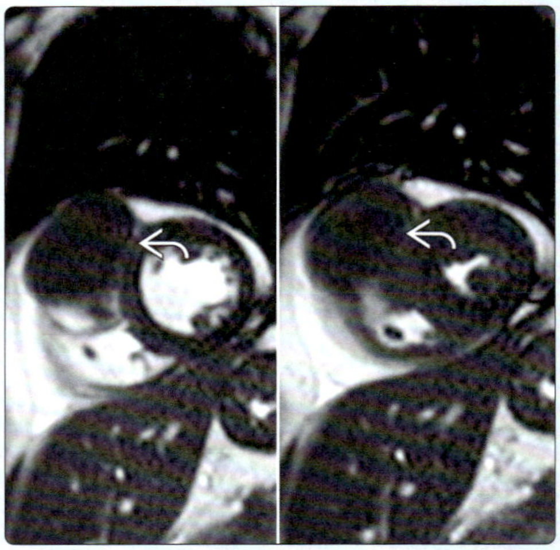

(Left) *Three-chamber cardiac-gated CT shows a large soft tissue mass within the left ventricular (LV) myocardium ➡. The mass is isodense to normal myocardium. Note the characteristic calcification ➡. Note also that the lesion is solitary and appears well defined with no associated pericardial effusion.* **(Right)** *Note the hypodense LV apical fibroma ➡ that extends adjacent to the left anterior descending coronary artery ➡, precluding total resection. Incomplete resection often proves sufficient.*

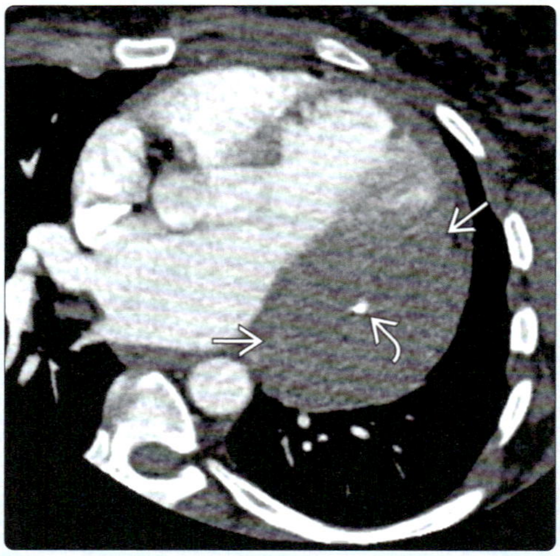

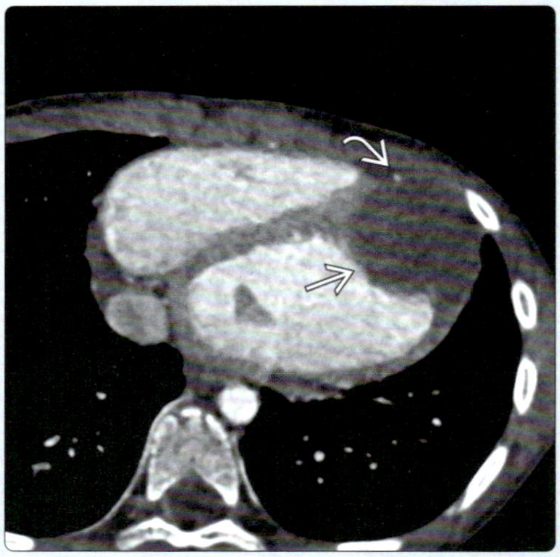

TERMINOLOGY

Synonyms

- Fibrous hamartoma

Definitions

- Benign congenital cardiac neoplasm composed of fibroblasts and abundant collagen

IMAGING

General Features

- Best diagnostic clue
  - Solitary myocardial mass most evident as area of altered contraction on cine imaging
- Location
  - Most commonly arises in left ventricular free wall, interventricular septum, or right ventricular free wall (in declining order)
    - Rare in atria
- Size
  - Diameter range: Typically 2-7 cm with mean of 5 cm in one pathology series
- Morphology
  - Most often solid, well-defined, oval mass
    - Less commonly has infiltrative appearance
    - Coarse calcifications seen in 15-20% on CT

Radiographic Findings

- Radiography
  - Cardiomegaly or focal bulge
  - Calcifications sometimes noted but less often than with CT

CT Findings

- NECT
  - Homogeneous mass; can have calcification
    - Solitary ventricular mass arising from myocardium with calcification strongly suggests diagnosis
- CECT
  - Heterogeneous enhancement

MR Findings

- T1WI
  - Isointense to myocardium
- T2WI
  - Often hypointense in adults, particularly centrally
    - T2 hypointensity is very uncommon in any other cardiac tumor and strongly suggests fibroma when seen
      - This is due to its extensive collagenous composition in adults
    - May be mildly T2 hyperintense in infants and children due to greater cellularity
  - T2 mapping can demonstrate low T2 values in lesion and are less subject to artifact than standard T2 images
- SSFP cine
  - Isointense ventricular wall mass that does not show contraction or deformity with contraction
- LGE
  - Shows intense LGE
    - Sometimes, may show peripheral enhancement with nonenhancing central core
- 1st-pass perfusion imaging
  - Fibromas do not usually show significant enhancement on 1st-pass perfusion imaging

Echocardiographic Findings

- Echocardiogram
  - Large, solid, noncontractile mass in myocardium
    - Calcification can be seen
    - May mimic focal hypertrophic cardiomyopathy

Imaging Recommendations

- Best imaging tool
  - Echocardiography is most often initially used for detection
  - MR is superior at tissue characterization
    - MR showing T2-hypointense, well-defined intramural ventricular mass with intense LGE is highly suggestive of fibroma
  - CT demonstrating intramural ventricular noncontractile mass containing calcification is also strongly suggestive of fibroma
- Protocol advice
  - LGE MR is very useful in differentiating from rhabdomyoma
    - Rhabdomyomas have similar low signal to normal myocardium on LGE imaging (whereas fibromas intensely enhance)
  - 1st-pass perfusion imaging is useful in differentiating from tumors that are more aggressive (e.g., metastases) or vascular (e.g., hemangiomas)

DIFFERENTIAL DIAGNOSIS

Rhabdomyoma

- Ventricular mass in young patients
  - At least 50% have tuberous sclerosis
  - Usually multiple (whereas fibroma is solitary lesion)
  - Does not calcify
- LGE MR shows signal intensity identical to normal myocardium (nulls or becomes dark), as opposed to intense enhancement of fibroma
- Often regresses spontaneously

Metastatic Disease

- Typically presents with multiple multifocal masses in patients with known primary malignancy
  - Multiplicity differentiates from fibroma, which is solitary lesion
- Most often isointense on T1, mildly hyperintense on T2, heterogeneous on LGE MR
- Often hypervascular on MR perfusion imaging (whereas fibroma is hypovascular)
- May be located anywhere (whereas fibroma is intramural and ventricular in origin)

Hypertrophic Cardiomyopathy

- Asymmetric septal variant can mimic focal mass
  - Some contraction may be evident on cine imaging
  - Isointense on T2 imaging (whereas fibroma is hypointense)

- LGE MR imaging shows characteristic right ventricular insertion site LGE or patchy midmyocardial LGE in majority of patients
- No calcification

Hemangioma

- When presenting as intramural mass, may simulate fibroma on CT and cine MR imaging
  - High signal on T2-weighted imaging is differentiating feature
    - Fibroma is classically hypointense on T2 imaging in adults and older children
  - Usually hypervascular on perfusion imaging (whereas fibroma is hypovascular)
  - Enhances intensely on LGE MR

Rhabdomyosarcoma

- Most common primary cardiac malignancy in childhood
- Large, heterogeneous, invasive mass that can occur anywhere in heart
- Shows poor boundary definition and infiltration on imaging

PATHOLOGY

General Features

- Etiology
  - May be hamartoma rather than neoplasm
- Genetics
  - When presenting as isolated abnormality, no defined genetic defect
- Associated abnormalities
  - Gorlin syndrome (a.k.a. basal cell nevus syndrome)
    - Premalignant condition with multisystem involvement
    - 4% of fibroma patients have Gorlin syndrome
    - 3% of Gorlin patients have fibromas

Gross Pathologic & Surgical Features

- Large, firm, white, fibrous masses within ventricular myocardium with discrete or (less commonly) infiltrative margins
  - 25% calcify
  - No necrosis, hemorrhage, or cystic change

Microscopic Features

- Infants
  - Fibroblast-rich (cellular) tumor with little collagen
    - May explain higher T2 signal that is often noted in infants and children
- Adolescents and adults
  - Predominantly collagenous
    - Abundance of collagen results in characteristic low signal on T2 MR imaging
    - Also likely explains marked hyperenhancement seen on LGE MR imaging
- Occasional mitoses, elastic tissue
- Even well-defined lesions on imaging may have microscopic foci of tumor interdigitation with normal myocardium
  - This may explain frequent occurrence of arrhythmias in patients with fibromas

CLINICAL ISSUES

Presentation

- Most common signs/symptoms
  - 1/3 present with arrhythmias or syncope
    - 2nd most common tumor associated with sudden death after atrioventricular node heterotopias
  - 1/3 present with heart failure or cyanosis
  - 1/3 of patients are asymptomatic, and lesion is discovered incidentally
- Other signs/symptoms
  - Lesions may result in murmurs due to disturbed flow

Demographics

- Age
  - 80-85% children; 15-20% adolescents and adults
    - Mean: 13 years
  - 1/3 are < 1 year at diagnosis
- Sex
  - No predilection
- Epidemiology
  - ~ 100 reported cases in 30 years

Natural History & Prognosis

- Can interfere with mechanical or electrical function
- Can be dormant; rarely regresses

Treatment

- Surgical excision is treatment of choice
  - Resection may necessarily be incomplete if tumor extensively involves ventricular wall or coronary arteries
  - Recurrence uncommon even after incomplete resection
- Controversial conservative approach if asymptomatic

DIAGNOSTIC CHECKLIST

Consider

- Fibroma in cases of solitary ventricular cardiac mass in child or adolescent

Image Interpretation Pearls

- Solitary ventricular mass
  - Dark on T2
  - Bright on LGE MR
  - Shows calcifications on CT

Reporting Tips

- Extent of ventricular myocardial involvement to determine resectability and reconstruction needed

SELECTED REFERENCES

1. Medina Perez M et al: Cardiac and pericardial neoplasms in children: radiologic-pathologic correlation. Radiographics. 43(9):e230010, 2023
2. Beroukhim RS et al: Accuracy of cardiac magnetic resonance imaging in diagnosing pediatric cardiac masses: a multicenter study. JACC Cardiovasc Imaging. 15(8):1391-405, 2022
3. Covington MK et al: Clinical impact of cardiac fibromas. Am J Cardiol. 182:95-103, 2022
4. Jones JP et al: Ventricular fibromas in children, arrhythmia risk, and outcomes: a multicenter study. Heart Rhythm. 15(10):1507-12, 2018
5. Tao TY et al: Pediatric cardiac tumors: clinical and imaging features. Radiographics. 34(4):1031-46, 2014
6. Araoz PA et al: CT and MR imaging of benign primary cardiac neoplasms with echocardiographic correlation. Radiographics. 20(5):1303-19, 2000

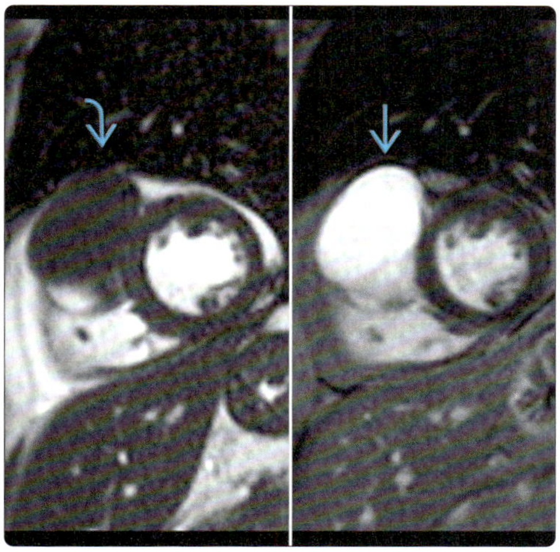

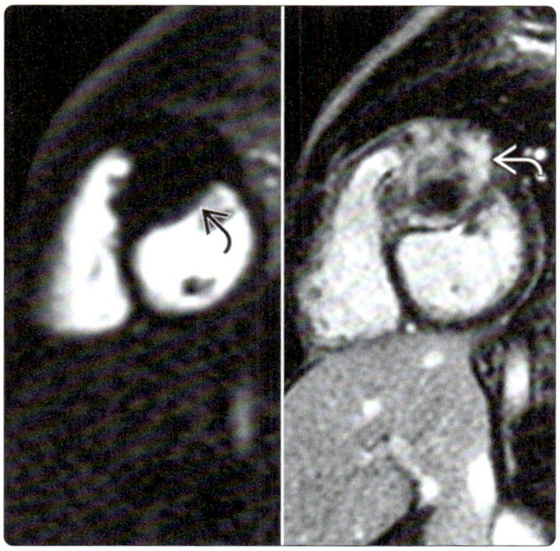

(Left) *Short-axis SSFP cine MR (left) demonstrates a well-defined, oval mass in the anterior RV representing a fibroma, which is isointense to the myocardium. Short-axis late gadolinium-enhanced (LGE) image (right) demonstrates characteristic intense hyperenhancement of the fibroma.* **(Right)** *MR perfusion (left) and LGE MR (right) of LV fibroma reveal absence of lesion hypervascularity on 1st-pass perfusion imaging and intense peripheral lesion enhancement on LGE MR with a central dark core.*

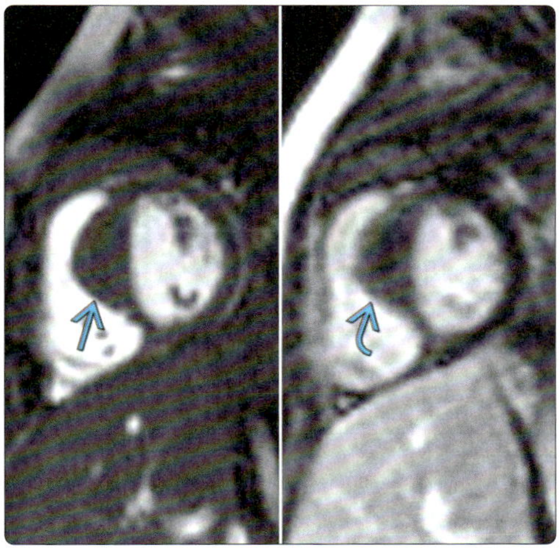

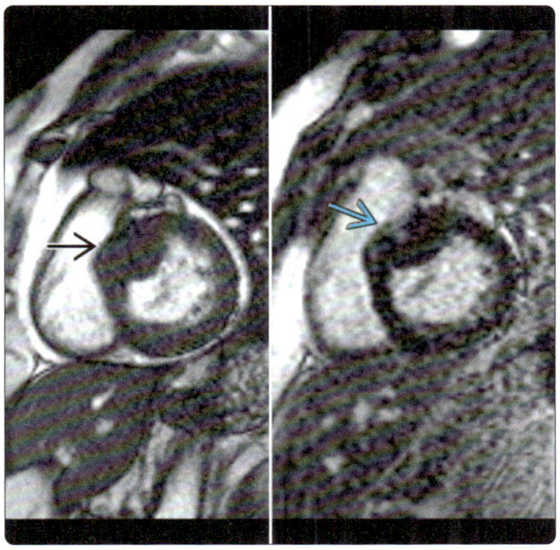

(Left) *Short-axis cine MR (left) shows a well-defined septal rhabdomyoma. LGE image (right) demonstrates that the rhabdomyoma nulls or has low signal similar to normal myocardium and different from enhancing fibromas.* **(Right)** *SAX cine (left) and LGE (right) MR images in a patient with asymmetric septal hypertrophic cardiomyopathy (HCM) resulting in a mass-like appearance are shown. Note the minimal enhancement of the septal insertion site, as commonly seen with HCM.*

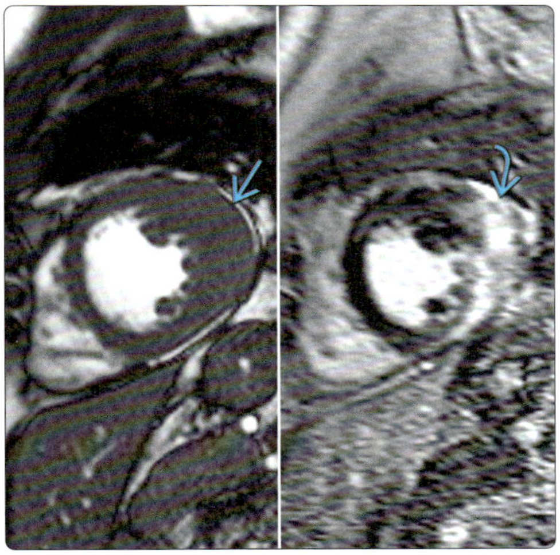

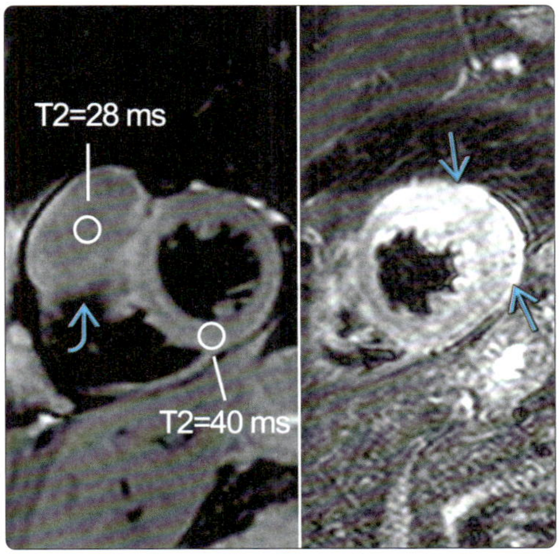

(Left) *Short-axis cine (left) and LGE (right) images show lymphoma infiltrating the lateral LV wall with poor border definition. LGE image shows typical heterogeneous enhancement.* **(Right)** *Short-axis T2-weighted images show a low T2 signal intensity fibroma (left) in the RV wall. Note that the lymphoma (right) infiltrating the LV lateral and anterior walls has high T2 signal. Fibroma T2 values were obtained with mapping technique.*

KEY FACTS

TERMINOLOGY

- Metastatic tumor deposition or extension of primary tumor into heart
- Metastases to heart occur via
  - Lymphatic spread
  - Direct extension
  - Hematogenous spread
  - Transvenous spread

IMAGING

- Initial manifestation may be lung, bone, or mediastinal metastases
- Pericardial effusion is common
- Mediastinal lymphadenopathy in 80% of cases of cardiac metastatic disease
- Pleural effusion in 50%
- Ascites
- Most metastases enhance with gadolinium

TOP DIFFERENTIAL DIAGNOSES

- Thrombus
- Primary cardiac neoplasm
  - Myxoma: Benign, most common
  - Malignant primary cardiac tumors are rare
- Myopericarditis

PATHOLOGY

- Immunohistochemical markers may be needed to distinguish from primary cardiac osteosarcoma

CLINICAL ISSUES

- Very poor prognosis

DIAGNOSTIC CHECKLIST

- Malignant pericardial effusion is often 1st sign of cardiac or pericardial metastatic disease
- Assess for signs of cardiac tamponade and coronary artery involvement

(Left) *Echocardiogram images show an echogenic mass in the right atrioventricular groove (AVG) invading into the right ventricle (RV) and right atrium (RA). A pericardial effusion (PEff) is present.* **(Right)** *Arterial (top left) and portal venous (top right) cardiac CTA images show the AVG mass encasing the right coronary artery and invading into the RA and RV. A nodular, metastatic PEff is seen. There is an incidental pulmonary embolus. The mass is isointense to myocardium on SSFP MR images (bottom).*

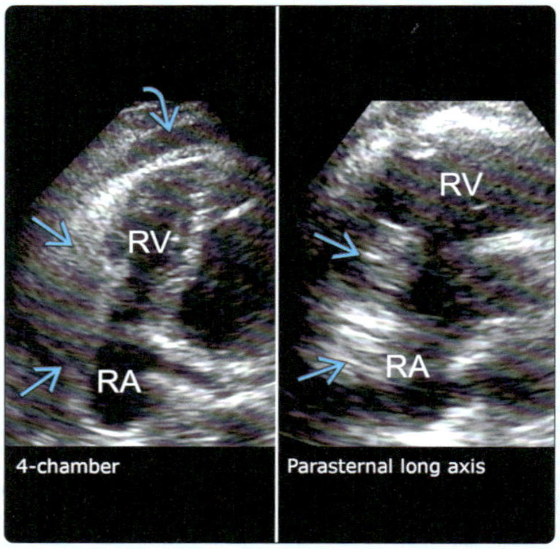

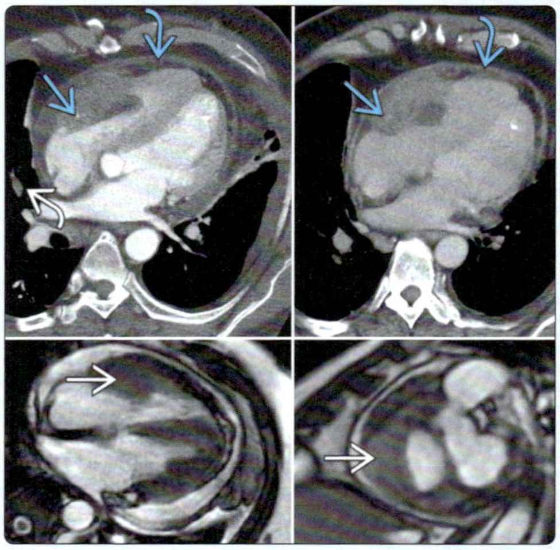

(Left) *Four-chamber CT (left) and PET/CT fused (right) images in the same patient show intense FDG uptake in the AVG mass and metastatic PEff. A large left external iliac lymph node shows intense FDG uptake. Biopsy of both lesions showed metastatic squamous cell carcinoma from a previous treated skin primary.* **(Right)** *Axial CT in a patient with metastatic melanoma shows a heterogeneously enhancing RA mass. Multiple subcutaneous and enhancing pulmonary metastases are present.*

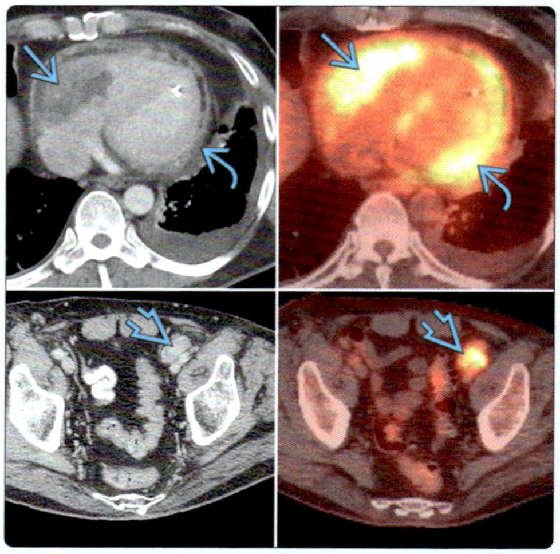

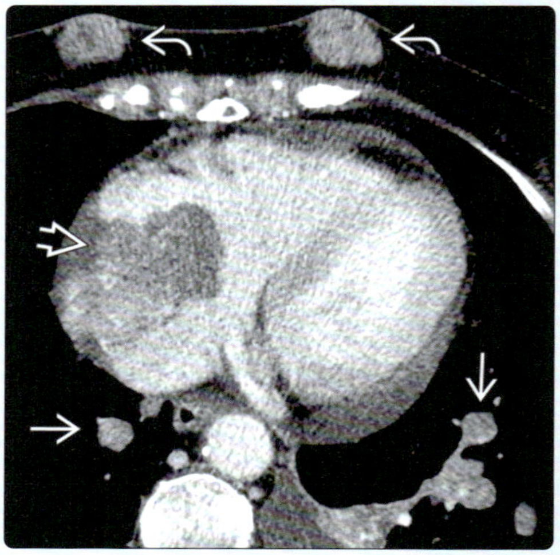

TERMINOLOGY

Definitions

- Metastatic tumor deposition or extension of primary tumor into heart
- Metastases to heart occur via
  - Lymphatic spread: Most common route; lung and breast cancer
  - Hematogenous spread: Typically melanoma
  - Direct extension: Usually lung cancer and thoracic malignancies; rarely mesothelioma
  - Transvenous spread: Several sources
    - Inferior vena cava (IVC): Hepatic, renal, adrenal, or pelvic tumors
    - Superior vena cava (SVC): Lung cancer; mediastinal tumors
    - Pulmonary veins: Lung cancer or metastases

IMAGING

General Features

- Best diagnostic clue
  - Pathologically, metastatic disease is 40x more common than primary cardiac tumor
  - Presence of multiple masses favors metastatic disease
  - Often associated with malignant pericardial effusion
- Location
  - Right atrium (RA) and right ventricle (RV) much more commonly affected than left atrium (LA) and left ventricle (LV)
  - Epicardium is most commonly affected layer
- Morphology
  - Often infiltrative or grows into cardiac chamber

Radiographic Findings

- Radiography
  - Frequently normal
  - Initial manifestation may be lung, bone, or mediastinal metastases
  - May mimic valvular heart disease
  - Cardiac silhouette enlargement (may be irregular) indicating pericardial effusion or cardiomegaly
    - Pericardial effusion may be diffuse or loculated
    - Cardiomegaly may be from mass(es) or chamber enlargement secondary to obstruction
  - Mediastinal lymphadenopathy in 80% of cases of cardiac metastatic disease
  - Secondary findings
    - Pulmonary edema, pleural effusion (50%), ascites
  - Rarely calcification (osteosarcoma metastasis)

CT Findings

- NECT
  - Massive cardiac involvement may lead to chamber enlargement
  - Calcifications are rare except in certain tumors
    - Osteosarcoma, chondrosarcoma
    - Tumors with psammomatous calcification
  - Fat in liposarcoma metastases
  - Associated signs of malignancy
    - Lung and bone metastases
    - Lymphadenopathy
    - Pericardial and pleural effusions
- CTA
  - Invasion of myocardium, pericardium, coronary arteries, valves, and mediastinal structures
  - Diffuse involvement or focal lesion
  - May better demonstrate solid and cystic components, hypervascular components, calcification
  - Lesions may be more conspicuous on portal venous-phase imaging
  - Metastases may enhance differently relative to myocardium
  - Can visualize direct invasion of lung cancer via pulmonary veins
  - Extension of renal or adrenal mass into RA via IVC
    - Inhomogeneous mixing of contrast-opacified and nonopacified blood in IVC may mimic tumor thrombus
    - Delayed imaging is essential
  - Retrospective cardiac gating may demonstrate valvular impairment from metastases
  - Perfusion or dual-energy CT can be used to assess biologic response to therapy

MR Findings

- T1WI
  - Usually slightly hypointense to myocardium
  - Melanoma and hemorrhagic metastases may be hyperintense on T1WI
- T2WI
  - High signal intensity relative to myocardium
- T1WI C+
  - Most metastases enhance with gadolinium
    - 1st pass and delayed enhancement should be performed
    - More sensitive than CT for lower grade enhancement
  - Differentiation from thrombus (chronic thrombus may appear to enhance peripherally)
    - Recommend delayed enhancement sequences with long inversion time (TI = 600 ms)
- Tissue characterization with fat-saturated images, diffusion, T2WI, and T1WI pre- and postcontrast administration
  - Some primary cardiac tumors (e.g., myxoma, fibroma) have typical MR properties
- Better assessment of subtle lesions and tissue invasion
  - Superior contrast resolution allows better detection of metastatic foci
- High signal intensity filling defects on T1W black-blood images when tumor invades chamber
  - Slow flow may artificially cause high-signal pseudofilling defects
- May detect and quantify hemodynamic consequences
  - Obstruction of RA inflow, pulmonary veins, RV or LV outflow tracts, or atrioventricular valves
  - Valvular regurgitation due to tumor infiltration
- MR findings associated with malignancy
  - 1 point: Sessile appearance, polylobate shape, pericardial effusion, heterogeneous enhancement
  - 2 points: Tumor infiltration, 1st-pass perfusion
  - MR mass score ≥ 5 has AUC = 0.976 for predicting malignant cardiac tumor
    - Does not differentiate between 1° tumors and mets

Echocardiographic Findings

- Echocardiogram
  - Recommended for initial evaluation of suspected pericardial effusion
    - Pericardial effusion in 50% of cases
  - No positive findings in 25%
  - Mass or myocardial thickening in 40%
  - May demonstrate associated thrombus
  - TTE often limited by acoustic window

Nuclear Medicine Findings

- PET/CT
  - Metastatic foci typically show increased FDG uptake vs. myocardium

Imaging Recommendations

- Best imaging tool
  - Echocardiography: Usually 1st imaging modality
  - Cardiac MR: Better assessment of extent of disease, low-level enhancement, and cardiac function
    - Superior contrast resolution increases sensitivity for metastatic foci and soft tissue invasion
  - CT: Best spatial resolution and anatomic delineation
- Protocol advice
  - CT scan with 90-second delay or MR can distinguish IVC tumor from contrast mixing artifact
  - Obtain comparable pre-and postcontrast MR images
  - Choose conventional cardiac imaging plane that best shows mass, then image 3 orthogonal planes

DIFFERENTIAL DIAGNOSIS

Thrombus

- Most commonly in atria and in areas of akinesia/dyskinesia
- Noninvasive, no true enhancement

Atrial Myxoma

- Most common benign primary tumor
- Typically in LA, attachment near foramen ovale

Other Primary Benign Tumors

- Rhabdomyoma, hemangioma, etc.

Primary Malignant Tumors

- Sarcomas, primary cardiac lymphoma, etc.
  - Very rare
  - May mimic metastases
  - Disease beyond heart and pericardial often absent

Myopericarditis

- Infectious, inflammatory, drug or radiation induced
- May cause enhancing, nodular pericardium, and epicardial enhancement on MR, mimicking metastases

PATHOLOGY

General Features

- Etiology
  - Most common neoplasms metastatic to heart and pericardium: Lung, breast, melanoma, lymphoma
  - Lung cancer: Primary tumor in 36% of patients with cardiac metastases
  - Leukemia and lymphoma: Primary malignancy in 20%
  - Malignant melanoma and lymphoma: Have highest propensity to metastasize to heart
- Associated abnormalities
  - Malignant pericardial effusions are overwhelmingly secondary to metastases
  - Extracardiac metastases are typically present
- Epicardium is most often involved with metastases

Gross Pathologic & Surgical Features

- Multiple infiltrating masses in epicardium, myocardium, and endocardium
- > 90% are epithelial in origin (e.g., lung, breast)
- Frequently associated sanguineous pericardial effusion

Microscopic Features

- Immune markers can help discriminate among different cell types
- Psammoma bodies in lung and ovarian cancers
- Osteosarcoma metastases are unique in that they contain bone elements
  - Calcium may not be readily visible on MR (signal voids)

CLINICAL ISSUES

Presentation

- Most common signs/symptoms
  - Asymptomatic in 50% of cases
- Other signs/symptoms
  - Obstructive symptoms depending on area of flow obstruction
  - Tamponade from malignant effusion or compressing tumor mass
  - Signs of heart failure

Demographics

- Epidemiology
  - 20-40x more frequent than primary cardiac neoplasms

Natural History & Prognosis

- Very poor prognosis

Treatment

- Palliative surgery, chemotherapy, or radiation
- Treatment of cardiac tamponade from malignant pericardial effusion

DIAGNOSTIC CHECKLIST

Image Interpretation Pearls

- Malignant pericardial effusion is often 1st sign of cardiac or pericardial metastatic disease
- Assess for signs of cardiac tamponade and coronary artery involvement
- Chronic thrombus may appear to enhance peripherally, mimicking cardiac mass

SELECTED REFERENCES

1. Lorca MC et al: Radiologic-pathologic correlation of cardiac tumors: updated 2021 WHO tumor classification. Radiographics. 44(6):e230126, 2024
2. Paolisso P et al: Cardiac magnetic resonance to predict cardiac mass malignancy: the CMR mass score. Circ Cardiovasc Imaging. 17(3):e016115, 2024
3. Lichtenberger JP 3rd et al: MR imaging of cardiac masses. Top Magn Reson Imaging. 27(2):103-11, 2018

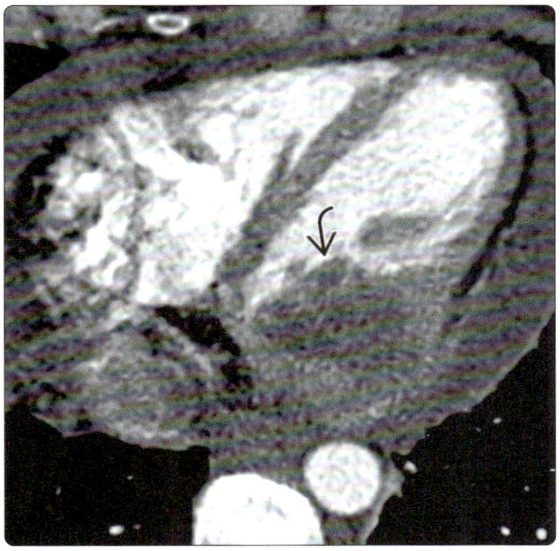

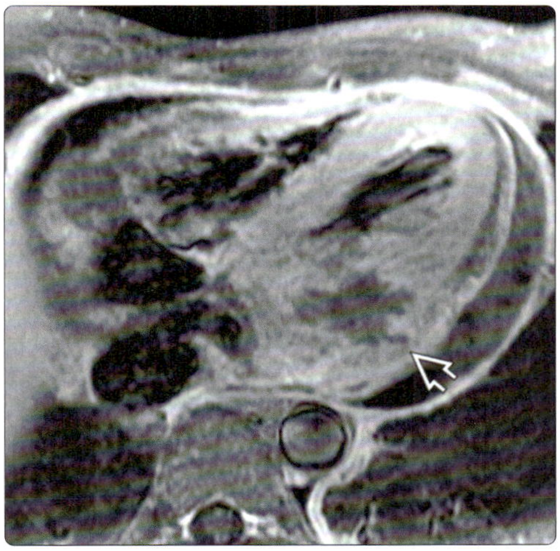

(Left) *Axial cardiac gated CT in a patient with metastatic sarcoma shows a centrally necrotic, enhancing mass of the inferolateral left ventricular wall with a large PEff.* **(Right)** *Axial T1 C+ FS MR in the same patient shows peripheral enhancement in the mass as well as diffuse pericardial enhancement, indicating a malignant PEff. PEff is often associated with malignant involvement of the heart.*

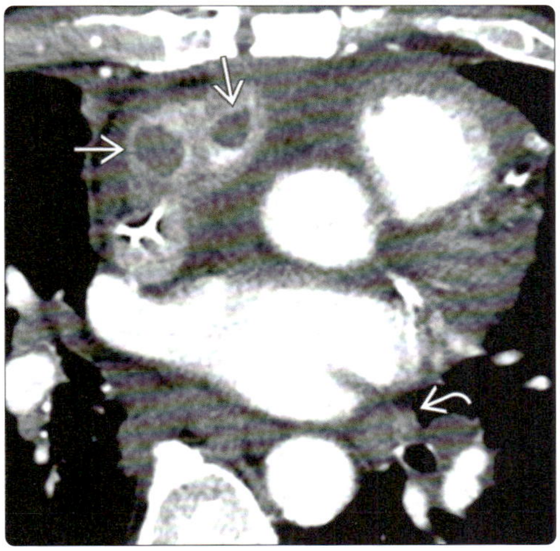

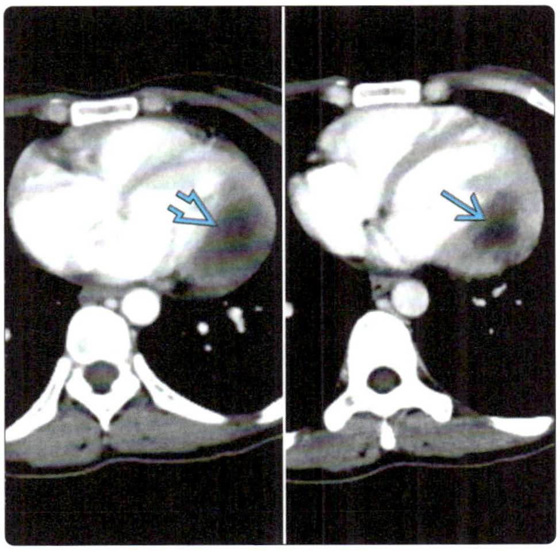

(Left) *Axial ECG gated CTA in a patient with metastatic pancreatic cancer shows low-attenuation masses in the right atrial appendage. Multiple cardiac masses favor metastatic disease. Lymphadenopathy and PEff are also present.* **(Right)** *Axial CECT during the arterial phase (left) in a young woman with cervical cancer shows a large left ventricular mass with central hypoattenuation and peripheral enhancement. At 45-second delay (right), peripheral enhancement increases with likely central necrosis.*

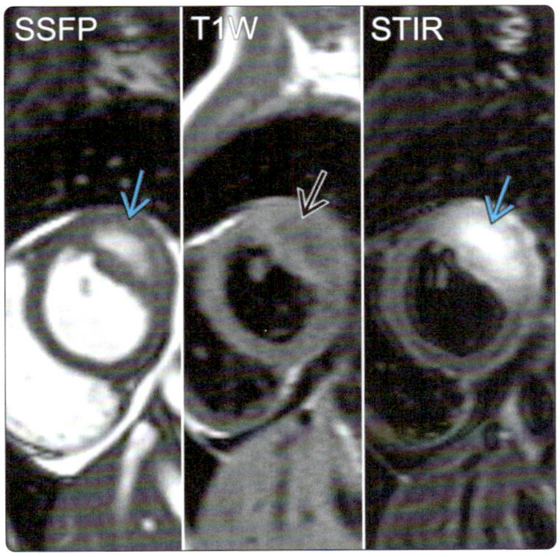

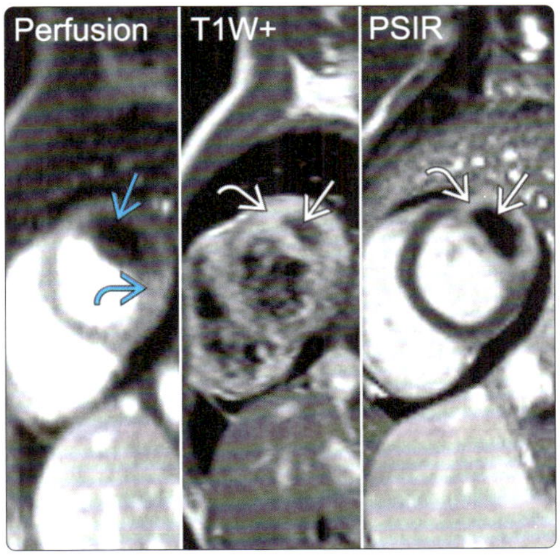

(Left) *Short-axis SSFP (left) and STIR (right) MR images in the same patient show central hyperintensity within the mass with more mild peripheral hyperintensity. T1 MR (center) shows the mass is centrally hypointense with mild peripheral hyperintensity.* **(Right)** *Perfusion MR (left) shows a large area of central hypoperfusion with mild rim perfusion. On T1W+ (center) and PSIR LGE (right) images, the peripheral enhancement and central necrosis are well delineated.*

Tumor Extension Into Atria

KEY FACTS

TERMINOLOGY

- Extracardiac tumor invading atria, typically through growth along venous structures

IMAGING

- Radiography
  - Findings mimic congestive heart failure
  - Enlargement of cardiac silhouette: Chamber dilation or pericardial effusion
- CT: Retrospectively gated cardiac CTA may show valvular involvement or prolapse into ventricle
- Cardiac MR: Best tool to differentiate bland thrombus from tumor thrombus
- Balanced cine SSFP: May show valvular involvement or prolapse into ventricle during cardiac cycle
- Imaging or reformatting in several planes is important in avoiding artifact and in surgical planning

TOP DIFFERENTIAL DIAGNOSES

- Thrombus
- Pseudothrombosis
- Myxoma
- Other primary cardiac tumors

CLINICAL ISSUES

- Heart failure, edema, dyspnea
- Syncope, arrhythmia

DIAGNOSTIC CHECKLIST

- Evaluate for associated bland thrombus, as intraatrial tumors disrupt flow dynamics
- Tumor extension into atria will often alter surgical planning and complicate radiation therapy
- Valvular involvement is important for operative planning

(Left) *Axial ECG gated CTA in a patient with pelvic leiomyosarcoma shows a lobulated mass extending through the inferior vena cava (IVC) into the right atrium. Note internal vascularity. This mass prolapses through the tricuspid valve into the right ventricle, and there is right heart enlargement.* **(Right)** *Axial CECT of the abdomen in the same patient shows the sarcoma invading the IVC. Delayed scan can differentiate a mass from a contrast mixing artifact.*

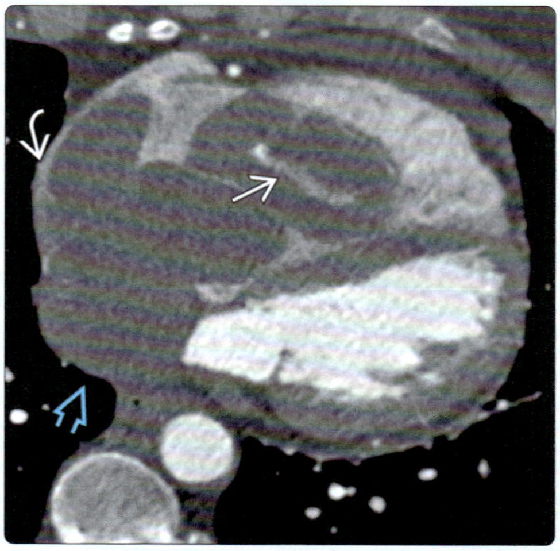

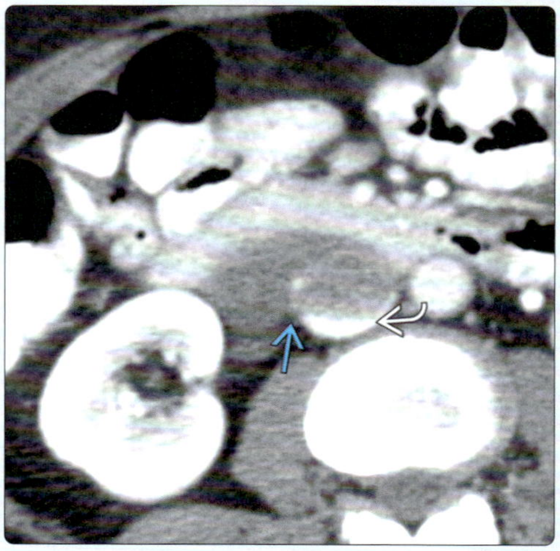

(Left) *Axial CECT in a patient with lung cancer shows a centrally necrotic pulmonary mass in the right middle lobe. Note the direct transvenous mass extension via right pulmonary veins into the left atrium.* **(Right)** *Sagittal CECT reformation in a patient with metastatic pancreatic cancer shows a tumor thrombus ascending into the right atrium via the IVC. Imaging or reformatting in multiple planes may help to avoid an artifact and can facilitate surgical planning in cases of a resectable tumor.*

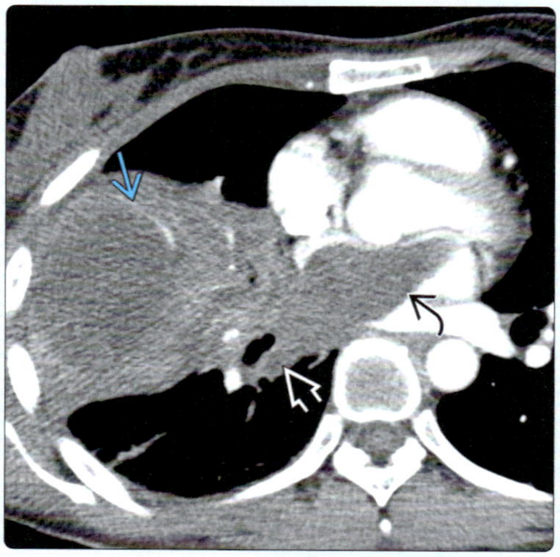

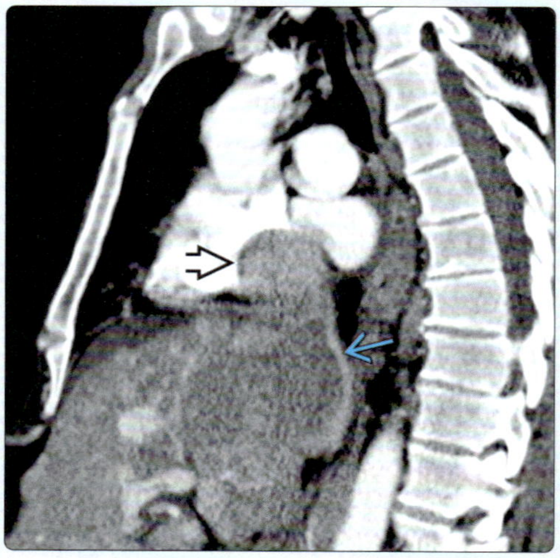

TERMINOLOGY

Synonyms

- Transvenous cardiac metastasis
- Cavoatrial extension

Definitions

- Extracardiac tumor invading atria, typically through growth along venous structures

IMAGING

General Features

- Best diagnostic clue
  - Intraatrial mass contiguous with extracardiac mass
- Location
  - Typically exophytic within atrial chamber
  - Transvenous extension of tumor from several sources
    - Superior vena cava (SVC): Lung cancer, mediastinal tumors
    - Inferior vena cava (IVC): Hepatic, renal, and adrenal tumors
    - Pulmonary veins: Lung cancer, pulmonary metastases
- Morphology
  - Tumor thrombus typically fills and expands involved venous structure
  - Tumors extending into atria often protrude into chamber and appear lobulated or pedunculated

Radiographic Findings

- Enlargement of cardiac silhouette may be secondary to chamber dilation from outflow obstruction or pericardial effusion
- Findings (e.g., pulmonary edema, pleural effusions) may mimic congestive heart failure

CT Findings

- NECT
  - Tumor thrombus is not well evaluated on NECT
  - Intravenous tumor may expand vein
  - Atrial dilation may occur if mass causes outflow obstruction
  - Primary mass may be detected
  - Portal vein enlargement and ascites
- CECT
  - Delayed phases (90 s) are needed for optimal right heart visualization
  - Better evaluation than NECT of both primary tumor and tumor extension into atria
  - May depict vascularity or enhancement of tumor thrombus
  - Massive collateral varices may enhance
- CTA
  - Allows detection of pulmonary emboli
- Cardiac gated CTA
  - May show valvular involvement or prolapse into ventricle during cardiac cycle if retrospectively gated
- Dual-energy CT
  - High iodine uptake in tumor thrombus than bland thrombus

MR Findings

- T1WI
  - Intraatrial tumor thrombus is typically hypointense relative to myocardium
- T2WI
  - Triple-inversion recovery images assess for edema or necrosis within tumor thrombus
- MRV
  - Evaluates intraluminal extent of disease
- Cine SSFP
  - Intraatrial mass may be pedunculated
  - May show valvular involvement or prolapse into ventricle during cardiac cycle
  - High spatial resolution images are useful for mobile, intrachamber masses
- 1st-pass perfusion may demonstrate vascularity
- LGE
  - Gadolinium may accumulate in regions of necrosis or fibrosis in tumor or as result of hyperemia of tumor
  - Tumor enhancement is important in differentiating tumor from bland thrombus that may be associated
- High inversion time (600-800 ms) turbo-type spoiled gradient-echo single-shot magnitude images may differentiate bland thrombus from tumor
  - Signal from bland thrombus is nulled at high inversion times
- Parametric mapping
  - Native T1 mapping shows intermediate values for bland thrombus; high values for tumor

Imaging Recommendations

- Best imaging tool
  - Transesophageal echocardiography (TEE) is often 1st study to evaluate IVC and atrial extension
  - Cardiac MR is best tool to differentiate bland thrombus from tumor thrombus
- Protocol advice
  - Imaging or reformatting in several planes is important in avoiding artifact and in surgical planning
  - Cine imaging is important to depict apparent attachment to atrial wall
  - Consider 2-minute delayed CT imaging or MR if venous contrast mixing artifact is possibility
  - MR: Dynamic perfusion, delayed enhancement, and MRV may help in differentiating bland thrombus from tumor thrombus and in defining exact anatomic boundaries of tumor

Echocardiographic Findings

- TEE is 1st imaging choice in suspected right atrial tumor extension
- May be contraindicated in cases complicated by significant esophageal varices

DIFFERENTIAL DIAGNOSIS

Thrombus

- Atrial fibrillation (left atrium) and central venous catheters (right atrium) are common causes
- Predilection for left atrial appendage in atrial fibrillation
- Myocardial scars are independent risk factors for intracardiac thrombus formation

- Intrachamber tumors may have associated bland thrombus

Pseudothrombosis

- Inhomogeneous mixing of contrast-opacified and nonopacified blood in IVC and right atrium may mimic mass on CT
- 2-minute delayed CT or MR for confirmation
- Higher iodine uptake than thrombus
- Characteristic laminar flow pattern from renal veins

Myxoma

- Most common primary cardiac tumor
- Typically located in left atrium, although location and morphology vary
- Characteristic stalk-like attachment to interatrial septum near foramen ovale

Other Primary Cardiac Tumors

- Malignant primary cardiac tumors are very rare
  - Sarcomas most commonly arise from right heart and may invade venous structures
  - Leiomyosarcoma is usually sessile and originates from posterior wall of left atrium, frequently invading pulmonary veins

Pseudolipoma

- Pseudolesion of IVC from pericaval fat above caudate lobe
- More common in chronic liver disease

PATHOLOGY

General Features

- Associated abnormalities
  - Tumor emboli to lungs may occur
  - Deep venous thrombosis

Staging, Grading, & Classification

- Varying amounts of penetration into walls of IVC and cardiac structures
- Tumor extension into atria typically indicates stage III or IV disease
  - Renal cell carcinoma (RCC): Spread into large veins to heart is T3c or stage III, although tumor invasion into cardiac structures may be considered stage IV
  - Lung cancer: Left atrial involvement is T4 disease, stage IIIB
    - 5-year survival rates from resection of selective locally invasive tumors: ~ 10-30%

CLINICAL ISSUES

Presentation

- Most common signs/symptoms
  - May remain asymptomatic until obstruction occurs
  - Syncope
  - Heart failure, edema, dyspnea
  - Stroke
  - Pansystolic murmur, diastolic rumble of tricuspid valve
- Other signs/symptoms
  - Budd-Chiari syndrome, ascites, hepatomegaly
  - SVC syndrome is possible
  - Symptoms may improve with left lateral decubitus position
  - Abdominal pain, anorexia, weight loss

Demographics

- Epidemiology
  - Intracardiac extension of tumors overall is rare
  - Most common tumors include
    - RCC
      - Most common cause of transvenous metastatic disease to heart
      - 4-10% have tumor thrombus; 1% has extension into right atrium
    - Hepatocellular carcinoma (HCC)
      - 2% have transvenous atrial extension at autopsy
    - Lung cancer
    - Adrenocortical carcinoma
    - Uterine cancers
    - Mediastinal masses
      - Thymic tumors
      - Thyroid carcinoma has also been reported
    - Vascular origin tumors
      - Leiomyoma, leiomyosarcoma

Natural History & Prognosis

- Poor prognosis in cases of malignant tumor extension
  - Median survival for HCC patients: 1-4 months
- Potential cardiac outflow obstruction

Treatment

- Penetration into walls of IVC and cardiac structures is variable, complicating surgical planning
- Dependent on histology, coagulopathy, portal hypertension
  - RCC: Radical nephrectomy and tumor thrombectomy
  - HCC: Thalidomide and surgical debulking
- Surgical reintervention may not be offered for recurrent or residual disease

DIAGNOSTIC CHECKLIST

Consider

- Tumor extension of extracardiac tumors when intraatrial mass approximates venous inflow structure

Image Interpretation Pearls

- Evaluate for associated bland thrombus, as intraatrial tumors may cause turbulent blood flow
- Pulmonary emboli may complicate intraatrial tumors

Reporting Tips

- Accurately localize tumor thrombus margins
- Tumor extension into atria will often significantly alter surgical planning and complicate radiation therapy
  - Apparent attachment of tumor thrombus to atrial wall is particularly important in surgical planning
- Valvular involvement is important for operative planning

SELECTED REFERENCES

1. Lorca MC et al: Radiologic-pathologic correlation of cardiac tumors: updated 2021 WHO tumor classification. Radiographics. 44(6):e230126, 2024
2. Karaosmanoglu AD et al: Tumor in the veins: an abdominal perspective with an emphasis on CT and MR imaging. Insights Imaging. 11(1):52, 2020
3. LeGout JD et al: Multimodality imaging of abdominopelvic tumors with venous invasion. Radiographics. 40(7):2098-116, 2020

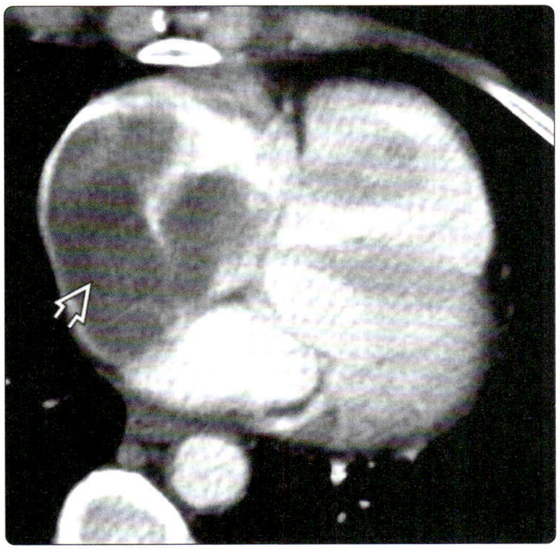

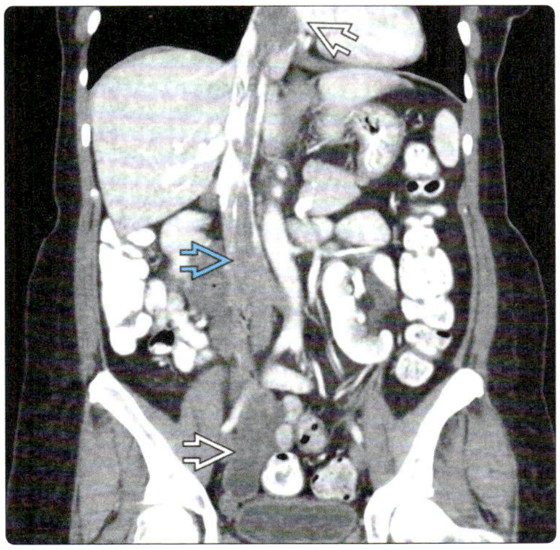

(Left) *Axial CECT in a patient with an invasive pelvic leiomyoma shows a lobulated mass in the right atrium ➡. Outflow obstruction may lead to chamber enlargement, and the right atrium is dilated in this case.* **(Right)** *Coronal reformation CECT in the same patient shows the extent of tumor thrombus within the IVC ➡ and the primary pelvic mass ➡. Extension into the right atrium is an important finding, as it significantly alters the surgical plan.*

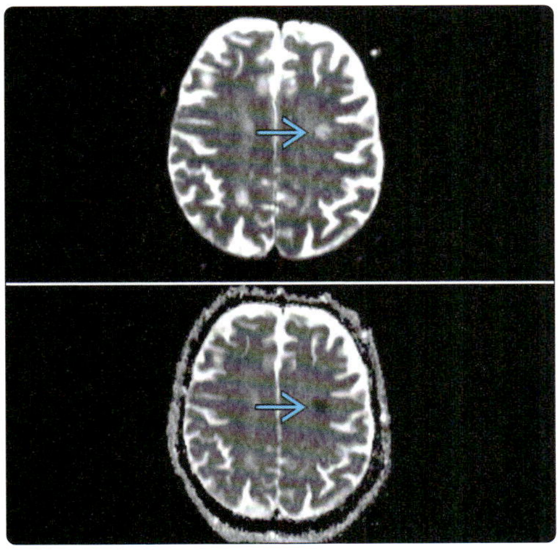

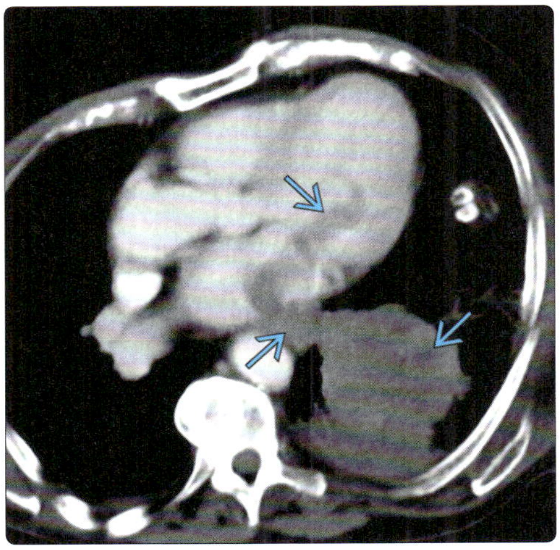

(Left) *Axial DWI (top) and ADC map (bottom) in an 86-year-old man who presented to the ED with slurred speech and elevated troponin show an acute infarct in the left frontal lobe ➡. Other infarcts were present suggestive of an embolic source.* **(Right)** *Due to a left atrial mass on echocardiogram, a chest CT was then performed, which showed a large left lower lobe (LLL) mass invading into the left inferior pulmonary vein with soft tissue in the left atrium prolapsing into the left ventricle (LV) ➡. Bx revealed squamous cell carcinoma.*

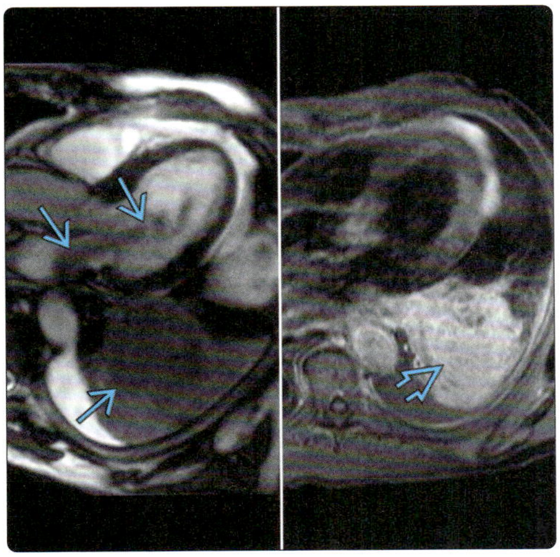

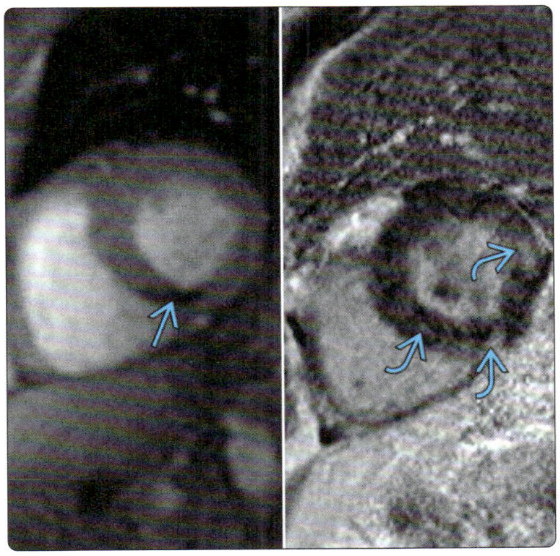

(Left) *SSFP image (left) shows the relatively isointense LLL mass invading into the left atrium with worm-like extension prolapsing into the LV during diastole ➡. T1W+ image (right) shows intense enhancement of the LLL mass ➡.* **(Right)** *Perfusion image (left) shows 1 of many focal areas of LV hypoperfusion ➡. PSIR image (right) shows nodular areas of LGE ➡, which were thought to be due to coronary emboli given distribution and elevated troponin levels. (Courtesy S. Kligerman, MD.)*

Cardiac Sarcomas

KEY FACTS

TERMINOLOGY

- Sarcomas are most common primary cardiac malignant tumor; angiosarcoma most common in right atrium and undifferentiated pleomorphic sarcomas most common in left atrium

IMAGING

- CECT
  - Right atrial angiosarcoma
    - Most commonly in right atrioventricular groove and encases right coronary artery; avidly enhances
    - Hemopericardium or intrapericardial tumor dissemination is common
  - Left atrial sarcomas
    - While there may be large, intracavitary component, subtle infiltration and thickening along left atrium wall and mitral valve apparatus (posterior > anterior leaflet) highlight diffuse infiltrative nature of this tumor
    - Invasion of pulmonary veins is uncommon and determines potential resectability
    - Differentiation between tumor types in left atrial sarcoma is often not possible
- MR
  - T1W: Heterogeneous; necrosis and hemorrhage
  - T2W: Heterogeneously hyperintense
  - Perfusion, T1W+ and LGE: Often intense enhancement

TOP DIFFERENTIAL DIAGNOSES

- Cardiac metastases
- Lymphoma
- Cardiac myxoma
- Thrombus

CLINICAL ISSUES

- Chest pain, dyspnea, weight loss, malaise
- Overall very poor prognosis

(Left) *Axial CT images show moderate hemopericardium. On the NECT (left), the right atrial (RA) mass is nearly invisible and slightly more conspicuous on the CTA.* **(Right)** *RA mass in the same patient encases the right coronary artery in the right atrioventricular groove and is hyperintense to myocardium on the SSFP and T2W images. Hemopericardium is best seen on T2W. The mass is predominantly hypointense on T1W with hyperintense foci due to blood products and shows enhancement postcontrast.*

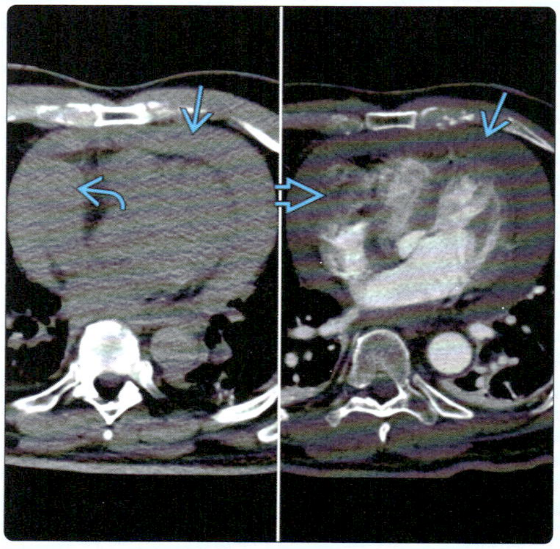

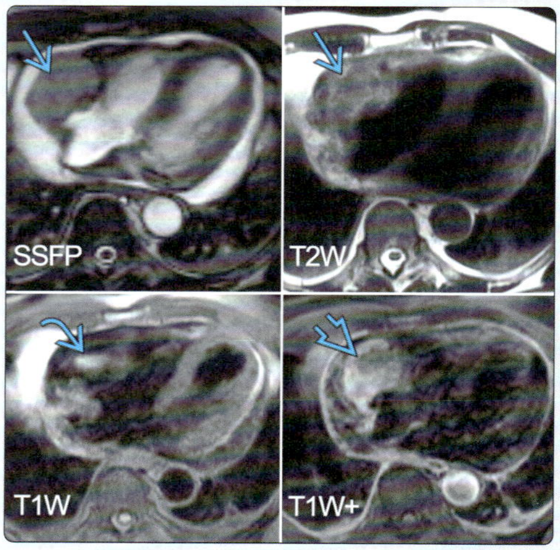

(Left) *Perfusion sequence shows intense perfusion of the RA mass 20 seconds after contrast injection. The mass shows extensive delayed enhancement. The imaging appearance is highly suggestive of a RA angiosarcoma.* **(Right)** *Axial PET/CT in the same patient shows intense FDG uptake in the RA mass. Image from cardiac catheterization (right) shows tumor neovascularity from the right coronary artery. Biopsy confirmed angiosarcoma.*

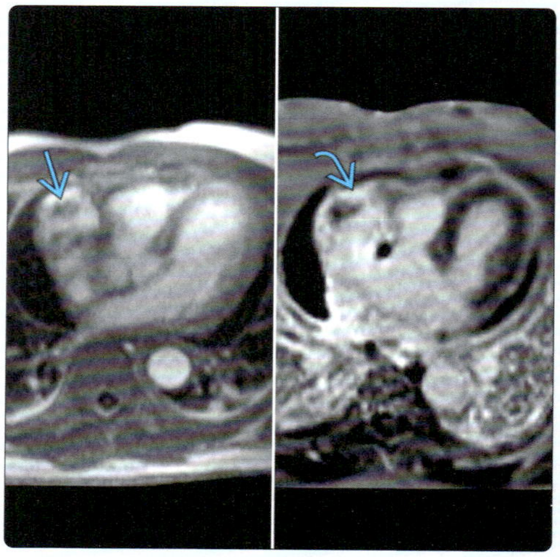

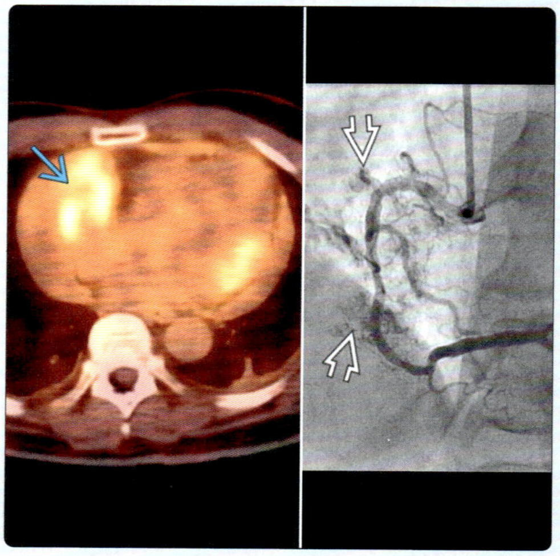

TERMINOLOGY

Definitions

- Sarcomas are most common primary cardiac malignant tumor
- Cardiac tumors that arise from one of connective tissues (mesodermal cell origin) of heart

Types of Cardiac Sarcoma

- Angiosarcoma (AS), undifferentiated pleomorphic sarcomas [(UPSs) previously classified as malignant fibrous histiocytoma], leiomyosarcoma, osteosarcoma, myxofibrosarcoma, synovial sarcoma, rhabdomyosarcoma

IMAGING

General Features

- Best diagnostic clue
  - Invasive or infiltrative mass involving cardiac wall &/or chambers without known primary malignancy
- Location
  - AS: Right atrium > left atrium
  - Other sarcomas (UPS, osteosarcoma, and leiomyosarcoma): Left atrium > right atrium> ventricles

Radiographic Findings

- Radiography
  - Often normal
  - **Cardiomegaly** is most common abnormality
  - Pulmonary metastases
  - Mass
  - Secondary findings due to obstructive physiology
    - Consolidation
    - Pericardial or pleural effusion
    - Pulmonary venous hypertension with cephalization
    - Congestive heart failure
    - Enlarged inferior vena cava and superior vena cava

CT Findings

- CECT
  - Discrete **soft tissue mass often infiltrative into myocardium**
    - Right atrial AS
      - Most commonly in right atrioventricular groove (AVG) and encases right coronary artery (RCA)
      - Avidly enhances
      - Often invades through right atrial or right ventricular wall
      - Tumor may infiltrate along tricuspid valve
      - Hemopericardium or intrapericardial tumor dissemination is common
    - Left atrial sarcomas
      - Arise from left atrium wall
      - While there may be large, intracavitary component, subtle infiltration and thickening along left atrium wall and mitral valve apparatus highlight infiltrative nature of this tumor
      - Invasion of pulmonary veins is common and determines potential resectability
      - Differentiation between histopathologic subtypes of left atrial sarcoma is often not possible
      - Osteoid matrix may be seen in osteosarcoma
      - Chondroid matrix may be seen in chondrosarcoma
      - Pericardial invasion and dissemination can occur
  - Additional findings
    - Pulmonary metastases may be present
    - Invasion into mediastinum or regional nodal disease can be seen
- Cardiac gated CTA
  - ± involvement of cardiac valve

MR Findings

- T1WI
  - **Heterogeneous, isointense**
    - Hypointense: Necrosis
    - Intermediate: Tumor
    - Hyperintense: Hemorrhage or macroscopic fat (e.g., liposarcoma)
- T2WI
  - **Heterogeneously hyperintense**
  - Assess for myocardial infiltration
- T1WI C+
  - **Heterogeneous enhancement**
    - Areas of necrosis or matrix will not enhance
- 1st-pass perfusion
  - Moderate to avid perfusion
  - Usually most intense with AS
- LGE
  - Intense heterogeneous enhancement
- Parametric mapping
  - Can quantify T1 and T2 values of mass
    - More useful when gadolinium cannot be administered
    - Different T1 and T2 values for tumor, thrombus, hemorrhage

Ultrasonographic Findings

- Echocardiography
  - Compression and distortion of anatomy by irregular echogenic mass
  - Abnormal physiology depending on tumor location and extent
  - Transesophageal echocardiography is useful in detection and guidance of transvenous biopsy

Imaging Recommendations

- Best imaging tool
  - Cardiac MR

DIFFERENTIAL DIAGNOSIS

Cardiac Metastasis

- 40-100x more common than primary sarcoma
- Often history of primary tumor
- Extracardiac primary needs to be excluded for any suspected primary cardiac malignancy

Lymphoma

- More commonly secondary with evidence of lymphoma elsewhere
- Right > left heart involvement
- Low signal intensity on T1-weighted images
- Perfusion and T1W+ enhancement usually less pronounced

Cardiac Myxoma

- Endoluminal lesion without mural involvement
- Well circumscribed and usually in left atrium
- Stalk connecting to interatrial septum

Thrombus

- Characteristic locations (e.g., left atrial appendage and left ventricular apex following myocardial infarction)
- Does not typical enhance
- No myocardial invasion
- Perform long inversion time LGE imaging to assess for thrombus

Other Primary Benign Tumors

- Rhabdomyoma, lipoma, hemangioma
- No signs of invasion
  - Lipoma has capsule and follows fat signal intensity on all pulse sequences
  - Hemangioma demonstrates avid enhancement on CT and hyperintensity on T2
  - Cardiac teratomas are very rare and usually in young children
    - Arise near roof of right atrium near aortic root

PATHOLOGY

General Features

- Sarcomas are most common primary cardiac malignant tumor
  - AS is most common sarcoma, 1/3 of all primary cardiac sarcomas, followed by UPSs and leiomyosarcoma
- Malignant tumor of mesenchymal cell origin
- Variable appearance
- Usually large, heterogeneous, invasive mass
- May replace myocardial wall
- Biopsies may be false-negative due to tumor being covered with thrombus
- Etiology: Unknown

Staging, Grading, & Classification

- Metastatic disease: 66-89% at presentation
  - **Lungs** > lymph nodes, bone, and liver

Gross Pathologic & Surgical Features

- Invasive mass or diffuse infiltration
- May be hemorrhagic and multilobular
- Cut surfaces typically firm and heterogeneous

Microscopic Features

- Microscopic features parallel corresponding soft tissue sarcoma
  - AS is immunoreactive for endothelial markers (ERG and CD31)
  - Leiomyosarcoma for smooth muscle markers (desmin and smooth muscle actin)

CLINICAL ISSUES

Presentation

- Most common signs/symptoms
  - Chest pain, dyspnea, weight loss, malaise
- Other signs/symptoms
  - Arrhythmia, peripheral edema, tamponade, and sudden death
  - Peripheral tumor embolization
- Clinical profile
  - Delayed diagnosis due to nonspecific symptoms

Demographics

- Age
  - Generally present between 40-60 years
  - Extremely rare in infants and children
- Sex
  - AS: M:F = 2:1
  - UPS and leiomyosarcoma: No predilection

Natural History & Prognosis

- AS has worse prognosis; 5-year survival rate of 10%
  - Recurrence and metastases within 1 year
- Better prognosis
  - Left atrial involvement
  - Low mitotic rate
  - No necrosis
  - No metastases at diagnosis

Treatment

- Surgery: Palliative; may prolong survival, especially in cases without metastatic disease
- Palliative radiation and chemotherapy are often not very helpful
- Left atrial autotransplantion
  - Left atrium is removed, tumor is removed from left atrium, bovine pericardium inserted, atrium is reimplanted into patient
  - Depending on number involved, pulmonary vein invasion may preclude surgery
  - Mean survival < 2 years with wide range
- Selective heart transplantation
  - No survival benefit in patients with right atrial AS

DIAGNOSTIC CHECKLIST

Consider

- Primary cardiac sarcoma in patient with locally invasive mass involving cardiac wall and chambers
- CT imaging of right atrial or ventricular tumors are difficult due to mixing artifact (contrast from superior vena cava with unopacified blood from inferior vena cava)
  - Delayed imaging is useful to accurately delineate mass
- Cardiac MR: Detailed information about location and extent of tumor

SELECTED REFERENCES

1. Lorca MC et al: Radiologic-pathologic correlation of cardiac tumors: updated 2021 WHO Tumor Classification. Radiographics. 44(6):e230126, 2024
2. Maleszewski JJ et al: The 2021 WHO Classification of Tumors of the Heart. J Thorac Oncol. 17(4):510-8, 2022
3. Tyebally S et al: Cardiac tumors: JACC CardioOncology state-of-the-art review. JACC CardioOncol. 2(2):293-311, 2020
4. Caspar T et al: Magnetic resonance evaluation of cardiac thrombi and masses by T1 and T2 mapping: an observational study. Int J Cardiovasc Imaging. 33(4):551-9, 2017
5. Esposito A et al: CMR in the assessment of cardiac masses: primary malignant tumors. JACC Cardiovasc Imaging. 7(10):1057-61, 2014

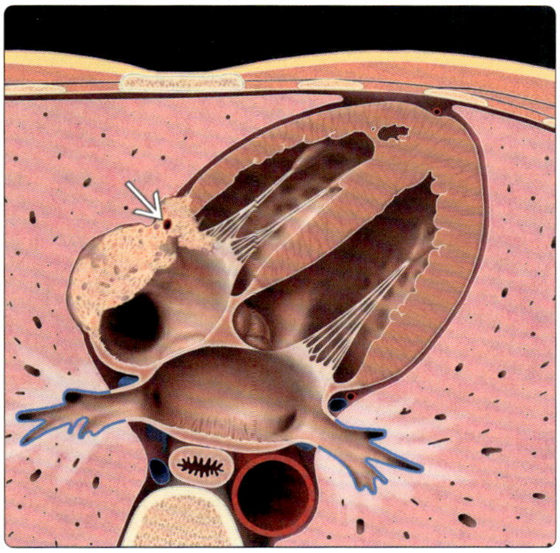

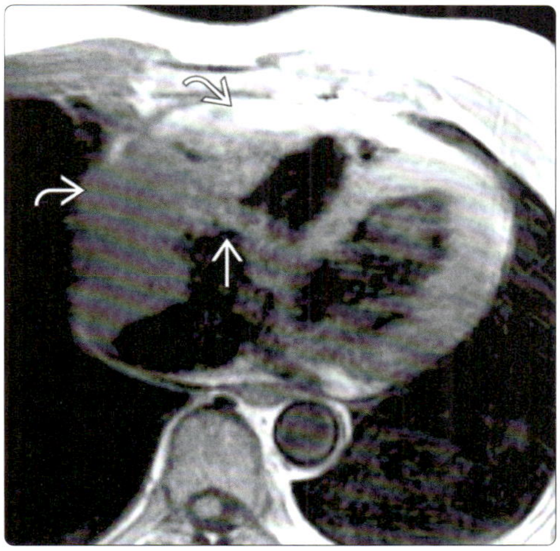

(Left) *Graphic demonstrates typical features of cardiac angiosarcoma arising from the lateral RA wall, infiltrating the mediastinal fat and tricuspid valve, and encasing the right coronary artery* ➡*.* **(Right)** *Axial T1 MR SE shows the typical appearance of a large primary cardiac angiosarcoma originating in the RA and invading the subepicardial fat and pericardium* ➡*, tricuspid valve* ➡*, and right ventricle.*

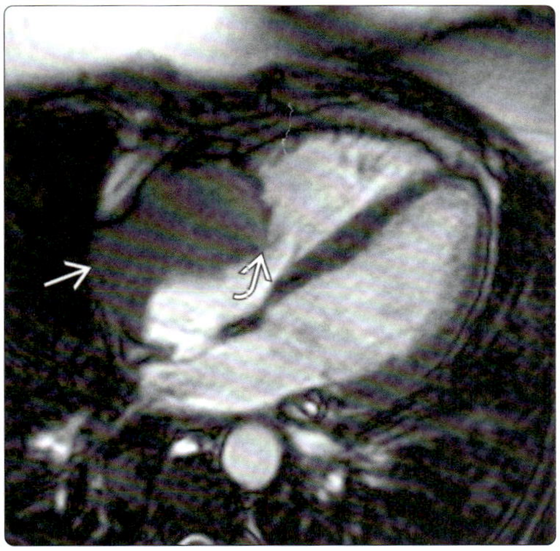

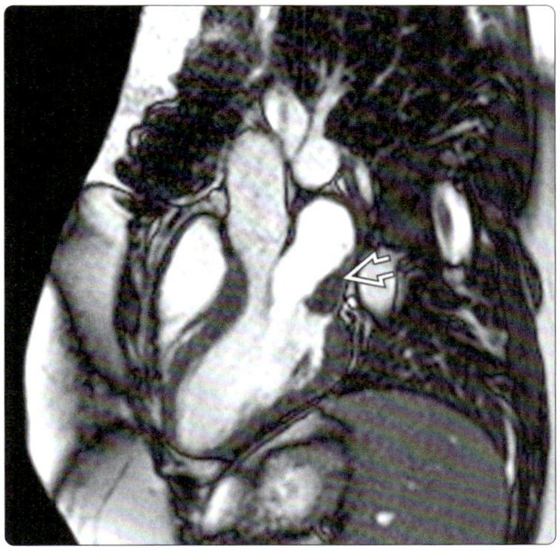

(Left) *Four-chamber SSFP MR shows a large mass* ➡ *originating from the free wall of the RA. Note extension and involvement of the tricuspid valve* ➡ *and invasion through epicardial fat. These features are highly suggestive of angiosarcoma.* **(Right)** *Left ventricular outflow tract SSFP MR shows a mass that is broadly adherent to the posterolateral left atrial wall* ➡ *and infiltrates the posterior leaflet of the mitral valve (PLMV).*

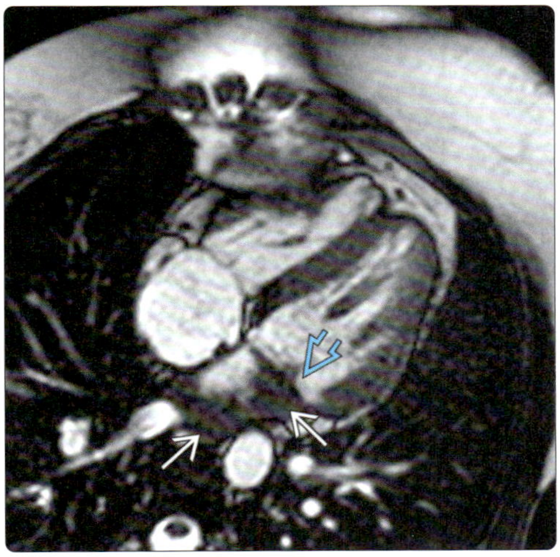

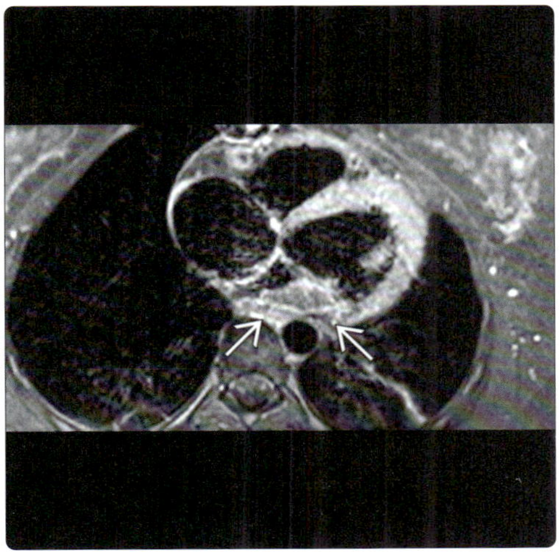

(Left) *Four-chamber SSSP MR in the same patient shows an infiltrative mass* ➡ *involving the posterior wall of the left atrium (LA) with extension into the mitral valve* ➡*.* **(Right)** *Four-chamber T1 C+ FS MR in the same patient demonstrates enhancement* ➡ *of the LA mass. This was a pathologically proven primary leiomyosarcoma in a 22-year-old woman. Leiomyosarcoma often invades the pulmonary veins.*

(Left) *Axial T1 MR shows foci of hemorrhage ➡ in a large RA sarcoma. There is pericardial thickening ➡ extending anterior, posterior, and medial to the mass, a finding suggestive of tumor spread to the pericardium.* **(Right)** *Four-chamber T1 C+ FS MR with fat saturation shows diffuse enhancement of a sarcoma ➡ in the right atrioventricular groove. The right coronary artery ➡ is encased by the mass.*

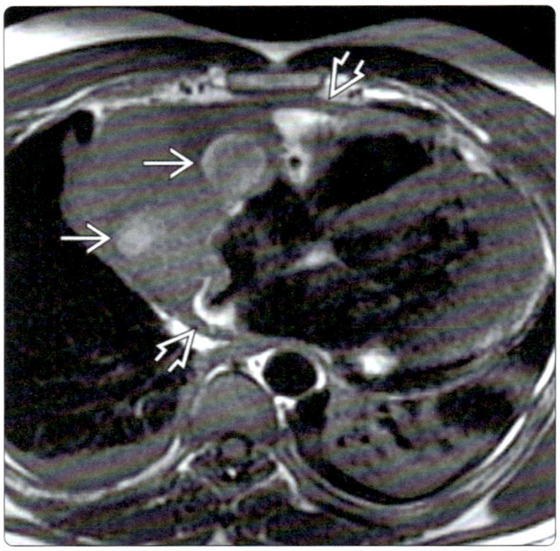

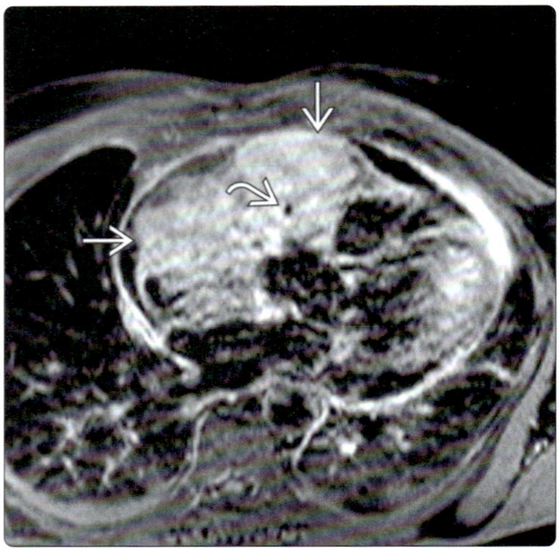

(Left) *CT shows a mass ➡ with osteoid matrix with infiltration of the left atrial wall and PLMV ➡. The mass encases 3 pulmonary veins ➡ with venous infarct ➡. A bone scan was performed (inset), which shows uptake throughout the mass ➡. LA osteosarcoma was confirmed on autopsy.* **(Right)** *Arterial (top) and delayed (bottom) images show an enhancing intracavitary left atrial mass ➡ with more pronounced enhancement along thickened posterior left atrial wall ➡ and PLMV ➡ from spindle cell sarcoma infiltration.*

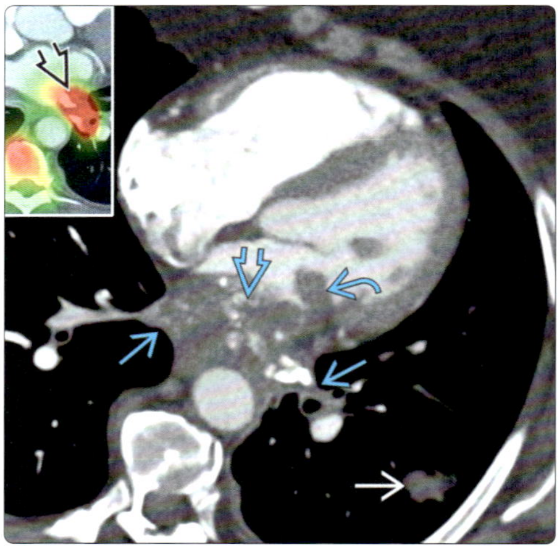

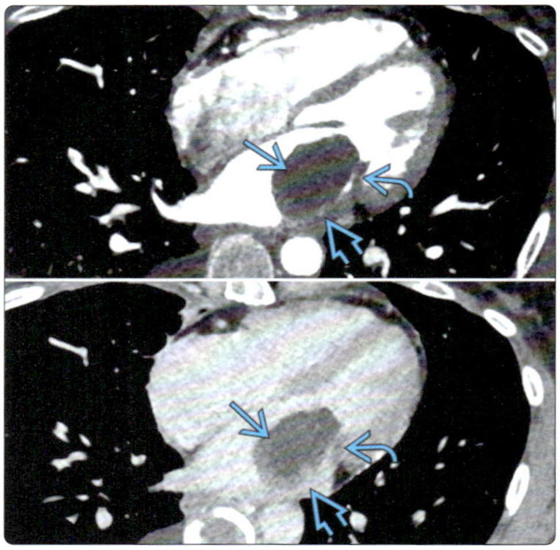

(Left) *Paraseptal long-axis (2-chamber) SSFP MR shows a pedunculated mass ➡ in the LA. This is an atypical example of a metastatic alveolar soft part sarcoma from the vulva in a 13-year-old girl that had invaded the left inferior pulmonary vein and extended into the LA.* **(Right)** *Three-chamber CECT demonstrates a large, lobulated mass ➡ originating from the posterior wall of the LA and extending to the mitral valve ➡ plane. Pathology revealed intimal sarcoma.*

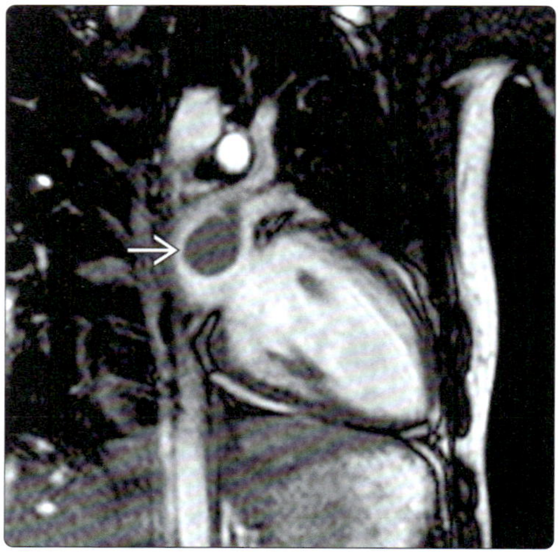

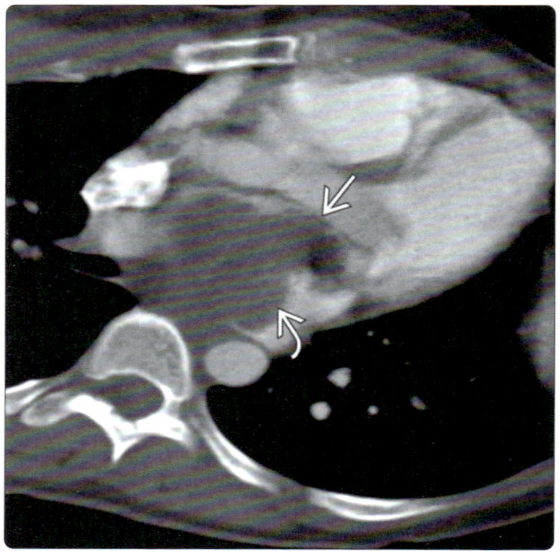

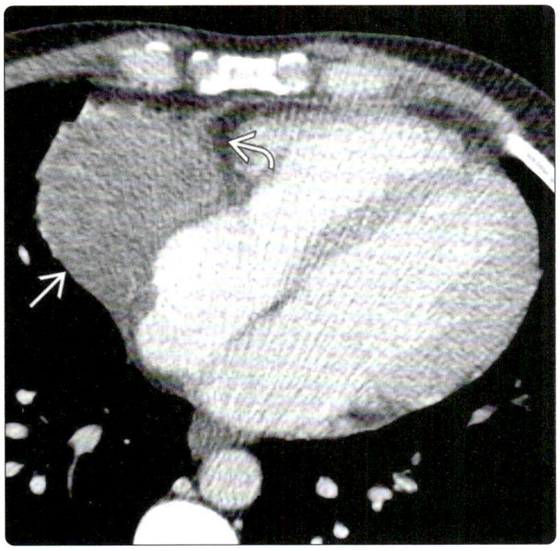

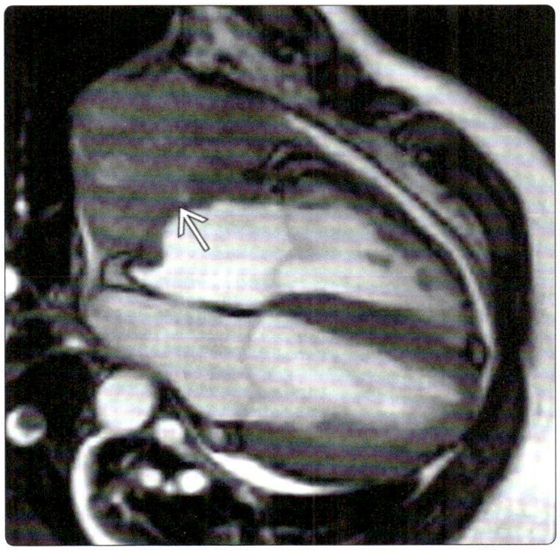

(Left) *Axial CECT in a patient with cardiac sarcoma shows a predominantly hypodense mass ➡ arising from the RA. The disruption of subepicardial fat ➡ and irregularity of adjacent pericardium are consistent with local invasion.* **(Right)** *Four-chamber view SSFP MR shows a large, heterogeneous sarcoma ➡ arising from the lateral wall of the RA. It invades through the subepicardial fat and abuts or invades the parietal pericardium.*

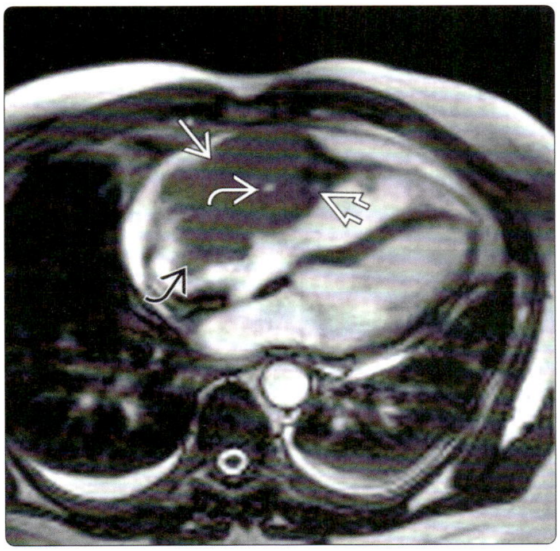

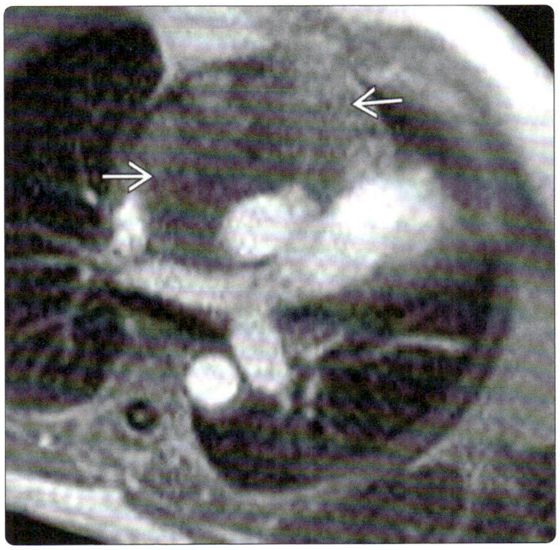

(Left) *Four-chamber view SSFP MR shows a large cardiac sarcoma ➡ centered around the right atrioventricular groove with invasion into the RA ➡ and right ventricle ➡. The mass encases the right coronary artery ➡.* **(Right)** *Four-chamber view MR perfusion in the same patient shows rapid early enhancement ➡ of the mass.*

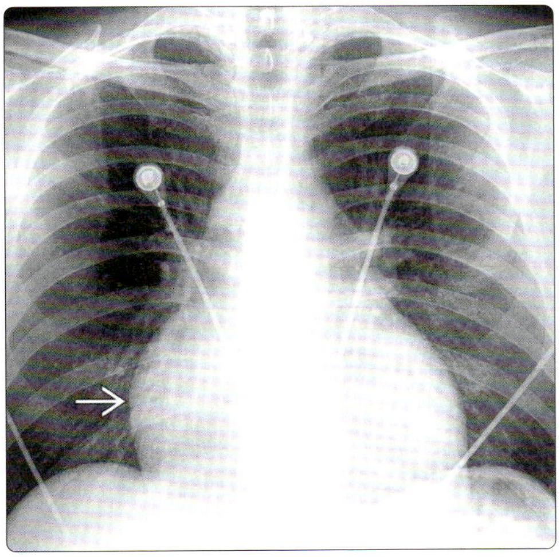

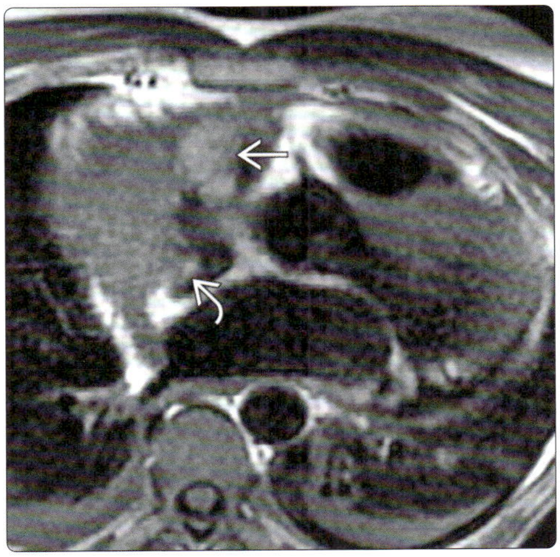

(Left) *AP chest radiograph of a patient with primary cardiac angiosarcoma shows enlargement of the RA ➡. Cardiomegaly is the most common abnormality detected on chest radiography in patients with cardiac sarcoma but is a nonspecific finding.* **(Right)** *Axial T1W FSE MR shows a large, infiltrative sarcoma in the RA. The hyperintense signal ➡ represents tumoral hemorrhage. Note invasion into the distal aspect of the superior vena cava ➡.*

KEY FACTS

TERMINOLOGY

- Primary sarcoma arising from intima of aorta

IMAGING

- Dominant polyploid mass leading to narrowing of aorta
- Soft tissue may extend beyond aortic wall
- Proximal and distal to dominant mass, variable degree of irregular aortic wall thickening
- Areas of intimal thickening can be noncontiguous from dominant mass
- Tumor extends pathologically beyond where it can be visualized due to intimal spread
- Enhancement with CT often absent or minimal
- Enhancement often subtle but present with MR
- Often limited atherosclerotic disease elsewhere in aorta
- FDG PET imaging will show noncontiguous uptake along tumor that is often mild

TOP DIFFERENTIAL DIAGNOSES

- Complex atheroma with mural thrombus
- Vasculitis
- Acute aortic syndrome

PATHOLOGY

- Polyploid endoluminal masses arising from intima but eventually grow into media and adventitia
- Malignant epithelioid cells extending over thrombus composed of fibrin, tumor, and areas of necrosis
  - Reason for mild uptake on FDG PET
- Very limited vascularity in mass
  - Reason for little enhancement on CT and MR

CLINICAL ISSUES

- Embolization of tumor into systemic arteries leading to claudication, abdominal pain, flank pain, etc.
- ~ 1/2 patients have metastases at time of diagnosis
- Very poor prognosis, even in absence of metastatic disease

(Left) *Axial CTs through the proximal (left), mid (center), and distal (right) descending thoracic aorta (DTA) in a 58-year-old man with intermittent chest pain shows an irregular filling defect* ➙ *with diffuse wall thickening proximally, a polyploid mass in the mid-DTA, and shaggy contours in distal DTA.* **(Right)** *CTA in the same patient shows the bizarre polyploid filling defect with irregular intimal thickening extending into the arch. The ascending aorta and abdominal aorta were normal. Surgical biopsy confirmed aortic intimal sarcoma.*

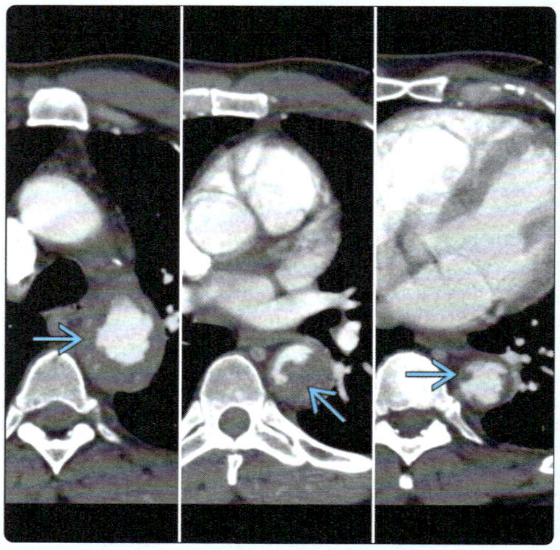

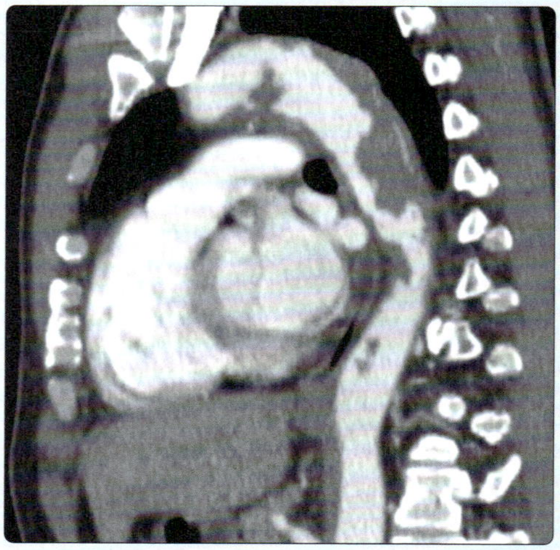

(Left) *CT images from a 61-year-old with leg and abdominal pain show a polyploid mass in the DTA* ➙*. Surrounding the mass, there is irregular intimal thickening* ➙*. Abdominal pain and leg pain were related to superior mesenteric artery* ➙ *and posterior tibial artery (not shown) emboli. The remainder of the thoracic and abdominal aorta were normal.* **(Right)** *Gross pathology and CT in the same patient show the polyploid mass in the DTA* ➙ *due to intimal sarcoma. The sarcoma extending throughout the entire DTA.*

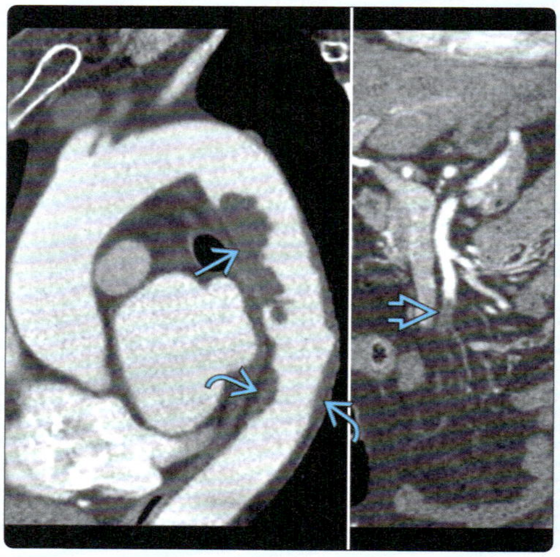

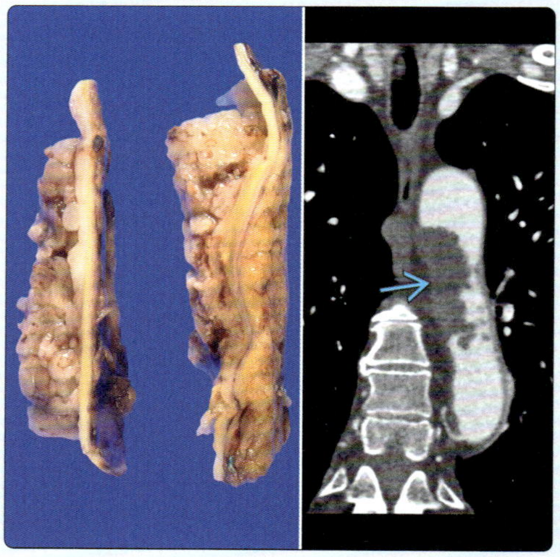

TERMINOLOGY

Abbreviations

- Aortic intimal sarcoma (AIS)

Definitions

- Primary sarcoma arising from intima of aorta

IMAGING

General Features

- Best diagnostic clue
  - Irregular polyplo d mass in aorta, often in absence of significant atherosclerotic disease
  - Irregular intimal thickening extending proximal and distal to mass
  - Evidence of systemic embolization
- Location
  - Thoracic aorta in 46% of patients
  - Abdominal aorta in 42% of patients
  - Both thoracic and abdominal aorta in 12% of patients

CT Findings

- Variable CT appearances of AIS along entire tumor
- Dominant polyploid mass leading to narrowing of aorta
- Soft tissue may extend beyond aortic wall
- Variable degree of irregular aortic wall thickening proximal and distal to dominant mass
  - Circumferential or focal thickening
  - Smooth in some areas and irregular/nodular in others
- Areas of intimal thickening may be discontinuous from dominant mass
- Enhancement often absent or minimal
- Often limited atherosclerotic disease elsewhere in aorta
- Aneurysmal dilation of aorta in region of AIS can occur
- Metastases may be present

MR Findings

- Similar morphology to CT findings
- Better assessment of possible spread of tumor along aortic wall and outside wall
- Often mild postcontrast enhancement

Nuclear Medicine Findings

- PET/CT
  - FDG PET imaging will show noncontiguous uptake along tumor that is often mild; most of tumor is actually fibrin clot

Imaging Recommendations

- Best imaging tool
  - Initial study is often CTA due to nonspecific symptoms
    - Given very characteristic AIS morphology, diagnosis can be made by CT alone
      - However, in one pathology series of 26 cases, AIS was not suspected clinically before surgery
  - PET is best 2nd study to help confirm primary tumor and assess for metastases
  - MR can help confirm diagnosis

DIFFERENTIAL DIAGNOSIS

Complex Atheroma With Mural Thrombus

- Diffuse atherosclerosis usually absent in AIS

Vasculitis

- Circumferential, enhancing wall thickening without mass

Acute Aortic Syndrome

- Large endoluminal mass not seen with acute aortic syndrome

PATHOLOGY

Gross Pathologic & Surgical Features

- Polyploid endoluminal masses arising from intima but eventually grow into media and adventitia
- Contiguous spread of tumor along intima distal to dominant mass

Microscopic Features

- Undifferentiated tumors are most common
  - Malignant epithelioid cells extending over thrombus composed of fibrin, tumor, and areas of necrosis
  - Very limited vascularity in mass
- Myxoid variant is less common
- Intimal spread of tumor may pathologically extend beyond where it can be visualized on imaging

CLINICAL ISSUES

Presentation

- Most common signs/symptoms
  - Nonspecific pain
  - Hypertension
  - Embolization of tumor into systemic arteries leading to claudication, abdominal pain, flank pain, etc.

Demographics

- Average age: 60 years; M > F

Natural History & Prognosis

- ~ 1/2 patients have metastases at time of diagnosis
- Very poor prognosis, even in absence of metastatic disease

Treatment

- Surgical resection attempted if possible
  - If entire tumor is removed, long-term survival possible
    - However, this is rarely achieved
- Chemotherapy, palliative surgery, and radiation
  - Survival still poor

DIAGNOSTIC CHECKLIST

Consider

- AIS in setting of irregular polyploid mass in descending thoracic aorta or abdominal aorta, especially when there is little or no atherosclerotic disease

SELECTED REFERENCES

1. Ropp AM et al: Intimal sarcoma of the great vessels. Radiographics. 41(2):361-79, 2021
2. Staats P et al: Intimal sarcomas of the aorta and iliofemoral arteries: a clinicopathological study of 26 cases. Pathology. 46(7):596-603, 2014

Lymphoma

KEY FACTS

TERMINOLOGY

- Primary cardiac lymphoma
- Secondary cardiac lymphoma
- Primary effusion lymphoma

IMAGING

- Ill-defined, infiltrative mass involving myocardium or pericardium, often with pericardial effusion
- Right atrium is most frequently involved
- Radiography
  - Enlarged cardiac silhouette
  - Lymphadenopathy
- Cardiac gated CT
  - Low-attenuation infiltrative myocardial masses
  - Often does not respect typical tissue boundaries
  - Encasement of coronary arteries
  - Pericardial effusion
  - May miss diffuse myocardial infiltration without cavitary component; delayed imaging (30 seconds) or dual energy can help
- MR
  - Superior tissue characterization
  - Usually significant enhancement post contrast
  - Multiple nodular, relatively hyperintense masses infiltrating myocardium

TOP DIFFERENTIAL DIAGNOSES

- Metastatic disease; thrombus;primary cardiac tumors

CLINICAL ISSUES

- Cardiac arrhythmia, heart failure

DIAGNOSTIC CHECKLIST

- Rapidly progressive and treatment-resistive congestive heart failure may be first presenting symptom

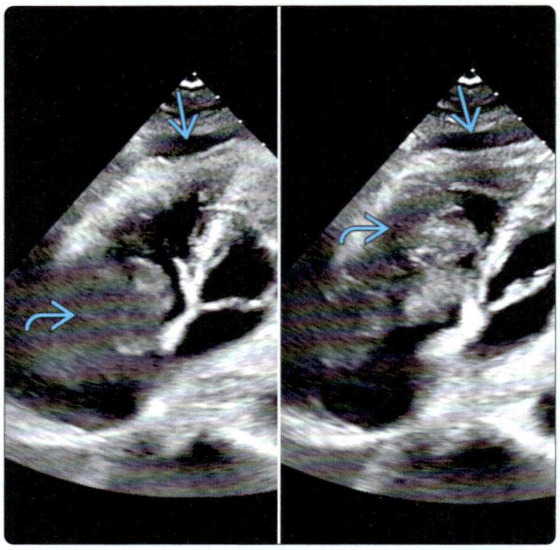

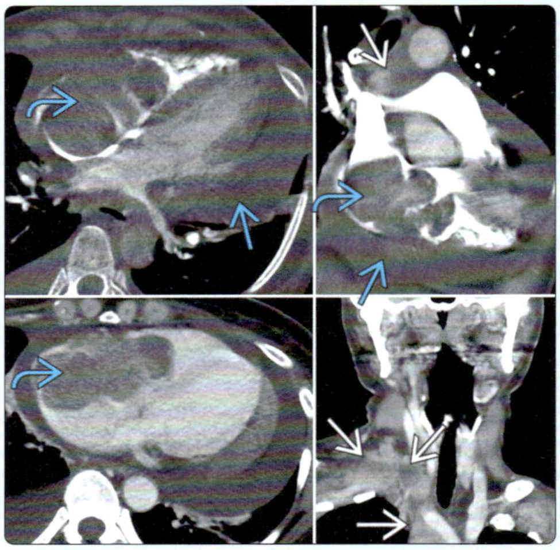

(Left) *Images during systole (left) show a large predominantly hypoechoic right atrial mass → prolapsing into the right ventricle during diastole (right) mimicking a myxoma. A pericardial effusion → is seen.* **(Right)** *Four-chamber (top left) and RVOT (top right) images show the right atrial mass → and moderate pleural and pericardial effusions →. The mass shows mild portal venous-phase (bottom left) enhancement. Bulky lymphadenopathy in the chest → and neck CT (bottom right) from lymphoma is seen.*

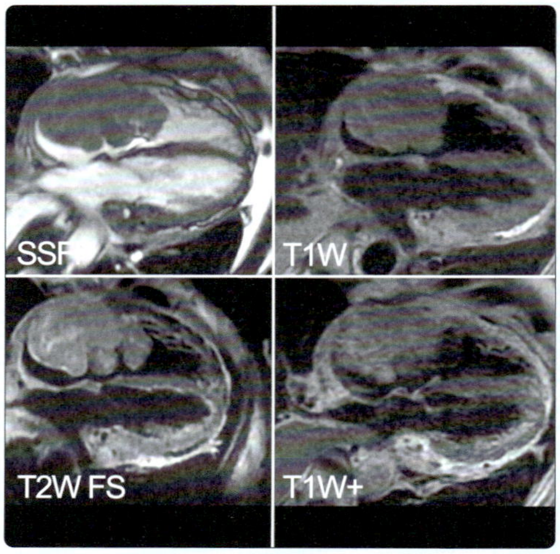

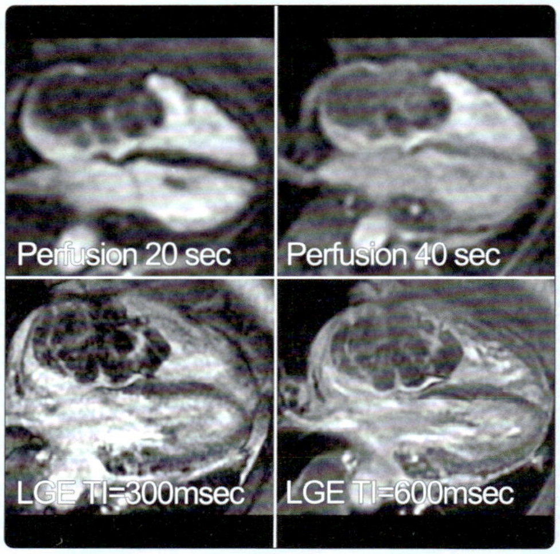

(Left) *The large right atrial mass is mildly hyperintense to the myocardium on SSFP (top left) and T2 (bottom left) sequences. The mass is isointense on T1 (top right) and shows mild enhancement after contrast (bottom right).* **(Right)** *First-pass perfusion images (top row) show progressive enhancement of the mass. On LGE sequence (bottom row) with a TI=300 msec and T1 = 600 msec, the signal in the majority of the mass is similar to the myocardium, although foci of enhancement are present.*

TERMINOLOGY

Definitions

- Primary cardiac lymphoma (PCL)
  - Confined to heart and pericardium without extracardiac disease; rare
  - Non-Hodgkin lymphoma
  - Majority occur in HIV/AIDS patients
- Secondary cardiac lymphoma (SCL)
  - Cardiac involvement in patients with systemic lymphoma
  - ~ 1/3 of lymphoma patients develop SCL (on pathology series)
- Primary effusion lymphoma (PEL)
  - Rare, HIV-associated non-Hodgkin lymphoma
  - Lymphomatous growth in liquid phase in body cavities, such as pericardium
  - Evidence of infection by human herpesvirus-8, which is associated with Kaposi sarcoma

IMAGING

General Features

- Best diagnostic clue
  - Ill-defined, infiltrative mass involving myocardium or pericardium, often with pericardial effusion
  - Extension along epicardial surface
  - Encasement of coronary arteries and aortic root
- Location
  - May involve any cardiac chamber and pericardium
    - Often infiltrative and does not respect boundaries
  - PCL is more common in right atrium
  - SCL most commonly has pericardial and extracardiac involvement
  - May lead to focal myocardial hypertrophy
    - Can mimic hypertrophic cardiomyopathy
  - Often with intracavitary component
    - Frequently nodular or lobulated
    - May present primarily as intracavitary mass
  - Epicardial involvement often encases coronary arteries, most notably right coronary artery
  - Can involve pericardial space exclusively, sometimes presenting with constriction
- Size
  - Variable but often large; fills most of affected cavity
- Morphology
  - Frequently manifests as ill-defined, infiltrative mass

Radiographic Findings

- May demonstrate lymphadenopathy
- Water bottle cardiac morphology due to pericardial effusion
- Signs of congestive heart failure
  - Right ventricular, left ventricular, or biventricular failure, depending on involved structures

CT Findings

- Tumor often hypo- or isoattenuating with respect to myocardium during arterial phase
  - May miss diffuse myocardial infiltration without cavitary component
  - Adding 30-second-delay scan helpful, as normal myocardium often enhances more than tumor
  - Dual-energy CT virtual monoenergetic images may improve lesion conspicuity
- Lobular mass with heterogeneous enhancement
- Other manifestations of lymphoma in secondary type

MR Findings

- DWI
  - Typically restricted diffusion
- Superior tissue characterization
- PCL
  - Multiple nodular, relatively hyperintense masses infiltrating myocardium
  - Diffuse infiltration of pericardium with hemorrhagic pericardial effusion
  - Usually heterogeneous enhancement
- T1- and T2-weighted sequences
  - Diffusely infiltrating, often isointense on T1W and isointense to hyperintense on T2W sequences
- Perfusion
  - Hypoperfusion to increased perfusion
- T1W+
  - Mild to moderate enhancement
- LGE
  - Present to varying degrees
  - Can mimic infiltrative cardiomyopathy
- Cine SSFP
  - Intracavitary masses better demonstrated
  - May demonstrate jets from flow obstruction
  - Ventricular and valvular function; volumes
  - Chamber enlargement if obstructing physiology
- Encasement of coronary arteries
- Monitoring of treatment success/remission and recurrence
- Pericardial effusions may result in tamponade

Echocardiographic Findings

- Transthoracic echocardiogram (TTE) for initial evaluation
- Hypoechoic mass: Not optimally visualized in standard echo planes
- Pericardial effusion

Imaging Recommendations

- Best imaging tool
  - MR provides comprehensive information
- Protocol advice
  - Cine images to assess for flow obstruction
  - T1-weighted spin-echo sequences pre- and post gadolinium (with identical spatial locations) to assess for abnormal enhancement
  - LGE imaging may improve contrast between unaffected and infiltrated myocardium

DIFFERENTIAL DIAGNOSIS

Metastatic Disease

- 40x more common than all primary cardiac neoplasms
- Lung cancer is most common, given prevalence
- Metastatic malignant melanoma has high incidence of cardiac involvement

Thrombus

- Bland or tumor thrombus should be considered in cardiac mass cases
- Nonaggressive, confined to chamber cavity
- Tumor thrombus results from extracardiac mass extending to atria via transvenous spread

Other Primary Cardiac Tumors

- Myxoma
  - Most common primary cardiac tumor
  - Characteristic stalk-like attachment to interatrial septum near foramen ovalis
  - Most commonly located in left atrium
  - Low-grade patchy enhancement
  - More hyperintense on T2 sequences than lymphoma
- Sarcoma
  - Most common primary cardiac malignancy
  - 2nd most common of all (benign or malignant) primary cardiac tumors after myxoma
  - May be distinguished by prominent enhancement
- Leiomyoma, rhabdomyoma, fibroma, hemangioma, lipoma

Nonneoplastic Disorders

- Hypertrophic cardiomyopathy

Pericardial Disease

- Infectious or inflammatory pericarditis
- Neoplastic pericardial disease

PATHOLOGY

General Features

- Etiology
  - Primary cardiac/pericardial involvement by T-cell phenotype has been described in post- (noncardiac) transplant patients
  - HIV/AIDS
    - Isolated cardiac tumors in HIV/AIDS patients are typically primary lymphomas
    - Primary cardiac non-Hodgkin lymphoma is 25-60x more common than in general population
    - Secondary cardiac tumors are often observed in widespread Kaposi sarcoma

Gross Pathologic & Surgical Features

- Multiple firm nodules
- Contiguous invasion of pericardium

Microscopic Features

- Immunophenotypic studies may allow differentiation of lymphoma from metastatic carcinoma or angiosarcoma

CLINICAL ISSUES

Presentation

- Most common signs/symptoms
  - Cardiac arrhythmia, heart failure, pericardial effusion
  - Dyspnea, chest pain, syncope
- Other signs/symptoms
  - Nonspecific ECG changes, such as atrioventricular block
  - May rapidly progress
  - May be occult until presenting with cardiac tamponade
  - Secondary lymphoma is frequently occult in vivo and detected post mortem
  - Sudden death

Demographics

- Age
  - PCL: Mean: 60 years
- Sex
  - Male predominance (2:1) in PCL
- Epidemiology
  - PCL has incidence of 0.06% in general population on pathology series
    - Only 1.3% of all primary cardiac tumors
    - 0.5% of extranodal lymphomas
  - SCL occurs in 20% of patients
    - May not be clinical relevant, most are discovered postmortem
  - Increasing prevalence due to Epstein-Barr virus-related lymphoproliferative disorders
    - Transplant recipients, particularly heart and lung transplant patients
  - PEL accounts for 4% of all HIV-associated non-Hodgkin lymphomas

Natural History & Prognosis

- Secondary lymphoma is frequently not apparent clinically
- T-cell lymphomas invade heart more frequently and are more aggressive than B-cell lymphomas
  - T-cell lymphomas are more likely to have cardiac manifestations
- Clinical outcome of PCL is variable
  - Early diagnosis and treatment improves prognosis and may result in complete remission
  - Prognosis of HIV-associated PCL is poor

Treatment

- PCL: Chemotherapy and monoclonal anti-CD20 antibody ± radiation
- Autologous stem cell transplant has been described
- Pericardial drainage if tamponade
- Surgical debulking in some cases

DIAGNOSTIC CHECKLIST

Consider

- Rapidly progressive and treatment-resistive congestive heart failure may be fist presenting symptom

Image Interpretation Pearls

- Other lymphomatous involvement in chest or abdomen will change diagnosis from primary to secondary

SELECTED REFERENCES

1. Lorca MC et al: Radiologic-pathologic correlation of cardiac tumors: updated 2021 WHO tumor classification. Radiographics. 44(6):e230126, 2024
2. Lichtenberger JP 3rd et al: Cardiac neoplasms: radiologic-pathologic correlation. Radiol Clin North Am. 59(2):231-42, 2021

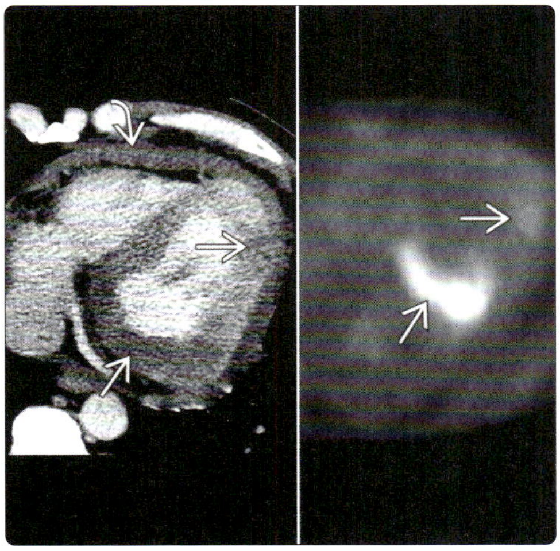

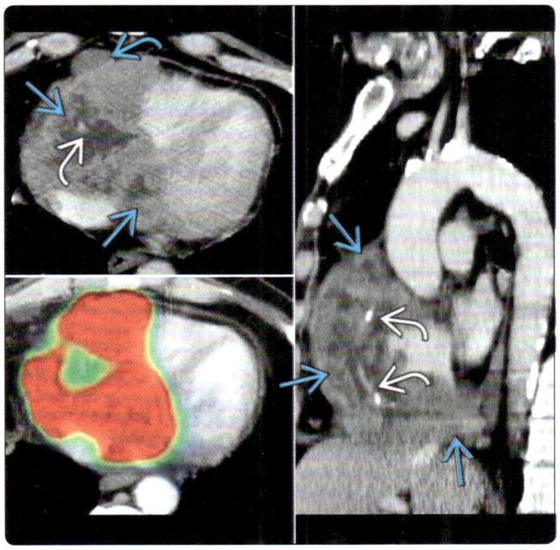

(Left) *Patient with HIV-associated primary cardiac lymphoma shows low-attenuation infiltrative masses within the left ventricular myocardium (left). Pericardial effusion is also present. FDG PET (right) shows increased uptake in the masses.* **(Right)** *Axial (top left) and sagittal (right) CT images show a heterogenous mass in the right atrioventricular groove with extensive cardiac infiltration. The right coronary artery is encased. PET/CT (bottom left) shows intense FDG uptake. A pericardial node is seen.*

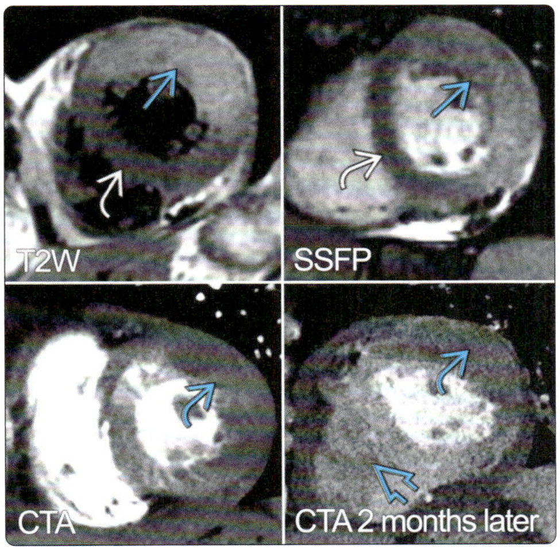

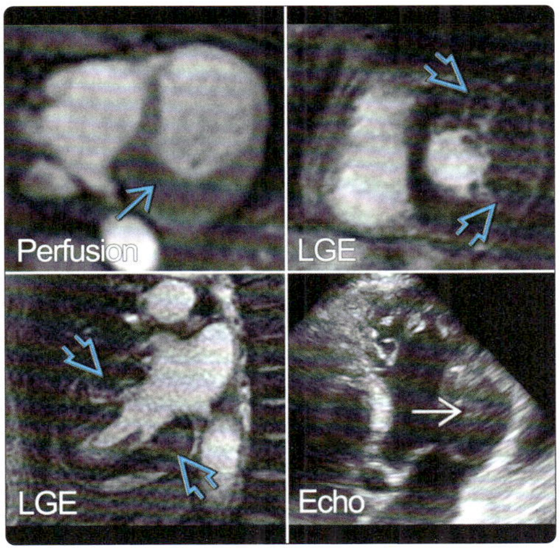

(Left) *T2 and SSFP images show asymmetric myocardial hypertrophy that is hyperintense compared to the normal myocardium. On CTA, the myocardium thickening is hypoattenuating. Two months later, there are new masses due to worsening lymphoma.* **(Right)** *The areas of lymphomatous infiltration show hypoperfusion. On LGE, the areas of hypertrophy show hazy enhancement mimicking hypertrophic cardiomyopathy. The masses are hypoechoic on echocardiogram.*

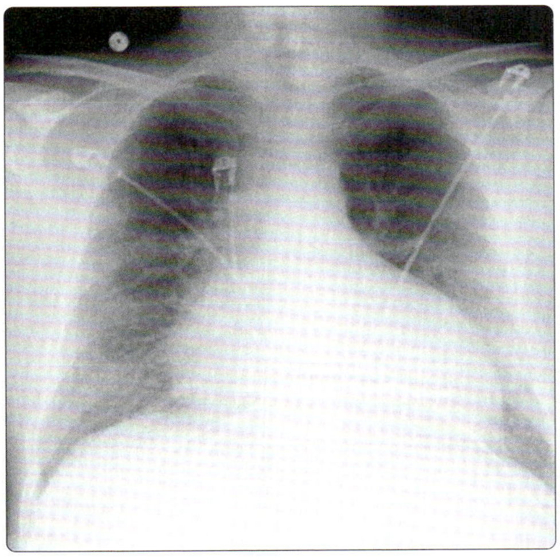

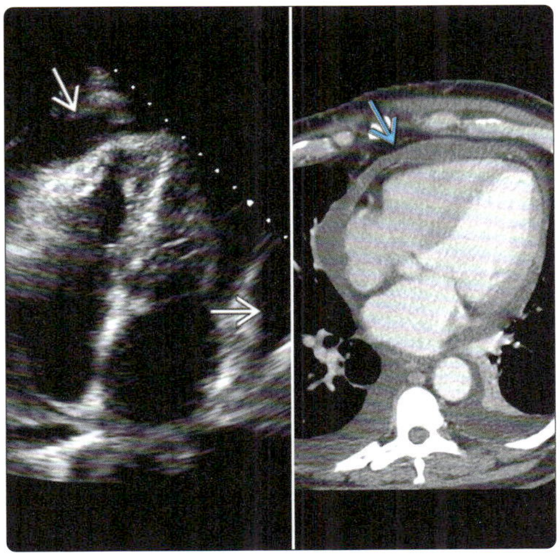

(Left) *AP radiograph shows a water bottle-shaped cardiac silhouette with mild pulmonary edema in a 53-year-old man with poorly controlled HIV.* **(Right)** *Four-chamber echocardiogram (left) shows a moderate pericardial effusion. Subsequent CT shows a small to moderate circumferential pericardial effusion with pericardial enhancement, bilateral pleural effusions, and moderate ascites (not shown). Cytology on the pericardial and ascitic fluid diagnosed primary effusion lymphoma (inset).*

Erdheim-Chester Disease

KEY FACTS

TERMINOLOGY

- Neoplastic non-Langerhans histiocytic multisystem disorder

IMAGING

- Epicardial soft tissue encasing right heart, aorta, &/or pleura
- CT
  - Hyperattenuating epicardial soft tissue around right atrium (RA) and right atrioventricular groove ~ 30-40%
    - Degree of enhancement is mild
  - Pericardial effusion or thickening ~ 45%
  - Circumferential periaortic soft tissue ~ 55%
  - Pleural thickening ± effusion
- MR
  - Soft tissue variable but often isointense to myocardium on T1W, T2W, and SSFP sequences
  - Often conspicuous 1st-pass perfusion, T1W+ enhancement, and intense LGE
  - Pericardial effusion common and may be large
    - Septal bounce due to tamponade
  - Myocardial invasion most commonly involves RA
- PET
  - FDG uptake often intense

TOP DIFFERENTIAL DIAGNOSES

- IgG4 disease
- Lymphoma
- Right atrial angiosarcoma
- Metastases
- Large vessel vasculitis

PATHOLOGY

- Xanthogranulomatous lesions composed of CD68(+)/CD1a(-) histiocytes admixed with inflammation and fibrosis
  - Fibrosis leads to intense uptake on LGE sequences

CLINICAL ISSUES

- Average age: 55 years; 75% men
- 5-year survival rate now 83%

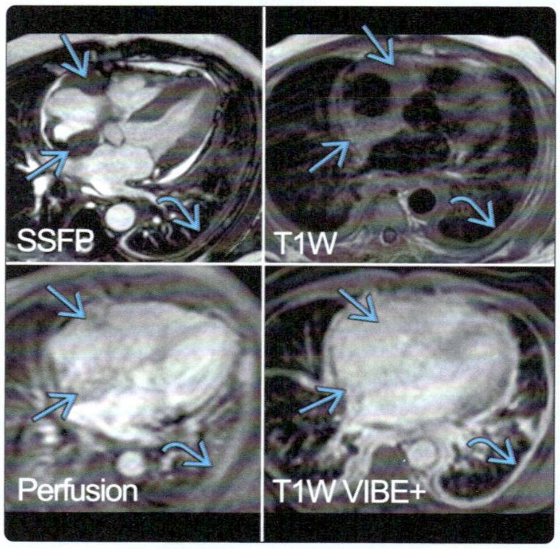

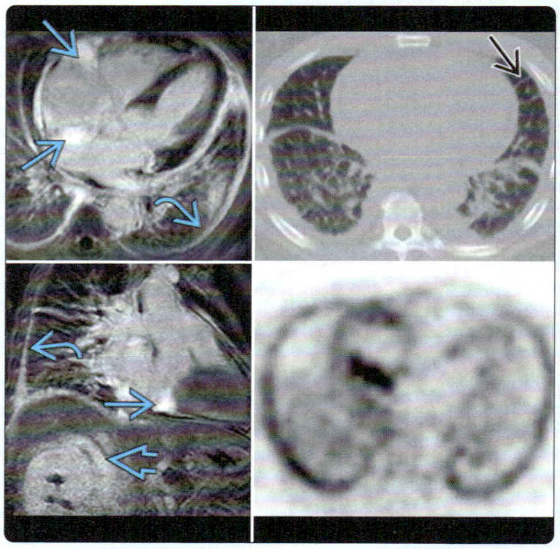

(Left) *MR images show abnormal epicardial soft tissue ➙ and pleural thickening ➙. The soft tissue is hypointense to the myocardium on SSFP, isointense to hyperintense on T1W sequences, and shows rapid perfusion and T1W+ enhancement.* **(Right)** *MR images (left) show intense LGE in the epicardium ➙ and pleura ➙. Additionally, there is similar soft tissue encasing the right kidney ➙. ECD was suggested and confirmed on biopsy. FDG PET (right) shows septal thickening ➙ and FDG uptake in the epicardial and pleural tissue.*

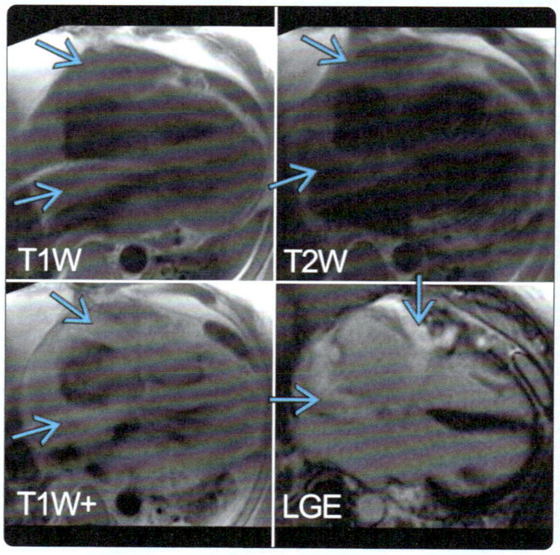

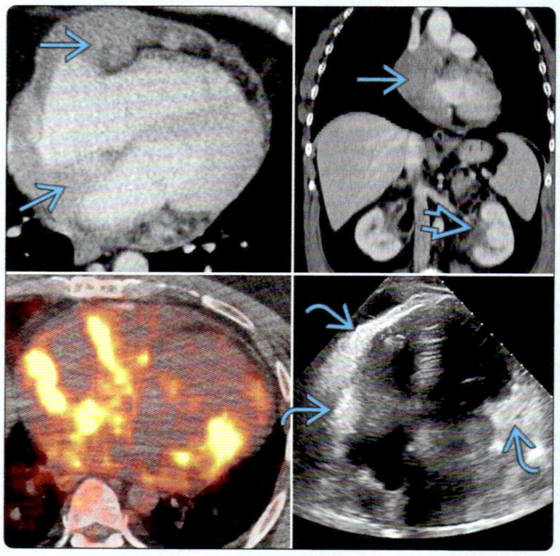

(Left) *Cardiac MR images in a 42-year-old man with ECD show epicardial and pericardial soft tissue encasing the heart ➙. Soft tissue is predominantly isointense to myocardium on T1W (top left), T2W (top right), and SSFP (video) sequences and shows prominent enhancement on T1W+ and LGE imaging.* **(Right)** *CT images (top) show high-attenuation epicardial and pericardial soft tissue encasing the heart ➙ and kidneys ➙. This tissue is FDG avid on PET/CT (bottom left). On echocardiogram, soft tissue is hyperechoic ➙.*

TERMINOLOGY

Abbreviations

- Erdheim-Chester Disease (ECD)

Definitions

- Rare neoplastic non-Langerhans histiocytic multisystem disorder

IMAGING

General Features

- Best diagnostic clue
  - Enhancing epicardial soft tissue encasing right heart aorta, pleura, &/or kidneys
- Location
  - Numerous locations throughout body
  - Most commonly in long bones and perirenal soft tissue
  - Cardiovascular system
    - Wide range of involvement from 22-55%
    - Epicardial space
      - Most common in right atrioventricular groove (AVG) and encasing right atrium (RA)
    - Myocardium invasion, most commonly invading RA
    - Pericardium
    - Aorta
- Morphology
  - Abnormal epicardial, pericardial, &/or periaortic soft tissue encasing structures

Radiographic Findings

- Cardiac enlargement from epicardial soft tissue ± pericardial effusion
- Pulmonary edema due to elevated right heart pressures from cardiac encasement
- May see pleural thickening and septal thickening

CT Findings

- Cardiac findings
  - Hyperattenuating epicardial soft tissue most notable around RA and right AVG ~ 30-40%
    - Often encases right coronary artery
      - Ischemia uncommon
      - Other coronary involvement rare
    - Soft tissue may involve pericardial recesses and envelop left heart in extensive disease
    - Soft tissue is hyperattenuating, but enhancement on CT is often mild
  - Myocardial invasion, if present, may be difficult to see on CT
  - Pericardial thickening or effusion in ~ 45%
- Aortic findings ~ 55%
  - Circumferential periaortic soft tissue
    - Soft tissue is hyperintense on noncontrast CT
    - Enhancement, if present, often mild
    - Dark rim between periaortic soft tissue and lumen often seen
      - Not specific of ECD
  - Most often diffuse but can be focal
    - If diffuse, can have homogeneous circumferential thickening or focal areas of more pronounced thickening
  - Areas of aneurysmal dilation or lumen stenosis not common
  - Areas of infiltrating soft tissue in periaortic fat, similar to perirenal infiltration, can occur
- Coronary and pulmonary artery (PA) involvement can occur but rare
- Thoracic findings
  - Pleural thickening ± effusion
  - Smooth septal thickening due to edema or fibrosis from ECD
- Abdominal findings
  - Retroperitoneal and perirenal soft tissue in 30%
  - Renal artery ± ureteral stenosis or obstruction
- Venous involvement less common

MR Findings

- Cardiac findings
  - Epicardial soft tissue in right AV groove and encasing RA; may extend superiorly into pericardial recesses and eventually along free wall of RV and left heart
    - SSFP: Soft tissue usually isointense to slightly hyperintense to myocardium
      - Diastolic septal bounce may indicate tamponade
    - T1W: Soft tissue often isointense to myocardium
      - Can be slightly hypointense or hyperintense
    - T2W: Soft tissue usually isointense but ranges from mildly hypointense to hyperintense
    - Perfusion: Conspicuous 1st-pass perfusion
    - T1W+: Intense enhancement of soft tissue
    - LGE: Very intense LGE
  - Pericardium
    - Pericardial effusion common and may be large
    - Soft tissue may infiltrate into pericardium
  - Myocardium
    - Myocardial invasion most commonly involves RA
- Aorta
  - T1W and T2W: Soft tissue often isointense to slightly hypointense to muscle
  - T1W+: Enhancement common
  - LGE: Intense enhancement
- Pleural involvement, if present, will show LGE and T1W+ enhancement
- Retroperitoneal and perirenal involvement similar imaging characteristics

Echocardiographic Findings

- Hyperechoic epicardial soft tissue encasing right heart
- Associated pericardial effusion, which may be large
  - Tamponade may be present

Nuclear Medicine Findings

- PET
  - FDG uptake in epicardial and periaortic tissue common

Imaging Recommendations

- Best imaging tool
  - Cardiac MR for cardiac involvement
  - CT or MR for aortic involvement
- Protocol advice
  - Follow cardiac mass protocol T1W, T2W, perfusion, T1W+, and LGE through abnormality

DIFFERENTIAL DIAGNOSIS

IgG4 Disease

- CT and MR signal characteristics can mimic ECD
- More likely to involve coronary arteries
  - Can lead to stenosis and aneurysm formation
- Aortic involvement can mimic ECD
  - More commonly focal or multifocal, whereas ECD often involves entire aorta
    - Abdominal aorta and iliac involvement > thoracic aorta
  - More commonly associated with aneurysm formation
  - More commonly associated with wall calcification

Lymphoma

- Can have similar morphology on CT and T1W, T2W, and SSFP imaging on MR
- Lymphoma more likely to invade along underlying structure of right heart
- 1st-pass perfusion, T1W+ enhancement, and LGE of lymphoma < < ECD
- Usually secondary with lymphadenopathy elsewhere

Right Atrial Angiosarcoma

- Often heterogenous signal characteristics on T1W and T2W imaging from necrosis
  - Areas of necrosis more conspicuous post contrast
- Often more hyperintense on T2W imaging
- LGE less intense with angiosarcoma
- More commonly invades cardiac chambers and valves
- Pericardial dissemination with hemopericardium common
- Metastases common

Metastases

- Underlying history of malignancy
- Likely to have metastases elsewhere in body
  - Less likely to just involve AVG and encase RA
- T2W and SSFP intensity usually greater than with ECD
- LGE metastases < ECD

Large Vessel Vasculitis

- Large vessel vasculitis (LVV), especially Takayasu, can involve aorta, coronary arteries, and PAs
- PA and coronary involvement more common with Takayasu
- LVV more common associated with stenosis and aneurysm
- Less likely to coat entire aorta like ECD
- Cardiac and pericardial involvement rare
- Retroperitoneal soft tissues involvement uncommon

PATHOLOGY

General Features

- Rare non-Langerhans cell histiocytosis
- Xanthogranulomatous lesions composed of CD68(+)/CD1a(-) histiocytes admixed with inflammation and fibrosis
  - Fibrosis leads to intense uptake on LGE sequences
- Considered histiocytic neoplasm
  - *BRAF* and *MAPK* mutations
- Can involve nearly any system in body

CLINICAL ISSUES

Presentation

- Most common signs/symptoms
  - Lower extremity bone pain most common symptom
  - Central diabetes insipidus due to pituitary involvement
    - Any pituitary deficiency possible
  - CNS, most common in posterior fossa
    - Ataxia, headaches, cognitive impairment
  - Pericardial involvement may cause tamponade
  - Hypertension due to renal or renovascular involvement
  - Xanthelasma: Yellowish plaques around eyelids
  - Orbital involvement can lead to exophthalmos, pain, or vision loss
  - Pulmonary involvement can lead to dyspnea
  - Sinus disease

Demographics

- Age
  - Average: 55 years
  - Rare pediatric cases
- Sex
  - 75% men

Natural History & Prognosis

- Improved prognosis given new advances in therapeutics
  - 5-year survival rate now 83%
- Cardiac involvement associated with worse outcomes in BRAF wildtype patients
- Advanced age of diagnosis, CNS, lung, and retroperitoneal involvement associated with worse outcomes overall

Treatment

- BRAF inhibitors
- MEK inhibitors
- mTOR inhibitors
- Conventional immunosuppressive and chemotherapeutic agents

DIAGNOSTIC CHECKLIST

Consider

- ECD in setting of epicardial soft tissue encasing right AVG and RA or aorta with associated prominent enhancement of 1st-pass perfusion, T1W+, and LGE sequences

SELECTED REFERENCES

1. Roset-Altadill A et al: Epicardial space: comprehensive anatomy and spectrum of disease. Radiographics. 44(4):e230160, 2024
2. Goyal G et al: Erdheim-Chester disease: consensus recommendations for evaluation, diagnosis, and treatment in the molecular era. Blood. 135(22):1929-45, 2020
3. Peng L et al: IgG4-related aortitis/periaortitis and periarteritis: a distinct spectrum of IgG4-related disease. Arthritis Res Ther. 22(1):103, 2020
4. Ghotra AS et al: Cardiovascular manifestations of Erdheim-Chester disease. Echocardiography. 36(2):229-36, 2019
5. Cohen-Aubart F et al: Phenotypes and survival in Erdheim-Chester disease: results from a 165-patient cohort. Am J Hematol. 93(5):E114-7, 2018
6. Villatoro-Villar M et al: Arterial involvement in Erdheim-Chester disease: a retrospective cohort study. Medicine (Baltimore). 97(49):e13452, 2018
7. Dion E et al: Imaging of thoracoabdominal involvement in Erdheim-Chester disease. AJR Am J Roentgenol. 183(5):1253-60, 2004

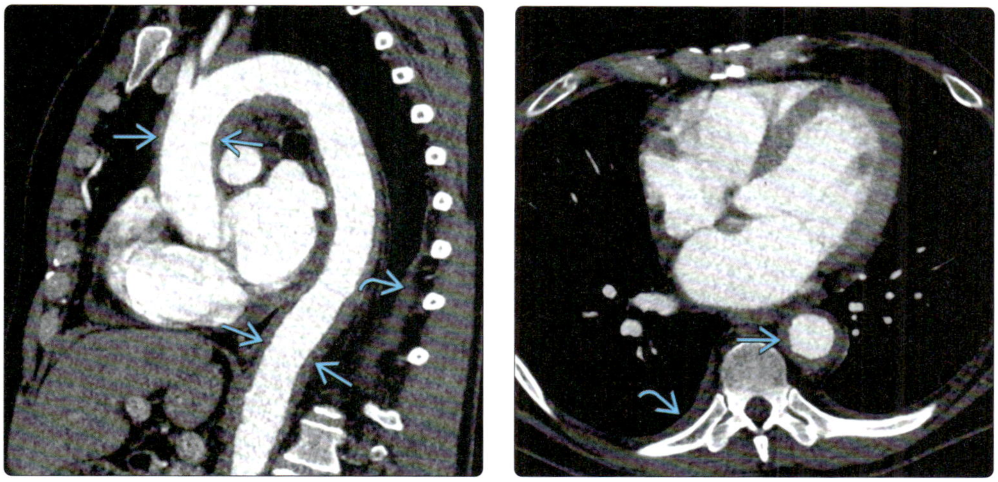

(Left) *CT of the aorta in a 65-year-old man with ECD shows long-segment, continuous circumferential thickening of the entire thoracic and superior abdominal aorta* ➙. *The pleura* ➙ *is also thickened. There is no aneurysm or stenosis, which would commonly be seen with a large-vessel vasculitis.* **(Right)** *Axial image shows the circumferential aortic thickening* ➙ *as well as pleural thickening* ➙. *The aortic wall thickening measures 59 HU.*

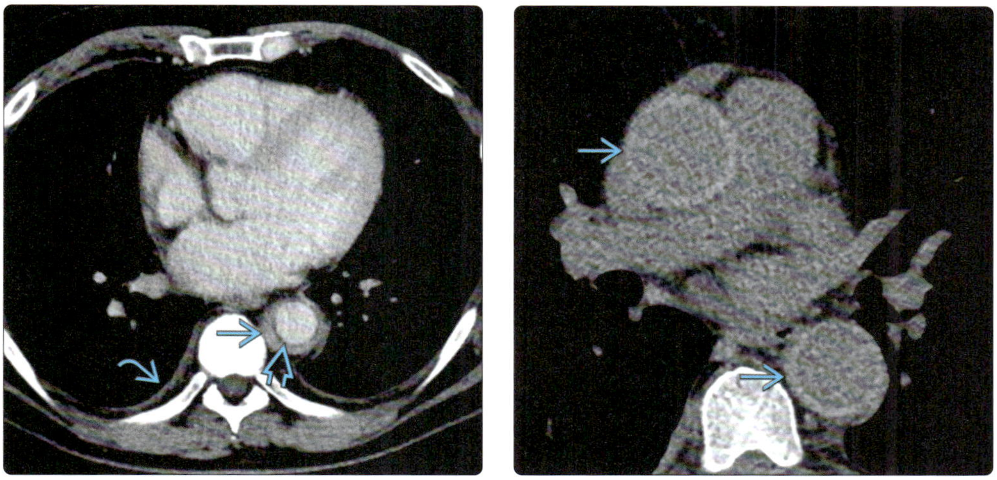

(Left) *Portal venous-phase CECT shows circumferential hyperattenuating soft tissue surrounding the aorta* ➙ *and pleural thickening* ➙. *While the periaortic thickening appears denser compared to the arterial-phase study, the attenuation measures 58 HU. The hypoattenuating rim* ➙ *between the aortic lumen and wall thickening can be seen with both ECD and IgG4 disease.* **(Right)** *NECT shows that the circumferential aortic wall thickening is hyperattenuating, measuring 60 HU, and could mimic an intramural hematoma* ➙.

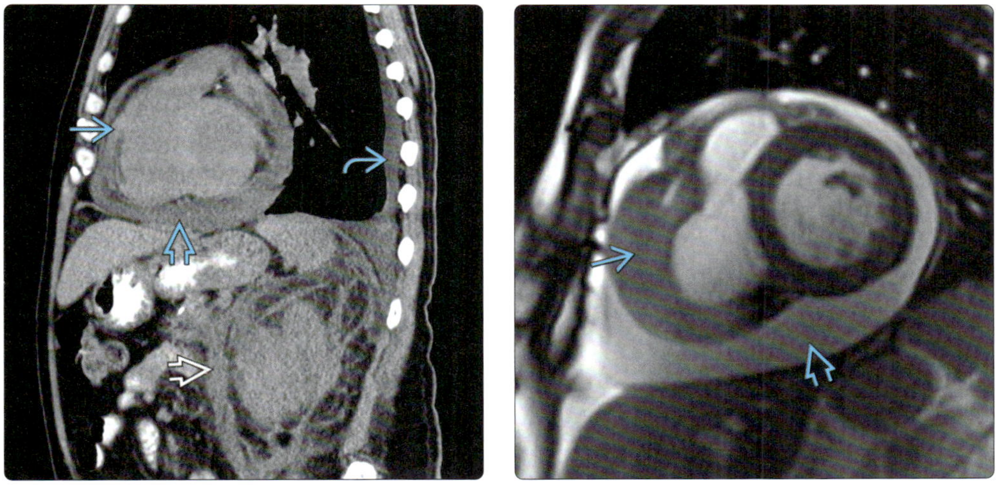

(Left) *Sagittal CT in a 70-year-old man with ECD shows a circumferential pericardial effusion* ➙ *with associated abnormal epicardial soft tissue* ➙. *A small pleural effusion with thickening* ➙ *and circumferential perirenal soft tissue* ➙ *are also shown.* **(Right)** *SSFP MR better shows the extent of the epicardial soft tissue* ➙ *in the right atrioventricular groove. A moderate pericardial effusion* ➙ *is also present. Histiocytes were present in the pericardial fluid from pericardiocentesis.*

Vascular Malformations

KEY FACTS

TERMINOLOGY

- Abnormality of vascular embryologic development
- High-flow vascular malformation (HFVM): Contains arterial feeders with high-velocity flow
  - Arteriovenous fistula (AVF)
    - Direct connections between arteries and veins without intervening capillary bed
  - Arteriovenous malformation (AVM)
    - Low-resistance nidus connected to multiple feeding arteries and draining veins
- Low-flow VM (LFVM): No arterial feeders with low-velocity flow
  - Can be isolated VM of combined venous and lymphatic malformation (LM)

IMAGING

- HFVM
  - Large feeding arteries and draining veins without intervening capillary network
  - Rapid arterial enhancement
  - Flow voids on MR
- LFVM
  - Solid mass with associated venous connections vs. numerous tortuous dilated venous structures without apparent solid component
  - May extend into various compartments
  - Phleboliths in 40%
  - Variable enhancement
    - Slow, progressive enhancement
    - Venous enhancement with washout
  - May have dysplastic draining vein
  - No flow voids on MR

TOP DIFFERENTIAL DIAGNOSES

- Hemangioma
- LM
- Paraganglioma

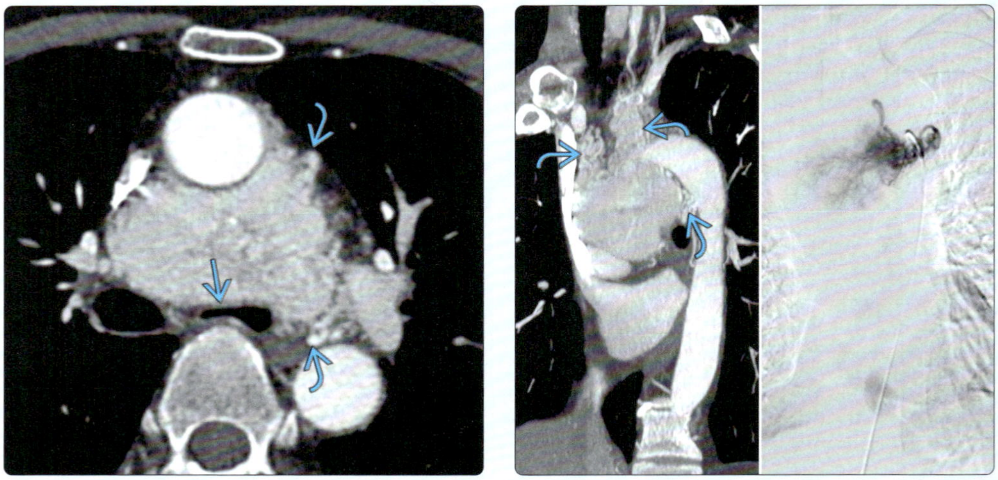

(Left) *Axial CTA in a 56-year-old man with incidental mass on CXR shows a large, avidly enhancing middle mediastinal mass with compression of left mainstem bronchus. Note numerous large feeding vessels.* **(Right)** *MIP (L) shows numerous large feeding arteries supplying the nidus. Bronchial artery angiogram (R) shows rapid arterial filling of the nidus. Without radiologist consultation, the mass was surgically biopsied, leading to extensive hemorrhage. Pathology showed a high-flow vascular malformation (VM).*

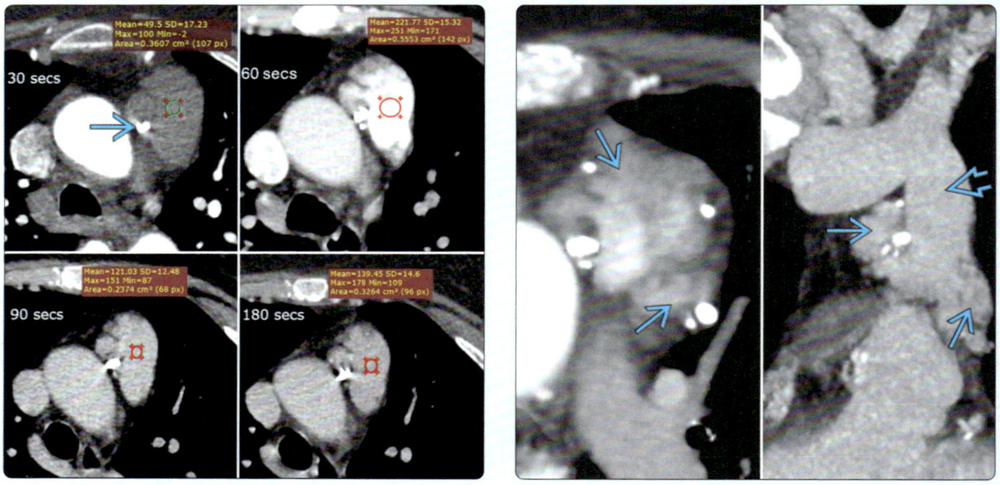

(Left) *Axial CT images obtained at 30, 60, 90, and 180 seconds after contrast show peak enhancement of a low-flow venous malformation at 60 seconds with mild persistent enhancement at 180 seconds. One of a few scattered phleboliths is seen.* **(Right)** *The mass with phleboliths drains into the left brachiocephalic vein via a large anomalous vein, which is not the left-sided superior vena cava. Slow-flow VMs of the mediastinum are commonly associated with anomalous draining veins.*

TERMINOLOGY

Abbreviations

- Vascular malformations (VMs)

Definitions

- Abnormality of vascular embryologic development
- Capillary, venous, arterial, or lymphatic components
  - Often mix of elements
- Often divided into high-flow VM (HFVM) and low-flow VM (LFVM)
- HFVM: Contains arterial feeders with high-velocity flow
  - Arteriovenous fistula (AVF)
    - Direct connections between arteries and veins without intervening capillary bed
  - Arteriovenous malformation (AVM)
    - Low-resistance nidus connected to multiple feeding arteries and draining veins
- LFVM: No arterial feeders with low-velocity flow

IMAGING

General Features

- Best diagnostic clue
  - HFVM: Large feeding arterial vessels supplying mediastinal nidus with draining veins
  - LFVM: Rounded mass in mediastinum with phleboliths with anomalous draining vein(s)
- Location
  - Mediastinum
    - Can occur anywhere in body
- Size
  - Variable

CT Findings

- HFVM
  - Mediastinal HFVMs are quite rare
  - Large feeding arteries and draining veins without intervening capillary network
  - May have large, arterially enhancing nidus, which can compress surrounding structures
- LFVM
  - Variable appearance
    - Solid mass with associated venous connections
    - Numerous tortuous dilated venous structures without apparent solid component
      - Fat often interspersed between vessels
  - May extend into various compartments
  - Phleboliths in 40%
    - Helps differentiate VMs from other malformations
  - Variable enhancement
    - Slow, progressive enhancement
    - Rapid or nodular enhancement with washout
  - May have dysplastic draining vein

MR Findings

- HFVM
  - T2 hyperintense
  - Feeding vessels from major arterial branches
    - Rapid perfusion and arterial enhancement
    - Well assessed with multiple MRA acquisitions
  - Flow voids common due to rapid blood flow
- LFVM
  - T2 hyperintense
  - Phleboliths as areas of signal void
  - Slow progressive enhancement > rapid enhancement and washout
  - Flow voids uncommon

DIFFERENTIAL DIAGNOSIS

Hemangioma

- Vascular tumor, not congenital
- Well-defined mass without large feeding arteries or veins

Lymphatic Malformation

- LFVM and lymphatic malformation (LM) may coexist within same mass
- Isolated LM has widely variable appearance

Paraganglioma

- HFVM with large, enhancing nidus can mimic paraganglioma
- ↑ PTH and calcium imbalance common in paraganglioma
- May have hypertension

PATHOLOGY

General Features

- LFVM
  - Dysplasias of small and large venous channels connected to adjacent veins
  - Variable amount of hamartomatous stroma
  - May be purely venous or mixed venous and LMs
- HFVM
  - Direct connection between arterial and venous systems
  - Mediastinal AVM not associated with hereditary hemorrhagic telangiectasia

CLINICAL ISSUES

Presentation

- Most common signs/symptoms
  - Mediastinal HFVM and LFVM often asymptomatic
  - May compress surrounding structures
  - HFVM can hemorrhage
- Other signs/symptoms
  - May be associated with syndromes, such as Sturge-Weber, Klippel-Trenaunay, Proteus syndrome, Maffucci, CLOVES
  - HFVM can lead to high-output cardiac failure

Treatment

- LFVM: May not require treatment in mediastinum
- HFVM: Interventional embolization

SELECTED REFERENCES

1. Ota Y et al: Vascular malformations and tumors: a review of classification and imaging features for cardiothoracic radiologists. Radiol Cardiothorac Imaging. 5(4):e220328, 2023
2. Hussein A et al: Imaging of vascular malformations. Radiol Clin North Am. 58(4):815-30, 2020
3. Merrow AC et al: 2014 revised classification of vascular lesions from the International Society for the Study of Vascular Anomalies: radiologic-pathologic update. Radiographics. 36(5):1494-516, 2016

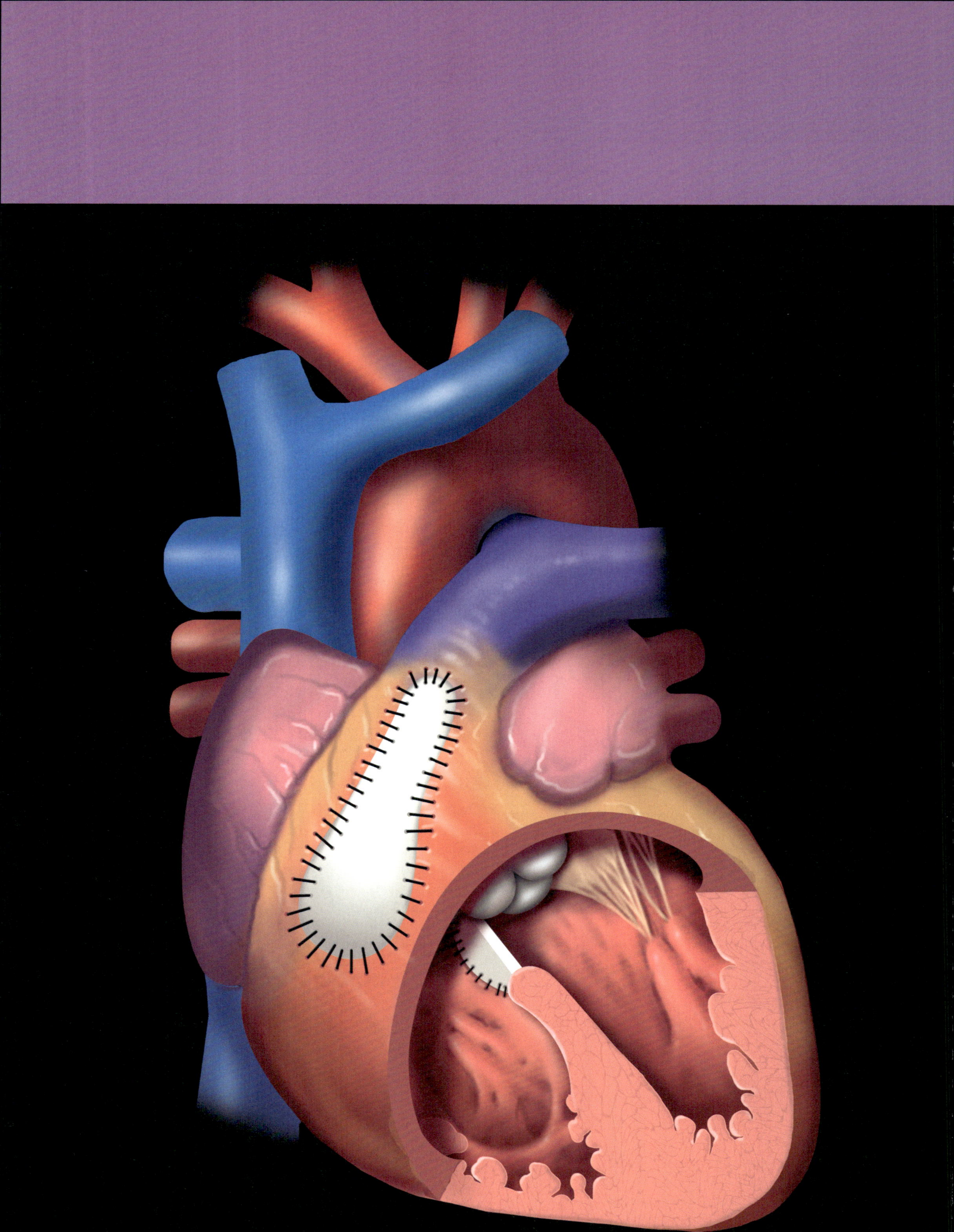

SECTION 7

Congenital Heart Disease

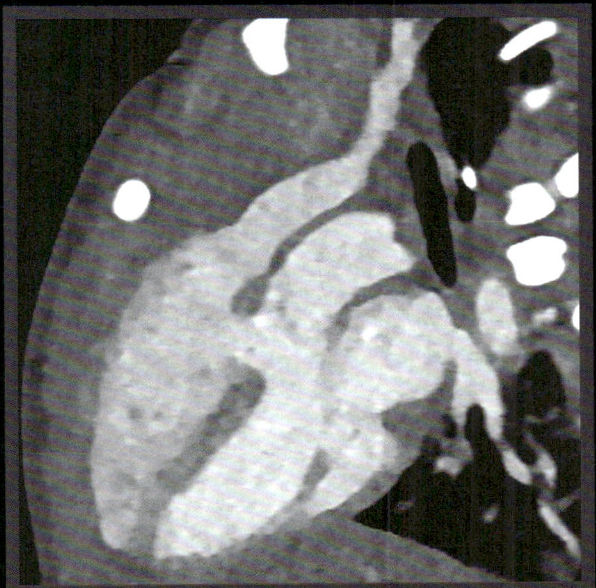

Introduction

Nearly 50 years ago, Van Praagh developed a system for classification of congenital heart disease (CHD) using a segmental anatomic model based on cardiac embryologic development: A simple notation using 3 letters separated by commas convey findings that can be understood among providers, a stepwise approach that allows the imager to organize even the most complicated cardiac malformations and more accurately assess structure, function, and dysfunction.

Van Praagh Segmental Approach

1st Step: Visceroatrial Situs

"Situs" refers to anatomic orientation of visceral organs across the left-right axis of the body. Visceroatrial situs is defined by the relationship between the atria and thoracoabdominal organs and categorized as follows.

- **Situs solitus** (S, -, -) represents the normal configuration with right-sided right atrium (RA) and liver and left-sided left atrium (LA), spleen, and stomach. There is a normal trilobed right lung with early takeoff of the right upper lobe bronchus from the main bronchus and eparterial bronchial position [i.e., the right pulmonary artery (RPA) travels immediately anterior to the right main bronchus]. There is a bilobed left lung defined by a more distal origin of the left upper lobe bronchus with hyparterial bronchial position [i.e., the left pulmonary artery (LPA) arches over the left main bronchus].
- **Situs inversus** (I, -, -) represents a mirror image configuration of **situs solitus**. The LA, spleen, and stomach are on the right. The RA and liver are on the left. There is a trilobed left lung with eparterial bronchus and a bilobed right lung with hyparterial bronchus.
- **Situs ambiguus** (A, -, -), or heterotaxy, is present when the **situs** is neither **solitus** nor **inversus**. There are 2 generally described subsets of **situs ambiguus**: Bilateral right-sidedness (asplenia syndrome, right isomerism) and bilateral left-sidedness (polysplenia syndrome, left isomerism). Patients with asplenia syndrome generally have bilateral trilobed lungs, a horizontal position to the liver, splenic agenesis, and severe CHD. In contrast, patients with polysplenia syndrome have bilateral bilobed lungs, multiple small splenules, interruption of the inferior vena cava (IVC) with azygos or hemiazygos continuation, and less severe CHD (e.g., atrial septal defect or ventricular septal defect).

Atrial situs can be reliably predicted by the bronchial branching pattern, as the RA is generally on the side of the trilobed lung, and the LA is generally on the side of the bilobed lung. However, cardiac chambers are not necessarily defined by their expected right-left location but more accurately by their structural characteristics. These designations can be determined by several features, including the shape of the atrial appendages and the venous contribution to the chamber (venoatrial concordance). The left atrial appendage is a finger-like, pointed projection with a narrow orifice, whereas the right atrial appendage has a broad opening and blunted shape. The cardiac chamber receiving systemic inflow via the IVC or coronary sinus is almost always the **morphologic** RA (so-called rule of venoatrial concordance). After determining the atrial arrangement, one should next determine the position of the liver, spleen, and stomach to identify the overall pattern of visceroatrial situs.

Cardiac position relative to the midline sternum is important to describe because discordant situs and cardiac position is associated with more severe congenital defects. These descriptors include **levocardia**, **dextrocardia**, or **mesocardia**, representing leftward, rightward, or midline cardiac orientation, respectively. These descriptors refer only to the position of the heart in the chest and do not imply internal cardiac chamber or other visceral arrangements.

2nd Step: Ventricular Loop Orientation

In week 4 of gestation, the primitive heart tube elongates and folds ventrally and caudally, either to the right or left, representing a critical maneuver in determining cardiac morphology. A normal D-loop (-, D, -) designation is applied when the morphologic right ventricle (RV) rotates rightward, and an L-loop (-, L, -) designation is applied when it rotates abnormally leftward.

Ventricular loop orientation is preceded by first identifying the **morphologic** RV and left ventricles (LVs) according to several distinguishing features of each. The morphologic RV is characterized by a muscular infundibulum separating the atrioventricular and ventriculoarterial valves, moderator band, coarse trabeculation, and papillary muscles that attach to both the septum and the free wall. The morphologic LV lacks a moderator band and instead has fibrous continuity of the atrioventricular and ventriculoarterial valves, fine trabeculae, a smooth interventricular septum, and papillary muscles that attach only to the free wall.

The hand rule is meant to help differentiate D-loop from L-loop. If the virtual right hand can be placed within the RV with the palm facing the ventricular septum, the thumb extending through the tricuspid valve, and the fingers within the RV outflow tract, then a D-loop exists. If this is only possible with the left hand, it indicates an L-loop.

When ventricular morphology is difficult to discern, the "loop rule" can be used, which maintains that the rotation is D-loop (i.e., the RV is to the right of the LV) in the presence of a right-sided aortic valve, and the rotation is L-loop (i.e., the RV is to the left of the LV) in the presence of a left-sided aortic valve.

3rd Step: Identification of Position and Origins of Great Vessels

In the normal configuration of the great vessels (-, -, S), the main pulmonary artery (MPA) is located anterior and to the left of the aorta (**solitus**). The opposite arrangement is referred to as **inversus** (-, -, I). A spectrum of other configurations may occur and are notated as D-transposition (-, -, D-TGA), L-transposition (-, -, L-TGA), D-malposition (-, -, D-MGA), and L-malposition (-, -, L-MGA).

In D-transposition, the aorta is located anterior and to the right of the MPA with the aorta originating from the morphologic RV and the MPA originating from the morphologic LV (ventriculoarterial discordance). In L-transposition, the aorta is located anterior and to the left of the MPA with the aorta originating from the morphologic RV and the MPA originating from the morphologic LV. In contrast to D-transposition, there is also atrioventricular discordance (i.e., the ventricular loop has an L-orientation). This creates a situation that has been termed congenitally corrected transposition, as oxygenated blood still flows to the systemic circulation, and deoxygenated blood still flows to the lungs.

Malpositions occur in the setting of a double-outlet ventricle and are diagnosed when the great vessels are parallel to each other and originate from a single ventricle. **Truncus arteriosus** occurs when a single great vessel arises from both ventricles.

Atrioventricular Connection

Five types of atrioventricular connections have been described: Concordant, discordant, ambiguous, double inlet, or absent. In concordant connection (normal), the LA connects to the LV, and the RA connects to the RV. In discordant connection (e.g., L-transposition), the RA connects to the LV, whereas the LA connects to the RV. An ambiguous connection occurs in the setting of heterotaxy syndrome. Double-inlet and absent connections are used in the setting of univentricular situations.

Associated Malformations

Associated malformations that are not addressed in the segmental approach are important to note, as they may influence the surgical approach. The size and type of atrial or ventricular septal defects and their effect on ventricular function should be assessed. Abnormalities of the aortic and pulmonary outflow tracts may include hypoplasia, interruption, stenosis, coarctation, and patent ductus arteriosus. When present, a left superior vena cava (SVC) typically enters into the RA via the coronary sinus. In 10% of patients, abnormal drainage occurs through an unroofed coronary sinus into the LA, creating a right-to-left shunt. Flow from the IVC may be interrupted with azygos or hemiazygos continuation. All pulmonary venous connections should be assessed for abnormalities in course or caliber.

Footsteps of Surgeon

Palliative Procedures

The **modified Blalock-Taussig shunt** (BTS) is used to augment pulmonary blood flow to decrease cyanosis as a bridge to definitive repair. Typically, a synthetic graft is interposed between the subclavian and pulmonary arteries. Thrombosis is the most common complication, occurring months to years following shunt creation. The shunt is typically taken down or ligated at the time of definitive repair.

Pulmonary arterial banding utilizes synthetic material about the pulmonary artery to decrease blood flow and protect the pulmonary arterioles from high-pressure states. It is also used to hypertrophy "train" the LV prior to a Jatene arterial switch procedure for repair of transposition. If the arterial switch procedure is performed without pulmonary arterial banding, the LV will often fail, as it has not been exposed to pressures required to pump blood systemically. Major complications of pulmonary arterial banding include pulmonary arterial dilation and pulmonic valve insufficiency.

Definitive Surgeries

The **bidirectional Glenn shunt** is used to augment pulmonary blood flow in the setting of right-sided heart hypoplasia or atresia (e.g., tricuspid atresia, hypoplastic right heart, Ebstein anomaly). The SVC is removed from the RA and is connected to the RPA, which allows deoxygenated blood from the upper extremity to bypass the heart and directly enter both lungs. The procedure requires a low-pressure system to perfuse the lungs, and, thus, must be performed after pulmonary vascular resistance drops (i.e., ~ 3-9 months following birth).

The bidirectional Glenn shunt is usually followed by a **Fontan procedure** in which venous return from the lower 1/2 of the body is diverted either around (conduit) or through (baffle) the right heart and directly into the pulmonary arteries via prosthetic tunnel from the IVC. Complications include shunt thrombosis, pulmonary arteriovenous malformations, or venovenous collaterals.

The **Norwood procedure** is a 3-stage surgery for treatment of patients with hypoplastic left heart syndrome. The goals of the surgery are to convert the RV into the systemic pumping chamber, create unobstructed systemic venous blood flow to the lungs, and divert pulmonary venous return to the RA. **Stage 1** is performed shortly after birth and uses a homograft from the MPA to reconstruct the hypoplastic aorta. The atrial septum is excised to create a single atrium and allow oxygenated pulmonary venous return to pass into the RV. Finally, the pulmonary blood flow is reestablished by a modified BTS or Sano shunt (i.e., RV to pulmonary artery conduit). **Stage 2** includes ligation of the modified BTS and placement of a bidirectional Glenn shunt. In **stage 3**, a Fontan procedure completely separates the systemic and pulmonary circulations.

Historically, repair for transposition of the great arteries (TGA) involved the use of intraatrial baffles (e.g., **Mustard** and **Senning** procedures) to redirect systemic venous blood to the LV and oxygenated pulmonary venous blood to the systemic RV. Complications included baffle stenosis, obstruction, or leak. The **Jatene arterial switch procedure with Lecompte maneuver** is now preferred for TGA repair. In this procedure, the aorta and pulmonary arteries are switched and reanastomosed to their respective ventricles. The Lecompte maneuver places the MPA anterior to the aorta to reduce the risk of coronary artery compression. Complications of the Jatene procedure include delayed pulmonary stenosis, aortic enlargement, and coronary artery stenoses.

The main goals of therapy in patients with tetralogy of Fallot include closing the ventricular septal defect and relieving RV outflow tract obstruction, typically via **transannular patch**. Early on, the response is adaptive and improves RV output but eventually leads to decompensation, pulmonic regurgitation, and RV dysfunction. In patients with **tetralogy of Fallot with pulmonary atresia**, early definitive surgical repair involves closure of the ventricular septal defect and placement of a valved conduit between the RV and MPA.

Aortic coarctation can be repaired either with open (direct excision, aortoplasty, bypass) or percutaneous approaches (angioplasty, stent). Complications associated with surgical repair include recurrent coarctation, aneurysm, and impaired growth of the left upper extremity. Complications of percutaneous techniques include aneurysm at the site of angioplasty, dissection, and vessel rupture.

Selected References

1. Canan A et al: Multimodality imaging of transposition of the great arteries. Radiographics. 41(2):338-60, 2021
2. Ranganath P et al: Computed tomography in adult congenital heart disease. Radiol Clin North Am. 57(1):85-111, 2019
3. Schallert EK et al: Describing congenital heart disease by using three-part segmental notation. Radiographics. 33(2):E33-46, 2013
4. Lu JC et al: Evaluation with cardiovascular MR imaging of baffles and conduits used in palliation or repair of congenital heart disease. Radiographics. 32(3):E107-27, 2012
5. Babar JL et al: Application of MR imaging in assessment and follow-up of congenital heart disease in adults. Radiographics. 30(4):1145, 2010
6. Lapierre C et al: Segmental approach to imaging of congenital heart disease. Radiographics. 30(2):397-411, 2010
7. Van Praagh R: Diagnosis of complex congenital heart disease: morphologic-anatomic method and terminology. Cardiovasc Intervent Radiol. 7(3-4):115-20, 1984

(Left) *Coronal CECT shows normal bronchial anatomy in situs solitus with early takeoff of the right upper lobe bronchus relative to the left upper lobe bronchus. The right bronchus is eparterial, whereas the left bronchus is hypoarterial.* **(Right)** *Composite image shows the right atrial appendage (left panel) with a broad opening and triangular shape. The left atrial appendage (right panel) has a narrow orifice located near the left superior pulmonary vein ostium.*

Normal Bronchial Anatomy

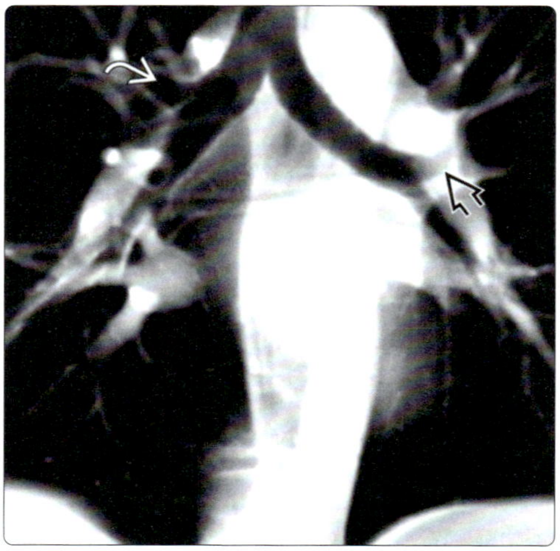

Atrial Appendage Morphology

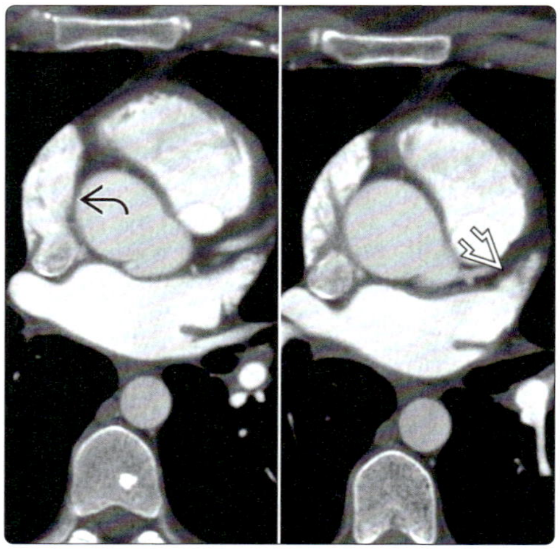

(Left) *Short-axis CTA at the midventricular level shows 2 papillary muscles attaching to the left ventricular free wall. No papillary muscles attach to the interventricular septum in the morphologic left ventricle (LV).* **(Right)** *Axial CTA shows a moderator band originating from the interventricular septum, a feature that identifies the ventricle as the morphologic right ventricle (RV). The cardiac loop is "L" in this case because the RV is to the left of the LV.*

Normal Left Ventricle

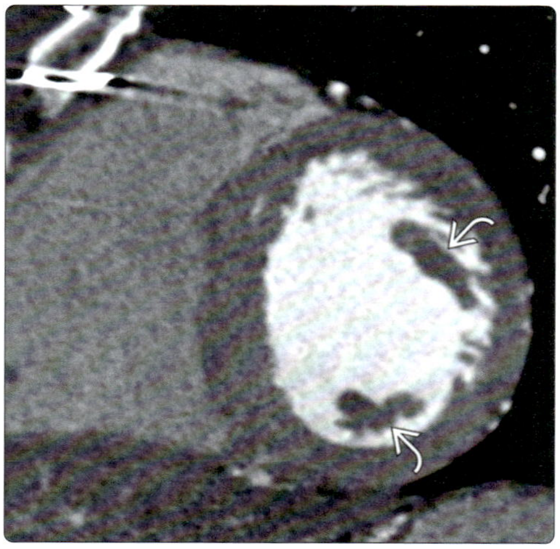

Right Ventricle Appearance in L-Loop

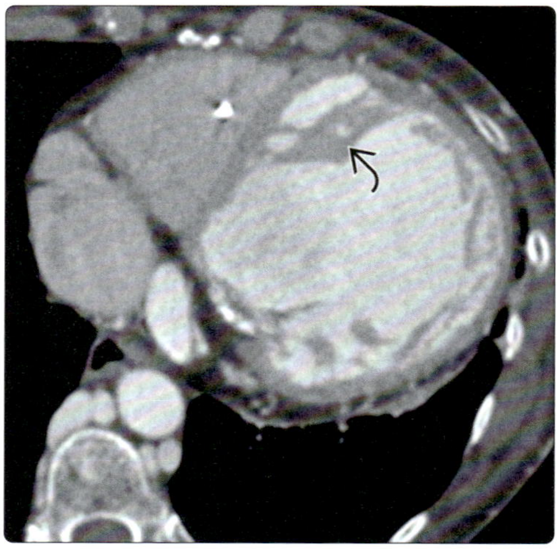

(Left) *Left ventricular outflow tract (3-chamber) view CTA shows fibrous continuity (connection) of the aortic valve and the mitral valve, which is a key feature for identification of the morphologic LV (aorta = Ao; left atrium = LA).* **(Right)** *Oblique coronal CECT shows a muscular infundibulum separating the pulmonic valve from the tricuspid valve, which is a key feature of the morphologic RV (right atrium = RA, main pulmonary artery = PA, aorta = Ao).*

Features of Morphologic Left Ventricle

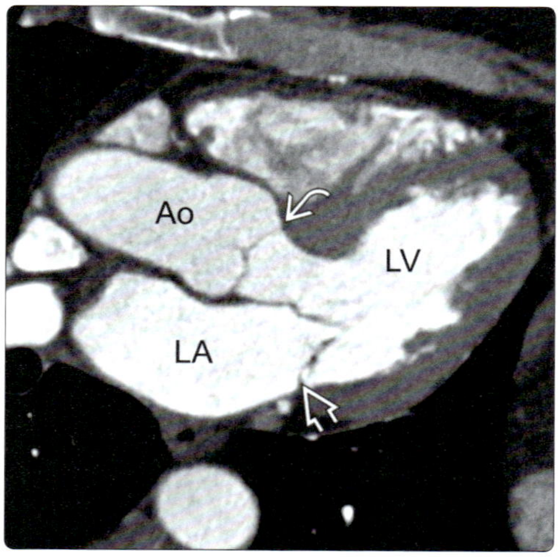

Features of Morphologic Right Ventricle

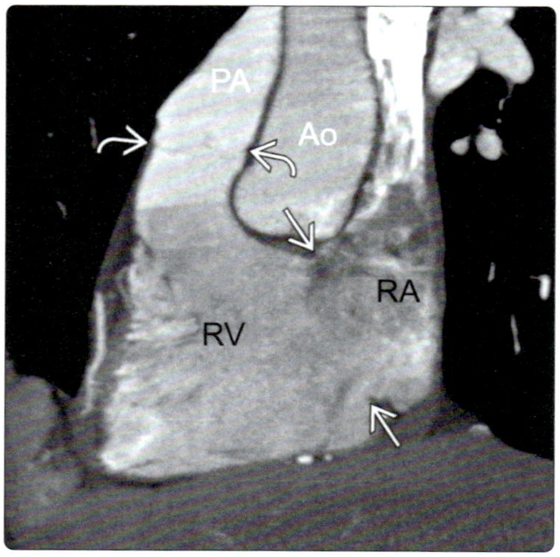

Situs Inversus

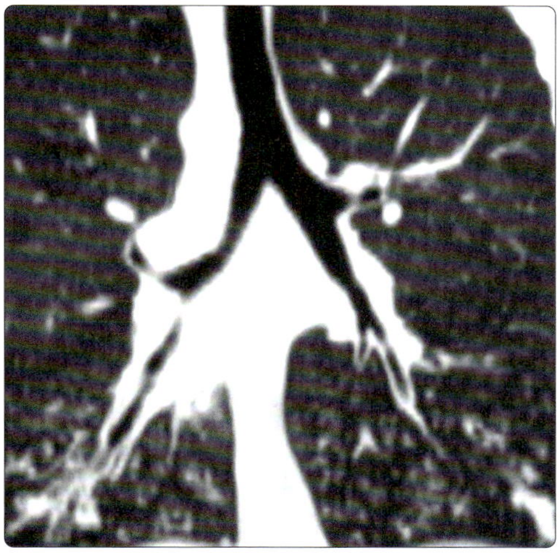

Situs Inversus

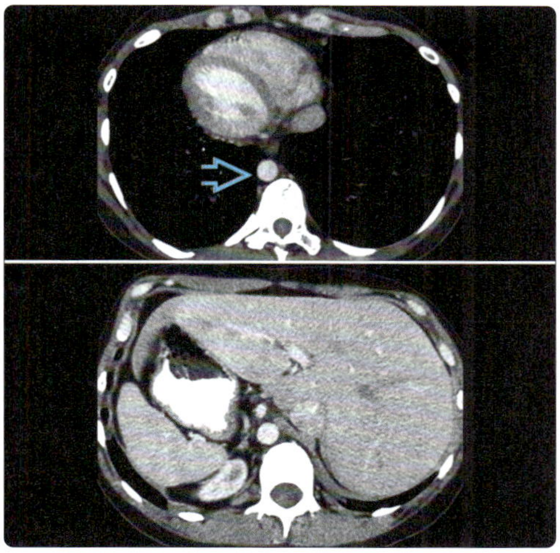

(Left) *Coronal CT shows situs inversus, lower lobe bronchiectasis, and tree-in-bud nodules in a patient with Kartagener syndrome. The right bronchus is hypoarterial & has late takeoff of the upper lobe bronchi, which is typical of the left lung, whereas the left bronchus is eparterial & has an early takeoff of upper lobe bronchus, which is more typical of right lung.* **(Right)** *Composite image in the same patient shows a right descending thoracic aorta (Ao), right-sided spleen, and left-sided liver in situs inversus totalis (I, -, -).*

Heterotaxy

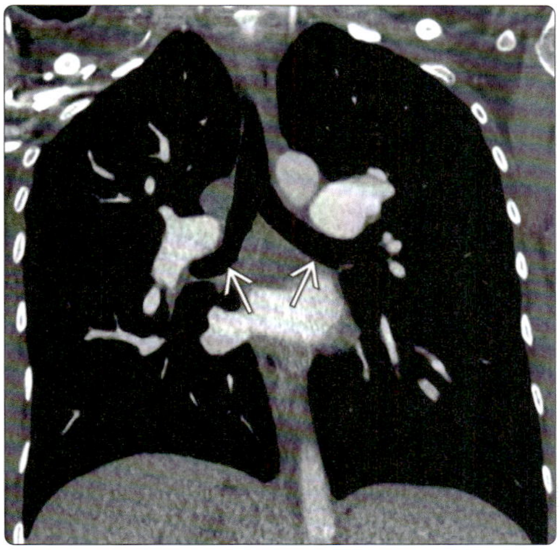

Heterotaxy

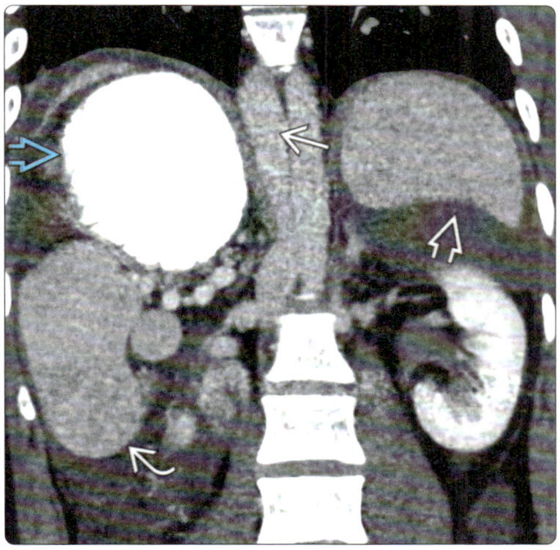

(Left) *Coronal CECT shows bilateral hyparterial bronchi with a bilateral left-sided bronchial branching pattern in this patient with heterotaxy syndrome.* **(Right)** *Coronal CT in a patient with known heterotaxy syndrome shows an extrahepatic inferior vena cava (IVC) continuing into the thorax as the azygos vein. Note the right-sided stomach and spleen and left-sided liver.*

Heterotaxy

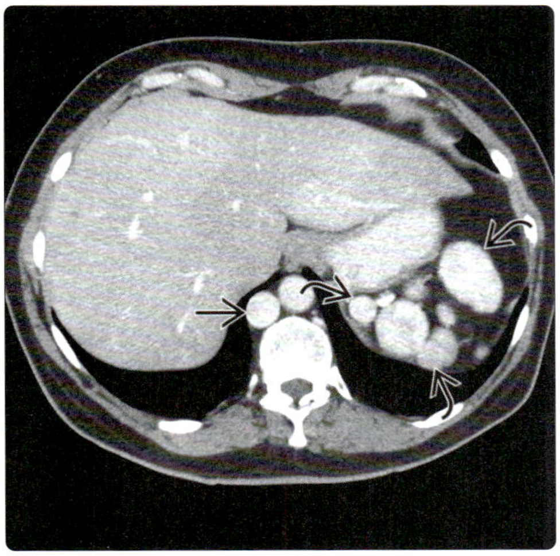

Heterotaxy

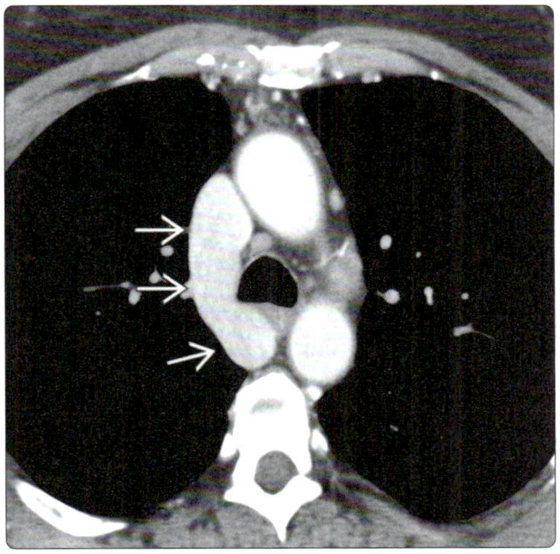

(Left) *Axial abdominopelvic CT shows an enlarged azygos vein and multiple spleens in heterotaxy syndrome with bilateral left-sidedness or polysplenia.* **(Right)** *Axial chest CT in the same patient shows a very enlarged and dilated azygos vein, in keeping with azygos continuation of the IVC in heterotaxy syndrome, a finding more often seen with bilateral left-sidedness.*

(Left) *Graphic shows the positions of the aortic (red) and pulmonary (blue) valves and arteries in the settings of solitus configuration, situs inversus totalis, D-transposition of great arteries (TGA), and L-transposition of great arteries (LGA).* **(Right)** *Composite image shows the relationship of the Ao and main pulmonary artery (PA) in a solitus (left) and inversus (right) configuration. In solitus, the Ao is located posterior and to the right of the PA. In inversus, the Ao is located posterior and to the left of the PA.*

Aortic/Pulmonic Valve Relation

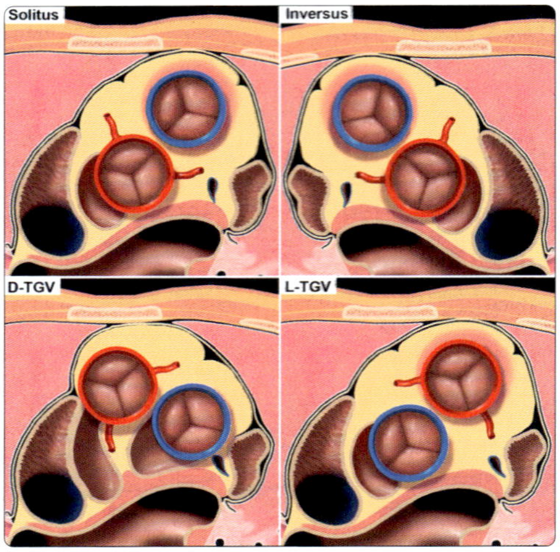

Aortic/Pulmonic Valve Relation

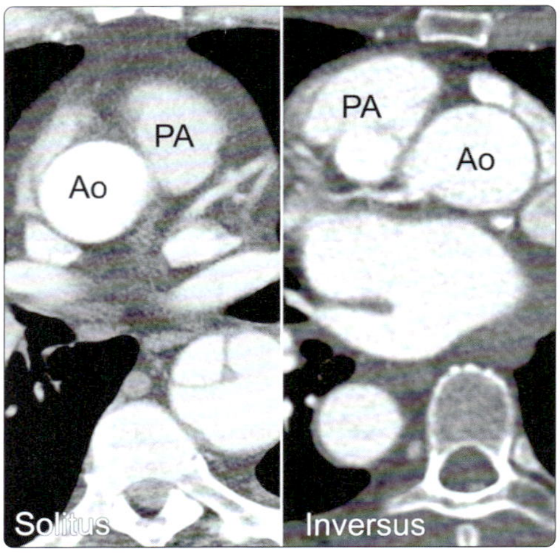

(Left) *Composite image shows the relationship of the Ao and main PA in D- (left) and L- (right) transposition. In D-TGA, the Ao is located anterior and to the right of the pulmonary artery. In L-TGA, the Ao is located anterior and to the left of the PA.* **(Right)** *Frontal chest radiograph shows globular cardiomegaly ⇨ with a narrow vascular pedicle →, the so-called egg-on-a-string configuration of the cardiomediastinal silhouette associated with TGA.*

Aortic/Pulmonic Valve Relation

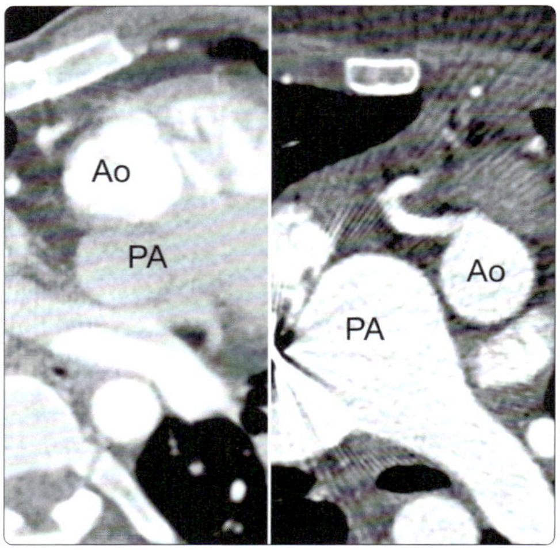

Transposition of Great Arteries

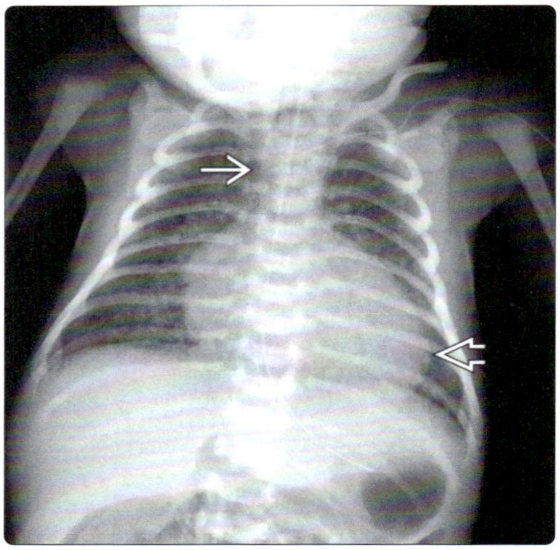

(Left) *Axial SSFP MR in a patient with repaired TGA by atrial switch procedure with intraatrial baffle → shows pulmonary venous drainage directed to the systemic right ventricle ⇨.* **(Right)** *Axial oblique MRA shows the classic findings of a Jatene arterial switch with the PA → lying anterior to the Ao ⇨ and the left and right PAs ↪ draping over the Ao. This is the preferred method for surgical correction of TGA.*

Transposition of Great Arteries

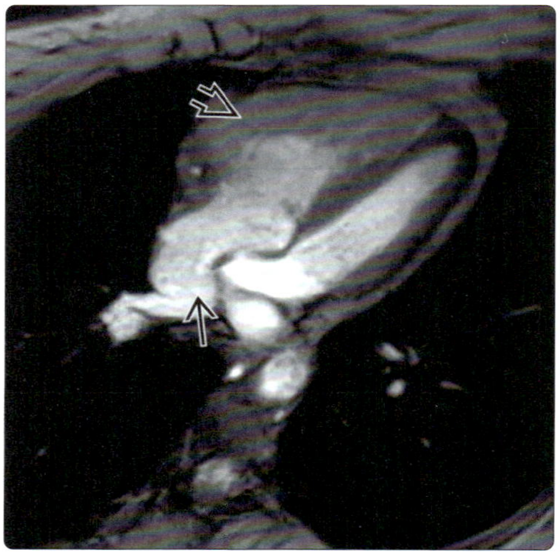

Status Post Jatene Procedure

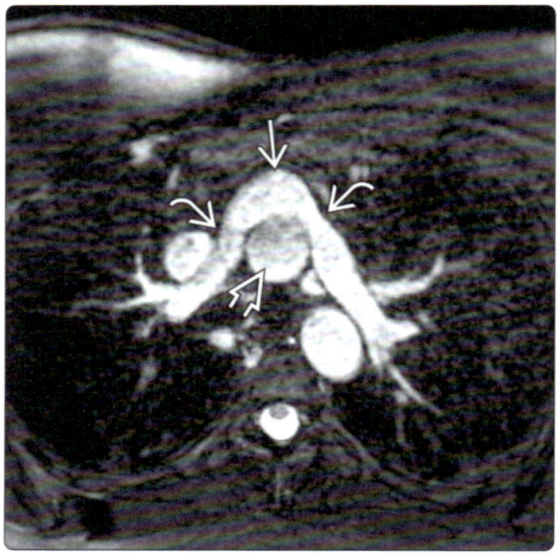

Tetralogy of Fallot

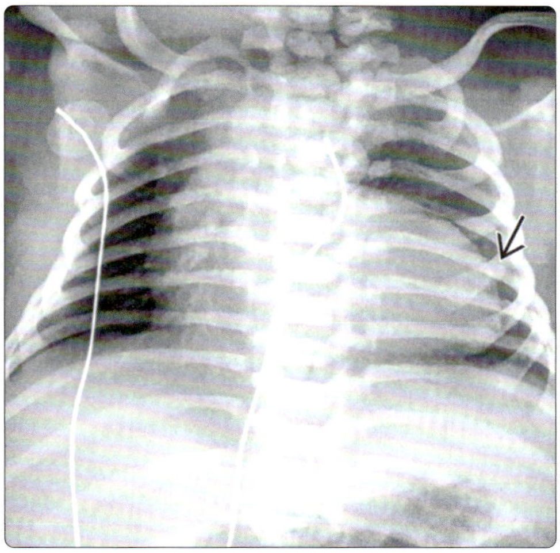

Tetralogy of Fallot

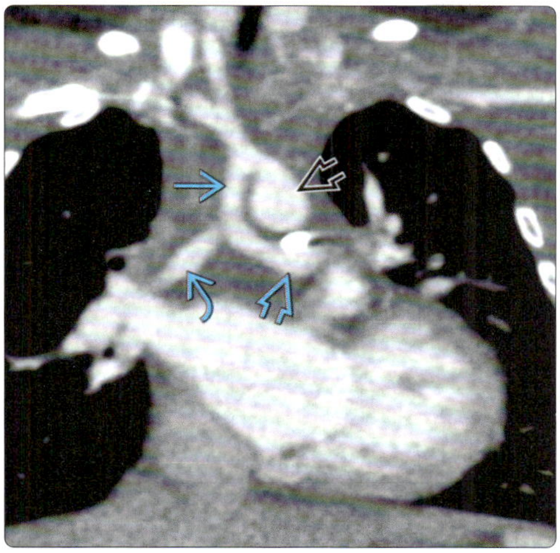

(Left) *Frontal chest radiograph in a neonate with known tetralogy of Fallot (TOF) shows the classic boot-shaped heart with upturned ventricular apex and right aortic arch. Note associated diminished pulmonary blood flow.* **(Right)** *CECT in a 4-month-old with TOF shows a modified Blalock-Taussig shunt (BTS) from the Ao to the right and left PAs. (Courtesy S. Kligerman, MD.)*

Hypoplastic Left Heart

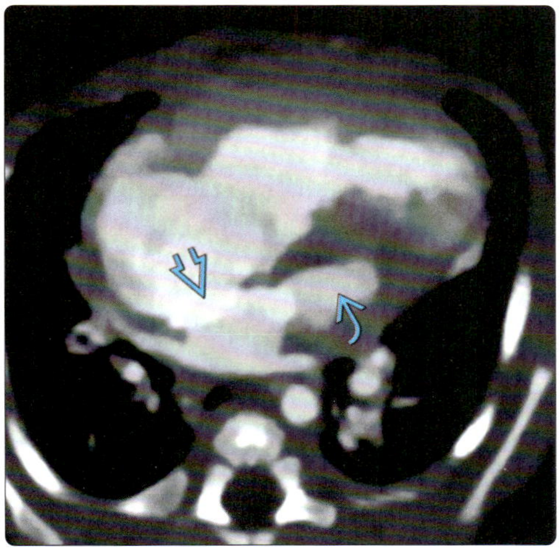

Hypoplastic Left Heart

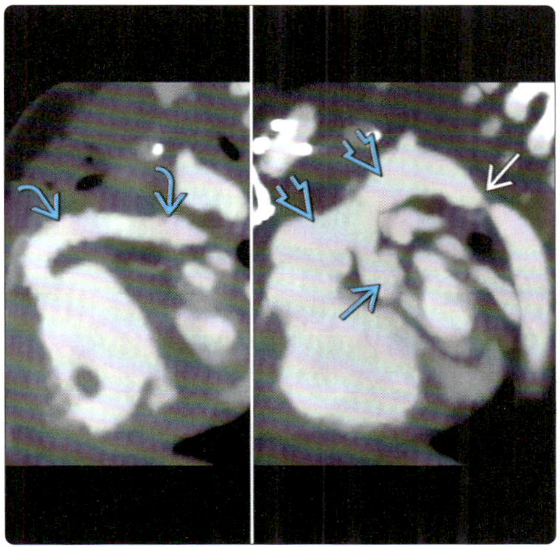

(Left) *Four-chamber CECT in a 2-month-old baby shows a hypoplastic left heart and a surgically created large atrial septal defect. The right atrium and RV are enlarged.* **(Right)** *Sagittal images from the same study show a Sano shunt (left) from the RV outflow tract to the main PA. Image slightly more midline (right) shows the result of a Norwood procedure, which uses the PA to reconstruct the hypoplastic Ao, which still connects to the small Ao root. Notice the aortic coarctation.*

Hypoplastic Left Heart

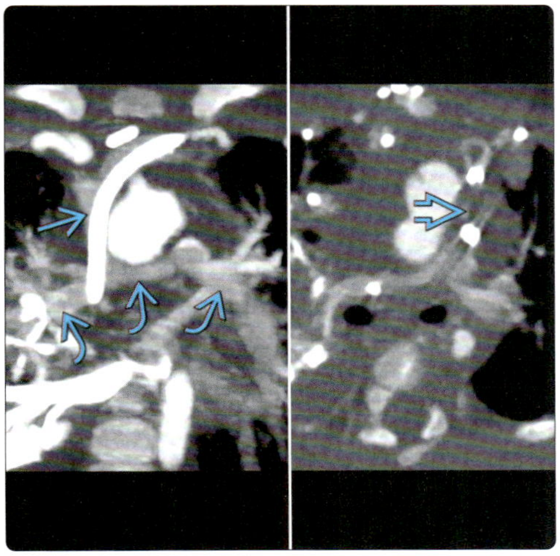

Hypoplastic Left Heart

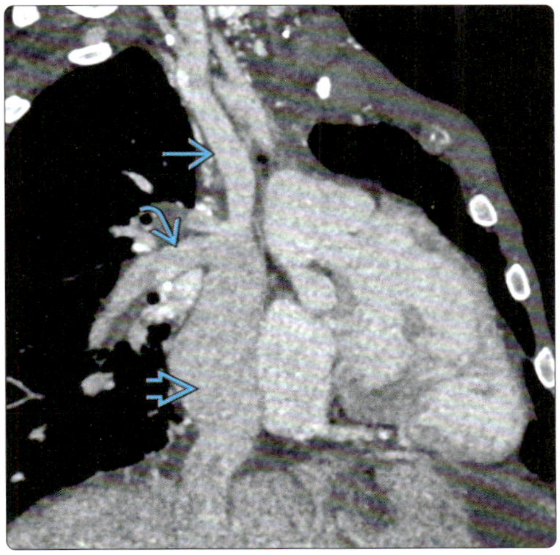

(Left) *Coronal-oblique MIP (left) in a hypoplastic left heart syndrome (HLHS) patient at 6 months of age immediately post-op shows the creation of a bidirectional Glenn shunt, which connects the superior vena cava to the PAs. Axial oblique image (right) shows ligation of the Sano.* **(Right)** *CECT in a 16-year-old patient with HLHS shows a Fontan circuit with the superior vena cava and IVC supplying the right and left (not seen) PAs. (Courtesy S. Kligerman, MD.)*

Introduction

Adults with congenital heart disease (CHD) will require regular imaging follow-up to assess cardiac structure and function as well as to monitor for disease progression or late complications. Early detection of altered hemodynamics related to both congenital repairs and age-related anatomic degeneration helps determine the need for intervention. Imaging protocols must be tailored to each individual patient according to his or her developmental or postoperative anatomy. Patients with CHD may undergo multiple imaging examinations over their lifetimes, many of which are associated with ionizing radiation (cardiac catheterization, CT, nuclear perfusion, stress tests, and chest radiography). Hence, cumulative radiation risk must be considered in selection of imaging modalities. Several options are available for imaging adults with CHD, each with distinct advantages and limitations.

Imaging Protocols

Echocardiography

According to the 2018 American Heart Association/American College of Cardiology Guidelines for the Management of Adults With Congenital Heart Disease, transthoracic (TTE) or transesophageal echocardiography (TEE) are considered 1st-line modalities for both initial and serial assessment for patients with adult CHD. Given its portability, widespread availability, and noninvasive technique, TTE can provide structural and functional information relatively quickly with less expense than CT and MR imaging. Contrast-enhanced echocardiography can be performed with introduction of echogenic microbubbles from agitated saline or other inert gases to evaluate shunts and improve endocardial resolution. Real-time, high-resolution images of intracardiac anatomy can be performed quickly, even in critical patients. However, echocardiography may be limited in its ability to provide details of certain extracardiac vascular anatomy, including coronary artery anatomy and course. Other limitations include the presence of metal, bone, air interfaces, or other patient factors (thoracic deformities, obesity, pulmonary disease), which may restrict the interrogation window or dampen the sonographic beam.

MR Imaging

Cardiovascular MR (CMR) imaging provides an alternate diagnostic option to echocardiography for evaluation of CHD. Both can be used for serial examinations, as they do not require ionizing radiation. With exquisite morphologic detail, CMR can address most imaging questions and plays a valuable role in noninvasive assessment of chamber size and function and valvular structure and function as well as extracardiac vasculature, shunts, and conduits with high spatial and temporal resolution. In fact, CMR is considered the gold standard for comprehensive evaluation of right ventricular structure and function. Exquisite tissue contrast afforded by CMR allows for assessment of the myocardium, including parametric mapping techniques for myocardial edema or fibrosis. Gadolinium contrast material provides information about ischemia, fibrosis, and masses (e.g., thrombi). Cine imaging allows for highly reproducible visualization of cardiac and valvular motion as well as comprehensive ventricular function. Phase-contrast mapping permits quantification of shunts and flow dynamics across valves.

Steady-state free precession (SSFP) is the workhorse CMR sequence, allowing simultaneous evaluation of cardiac structure and motion without the need for contrast. Data are acquired over many cardiac cycles in a single 10- to 5-second breath hold. Spatial and temporal resolution afforded by SSFP allows quantification of ventricular mass, chamber volume, and ejection fraction with measurements made on contiguous short-axis images. Tissue characterization techniques, such as black-blood spin-echo sequences, apply excitation and refocusing pulses, which excludes signals produced from moving protons (flowing blood) but require longer acquisitions. Phase-contrast imaging involves short-axis acquisition in vascular planes, allowing directional flow calculation through the prescribed imaging plane and assessment of flow jets, stenoses, regurgitation, and shunts. 4D flow techniques allow quantification of directional flow assessment. 3D slab imaging allows segmental evaluation of the heart, acquiring thinner slices, which allow for post processing of MR data.

Commercially available software allows the imager to reconstruct CMR data sets and create measurements of anatomy as well as function, including stroke volumes, ejection fraction, and wall motion. 3D and volumetric reconstructions allow visualization of complex postoperative anatomy, including surgical shunts and conduits.

CT

Cardiac CT (CCT) can serve a complementary role in the diagnostic evaluation of adults with CHD and is the preferred option when CMR is contraindicated or unavailable. Very small anatomic structures can be imaged given the high spatial resolution of CCT, including the noninvasive evaluation of coronary artery anomalies and patency. In addition to cardiac morphology, CCT allows for assessment of other extracardiac vascular structures. Functional information can be obtained with newer generation scanners but requires longer exposure times applied over the entire cardiac cycle. Unlike CMR, CCT is very fast, and the entire heart may be imaged within a second or seconds, especially with advanced multidetector and dual-source CT technology. The primary disadvantage of CCT over echocardiography and CMR is the exposure of patients to ionizing radiation. Medications (β-blockers and nitroglycerin) may be necessary to control heart rate and optimize coronary artery evaluation. Iodinated contrast material is used, which carries its own risks of allergy and nephrotoxicity.

Scanners with a 64-detector row or higher with cardiac gating capability are necessary to collect rapid and high-quality, thin-section data sets. Tube voltage, current, and pitch parameters should be adjusted based on patient body size with pediatric protocols varying from 80-120 kVp 30-80 mA, pitch 2.0 to adult protocols using up to 220 mA, 100-140k Vp, and lower pitch. Automated anatomy-based or ECG-based dose-modulation techniques can be added for dose reduction. A precontrast scan may be added to identify surgical material, degenerative changes, or calcifications and are particularly useful in suspected acute aortic pathology, such as intramural hematoma or for determination of coronary artery calcium scores. In some instances, delayed venous-phase scans (60-90 seconds) may be added to assess the patency of the inferior limb of Fontan pathways.

- **High-pitch helical** scanning (pitch values up to 3.4) requires dual-source scanner ability to scan chest and entire aorta to femoral arteries in 1-2 seconds, all while maintaining very low effective radiation dose (often submillisievert); this can be performed ± ECG gating; temporal resolution of as low as 75 ms is possible with

this technology and may eliminate need for ECG gating and β-blockade in some instances
- **Volumetric** scanning utilizes multidetector row CT configuration with large coverage in single heartbeat (320 or 640 slices, z-axis coverage of 8-16 cm); temporal resolution is less robust than ultra-high-pitch options
- **Prospectively triggered** sequential scanning (step-and-shoot) techniques acquire CT data in interrupted sequential slabs, turning tube current on and off between successive table positions; excellent anatomic detail can be obtained, but misregistration with motion (stair-step) artifacts limit its utility; function, wall motion, or chamber dimensional information can be derived; inhomogeneous contrast opacification may occur as 1-2 heartbeats typically pass between successive slabs for table movement
- **Adaptive sequential** scanning is variation of prospective acquisition, wherein acquisition of data occurs in various points in cardiac cycle and is post processed together with ECG data; this allows for assessment of cardiac motion but still requires regular rhythm with added cost of higher radiation
- **Retrospectively gated helical** acquisition techniques employ oversampling of data at every level to increase temporal coverage; ECG data is recorded throughout, and 3D data set over entire heart cycle is post processed ("retrospective"); this allows for assessment of valve motion and myocardial function, despite arrhythmia, but requires high radiation dose; radiation dose can be reduced in this technique by using tube current modulation, wherein maximal tube current is delivered in preselected phases and lower radiation dose is utilized for remaining cardiac phases

CT data can be transferred to dedicated software programs to allow reformatting targeted to the structure or physiologic variable in question. Example reformats include oblique planar reconstruction into cardiac projections (short axis, vertical long axis, 3 chamber, 4 chamber), valve planes, linear or curved vessel projections, maximum or minimum intensity projection (MIP, minIP), shaded surface display, volume rendering, and occasional functional data.

Patient Preparation and Contrast Injection

Deliberate preparation of both pediatric and adult patients for CCT ensures patient safety, reduces radiation dose, and optimizes image quality. All patients should be screened for allergy to contrast media and renal insufficiency. Young children may require sedation. Elevated heart rates generally contribute to reduced image quality, which can be improved with administration of β-blockers prior to the scan. However, evolving CT technology and image speed has produced high-quality image reconstruction despite motion, allowing β-blockade to be avoided in patients with CHD, as the ability to evaluate intracardiac abnormalities and coronary artery course is preserved. Nitroglycerin may be required for adequate assessment of coronary artery stenosis. Patients should be screened for use of phosphodiesterase inhibitors (e.g., Viagra-like drugs), as the combination with nitroglycerin can precipitate fatal hypotension. Iodinated intravascular contrast material is injected at body-sized adjusted doses and varying rates, generally through upper extremity veins using power-injectable IV access of at least 20-g caliber. Saline bolus chasing techniques may be applied to avoid streak artifacts from undiluted contrast in the right ventricle. Automated bolus-tracking techniques allow triggering of scans at various threshold attenuation values measured from regions of interest placed on the left ventricle (pediatric) or ascending aorta (adults). Test bolus techniques use a plot of the arrival of a small bolus of contrast material within the aorta or pulmonary artery to determine the optimal timing of the scan. These techniques may need to be adjusted for evaluation of complex anatomy, e.g., in patients with single-ventricle functional configuration, wherein adjustments to contrast injection and scan triggering (pulmonary artery) are required.

CMR examinations require extensive planning and protocol preparation on the part of the imager. The sequences should be selected to answer the specific clinical question. Contraindications to the use of CMR include the presence of ferromagnetic implants or certain pacemakers. It is now possible to scan patients with several pacemakers and implantable cardioverter defibrillators (ICDs), provided adequate safety procedures and operational conditions are followed. Magnetic field limitations include image degradation by metallic susceptibility artifacts within the field of view (e.g., sternotomy wires or other implants) as well as cardiopulmonary motion artifacts, which may require cardiac or respiratory triggering in addition to patient cooperation with breath-holding maneuvers over several sequences.

Summary

As treatments for CHD have advanced over the past decades, so have the number of patients who survive to adulthood. Patients with mild disease may remain asymptomatic throughout childhood, ultimately receiving the 1st diagnosis as adults when they present with symptoms of acquired cardiopulmonary alterations resulting from chronic CHD and other age-related comorbidities. Many such patients may be encountered in community healthcare settings, and, thus, general imagers must be prepared to diagnose CHD and associated complications. In addition, the imager must understand the complex pathophysiology of each congenital abnormality, recognize the sequelae of surgical interventions, and prescribe specific imaging protocols to permit systematic assessment of cardiovascular anatomy, dynamics, and related complications that may require intervention.

Selected References

1. Egidy Assenza G et al: AHA/ACC vs ESC guidelines for management of adults with congenital heart disease: JACC Guideline Comparison. J Am Coll Cardiol. 78(19):1904-18, 2021
2. Ranganath P et al: Computed tomography in adult congenital heart disease. Radiol Clin North Am. 57(1):85-111, 2019
3. Stout KK et al: 2018 AHA/ACC guideline for the management of adults with congenital heart disease: executive summary: a report of the American College of Cardiology/American Heart Association Task Force on clinical practice guidelines. J Am Coll Cardiol. 73(12):1494-563, 2018
4. De Cecco CN et al: Pictorial review of surgical anatomy in adult congenital heart disease. J Thorac Imaging. 32(4):217-32, 2017
5. Gaydos SS et al: Imaging in adult congenital heart disease. J Thorac Imaging. 32(4):205-16, 2017
6. Suranyi P et al: An overview of cardiac computed tomography in adults with congenital heart disease. J Thorac Imaging. 32(4):258-73, 2017
7. Ghadimi Mahani M et al: CT for assessment of thrombosis and pulmonary embolism in multiple stages of single-ventricle palliation: challenges and suggested protocols. Radiographics. 36(5):1273-84, 2016
8. Lapierre C et al: Segmental approach to imaging of congenital heart disease. Radiographics. 30(2):397-411, 2010

Sinus Venosus Atrial Septal Defect

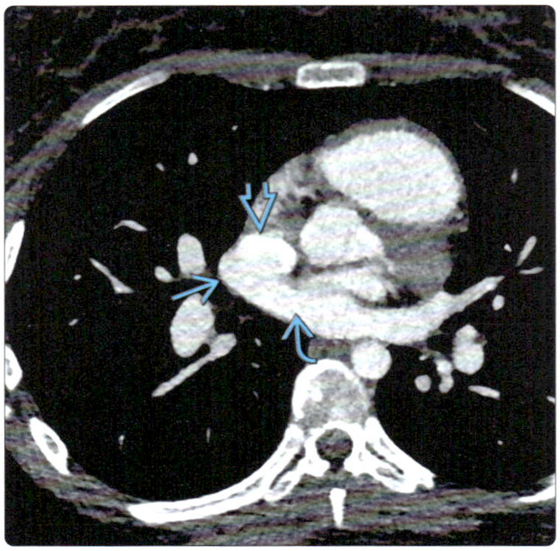

Sinus Venosus Atrial Septal Defect and Partial Anomalous Pulmonary Venous Return

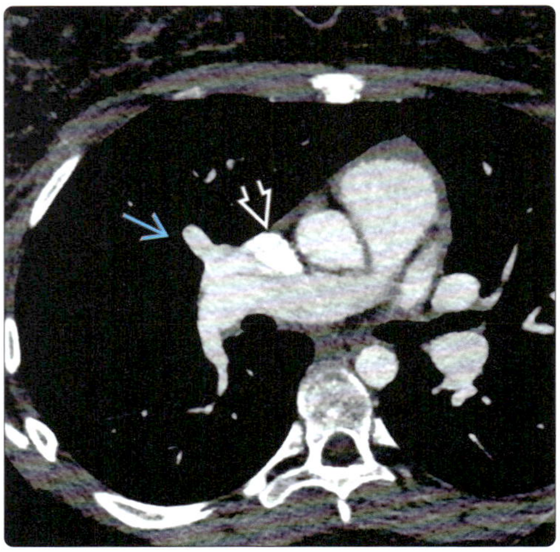

(Left) *Axial CECT in a 44-year-old woman with progressive dyspnea on exertion shows an abnormal connection between the right superior pulmonary vein, superior vena cava (SVC), and left atrium in keeping with partial anomalous venous return from the right upper lobe and associated sinus venosus atrial septal defect (ASD).* **(Right)** *Axial CECT in the same patient better depicts the abnormal connection between the right superior pulmonary vein and SVC, producing a left-to-right shunt.*

Patent Ductus Arteriosus

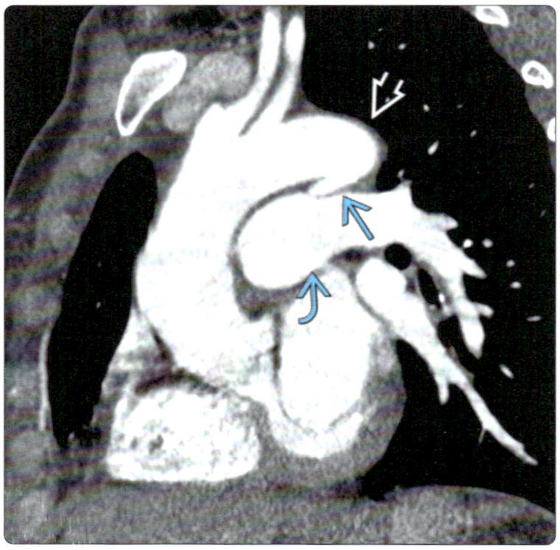

Coarctation

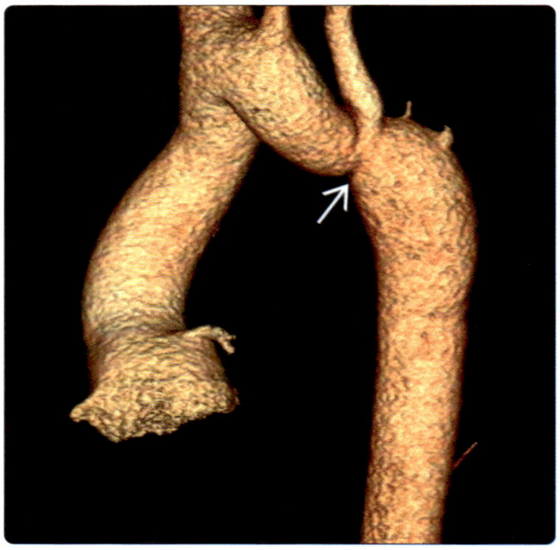

(Left) *Sagittal oblique reformatted CECT in a 52-year-old woman with progressive dyspnea depicts the morphology and size of a patent ductus arteriosus, which connects the aortic arch and main pulmonary artery (PA).* **(Right)** *3D volume-rendered CTA of the aorta details the appearance of the aorta as well as the degree of stenosis at the site of prior coarctation repair. Post processing of CT or MR data to create 3D reconstructions often aids in surgical planning.*

Tetralogy Repair

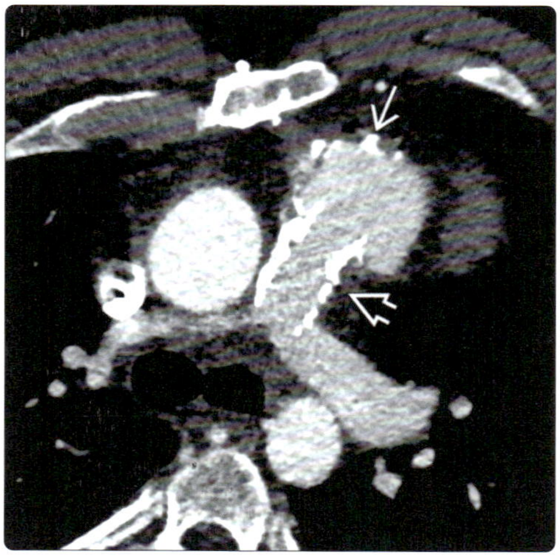

Tetralogy Repair

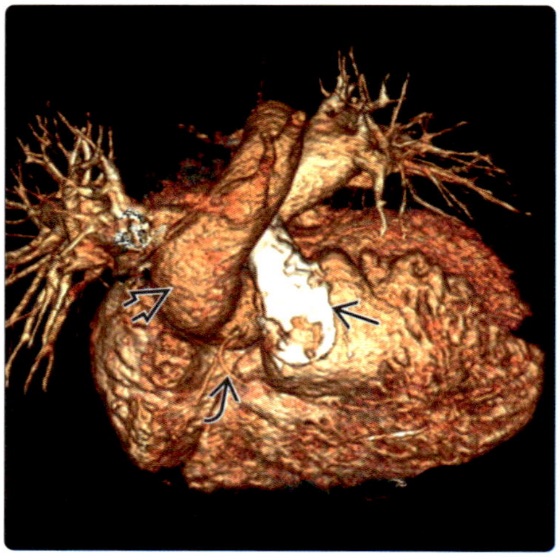

(Left) *Axial CECT in a patient with remote Tetralogy of Fallot (TOF) repair shows high-attenuation material around the right ventricular outflow tract (RVOT), representing the RVOT patch and size discrepancy of the repaired main PA.* **(Right)** *3D volume-rendered CT reformat in the same patient shows the relationship of the RVOT patch to the surrounding anatomy, including the ascending aorta and coronary arteries.*

Tetralogy Repair

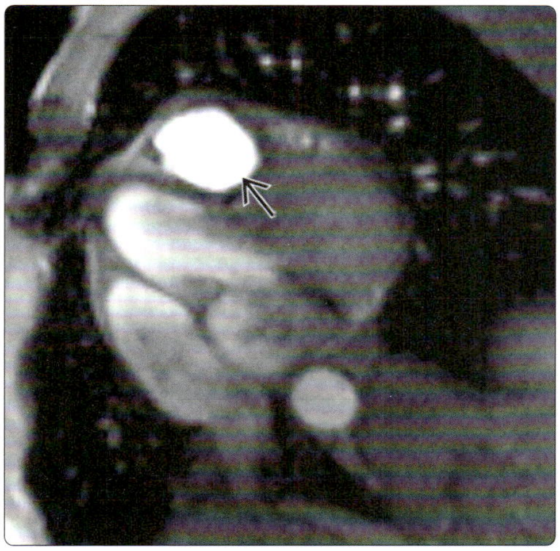

Tetralogy Repair

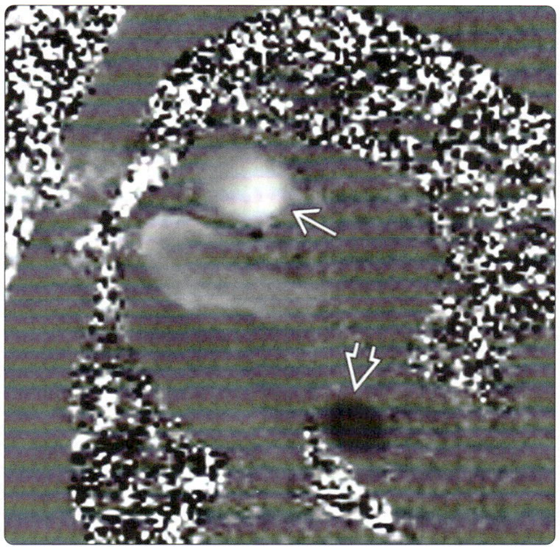

(Left) *Axial oblique phase-contrast MR (magnitude) in plane with the pulmonic valve ➙ in a patient with repaired TOF with RVOT patch is shown.* **(Right)** *Corresponding axial oblique phase-contrast MR in the same patient shows antegrade (cranial) flow ➙ through the pulmonic valve (white signal). The descending aorta shows antegrade (caudal) flow that is in the opposite direction (black signal) ➙. Phase-contrast MR allows the evaluation of jet flows, valve regurgitation or stenosis, and cardiac shunts.*

Fontan

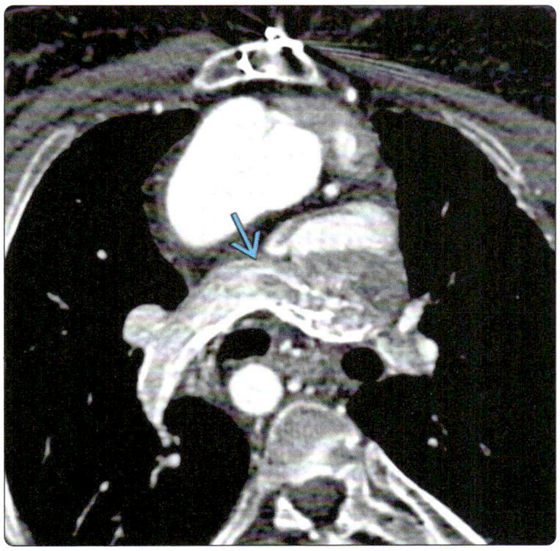

Fontan

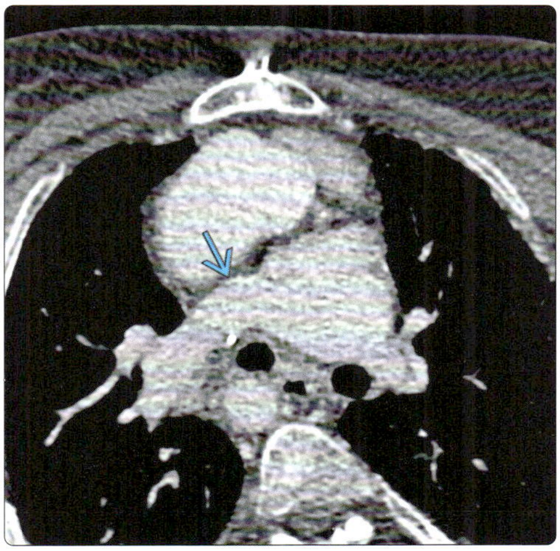

(Left) *Early-phase CECT in a girl with heterotaxy, D-transposition of the great arteries, & double-outlet right ventricle treated with Fontan procedure shows streaky mixing artifact ➙ within PAs.* **(Right)** *Axial delayed (90 seconds) CECT (same patient) shows homogeneous enhancement of PAs ➙, excluding central thrombus. Patients with single ventricle palliation require protocol modifications, such as delayed imaging or dual injection of contrast into upper and lower extremity veins to prevent false-positives.*

Truncus Arteriosus

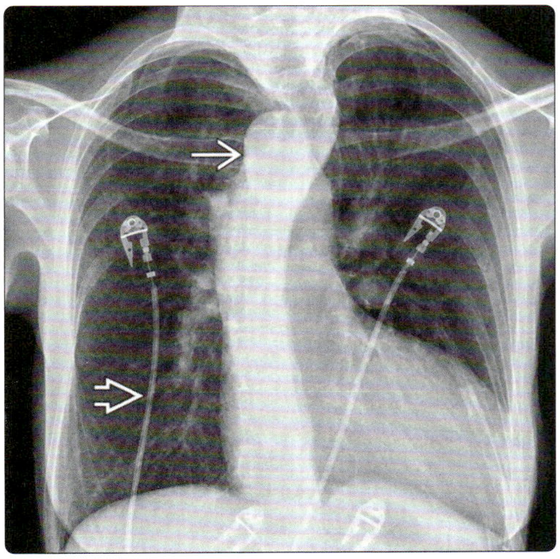

Truncus Arteriosus

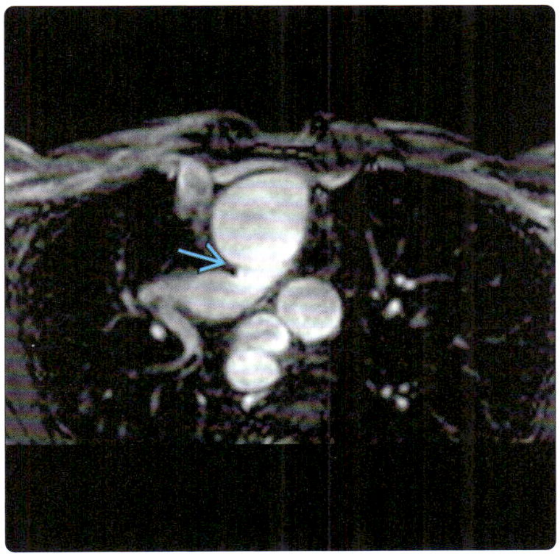

(Left) *Frontal chest radiograph in a patient with unrepaired truncus arteriosus and a ventricular septal defect (VSD) shows a right-sided aortic arch ➙, narrow superior cardiomediastinal silhouette, vascular pruning ➙, and cardiomegaly.* **(Right)** *Axial MR in the same patient shows the right PA arising from the posterior aspect of ascending truncus ➙. The left PA arises from the underside of the aortic arch (not shown). This configuration is consistent with the type A3 Van Praagh truncus classification.*

Tetralogy of Fallot

KEY FACTS

TERMINOLOGY

- Underdevelopment of pulmonary infundibulum due to unequal partitioning of conal truncus resulting in subvalvular or valvular right ventricular (RV) outflow tract stenosis, subaortic ventricular septal defect (VSD), overriding aorta, and RV hypertrophy

IMAGING

- Echocardiography is 1st-line to diagnose and monitor
- Classic radiographic appearance: Boot-shaped heart
- CTA or cardiac MR for pulmonary artery (PA) anatomy, aortopulmonary collateral arteries
- Cardiac catheterization and angiography for PA pressure measurements and percutaneous interventions

PATHOLOGY

- ↓ pulmonary blood flow → greater right-to-left shunting → cyanosis (classic blue "tet")
- Normal or ↑ pulmonary flow → congestive heart failure (pink "tet")
- Frequent associations: Right-sided aortic arch with mirror image branching, atrial septal defect (ASD), left superior vena cava, absent pulmonary vein (PV), coronary anomalies

CLINICAL ISSUES

- Most common cyanotic congenital heart disease

DIAGNOSTIC CHECKLIST

- Goals of preoperative imaging
  - Identify level and degree of obstruction
  - Identify pulmonary vascular anatomy: PV or PA stenosis/atresia
  - Locate alternative sources of pulmonary blood flow: Major aortopulmonary collateral arteries, PDA
  - Configuration of aortic arch and branches
  - Cardiac shunts: VSD, ASD
  - Other congenital abnormalities and anatomy of tracheobronchial tree

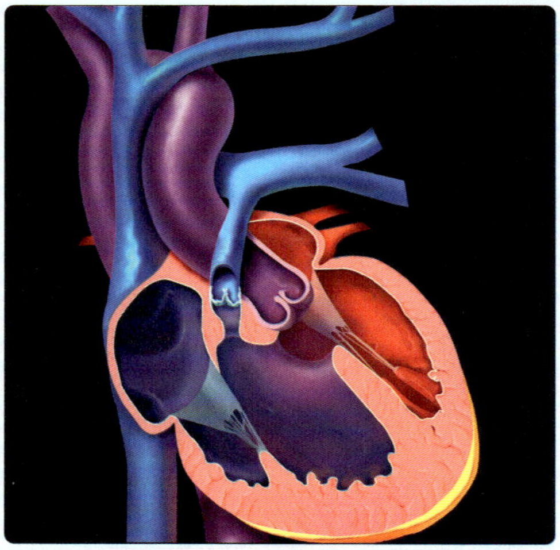

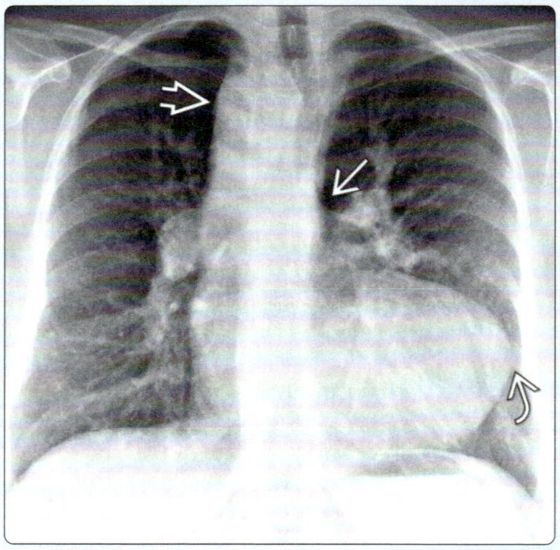

(Left) *Graphic shows subvalvular and valvular pulmonary stenosis with a hypoplastic pulmonary artery, a membranous ventricular septal defect, muscular right ventricular (RV) hypertrophy, and an overriding aorta (Ao) receiving mixed blood from the RV and left ventricle (LV), indicating tetralogy of Fallot (TOF).* **(Right)** *PA radiograph of an adult with untreated TOF shows a right aortic arch, a narrow vascular neck due to pulmonary atresia, and an elevated cardiac apex due to RV hypertrophy (coeur en sabot appearance).*

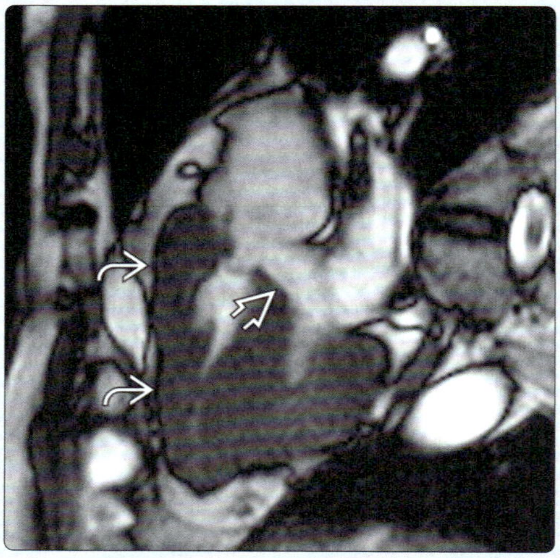

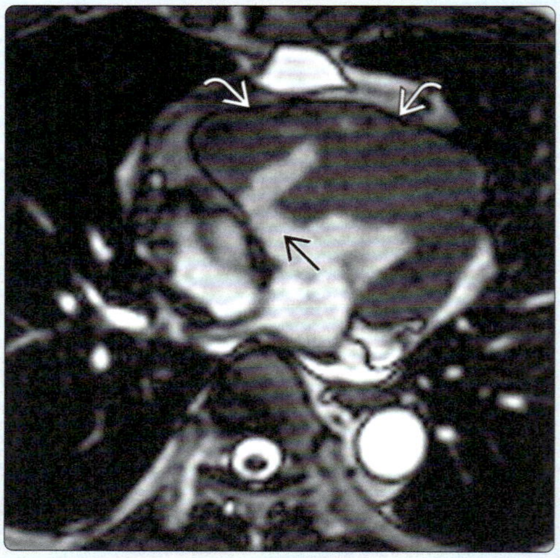

(Left) *LV outflow tract SSFP CMR shows typical features of TOF with membranous ventricular septal defect, Ao overriding interventricular septum, and RV hypertrophy.* **(Right)** *Axial SSFP CMR shows RV hypertrophy and a membranous ventricular septal defect. CMR is ideally suited to identify anatomy of pulmonary arteries and depict other sources of pulmonary arterial blood flow (e.g., aortopulmonary arterial collaterals or patent ductus arteriosus) prior to definitive operative repair.*

TERMINOLOGY

Abbreviations

- Tetralogy of Fallot (TOF)

Definitions

- Subvalvular or valvular right ventricular (RV) outflow tract (RVOT) stenosis, subaortic ventricular septal defect (VSD), overriding aorta, and RV hypertrophy
  - Main pulmonary artery (PA) and its branches can also be obstructed at various levels

IMAGING

General Features

- Best diagnostic clue
  - Infundibular stenosis of RVOT + VSD

Radiographic Findings

- Radiography
  - Classic radiographic appearance: Boot-shaped heart (a.k.a. coeur en sabot)
  - RV hypertrophy and concave PA segment
  - Right-sided aortic arch in 25% of cases
  - Normal or decreased pulmonary vascularity (oligemia)
  - Normal heart size

CT Findings

- CT is utilized when echocardiography does not provide all anatomic information
- CTA with volume rendering: Depicts PA anatomy, especially in patients with severe stenosis/atresia
- Identifies location and degree of branch pulmonary stenoses
- May demonstrate major aortopulmonary collateral arteries (MAPCAs)
  - Evaluation of vascular supply to each pulmonary segment; relative contribution of PAs and MAPCAs
- Establish extent of pulmonary hypoplasia
- Identify coronary anatomy

MR Findings

- Used when anatomy is not well demonstrated by echocardiography
  - Extracardiac anatomy; PA anatomy; may be stenotic, hypoplastic, or atretic
  - Evaluation of MAPCAs; presence, origin, and course
  - Presence of central PAs
  - Associated anomalies
- Relative contribution of MAPCAs and PAs to supply lungs
- Establish extent of pulmonary hypoplasia
  - Measurement of PAs
  - Nakata index: Area of right and left PAs divided by body surface area (BSA); π x 2/diameter/BSA
    - Normal: 330 ± 30 mm/m²
    - > 100 mm/m² have better survival after complete correction

Ultrasonographic Findings

- In utero: Dilated aorta overriding interventricular septum, ± perimembranous VSD and RVOT narrowing
- No RV hypertrophy in 2nd trimester

Echocardiographic Findings

- 1st-line imaging modality to diagnose and monitor (especially in pediatric population)
- Provides good information on preoperative anatomy
- Degree of RVOT obstruction, function of pulmonary valve (PV), anatomy of branch PAs
- VSD location, additional muscular VSDs
- Degree of aortic override, position of arch

Angiographic Findings

- Cardiac catheterization and angiography indications are limited to severe forms of TOF in which collaterals are present or if procedure is required
  - Coronary anatomy, anatomy/distribution of MAPCAs
  - PA branch stenosis: Balloon angioplasty with stent placement
  - Transcatheter PV replacement (e.g., Melody valve)

Imaging Recommendations

- Echocardiography for initial diagnosis and monitoring
- CTA or CMR for evaluation of RVOT and PA anatomy
- Cardiac catheterization for PA pressure measurements and percutaneous interventions

DIFFERENTIAL DIAGNOSIS

Pulmonary Atresia With Ventricular Septal Defect

- Considered subset of TOF
  - Type A: Only native PAs
  - Type B: Pulmonary blood flow via both native PAs and MAPCAs
  - Type C: Only MAPCAs, no native PAs

Tricuspid Atresia With Ventricular Septal Defect

- Muscular or membranous partition between right atrium and RV
- Obligatory shunting from right atrium → left atrium → left ventricle (LV) → RV
- Decreased pulmonary flow → severe cyanosis at birth
- Increased pulmonary flow when associated with transposition of great arteries

Trilogy of Fallot

- PV stenosis, RV hypertrophy, and atrial septal defect (ASD) with right-to-left shunt due to increased right-sided pressures

Pentalogy of Fallot

- Tetralogy with additional ASD

Double-Outlet Right Ventricle

- Wide, nonrestrictive subaortic conus
- Mitral-aortic fibrous discontinuity
- Overriding aorta (50%)

PATHOLOGY

General Features

- Genetics
  - Chromosomal abnormalities in 11% (chromosome 22), other congenital anomalies in 16%; syndromic in 8%
- Frequent associations

- Right-sided aortic arch with mirror image branching (25%)
- PA branch stenosis or hypoplasia
- Absent PV: Severe PV regurgitation → aneurysmal dilatation of PAs → tracheobronchial compression → severe respiratory distress
- ASD (5%)
- Patent foramen ovale
- Left superior vena cava (11%)
- Coronary anomalies (5%): Left anterior descending (LAD) artery arising from right coronary artery (RCA) or RCA arising from LAD and crossing RVOT (anterior to RV infundibulum) with implications for surgical repair
- Down syndrome (trisomy 21)
- Tracheoesophageal fistula, scoliosis, forked ribs

- Embryology
  - Anterosuperior deviation of conal septum and unequal partitioning of conal truncus
  - Primary hypoplasia of infundibular septum
- Hemodynamics: RVOT obstruction → pressure overload
- Pulmonary flow is maintained by
  - Patent ductus arteriosus (PDA) if main PA and its branches are intact
  - MAPCAs when PAs are absent or severely hypoplastic
- Balance between RVOT obstruction and VSD
  - Decreased pulmonary blood flow → greater right-to-left shunting → cyanosis (classic blue "tet")
  - Normal or increased pulmonary flow → congestive heart failure (pink "tet")

Staging, Grading, & Classification

- Category: Cyanotic, normal heart size, decreased pulmonary vascularity
- Adult Congenital Heart Disease Anatomy and Physiology (ACHD AP) classification
  - Congenital heart disease (CHD) anatomy
    - Repaired TOF: Grade II (moderate complexity)
    - Unrepaired TOF: Grade III (great complexity)
  - Physiologic stage
    - A: No hemodynamic sequelae or arrhythmia, normal exercise capacity
    - B: Mild hemodynamic sequelae, mild valvular disease, small shunt, arrhythmia not requiring treatment
    - C: ≥ moderate valvular and ventricular dysfunction, hemodynamically significant shunt, pulmonary hypertension
    - D: Refractory arrhythmia, severe hypoxemia, severe pulmonary hypertension, Eisenmenger syndrome

CLINICAL ISSUES

Presentation

- Varying degrees of cyanosis at birth
- Exertional hypercyanotic episodes ("tet" spells) relieved by typical squatting position
  - Squatting pinches femoral arteries → increased systemic resistance → increased pulmonary flow
- Clubbing of fingers and toes
- Congestive heart failure (large VSD)
- Bacterial endocarditis, stroke (paradoxical embolus), hyperviscosity syndrome (polycythemia)

Demographics

- Epidemiology
  - Incidence: 3-5 per 10,000 live births
  - Most common cyanotic CHD
  - 4th most common congenital heart anomaly (5-7% of all CHD)
  - Most frequent complex CHD in adulthood

Natural History & Prognosis

- 10% of untreated patients live > 20 years
- Short term: Excellent results after early complete repair
  - Early mortality rate < 2%
- Long term: Determined by RV diastolic dysfunction, PV regurgitation, PV or conduit stenosis, arrhythmias (15-20%), sudden cardiac death (2% per decade)

Treatment

- Palliative shunt to increase pulmonary blood flow, followed by complete repair
  - Classic or modified Blalock-Taussig (BT) shunt
  - Central shunts (Waterston-Cooley, Potts)
- Definitive repair: Repair of RVOT obstruction + VSD closure
  - 3-11 months of age
  - Timing for surgery and type of repair depends on level of RVOT obstruction and patient's clinical condition
- PV replacement after TOF repair: Surgical or transcatheter
  - Moderate or severe PR in symptomatic patients: Class I indication for PV replacement
  - Asymptomatic patients with moderate or severe PR; consider if at least 2 of following present (class IIa)
    - Mild or greater RV or LV dysfunction
    - Severe RV dilation (RV end-diastolic volume index ≥ 160 mL/m², RV end-systolic volume index ≥ 80 mL/m²)
    - RV end-diastolic volume ≥ 2x LV end-diastolic volume
    - RV systolic pressure ≥ 2/3 systemic pressure
    - Objective reduction in exercise capacity

DIAGNOSTIC CHECKLIST

Reporting Tips

- Goals of preoperative imaging
  - Identify obstruction level and degree
  - Identify pulmonary vascular anatomy: PV or PA stenosis/atresia
  - Locate alternative sources of pulmonary blood flow: MAPCAs, PDA
  - Configuration of aortic arch and branches
  - Cardiac shunts: VSD, ASD
  - Other congenital abnormalities and anatomy of tracheobronchial tree

SELECTED REFERENCES

1. Moscatelli S et al: Multimodality imaging assessment of tetralogy of Fallot: from diagnosis to long-term follow-up. Children (Basel). 10(11), 2023
2. Ranganath P et al: Computed tomography in adult congenital heart disease. Radiol Clin North Am. 57(1):85-111, 2019
3. Stout KK et al: 2018 AHA/ACC guideline for the management of adults with congenital heart disease: executive summary: a report of the American College of Cardiology/American Heart Association Task Force on clinical practice guidelines. J Am Coll Cardiol. 73(12):1494-563, 2018
4. Lapierre C et al: Tetralogy of Fallot: preoperative assessment with MR and CT imaging. Diagn Interv Imaging. 97(5):531-41, 2016
5. Orwat S et al: Imaging of congenital heart disease in adults: choice of modalities. Eur Heart J Cardiovasc Imaging. 15(1):6-17, 2014

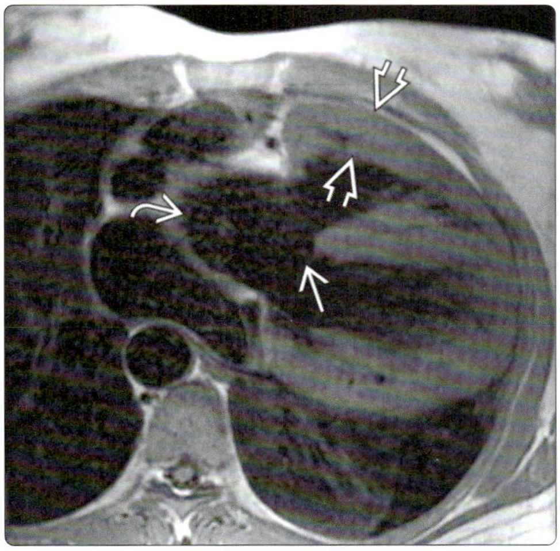

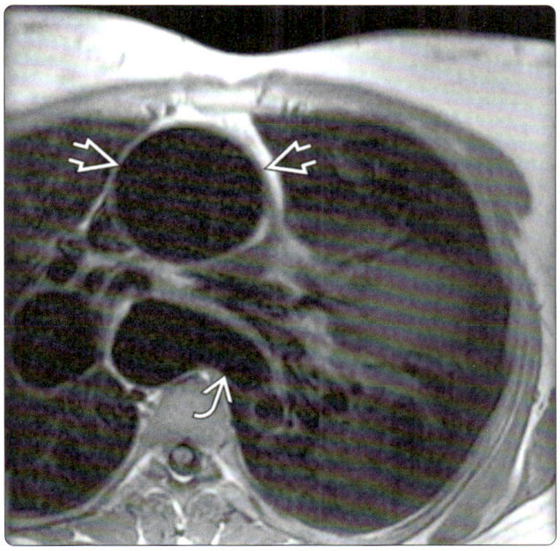

(Left) *Axial black-blood spin-echo shows a large membranous ventricular septal defect and markedly thickened RV myocardium, similar in thickness to LV myocardium. Note enlarged Ao overriding ventricular septal defect.* **(Right)** *Axial spin-echo MR (same patient) demonstrates an enlarged Ao and atretic pulmonary artery with tiny pulmonary valve remnant (not shown). Large arterial branches arise from descending thoracic Ao to perfuse lungs, consistent with TOF with pulmonary atresia (pseudotruncus).*

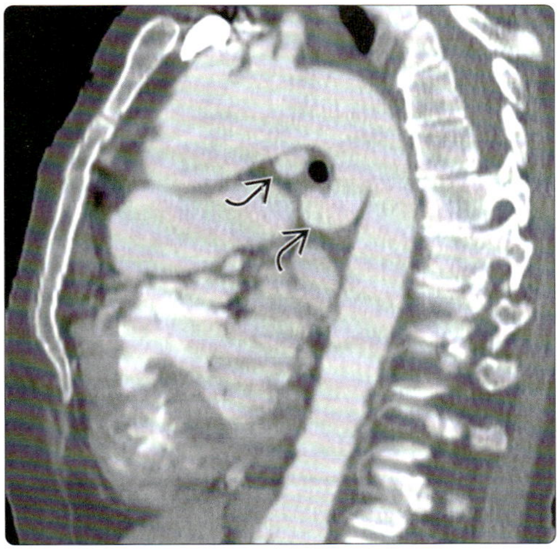

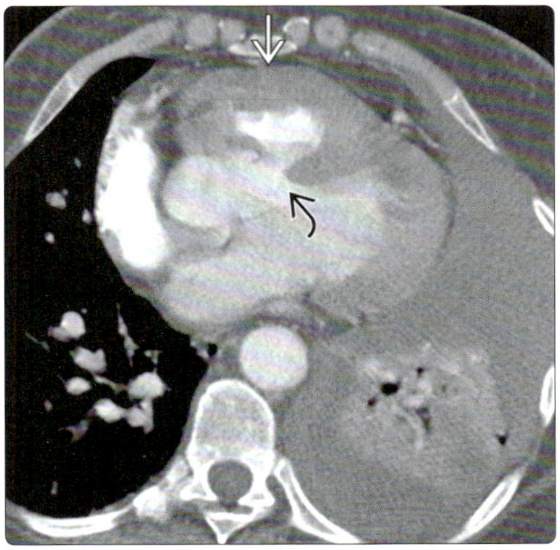

(Left) *Sagittal CTA in a 51-year-old woman with unrepaired TOF shows large aortopulmonary collaterals. These collaterals develop in patients with atresia or hypoplasia of the central pulmonary arteries and function to bring blood to the lungs.* **(Right)** *Axial CTA in the same patient shows the Ao overriding the interventricular septum. Note the membranous type ventricular septal defect and RV hypertrophy due to pulmonary artery infundibular stenosis.*

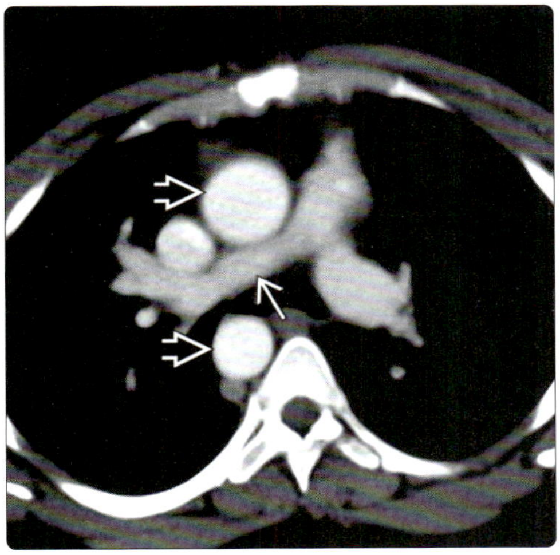

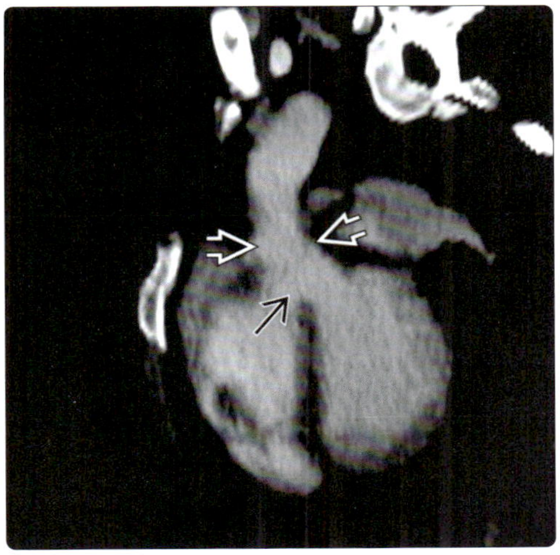

(Left) *Axial oblique CECT shows mild long-segment narrowing of the right pulmonary artery. The aortic arch is right-sided.* **(Right)** *Oblique CECT in the same patient shows a membranous ventricular septal defect and an Ao that overrides the interventricular septum. There is RV hypertrophy. The constellation of these 4 findings comprises TOF.*

Tetralogy of Fallot: Postsurgical and Palliation, Blalock-Taussig Shunt

KEY FACTS

TERMINOLOGY

- **Palliative procedure** to increase pulmonary blood flow
  - Modified Blalock-Taussig (BT) shunt; graft between subclavian artery and ipsilateral pulmonary artery (PA)
- **Definitive repair**: Closure of ventricular septal defect (VSD) and repair of right ventricular outflow tract (RVOT) obstruction

IMAGING

- **Complications of palliative surgery**
  - Shunt occlusion (11%)
  - Perigraft seroma (2.5-9.5%)
- **Complications of definitive repair**
  - Early complications: Rare, 3- to 6-year survival rate is 96%
  - Late complications: 10-30 years after surgery
  - Pulmonary regurgitation (PR) ± RV dilation &/or dysfunction
  - Residual RVOT obstruction ± branch PA stenosis
  - Residual VSD (2-5%)
  - Tricuspid regurgitation: Usually with PV regurgitation
  - RVOT aneurysm/pseudoaneurysm
  - RV to PA conduit stenosis/regurgitation of conduit valve
- **Imaging recommendations**
- Echocardiography is 1st-line imaging for postoperative follow-up
- Volume-rendered cardiac gated CT for evaluation of PAs, RVOT, RV function, and BT shunts
- Cardiac MR is gold standard for serial follow-up of repaired tetralogy of Fallot (TOF) complications
  - Quantification of PR, RV size, and RV function

CLINICAL ISSUES

- Treatment
  - Severe PR and RV dilation: Pulmonary valve replacement (PVR)
    - Optimal timing for surgical PVR is decided according to MR-derived quantitative analysis of RV-indexed volumes

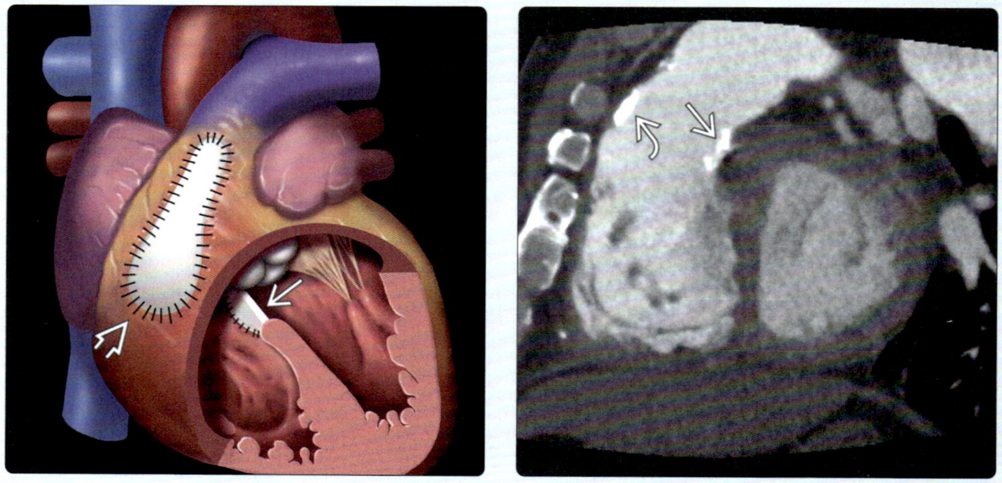

(Left) *Graphic shows definitive repair of tetralogy of Fallot (TOF) with a ventricular septal defect (VSD) patch ➡ and right ventricular outflow tract (RVOT) patch ➡ plasty. Preexisting palliatively placed Blalock-Taussig (BT) shunts are typically ligated at the time of definitive repair.* **(Right)** *Reconstructed RVOT cardiac CT status post definitive repair of TOF shows partially calcified RVOT patch ➡ and extension of the calcified VSD patch ➡.*

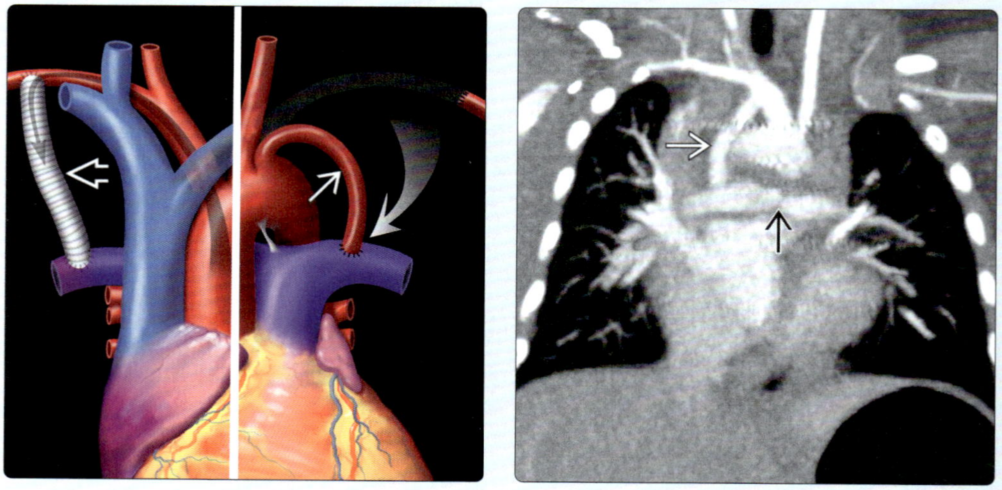

(Left) *Graphic shows a modified BT shunt ➡ connecting the subclavian artery (SCA) and pulmonary artery. Note the original BT shunt ➡ with the distal ligated SCA. Mobilized proximal SCA is anastomosed to the pulmonary artery.* **(Right)** *Coronal CTA shows stenosis at the pulmonary artery branch confluence ⇨ and patent right-sided modified BT shunt ➡ (proximal anastomosis to brachiocephalic trunk) in a patient with TOF.*

TERMINOLOGY

Abbreviations

- Tetralogy of Fallot (TOF)
- Blalock-Taussig (BT)

Synonyms

- BT shunt, BT procedure, "blue baby" operation

Definitions

- **Definitive repair**: Closure of ventricular septal defect (VSD) and repair of right ventricular outflow tract (RVOT) obstruction
  - Pulmonary valvotomy for mild RVOT obstruction
  - Placement of transannular patch ± division/resection of obstructing muscle bundles
  - Placement of graft conduit between right ventricle (RV) and pulmonary artery (PA) if anomalous coronary artery prevents access to RV infundibulum or complete pulmonary valve (PV) atresia
- Previous palliative shunts are usually taken down
- **Palliative procedure** to increase pulmonary blood flow
- Original BT shunt sacrifices subclavian artery (distal ligation)
  - Proximal portion of subclavian artery routed inferiorly to end-to-side anastomosis with ipsilateral branch PA
- Modified BT shunt uses synthetic graft, usually polytetrafluoroethylene (Gore-Tex)
  - Proximal anastomosis is end-to-side between graft (end) and subclavian artery or brachiocephalic trunk (side)
  - Distal anastomosis is end-to-side between distal graft (end) and ipsilateral PA (side)
- Ductus arteriosus stenting
- Waterson-Cooley shunt: Ascending aorta to right PA
- Potts shunt: Descending aorta to left PA (no longer performed)

IMAGING

General Features

- **Complications of palliative surgery**
  - Subclavian artery occlusion distal to graft anastomosis
  - Shunt occlusion in 11% of cases
    - More common in smaller grafts (4 mm)
  - Perigraft seroma in 2.5-9.5% of cases
- **Complications of definitive repair**
  - Early complications: Rare, 3- to 6-year survival rate is 96%
  - Late complications: 10-30 years after surgery
  - Pulmonary regurgitation (PR) ± RV dilation &/or dysfunction
    - Most common and important complication due to treatability and contribution to development of majority of long-term complications
  - Residual RVOT obstruction ± branch PA stenosis
  - Residual VSD (2-5%) or atrial septal defect
  - Tricuspid regurgitation: Usually with PV regurgitation
  - RVOT aneurysm/pseudoaneurysm
  - RV to PA conduit stenosis/regurgitation of conduit valve

Radiographic Findings

- RV hypertrophy with filling of retrosternal clear space
- May demonstrate calcifications along anterior RV wall on lateral radiograph
- May show systemic aortopulmonary collaterals
- **BT shunt**: Increased pulmonary blood flow
  - Rib notching ipsilateral to traditional shunt

CT Findings

- High-density material at RVOT corresponds to patch and is potentially transannular, spanning into PA
  - May have pledgets at suture site
  - May calcify
  - Patch is usually more thinner than native wall and akinetic
- RVOT aneurysm/pseudoaneurysm
- RV dilation + increased myocardial thickness
- Calcified VSD patch with hyperdense pledgets at suture site
  - Best seen on oblique left ventricular long-axis view
- Tube graft from RVOT patch or RA to distal main PA
  - Narrowing of conduit due to calcification or obstruction at anastomosis site with PA
- Detection of aortopulmonary collateral arteries
- **BT shunt**: Tubular contrast-filled structure connecting subclavian and ipsilateral PAs
  - Occluded shunts are difficult to visualize due to absence of contrast; multiplanar reconstructions helpful
- Cardiac gated CTA
  - Preferred due to motion-free imaging of heart
  - Retrospective ECG gated: Quantification of RV function, visualization of wall motion abnormalities
  - Volume rendering images are excellent in depicting morphology of RVOT

MR Findings

- Best modality for serial follow-up of repaired TOF complications
- Best diagnostic tool for evaluation of PR, RV size, and RV function
  - Degree of PR and RV dilation increases over time and makes MR best tool for **longitudinal** follow-up
- **SSFP cine**
  - PR: Diastolic regurgitant jet across pulmonary valve
  - Residual VSD: Flow jet across VSD patch to RV
  - Functional assessment of RV
    - Ejection fraction (EF), end-systolic and end-diastolic volumes (including indexed volumes), muscle mass, and regional wall motion abnormalities
  - RVOT obstruction: Narrowing with turbulent flow jet at level of stenosis
  - RVOT aneurysm: Outward movement of wall during systole
  - Tricuspid regurgitation: Flow jet emanating from tricuspid valve during systole
  - Conduit stenosis: Narrowing of conduit with jet flow
  - **BT shunt**: Tubular structure with flow void connecting subclavian and ipsilateral PAs
    - Bright signal on gradient-echo or SSFP sequences
    - May contain high signal on spin-echo or FSE or low signal on SSFP if occluded
- **Phase-contrast imaging** allows quantification of flow
  - Quantification of regurgitant fraction, systemic and pulmonary flows
  - Quantification of shunt: Qp/Qs
- **Delayed enhancement**

- Delayed enhancement of RVOT patch
- Abnormal hyperenhancement of myocardium indicates ventricular fibrosis
  - Fibrosis in adults correlates with adverse clinical outcome (ventricular dysfunction, exercise intolerance, and arrhythmia)

Echocardiographic Findings

- Routine imaging tool of choice for TOF repair follow-up
- Visual estimation of RV size and function
- PR, tricuspid regurgitation, residual VSD
- Isolated RV restriction late after repair in 50% of patients
- May demonstrate BT shunt graft patency and pressure gradients across graft ± stenosis

Angiographic Findings

- If intervention is needed
  - Balloon angioplasty of branch pulmonary stenosis
  - Transcatheter PV replacement (e.g., Melody valve)

CLINICAL ISSUES

Natural History & Prognosis

- High survival in 1st and 2nd decades after definitive repair
- Survival drops considerably in 3rd decade due to long-term complications
- PR is most common and important complication due to treatability and contribution to development of majority of long-term complications
  - Disruption and loss of normal pulmonary valve function due to RVOT repair
  - PR → RV overload → progressive RV dilation → RV dysfunction → heart failure
- Symptoms of RV volume overload may be inapparent until significant RV failure is present
- Arrhythmias may be due to myotomies/resection of muscle bundles or due to severe PR and RV dilation
  - Atrial flutter is more common than atrial fibrillation
  - May lead to sudden cardiac death
- Aortic root dilation is common in adults with remote repair of TOF
  - ~ 2% will require aortic valve or root replacement
- Pregnancy may be feasible in some cases with modern TOF repairs

Treatment

- Moderate to severe PR (regurgitant fraction ≥ 25%) in symptomatic patients: PV replacement (surgical vs. transcatheter)
  - Has been shown to reduce RV dilation and improve RV function
  - Should be performed before irreversible RV dysfunction ensues
  - Optimal timing for PV replacement (PVR) is decided based on MR-derived quantitative analysis of RV-indexed volumes
  - PVR is reasonable in asymptomatic patients with moderate to severe PR and at least 2 of following, according to 2018 ACHD guideline
    - Mild or greater RV or LV dysfunction (RVEF < 47%, LVEF < 55%), severe RV dilation (RV EDV indexed > 160 mL/m², RV ESV indexed > 80mL/m²), RV end-diastolic volume ≥ 2x LV end-diastolic volume, RV systolic pressure ≥ 2/3 of systemic pressure, progressive objective reduction in exercise capacity
  - Can be performed via transcatheter or surgically
- Complications of PVR: Thrombus, pannus, pseudoaneurysm, hypoattenuating leaflet thickening (HALT)
- Ventricular arrhythmia treatment includes medical therapy, radiofrequency ablation, &/or implantable cardioverter defibrillator
- Pulmonary stenosis may be balloon dilated
  - MAPCAs are occasionally coiled at same time

DIAGNOSTIC CHECKLIST

Consider

- CTA and MRA for PA and RVOT anatomy assessment
- CTA also allows identification of aortopulmonary collaterals in case of insufficient BT shunt
- Cardiac MR is gold standard for functional assessment of postoperative PV regurgitation and RV dysfunction
  - Physiologic stages A and B: CTA/cardiac MR every 24-36 months; stages C and D: Every 12-24 months
- Echocardiography best for intracardiac assessment of VSD

Reporting Tips

- Checklist for CT or MR evaluation after TOF repair
  - PR: Quantification of regurgitant fraction
  - Quantification of RV volume and function (EDV, ESV, EF)
  - RVOT obstruction, aneurysm/dyskinesia: Localization, extent, and degree of stenosis
  - Residual VSD: Quantification of shunt (Qp/Qs)
  - Conduit calcifications/stenosis: Localization, extent, and degree
  - PA stenosis: Localization, extent, and degree
  - Aortic root dilation and aortic regurgitation
  - BT shunt: Patency, localization, flow

SELECTED REFERENCES

1. Canan A et al: Pre- and postprocedure imaging of transcatheter pulmonary valve implantation. Radiographics. 42(4):991-1011, 2022
2. Chau AK: Transcatheter pulmonary valve replacement in congenital heart diseases. Pediatr Investig. 6(4):280-90, 2022
3. Ranganath P et al: Computed tomography in adult congenital heart disease. Radiol Clin North Am. 57(1):85-111, 2019
4. Mercer-Rosa L et al: Perioperative factors influence the long-term outcomes of children and adolescents with repaired tetralogy of Fallot. Pediatr Cardiol. 39(7):1433-9, 2018
5. Stout KK et al: 2018 AHA/ACC guideline for the management of adults with congenital heart disease: a report of the American College of Cardiology/American Heart Association Task Force on Clinical Practice Guidelines. J Am Coll Cardiol. 73(12):e81-e192, 2018
6. Vaujois L et al: Imaging of postoperative tetralogy of Fallot repair. Diagn Interv Imaging. 97(5):549-60, 2016
7. Ahmed S et al: Role of multidetector CT in assessment of repaired tetralogy of Fallot. Radiographics. 33(4):1023-36, 2013
8. Yuan SM et al: The Blalock-Taussig shunt. J Card Surg. 24(2):101-8, 2009

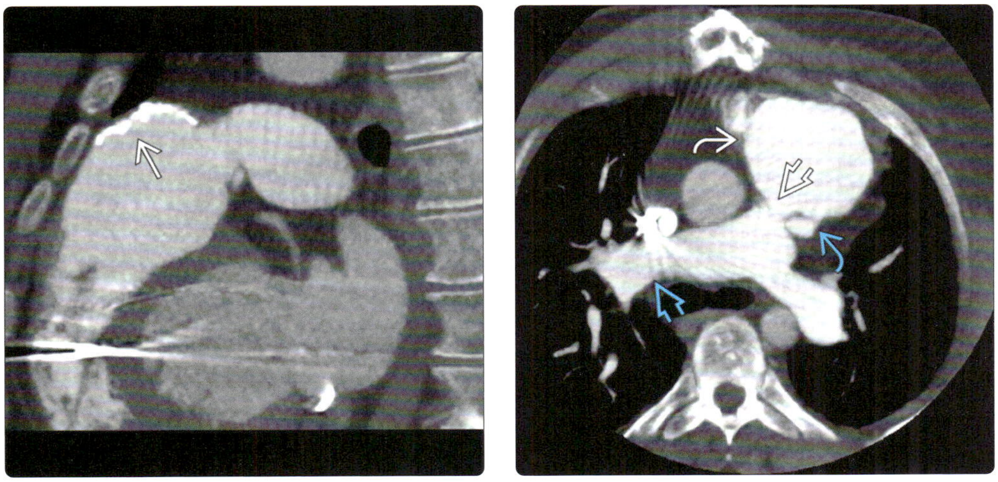

(Left) *Reconstructed sagittal RVOT cardiac CT status post definitive repair shows a RVOT patch → and aneurysmal dilation of the RVOT.* **(Right)** *Axial cardiac CT in the same patient shows aneurysmal dilation of the RVOT → and a small contrast outpouching with a narrow neck, consistent with pseudoaneurysm →. Also note mild narrowing → at the origin of the main pulmonary artery and the poststenotic dilation of the right pulmonary artery →.*

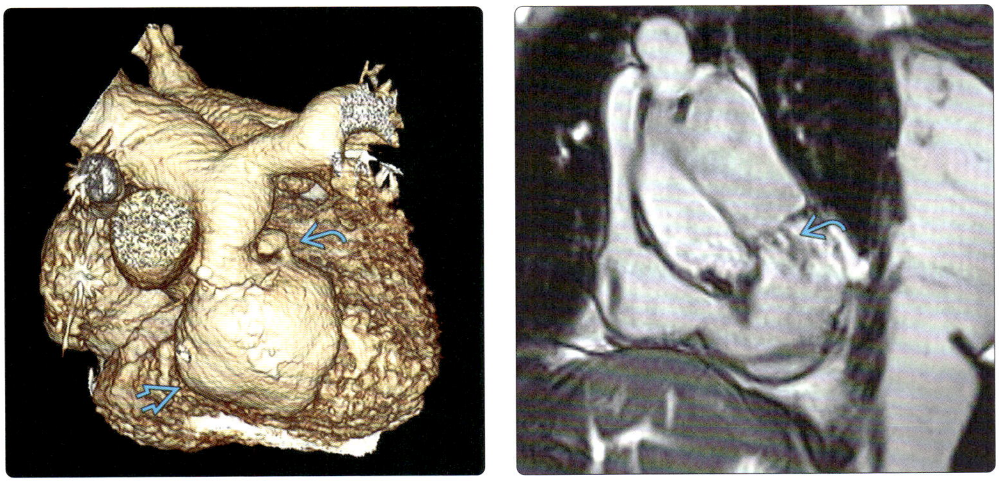

(Left) *3D volume-rendering CT in the same patient demonstrates the aneurysmal dilation → of the RVOT and pseudoaneurysm →.* **(Right)** *RV vertical long-axis SSFP cine MR in a patient status post definitive repair shows a flow void jet → of pulmonary regurgitation extending back into the RV in diastole, consistent with pulmonic regurgitation. Cardiac MR is used to guide the timing of pulmonary valve (PV) replacement by quantifying pulmonary regurgitant fraction and RV function and size.*

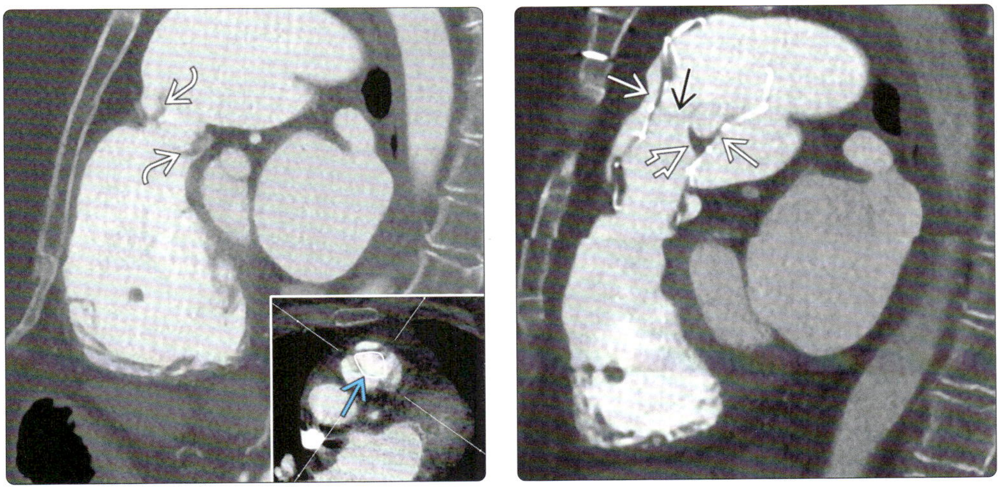

(Left) *Sagittal cardiac CTA shows thickened PV leaflets → in a patient with history of PV stenosis and prior valvotomy. Short-axis view of the PV (inlet) shows incomplete coaptation and large regurgitation orifice →.* **(Right)** *Sagittal CECT in the same patient after implantation of a Harmony valve → shows hypoattenuating leaflet thickening (HALT) → of the prosthetic valve. Note the classical crescent shape thickening of the leaflet. The anterior leaflet → appears normal.*

D-Transposition of Great Arteries

KEY FACTS

TERMINOLOGY

- Atrioventricular concordance and ventriculoarterial discordance
  - Aorta arises from right ventricle (RV); pulmonary artery (PA) arises from left ventricle (LV)
- Category: Cyanotic, cardiomegaly, increased pulmonary vascularity

IMAGING

- Chest radiography: May be normal in neonates
  - Egg on string appearance of heart
  - Narrow superior mediastinum
- CTA and MR
  - Direct visualization of abnormal anatomy
- Echocardiogram: Optimal for preoperative diagnosis

TOP DIFFERENTIAL DIAGNOSES

- Congenitally corrected transposition
- Criss-cross heart
- Truncus arteriosus
- Total anomalous pulmonary venous return

CLINICAL ISSUES

- Symptoms: Peripheral cyanosis; tachypnea, weakness, and fatigue; failure to thrive
- Treatment
  - Prostaglandin E1 keeps ductus arteriosus open
  - Balloon atrial septostomy (Rashkind)
  - Jatene arterial switch with transposition of coronary arteries
  - Atrial switch with rerouting of venous flow in atria with pericardial baffle (Mustard) or reorientation of atrial septum (Senning)
  - Rastelli procedure: Intracardiac baffle to tunnel LV to aorta + extracardiac conduit to connect RV to PA

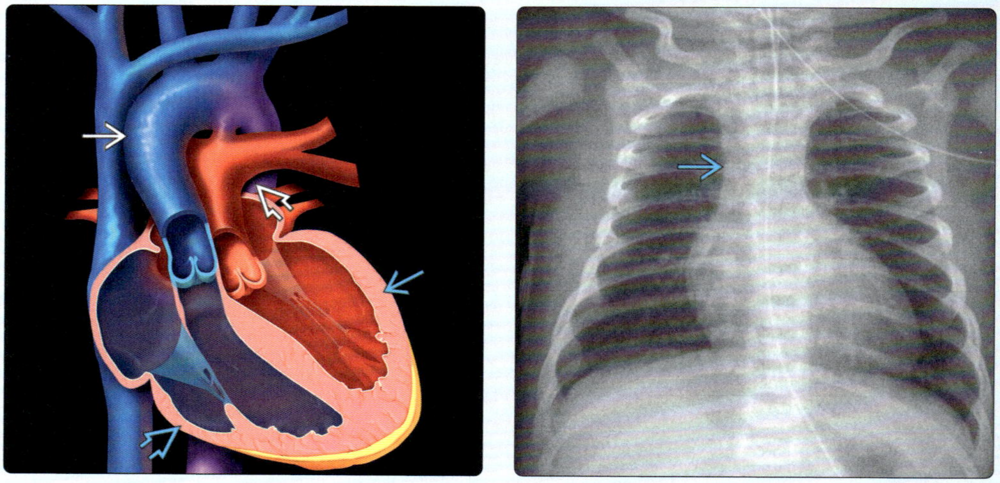

(Left) *Graphic shows the atrioventricular (AV) concordance and ventriculoarterial (VA) discordance of D-TGA. The aorta is anterior and connected via the infundibulum to the right ventricle (RV). Pulmonary trunk is posterior and connected to the left ventricle (LV).* **(Right)** *Egg on a string appearance of the cardiomediastinal silhouette in D-TGA is shown. The superior mediastinum is narrow, given the parallel orientation of the great vessels. The heart is globular in shape.*

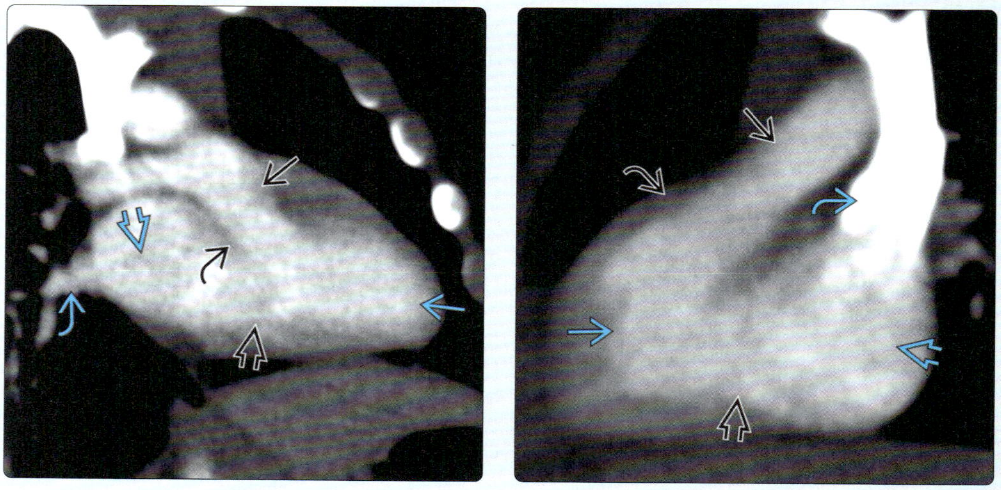

(Left) *CTA in a 3-day-old shows flow from the pulmonary veins → left atrium (LA) → mitral valve → LV → main pulmonary artery. This is the LV because of the shared intervalvular fibrosa.* **(Right)** *Image shows flow from the superior vena cava (SVC) → right atrium → tricuspid valve → RV → ascending aorta. This is the RV because the conus separates inflow and outflow valves. AV concordance and VA discordance = D-TGA. (Courtesy S. Kligerman, MD.)*

TERMINOLOGY

Abbreviations

- Dextro transposition of great arteries (D-TGA)
  - **D** = **d**extro = right

Definitions

- Ventriculoarterial discordance with atrioventricular (AV) concordance
  - Aorta arises from right ventricle (RV); pulmonary trunk arises from left ventricle (LV)
  - LV connects to left atrium (LA); RV connects to right atrium (RA)
- Anatomic arrangement represented by designation "S, D, D" (Van Praagh segmental approach)
  - S: Visceroatrial situs solitus
    - RA, liver on right
    - LA, stomach, spleen on left
    - Right-sided trilobed lung with eparterial bronchus
    - Left-sided bilobed lung with hypoarterial bronchus
  - D: D-looped ventricles
    - Morphologic RV on right
      - ▫ Morphologic RV: Infundibulum (conus) separates AV and ventriculoarterial valves; moderator band; prominent trabeculations; more apical location of tricuspid valve
    - Morphologic LV on left
      - ▫ Morphologic LV: Fibrous continuity between AV and ventriculoarterial valves; no moderator band; less prominent trabeculations
  - D: D-transposed great arteries
    - Ascending aorta located anterior and to right of pulmonary artery (PA)
    - Great vessels parallel instead of crossing
- Category: Cyanotic, cardiomegaly, increased pulmonary vascularity
- Hemodynamics
  - RV → systemic circulation: Pressure overload
  - LV → pulmonary circulation: Volume overload
  - 2 parallel circuits
    - Incompatible with life without flow admixture
      - ▫ Patent ductus arteriosus (PDA), ventricular septal defect (VSD), patent foramen ovale (PFO)

IMAGING

General Features

- Best diagnostic clue
  - Aortic valve located to right of and anterior to pulmonic valve
  - Aorta and pulmonary trunk lie parallel in sagittal plane

Radiographic Findings

- Radiography
  - May be normal in neonates
  - Egg on string appearance of heart
    - Cardiomegaly: Biatrial enlargement from increased pulmonary flow
    - Narrow pedicle due to parallel anteroposterior orientation of transposed great arteries + stress-induced thymic atrophy + hyperinflated lungs
  - Increased pulmonary flow: After closure of ductus arteriosus

CT Findings

- Cardiac gated CTA
  - CTA is excellent for rapidly assessing anatomy
    - Low-radiation-dose protocols are utilized, especially in children
  - Morphology: AV concordance and ventriculoarterial discordance
  - Defines coronary anatomy and course
    - Usual pattern: Left main coronary (LCA) originates from left facing sinus; right coronary artery (RCA) from right posterior
    - Usual pattern with left circumflex (LCx) originating from RCA and retropulmonary course
    - Inverted pattern: LCA from right posterior and RCA from left facing sinus
    - Inverted RCA and LCx: Artery from left facing sinus bifurcates into left anterior descending (LAD) and RCA; LCx from right posterior sinus
    - Single coronary from right posterior sinus, dividing into LCA and RCA
    - Single coronary from left facing sinus, dividing into LCA and RCA

MR Findings

- T1WI
  - MR is not used typically for preoperative evaluation
    - Indeterminate or suboptimal echocardiography
    - Delineate pulmonary vasculature
    - Quantification of LV mass, function following pulmonary banding
    - Associated anomalies
  - Morphologic evaluation
    - AV concordance and ventriculoarterial discordance
      - ▫ Ascending aorta is anterior and to right of main PA
      - ▫ Ascending aorta and main PA in same sagittal plane
    - Associated cardiac and extracardiac abnormalities
- Cine SSFP
  - Morphologic features
  - Quantification of biventricular volumes and function
  - Visualization of valvular abnormalities
- MR angiography
  - Vascular anatomy and connections
- Noncontrast 3D angiography
  - Evaluation of coronary arterial anatomy and patency
- Phase-contrast MR
  - Stenoses and regurgitation quantification

Echocardiographic Findings

- Echocardiogram
  - 1st-line imaging for preoperative assessment
    - Identification of atria, ventricles, and their connections
    - Identification of PFO, VSD
- Proximal coronary artery anatomy

Angiographic Findings

- Conventional
  - Cardiac catheterization for Rashkind procedure (balloon atrial septostomy)

Imaging Recommendations

- Echocardiography allows for complete preoperative diagnosis in majority of cases
- MR or CT assists in preoperative evaluation

DIFFERENTIAL DIAGNOSIS

Congenitally Corrected Transposition

- AV and ventriculoarterial discordance
  - Ascending aorta is anterior and to left of PA
  - Morphologic RV is to left of morphologic LV
- Category: Dependent on associated anomalies
  - LV outflow tract (subpulmonic) obstruction (LVOTO): Cyanotic
  - VSD: Acyanotic

Criss-Cross heart

- Twisted AV connections
- Discordance between AV alignment and AV connections
- Axes of AV inlets cross each other in transverse plane
- Majority have AV concordance; discordance may be seen

Truncus Arteriosus

- Common arterial vessel giving rise to aorta, pulmonary trunk, and coronaries
- Cyanosis, cardiomegaly, increased pulmonary vascularity
- Cardiac anomaly most commonly associated with right aortic arch

Total Anomalous Pulmonary Venous Return

- Abnormal connection of pulmonary veins to RA, coronary sinus, or systemic veins
- Type 1: Supracardiac; type 2L: Cardiac; type 3: Infracardiac
- Severe cyanosis at birth
- Supracardiac type: Cardiomegaly, increased pulmonary vascularity, snowman appearance

PATHOLOGY

General Features

- Etiology
  - Embryology
    - Faulty separation of aorta and PA from primitive bulbus cordis (conotruncus)
  - Associated with maternal diabetes
- Associated abnormalities
  - Abnormalities of heart and aorta
    - VSD (15-25%)
    - ASD
    - LV outflow (pulmonary) stenosis
    - RV hypoplasia
    - Aortic coarctation, interruption
    - Overriding AV valves
    - Left juxtaposed atrial appendages
    - Aortopulmonary collaterals
  - Abnormalities of PAs
    - Pulmonary atresia
    - Pulmonary stenosis
  - Isolated abnormality: 90% of cases

Staging, Grading, & Classification

- With intact septum; with VSD; with VSD and LVOT obstruction; intact septum and LVOTO

Gross Pathologic & Surgical Features

- Infundibulum of RV connected to aortic valve, anterior and slightly to right of midline (D-loop)
- LV connected without infundibulum to pulmonary valve, posterior and slightly to left of aortic valve

CLINICAL ISSUES

Presentation

- Most common signs/symptoms
  - Peripheral cyanosis
    - Depends on mixing between 2 sides, size of ASD, relative resistance in pulmonary and systemic circulation and coexistent pulmonic stenosis
- Other signs/symptoms
  - Tachypnea, weakness, and fatigue
  - Failure to thrive
  - Syncope and clubbing may develop if left untreated

Demographics

- Sex
  - M > F
- Epidemiology
  - Incidence: 315 in 1 million live births
  - 5% of congenital heart diseases
  - 2nd most common cyanotic congenital cardiac disorder diagnosed in 1st year of life

Natural History & Prognosis

- Early death without communicating shunt
- Large VSD: Congestive heart failure in neonatal period
- Large VSD and subpulmonic stenosis: Mild symptoms; may survive without treatment
- Transposition with early arterial switch: Good prognosis
- Long-term prognosis determined by potential coronary abnormalities

Treatment

- Prostaglandin E1 keeps ductus arteriosus open
- Balloon atrial septostomy (Rashkind)
- Arterial switch with transposition of coronary arteries (Jatene)
  - Definitive procedure done in 1st few weeks of life
- Atrial switch: Rerouting of venous flow in atria to contralateral AV valve and ventricle with pericardial baffle (Mustard) or reorientation of atrial septum (Senning)
  - Used to be definitive procedure before advent of arterial switch; now performed only if arterial switch not possible
- Rastelli procedure: Intracardiac baffle to tunnel LV to aorta + extracardiac conduit to connect RV to PA
  - In D-TGA with VSD and pulmonic stenosis

SELECTED REFERENCES

1. Canan A et al: Multimodality imaging of transposition of the great arteries. Radiographics. 41(2):338-60, 2021
2. Swanson SK et al: Interpretation and reporting of coronary arteries in transposition of the great arteries: cross-sectional imaging perspective. J Thorac Imaging. 33(4):W14-21, 2018

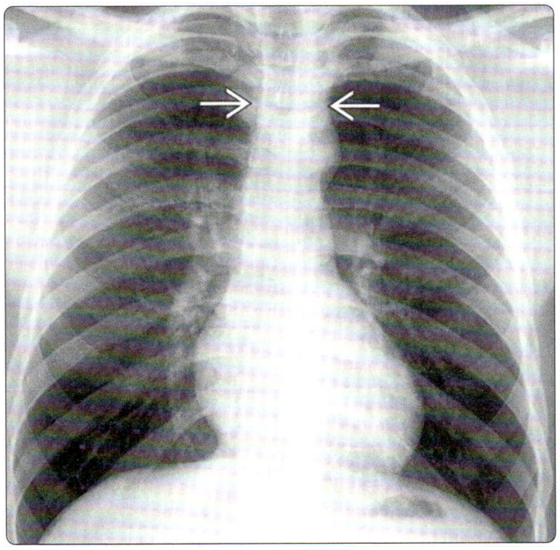

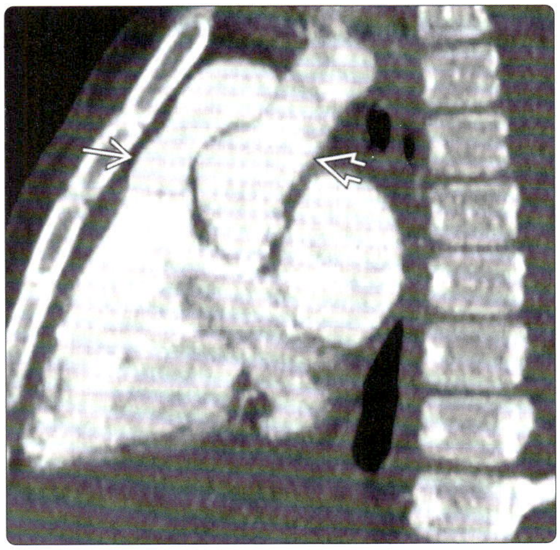

(Left) *PA chest radiograph demonstrates a narrowed superior mediastinum in D-TGA.* **(Right)** *Sagittal cardiac CT in the same patient shows the typical anteroposterior relationship of the pulmonary artery and the ascending aorta, which are running in the same sagittal plane with lack of normal spiraling around each other.*

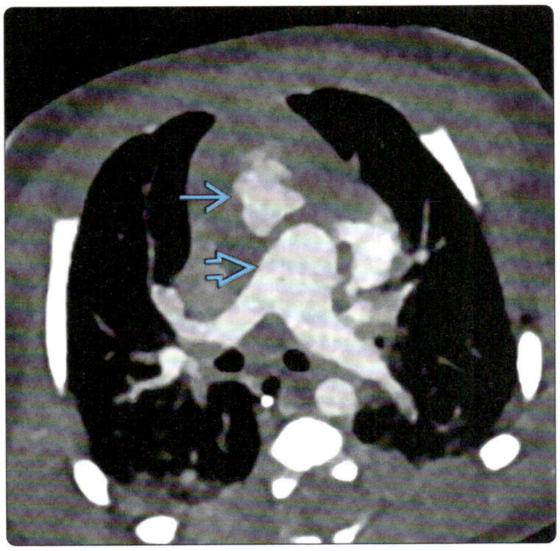

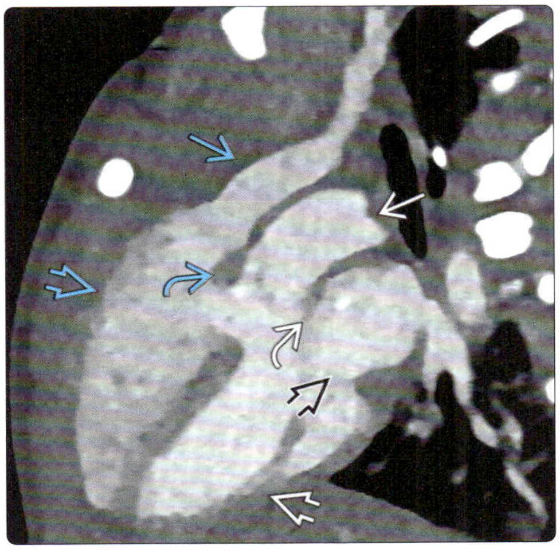

(Left) *Axial oblique reconstructed cardiac CT shows the ascending aorta located anterior and to the right of the pulmonary trunk, a characteristic arrangement seen in D-TGA.* **(Right)** *Sagittal oblique CTA in D-TGA shows an anteriorly placed aorta originating from the RV, inferred by a muscular band adjacent the aortic valve. Pulmonary trunk originates from the LV, inferred by fibrous continuity between the pulmonary valve and the AV valve.*

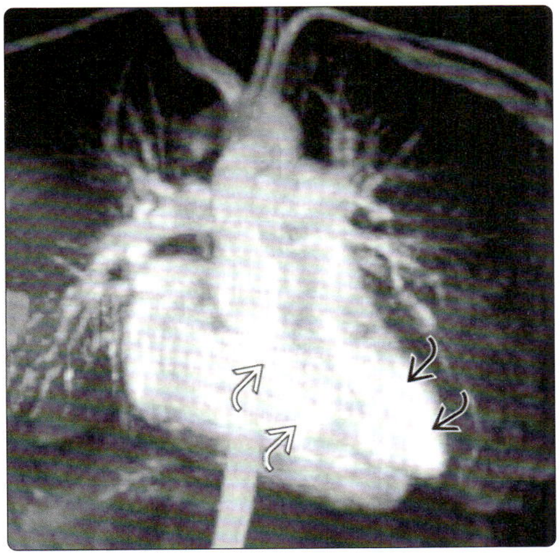

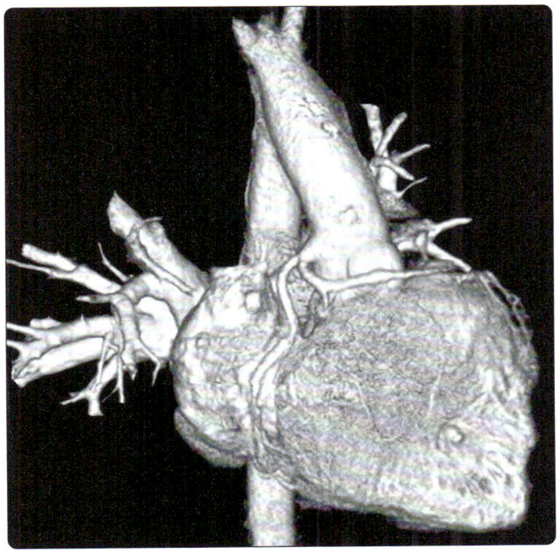

(Left) *Coronal MIP MRA demonstrates the malposition of the ventricles relative to the great vessels. The RV is related to the ascending aorta, and the LV gives origin to the pulmonary artery.* **(Right)** *Coronal cardiac CT shows anteriorly placed D-loop aorta, which is connected with the RV.*

L-Transposition of Great Arteries

KEY FACTS

TERMINOLOGY

- Synonym: Congenitally corrected transposition of great arteries
  - Most patients have concomitant congenital abnormalities

IMAGING

- Inversion of ventricles and great arteries: Atrioventricular (AV) and ventriculoarterial discordance
- Great vessels lie parallel and almost in same coronal plane; aortic valve anterior and slightly to left (L-loop) of pulmonary valve
- Hemodynamics
  - Right atrium → mitral valve → right-sided morphologic left ventricle → pulmonary circulation
  - Left atrium → tricuspid valve → left-sided morphologic right ventricle → systemic circulation
- Echocardiography allows for complete preoperative diagnosis in majority of cases
- CT and MR are complementary, noninvasive, cross-sectional tests for more complex abnormalities
- {S, L, L} heart
- Atrial situs solitus, L-loop, L-TGA
- {I, D, D} heart
- Atrial situs inversus, D-loop, D-TGA
- Mirror image of {S, L, L} heart

PATHOLOGY

- Concomitant ventricular septal defect (VSD): 80%

CLINICAL ISSUES

- Most common presentation
  - Heart failure (VSD, systemic AV valve dysfunction)
  - Cyanosis (subpulmonary stenosis)
- Incidence: 1 in 13,000 live births, 1% of congenital heart disease, M > F
- Prognosis: Determined by presence of AV valve dysfunction
- Surgical treatment focuses on associated abnormalities

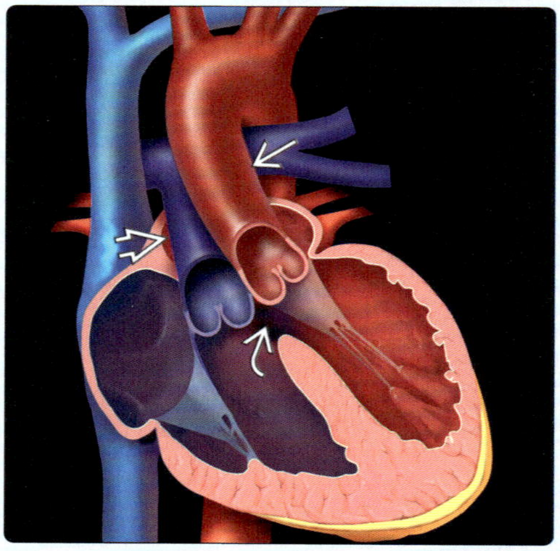

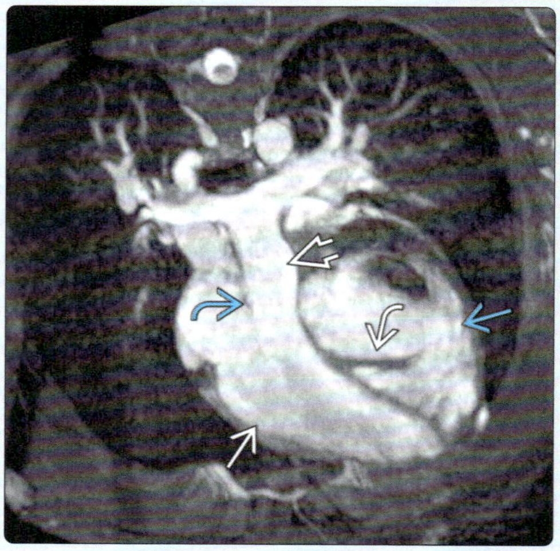

(Left) *Graphic of L-transposition of great arteries (TGA) shows a left-sided aorta connected to a left-sided morphologic right ventricle (RV). The right-sided pulmonary artery is connected to right-sided left ventricle (LV). There is a high ventricular septal defect (VSD).* **(Right)** *MRA shows the LV supplying the pulmonary artery (PA). The RV is recognized by its partially visualized moderator band. Fibrous continuity of the inflow and outflow valves denotes the LV. (Courtesy S. Kligerman, MD.)*

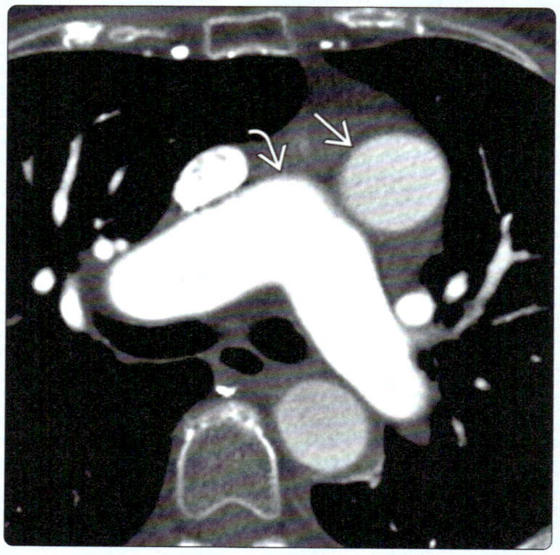

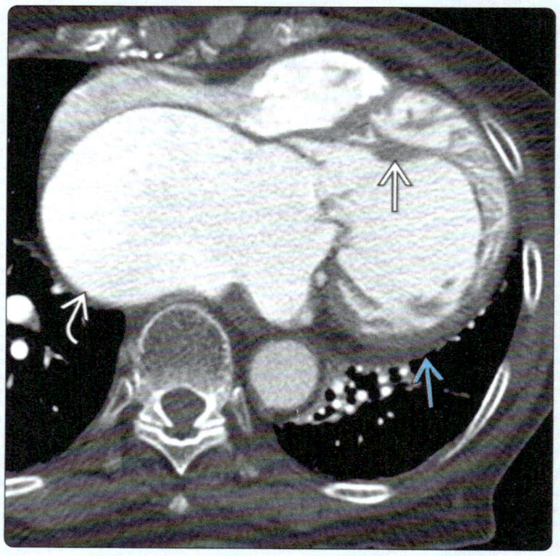

(Left) *Axial CTA shows the abnormal location of the ascending aorta, anterior and to the left of the PA, consistent with L-TGA.* **(Right)** *Axial CTA in the same patient shows a markedly dilated left-sided morphologic RV (identified by the moderator band and a large amount of trabeculation) and systemic left atrium (LA). Dilation of the systemic atrium and ventricle from ventricular failure is not uncommon in L-TGA.*

TERMINOLOGY

Abbreviations

- Levo transposition of great arteries (L-TGA)

Synonyms

- Congenitally corrected TGA
- Discordant transposition
- Ventricular inversion

Definitions

- Inversion of ventricles and great arteries: Atrioventricular (AV) and ventriculoarterial (VA) discordance
- Segmental approach to congenital heart disease (3 steps)
  - Visceroatrial situs: Atria relative to nearby anatomy
    - Situs solitus (S): Normal
    - Situs inversus ( ): Inverted
    - Situs ambiguus (A): Ambiguous
  - Ventricular topology: Orientation of ventricular loop
    - Dextro-loop (D): Rightward
    - Levo-loop (L): Leftward
  - Great arterial pos tion
    - Solitus (S): Normal
    - Inversus (I): Inverted
    - L-transposition (L)
    - D-transposition (D)

IMAGING

General Features

- Best diagnostic clue
  - Great vessels lie parallel and almost in same coronal plane; aortic valve anterior and slightly to left (L-transposed) of pulmonic valve
- Location
  - Hemodynamics
    - Superior/inferior vena cava → right atrium → mitral valve → morphologic left ventricle (LV) on right side→ pulmonary artery
    - Pulmonary veins → left atrium → tricuspid valve → morphologic right ventricle (RV) on left side → systemic circulation
    - Hemodynamics dependent on associated anomalies
- Morphology
  - {S, L, L} heart
    - Atrial situs solitus, L-loop, L-TGA
      - Right-sided morphologic LV characterized by fibrous cont nuity between mitral and pulmonic valves, smooth wall, and absent outflow chamber to pulmonary valve
      - Left-sided morphologic RV characterized by tricuspid valve, muscular infundibulum between tricuspid and aortic valves; trabeculated wall and moderator band
  - {I, D, D} heart
    - Atrial situs inversus, D-loop, D-TGA
      - Mirror image of {S, L, L} heart
      - Almost always associated with cardiac malposition: Mesocardia, dextroversion, true dextrocardia (25%)

Radiographic Findings

- Radiography
  - Variable findings
  - Dextrocardia (25% of cases)
  - Bulge along left heart border due to leftward aorta, RV outflow tract, and juxtaposed left atrial appendage
  - Other findings from associated anomalies

CT Findings

- Aortic valve is anterior and to left of pulmonic valve
- Aorta connects to morphologic RV, which is located to left of morphologic LV
  - Hypertrophied RV can mimic morphologic LV
  - 3D and multiplanar reformats depict abnormal AV and VA relationships
- Retrospective ECG-gated CT for functional evaluation
- Good test for showing coronary artery morphology and course

MR Findings

- T1WI
  - Multiplanar cardiac gated T1WI and 3D gadolinium MRA for segmental cardiac analysis and anatomic evaluation
  - MRA for coronary ostia and course
- SSFP cine
  - Aorta located anterior and to left of pulmonic valve
  - Aorta connects to morphologic RV, which is located to left of morphologic LV
    - Morphologic RV: Muscular infundibulum between semilunar and AV valves; moderator band; prominent trabeculations; tricuspid valve is more apical than mitral valve.
    - Morphologic LV: Fibrous continuity between semilunar and AV valves; no trabeculations in septum
  - Hypertrophied RV can mimic morphologic LV, so careful evaluation of connections and morphology is essential
  - RV hypertrophy due to systemic resistance; eventually RV fails and dilates
  - Coronary artery origin and course can be shown
  - Inverted form, {I, D, D}
    - Aorta anterior and right of PA
    - Aorta connected to morphologic RV, located on right of LV
    - PA connected to morphologic LV, located on left of RV

Echocardiographic Findings

- Echocardiogram
  - Segmental cardiac analysis: Identification of atria, ventricles, great arteries, and their connections
  - Continuity between right-sided mitral and pulmonary valve annuli
  - Discontinuity between AV and aortic valve annuli (separated by muscular ring) defines systemic ventricle as morphologic RV and, therefore, AV valve as tricuspid valve
  - Abnormally straight, vertical course of interventricular septum
  - Coronary ostia assessed on short-axis imaging of cardiac base

Imaging Recommendations

- Protocol advice

- Echocardiography allows for complete preoperative diagnosis in majority of cases
- CT and MR are complementary; for more complex abnormalities
  - MR: Preferred over CT given radiation risks
  - CT: Best test to define coronary anatomy

DIFFERENTIAL DIAGNOSIS

Congestive Heart Failure, Increased Pulmonary Blood Flow

- Isolated ventricular septal defect (VSD)
- Double-inlet ventricle
- Tricuspid atresia with increased pulmonary blood flow
- Double-outlet RV with subaortic VSD

Cyanosis, Decreased Pulmonary Blood Flow

- Tetralogy of Fallot

Atrioventricular Discordance With Ventriculoarterial Concordance

- Isolated ventricular inversion with each ventricle connected to its appropriate great artery and physiology resembling D-transposition

PATHOLOGY

General Features

- Genetics
  - No genetic factors or chromosomal abnormalities
  - Not commonly associated with significant extracardiac malformations
- Associated abnormalities
  - VSD: 80% of cases
  - LV outflow tract (subpulmonary) obstruction: 30%
  - Left-sided tricuspid valve dysplasia, Ebstein-like anomaly, regurgitation: 30%
  - Can be associated with atrial situs inversus: Dextrocardia {I, D, D}
  - Pulmonary stenosis: 40-50% mainly subvalvular but also valvular
  - Rare: Ventricular hypoplasia, AV canal, straddling AV valves, aortic atresia, coarctation, or interruption
- Ventricular arrangement is not simply mirror image of normal
- Ventricles and great arteries form L-loop
- Interventricular septum is more vertical in orientation than normal
- Coronary distribution is mirror image of normal distribution (right-sided coronary artery bifurcates into circumflex and anterior descending arteries)
- Embryology: Primitive cardiac tube loops to left (L-loop), leading to ventricular inversion and left-sided position of ascending aorta
- Pathophysiology
  - Determined by associated anomalies: VSD, subpulmonary stenosis, AV valve dysfunction
  - Late sequel: Left-sided RV is not able to sustain systemic circulation

Gross Pathologic & Surgical Features

- Right-sided morphologic LV connected without infundibulum to pulmonic valve, which is posterior and to right of aortic valve
- Infundibulum of systemic morphologic RV connected to aortic valve, which is slightly anterior and to left of pulmonic valve (L-loop)
- Pulmonary artery and ascending aorta lie nearly parallel in coronal plane
- Interruption of conduction system of heart due to malalignment between atrial and ventricular septa: Disconnection between AV node and bundle of His → 3rd-degree heart block

CLINICAL ISSUES

Presentation

- Most common signs/symptoms
  - Heart failure (VSD, systemic AV valve dysfunction)
  - Cyanosis (subpulmonary stenosis)
  - Rarely completely asymptomatic; often present as incidental finding on chest radiograph (straight upper left heart border)
- Other signs/symptoms
  - Conduction disturbances: Bradycardia (heart block) and tachydysrhythmia
  - Decreased exercise tolerance due to dysfunction of systemic ventricle (morphologic RV)

Demographics

- Epidemiology
  - Incidence: 1 in 13,000 live births
  - 1% of congenital heart disease
  - M > F

Natural History & Prognosis

- Determined by presence of AV valve dysfunction
- Guarded prognosis due to progressive systemic AV valve and RV dysfunction: 50% mortality rate after 15 years
- Patients with true congenitally corrected transposition may have normal life expectancy

Treatment

- Surgical treatment focuses on associated abnormalities
  - Congestive heart failure from VSD shunt: Pulmonary artery banding or VSD closure
  - Cyanosis from subpulmonary stenosis: Systemic to PA shunt (Blalock) or LV to PA conduit (Rastelli)
  - Pulmonary venous hypertension from tricuspid valve dysfunction: Tricuspid valvuloplasty
- Double-switch operation to prevent late systemic ventricular (RV) failure
  - Venous switch (Senning) reroutes atrial blood into appropriate ventricles
  - Ventricular (Rastelli) or arterial switch: Morphologic LV becomes systemic ventricle
- Pacemaker insertion

SELECTED REFERENCES

1. Canan A et al: Multimodality imaging of transposition of the great arteries. Radiographics. 41(2):338-60, 2021

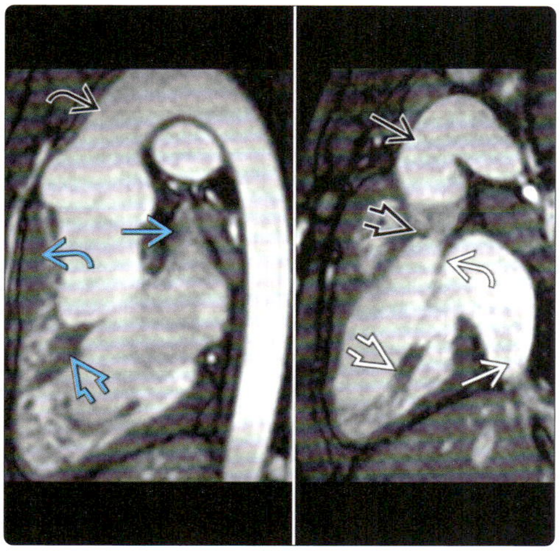

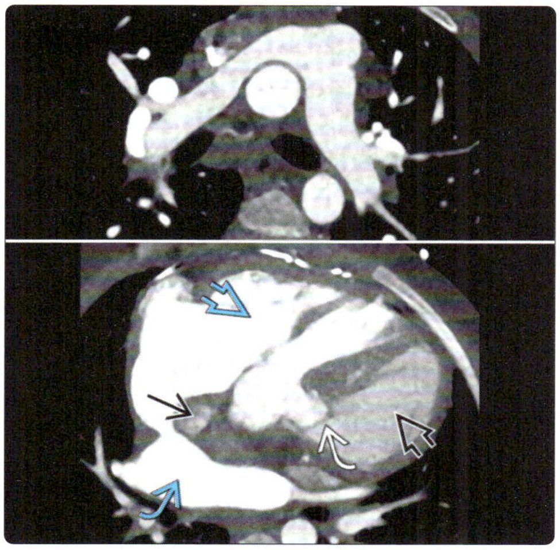

(Left) *MRA (left) shows flow from pulmonary veins → LA → RV (moderator band , conus) → aorta . MRA (right) shows flow from the inferior vena cava → RA → LV (papillary muscles and fibrous continuity of the valves → PA). Note subvalvular pulmonic stenosis .* **(Right)** *Double switch in L-TGA shows arterial (top) and atrial switch (bottom). Pulmonary vein flow is directed to the LV , and superior vena cava flow is directed toward the RV . A VSD is covered by an overgrown valve leaflet . (Courtesy S. Kligerman, MD.)*

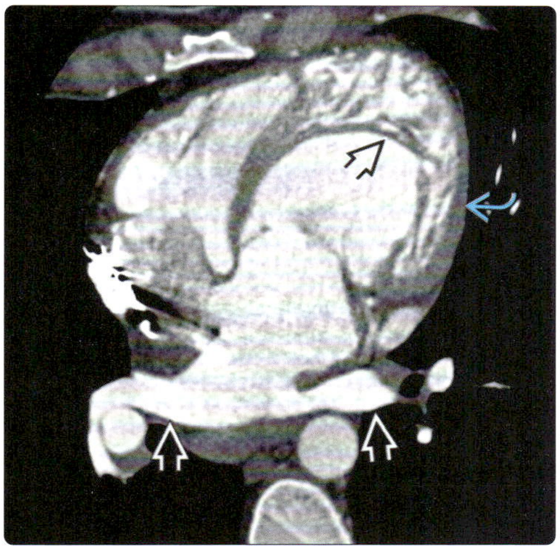

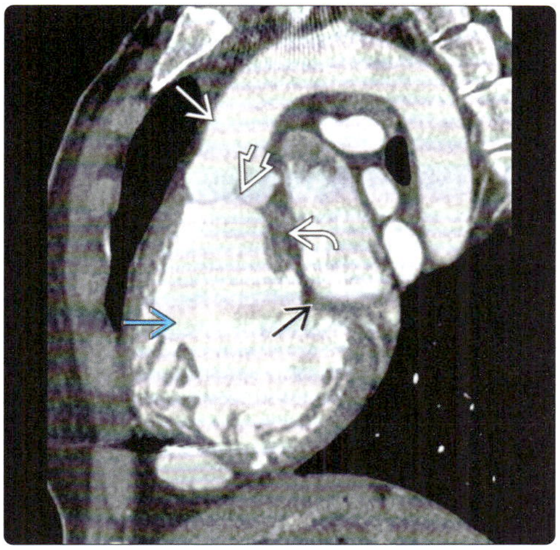

(Left) *Four-chamber cardiac CT shows a normal LA receiving pulmonary venous inflow . However, the LA empties into the anatomic RV , which can be recognized by its increased trabeculation and moderator band .* **(Right)** *RV outflow tract view of a CTA shows the morphologic RV draining into the aorta . The morphologic RV shows separation of the inflow valve plane and outflow tract by a muscular infundibulum .*

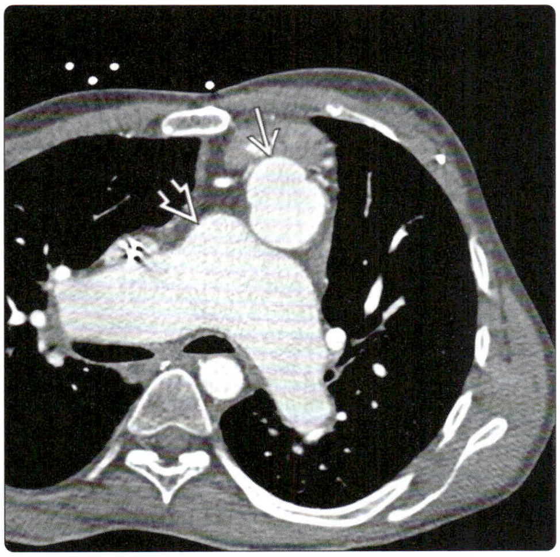

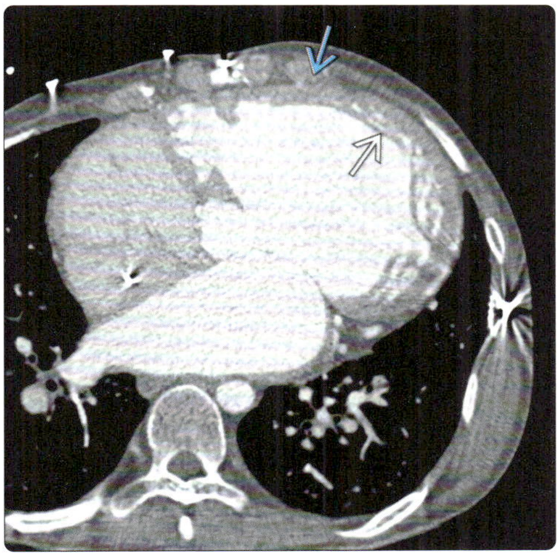

(Left) *Axial CECT shows the typical location of the ascending aorta in L-TGA (i.e., anterior and to the left of the PA). In normal patients, the ascending aorta should be at relatively the same AP level as the PA.* **(Right)** *Axial CECT shows a severely dilated left-sided morphologic RV (as suggested by the large degree of trabeculation). Failure of the morphologic RV is common in L-TGA, given the chronic exposure to systemic arterial pressure.*

TGA Repair: Arterial and Atrial Switch

KEY FACTS

TERMINOLOGY

- AtrSO and ASO are surgeries performed for treatment of D-TGA
- AtrSO: Redirection of blood flow at atrial level using baffles
  - Senning: Right atrial tissue; Mustard: Pericardium/synthetic material
- ASO: Reimplantation of great vessels to respective ventricles and coronary buttons to neoaortic root
  - Distal pulmonary artery (PA) is brought anterior to aorta = Lecompte maneuver

IMAGING

- Echocardiography is 1st-line imaging test
- MR provides comprehensive information
- CT when MR cannot be performed, especially with devices
- AtrSO complications
  - Baffle stenosis: Images perpendicular and parallel to venous pathways
    - Narrowed baffles; high-pressure gradients; collateral vessels; reversed flow in azygos
  - Baffle leak is difficult to identify on CT
    - High-resolution bFFP, time-resolved MRA, or perfusion imaging required in MR; quantified directly or Qp:Qs
  - Systemic ventricular failure: RV dilated, hypertrophied, dysfunctional
    - Tricuspid regurgitation quantified with MR
- ASO complications
  - PA stenosis, more in branch PAs, L > R
    - Due to elliptical orifice, 2 measurements given in CT and MR
    - MR shows high-velocity jets (> 350 cm/sec), vortices
  - Neoaortic root dilatation is common
    - Double oblique measurement; Z-scores > 2.5
  - Coronary artery stenosis/occlusion
    - CTA/MRA provide anatomic information
    - MR perfusion/dobutamine for ischemia

(Left) *Axial cardiac CT in a patient with D-transposition of great arteries (TGA) post arterial switch shows the classic orientation of the aorta and pulmonary artery (PA). Lecompte maneuver results in anterior position of main and branch PAs, which hug the ascending aorta.* **(Right)** *Anterior 3D VR derived from the cardiac CT in the same patient shows the relationship of PAs and ascending aorta, which is classic for Jatene procedure (arterial switch). Also note the dilated aortic root.*

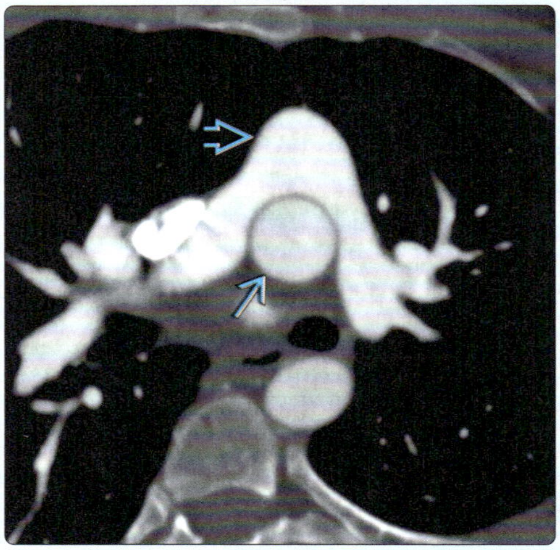

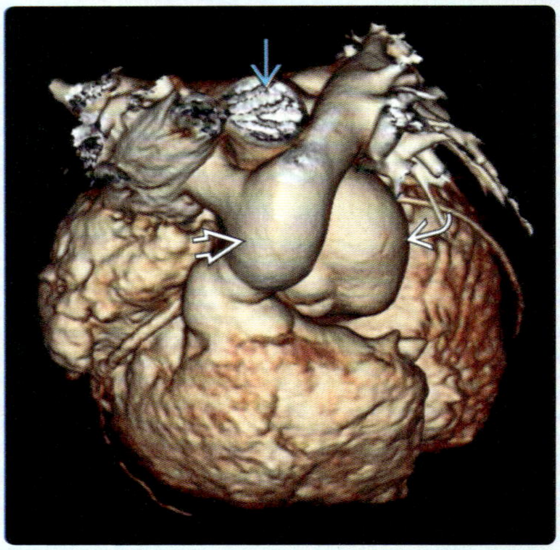

(Left) *Axial oblique MIP shows anterior pulmonary valve and posterior aortic root. Right and left coronary arteries originate from the posteriorly oriented cusp. Note diminutive and occluded left anterior descending artery. Coronary artery occlusion is the most common cause of mortality.* **(Right)** *Axial CTA in a patient after arterial switch shows the classic appearance of PA branches straddling ascending aorta. Note patent stents within bilateral branch PA to treat PA stenosis, which is common after Lecompte maneuver.*

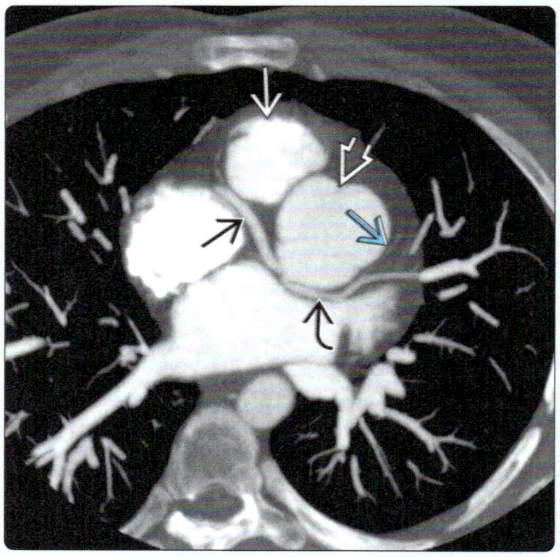

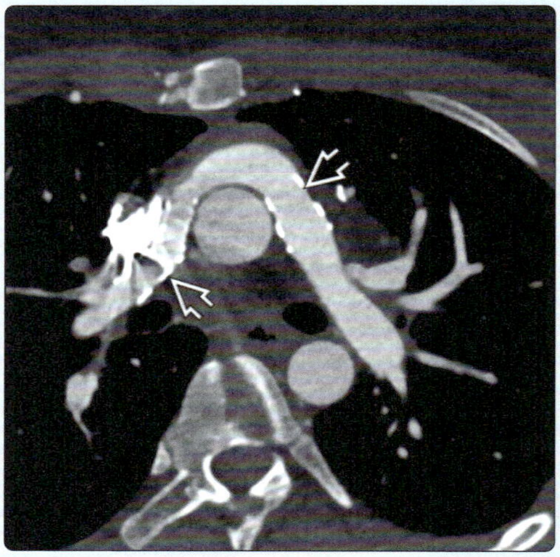

TERMINOLOGY

Abbreviations

- Atrial switch operation (AtrSO)
- Arterial switch operation (ASO)

Synonyms

- AtrSO: Mustard, Senning procedure
- ASO: Jatene procedure

Definitions

- AtrSO and ASO are surgeries performed for treatment of D-TGA
- AtrSO: Redirection of blood flow at atrial level using baffles
  - Pulmonary venous flow redirected through baffle to tricuspid valve, right ventricle (RV), aorta
  - Systemic venous flow redirected through baffle to mitral valve, left ventricle (LV), and pulmonary artery (PA)
  - Senning procedure: Right atrial wall used as baffle
  - Mustard procedure: Pericardium or synthetic material used as baffle
  - Used to be definitive treatment option; no longer performed due to complications
- ASO: Resection of aorta and PA and reimplantation to LV and RV, respectively; coronary buttons harvested with patch of aorta and reimplanted to neoaortic root
  - Distal PA is brought anterior to aorta = Lecompte maneuver
  - Definitive procedure; performed in 1st few weeks of life

IMAGING

General Features

- Best diagnostic clue
  - AtrSO: Baffles are seen redirecting flow; pulmonary vein (PV) baffle redirects flow to right heart; systemic baffles redirect flow to left heart
  - ASO: PA anterior and draping aorta

CT Findings

- Excellent spatial resolution allows for detailed anatomic assessment
  - May be preferable to MR in patients with implanted cardiac devices
- Quantification of ventricular volumes, function, and mass
  - Can be used if MR contraindicated
- AtrSO
  - Baffle stenosis evaluation required before pacemaker placement to avoid worsening of stenosis
    - Delayed-phase imaging may be required
    - Assessment of baffle patency and collateral vessels
  - Baffle leak difficult to identify in CT
    - Positive or negative contrast jet across leak is essential: Use biphasic contrast
    - Globular shape of subpulmonic LV is clue (usually banana/crescent shape)
- ASO
  - Accurate for assessing branch PAs and possible stenosis
  - Neoaortic root dilatation/abnormal Z-score
  - Coronary artery anatomy and stenosis assessment

MR Findings

- AtrSO
  - Pulmonary venous flow redirected through baffle to tricuspid valve, RV, aorta
  - Systemic venous flow directed through baffle to mitral valve, LV, and PA
  - Complications
    - Baffle stenosis
      - Can be seen in black-blood, bSSFP cine, or MRA
      - Requires thin-section image parallel and perpendicular to venous pathways
      - Systemic venous pathways best in coronal oblique; PV baffles best in axial images
      - bSSFP: Focal narrowing of baffle with dephasing; dynamic changes in caliber
      - Proximal venous pathways are dilated, including azygos vein
      - Phase contrast (PC) MR: Detection and quantification of pressure gradient; 4D PC preferable if available
      - Reversal of flow in azygos vein in PC MR
    - Baffle leak
      - Low sensitivity and specificity in detection
      - High-temporal-resolution cine SSFP in multiple planes, time-resolved MRA, and 1st-pass perfusion imaging may show flow across baffle
      - Easier to identify using 4D PC vs. 2D PC
      - Quantifies leak either directly through leak or Qp:Qs (R-L shunt > 1.2 or L-R shunt < 0.8 significant)
    - Failure of morphologic RV (systemic ventricle)
      - RV hypertrophied, dilated with systolic dysfunction
      - Accurate quantification by MR
    - Tricuspid valve regurgitation
      - Direct or indirect quantification
    - LGE seen in 61%
      - RV insertion points; focal full thickness of anterior RV; small foci in trabeculations; basal septal
      - Correlates with age, RV dysfunction, clinical events
    - LV (pulmonary) outflow obstruction
    - Atrial or baffle thrombus
- ASO
  - Aorta reconnected to LV; PA reconnected to RV
  - PA and branches draped anterior to aorta (Lecompte maneuver)
  - Complications
    - PA branch stenosis
      - Smaller caliber; 2 measurements due to elliptical orifice
      - High velocities (> 350 cm/sec) and vortices in 4D flow
      - Continuous diastolic flow in narrower artery
      - Differential pulmonary flow; lower flow in affected lung L > R
    - Dilatation of neoaortic root
      - Measured in double oblique reconstruction; Z-scores > 2.5
      - Aortic regurgitation quantified by 2D/4D flow; holodiastolic flow reversal in descending aorta; increased aortic stiffness, decreased distensibility
      - Airway compression

- Coronary arterial stenosis
  - Noncontrast MRA can evaluate coronary arterial anatomy
  - Stress perfusion MR/dobutamine can evaluate myocardial ischemia
  - Subendocardial and transmural LGE can be seen with myocardial infarction in 1.8%
- Pulmonary regurgitation; pulmonary hypertension

Ultrasonographic Findings

- 1st-line imaging modality in evaluation of complications
- Baffle stenosis: Limited evaluation of entire baffle and venous system
- Baffle leak: Agitated saline injection shows shunt
- Limited evaluation of systemic, morphologic RV in AtrSO due to retrosternal location

Angiographic Findings

- Rarely used for diagnosis
- Required for diagnosis of baffle leak

Imaging Recommendations

- Best imaging tool
  - Echocardiography is 1st-line imaging for evaluation of AtrSO and ASO
  - MR is definitive imaging modality for comprehensive anatomic and functional evaluation of AtrSO and ASO
  - CT is useful for detailed anatomic evaluation, when MR is contraindicated or expected to have artifacts, and for assessment of coronary arteries and collateral vessels

CLINICAL ISSUES

Natural History & Prognosis

- Complications of AtrSO
  - Arrhythmias: Injury to sinoatrial (SA) node during surgery, especially with Mustard procedure
  - Baffle stenosis (in 20% of patients); more common in systemic baffles; superior vena cava > inferior vena cava
  - Baffle leak (in 20% of patients); usually small and insignificant
    - Significant leaks can cause cyanosis, paradoxical embolism, and stroke
  - Systemic ventricular failure: 7-10% fail at 10 years
    - Primarily remodeling due to systemic afterload; also coronary flow mismatch, suboptimal conduction
  - Tricuspid regurgitation (TR)
    - Due to altered geometry of tricuspid valve anulus or septal leaflet due to systemic pressures
  - Myocardial fibrosis
- Complications of ASO
  - Arrhythmia
  - PA stenosis: Branch/supravalvular: 5-40%
    - Neopulmonary root compressed between sternum and aorta
    - Smaller branch PAs more often involved, L > R where branch crosses ascending aorta
  - Pulmonary hypertension
    - From PA stenosis, ventricular septal defect (VSD), or aortopulmonary collaterals
    - Pulmonary regurgitation can be seen
  - Neoaortic root dilatation (in 76% of patients)
    - Maladaptation of neoaortic wall, PA banding, VSD, aortopathy, angular shape of arch
  - Neoaortic valve regurgitation
    - Moderate to severe in 8%
    - Associated with increased diameter of neoaortic root; ASO after 1st year of life; history of VSD repair or PA banding
    - Can result in LV dilatation and dysfunction
  - Subaortic obstruction
  - Coronary stenosis/occlusion: 2-1%
    - Surgical injury (suture line fibrosis), intimal thickening, kinking, compression by PAs, neoaortic dilatation
    - Most common cause of early mortality
  - Aortopulmonary collaterals: Rare, can be seen before or after ASO

Treatment

- Baffle stenosis in AtrSO
  - Significant stenosis requires percutaneous balloon dilatation with stent placement or surgical intervention
- Baffle leak in AtrSO
  - Requires percutaneous or surgical closure
- Systemic RV failure in AtrSO
  - Medical therapy
    - Not well studied
    - Angiotensin receptor/neprilysin inhibitor and sodium-glucose cotransporter 2 (SGLT2) inhibitors may improve functional status
  - Pacemakers and implantable cardioverter-defibrillator placement
    - Biventricular pacing
    - Implantable cardioverter defibrillator (ICD) implantation considered for secondary prevention of sudden cardiac death
      - Systemic RV dysfunction ejection fraction < 35%
      - NYHA functional class II/III
      - Severe systemic atrioventricular valve regurgitation
      - Wide QRS duration ≥ 140 ms
  - Tricuspid valve repair/replacement for TR
  - Heart transplant of ventricular assist devices
- PA stenosis in ASO
  - Balloon angioplasty; surgical reconstruction; PA stenting
- Neoaortic root dilation or AV regurgitation in ASO
  - Usually mild and requires no treatment
  - Surgical repair required in > 11% at 30 years
- Aorticopulmonary collateral vessels; coiling

SELECTED REFERENCES

1. Han BK et al: Technical recommendations for computed tomography guidance of intervention in the right ventricular outflow tract: native RVOT, conduits and bioprosthetic valves: a white paper of the Society of Cardiovascular Computed Tomography (SCCT), Congenital Heart Surgeons' Society (CHSS), and Society for Cardiovascular Angiography & Interventions (SCAI). J Cardiovasc Comput Tomogr. 18(1):75-99, 2024
2. Zhu MZL et al: Outcomes of neo-aortic valve and root surgery late after arterial switch operation. J Thorac Cardiovasc Surg. 167(4):1391-401.e3, 2024
3. Sabbah BN et al: Heart failure in systemic right ventricle: mechanisms and therapeutic options. Front Cardiovasc Med. 9:1064196, 2022
4. Canan A et al: Multimodality imaging of transposition of the great arteries. Radiographics. 41(2):338-60, 2021

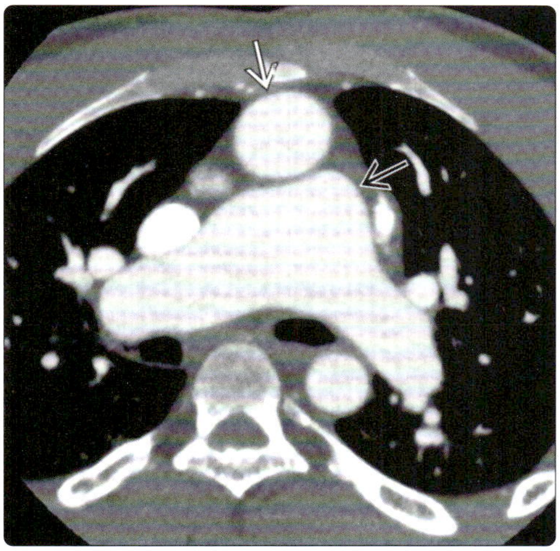

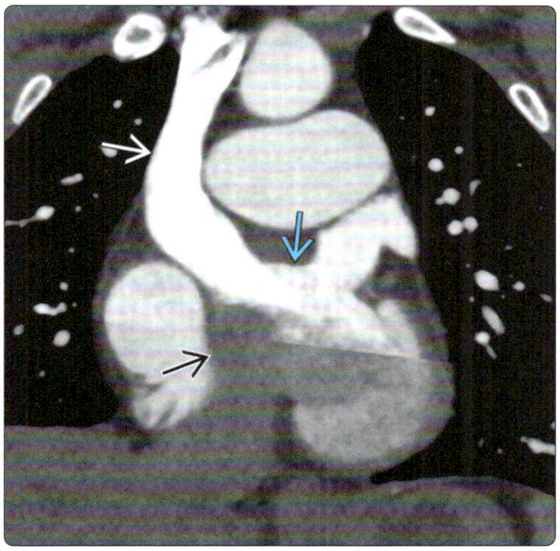

(Left) *Axial CT in a 31-year-old man with D-TGA status post atrial switch shows the ascending aorta ➔ located anterior to the main PA ⇨.* **(Right)** *Coronal oblique CT in the same patient demonstrates systemic venous baffles. During atrial switch operation, superior vena cava (SVC) ➔ and inferior vena cava (IVC) ⇨ are directed to left atrium ⇨. Image was obtained during arterial phase, which resulted in absence of contrast within the IVC. A delayed phase is necessary to complete the assessment of IVC baffle.*

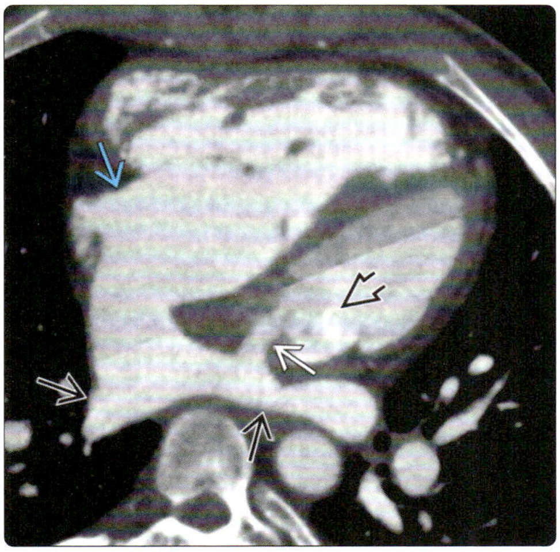

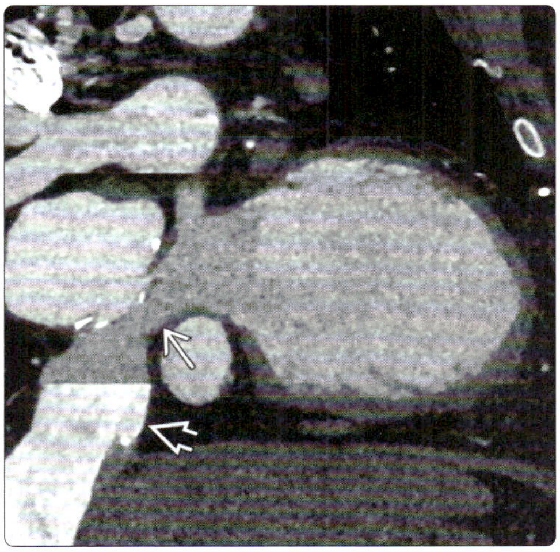

(Left) *Axial oblique CT in the same patient shows patent pulmonary venous baffles. Note that all pulmonary veins ⇨ are directed into right atrium ⇨. Also, a baffle leak ➔ from left pulmonary vein into the left atrium ⇨ is noted.* **(Right)** *Coronal oblique CTA shows narrowing of the IVC baffle ➔ at the junction of left atrium. Note the dilated suprahepatic IVC ➔. Delayed phase CT is helpful for evaluation of IVC baffles.*

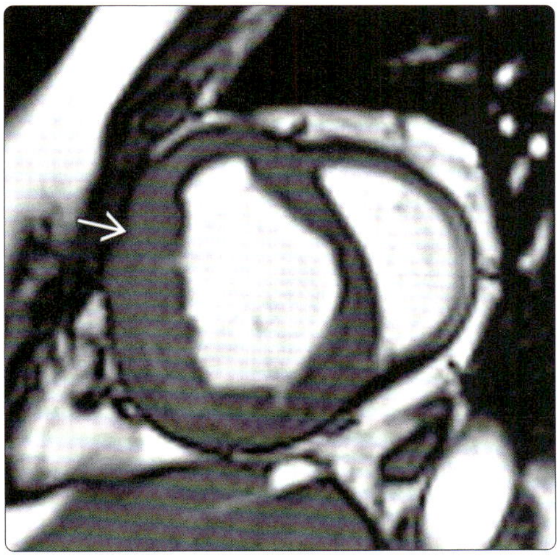

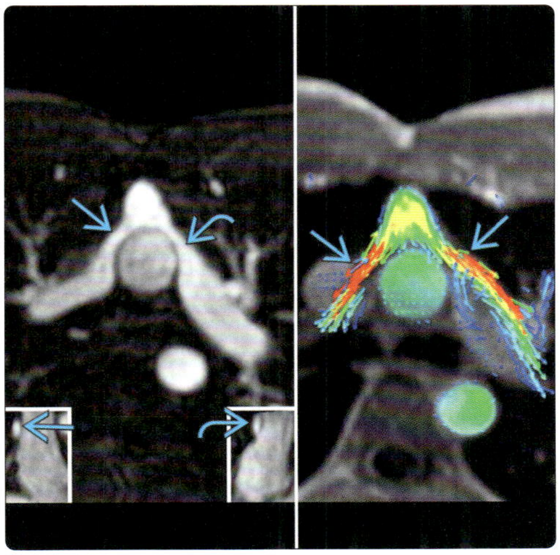

(Left) *Systolic SSFP MR shows a hypertrophied and dilated systemic right ventricle (RV) ➔ with leftward bowing of the interventricular septum. RV dilation and failure are common long-term complications of atrial switch.* **(Right)** *MRA (left) post arterial switch shows narrowing of the right PA ⇨ and left PA ⇨, which measure 12 x 6 mm and 13 x 5 mm, respectively (insets). 4D flow at the same level (right) shows increased velocity due to stenosis with peak gradient > 30 mmHg for both PAs.*

Truncus Arteriosus

KEY FACTS

TERMINOLOGY

- Common arterial vessel arising from heart
  - Gives rise to aorta, pulmonary arteries (PAs), and coronary arteries
- Category: Cyanotic, cardiomegaly, and increased pulmonary vascularity

IMAGING

- Classic radiographic appearance: Cardiomegaly, right aortic arch, narrow mediastinum, and increased pulmonary vascularity
- Diagnosis typically made with echocardiography
- MR/CTA for preoperative delineation of anatomy
- MR/CTA for postoperative assessment of conduit and stents

TOP DIFFERENTIAL DIAGNOSES

- Hemitruncus
- Aortopulmonary window

PATHOLOGY

- Strong association with chromosome 22q11.2 (DiGeorge) syndrome

CLINICAL ISSUES

- 2% of all congenital cardiac anomalies
- Most common congenital heart condition associated with right aortic arch
- Symptoms include progressive congestive heart failure and increasing cyanosis
- Treatment
  - Early complete repair (at 2-6 weeks of life) is favored
  - PAs detached from arterial trunk and conduit placed between PAs and right ventricle; patch closure of ventricular septal defect (VSD)
  - Complications: Conduit stenosis or regurgitation, branch PA stenosis, truncal stenosis or regurgitation
  - Conduit revisions ± replacement usually necessary

(Left) *Graphic demonstrates a type 1 truncus giving rise to the aorta and a main pulmonary artery (PA). Note the common truncal valve overriding the high ventricular septal defect. A right aortic arch is present.* **(Right)** *Posteroanterior chest radiograph of a patient with truncus arteriosus shows cardiomegaly, right aortic arch, and increased pulmonary vascularity. Cyanosis is due to flow admixture within the ventricles and the truncus.*

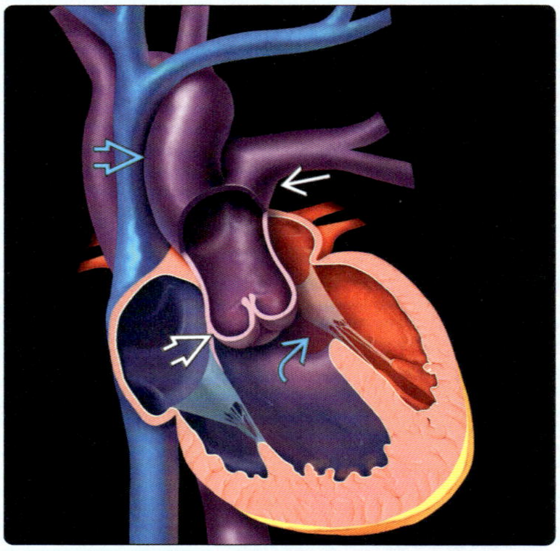

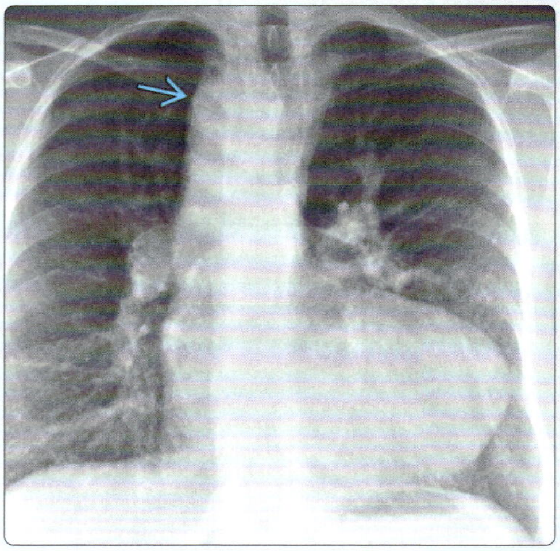

(Left) *Coronal oblique reconstructed CTA shows a common trunk for the ascending aorta and the main PA (MPA), consistent with truncus arteriosus. A common truncal valve and ventricular septal defect (VSD) are also seen.* **(Right)** *Axial oblique reconstructed CTA shows a common trunk for the ascending aorta and the MPA, consistent with truncus arteriosus.*

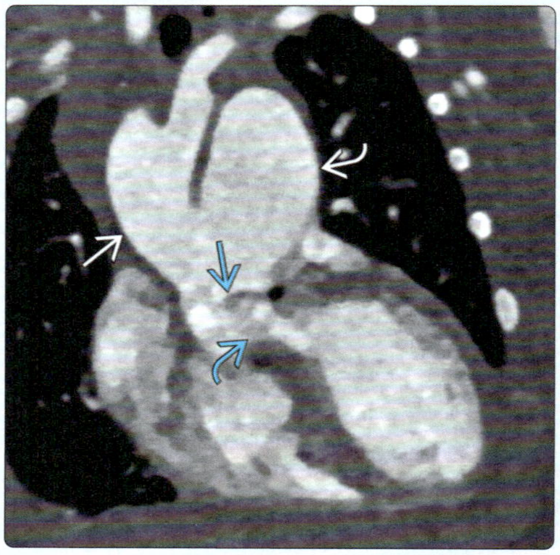

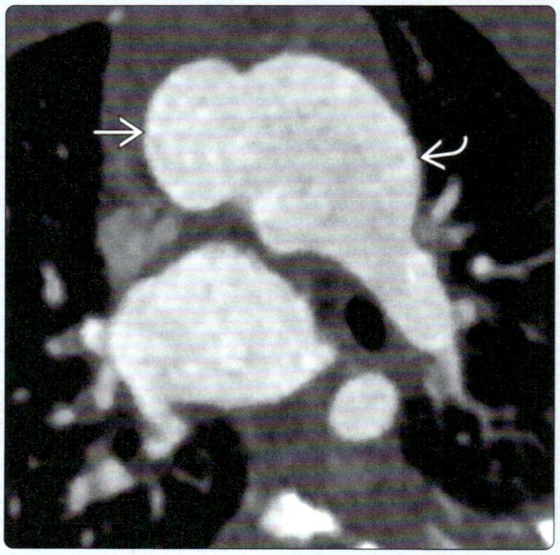

TERMINOLOGY

Abbreviations

- Truncus arteriosus (TA)

Definitions

- Common arterial trunk arising from heart
  - Gives rise to aorta, pulmonary arteries (PAs), and coronary arteries
- Category: Cyanotic, cardiomegaly, and increased pulmonary vascularity
- Hemodynamics
  - Both ventricles are connected to pulmonary and systemic circulations
  - Flow admixture across ventricular septal defect (VSD) and within truncus → cyanosis
  - Postnatal drop in pulmonary vascular resistance → relative increase in pulmonary blood flow → volume overload of pulmonary circulation

IMAGING

General Features

- Best diagnostic clue
  - Common arterial trunk arising from both ventricles

Radiographic Findings

- Radiography
  - Cardiomegaly
  - Right aortic arch
  - Narrow mediastinum due to thymic agenesis
  - Increased pulmonary vascularity
  - Atelectasis
    - Dilated PAs may compress neighboring bronchi

CT Findings

- CTA
  - Preoperative
    - Common arterial trunk arising from both ventricles
      - Larger than normal thoracic aorta
    - Relationship of branch PAs to truncus
      - See classification listed
    - Evaluate coronary anatomy
      - Normal origin in 2/3
      - LAD is often small and displaced to left
      - Large conus branch supplies RVOT and septum
      - Left-dominant circulation in 27%

MR Findings

- MRA
  - Evaluate global anatomy, patency of conduit, vessel sizes
  - Common arterial trunk arising from both ventricles
- MR cine
  - Truncal valve: Morphology, stenosis, regurgitation
  - Ventricular function and volumes
  - Associated anomalies
- Phase-contrast MR
  - Quantification of truncal stenosis/regurgitation
  - Shunt fraction to quantify of L-to-R shunt via VSD
  - Flow, velocities, and gradients across stenotic lesions
  - Extent of collateralization
- General
  - More effective than echocardiography to evaluate
    - Branch PAs
    - Aortopulmonary collateral vessels
    - Complex abnormalities of aortic arch or pulmonary veins
  - Evaluate for postoperative complications

Echocardiographic Findings

- Echocardiogram
  - Typically used for diagnosis and surgical planning
  - Common arterial trunk originating from both ventricles
  - High (outlet) VSD immediately below truncal valve
    - Biventricular (68-83%); over RV (11-29%); over LV (4-6%)
  - Common truncal valve with 2 (9%), 3 (69%), or 4 (22%) cusps
- Color Doppler
  - Bidirectional flow across VSD
  - Truncal valve regurgitation

Angiographic Findings

- Conventional
  - Cardiac catheterization with angiography
    - Define truncal anatomy
    - Evaluate truncal valve insufficiency
    - Hemodynamic study is gold standard for calculation of pulmonary vascular resistance

DIFFERENTIAL DIAGNOSIS

Hemitruncus Arteriosus

- One branch of PA (usually RPA) originates from ascending aorta, and other (LPA) originates from normal MPA
- a.k.a. anomalous origin of RPA (AORPA) from ascending aorta
- All systemic blood from RV goes to left lung → pulmonary hypertension
- Oxygenated blood to right lung → pulmonary hypertension due to systemic pressures

Aortopulmonary Window

- a.k.a. aortopulmonary septal defect
- Direct communication between ascending aorta and PA
- Incomplete division of embryonic common trunk
- Separate origin of MPA and aorta from ventricles

PATHOLOGY

General Features

- Etiology
  - Embryology
    - Lack of separation of primitive bulbus cordis into aorta and MPA
    - Associated persistence of primitive aortic arches
  - Pathophysiology
    - Congestive heart failure vs. cyanosis (degree of cyanosis is determined by balance of pulmonary and systemic resistance)
      - Marked increase in pulmonary blood flow in early neonatal period due to drop in pulmonary vascular resistance → slight improvement in cyanosis but worsening congestive heart failure

- Development of pulmonary vascular obstructive disease leads to improvement in congestive heart failure but worsening cyanosis
- Genetics
  - Strong association with chromosome 22q11.2 (DiGeorge) syndrome
  - CATCH-22: Craniofacial anomaly, absent thymus, hypocalcemia, heart defect
  - Velocardiofacial (Shprintzen) syndrome
- Associated abnormalities
  - Malalignment VSD present in almost all cases
    - Subarterial, large, nonrestrictive
  - Right aortic arch
  - Interrupted aortic arch (11-14%)
  - Atrial septal defect
  - Aberrant subclavian artery
  - Left superior vena cava
  - Other
    - Abnormalities of mitral valve, coronary arteries, pulmonary veins

Staging, Grading, & Classification

- Collett and Edwards classification system
  - Type I: PAs arise from short pulmonary trunk (48-68%)
  - Type II: PAs arise separately from posterior aspect of truncus (29-48%)
  - Type III: PAs arise separately from lateral aspect of truncus (6-10%)
  - Type IV: No PAs; lung supply by large MAPCAs; considered to be form of pulmonary atresia with VSD (pseudotruncus)
- Van Praagh and Van Praagh classification
  - Type 1: PAs arise from short pulmonary trunk
  - Type 2: PAs arise separately from posterior aspect of truncus
  - Type 3: One branch PA arises from truncus, other from patent ductus arteriosus (PDA or aorta)
  - Type 4: Hypoplastic/interrupted arch; large PDA
  - A: Presence of VSD; B: No VSD
- Society of Thoracic Surgeons classification
  - Truncus with confluent or near-confluent PAs (types A1, A2, I, II, III)
  - Truncus with absence of 1 PA (type A3)
  - Truncus with interrupted aortic arch or severe coarctation (type A4)

Gross Pathologic & Surgical Features

- PAs
  - Usually from left posterolateral
  - When separate, left is higher than right
  - LPA to right of RPA in interruption
- Common trunk has medial wall abnormalities, like Marfan

CLINICAL ISSUES

Presentation

- Most common signs/symptoms
  - Progressive congestive heart failure in young infant
  - Increasing cyanosis
- Other signs/symptoms
  - T-cell immunodeficiency (thymic agenesis in DiGeorge syndrome)
  - Neonatal tetany (absent parathyroid glands in DiGeorge syndrome)

Demographics

- Epidemiology
  - 2% of all congenital cardiac anomalies
  - 94 per 1 million live births
  - Most common congenital heart condition associated with right aortic arch

Natural History & Prognosis

- Mortality if untreated
  - 6 months: 65%; 12 months: 75%
- Intractable congestive heart failure
  - Marked increase in pulmonary flow after drop in pulmonary vascular resistance
  - Aggravated by presence of truncal valve regurgitation (50% of cases)
- Eventual shunt reversal with progressive cyanosis and sudden death
  - Pulmonary vascular obstructive disease with Eisenmenger physiology can develop as early as 6 months of age
- Postoperative course determined by function of conduit and morbidity of conduit replacement

Treatment

- Palliative: Banding of MPA
  - Initial palliation with PA banding often unsatisfactory
    - Early development of pulmonary arterial hypertension
- Surgical repair
  - Patch closure of VSD
  - Correction of aortic coarctation/interruption
  - Early complete repair (at 2-6 weeks of life) is favored by most surgeons
    - PAs detached from arterial trunk and conduit placed between PAs and RV
    - Complications
      - PA-RV conduit stenosis or regurgitation
      - Branch PA stenosis
      - Neoaortic valve (truncal) stenosis or regurgitation
      - VSD patch leak
      - Obstruction of aortic arch
    - Conduit revisions ± replacement usually necessary by 10-12 years
      - Patient outgrows fixed conduit size
      - Stenosis, neointimal hyperplasia
      - Anastomotic pseudoaneurysm
      - Calcification
      - Conduit valve dysfunction

SELECTED REFERENCES

1. Kumar P et al: Role of CT in the pre- and postoperative assessment of conotruncal anomalies. Radiol Cardiothorac Imaging. 4(3):e210089, 2022
2. Chikkabyrappa S et al: Common arterial trunk: physiology, imaging, and management. Semin Cardiothorac Vasc Anesth. 1089253218821382, 2018
3. Fratz S et al: Guidelines and protocols for cardiovascular magnetic resonance in children and adults with congenital heart disease: SCMR expert consensus group on congenital heart disease. J Cardiovasc Magn Reson. 15:51, 2013
4. Saremi F et al: Right ventricular outflow tract imaging with CT and mRI: part 1, morphology. AJR Am J Roentgenol. 200(1):W39-50, 2013

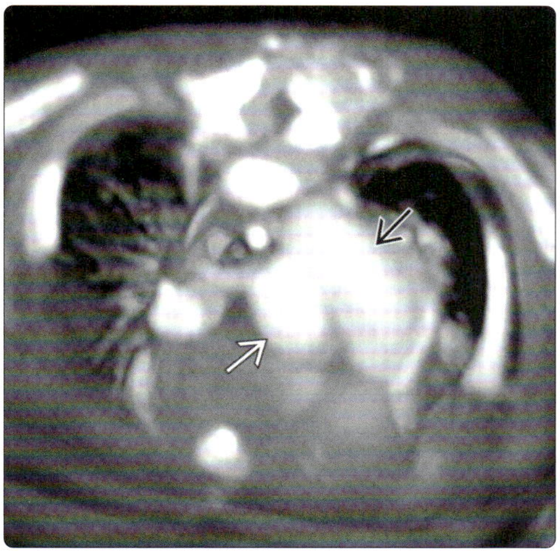

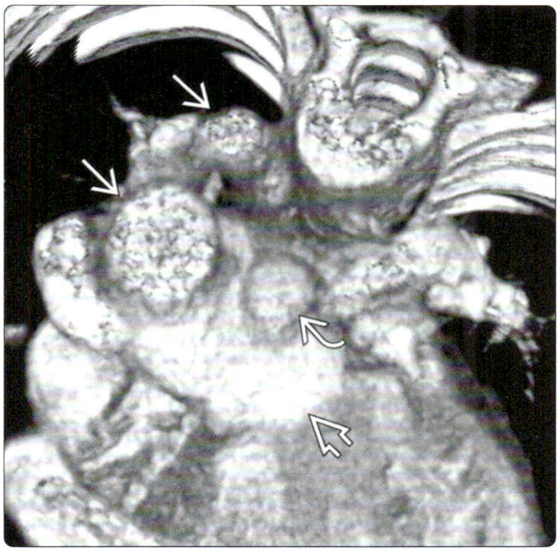

(Left) *Oblique CTA shows a connection between the aorta* ⇨ *and PA* ➡ *in this 3-day-old infant with an aortopulmonary window.* **(Right)** *Oblique volume-rendered reconstruction of CTA shows truncus* ➡*, giving rise to the right aortic arch* ➡ *and pulmonary trunk* ➡*.*

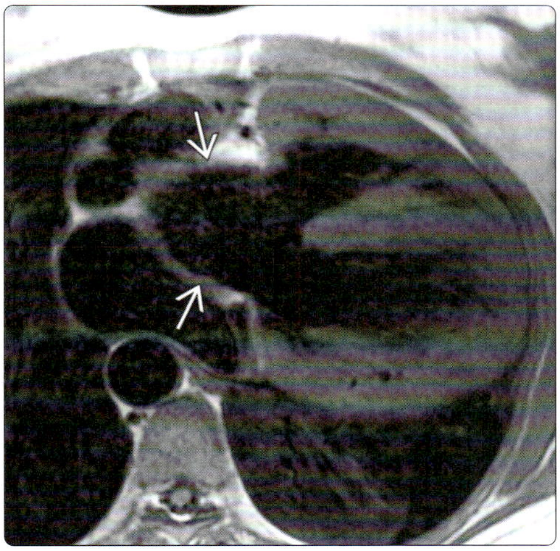

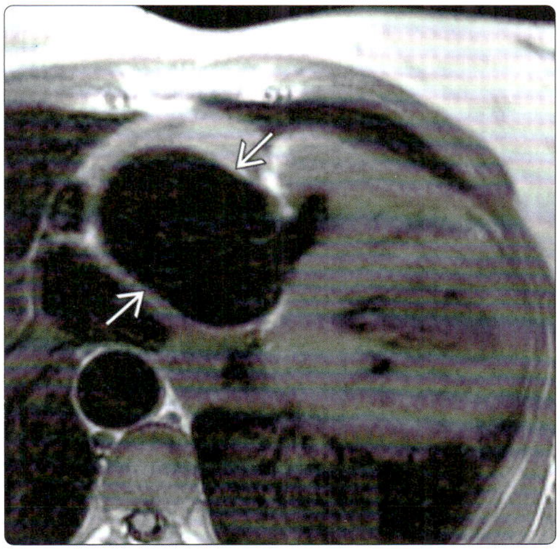

(Left) *Axial black-blood MR in a patient with truncus arteriosus shows a common arterial trunk arising from both ventricles* ➡*.* **(Right)** *Axial black-blood MR in the same patient demonstrates dilation of the truncus* ➡ *secondary to truncal valve dysfunction (regurgitation), which may necessitate valvuloplasty or placement of a prosthesis. Truncus arteriosus represents a lack of separation of the primitive bulbus cordis into the aorta and the MPA.*

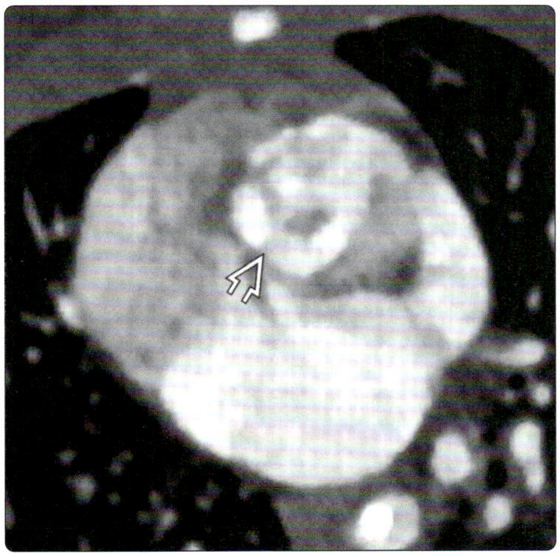

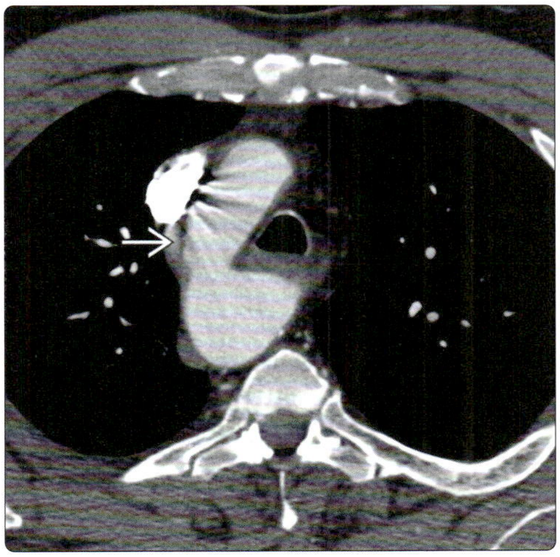

(Left) *Axial oblique reconstructed CTA in a patient with truncus arteriosus shows a truncal valve* ➡*.* **(Right)** *Axial CECT in the same patient shows the right aortic arch* ➡*. Truncus arteriosus is the congenital heart condition most commonly associated with a right aortic arch. Other anomalies, such as atrial septal defect, aberrant subclavian arteries, and left superior vena cava, may be present.*

KEY FACTS

TERMINOLOGY

- Congenital malformation characterized by failed development of pulmonary valve orifice
- 2 distinct types based upon status of interventricular septum
- Category: Cyanotic, cardiomegaly, decreased ± irregular pulmonary vascularity

IMAGING

- Best diagnostic clue: RVOT ± pulmonary valve atresia
- Chest radiography: Decreased pulmonary circulation
  - PA-VSD: Boot-shaped heart
  - PA-IVS: Right atrial enlargement
- Initial diagnosis with echocardiography
- CT for anatomic assessment and coronary sinusoid assessment in PA-IVS
- MR for anatomic assessment and shunt evaluation
- Cardiac catheterization for hemodynamic assessment, selective injection studies, and catheter-based interventions

TOP DIFFERENTIAL DIAGNOSES

- Ebstein anomaly
- Tricuspid atresia with VSD

CLINICAL ISSUES

- Progressive cyanosis after birth with closure of ductus arteriosus
- Congestive heart failure with large and unobstructed high-flow multiple aortopulmonary collateral arteries
- Prognosis depends on feasibility of surgery
- Treatment
  - Prostaglandin E1 to keep ductus arteriosus open
  - Management of congestive heart failure
  - PA-VSD: Staged complete repair with unifocalization of major aortopulmonary collateral arteries (MAPCAs)
  - PA-IVS: Type of repair depends on RV size and RV dependency on coronary circulation

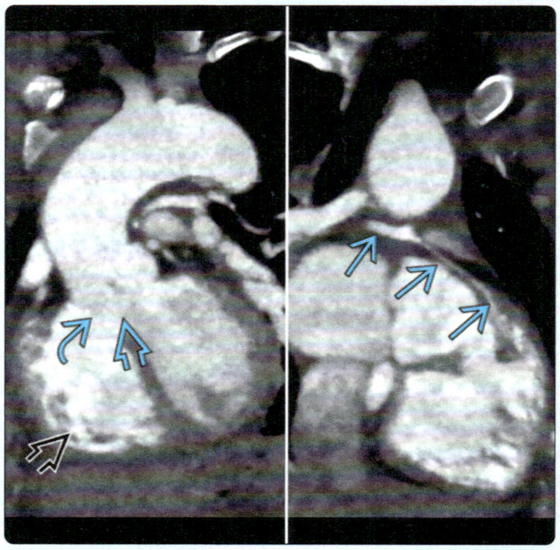

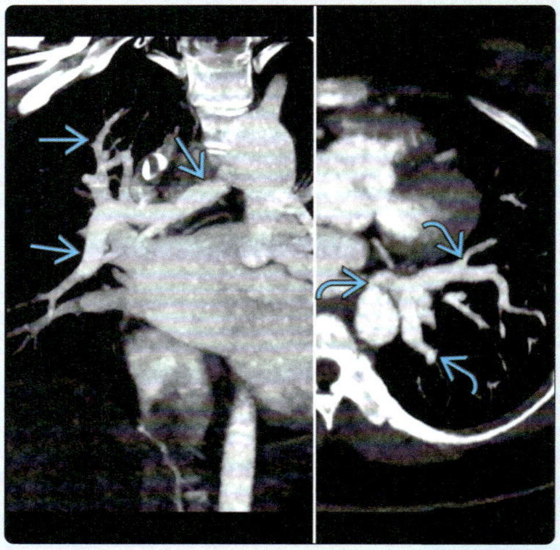

(Left) *CT images in an 18-year-old show uncorrected findings of tetralogy of Fallot (TOF), including perimembranous ventricular septal defect (VSD), overriding aorta, right ventricular (RV) hypertrophy, and severe hypoplasia of the pulmonary artery.* **(Right)** *CT images show major aorticopulmonary collateral arteries (MAPCAs) arising from the proximal descending thoracic aorta supplying the right lung and from the middescending thoracic aorta supplying the left lung. Additional MAPCAs were present.*

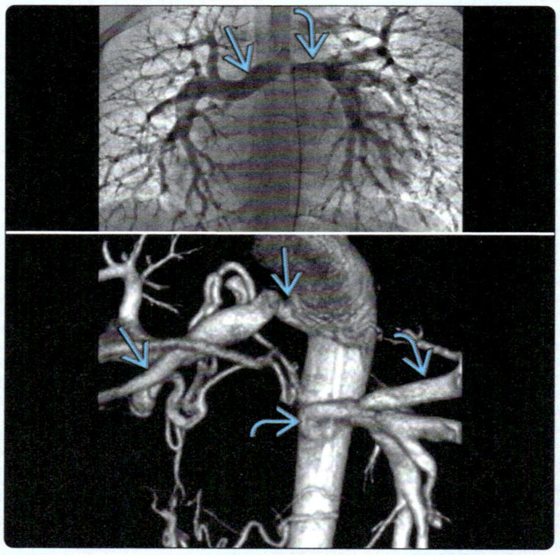

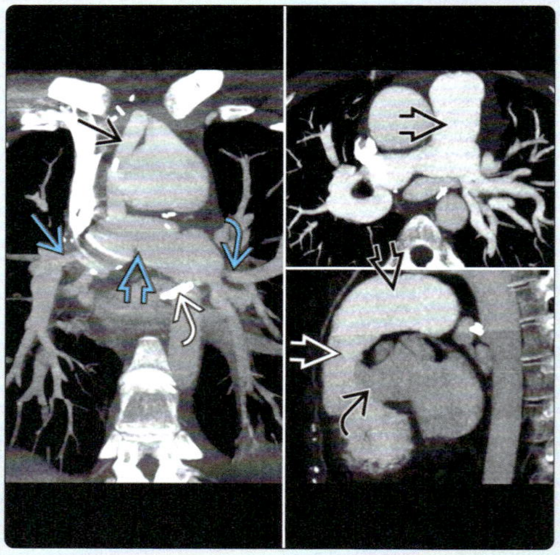

(Left) *Catheter aortic angiogram images (top) and 3D volume-rendered image from the angiogram (bottom) show the MAPCAs supplying the right and left lung.* **(Right)** *Patient underwent 2-stage unifocalization with MAPCA ligation. The large MAPCAs, were then anastomosed to a PA conduit (left), which was supplied by a modified BT shunt. Months later (right), the VSD was closed, a neo-RVOT was created and attached to a neo-PA, PA conduit, and unifocalized MAPCAs. The BT shunt was ligated.*

TERMINOLOGY

Abbreviations

- Pulmonary atresia with ventricular septal defect (PA-VSD)
- Pulmonary atresia with intact ventricular septum (PA-IVS)

Definitions

- Absence of communication between right ventricle (RV) and main pulmonary artery (MPA)
- 2 distinct types based on interventricular septum
  - PA-IVS
    - Complete atresia of pulmonary valve
    - RV hypoplasia (single ventricle physiology) or dilation
    - Normal-sized PAs
    - Lungs supplied by patent ductus arteriosus (PDA) and patent foramen ovale (PFO)
    - Coronary sinusoids (coronary-cameral fistula)
      - Coronary artery to RV connections in 50% at birth
    - Tricuspid valve hypoplasia/dysplasia
  - PA-VSD
    - Usually severe form of tetralogy of Fallot (TOF)
    - Ranges from imperforate pulmonary valve to hypoplastic/absent PAs and branches
    - Major aortopulmonary collateral arteries (MAPCAs) supply 1 or both lungs
    - 2 functional ventricles exist
    - RV blood exits through overriding aorta and supplies systemic and pulmonary circuit

IMAGING

General Features

- Best diagnostic clue
  - Atresia of RV outflow tract (RVOT) ± pulmonary valve

Radiographic Findings

- PA-VSD
  - Boot-shaped configuration of heart
  - Right aortic arch is common
  - Diminutive PA shadow
  - Decreased size of pulmonary vasculature
  - May be able to visualize MAPCAs
- PA-IVS
  - Massive right atrial dilation
  - Diminutive PA shadow
  - Decreased size of pulmonary vasculature

CT Findings

- CTA
  - PA-VSD
    - Findings of TOF
      - Perimembranous VSD, overriding aorta, RV hypertrophy
      - Severe pulmonary stenosis with severely hypoplastic to agenesis of RVOT, pulmonic valve, ± central PAs
    - Assess anatomy and distribution of MAPCAs
  - PA-IVS
    - Large right atrium (RA) and small, hypertrophied RV
    - Tricuspid valve hypoplasia to agenesis
    - Atresia of pulmonary valve
    - Assess for presence and origin of coronary sinusoids
      - Left anterior descending (LAD) and right coronary artery (RCA) most common
    - Assessment of RV-dependent coronary circulation (RVDCC)
      - Areas of coronary stenosis or absent aortic ostia
  - Evaluate patency of shunts/conduits postoperatively

MR Findings

- MR cine
  - Assessment of anatomy and anomalies
  - Quantification of RV volumes and function
- MRA
  - ECG and respiratory-gated whole-heart MRA angiography
    - Assess vascular anatomy, size, and origin of MAPCAs
- Phase contrast
  - PA flow/differential branch flow
  - Quantification of gradients through stenosed vessels

Echocardiographic Findings

- Echocardiogram
  - PA-VSD, MAPCAs
    - Characteristics of intracardiac anatomy, position and size of VSD, overriding aortic root
    - Development of branch PAs, confluence
  - PA-IVS
    - Morphology of interatrial septum
      - Evaluate for restricted flow across PFO
    - Size of RV and tricuspid anulus (expressed as z-score), degree of tricuspid regurgitation
      - Important for surgical planning
    - Presence and location of coronary sinusoids

Angiographic Findings

- Conventional
  - PA-VSD, MAPCAs
    - Selective injection with pressure recordings of all MAPCAs, imaging of true PAs
  - PA-IVS
    - Suprasystemic pressure recordings in RV
    - Detailed imaging of coronary sinusoids, including stenoses
    - Assessment of RVDCC is diagnosed by cardiac catheterization (25%)
      - Presence of any coronary-cameral fistula with coronary obstruction (severe stenosis, interruption, atresia) proximal to fistula
      - Angiographic evidence of RV perfusion of myocardium through fistulous communication

Imaging Recommendations

- Best imaging tool
  - Initial diagnosis with echocardiogram
  - CT or MR for anatomic assessment
  - Cardiac catheterization for hemodynamic assessment

DIFFERENTIAL DIAGNOSIS

Ebstein Anomaly

- May mimic PA-IVS with large tricuspid anulus and massive tricuspid regurgitation

Tricuspid Atresia With Ventricular Septal Defect

- Can have PA-VSD but often classified differently
- Muscular or membranous partition between RA and RV
- Obligatory shunting from RA → left atrium (LA) → left ventricle (LV) → RV
- Decreased pulmonary flow → severe cyanosis at birth

PATHOLOGY

General Features

- Etiology
  - Pathophysiology of PA-VSD, MAPCAs
    - Balance between flow though PAs and MAPCAs determines pulmonary perfusion
      - PA flow at subsystemic pressures, restricted by narrow caliber and eventual closure of PDA
      - Flow through MAPCAs → increased lung perfusion at systemic pressures (unless restricted by stenosis)
      - Degree of cyanosis is determined by intracardiac admixture and amount of pulmonary flow
      - Large amount of pulmonary blood flow through unrestricted MAPCAs → congestive heart failure
  - Pathophysiology of PA-IVS
    - Obligatory right-to-left shunt through PFO/ASD
    - Hypoplastic, heavily trabeculated RV with suprasystemic pressures
    - Pulmonary blood flow through PDA
    - Coronary sinusoids: At least 1 fistulous connection between diminutive RV and coronary circulation
      - 2 forms: RVDCC or independent coronary circulation coronary perfusion is thus dependent of high RV pressures and contractility
    - RVDCC (25-30%)
      - Coronary arteries proximal to coronary cameral fistula have stenoses or coronary arteries arise directly from RV (no aortic origin)
      - Coronary perfusion is dependent upon RV filling and contractility
      - Even minor changes in RV preload or surgical RV decompression → coronary ischemia
    - RV-independent coronary circulation
      - Fistulous connections between RV and coronary artery present but no coronary stenosis and normal coronary origin from aorta
      - Coronary artery has dual supply from RV and aorta
      - Fistulas may regress over time, and RV decompression possible
- Associated abnormalities
  - PA-IVS
    - Tricuspid hypoplasia
    - Absent central PAs
  - PA-VSD
    - Associated findings with TOF, such as right aortic arch

Gross Pathologic & Surgical Features

- Presence and confluence of central portions of true PAs are important for surgical repair

CLINICAL ISSUES

Presentation

- Most common signs/symptoms
  - Progressive cyanosis after birth with closure of ductus arteriosus
  - Congestive heart failure with large and unobstructed high-flow MAPCAs
- Other signs/symptoms
  - Failure to thrive, polycythemia, and clubbing

Demographics

- Epidemiology
  - PA-VSD: 2.5-3.4% of congenital cardiac anomalies
  - PA-IVS: 0.7-3.1% of congenital cardiac anomalies

Natural History & Prognosis

- Progressive cyanosis
  - Development of pulmonary vascular disease → irreversible pulmonary hypertension
- Life expectancy < 10 years if untreated
- Increased survival into adulthood for PA-VSD
- Prognosis depends on feasibility of surgery

Treatment

- Depends on native pulmonary vasculature and collaterals
- Prostaglandin E1 to keep ductus arteriosus open
- Palliative
  - Systemic-to-PA shunt [Blalock-Taussig (BT), modified BT, Waterston-Cooley, Potts, central or Melbourne shunt]
  - Initial banding of high-flow MAPCAs
- PA-VSD: Staged complete repair
  - Unifocalization of MAPCAs and true PAs
  - Early 1-stage repair in infancy with incorporation of all MAPCAs in PA conduit
  - Complete repair with incorporation of MAPCAs and PAs in conduit, connected to reconstructed RVOT (RV-PA conduit), closure of VSD
    - High pressure in pulmonary system from residual stenosis/hypoplasia and pulmonary vascular disease limit feasibility
  - Catheter-based interventions
    - Angioplasty with stenting of stenoses, embolization of superfluous ± bleeding MAPCAs
- PA-IVS: Type of repair dependent on RV size and RVDCC
  - RV-independent coronary circulation
    - Restricted flow across PFO: Balloon atrial septostomy
    - Catheter-based or surgical pulmonary valvotomy
    - Severely hypoplastic RV: Cavopulmonary (Glenn) shunt → univentricular repair (Fontan)
  - RVDCC
    - Cavopulmonary (Glenn) shunt, staged completion of univentricular repair (Fontan)

SELECTED REFERENCES

1. Alex A et al: Major aortopulmonary collateral arteries. Radiol Cardiothorac Imaging. 4(1):e210157, 2022
2. Kumar P et al: Role of CT in the pre- and postoperative assessment of conotruncal anomalies. Radiol Cardiothorac Imaging. 4(3):e210089, 2022
3. Spigel ZA et al: Right ventricle-dependent coronary circulation: location of obstruction is associated with survival. Ann Thorac Surg. 109(5):1480-7, 2020
4. Wright LK et al: Long-term outcomes after intervention for pulmonary atresia with intact ventricular septum. Heart. 105(13):1007-13, 2019
5. Presnell LB et al: An overview of pulmonary atresia and major aortopulmonary collateral arteries. World J Pediatr Congenit Heart Surg. 6(4):630-9, 2015
6. Rajeshkannan R et al: Role of 64-MDCT in evaluation of pulmonary atresia with ventricular septal defect. AJR Am J Roentgenol. 194(1):110-8, 2010

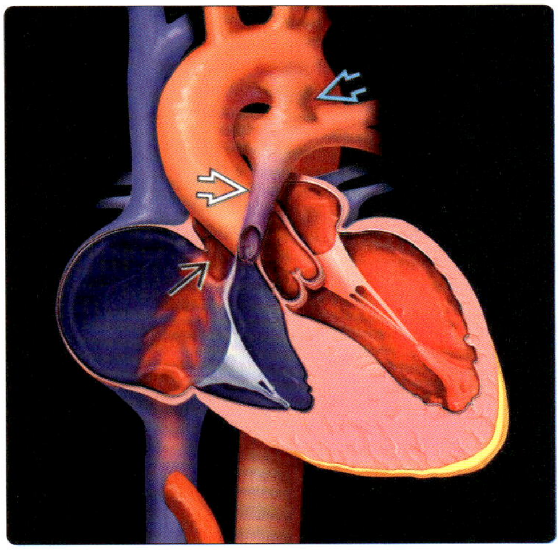

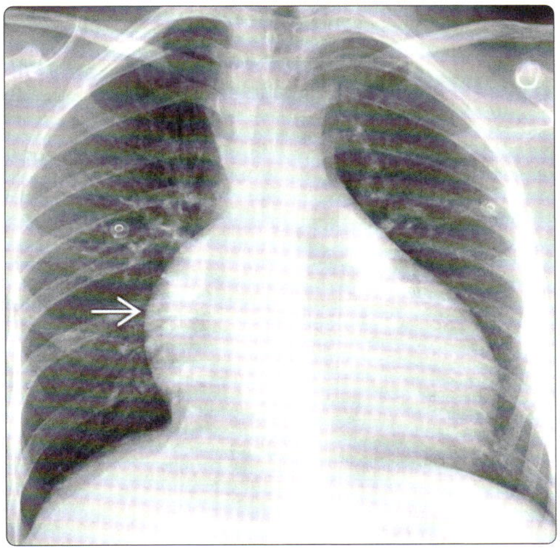

(Left) *Graphic demonstrates pulmonary atresia ➡ with intact ventricular septum (PA-IVS). A patent foramen ovale (PFO) ➡ is present. The right atrium (RA) is dilated, and the RV is hypoplastic and hypertrophied. The PAs are perfused via a patent ductus arteriosus (PDA) ➡.* **(Right)** *Radiograph in a patient with PA-IVS shows marked right atrial dilation ➡ resembles Ebstein anomaly. PA-IVS is characterized by an obligatory right-to-left shunt through a PFO, and the PAs are supplied by a PDA.*

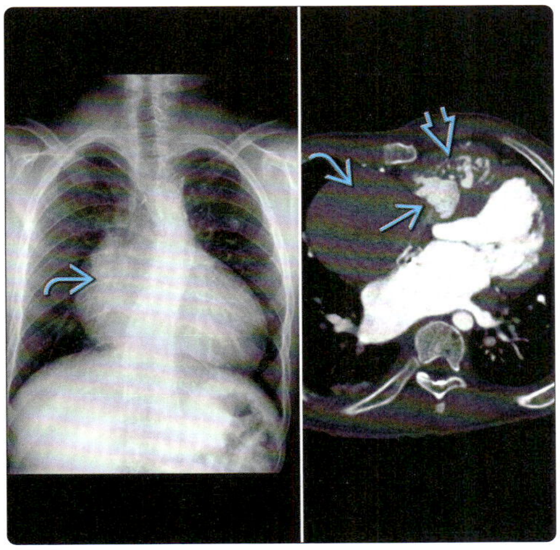

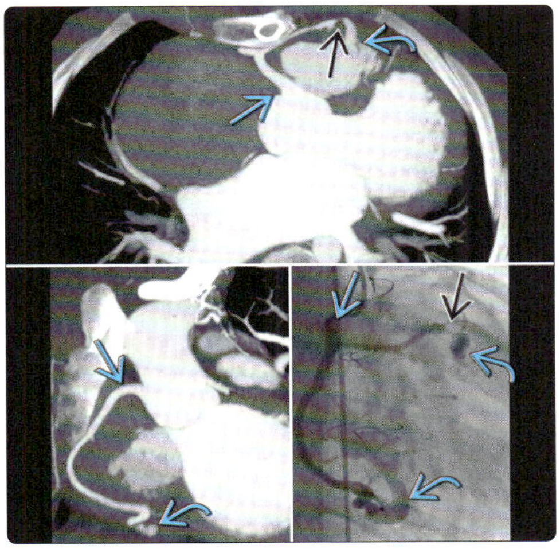

(Left) *PA CXR (left) and 4-chamber CT (right) in an patient with PA-IVS s/p Fontan show marked RA enlargement ➡ with paucity of pulmonary vasculature on CXR. The RV is small and hypertrophied ➡, as is the tricuspid valve (TV) ➡.* **(Right)** *CT (top and left) and angiogram (bottom right) show the RCA arising from the aorta ➡ with multiple RCA coronary-cameral fistulae (CCF) ➡. Multiple LAD CCF are also present (not shown). This and the stenosis adjacent to the CCF ➡ create an RV-dependent coronary circulation (RVDCC).*

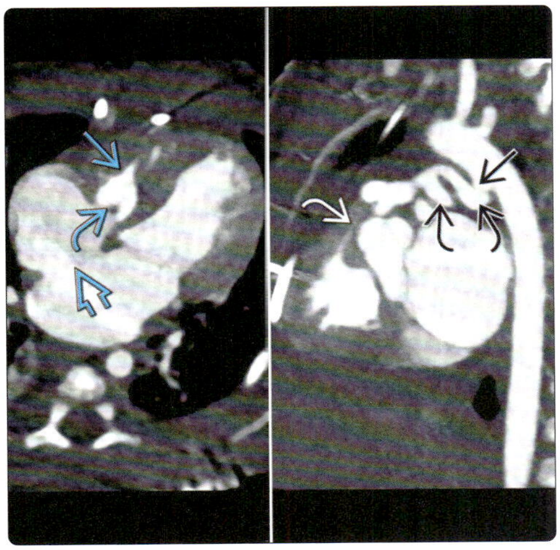

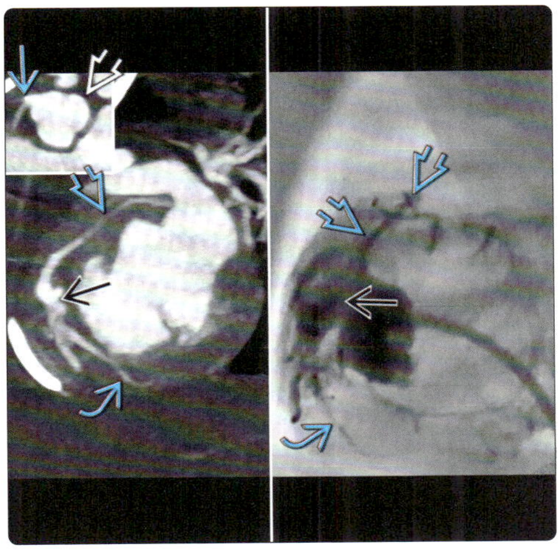

(Left) *Four-chamber image (left) in a newborn with PA-IVS shows a hypoplastic TV ➡, hypoplastic RV ➡, and a secundum atrial septal defect (ASD) ➡ but no VSD. RVOT image (right) shows agenesis of the RVOT ➡. The small PAs ➡ are supplied by a PDA ➡.* **(Right)** *CT (left) and angiography (right) images show the left main (LM) circulation ➡ arising from the RV chamber ➡. No LM originates from the left sinus of Valsalva ➡ (inset) creating a RVDCC. Although the RCA arises from the right sinus ➡ (inset), RCA CCF ➡ are seen.*

Hypoplastic Left Heart Syndrome

KEY FACTS

TERMINOLOGY

- Hypoplasia/atresia of ascending aorta, aortic valve, left ventricle (LV), and mitral valve

IMAGING

- Radiography
  - Cardiomegaly
  - Pulmonary venous congestion with interstitial fluid
- CT or MR
  - Atresia or hypoplasia of ascending aorta and LV
  - Severe obstruction of flow to systemic circulation (ductus dependent)
  - Retrograde flow in hypoplastic aortic arch and ascending aorta for cranial and coronary perfusion
  - Volume overload in pulmonary circulation
  - Left-to-right shunting through patent foramen ovale
  - Identification of postoperative complications and sequelae
- Echocardiogram or MR
  - Prenatal diagnosis commonly made

TOP DIFFERENTIAL DIAGNOSES

- Critical aortic stenosis, infantile coarctation, interrupted aortic arch

PATHOLOGY

- Due to abnormal partitioning of primitive conotruncus into left and right ventricular outflow tracts → hypoplasia/atresia of aortic valve

CLINICAL ISSUES

- Cyanosis (flow admixture in right heart)
- Cardiogenic shock after closure of patent ductus arteriosus
- Congestive heart failure (volume overload in pulmonary circulation)
- Treatment: Prostaglandin E1 to keep patent ductus arteriosus open, palliative surgical repair, cardiac transplantation

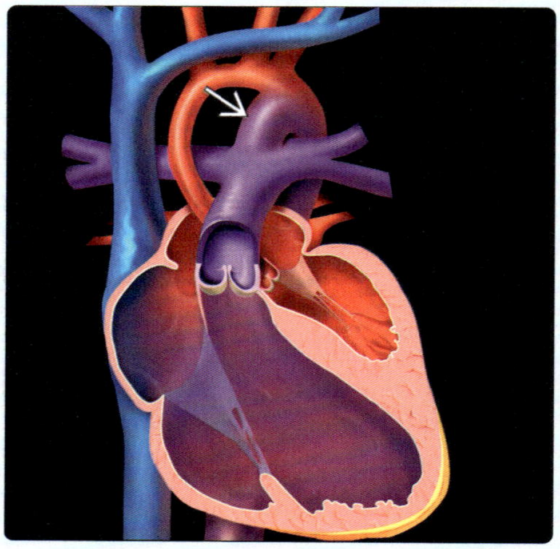

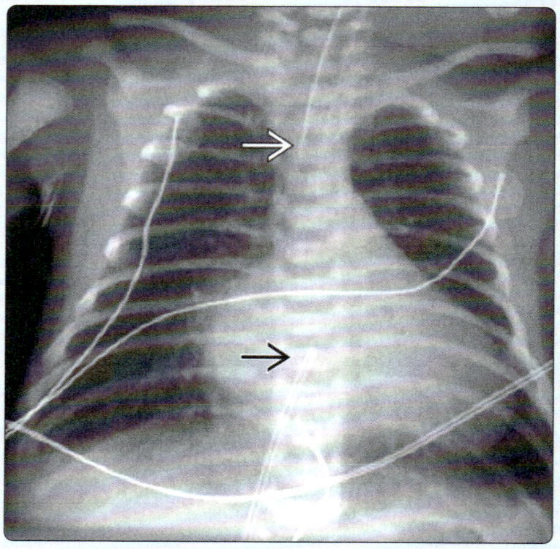

(Left) *Graphic of hypoplastic left heart syndrome (HLHS) shows hypoplasia of the left atrium, left ventricle, aortic valve, and ascending aorta. The systemic flow depends on the patency of the ductus arteriosus* ➔. **(Right)** *AP radiograph in a patient with HLHS during the 1st day of life shows cardiomegaly, vascular congestion, and hyperinflation. Endotracheal tube* ➔ *projects over the thoracic trachea, and the umbilical venous catheter* ➔ *extends into the right atrium.*

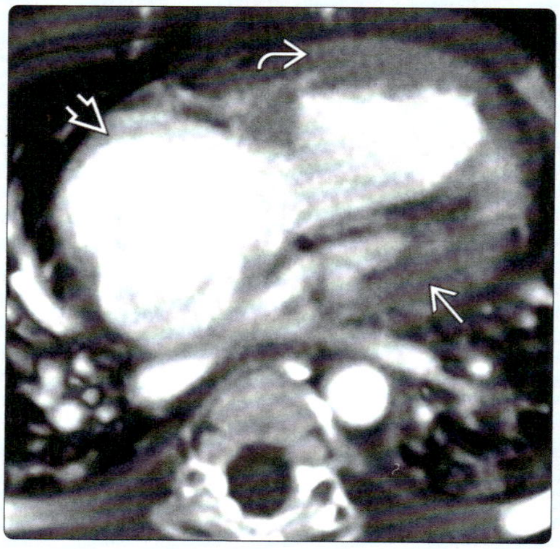

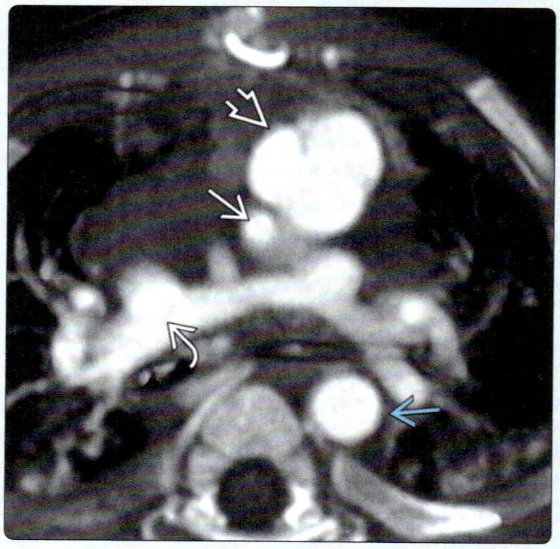

(Left) *Axial CTA in a patient with left HLHS shows hypoplasia of the left ventricle* ➔ *with marked dilatation of the right atrium* ➔ *and ventricle* ➔. **(Right)** *Axial CTA in the same patient shows hypoplastic ascending aorta* ➔*, a large pulmonary artery (PA)* ➔ *serving as cardiac output conduit, and a right-sided cavopulmonary shunt (Glenn)* ➔. *Note the descending aorta* ➔ *is relatively larger than the hypoplastic ascending aorta.*

TERMINOLOGY

Abbreviations

- Hypoplastic left heart syndrome (HLHS)

Synonyms

- Aortic atresia
- Mitral atresia

Definitions

- Hypoplasia/atresia of ascending aorta, aortic valve, left ventricle (LV), and mitral valve
  - Secondary findings: Patent ductus arteriosus (PDA), juxtaductal coarctation
- Most severe congenital heart lesion presenting in neonatal period with congestive heart failure, cardiogenic shock, and cyanosis
- Category: Cyanotic, cardiomegaly, increased pulmonary vascularity
- Hemodynamics
  - Severe obstruction of flow to systemic circulation (ductus dependent)
  - Retrograde flow in hypoplastic aortic arch and ascending aorta for cranial and coronary perfusion
  - Volume overload in pulmonary circulation
  - Left-to-right shunting through patent foramen ovale (PFO)
  - Flow admixture in right atrium → severe cyanosis

IMAGING

General Features

- Best diagnostic clue
  - Hypoplasia of ascending aorta and LV

Radiographic Findings

- Radiography
  - Cardiomegaly
    - Size and shape may vary, depending on degree of LV/aortic hypoplasia, compensatory right heart changes, degree of thymic atrophy
    - Cardiac silhouette can also be small or normal in size
  - Pulmonary venous congestion with interstitial edema, due to restrictive interatrial communication elevating left atrium (LA) pressure
    - Can also be normal, pulmonary arterial hypertension [nonrestrictive atrial septal defect (ASD)], or mixed pattern
  - Narrow mediastinum due to thymic atrophy

CT Findings

- CTA
  - Hypoplastic LV
    - Size of LV is variable (slit-like to nearly normal size)
  - Hypoplasia/atresia of aortic valve
  - Hypoplasia/atresia of mitral valve
  - Hypoplastic ascending aorta/arch
  - Dilated right atrium, right ventricle, pulmonary artery (PA)
  - PDA, PFO, ASD

MR Findings

- SSFP cine
  - Morphology of hypoplastic left heart
  - Ventricular volume measurements in marginally hypoplastic left heart to determine feasibility of biventricular repair
  - Functional assessment of univentricular heart to determine suitability for Fontan operation
- Phase-contrast MR
  - Measurement of flow through aortic isthmus, PDA, and foramen ovale
  - Can predict response to intraoperative test closure of ASD and PDA to determine feasibility of biventricular repair
- MRA
  - Evaluation of vascular anatomy

Echocardiographic Findings

- Echocardiogram
  - HLHS increasingly diagnosed prenatally
    - Retrograde flow in diminutive ascending aorta
    - LV growth arrest becomes manifest between 18-22 weeks of gestation
  - Postnatal diagnosis with echo sufficient for treatment planning
    - Diminutive ascending aorta < 5 mm
    - Small, thick-walled LV
    - Mitral valve size is expressed as Z-score: Important parameter to decide whether biventricular repair is possible in marginally hypoplastic LVs
    - Dilatation of right-sided chambers and PA
    - Size and location of ductus arteriosus
    - Patency of foramen ovale or presence of ASD
    - Abnormal ventricular wall motion (ischemic damage, fibroelastosis)
- Color Doppler
  - Hemodynamics of aortic root
  - Left-to-right shunt through foramen ovale
  - Tricuspid regurgitation

Angiographic Findings

- Conventional angiography
  - Cardiac catheterization with angiography
    - Can be done via umbilical artery catheter
    - Retrograde flow in hypoplastic ascending aorta, filling of PAs via ductus arteriosus

Imaging Recommendations

- Primary diagnosis is made with echocardiography in majority of cases
- CT/MR can be performed if echocardiography is suboptimal

DIFFERENTIAL DIAGNOSIS

Critical Aortic Stenosis, Infantile Coarctation, Interrupted Aortic Arch

- Pressure overload of normally developed LV

Cranial (Vein of Galen) or Hepatic Arteriovenous Malformation

- Structurally normal heart, volume overload of all chambers

Cardiomyopathy, Endocardial Fibroelastosis

- Globally enlarged, structurally normal heart; myocardial dysfunction

Anomalous Left Coronary Artery From Pulmonary Artery

- Left coronary originates from PA, LV infarction

Severe Arrhythmias: Paroxysmal Supraventricular Tachycardia

- Characteristic electrocardiogram

PATHOLOGY

General Features

- Genetics
  - No clear genetic defect in most
  - Extracardiac malformations uncommon
- Underdevelopment of left-sided cardiac structures
  - Hypoplasia or atresia of aortic and mitral valves
  - Hypoplasia of LV and ascending aorta
- Compatible with normal fetal hemodynamics → no fetal compromise
- Embryology
  - Abnormal partitioning of primitive conotruncus into left and right ventricular outflow tracts → hypoplasia/atresia of aortic valve
  - Diminished prenatal antegrade flow through aorta → underdevelopment of LV and ascending aorta
- Pathophysiology
  - Severe obstruction to outflow of diminutive LV
  - Pulmonary venous flow shunts through foramen ovale into right atrium
  - Dilated right-sided cardiac chambers and PA
  - Systemic perfusion via PDA

Gross Pathologic & Surgical Features

- Severe hypoplasia of left-sided cardiac chambers and ascending aorta
- Large main PA, ductus arteriosus
- Localized aortic coarctation (80%)
- Endocardial fibroelastosis in small, thick-walled LV

CLINICAL ISSUES

Presentation

- Most common signs/symptoms
  - No circulatory symptoms immediately at birth but rapid deterioration
    - Cyanosis (flow admixture in right heart)
    - Congestive heart failure (volume overload in pulmonary circulation)
    - Hypoxia → pulmonary hypertension, persistent fetal circulation
    - Cardiogenic shock after closure of PDA
- Other signs/symptoms
  - Poor systemic perfusion, metabolic acidosis
    - Acute tubular necrosis, renal failure
    - Necrotizing enterocolitis

Demographics

- Epidemiology
  - 1-3 per 10,000 live births; M:F = 2:1
  - 4th most common congenital heart lesion presenting at < 1 year of age (7-9%)

Natural History & Prognosis

- Death within days/weeks when untreated
- Poor prognosis without treatment; has improved substantially in recent years
  - However, even with surgery, < 33-40% survive to 15 years of age without transplant
- Determined by complications, residua and sequelae of staged Norwood repair and Fontan operation (right ventricular dysfunction, venous hypertension)
- Significant tricuspid regurgitation after surgical palliation correlates with poor outcome

Treatment

- Medical: Prostaglandin E1 to keep PDA open
- Prenatal: US-guided balloon dilatation of aortic valve in mid-/late fetal period is now possible
  - Change in fetal hemodynamics may enhance prenatal growth of left-sided cardiac structures
- Rashkind balloon atrial septostomy (in case of flow restriction across foramen ovale)
- Palliative repair
  - Stage I (3 weeks)
    - Goal: Create unobstructed systemic flow and provide pulmonary blood flow
    - Norwood: Atrial septectomy, construction of aorta from PA, creation of pulmonary flow (modified Blalock-Taussig or Sano shunt)
      - Damus-Kaye-Stansel anastomosis: Variation of Norwood with side-to-side anastomosis between PA and hypoplastic ascending aorta
    - Modified Blalock-Taussig: Shunt between subclavian artery and PA
    - Sano shunt: Right ventricle to PA conduit
  - Stage II: Superior cavopulmonary connection (4-6 months)
    - Goal: Decreased right ventricular volume overload by redirecting systemic venous return from upper body to PA directly
    - Bidirectional Glenn: Superior vena cava (SVC) to right PA anastomosis
    - Hemi-Fontan: Homograft between SVC and right PA
  - Stage III: Total cavopulmonary connection (1.5-2 years)
    - Goal: Redirection of total systemic venous return to lungs
    - Fontan: Fenestrated venous conduit through right atrium of inferior caval flow to right PA
- Marginally hypoplastic LV: Biventricular repair may be feasible
  - LV volume is commonly underestimated with echocardiography
  - Functional MR (SSPE cine: Ventricular volumes and function; PC-MRA: Flow volumes) is more accurate
- In some centers: Cardiac transplantation

SELECTED REFERENCES

1. Cheasty E et al: The use of cardiovascular CT for the follow up of paediatric hypoplastic left heart syndrome. J Cardiovasc Comput Tomogr. 14(5):e18-19, 2018
2. Roeleveld PP et al: Hypoplastic left heart syndrome: from fetus to fontan. Cardiol Young. 28(11):1275-88, 2018
3. Bardo DM et al: Hypoplastic left heart syndrome. Radiographics. 21(3):705-17, 2001

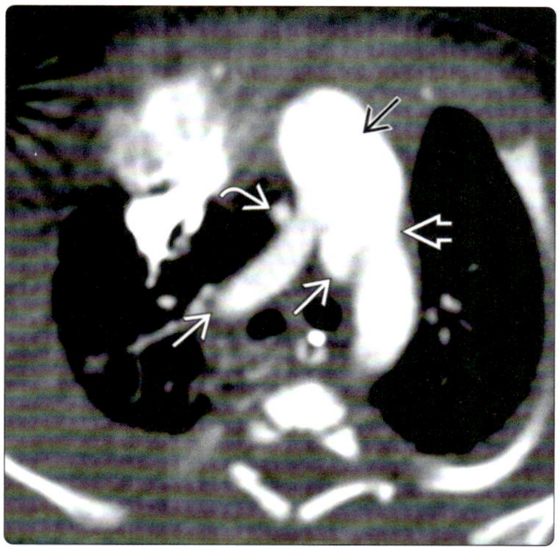

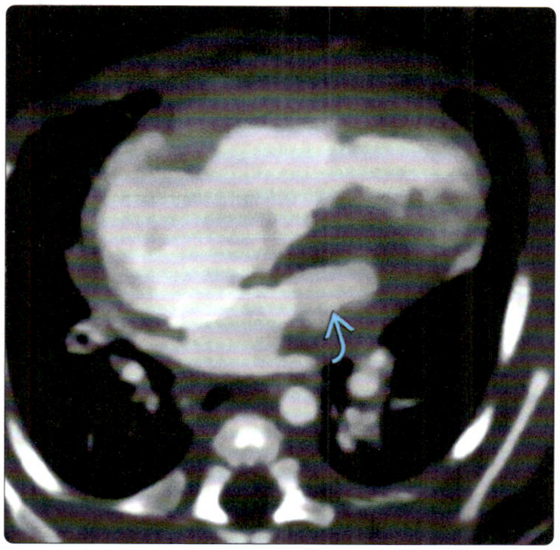

(Left) *Axial CTA shows hypoplastic ascending aorta. The large main PA connects via the ductus arteriosus to the descending aorta. Notice the take-off of both branch PAs from the main PA.* **(Right)** *Four-chamber CECT in a 2-month-old baby with HLHS shows a large right ventricle and diminutive left ventricle. A large iatrogenic atrial septal defect (ASD) is present.*

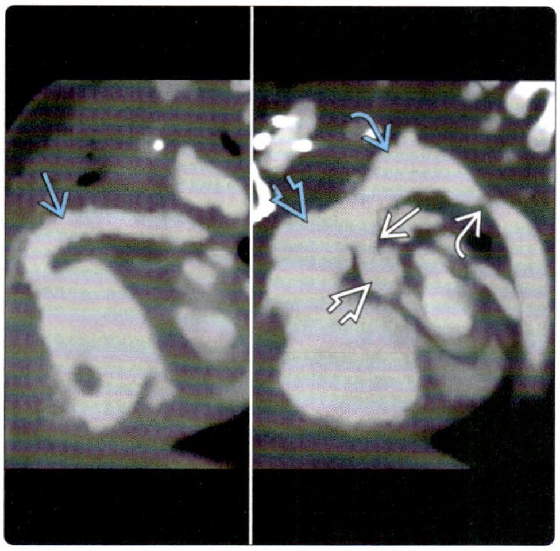

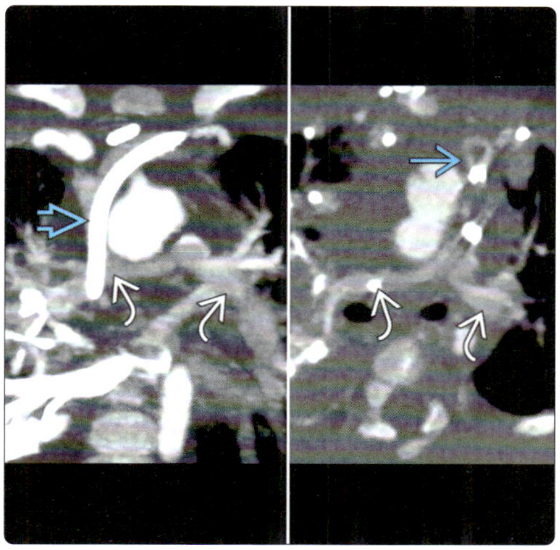

(Left) *Images show a Sano shunt connecting the right ventricle to the PAs (left) in the same patient. A Norwood procedure (right) has been performed connecting the main PA to the aorta. Notice the aortic coarctation. The hypoplastic aortic root and ascending aorta can be seen.* **(Right)** *At 6 months of age, a bidirectional Glenn shunt has been placed connecting the superior vena cava to the PAs. The Sano has been ligated. (Courtesy S. Kligerman, MD.)*

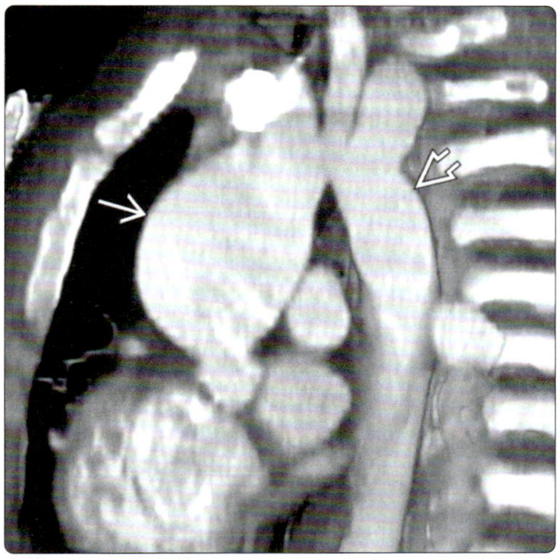

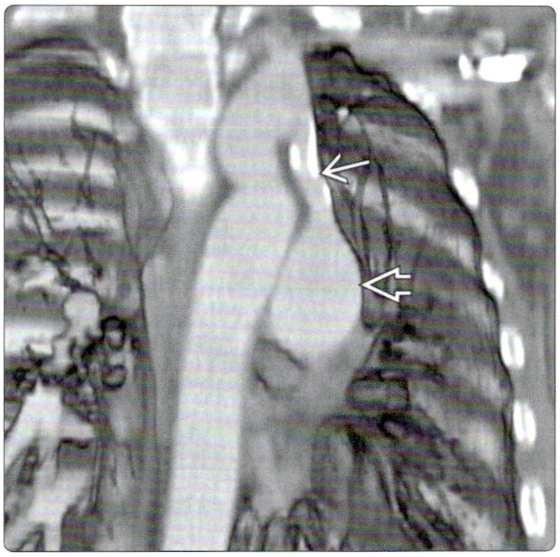

(Left) *Sagittal oblique VR CTA shows a markedly dilated PA, which provides flow to the systemic circulation status post Norwood surgery.* **(Right)** *Coronal oblique VR CTA shows a modified Blalock-Taussig (BT) shunt perfusing the pulmonary arterial circulation in the same patient. In the Norwood surgery, the main PA is used to widen the ascending aorta. Flow to the pulmonary arterial circulation must be surgically created either with a modified BT shunt or Sano shunt.*

KEY FACTS

TERMINOLOGY

- Absent tricuspid valve with hypoplastic right ventricle (RV) and atrial septal defect (ASD)
- Surgical correction with Fontan (3-stage surgical correction)

IMAGING

- ASD in all cases, ventricular septal defect (VSD) in most cases; small/hypoplastic RV present in all cases
- Associated hypoplastic in RV, ASD, and most cases of VSD; if VSD not present, look for patent ductus arteriosus (PDA)
- Lack of normal tricuspid valve with muscular or membranous obstruction of right atrium (RA) to RV (epicardial fat or muscular/membranous separation between RA and RV)
- Evaluate for associated lesions, such as pulmonary outflow obstruction, ventricular arterial discordance, and pulmonary artery hypoplasia
- MR most helpful in adults after corrective surgery to assess for complications

PATHOLOGY

- Surgical management is 3-staged procedure
  - Stage 1: Maintain adequate pulmonary flow
    - Pulmonary artery banding for increased pulmonary flow (i.e. large VSD, type Ic)
    - PDA stent or classic Blalock-Taussig (BT) or modified BT shunt for decreased pulmonary flow
  - Stage 2: Glenn and removal of shunt
  - Stage 3: Total cavopulmonary connection (Fontan completion)
- Type I (70-80%): Normal alignment of great vessels
- Type II (12-25%): D-transposition
- Type III (3-6%): Malalignment of great vessels other than D-transposition
- Type IV: Truncus arteriosus

CLINICAL ISSUES

- Initially, medical management to ensure pulmonary blood flow by maintaining PDA

(Left) AP radiograph in a newborn shows a right aortic arch (AA), decreased pulmonary vascularity with small central pulmonary artery (PA) branches, and a mildly enlarged right atrial (RA) contour. (Right) CT images show tricuspid atresia (TA), atrial and ventricular septal defects, and a hypoplastic right ventricle (RV). There is pulmonary atresia with the right and left PAs being supplied by major aorticopulmonary collateral arteries (MAPCAs). This would be classified as type Ia TA.

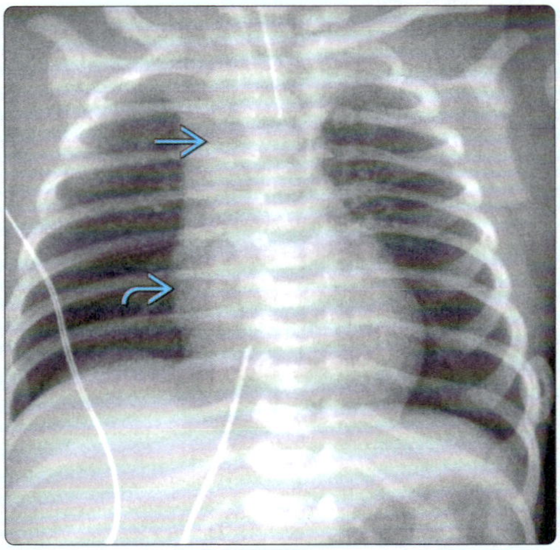

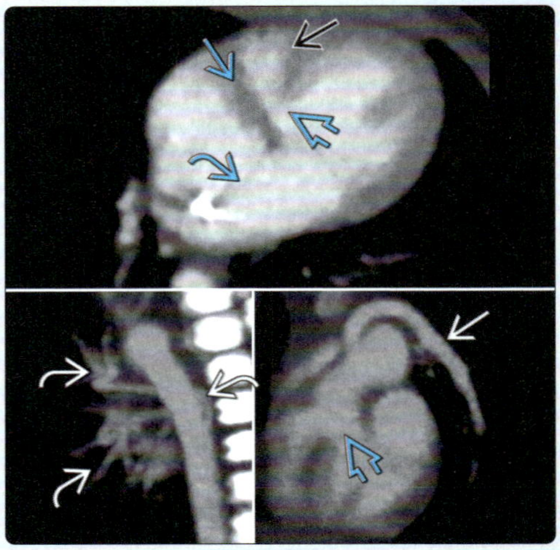

(Left) CTs in an 18-month-old show TA anatomy with medialized right coronary artery and right AA. Patient is status post unifocalization of MAPCAs to a pulmonary homograft patch, supplied by a modified Blalock-Taussig (BT) shunt. (Right) CTA at 3 years old (L) shows BT shunt ligation with placement of bidirectional Glenn supplying PA homograft and left larger than right unifocalized MAPCAs. At 4 years (R), extracardiac Fontan was placed with persistent asymmetry in PA size.

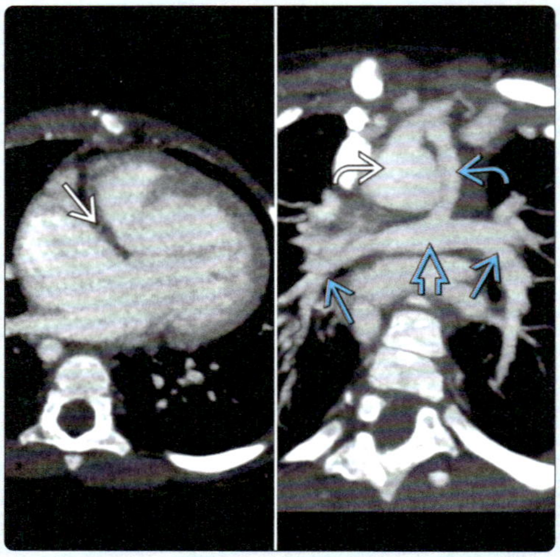

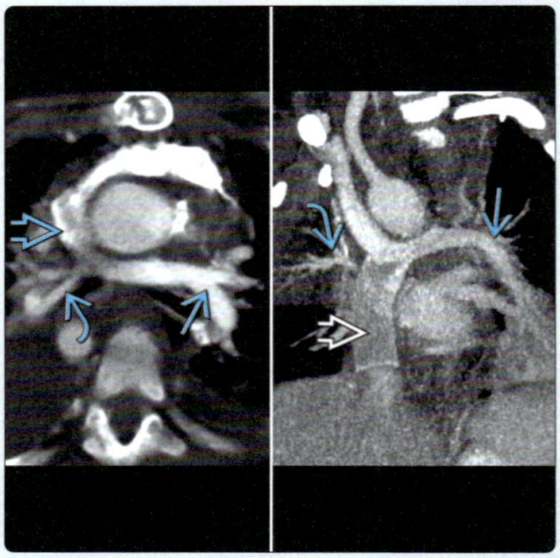

TERMINOLOGY

Definitions

- Congenital absence of tricuspid valve (TV) resulting in lack of communication between right atrium (RA) and right ventricle (RV)
- Associated atria septal defect (ASD) in 100% of cases results in cyanosis
- 3rd most common cyanotic heart defect

IMAGING

General Features

- Best diagnostic clue
  - Absence of TV with hypoplastic RV
  - ASD in all cases and, in most cases, ventricular septal defect (VSD)
  - Other associated cardiac defects in decreasing order of frequency include pulmonary outflow obstruction, ventricular arterial (V-A) discordance, pulmonary artery (PA) hypoplasia, aortic or subaortic stenosis, aortic coarctation, interrupted aortic arch, and coronary anomalies
- Location
  - Absent TV
- Morphology
  - Different morphologic types of tricuspid atresia
    - Muscular (80% of cases): Muscular floor of RA
    - Membranous (10% of cases): Membranous floor of RA
    - Valvular (5% of cases): Tiny, fused valve leaflets
    - Ebstein subtype: Downward/apical displacement and fusion of TV leaflets
  - Small/hypoplastic RV present in all cases
  - ASD present in all cases
  - VSD present in most cases (95%)
    - Trabecular muscular
  - Pulmonary outflow obstruction present in most cases (75%)
  - V-A discordance present in 28% of cases
  - PA hypoplasia present in 17% of cases
    - May be associated with major aorticopulmonary collateral arteries (MAPCAs)
  - Aortic or subaortic stenosis in 11% of cases
  - Aortic coarctation or interruption in 8% of cases
  - Coronary anomaly in 3% of cases

Radiographic Findings

- Absence of normal right heart border
- Pulmonary flow and heart size varies
  - Normal or decreased in absence of VSD or small restrictive VSD
  - Increased in presence of large VSD

CT Findings

- Absent normal TV with muscular or membranous obstruction of RA → RV flow
  - Associated hypoplastic in RV, ASD, and in most cases of VSD; if VSD absent, look for patent ductus arteriosus (PDA) (type Ia)
  - Evaluate for associated lesions, such as pulmonary outflow obstruction, V-A discordance, and PA hypoplasia
  - Evaluate for MAPCAs in pulmonary hypoplasia/atresia
- Most patients with tricuspid atresia have Fontan palliation
- CT is most helpful status post corrective surgery to assess anatomy and for complications
  - Ventricular dysfunction, Glenn obstruction, Fontan thrombosis or stenosis, venovenous collaterals
- Delayed imaging is preferred for evaluation of Fontan patency

MR Findings

- Lack of normal TV with muscular or membranous obstruction of RA to RV
  - Associated hypoplastic in RV, ASD, and most cases of VSD; if VSD not present, look for PDA
  - Evaluate for associated lesions
- Most patients with tricuspid atresia have Fontan palliation
- MR most helpful after corrective surgery to assess for complications

Ultrasonographic Findings

- Imaging modality of choice
- Fetal ultrasound shows absent TV, RV hypoplasia, ASD, and most cases of VSD
  - Evaluate presence and size of VSD
  - Evaluate relationship of great arteries
  - Evaluate for reverse flow in PDA (left-to-right)
    - Inadequate pulmonary flow
      - Postnatal prostaglandin therapy to maintain ductal patency
- Postnatal ultrasound shows absent TV, RV hypoplasia, ASD, and most cases of VSD
  - Evaluate presence and size of VSD, ASD, and degree of shunting
  - Evaluate pulmonary outflow obstruction
  - Evaluate relationship of great arteries

Imaging Recommendations

- Best imaging tool
  - Fetal and postnatal echocardiography is best imaging tool
- Protocol advice
  - CT with delayed imaging allows for evaluation of Fontan patency and pulmonary circulation

DIFFERENTIAL DIAGNOSIS

Tetralogy of Fallot

- Most common cyanotic congenital heart disease
  - VSD, overriding aorta, RV hypertrophy, and RV outflow tract obstruction
  - Pulmonary atresia can occur
- TV is usually normal

Tricuspid Stenosis

- Narrowing of opening of TV
- Most common cause is rheumatic fever

Pulmonary Valve Atresia

- Lack of normal pulmonary valve development
  - Intact ventricular septum (PDA dependent)
    - Small, hypertrophied RV
    - Coronary sinusoids often present
    - TV hypoplastic but usually present
  - With VSD

  - Usually severe form of tetralogy of Fallot
  - Can have TV and pulmonary atresia

PATHOLOGY

General Features

- Lack of normal TV development with RV hypoplasia, ASD, and most cases of VSD

Staging, Grading, & Classification

- Unified classification of tricuspid atresia
  - Type I: Normal anatomy of great arteries (70-80%)
  - Type II: D-transposition (12-25%)
  - Type III: Malposition of great arteries other than transposition (3-6%)
    - L-transposition, double-outlet RV or left ventricle, etc.
  - Type IV: Persistent truncus arteriosus
    - Very rare and may be classified as type III
  - Each type then divided into subgroups based on PAs
    - Subgroup a: Pulmonary atresia
    - Subgroup b: Pulmonary stenosis or hypoplasia
    - Subgroup c: Normal PAs

Gross Pathologic & Surgical Features

- Passage of blood from RA into left atrium through atrial septal communication
  - Cyanosis is always present
  - In cases in which PDA is only source of blood to PAs (ductal dependent)
    - Prostaglandin E1 is needed to main patency of ductus arteriosus
- Surgical management is 3-staged procedure
  - Stage 1: Maintain adequate pulmonary flow
    - PA banding for increased pulmonary flow
    - PDA stent or classic Blalock-Taussig (BT) or modified BT shunt for decreased pulmonary flow
  - Stage 2: Glenn and removal of shunt
  - Stage 3: Total cavopulmonary connection (Fontan completion)

CLINICAL ISSUES

Presentation

- Most common signs/symptoms
  - Cyanosis always present at birth
  - In absence of restricted pulmonary flow, symptoms of heart failure are seen 2-3 weeks after birth
  - In patients with restrictive atrial communication, central venous congestion can be detected
  - Decreased femoral pulses in setting of associated aortic coarctation
- Other signs/symptoms
  - In absence of surgical correction, prognosis is very poor

Demographics

- No sex predilection
- 0.5-1.2 per 10,000 live births

Treatment

- Care at tertiary medical center with experience in managing complex congenital heart disease
- Initially, medical management to ensure pulmonary blood flow and hemodynamic stability
  - Maintain patency of PDA for pulmonary flow, if needed
- Staged single ventricle palliative surgical repair
  - Neonatal period: Maintain adequate pulmonary flow
    - If decreased pulmonary flow (types Ia and Ib): PDA stent or classic or modified BT shunt
    - If increased pulmonary flow (type Ic): PA banding
  - In setting of associated transposition of great arteries
    - If associated subaortic obstruction with restrictive VSD: Enlargement of VSD or anastomosis between main PA and ascending aorta (Damus-Kaye-Stansel)
    - If aortic coarctation: Repair of coarctation
    - Nonrestrictive VSD: Pulmonary banding
  - 3-6 months of age: Bidirectional Glenn and removal of shunt (i.e., BT, modified BT)
  - 2-5 years of age: Fontan procedure (total cavopulmonary connection)
    - Classic: Direct RA to PA connection
    - Lateral tunnel
    - Extracardiac conduit ± fenestration between conduit and RA allows right-to-left shunt (helps systemic ventricular preload)
  - Long-term follow-up includes monitoring cardiac function, exercise tolerance, endocarditis prophylaxis, and routine vaccinations

DIAGNOSTIC CHECKLIST

Image Interpretation Pearls

- Absent TV with epicardial fat or muscular/membranous separation between RA and RV
- Hypoplastic RV + ASD
- Most of time, VSD
- Evaluate postsurgical heart after Fontan palliation
  - Evaluate surgical anatomy
  - Evaluate single ventricle chamber size and function
  - Evaluate patency of Glenn and Fontan
  - Evaluate for venovenous collaterals
- In patients with cyanosis after Fontan (oxygen saturation < 90% at rest) common, causes to evaluate include: Venovenous connections, Fontan fenestration, pulmonary arteriovenous malformations, Fontan circuit obstruction, and other unexpected intracardiac shunts

SELECTED REFERENCES

1. Writing Group et al: ACC/AHA/ASE/HRS/ISACHD/SCAI/SCCT/SCMR/SOPE 2020 appropriate use criteria for multimodality imaging during the follow-up care of patients with congenital heart disease: a report of the American College of Cardiology Solution Set Oversight Committee and Appropriate Use Criteria Task Force, American Heart Association, American Society of Echocardiography, Heart Rhythm Society, International Society for Adult Congenital Heart Disease, Society for Cardiovascular Angiography and Interventions, Society of Cardiovascular Computed Tomography, Society for Cardiovascular Magnetic Resonance, and Society of Pediatric Echocardiography. J Am Soc Echocardiogr. 33(10):e1-48, 2020
2. Stout KK et al: 2018 AHA/ACC guideline for the management of adults with congenital heart disease: a report of the American College of Cardiology/American Heart Association Task Force on clinical practice guidelines. J Am Coll Cardiol. 73(12):e81-192, 2018

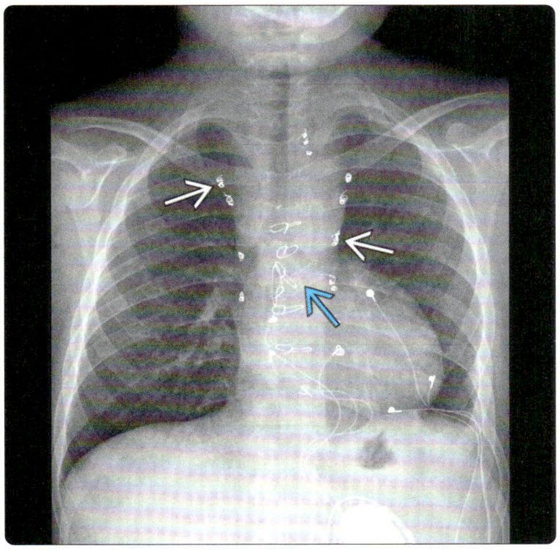

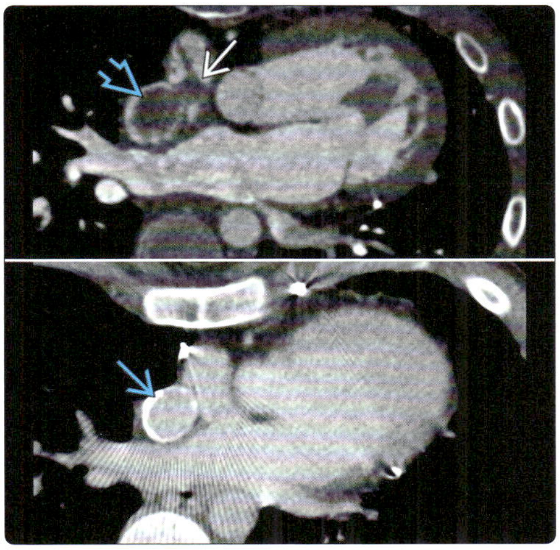

(Left) *PA chest x-ray in a patient with history of TA status post Fontan conduit shows a left PA stent from repair of PA branch stenosis and mediastinal coils from embolization of mediastinal venovenous collaterals.* **(Right)** *Arterial-phase CT images (top) show a fenestrated extracardiac Fontan in a patient with TA. Notice unopacified blood entering the RA due to fenestration. Delayed phase (bottom) allows evaluation of the extracardiac conduit, which is free of thrombus.*

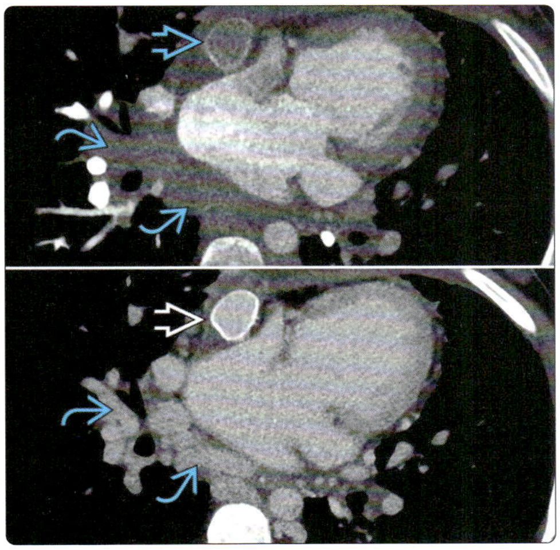

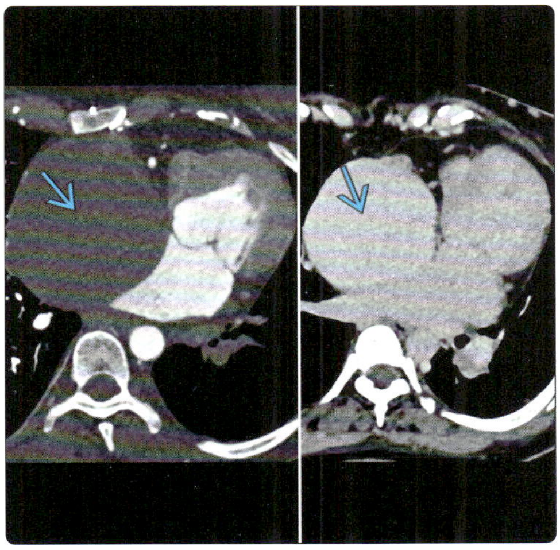

(Left) *Arterial CT (top) shows TA and an unopacified extracardiac Fontan, which fills with contrast on delayed phase (bottom). Abnormal mediastinal and hilar soft tissue, which looks like lymphadenopathy on arterial phase, is due to large venovenous collaterals that can lead to hypoxia.* **(Right)** *Axial CT during arterial (L) and delayed (R) phases in a patient with TA post Fontan shows RA dilation. The RA is unopacified during arterial phase and thus difficult to assess. Delayed-phase imaging shows absence of thrombus.*

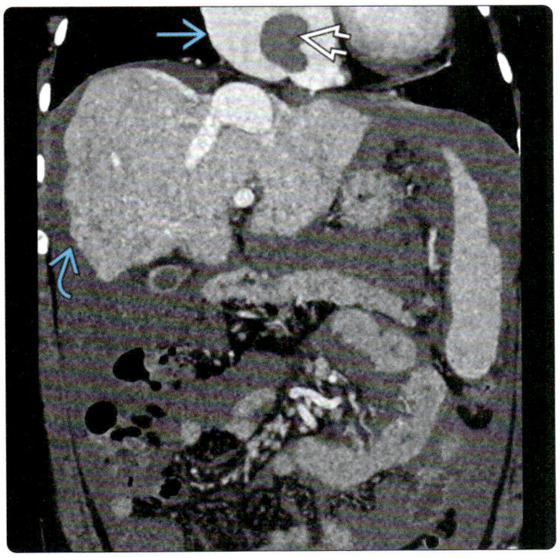

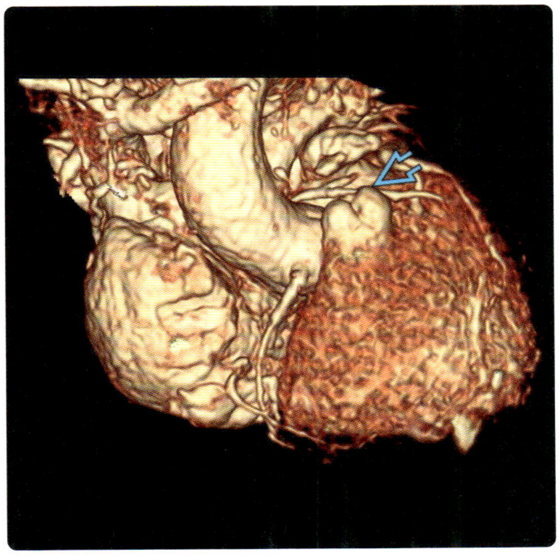

(Left) *Coronal CT during delayed phase in a patient with a classic Fontan surgical correction shows a dilated RA with intracavitary thrombus formation. Also notice cirrhotic liver morphology and ascites.* **(Right)** *Volume-rendered oblique MR angiogram in a patient with TA shows changes resulting from prior PA banding.*

Glenn and Fontan Shunts

KEY FACTS

TERMINOLOGY

- Fontan procedure is surgical strategy to repair certain types of congenital heart disease
  - Diversion of systemic venous return to lungs without going through heart
  - Allows single functional ventricle to supply high resistance systemic circulation
    - Classic Fontan: Right atrium to pulmonary artery (PA) ± direct anastomosis
    - Lateral tunnel ± fenestration
    - Extracardiac conduit ± fenestration
- Glenn shunt
  - Unidirectional = superior vena cava (SVC) to right PA anastomosis (side-to-end) with unilateral lung perfusion (ligation of distal SVC with anastomosis to divided right PA)
  - Bidirectional (a.k.a. modified Glenn or hemi-Fontan) = SVC to undivided right PA anastomosis (end-to-side) with bilateral lung perfusion

IMAGING

- Connection of systemic venous return to PA
- SVC to right PA (unidirectional vs. bidirectional)
- IVC to right PA

TOP DIFFERENTIAL DIAGNOSES

- Hypoplastic left heart
- Tricuspid atresia

CLINICAL ISSUES

- Most common signs/symptoms
  - Cyanosis
  - Arrhythmias
  - Heart failure
  - Atrioventricular valve dysfunction
  - Thrombosis

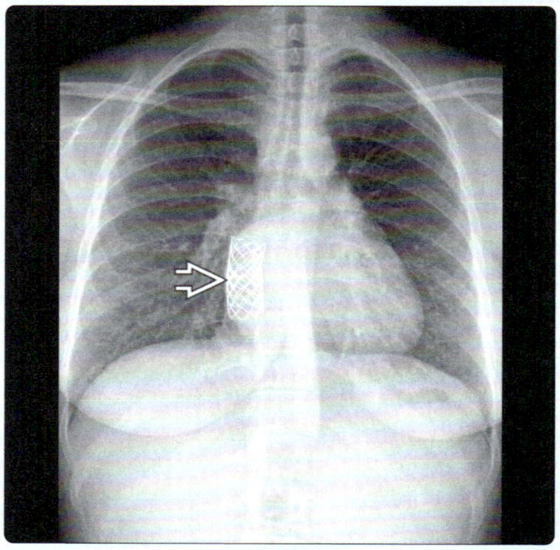
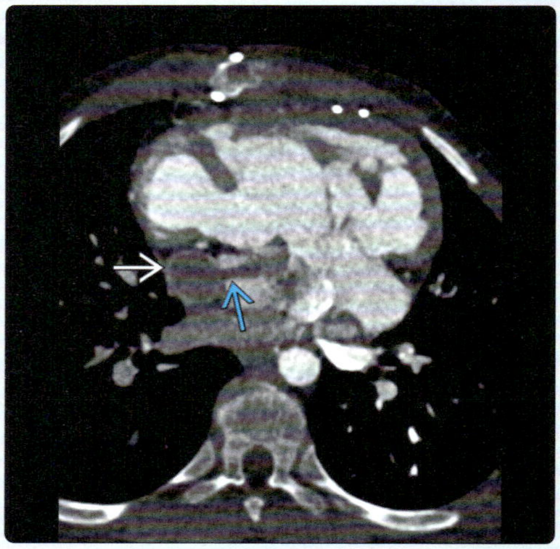

(Left) *Frontal radiograph of the chest shows surgical changes of Fontan with stented extracardiac conduit* ➡. **(Right)** *Axial CT angiogram in a patient with tricuspid atresia and surgical changes with a fenestrated extracardiac Fontan conduit* ➡ *is shown. Note the unopacified blood jet into the single atrium due to Fontan fenestration* ➡.

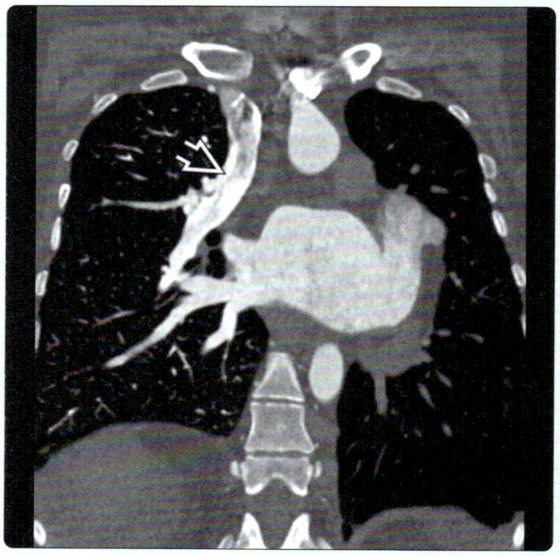
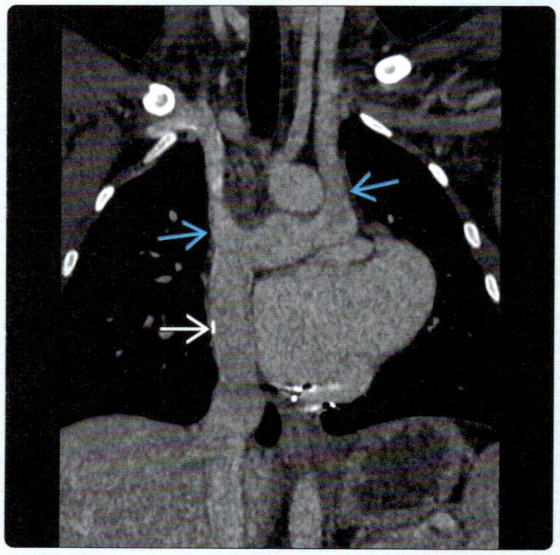

(Left) *Coronal CT angiogram shows unidirectional Glenn* ➡ *[superior vena cava (SVC) to divided right pulmonary artery (PA) anastomosis].* **(Right)** *Coronal delayed CT angiogram in a patient with single ventricle and persistent left SVC shows surgical changes of extracardiac Fontan conduit* ➡ *and bilateral cavopulmonary anastomosis* ➡.

TERMINOLOGY

Synonyms

- Cavopulmonary connection (superior and inferior)
  - Hemi-Fontan shunt (bidirectional Glenn or modified Glenn)
  - Fontan procedure (total cavopulmonary connection)

Definitions

- Fontan procedure is surgical strategy to repair certain types of congenital heart disease
  - Done in combination with other procedures depending on cardiac anomaly
  - Common indications include
    - Hypoplastic left heart syndrome
    - Tricuspid atresia
    - Pulmonary atresia with intact ventricular septum
    - Double-inlet left ventricle
    - Unbalanced atrioventricular canal defects
- Fontan procedure
  - Diversion of systemic venous return to lungs without going through heart
  - Allows single functional ventricle to supply high-resistance systemic circulation
- Palliative surgeries prior to Fontan completion (common since 1990s)
  - Systemic to pulmonary shunts
    - Blalock-Taussig (BT) shunt
    - Potts shunt
    - Waterston shunt
  - Atrial septectomy or septostomy
  - Norwood procedure (in setting of hypoplastic left heart)
    - Constructing neoaorta
    - Systemic to pulmonary artery (PA) shunt (BT shunt or Sano shunt)
    - Atrial septal resection
- Glenn shunt
  - Unidirectional = superior vena cava (SVC) to right PA anastomosis (side-to-end) with unilateral lung perfusion (ligation of distal SVC with anastomosis to divided right PA)
  - Bidirectional (a.k.a. modified Glenn or hemi-Fontan) = SVC to undivided right PA anastomosis (end-to-side) with bilateral lung perfusion
- Fontan completion
  - Classic Fontan (aortopulmonary Fontan): Right atrium (RA) to PA direct anastomosis
  - Inferior vena cava (IVC) to right PA anastomosis (end-to-side) ± fenestration
    - Lateral tunnel: IVC is connected to PA via lateral tunnel within RA comprised of posterior RA wall and prosthetic patch
    - Extracardiac conduit: Graft placed entirely outside RA, connecting transection IVC and PA; RA is bypassed
  - Kawashima procedure: Used in setting of single ventricle with interrupted IVC with azygous continuation; blood from SVC and azygos vein are diverted into PA

IMAGING

General Features

- Best diagnostic clue
  - Connection of systemic venous return to PA
    - SVC to right PA (unidirectional vs. bidirectional)
    - IVC to right PA
      - Lateral tunnel conduit (intraatrial)
      - Extracardiac conduit (intrapericardial)
      - ± fenestration between conduit and RA allows right-to-left shunt (helps systemic ventricular preload)
    - "Classic" atriopulmonary connection (right aortic arch to main PA) is no longer used due to atrial dilation, arrhythmias, and thrombus formation
  - Single ventricle supplies systemic circulation
- Location
  - SVC to PA connection
  - IVC to PA connection

Radiographic Findings

- End-to-side SVC to right pulmonary connection
  - Unidirectional vs. bidirectional
- IVC to right PA connection ± fenestration
  - Intracardiac lateral tunnel
  - Extracardiac

CT Findings

- Evaluate postsurgical anatomy
  - Evaluate cavopulmonary connections (exclude thrombus or stenosis)
  - Single ventricle size and function
  - Valvular function
  - Evaluate for venovenous collaterals
  - Evaluate for associated pulmonary arteriovenous malformation (AVM)
- Delayed scans are preferred to opacify cardiac chambers and pulmonary circulation

MR Findings

- Evaluate postsurgical anatomy
  - Evaluate cavopulmonary connections (exclude thrombus or stenosis)
  - Single ventricle size and function
  - Valvular function and intracardiac shunting
  - Evaluate for venovenous collaterals

Ultrasonographic Findings

- Imaging modality of choice
- Fetal ultrasound to diagnose congenital anomalies
- Postnatal ultrasound to diagnose congenital anomalies and evaluate surgical correction and complications
  - Ventricular size and function
  - Patency of Fontan circulation
  - Thrombus formation
  - Valvular function
  - Intracardiac shunting

Imaging Recommendations

- Best imaging tool

- Echocardiography is 1st-line imaging of choice for evaluation of Fontan patency, ventricular and valvular function
- Cardiac MR with time-resolved MR angiography for evaluation of Fontan patency, ventricular volumes, and function and collateral formation
- Cardiac CT is good alternative when MR cannot be performed
- Protocol advice
  - Delayed imaging CT for evaluation of Fontan patency and pulmonary circulation

DIFFERENTIAL DIAGNOSIS

Hypoplastic Left Heart

- Underdevelopment of left heart structures
- Repaired with Norwood + Fontan procedures

PATHOLOGY

General Features

- Glenn (superior cavopulmonary connection)
  - End-to-side anastomosis of SVC to right PA
- Fontan (inferior cavopulmonary connection)

CLINICAL ISSUES

Presentation

- Most common signs/symptoms
  - Cyanosis
    - Common saturation after Fontan is 90-95%; when > 90%, cardiac catheterization is in search for
      - Unknown fenestration
      - Systemic venous collaterals
      - Fontan obstruction
      - Pulmonary AVM or other shunts
  - Arrhythmias
    - Supraventricular arrhythmias
      - Most common: Intraatrial reentry tachycardia, atrial flutter, and sinus node dysfunction
    - More common in atriopulmonary Fontan
    - Treatment options include ablation, pacemaker, antiarrhythmic, and anticoagulation
  - Heart failure
    - Medical therapy, biventricular pacing or transplant
  - Atrioventricular valve dysfunction
  - Thrombosis
    - High risk of systemic and pulmonary thromboembolic disease
      - Low flow in Fontan circulation
      - Alterations in clotting and fibrinolysis factors
      - Systemic thromboembolic events are more common in fenestrated Fontan
  - Bleeding
  - Venous insufficiency
  - Restrictive lung disease
  - Plastic bronchitis
    - Mucofibrinous bronchial casts due to intrapulmonary lymphatic overload and leakage
  - Protein-losing enteropathy
    - Secondary to chronic venous congestion, lymphatic overload, and poor perfusion of gastrointestinal mucosa
  - Liver disease
    - Due to passive hepatic congestion leading to cirrhosis
  - Others, including neurologic, renal, and psychiatric

Treatment

- Medical management and lifelong follow-up by cardiologist
- Staged single ventricle palliative surgical repair in neonatal period depending on congenital defect; can include
  - ± reconstructing aorta
  - ± allow adequate pulmonary venous return via atrial septectomy
  - BT and modified BT (mBT) or Sano shunt vs. pulmonary banding to maintain adequate pulmonary flow
- 3-6 months of age: Bidirectional Glenn and removal of shunt (i.e., BT, mBT)
- 2-5 years of age: Fontan procedure (total cavopulmonary connection)
- Catheter-based or surgical reintervention for complications, such as
  - Arrhythmias, Fontan obstruction (dilation or stenting), venovenous collaterals closure, fenestration (closure or creation), pulmonary AVM closure, residual atrial septal defect closure, and pulmonary venous compression

DIAGNOSTIC CHECKLIST

Consider

- Patency of Fontan and upper cavopulmonary connection
- Presence or absence of fenestration
- Venovenous collaterals
- Ventricular volumes and function
- Atrioventricular valve function

Reporting Tips

- Surgical anatomy and patency of surgical connections (document presence or absence of Fontan fenestration)
- Ventricular volumes and function
- Valvular function
- Presence or absence of venovenous collaterals and other unexpected intracardiac or extracardiac shunts

SELECTED REFERENCES

1. Writing Group et al: ACC/AHA/ASE/HRS/ISACHD/SCAI/SCCT/SCMR/SOPE 2020 appropriate use criteria for multimodality imaging during the follow-up care of patients with congenital heart disease: a report of the American College of Cardiology Solution Set Oversight Committee and Appropriate Use Criteria Task Force, American Heart Association, American Society of Echocardiography, Heart Rhythm Society, International Society for Adult Congenital Heart Disease, Society for Cardiovascular Angiography and Interventions, Society of Cardiovascular Computed Tomography, Society for Cardiovascular Magnetic Resonance, and Society of Pediatric Echocardiography. J Am Soc Echocardiogr. 33(10):e1-48, 2020
2. Stout KK et al: 2018 AHA/ACC guideline for the management of adults with congenital heart disease: a report of the American College of Cardiology/American Heart Association Task Force on Clinical Practice Guidelines. J Am Coll Cardiol. 73(12):e81-192, 2018
3. Ghadimi Mahani M et al: CT for assessment of thrombosis and pulmonary embolism in multiple stages of single-ventricle palliation: challenges and suggested protocols. Radiographics. 36(5):1273-84, 2016

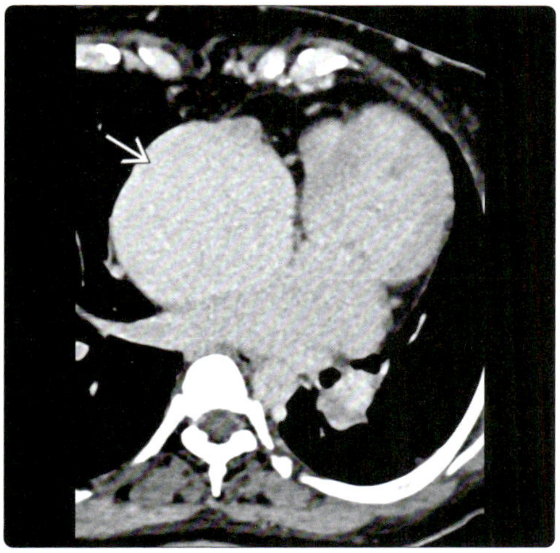

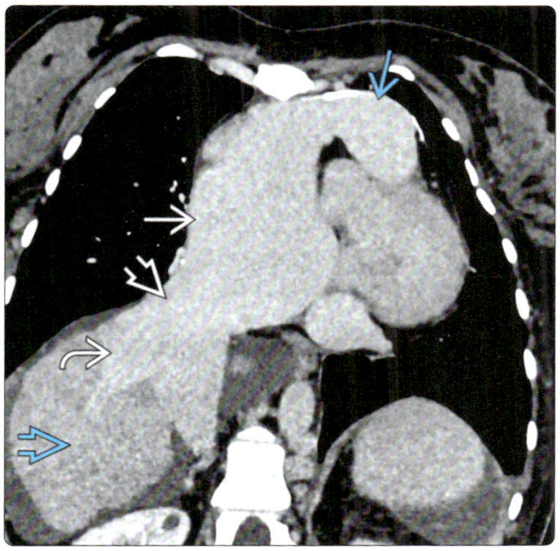

(Left) *Axial and coronal delayed CT images in a patient with tricuspid atresia show surgical changes of classic Fontan (right atrium to PA anastomosis) with a dilated right atrium.* **(Right)** *Axial and coronal delayed CT images in a patient with tricuspid atresia show surgical changes of classic Fontan with right atrial to main PA anastomosis. Also notice the dilated inferior vena cava and hepatic veins as well as a cirrhotic liver.*

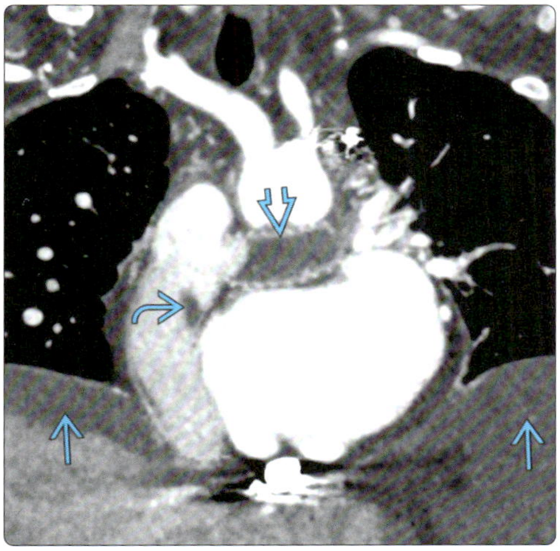

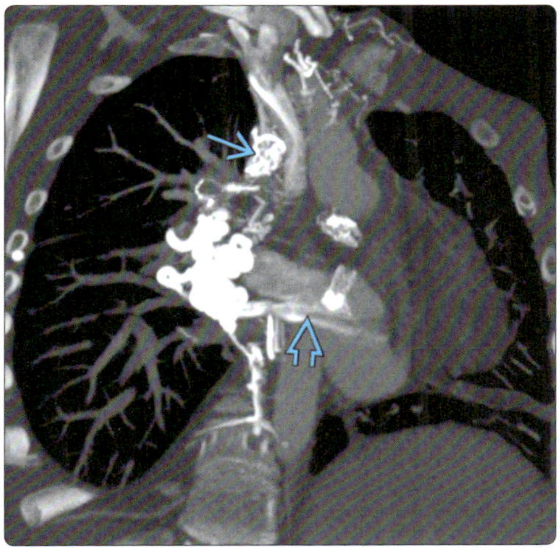

(Left) *Coronal oblique CT in a patient with hypoplastic right heart shows thrombus in the extracardiac Fontan and clot occluding the left PA graft. The liver is cirrhotic due to passive hepatic congestion with ascites. (Courtesy S. Kligerman, MD.)* **(Right)** *Coronal oblique CT in a 20-year-old with extracardiac Fontan shows large venovenous collaterals due to elevated Fontan pressures. Systemic venous collaterals drain into the left atrium via right inferior pulmonary vein, creating an R-to-L shunt. (Courtesy S. Kligerman, MD.)*

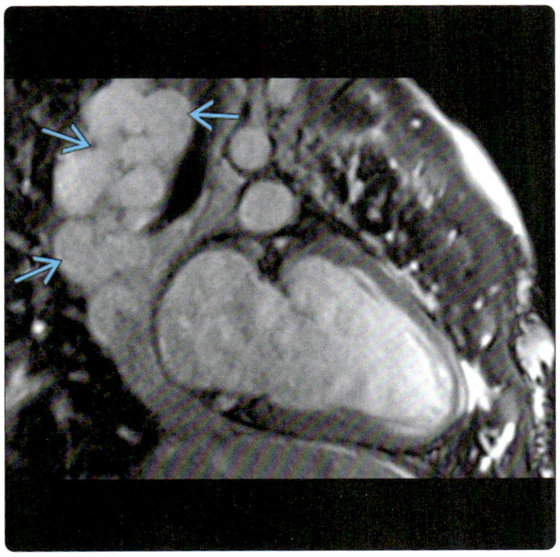

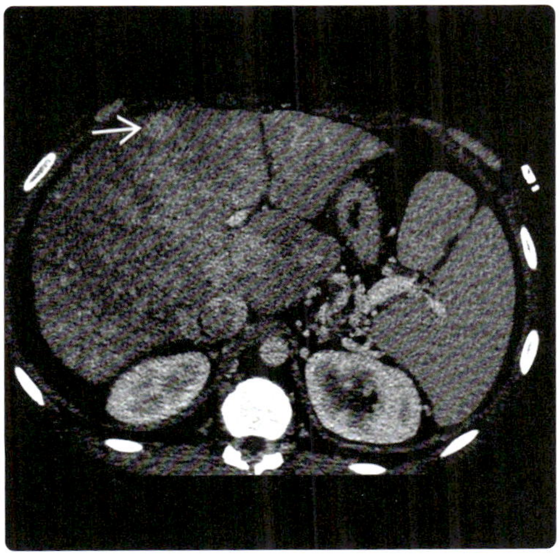

(Left) *Two-chamber view of the left heart in a patient with tricuspid atresia after Fontan shows large mediastinal venovenous collaterals.* **(Right)** *Axial CT of the upper abdomen in a patient with a single ventricle and Fontan palliation shows heterogeneous enhancement of the liver parenchyma and enhancing nodule in hepatic segment IV, consistent with focal nodular hyperplasia.*

Ebstein Anomaly

KEY FACTS

IMAGING

- Classic plain film appearance: Massive right-sided cardiomegaly (box-shaped heart)
- Small vascular pedicle
- Apical displacement of septal tricuspid leaflet (≥ 8 mm/m² body surface area)
  - Hemodynamics: Severe tricuspid valve regurgitation
  - Volume overload to right heart
- Right-to-left shunting through patent foramen ovale leads to cyanosis

TOP DIFFERENTIAL DIAGNOSES

- Uhl anomaly and arrhythmogenic right ventricular dysplasia (ARVD)
  - Similar but distinct entities: Congenital absence (Uhl) or fibrofatty infiltration (ARVD) of right ventricle myocardium
- Large atrial septal defect

PATHOLOGY

- Downward displacement of septal and posterior leaflets of tricuspid valve
  - Although anulus remains in normal position, proximal portions of leaflets are attached to ventricular walls, displacing leaflet hinge points toward apex
- 3 compartments: Right atrium, atrialized noncontracting inlet portion, and functional outlet portion of right ventricle

CLINICAL ISSUES

- Wide spectrum of findings and ages at 1st presentation; some patients are asymptomatic
- Presence of cyanosis depends on balance between right and left atrial pressure
- Accessory atrioventricular conduction pathways (preexcitation) → tachyarrhythmias, which can be unexpected and fatal

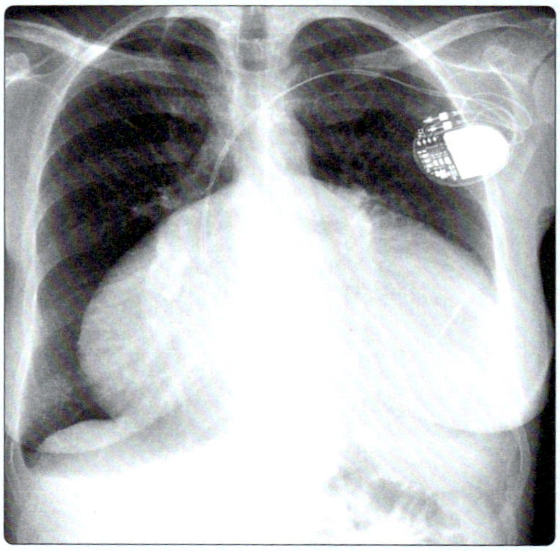

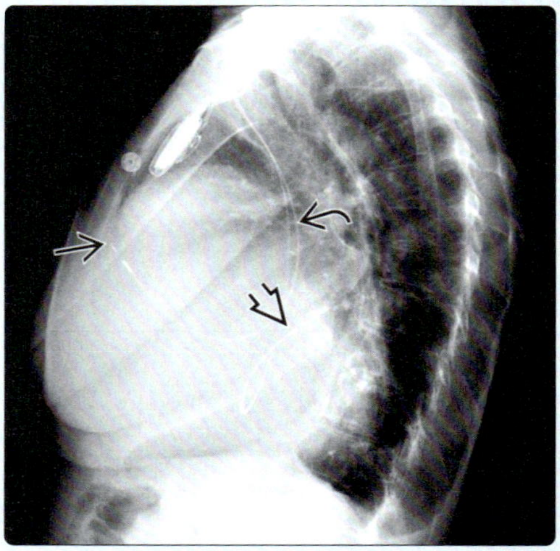

(Left) *PA radiograph shows a markedly enlarged, box-shaped heart. Note narrow vascular pedicle and normal to decreased pulmonary vasculature. Pacemaker lead positions demarcate massive right atrial (RA) and ventricular (RV) enlargement.* **(Right)** *Lateral radiograph shows an enlarged right heart filling the retrosternal space. Large distance between pacer leads in superior vena cava (SVC) → and lead tip at anterior RA wall → shows degree of RA enlargement. Displaced small left ventricle is posterior to RV lead tip →.*

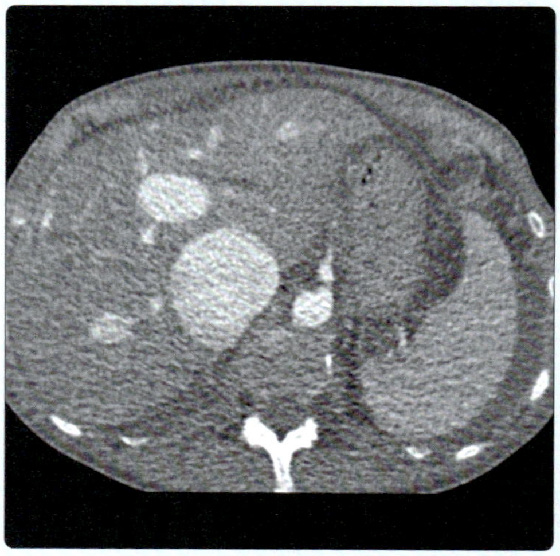

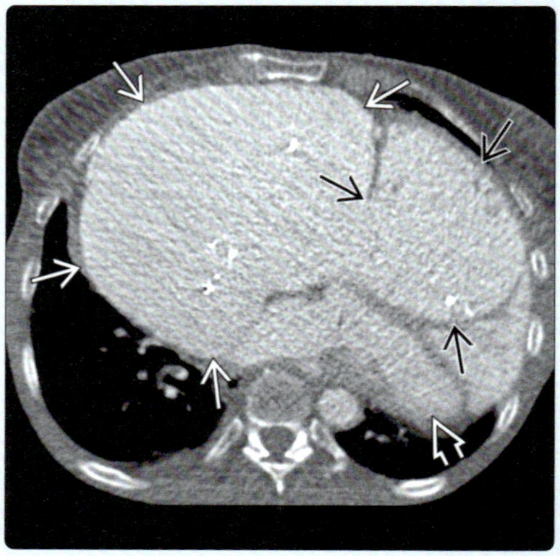

(Left) *Axial CTA demonstrates a congested liver with a markedly enlarged inferior vena cava (IVC) and hepatic veins due to tricuspid regurgitation.* **(Right)** *Axial CTA in the same patient shows a massively dilated RA →, an atrialized portion of the RV →, and a posteriorly displaced, small-appearing but normal-sized left ventricle →.*

TERMINOLOGY

Definitions

- Apical displacement of septal and posterior leaflets of tricuspid valve
  - Although anulus remains in normal position, proximal portions of leaflets are attached to ventricular walls, effectively displacing leaflet hinge points toward apex
- Classic plain film appearance: Massive right-sided cardiomegaly (box-shaped heart)
- Category: Cyanotic, (severe) cardiomegaly, normal or decreased pulmonary vascularity
- Hemodynamics: Severe tricuspid valve regurgitation
  - Volume overload to right heart
  - Right-to-left shunting through patent foramen ovale (PFO) leads to cyanosis

IMAGING

General Features

- Best diagnostic clue
  - Apical displacement of septal tricuspid leaflet (≥ 8 mm/m² body surface area)
- Location
  - Tricuspid valve

Radiographic Findings

- Radiography
  - Severe right-sided cardiomegaly
    - Heart size can be near normal in newborn period but can also be massively enlarged at birth
    - Heart increases gradually in size over time, reaching massive proportions in untreated cases during adulthood (wall-to-wall heart)
    - Cardiothoracic ratio used as follow-up parameter
  - Small vascular pedicle
  - May mimic large pericardial effusion

CT Findings

- CTA
  - Right chamber enlargement with "atrialized" portion of right ventricle (RV)
  - Normal-sized left atrium and ventricle; latter often displaced into posterior left chest
  - May demonstrate apical displacement of septal tricuspid valve leaflet and sail-like anterior leaflet
- Dynamic cine CT can be used for functional analysis of ventricular contraction in patients with contraindications for MR
  - Signs of RV volume overload on cine imaging: Ventricular septal straightening during diastole only

MR Findings

- T1WI
  - Right chamber best seen on long-axis imaging
- MRA
  - Associated cardiac abnormalities
- SSFP cine
  - ECG-gated, SSFP cine MR
    - Morphology demonstrated in cine images: Apical displacement of septal leaflet; atrialized RV; tricuspid regurgitation
    - Ventricular volumes, volume of atrialized RV ejection fraction, tricuspid regurgitation fraction
    - Left ventricular function affected by RV dilatation, diastolic bowing of septum, mitral valve prolapse
- Phase contrast
  - Flow/shunt calculations
  - Degree of tricuspid regurgitation (regurgitant volume)

Echocardiographic Findings

- Echocardiogram
  - Right chamber enlargement, atrialized portion of RV
  - Enlarged tricuspid anulus (expressed in Z-score)
  - Apical displacement of septal tricuspid leaflet (> 15 mm in children < 14 years; > 20 mm in adults, or ≥ 8 mm/m² body surface area)
- Color Doppler
  - Tricuspid regurgitation
  - PFO with right-to-left shunting

Angiographic Findings

- Conventional
  - Characteristic notch at inferior RV border at insertion of displaced anterior tricuspid leaflet
  - Seldom required for primary diagnosis

Nuclear Medicine Findings

- Radionuclide imaging
  - Decreased left ventricular ejection fraction in 50%

Imaging Recommendations

- Protocol advice
  - Anatomic and functional assessment with echocardiogram or MR in infants
  - Cine MR in (young) adults

DIFFERENTIAL DIAGNOSIS

Large Atrial Septal Defect

- Acyanotic
- Increased pulmonary vascularity
- Left-to-right flow through atrial septal defect

Pericardial Effusion

- Acyanotic
- Easy differentiation with ECG

Tricuspid Regurgitation

- Primary: Due to dysplastic valve
- Secondary: Due to pulmonary atresia with intact ventricular septum

Uhl Anomaly and Arrhythmogenic Right Ventricular Dysplasia

- Similar but distinct entities with congenital absence (Uhl) or fibrofatty infiltration [arrhythmogenic RV dysplasia (ARVD)] of RV myocardium
- May be differentiated from Ebstein anomaly with spin-echo and cine MR

Right-Sided Obstructive Cyanotic Heart Lesions With Decreased Pulmonary Vascularity

- Tetralogy of Fallot
- Pulmonary atresia

- With ventricular septal defect and aortopulmonary collaterals
- With intact ventricular septum
  - Ebstein anomaly and pulmonary atresia with intact ventricular septum are 2 lesions that cause most severe cardiomegaly
- Tricuspid atresia
- Transposition of great arteries (TGA) with pulmonary stenosis
- Double-outlet RV with pulmonary stenosis

PATHOLOGY

General Features

- Genetics
  - Most often sporadic
- Associated abnormalities
  - PFO, secundum atrial septal defect in 90%
- Massive right-sided chamber enlargement
- 3 compartments: Right atrium, atrialized noncontracting inlet portion, and functional outlet portion of RV
- Ebstein anomaly frequently involves left-sided tricuspid valve in congenitally corrected (L) TGA
- Embryology
  - Insufficient separation of tricuspid valve leaflets and chordae tendineae from RV endocardium
- Pathophysiology
  - Massive tricuspid regurgitation
  - Volume overload to right side of heart
  - Right-to-left shunt through PFO → cyanosis
  - Left ventricular diastolic dysfunction may result from massive right-sided cardiac enlargement
  - Arrhythmias due to conduction abnormalities

Gross Pathologic & Surgical Features

- Thickened valve leaflets, adherent to underlying myocardium
- Downward displacement of septal and posterior tricuspid leaflets
- Normally placed, redundant, sail-like anterior tricuspid leaflet
- May occur on left side of heart with congenitally corrected (L) transposition

CLINICAL ISSUES

Presentation

- Most common signs/symptoms
  - Wide spectrum of findings and ages at 1st presentation; some patients are asymptomatic
  - Chronic right heart failure
    - Decreased exercise tolerance [classified as New York Heart Association (NYHA) classes I-IV]
  - Presence of cyanosis depends on balance between right and left atrial pressure
    - Physiologic drop in pulmonary vascular resistance in neonatal period → decrease in right-to-left shunting through PFO → gradual improvement in cyanosis in 1st weeks of life
    - Polycythemia
- Other signs/symptoms
  - Hydrops fetalis in neonatal cases
  - Severe cardiomegaly in fetal life → pulmonary hypoplasia
  - Thrombosis, paradoxical embolus
  - Arrhythmias
    - Atrial fibrillation, atrial flutter
    - Accessory atrioventricular conduction pathways (preexcitation) → tachyarrhythmias, which can be unexpected and fatal

Demographics

- Age
  - 1st presentation can range from newborn period through old age (average: 14 years)
- Epidemiology
  - < 1% of congenital cardiac anomalies; incidence: 1/210,000 live births
  - M:F = 1:1

Natural History & Prognosis

- Sudden death due to fatal atrial arrhythmias
- Uncomplicated pregnancies possible in women with hemodynamically well-balanced lesions
- Prognosis is dependent on hemodynamic significance of tricuspid regurgitation, presence of cyanosis

Treatment

- Supportive treatment in cyanotic neonate: Oxygen, nitric oxide ventilation to lower pulmonary resistance
- Systemic to pulmonary (Blalock-Taussig and central) shunts are ineffective
- Some patients benefit from total right-sided heart bypass procedures (Glenn → Fontan surgical treatment pathway)
- Tricuspid valve replacement &/or reconstruction (valvuloplasty) is definitive repair procedure
  - Valvuloplasty and bioprosthesis placement are preferable to mechanical valve (allow growth; no need for lifelong anticoagulation)
  - Valvuloplasty uses tissues from existing valve (redundant anterior tricuspid leaflet)
  - Bioprosthesis: Homograft or xenograft (porcine valve)
- Indications for valve repair
  - NYHA classes III and IV
  - NYHA classes I and II with cardiothoracic ratio > 0.65
  - Significant cyanosis (arterial saturation < 80%) &/or polycythemia (Hb > 16 g/dL)
  - History of paradoxical embolus
  - Arrhythmia due to accessory atrioventricular pathway
- Arrhythmia treatments
  - Radiofrequency ablation
  - Antiarrhythmic drugs
  - Permanent pacemaker implantation

SELECTED REFERENCES

1. Pasqualin G et al: Ebstein's anomaly in children and adults: multidisciplinary insights into imaging and therapy. Heart. 110(4):235-44, 2024
2. Qureshi MY et al: Cardiac imaging in Ebstein anomaly. Trends Cardiovasc Med. 28(6):403-9, 2018
3. Tobler D et al: Right heart characteristics and exercise parameters in adults with Ebstein anomaly: new perspectives from cardiac magnetic resonance imaging studies. Int J Cardiol. 165(1):146-50, 2013

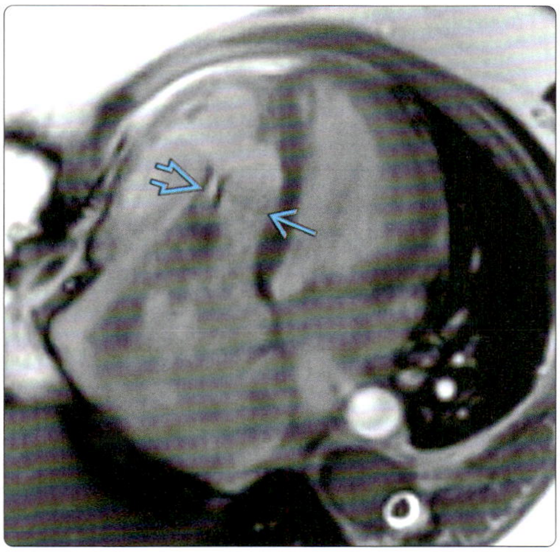

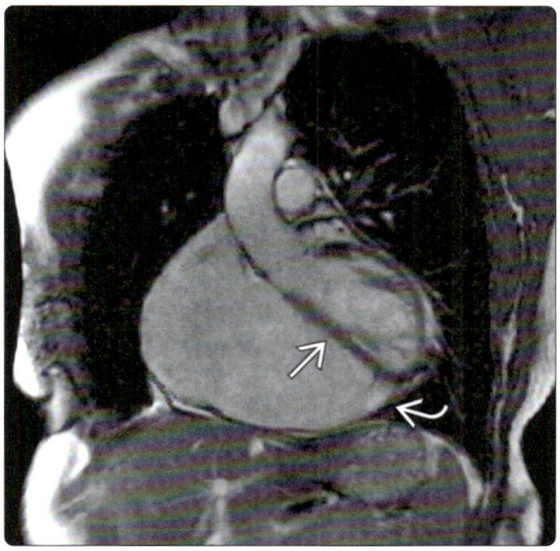

(Left) *Four-chamber SSFP MR shows anterior displacement of the septal leaflet with severe tricuspid regurgitation and systolic inversion of the septum in a patient with Ebstein anomaly.* **(Right)** *Coronal oblique SSFP MR in the same patient demonstrates an enlarged RA and RV. The inferior portion of the left heart border seen on the radiograph actually represents an enlarged left ventricle. Note also flattening of the ventricular septum.*

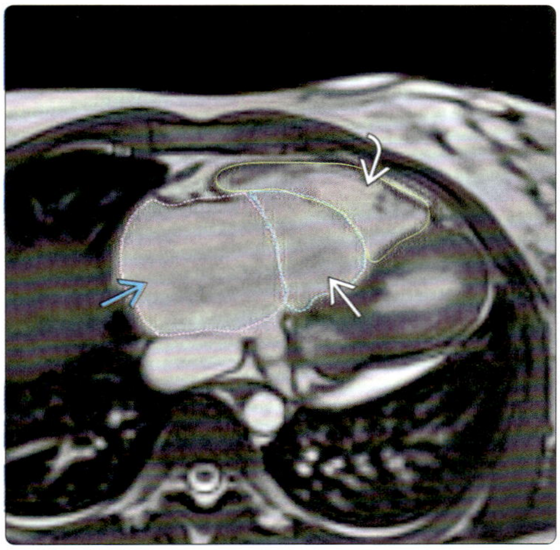

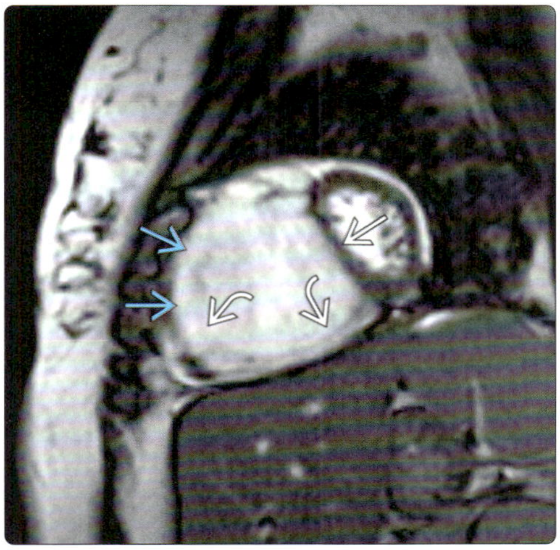

(Left) *Axial SSFP MR displays contouring for quantifying right-sided volumes: Purple contours delineate the RA, blue contours outline the atrialized RV (aRV), and yellow contours define the RV. The ratio of total right-sided volumes:left-sided volumes is used to assess the severity of an Ebstein anomaly.* **(Right)** *Short-axis SSFP MR shows the boundaries of the aRV and functional RV (fRV) with septal flattening.*

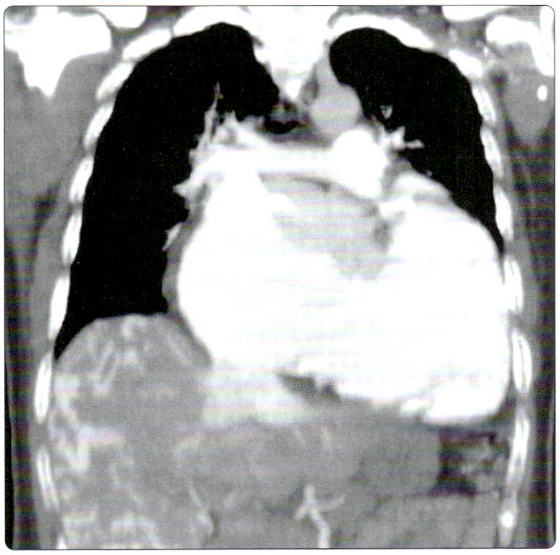

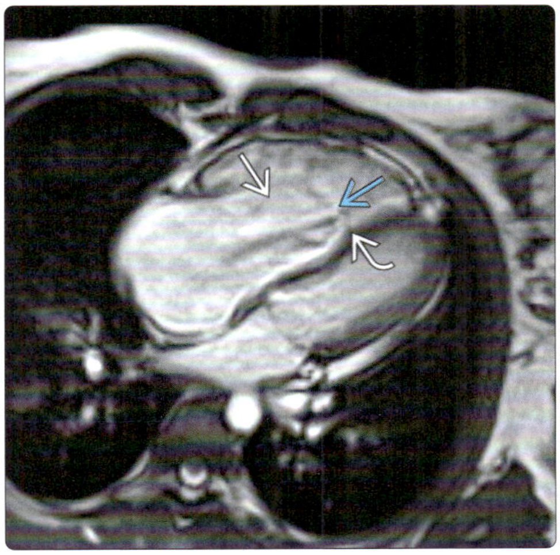

(Left) *Coronal CTA depicts massive dilatation of right-sided cardiac chambers. Note reflux of contrast into passively congested dilated and tortuous hepatic veins due to tricuspid regurgitation and systemic venous hypertension.* **(Right)** *Four-chamber SSFP MR reveals apical displacement of the septal tricuspid valve, aRV, and a dephasing jet indicative of tricuspid regurgitation.*

Cor Triatriatum

KEY FACTS

TERMINOLOGY

- Usually refers to cor triatriatum sinister (CTS)
  - Congenital anomaly with fibromuscular diaphragm or membrane dividing left atrium into posterior and anterior chambers
    - Posterior (proximal) chamber receives pulmonary veins
    - Anterior (distal) chamber gives rise to left atrial appendage (LAA) and mitral valve
    - Communication between chambers through defect of varying size
- Cor triatriatum **dexter**: Analogous abnormality in right atrium

IMAGING

- Arterial-phase CT demonstrates membrane of varying size dividing left atrium into posterior and anterior chambers
  - CTS: Membrane attaches between LAA and pulmonary vein ostia
  - Distinguished from supravalvular ring by being superior/posterior to LAA
  - Paraseptal long-axis reconstructions helpful in visualizing insertion site with respect to LAA ostium

TOP DIFFERENTIAL DIAGNOSES

- Submitral ring or web
  - Web connects between LAA and mitral anulus
- Total anomalous pulmonary venous return
  - Common posterior collecting vein receives pulmonary veins and does not connect to left atrium
  - Supracardiac, infracardiac, or cardiac right-sided drainage site may be identified
- Aberrant atrial band
  - Bands and band-like structures can occur within cardiac chambers
  - Congenital left atrial band is found in 2% of autopsies

(Left) *Axial oblique cardiac CT shows a thin membrane ➔ dividing the left atrium into an anterior and posterior component. The posterior portion of the left atrium receives the pulmonary veins ➔, and the anterior chamber connects to the left atrial appendage ➔.* **(Right)** *Vertical long-axis (2-chamber) cardiac CT in the same patient shows the pulmonary vein draining into the posterior chamber ➔. The membrane ➔ inserts between the pulmonary vein ostia and left atrial appendage ostium ➔.*

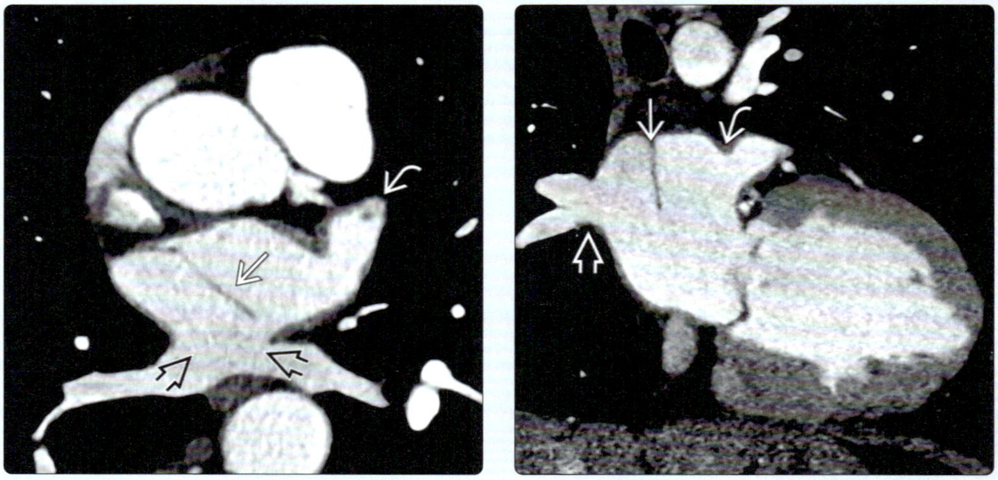

(Left) *Vertical long-axis (2-chamber) cine MR demonstrates a thin membrane ➔ within the left atrium, dividing it into anterior and posterior chambers. Note the incomplete nature of the membrane allowing communication between the chambers. Also note the left atrial enlargement.* **(Right)** *Horizontal long-axis (4-chamber) cine MR in a patient with cor triatriatum dexter is shown. Thin membrane ➔ divides the right atrium into 2 chambers.*

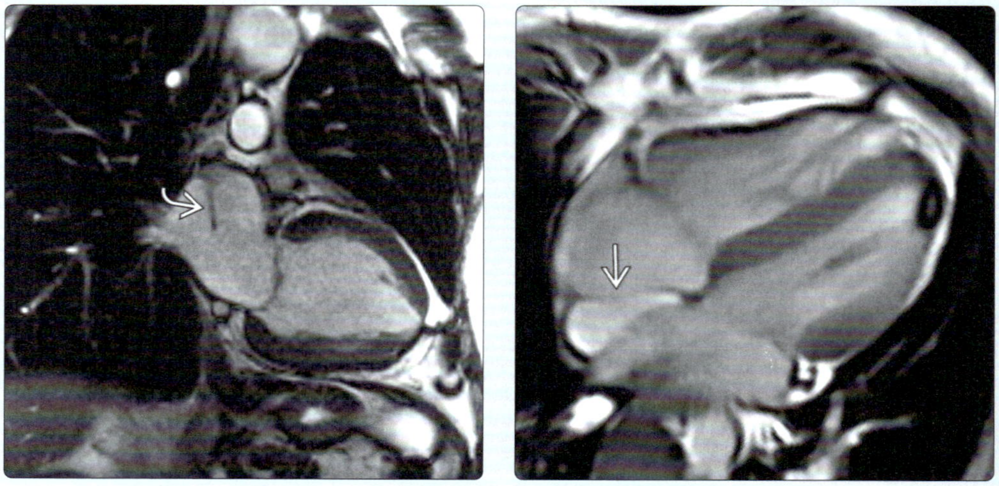

TERMINOLOGY

Synonyms

- Usually refers to cor triatriatum sinister (CTS)
- Cor triatriatum dexter: Analogous abnormality in right atrium

Definitions

- CTS: Fibromuscular diaphragm or membrane dividing left atrium into 2 chambers
  - Posterior (proximal or accessory) chamber receives all or part of pulmonary veins
  - Anterior (distal or left atrium) chamber connects to left atrial appendage (LAA) and mitral valve
  - Communication between chambers through defect of varying size in membrane
  - Accessory chamber may connect to right atrium only or have total anomalous pulmonary venous return/connection (TAPVR/C)
- Cor triatriatum **dexter**: Analogous abnormality in right atrium; due to persistence of right valve of sinus venosus
  - 2 right atrial chambers
    - Sinus venarum receiving superior vena cava (SVC) and inferior vena cava (IVC)
    - Trabeculated portion connecting to tricuspid valve
  - May mimic Ebstein anomaly

IMAGING

General Features

- Best diagnostic clue
  - Membrane of varying size dividing left atrium into posterior and anterior chambers
- Location
  - CTS: Membrane attaches between LAA and pulmonary vein ostia

CT Findings

- CECT
  - Best seen on arterial-phase gated CT
    - Paraseptal long-axis reconstructions helpful in visualizing insertion site with respect to LAA ostium
  - Signs of pulmonary venous obstruction due to gradient across membrane (mimics mitral stenosis)
    - Left atrium and right chambers may be dilated
    - Pulmonary venous hypertension (PVH) and interstitial edema
    - May develop main pulmonary artery dilation secondary to chronic PVH

MR Findings

- Findings on black-blood or cine images similar to CT
- Cine imaging or phase-contrast images may demonstrate jet across membrane

Echocardiographic Findings

- Echocardiogram
  - Transesophageal echocardiography preferred for membrane visualization
  - May show high-velocity Doppler flow in distal atrial chamber and at mitral orifice
  - Diastolic fluttering of mitral valve leaflets
  - Distinguished from supravalvular ring by being superior/posterior to LAA

DIFFERENTIAL DIAGNOSIS

Submitral Ring or Web

- Web connects between LAA and mitral anulus

Total Anomalous Pulmonary Venous Return

- Common posterior collecting vein receives pulmonary veins and does not connect to left atrium
- Supracardiac, infracardiac, or cardiac right-sided drainage site may be identified

Aberrant Atrial Band

- Bands and band-like structures can occur within cardiac chambers

PATHOLOGY

General Features

- Etiology
  - Congenital malformation due to failure of incorporation of common pulmonary vein into left atrium

Staging, Grading, & Classification

- Loeffler classification
  - Group 1: No opening
  - Group 2: 1 or more small openings
  - Group 3: Single large opening
- Other classifications exist taking into account isolated CTS vs. complex CTS, nonobstructive vs. obstructive, atrial level communications, pulmonary venous anatomy [normal vs. partial anomalous pulmonary venous connection (PAPVC) and total anomalous pulmonary venous connection (TAPVC)], and in complex-type single vs. 2-ventricle circulation

CLINICAL ISSUES

Presentation

- Most common signs/symptoms
  - Dyspnea, palpitations, and orthopnea as result of obstruction by intraatrial membrane
    - Symptom severity depends on fenestration size
      - Larger defects asymptomatic or present with only mild symptoms
  - Pulmonary hypertension and right-sided heart failure
- Symptoms may mimic mitral valve stenosis
- May present with PVH

Treatment

- Surgical resection or percutaneous catheter disruption for symptomatic patients

SELECTED REFERENCES

1. Mashadi AH et al: Cor triatriatum sinister: long-term surgical outcomes in children and a proposal for a new classification. J Card Surg. 37(12):4526-33, 2022
2. Tamkeviciute L et al: Multimodality imaging of cor triatriatum sinister in an adult. Radiol Cardiothorac Imaging. 2(6):e200367, 2020
3. Rajiah P et al: Bands in the heart: multimodality imaging review. Radiographics. 39(5):1238-63, 2019

KEY FACTS

TERMINOLOGY

- Synonym: Situs ambiguous
- Heterotaxy: Abnormal arrangement of thoracoabdominal viscera across left-right body axis
- Isomerism: Dominance or duplication of normally right- or left-sided structures

IMAGING

- Radiography: Opposite orientation of cardiac apex & stomach; findings of congenital heart disease (CHD)
- CT & cardiovascular MR: Detail relationships of thoracoabdominal viscera; characterization of intracardiac anomalies, abnormal systemic &/or pulmonary venous connections
- Echocardiogram: Characterization of intracardiac anomalies, abnormal systemic &/or pulmonary venous connections
- Upper GI study: Exclude malrotation
- Echocardiography, followed by MR

TOP DIFFERENTIAL DIAGNOSES

- Technical error: Mislabeled images
- Situs inversus totalis
- Situs solitus with dextrocardia
- Situs inversus with levocardia

CLINICAL ISSUES

- Prognosis determined by complexity of associated CHD
- 1st-year mortality: 85% asplenia, 65% polysplenia
  - Associated with higher mortality across CHD subgroups
- Asplenia: Neonate with severe cyanosis, susceptibility to infection
- Polysplenia: Variable, often asymptomatic adult

DIAGNOSTIC CHECKLIST

- Asymmetric arrangement of thoracic & abdominal structures as clue to diagnosis
- Rigorous application of segmental analysis on cross-sectional study for complex cases

(Left) *3D reconstruction of MDCT tracheobronchial tree shows symmetric long mainstem bronchi with late takeoff of the upper lobe bronchi ➔ bilaterally, indicating bilateral left-sidedness or left isomerism.* **(Right)** *Axial CTA in the same patient shows an enlarged azygos vein ➔ due to interrupted inferior vena cava and bilateral pulmonary arteries ➔ arching over the mainstem bronchi, indicating bilateral hyparterial bronchi. This latter relationship is often best appreciated on coronal views.*

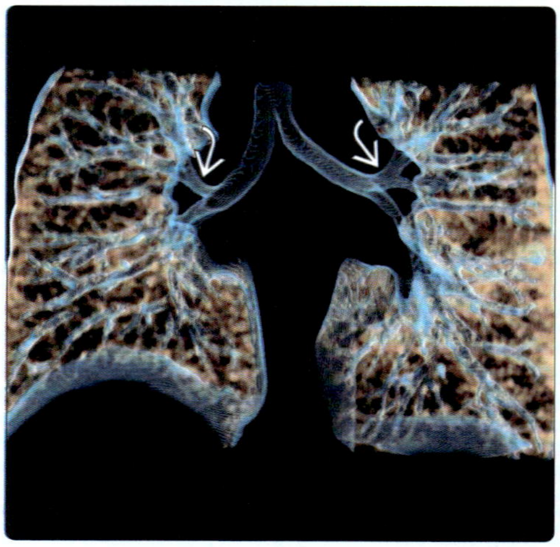

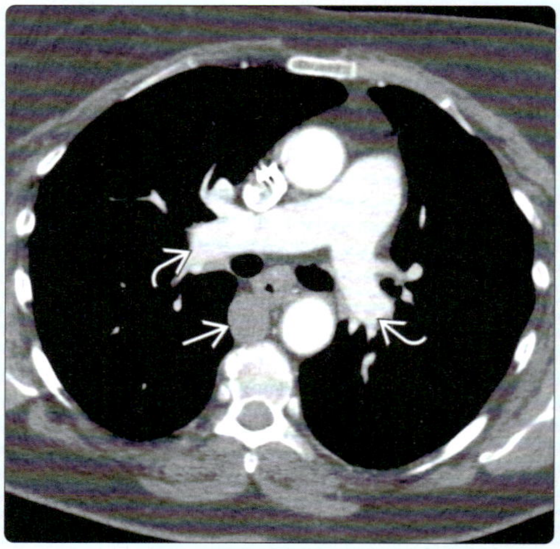

(Left) *Sagittal HRCT in the same patient shows the right lung with a major fissure ➔ and absence of a minor fissure, indicating bilobed right lung.* **(Right)** *Sagittal HRCT of the left lung also shows only a major fissure ➔, indicating bilateral bilobed (left) lungs, consistent with left isomerism or polysplenia.*

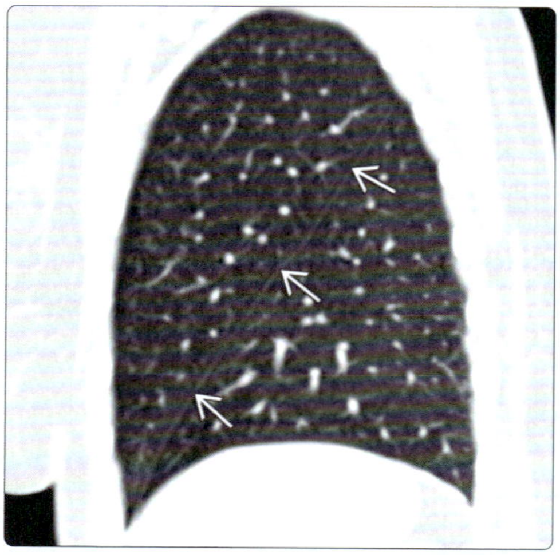

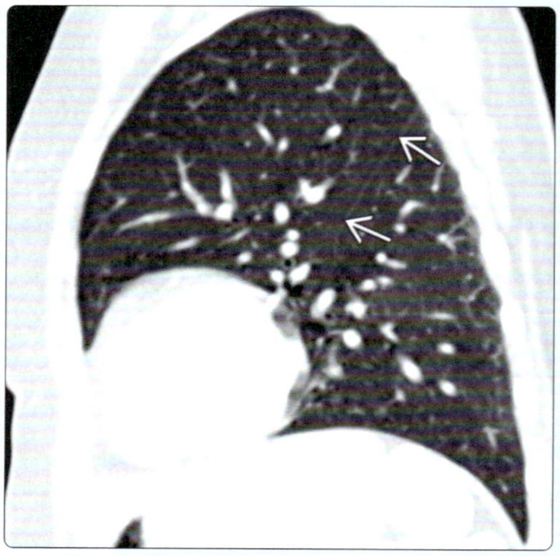

TERMINOLOGY

Synonyms

- Heterotaxy, visceral heterotaxy, situs ambiguous, right/left isomerism, cardiosplenic syndromes

Definitions

- Abnormal arrangement of thoracoabdominal viscera across left-right body axis
  - Exclusive of mirror-image thoracoabdominal arrangement (situs inversus totalis)
- Isomerism: Dominance or duplication of normally right- or left-sided structures
  - Right isomerism (asplenia syndrome, bilateral right-sidedness)
  - Left isomerism (polysplenia syndrome, bilateral left-sidedness)

IMAGING

General Features

- Best diagnostic clue
  - Asymmetric arrangement of thoracic & abdominal structures
  - All imaging findings need not be present for diagnosis

Radiographic Findings

- Opposite orientation of cardiac apex & stomach; bilateral left- or right-sided bronchial arrangement & lobar segmentation; findings of congenital heart disease (CHD); transverse liver
- Right isomerism
  - Bronchi: 1st-order branch located superior to main pulmonary artery (eparterial); symmetric short course before takeoff of upper lobe bronchus
  - Lungs: Bilateral minor fissures (trilobed lungs)
  - Cardiomegaly, pulmonary edema
- Left isomerism
  - Bronchi: 1st-order branch located inferior to main pulmonary artery (hyparterial); symmetric long course before takeoff of upper lobe bronchus
  - Lungs: No minor fissure on either side (bilobed lungs)
  - Prominent azygos shadow on frontal radiograph from interrupted inferior vena cava (IVC)
- Both syndromes
  - Cardiac malposition (40% meso-/dextrocardia)
  - Right-sided stomach with levocardia, left-sided stomach with dextrocardia, or midline stomach
  - Transverse liver

CT Findings

- Right- or left-sidedness described by both spatial arrangement relative to midline & by structural features
  - Right sided
    - Atrium: Blunt/trapezoidal-shaped appendage with broad orifice, pectinate muscles extend beyond appendage; crista terminalis
  - Left sided
    - Atrium: Tubular/finger-like appendage with narrow orifice, pectinate muscles confined within appendage
  - Rule of venoatrial concordance: Chamber that receives direct drainage of suprahepatic IVC or coronary sinus is right atrium
  - Other: Preduodenal portal vein, absent gallbladder, extrahepatic biliary atresia, short pancreas
- Right isomerism
  - Bilateral right atrial appendages, eparterial bronchi, trilobed lungs; absence of spleen
  - Abnormalities of systemic venous connections
    - Bilateral superior vena cava (SVC) (36%), absent coronary sinus; VC & aorta on same side
  - Abnormalities of pulmonary venous connections: Total anomalous pulmonary venous return (TAPVR) (> 80%); often obstructed, below diaphragm (type III)
  - Associated with severe cyanotic CHD [atrioventricular septal defect, common atrioventricular valve, double outlet right ventricle (DORV), transposition of great arteries (TGA), pulmonary stenosis/atresia]
- Left isomerism
  - Bilateral left atrial appendages, hyparterial bronchi, bilobed lungs
  - Multiple spleens, anisosplenia (i.e., 1 or more larger & 1 or more smaller spleens), multilobed spleen
  - Abnormalities of systemic venous connections
    - Bilateral SVC (41%), connect to coronary sinus
    - Azygos or hemiazygos continuation of IVC (> 70%)
    - Hepatic veins drain separately into common atrium
  - Associated with less severe CHD & specifically left-to-right shunts [atrial septal defect (ASD), partial anomalous pulmonary venous return, & atrioventricular canal]

MR Findings

- Nonionizing alternative to CT, allowing assessment of morphology & function
- SSFP cine
  - Assess ventricular volumes & function to determine suitability for biventricular vs. univentricular (Fontan) repair
- MRA
  - Gadolinium-enhanced 3D MRA: Comparable to CTA
  - Ultrafast, time-resolved, gadolinium-enhanced MRA with repeated acquisitions allows for dynamic circulation study
  - Phase-contrast MRA for flow/shunt quantification
- Late gadolinium enhancement: Assess myocardial fibrosis

Echocardiographic Findings

- Often definitive test for characterization of intracardiac anomalies, abnormal systemic &/or pulmonary venous connections

Other Modality Findings

- Upper GI study to assess for associated malrotation

Imaging Recommendations

- Protocol advice
  - Echocardiography, followed by MR
  - CTA for anatomic study in postoperative patients

DIFFERENTIAL DIAGNOSIS

Technical Error: Mislabeled Images

- Discussion with technologists prior to interpretation

Situs Inversus Totalis (I, L, L)

- Mirror image of normal
- Low association with CHD (3-5%)
- Association with immotile cilia (Kartagener) syndrome: Sinusitis, bronchiectasis, infertility

Situs Solitus With Dextrocardia

- Heart mass positioned predominantly to right of midline, independent of cardiac apex orientation
- e.g., right pulmonary venolobar (scimitar) syndrome, left-sided mass lesions (diaphragmatic hernia, congenital pulmonary airway malformation of lung)

Situs Inversus With Levocardia

- Situs inversus with heart mass positioned normally to left of midline (isolated levocardia)
- Extremely rare; nearly 100% association with CHD

PATHOLOGY

General Features

- Genetics
  - No specific genetic defect in most; presumed multifactorial inheritance
- Associated abnormalities
  - Spectrum of abnormalities with overlap between distinct right & left isomerism subtypes
    - Classic right isomerism: Bilateral right atrial appendages, right bronchopulmonary branching pattern, asplenia
    - Classic left isomerism: Bilateral left atrial appendages, left bronchopulmonary branching pattern, polysplenia
  - Deviation from classic patterns in > 20% of cases
- Embryology: Early embryologic disturbance (5th week of gestation) leading to complex anomalies
- Pathophysiology: Determined by complexity of associated CHD

Staging, Grading, & Classification

- Segmental approach to analysis of complex cardiac anomalies summarized by 3-letter code: (S/A/I, D/L, D/L)
  - Visceroatrial situs designated by S (solitus = normal), A (ambiguous), or I (inversus = mirror image of normal)
    - Situs ambiguous (heterotaxy): Any arrangement other than situs solitus or inversus
    - Defined by relationships of atria to abdominal viscera
      - Problematic, as atrial appendage morphology indefinable by imaging in up to 15% of cases
  - Ventricular loop: D (normal) or L (inverted)
  - Orientation of great arteries: S (solitus), I (inversus), D- or L-TGA/malposition of great arteries (transposition/malposition)
- Connections (atrioventricular, ventriculoarterial): Concordant, discordant, ambiguous, double inlet, absent
- Associated abnormalities: DORV, TAPVR

CLINICAL ISSUES

Presentation

- Most common signs/symptoms
  - Asplenia: Neonate with severe cyanosis, susceptibility to infection
  - Polysplenia: Variable, often asymptomatic adult
  - Malrotation leading to volvulus

Demographics

- Epidemiology
  - Prevalence: 1 per 22,000-24,000; 1-3% of CHD
  - Asplenia more common in boys; equal sex ratio for polysplenia

Natural History & Prognosis

- 1st-year mortality: 85% asplenia, 65% polysplenia
- Heterotaxy associated with higher mortality across CHD subgroups
- Postoperative: Development of pulmonary to systemic venous collaterals, arteriovenous malformations, pulmonary vein stenosis

Treatment

- Supportive: Prostaglandins, antibiotic & vaccine prophylaxis
- Asplenia/polysplenia with pulmonary overcirculation: Pulmonary artery banding
- Asplenia with obstructed pulmonary flow & TAPVR: Delicate balance between pulmonary arterial inflow & venous outflow
  - Systemic to pulmonary artery (Blalock-Taussig or central) shunt, concurrent TAPVR repair
- Univentricle physiology: Initial Glenn or hemi-Fontan, completion-modified Fontan
  - Polysplenia: Incorporation of azygos vein to cavopulmonary anastomosis (Kawashima operation)
- Ladd procedure for volvulus

DIAGNOSTIC CHECKLIST

Image Interpretation Pearls

- Asymmetric arrangement of thoracic & abdominal structures as clue to diagnosis
- Rigorous application of segmental analysis on cross-sectional study for complex cases

SELECTED REFERENCES

1. Akalın M et al: Heterotaxy syndrome: prenatal diagnosis, concomitant malformations and outcomes. Prenat Diagn. 42(4):435-46, 2022
2. Yim D et al: Disharmonious patterns of heterotaxy and isomerism: how often are the classic patterns breached? Circ Cardiovasc Imaging. 11(2):e006917, 2018
3. Franklin RCG et al: Nomenclature for congenital and paediatric cardiac disease: the International Paediatric and Congenital Cardiac Code (IPCCC) and the Eleventh Iteration of the International Classification of Diseases (ICD-11). Cardiol Young. 27(10):1872-938, 2017
4. Abdullah NL et al: Clinics in diagnostic imaging (160). Levocardia with abdominal situs inversus. Singapore Med J. 56(4):198-201; quiz 202, 2015
5. Lin AE et al: Laterality defects in the national birth defects prevention study (1998-2007): birth prevalence and descriptive epidemiology. Am J Med Genet A. 164A(10):2581-91, 2014
6. Wolla CD et al: Cardiovascular manifestations of heterotaxy and related situs abnormalities assessed with CT angiography. J Cardiovasc Comput Tomogr. 7(6):408-16, 2013
7. Jacobs JP et al: Heterotaxy: lessons learned about patterns of practice and outcomes from the congenital heart surgery database of the society of thoracic surgeons. World J Pediatr Congenit Heart Surg. 2(2):278-86, 2011
8. Kim SJ: Heterotaxy syndrome. Korean Circ J. 41(5):227-32, 2011
9. Babar JL et al: Application of MR imaging in assessment and follow-up of congenital heart disease in adults. Radiographics. 30(4):1145, 2010
10. Maldjian PD et al: Approach to dextrocardia in adults: review. AJR Am J Roentgenol. 188(6 Suppl):S39-49; quiz S35-8, 2007

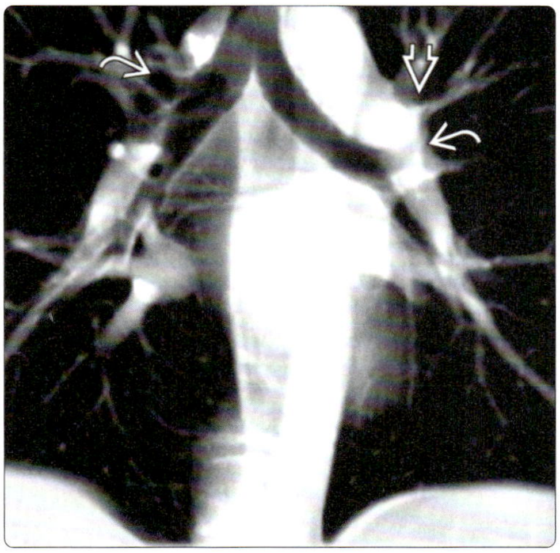

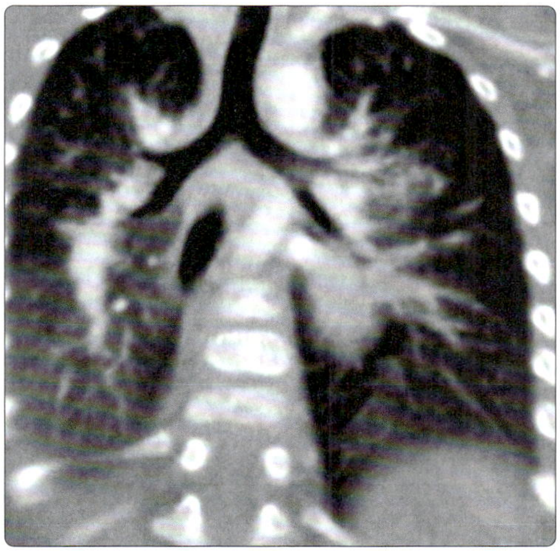

(Left) *Coronal CT MPR shows the normal asymmetry with a short right and a long left mainstem bronchi (upper lobe bronchi). The left pulmonary artery arches over the (hyparterial) bronchus; the right does not (eparterial bronchus).* **(Right)** *Coronal CTA MPR in the same patient shows abnormally symmetric short mainstem bronchi with early takeoff of upper lobe bronchi bilaterally. Note that neither bronchus has a pulmonary artery arching over it (bilateral eparterial bronchi), indicating right isomerism/asplenia.*

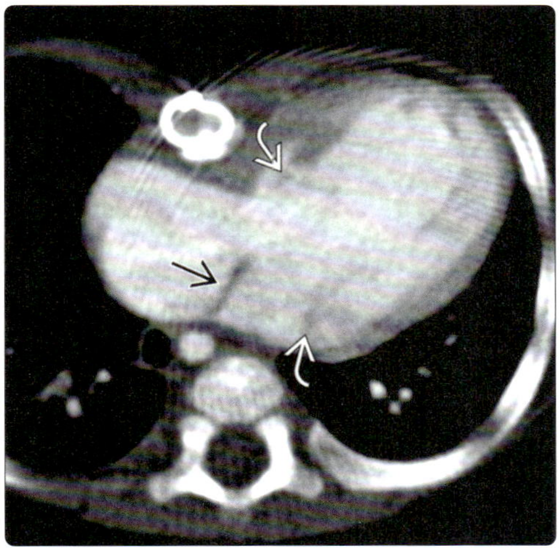

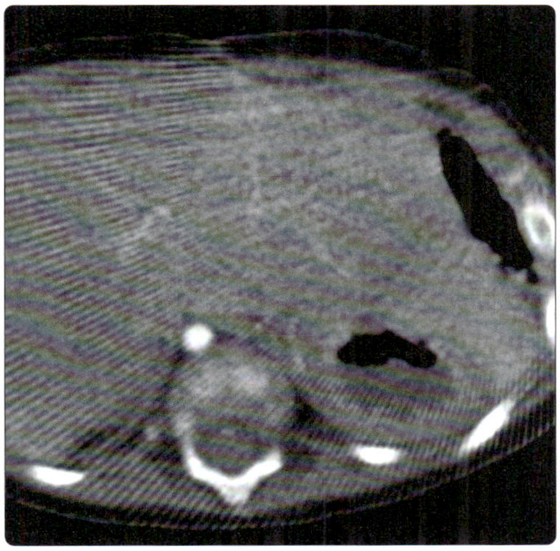

(Left) *Axial CTA shows a univentricular heart (single ventricle) with a common atrium and a common atrioventricular valve . Note a remnant of the atrial septum . Also note a pectus deformity and median sternotomy wires.* **(Right)** *Axial CTA through the abdomen in the same patient shows absence of the spleen, consistent with asplenia.*

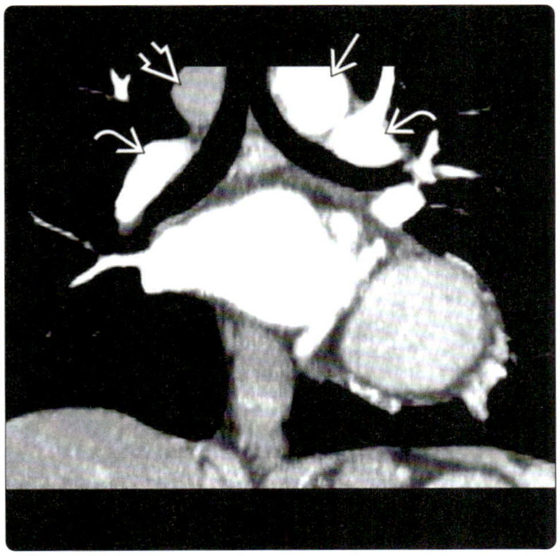

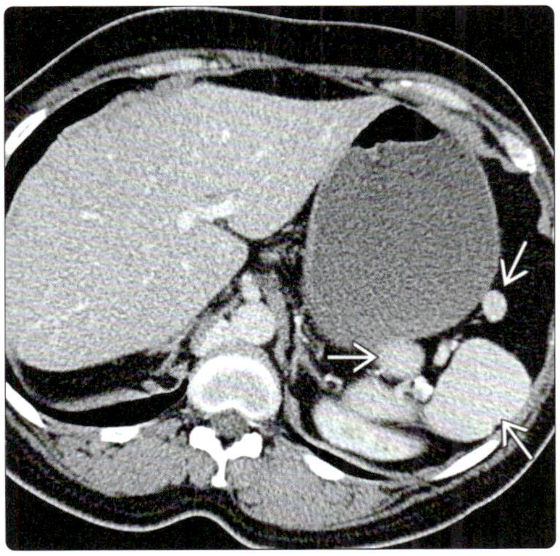

(Left) *Coronal CTA shows symmetric long bilateral hyparterial bronchi with bilateral pulmonary arteries arching over their respective bronchi , indicating bilateral left-sidedness. Note the enlarged azygos arch due to azygos continuation of the inferior vena cava. Also note the aorta giving a bilateral double-barrel appearance.* **(Right)** *Axial CT in the same patient shows multiple spleens, consistent with left isomerism and polysplenia .*

(Left) *Frontal radiograph shows dextrocardia , a right aortic arch , and a bridging or midline liver . The left hemidiaphragm was elevated due to phrenic nerve injury at the time of surgery for tricuspid and pulmonic valve atresia in this patient with heterotaxy and asplenia.* **(Right)** *Coronal CECT in the same patient shows dextrocardia , a bridging liver , and asplenia. Note the Fontan shunt directed from the inferior vena cava to the main pulmonary artery.*

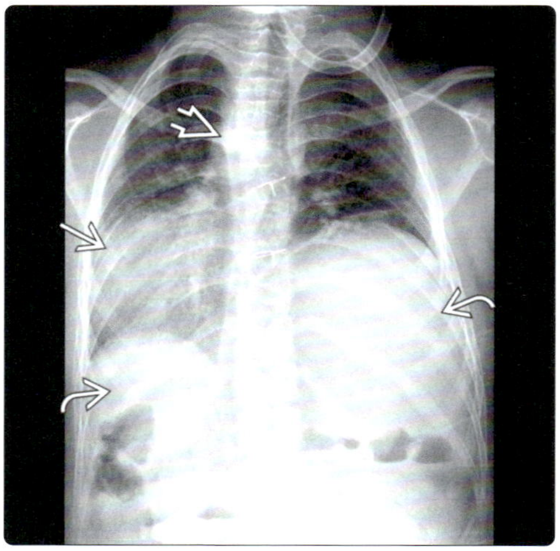

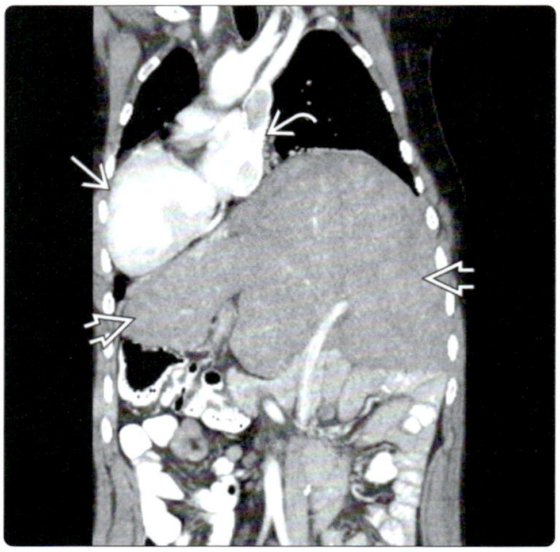

(Left) *Axial MR shows dextrocardia , azygos continuation of an interrupted inferior vena cava, and an atrial septal defect . The most common cardiac malformations in polysplenic patients include atrial septal defect, partial anomalous pulmonary venous return, and atrioventricular canal.* **(Right)** *Axial MR in the same patient shows polysplenia , bridging liver, and azygos continuation of an interrupted inferior vena cava.*

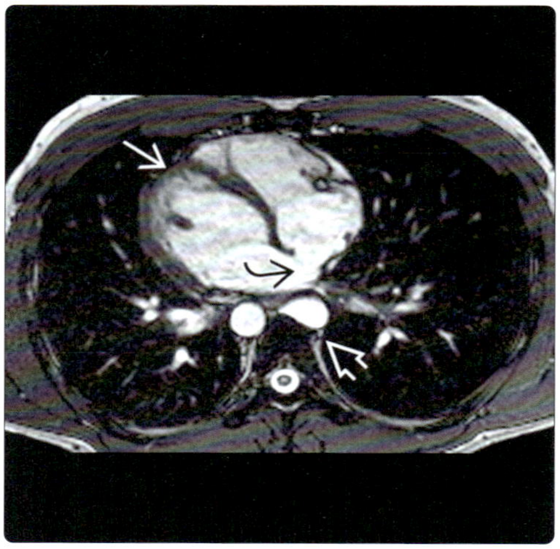

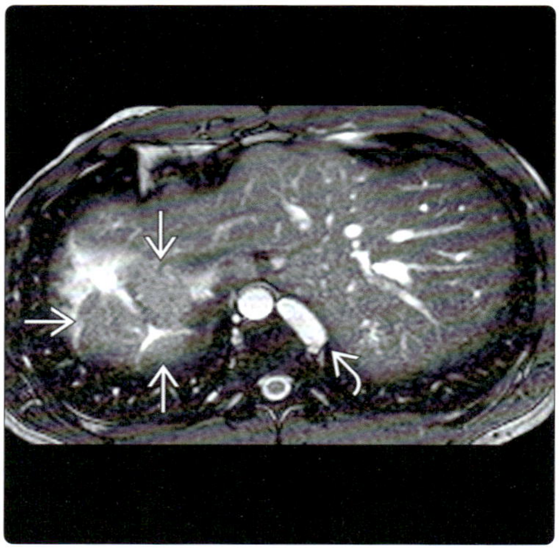

(Left) *Axial MR shows hemiazygos continuation of an interrupted inferior vena cava and polysplenia . The liver, stomach, and cardiac apex were in their expected positions.* **(Right)** *Axial CECT in the same patient shows a normal-sided stomach and liver. There is an enlarged hemiazygos vein and polysplenia . Cardiac anomalies are usually less severe and present later in polysplenic patients compared to those with asplenia.*

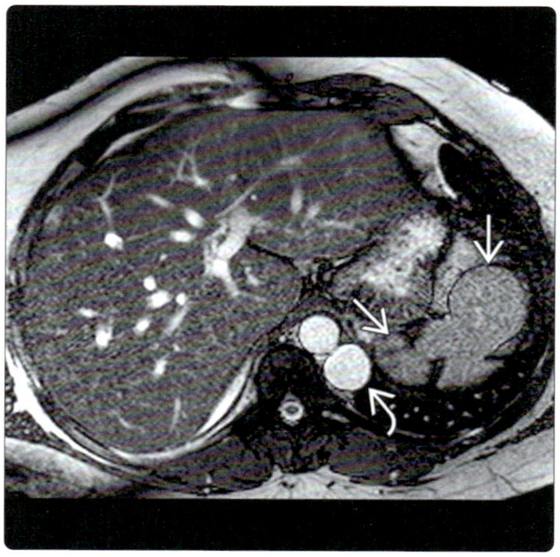

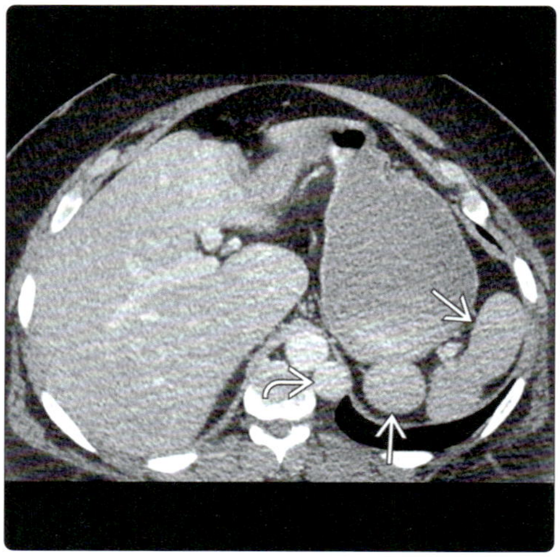

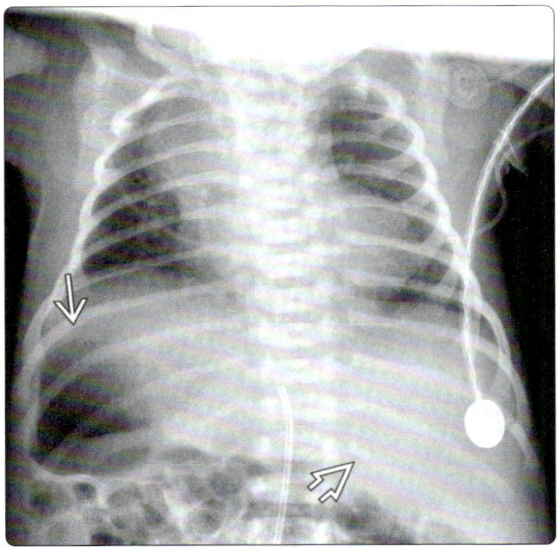

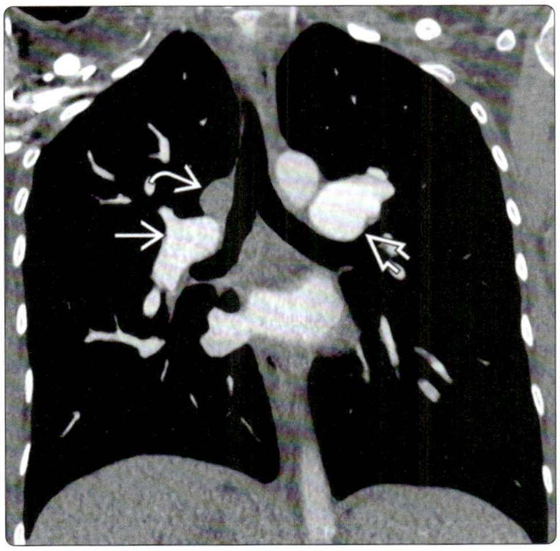

(Left) *Frontal radiograph shows a normal cardiac situs, a right stomach ➡, and a left-sided liver ➡ in this infant with asplenia.* **(Right)** *Coronal CECT shows bilateral hyparterial bronchi under the right ➡ and left ➡ pulmonary arteries. Note the enlarged azygos vein ➡ from collateral flow due to an interrupted inferior vena cava. Axial CT (not shown) more inferiorly demonstrated polysplenia and a horizontal liver.*

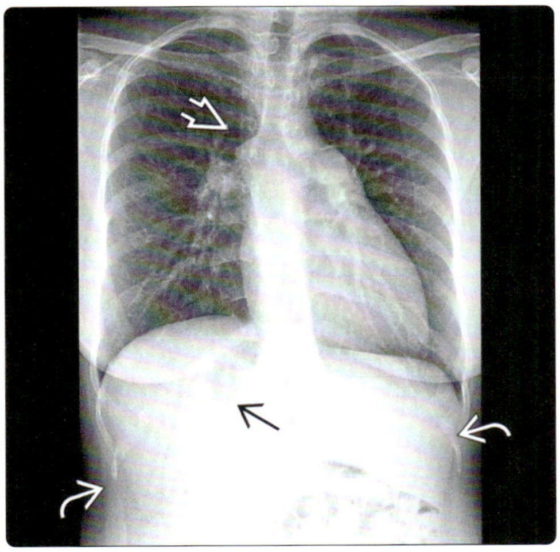

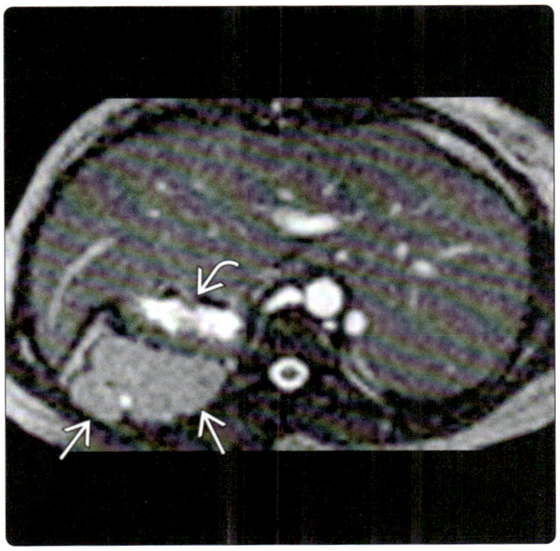

(Left) *Frontal radiograph shows an enlarged azygos vein ➡ from inferior vena cava interruption. The cardiac situs is normal, but the gastric bubble ➡ is right sided. There is a horizontal liver ➡.* **(Right)** *Axial MR in the same patient shows a horizontal liver, polysplenia ➡, a right stomach ➡, and absence of an intrahepatic inferior vena cava.*

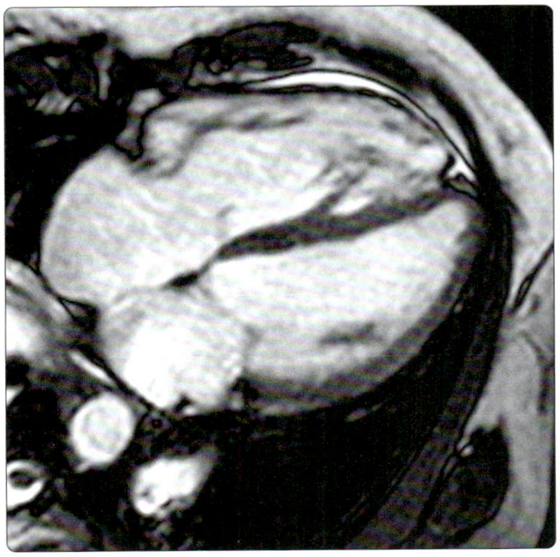

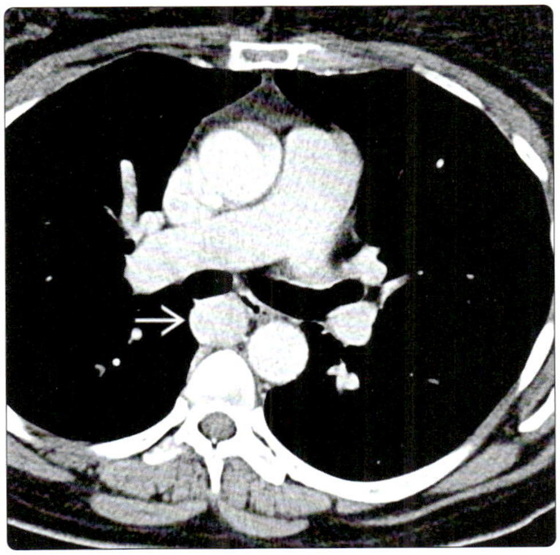

(Left) *Four-chamber cine MR in the same patient shows an enlarged right atrium and right ventricle due to a fenestrated atrial septal defect. The Qp:Qs ratio was calculated at 1.6 (normal is 1). Left-to-right shunts are the most common cardiac anomalies associated with polysplenia.* **(Right)** *Axial CECT shows an enlarged azygos vein ➡ due to an interrupted inferior vena cava. Lower images (not shown) revealed polysplenia.*

Intracardiac Shunts

An intracardiac shunt is an abnormal communication between the pulmonary and systemic circulations at the level of the heart, which results in mixing of venous and arterial blood. Shunting occurs from the higher-pressure system to the lower-pressure system. Isolated intracardiac communications [atrial septal defects (ASDs) and ventricular septal defects (VSDs)] typically result in left-to-right flow and may elude detection for many years. Conversely, intracardiac shunts resulting in right-to-left flow are detected earlier due to the presence of cyanosis. Longstanding left-to-right shunts can increase the right-sided pressures to a point where there is flow reversal across the shunt (Eisenmenger syndrome).

Intracardiac shunts are most commonly congenital and result from abnormal morphogenesis of the atrial or ventricular septa. Intracardiac shunts are the most common congenital heart defects. Acquired shunts are less common and can result from ischemia, trauma, infection, or iatrogenesis.

Although shunts are typically first detected and characterized by echocardiography, the role of cardiac MR and cardiac CT continues to grow. Both CT and MR have good spatial resolution to anatomically characterize the shunt, their relationship with other anatomical structures, and detection of associated anomalies. With the use of phase-contrast imaging on cardiac MR, blood flow can be reliably quantified in the systemic and pulmonary systems, allowing determination of the degree of shunting. Cardiac MR and CT can also accurately quantify ventricular volumes and function, although MR is considered the gold standard.

A pulmonary to systemic flow ratio (Qp:Qs) > 1.5 is considered significant and can result in right heart overload and eventual failure. Given that cardiac CT cannot directly measure blood flow and exposes the patient to ionizing radiation, it is used mainly for anatomic evaluation or when other imaging modalities are limited or unavailable.

Treatment options depend on multiple factors, including the patient's symptoms, ventricular volumes and function, pulmonary arterial pressure, Qp:Qs ratio, location of the defect, size of the defect and surrounding septa, the number of defects, associated anomalies, and others factors.

Types of Intracardiac Shunts

Atrial Septal Defects

ASDs result from abnormal communication at the level of the atria. They may be single or multiple and can vary in size and shape. Based on location, an ASD is classified as ostium secundum, ostium primum, or sinus venosus. An unroofed coronary sinus, although not a direct communication between the left and right atria, is considered a 4th type of ASD. ASDs typically result in enlargement of the right atrium, right ventricle, and pulmonary arteries.

Ostium secundum ASD is the most common (75% of all ASDs) defect and is centered in the fossa ovalis. It results from excessive apoptosis of the septum primum or incomplete formation of the septum secundum leading to a permanent interatrial communication. This is unlike a patent foramen ovale (PFO), which is a persistent fetal interatrial communication into adulthood. In cases of a PFO, there is normal development of the septum primum flap and septum secundum; however, there is lack of fusion of these 2 structures, resulting in interatrial communication. In some cases, it can be difficult to differentiate a large PFO from a small secundum ASD on imaging.

Ostium primum ASD (15-20% of ASDs) is considered the mildest form of an endocardial cushion defect and results from failed fusion between the free edge of the septum primum and the atrioventricular cushions. This defect is located immediately adjacent to the mitral valve anulus.

Sinus venosus ASD (5-10% of all ASDs) is a defect located either in the superior interatrial septum or in the inferior interatrial septum. A superior sinus venosus ASD is typically associated with partial anomalous pulmonary venous return of the right superior pulmonary vein into the superior vena cava. An inferior sinus venosus ASD may be associated with partial anomalous pulmonary venous return to the intrapericardial segment of the inferior vena cava or right atrium.

Unroofed coronary sinus ASD is the rarest (accounts for < 1% of all ASDs) and results from abnormal septation between the left atrium and the adjacent coronary sinus. This results in left to right shunting from the left atrium to the coronary sinus to the right atrium and is thus considered a form of ASD. It is often associated with a left-sided superior vena cava.

Ventricular Septal Defects

VSDs result from abnormal communication at the level of the ventricles. These defects are the most common congenital abnormality found in children and may close spontaneously in a large percentage of patients. VSDs may be single or multiple and can vary in size and shape. Depending on their location, they can be classified as perimembranous, subarterial/outflow, muscular, and inflow. VSDs result in enlargement of the right ventricle, pulmonary artery, left atrium, and left ventricle.

Perimembranous central VSD is the most common type and accounts for 80% of all VSDs. This type of defect is located below the crista supraventricularis, anterior to the septal leaflet of the tricuspid valve, and is bounded by muscular and membranous septum. This defect may close spontaneously by apposition of the septal leaflet of the tricuspid valve over the defect.

Outlet VSD accounts for 5% of all VSDs. This defect is located above the crista supraventricularis and is bounded by the fibrous anulus of the semilunar valve &/or muscular tissue. It may be associated with aortic valve prolapse and regurgitation.

Muscular VSD accounts for 10% of all VSDs. This defect is located in the trabecular portion of the interventricular septum; therefore, the defect is bounded only by muscle.

Inlet VSD accounts for 5% of all VSDs and is almost exclusively associated with endocardial cushion defects. This defect is located anterior to the tricuspid valve anulus and extends to the muscular &/or membranous septum.

Atrioventricular Septal Defects

Atrioventricular septal (canal) defect, also known as an endocardial cushion defect, is secondary to abnormal development of the endocardial cushion, which results in a spectrum of interatrial and interventricular communications associated with atrioventricular valve abnormalities. In turn, endocardial cushion defects result in enlargement of the right atrium, right ventricle, pulmonary artery, left atrium, and left ventricle.

Partial atrioventricular canal defect results in a defect in the anterior and inferior aspect of the atrial septum (i.e., an ostium primum ASD) and is associated with a cleft in the anterior leaflet of the mitral valve.

Intermediate atrioventricular canal defect results in a defect in the anterior and inferior aspect of the atrial septum (i.e., an ostium primum ASD), a small inlet VSD, and a cleft in the mitral and tricuspid valves.

Complete atrioventricular canal defect results in a large defect in the anterior and inferior aspect of the atrial septum, a large VSD, and a common atrioventricular valve.

Embryology

The development of the interatrial septum starts during the 5th week of gestational life. The common atrium divides into left and right atria through the formation of 2 separate overlapping septa (i.e., septum primum and septum secundum). Interatrial communication during fetal life is normal through the foramen ovale. However, persistence of interatrial communication beyond the first 2 years of life as a valve mechanism is abnormal and occurs in ~ 30% of the population. This condition is known as a PFO. Deficient morphogenesis of the septum primum or septum secundum results in an ASD.

The development of the interventricular septum starts during the 5th week of gestational life. The common ventricle divides into left and right ventricles through the fusion of 3 independent septa (i.e., muscular septa, outlet septa, and inlet septa). Incomplete fusion of these septa results in a VSD.

The endocardial cushions are responsible for the formation of the inferior and anterior portion of the interatrial septum, the inlet portion of the ventricular septum, and the atrioventricular valves. Incomplete development of the endocardial cushions results in a spectrum of abnormalities as described above.

Clinical Implications

Small isolated intracardiac shunts may be asymptomatic for many years and only incidentally detected on physical exam. In contrast, large shunts present early with shortness of breath, exercise intolerance, palpitations, syncope, and heart failure. Shunt complications include pulmonary hypertension, right-sided heart failure, arrhythmias, stroke from paradoxical embolism, and Eisenmenger syndrome. In the setting of acquired (traumatic, ischemic, and infectious) VSDs, the underlying etiology of the VSD is paramount and can alter management on a case-by-case basis.

Treatment options depend on many factors and range from medical management to surgical or endovascular closure of the defect. Defects > 36 mm are typically not amenable for endovascular closure. In cases of ASD, a rim size > 3-4 mm is usually required for successful deployment and seating of the closure device, although newer devices and techniques may require less of a rim.

Imaging Protocols

When evaluating a patient with an intracardiac shunt, it is important to determine the location and size of the defect, identify associated abnormalities, quantify ventricular volumes and function, and calculate the Qp:Qs ratio. All of this information can be obtained with cardiac MR.

Cardiac MR

Cardiac MR protocol to assess for intracardiac shunts includes basic localizer images followed by single, balanced steady-state free precession (SSFP) images in the paraseptal long-axis and modified 4-chamber views. These images are then used to prescribe images covering the entire heart in the short-axis plane, often with coverage of the entire heart in the 4-chamber plane. Ideally, thin cuts without spacing should be performed in the regions of concern. These images allow for morphologic assessment of the heart, quantification of ventricular volumes and function, and detection of small dephasing jets.

Additional orthogonal balanced SSFP views of the suspected jets can be obtained to confirm, if in doubt. Balanced SSFP images in the 3-chamber and orthogonal (left ventricular outflow tract) planes are then performed for prescribing phase-contrast images of the aorta. Balanced SSFP images in a right ventricular outflow tract plane and orthogonal plane "driveway" view are also performed for prescribing phase-contrast images of the pulmonary artery. The obtained phase-contrast images are used to determine the Qp:Qs ratio using dedicated postprocessing software. With 4D flow sequences, the flow can be quantified in an entire imaging volume without the need for dedicated planning for individual structures. Triple inversion recovery black-blood images in the short axis can be used to assess myocardial edema in the setting of traumatic, infectious, or ischemic VSDs. 3D whole-heart images may be obtained for morphologic assessment of the defect and for detection of associated anomalies in congenital cases. Finally, late gadolinium enhancement images can be useful to detect myocardial scar in the setting of a traumatic or ischemic VSD.

Cardiac CT

Cardiac CT can be used in cases of intracardiac shunts where there is need for better anatomic delineation or in cases in which cardiac MR &/or echocardiography are contraindicated or limited. Cardiac CT allows the detection and sizing of the defects. Particularly, the analysis of the surrounding rim is easily performed with CT due to the high-resolution isovolumetric nature of the datasets. Preoperative evaluation of coronary artery disease can be an advantage of cardiac CT over other cardiac MR and echocardiography. Cardiac CT can also be very helpful when evaluating associated injuries &/or complications in cases of acquired VSDs. Cardiac CT cannot reliably measure Qp:Qs.

ECG-gated cardiac allows for the assessment biventricular function, volumes, and morphology when images are acquired using a low-pitch, retrospective scan or an axial scan during a single heartbeat using a CT scanner with a large z-axis. Overall, cardiac CT has excellent spatial resolution that allows accurate sizing of the defect and visualization of the surrounding structures for treatment planning.

Selected References

1. Lopez L et al: Classification of ventricular septal defects for the eleventh iteration of the international classification of diseases-striving for consensus: a report from the International Society for Nomenclature of Paediatric and Congenital Heart Disease. Ann Thorac Surg. 106(5):1578-89, 2018
2. Rojas CA et al: Ventricular septal defects: embryology and imaging findings. J Thorac Imaging. 28(2):W28-34, 2013
3. Johri AM et al: Imaging of atrial septal defects: echocardiography and CT correlation. Heart. 97(17):1441-53, 2011
4. Rajiah P et al: Cardiac MRI: Part 1, cardiovascular shunts. AJR Am J Roentgenol. 197(4):W603-20, 2011

Atrial Septal Defects

KEY FACTS

TERMINOLOGY

- Atrial septal defect (ASD)
- Interatrial septum defects that allow left-to-right shunt

IMAGING

- Radiography
  - Enlarged right ventricle and right atrium with shunt vascularity
- Cardiac gated CTA
  - Direct visualization of ASD
  - Evaluation of right atrial and ventricular volumes, associated abnormalities
- MR
  - Direct visualization of ASD
  - Determination of shunt volume and direction
  - Evaluation of right atrial and ventricular volumes, associated abnormalities
- Possible visualization of mitral valve prolapse

TOP DIFFERENTIAL DIAGNOSES

- Ventricular septal defect
- Patent ductus arteriosus
- Pulmonary artery hypertension

CLINICAL ISSUES

- Usually asymptomatic in early life
- Becomes symptomatic with advancing age
- 90% of patients become symptomatic by 40 years
  - Exertional dyspnea, fatigue, palpitations, congestive heart failure
- Surgical repair
  - Open repair with extracorporeal support most common
  - Minimally invasive approaches
- Percutaneous transcatheter therapy
  - Small ostium secundum defects most amenable with rim > 5 mm
  - Fewer complications vs. surgical repair

(Left) *PA and lateral radiographs in a 46-year-old woman with dyspnea show massive enlarged central pulmonary arteries with cephalization of blood flow. On the lateral radiograph, there is marked enlargement of the right ventricle (RV)* ➡. **(Right)** *Anatomic (left) and Doppler (right) images from an echocardiogram show a large ostium secundum atrial septal defect (ASD)* ➡. *On atrial systole, there is right-to-left flow across the ASD* ➡ *due to severe pulmonary hypertension. The right heart is enlarged.*

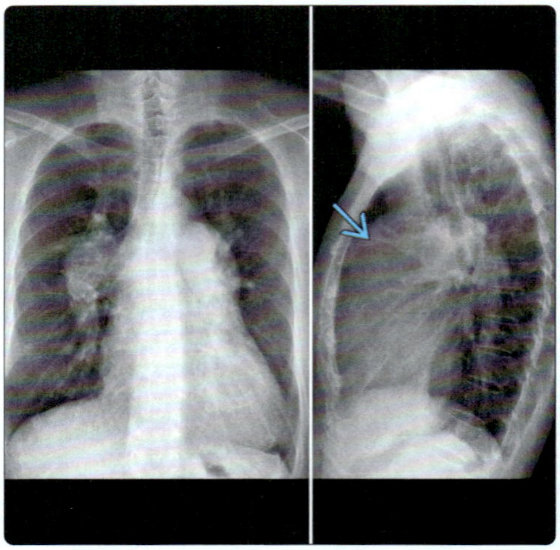

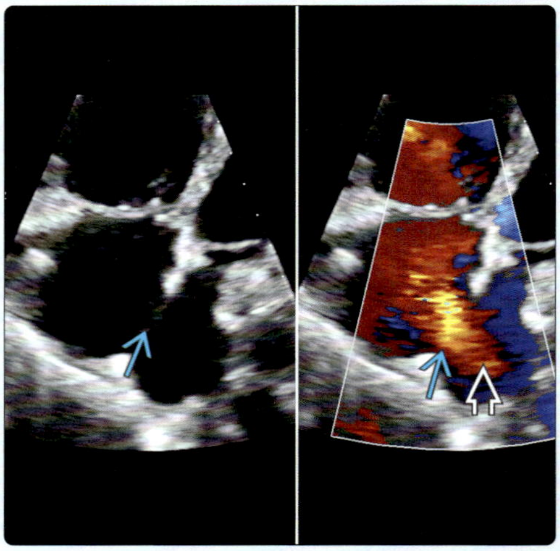

(Left) *Gated CT in the same patient shows the large secundum ASD* ➡ *with right-to-left flow* ➡, *consistent with Eisenmenger physiology. The RV is severely dilated and hypertrophied, and the right atrium (RA) is dilated.* **(Right)** *4D flow MR in the same patient nicely shows the right-to-left flow* ➡ *across the ASD during atrial contraction. Left-to-right flow was present during atrial diastole. Given bidirectional flow across the ASD, the Qp:Qs was 1.06. Due to Eisenmenger physiology, the patient was referred for heart-lung transplant.*

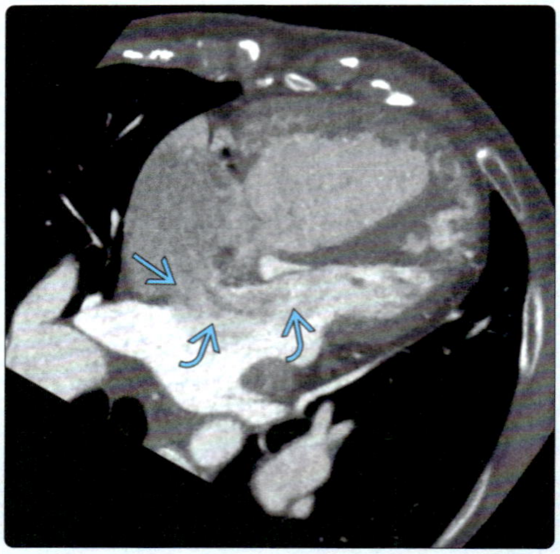

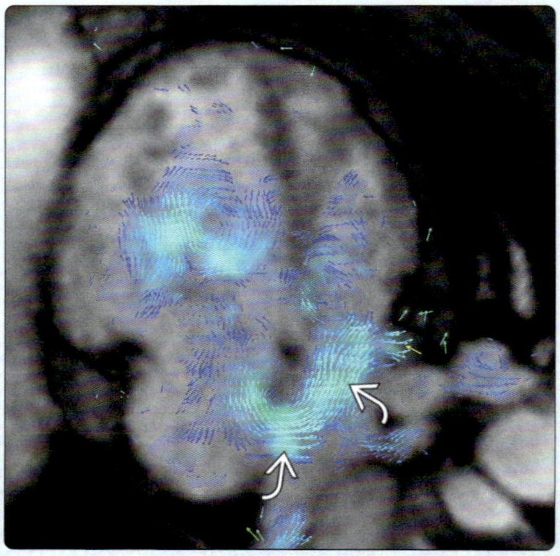

TERMINOLOGY

Abbreviations

- Atrial septal defect (ASD)

Definitions

- Interatrial septum defects allow interatrial communication

IMAGING

General Features

- Best diagnostic clue
  - Direct visualization of defect on cardiac MR or CT
- Location
  - Ostium primum defect (15-20%)
    - Anterior/inferior interatrial septum
    - May involve atrioventricular valves
  - Ostium secundum defect (75%)
    - Mid interatrial septum
    - Oval defect bordered by fossa ovalis
  - Sinus venosus defect (SV-ASD) (5-10%)
    - Superior interatrial septum near superior vena cava (SVC) or inferior interatrial septum near inferior vena cava (IVC)
    - Superior or inferior to fossa ovalis
  - Unroofed coronary sinus (UCS) (< 1%)
    - Communication between left atrium (LA) and coronary sinus (CS)
      - Type I: Complete unroofing of CS and persistent left SVC (PLSVC)
      - Type II: Complete unroofing of CS without PLSVC
      - Type III: Partial unroofing of midportion CS
      - Type IV: Partially unroofing of terminal portion CS
    - Interatrial septum intact
  - Biatrial drainage of right SVC (a.k.a. cavopulmonary venous defect or venovenous bridge) (< 1%)
    - Defect between right SVC and right upper &/or middle pulmonary vein
      - Pulmonary veins retain their normal connection to LA resulting in left-to-right shunt
      - Associated narrowing of SVC-right atrial junction results in predominantly right-to-left shunt
    - Interatrial septum is intact as such

Radiographic Findings

- Radiography
  - Enlargement of right atrium (RA) and right ventricle (RV) depends on size of ASD
  - LA typically normal in size
    - Differentiates ASD from ventricular septal defect (VSD) and patent ductus arteriosus (PDA)
  - **Shunt vascularity**
  - Findings of pulmonary hypertension
    - Enlarged pulmonary trunk and pulmonary arteries
    - Enlarged RA and RV

CT Findings

- Cardiac gated CTA
  - Direct visualization and sizing of ASD
  - Enlarged RA and RV
  - Enlarged pulmonary arteries
  - Associated abnormalities
    - Partial anomalous pulmonary venous return (PAPVR)
      - Strongest association with SV-ASD
      - Pulmonary vein draining into SVC
      - Usually involves vein draining right upper lobe &/or right middle lobe
    - Left-sided SVC
      - Associated with type I UCS

MR Findings

- Cine MR
  - Direct visualization and sizing of ASD
  - Assessment of shunt volume and direction
  - Enlarged RA and RV
  - Enlarged pulmonary arteries
  - Associated anomalies
    - PAPVR
- Phase-contrast MR
  - Shunt volume and fraction calculation through Qp:Qs
  - Direct quantification of shunt: En face view
  - Typically 2D flow; 4D flow allows quantification from single imaging volume
- MR angiography
  - Associated vascular abnormalities

Echocardiographic Findings

- Echocardiogram
  - Direct visualization of ASD
  - Possible visualization of associated atrioventricular valve abnormalities
- Doppler
  - Shunt volume, shunt ratios, and pulmonary artery pressures can be measured

Angiographic Findings

- Cardiac catheterization
  - Performed when echocardiography is inconclusive or to evaluate associated abnormalities
  - Shunt fraction

Imaging Recommendations

- Best imaging tool
  - Echocardiogram, MR, and CT are complementary

DIFFERENTIAL DIAGNOSIS

Patent Foramen Ovale

- Lack of fusion between septum secundum and flap of septum primum
- Present in ≤ 1/3 of population
- Normal communication between LA and RA in fetal life
- Tunnel configuration of interatrial communication
  - Left-to-right shunt directed to inferior RA
  - Right-to-left shunt directed to roof of LA
- Considered clinically relevant in patients with cryptogenic stroke and arterial hypoxemia that may require closure

Ventricular Septal Defect

- Defect in interventricular septum (perimembranous central, outlet, trabecular muscular, and inlet)
- Left-to-right intracardiac shunt
- Enlarged cardiac silhouette: LA and left ventricle (LV)

- Shunt vascularity

Patent Ductus Arteriosus

- Persistent connection between descending thoracic aorta and proximal left pulmonary artery
- Left-to-right extracardiac shunt
- Enlarged cardiac silhouette: LA and LV
- Enlarged aortic arch: Distinguishes PDA from VSD
- Shunt vascularity

Pulmonary Hypertension

- Mean pulmonary pressure > 20 mmHg

PATHOLOGY

General Features

- Etiology
  - Ostium secundum
    - Incomplete development of septum primum or septum secundum at fossa ovalis
  - Ostium primum
    - Incomplete fusion of septum primum and septum secundum with endocardial cushion
  - SV
    - Interatrial connection near the upper or lower SVC-right atrial junction
- Genetics
  - Ellis van Creveld
    - Skeletal dysplasia with common atrium
    - Autosomal recessive pattern of inheritance
  - Holt-Oram syndrome
    - ASD and upper extremity anomalies
    - Autosomal dominant pattern of inheritance
  - Trisomy 21
    - Associated with ostium primum and endocardial cushion defects
  - Other syndromes
    - Familial ASD associated with progressive atrioventricular block
      - Autosomal dominant pattern of inheritance
- Associated abnormalities
  - Mitral valve abnormalities
    - Double-orifice mitral valve
      - 2% of ostium primum defects
    - Mitral valve cleft
  - PAPVR return with SV-ASD
  - PLSVC with type I UCS

CLINICAL ISSUES

Presentation

- Most common signs/symptoms
  - May be asymptomatic in early life
    - Some patients may be symptomatic
      - Dyspnea, fatigue, and congestive heart failure
  - Typically become symptomatic with advancing age
    - 90% of patients with ASD symptomatic by age 40
  - Pulmonary arterial hypertension (PAH)
    - Dyspnea on exertion, fatigue, syncope, chest pain
  - Eisenmenger syndrome
    - May develop in large shunts that lead to PAH and increase right heart pressures
    - Shunt reversal: Left-to-right becomes right-to-left shunt
    - Cyanosis, polycythemia, clubbing
    - Precludes repair

Demographics

- Epidemiology
  - Most common congenital cardiac anomaly in adults, 10% of all congenital cardiac anomalies

Natural History & Prognosis

- 20% close spontaneously during 1st year of life
  - Spontaneous closure in adulthood is unlikely
- 1% become symptomatic during 1st year of life
  - 0.1% mortality
- Defects may result in PAH
  - May be reversible if treated early
  - Development of Eisenmenger syndrome
- 25% lifetime mortality rate if unrepaired

Treatment

- Medical therapy
  - Limited to atrial arrhythmias and volume overload
- Defect closure (surgical or endovascular)
  - Indications
    - Right ventricular overload without pulmonary hypertension, ± symptoms
    - Patients with documented orthodeoxia-platypnea
      - Arterial desaturation (orthodeoxia) and dyspnea (platypnea) in upright position with improvement in supine position
    - Patients with paradoxical embolism
    - At time of mitral valve repair (patients with primum ASD)
  - Contraindications
    - Eisenmenger syndrome, severe PAH
  - Open repair with extracorporeal support most common
    - Direct closure and patch repair
  - Minimally invasive approaches
    - No difference in morbidity and mortality
  - Percutaneous transcatheter therapy
    - Fewer complications and decreased hospitalization time vs. surgical repair
    - Success rates: ± 96%
    - Small ostium secundum defects most amenable with rim > 5 mm

DIAGNOSTIC CHECKLIST

Consider

- ASD in setting of enlarged right-side chambers with normal LA and shunt vascularity on chest radiography

SELECTED REFERENCES

1. Panjwani B et al: CT and MR imaging for atrial septal defect repair. Semin Roentgenol. 59(1):103-11, 2024
2. Ranganath P et al: Computed tomography in adult congenital heart disease. Radiol Clin North Am. 57(1):85-111, 2019
3. Sun L et al: Evaluation of unroofed coronary sinus syndrome using cardiovascular CT angiography: an observational study. AJR Am J Roentgenol. 211(2):314-20, 2018

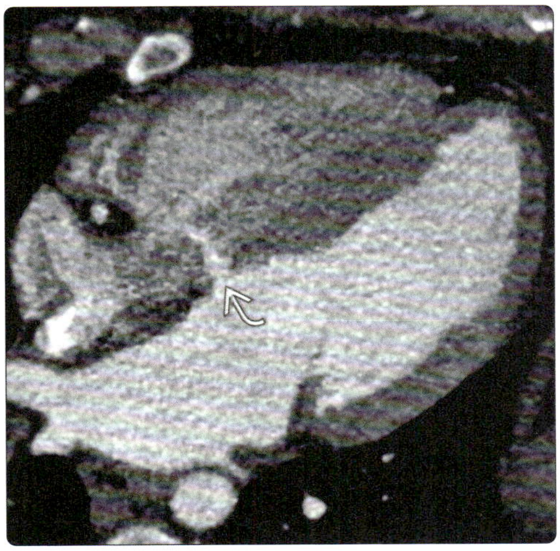

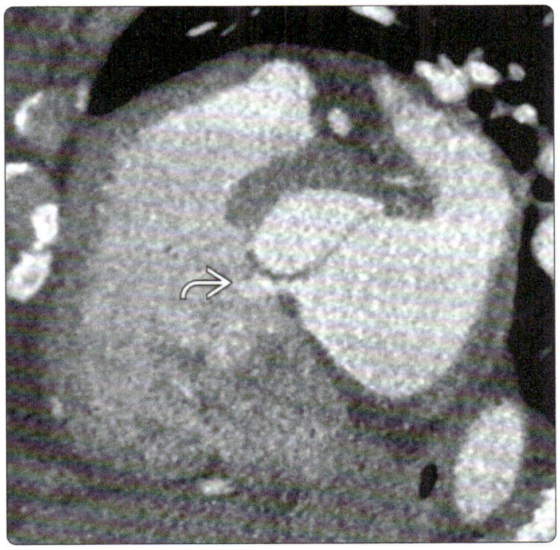

(Left) *Four-chamber cardiac CT demonstrates a small defect in the interatrial septum immediately posterior to the atrioventricular valves, compatible with an ostium primum ASD* ➨*.* **(Right)** *Short-axis cardiac CT in the same patient demonstrates a small defect in the superior and anterior interatrial septum, compatible with an ostium primum ASD* ➨*. There is no enlargement of the right heart secondary to the small size of the defect.*

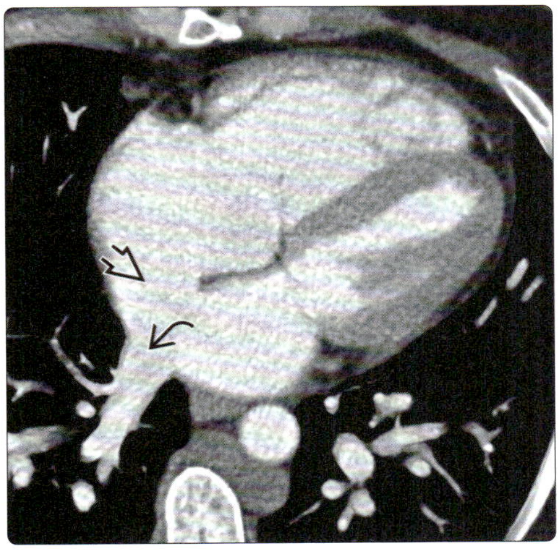

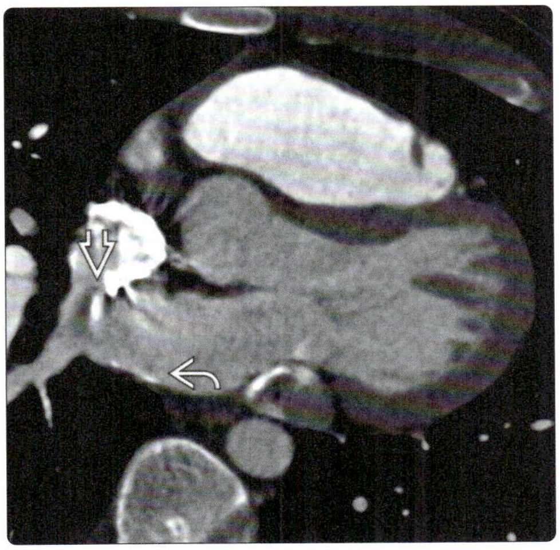

(Left) *Four-chamber cardiac CT demonstrates a large defect in the posterior and inferior interatrial septum* ➨ *at the level of the right inferior pulmonary vein insertion* ➨*, indicating inferior sinus venosus ASD.* **(Right)** *Three-chamber cardiac CT shows a defect in the superior interatrial septum at the superior vena cava-right atrial junction, indicating a superior sinus venosus ASD* ➨*. Note the high-density contrast material in the dependent left atrium, the fallen contrast sign* ➨*.*

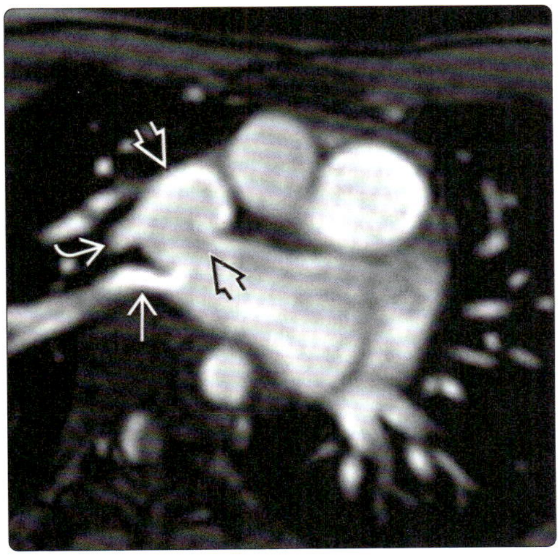

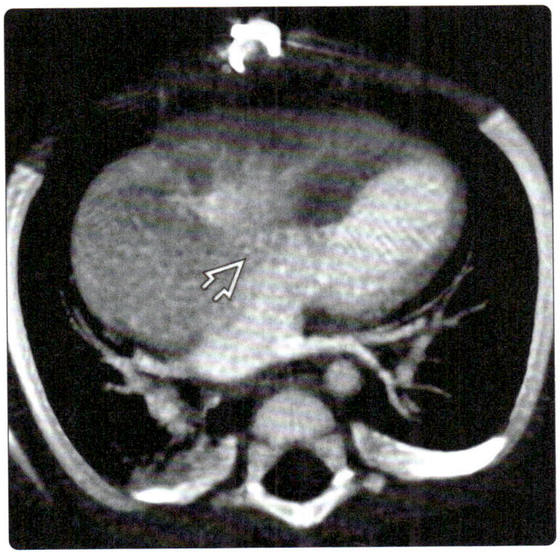

(Left) *Axial oblique cine MR demonstrates a large superior sinus venosus ASD* ➨ *with partial anomalous pulmonary venous return* ➨ *to the superior vena cava (SVC)* ➨*. Note the right inferior pulmonary vein entering the left atrium* ➨*.* **(Right)** *Four-chamber CTA of the chest demonstrates free communication between the 4 cardiac chambers at the crux of the heart* ➨*, indicating endocardial cushion defect. Note the contrast shunting from the left heart into the RV.*

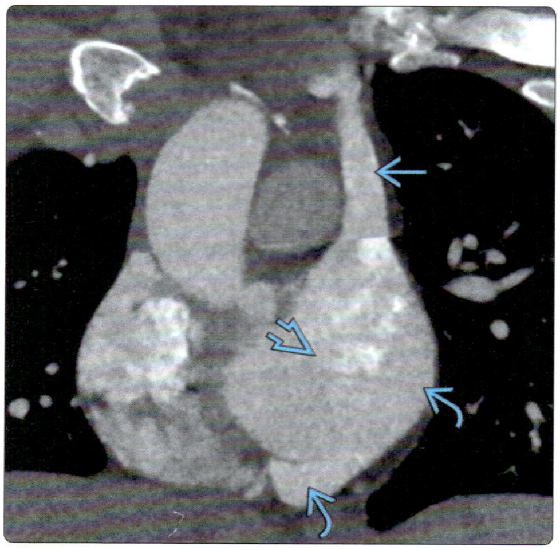

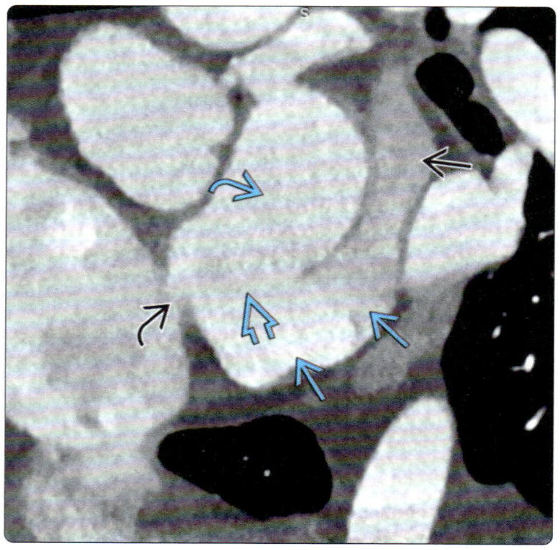

(Left) *Coronal oblique CECT in a patient with a type I unroofed coronary sinus (UCS) with a left-sided SVC ➡ shows a complete defect between the coronary sinus ➡ and the left atrium ➡.* **(Right)** *Short-axis CT in a patient with a type II UCS shows an enlarged great cardiac vein (GCV) ➡ with a UCS ➡, which communicates with the left atrium ➡ through a large defect ➡. There is no left-sided SVC. A moderate size patent foramen ovale (PFO) ➡ is present.*

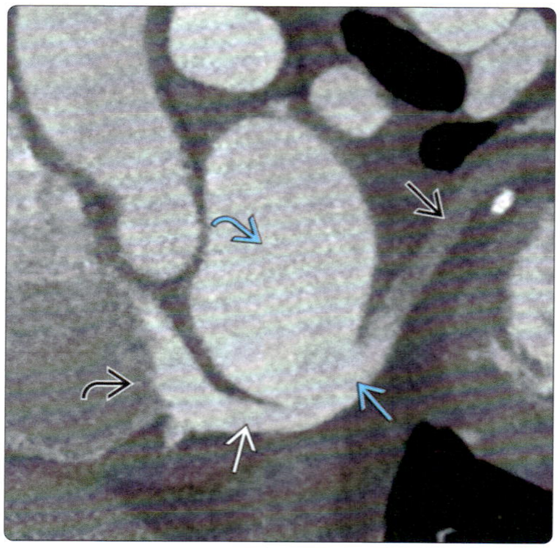

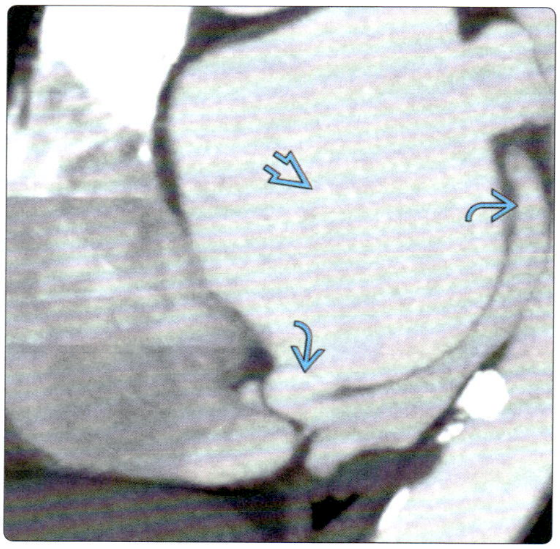

(Left) *Short-axis CECT shows a type III UCS with a partially unroofed midportion of the coronary sinus ➡, which continues distal to the defect ➡ and drains into the right atrium ➡. Note the left atrium ➡ and GCV ➡.* **(Right)** *Coronal oblique MIP in a patient with UCS type IV shows partial unroofing of the distal coronary sinus near the thebesian valve. Note the left atrium ➡ and GCV ➡.*

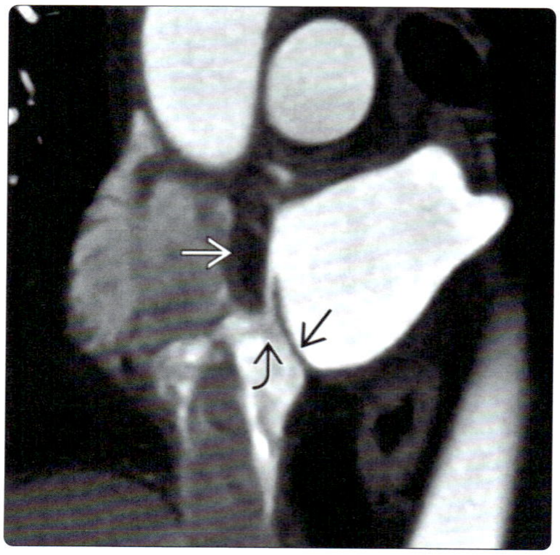

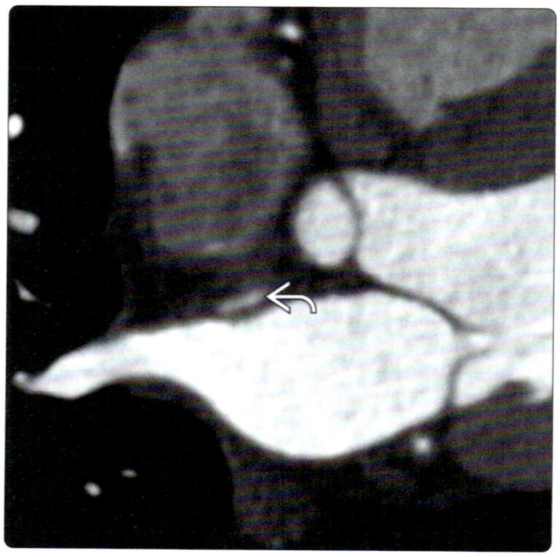

(Left) *Short-axis cardiac CT shows a PFO with lack of fusion between septum secundum ➡ and the flap valve of septum primum ➡. Shunting of high-attenuated blood from the left atrium to the right atrium ➡ is present.* **(Right)** *Four-chamber cardiac CT demonstrates the interatrial tunnel of a PFO ➡. This is a common finding, and PFO can be called only if contrast enters the right atrium.*

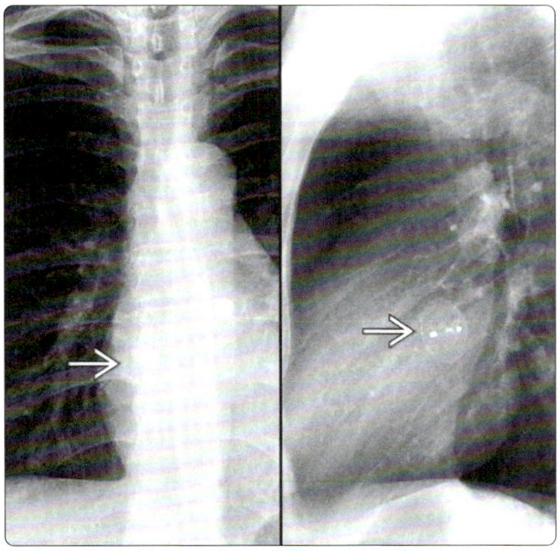

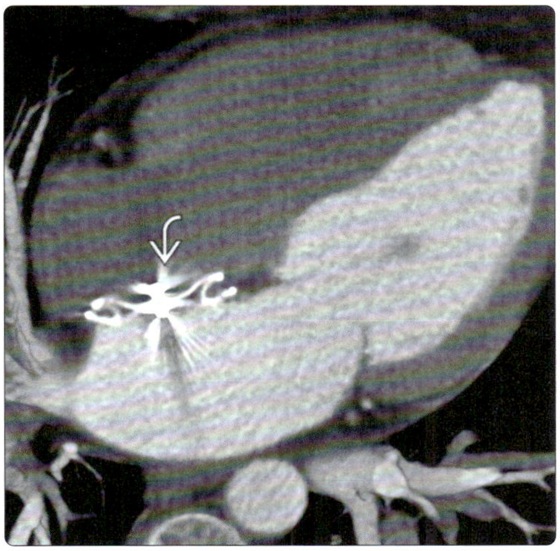

(Left) *PA and lateral chest radiographs in a patient following percutaneous closure of an ASD demonstrate an atrial septal occluder ➔ projecting over the expected position of the interatrial septum.* **(Right)** *Four-chamber cardiac CT demonstrates a normally seated, self-centering Amplatzer Septal Occluder device ➔ (AGA; Plymouth, MN) in place from endovascular closure of an ostium secundum ASD.*

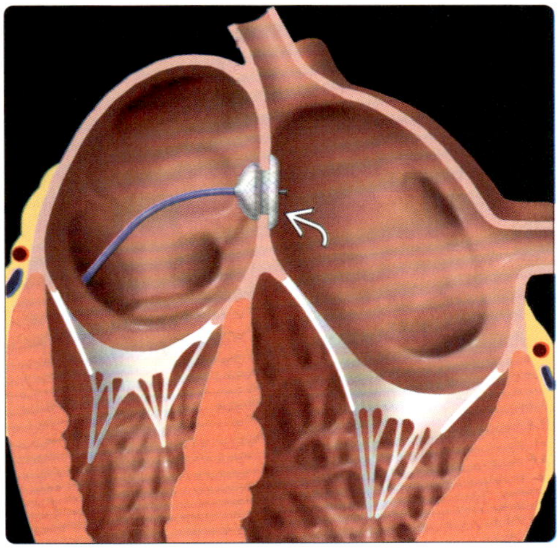

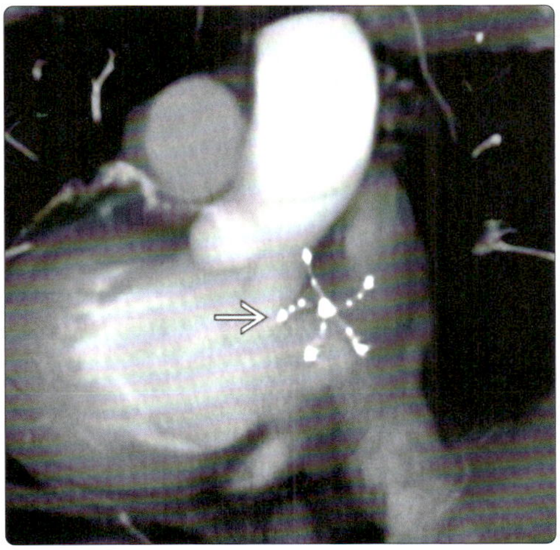

(Left) *Graphic shows the placement of an atrial septal occluder introduced into the right atrium via the inferior vena cava approach. The device is placed and expanded within the ASD ➔ so that its double-disc morphology secures it within the defect, resulting in closure.* **(Right)** *Coronal oblique cardiac CT shows a normally seated, self-centering CardioSEAL STARFlex Septal Occluder device ➔ (NMT Medical; Boston, MA) in place from endovascular closure of an ostium secundum ASD.*

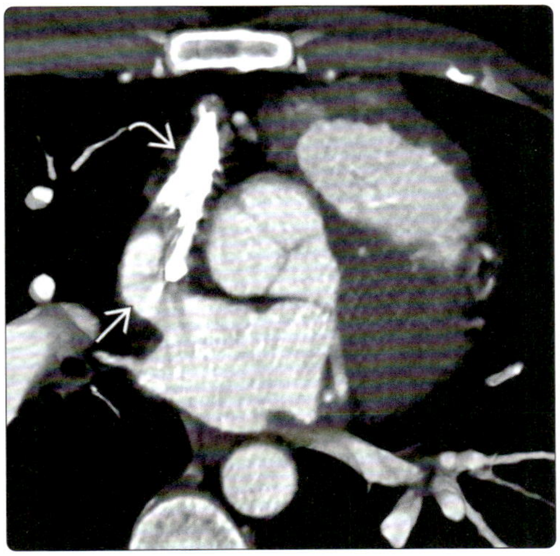

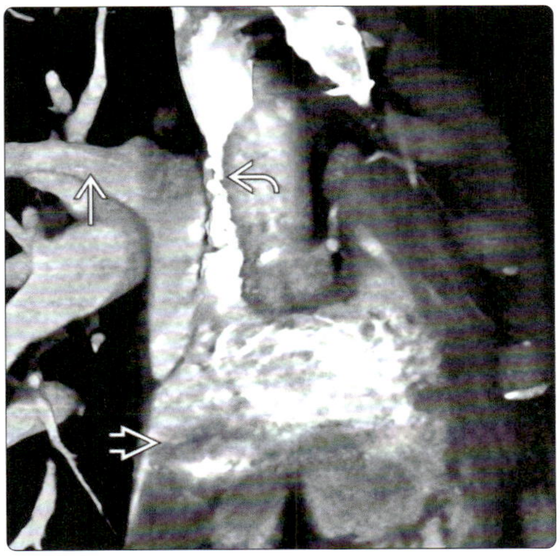

(Left) *Axial oblique cardiac CT in a patient with superior sinus venosus defect after surgical repair (Warden procedure) shows high-density contrast flowing through reconstructed SVC ➔ into the right atrium. The abnormal venous return of the right upper lobe has been baffled ➔ back into the left atrium.* **(Right)** *Coronal oblique cardiac CT (same patient) shows high-density contrast flowing through the reconstructed SVC ➔ into the right atrium ➔. The abnormal venous return of the right upper lobe ➔ has been baffled back into left atrium.*

Ventricular Septal Defects

KEY FACTS

TERMINOLOGY

- Ventricular septal defect (VSD)
  - Perimembranous central
  - Muscular
  - Inlet
  - Outlet

IMAGING

- Chest radiographs may be normal with small defects
- Cardiac enlargement with larger defects
  - Left atrial enlargement: Distinguishes VSD and patent ductus arteriosus (PDA) from atrial septal defect (ASD)
- Aortic arch normal in size: Distinguishes VSD from PDA
- Findings of pulmonary artery hypertension
- Direct visualization of VSD on echocardiography (ECG), CT, and MR
  - ECG: Identifies and characterizes most VSDs
  - MR: Ventricular volumes and function; direction and quantification of shunt

TOP DIFFERENTIAL DIAGNOSES

- ASD
- PDA
- Myocardial crypt

PATHOLOGY

- Congenital most common
- 4 types depending on location of defect: Perimembranous central, outlet, trabecular muscular, and inlet

CLINICAL ISSUES

- Patients with small defects may be asymptomatic
  - Perimembranous defects often close by overgrowth of septal leaflet of tricuspid valve that extends over VSD
- Small VSDs typically close spontaneously
- Large VSDs require surgical correction
- Large or longstanding defects may result in pulmonary hypertension and Eisenmenger syndrome
- Treatment can be medical or surgical

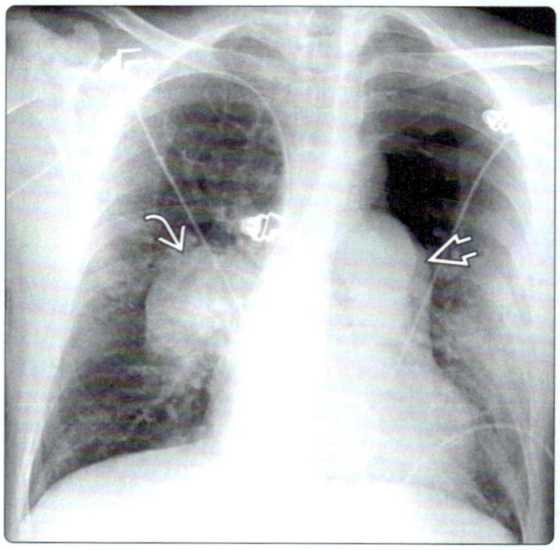
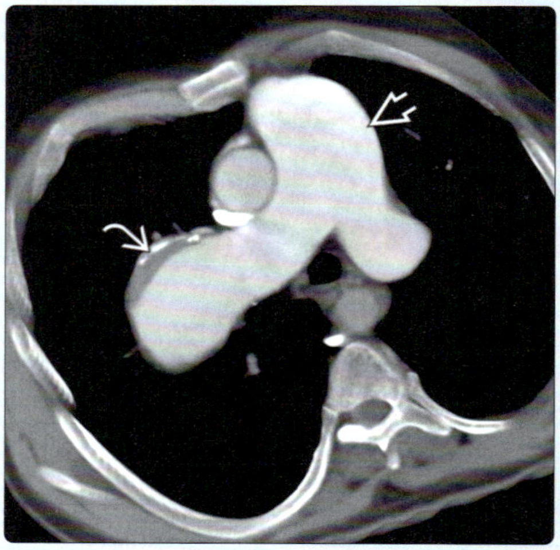

(Left) *AP radiograph of the chest demonstrates severe enlargement of the main* ➔ *and central pulmonary arteries (PAs), most conspicuous on the right* ➔*.* **(Right)** *Axial oblique cardiac CT in the same patient demonstrates massive enlargement of the pulmonary trunk* ➔ *and main PAs. Intimal calcification* ➔ *and a small amount of adjacent mural thrombus is due to atherosclerotic disease from near systemic PA pressures.*

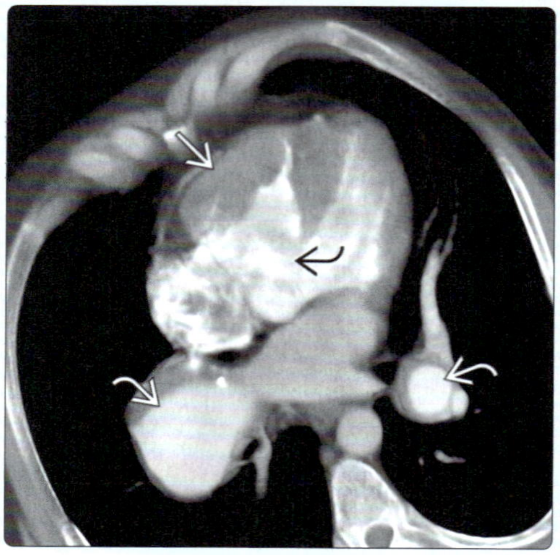
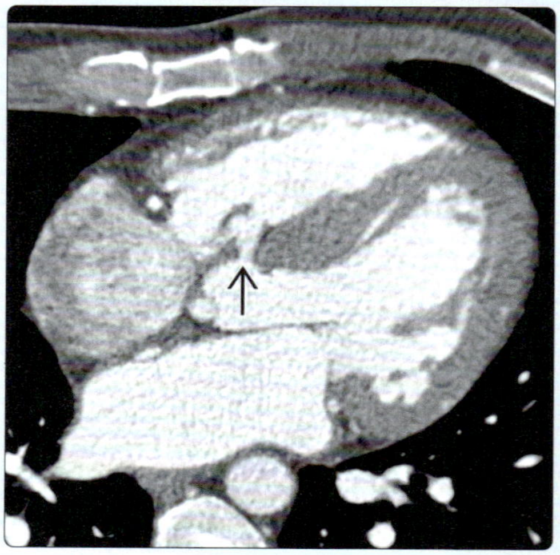

(Left) *Axial oblique cardiac CT in the same patient demonstrates a large perimembranous central ventricular septal defect (VSD)* ⇨ *associated with right ventricular muscular hypertrophy* ➔ *and massive enlargement of the PAs* ➔*. Note that there is no enlargement of the cardiac chambers.* **(Right)** *Axial cardiac gated CTA demonstrates a perimembranous central VSD* →*.*

TERMINOLOGY

Abbreviations

- Ventricular septal defect (VSD)

IMAGING

General Features

- Best diagnostic clue
  - Defect in ventricular septum resulting in direct communication of ventricles
  - Congenital or acquired
  - Enlargement of right ventricle, pulmonary vasculature, left atrium, and left ventricle on chest radiography
- Location
  - Perimembranous central (75%), inlet (8-10%), trabecular muscular (5-10%), outlet (5%)
- Morphology
  - In infants and children, defects can be classified by size and ratio of pulmonary:systemic blood flow (Qp:Qs)
    - Small/restrictive (< 4 mm, Qp:Qs < 1.5)
    - Moderate (4-6 mm, Qp:Qs 1.5-2.3)
    - Large (> 6 mm, Qp:Qs > 2.3)
  - In adults, defects can be classified according to size with respect to aortic anulus diameter
    - Small (< 25% of aortic anulus diameter)
    - Moderate (25-75% of aortic anulus diameter)
    - Large (> 75% of aortic anulus diameter)
  - Multiple defects may occur
    - More common in muscular septum (Swiss cheese VSD)

Radiographic Findings

- Radiography
  - Chest radiographs may be normal in patients with small defects
  - **Moderate-sized defects**
    - Mild to moderate enlargement of cardiac silhouette
      - Right atrial and ventricular dilation best seen on frontal and lateral views, respectively
    - Enlarged pulmonary vasculature
  - **Large defects**
    - Enlargement of cardiac silhouette
    - Aortic arch normal in size; enlarged with patent ductus arteriosus (PDA)
    - Enlargement pulmonary vasculature
    - Pulmonary edema and pleural effusions

CT Findings

- Cardiac gated CTA
  - **Direct visualization of VSD**
  - Location, size, and number of defects

MR Findings

- SSFP cine
  - Visualization of VSD, morphology, valvular function
  - Quantification of ventricular volume, mass, function
- Phase-contrast MR
  - Shunt volume, direction, fraction

Echocardiographic Findings

- Echocardiogram
  - Most VSDs identified and sufficiently characterized by echocardiography (ECG)
  - Direct visualization of defects and direction and velocity of shunting on Doppler/duplex sonography
- Color Doppler
  - Helpful in detecting small defects

Angiographic Findings

- Small defects
  - Normal right heart pressures
  - Normal pulmonary vascular resistance
  - Qp:Qs mildly elevated
- Large defects
  - Pulmonary and systemic systolic pressures can equilibrate
- **Eisenmenger syndrome**
  - ↑ systolic and diastolic pulmonary artery pressures
  - Desaturation of blood in left ventricle
  - Minimal left-to-right shunting or reversal of shunt

Imaging Recommendations

- Best imaging tool
  - Echocardiogram as 1st-line assessment
  - Cardiac MR or ECG-gated cardiac CTA to anatomically assess defect
  - Cardiac MR to quantify shunt

DIFFERENTIAL DIAGNOSIS

Atrial Septal Defect

- Defect in atrial septum and not ventricular septum
- Left-to-right shunt
- Left atrium may be normal in size in smaller defects

Patent Ductus Arteriosus

- Persistent connection between descending thoracic aorta and proximal left pulmonary artery
- Left-to-right shunt
- Enlargement of aortic arch: Distinguishes PDA from VSD

Ventricular Septal Crypt

- Deep crypts or clefts can occur in interventricular septum
- However, no left-to-right flow

Numerous Other Causes of Pulmonary Hypertension

- Congenital heart disease is one of many causes of pulmonary hypertension (PH)
- Detailed evaluation of patients with PH often include CT and MR

PATHOLOGY

General Features

- Etiology
  - **Congenital**: Most common etiology
  - **Traumatic**: Blunt or penetrating chest trauma
    - Common location of defect is in anteroseptum
    - Represents myocardial rupture
  - **Postmyocardial infarction**
    - Common location of defect is in inferoseptum
    - Represents myocardial rupture
  - **Endocarditis and iatrogenic**
    - Common perimembranous central location of defect

- Can result in Gerbode-type defect with communication of left ventricle and right atrium
- Associated abnormalities
  - Tetralogy of Fallot, truncus arteriosus, and double-outlet right ventricle
  - Coarctation and tricuspid atresia less common

Staging, Grading, & Classification

- 4 types depending on location of defect from right ventricle perspective
- Perimembranous central: Located below crista supraventricularis-septal band (below commissure right and noncoronary leaflets of aortic valve and behind septal leaflet of tricuspid valve)
  - Bound by both membranous and muscular tissue
  - Can be associated to misalignment of aortopulmonary septum (tetralogy of Fallot and interrupted aortic arch)
  - 1/3 close spontaneously by apposition of septal leaflet of tricuspid valve
  - Gerbode defect (left ventricle to right atrium communication) is located at atrioventricular (AV) component of membranous septum
  - AV conduction system courses inferior to defect
  - Associated with aortic valve prolapse and regurgitation
- Trabecular muscular: In trabecular portion of interventricular septum
  - Bound by muscle; 2/3 located in apical region
- Outlet: Below semilunar valve and at or above crista supraventricularis-septal band
  - Bound by fibrous anulus of semilunar valves &/or muscular tissue
  - Associated with aortic valve prolapse and regurgitation
  - AV conduction system courses inferior to defect
  - Associated with malalignment of muscular outlet septum
- Inlet: Associated with endocardial cushion defects and trisomies 18 and 21
  - Bound by tricuspid valve anulus
  - Extends to muscular septum ± membranous septum
  - Associated with malalignment of atrial septum and ventricular septum

CLINICAL ISSUES

Presentation

- Most common signs/symptoms
  - **Patients with small defects may be asymptomatic**
  - Development of symptoms depends on several factors
    - Size and location
    - Pulmonary arterial pressure
    - Left ventricular outflow resistance
  - Most common symptoms
    - Shortness of breath, tachypnea, tachycardia, and failure to thrive
  - PH
    - Dyspnea on exertion, fatigue, syncope, and chest pain
  - Eisenmenger syndrome
    - Symptoms related to polycythemia
    - Headache, fatigue, and marked dyspnea
  - Physical examination
    - Holosystolic or pansystolic murmur

Demographics

- Epidemiology
  - VSD accounts for 20% of all congenital cardiac anomalies

Natural History & Prognosis

- Defects that spontaneously close or ↓ in size early in life usually require no treatment
- Small VSDs typically close spontaneously
  - Inlet VSDs rarely close spontaneously
- Large VSDs require surgical correction
- Defects may result in PH
  - May be reversible if treated early
  - Development of Eisenmenger syndrome
    - Reversal of left-to-right shunt

Treatment

- Medical management
  - Treatment of congestive heart failure
    - Diuretics and afterload reduction
  - Treatment of Eisenmenger syndrome
    - Partial exchange transfusion
  - Endocarditis prophylaxis
- Surgical management
  - Pulmonary artery banding
    - May enable postponement of surgery
    - Constriction of VSD may be seen
  - Surgical closure
    - Indications
      - ☐ Symptomatic patients; large defects
      - ☐ Qp:Qs > 2 and clinical evidence of left ventricular volume overload
      - ☐ Prior history of endocarditis
      - ☐ Qp:Qs > 1.5 with pulmonary artery pressure < 2/3 of systemic pressure and pulmonary vascular resistance < 2/3 of systemic vascular resistance
      - ☐ Qp:Qs > 1.5 in left ventricular systolic dysfunction
    - Contraindications
      - ☐ Severe irreversible PH
  - Minimally invasive surgical closure
    - Typically for perimembranous VSD
  - Percutaneous transcatheter device occlusion
    - Typically for perimembranous and muscular VSDs
    - Complications include complete heart block, aortic and tricuspid regurgitation
  - Heart-lung transplant in Eisenmenger syndrome

DIAGNOSTIC CHECKLIST

Consider

- VSD in patient with left atrial and ventricular enlargement and ↑ pulmonary vasculature on chest radiography

Image Interpretation Pearls

- Right cardiac enlargement is less common than with ASDs

SELECTED REFERENCES

1. Kumar P et al: Role of CT in the pre- and postoperative assessment of conotruncal anomalies. Radiol Cardiothorac Imaging. 4(3):e210089, 2022
2. Lopez L et al: Classification of ventricular septal defects for the eleventh iteration of the International Classification of Diseases-Striving for Consensus: a report from the International Society for Nomenclature of Paediatric and Congenital Heart Disease. Ann Thorac Surg. 106(5):1578-89, 2018

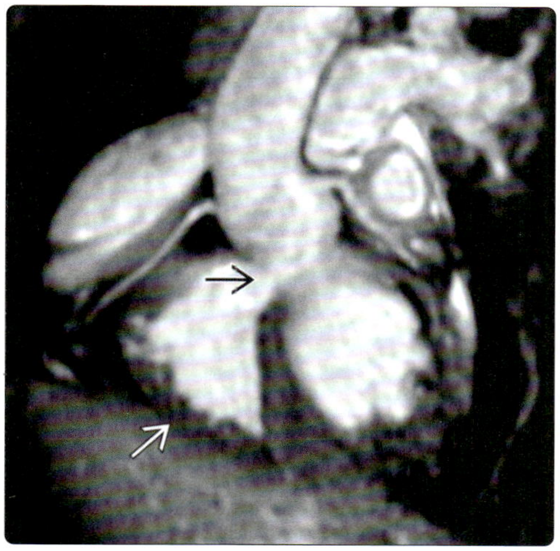

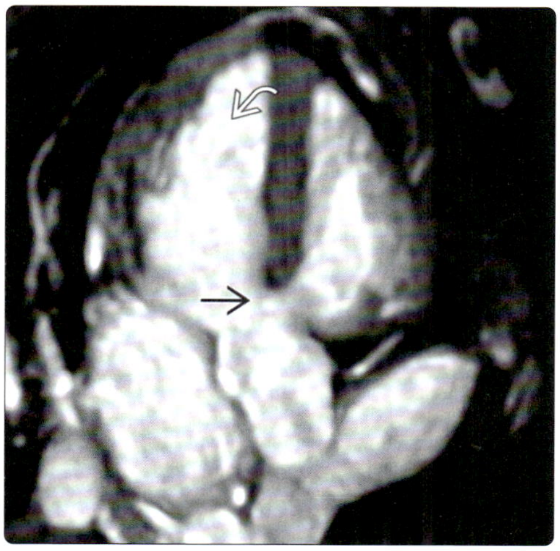

(Left) *Coronal oblique MR (3D bSSFP) demonstrates a moderately sized outlet VSD in this patient with tetralogy of Fallot. Also note right ventricular hypertrophy.* **(Right)** *Axial oblique MR (3D bSSFP) demonstrates a moderately sized outlet VSD. Note that the enlargement of the right ventricle is only mild.*

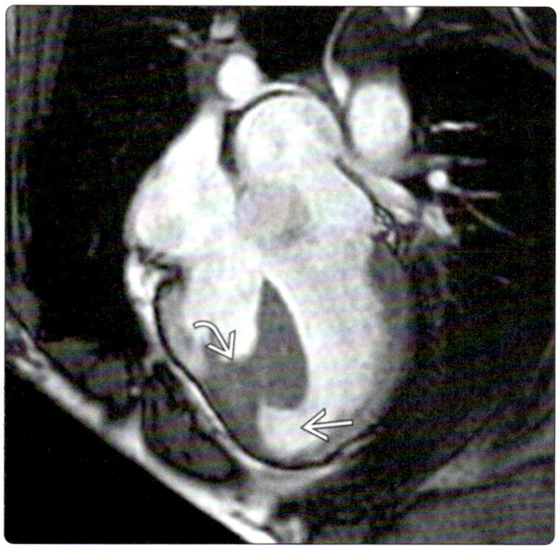

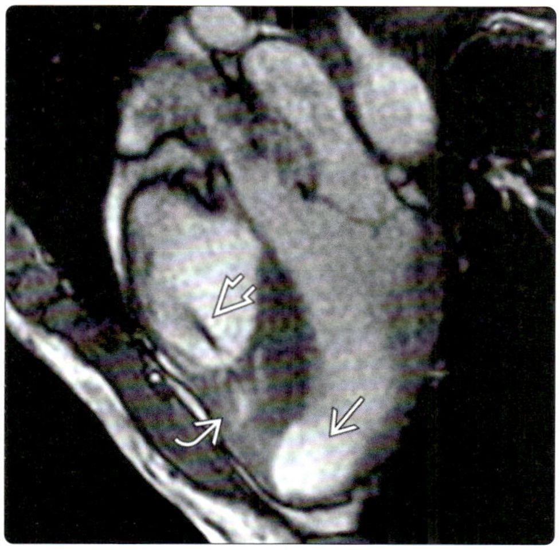

(Left) *Four-chamber MR cine single image during systole demonstrates a large apical muscular VSD associated with coarse trabeculations in the midright ventricle.* **(Right)** *Three-chamber MR cine single image in the same patient during systole shows a large, apical muscular VSD associated with coarse trabeculations in the midright ventricle and small intrachamber jet compatible with a dual-chamber right ventricle.*

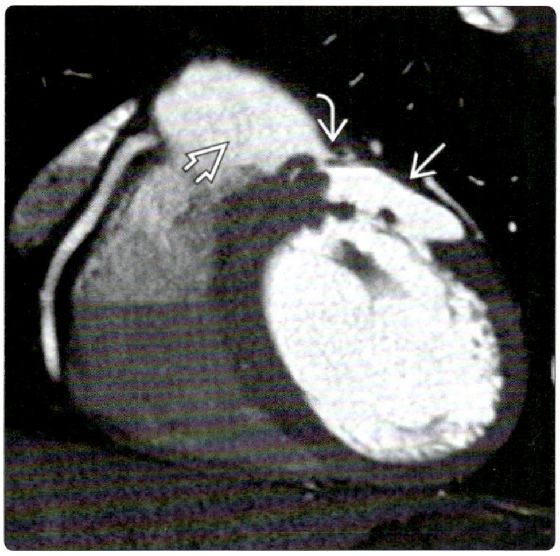

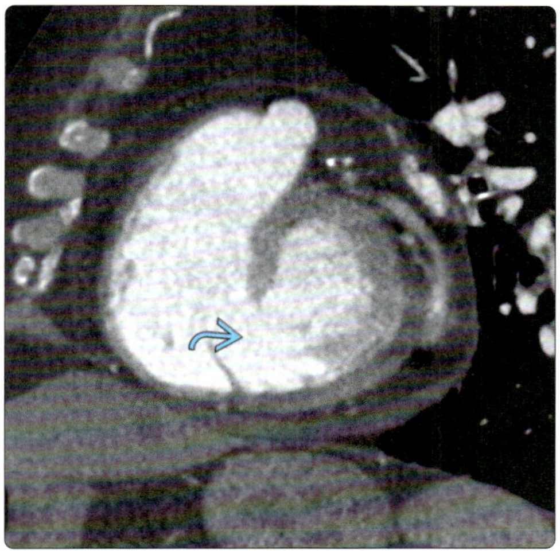

(Left) *Short-axis cardiac CT in a patient with a history of blunt trauma shows a large defect in the basal anterosuperior wall of the left ventricle extending to the right ventricular outflow tract (RVOT), compatible with a traumatic VSD.* **(Right)** *Patient with severe dyspnea 11 days after myocardial infarction shows a large inferolateral postinfarct VSD. Due to the size of the defect and lack of surrounding viable tissue, repair was not attempted. Patient was sent to hospice.*

(Left) *Sagittal reformatted cardiac gated CTA shows a small-outlet VSD* ➨*. VSDs account for ~ 20% of congenital cardiac anomalies.* **(Right)** *Axial cardiac gated CTA demonstrates a defect* ➨ *within the high aspect of the interventricular septum near the noncoronary cusp of the aorta, allowing for flow communication between the left and right ventricles.*

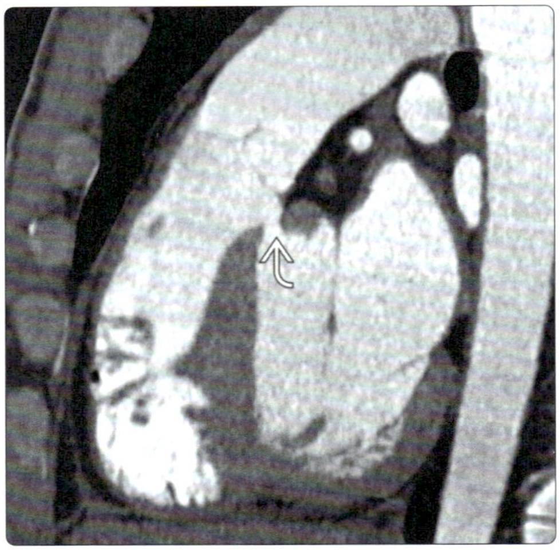

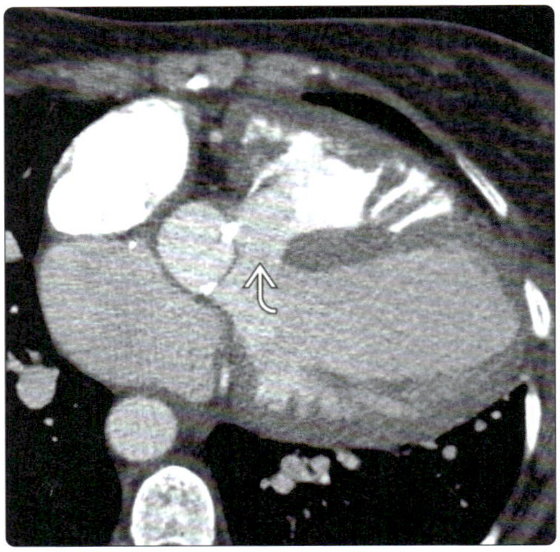

(Left) *CECT shows a small-outlet VSD* ➨ *with left-to-right flow in a 74-year-old man with severe pulmonary hypertension. The main PA measures 5.1 cm. The right ventricle is dilated and hypertrophied* ➨*. Severe emphysema also contributes to pulmonary hypertension.* **(Right)** *4D flow during systole (left) shows left-to-right flow across the VSD* ➨ *with right-to-left flow* ➨ *during early diastole due to elevated right heart pressures. The patient also had moderate pulmonic regurgitation from the VSD jet hitting the pulmonary vein.*

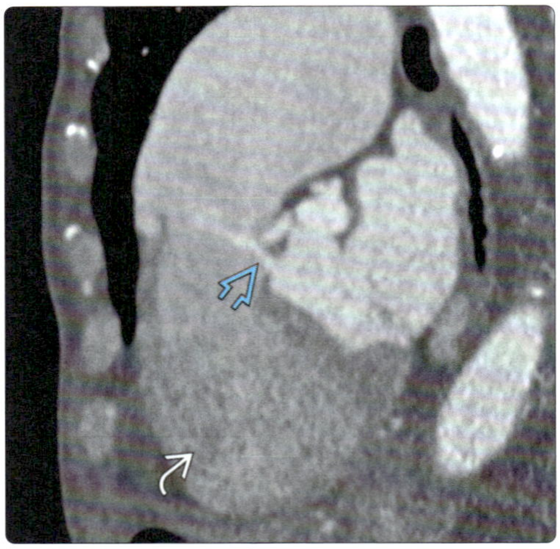

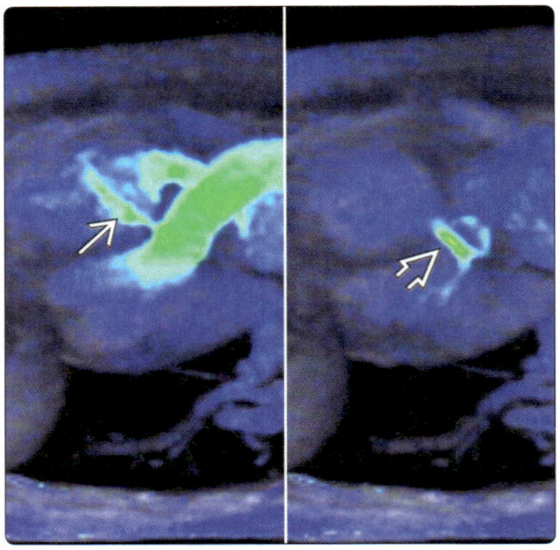

(Left) *Echocardiogram in the same patient shows left-to-right flow across the VSD during systole* ➨ *and right-to-left flow across the VSD during early diastole* ➨*.* **(Right)** *4D flow MR (left) and echo (right) images in a patient with D-transposition status post atrial switch shows a high-velocity jet* ➨ *from the left ventricular outflow tract (LVOT)* ➨ *into the right atrium* ➨ *due to a Gerbode defect.*

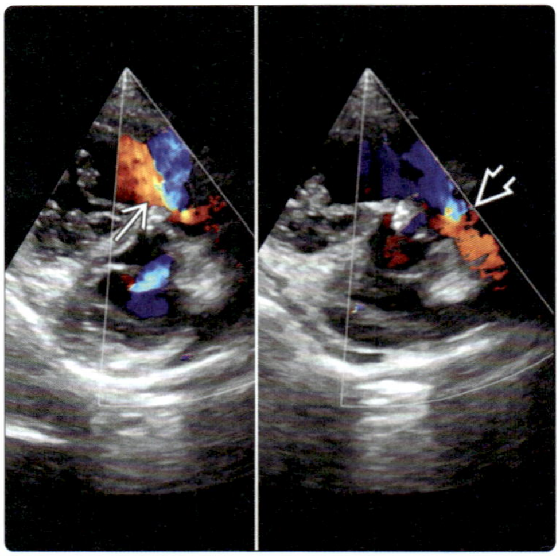

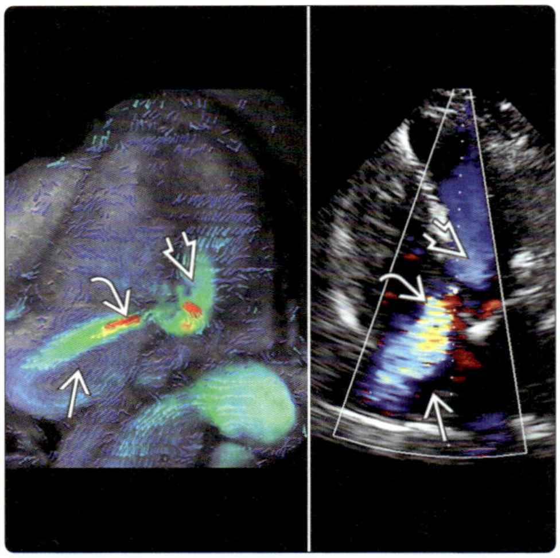

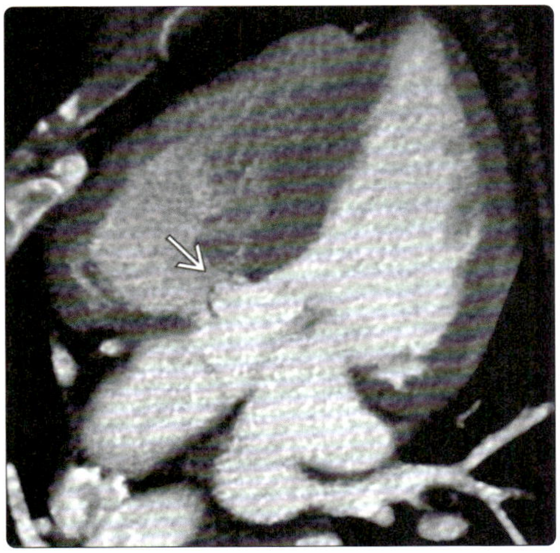

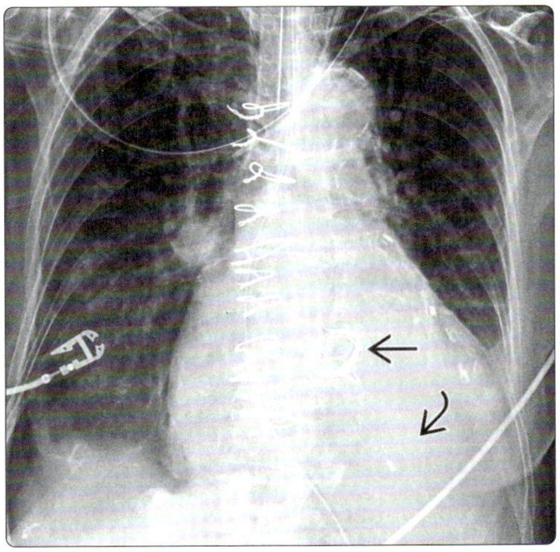

(Left) *Axial oblique cardiac CT demonstrates a small aneurysm of the interventricular septum ➡ secondary to spontaneous closure of perimembranous central VSD. No residual shunting was noted.* **(Right)** *Portable chest radiograph obtained following percutaneous device closure of a VSD shows an occluder device ➡ in the expected position of the interventricular septum. Note that it is made of the sternotomy wires in this patient with a previous aortic and mitral valve replacements ➡.*

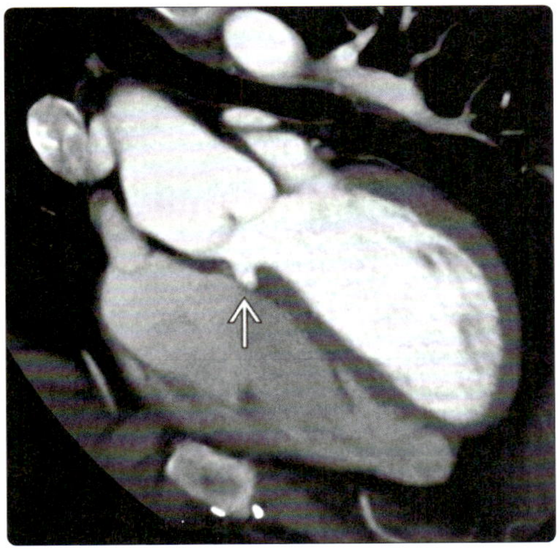

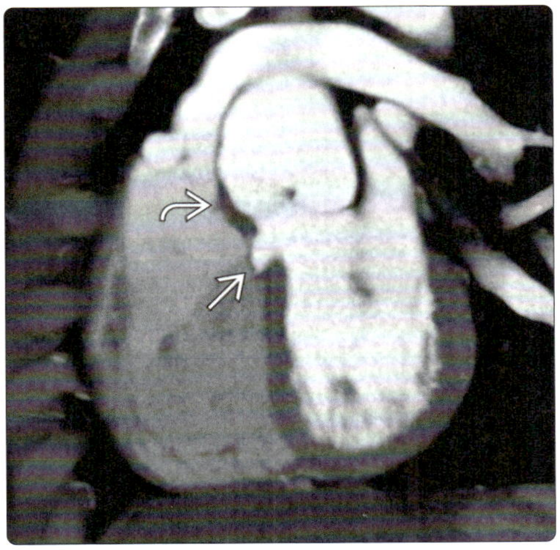

(Left) *Four-chamber cardiac CT in a patient with history of D-transposition of the great vessels and perimembranous VSD repair shows a small outpouching of contrast in the region of the perimembranous septum ➡, consistent with postsurgical change.* **(Right)** *Short-axis cardiac CT in the same patient shows a small outpouching of contrast ➡ below the crista supraventricularis ➡, consistent with postsurgical change from prior perimembranous central VSD repair. No residual shunting was noted.*

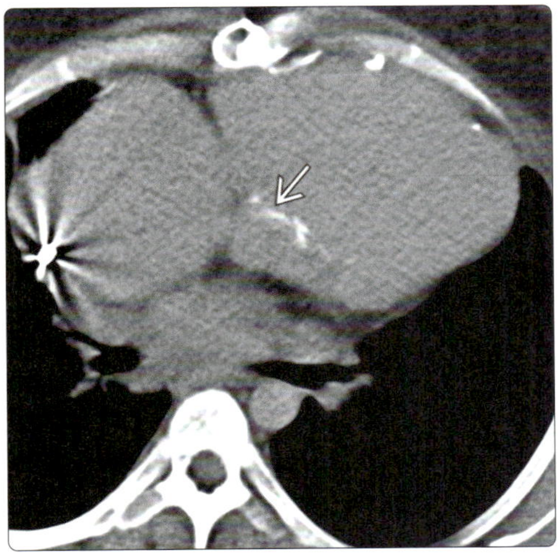

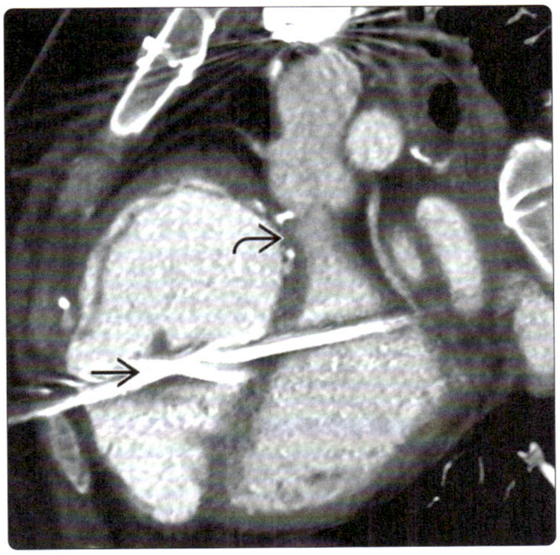

(Left) *Axial CT in a patient with history of tetralogy of Fallot demonstrates high-density material in the region of the LVOT and interventricular septum ➡ from prior patch repair of a large-outlet VSD.* **(Right)** *Short-axis cardiac CT in the same patient demonstrates high-density material in the region of the LVOT and interventricular septum ➡ from prior patch repair of a large-outlet VSD. Metallic artifact from an ICD wire ➡ is noted in the right ventricle.*

Endocardial Cushion Defect

KEY FACTS

TERMINOLOGY

- Synonyms: Atrioventricular (AV) septal defect; AV canal (AVC) defect; common AVC (CAVC); common AV orifice; atrioventricularis communis
- Broad spectrum of defects characterized by involvement in atrial septum, ventricular septum, and AV valves

IMAGING

- Echocardiography
  - Defines lesion in infants and young children
- MR
  - Direct visualization of defects
  - Evaluation of chamber size and function
  - Shunt direction and quantification

TOP DIFFERENTIAL DIAGNOSES

- Atrial septal defect
- Ventricular septal defect
- Patent ductus arteriosus
- Gerbode defect

PATHOLOGY

- Partial AVC: Ostium primum atrial septal defect + varying degrees of left AV valve malformation
- Intermediate AVC: Ostium primum atrial septal defect + inflow ventricular septal defect (restrictive) + left AV valve malformation + right AV valve malformation
- Complete AVC: Ostium primum atrial septal defect + inflow ventricular septal defect (nonrestrictive) + common AV valve

CLINICAL ISSUES

- Large AVC defects present early in life with tachypnea, tachycardia, failure to thrive
- Small partial AVC defect can be asymptomatic early in life
- Medical management of congestive heart failure
- Surgical closure of atrial- and ventricular-level defects
  - Surgical correction of AV valve clefts

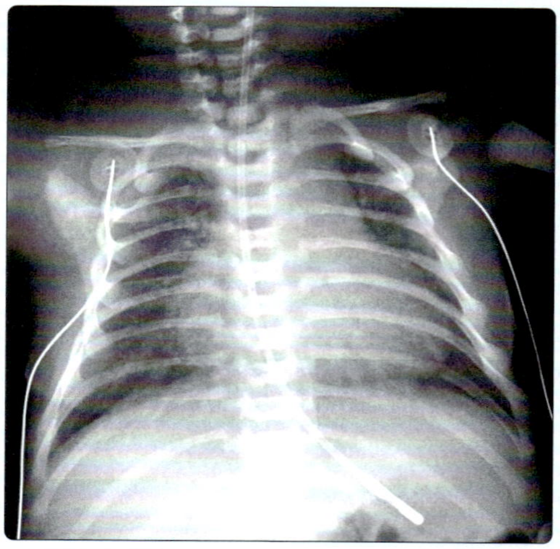
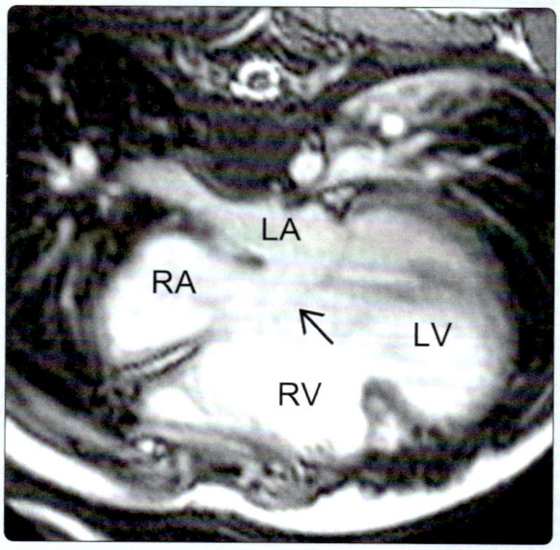

(Left) *AP radiograph in a patient with Down syndrome and known complete atrioventricular canal (AVC) shows an enlarged cardiac silhouette and increased pulmonary vascularity. Note that only 11 sets of ribs are present.* **(Right)** *Four-chamber SSFP cine MR demonstrates global cardiomegaly in a patient with a complete AVC. Note a single common AV valve ➔ and open communication between the right atrium (RA), left atrium (LA), right ventricle (RV), and left ventricle (LV).*

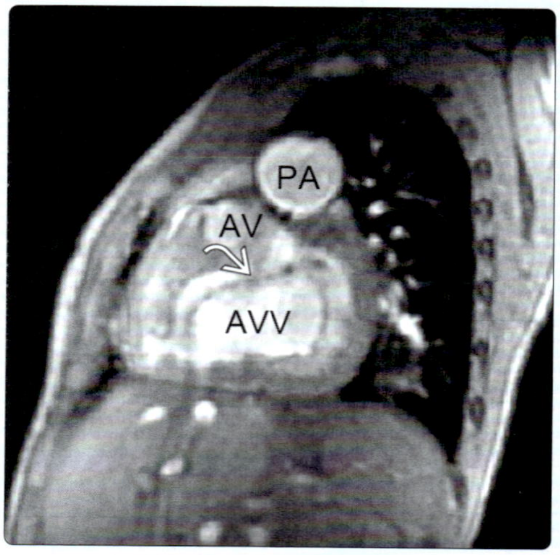

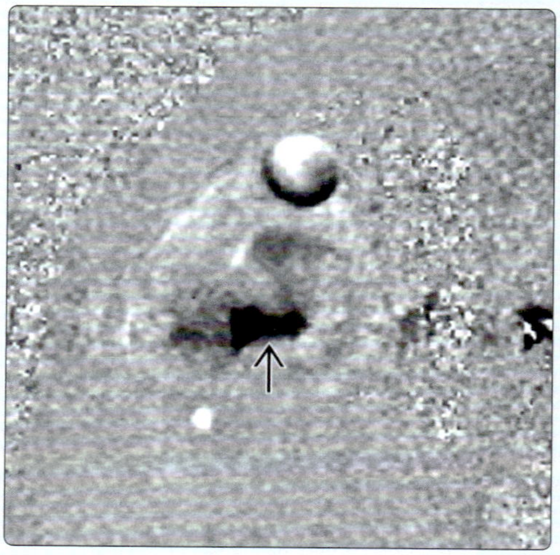

(Left) *Double oblique single cine MR through the valve plane in a patient with complete AVC demonstrates a single common AV valve. (Note in this anterior leaflet ➔ graphic, AV = aortic valve; PA = pulmonary artery.)* **(Right)** *Short-axis velocity-encoded PC MR at the level of the atria demonstrates black signal at the site of common AV valve (incomplete) coaptation during systole, indicative of AV valve regurgitation ➔.*

TERMINOLOGY

Abbreviations

- Endocardial cushion defect (ECD)

Synonyms

- Atrioventricular (AV) septal defect; AV canal (AVC) defect

Definitions

- Broad spectrum of defects secondary to deficiency of structures that originate from endocardial cushions (AV septum and septal portions of AV valves)

IMAGING

General Features

- Best diagnostic clue
  - Spectrum of intracardiac shunting ranging from interatrial communication with mitral valve cleft to single AV valve with atrial septal defect (ASD) and unrestricted ventricular septal defect (VSD)
  - Associated chamber and pulmonary arterial enlargement depending on degree of shunting
  - Elongated left ventricular outflow tract (LVOT)
- Location
  - Partial AVC
    - Defect in anteroinferior aspect of atrial septum (ostium primum ASD)
    - Coexists with cleft in anterior leaflet of mitral valve
    - 5-leaflet AV valve (single fibrous AV anulus) can be present with separate valve orifices to right and left ventricles
  - Intermediate AVC
    - Large defect in anteroinferior aspect of atrial septum (ostium primum ASD)
    - Small defect (restrictive) in ventricular septum immediately anterior to AV valve (inlet VSD)
    - Coexists with cleft in mitral and tricuspid leaflets
  - Complete AVC
    - Large defect in anterior inferior part of atrial septum (ostium primum ASD)
    - Large defect (unrestrictive) in ventricular septum immediately anterior to AV valve (inlet VSD)
    - Common AV valve: If valve opens toward 1 ventricle, hypoplasia of 1 ventricle can be present

Radiographic Findings

- Chest radiograph: Large heart with shunt vascularity
  - When mitral insufficiency is severe, left atrium can be large and cause left lower lobe to collapse

Echocardiographic Findings

- Echocardiogram
  - Defines lesion in infants and young children
    - Primum defects have echo dropout in lower portion of septum, cleft in mitral valve
    - Anterior and superior displacement of aorta due to common AV valve

MR Findings

- Phase-contrast and cine MR
  - Location, number, and size of defects; enlargement of pulmonary vasculature
  - Associated mitral or tricuspid insufficiency
  - Atrial and ventricular volumes and function
  - Shunt volume and direction; LVOT elongation ± obstruction
  - Postoperative evaluation to determine residual shunting &/or valvular insufficiency

CT Findings

- Cardiac gated CTA
  - Not done for diagnosis but identifies ASD and VSD and can quantify ventricular volumes and function
  - Surgical changes of AVC repair can be seen as high-density surgical material (patch) in anterior-inferior aspect of atrial septum, inlet portion of interventricular septum, &/or along AV valves

Angiographic Findings

- Conventional
  - Cardiac catheterization is not usually performed to characterize anatomy but to measure pulmonary vascular resistance
    - Left ventriculogram shows cleft in mitral valve, shunts, respective size of ventricles, and LVOT obstruction
  - Gooseneck deformity
    - Apical displacement of AV valves
    - Anteriorly located and narrow LVOT

Imaging Recommendations

- Best imaging tool
  - Echocardiography: Easily accessible and more commonly used to define these lesions
  - Role of MR is growing due to precise and reproducible quantification of chamber volume and function as well as quantification of shunting

DIFFERENTIAL DIAGNOSIS

Ventricular Septal Defect

- Defect only in ventricular septum

Atrial Septal Defect

- Defect only in atrial septum

Patent Ductus Arteriosus

- Communication between high-pressure aorta and lower pressure pulmonary artery

Gerbode Defect

- Defect along AV portion of membranous interventricular septum resulting in high-gradient shunt from left ventricle into right atrium
- Normal tricuspid valve anulus is apical in location in relation to mitral valve anulus, resulting in short segment of membranous septum where there is left ventricle on one side and right atrium on other

SELECTED REFERENCES

1. Sainathan S et al: National outcomes of the Fontan operation with endocardial cushion defect. J Card Surg. 37(10):3151-8, 2022
2. Backer CL et al: Shunt lesions part I: patent ductus arteriosus, atrial septal defect, ventricular septal defect, and atrioventricular septal defect. Pediatr Crit Care Med. 17(8 Suppl 1):S302-9, 2016
3. Calkoen EE et al: Atrioventricular septal defect: from embryonic development to long-term follow-up. Int J Cardiol. 202:784-95, 2016

KEY FACTS

TERMINOLOGY

- Persistent postnatal patency of normal prenatal connection from pulmonary artery to proximal descending aorta
- Category: Acyanotic, increased pulmonary blood flow
- Patent ductus arteriosus (PDA) is frequently essential part of complex congenital heart disease
  - Hypoplastic left heart syndrome, preductal coarctation, interrupted aortic arch: Conduit for systemic perfusion (R → L flow)
  - D-transposition: Necessary for admixture between systemic and pulmonary circuits (L → R flow)
  - Pulmonary atresia and other severe cyanotic heart diseases with right-sided obstruction: Conduit for pulmonary perfusion (L → R flow)

IMAGING

- Cardiomegaly (left atrium and left ventricle)
- Increased pulmonary vascularity
- Enlarged proximal aortic arch

TOP DIFFERENTIAL DIAGNOSES

- Other causes of L → R shunting
  - Septal defects, atrioventricular canal, partial anomalous pulmonary venous return
- Persistent fetal circulation syndrome

PATHOLOGY

- Postnatal persistence of normal prenatal ductus arteriosus beyond 3 months of life

CLINICAL ISSUES

- Irreversible pulmonary hypertension (Eisenmenger physiology) results in shunt reversal and cyanosis

DIAGNOSTIC CHECKLIST

- Detailed description of PDA influences percutaneous closure technique (coils vs. occluder devices)

(Left) *Graphic shows a patent ductus arteriosus (PDA) ➡ connecting the aortic isthmus to the left pulmonary artery (PA), resulting in a L → R shunt and dilated left ventricle. The high-pressure jet and L → R shunt can lead to pulmonary trunk enlargement (not shown).* **(Right)** *Oblique coronal MIP MRA shows a large abnormal connection between the PA ➡ and the distal aortic arch ➡, indicating PDA ➡. Note the higher signal intensity (Gd) blood passing from the aorta into the pulmonary circulation.*

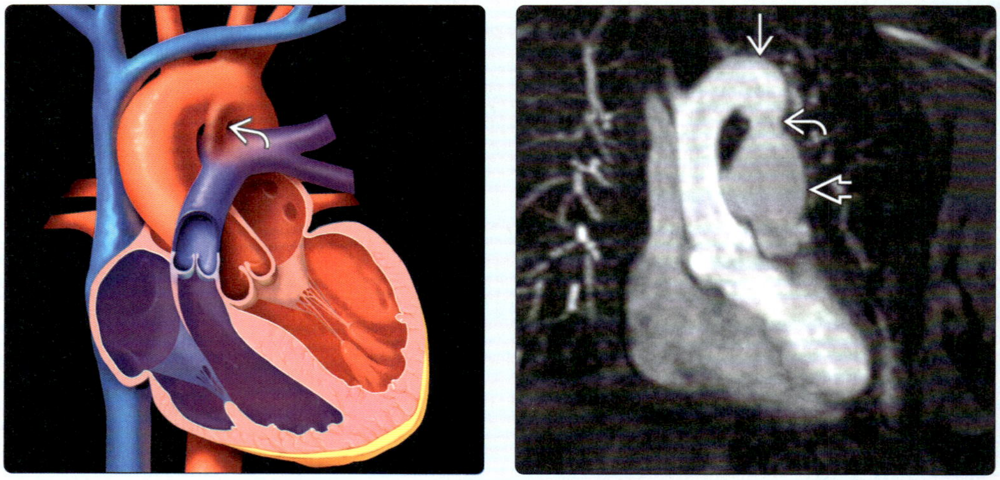

(Left) *RVOT SSFP cine MR shows a spin-dephasing flow-void artifact ➡. The jet is due to a small PDA ➡ and is directed from the aorta retrograde into the main PA. The jet is constant throughout systole and diastole due to the pressure gradient between the aorta and PA.* **(Right)** *MRA VRT shows a small PDA ➡ connecting the proximal descending aorta to the proximal left main PA. Note the enlargement of the pulmonary trunk ➡, which can cause extrinsic left main coronary artery compression.*

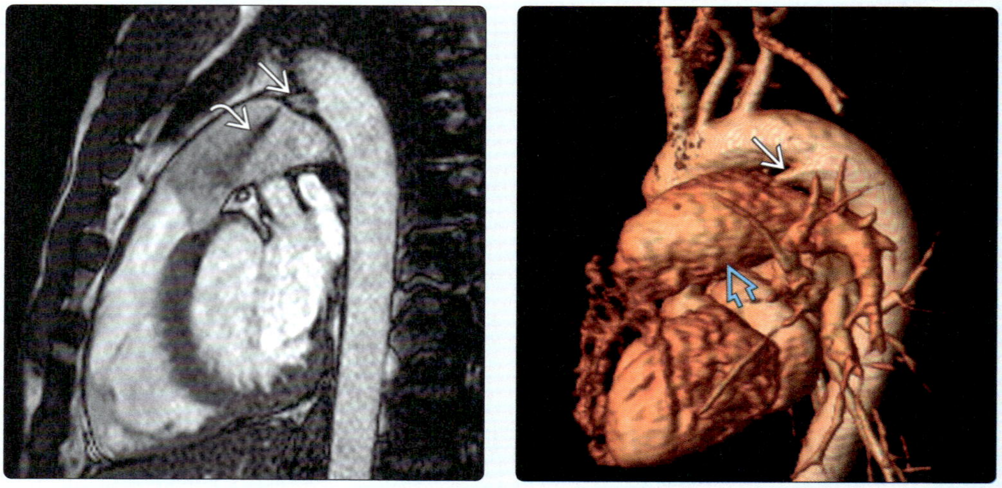

TERMINOLOGY

Abbreviations

- Patent ductus arteriosus (PDA)

Synonyms

- Persistent arterial duct, patent ductus Botalli, patent Botallo duct

Definitions

- Persistence of normal prenatal connection between proximal left pulmonary artery (PA) to aortic isthmus beyond 3 months of life
- Category: Acyanotic, increased pulmonary blood flow
- Hemodynamics: L → R shunt between aorta and PA
- PDA is frequently essential part of complex congenital heart disease
  - Hypoplastic left heart syndrome, preductal coarctation, interrupted aortic arch: Conduit for systemic perfusion (R → L flow)
  - Pulmonary atresia and other severe cyanotic heart diseases with right-sided obstruction: Conduit for pulmonary perfusion (L → R flow)
  - D-transposition: Necessary for admixture between systemic and pulmonary circuits (L → R flow)
- PDA is part of persistent fetal circulation syndrome: R → L flow
  - Severe lung disease (meconium aspiration, surfactant deficiency disease, neonatal pneumonia)
  - Primary pulmonary hypertension of neonate

IMAGING

General Features

- Best diagnostic clue
  - Connection of aorta and PA near normal ductus bump
  - Flow jet from aorta into PA

Radiographic Findings

- Radiography
  - Cardiomegaly (left atrium and left ventricle)
  - Increased pulmonary vascularity and main PA enlargement
  - Enlarged proximal aortic arch

CT Findings

- CECT
  - Can be incidentally discovered in routine NECT or CECT
  - Small tubular structure, between aorta and PA
    - May be calcified
  - Vascular jets may be seen with vascular window settings (width: 280; length: 400 HU)
    - Positive jet: Enhanced jet from aorta to PA (in studies timed for aorta)
    - Negative jet: Unenhanced blood flowing from aorta to PA (in studies timed for PA)
- CTA
  - 3D volume renditions of aortic arch depict PDA
  - Excellent for sizing of ductus prior to cardiac catheterization for placement of occluder device
  - Endoscopic 3D view shows orifice of PDA and spatial relationship to adjacent structures
  - Relationship between PDA and left main bronchus useful prior to transcatheter closure
  - May demonstrate marked dilation of main PA and compression of coronary arteries
  - Heavy, calcified, distorted, or aneurysmal ductus are not candidates for surgery

MR Findings

- Cardiac gated T1 (black-blood) imaging
  - Sagittal oblique plane through aortic arch depicts ductus
- Cine steady-state free precession (SSFP) MR
  - May demonstrate flow jet from aorta into PA or, if Eisenmenger physiology occurred, bidirectional jets
    - Jet not seen if pulmonary vascular resistance is high and flow is slow
  - Additional findings seen in Eisenmenger syndrome: Right ventricular (RV) hypertrophy, septal flattening, high-velocity pulmonary regurgitation, tricuspid regurgitation
    - RV volumes and function can be quantified
  - Associated congenital anomalies can be evaluated
- 3D gadolinium or noncontrast MRA with multiplanar reformations and volume-rendered reconstructions for direct visualization and sizing
- Phase-contrast imaging for quantification of L → R shunt
  - Percentage of L → R shunt = (Qs-Qp)/Qs, since this is measured proximal to shunt
    - Qp/Qs > 1.75 is clinically significant threshold for surgery
  - Direct shunt quantification can be performed by PC MR perpendicular to direction of PDA flow (en face view)
    - Usually PDA flow is directed toward main PA
  - 4D flow PC MR: Improved visualization and quantification of shunt
- Aneurysm of ductus more common in children

Echocardiographic Findings

- Suprasternal notch view: Direct visualization of ductus

DIFFERENTIAL DIAGNOSIS

Other Causes of L → R Shunting

- Septal defects, atrioventricular canal, partial anomalous pulmonary venous return

Persistent Fetal Circulation Syndrome

- Pulmonary hypertension (primary or secondary to severe lung disease)
- Patent foramen ovale, PDA secondary to profound irreversible hypoxia

Ductus Diverticulum

- Focal outpouching from aortic isthmus
- Has no connection to PA

PATHOLOGY

General Features

- Etiology
  - Prematurity: Persistent postnatal hypoxia → failure of ductus constriction
  - Term infant: Association with maternal rubella
  - Syndrome: Trisomy 21, 4p, Holt-Oram, incontinentia pigmenti

- Genetics
  - No specific genetic defect identified in most cases of isolated PDA
- Normal neonate: Ductus arteriosus closes functionally 18-24 hours after birth and anatomically at 1 month
- PDA is postnatal persistence of normal prenatal structure beyond 3 months of life
- Embryology
  - Ductus originates from primitive 6th left aortic arch
- Pathophysiology (for simple PDA)
  - L → R shunt, aorta to PA
  - Volume overload of left heart chambers → failure, pulmonary edema
  - Eisenmenger physiology: Pulmonary hypertension and RV pressure overload → reversal of shunt (R → L) and cyanosis (late finding)
  - Diastolic flow reversal in aorta → renal and intestinal hypoperfusion: Renal dysfunction, necrotizing enterocolitis

Staging, Grading, & Classification

- Morphologic classification by angiography
  - Type A: Narrowest diameter at pulmonary insertion
  - Type B: Narrowest diameter at aortic insertion
  - Type C: Same diameter throughout
  - Type D: Multiple constrictions
  - Type E: Bizarre conical configuration and constriction away from PA

Gross Pathologic & Surgical Features

- Patent arterial duct, most often wider on aortic side
  - Length: 2-8 mm; diameter: 4-12 mm
  - Makes acute angle with aorta in simple PDA; blunt angle with associated congenital heart disease
- Contractile tissue mainly on pulmonary side, spirally arranged muscle bundles in media
  - Prostaglandin E1 present in fetal life maintains relaxation
  - Increased oxygen pressure causes constriction
- Thickening of intima with mucoid degeneration
- Closed ductus forms ligamentum arteriosum, often calcifies
- Can be right sided

CLINICAL ISSUES

Presentation

- Most common signs/symptoms
  - Characteristic continuous, machinery-like murmur
  - Bounding peripheral pulses
  - Congestive heart failure
  - Special situation: Premature infant recovering from surfactant deficiency disease
    - Decrease in hypoxia
    - Drop in pulmonary vascular resistance
    - Increase in shunt flow through ductus arteriosus leading to pulmonary edema
- Other signs/symptoms
  - Subacute bacterial endocarditis
  - Ductal aneurysm
    - Can result from premature narrowing of ductus on pulmonary side
  - Massive PA enlargement can cause left main coronary artery compression and myocardial ischemia

Demographics

- Epidemiology
  - 10-12% of congenital heart disease cases
  - 1 per 2,500-5,000 live births
  - More common in females (2:1)
  - Associated with prematurity (21-35%)

Natural History & Prognosis

- Irreversible pulmonary hypertension (Eisenmenger physiology) → shunt reversal and cyanosis
- Isolated PDA: Excellent prognosis with early closure
- When associated with complex heart disease: Prognosis determined by underlying disorder
- Persistent fetal circulation, pulmonary hypertension: Treatment with extracorporeal membrane oxygenation is often necessary to disrupt vicious cycle
  - Hypoxia → pulmonary vasoconstriction → decreased pulmonary flow → more severe hypoxia

Treatment

- To close ductus in premature infants: Indomethacin (prostaglandin inhibitor)
- To keep ductus open (cyanotic heart disease): Prostaglandin E1
- Term infants, older children: Surgical clipping or ligation
  - Video-assisted &/or robotic guidance
  - Complications: Inadvertent ligation of aortic isthmus, PA, or recurrent laryngeal nerve
- Endovascular closure with duct occluder devices &/or coils
  - Small ductus (< 4 mm): Gianturco coils
  - Large ductus (> 4 mm): Ivalon plug, Rashkind and Amplatzer duct occluders (ADOs)
  - Complications: Protrusion of occluder device into left PA orifice (→ decreased left lung perfusion), peripheral embolization
  - Incomplete closure in 10-20%

DIAGNOSTIC CHECKLIST

Reporting Tips

- Detailed description of PDA influences percutaneous closure technique (coils vs. occluder devices)
  - Length and diameter at aortic and PA ends; diameter and location of narrowest site; angle ductus makes with descending thoracic aorta; presence of associated calcification
  - ± presence of complications (e.g., pulmonary hypertension)

SELECTED REFERENCES

1. Lee SJ et al: The patent ductus arteriosus in adults with special focus on role of CT. Diagnostics (Basel). 11(12), 2021
2. Agrawal H et al: New patent ductus arteriosus closure devices and techniques. Interv Cardiol Clin. 8(1):23-32, 2019
3. Goitein O et al: Incidental finding on MDCT of patent ductus arteriosus: use of CT and MRI to assess clinical importance. AJR Am J Roentgenol. 184(6):1924-31, 2005

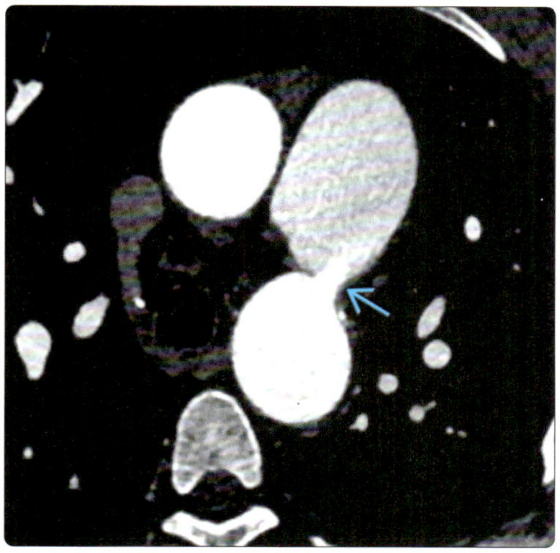

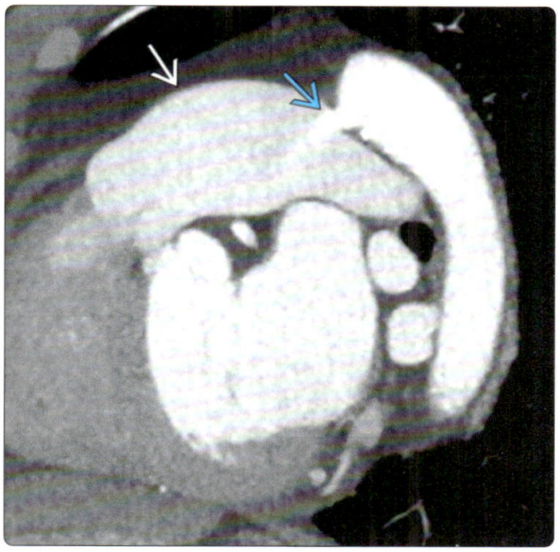

(Left) *Axial CECT shows a PDA connecting the descending aorta and the main PA. Note the high-attenuation blood flow from the aorta into the PA, indicating L → R shunt.* **(Right)** *Sagittal CECT in the same patient shows the PDA resulting in L → R shunt. Note that the main PA is dilated.*

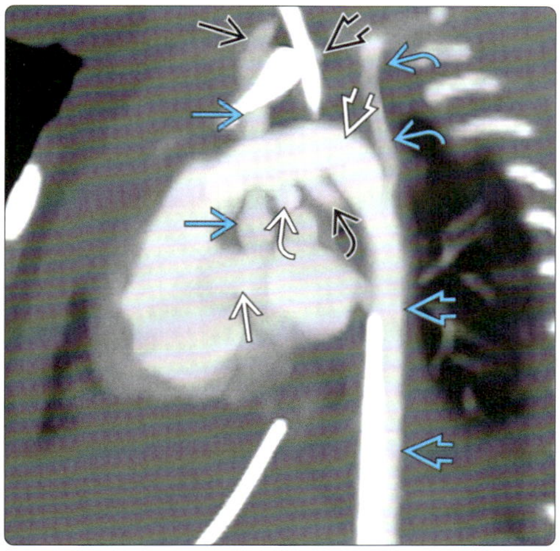

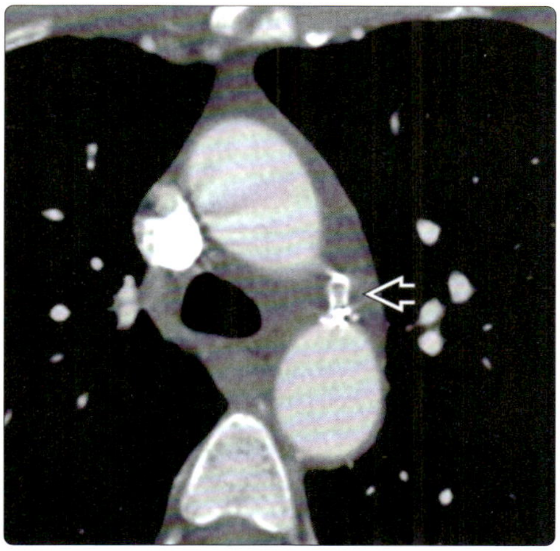

(Left) *Newborn with type B interrupted aortic arch has a hypoplastic ascending aorta supplying right innominate and left common carotid arteries. The left subclavian artery arises from the descending aorta, which is supplied by the PA via a large PDA. A large ventricular septal defect is present. Left PA and right PA branches are seen.* **(Right)** *Axial CECT in a patient with a PDA shows the expected posttreatment CT appearance of self-expandable Nitinol wire mesh device (Amplatzer duct occluder).*

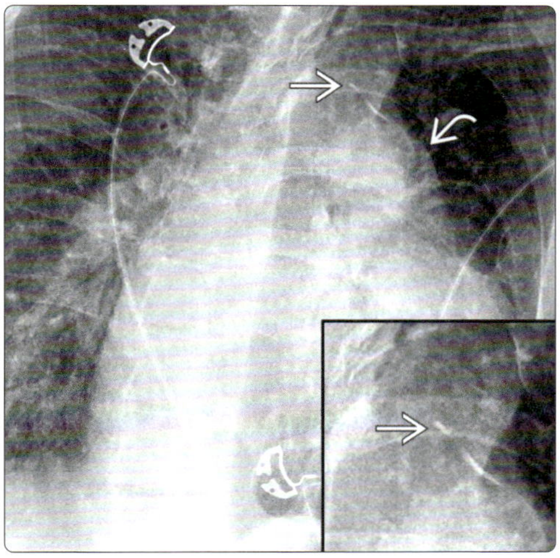

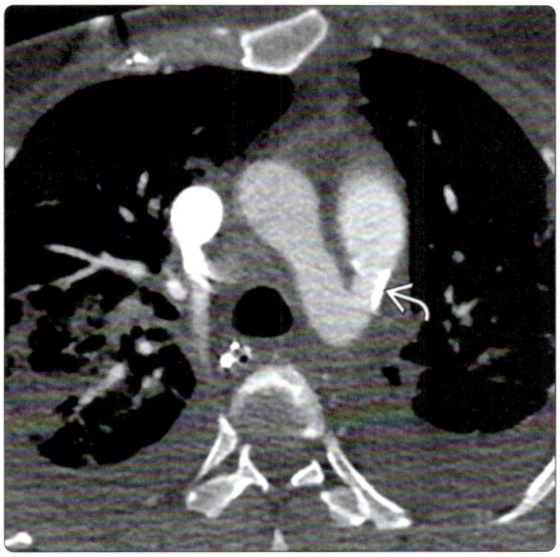

(Left) *Frontal radiograph shows cardiomegaly and enlargement and convexity of the main PA segment, indicating the presence of pulmonary trunk enlargement. Note the calcification (see also the magnified inset) immediately superior to the main PA in the expected location of the ductus arteriosus.* **(Right)** *Axial CECT in the same patient shows a widely PDA. Note the wall calcification corresponding to the chest radiograph finding.*

Aortopulmonary Window

KEY FACTS

TERMINOLOGY

- Abnormal communication between ascending aorta and main pulmonary artery &/or right pulmonary artery

IMAGING

- Radiography: Cardiomegaly, increased pulmonary vascular markings
- CTA: Communication between ascending aorta and main pulmonary artery with separate aortic and pulmonary valves
- MR: Morphology, ventricular function, and shunt assessment (Qp:Qs ratio)
- Echocardiogram is 1st-line imaging modality; CT and MR complementary to echocardiography

TOP DIFFERENTIAL DIAGNOSES

- Truncus arteriosus
- Patent ductus arteriosus type B (window)
- Hemitruncus: AORPA/AOLPA

PATHOLOGY

- Failure of complete closure of aortopulmonary septum during conotruncal development
- Commonly associated with ventricular septal defect, coarctation of aorta, and patent ductus arteriosus
- Type I proximal (most common), type II distal, type III total, type IV intermediate

CLINICAL ISSUES

- Congestive heart failure
- Over time may develop pulmonary hypertension
- Treatment: Surgical repair or percutaneous closure device

DIAGNOSTIC CHECKLIST

- Measure aortopulmonary window size
- Distance from semilunar valves and coronary arteries ostiums to defect
- Length of proximal and distal rims

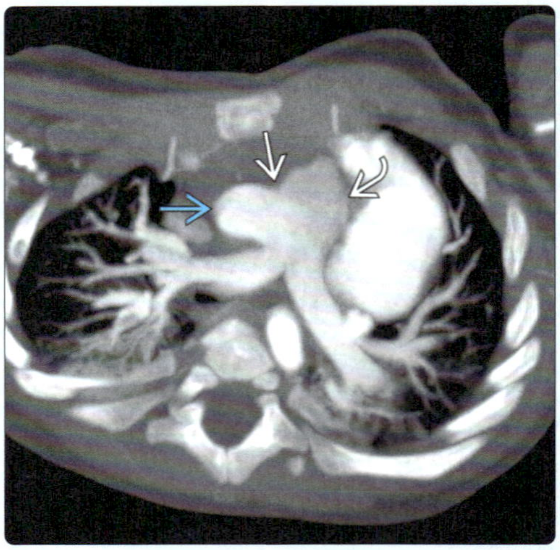

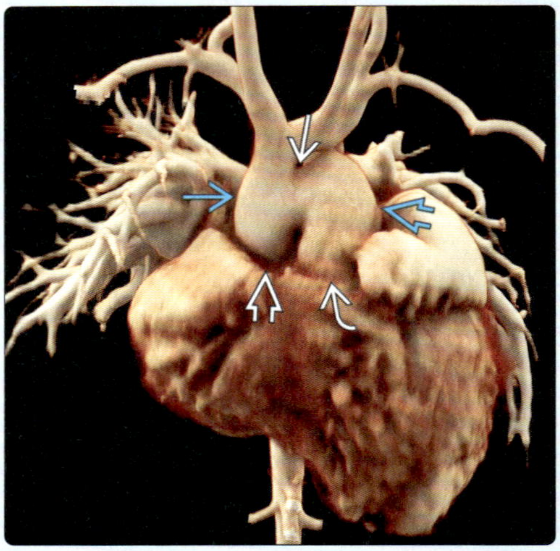

(Left) *Axial oblique MIP chest CT angiography in a newborn shows a communication → between the ascending aorta → and main pulmonary artery →, consistent with an aortopulmonary (AP) window.* **(Right)** *CTA cinematic rendering reconstruction demonstrates a distal AP window → (type II) between the ascending aorta → and main pulmonary artery →. Note the proximal separation of aortic → and pulmonary → valves.*

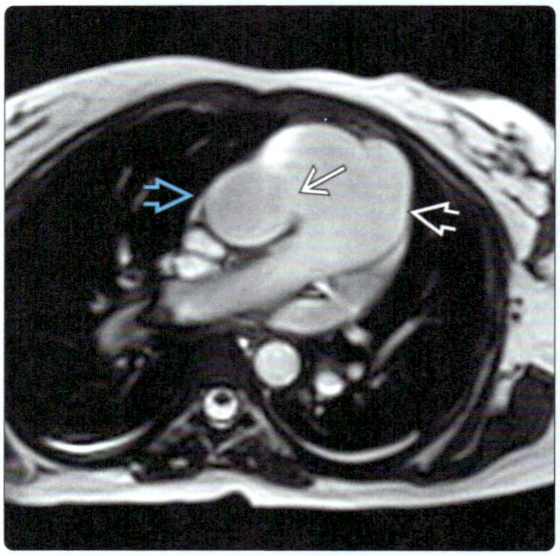

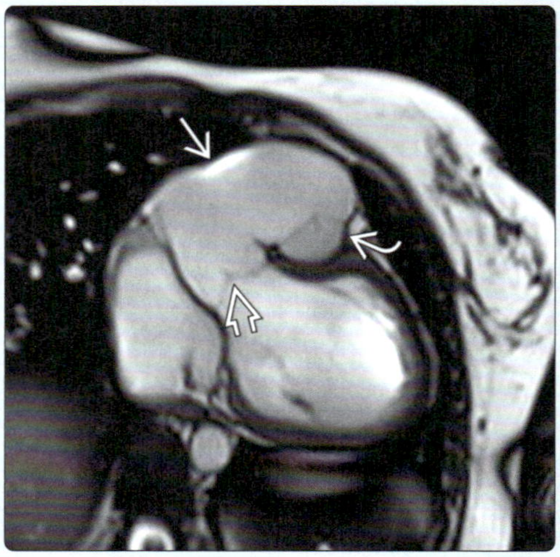

(Left) *Axial SSFP cardiac MR shows large communication → between the ascending aorta → and main pulmonary artery →, consistent with a large AP window. Note the severely dilated main pulmonary artery due to a left-to-right shunt.* **(Right)** *Left ventricular outflow tract SSFP cardiac MR shows a large proximal AP window (type I) →. Note the separated aortic → and pulmonary → valves. The defect begins just above the level of the sinus of Valsalva.*

TERMINOLOGY

Abbreviations

- Aortopulmonary window (AP window, APW)

Synonyms

- Aortopulmonary septal defect
- Ventral aortopulmonary communication

Definitions

- Abnormal communication between ascending aorta and main pulmonary artery (PA) &/or right PA

IMAGING

General Features

- Best diagnostic clue
  - Communication between ascending aorta and PA + separate aortic and pulmonary valves
- Location
  - Ascending aorta and main/right PA
  - Proximal, distal, or complete AP septal defect
- Size
  - Variable: Type III > type I > type II; > type IV
- Morphology
  - Lack of separation between ascending aorta and PA with separate aortic and pulmonary valves

Radiographic Findings

- Cardiomegaly due to left-sided volume overload
- Enlarged main PA
- Increased pulmonary vascular markings
- Signs of pulmonary hypertension
- Signs of congestive heart failure

CT Findings

- NECT
  - No wall between ascending aorta and main PA
  - Dilated main PA due to left-to-right shunt
- CTA
  - Communication between ascending aorta and main PA
    - Better seen in axial and coronal planes
    - Measurement of defect size, location, distance to semilunar valves, size of great vessels, and extracardiac findings
    - MPR, MIP, VRT reconstructions provide detailed information on anatomy of defect for surgical planning
    - Cinematic rendering shows photorealistic images of defect
  - Separate aortic and pulmonary valves
  - Dilated left ventricle (LV) and left atrium (LA) due to left-sided volume overload

MR Findings

- SSFP cine
  - Axial, coronal, and LV outflow tract views are best to show defect
  - Cine shows turbulent flow artifacts at level of APW (especially in 3T scanners)
  - LV and right ventricle (RV) function assessment to determine end-diastolic (ED), ED and stroke volumes, and ejection fraction
    - LV shows increased ED volume (volume overload) due to left-to-right shunt at level of ascending aorta-main PA
  - Measuring APW size during end-systolic phase
- Black blood SE
  - T1 and T2, DIR and TIR to visualize defect
- Phase-contrast flow
  - Provides reliable estimation of shunt volume and fraction with QP:QS ratio
    - QP:QS > 1.5:1 = significant left-to-right shunt
  - Direct shunt quantification: Perpendicular to flow at level of APW (through-plane)
  - Indirect shunt quantification
    - Aortic and PA flow measurement
    - **Proximal to shunt**: Flow in aorta is > PA
      - Flow in aorta includes additional shunt volume, which is recirculating through lung and left heart chambers, resulting in dilated LA and LV
      - Flow in PA includes only systemic venous return from inferior and superior venae cavae and coronary sinus
      - Thus, Qp reflects aortic flow, and Qs reflects PA flow if measured before shunt
    - **Distal to shunt**: Flow in PA is > aorta
      - Flow in aorta: Includes remaining flow in aorta
      - Flow in PA: Includes additional shunt volume
      - Thus, Qp reflects PA flow, and Qs reflects systemic flow (similar to intracardiac shunts)
    - Measurement proximal to shunt: QP = aortic flow, QS = PA flow
    - Measurement distal to shunt: QP = PA flow, QS = aortic flow
- 4D flow
  - Qualitative and quantitative assessment of flow in entire heart and great vessels at same time
  - Improved visualization and quantification of complex shunt

Ultrasonographic Findings

- Subcostal and parasternal short-axis view to evaluate location and size of APW, distant from semilunar valves
- Suprasternal view: Visualization of APW plus aortic arch view for evaluation of other abnormalities, such as hypoplastic aortic arch
- Color Doppler: Confirms defect and demonstrates communication between ascending aorta and PA

Imaging Recommendations

- Best imaging tool
  - Echocardiogram is 1st-line imaging modality
  - MR and CT complementary to echocardiography
    - Provide comprehensive information on vasculature and adjacent structures
- Protocol advice
  - CTA: In newborn and infants, use weight-based dose of contrast
    - Contrast injection: Variable rate, dependent on patient weight/size, IV access

- Bolus tracking: ROI at level of main PA
  - In newborn and extremely small patients: Start acquisition immediately after injection or manual triggering when contrast arrives in right heart
- Reconstruction: Thinnest possible slice thickness

DIFFERENTIAL DIAGNOSIS

Truncus Arteriosus

- Single aortopulmonary trunk with single semilunar valve
- Main PA or branches originates directly from trunk

Patent Ductus Arteriosus Type B (Window)

- Large communication between aorta and PA at level of ductus arteriosus
- Located distal to origin of supraaortic vessels

Hemitruncus

- Anomalous origin of branch PA from aorta; AORPA (right)/AOLPA (left)
- Separated aortic and main PA
- Single branch from main PA
- One pulmonary aortic branch anomalous originates from ascending aorta

PATHOLOGY

General Features

- Etiology
  - Failure of complete closure of aortopulmonary septum during conotruncal development
- Genetics
  - No genetic factors are associated
  - No association with DiGeorge syndrome, unlike other conotruncal anomalies
- Associated abnormalities
  - Associated with other congenital heart diseases in 44%
  - Commonly associated with ventricular septal defect, coarctation of aorta, and patent ductus arteriosus
  - VACTERL, CHARGE, CATCH-22

Staging, Grading, & Classification

- Mori classification: Types I, II, and III
  - Ho et al. added intermediate type IV
- **Type I** (proximal): Most common (70-96%); located just above sinus of Valsalva
  - Small or no proximal rim
  - High risk for coronary occlusion or semilunar valve dysfunction with percutaneous closure devices
- **Type II** (distal): 14-25%; communication between ascending aorta and origin of right PA
  - Large proximal rim with small or no distal rim
- **Type III** (total): 5%; complete absence of aortopulmonary septum
  - No proximal and distal rims
- **Type IV** (intermediate); small defect with adequate proximal and distal rims
  - Best defect suitable for percutaneous closure devices

CLINICAL ISSUES

Presentation

- Most common signs/symptoms
  - Due to pulmonary overcirculation as pulmonary vascular resistance falls over 1st few weeks of life
  - Diaphoresis, tachypnea, tachycardia, poor weight gain, frequent pulmonary infection
  - Eventually congestive heart failure
- Other signs/symptoms
  - Pulmonary hypertension may develop with time
  - Cyanosis may be present when shunt becomes bidirectional or right-to-left (Eisenmenger)

Demographics

- Sex
  - F > M
  - 70-80% female in reported series
- Epidemiology
  - 0.1% of all congenital heart disease

Natural History & Prognosis

- Pulmonary overcirculation leads to progressive pulmonary vascular disease with pulmonary hypertension
- Usually fatal if untreated
- Early repair has excellent long-term prognosis

Treatment

- Surgical repair
- Percutaneous closure devices
  - Small defects, suitable for device closure
  - If no interference with semilunar valves

DIAGNOSTIC CHECKLIST

Consider

- Type of APW
- Size of defect
- Signs of pulmonary overcirculation

Reporting Tips

- Measure size of communication
- Length of proximal and distal rims
- Distance from semilunar valves and coronary artery ostia to defect

SELECTED REFERENCES

1. Prabhu S et al: Tetralogy of Fallot with pulmonary atresia and aortopulmonary window may mimic common arterial trunk. Cardiol Young. 32(3):410-14, 2022
2. Bin-Moallim M et al: Aortopulmonary window: types, associated cardiovascular anomalies, and surgical outcome. Retrospective analysis of a single center experience. J Saudi Heart Assoc. 32(2):127-33, 2020
3. Chelu RG et al: Evaluation of atrial septal defects with 4D flow MRI-multilevel and inter-reader reproducibility for quantification of shunt severity. MAGMA. 32(2):269-79, 2018
4. Law MA et al: Aortopulmonary septal defect. Statpearls, 2018
5. Awasthy N et al: Aortopulmonary window with crisscross pulmonary arteries: anatomically type 1, physiologically type 2. J Cardiovasc Echogr. 27(4):143-4, 2017
6. Rajiah P et al: Cardiac MRI: Part 1, cardiovascular shunts. AJR Am J Roentgenol. 197(4):W603-20, 2011
7. Kimura-Hayama ET et al: Uncommon congenital and acquired aortic diseases: role of multidetector CT angiography. Radiographics. 30(1):79-98, 2010

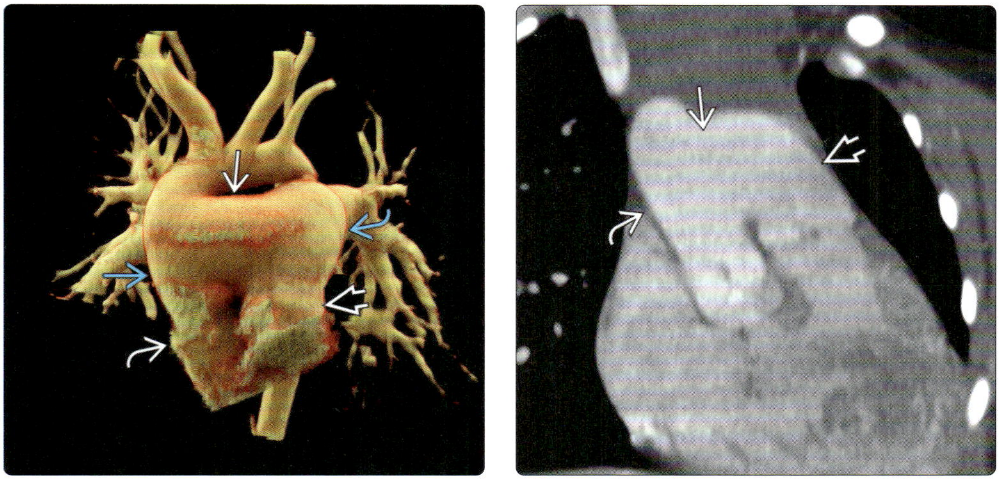

(Left) *CTA cinematic rendering technique shows a large AP window (type III) between the ascending aorta and main pulmonary artery. Note the proximal separation of aortic and pulmonary valves.* **(Right)** *Coronal oblique MPR CTA shows a large communication between the main pulmonary artery and ascending aorta, which is consistent with a type III AP window.*

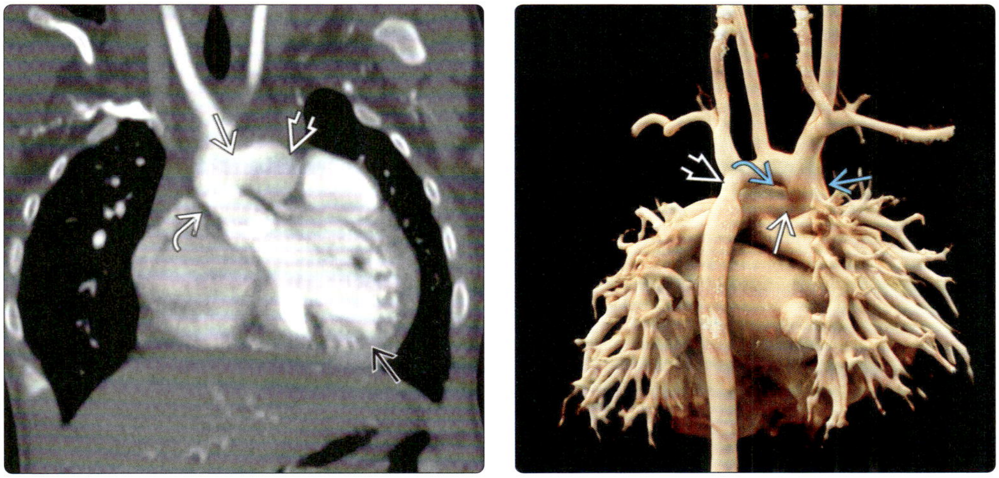

(Left) *Reconstructed coronal oblique image from a CTA shows communication between the main pulmonary artery and ascending aorta, which is consistent with an AP window. Note the dilated left ventricle due to left heart volume overload.* **(Right)** *Posterior oblique cinematic rendering CTA demonstrates an AP window between the ascending aorta and main pulmonary artery. Note the associated coarctation of aorta. The other common associated abnormalities are ventricular septal defect and patent ductus arteriosus.*

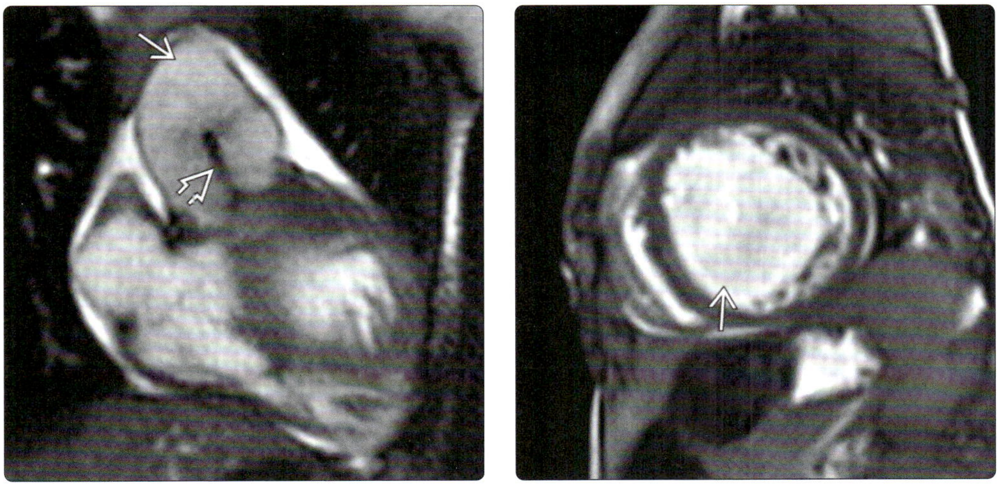

(Left) *Coronal oblique SSFP cardiac MR shows a distal AP window with a proximal rim, which is consistent with a type II AP window.* **(Right)** *Short-axis SSFP cardiac MR demonstrates severe dilatation of the left ventricle due to volume overload. Cardiac MR allows visualization and assessment of a defect and quantification of ventricular functions (left ventricle and right ventricle volumes, ejection fraction) and shunt volumes (Qp:Qs ratio).*

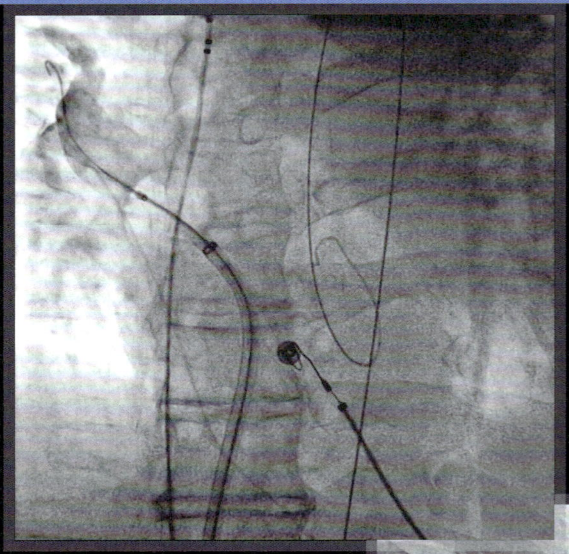
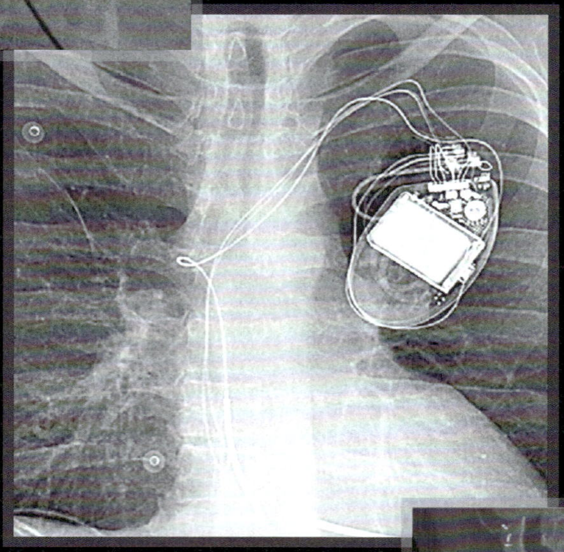
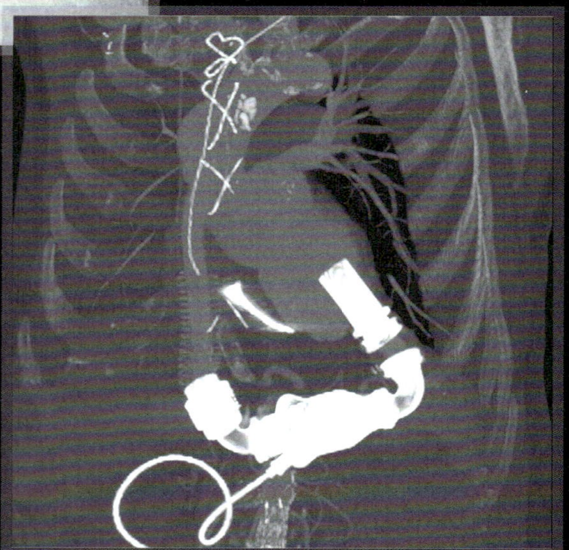

SECTION 8

Interventional and Electrophysiological Procedures

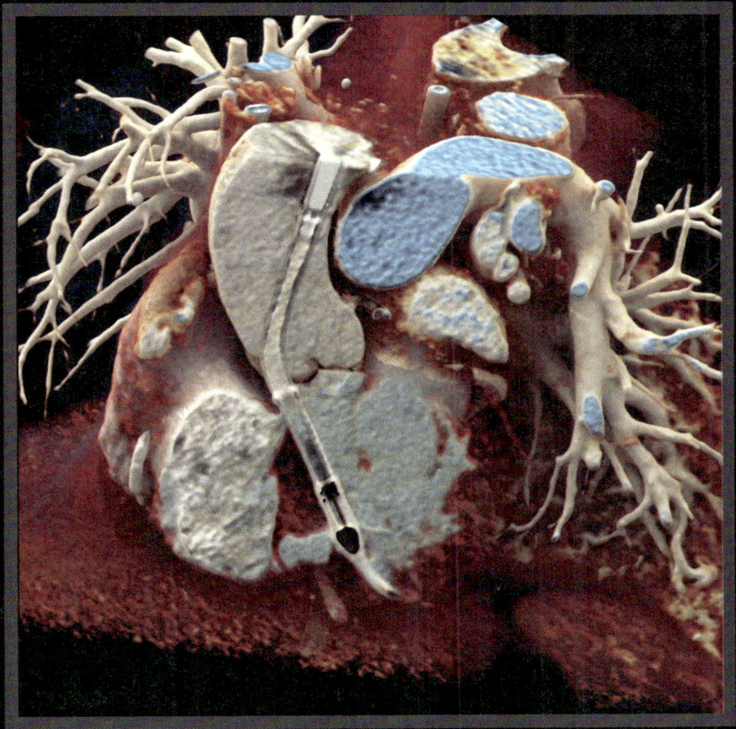

KEY FACTS

TERMINOLOGY

- Transcatheter aortic valve replacement (TAVR)

IMAGING ANATOMY

- Aortic annular plane is ovoid and in double-oblique orientation, which is better assessed with 3D imaging

ANATOMY IMAGING ISSUES

- Best imaging modality: Full-cardiac-cycle contrast-enhanced CT imaging

PATHOLOGY ISSUES

- Correct assessment of valvular area has been shown to have better outcomes in terms of reduced risk of annular rupture and paravalvular regurgitation (PAR)
- Adverse root features
  - Low coronary height
  - Bicuspid morphology
  - Moderate and severe left ventricular outflow tract (LVOT) calcification

CLINICAL IMPLICATIONS

- TAVR is treatment modality of choice for high and intermediate surgical risk patient
- Selection of valve size, access site, and type of device delivered should be based upon anatomic and clinical features and discussed in multidisciplinary heart team
- Serious complications
  - Annular rupture: Complication with high mortality and morbidity
  - Coronary occlusion
- Other complications
  - Interruption of electrical conduction system and necessity for permanent pacemaker implantation
  - Paravalvular regurgitation
  - Patient-prosthesis mismatch: Severe in 12% of patients, moderate in 24% of patients
  - Long-term complications: Prosthetic valve thrombosis, fibrosis, calcification, and dysfunction

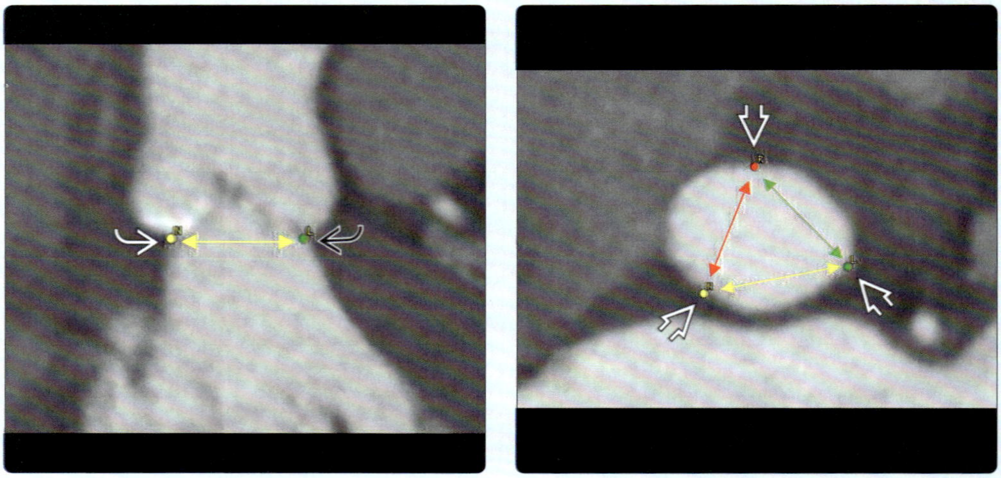

(Left) *Double-oblique reformatted contrast-enhanced CT shows the lowest points from the left (L) and noncoronary (N) cusp. The yellow line marks the annular plane reconstruction image.* **(Right)** *Double-oblique reformatted contrast-enhanced CT shows the annular plane. It is highlighted by the 3 basal points, which determine the correct plane and level of the aortic root. Three different colored arrows were inserted as a reference for the annular segmentation images.*

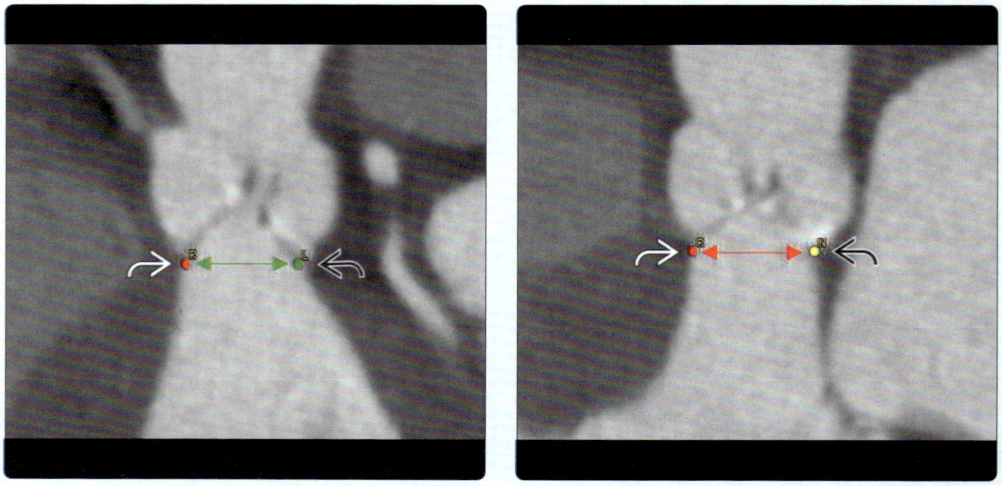

(Left) *Double-oblique reformatted contrast-enhanced CT highlights the corresponding basal points for annular segmentation on the right (R) and left (L) coronary cusp. The green arrows are a reference for the annular plane.* **(Right)** *Double-oblique reformatted contrast-enhanced CT demonstrates the lowest points for the annular plane on the right (R) and the noncoronary (N) cusp. The red line is a reference for the annular plane.*

TERMINOLOGY

Abbreviations

- Transcatheter aortic valve replacement (TAVR)

Synonyms

- Transcatheter aortic valve implantation (TAVI)
- Percutaneous aortic valve replacement

Definitions

- TAVR is percutaneous deployment of bioprosthetic valve in aortic root
  - Endovascular access point for delivery of valve is commonly femoral artery; however, other options include left ventricular (LV) transapical approach
  - Treatment of choice for patients with aortic stenosis at high or intermediate surgical risk and as alternative for those at low surgical risk

IMAGING ANATOMY

General Anatomic Considerations

- Aortic root is direct continuation of LV outflow tract (LVOT) and extends from basal attachment of aortic valve cusps within LV to their peripheral attachment at level of sinotubular junction
- Anulus is noncircular 3D structure at base of aortic root; its orientations varies from patient to patient and could be better evaluated by double-oblique images

Critical Anatomic Structures

- Annular plane is crucial to determine correct plane of aortic anulus with double-oblique orientation; plane is defined by 3 lowest insertion points of aortic valve leaflets
- Measure annular area, perimeter, and long and short diameters
  - There is well-known dynamism with frequently larger systolic annular area; thus, recommended to assess annular size in systolic phase between 20-40% of RR interval or before mitral valve opening
- Measure coronary heights and state any anomaly of coronary artery origin or course
- Determine sinotubular junction diameter and height, sinus of Valsalva diameters (3), LVOT area, and grade level of calcification in this location

Imaging Recommendations

- Best diagnostic tool: Full-cardiac-cycle contrast-enhanced cardiac CT
  - Useful in aortic root assessment and evaluation of endovascular access site; full cardiac cycle is needed for complete image assessment
  - Contrast-enhanced cardiac CT should be obtained by electrocardiogram synchronization and retrospective reconstruction; noncontrast synchronized phase could be added to calculate calcium score of aortic valve, which correlates with severity of aortic stenosis
  - For better contrast timing, test bolus technique or bolus triggering with preselected minimum HU should be implemented (usually 150 HU)
  - Using same contrast bolus, assessment of anticipated access sites can be determined, including femoral arteries and proximal supraaortic vessels
  - Reconstruction of cardiac images should meet 0.60-0.75 mm in spatial resolution; for evaluation of access site, CT can be reconstructed with 1 mm
- Cardiac magnetic resonance
  - Good alternative to CT in patients with iodine contrast contraindications with high inherent contrast resolution images, but is time-consuming and variably available modality with lower spatial resolution than CT
  - MR image quality may be limited by high-susceptibility artifacts, magnetic field-incompatible devices, patient claustrophobia, and arrhythmias
  - Cardiac MR-guided TAVR is noninferior to CT-guided TAVR in terms of successful device implantation in recent data
  - Can evaluate valve function, hemodynamics, and ventricular function and perform advanced tissue characterization, assessing for common coexisting cardiomyopathies, such as amyloidosis
  - Group 2 gadolinium-based contrast media (GBCM) can be safely administered, even in patients with severe renal dysfunction
  - Ferumoxytol, iron-containing blood-pool contrast media can be effective alternative to GBCM: Due to prolonged vascular presence, high-resolution ECG gated images of aortic root can be obtained without concerns of missing contrast bolus or breath holding
  - MR cannot assess calcifications in access vessels
    - Luminal assessment by MR can be combined with calcification from noncontrast CT
- Echocardiography
  - Key modality for diagnosing aortic stenosis and stenosis severity, left ventricle size and function, and detection of other valvular pathology
  - Standard 2D TTE/TEE imaging lacks 3D representation of anulus, and anulus measurements with this modality have been associated with excess post-TAVI paravalvular leak when compared to TAVI guided by CT-derived anulus area dimensions
  - 3D echocardiography may be used as alternative for aortic anulus measurements

CLINICAL IMPLICATIONS

Clinical Importance

- Clinical indication: Severe symptomatic aortic stenosis at intermediate or high surgical risk
- Adverse root features
  - Low coronary height: Distance from annular plane to coronary ostia when < 10-12 mm ↑ risk of coronary obstruction caused by displacement of native aortic leaflets with new device
  - Severe LVOT and annular calcification
    - Interferes with device deployment and ↑ risk of anulus rupture
    - Calcification can be classified as none, mild, moderate, and severe
  - Bicuspid aortic valve (BAV)
    - BAV morphology is better assessed by CT
    - In past, aortic valve replacement in setting of BAV was associated with poorer outcomes with ↑ incidence of paravalvular leak and anulus rupture

        - With inclusion of lesser surgical risk populations, more younger patients have been included with ↑ BAV prevalence, and, fortunately, with advancements in device technology, success of TAVR for treatment of aortic stenosis with underlying BAV has improved
    - Sinus of Valsalva diameter < 30 mm; most patients that developed coronary occlusion with TAVI procedure had diameter < 30 mm
    - Long leaflet length and bulky calcifications; ↑ risk of coronary occlusion
- Device selection for each patient: Patient-specific approach to prevent complications, such as annular ruptures and paravalvular regurgitation (PAR)
    - Type: Self-expanding vs. balloon-expandable devices
        - Balloon-expandable devices exert more radial force and have ↑ risk of annular rupture, particularly when combined with adverse pattern of calcification
        - Self-expanding devices exert less radial force and require greater degree of oversizing
    - Valve sizing
        - In order to avoid regurgitation, oversizing 2-10% by area is expected when using balloon-expandable valves (SAPIEN 3 THV)
        - Annular perimeter is most frequently used in cases of self-expanding devices, anticipating 10-25% of oversizing
    - Sizing for valve-in-valve procedures
        - Internal diameter needs to be determined at surgical valve inflow as it may differ from label size; too small inner diameter can lead to patient prosthesis mismatch or under expansion of THV, resulting in high gradients
- Selection of ideal endovascular access site for delivering device
    - Most commonly used access route is transfemoral (retrograde); however, other options include subclavian (retrograde), transaortic (retrograde), and transapical (anterograde) access
    - Level of vascular calcification, tortuosity, and minimal luminal vessel diameter appropriate for each device should be considered; evaluation can be done using MPR reconstructions from CT dataset
- Prediction of angiographic projection angles
    - There are significant variations in patient's anatomy; aortic valve is most commonly oriented in cranial and anterior position with slight tilt to right
    - Interventionist cardiologist requires fluoroscopy projection oriented orthogonal to native valve plane, using multiple aortograms to achieve that plane
    - Patient´s aortic root orientation can be extracted from CT datasets, and all of those projections can be simulated prior to procedure, reducing need for repeat aortograms with shorter radiation exposure and less contrast use
        - Common projections are **(a)** craniocaudal without right anterior oblique (RAO) or left anterior oblique (LAO) angulation, **(b)** straight RAO to LAO as needed without cranial or caudal angulation, and **(c)** LAO 30° with cranial or caudal angulation as needed
- Complications
    - Short term
        - Annular rupture in balloon-expandable devices; < 1% of patients; associated with aggressive oversizing (≥ 20%) and higher degree of LVOT calcification, especially in nodular formation under noncoronary cusp
            - Other factors associated with this risk: Prior radiation therapy and female sex
        - Coronary occlusion: Infrequent but serious complication with high mortality (40.9% of patients at 30 days) and morbidity
        - Vascular injuries due to delivery system: Dissection, intramural hematomas, rupture, embolism
        - Conduction disease with need for permanent pacemaker implantation
            - Direct mechanical effect over electrical system (atrioventricular node/His bundle) can cause conduction tissue damage, resulting in left bundle branch block and atrioventricular block
            - Associated with self-expanding devices and low deployment; longer membranous interventricular septum; lower probability of having trauma by device
        - PAR
            - Has direct relationship with underestimation of annular size, aortic root calcification, and suboptimal device implantation; moderate and severe regurgitation is linked to poorer outcomes at 30 days and higher 1-year mortality
    - Long term
        - Valve degeneration and dysfunction
            - Prosthetic valve thrombosis, fibrosis, calcification, and then dysfunction
            - Pannus formation at valve inflow
        - Prosthesis-patient mismatch (PPM)
            - Defined by effective valve orifice area indexed (EOAI) to body surface area (BSA)
            - Severe PPM for TAVR is estimated ~ 12% and associated with ↑ heart failure hospitalization and mortality

SELECTED REFERENCES

1. Reindl M et al: Cardiac magnetic resonance imaging versus computed tomography to guide transcatheter aortic valve replacement: a randomized, open-label, noninferiority trial. Circulation. 148(16):1220-30, 2023
2. Wilson R et al: Transcatheter aortic and mitral valve replacements. Radiol Clin North Am. 57(1):165-78, 2019
3. Akinseye OA et al: Clinical outcomes of coronary occlusion following transcatheter aortic valve replacement: a systematic review. Cardiovasc Revasc Med. 19(2):229-36, 2018
4. Blanke P et al: Valvular Diseases and Interventions. In Budoff M et al: Atlas of Cardiovascular Computed Tomography. 2nd ed. Springer, 2018
5. Herrmann HC et al: Prosthesis-patient mismatch in patients undergoing transcatheter aortic valve replacement: from the STS/ACC TVT registry. J Am Coll Cardiol. 72(22):2701-11, 2018
6. Pollari F et al: Risk factors for paravalvular leak after transcatheter aortic valve replacement. J Thorac Cardiovasc Surg. 157(4):1406-15, 2018
7. Expert Panel on Cardiac imaging and vascular imaging:. et al: ACR Appropriateness Criteria® imaging for transcatheter aortic valve replacement. J Am Coll Radiol. 14(11S):S449-55, 2017
8. Hell MM et al: Prediction of fluoroscopic angulations for transcatheter aortic valve implantation by CT angiography: influence on procedural parameters. Eur Heart J Cardiovasc Imaging. 18(8):906-14, 2017
9. Rodriguez-Gabella T et al: Aortic bioprosthetic valve durability: incidence, mechanisms, predictors, and management of surgical and transcatheter valve degeneration. J Am Coll Cardiol. 70(8):1013-28, 2017
10. Soon J et al: Multimodality imaging for planning and follow-up of transcatheter aortic valve replacement. Can J Cardiol. 33(9):1110-23, 2017

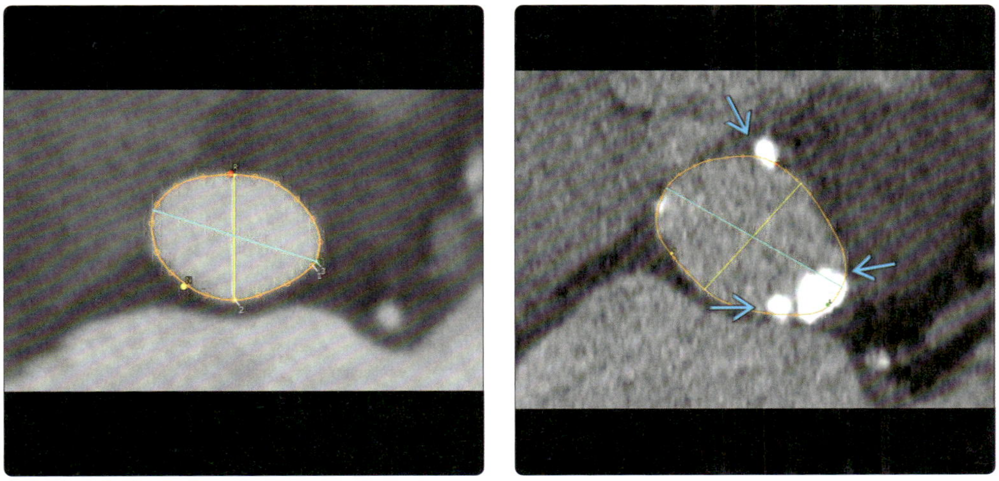

(Left) *Double-oblique reformatted CECT at the level of the anulus shows the area, perimeter, and maximum and minimum diameters measured with semiautomatic tools.* **(Right)** *Double-oblique reformatted CECT at the level of the anulus shows severe, protruding, and multiple calcifications at the annular level.*

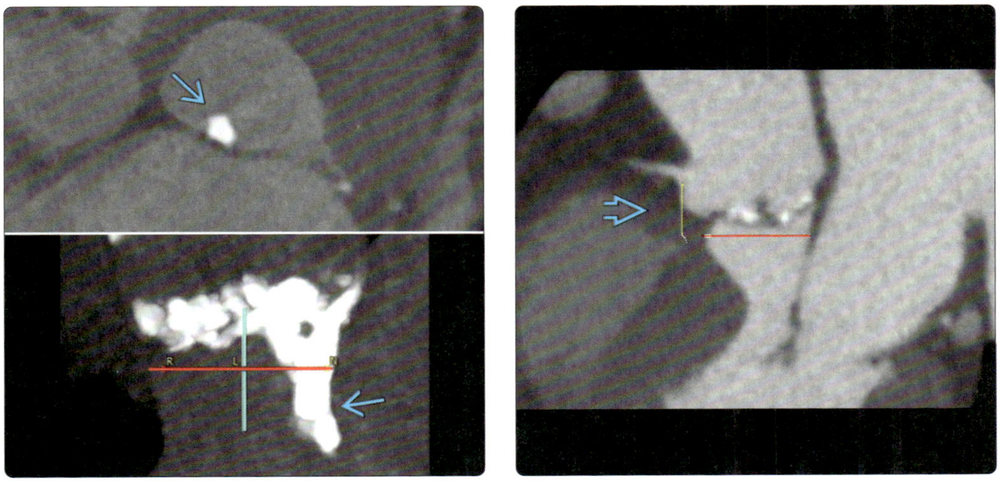

(Left) *MPR reformatted contrast-enhanced CT (top) displays severe, protruding calcification under the level of the anulus. MIP reconstruction (bottom) shows extension to the left ventricular outflow tract.* **(Right)** *Double-oblique reformatted CECT shows low right coronary height , ~ 8.9 mm.*

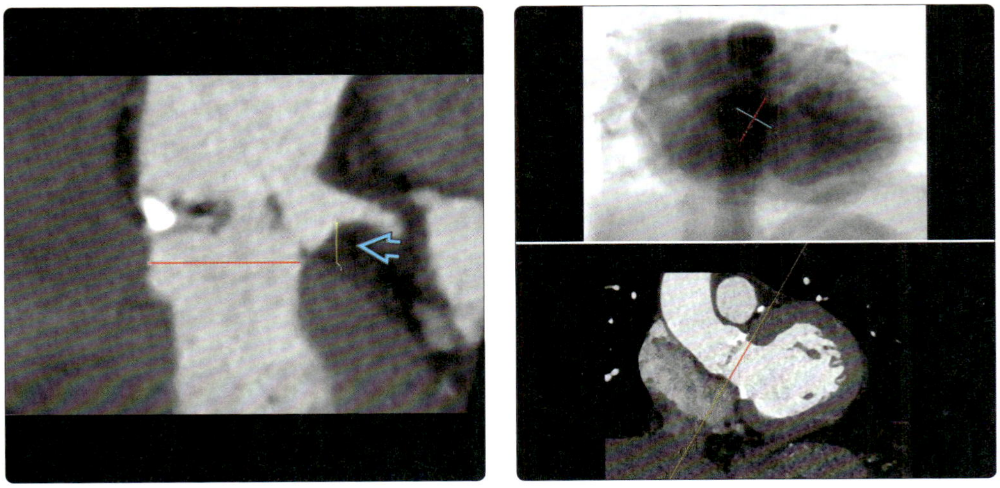

(Left) *Double-oblique reformatted contrast-enhanced CT displays the left coronary height of only 6.9 mm . Notice also the low height of the sinus of Valsalva.* **(Right)** *Double-oblique reformatted contrast-enhanced CT (bottom) and predicted fluoroscopic view (top) of the annular plane for the device deployment shows the right coronary cusp projection at left anterior oblique 4° and caudal 6°. The red line shows the annular plane.*

KEY FACTS

IMAGING ANATOMY

- Important to be familiar with normal appearance of commonly implanted transcatheter aortic valve replacement (TAVR) valves

PATHOLOGY ISSUES

- Thrombosis
  - Hypoattenuated leaflet thickening (HALT)
- Structural valve degeneration
  - Pannus, leaflet calcification
  - Incorrect device positioning, fracture, or underexpansion
- Embolization or migration of device
- Patient-prosthesis mismatch; paravalvular leak
- Device infection
- Vascular complications
  - Iliofemoral: Access site hematoma, pseudoaneurysm, arterial dissection, arterial avulsion, arterial stenosis/thrombosis/occlusion
  - Aortic: Aortic dissection, aortic rupture

PATHOLOGY IMAGING ISSUES

- Echocardiography is most used and relevant imaging modality for assessing prosthetic valve function
- Routine cardiac CT imaging for complications is not advised; main role is redo TAVR planning and further assessment of abnormalities identified on echocardiography
  - Indications for CT include
    - Concerning echocardiographic findings: Elevated transvalvular gradient, increased leaflet thickness, reduced cusp mobility
    - Unclear echocardiographic or clinical findings
    - New or progressing functional impairment of valve
- Cardiac MR has complementary role
  - Assessment of prosthetic valve regurgitation severity, when echocardiographic assessment is difficult or inconclusive
  - Paravalvular leak
  - Assessment of left ventricular reverse remodeling

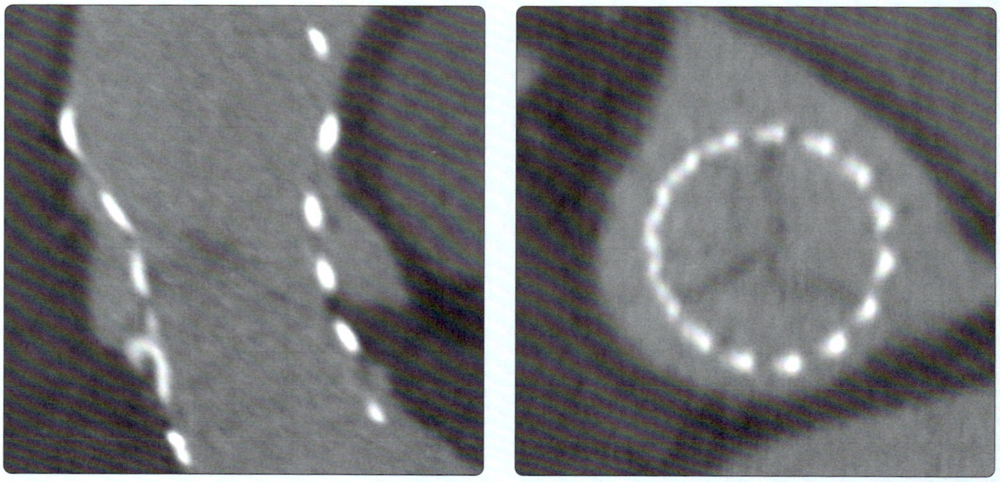

(Left) *Contrast-enhanced cardiac CT shows a normal appearance of a self-expanding Evolut device in the coronal plane.* **(Right)** *Contrast-enhanced cardiac CT shows a normal appearance of a self-expanding Evolut device in the axial plane. This is a diastolic image as the bioprosthetic valve leaflets are closed.*

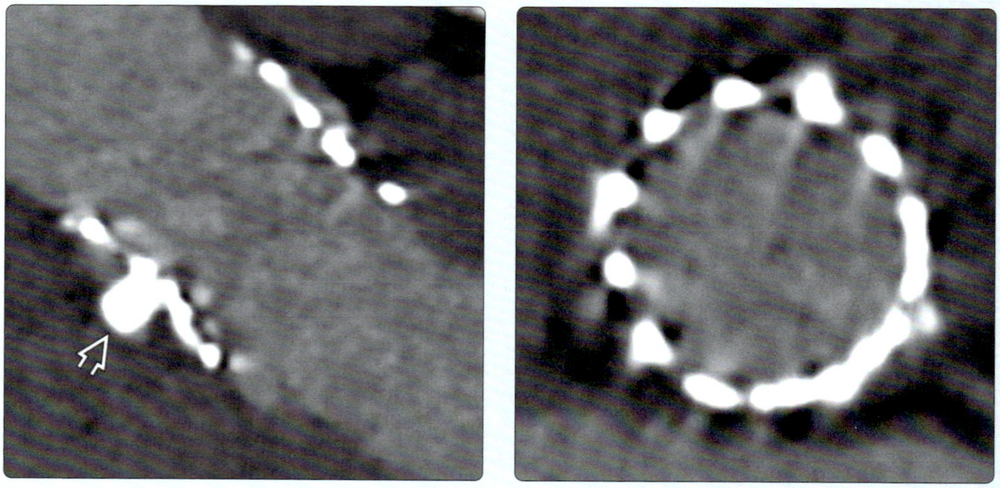

(Left) *Coronal CT shows the normal appearance of the SAPIEN 3 device with displacement of the native leaflet's calcifications ➡ toward the sinus of Valsalva. Transcatheter aortic valve replacement (TAVR) procedure does not require the removal of the calcified native aortic valves.* **(Right)** *Axial representation of the annular plane is shown with the device fully expanded and with the typical circular shape.*

TERMINOLOGY

Abbreviations

- Transcatheter aortic valve replacement (TAVR)

Definitions

- Clinical and imaging assessment following TAVR valve deployment

IMAGING ANATOMY

General Anatomic Considerations

- Normal appearance of commonly implanted TAVR valves
  - Balloon-expandable valve
    - SAPIEN X4-Edwards Lifesciences
      - On-balloon delivery system with rotation control, cobalt-chromium stent, bovine pericardial leaflets with RESILIA tissue to reduce valve degeneration; outer skirt reduces risk of paravalvular leak (PVL)
      - Normal postoperative appearance is circular and unfolded device, situated ~ 2 mm below annular plane
      - Native calcified leaflets are displaced toward aortic sinus of Valsalva
  - Self-expanding valve
    - Evolut FX-Medtronic
      - Autoexpandable device with cup-shaped nitinol stent with porcine pericardial leaflets and tall porcine pericardial sealing skirt and wrap to reduce PVL; 3 radiopaque dot markers aid deployment
      - Deployment of this valve results in noncircular expansion of device as it adapts to anatomy of root without modifying it, respecting calcifications of annular plane
  - Other valve systems
    - Portico Navitor-Abbot
      - Self-expanding system with nitinol frame, bovine pericardial leaflets, and porcine pericardium sealing cuff
      - Can be fully repositioned, recaptured, and retrieved prior to full deployment
      - Large sizing allows for treatment of anulus perimeter up to 85 mm
- Leaflets can be recognized by CT as fine, hypodense, and semicircular structures within lumen
  - Assessment of leaflet motion remains challenging due to limited temporal resolution of CT

CLINICAL IMPLICATIONS

Clinical Importance

- **Anatomic complications**
  - **Valve thrombosis**
    - Suspected when postprocedural echocardiography identifies rise in transvalvular gradient
      - Leaflet thickness ≥ 2 mm and abnormal leaflet motion
    - Incidence of thrombosis estimated at 5-10% in post-TAVR follow-up studies
      - Most often occurs in 1st year after TAVR
    - CT provides comprehensive approach to recognition of **hypoattenuated leaflet thickening (HALT)**
      - Seen mainly as low-attenuation meniscoid thickening along aortic surface of leaflets from base to tip
      - Accepted as hallmark of subclinical leaflet thrombosis; each leaflet is graded (grades 1-4) by percentage of leaflet involved
      - If associated with restricted leaflet motion (> 50%), called **hypoattenuation affecting motion (HAM)**
      - Mostly asymptomatic, no ↑ gradient on echocardiography
      - Resolution after therapeutic anticoagulation
    - Despite optimal IV contrast-enhanced full-cardiac-cycle CT, limited temporal resolution makes diagnosis challenging
  - **Incorrect device position**
    - Detected using postprocedure echocardiographic and fluoroscopic evaluation or CT
    - Deployment should cover annular plane, and top of native leaflets should not pass distal portion of device
    - Similarly, device should be positioned in distal left ventricular outflow tract (LVOT), not making contact with mitral apparatus
    - Device fracture or underexpansion
      - Can be assessed on ECG gated full-cardiac-cycle noncontrast images
  - **Embolization or late migration of TAVR device**
    - Embolization related to movement of device toward aorta, occurs with 1st hour post deployment
    - Late migration refers to movement of device into LVOT or further into left ventricle with further consequences: Prosthetic valve regurgitation, native valve restenosis, and impingement of mitral valve
  - **Patient-prosthesis mismatch**
    - Defined by relation of effective orifice area to total body surface area
      - Severe if < 0.65 cm^2/m^2 with implications to long-term patient prognosis
    - Cause of high gradient measured by echo
  - **PVL**
    - Consists of regurgitation, frequently between aortic root and device
      - Contrast-filled channel connecting aortic root and LVOT on CT
    - Frequently as result of underdeployment of device or calcification of ring
    - Can be treated with repeated ballon expansion to permit proper expansion
    - Some new devices, such as Evolut and Navitor, can be repositioned before final full deployment
    - Associated with ↑ mortality
    - Better assessed by echocardiography
    - CT or MR may have complimentary role in identifying location and mechanism of valvular regurgitation
  - **Aortic valve regurgitation**
    - Mostly due to improper valve deployment or sizing; detected at immediate postprocedure work-up
    - Late-term regurgitation due to degeneration of leaflets
    - Centrally positioned regurgitant flow on echocardiography
  - **Device infection**

- Initially suspected in appropriate clinical setting, such as febrile illness
- Echocardiography may detect features of device-related infection, such as vegetation
- CT provides detailed assessment of periaortitis, aortic root abscesses, and vegetations
  - Vegetation: Irregular, hypoattenuating masses; adherent to prosthetic leaflets
  - Aortic root infection/abscess: Earliest visible change is edema and thickening along intervalvular fibrosa
- 18F-FDG PET/CT can be used in patients with suspected device infection

- **Pannus**
  - Ingrowth of fibrous tissue at inflow of bioprosthetic valve as opposed to valve outflow with thrombus
    - Usually occurs >1 year post-TAVR implant
  - Can significantly reduce inflow orifice area with concomitant rise in transvalvular gradient
  - No resolution with therapeutic anticoagulation

Vascular Complications

- Reported in 4.2-5.6% of TAVRs
  - Overall incidence is ↓ due to improved vascular access and closure technique, smaller access sheaths and delivery systems, ↑ operator experience, improved patient selection
- Main risk factors are small vessel diameter (females), renal failure, extensive iliofemoral arterial calcification
- Associated with worse outcomes, including longer length of hospital stay, higher cost of care, and poor quality of life
- Main iliofemoral complications: Hematoma, pseudoaneurysm, dissection, stenosis/thrombosis/occlusion, and perforation/avulsion
- Aortic complications include dissection and rupture

IMAGING

Echocardiography

- Most used and relevant imaging modality for assessing prosthetic valve function
  - Assessment of leaflet motion, limitation of valve opening/closing, and leaflet thickening
- Can determine changes in hemodynamic parameters (peak velocity, mean pressure gradient, effective orifice area, and presence of regurgitation) through Doppler evaluation
- Performed during and immediately following device deployment
  - Then again prior to hospital discharge to obtain baseline TAVR valve hemodynamics; also at 6 and 12 months, then yearly
- Immediate post-TAVR aortic regurgitation should be characterized in terms of location, severity, and cause
- Evaluation of cardiac function post TAVR must include left ventricle size, ejection fraction, stroke volume, and cardiac index for left and right side

ECG Gated Cardiac CT

- Routine cardiac CT imaging is not advised for assessment of complications
  - Main role is in HALT, pannus and prosthesis expansion assessment, and in redo TAVR planning
- Indications for CT include
  - Concerning echocardiographic findings: Elevated transvalvular gradient, ↑ leaflet thickness, ↓ cusp mobility
  - Unclear echocardiographic or clinical findings
  - New or progressing functional impairment of valve
- Only reliable method in evaluation of device fractures and device expansion
- CT plays auxiliary role in setting of suspected infection, thrombosis, PVL, and valve degeneration
- Can assist in evaluation mobility and opening of leaflets
- Detection of postprocedural position of device, device fracture, leaflet calcification, and pannus
- New nomenclature has been created to name CT post TAVR findings: HALT and HAM
- Protocol advice: Should be planned as contrast-enhanced retrospective ECG gated acquisition with reconstructions of entire cardiac cycle
- CT planning for redo TAVR (valve-in-valve TAVR)
  - Commissural alignment: Alignment of bioprosthetic valve commissures with commissures of host valve
  - Coronary alignment: Aligning bioprosthetic valve commissure with coronary ostia in cases of coronary eccentricity
  - Risk of coronary obstruction or sinus sequestration in redo TAVR procedure

Cardiac MR

- MR has adjunct role
  - Assessment of prosthetic valve regurgitation severity, when echocardiographic assessment is difficult or inconclusive
  - PVL
- TAVR valve itself is difficult to assess due to its paramagnetic properties
- However, prosthetic valve regurgitation volumes and fraction can be determined
  - Visualized in SSFP cine MR
  - Quantified using velocity-encoded phase-contrast MR
- Can assess left ventricle reverse remodeling; reduction in left ventricle mass and volume along with improvement in cardiac function

SELECTED REFERENCES

1. Bapat VN et al: A guide to transcatheter aortic valve design and systematic planning for a redo-TAV (TAV-in-TAV) procedure. JACC Cardiovasc Interv. 17(14):1631-51, 2024
2. He A et al: Cardiac computed tomography post-transcatheter aortic valve replacement. J Cardiovasc Comput Tomogr. 18(4):319-26, 2024
3. Garcia S et al: Clinical impact of hypoattenuating leaflet thickening after transcatheter aortic valve replacement. Circ Cardiovasc Interv. 15(3):e011480, 2022
4. Blanke P et al: Computed tomography imaging in the context of transcatheter aortic valve implantation (TAVI)/transcatheter aortic valve replacement (TAVR): an expert consensus document of the Society of Cardiovascular Computed Tomography. JACC Cardiovasc Imaging. 12(1):1-24, 2019
5. Sellers SL et al: Transcatheter aortic heart valves: histological analysis providing insight to leaflet thickening and structural valve degeneration. JACC Cardiovasc Imaging. 12(1):35-145, 2019
6. Soon J et al: Multimodality imaging for planning and follow-up of transcatheter aortic valve replacement. Can J Cardiol. 33(9):1110-23, 2017

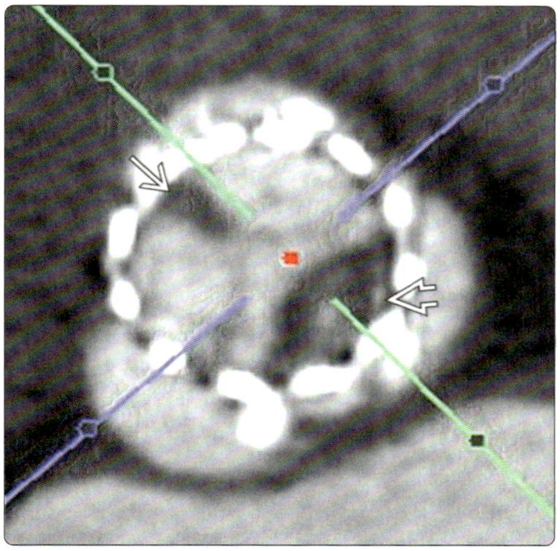

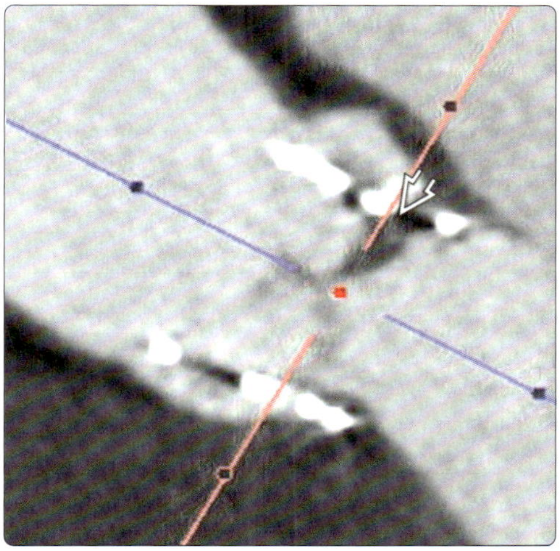

(Left) *Contrast-enhanced cardiac CT shows grade 3 hypoattenuated leaflet thickening (HALT)* ➡ *involving the prosthetic leaflet adjacent to left cusp. There is further grade 1 HALT of leaflet nearest noncoronary cusp* ➡. **(Right)** *Cardiac CT from the same valve in the coronal plane orientated through the leaflet nearest the left coronary cusp* ➡ *shows the meniscoid thickening from base of the leaflet to allow for accurate grading of HALT. In this case, there is grade 3 HALT (75% of the leaflet involved).*

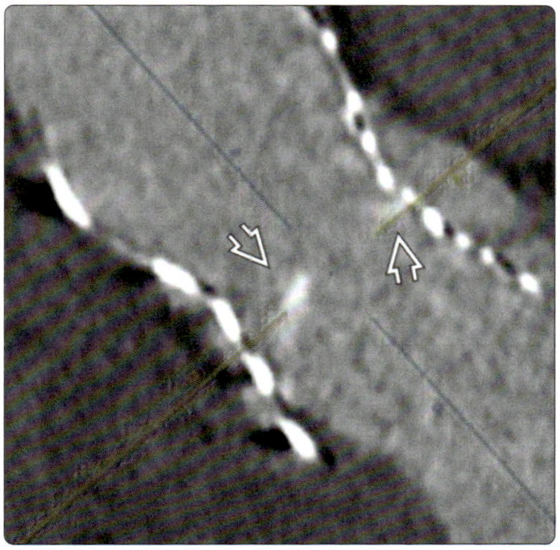

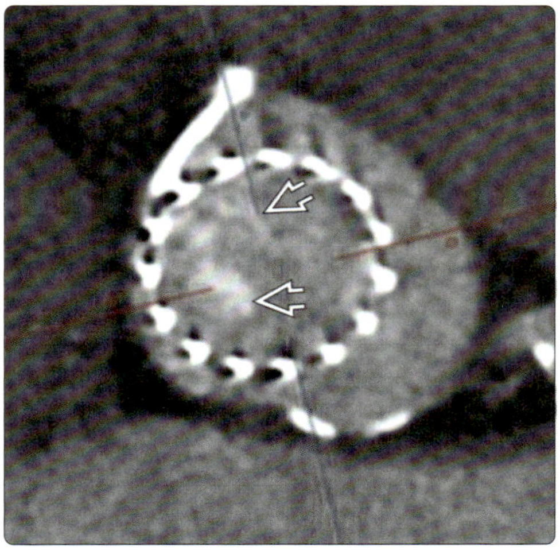

(Left) *Long-axis MPR CT reconstruction shows linear calcifications* ➡ *on the device's leaflets. This patient was referred due to high gradient values on echo.* **(Right)** *Short-axis MPR CT reconstruction shows linear calcifications* ➡ *on the device's leaflets. This patient was referred due to high gradient values on echocardiography. Late-term degeneration of the leaflets due to calcification or fibrosis results in prosthesis dysfunction.*

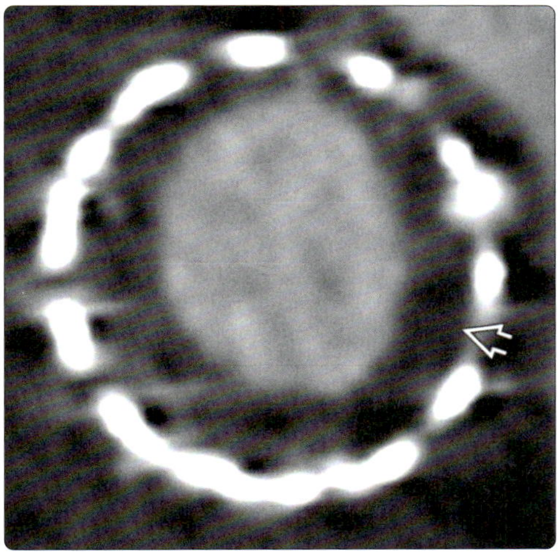

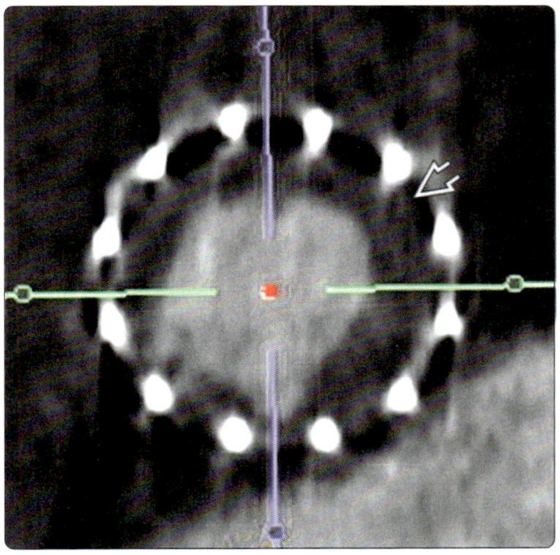

(Left) *Contrast-enhanced CT shows circumferential low-attenuation thickening of the valve inflow in keeping with pannus formation* ➡. *This narrows the effective orifice or the prosthetic valve.* **(Right)** *Contrast-enhanced CT shows circumferential low-attenuation thickening of the valve inflow* ➡ *in a balloon-expandable device, narrowing the effective valve orifice.*

KEY FACTS

TERMINOLOGY

- Mitral valve (MV) apparatus is composed of anterior and posterior leaflet, chordae tendineae, anterolateral and posteromedial papillary muscles, and mitral anulus
- Mitral stenosis (MS) is most commonly due rheumatic fever, which involves leaflet and subvalvular thickening, commissural fusion, leaflet calcification, and reduced leaflet mobility
- Primary mitral regurgitation (PMR) is due to intrinsic pathology of MV apparatus
- Secondary mitral regurgitation (SMR) is due to pathology of atria or ventricle

TRANSCATHETER THERAPIES

- Transcatheter edge to edge repair (TEER) is reasonable in symptomatic, severe patients with PMR who are at high or prohibitive surgical risk (class II)
- TEER is limited to suitable anatomies
- Transcatheter MV implantation (TMVI) is promising intervention with range of dedicated systems, which are subject of pivotal trials
- Left ventricular outflow tract obstruction (LVOTO) is major complication of TMVI associated with poor outcomes

IMAGING ANATOMY

- Full-cardiac cycle imaging allows use of diastole for largest mitral anulus, systole for smallest neo-LVOT, and both phases for quantifying chamber volumes and ejection fraction
- In native valves, mitral anulus is traced to form saddle-shaped anulus, while simplified D-shaped anulus is formed by excluding anterior horn
- CT allows accurate assessment of amount and distribution of valve calcium
- LVOTO risk can be estimated by calculating neo-LVOT area

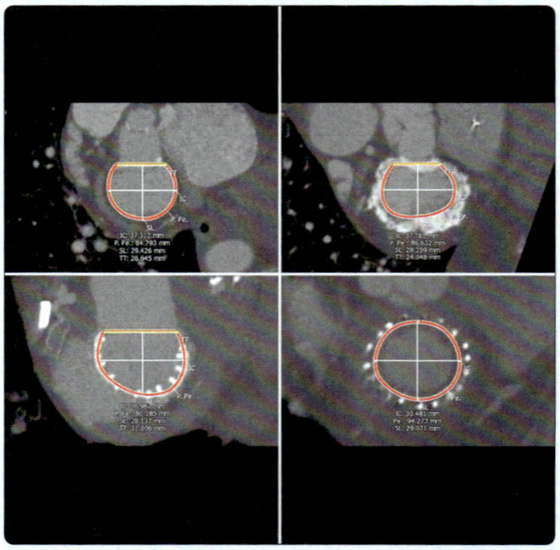

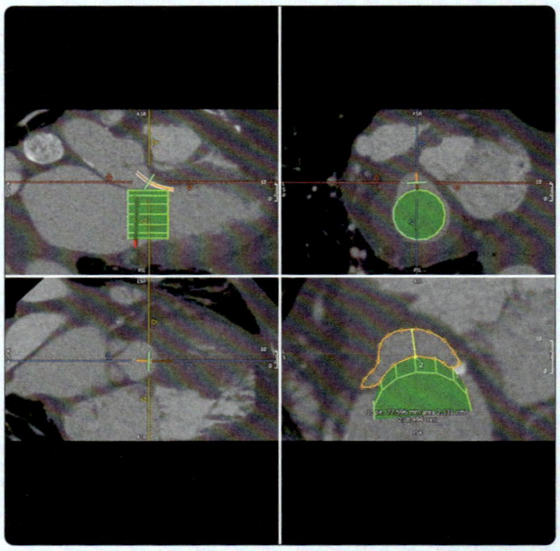

(Left) *Determination of the mitral annular area and intercommissural (lateromedial), septal-to-lateral (anteroposterior), and trigone-to-trigone distances are demonstrated in cases of a native noncalcified valve, mitral annular calcification, failing incomplete annuloplasty ring, and degenerated surgical bioprostheses.* **(Right)** *CT of neo-left ventricular outflow tract (LVOT) area estimated after simulation of the transcatheter heart valve suggests a low risk of LVOT obstruction.*

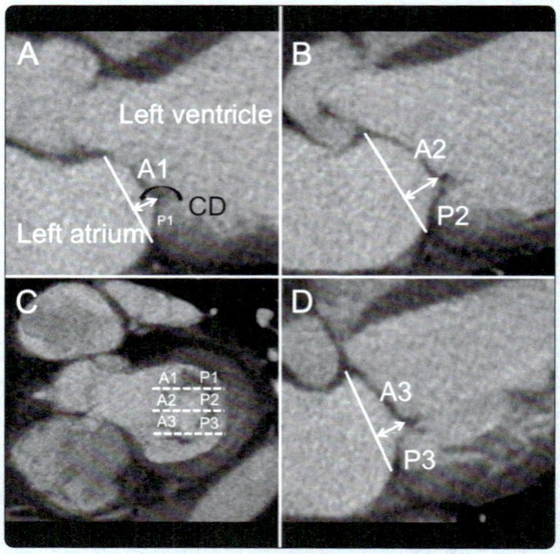

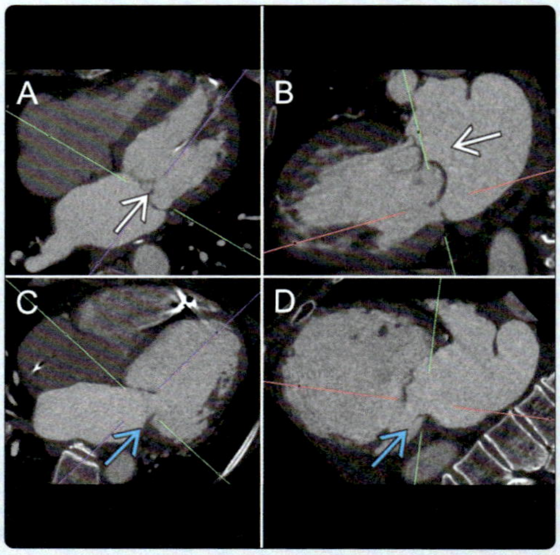

(Left) *Based on short-axis view of mitral valve (MV) at level of leaflets and commissures, orthogonal planes across leaflet segments (A1-P2, A2-P2, P3-P3) can be used to derive apical views of MV apparatus for measurement of coaptation depth (CD) and leaflet angles.* **(Right)** *Man with NHYA class II dyspnea, prior CABG, + LVEF of 35% has MV prolapse ➡. Secondary functional mitral regurgitation in woman with NHYA class II-III symptoms, nonischemic dilated cardiomyopathy, LVEF of 25%, and short posterior mitral leaflet ➡ is shown.*

TERMINOLOGY

Mitral Valve Disease

- Mitral valve (MV) apparatus is composed of anterior and posterior leaflet, chordae tendineae, anterolateral and posteromedial papillary muscles, and mitral anulus
- Mitral regurgitation (MR) is most common disorder involving MV and can be classified as either primary or secondary
- Primary MR (PMR) is due to intrinsic pathology of MV apparatus
  - Barlow disease (MV prolapse) is most common cause
  - Other causes include infective endocarditis, rheumatic fever, and radiation heart disease
- Secondary MR (SMR) is due to pathology of atria or ventricle
  - Atrial functional MR (AFMR) involves leaflet malcoaptation from left atrial and annular dilatation (e.g., chronic atrial fibrillation)
  - Ventricular functional MR (VFMR) involves left ventricular remodeling with asymmetrical or symmetrical leaflet tethering (e.g., ischemic or dilated cardiomyopathies, respectively)
- Mitral stenosis (MS) is most commonly due rheumatic fever, which involves leaflet and subvalvular thickening, commissural fusion, leaflet calcification, and reduced leaflet mobility
- MS related to mitral annular calcification (MAC) is distinct entity

Guideline-Directed Care

- American (2020) and European (2021) guidelines help address diagnostic and therapeutic challenges of MV disease (MS, PMR, and SMR)
- MS: Percutaneous mitral commissurotomy (PMC), also called balloon valvuloplasty, is recommended in symptomatic, severe MS with favorable anatomy (class I) and asymptomatic, severe MS with elevated pulmonary pressures (> 50 mm Hg at rest) (class II)
- MS: If PMC is not suitable for anatomic reasons, then MV surgery is recommended (class I)
- PMR: Surgery is recommended in symptomatic, severe chronic PMR (class I) or asymptomatic, severe PMR with ventricular dysfunction (left ventricular ejection fraction < 60% &/or left ventricular end-systolic diameter > 40 mm) (class I)
- PMR: Surgical MV repair is preferred over valve replacement provided successful and durable repair is likely
- PMR: Transcatheter edge-to-edge repair (TEER) is reasonable in symptomatic, severe patients at high or prohibitive surgical risk (class II)
- SMR: Guideline-directed medical therapy (GDMT) is initial treatment (class 1) in chronic SMR
- SMR: If, despite GDMT, symptoms and severe MR persist, then MV intervention (surgery or TEER) may be considered by heart team
- SMR: If this patient group meets criteria for chronic resynchronization therapy (CRT), then CRT should be performed prior to intervention

Transcatheter Edge-to-Edge Repair

- TEER is limited to suitable anatomies: Less suitable anatomies include small MV area, previous annuloplasty, MAC, preexisting stenosis, short posterior leaflet, and complex Barlow disease
- MitralClip (Abbott) in SMR was subject of randomized trials (EVERST II, COAPT, and MITRA-FR), which led to current view that TEER in selected patients may reduce hospitalizations for heart failure and mortality
- Other TEER devices include PASCAL (Edward Lifesciences) and DragonFly (Hangzhou Valgen Medtech Co, Ltd.)
- CLASP IIF randomized trial is currently evaluating safety and effectiveness of PASCAL compared to MitraClip in SMR

Transcatheter Mitral Valve Implantation

- Less invasive than MV surgery, and compared to TEER, may potentially treat stenosis and offer greater MR reduction
- Range of dedicated transcatheter mitral valve implantation (TMVI) systems have been developed with either transseptal or transapical access
- Multistep devices, in which anchoring member is placed 1st followed by low-profile valve prosthesis, include SAPIEN M3 (Edwards Lifesciences), HighLife (HighLife SAS), and Saturn (InnovHeart)
- Single-step devices include Intrepid (Medtronic), Tendyne (Abbott Structural), EVOQUE Eos (Edwards Lifesciences), AltaValve (4C Medical), CardioValve (Venus MedTech), and Cephea (Abbott Structural)
- Pivotal TMVI trials, which include SUMMIT (Tendyne), MITRAL [valve in MAC with aortic transcatheter heart valves (THVs)], APOLLO (Intrepid), and ENCIRCLE (SAPIEN M3) will help establish role of TMVI in growing landscape of safe and effective transcatheter technologies
- Potential complications include left ventricular outflow tract obstruction (LVOTO), thrombosis, paravalvular leak, and migration/embolization
- LVOTO is major complication associated with poor outcomes
  - Methods to prevent LVOTO include septal reduction and leaflet laceration
    - Septal scoring along midline endocardium (SESAME) is novel percutaneous septal myotomy technique
    - Laceration of anterior mitral leaflet to prevent outflow obstruction (LAMPOON) is transcatheter electrosurgical procedure to split anterior mitral leaflet
- TMVI can be performed in noncalcified native valves as well as in MAC [valve-in-MAC (ViMAC)], failing bioprostheses [valve-in-valve, (ViV)], or failing surgical rings [valve-in-ring (ViR)]
  - ViMAC, ViV, and ViR cases use aortic THVs and are placed via 3 approaches: Transseptal, transapical, and transatrial
  - MAC patients often have mixed valve disease, may be challenging surgical candidates, and frequently are ineligible for TMVI due to pattern of calcification

Other Transcutaneous Treatments

- Role of other transcatheter interventions in MR continues to be established
- e.g., ring annuloplasty combined with atrial fibrillation ablation may offer effective treatment for AFMR

IMAGING ANATOMY

Echocardiography

- Transthoracic echocardiography is initial test to diagnose MV disease, determine severity, assess chambers, and estimate hemodynamics
- Transesophageal echocardiography is performed to further assess MV anatomy and exclude left atrial thrombus
- Echocardiography also remains pivotal for periprocedural guidance and postprocedural follow-up

Cardiac MR

- Has emerging role in management of MR by accurately assessing MR severity and evaluating chamber size and function
- Compared to echocardiography, offers better prediction of outcome and chamber remodeling post MV surgery

CT

- Offers excellent spatial resolution and is essential for preprocedural TMVI planning to enable safe and successful procedure
- Full-cardiac-cycle CT imaging is suggested given dynamic changes of MV apparatus and left ventricle
  - This can be achieved either through retrospective ECG-triggered data acquisition or prospectively ECG-triggered data acquisition with whole-heart detector coverage
- Full-cardiac-cycle imaging allows use of diastole for largest mitral anulus, systole for smallest neo-LVOT, and both phases for quantifying chamber volumes and ejection fraction
- Multiplanar reconstruction (MPR) analysis is used to simulate standard views (2-chamber, commissural, 3-chamber, 4-chamber, and short-axis)
- CT is crucial for accurately measuring mitral annular dimensions, including area, perimeter, intercommissural distance, and septal-to-lateral distance, which are used to guide valve sizing
- In native valves, mitral anulus is traced to form saddle-shaped anulus, while simplified D-shaped anulus is formed by connecting medial and lateral trigones, thereby excluding anterior horn
- In failed surgical rings and bioprosthetic valves, anulus is measured by tracing along contour of annuloplasty ring and prosthetic sewing ring, respectively
- CT allows accurate assessment of amount and distribution of valve calcium
  - Scoring system incorporating calcium thickness, annular distribution, trigone involvement, and leaflet involvement is used to grade severity and predict valve embolization/migration
- LVOTO risk can be estimated using neo-LVOT area, which is calculated by simulating correctly sized THV at end-systole and tracing smallest space between interventricular septum anteriorly and displaced anterior MV leaflet posteriorly
  - Neo-LVOT area < 170 mm^2 has been suggested to be high risk for LVOTO
  - If leaflet laceration is planned, then skirt neo-LVOT has been proposed in which neo-LVOT at level of THV skirt is measured and area < 150 mm^2 has been used to predict LVOTO risk
  - In failed surgical bioprosthetic valves, neo-LVOT should be measured at level of "neo-skirt" of surgical valve, which, depending on valve type, may be shorter then stent posts
- Other CT measurable anatomic factors for LVOTO include septal hypertrophy, narrow aortomitral angle, long anterior mitral leaflet, and small ventricle
- CT is also valuable for planning access, guiding location of puncture, achieving optimal coaxial trajectory for TMVI device deployment, identifying relative position of important surrounding structures, and coronary artery assessment

SELECTED REFERENCES

1. Coisne A et al: ACC/AHA and ESC/EACTS guidelines for the management of valvular heart diseases: JACC guideline comparison. J Am Coll Cardiol. 82(8):721-34, 2023
2. Guerrero ME et al: Diagnosis, classification, and management strategies for mitral annular calcification: a heart valve collaboratory position statement. JACC Cardiovasc Interv. 16(18):2195-210, 2023
3. Lander MM et al: Mitral interventions in heart failure. JACC Heart Fail. 11(8 Pt 2):1055-69, 2023
4. Maher T et al: Mitral regurgitation: advanced imaging parameters and changing treatment landscape. Heart Fail Clin. 19(4):525-30, 2023
5. Urena M et al: Transcatheter mitral valve implantation for native valve disease. EuroIntervention. 19(9):720-38, 2023
6. Akodad M et al: Multimodality imaging to assess leaflet height in mitral bioprosthetic valves: implications for mitral valve-in-valve procedure. JACC Cardiovasc Imaging. 15(9):1663-5, 2022
7. Vahanian A et al: 2021 ESC/EACTS guidelines for the management of valvular heart disease. Eur Heart J. 43(7):561-632, 2022
8. Zoghbi WA et al: Atrial functional mitral regurgitation: a JACC cardiovascular imaging expert panel viewpoint. JACC Cardiovasc Imaging. 15(11):1870-82, 2022
9. Hensey M et al: Transcatheter mitral valve replacement: an update on current techniques, technologies, and future directions. JACC Cardiovasc Interv. 14(5):489-500, 2021
10. Otto CM et al: 2020 ACC/AHA guideline for the management of patients with valvular heart disease: executive summary: a report of the American College of Cardiology/American Heart Association Joint Committee on Clinical Practice Guidelines. Circulation. 143(5):e35-71, 2021
11. Urena M et al: Current indications for transcatheter mitral valve replacement using transcatheter aortic valves: valve-in-valve, valve-in-ring, and valve-in-mitral annulus calcification. Circulation. 143(2):178-96, 2021
12. Guerrero M et al: A cardiac computed tomography-based score to categorize mitral annular calcification severity and predict valve embolization. JACC Cardiovasc Imaging. 13(9):1945-57, 2020

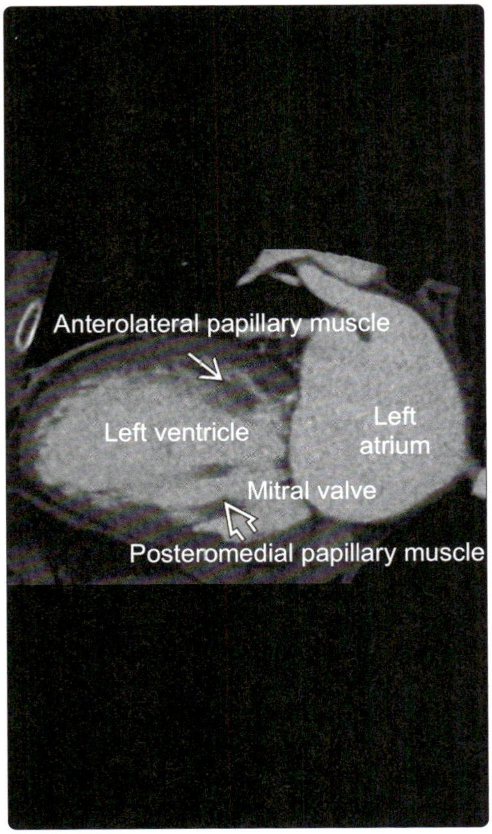

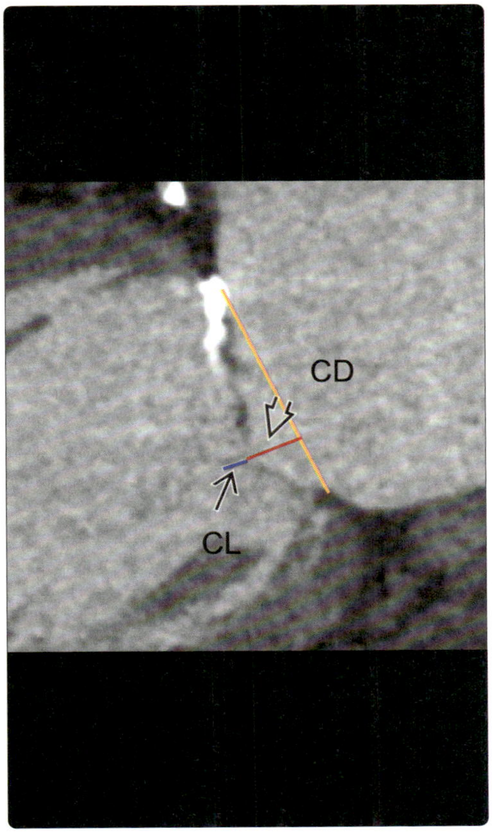

(Left) *Two-chamber view demonstrates left heart chamber structures. Note the anterolateral ➡ and posteromedial ➡ papillary muscles.* **(Right)** *CT of the MV demonstrates the measurement of coaptation length and depth for MitraClip device deployment. CD = coaptation depth ➡; CL = coaptation length ➡.*

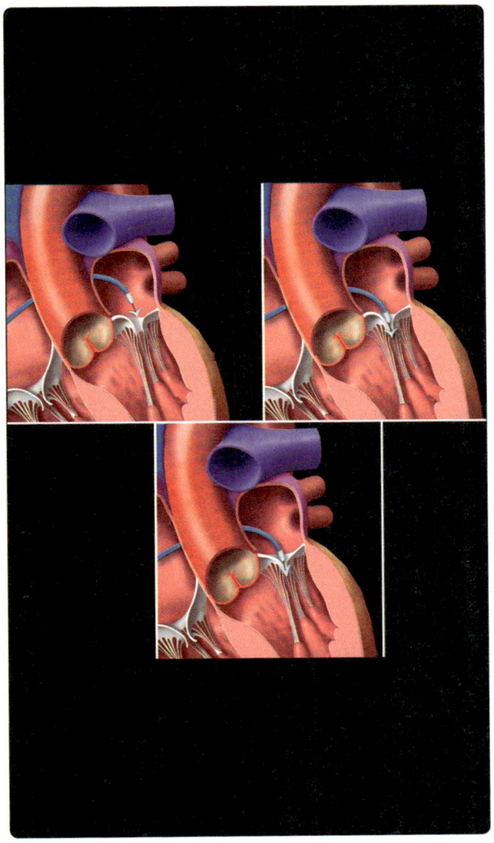

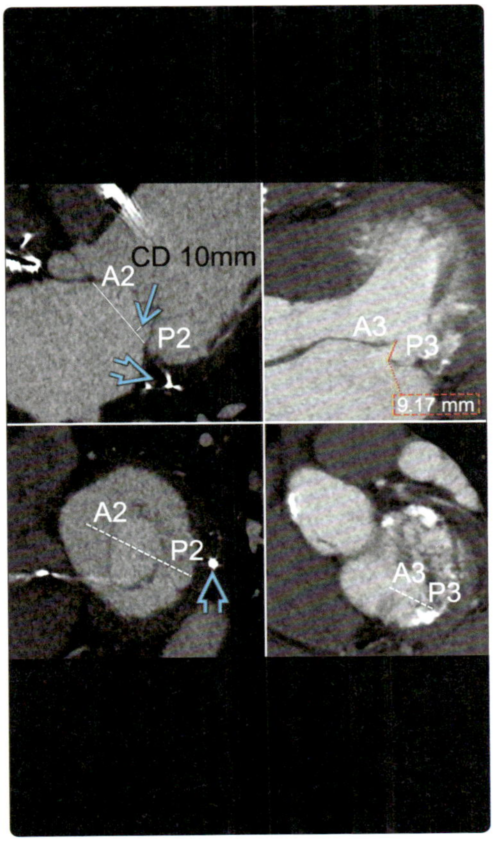

(Left) *Graphic shows deployment of the MitraClip device. (Reprinted with permission from JACC.)* **(Right)** *Observe CT planning for a MitraClip device use in a patient (left top and bottom) with secondary functional mitral regurgitation due to a nonischemic dilated cardiomyopathy (coaptation depth 10 mm ➡) and in another patient (right top and bottom) with mitral valve prolapse. Anatomy in the 1st patient was suitable for MitraClip, but large flail gap and calcification of posterior mitral anulus was prohibitive in the 2nd patient. Note the left ventricular lead ➡ in both patients.*

Transcatheter Mitral Valve Replacement: Procedure Planning and Follow-Up

KEY FACTS

TERMINOLOGY

- Catheter-based mitral valve (MV) replacement that is alternative to surgical MV replacement

IMAGING ANATOMY

- MV apparatus has valve, anulus, and subvalvular apparatus
- Mitral anulus has complex saddle shape

CLINICAL IMPLICATIONS

- Performed in mitral regurgitation with failed medical therapy, high surgical risk, and unfavorable anatomy for repair; calcific mitral stenosis, and failed bioprosthetic valves or rings

TYPES

- Native valve, valve-in-mitral annular calcification (MAC), valve-in-valve, valve-in-ring

CT PARAMETERS

- Assessment of MV disease
- Mitral anulus measurement: D-shaped anulus using 3D cubic spline; diameters, perimeter, and area measured in systole and diastole
- Device-sizing based on anulus measurements
- Risk of neo-left ventricular outflow tract (LVOT) obstruction: Assessed by measuring neo-LVOT diameter using virtual prosthesis; lower risk if area > 200 m²
- For small neo-LVOT, septal thickness can be ↓ by alcohol septal ablation or SESAME procedure; elongated anterior mitral leaflet can be managed by LAMPOON procedure
- CT-based MAC score is provided for valve-in-MAC; higher score = better anchoring of TMVR
- Relationship to left circumflex (LCx) coronary artery and coronary sinus assessed; fluoroscopic angles provided for compromise and septolateral views

POSTPROCEDURAL EVALUATION

- Neo-LVOT obstruction, pseudoaneurysm, paravalvular leak , compression of LCx or coronary sinus are complications

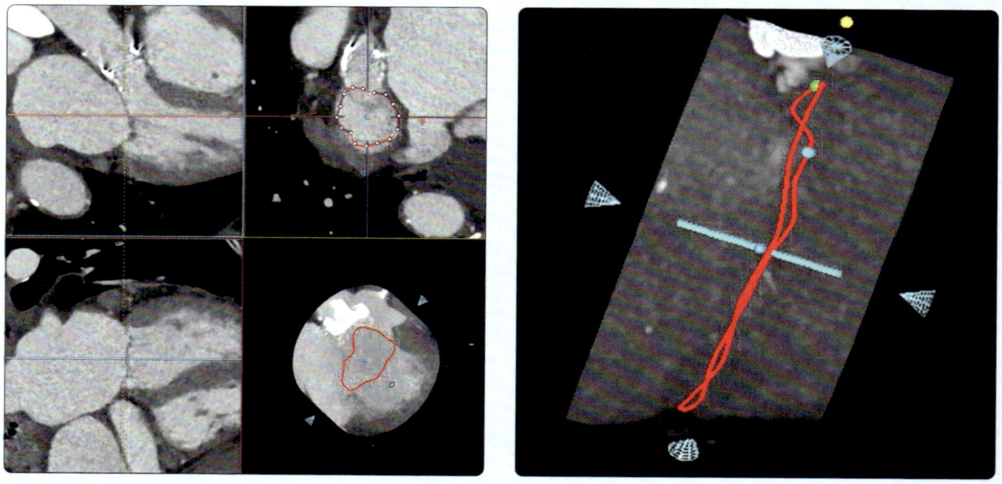

(Left) *Mitral anulus is ideally measured using a dedicated software program that allows placement of multiple seed points at the hinge points of the mitral anulus as the imaging plane is rotated around the central axis of left ventricle (LV) and extends beyond any single image plane.* **(Right)** *A cubic spline of the mitral anulus is created from the seed points. This represents the 3D perimeter of the saddle-shaped mitral anulus.*

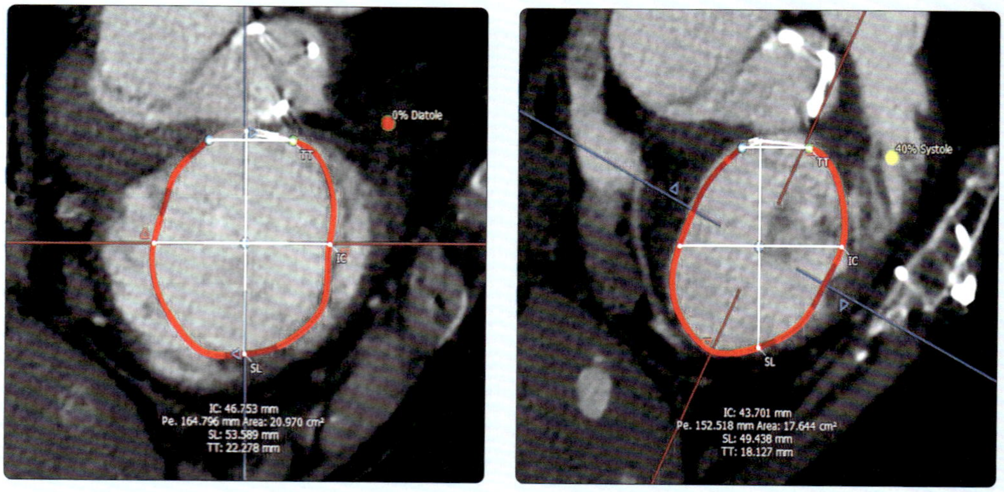

(Left) *A D-shaped anulus is reconstructed in the end-diastolic phase by identifying trigones and placing a virtual trigone-trigone line. From this model, the diameters (intercommissural, trigone-to-trigone, septolateral), perimeter, and the area of the mitral anulus are measured.* **(Right)** *Similar measurements of the mitral anulus (diameter, perimeter, area) are also made in systole, since the mitral anulus is dynamic with varying measurements at different cardiac phases. Using these measurements, a specific device size is selected.*

Transcatheter Mitral Valve Replacement: Procedure Planning and Follow-Up

TERMINOLOGY

Abbreviations

- Transcatheter mitral valve replacement (TMVR)

Definitions

- Catheter-based mitral valve (MV) replacement that is alternative to surgical MV replacement

IMAGING ANATOMY

General Anatomic Considerations

- MV has anterior and posterior leaflets
  - Each with 3 cusps/scallops (A1, A2, A3 and P1, P2, P3)
  - Medial and lateral trigones
  - Medial and lateral commissures
- Mitral anulus: Complex saddle shape
- Subvalvular apparatus has chordae tendinae and papillary muscles (anterolateral and posteromedial)

CLINICAL IMPLICATIONS

Indications for TMVR

- Native mitral regurgitation (primary or secondary) in patients with
  - Failed goal-directed medical therapy
  - High surgical risk
  - Unfavorable anatomy for transcatheter MV repair
- Calcific mitral stenosis
- Failed surgical MV rings or bioprosthesis

Types of TMVR Procedures

- Native valve: Prosthesis placed in native MV
- Valve-in-mitral annular calcification (MAC): Prosthesis placed in native valve with MAC
- Valve-in-valve: Prosthesis placed in preexisting bioprosthetic valve
- Valve-in-ring: Prosthesis placed in preexisting mitral annuloplasty ring (complete or incomplete)

TMVR Devices

- Several (> 30) devices are currently available or being tested
  - Common valves used: SAPIEN 3, Tendyne, Intrepid, Tiara, CardiAQ-Edwards
  - SAPIEN 3 valve used off-label for valve-in-MAC

IMAGING

Echocardiography

- Transthoracic echocardiography is 1st-line imaging modality for evaluation of MV disease and postprocedural follow-up
- Transesophageal echocardiography (TEE) used for detailed evaluation and assessment of left atrial appendage
- TEE and intracardiac echocardiography (ICE) used for procedural guidance

CT

- Imaging modality of choice for preprocedural evaluation, including virtual prosthesis, neo-left ventricular outflow tract (LVOT), and extracardiac structures
- CT protocol optimized for evaluation of MV
  - Retrospective ECG gating without tube-current modulation or prospective ECG-triggered acquisition in volume scanners
    - Anulus is dynamic: Measurements required in systole and diastole
  - Triphasic contrast injection protocol with bolus trigger in ascending aorta
- Assessment of MV disease: Complementary information to echocardiography
  - Mitral stenosis: Thickened leaflets; ± calcification; restricted diastolic opening
  - Mitral regurgitation: Incomplete systolic coaptation; annular dilation, leaflet tenting and tethering of posterior leaflet in functional MR; thickened and bowing of leaflets in MV prolapse
- MAC
  - Spares leaflet commissures and anterior leaflet
  - Large amount of MAC: Increases surgical risk but increases device anchoring for TMVR
  - CT-based MAC score: Evaluated in 3D volumetric view with superimposed hockey puck-shaped mitral anulus
    - Average calcium thickness (< 5 mm = score 1; 5-9.99 mm = score 2; ≥ 10 mm = score 3)
    - Degree of anulus circumference involved (< 180°= score 1; 180-270° = score 2; > 270° = score 3)
    - Calcification of trigones (1 = score 1; both = score 2)
    - Calcification of leaflets (1 leaflet = score 1; 2 leaflets = score 2)
    - Severe MAC = score ≥ 7; lower risk of device embolization or migration
- Mitral anulus measurements
  - Native anulus has complex saddle shape to account for anterior horn/aortomitral continuity
  - D-shaped anulus is used for reproducible measurements
    - Excludes anterior horn with virtual line between medial and lateral trigones
  - Anulus can be measured in short-axis plane derived from 2 long-axis views at level of mitral anulus
  - Dedicated software allows placement of seed points (12-16) at hinge points of mitral anulus when rotating around left ventricle (LV) central axis to form cubic spline of 3D anulus plane
    - Trigones are identified, and virtual TT line is drawn between trigones, forming D-shaped anulus
    - TT distance, septolateral distance, intercommissural distance, and perimeter areas measured
  - Measurements are based both in end-systole and end-diastole due to dynamism of mitral anulus
- Device sizing
  - Based on anulus measurements
    - e.g., SAPIEN 3 is available in 20, 23, 26, and 29 mm diameters
    - e.g., CardiAQ Edwards is available in 43, 46, and 50 mm diameters
- Neo-LVOT assessment
  - Placing TMVR device causes anterior deflection of anterior mitral leaflet (AML), which narrows and elongates LVOT = neo-LVOT
  - Obstruction of neo-LVOT is important cause of morbidity and mortality after TMVR

- CT can assess risk of neo-LVOT obstruction by simulating virtual prosthesis, which is 3D model that matches shape and dimensions of planned TMVR device
- Based on anulus dimensions, virtual prosthesis is positioned along central axis of mitral anulus with 20% located in atrium and 80% in LV
- In end-systolic images, centerline is created through neo-LVOT
- From curved MPR through neo-LVOT, smallest cross-sectional area of neo-LVOT is generated
- Ideal candidates for TMVR will have neo-LVOT area > 200 m²; < 170 mm² predicts neo-LVOT obstruction
  - Measurement at end-systole is overly conservative and may unnecessarily exclude patients; measure throughout systole
- Higher risk with greater flaring, protrusion, and skirt size of device
- Higher risk with septal hypertrophy, elongated AML, and higher aortomitral angles

- Interventions for small neo-LVOT
  - Hypertrophied basal septum
    - Alcohol septal ablation is used to decrease septal thickness
    - SESAME (SEptal Scoring Along Midline Endocardium) = transcatheter basal septal myotomy
    - CT used for assessment of neo-LVOT pre- and postseptal ablation or SESAME
  - Elongated AML
    - Measured from tip of A2 scallop to junction between AML and posterior aortic wall; > 30 mm
    - LAMPOON procedure = Laceration of AML to Prevent Outflow ObstructioN
      - Laceration of AML opens channels through which blood can traverse neo-LVOT through skirt of SAPIEN valve
    - In patients with small neo-LVOT with long AML, neo-LVOT dimension is measured with skirt of valve alone, predicting size of neo-LVOT after LAMPOON
- Atrioventricular shelf
  - Seen adjacent to PML insertion point in functional MR due to remodeling of basal myocardium
  - Changes shape during cardiac cycle; more apparent in diastole
  - Persistent shelf is important for devices, such as Tiara, which uses basal inferolateral myocardium for anchoring
- Subvalvular apparatus and other measurements
  - Distance from mitral anulus to papillary muscle heads in 2-chamber: Less subvalvular interference by prosthesis with larger distance
  - Distance between papillary muscles in short-axis view
  - Distance between left atrial appendage (LAA) ostium and mitral anulus plane: Less chance of LAA ostial occlusion when larger distance
- Relationship to adjacent structures
  - Coronary sinus: Important landmark for device deployment
  - Left circumflex coronary artery: Risk of compression with device oversizing
- Procedural fluoroscopic angles
  - Compromise view: Best view of potential LVOT compromise
  - Septolateral view: Best to align deployment along mitral anulus axis
  - TT view: Not clinically feasible due to C-arm restraints
- Valve-in-MAC
  - Ideally requires calcification > 75% of circumference for anchoring
  - When contouring, anulus shape can be kept smooth, rather than intricately contoured
  - Higher periprocedural complication risk, including mortality, LVOT obstruction, valve embolization, and stroke
- Valve-in-valve
  - Valve anulus dimensions = mitral anulus dimensions
  - Aortomitral angle using seating of surgical valve; surgical prosthesis may not sit perfectly in anulus
- Valve-in-ring
  - Ring dimensions = mitral anulus dimensions for planning
  - Complete/incomplete ring
- Transapical approach
  - Volumetric images of whole chest help determine which intercostal space is closest to LV apex
  - Optimal fluoroscopic angles for transapical coaxial deployment
- 3D printing
  - Device sizing, bench testing
  - Landing zone, apposition and expansion in MAC: Risk of neo-LVOT obstruction and paravalvular leak (PVL)

POSTPROCEDURAL ASSESSMENT

Echocardiography

- 1st-line imaging modality
- Normal TMVR: Unrestricted, free mobility of valve leaflets

CT

- Used for further characterization of echocardiographic findings
- Neo-LVOT obstruction
  - Typically diagnosed during procedure
  - Rarely seen in imaging; valve projects into and narrows LVOT
- Pseudoaneurysm
  - LV pseudoaneurysm is rare, life-threatening complication
  - At prosthesis anchor points or LV apex
- PVL: Free channel of contrast that connects left atrium and LV
- Device embolization/migration
- Obstruction of left circumflex coronary artery or coronary sinus

SELECTED REFERENCES

1. Guerrero M et al: A cardiac computed tomography-based score to categorize mitral annular calcification severity and predict valve embolization. JACC Cardiovasc Imaging. 13(9):1945-57, 2020
2. Ranganath P et al: CT for pre- and postprocedural evaluation of transcatheter mitral valve replacement. Radiographics. 40(6):1528-53, 2020
3. Blanke P et al: Mitral annular evaluation with CT in the context of transcatheter mitral valve replacement. JACC Cardiovasc Imaging. 8(5):612-5, 2015

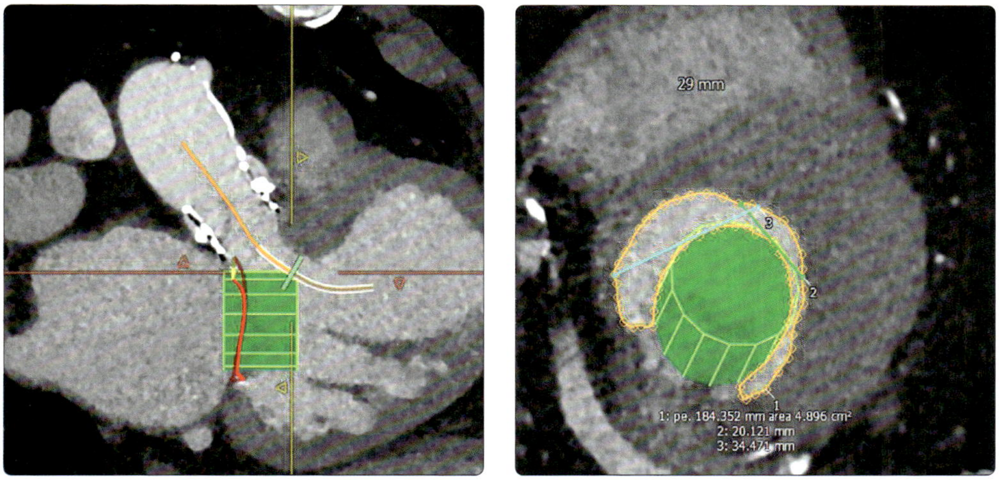

(Left) *Neo-LV outflow tract (LVOT) is estimated in an end-systolic image by placing a virtual prosthesis in the mitral anulus. In this patient, a 29-mm SAPIEN 3 valve was virtually implanted with 20% in the left atrium and 80% in the LV. Subsequently, a centerline is drawn through the LVOT (orange line).* **(Right)** *From a curved MPR of the LVOT, the shortest diameter is identified. Measurements of the LVOT (area and perimeter) are made in this view. In this patient, the area is 489 mm², which is sufficient for safely implanting a TMVR device.*

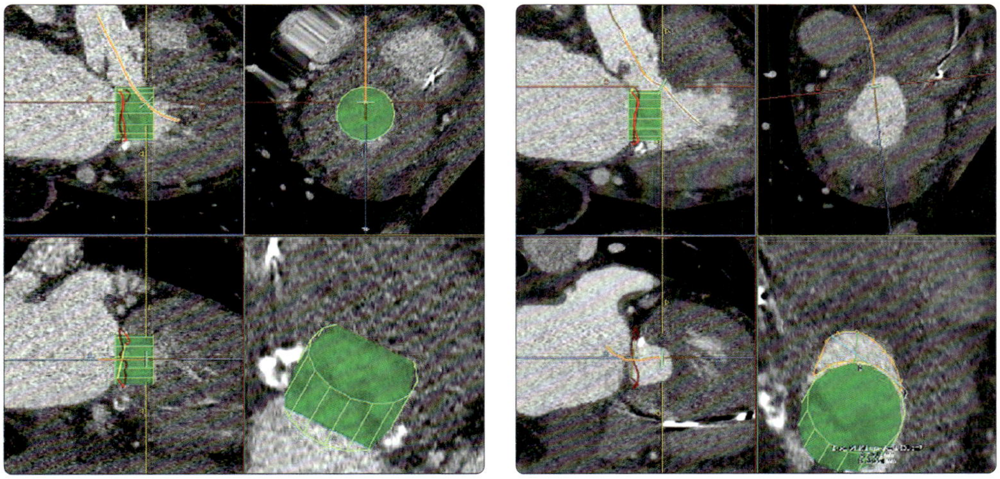

(Left) *Measurements of the LVOT in a patient with severely hypertrophied basal ventricular septum shows obliteration of neo-LVOT with virtual placement of a 29-mm SAPIEN 3 valve prosthesis.* **(Right)** *Due to the need for TMVR, this patient underwent alcohol ablation of the ventricular septum. Following this, a repeat CT showed that the thickness of the basal septum has decreased. The neo-LVOT now measures 190 mm², which is amenable for TMVR placement.*

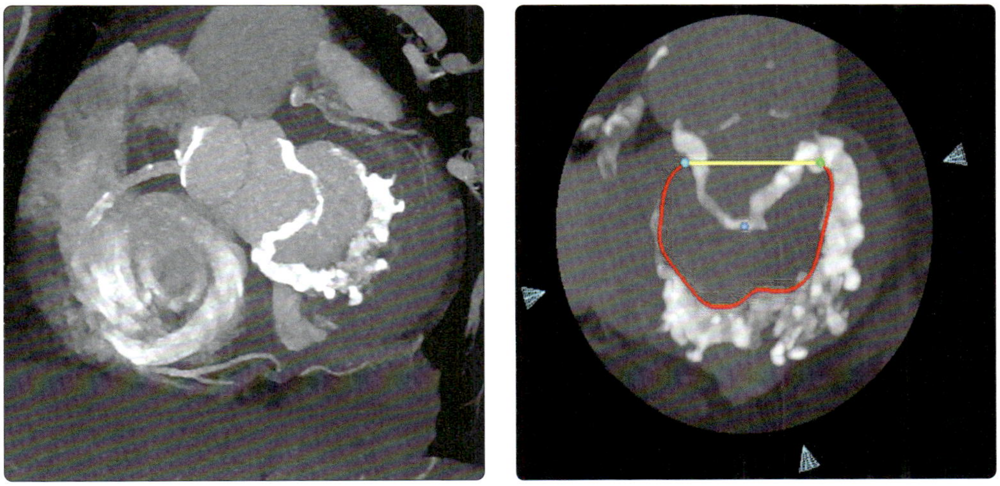

(Left) *Short-axis MIP reconstruction shows the extent and amount of mitral annular calcification (MAC). This patient had extensive MAC with a CT MAC score of 10, which is good for anchoring of a SAPIEN device.* **(Right)** *Measurement of the mitral anulus by 3D extrapolation of a D-shaped mitral anulus in MAC is shown.*

KEY FACTS

TERMINOLOGY

- Pacemakers: Electronic devices connected to endocardium or epicardium of heart by pacing wires or capsule-like electronic device without traditional pocket and wires (i.e., leadless pacemaker) that use electrical impulses to regulate cardiac rate or rhythm
- Implantable cardioverter-defibrillators (ICDs): Electronic devices that administer electric shocks to heart to restore normal cardiac rhythm if defined rapid ventricular arrhythmias are sensed

IMAGING

- ICD leads are thicker than pacemaker leads
- Generator will overlie left or right anterior chest wall in most cases
- CT allows for more detailed evaluation of lead integrity
- Leads may fracture, typically between 1st rib and clavicle

PATHOLOGY

- ACC/AHA guidelines for ICD therapy include as class I indications
  - Cardiac arrest due to ventricular fibrillation (VF) or tachycardia (VT)
  - Spontaneous sustained VT
  - Syncope with inducible VT or VF in electrophysiological (EP) study
  - Nonsustained VT in setting of ischemic heart disease and inducible VF or VT in EP study
- Indications for permanent pacing therapy include (among others)
  - Certain atrioventricular blocks
  - Sinus node dysfunction with bradycardia ± symptoms
  - Hypertrophic or dilated cardiomyopathies with sinus node dysfunction
  - Neurocardiogenic syncope

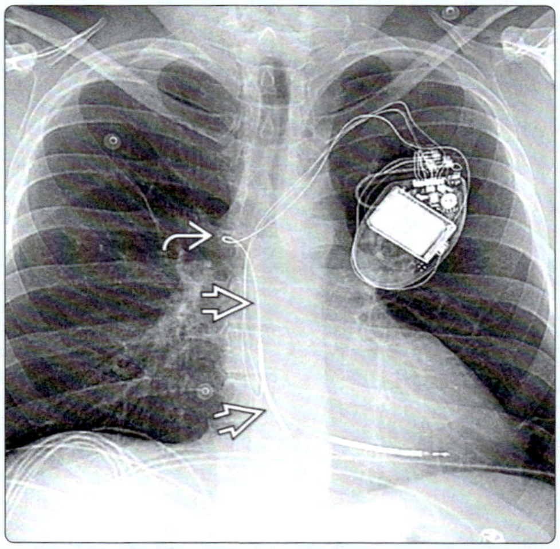

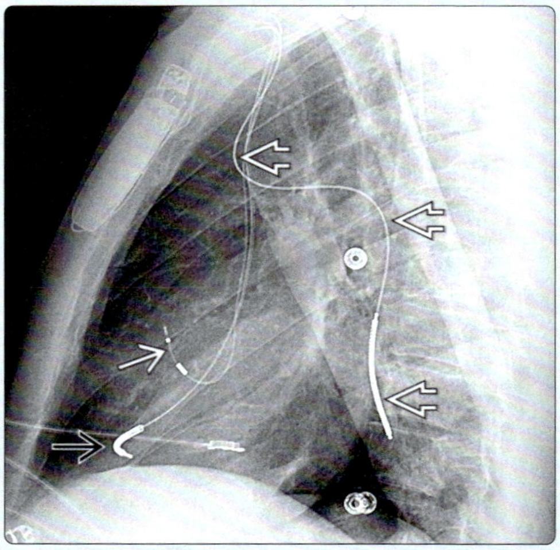

(Left) *Frontal radiograph shows a high-voltage defibrillator lead in the azygos vein. The characteristic redundant appearance of the lead at the en face portion of the azygos vein is essentially diagnostic of an azygos position.* **(Right)** *Lateral radiograph shows the typical course of a lead in the azygos vein. The advantage of this position is a discharge across the left ventricular mass. A right atrial appendage lead and right ventricular lead are also present and in place.*

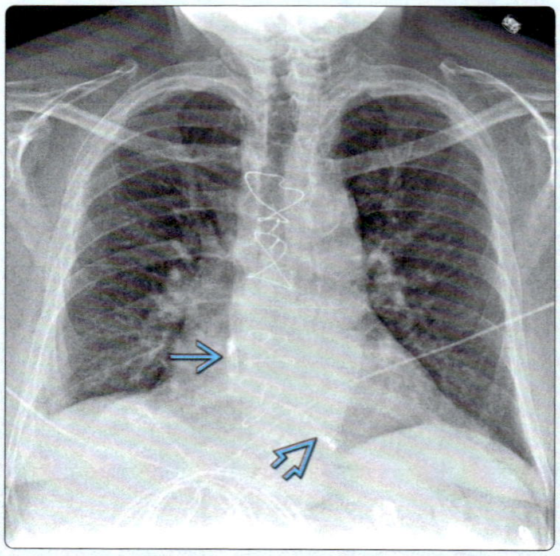

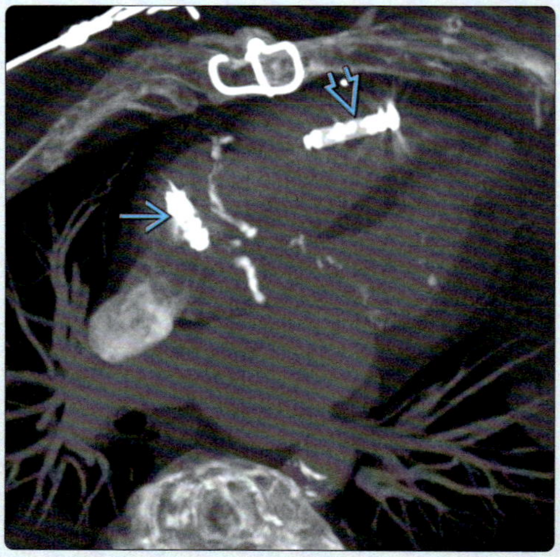

(Left) *AP chest radiograph shows a right atrial and right ventricular dual-chamber leadless pacemaker system, which safely provides atrial pacing and reliable atrioventricular synchrony for 3 months after implantation.* **(Right)** *Reconstructed 4-chamber MIP CT shows a leadless right atrial and right ventricular dual-chamber leadless pacemaker system.*

TERMINOLOGY

Abbreviations

- Implantable card overter-defibrillator (ICD)

Definitions

- Pacemakers (PMs)
  - Permanently implanted, battery-operated electronic devices that use electrical impulses to regulate cardiac rate or rhythm
    - Connected to endocardium or epicardium of heart by pacing wires or capsule-like electronic device without traditional pocket and wires [i.e., leadless pacemaker (LP)]
    - Substitute for natural pacemaker (sinus node)
- ICDs
  - Permanently implanted, battery-operated electronic devices that administer electric shocks via intracardiac or epicardial leads to heart to restore normal cardiac rhythm if defined rapid ventricular arrhythmias are sensed

IMAGING

General Features

- Location
  - Usually right or left pectoral pocket containing device generator
  - Older devices and epicardial pacing or defibrillator devices in abdominal wall tissue
  - Temporary leads may have leads through right internal jugular vein, right subclavian vein, or femoral vein and connect to extracorporal device
  - Leads typically extend through superior vena cava and right or left innominate and subclavian veins
  - Older leads may extend through subcutaneous tissue from abdominal wall
  - Epicardial leads typically perforate pericardium anteriorly
  - Temporary pacing wires are placed surgically over right ventricular and right atrial surface and may be removed
  - Lead tip locations
    - Right atrium, commonly atrial appendage
    - Right ventricle near apex
    - Left ventricle
      - Via coronary sinus in great cardiac vein or its tributaries (transvenous leads)
      - Via pericardium within epicardial myocardium (epicardial leads)
  - Subcutaneous ICD: Lead in subcutaneous tissue of anterior chest wall, 1-2 cm to left of sternum
  - Right ventricle LP location
    - Linear radiopaque device implanted via femoral venous access and actively fixated to right ventricular myocardium
  - Wireless cardiac stimulation system for left ventricle (WiCS-LV) pacer located in LV myocardium provides wireless pacing of LV endocardium by transmitting ultrasonic energy from pulse generator transmitter implanted subcutaneously over ribcage to receiver electrode/pacer implanted in LV myocardium
- Morphology
  - Single-chamber pacing
    - 1 lead: Either in right atrium or in right ventricle
  - Dual-chamber pacing
    - 2 leads: 1 in right atrium and 1 in right ventricle
  - Biventricular pacing
    - 3 leads: 1 in right atrium, 1 in right ventricle, and 1 via coronary sinus in great cardiac vein or tributary
  - Epicardial pacing
    - 2 screw-in leads in LV myocardium
    - Device location: Abdominal wall
  - Epicardial defibrillator
    - Leads implanted over anterior right ventricle, right atrium, and posterior lateral left ventricle
    - Device location: Abdominal wall
  - ICD
    - 1 multifunctional lead
      - Defibrillator shock coils at right ventricle level ± superior vena cava coil
      - Sensing electrode at lead tip of right ventricle
    - ± coronary sinus lead and right atrial lead if also biventricularly paced

Radiographic Findings

- May demonstrate
  - Lead fractures
  - Tip dislodgement
  - Device migration, retained lead fragments

CT Findings

- CECT
  - CT may demonstrate complication from device placement
    - Hemothorax
    - Pneumothorax or pneumopericardium
    - Chamber or coronary sinus rupture with hemopericardium ± tamponade
    - Device infection; however, is best assessed with 18F-FDG PET/CT due to high sensitivity, specificity, positive predictive value, and negative predictive value
  - ECG gating, sharp reconstruction kernels, metal artifact reduction algorithms, and iterative reconstruction algorithms improve visualization
  - Interaction of CT with pacemaker/ICD: Transient oversensing in majority of devices
    - Temporary inhibition of pacing has been reported from pacemakers and cardiac resynchronization therapy (CRT) pacemakers
    - Temporary inhibition of pacing therapy, inhibition of shock therapy, and inappropriate shock therapy have been reported with ICD and CRT defibrillators
    - Distance between beam and device is maximized and placement of device directly into x-ray beam is avoided
    - Programming may reduce interference during CT scan
      - Pacemaker: Asynchronous pacing mode
      - ICD: Turn off tachy mode or program tachy mode to electrocautery protection mode or to off electrocautery

MR Findings

- MR was traditionally considered contraindication in patients with pacemakers/ICDs

- However, MR can now be safely performed in these patients
  - Both in MR-conditional as well as legacy devices, which were nonconditional
  - Proper evaluation of device, safety precautions, and device programming must be done
    - Pacemakers: **PM-dependent**: Set to asynchronous pacing mode; **non-PM dependent**: Disable pacing and sensing
    - ICD: **PM-dependent**: Do not scan; **non-PM dependent**: Disable pacing and sensing
    - Legacy device: Set to VVI/DDI mode with undesired behavior programmed off
    - Following scan, device is reprogrammed to its baseline level
- Artifacts are expected in cardiac MR due to proximity of these devices and their leads
  - ICDs produce larger susceptibility and off-resonance artifact than PMs
- Strategies to reduce artifacts from devices
  - Minimize inhomogeneity: Move generator up and away from heart; optimize shimming
  - Technical parameters: Shortest echo time; highest bandwidth; lower voxel size; parallel imaging; reconstruction algorithms to correct phase errors
  - Use appropriate sequences to minimize artifacts
    - Spin-echo sequences wherever possible, especially for morphologic imaging
    - Cine imaging: Nonbalanced, gradient-echo sequence has less artifacts than commonly used SSFP cine sequence
    - LGE: Use wideband sequence (higher bandwidth) to avoid artifactual areas of high signal
      - Inadequate inversion of myocardium due to offset in myocardial frequency of 2-6 kHz, which is outside bandwidth of inversion pulse (1.1 kHz)
      - Using wideband adiabatic inversion pulse (bandwidth 3.8 kHz) inverts myocardial signal
  - T1 mapping and perfusion will also benefit from wideband pulses to minimize artifact

DIFFERENTIAL DIAGNOSIS

Other Electronic Devices

- Deep brain stimulator: Leads toward cranium
- Vagal nerve stimulator: Leads terminate in lower neck
- Spinal cord stimulators: Leads in epidural space of thoracolumbar spine
- Diaphragmatic pacemaker; gastric stimulator; bladder pacemaker

PATHOLOGY

General Features

- Class I indications included in American College of Cardiology(ACC)/American Heart Association (AHA) guidelines for ICD therapy
  - Cardiac arrest due to ventricular fibrillation or tachycardia not due to transient cause
  - Spontaneous sustained ventricular tachycardia
  - Syncope with inducible ventricular tachycardia or ventricular fibrillation in electrophysiologic study
  - Nonsustained ventricular tachycardia in setting of ischemic heart disease and inducible ventricular fibrillation or tachycardia in electrophysiologic study
- Other indications for ICD treatment include (among others)
  - Ventricular tachycardia while awaiting transplant
  - Familial conditions, such as hypertrophic cardiomyopathy or long QT syndrome
- Indications for permanent pacing therapy include
  - Acquired atrioventricular block with bradycardia, arrhythmia, asystole > 3 seconds, or after surgery or ablation procedures
  - Bifascicular or trifascicular atrioventricular blocks
  - Sinus node dysfunction with bradycardia ± symptoms
  - Hypertrophic or dilated cardiomyopathies with sinus node dysfunction
  - Neurocardiogenic syncope
- Indications for right ventricular leadless pacer
  - To minimize long-term lead-related risks in treatment of sick sinus syndrome, chronic, symptomatic 2nd- and 3rd-degree arteriovenous block, recurrent Adams-Stokes syndrome, and symptomatic, bilateral bundle-branch block

CLINICAL ISSUES

Presentation

- Complications of non-LP/ICDs
  - Cardiac perforation or coronary sinus transection
  - Pneumothorax &/or pneumopericardium
  - Dislodgement of leads
  - Hemothorax, pleural effusions
  - Infection of pacer generator or ICDs &/or leads
  - Stimulation of diaphragm via phrenic nerve
  - Device migration
- Old leads frequently left in place when generator replaced

DIAGNOSTIC CHECKLIST

Consider

- Carefully follow course of leads, as fractures may be nondisplaced and subtle
- Compare lead position with initial postplacement radiograph to exclude lead migration

Image Interpretation Pearls

- Beam hardening artifact may mimic right ventricular perforation by lead tip
  - Absence of pericardial fluid in absence of clinical symptoms suggests absence of free perforation

SELECTED REFERENCES

1. Waqanivavalagi SWFR: Temporary pacing following cardiac surgery - a reference guide for surgical teams. J Cardiothorac Surg. 19(1):115, 2024
2. Knops RE et al: A dual-chamber leadless pacemaker. N Engl J Med. 388(25):2360-70, 2023
3. Garg J et al: Leadless cardiac pacemakers: paradigm shift in cardiac pacing. Heart Rhythm. 16(1):72-3, 2019

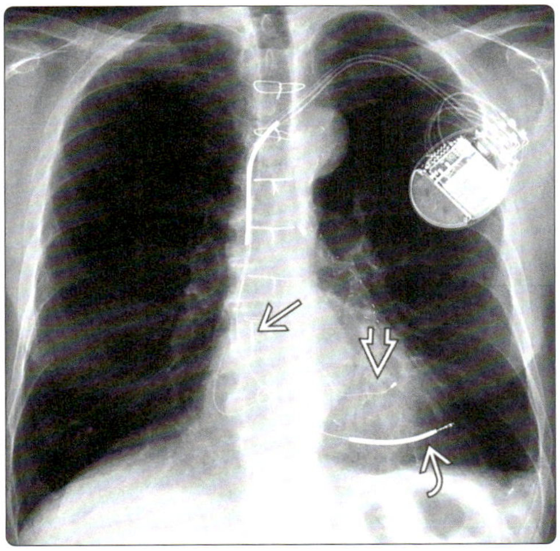

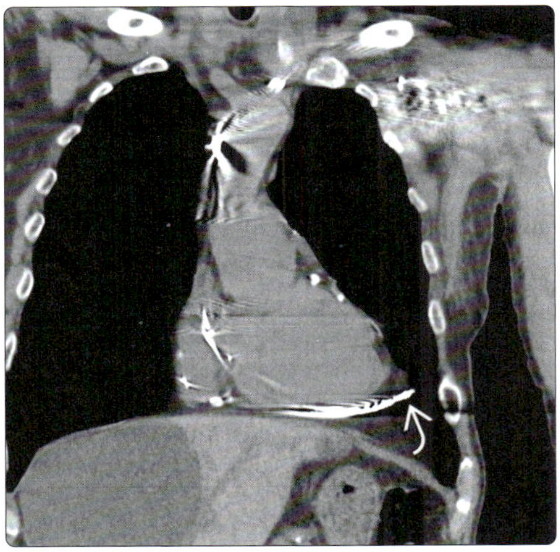

(Left) *PA radiograph shows a 3-lead automated implantable cardiac defibrillator (AICD) with 1 lead in the right atrium, 1 lead in the right ventricle, and 1 lead in the coronary sinus. The right ventricular lead extends more laterally than expected beyond confines of cardiac silhouette, which is worrisome for cardiac perforation.* **(Right)** *Coronal oblique CT shows that the right ventricular lead has perforated through the right ventricle and pericardium and lies within the epicardial fat. No pericardial effusion is noted.*

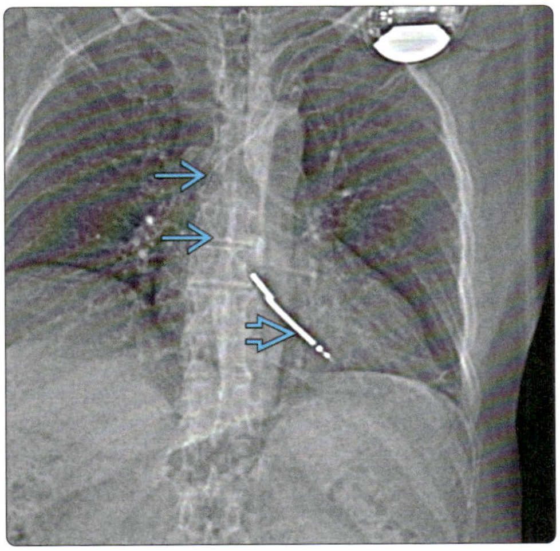

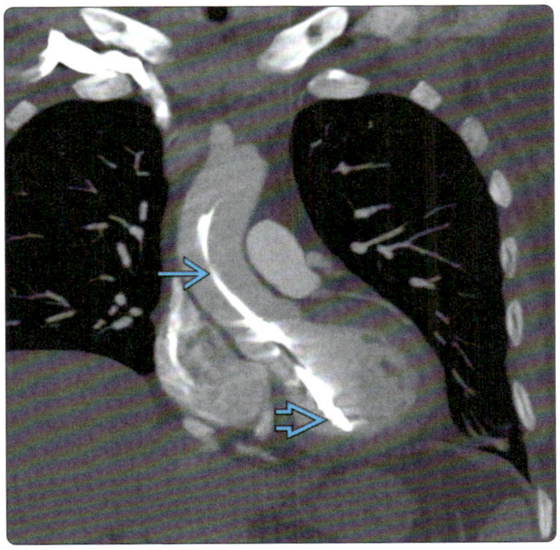

(Left) *AP chest radiograph shows an unusual course of an AICD lead more leftward than the anticipated course of superior vena cava and a more leftward course over the cardiac silhouette with the tip projecting over the inferior portion of the cardiac silhouette.* **(Right)** *Coronal CTA MIP shows the malpositioned AICD lead entered through the left subclavian artery and aorta with the lead tip malpositioned within the posterior margin of the posteromedial papillary muscle of the left ventricle.*

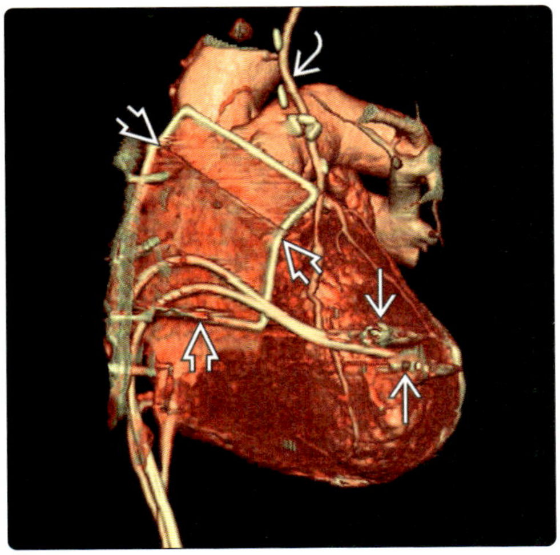

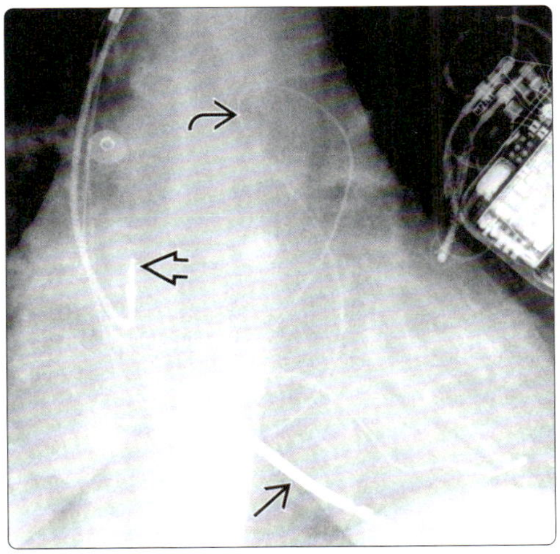

(Left) *Oblique cardiac CT shows epicardial defibrillator patches and screw-in epicardial leads in the left ventricular myocardium. Note the left internal mammary artery bypass graft.* **(Right)** *PA radiograph after development of chest pain demonstrates prolapse of the epicardial vein lead into the right ventricle and main pulmonary artery, although the tip is in its original position. The right atrial and right ventricular leads are unchanged and within the expected locations for such leads.*

Introduction

Preprocedural imaging has become integral in electrophysiology (EP) to minimize the risks of difficult EP procedures. Common EP procedures are ablation for atrial fibrillation (AF), ventricular tachycardia, and cardiac resynchronization therapy (CRT). Postprocedural imaging is also imperative to detect complications. CT and MR are emerging as valuable noninvasive imaging modalities to provide this information, including establishing the etiology, identifying the substrate, prognosis/risk stratification, preprocedural evaluation/mapping, guidance during intervention, and postprocedural assessment.

Establishing Etiology

MR can help in establishing the etiology of an arrhythmia with cine SSFP imaging demonstrating the morphology and quantifying functional parameters. The etiology of an arrhythmia (different cardiomyopathies) may be established based on the LGE pattern. Parametric mapping techniques (T1, T2, T2*, ECV) also help in tissue characterization. When MR is contraindicated, CT may be used to provide some information using morphology, iodine late enhancement (ILE) and ECV measurement. ILE in CT has lower contrast:noise ratio (CNR) compared to MR. Multienergy CT techniques can improve the performance of CT.

Identifying Substrate

Scarring or fibrosis identified with LGE MR likely contains the focus or substrate for an arrhythmia. The scar border zone is critical in the perpetuation of an arrhythmia. MR is generally better in identifying substrates in the ventricles than the thin-walled atria. Using MR, myocardial disease is identified in 74% of patients, compared to 51% using non-MR techniques and 50% that are reassigned as a new or alternative diagnosis. CT can also identify scars but with lower CNR.

Prognosis/Risk Stratification

Several MR biomarkers are prognostic indicators of future adverse cardiovascular events. Scar burden (scar percentage, transmurality), total scar size, scar core size, scar heterogeneity, and periinfarct gray zone are predictors of an arrhythmia. MR is a risk stratification tool for implantable cardioverter defibrillator (ICD) selection, based on the extent of the scar and ventricular function. Fibrosis also predicts appropriate device therapy in patients with an ICD.

Preprocedural Evaluation and Mapping

Atrial Fibrillation/Flutter Ablation

CT and MR provide knowledge on the anatomy of the pulmonary veins (PV), which is essential to ensure that all the ectopic foci are ablated. Variations can be seen in the number, branching pattern, and length. Accessory ostium (1.6-19%) and common ostium (2.4-25%) are the common variations. Ostial orientation and distances of the branches from the ostia is essential to avoid branch vessel stenosis. PV stenosis and left atrial (LA) thrombus are contraindications for the procedure. The relationship of the left atrium to the esophagus and phrenic nerve, and the thickness of the LA wall and adjacent fat, help in minimizing complications.

MR can evaluate LA volume and function, which indicate persistent AF. The extent of LGE is a predictor of the type and the recurrence of AF. LGE MR is used in some centers for guidance of ablation. Postcontrast T1 MR has also been used for the same purpose.

Left Atrial Appendage Closure

CT is useful in identifying contraindications, providing measurements for accurate device sizing, and minimizing manipulation. LA appendage (LAA) thrombus and pericardial abnormalities are contraindications. For accurate sizing of the device, the LAA ostial diameter, LAA landing zone, LAA length from the landing zone, LAA depth, and the shape of the LAA are evaluated. Atrial septal anatomy, PV anatomy, left atrium size, and accessory LAA/diverticula morphology can also be assessed. CT also provides optimal fluoroscopic angulations for the procedure.

Ventricular Tachycardia Ablation

MR and, occasionally, CT can provide information on scars, which can be used to establish etiology and provide a target for ablation. Similar to AF, thrombus is a contraindication for the procedure. The amount of epicardial fat and endocardial trabeculations also helps in determining suitability for epicardial and endocardial access.

Cardiac Resynchronization Therapy/Implantable Cardioverter Defibrillator

CT and MR provide knowledge about coronary venous anatomy prior to CRT, which is essential for venous access and to minimize fluoroscopy time. CRT is not possible if there are no coronary sinus tributaries, either as a normal variation or due to thrombosis. Extensive scarring, especially in the lateral left ventricular wall, indicates that CRT will not be successful. The presence of septolateral delay in strain imaging, such as velocity-encoded or feature-tracking MR, is a predictor of good CRT response.

Procedural Guidance

Procedural guidance is typically performed using fluoroscopy or a transesophageal echocardiograph. CT or MR data are loaded on to electroanatomic mapping systems. Interventional MR-guided EP procedures offer the potential for enhanced arrhythmia substrate assessment, improved procedural guidance, real-time assessment of ablation formation, and decreased complications.

Postprocedural Evaluation

CT and MR can evaluate complications of AF ablation, particularly PV stenosis/occlusion and thrombus. Rare complications, such as esophagoatrial fistula, can be evaluated best with CT. Cardiac perforation, cardiac tamponade, pericarditis, and vascular insults are other complications. MR can help in ablation of recurrent AF by identifying gaps in LGE. LGE correlates negatively with AF recurrence. LA volumes and function improve after successful ablation.

MR can be used to evaluate the adequacy of ventricular tachycardia ablation. Ablation lesion has high signal with a central low-signal core in LGE. Complications, such as a steam pop injury, can be seen.

CT is useful in evaluation of complications of an LAA device, including incomplete LAA closure, peridevice leak, device-related thrombus, and device dislodgement/embolization.

Selected References

1. Sultana S et al: Role of computed tomography in cardiac electrophysiology. Radiol Clin North Am. 62(3):489-508, 2024
2. Chubb H et al: Cardiac electrophysiology under MRI guidance: an emerging technology. Arrhythm Electrophysiol Rev. 6(2):85-93, 2017

Thrombus, Cardiac CT

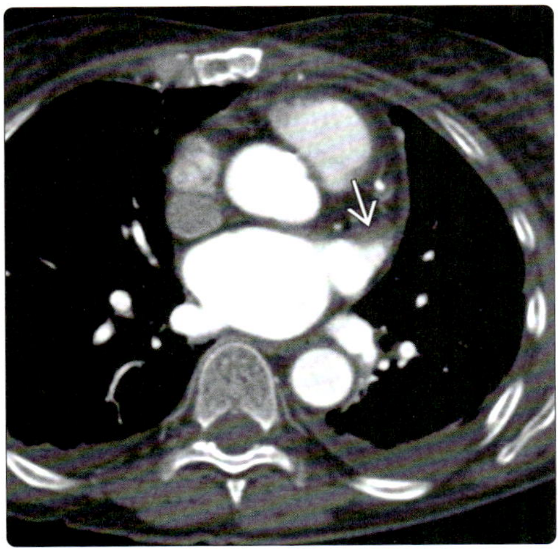

Thrombus, Two-Chamber CT

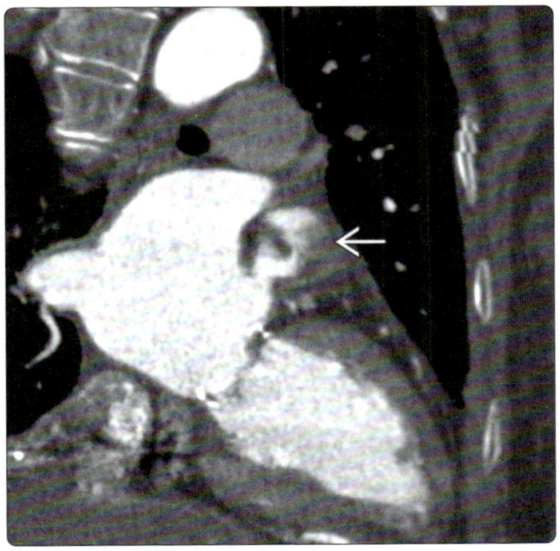

(Left) *Axial cardiac CT in a patient with atrial fibrillation being evaluated for radiofrequency ablation (RFA) shows a thrombus* ➡ *in the tip of the left atrial appendage, which is a contraindication for the procedure.* **(Right)** *Two-chamber reconstructed CT in the same patient demonstrates a thrombus* ➡ *in the tip of the left atrial appendage. Note that detection of a left atrial thrombus before ablation for atrial fibrillation is imperative to avoid distal systemic embolization of the thrombus.*

Left Inferior Pulmonary Vein, Cardiac CT

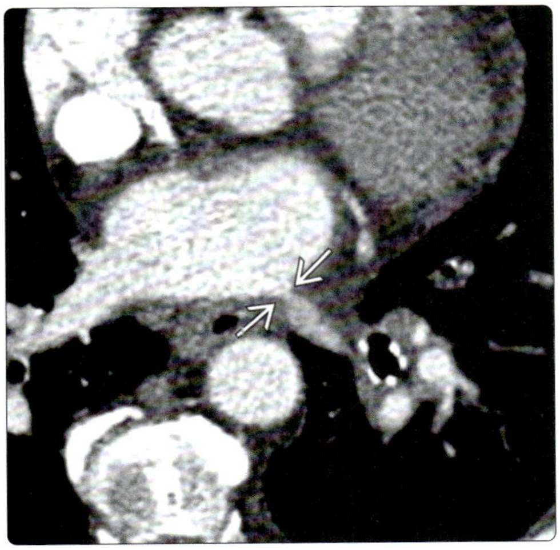

Pulmonary Vein Obliteration, CT

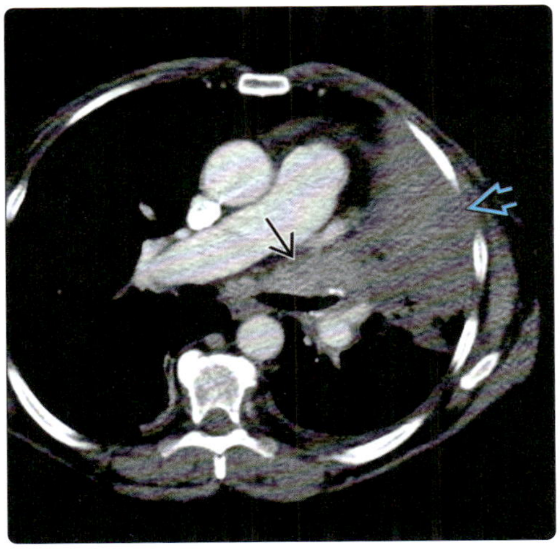

(Left) *Axial cardiac CT shows narrowing at the ostium of the left inferior pulmonary vein* ➡*, which developed as a complication of RFA of the pulmonary ostia.* **(Right)** *Axial CT in the same patient shows left superior pulmonary vein obliteration* ⇨ *and consequent left upper lobe infarction and hemorrhage* ⇨*. This vein was stented (not shown), and the left upper lobe consolidation eventually resolved.*

Dilated Left Ventricle, SSFP Cine MR

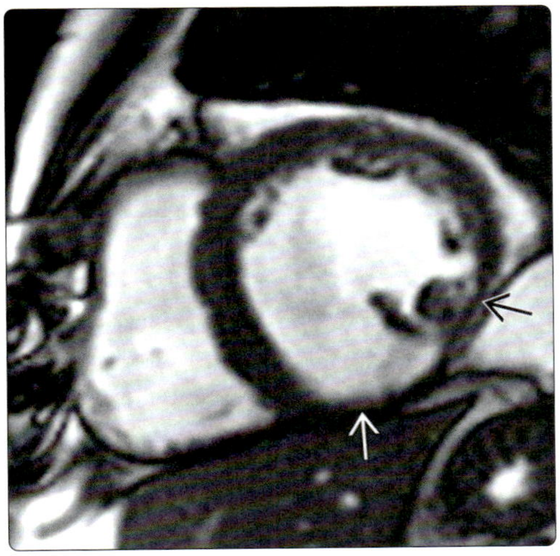

Left Ventricular Myocardium, Short-Axis MR

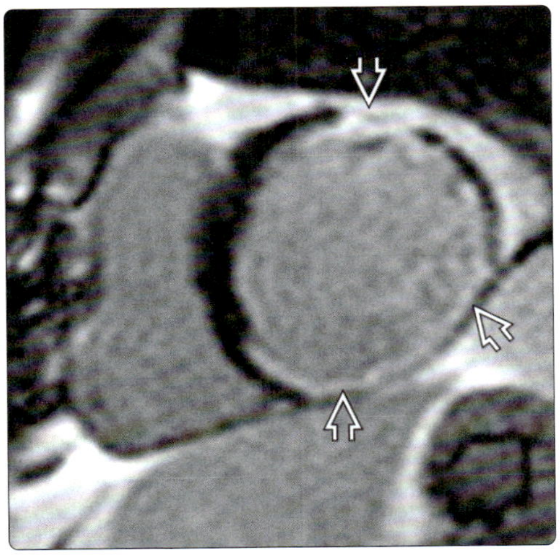

(Left) *Short-axis SSFP cine MR at end-diastole shows dilation of the left ventricle with thinning of the inferior* ➡ *and lateral* ⇨ *walls.* **(Right)** *Delayed postcontrast short-axis MR shows a large degree of LGE involving the left ventricular myocardium* ➡*. The pattern is subendocardial to transmural involving lateral, inferior, and anterior segments, indicative of myocardial infarction. Given the large degree of scarring, the patient would be at risk for a poor response to cardiac resynchronization therapy.*

KEY FACTS

TERMINOLOGY

- Pulmonary veins (PVs) drain oxygenated blood from lungs into left atrium
  - Electrical foci inside PVs may trigger atrial fibrillation, which is common arrhythmia
  - Catheter-based PV isolation is widespread treatment for atrial fibrillation and benefits from preprocedure PV imaging to guide ablation procedures
- Normal PV anatomy: 2 left and 2 right PVs drain into left atrium
- Anomalies of PV return
  - PVs may drain into structures other than left atrium (most frequently right atrium or superior vena cava)
  - Scimitar syndrome: PV return from right lung to right atrium
- Variants of PV return
  - Any variant in which all PVs drain to left atrium, but there are < or > 2 right and 2 left PV ostia

IMAGING

- Transesophageal echocardiography can visualize PVs, but complete visualization of anatomy is difficult
- CTA and MRA are equally effective in defining PV anatomy prior to ablation; choice depends on local expertise and patient preference

CLINICAL ISSUES

- PV ostia are often strongly tapered (especially lower left); diagnosis of PV stenosis requires comparison of pre- and postablation images
- Variants of PV anatomy are present in 25-40% of patients undergoing PV ablation
- CT and MR images of PV anatomy are often fused with electroanatomic mapping systems to facilitate catheter guidance during atrial fibrillation ablation
- PV stenosis can occur following PV ablation but has become infrequent with modern ablation techniques

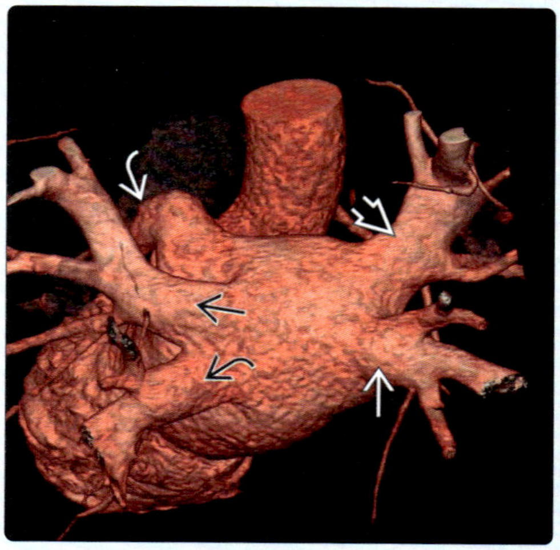

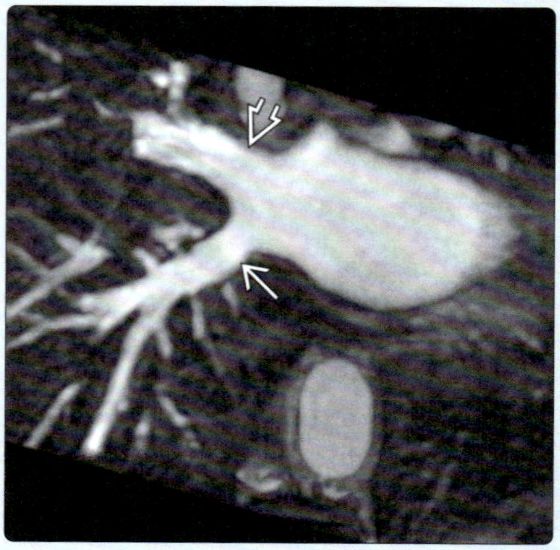

(Left) *3D reconstruction of normal pulmonary vein (PV) anatomy by multidetector-row CECT, viewed from a posterior aspect, shows that the right upper ➡, right lower ➡, left upper ➡, and left lower ➡ PVs enter the left atrium separately. The left atrial appendage ➡ is seen as well.* **(Right)** *MR angiography shows the left upper ➡ and left lower ➡ PVs demonstrating that PVs can also be visualized on 2D imaging.*

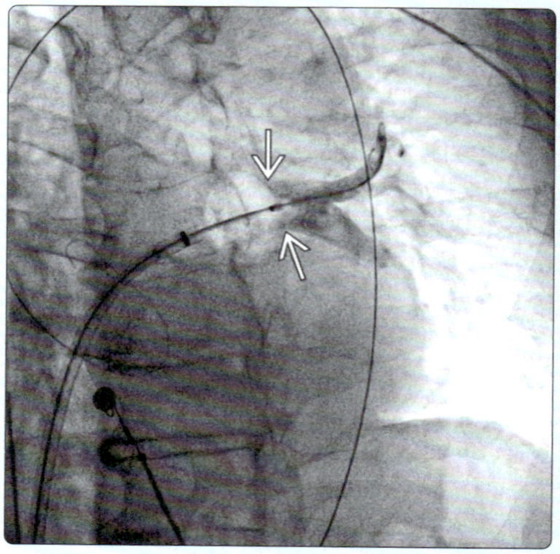

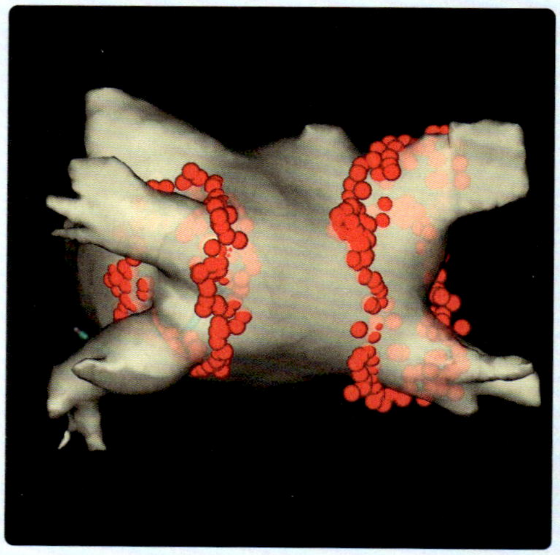

(Left) *PVs are seen during a cryoballoon ablation procedure. The left upper PV ostium ➡ is blocked by a balloon, and contrast is injected to ensure complete blockage.* **(Right)** *Fusion of 3D anatomic imaging (in this case, CTA) and electrophysiologic mapping shows the location of high-frequency energy applied to the left atrial wall (red dots). Several commercially available systems can be used for image fusion using DICOM data sets for anatomic reference and superimposing current catheter position.*

TERMINOLOGY

Definitions

- Pulmonary veins (PVs) drain oxygenated blood from lungs into left atrium
  - Electrical foci inside PVs may trigger atrial fibrillation, which is common arrhythmia
  - Catheter-based PV isolation is widespread treatment for atrial fibrillation
- PV anatomy is important to guide ablation procedures
- Normal PV anatomy: 2 left and 2 PVs drain into left atrium
- Variants of PV anatomy are common and include supernumerary veins draining into left atrium or single ostia for left or right PVs
- Anomalies of PVs are defined as any pattern where PVs drain into structures other than left atrium [most frequently inferior vena cava (IVC), right atrium, or superior vena cava]
  - Scimitar syndrome is infrequent PV anomaly where PVs from right middle and lower lobe drain into IVC or right atrium

IMAGING

General Features

- In normal PV anatomy (75-80% of individuals), 2 right and 2 left PVs have separate ostia into posterior wall of left atrium
- Right superior PV is usually largest
- Most frequent variants are presence of middle right PV and common left PV trunk
- Most frequent anomaly is drainage of right superior PV into superior vena cava, often associated with atrial septal defect
- PV stenosis (PVS) may occur after ablation; however, PV ostia often show tapering even before ablation
  - Comparison of pre- and postablation images is mandatory to diagnose PVS

Echocardiographic Findings

- In transesophageal echocardiography, ostia of PVs can be identified by skilled operators, but complete visualization of anatomy is difficult

Angiographic Findings

- Invasive angiography
  - PVs can be visualized by invasive angiography after transseptal passage and balloon occlusion
  - Performed during ablation process to verify balloon position (cryoablation) or catheter tip position (high-frequency current ablation)

CT Findings

- CTA
  - EKG gated cardiac CT is needed (prospective or retrospective)
  - Identifies PV anatomy with high resolution
  - Reformatted images allow measurement of PV diameters
    - 3D reconstructions are helpful for interpretation
  - CT images may be fused with electroanatomic imaging systems (e.g., CARTO for catheter guidance during ablation)
  - Detects left atrial volume and relationship of esophagus
  - Identifies contraindications for ablation procedure, such as left atrial thrombus (LAT)
    - Delayed imaging or prone position may help to exclude thrombus
  - Assesses complications after procedure
    - PVS
      - Incidence of severe PVS between 0.29-3.4%
      - More common with left-sided veins
      - Can cause unilateral pulmonary edema or venous infarct
    - Atrioesophageal fistula (AEF)
      - Extremely rare but deadly complication
      - Total incidence: 0.025%; radiofrequency > cryoballoon
      - Diagnosis most commonly made with CT
      - Esophageal thickening with small amount of extraluminal air adjacent to left atrium
      - Head CT with multiple strokes or pneumocephaly

MR Findings

- MRA
  - PV anatomy is readily identified
  - Reformatted images allow measurement of PV diameters

Imaging Recommendations

- Best imaging tool
  - CTA and MRA are equally effective to define PV anatomy prior to ablation
    - Choice will depend on local expertise and patient preference

CLINICAL ISSUES

Presentation

- Variants of PV anatomy are present in 25-40% of patients undergoing PV ablation
- PVS following PV ablation infrequent but does occur
  - Treated with PV stenting
    - Restenosis in 17%
    - Occluded PV not amenable
  - Unilateral pulmonary edema, venous infarction, and pulmonary hypertension can occur
- AEF with very high mortality of 50-83%
- LAT contraindication for ablation

DIAGNOSTIC CHECKLIST

Image Interpretation Pearls

- PV ostia are often tapered; therefore, diagnosis of PVS requires comparison of pre- and postablation images

SELECTED REFERENCES

1. Saad H et al: Radiologic manifestations of pulmonary vein ablation complications: a pictorial review. J Thorac Imaging. 36(5):W89-95, 2021
2. Fender EA et al: Assessment and management of pulmonary vein occlusion after atrial fibrillation ablation. JACC Cardiovasc Interv. 11(16):1633-9, 2018

(Left) *CECT shows normal PV anatomy. A multiplanar reconstruction in axial orientation shows the left upper PV ➡ and right upper PV ➡. Note the left atrium ➡ and small cross section of the left atrial appendage.* **(Right)** *Multiplanar reconstruction, again in axial orientation but several centimeters caudal, shows the left atrium ➡ and the left lower ➡ and right lower ➡ PVs.*

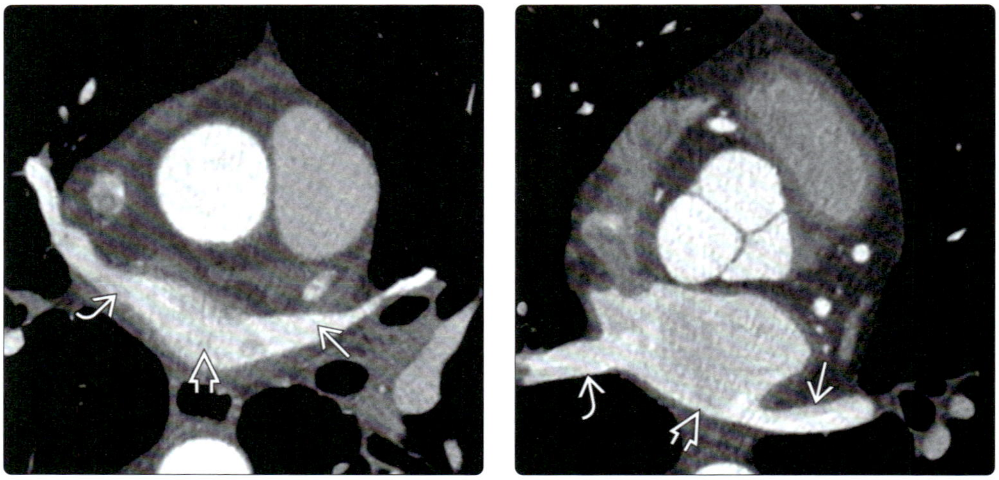

(Left) *CECT demonstrates the anatomy of all 4 PVs. Eight-mm MIP multiplanar reconstruction shows the ostia of all 4 PVs ➡.* **(Right)** *3D reconstruction of the left atrium and PVs shows the heart from a posterior view. The descending aorta and the spine have been removed. Note the normal anatomy of the left and right PVs with separate ostia.*

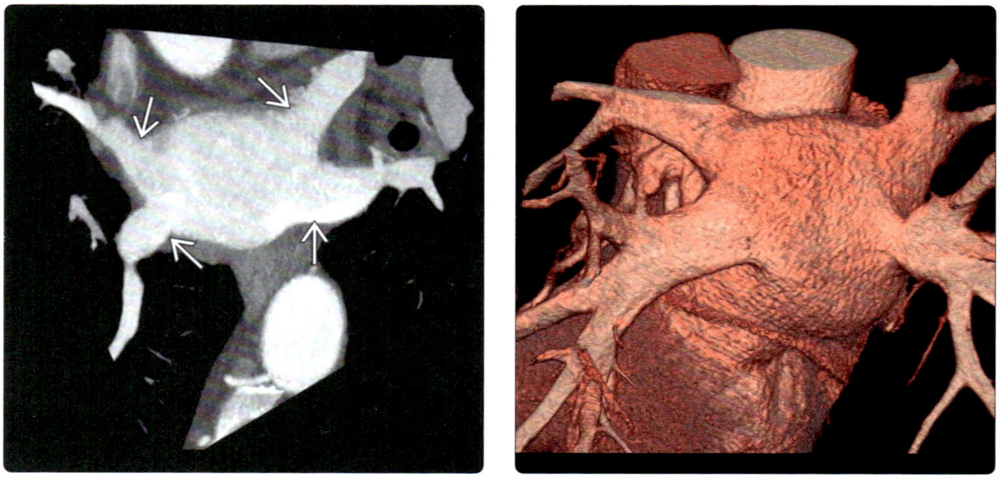

(Left) *MIP MRA shows normal anatomy of the 4 PVs with separate ostia into the left atrium ➡. Slight tapering of the lower left pulmonary artery is frequently seen even in healthy individuals.* **(Right)** *This 3D reconstruction of normal PV anatomy is based on MRA.*

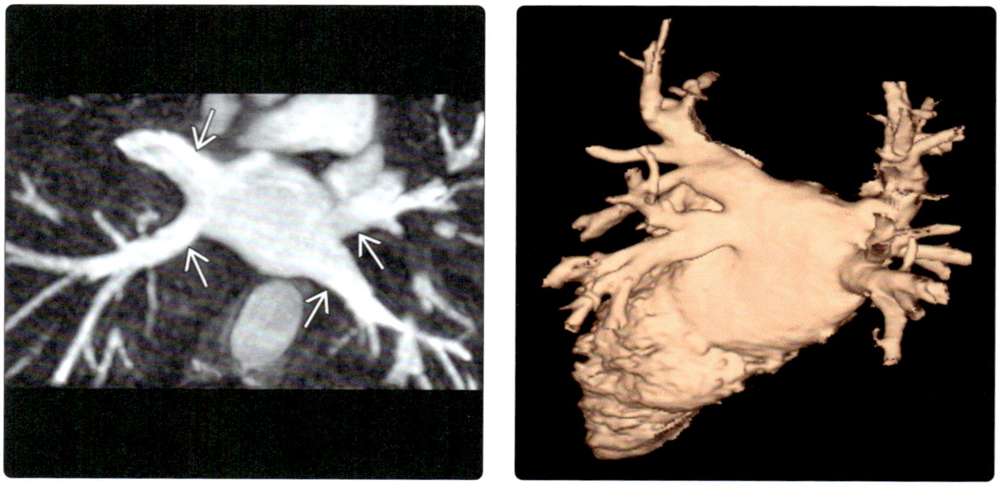

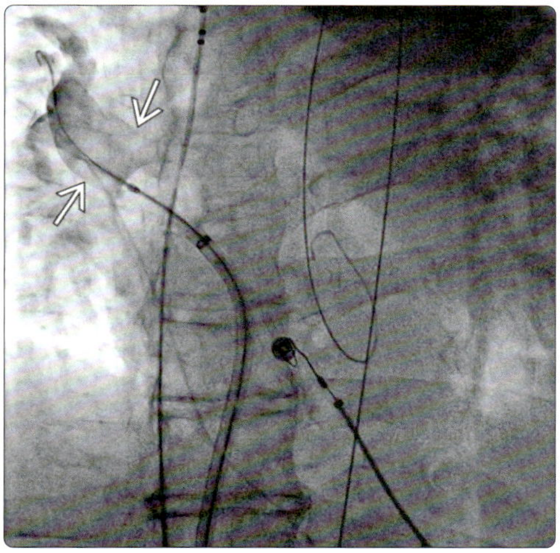

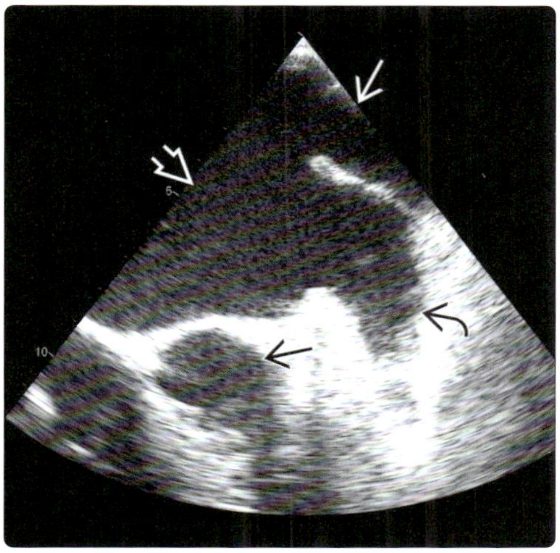

(Left) *Angiography shows the right upper PV during a cryoballoon ablation procedure. The ostium of the right upper PV is blocked by a balloon, and contrast is injected.* **(Right)** *Transesophageal echocardiography demonstrates the ostium of the left upper PV, left atrial appendage, left atrium, and aorta.*

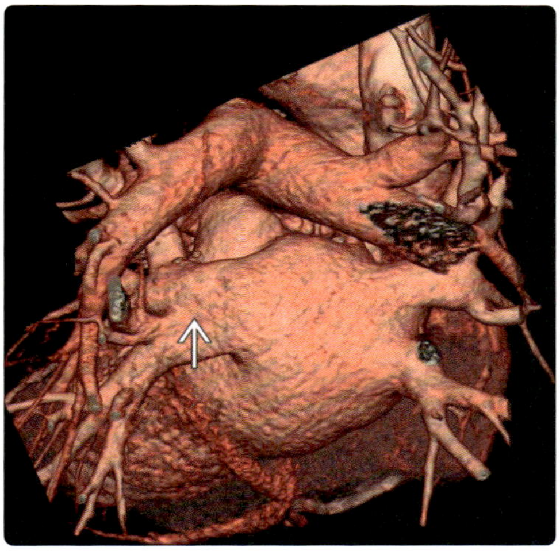

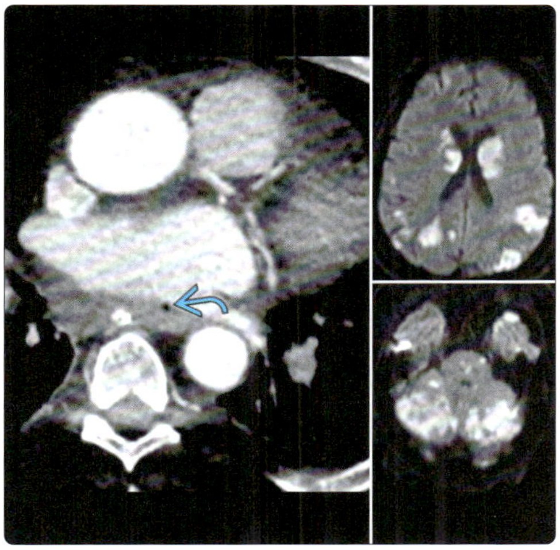

(Left) *CECT 3D reconstruction shows a common ostium of the left superior and inferior PVs, which is one of the most frequent variants of PV anatomy. The right-sided PVs demonstrate normal anatomy.* **(Right)** *CTA (left) 20 days after PV ablation shows esophageal thickening and a punctate focus of air between the esophagus and atrial wall, which are the only signs of an atrioesophageal fistula in the chest. DWI images (right) 1 day later show numerous bilateral infarcts.*

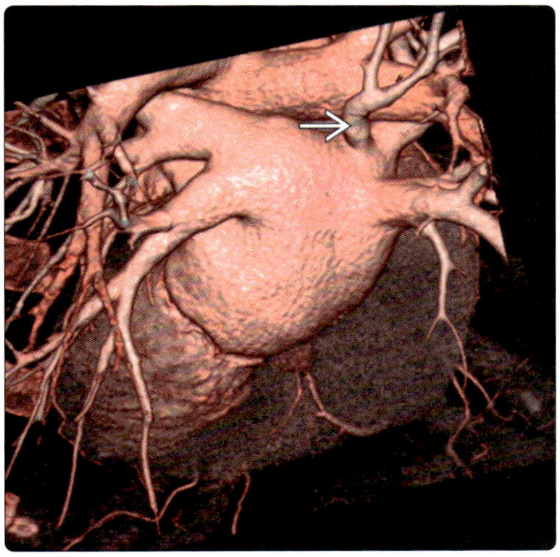

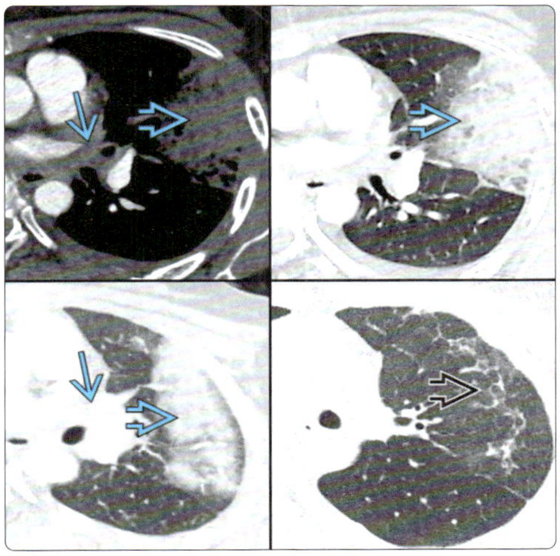

(Left) *CECT 3D reconstruction shows accessory PV close to ostium of the right upper PV.* **(Right)** *Outside CTPA in a young woman 1 (top) and 3 (bottom left) months after PV ablation shows left superior PV occlusion with left upper lobe (LUL) venous infarct. Infarct shows signs of organization at 3 months. Occlusion was not detected on either study, and consolidation was called pneumonia. Study 6 months after ablation (bottom right) shows residual band-like LUL scarring and hazy ground glass due to healing venous infarct.*

Left Atrial Thrombus

KEY FACTS

TERMINOLOGY

- Thrombus formation in left atrial appendage (LAA) or, occasionally, in body of left atrium
- Usually due to atrial fibrillation or mitral valve stenosis

IMAGING

- Best diagnostic clue: Filling defect within LAA persistent on delayed enhanced imaging
- Transesophageal echocardiography (TEE) is considered gold standard for excluding LAA thrombus
- Cardiac CTA
  - Delayed scans allow for differentiation of slow mixing and LAA thrombus
  - Sharper interface between filling defect and contrast opacified lumen is suggestive of thrombus
  - Low HU filling defect suggests thrombus
  - HU > 80 in LAA more likely represents slow mixing
  - Thrombus has lower LAA:aorta HU ratio (< 0.25)
- Cardiac MR
  - White-blood imaging in multiple planes helps outline thrombus, especially in body of left ventricle
  - Gadolinium-enhanced MR is inferior to TEE for detection of LAA thrombus
  - No enhancement on LGE MR and persistent low signal at long inversion times is consistent with thrombus

TOP DIFFERENTIAL DIAGNOSES

- Pseudothrombus (on CTA)
- Tumors
- Surgical exclusion of LAA

CLINICAL ISSUES

- Treatment
  - Anticoagulant therapy (warfarin) substantially reduces embolic event risk
  - Surgical: Maze procedure and similar operations
  - LAA obliteration

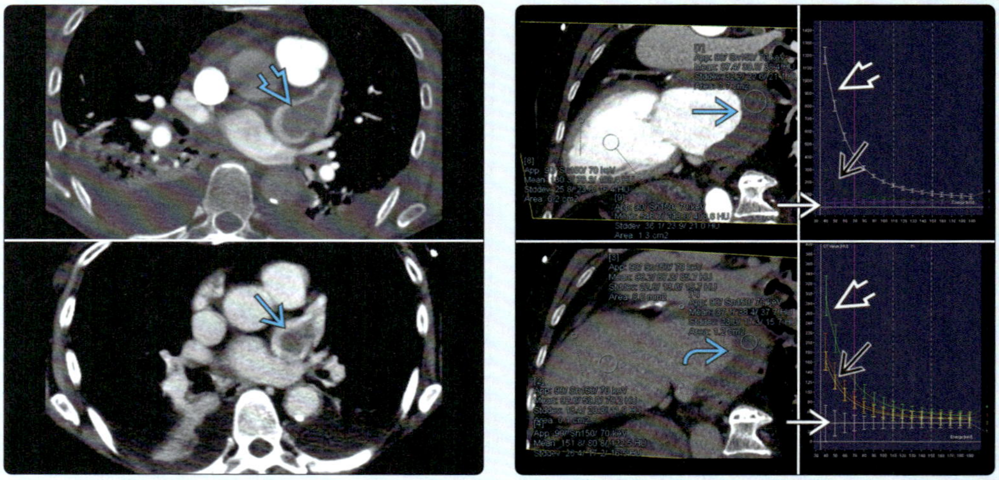

(Left) *CTPA image (top) shows a left atrial appendage (LAA) thrombus ⇨. On delayed phase (bottom), the thrombus appears smaller ⇨, suggesting some peripheral hypoattenuation on CTPA was due to slow flow.* **(Right)** *Dual-energy CTA shows a large left atrial thrombus on low ⇨ (top) and high keV ↪ (bottom) recons. While the blood pool ➡ and myocardial ⇨ HU curves both show high attenuation that ↓ with ↑ keV, the thrombus attenuation curve ➡ shows low HU without change across keV, signifying no enhancement.*

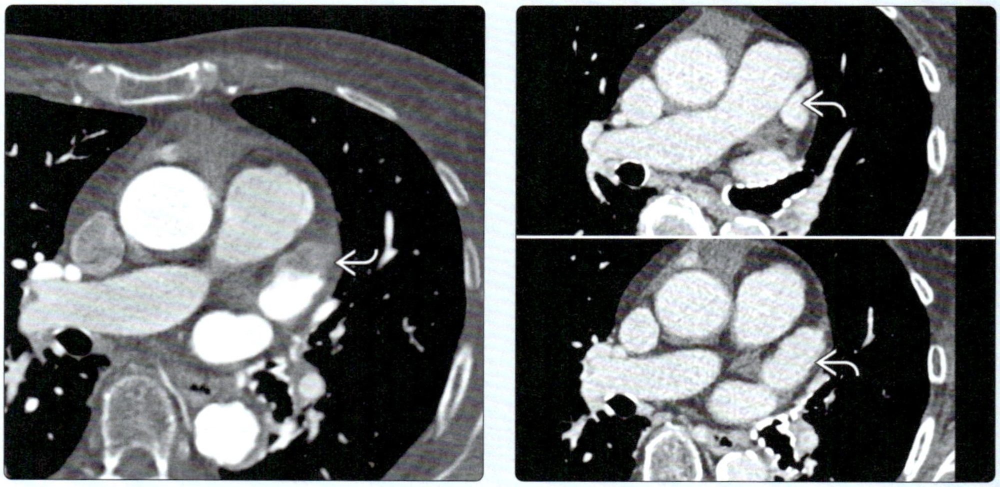

(Left) *Axial cardiac CT shows a relatively well-defined filling defect ➡ in the nondependent portion of the LAA, suggesting a possible thrombus.* **(Right)** *Delayed CT images in the same patient show complete contrast filling of the LAA ➡, indicating absence of thrombus and slow mixing across the LAA. This case illustrates the value of delayed scans to confirm the presence or absence of LAA thrombus.*

TERMINOLOGY

Definitions

- Thrombus formation in left atrial appendage (LAA) or in body of left atrium
  - Usually due to atrial fibrillation (AF) or mitral valve stenosis or other slow-flow states

IMAGING

General Features

- Best diagnostic clue
  - Filling defect within LAA on enhanced scans that persists on delayed phase
  - Persistent on delayed CECT
- Location
  - Usually in LAA; most common source of thrombus in patients with AF
  - Occasionally in body of left atrium
- Size
  - Variable
- Morphology
  - Chronic, broad-based thrombus may develop neovascularization, which will lead to low-grade enhancement on postcontrast MR
    - May present diagnostic challenge when differentiating chronic thrombus from malignancy

Radiographic Findings

- Not visible on radiograph unless if calcified
- May see signs of left atrial enlargement
  - Double density sign
  - Splaying of carina
  - Enlargement of LAA

CT Findings

- CTA
  - Thoracic CTA may incidentally show LAA thrombus
    - Thin-cut reconstructions and delayed scans are most helpful in demonstrating persistent filling defect
    - Lack of filling during arterial-phase imaging can mimic thrombus
      - □ LAA is last part of heart to fill with contrast
- Cardiac gated CTA
  - Mean sensitivity of 96% and specificity of 92% for detection of LAA thrombus
  - High negative predictive value (NPV) (96-100%)
  - Slow-mixing artifact may mimic LAA thrombus
    - LAA thrombus appears round or oval in shape, whereas filling defects appear triangular with homogeneous signal intensity
    - Sharper interface between filling defect and contrast-opacified lumen is suggestive of thrombus
    - Delayed scans allow for differentiation of slow-mixing artifact from LAA thrombus
      - □ Thrombus persists on delayed images
  - Qualitative assessment of LAA thrombus
    - Low HU filling defect is suggestive of thrombus
    - HU > 80 in LAA more likely represents slow mixing
    - LAA:ascending aorta HU ratio
      - □ LAA:aorta HU ratio is inversely associated with presence of spontaneous echo contrast and thrombus
      - □ Cut-off value for LAA:aorta HU ratio for detection of thrombus ~ < 0.25 with high NPV
  - When differentiating thrombus from malignancy, CTA enhancement is less helpful than MR enhancement
  - May show findings of underlying mitral valve disease
  - Retrospective-gated study may show absence of atrial kick in patients with AF
  - Cardiac CTA is useful for anatomic metrics and exclusion of thrombus prior to percutaneous occlusion device implantation
    - Follow-up scans may be used to confirm proper device placement and exclude residual perfusion
  - Multienergy (spectral, dual-energy, photon-counting) CT may reduce false-positive findings
    - Iodine concentration images shown to have better diagnostic performance compared to conventional arterial-phase images

MR Findings

- Cine-SSFP imaging in multiple planes is helpful for outlining thrombus
- T1 and T2 signal depends on age of thrombus
  - Acute: Intermediate on T1 and T2
  - Subacute: Low on T1; high on T2
  - Chronic: Low on T1 and T2
- Perfusion and early gadolinium enhancement imaging: No contrast uptake
- LGE sequence: Thrombus has low signal at myocardial inversion time
- LGE at long inversion times (i.e., 600 ms): Low signal due to high T1 of thrombus; reliably distinguishes thrombus from other neoplasms
- Chronic vascularized thrombus: May show peripheral enhancement
- T1 mapping: Intermediate native T1 values

Echocardiographic Findings

- Echocardiogram
  - Transesophageal echocardiography is considered reference standard for excluding LAA thrombus
    - Spontaneous echo contrast or "smoke" and other artifacts may hamper identification or exclusion of LAA thrombus
  - Visualization of LAA thrombus may be improved with use of thrombus-targeting US contrast agent (MRX-408A1)

Imaging Recommendations

- Best imaging tool
  - Transesophageal echocardiography
  - Cardiac CT with delayed phase scan is useful tool
- Protocol advice
  - CTA delayed scan reduces false-positive findings from slow mixing, may show reverse gradient

DIFFERENTIAL DIAGNOSIS

Pseudothrombus (on CTA)

- Low attenuation within LAA due to slow mixing of contrast containing blood with nonopacified blood

- More common in AF and poor LAA ejection fraction
- Can be differentiated on CT from actual thrombus by using delayed phase or prone imaging

Myxoma

- High-signal T2 imaging
- Usually attached to fossa ovalis, which is atypical location for thrombus
- Usually shows some degree of enhancement on CT or MR

Papillary Fibroelastoma

- Can occur along and endocardial surface, including LA
- Can mimic thrombus on anatomic imaging
  - Often appears frond-like
- Intense LGE

Surgical Exclusion of Left Atrial Appendage

- Performed after valve surgery to prevent LAA thrombosis
- Can appear similar to LAA thrombus

PATHOLOGY

General Features

- Etiology
  - Virchow triad: Endothelial damage, blood stasis, and hypercoagulability
  - AF
    - 91% of AF-related thrombus is located in LAA
    - LAA thrombus in AF is larger and has higher mortality compared to other thromboembolic sources
  - Mitral valve disease of any cause
  - Left atrial thrombus formation on atrial septal defect occluder systems has been reported
- Associated abnormalities
  - Often source of neurologic events, large artery occlusion
    - Cardiac (left atrial or ventricular) thrombus must be excluded in absence of otherwise identifiable source of embolic (cryptogenic) stroke or transient ischemic attack
    - If negative, patent foramen ovale (PFO) and deep vein thrombosis (DVT) need to be excluded
    - Lower extremity US and pelvic MR venography are used to exclude DVT in patients with PFO and cryptogenic stroke

CLINICAL ISSUES

Presentation

- Most common signs/symptoms
  - Asymptomatic; cryptogenic stroke; other embolic events
- Other signs/symptoms
  - Symptoms or imaging findings from underlying disease
    - AF; mitral valve disease
  - In rheumatic mitral stenosis
    - Coarse F waves on ECG associated with LAA dysfunction
    - Presence indicates higher thromboembolic risk

Demographics

- M = F
- Age range parallels that of underlying conditions

Natural History & Prognosis

- May resolve spontaneously, persist without complication
- May embolize to brain → transient ischemic attack or stroke
- Recurrence common if underlying cause not treated

Treatment

- Anticoagulant therapy (warfarin) substantially reduces embolic event risk in AF from LAA thrombus
  - Needs frequent international normalized ratio (INR) monitoring and carries bleeding risk
- Other drugs may have clinical roles in select cases
  - Dabigatran, rivaroxaban, apixaban, and edoxaban
  - Antiplatelet therapy ± low-dose warfarin, etc.
- Surgical: Maze procedure and similar operations
- Catheter-based radiofrequency ablation (pulmonary vein isolation)
  - Prevention of thrombus formation
- LAA obliteration: Surgical/catheter-based occlusion device
  - For stroke prevention in high-risk patients with contraindication for oral anticoagulation
  - Surgical: Atriclip, Lariat
  - Catheter-based devices: Watchman, Amplatzer Amulet

DIAGNOSTIC CHECKLIST

Consider

- 1-minute delayed gated scan to follow CTA or CTV if filling defect is noted on initial images
  - Slow mixing of opacified and nonopacified blood across neck of LAA may mimic thrombus
  - Delayed scan allows for more complete mixing
  - If filling defect persists, thrombus is present
  - If LAA fills with contrast, there is slow-flow artifact
    - Equivalent to smoke on transesophageal echocardiography
  - Lower HU density and LAA:aorta HU ratio is associated with thrombus rather than mixing artifact
- No enhancement on LGE MR and persistent low signal at long inversion times is consistent with thrombus

SELECTED REFERENCES

1. Cresti A et al: Left atrial thrombus-are all atria and appendages equal? Card Electrophysiol Clin. 15(2):119-32, 2023
2. Li W et al: Detection of left atrial appendage thrombus by dual-energy computed tomography-derived imaging biomarkers in patients with atrial fibrillation. Front Cardiovasc Med. 9:809688, 2022
3. Qureshi A et al: Imaging and biophysical modelling of thrombogenic mechanisms in atrial fibrillation and stroke. Front Cardiovasc Med. 9:1074562, 2022
4. Rajiah P et al: Pre- and postprocedural CT of transcatheter left atrial appendage closure devices. Radiographics. 41(3):680-98, 2021
5. Li W et al: Detection of left atrial appendage thrombi by third-generation dual-source dual-energy CT: iodine concentration versus conventional enhancement measurements. Int J Cardiol. 292:265-70, 2019

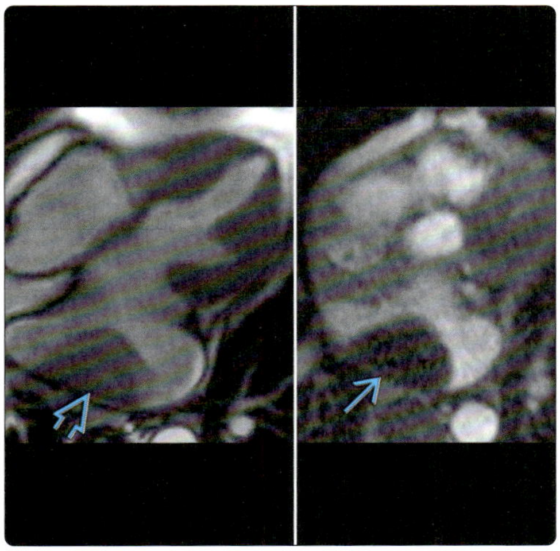

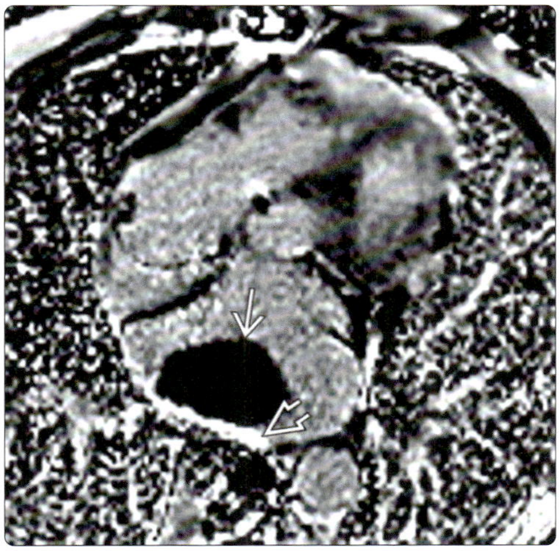

(Left) *SSFP MR (left) in a patient with a history of cardiac transplant shows a heterogeneous, but predominantly isointense, mass along the posterior wall of the left atrium* ⇨. *The left atrium is moderately dilated. Perfusion MR (right) shows absent perfusion in the mass* →. **(Right)** *Four-chamber LGE image shows no enhancement within the hypointense thrombus* ➡. *However, there is LGE along the left atrial wall and posterior rim of the thrombus* ⇨ *due to its chronicity.*

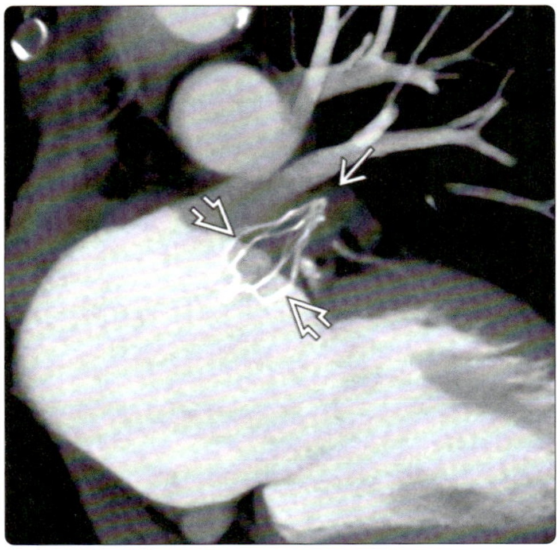

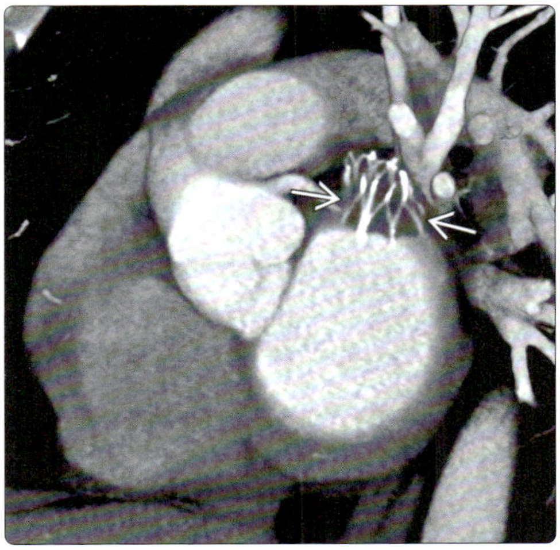

(Left) *Long-axis contrast-enhanced CTA shows occlusion of the LAA* ➡ *by an LAA closure (Watchman) device* ⇨. **(Right)** *Volume-rendered contrast-enhanced CTA in the same patient shows occlusion of the LAA by an LAA closure (Watchman) device* ➡. *An LAA closure device is used in patients with atrial fibrillation in order to decrease the risk of distal embolization.*

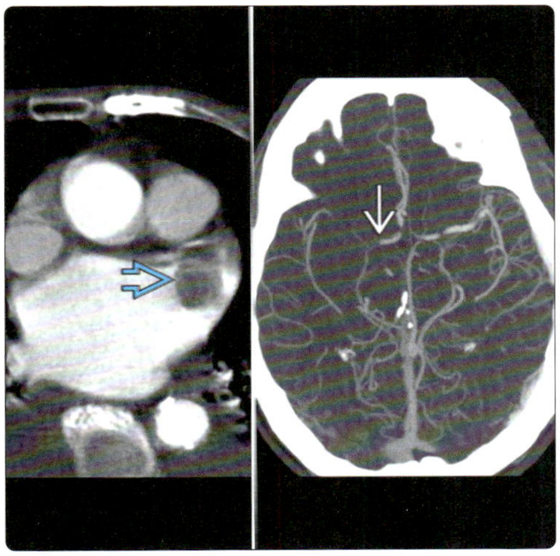

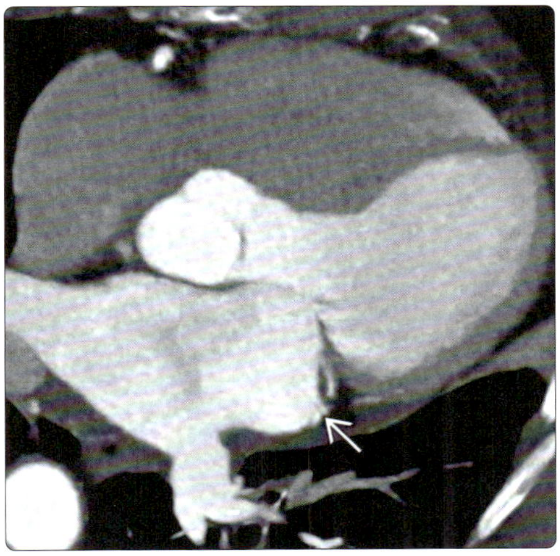

(Left) *Inferiormost axial neck CTA in a patient with a middle cerebral artery (MCA) stroke shows a large thrombus in the LAA* ⇨. *Axial MRA shows abrupt cutoff of the MCA secondary to embolism* ➡. **(Right)** *MIP cardiac CTA shows a small outpouching* ➡ *along the lateral aspect of the left atrium with internal trabeculation, consistent with an accessory LAA. An accessory LAA can theoretically increase the risk of left atrial thrombus formation in the setting of atrial fibrillation or atrial flutter.*

Left Atrial Appendage Imaging Pre- and Post Occluder Device Placement

KEY FACTS

CLINICAL IMPLICATIONS

- Left atrial appendage (LAA) is common site of thrombus formation in patients with nonvalvular-related atrial fibrillation (AF)
  - Even with successful therapy for AF, patients are placed on anticoagulation due to continued risk of systemic embolization; however, some patients cannot safely take anticoagulation medication
- Various open, minimally invasive, and endovascular therapies can be used to occlude LAA
  - Open technique involves median sternotomy and suture ligation or clipping of LAA
  - Minimally invasive technique involves placement of clip around neck of LAA using video-assisted thoracoscopic surgery (VATS)
  - Endovascular technique involves placement of device in LAA with subsequent occlusion
    - Most commonly used devices are Watchman device and Amplatzer plug
  - High success rate and relatively low complication rate

IMAGING

- Echocardiography: Transesophageal echocardiography (TEE) primary method to evaluate LAA anatomy prior to minimally invasive and endovascular therapy for LAA occlusion
- ECG gated cardiac CTA with contrast
  - Provides more accurate measurements than TEE
  - Device sizing by CT is in most agreement with actual device sizing
  - **Preprocedural CT evaluation**: Provide atrial map prior to AF ablation procedure; evaluation of LAA morphology and measurements of LAA size; detection of LAA thrombus; identification of interatrial septal abnormalities; assessment of relationship to surrounding structures
  - **Postprocedural CT evaluation**: Confirmation of correct positioning of device; identification of peridevice leak, assessment of complications

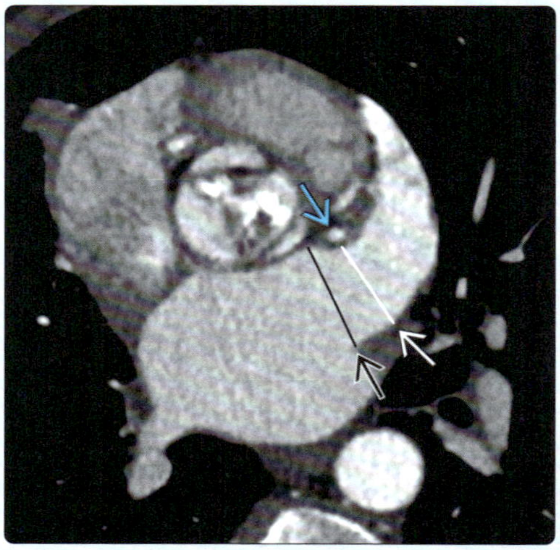

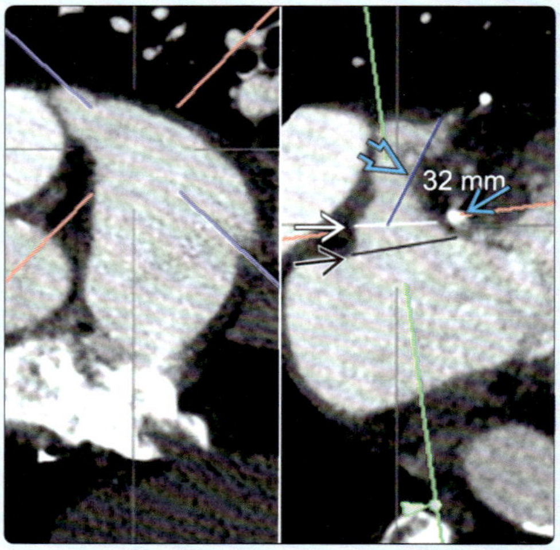

(Left) *Cardiac CT in a patient with aortic stenosis and atrial fibrillation shows the anatomic delineation of the ostium (black line →), neck (white line →), and lobar portions of the left atrial appendage (LAA). The proximal left circumflex (LCx) coronary artery → helps demarcate the boundary of the neck of the LAA.* **(Right)** *Pre-Watchman device ECG gated CTA shows the proximal LCx →, LAA ostium (black line →), and neck (→ white line). LAA length (blue line →) is an important measurement for certain endovascular devices.*

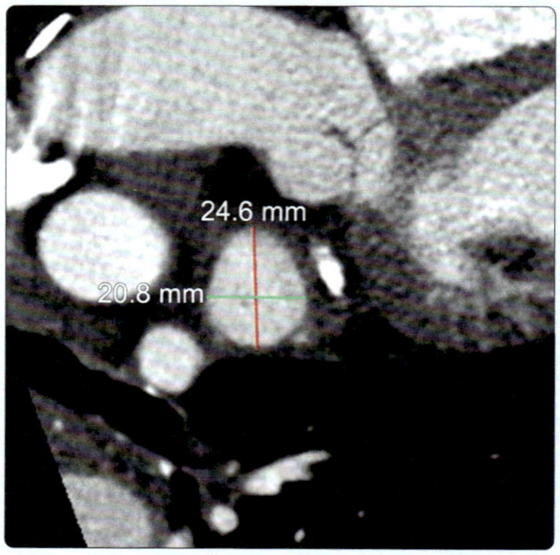

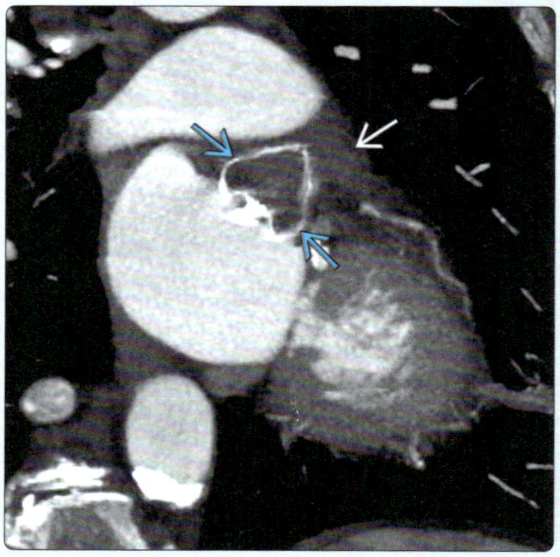

(Left) *Transverse MPR CECT through the neck of the LAA shows the maximum diameter to be 25 mm, which correlates to a 27-mm Watchman device. Transesophageal echocardiography (TEE) measurements also sized the device at 27 mm.* **(Right)** *Two-chamber MIP CECT shows the Watchman device → in place with complete occlusion of the distal LAA →. Watchman device aligns to the long axis of the lobar portion of LAA, hence it is seated in the neck of the LAA (a.k.a. landing zone) instead of true ostium.*

TERMINOLOGY

Abbreviations

- Left atrial appendage (LAA)

IMAGING ANATOMY

General Anatomic Considerations

- LAA = finger-like projection extending anteriorly from left atrium (LA)

Critical Anatomic Structures

- **LAA ostium**
  - Opening from LA to LAA; usually ovoid in shape
  - Separated from origin of left superior pulmonary vein (LSPV) by lateral ridge
    - Thin ridge may cause impairment of pulmonary vein (PV) return or interfere with future ablation procedures
  - Eccentric LAA ostium can lead to device leakage
- **LAA neck**
  - Tubular junction between ostium and lobar portion
  - Proximal left circumflex (LCx) coronary artery helps to delineate boundary of neck of LAA
  - > 1/2 of patients have variable-sized pits or troughs
  - Secondary lobe originating from neck or severe angulation of neck complicates measurements and effective occlusion
- **Lobar portion**
  - Most variable portion of LAA
    - Various LAA morphologies are present with variable classification schemes
      - Chicken wing: Multilobed with obvious bend; less likely to develop thrombosis
      - Cactus: Multilobed with dominant lobe but no bend
      - Windsock: Single lobed without bend
      - Cauliflower: Multilobed, no bend or dominant lobe
    - Includes pectinate muscles, which may mimic thrombus
      - Thin wall areas between pectinate muscles ↑ risk of perforation
  - Main lobe needs to be long enough to allow device insertion

Anatomic Relationships

- **LAA ostium**: Adjacent to mitral valve and LSPV, which can be compressed &/or distorted by device
- **LAA neck**: Adjacent to LCx and LAD, which can be damaged during procedure
- **Lobar portion**: Distal portion of appendage near pulmonary artery, LAD, and phrenic nerve, which can be damaged during procedure

CLINICAL IMPLICATIONS

Clinical Importance

- LAA is common site of thrombus formation in patients with nonvalvular-related atrial fibrillation (AF)
- Mainstay of therapy is ablation or cardioversion
- Even with successful therapy, patients are placed on anticoagulation due to continued risk of systemic embolization
  - However, many patients cannot tolerate anticoagulant therapy or are noncompliant
- In certain patients, decision is made to occlude LAA
  - Open, minimally invasive, and endovascular techniques can be used
- Open technique involves median sternotomy with suture ligation or clipping of LAA
  - Often performed when sternotomy is being performed for additional reasons, such as coronary artery bypass grafting (CABG), valve repair, etc.
- Minimally invasive technique involves clip closure (Atriclip) of LAA via video-assisted thoracoscopic surgery (VATS)
- Newer endovascular devices allow for occlusion of LAA
- **Watchman Flx and Watchman Flx Pro devices**
  - LAA closure (LAAC) device
  - Self-expanding, nitinol, multistrut frame with permeable polyethylene terephthalate membrane cap facing LA
  - Studied in multiple randomized trials, which showed noninferiority to anticoagulation
  - Large study showed complication rate of 5.7% with most complications being minor
    - Pericardial effusion is most common complication (3.4% of patients)
    - 2nd most common complication is major bleeding requiring blood transfusion (1.4% of patients)
  - Technical success rates > 95%
  - Variable sizes ranging from 20-40 mm
- **Amplatzer Amulet device**
  - Self-expanding, nitinol mesh plug with distal lobe and proximal disk with polyester fabric, connected by waist
  - Similar success and complication rate as Watchman devices
  - ↑ rate of LAA occlusion compared to Watchman devices
- **LARIAT device**
  - Combined transcatheter endocardial and epicardial approach
  - LAA is snared via epicardial approach and subsequently closed by suture ligations
  - Can be used in some cases where LAA morphology precludes endovascular approach
  - High technical success rate
  - Initial studies showed relatively high serious adverse event rate, including emergent cardiac surgery
  - More recent studies have showed lower serious complication rate

Function and Dysfunction

- Although technical success rates are high, some degree of persistent filling of LAA is seen in ~ 1/3 of patients 12 months after undergoing closure of LAA
  - However, largest study looking at complications post device placement shows no ↑ risk of thromboembolism in patients with residual filling of LAA compared to those with complete occlusion

IMAGING

Echocardiography

- 2D or 3D transesophageal echocardiography (TEE) most widely used method to assess for LAA thrombus
  - Highly sensitive and specific for thrombus detection

- Doppler measurement of blood velocity in LAA appendage can assess stroke risk
- Blood velocities < 40 cm/s in LAA are associated with ↑ risk of stroke

- TEE is primary method to evaluate LAA anatomy prior to minimally invasive and endovascular therapy for LAA occlusion
    - Contrast agents can help elucidate anatomy
    - For Watchman devices, LAA diameter is measured at angles 0°, 45°, 90°, and 135°
    - Largest diameter used to Watchman device sizing

ECG Gated Cardiac CTA With Contrast

- ECG gated cardiac imaging has become common study ordered for assessment of LA and LAA due to high spatial and temporal resolution
    - More accurate measurements than TEE
    - Device sizing by CT agrees most with actual device sizing
        - Watchman device selection by CT-derived measurements is 100% accurate
    - Newer data suggests use of 3D CT printing technology may facilitate device size selection
        - 3D physical model of LAA customized to each patient is created, then physical device is implanted ex vivo to decide exact device size
    - Better assessment of relationship to surrounding structure than TEE
- **Preprocedural CT evaluation**
    - Provides atrial map prior to AF ablation procedure
        - Assesses number and morphology of PVs
    - Provides accurate measurements of LAA size and morphology prior to occlusion
    - Assessment of relationship to surrounding structures
    - Identification of contraindications
        - Thrombus is absolute contraindication for both AF ablation and LAA occlusion procedures
    - Detection of interatrial septal abnormalities
        - Transseptal puncture used during procedure
    - Assessment of coplanar viewing angles
    - Assessment of pericardial access route and relationship with surrounding structures (left internal mammary artery, inferior epigastric artery, phrenic nerve) for LARIAT device
- **Postprocedural CT evaluation**
    - Confirmation of correct positioning of device and assessment for LAA occlusion
    - Identification of peridevice leak
        - CT has greater sensitivity for leak than TEE
        - Contrast rim around device and distal flow
        - Thromboembolic stroke risk related to size of leak
        - < 3-mm peridevice gap is acceptable without substantial additional risk of stroke
    - Assess for other complications
        - Device embolization
        - Thrombus on atrial side of device
            - In patients undergoing follow-up LAA imaging, rate 7.2% per year
            - Significant ↑ risk of stroke
        - Pericardial effusion or hemopericardium that can lead to tamponade; device erosion through LAA
- **Important measurements**
    - Watchman Flx devices
        - Device is slightly oversized compared to LAA max ostial diameter
        - Aligns to long axis of lobar portion, hence device does not necessarily match to true ostium of LAA
        - Transverse measurements, area and perimeter of landing zone
            - Landing zone: Plane near true ostium, orthogonal to long axis of lobar portion in which device would be seated
        - Maximum length of lobar portion from tip of LAA to landing zone
    - Amplatzer and Amulet cardiac plugs
        - Need to measure 2 transverse diameters
        - Transverse measurements of ostium of LAA, where disc is seated
        - Transverse measurements 10 mm distal to ostium, where lobe is seated
    - LARIAT device
        - Exclusion criteria: Presence of pericardial thickening; calcification or adhesions of pericardial access; large LAA width (> 40 mm); retropulmonary artery; pectus deformity; previous coronary bypass grafting

Imaging Protocols

- ECG-gated cardiac CTA with contrast
- Retrospective or prospective acquisition can be performed
    - Ostium of LAA size and morphology changes during cardiac cycle
        - Best assessed with retrospective gating
    - If prospective ECG triggering is used, acquisition should be timed for systolic phase
    - Consider delayed-phase image (40-60 s) to assess for LAA thrombus
- 3D postprocessing required for device-specific measurements

Imaging Pitfalls

- Due to passive filling and dilation, tip of LAA may be last cardiac structure to opacify
- Low-dose delayed imaging scan is very useful to differentiate thrombus from slow filling in patients undergoing atrial mapping

SELECTED REFERENCES

1. Kewcharoen J et al: Adverse events associated with Amplatzer left atrial appendage occlusion delivery system: a Food and Drug Administration MAUDE database study. J Cardiovasc Electrophysiol. 34(11):2382-5, 2023
2. Shrestha B et al: National yearly trend of utilization and procedural complication of the Watchman Device in the United States. Cureus. 14(6):e25567, 2022
3. Lakkireddy D et al: Amplatzer amulet left atrial appendage occluder versus Watchman Device for stroke prophylaxis (Amulet IDE): a randomized, controlled trial. Circulation. 144(19):1543-52, 2021
4. Rajiah P et al: Pre- and postprocedural CT of transcatheter left atrial appendage closure devices. Radiographics. 41(3):680-98, 2021
5. Calkins H et al: 2017 HRS/EHRA/ECAS/APHRS/SOLAECE expert consensus statement on catheter and surgical ablation of atrial fibrillation. Europace. 20(1):e1-160, 2018
6. Eng MH et al: Computed tomography for left atrial appendage occlusion case planning. Interv Cardiol Clin. 7(3):367-78, 2018
7. Fauchier L et al: Device-related thrombosis after percutaneous left atrial appendage occlusion for atrial fibrillation. J Am Coll Cardiol. 71(14):1528-36, 2018
8. Xu B et al: Computed tomography measurement of the left atrial appendage for optimal sizing of the Watchman device. J Cardiovasc Comput Tomogr. 12(1):50-5, 2018

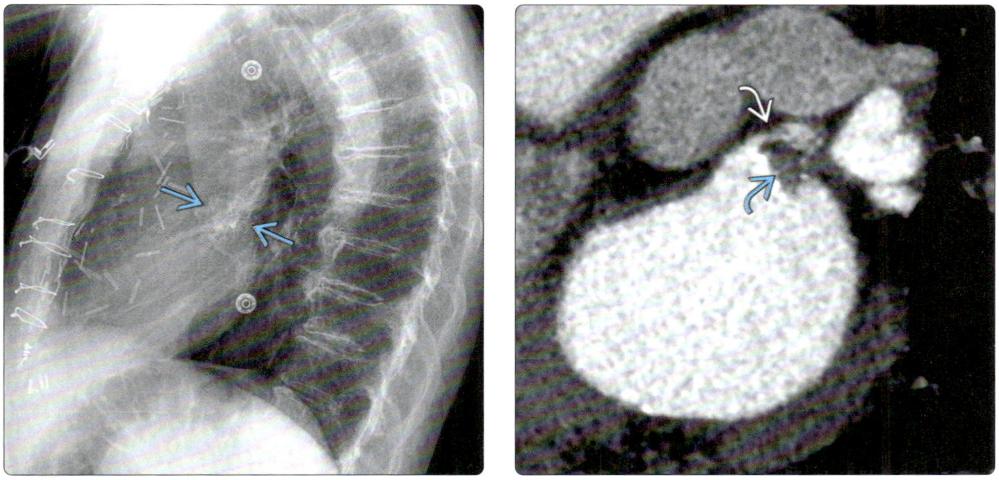

(Left) *Lateral radiograph shows the expected location and appearance of the Watchman device.* **(Right)** *ECG gated CTA in a 67-year-old man with atrial fibrillation status post Watchman device placement shows a small channel of persistent contrast opacification through the neck of the LAA due to incomplete closure. There is persistent filling of the LAA. CT has a greater sensitivity to detect peridevice leak than TEE.*

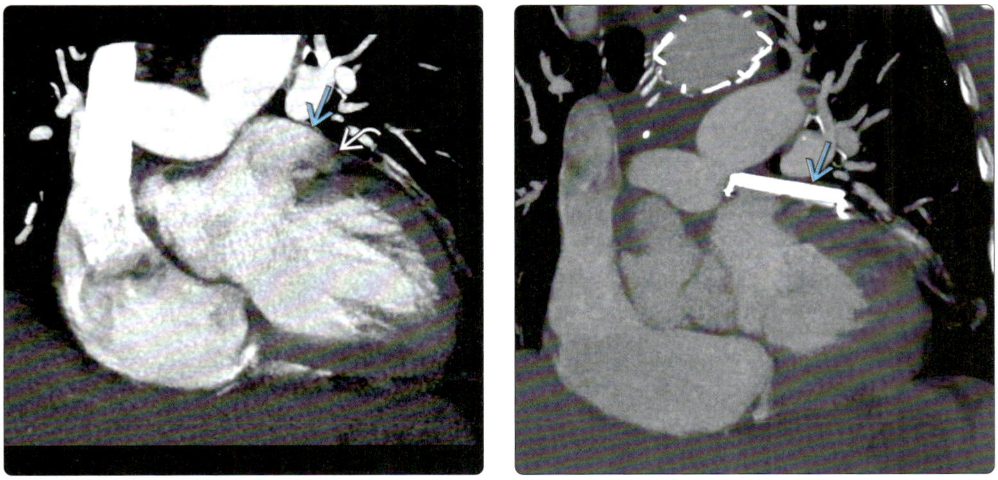

(Left) *Coronal oblique CECT in a woman with a ruptured type A aortic dissection (not shown) demonstrates a nearly completely opacified LAA. Lack of opacification of the tip of the LAA was secondary to poor filling.* **(Right)** *Due to the high risk of stroke in this patient and contraindication to anticoagulation, the LAA was occluded using an Atriclip device during the operation to fix the ruptured type A aortic dissection.*

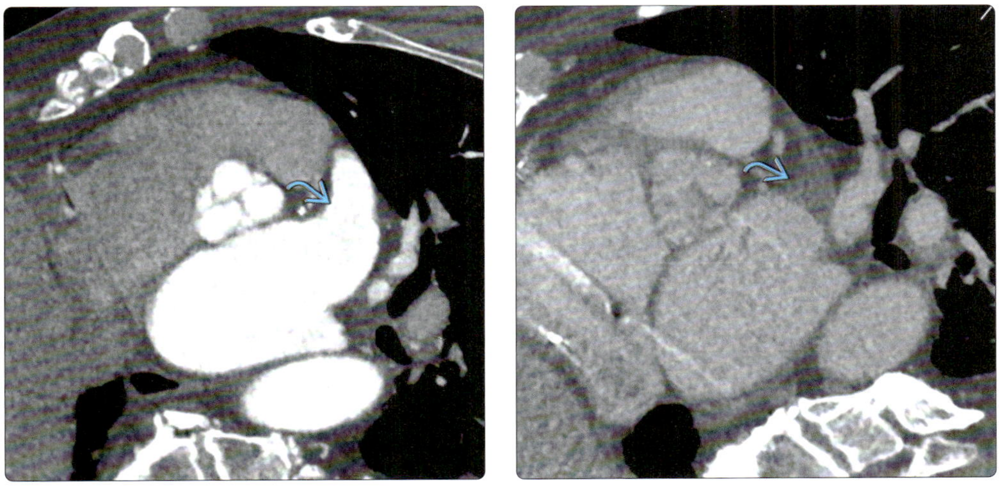

(Left) *Sagittal oblique ECG gated CTA for Watchman device placement in a patient with atrial fibrillation, mitral regurgitation, and a contraindication to anticoagulation shows an opacified LAA.* **(Right)** *Although this patient was initially scheduled to undergo endovascular occlusion of the LAA, the decision was made to perform an open sternotomy to repair his mitral valve due to severity of the mitral regurgitation. During this open procedure, the LAA was oversewn and occluded.*

Introduction

Cardiac CT is becoming increasingly important for procedure planning prior to ventricular tachycardia (VT) ablation. CT aids in diagnosis, identification of ablation substrates, detailed electroanatomic mapping, and provides vital prognostic information. Technical advancements have expanded the utility of CT, particularly for patients who experience excessive artifacts on MR or have safety concerns. Emerging techniques, such as multienergy CT, are further enhancing the assessment of delayed enhancement and tissue characterization, offering a comprehensive evaluation in these complex cases.

Diagnostic Role

Cardiac CT techniques, such as late iodine enhancement (LIE), allow tissue characterization analogous to late gadolinium enhancement (LGE) in cardiac MR. While CT offers superior spatial resolution and near-isotropic imaging, CT has a lower contrast:noise ratio compared to MR.

Preprocedural Planning

Intracardiac thrombus is considered a contraindication to VT ablation, particularly if the thrombus is mobile. Mobile thrombi pose an elevated risk of embolization during the procedure, which can lead to severe complications, such as stroke. In some cases, where the thrombus is laminated, adhering to the heart wall and less likely to dislodge, ablation might still be considered, sometimes using an epicardial-only approach. On cardiac CT, thrombi typically appear as low-attenuation, nonenhancing masses within the cardiac chambers that persists in delayed phase.

Epicardial access requires an intact epicardium; thus, patients with rare conditions, such as congenital absence of the pericardium, are not eligible for this procedure. Additionally, identifying and describing pericardial calcifications or adhesions before VT ablation is important, as it can significantly limit catheter maneuverability and hinder the procedure. Utilizing CT to assess the detailed anatomy of the pericardium in relation to nearby structures allows for precise planning of needle trajectory, thereby minimizing the risk of inadvertent damage to the right ventricle, blood vessels, diaphragm, and intraabdominal organs.

Although not an absolute contraindication, an epicardial fat pad of < 10 mm is desirable. Thick fat attenuates the amplitude of electrograms, which can be confused with scarring and make ablation ineffective. Excessive trabeculations may cause poor contact with catheter electrodes in an endocardial approach. CT can also provide venous anatomy, which is essential for access planning. Occluded or anatomically prohibitive veins, such as an interrupted inferior vena cava (IVC), limit endocardial access.

Identification of Ventricular Tachycardia Substrate

Myocardial fibrosis is a key substrate for reentrant circuits that commonly generate VT in patients with structural heart disease. Scarring from myocardial infarction can be identified by segmental wall thinning (< 5 mm in diastole, most cases being < 2 mm), hypoperfusion in arterial phase, fatty metaplasia, or LIE. A nonischemic scar is midmyocardial, subepicardial, or diffuse subendocardial. Strong correlation exists between focal delayed enhancement and fibrosis or scarring on histology. To guide VT ablation, LIE is described according to the segmental left ventricle (LV) anatomy, including distribution in subendocardial, midwall, or subepicardial locations, and the degree of transmurality (10-25%, 25-50%, 50-75%, 75-90%).

3D maps of LV wall thickness are invaluable for guiding electroanatomic mapping and optimizing ablation procedures. Ridges, i.e., areas where wall thickness varies by > 1 mm within a thin segment (< 5 mm), represents reentrant circuits.

Given the higher recurrence rates of VT during the inflammatory phase of cardiomyopathies, such as sarcoidosis, FDG PET/CT can be highly effective when combined with CT and MR to determine the extent of myocardial scarring and differentiate between chronic scarring and acute inflammation, thereby guiding appropriate treatment strategies.

Assessing Prognosis

The presence and extent of ventricular scarring identified by LGE are strongly associated with an increased risk of sudden cardiac death (SCD), recurrent VT, and appropriate implantable cardioverter defibrillator (ICD) discharge in patients with impaired LV systolic function. Since CT derived myocardial delayed enhancement (MDE) serves as a surrogate for LGE, the characterization of specific scar features, such as pattern, border zone size, transmurality, heterogeneity, and the number of core islands, can further refine the risk assessment for adverse arrhythmic events. This highlights the critical prognostic value of accurately identifying, characterizing, and quantifying MDE in these patients.

Emerging Imaging Techniques

Cardiac CT has become increasingly valuable in evaluating patients before VT ablation due to its 3D imaging capabilities and superior spatial resolution. This technology significantly enhances electroanatomic mapping of the myocardium, supporting both standard catheter ablation and advanced techniques, such as stereotactic ablative body radiotherapy (SABR). Additionally, cardiac CT is essential for patients where MR safety concerns preclude the use of MR. While CT-detected LIE often resembles LGE distribution in scarring, its detection is hindered by the lower contrast:noise ratio of CT. To improve LIE imaging, protocols often involve acquiring images at 5 minutes post contrast with a higher contrast load and lower kVp settings (e.g., 80 kVp).

Furthermore, multienergy CT improves the distinction between scar tissue and preserved myocardium by using lower virtual monoenergetic images (40-60 keV) for better contrast:noise ratio, compared to 120 kVp images, and iodine density maps for enhanced visualization of LIE. Electrocardiographic imaging generates noninvasive epicardial voltage and activation maps from a large number (250) of electrodes placed on a torso vest followed by a noncontrast CT. This predicts arrhythmogenic substrate through voltage and activation maps prior to the patient going to electrophysiology (EP) lab.

Selected References

1. Bugenhagen S et al: Utility of CT and MRI in cardiac electrophysiology. Radiographics. 44(9):e230222, 2024
2. Deneke T et al: Pre- and post-procedural cardiac imaging (computed tomography and magnetic resonance imaging) in electrophysiology: a clinical consensus statement of the European Heart Rhythm Association and European Association of Cardiovascular Imaging of the European Society of Cardiology. Europace. 26(5), 2024
3. Sultana S et al: Role of computed tomography in cardiac electrophysiology. Radiol Clin North Am. 62(3):489-508, 2024

Contraindications to Catheter VT Ablation: Mobile Left Ventricular Thrombus

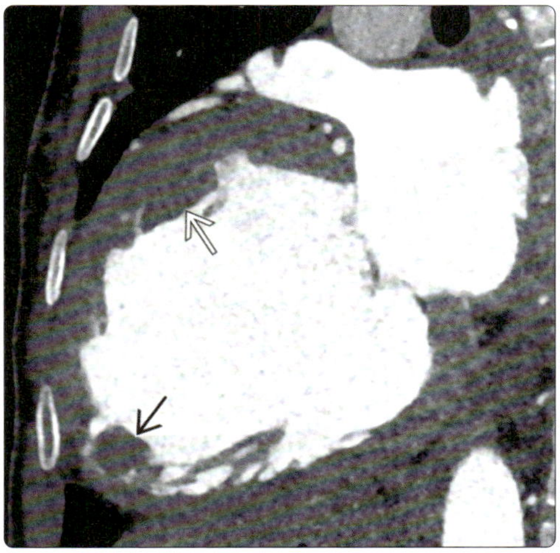

Contraindications to Catheter VT Ablation: Pericardial Calcifications

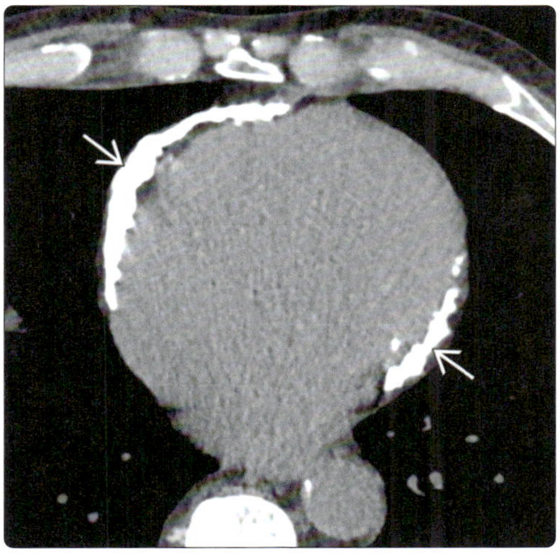

(Left) *Two-chamber cardiac CT in a patient with ventricular tachycardia (VT) shows a round thrombus → loosely attached to a thinned, hypoattenuating area at the left ventricular apex. Another thrombus → is loosely attached to the anterior wall. Catheter engagement in this scenario poses a high embolization risk.* **(Right)** *Axial noncontrast cardiac CT in another VT patient reveals thick pericardial calcifications → that limit the epicardial approach for ablation.*

Identifying VT Substrate #1

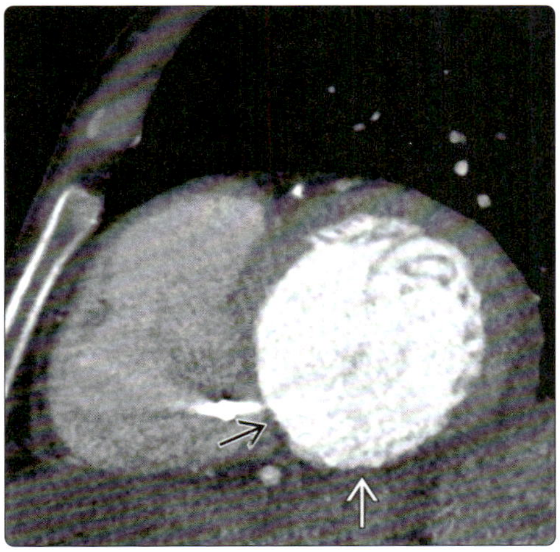

Identifying VT Substrate #1

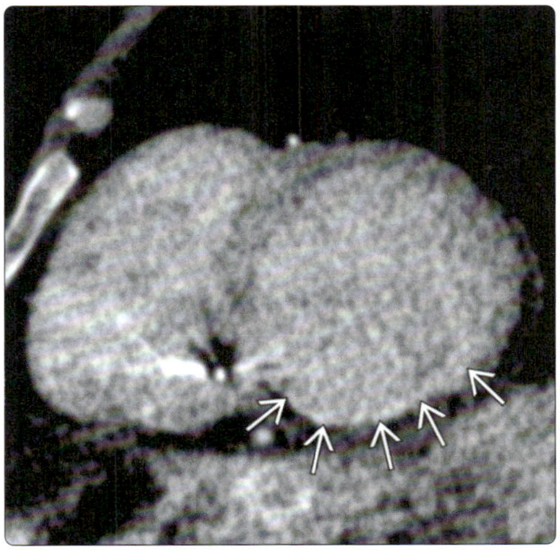

(Left) *Short-axis arterial-phase cardiac CT in a VT patient shows wall thinning and fatty metaplasia of the basal inferior → and inferoseptal → segments of the left ventricle, consistent with sequela of a prior myocardial infarction.* **(Right)** *Short-axis 5-minute delayed-phase cardiac CT in the same patient shows subendocardial-delayed enhancement along the myocardial scar →. The low contrast:noise ratio prompts careful window setting adjustments for adequate visualization.*

Supporting Electroanatomic Mapping #1

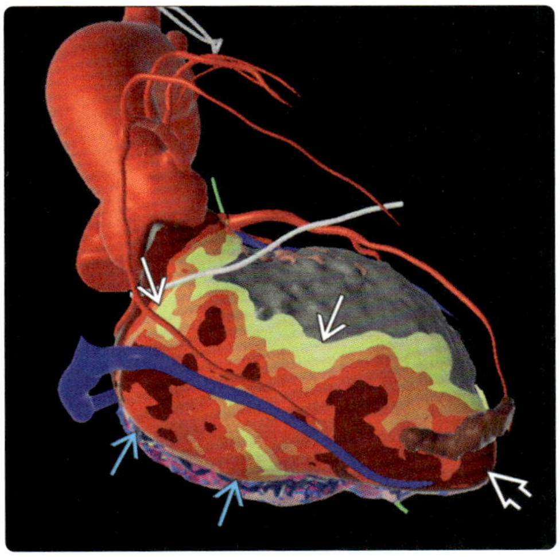

Supporting Electroanatomic Mapping #1

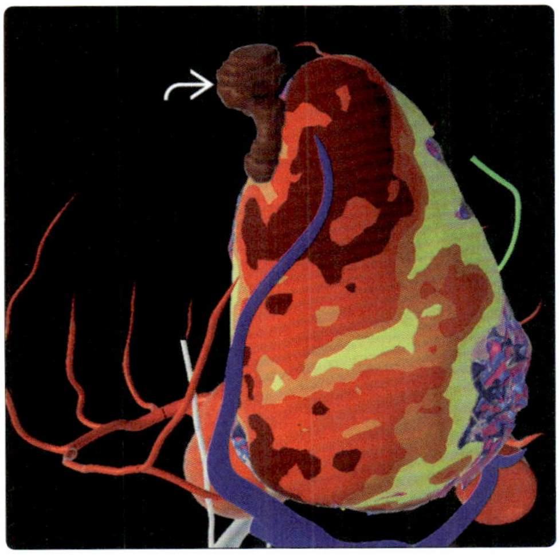

(Left) *Right anterior oblique 3D cardiac CT model in the same patient highlights wall thinning in the septum → and inferior → and apical → segments of the left ventricle. Thinned regions are color coded from yellow (less severe) to dark red (more severe).* **(Right)** *Inferior view of the same 3D model shows extensive thinning of the inferior and inferoseptal left ventricular walls with an incidental thrombus in the right ventricular apex →. This model aids in catheter navigation.*

Identifying VT Substrate #2

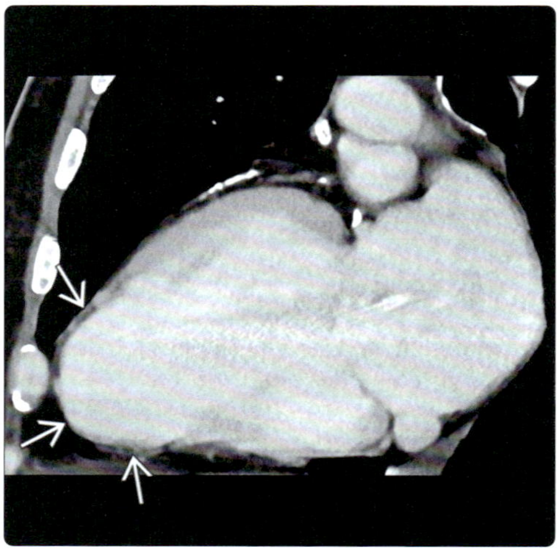

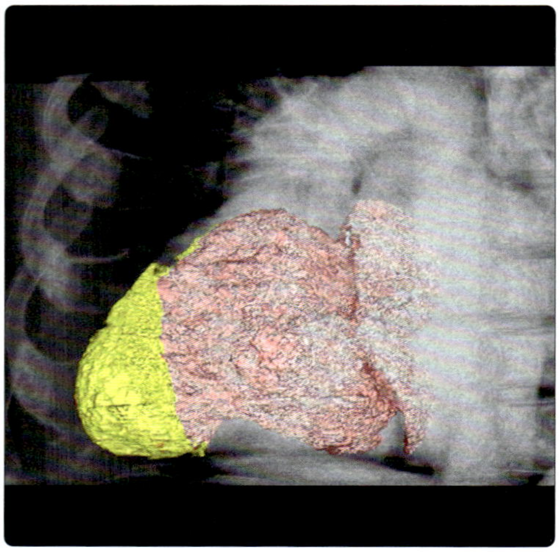

(Left) *Two-chamber delayed-phase cardiac CT in a patient with VT shows wall thinning and fatty metaplasia involving the apical segments of the left ventricle, consistent with a scar from a prior myocardial infarction.* **(Right)** *Left anterior oblique 3D volume-rendered reconstruction of the same cardiac CT with color-coded segmented areas shows apical wall thinning in yellow and preserved myocardium in red.*

Identifying VT Substrate #2

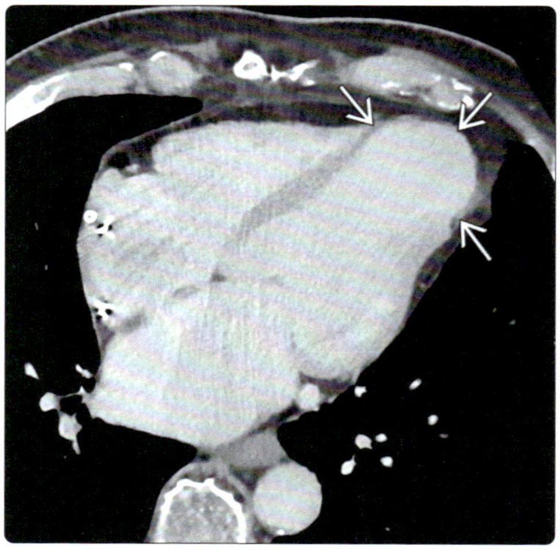

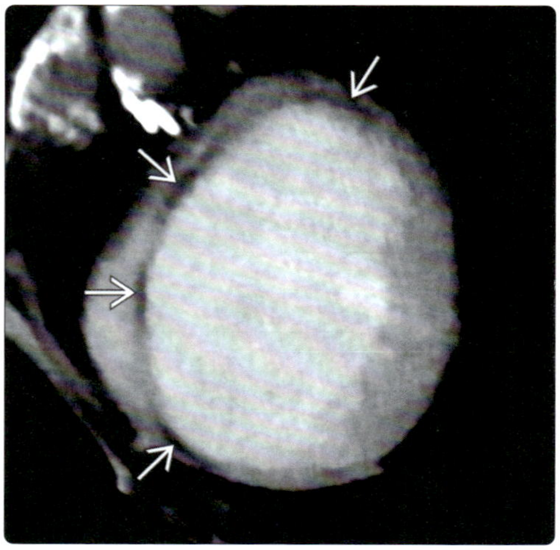

(Left) *Four-chamber delayed-phase cardiac CT in the same patient shows wall thinning and fatty metaplasia in the apical segments of the left ventricle.* **(Right)** *Short-axis delayed-phase cardiac CT in the same patient more clearly displays hypoattenuating foci within the thinned left ventricular apex, consistent with fatty metaplasia.*

Supporting Electroanatomic Mapping #2

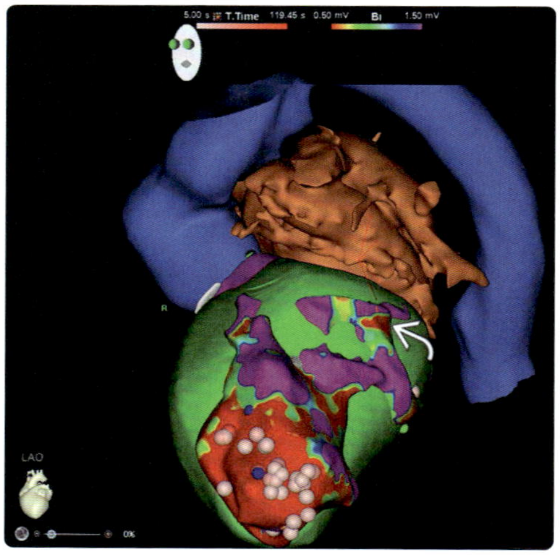

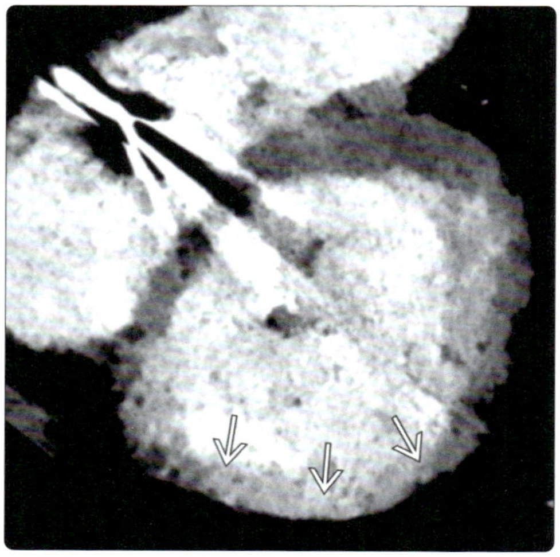

(Left) *3D model generated from the same cardiac CT data, overlaid with a rainbow-colored invasive electrical activity map, shows potential scar tissue in red. This scar tissue colocalizes with the apical scar, and an additional area of interest is noted in the basal inferolateral wall of the left ventricle.* **(Right)** *Delayed-phase short-axis view of the same cardiac CT using virtual monoenergetic imaging at 50 keV reveals a transmural area of delayed enhancement in the basal inferior and inferolateral segments, indicative of scarring.*

Emerging Imaging Techniques #1

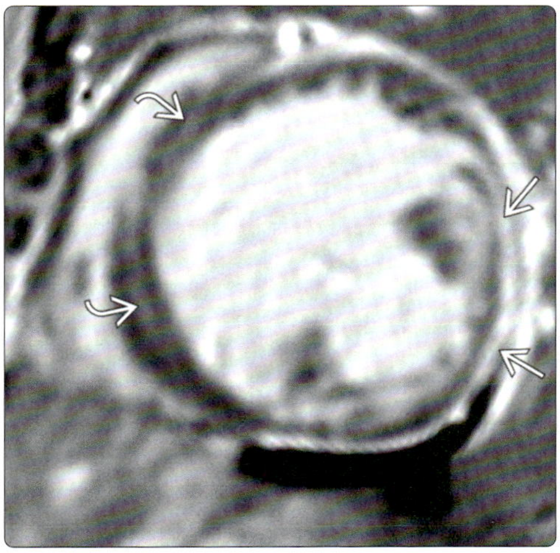

Emerging Imaging Techniques #1

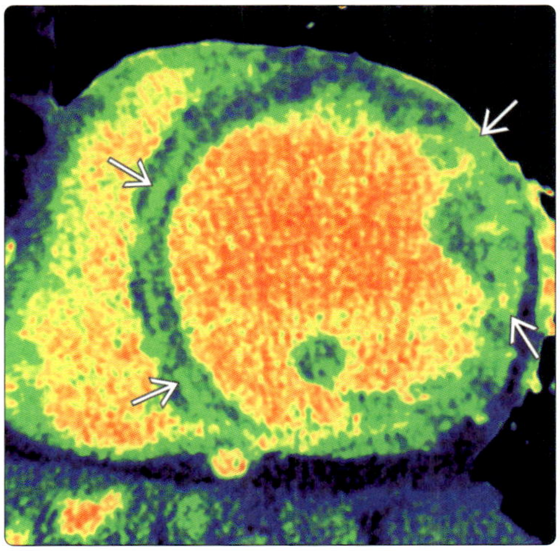

(Left) *Short-axis midventricular LGE MR in a patient with cardiac sarcoidosis and recurrent VT reveals midwall enhancement in the septum* ↪ *and subepicardial enhancement in the lateral segments* ➔*, consistent with nonischemic scarring.* **(Right)** *Short-axis delayed-phase multienergy CT, performed a few days after the cardiac MR, shows iodine concentration on colored maps matching the distribution of LGE* ➔*. Note the higher spatial resolution of CT compared to MR.*

Emerging Imaging Techniques #2

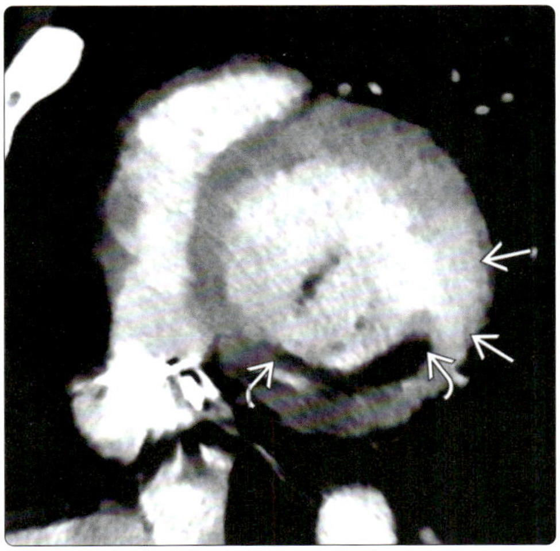

Emerging Imaging Techniques #2

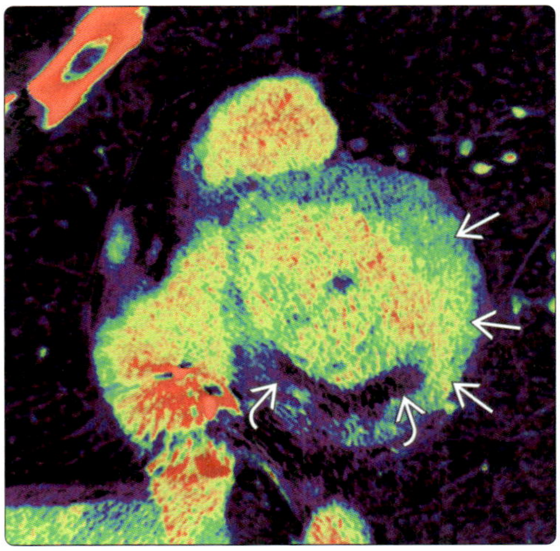

(Left) *Short-axis delayed enhancement multienergy cardiac CT, reconstructed at 50 keV, in a patient with VT shows subendocardial fatty metaplasia along the basal inferior wall* ↪ *and transmural delayed enhancement in the basal lateral segments* ➔*.* **(Right)** *The corresponding overlaid iodine/water material decomposition mapping enhances the differentiation between areas of fatty metaplasia in the inferior wall* ↪ *and delayed enhancement in the lateral segments* ➔*.*

Emerging Imaging Techniques #2

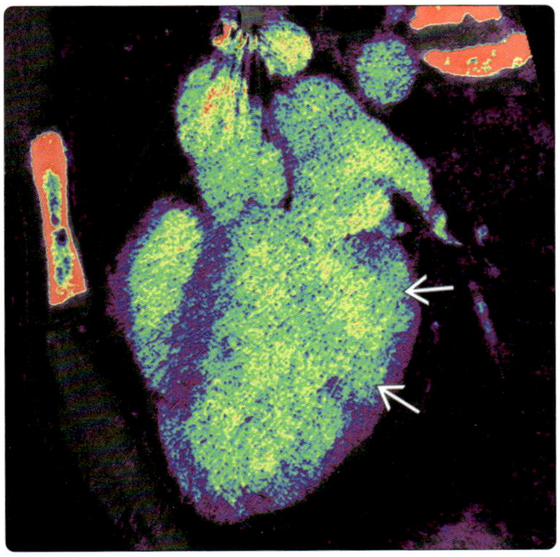

Emerging Imaging Techniques #2

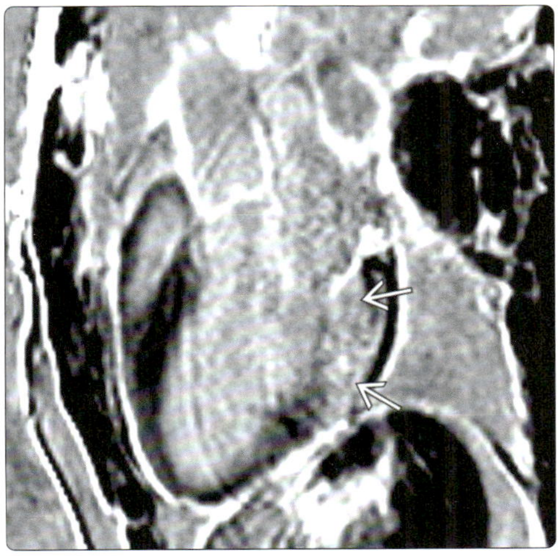

(Left) *Three-chamber delayed-phase color-overlayed iodine/water material decomposition mapping of the same multienergy cardiac CT reveals an area of delayed enhancement along the basal and midventricular inferolateral segments* ➔*.* **(Right)** *Three-chamber LGE cardiac MR in the same patient, obtained a few months before the multienergy cardiac CT, reveals a nonischemic enhancement pattern in a distribution similar to the delayed enhancement* ➔ *seen on CT.*

MR Prior to Ablation of Scar in Ventricle

KEY FACTS

TERMINOLOGY

- Monomorphic ventricular tachycardia (VT) is potentially lethal arrhythmia that can degenerate to ventricular fibrillation
- Arrhythmogenic substrate for VT in patients with structural heart disease is typically scar l tissue, which slows myocardial conduction and allows formation of self-sustaining reentrant circuit
- Electroanatomic mapping (EAM) is invasive catheter-based procedure performed by electrophysiologists to sample local electrograms from endocardial (and sometimes epicardial) surfaces of left &/or right ventricles to characterize local electrical conduction properties and identify regions involved in VT circuit
- VT ablation is invasive procedure that uses intracardiac catheters to map VT circuit and deliver energy locally to modify/eliminate arrhythmogenic substrate and prevent VT recurrence

CARDIAC MR IN VENTRICULAR TACHYCARDIA ABLATION

- Cardiac MR with LGE sequences prior to VT ablation can identify myocardial substrate, i.e., scarring
- Integrating detailed 3D LGE maps into EAM provides additional anatomic guidance for substrate-guided VT ablations and may help reduce VT recurrence rates
- MR provides information needed for procedural access, including scar location, patency of veins, epicardial fat thickness, endocardial trabeculations, relationship to vital structures, contraindications
- MR of VT patients with cardiac devices requires device reprogramming before and after cardiac MR by electrophysiologist or electrophysiology-trained nurse/technician, monitoring throughout exam, and sequences optimized to reduce device artifacts
- Devices, particularly internal cardioverter-defibrillators (ICDs), create large artifacts on cardiac MR LGE imaging that can be reduced by wideband LGE sequences

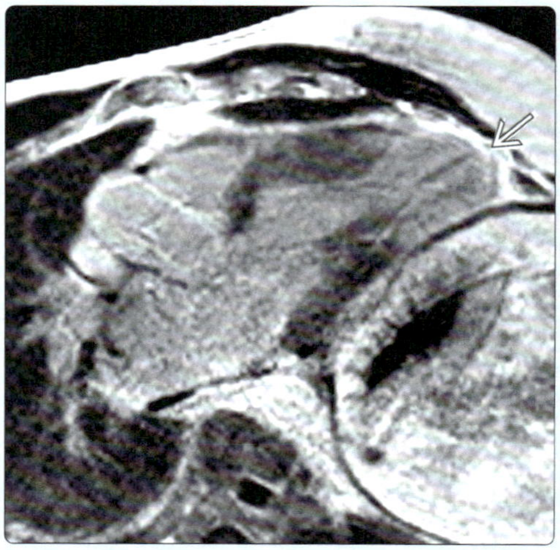

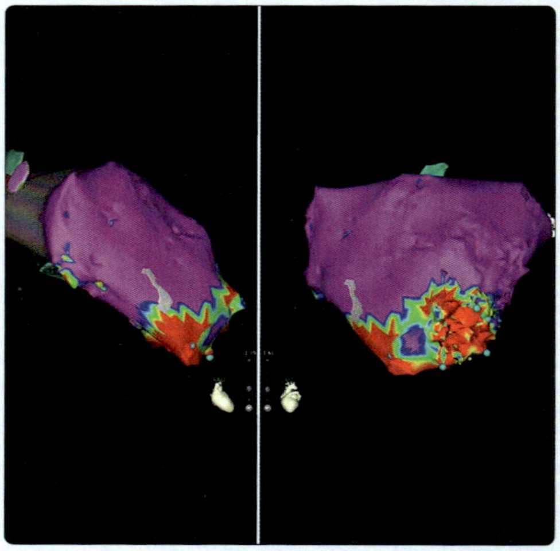

(Left) *Three-chamber LGE MR in a 53-year-old with recurrent ventricular tachycardia (VT) prior to ablation shows diffuse thinning of apex of the left ventricle (LV) with transmural LGE, compatible with full-thickness scarring →. Patient had internal cardioverter-defibrillators (ICDs) at the time of MR and elevated left hemidiaphragm.* **(Right)** *EAM of the LV in the same patient undergoing EP ablation shows a large region of low voltage in apex (red) corresponding to the area of LGE with scattered blue dots representing sites of abnormal electrograms.*

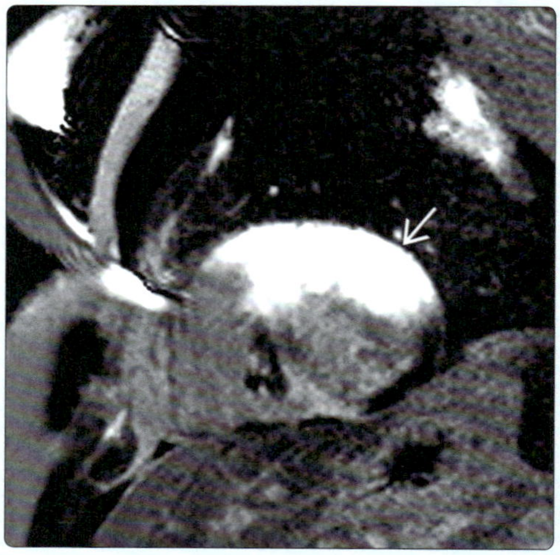

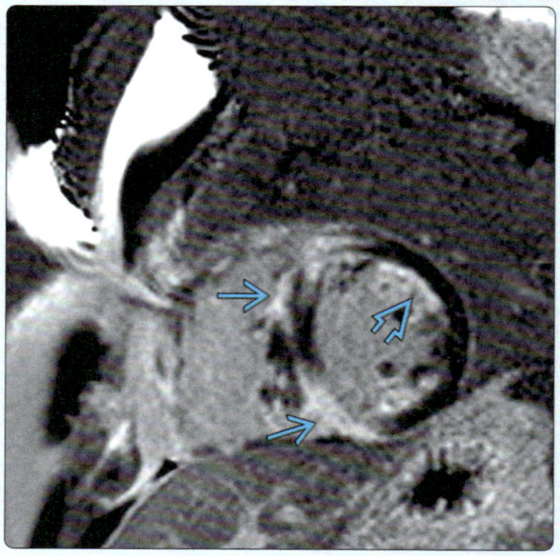

(Left) *Standard short-axis LGE shows a typical ICD-related artifact. The anterior wall of the LV has an artificially high signal → due to inappropriate nulling in this region of magnetic field distortion related to the ICD.* **(Right)** *Wideband short-axis LGE in the same patient shows diagnostic imaging of the entire LV. The anterior wall nulling is now accurate. Abnormal areas of enhancement can be seen in the septum → and lateral wall → in this patient with suspected sarcoidosis.*

CLINICAL IMPLICATIONS

Clinical Importance

- In patients with ventricular tachycardia (VT) or ventricular fibrillation (VF), cardiac MR can be used to identify scar tissue that may be source of arrhythmias and target for ablation procedures

CLINICAL ISSUES

Pathophysiology and Clinical Characterization of Ventricular Tachycardia

- VT is important cause of sudden cardiac death
  - Often result of abnormal myocardial tissue that creates reentrant circuits
  - Prior myocardial infarction is most common cause for myocardial scarring that results in VT
- Arrhythmogenic substrate is abnormal myocardial tissue that serves as slow conducting pathway, or channel, that permits reentry, usually traveling within areas of scar
- Sustained VT from structural heart disease (scar) is often monomorphic, i.e., with stable EKG morphology

Treatment of Ventricular Tachycardia

- Catheter ablation of VT can be curative, but recurrence rates vary depending on etiology, extent of underlying substrate, and ablation techniques used
- Goal of VT ablation is to eliminate reentrant circuit identified through electroanatomic maps (EAM) by rendering slow conducting tissue nonconductive (and thus VT noninducible) via delivery of energy, most often in form of heat using radiofrequency energy

CARDIAC MR IN VENTRICULAR TACHYCARDIA ABLATION

Scar Imaging and Ablation Guidance

- Purposes of MR
  - Anatomic mapping of blood pool for merging with EAM (MRA)
  - Detection and characterization of myocardial scar (LGE)
  - Procedural access
- Imported preprocedural LGE scar data can reduce procedural time and may improve both acute noninducibility and short- and long-term clinical outcomes
  - 3D, free-breathing LGE has higher spatial resolution and signal-to-noise ratio for EAM
- Scar mapping AND characterization
  - Low voltage (scar) on endocardial voltage maps corresponds abnormal LGE on MR
    - Greater scar transmurality on LGE MR = lower voltage at EAM
    - Midmyocardial scar may evoke normal voltage at EAM (MR helpful)
  - Border zone: Has lower signal intensity than central core
    - Signal 2-3 SD above normal myocardium V scar, which is > 3 SD of normal myocardium
    - Mixture of scar and surviving muscle bundles: Correlates with channels in voltage maps
    - Identifies high-risk patients
  - Other electrical abnormalities associated with arrhythmogenesis are also found in areas with LGE, such as fractionated electrograms, isolated potentials, and slow conducting channels
  - Identifies active inflammation (e.g., cardiac sarcoidosis) = requires steroid therapy prior to ablation
- Procedural access evaluation: Endocardial vs. epicardial vs. hybrid
  - Subendocardial: Endocardial approach; midmyocardial, subepicardial, full-thickness require epicardial/combined approach
  - Relationship to adjacent vital structures, e.g., coronary arteries, phrenic nerve
  - Contraindications: Thrombus or pseudoaneurysm
  - Altered venous anatomy that may challenge access can be identified with MRA (e.g., occluded veins, interrupted inferior vena cava)
  - Endocardial ablation may be challenging with excessive trabeculations
  - Epicardial ablation may be challenging with excessive epicardia fat pad (> 10 mm)

Ischemic and Nonischemic Myocardial Scar

- Ischemic scars always involve endocardium and are typically approached by endocardial ablation technique
- Nonischemic scars may be midwall, subepicardial, or transmural; identification of subepicardial scar with LGE MR prior to ablation is useful as success rates are improved by epicardial ablation in these patients
- Scars that are deep within myocardial wall may require specialized targeting techniques, including epicardial or combined approaches

Use of Cardiac MR in Patients With Devices

- Many patients being evaluated for VT ablation will have implantable cardioverter defibrillator (ICD)
- Cardiac MR can be safely performed in patients with ICDs, even if devices are not designed to be MR compatible, provided appropriate precautions are taken
- Requires electrophysiologist or electrophysiology nurse/technician to adjust device settings prior to exam, disabling sensing and intervention features that could mistake EKG changes caused by changing magnetic field in MR environment for true arrhythmias and result in shocks
- Pacemaker-dependent patients will typically have pacer set on asynchronous (nonsensing) mode
- Segmented GRE cine images often used in place of SSFP cine images for functional evaluation due to reduced device-related banding artifacts
- Incomplete myocardial nulling and artifactual high signal can be on standard LGE sequences; wideband LGE sequence can reduce ICD-related artifacts on LGE

SELECTED REFERENCES

1. Bugenhagen S et al: Utility of CT and MRI in cardiac electrophysiology. Radiographics. 44(9):e230222, 2024
2. Kim D et al: SCMR expert consensus statement for cardiovascular magnetic resonance of patients with a cardiac implantable electronic device. J Cardiovasc Magn Reson. 26(1):100995, 2024
3. Dabbagh GS et al: Magnetic resonance mapping of catheter ablation lesions after post-infarction ventricular tachycardia ablation. JACC Cardiovasc Imaging. 14(3):588-98, 2021
4. Zghaib T et al: Standard ablation versus magnetic resonance imaging-guided ablation in the treatment of ventricular tachycardia. Circ Arrhythm Electrophysiol. 11(1):e005973, 2018

KEY FACTS

TERMINOLOGY

- Cardiovascular devices and implants are broadly grouped into major categories
  - Pacemakers
    - Single-chamber pacemaker
    - Dual-chamber pacemaker
    - Biventricular pacemaker
    - Epicardial pacing leads
    - Leadless pacemaker device
  - Defibrillators
    - Implantable cardioverter defibrillators (ICDs)
    - Subcutaneous ICD
  - Recorders
    - Loop recorders
  - Valve replacement and repair
    - Mechanical valves
    - Bioprosthetic valves
    - Transcatheter valve replacement
    - Valve clips
    - Valve ring
  - Closure devices
    - Atrial septal defect occluders
    - Watchman device (left atrial appendage closure)
    - Patent puctus arteriosus occluders
  - Ventricular assist devices
    - Left ventricular assist device
    - Right ventricular assist device
    - Impella
  - Intraaortic balloon pump
  - Vascular stents
    - Coronary artery, aortic, venous stents, stented valves
  - ICU monitoring devices
    - CardioMEMS
    - Extracorporeal membrane oxygenation catheters

Cardiac Valve Positions

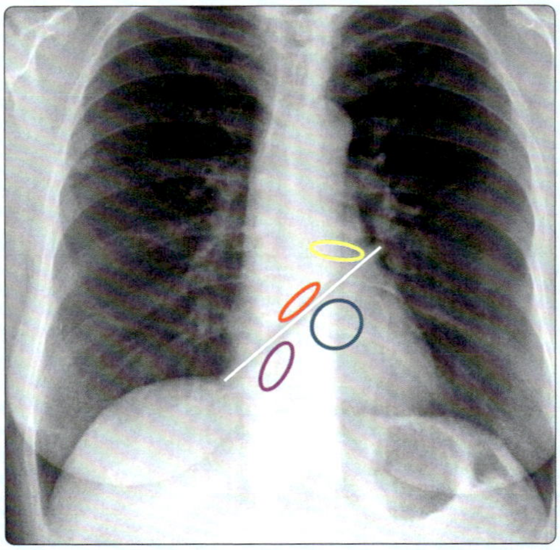

Cardiac Valve Positions

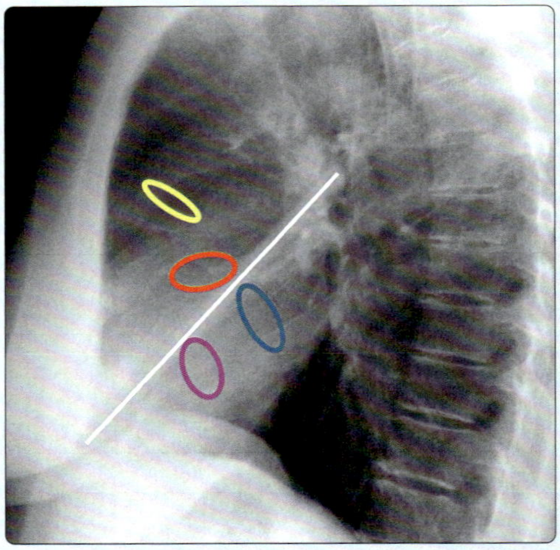

(Left) *On PA view, a line from the left atrial appendage to the right cardiophrenic angle helps locate valves: Aortic (red) is centrally located over the spine, mitral (blue) is below and to the left, and tricuspid (purple) is below the right paramedian. Pulmonic (yellow) is the highest valve above the line and near the left border.* **(Right)** *On the lateral view, the aortic valve is more in profile compared to the PA view, while the mitral valve is more en face. The pulmonic valve is the most superior, and the tricuspid valve is the most inferior.*

Bioprosthetic Valve Function in Cardiac CT

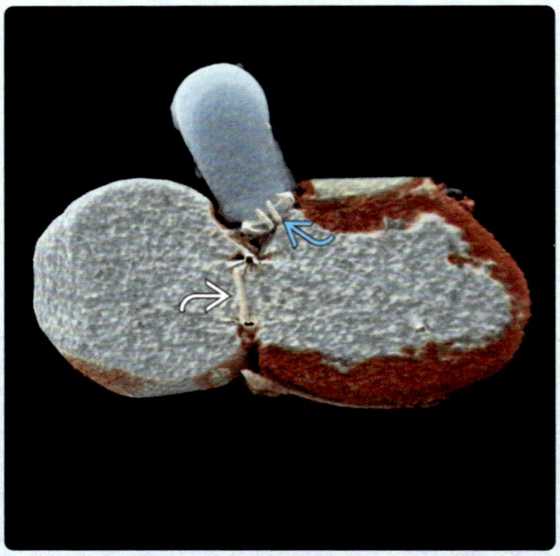

Bileaflet Tilting Disc Mechanical Valve Replacement

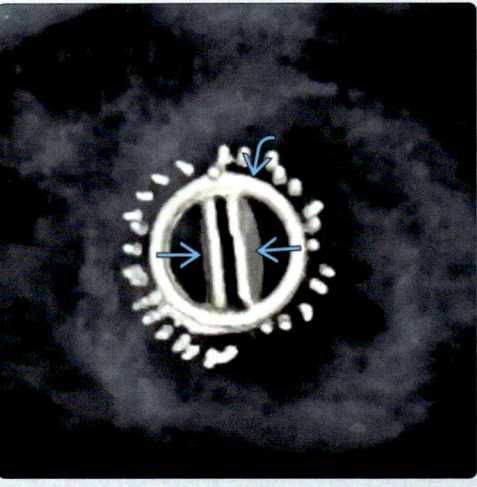

(Left) *Cinematic rendering of a cardiac CT shows bioprosthetic valves in the aortic and mitral positions during systole with the mitral valve's mechanical leaflets closed and the aortic valve's mechanical leaflets open. Opening and closing angles of leaflets are measured when assessing prosthetic valve function.* **(Right)** *3D CECT shows an aortic mechanical valve en face, highlighting the metal ring, and the bileaflet tilting the mechanical disc prosthesis in systole with the valve fully open.*

TERMINOLOGY

Definitions

- Cardiac conduction devices
  - Pacemaker: Device implanted to regulate heart rhythm by sending electrical impulses to stimulate heart muscle
    - Single-chamber pacemaker: Uses 1 lead, usually in either right atrium (RA) or ventricle
    - Dual-chamber pacemaker: Uses leads in both atrium and ventricle
    - Biventricular pacemaker [cardiac resynchronization therapy (CRT)]: Utilizes leads across both ventricles to synchronize heartbeats in heart failure patients
    - Leadless pacemaker: Self-contained pacemaker implanted directly in heart, typically in right ventricle (RV) with no external leads or wires
    - Epicardial leads: Electrodes surgically attached to heart's outer surface; used for pacing or sensing when transvenous access is not feasible
    - Septal pacemaker: Pacemaker lead positioned in ventricular septum, aiming to mimic natural heart conduction and to activate both ventricles at same time
- Automatic implantable cardioverter defibrillators (ICDs)
  - Device that detects and treats life-threatening arrhythmias by delivering shocks to restore normal heart rhythm
  - Subcutaneous ICD: Extrathoracic device provides defibrillation via subcutaneous lead along sternum; lacks pacemaker therapy and remote monitoring; offers limited capabilities
  - LifeVest wearable cardioverter defibrillator: External automatic defibrillation for patients at high risk of sudden cardiac arrest who may not yet qualify for, or are awaiting, permanent implantable defibrillator
- Cardiovascular monitoring device
  - Implantable pulmonary artery (PA) pressure monitoring device (CardioMEMS): Implantable PA sensor that continuously monitors PA pressure, aiding in proactive heart failure management and reduction of heart failure hospitalizations
  - Implantable loop recorders: Subcutaneous devices that continuously monitor cardiac rhythms for evaluating recurrent unexplained palpitations or syncope
- Cardiac valve-repairing or replacement devices
  - Surgical valve replacement: Traditional open-heart procedure to replace damaged valves with mechanical or bioprosthetic valves
  - Transcatheter valve replacement: Minimally invasive procedure to replace valve using catheter-delivered prosthetic valve [e.g., transcatheter aortic valve replacement, transcatheter mitral valve replacement, transcatheter pulmonary valve replacement, transcatheter tricuspid valve (TV) replacement]
  - Annuloplasty rings: Used to repair and reshape valve anulus, improving valve function without replacement (tricuspid and mitral ring devices)
  - Mitral and tricuspid clips are minimally invasive transcatheter therapies designed to treat mitral or tricuspid regurgitation, respectively; these devices function by approximating valve leaflets, thereby reducing regurgitation and improving valve function
- Left atrial appendage occlusion
  - Implants or devices designed to prevent stroke in atrial fibrillation patients by sealing or excluding left atrial appendage, site prone to thrombus formation
    - Watchman device: Parachute-shaped implant designed to seal left atrial appendage and reduce stroke risk in patients with atrial fibrillation
    - AtriClip device: Surgical implant used to mechanically occlude left atrial appendage, typically during open-heart surgery, to reduce stroke risk in atrial fibrillation patients
    - Amplatzer Amulet device: Self-expanding implant designed to seal left atrial appendage, reducing stroke risk in atrial fibrillation patients, with design optimized for diverse anatomic variations
    - LARIAT device: Transpericardial catheter-deployed system used to externally suture-ligate and close left atrial appendage, offering nonimplant alternative for stroke prevention in atrial fibrillation patients
- Septal defect occlusion devices
  - Implantable cardiac devices used to close ventricular or atrial septal defects (ASDs) or patent foramen ovale (PFO), thereby preventing paradoxical embolism and left-to-right shunting
  - Common ASD and PFO occlusion devices
    - Amplatzer Septal Occluder
      - Self-expanding, double-disc device made of nitinol mesh with polyester fabric
      - Delivered via catheter; discs expand on either side of septal defect to secure closure
    - GORE HELEX Septal Occluder
      - Single-disc device with central wire frame covered by expanded polytetrafluoroethylene (ePTFE) membrane
      - Disc conforms to septal wall and central frame provides support
    - CardioSEAL/STARFlex devices
      - Double umbrella-like structure with central connecting hub
      - Umbrellas open on either side of defect and hooks anchor device
- Cardiopulmonary assist devices
  - Intraaortic balloon pump: Improves coronary perfusion and reduces cardiac workload by helium inflating intraaortic balloon during diastole and deflating in systole, used to temporarily support acutely weakened left ventricle (LV) in cardiogenic shock and acute myocardial infarction
  - Left or right ventricular assist devices (LVAD or RVAD): Mechanical pumps implanted to support function of failing LV by delivering blood from LV to aorta, typically used as bridge to transplantation, destination therapy, or bridge to recovery in patients with advanced heart failure
    - Impella: Temporary percutaneous placed catheter-based device that extends from aorta into LV and supports cardiac output by actively pumping blood from LV into ascending aorta
  - Extracorporeal membrane oxygenation (ECMO): Life-support system that provides cardiac and respiratory support by oxygenating blood outside body and returning it; used in severe cardiac or respiratory failure

- Venoarterial ECMO
  - Provides both cardiac and respiratory support
  - Blood is drained from venous system (typically femoral vein) and oxygenated in ECMO circuit
  - Oxygenated blood is reinfused into arterial system (typically via femoral or axillary artery) to bypass both heart and lungs
  - Indications: Cardiogenic shock, cardiac arrest, combined failure
- Venovenous ECM
  - Provides respiratory support only
  - Blood is drained from venous system (typically via femoral vein) and oxygenated in ECMO circuit
  - Oxygenated blood is reinfused into venous system (typically via internal jugular vein), returning to heart for systemic circulation
  - Indications: Severe respiratory failure, acute respiratory distress syndrome, bridging to recovery

- Miscellaneous: Other cardiac and extracardiac devices that may be encountered on cardiothoracic and chest imaging
  - Embolization coils
    - Most commonly encountered in treatment of thoracic vascular abnormalities, such as pulmonary arteriovenous malformations (PAVMs), bronchial artery embolization for hemoptysis, and thoracic aneurysms or fistulas
    - Coils appear as small, dense radiopaque structures within thoracic cavity
  - Coronary artery bypass graft (CABG) markers and surgical clips
    - Radiopaque markers placed at ostia of aortocoronary grafts to facilitate catheter insertion of graft ostia at future coronary angiography
  - Cardiac stents (coronary stents, PA stents, venous stents, aortic coarctation stents)
  - Deep brain stimulator (DBS)
    - Implanting electrodes within specific brain regions to modulate neural activity, primarily for treating movement disorders, such as Parkinson disease, essential tremor, and dystonia
    - Comprised of intracranial electrodes connected via subcutaneous leads to implanted pulse generator (IPG), typically positioned in anterior chest wall
  - Hypoglossal nerve stimulator
    - Implantable device used to treat obstructive sleep apnea (OSA) by stimulating hypoglossal nerve
  - Vagus nerve stimulator
    - Implantable device used primarily for treatment of refractory epilepsy and depression
  - Diaphragmatic pacemaker
    - Device that electrically stimulates phrenic nerve or diaphragm to induce respiration in patients with respiratory failure due to central or peripheral causes, such as spinal cord injuries or central hypoventilation syndrome

IMAGING ANATOMY

General Anatomic Considerations

- Pacemakers
  - Generator
    - Implanted in subcutaneous or subpectoral space, typically in left infraclavicular; may be placed in right infraclavicular in specific clinical scenarios
    - Cardiac generator may feature Bluetooth capability, enabling wireless transmission of monitoring and performance data to physicians
      - Caveat: Pacemaker's Bluetooth antenna may mimic fractured wire on imaging
  - Leads
    - Single-chamber pacemaker
      - Single lead introduced via subclavian vein, traversing superior vena cava (SVC) to terminate within RA or RV
    - Dual-chamber pacemaker
      - 2 leads terminate in right atrial appendage and right ventricular apex or at interventricular septum
    - Biventricular pacemaker
      - Also known as CRT
      - At least 1 right ventricular lead and 1 left ventricular lead with possibility of additional right atrial lead
      - Typically, normal dual-chamber system includes additional lead advanced through coronary venous sinus into posterolateral vein overlying LV
    - Leadless pacemaker
      - Small, bullet-shaped devices implanted directly into RV via femoral approach
      - Smaller than AAA battery, can be mistaken for implantable loop recorders on PA radiographs but are distinguishable on lateral views
      - Provide single-chamber ventricular pacing without defibrillation capability
      - Dual-chamber devices will show devices in both RA and RV with wired interconnection or wireless pairing
    - Epicardial leads
      - Electrodes surgically attached to outer surface of heart (epicardium)
    - Septal pacemaker
      - Right ventricular lead positioned on interventricular septum rather than apex
      - On chest x-ray, lead tip is seen left of spine in midseptal region with more anterior course on lateral views
- ICDs
  - Generator
    - Typically implanted subcutaneously or subpectorally in infraclavicular region
    - Occasionally implanted on right side in cases of left-sided contraindications (e.g., venous obstruction or prior mastectomy)
    - Larger generator compared to pacemakers, reflecting defibrillator components
  - Leads
    - Travel via subclavian vein through brachiocephalic vein and SVC to heart
    - Shock coil
      - Appear as thicker radiopaque segments
      - Right ventricular shock coil: In RV near apex or along interventricular septum

  - ◻ SVC coil (in dual-coil systems): In SVC near junction with RA
- – ± pacing leads (if present)
  - ◻ Terminate in right atrial appendage (atrial pacing) or right ventricular near apex (ventricular pacing)
  - ◻ Additional coronary sinus leads in dual-chamber or biventricular ICDs
- Subcutaneous ICDs
  - Generator
    - Subcutaneously implanted laterally in chest along left midaxillary line
  - Lead
    - Positioned subcutaneously along left parasternal margin without entering vasculature
    - Subcutaneous lead appears as linear radiopaque structure running along sternum
- Valve repair and replacement devices
  - Surgical valve replacement
    - Mechanical valves
      - ◻ Appear as distinct structures at valve position with variable radiopaque components (aortic, mitral, tricuspid, or pulmonary)
      - ◻ Configuration varies with valve type; e.g., mechanical bileaflet valves show 2 semicircular discs
    - Bioprosthetic valves
      - ◻ Made of tissue-based porcine or bovine radiolucent leaflets but may have radiopaque markers, wires, or rings
  - Transcatheter valve replacement
    - Leaflets are bioprosthetic
    - Positioned within native anulus or within previously placed prosthetic valve (valve-in-valve procedure)
    - Radiopaque circular/tubular or hourglass-shaped stent
  - Annuloplasty rings
    - Mitral annuloplasty rings
      - ◻ At left atrioventricular (AV) junction, stabilizing and reshaping mitral valve anulus
      - ◻ Partial or complete radiopaque circular structure
      - ◻ Ring shape can vary depending on specific design (rigid, flexible, or semirigid)
    - Tricuspid annuloplasty rings
      - ◻ Positioned within right AV groove, stabilizing TV anulus between RA and RV
      - ◻ Appears as radiopaque structure along right cardiac border, often less circular than mitral annuloplasty ring; may appear more subtle due to its position closer to spine and diaphragm
  - Mitral and tricuspid clips
    - Clip has 2 movable arms and grippers that grasp leaflets to form double orifice valve; appears as Y-shaped 15-18 mm long metallic structure at location of mitral or TV center
- Septal occlusion devices
  - Circular double disk-like structure visible over interatrial septum (ASD) or ventricular septum (ventricular septal defect)
- Left atrial appendage occlusion devices
  - Metallic, radiopaque structure within left atrial appendage segment of left heart border of cardiac silhouette
- Intraaortic balloon pump
  - Radiopaque linear structure within descending thoracic aorta; some systems show only radiopaque proximal and distal markers; may see gas-filled tubular balloon if image obtained during diastolic filling; helium is used because it is inert, has low viscosity, and can be rapidly absorbed into bloodstream
  - Balloon catheter tip is expected between aortic knob and carina on chest x-ray, just distal to origin of left subclavian artery on CT
- LVADs
  - Inflow cannula
    - Sewn into left ventricular apex, drawing blood from LV
    - Radiopaque tube extending into cardiac silhouette, terminating at left ventricular apex
  - Pump housing
    - Typically implanted in epigastric abdominal wall or within upper abdomen
    - Appears as radiopaque circular or oval structure in lower thoracic or upper abdominal region
  - Outflow graft
    - Anastomosed to ascending aorta, bypassing failing LV to maintain systemic perfusion
    - Radiopaque structure coursing anteriorly and superiorly from device toward ascending aorta
  - Driveline
    - Exits abdominal wall to connect internal device to external controller and power source
- Impella device
  - Catheter
    - Inserted percutaneously through femoral or axillary artery for left-sided devices or femoral vein for right-sided devices; catheter contains driveline
    - Appears as radiopaque catheter with tubular structure traversing aortic or pulmonic valve; catheter path through femoral or axillary artery into ascending aorta and crossing aortic valve to terminate in LV, or femoral vein, inferior vena cava (IVC), RA, RV, and crossing pulmonic valve to terminate in PA
    - Tip of left-sided systems contains inlet and is positioned within LV, outflow is positioned in ascending aorta
    - Right systems may be positioned via femoral or jugular venous approach; inlets are positioned in venae cavae or RA, and tip containing outlet is positioned within PA
  - Pump housing
    - Distal thicker tubular structure at catheter, positioned across aortic valve (left-sided devices) or pulmonic valve (right-sided devices)
  - Inflow port
    - Positioned in LV or RV
  - Outflow port
    - Positioned in ascending aorta (left-sided devices) or PA (right-sided devices)
- ECMO
  - Venoarterial ECMO

- Venous cannula tip should be near RA
- Arterial cannula visible in femoral artery, coursing toward descending thoracic aorta
  - Venovenous ECMO
    - Both cannula tips should be near RA (1 in IVC, other in SVC)
    - Cannulas must not interfere with TV function
- Deep brain stimulation (DBS)
  - Pulse generator
    - Radiopaque device located in right or left anterior chest wall; size and shape comparable to cardiac pacemakers
  - Leadshe
    - Leads are tunneled subcutaneously from cranial electrodes, descending along neck and chest to connect with generator
- Hypoglossal nerve stimulator
  - Stimulator implant
    - Positioned subcutaneously, typically in upper chest (similar to pacemaker)
  - Stimulation electrode
    - Placed around branch of hypoglossal nerve in submandibular neck
  - Respiratory sensor
    - Inserted subcutaneously in intercostal space near diaphragm; detects respiratory effort to synchronize nerve stimulation
- Vagus nerve stimulator
  - Pulse generator
    - Appears as radiopaque oval or rectangular device in upper chest wall, similar to pacemaker
  - Leads/electrodes
    - Radiopaque lead extending superiorly from chest wall to left side of neck, terminating near carotid sheath at level of vagus nerve
- Diaphragmatic pacemaker
  - Pulse generator
    - Radiopaque rectangular or oval device in anterior chest wall, similar to cardiac pacemakers
  - Electrodes
    - Leads terminating near diaphragm or phrenic nerve in neck or thoracic cavity
- CABG markers and clips
  - Radiopaque metallic markers and clips appear along cardiac silhouette and mediastinum
    - Ostial markers: Incomplete or complete ring-like structure at ascending aortic ostium of aortocoronary grafts
    - Hemostasis: Along course of grafts atraumatic, titanium clips are used to control bleeding from vessels, grafts, and side branches of internal mammary artery grafts
    - Facilitating anastomosis: U clips allow interrupted anastomotic sutures and prevent purse-string effect and hence improve patency rate
- CardioMEMS
  - Small, radiopaque structure usually overlying left lower lobar PA
  - Nitinol loops on both ends expand to securely anchor device
- Implantable loop recorders
  - Small, cylindrical devices, typically 4-8 cm in length, resembling USB drive
  - Positioned within subcutaneous tissue, superficial to ribs and pectoral muscles
  - Aligned in midline or left lateral to sternum to optimize sensing cardiac electrical activity

CLINICAL IMPLICATIONS

Clinical Importance

- Pacemakers and defibrillators
  - It is crucial to thoroughly evaluate all components of pacemakers or cardiac defibrillators, starting from cardiac generator to distal tip, for fractures, malposition, secure connection vs. disengagement of generator leads, and presence of abandoned leads; compatibility with MR should also be assessed when indicated
- Valves
  - Identifying replaced or repaired valve on chest radiography is done based on its location with respect to cardiomediastinal silhouette
    - PA view: Right cardiac border is formed by SVC and RA, while left is shaped by left atrial appendage and LV, with no contribution from RV
    - Lateral view: Anterior retrosternal space is occupied by RV/right ventricular outflow tract, while posterior silhouette includes left atrium, LV, and IVC
  - CT is useful for assessing valve function, position, leaks, opening/closing angles, or complications, such as hypoattenuating valve thickening (HALT)
- Closure devices
  - Evaluate occluders for residual defects, leaks, and proper positioning
- Ventricular assist devices
  - Assess device position and components for complications, such as thrombus formation, graft cannula narrowing, kinking, or malposition

SELECTED REFERENCES

1. Stankovic I et al: Imaging in patients with cardiovascular implantable electronic devices: part 1-imaging before and during device implantation. A clinical consensus statement of the European Association of Cardiovascular Imaging (EACVI) and the European Heart Rhythm Association (EHRA) of the ESC. Eur Heart J Cardiovasc Imaging. 25(1):e1-32, 2023
2. Rhodes NG et al: Radiology of intra-aortic balloon pump catheters. Radiol Cardiothorac Imaging. 4(2):e210120, 2022
3. Rajiah P et al: Pre- and postprocedural CT of transcatheter left atrial appendage closure devices. Radiographics. 41(3):680-98, 2021
4. Saleh AS et al: Pacemaker bluetooth antenna misinterpreted as fractured wire. Radiol Cardiothorac Imaging. 2(1):e190085, 2020
5. Cressman S et al: Chest radiographic appearance of minimally invasive cardiac implants and support devices: what the radiologist needs to know. Curr Probl Diagn Radiol. 48(3):274-88, 2019

Orientation of Valve Prostheses

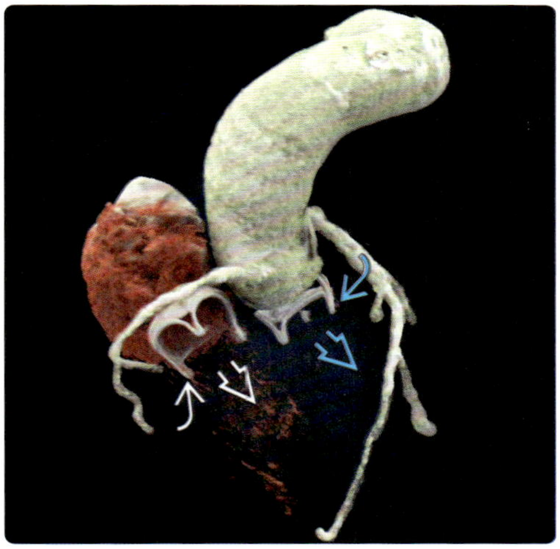

Surgical Bioprosthetic Valve Replacements

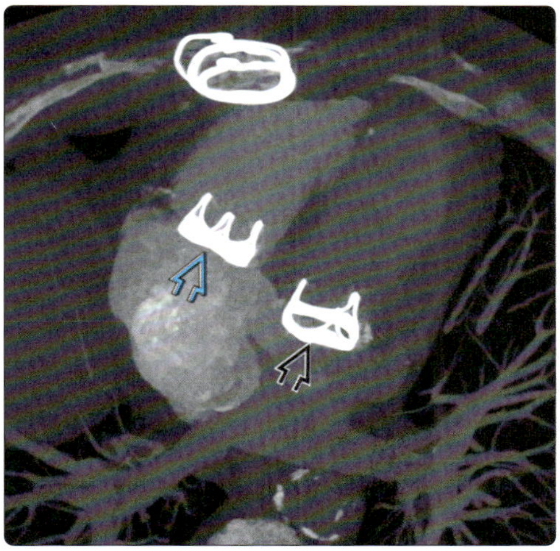

(Left) *Cinematic rendering of a cardiac CT shows prosthetic valve orientation with crowns directed toward the outflow: Mitral crown to the left ventricle (LV) and tricuspid crown to the right ventricle (RV). This helps in understanding valve orientation and blood flow on radiographs.* **(Right)** *Four-chamber cardiac CT MIP confirms tricuspid and mitral valve positions. The valve struts point toward the LV and the RV, respectively. No radiopaque leaflets are seen as these are bioprosthetic valves.*

Surgical Bioprosthetic Pulmonic Valve Replacement

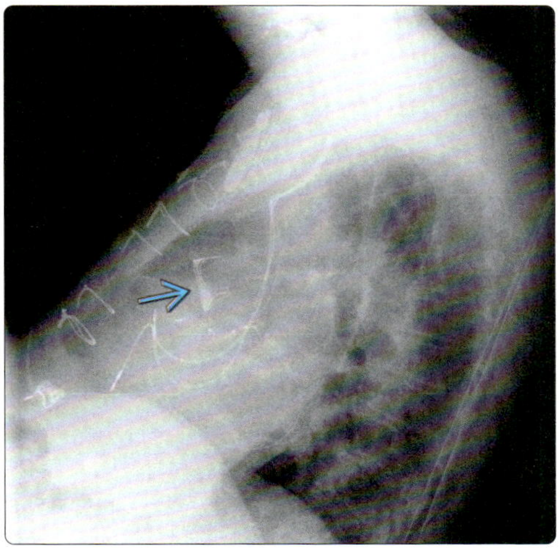

Transcatheter Pulmonary Valve Replacement

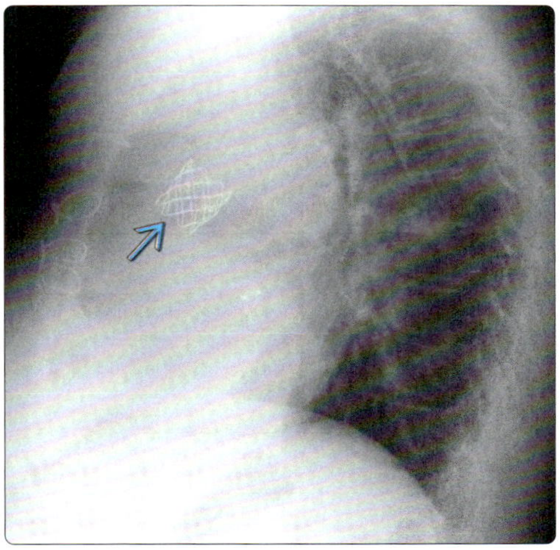

(Left) *Lateral chest radiograph shows an anterosuperior valve with struts pointing toward the pulmonary artery, indicating a pulmonary valve prosthesis. These appear slightly posterior to the sternum and at the superior aspect of the right ventricular outflow tract.* **(Right)** *Lateral chest radiograph shows the characteristic net-like appearance of a transcatheter pulmonic valve. These may have bovine (Melody) or porcine (Harmony) leaflets in self-expanding platinum-iridium or nickel-titanium (Nitinol) wire frames.*

Transcatheter Pulmonary Valve Replacement

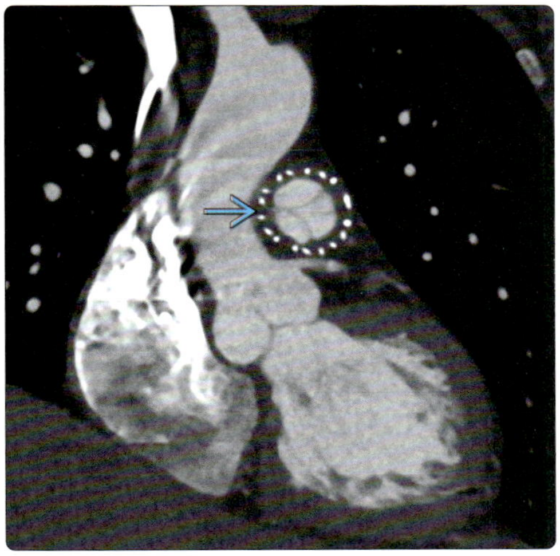

Mitral Valve-in-Valve

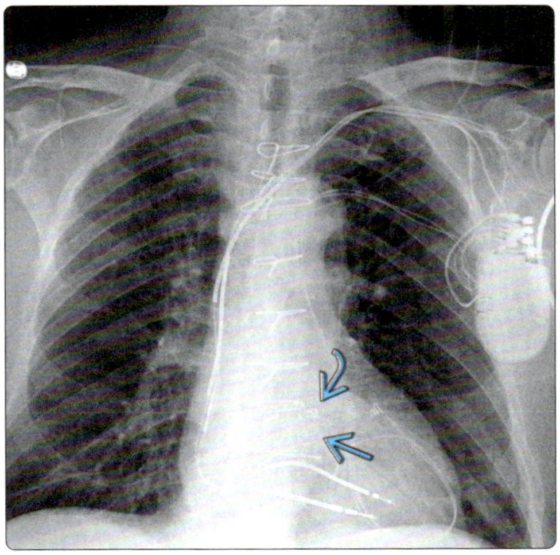

(Left) *Coronal oblique cardiac CTA shows the characteristic appearance of a transcatheter pulmonary valve replacement (TPVR) with bioprosthetic leaflets in a patient with a history of tetralogy of Fallot.* **(Right)** *Frontal radiograph shows a transcatheter mitral valve replacement (TMVR) placed within a failed bioprosthetic valve (valve-in-valve procedure).*

Transcatheter Aortic Valve Replacement

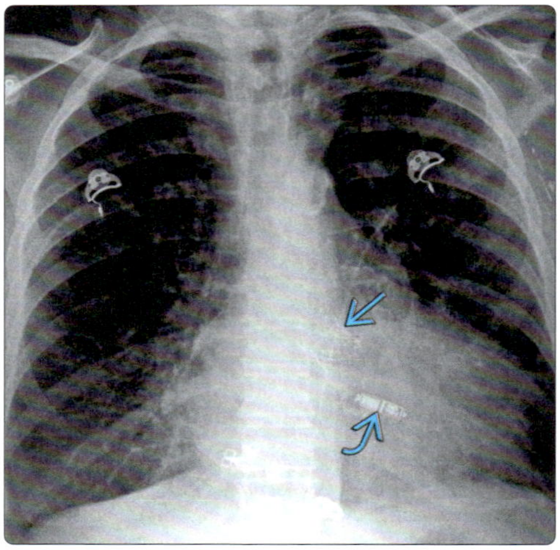

Transcatheter Aortic Valve Replacement Deployment

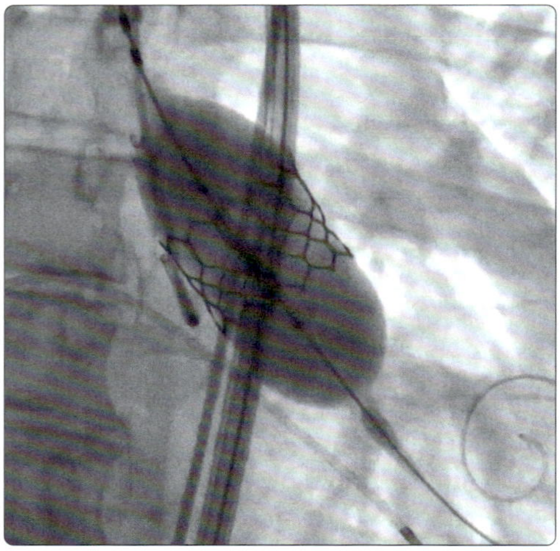

(Left) *Frontal chest x-ray shows the characteristic appearance of a transcatheter aortic valve replacement (TAVR) ➡ with its orientation pointed toward the right shoulder, along with a leadless pacemaker ➡.* **(Right)** *Angiographic image shows the deployment of the transcatheter valve at the expected location of the aortic valve.*

Interatrial Septal Occluder Device

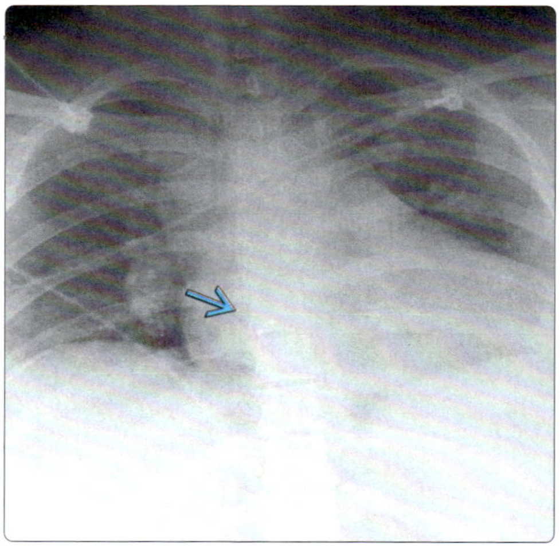

Interatrial Septal Occluder Device

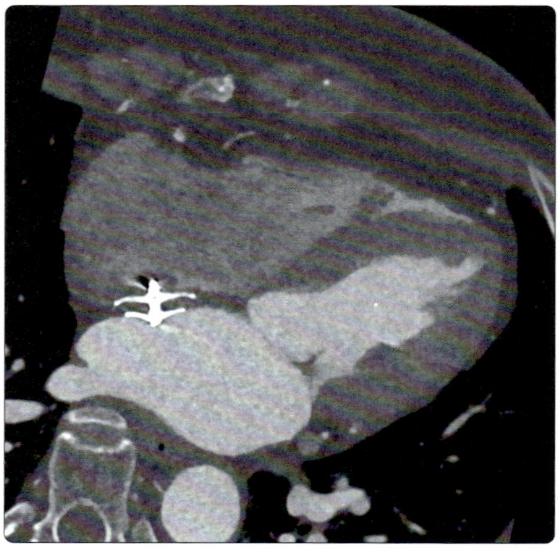

(Left) *AP chest radiograph shows a faint metallic density ➡ at the expected interatrial septum with a mesh-like disc structure adjacent to it (poorly seen), consistent with an interatrial septal occluder.* **(Right)** *Axial cardiac CTA shows a double disc-shaped density in the interatrial septum, consistent with an Amplatzer occluder device. Differential contrast density between the left and right heart shows no transseptal contrast flow, indicating absence of residual shunt.*

MitraClip Devices

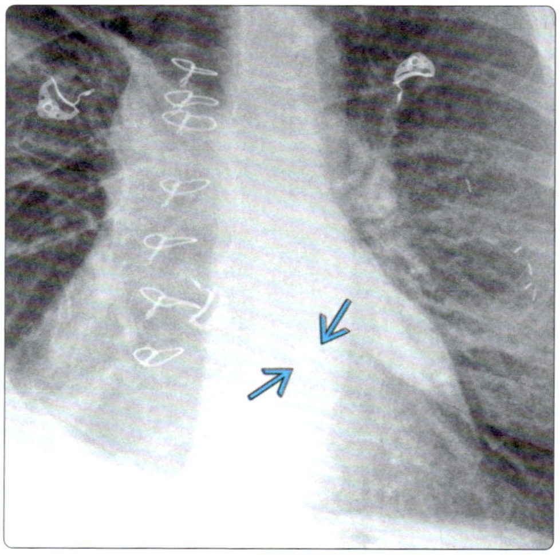

Tricuspid Valve Clips

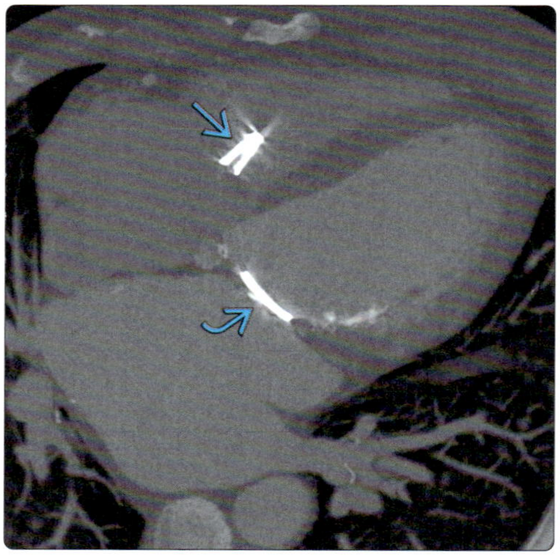

(Left) *Frontal chest X-ray shows 2 symmetrical metallic densities ➡ at the expected location of the mitral valve, consistent with MitraClip devices. These densities may overlap or appear as paired dots or a single dense structure, depending on the number of clips placed and the angle of imaging.* **(Right)** *Axial cardiac CT MIP shows tricuspid clips ➡ as small, radiopaque metallic densities centrally placed at the tricuspid valve, along with the inferior margin of a mitral annuloplasty ring ➡.*

Single-Chamber Cardiac Pacemaker

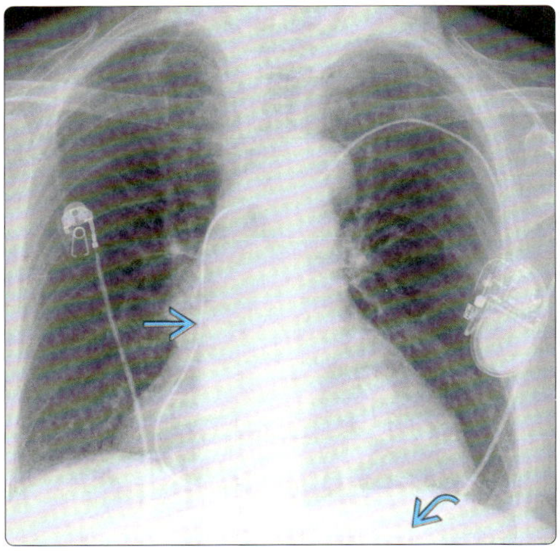

Dual-Chamber Cardiac Pacemaker and Defibrillator

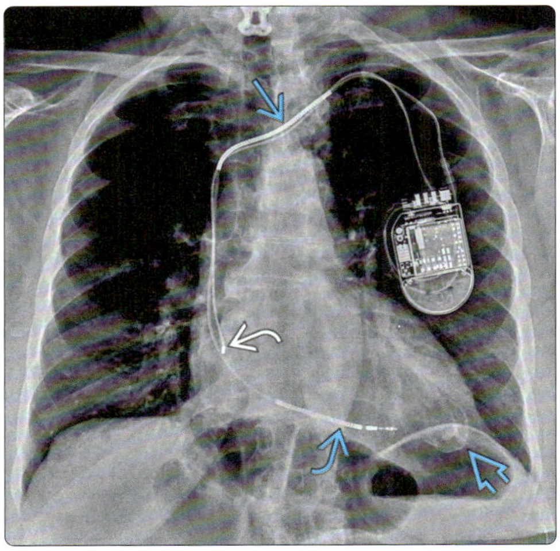

(Left) *Frontal chest x-ray shows a left chest wall cardiac pacemaker with a single lead terminating in the RV near the cardiac apex. Typical single-chamber pacemakers may have leads terminating in the RV or right atrium.* **(Right)** *Chest x-ray shows a dual-chamber cardiac defibrillator with a shock coil in the brachiocephalic vein extending to superior vena cava and one in the RV, plus a pacing lead terminating in the right atrial appendage. Note calcified apical LV aneurysm, which may be associated with arrhythmogenic fibrosis.*

Biventricular Pacemaker and Defibrillator

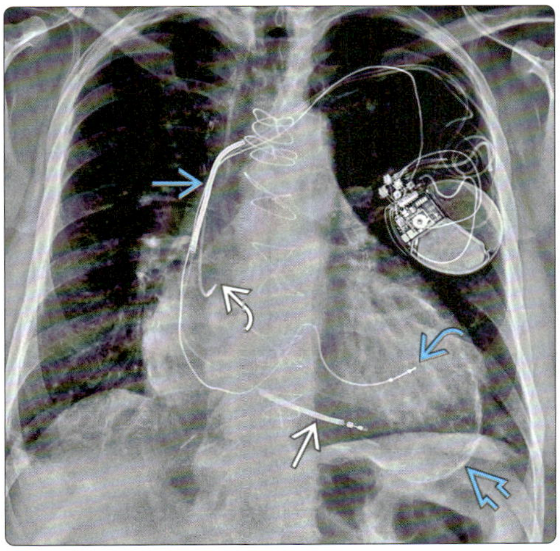

Abandoned Epicardial Leads

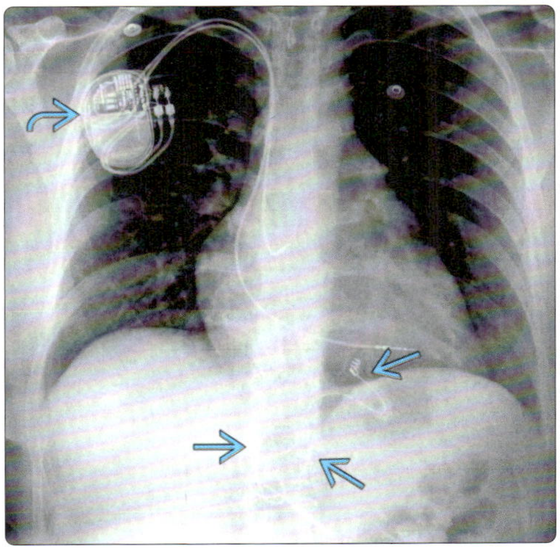

(Left) *Frontal chest x-ray in a patient with a calcified apical aneurysm shows a biventricular cardiac pacemaker and defibrillator with shock coils in superior vena cava and right ventricular apex. Three leads are visualized: 1 in the right atrial appendage, 1 in the right ventricular apex, and a curved lead in a coronary sinus tributary.* **(Right)** *Chest x-ray shows abandoned epicardial leads with the tips over the anteroinferior cardiac silhouette. A newer dual-chamber pacemaker is in place.*

Epicardial Pacemaker

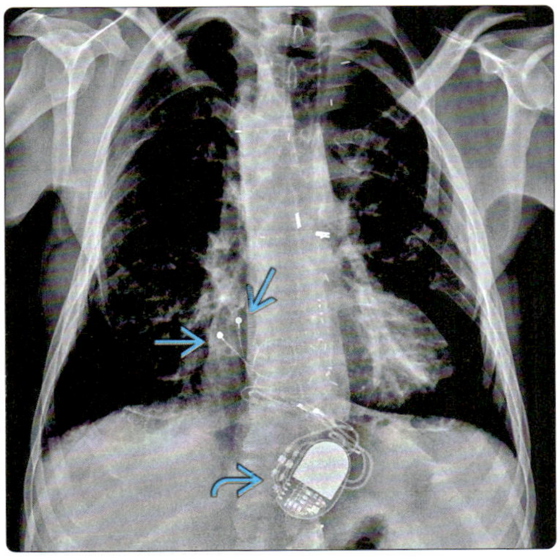

Subcutaneous Cardiac Defibrillator

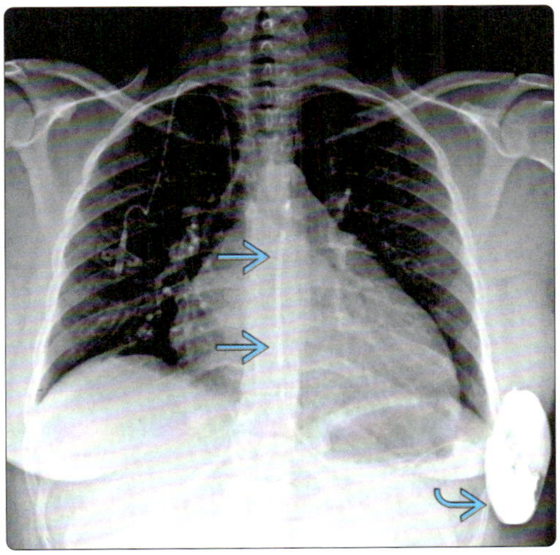

(Left) *Chest radiograph shows epicardial leads projecting over the right cardiac silhouette, connected to a pacemaker.* **(Right)** *Frontal chest radiograph shows a subcutaneous cardiac defibrillator in the left lateral chest wall with a shock lead in the subcutaneous parasternal position. Lateral views may be useful to confirm the extrathoracic location of the lead.*

(Left) *Frontal chest radiograph shows a dual-chamber pacemaker with leads terminating in the right atrium and the RV, likely at the ventricular septum. RV leads can terminate either near the apex or at the septum, as in this case. The Bluetooth antenna of the pacemaker is also visible.* **(Right)** *Magnified view of the pacemaker shows the device with a Bluetooth antenna wire, which can resemble a fractured lead.*

Dual-Chamber Pacemaker

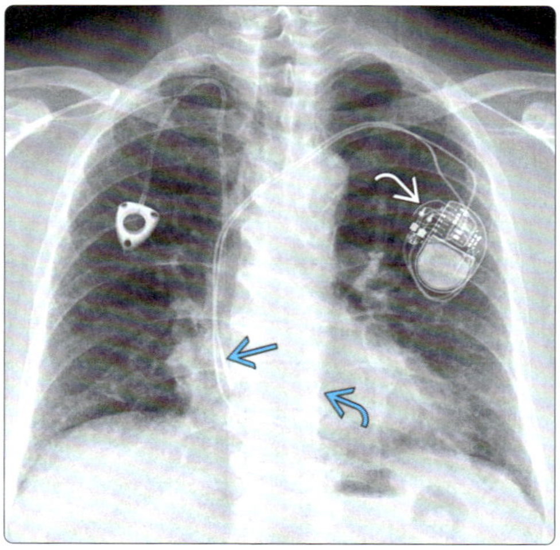

Bluetooth Antenna Pacemaker

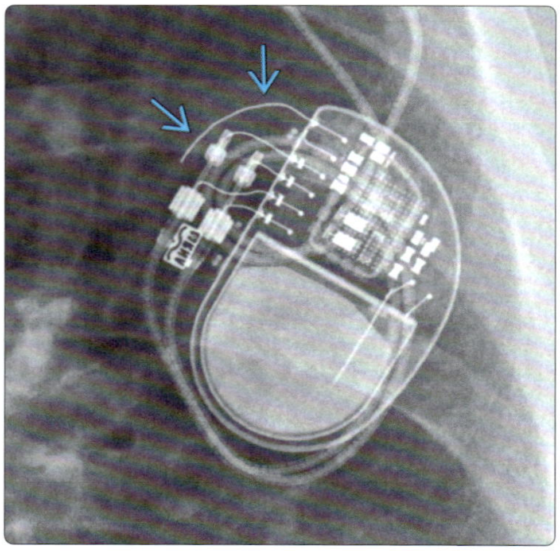

(Left) *PA chest radiograph shows external interconnected electronics and electrodes and defibrillator pads, consistent with a wearable cardioverter defibrillator (WCD), LifeVest.* **(Right)** *Lateral chest x-ray shows a wearable external defibrillator vest with electrodes positioned over the chest wall. A WCD may be used for noninvasive cardiac monitoring and defibrillation in the setting of acute myocardial infarction in patients with a left ventricular ejection fraction of 35% or less.*

Wearable Cardioverter Defibrillator: LifeVest

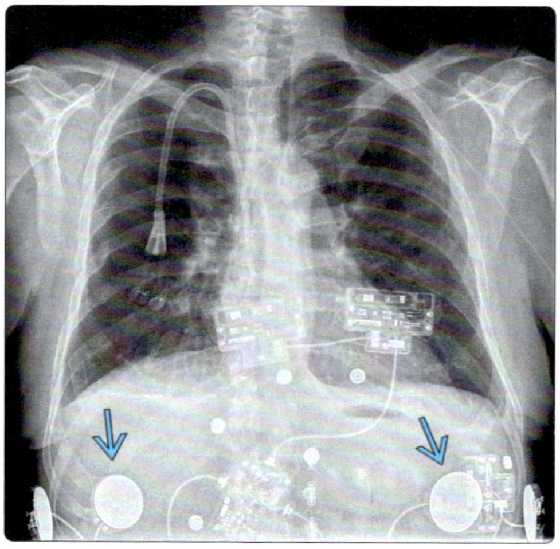

Wearable Cardioverter Defibrillator: LifeVest

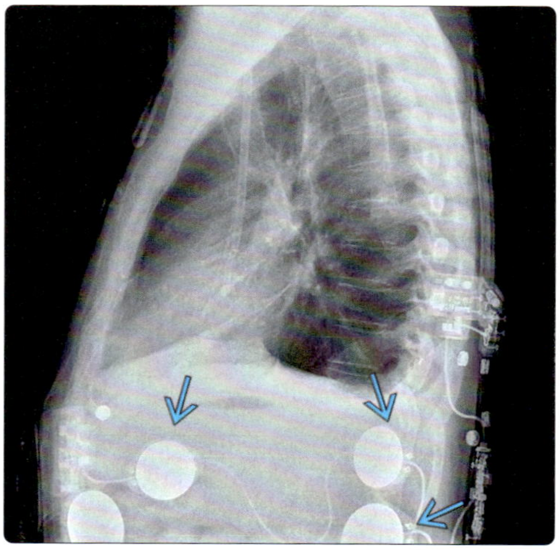

(Left) *Frontal chest x-ray demonstrates a leadless pacemaker, visible as a bullet-shaped device positioned within the RV, without transvenous leads. These self-contained generators with integrated electrodes minimize complications related to conventional leads (lead fracture, venous stenosis/occlusion) and pocket complications, such as infection.* **(Right)** *Magnified view in the same patient shows the tubular shape of the leadless pacemaker positioned within the RV.*

Leadless Pacemaker

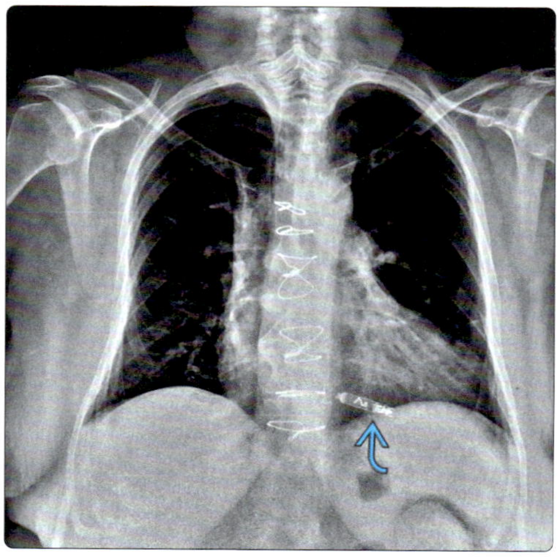

Leadless Pacemaker

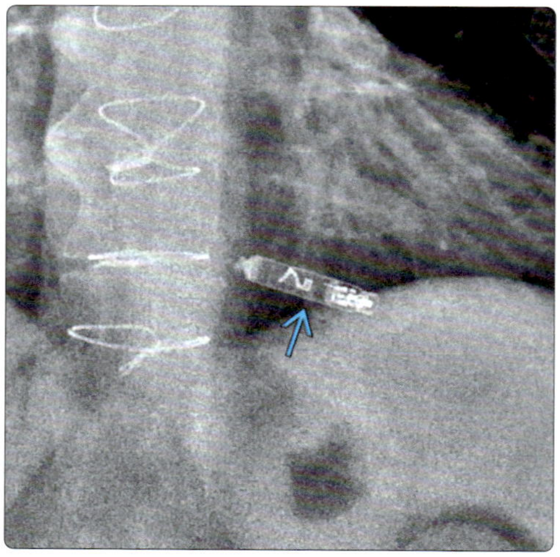

Leadless Pacemaker

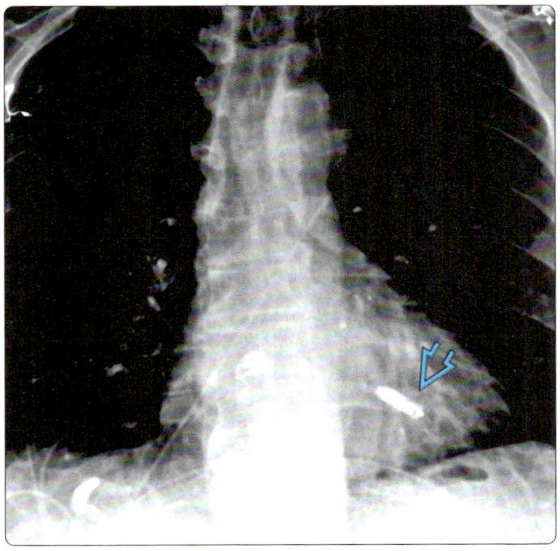

Leadless Pacemaker

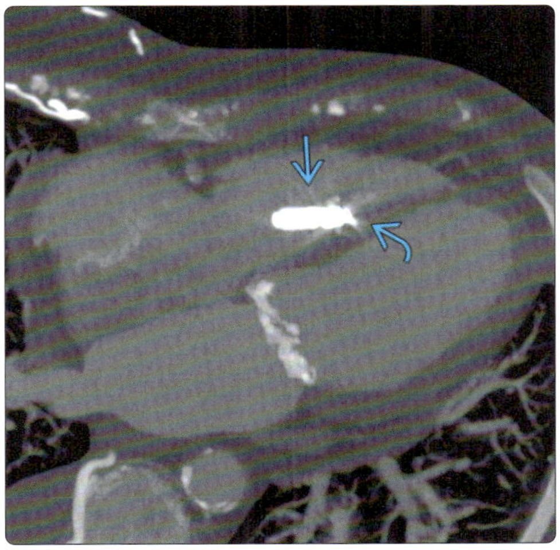

(Left) *Frontal chest radiograph shows a leadless pacemaker device projected over the RV* . **(Right)** *MIP cardiac CT shows a bullet-shaped leadless pacemaker device in the RV* *, securely hooked into the interventricular septum* *. The devices are transcatheter-delivered, and once in an electrophysiologically effective position, the pacemaker tines are deployed or a helix wire is rotated into the myocardium, securing the device in place.*

Subcutaneously Implanted Loop Recorder

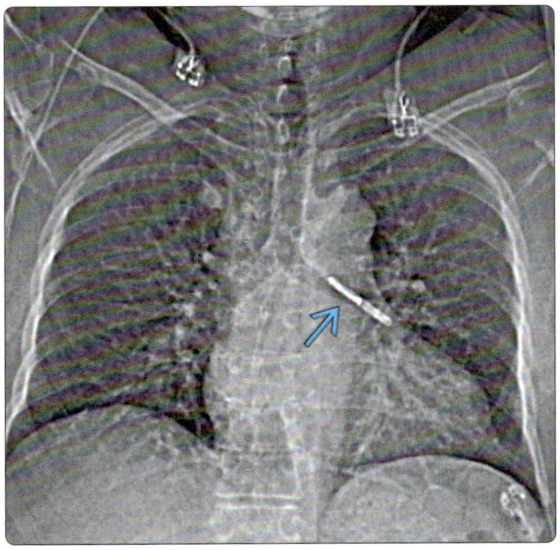

Subcutaneously Implanted Loop Recorder

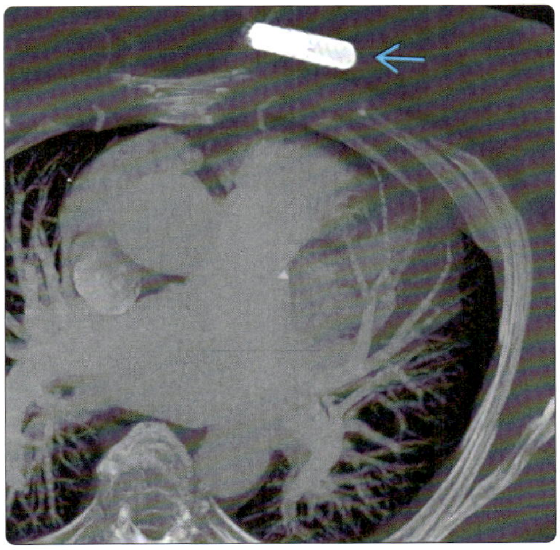

(Left) *Frontal chest radiograph demonstrates a subcutaneously implanted loop recorder* *in the left anterior chest wall, identifiable as a tubular device (typically smaller than a AAA-sized battery).* **(Right)** *Axial cardiac CTA MIP shows the classic appearance of the implanted loop recorder positioned subcutaneously in the left chest wall* .

Subcutaneously Implanted Loop Recorder

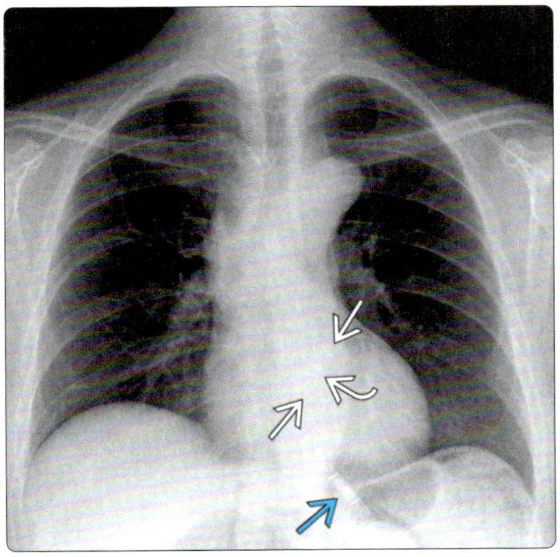

Subcutaneously Implanted Loop Recorder

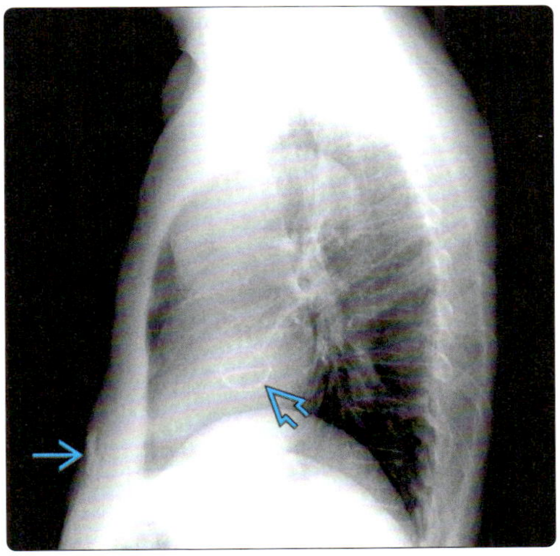

(Left) *Frontal radiograph shows an implantable loop recorder* *at left lower chest wall, which may appear similar to a leadless pacemakers, although in this patient, it is lower than the RV location where a leadless pacemaker would be expected. Note the prosthetic aortic valve* *with mechanical bileaflet tilting discs* . **(Right)** *Lateral radiograph confirms the implantable loop recorder* *in the extrathoracic left lower chest wall tissue anterior to the sternum. Note the bileaflet mechanical aortic valve prosthesis* .

Left Atrial Appendage Clip (AtriClip)

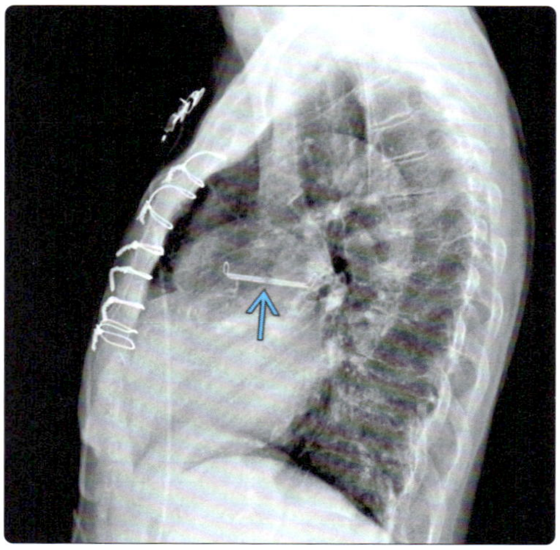

Left Atrial Appendage Clip (AtriClip)

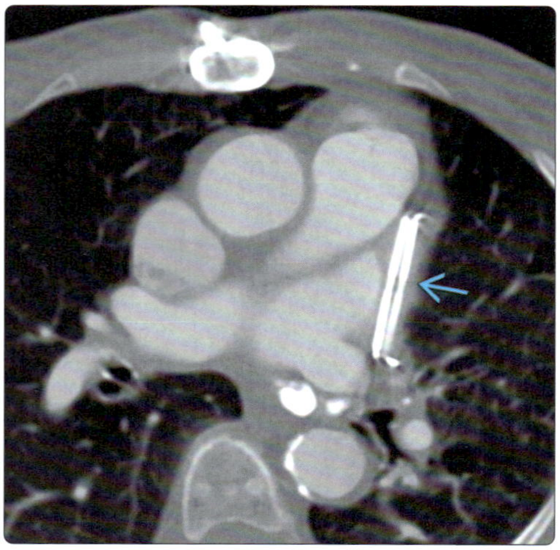

(Left) *Lateral radiograph shows a surgically placed left atrial appendage clip* ➙ *(AtriClip) positioned at the base of the left atrial appendage (LAA) to exclude the LAA from blood flow, thereby preventing thrombus formation and embolization.* **(Right)** *Cardiac CT shows the clip* ➙ *at the ostial LAA completely occluding the appendage.*

Left Atrial Appendage Occluder (Watchman)

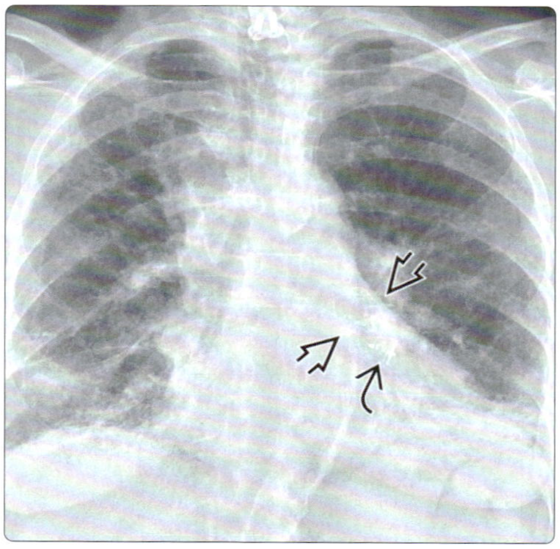

Left Atrial Occluder (Watchman) Device

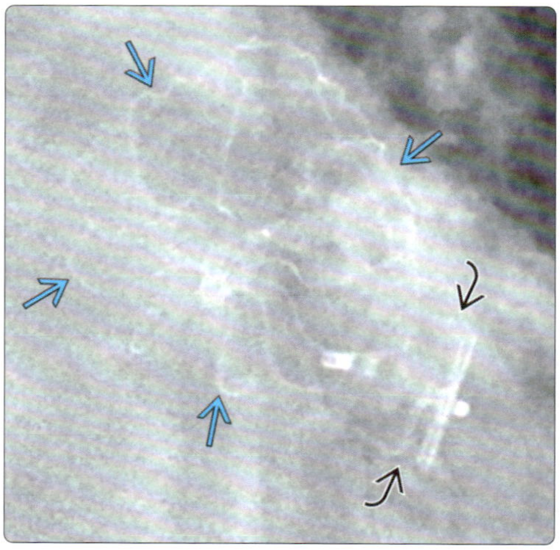

(Left) *Frontal chest radiograph shows wire mesh from a Watchman device positioned in the LAA* ⇨*, excluding it from the left atrium to prevent thrombus embolization, and a secondary cardiac plug* ⇨*.* **(Right)** *Magnified view in the same patient shows the classic location and umbrella-like shape of the Watchman device* ➙ *positioned in the LAA. Note an additional Amplatzer cardiac plug device* ⇨ *used as a secondary closure device to seal a significant peridevice leak detected on follow-up imaging.*

Sealed Watchman Device

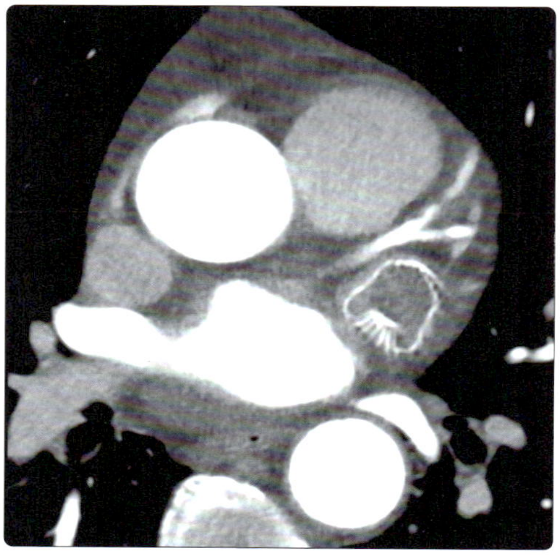

Incomplete Closure of Left Atrial Appendage

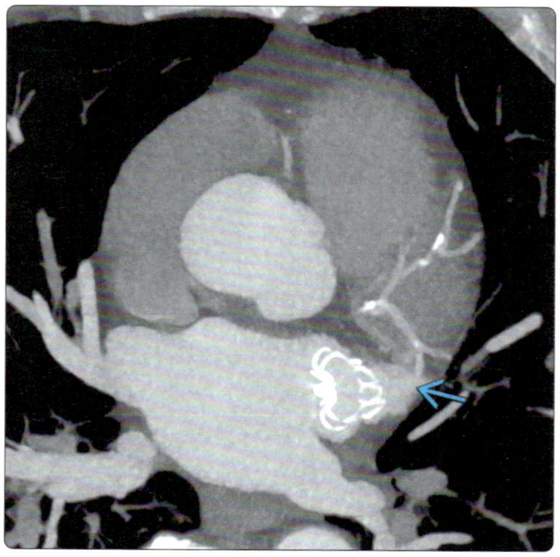

(Left) *Axial cardiac CT shows a parachute-like Watchman device securely positioned in the LAA, indicating successful endothelialization with no peridevice leak.* **(Right)** *Cardiac CTA shows free flow of contrast in the LLA* ➙ *beyond the Watchman device, consistent with the absence of neoendothelialization.*

Left Ventricular Assist Device

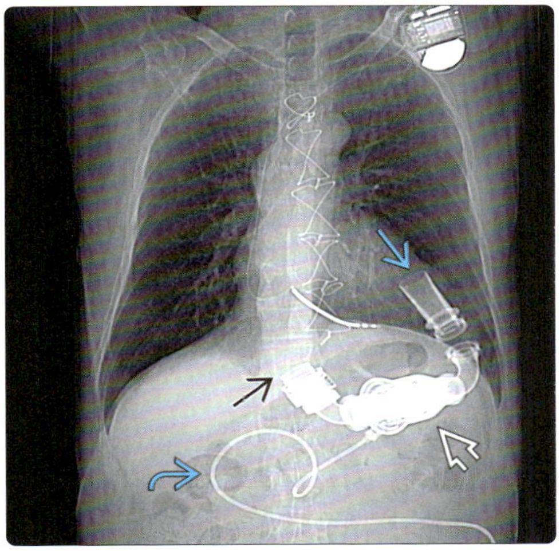

Left Ventricular Assist Device

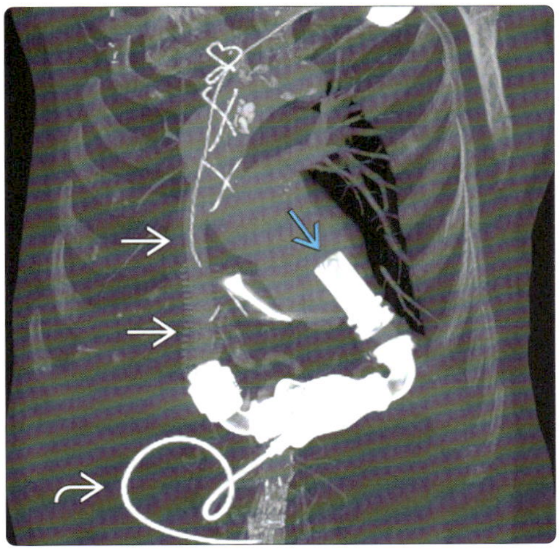

(Left) *Frontal chest radiograph shows a left ventricular assist device (LVAD) with an inflow cannula* ⇨ *in the LV, outflow cannula* ⇨ *connected to the ascending aorta, and a pump* ➡ *in the expected position with its driveline* ⇨ *extending to the abdominal wall.* **(Right)** *Coronal CTA shows a LVAD with an inflow cannula* ⇨ *drawing blood from the LV and pumping it through the outflow cannula via a graft* ➡ *into the ascending aorta. The driveline* ➡ *extends downward toward the abdominal wall.*

Impella Left Ventricular Assist Device

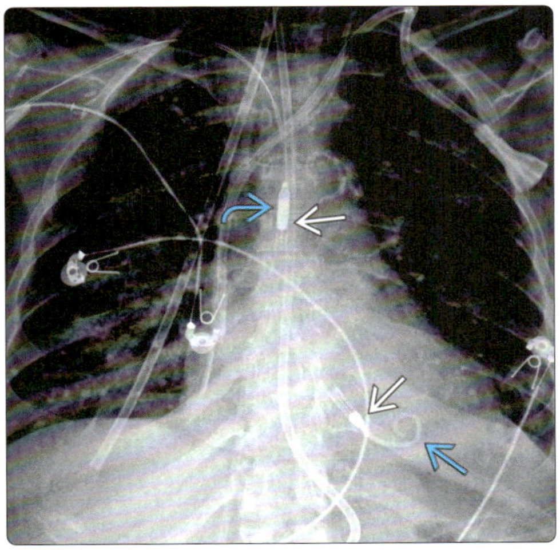

Impella Left Ventricular Assist Device

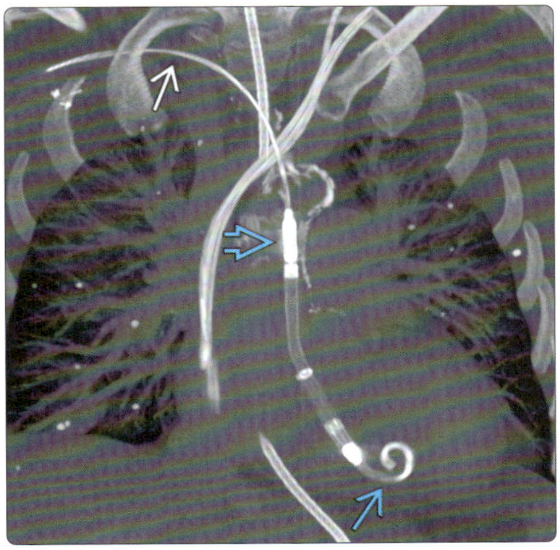

(Left) *Frontal chest x-ray shows a right axillary-approach percutaneous LVAD (Impella) in the appropriate position with an inlet pigtail* ⇨ *projecting over the LV apex and the outlet within the ascending aorta* ⇨*. The Impella housing is visible between the 2 radiodense ends of the device* ➡*.* **(Right)** *Coronal MIP CCTA shows an axillary-approach* ➡ *percutaneous Impella LVAD with the inlet and pigtail* ⇨ *extending over the LV apex and the outlet* ⇨ *located in the ascending aorta.*

Impella Left Ventricular Assist Device

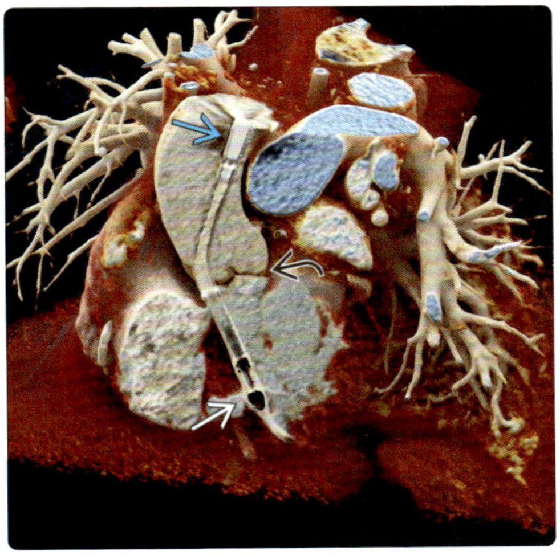

Left Ventricular Assist Device and Right Ventricular Assist Device

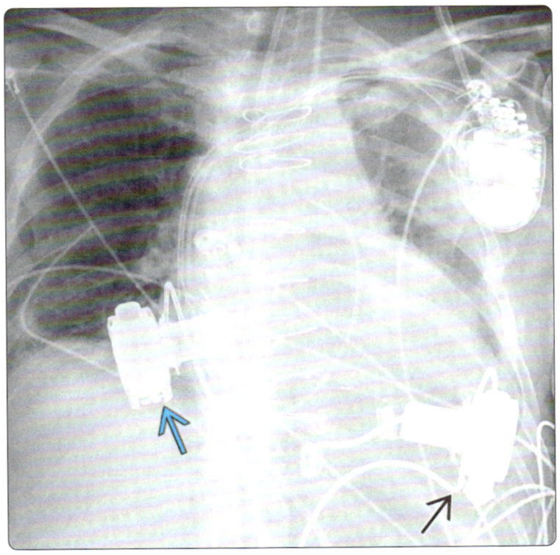

(Left) *Cinematic rendering coronal oblique view shows the relationship of the Impella inlet* ➡ *and outlet* ⇨ *to the aortic valve* ⇨*. The aortic valve should be between the inlet and outlet of the device.* **(Right)** *Frontal chest radiograph shows both a LVAD and a right ventricular assist device (RVAD)* ⇨ *with the LVAD* ⇨ *connecting the LV to the ascending aorta and the RVAD connecting the RV to the pulmonary artery. Drivelines tunnel through the abdominal wall before exiting subcostal skin and connecting to the controller unit.*

Intraaortic Balloon Pump Catheter

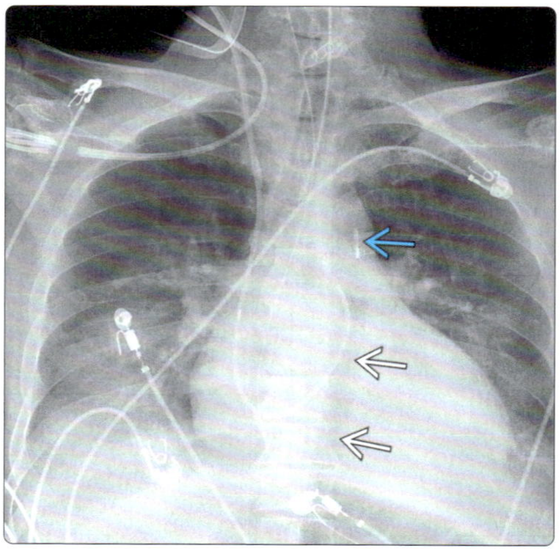

Intraaortic Balloon Pump Catheter

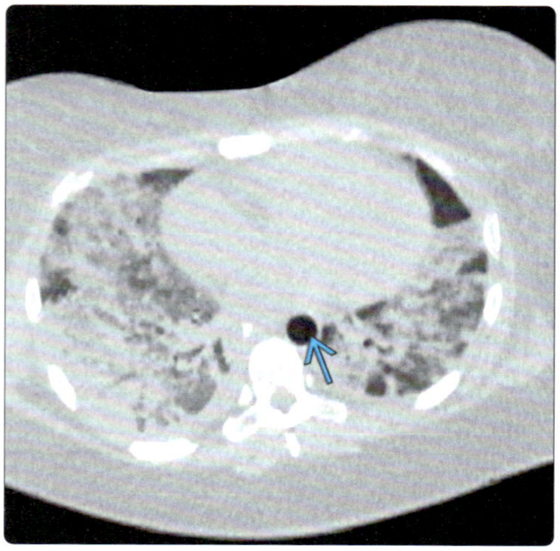

(Left) *Femoral-approach catheter with a cephalad tip ➞ marker is visible within the proximal descending aorta between the top of the aortic knob and the carina. Proper placement is important to prevent occlusion of branch arteries, such as the left subclavian artery. The lucency ➞ is due to helium currently within the balloon in diastole. The caudal marker (not shown) projects over superior margin of L2.* **(Right)** *CT shows a helium-inflated balloon ➞ in the descending thoracic aorta during diastole, which aids coronary perfusion.*

CardioMEMS

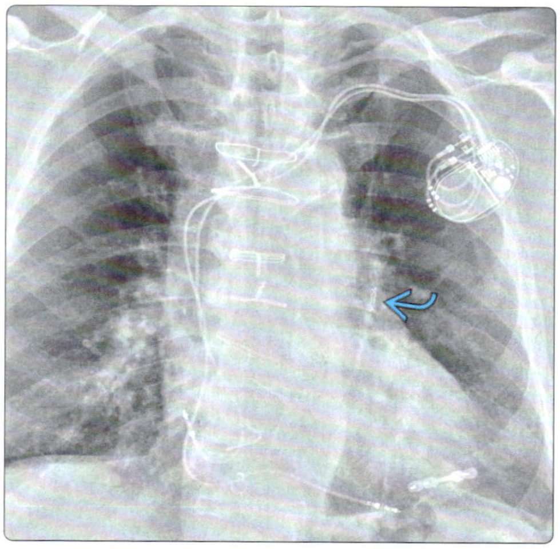

CardioMEMS

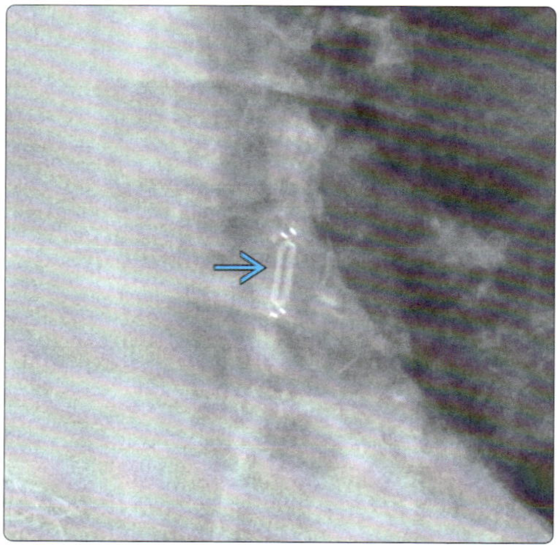

(Left) *Frontal chest radiograph shows a CardioMEMS device ➞ properly positioned in the left lower lobe pulmonary artery, appearing as a radiopaque structure within the vessel.* **(Right)** *Magnified view demonstrates the implantable CardioMEMS monitoring device ➞, characterized by its distinctive configuration (loops better appreciated on CT) positioned in the left lower pulmonary artery (as in this case) or potentially in the right lower pulmonary artery.*

CardioMEMS

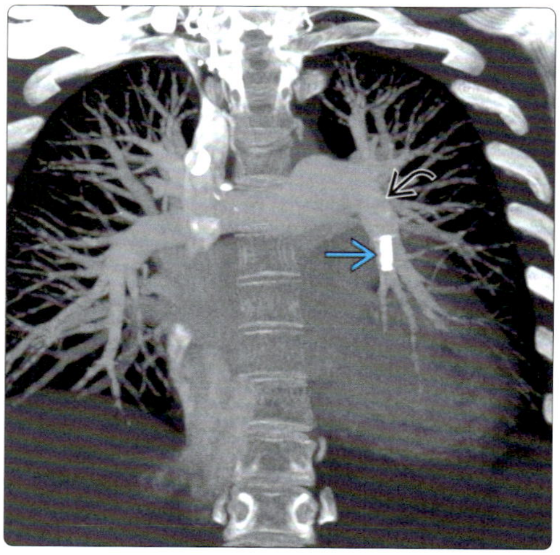

CardioMEMS

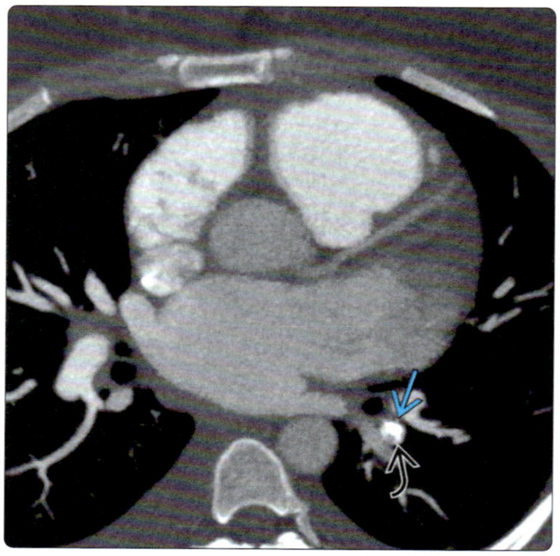

(Left) *Coronal MIP CTA demonstrates an appropriately positioned CardioMEMS device within the left lower lobe pulmonary artery ➞ without causing blood flow obstruction. Note the nitinol loops at each end of the device ➞.* **(Right)** *Axial cardiac CTA demonstrates the CardioMEMS device extending into a segmental left lower lobe pulmonary artery. Imaging confirms its secure position within the pulmonary artery ➞ with normal contrast flow ➞ beyond the device.*

Pacemaker Mimicker: Deep Brain Stimulator

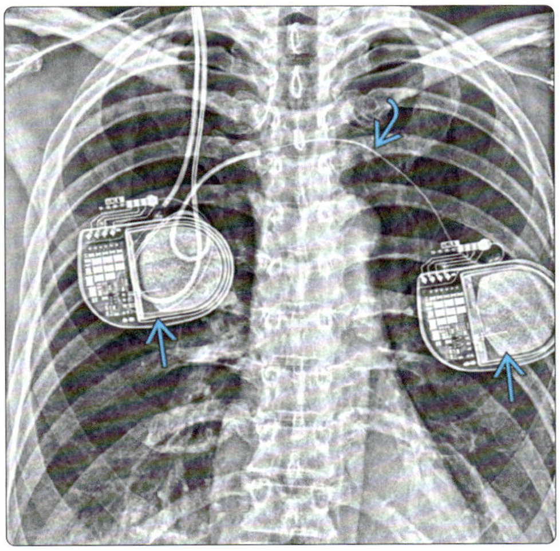

Pacemaker Mimicker: Deep Brain Stimulator

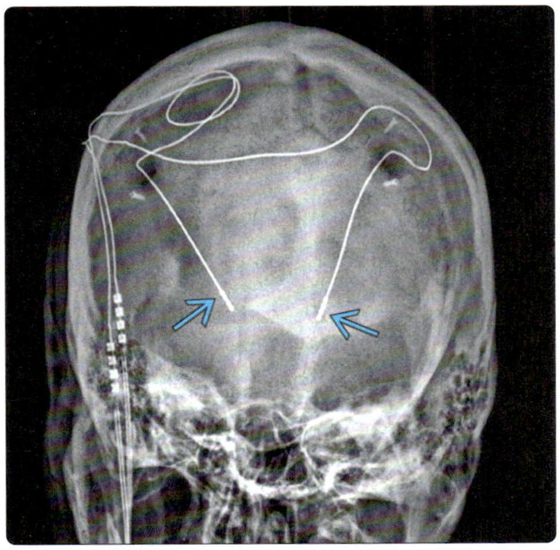

(Left) *Frontal chest x-ray shows bilateral deep brain stimulator pulse generators on the anterior chest wall with the left lead crossing the midline to join the right. Both leads ascend cephalad via deep brain stimulator lead tunneling.* **(Right)** *Skull x-ray shows bifrontal-approach leads terminating in the expected location of the subthalamic nuclei, consistent with deep brain stimulation for Parkinson disease.*

Hypoglossal Nerve Stimulator

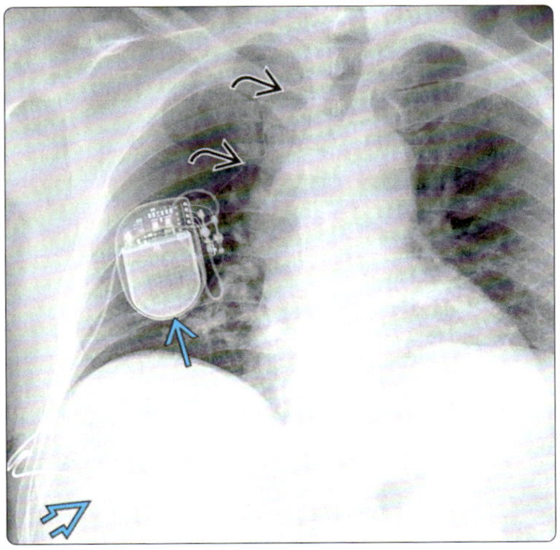

Hypoglossal Nerve Stimulator

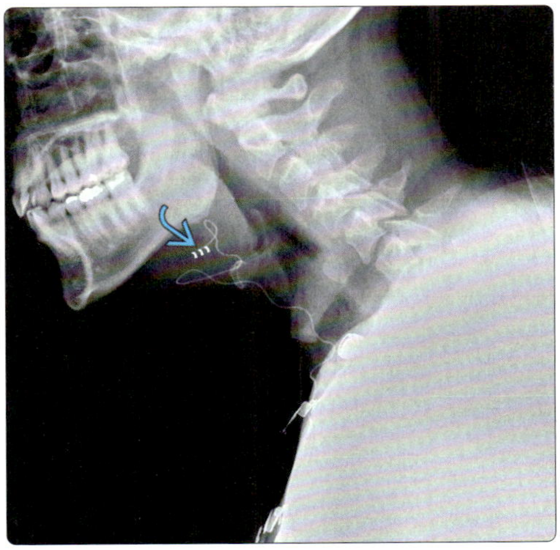

(Left) *Frontal chest and neck x-ray shows a hypoglossal nerve stimulator with the generator in the right anterior chest wall, a thin lead ascending into the neck, and a respiratory sensing lead within the intercostal muscles.* **(Right)** *Lateral neck x-ray shows the hypoglossal nerve stimulator lead tip tunneled to the submandibular region, wrapping around the hypoglossal nerve branches.*

Vagus Nerve Stimulator

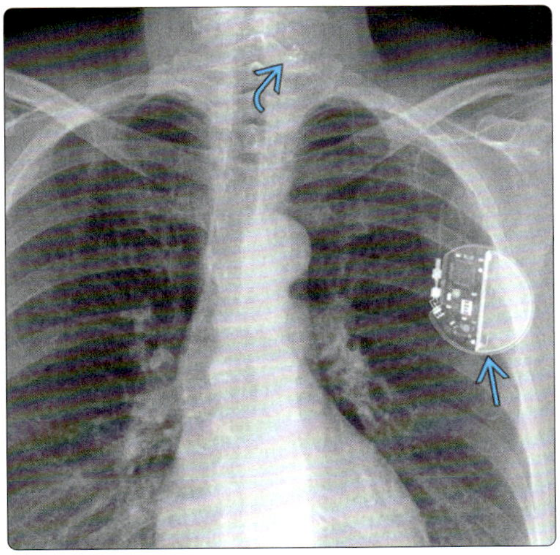

Pacemaker Mimicker: Vagus Nerve Stimulator

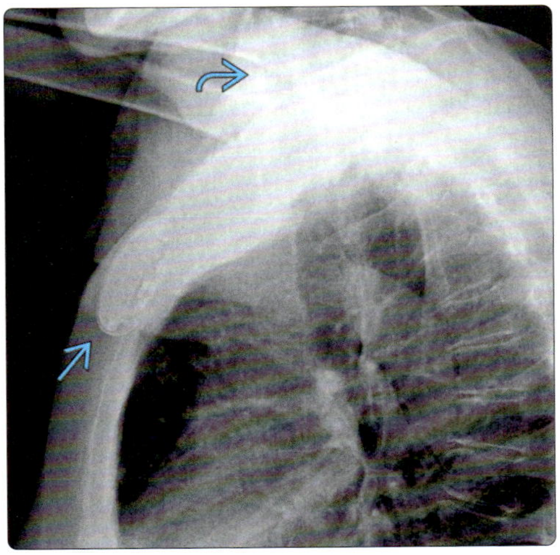

(Left) *Radiograph demonstrates a vagus nerve stimulator with the generator implanted in the left anterior chest and the lead coursing superiorly to wrap around the left vagus nerve in the neck (usually at the level of the carotid sheath).* **(Right)** *Lateral chest radiograph shows the subcutaneous vagus nerve stimulator with the lead ascending cranially to the level of the left carotid sheath to stimulate the vagus nerve.*

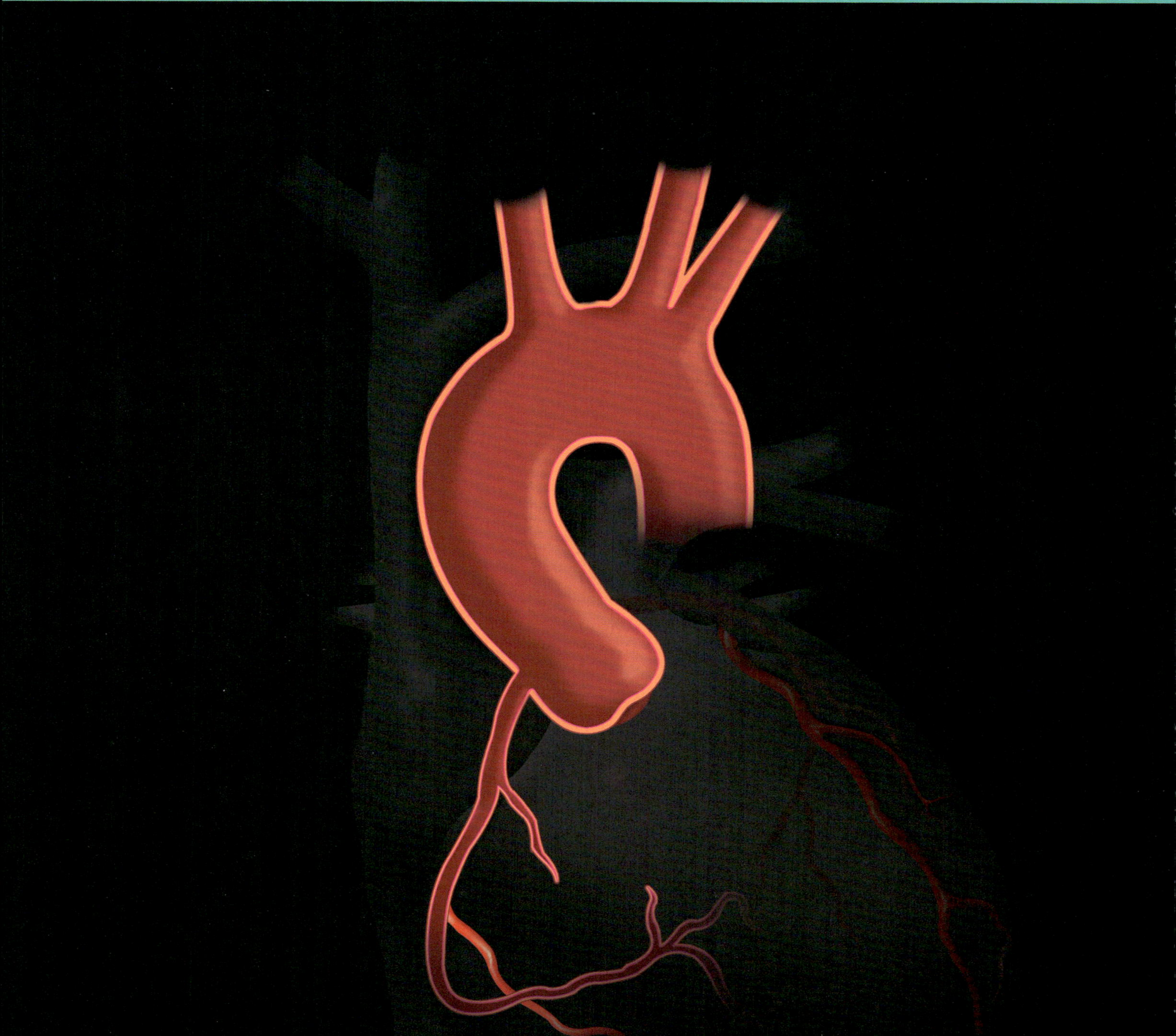

SECTION 9

Aorta

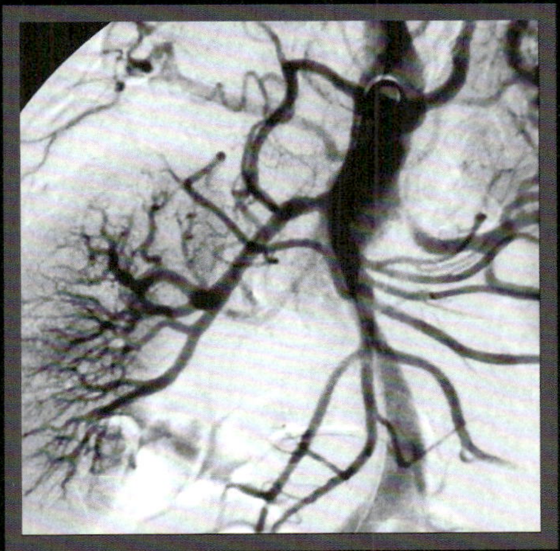

Introduction

The aorta develops as a culmination of embryologic steps based around 6 pharyngeal arches that develop and regress at varying times. Arches 1, 2, and 5 regress, while arch 3 gives rise to the carotids, arch 4 gives rise to the aortic arch (AA) and subclavian arteries (SCAs), and arch 6 gives rise to the pulmonary artery and left ligamentum arteriosus. The aorta has 3 layers, the intimate, media and adventitia, that allow the aorta to carry high volumes of blood while maintaining systemic pressure. The middle layer (media) has an inner layer of circumferentially oriented muscular fibers (inner 2/3) and outer layer of longitudinal fibers (outer 1/3). The net result is a potential natural cleavage plane within the media, which is affected in acute aortic syndrome (AAS). Genetic mutations tend to manifest in early adulthood with atypical presentations of ascending aortic aneurysms. The aorta can be affected by infection, inflammation, neoplasms, or metabolic disorders.

Radiography may incidentally detect an aortic abnormality but is rarely used for 1st-line imaging for suspected aortic pathology. That role has been assumed by echocardiography in the asymptomatic patient due to wide availability and relatively lower cost than CT or MR. In symptomatic patients or patients with high risk for aortic disease, CT, MR, and echocardiography have been shown to be nearly equal in sensitivity and detection of disease, especially AAS. In many emergency departments, CT has gained in popularity owing to its proximity to the department and speed of image acquisition. CT is also very easily understood by all members of the care team. Increasingly, PET/CT is being used for problem solving with an abnormal aortic finding, such as a potential thrombus vs. tumor, or vasculitis vs. atypical atherosclerosis.

Imaging Approach

The aorta is divided into 5 distinct segments: The root, which extends from the aortic anulus to the sinotubular junction; the tubular ascending aorta, which extends from the sinotubular junction to the takeoff of the right brachiocephalic artery; the arch, which extends from the takeoff of the right brachiocephalic artery to the left SCA; the descending thoracic aorta, which extends from the left SCA to the diaphragm; and the abdominal aorta, which extends from the diaphragm to the aortic bifurcation. Normal sizes are different for each segment and vary with the body habitus of the patient. In children, measurements are usually obtained by echocardiogram and compared to the body surface area to obtain a population-derived Z-score. In adults, measurements also tend to vary by sex and body surface area. In normal patients without cardiovascular disease, the mean size of the aorta at the sinuses of Valsalva and ascending aorta is ~ 3 cm, but should not exceed 4 cm or fall below 2 cm. The isthmus and descending aorta tend to be closer to 2.5 cm and should not exceed 3.2 cm or fall below 1.8 cm. Measurements should be performed orthogonal to the long axis of the vessel (not on transverse images alone).

Isolated ascending aortic enlargement is unusual in hypertension alone and tends to be indicative of other conditions, most notably bicuspid aortopathy, Marfan syndrome, Loeys-Dietz syndrome, inherited aortopathies, conotruncal abnormalities, and large vessel vasculitis. Atherosclerosis-related aneurysms tend to be fusiform. A saccular outpouching should invoke consideration of a pseudoaneurysm, which may be the sequela of prior trauma, infection, or penetrating atherosclerotic ulcer. However, at the level of the aortic isthmus ductus, aneurysms often have a saccular morphology.

AAS, including aortic dissections, intramural hematomas (IMH), and penetrating atherosclerotic ulcers (PAU) occur within the media. Normally, the 3 layers of the aortic wall are seen as a thin structure (< 2 mm). Any aortic wall thickening must be critically assessed for the potential of AAS. These conditions tend to present with chest pain and can be lethal. The blood in the wall (especially with IMH and PAU) is high attenuating on NECT or high signal on black-blood MR. Blood within the wall should be eccentric and not involve all 360° of the aorta on a transverse plane. Aortic dissection represents the most common AAS. Imaging must focus on assessing extension of the flap and delineating between the true and false lumina. In the era of endovascular repair, the presence of fenestrations is also quite important.

Vasculitis, conversely, often presents with circumferential thickening of the aortic wall and may have concomitant soft tissue stranding and lymphadenopathy. FDG PET will show uptake in vasculitis, which may help distinguish vasculitis from AAS. MR may be useful as vasculitis will show high T2 signal and contrast enhancement, whereby AAS will not. Enhancement is often best appreciated on delayed (venous-phase) imaging post IV contrast. Occasionally, periaortitis can mimic vasculitis as periaortitis can also affect the perivascular soft tissues, while vasculitis is limited to the vascular wall. These conditions, including IgG4 and Erdheim-Chester disease, often involve other organs, which can help suggest the diagnosis. However, in cases where they are confined to the vascular wall, they may be indistinguishable from vasculitis. On MR, a fat plane between the thickening and aorta may be seen. Fat surrounding the aorta should be seen as homogeneously low attenuating or uniform in signal intensity. When effaced, stranding may be indicative of a ruptured aneurysm, infection, or traumatic injury. Adjacent processes may also result in periaortic fat effacement, but any stranding should prompt a 2nd look at the aorta.

The most common aortic mass is an intraluminal thrombus. Increasingly, the thoracic aortic mobile thrombus (TAMT) is being recognized as an embolic source in patients without any predisposing condition. These lesions are often seen near the isthmus. Although the etiology of the TAMT is unknown, some authors have postulated that they come from developmental scars related to ductal resorption. TAMTs should not enhance. An aortic mass that enhances should raise suspicion for neoplasm. Aortic neoplasms are unusual. Most often, they are metastases from a lung or breast adenocarcinoma. Primary aortic intimal sarcomas are very rare and have the appearance of a focal intraluminal polyploid mass with aortic wall thickening proximal and distal to the main component of the mass. Extraluminal extension and adjacent lymphadenopathy can be helpful in distinguishing neoplasm from TAMT.

Congenital aortic conditions can be symptomatic, especially when associated with a double AA or its variants. The double arch and its variants tend to present with respiratory syndromes from the vascular ring, especially when 1 part of the ring is atretic. The atretic cords cannot be visualized on CT or MR but can be inferred when there are signs of a vascular ring with compression on the trachea and esophagus. Another relatively common variant is the right AA. The 2 main variants include the right arch with mirror image branching and the right arch with an aberrant left SCA that passes posterior to the esophagus. The former tends to be seen with congenital heart disease and is not a vascular ring. The latter tends to be seen in isolation and is usually asymptomatic, except in a case of a large ductus diverticulum that can lead to focal compression. Both CT and MR are useful in delineation of these entities.

Acute aortic occlusion is rare but can be seen in hypercoagulable states with clot expanding and obstructing the aorta. More chronic occlusions (either congenital as in a coarctation or acquired from atherosclerosis) will manifest with narrowing and collateral vessel formation. On MR, velocity-encoded sequences can be used to estimate gradients of the stenosis based on using the peak velocity and a modified Bernoulli equation. Rare congenital lesions can result in unusual aortic locations, which may simulate a mass on physical examination (e.g., cervical arch) or on radiography (e.g., pseudocoarctation). Knowledge of these variants will help prevent needless work-up or, worse, biopsy.

CT is the preferred modality for imaging traumatic aortic injury, direct and indirect signs. Direct signs include flaps, contrast extravasation, eccentric filling defects, abrupt change of aortic caliber, and lobulated or saccular configuration. Effacement of the periaortic fat is the only indirect sign, and, when encountered in isolation, follow-up CT or MR is usually performed in 24-36 hours.

Conclusion

The aorta is a complex organ that represents the intersection of development, genetic make-up, physiologic forces, and aging. Diagnosis of aortic pathology rests on echocardiographic, CT, or MR findings. In the modern era, radiography and angiography are rarely used as 1st-line imaging.

Selected References

1. Isselbacher EM et al: 2022 ACC/AHA guideline for the diagnosis and management of aortic disease: a report of the American Heart Association/American College of Cardiology Joint Committee on Clinical Practice Guidelines. Circulation. 146(24):e334-482, 2022
2. Bhave NM et al: Multimodality imaging of thoracic aortic diseases in adults. JACC Cardiovasc Imaging. 11(6):902-19, 2018
3. Hanneman K et al: Congenital variants and anomalies of the aortic arch. Radiographics. 37(1):32-51, 2017
4. Raptis CA et al: Acute traumatic aortic injury: practical considerations for the diagnostic radiologist. J Thorac Imaging. 30(3):202-13, 2015

Intramural Hematoma

CT and PET in Large Vessel Vasculitis

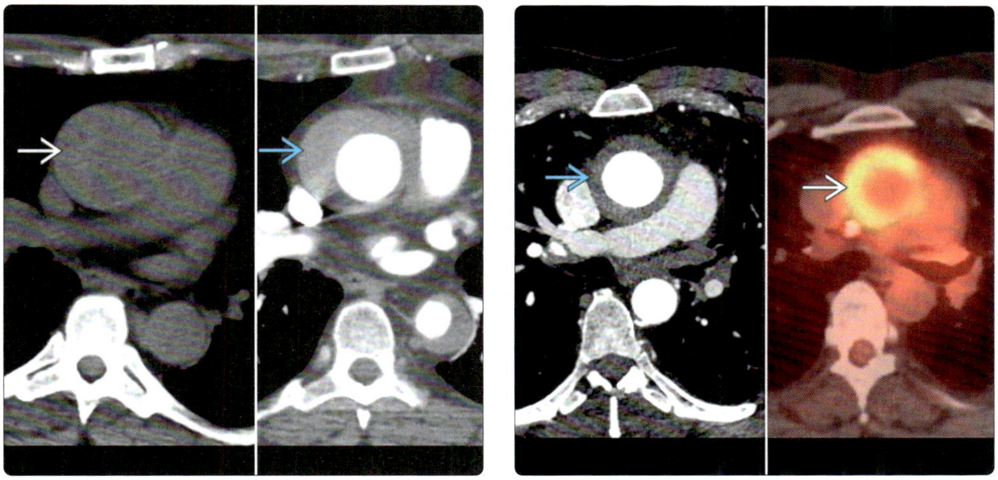

(Left) Axial NECT in a patient with pain shows subtle increased attenuation within the aortic wall ➡. CECT confirms an intramural hematoma ➡. The eccentric involvement helps distinguish from a vasculitis. **(Right)** *Axial CT shows circumferential wall thickening of the ascending aorta ➡. Although the wall thickening was hyperintense on NECT (not shown), the circumferential extent is atypical for acute aortic syndrome. PET shows avid uptake ➡ in the wall due to a large vessel vasculitis.*

Congenital Vascular Rings

Aortic Thrombus

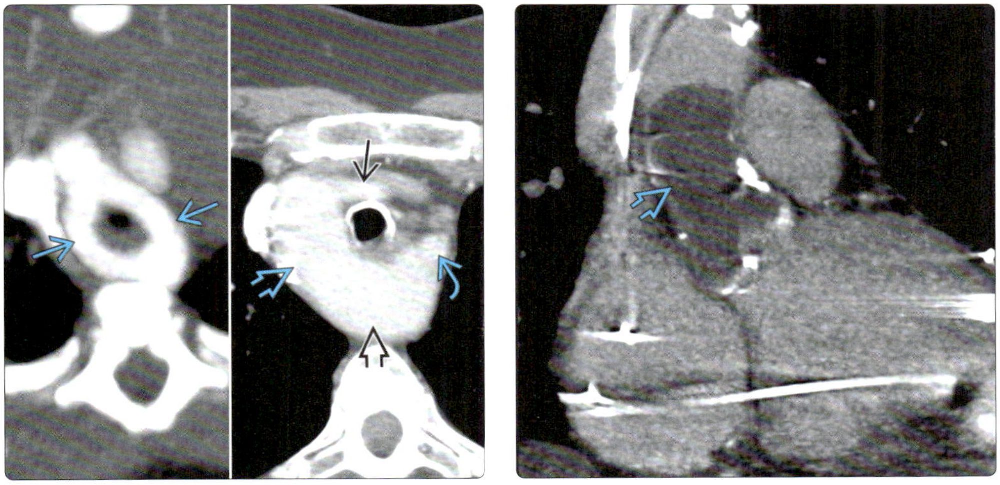

(Left) *4-mm MIP in a 2-day-old shows a double aortic arch ➡ surrounding a mildly narrowed esophagus. CT in a 68-year-old man shows a right aortic arch ➡. An aberrant left subclavian artery ➡ courses posterior to the esophagus with a 3.8-cm ductus diverticulum ➡. The left carotid courses anteriorly ➡.* **(Right)** *Coronal oblique CT in a woman with coronary bypass and ischemic cardiomyopathy shows thrombus filling the aortic root and ascending aorta ➡. This may have been related to coagulopathy and decreased cardiac output.*

TERMINOLOGY

Definitions

- Aortic root
  - Anulus to sinotubular junction (STJ)
- Ascending aorta (AsAo)
  - Extends up to origin of brachiocephalic trunk
- Aortic arch or transverse aorta
  - From brachiocephalic trunk to ligamentum arteriosum
  - Ligamentum arteriosum is remnant of ductus arteriosus and typically lies immediately distal to origin of left subclavian artery (SCA)
- Aortic isthmus
  - Segment of distal aortic arch between left subclavian origin and ligamentum arteriosum
- Descending thoracic aorta (DsAo)
  - Ligamentum arteriosum to diaphragmatic hiatus

IMAGING ANATOMY

Overview

- Thoracic aorta divided into 4 segments from proximal to distal
  - Aortic root
  - AsAo
  - Aortic arch
  - DsAo
- Aortic root extends from aortic anulus to STJ
  - Aortic anulus
    - Virtual ring at base of aortic root defined by lowest attachment point of aortic cusps; cusp attachment site has complex crown shape
    - Typically elliptical shape
    - Important for sizing of aortic valve replacement
  - Sinuses of Valsalva (SoVs)
    - 3 sinuses defined by coronary origins
    - Left coronary artery arises from left coronary sinus
    - Right coronary artery arises from right coronary sinus
    - Interatrial septum points toward noncoronary sinus, which is typically located posteriorly and to right on axial images
    - SoV typically greatest caliber segment of thoracic aorta
  - STJ
    - Anatomic landmark dividing aortic root from tubular AsAo
    - Narrower than SoVs
- AsAo extends from STJ to origin of brachiocephalic trunk
  - Typically greatest in diameter and nearly orthogonal to axial plane at right pulmonary artery level, which is convenient and standard level of measurement
- Aortic arch extends from brachiocephalic trunk to ligamentum arteriosum
  - Distal arch or aortic isthmus short (~ 2-cm) segment between left subclavian origin and remnant of ductus arteriosus
  - Aortic isthmus typically narrower than adjoining aortic segments
  - If ligamentum arteriosum cannot be identified, aortic arch can also be defined as extending past left subclavian origin
  - Ductus diverticulum (or "bump"): Focal, smooth bulge at site of obliterated ductus arteriosus along undersurface of isthmus
    - Normal variant that can be mistaken for traumatic aortic injury, which also occurs at this location
    - May become aneurysmal (> 3 cm)
- Aortic arch branch vessels to head, neck, upper extremities, and chest wall termed great vessels
  - Brachiocephalic trunk (innominate artery): 1st and largest of great vessels of aortic arch; divides into right common carotid artery (CCA) and SCA
    - Right SCA branches include right internal mammary, vertebral artery (VA), thyrocervical, costocervical, and long thoracic arteries, and it continues as axillary artery after margin of 1st rib
    - Right CCA divides into internal carotid artery (ICA) and external carotid artery (ECA) in neck
  - Left CCA is 2nd great vessel from arch
    - Divides into ICA and ECA
  - Left SCA is 3rd and final great vessel from arch
    - Gives off internal mammary, VA, thyrocervical, costocervical, and long thoracic arteries and continues as axillary artery
  - Rare (3%) thyroid ima or thyroidea ima with inferior thyroid artery arises directly from aortic arch or innominate artery as opposed to normal origin from thyrocervical trunk
- DsAo extends from distal arch to diaphragmatic hiatus, where it continues as abdominal aorta
  - Descending aorta typically smaller in caliber than AsAo
  - Aortic spindle: Bulge in proximal descending aorta just distal to isthmus
    - Commonly seen in children but can persist into adulthood
- Descending aorta gives off important small arteries
  - Bronchial arteries
  - Intercostal arteries
    - Supreme intercostals supply T1-T3; arise from costocervical trunk of SCAs
    - Paired intercostals arise directly from descending aorta from T4-T12
  - Thoracic spinal cord supply comes from DsAo
    - Anterior spinal artery supplied from intercostal and bronchial arteries at T4-T5
    - Artery of Adamkiewicz arises from intercostal arteries at T6-T12 (75%)
  - Esophageal, pericardial, superior phrenic, and other miscellaneous mediastinal branches
- Central venous anatomy
  - Jugular veins
    - Internal jugular veins drain head and neck; joined by external jugular veins draining face and scalp
  - Subclavian veins
    - Originate at axillary vein transition at 1st rib margin
    - Typically valveless; joined by cephalic vein
  - Brachiocephalic veins
    - Formed by junction of subclavian and internal jugular veins
    - Right: Short and vertical; left: Longer and crosses mediastinum anterior to great vessels

- Tributaries: Internal mammary, vertebral, pericardiophrenic, 1st intercostal, inferior thyroidal
- Superior vena cava (SVC)
  - Formed by right and left brachiocephalic veins
  - 6-8 cm long, up to 2 cm in diameter
  - Azygos vein joins above pericardium; SVC enters right atrium

Anatomy Relationships

- Aortic arch variants
  - Right aortic arch (< 0.1%); 2 types
    - Mirror-image branching (65%); associated with cyanotic congenital heart disease in 90%
    - Aberrant left SCA or other great vessel origin (35%); not associated with cyanotic congenital heart disease
    - Dilated origin of aberrant left SCA in 60%; Kommerell diverticulum; if also ligamentum arteriosum → vascular ring and tracheal compression
  - Double (duplicated) aortic arch (< 0.1%)
    - Arises from 3rd rather than 4th branchial arch
    - High location in chest, near lung apex
    - May have anomalous great vessel origins
  - Coarctation (< 0.1%)
    - Congenital narrowing of aortic arch, usually distal to left subclavian origin
    - May be preductal (infantile), juxtaductal, or post ductal (adult)
    - Common with other congenital aortic pathology, such as bicuspid aortic valve and Turner syndrome
- Great vessel origin variants
  - Bovine arch (20%): Left CCA may have common origin with or arise from innominate artery
  - 4-vessel arch (5%): Left VA may arise directly from aortic arch between left CCA and left SCA rather than from left SCA
  - Aberrant right SCA: Right SCA may arise separately from aortic arch, distal to left SCA
    - Diverticulum of Kommerell: Dilatation at origin of aberrant right SCA; can be associated with dysphagia (dysphagia lusoria) when large

ANATOMY IMAGING ISSUES

Imaging Recommendations

- Thoracic aorta imaged with catheter angiography, transthoracic or transesophageal echocardiography, and CT or MR angiography
- CT angiography: Protocol may include noncontrast, arterial, and delayed-phase imaging
  - Noncontrast images helpful in cases of extensive calcium, prior surgery, or suspicion for intramural hematoma
  - Delayed images better delineate mediastinal anatomy and are also helpful in postsurgical patients when concern for endoleak
  - Noncontrast and delayed images often not necessary for routine follow-up of known aortic aneurysm
  - Thin-section (≤ 1.25-mm) reconstruction preferred
  - ECG-gated or high-pitch dual-source CT preferred for accurate evaluation of aortic root due to cardiac motion artifact if root pathology suspected or followed
- MR angiography: Contrast angiography preferred
  - Noncontrast sequences often give diagnostic study and are test of choice when contraindication to iodinated and gadolinium contrast agent
- In general, for follow-up exams, best to employ consistent imaging modality and measurement technique
- "Candy cane" oblique view places thoracic aorta in profile and is commonly employed for catheter, CT, and MR angiography
- Aortic measurement should be performed in plane orthogonal to longitudinal axis of aorta
  - Measurements made in axial plane may be oblique to aorta and less accurate and reproducible

Transcatheter Aortic Valve Implantation/Replacement Assessment

- For severe aortic stenosis in nonsurgical patients
- Transfemoral or transapical approach may be chosen
- CT angiography plays increasing role in sizing of aortic anulus and determining suitability of iliofemoral approach
- Indications and criteria evolving
- PARTNER trial exclusion criteria
  - Native aortic anulus size < 18 mm or > 25 mm
  - Iliofemoral vessels too calcified or small to accommodate 22-Fr or 24-Fr introducer sheath (minimum luminal diameter of 7-8 mm, respectively)
  - Severe aortic or iliofemoral disease that would preclude safe placement, such as aneurysm, tortuosity, extensive atheroma, or dissection
  - Bulky, calcified aortic valve leaflets in close proximity to coronary ostia

SELECTED REFERENCES

1. Feldstein E et al: A novel variant of the aortic arch great vessels. Clin Neurol Neurosurg. 214:107172, 2022
2. Smith CR et al: Transcatheter versus surgical aortic-valve replacement in high-risk patients. N Engl J Med. 364(23):2187-98, 2011
3. Hiratzka LF et al: 2010 ACCF/AHA/AATS/ACR/ASA/SCA/SCAI/SIR/STS/SVM guidelines for the diagnosis and management of patients with thoracic aortic disease. Circulation. 121(13):e266-369, 2010. Erratum in: Circulation. 122(4):e410, 2010
4. Agarwal PP et al: Multidetector CT of thoracic aortic aneurysms. Radiographics. 29(2):537-52, 2009
5. Leipsic J et al: The evolving role of MDCT in transcatheter aortic valve replacement: a radiologists' perspective. AJR Am J Roentgenol. 193(3):W214-9, 2009
6. Davies M et al: Developmental abnormalities of the great vessels of the thorax and their embryological basis. Br J Radiol. 76(907):491-502, 2003

THORACIC AORTA AND GREAT VESSELS

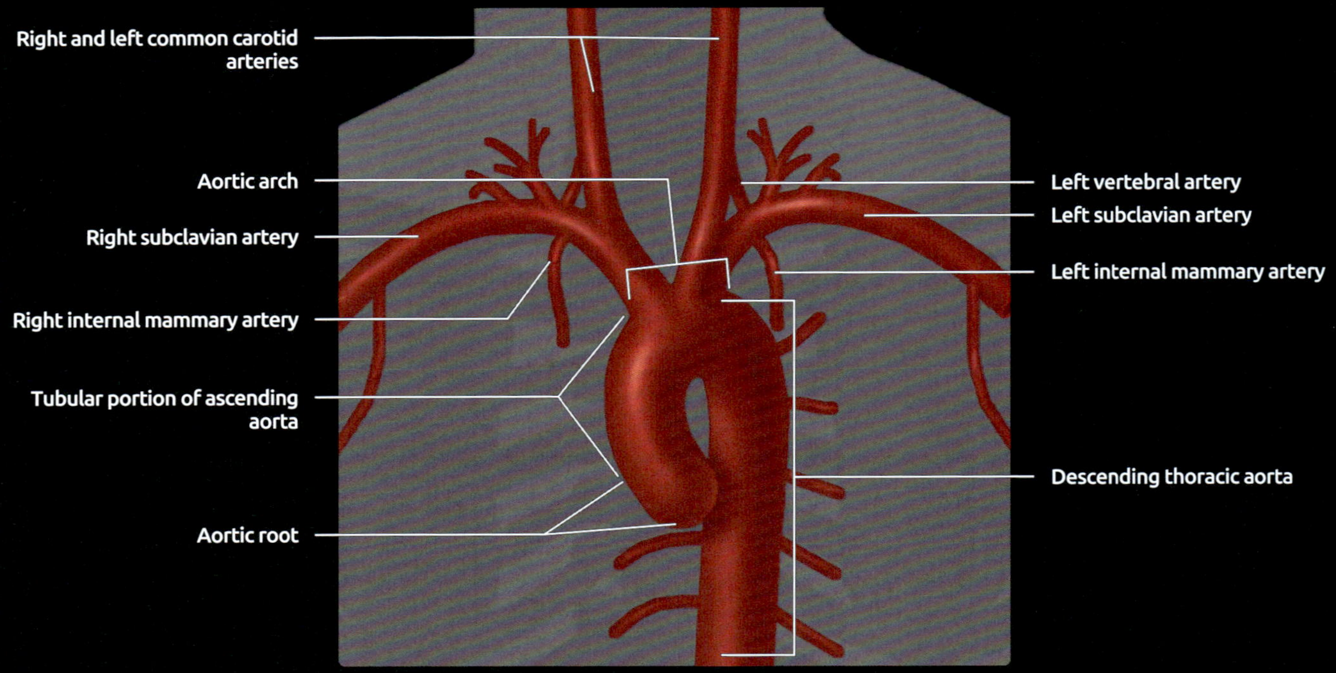

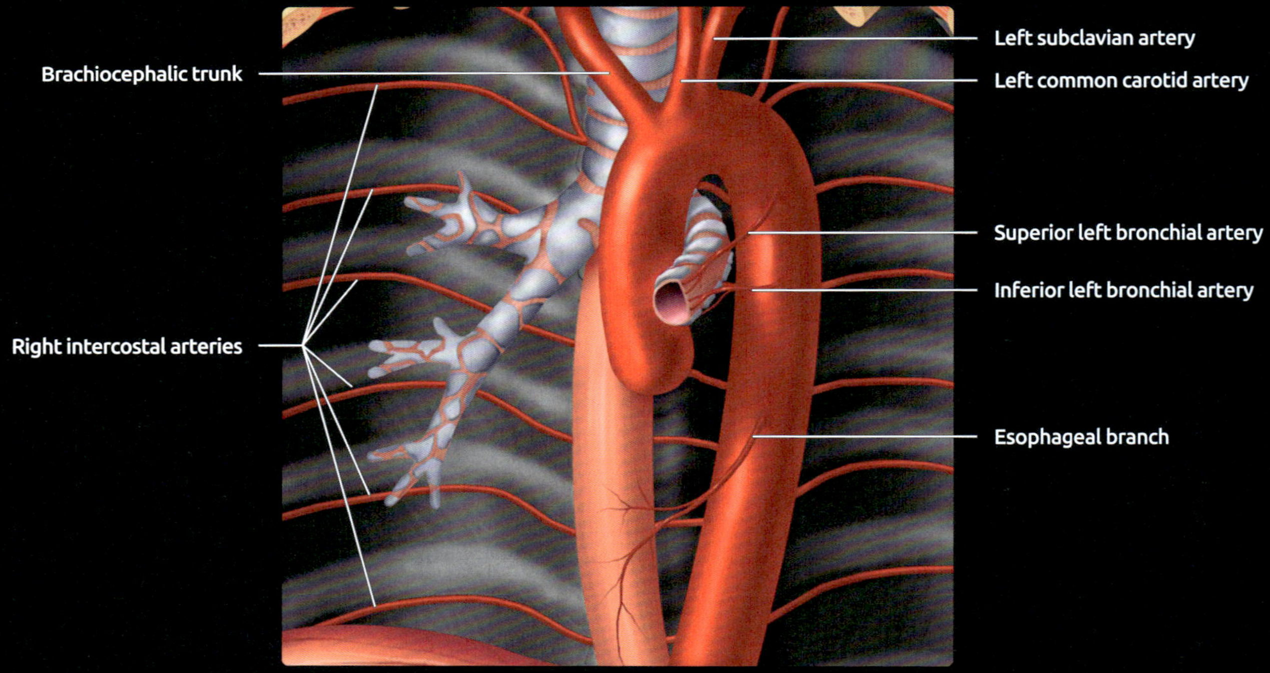

(Top) *Graphic depicts the thoracic aorta and great vessel origins.* **(Bottom)** *Graphic depicts the branches of the descending thoracic aorta, including the intercostal, esophageal, and bronchial arteries. Typically, there are both superior and inferior left bronchial arteries and a single right bronchial artery (not pictured). Note that the left mainstem bronchus is bent anterior to allow depiction of the bronchial arteries.*

NORMAL ANATOMY OF THORACIC AORTA AND GREAT VESSELS

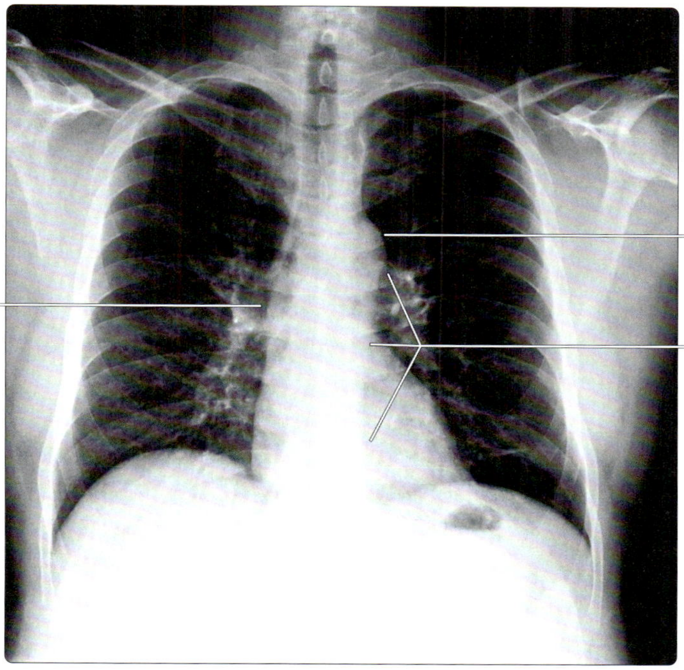

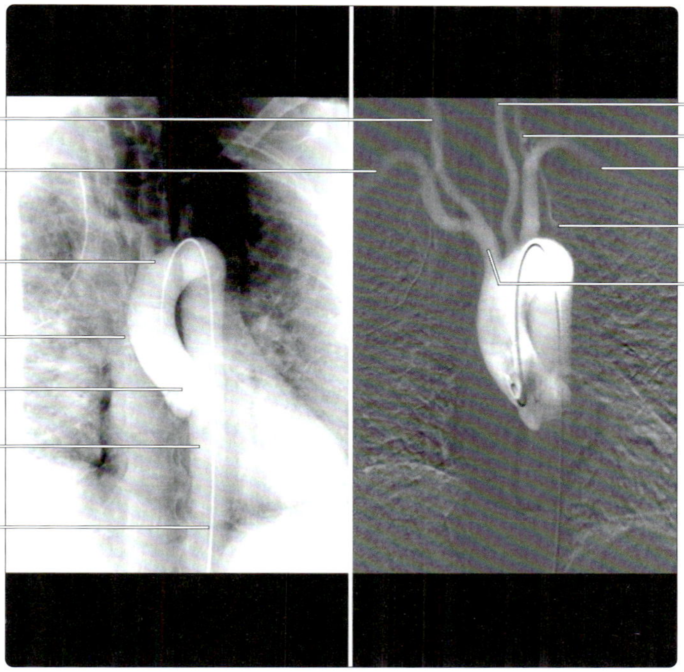

(Top) *Frontal chest radiograph shows a normal thoracic aorta. The aortic knob shadow is created by a superimposition of the aortic arch and proximal descending aorta. The lateral margin of the descending thoracic aorta should always be visible, but the medial margin is usually not perceptible. The lateral margin of the ascending aorta is visible as part of the right mediastinal border.* **(Bottom)** *Corresponding frontal projection of a catheter angiogram (left) and digital subtraction image (right) of the thoracic aorta illustrate normal anatomy of the aorta and great vessel origins.*

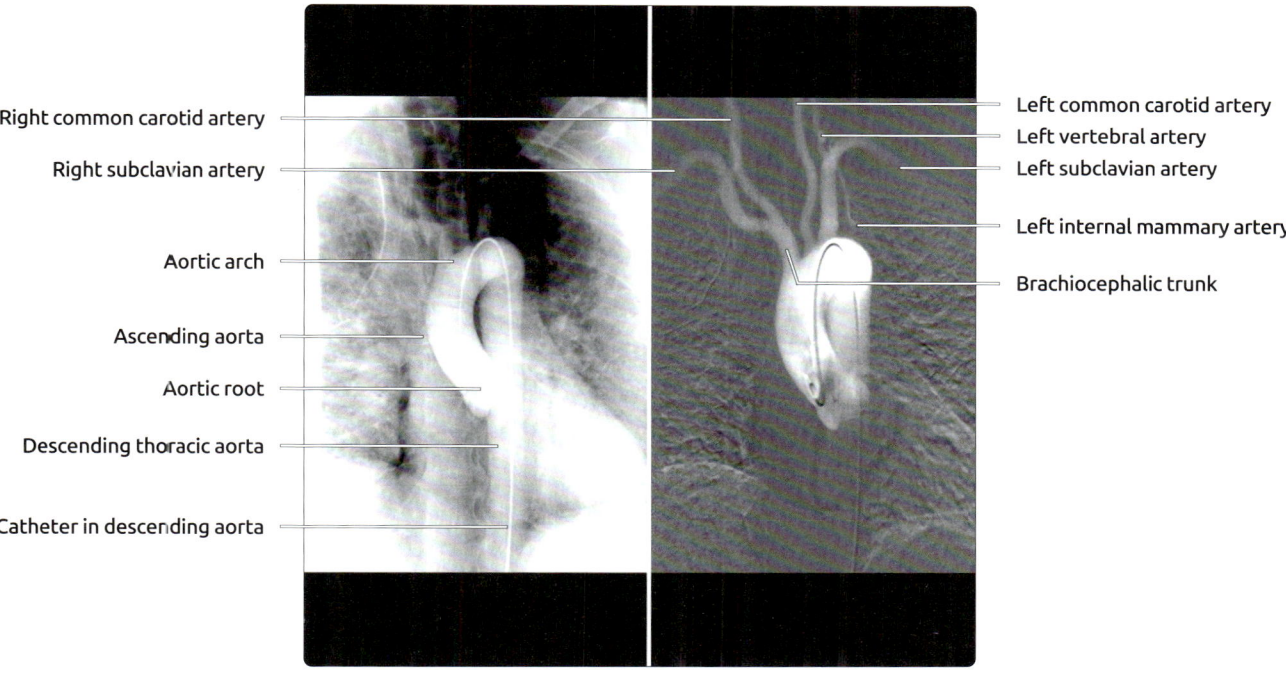

AORTIC ROOT CT ANATOMY

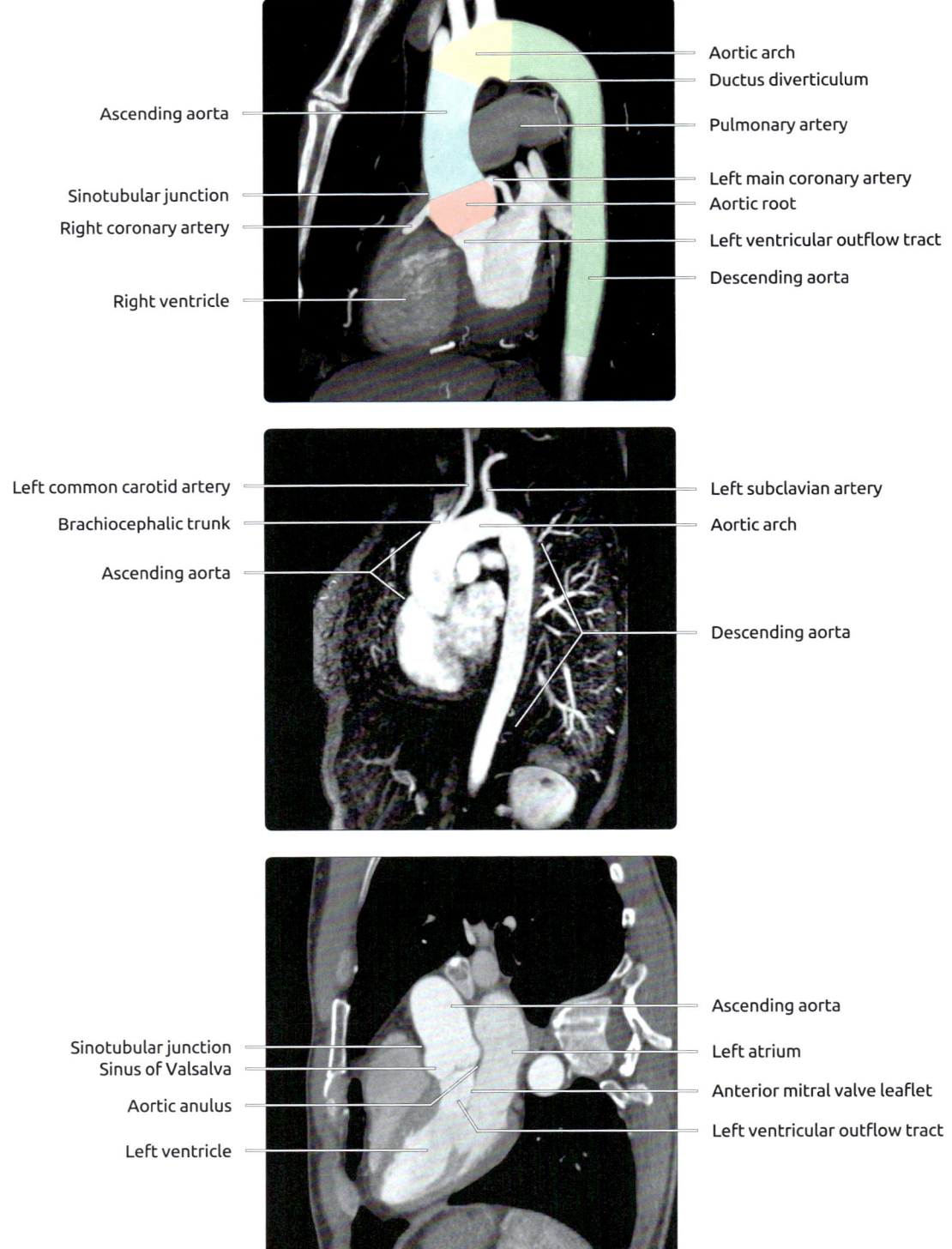

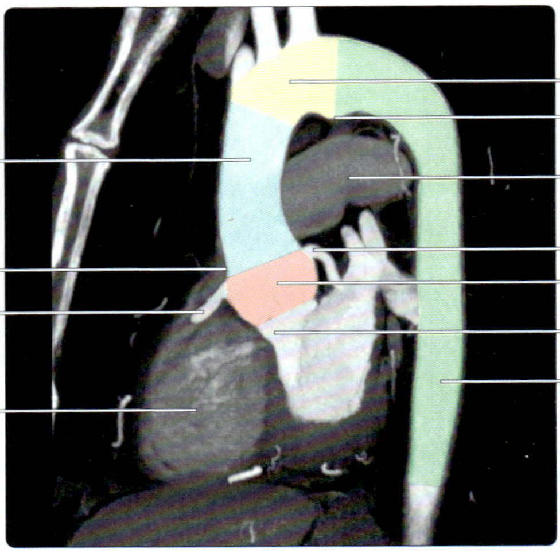

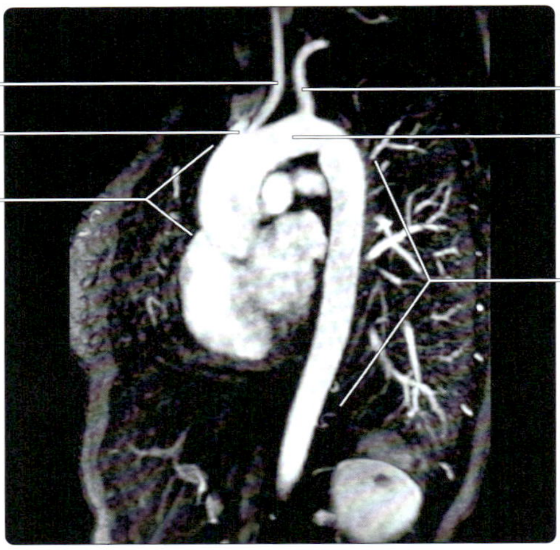

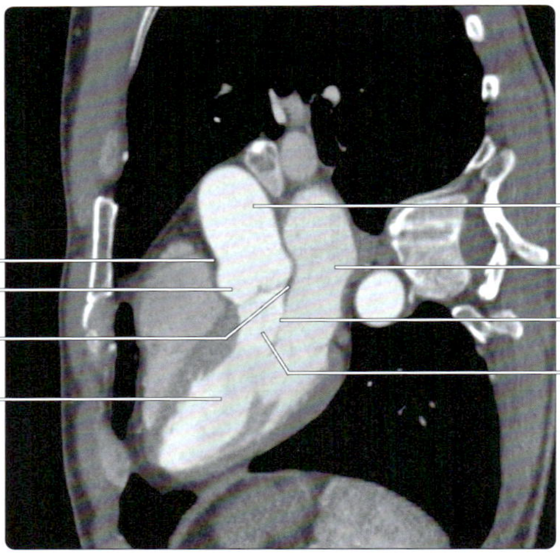

(Top) *"Candy cane" oblique MPR depicts the segments of the thoracic aorta. The aortic root (red) extends from the aortic anulus to the sinotubular junction. The ascending aorta (blue) extends to the origin of the brachiocephalic trunk. The aortic arch (yellow) extends to the ligamentum arteriosum. The descending thoracic aorta (green) extends to the diaphragmatic hiatus, where it continues as the abdominal aorta. Note the smooth outpouching along the inferior surface of the aortic arch at the remnant of the ductus arteriosum. This is a normal ductus diverticulum and should not be mistaken for a traumatic aortic injury.* **(Middle)** *"Candy cane" view of an MRA shows a thoracic aorta.* **(Bottom)** *Three-chamber view from a CT angiogram depicts the anatomy of the left ventricular outflow tract and aortic root.*

AORTIC ROOT CT ANATOMY

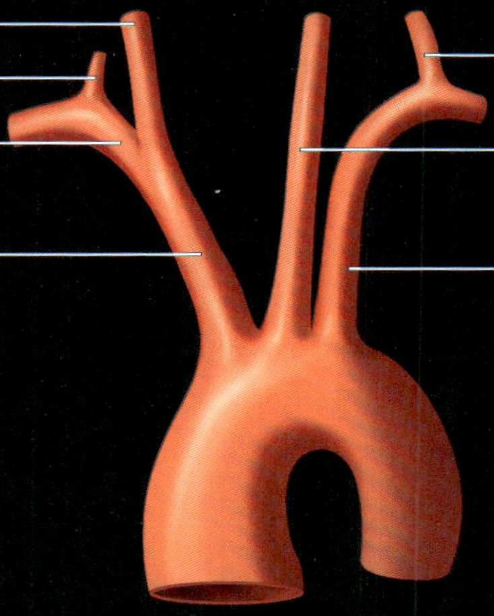

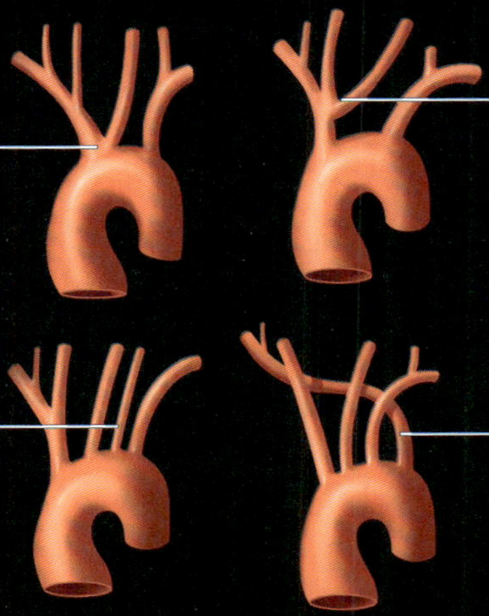

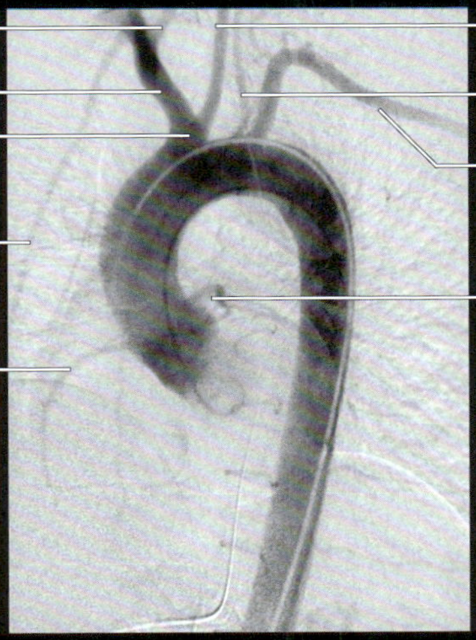

(Top) *Graphic depicts the most common configuration of the aortic arch, the 3-vessel arch.* **(Middle)** *Graphic depicts common aortic arch variants. In the most common variant (upper left), the brachiocephalic trunk and left common carotid artery share a common origin. In the 2nd most common variant (upper right), the left common carotid artery arises from the brachiocephalic trunk. The left vertebral artery may arise directly from the aortic arch (lower left), between the left common carotid and subclavian arteries. The aberrant right subclavian artery arises from the distal aortic arch after the takeoff of the left subclavian artery (lower right), courses behind the trachea and esophagus to the right, and therefore may cause dysphagia (termed dysphagia lusoria).* **(Bottom)** *Digital subtraction catheter angiogram in the "candy cane" oblique view demonstrates 2 common aortic arch variants: Common origin of the brachiocephalic trunk and left common carotid (bovine arch) and a left vertebral artery arising directly from the aortic arch.*

STANDARD MEASUREMENTS

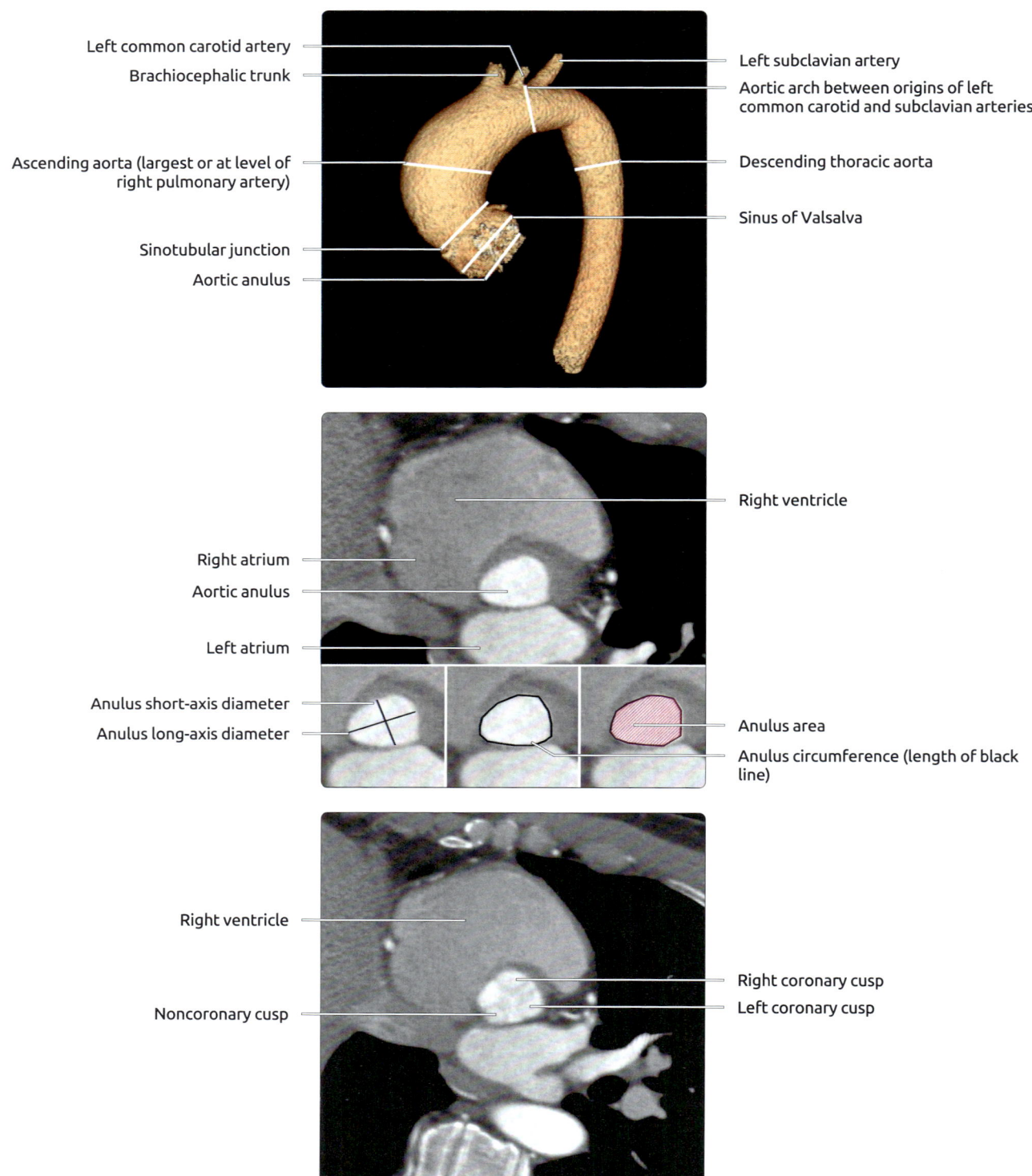

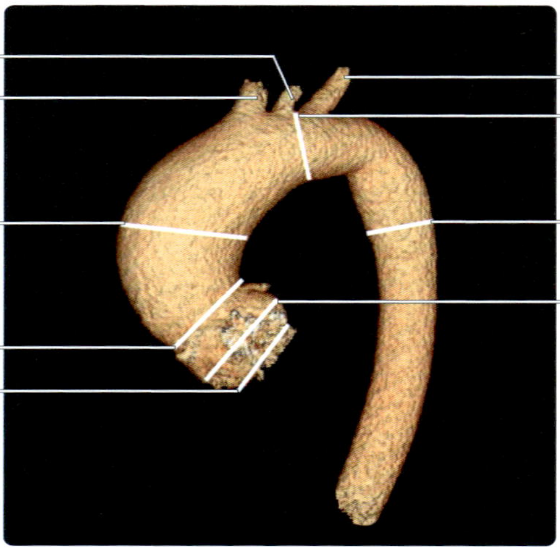

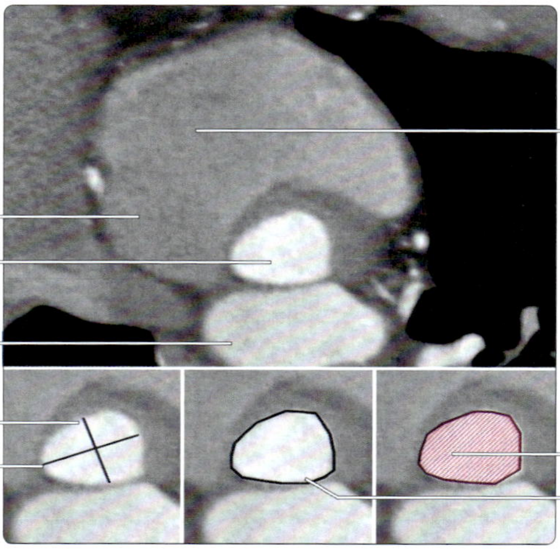

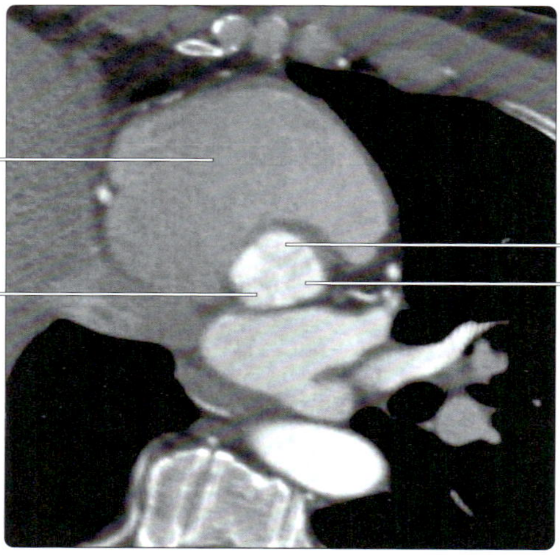

(Top) *Volume-rendered 3D CTA in "candy cane" view from a patient with a bicuspid aortic valve shows characteristic aneurysmal bowing of the ascending aorta. White lines denote standard aortic measurement planes, orthogonal to the long axis of the respective aortic segment. From proximal to distal, they include aortic anulus, sinus of Valsalva, sinotubular junction, ascending aorta at the level of the right pulmonary artery, aortic arch between the origins of the left subclavian and common carotid arteries, and the descending aorta.* **(Middle)** *Multiplanar reformation of the aortic anulus shows the typical ovoid shape of the anulus. Accurate measurement of the anulus is important for sizing aortic valve replacements. Long- and short-axis diameters are reported. Annular circumference and area may also be helpful.* **(Bottom)** *Image immediately above the aortic anulus depicts portions of the aortic valve cusps. The anulus is measured as a virtual ring defined by the attachment of the lowest points of each aortic cusp.*

AORTIC ROOT SHORT-AXIS PLANES

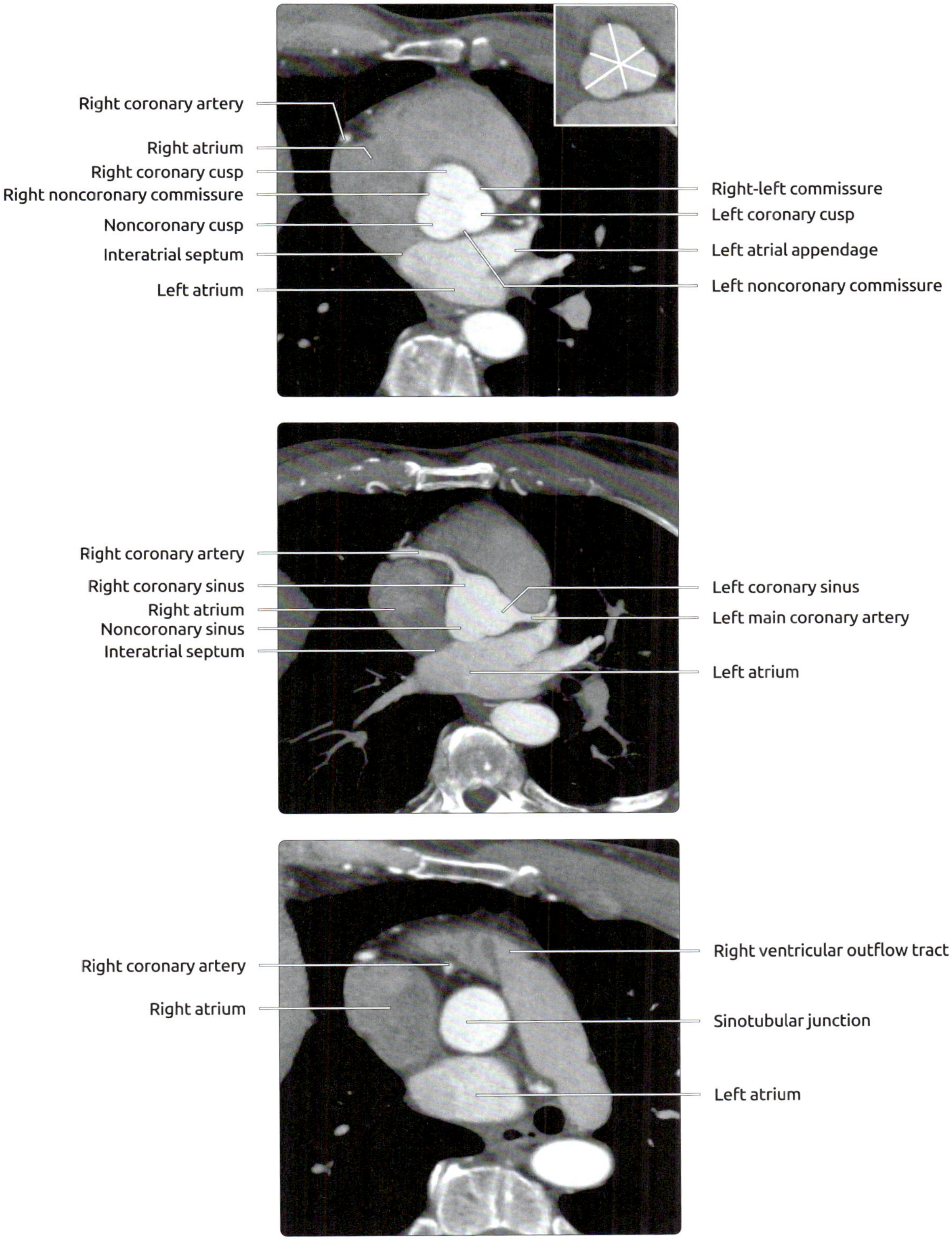

(Top) *Multiplanar reformat through the sinus of Valsalva is shown. The sinus of Valsalva diameters are measured from commissure to cusp. Note that the interatrial septum points toward the noncoronary cusp in all projections. Inset shows the 3 diameter measurements (commissure to contralateral sinus) obtained in this plane.* **(Middle)** *Oblique MIP through the sinus of Valsalva depicts the coronary origins.* **(Bottom)** *Oblique MPR, orthogonal to the aorta at the level of the sinotubular junction, shows that the sinotubular junction is of lower caliber than the sinus of Valsalva. Aortic diameters are most accurately and reproducibly measured in the plane orthogonal to the centerline of the aorta.*

STANDARD PLANES OF AORTA

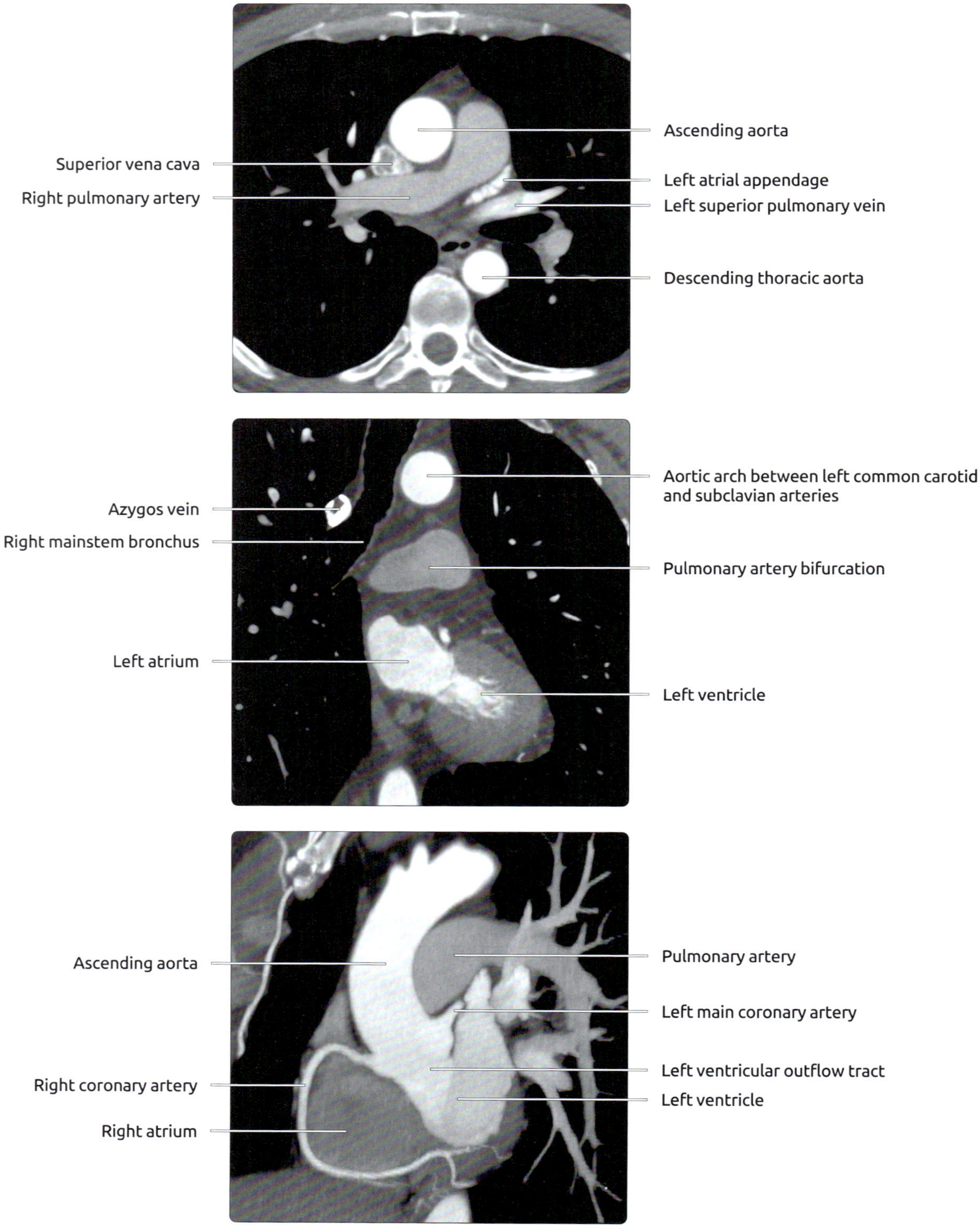

(Top) *Axial CT at the level of the right pulmonary artery shows the ascending and descending aorta. The ascending aorta is often greatest in diameter and nearly orthogonal to the axial plane at this level.* **(Middle)** *MPR orthogonal to the aortic long axis at the level of the aortic arch, between the origins of the left common carotid and left subclavian arteries, is the standard plane for aortic arch diameter measurement.* **(Bottom)** *Oblique MIP in C view depicts the course of the right coronary artery and the origins of the left and right coronary arteries from the sinus of Valsalva.*

TAVI/R PLANNING

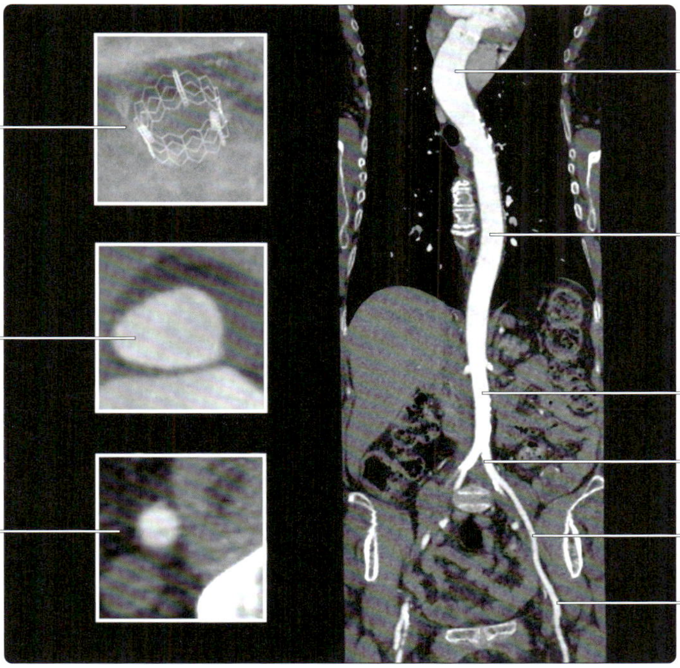

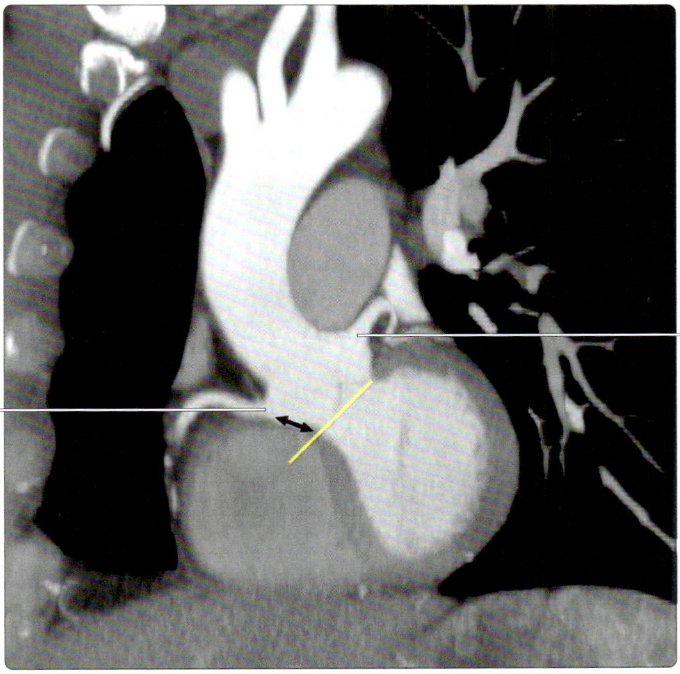

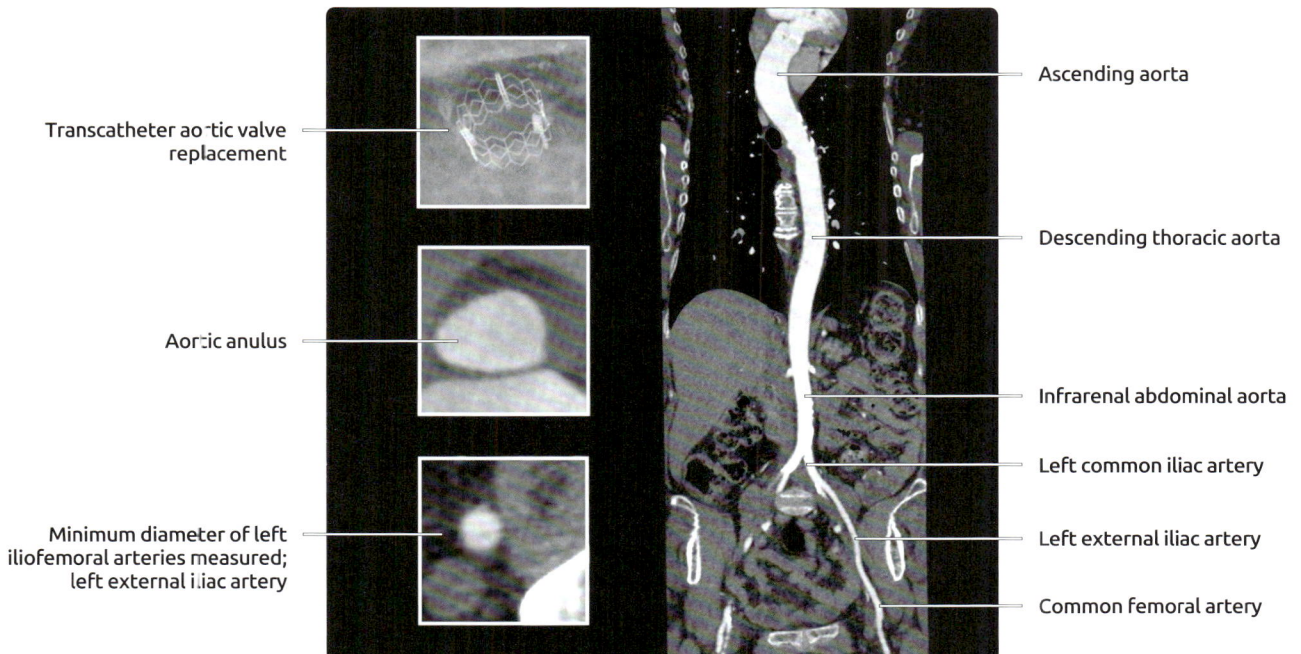

(Top) *Curved multiplanar reformation high-pitch gated CTA shows the entire aorta and left iliofemoral system (right). Coned-down lateral radiograph shows a transcatheter aortic valve replacement (TAVR) (upper left inset). CTA is increasingly used for TAVR planning. The dimensions of the aortic anulus (mid left inset) are critical for valve sizing. The minimum luminal diameter of the iliofemoral arteries (lower left inset) and the degree of tortuosity and calcification of the aorta and iliofemoral system (right) determine whether a transfemoral approach is possible.* **(Bottom)** *Oblique MIP depicts the coronary artery origins. Obstruction of the coronary ostia by displaced aortic valve leaflets is an infrequent but reported complication of TAVR, so the distance from the aortic anulus plane (yellow line) to the closest coronary ostium is provided. In this case, the distance to the right coronary ostium corresponds to the double-headed black arrow.*

Coarctation of Aorta

KEY FACTS

TERMINOLOGY

- Congenital narrowing of aorta, most commonly occurring just distal to left subclavian artery origin

IMAGING

- Chest radiograph: Inferior rib notching, figure 3 sign
- CTA: Focal, shelf-like narrowing of posterior/lateral aorta just distal to left subclavian origin
- MR
  - Contrast-enhanced 3D MR angiography (MRA) for vessel morphology and depiction of enlarged collateral arteries
  - Velocity-encoded cine is used to estimate pressure gradients and flow volumes
- Angiography
  - Morphology of coarctation and collateral vessels
  - Measurement of pressure gradients

TOP DIFFERENTIAL DIAGNOSES

- Pseudocoarctation
- Takayasu arteritis
- Interrupted aortic arch

PATHOLOGY

- Associations
  - Bicuspid aortic valve, ventricular septal defect, patent ductus arteriosus
  - Turner syndrome

CLINICAL ISSUES

- Surgical correction used for infants
- Balloon angioplasty used for children and adults
- Stent placement typically for recoarctation

DIAGNOSTIC CHECKLIST

- Search for subtle signs of coarctation in any young patient with hypertension

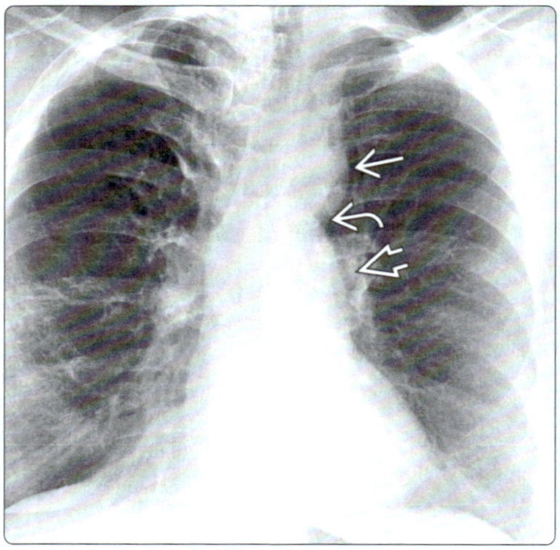

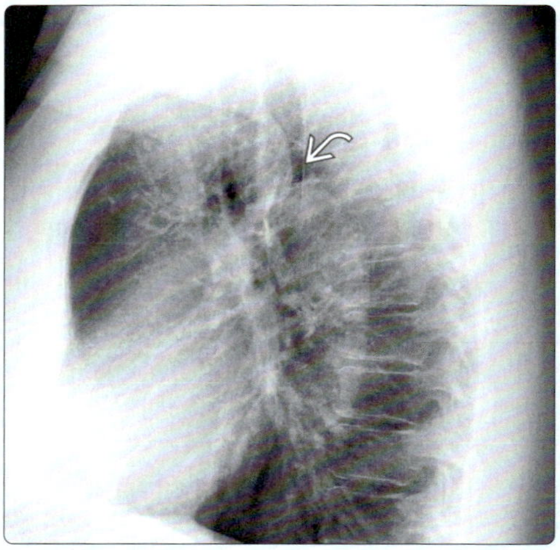

(Left) *PA radiograph of the chest demonstrates the classic figure 3 morphology in a patient with aortic coarctation. Note the area of stenosis, dilated subclavian artery, and poststenotic dilatation.* **(Right)** *Lateral radiograph of the chest in the same patient reveals an indentation along the aortic isthmus, representing the stenosis. While the figure 3 sign is not frequently seen, its presence suggests the diagnosis and should prompt additional evaluation.*

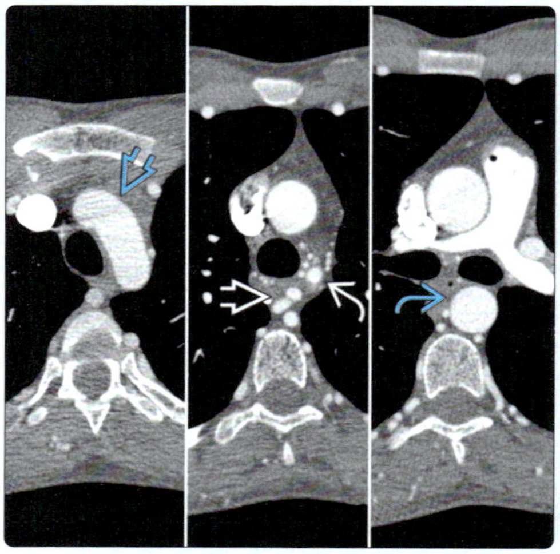

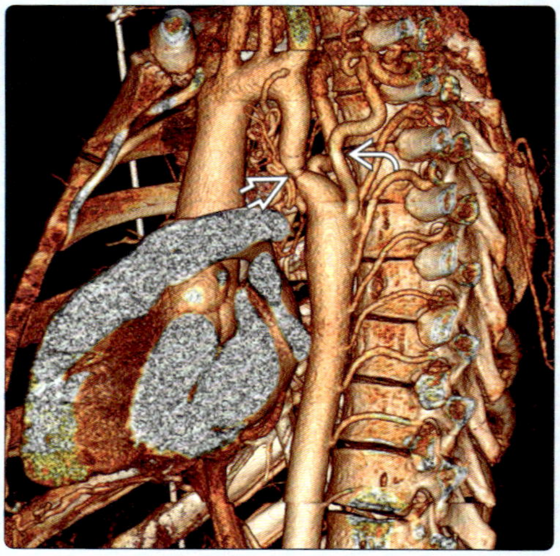

(Left) *Axial CTA of the aorta shows a classic coarctation. Note the relatively normal caliber of the aorta proximal and distal to the critical stenosis. There are extensive mediastinal collaterals seen as serpiginous vessels around the coarctation and dilated internal mammary arteries, which also reflect collateral flow.* **(Right)** *Oblique CTA 3D reformation in the same patient shows the coarctation. Note the intercostal arteries, which appear dilated due to collateralization.*

TERMINOLOGY

Definitions

- Congenital narrowing of aorta, most commonly occurring just distal to left subclavian artery origin

IMAGING

Radiographic Findings

- Radiography
  - **Inferior rib notching (Roesler sign)**
    - Related to enlargement of intercostal arteries serving as collaterals
    - Rare before 5 years of age
    - Affects ribs 3-8; ribs 1 and 2 are not affected, as they arise from costocervical trunk and do not anastomose with distal aorta
  - **Figure 3 sign in up to 50% of cases**
    - Dilated left subclavian artery produces proximal convexity
    - Indentation at coarctation
    - Poststenotic descending aorta produces distal convexity
  - **Ill-defined or obscured aortic arch**
  - Mediastinal widening

CT Findings

- CTA
  - Excellent morphologic characterization
    - Defines location and severity of stenosis
    - Focal, shelf-like narrowing of posterior/lateral aorta just distal to left subclavian origin
    - Enlarged collateral arteries indicate hemodynamic significant obstruction at coarctation site
  - Gradient cannot be calculated

MR Findings

- Allows morphologic and functional assessment
- Morphology
  - Achieved with several MR protocols: HASTE, SSFP (TrueFISP, FIESTA), contrast-enhanced MR angiography (MRA)
  - "Gothic" or angulated aortic morphology after coarctation surgery is associated with high risk of arterial hypertension
  - Useful to assess for complications: Aneurysm, pseudoaneurysm, recoarctation
  - **Contrast-enhanced MRA**
    - Planimetry: Determine orthogonal diameters and areas from proximal to distal to ductus
    - **Indexed minimal aortic cross-sectional area (cm^2/m^2)**
      - □ Best predictor of severity
      - □ < 0.33 cm^2/m^2 indicates severe coarctation (gradient ≥ 20 mmHg)
    - Demonstrates enlarged collateral arteries
- **Velocity-encoded cine MR**
  - **Heart rate-corrected deceleration time ($sec^{-0.5}$)**
    - Adjusted to heart rate
      - □ Deceleration time = [(flow at end of deceleration) - (peak systolic flow)]/(deceleration time)
    - Excellent predictor of severity
    - ≥ 0.30 $sec^{-0.5}$ indicates severe coarctation (gradient ≥ 20 mmHg)
  - Amount of collateral flow
    - Percentage increase in flow between aorta immediately distal to coarctation and just above diaphragmatic crura due to collateral flow
      - □ Normal subjects: 7% ± 6% decrease
      - □ Coarctation (gradient < 20 mmHg): No increase
      - □ Coarctation (gradient ≥ 20 mmHg): 83% ± 50% mean increase
  - May be used to quantify aortic valve stenosis and regurgitation
- **Combination of indexed minimal cross-sectional area and heart rate-corrected deceleration time best predicts hemodynamically significant coarctation**
- Cine MR
  - Gold standard to assess left ventricular hypertrophy (myocardial thickness and mass)
  - Enables characterization of bicuspid aortic valve
- 4D flow MR
  - Vortical flow pattern in regions of poststenotic dilatation

Angiographic Findings

- Vessel morphology and direct measurement of pressure gradient (ΔP)
  - < 20 mmHg: Mild coarctation
  - ≥ 20 mmHg: Suggests need for intervention

Imaging Recommendations

- Best imaging tool
  - MR and MRA often fully characterize and determine needs of treatment
  - Angiography remains gold standard; used when MR is inconclusive

DIFFERENTIAL DIAGNOSIS

Pseudocoarctation

- Older adult with elongation and kinking of aorta related to atherosclerosis
- No hemodynamically significant stenosis or collateral vessels

Takayasu Arteritis

- Inflammatory narrowing of unknown etiology
- Narrowing &/or occlusion of aorta and branch vessels, rarely isolated to aortic isthmus

Interrupted Aortic Arch

- Complete absence of continuity between 2 segments of aorta
- Nearly always manifests in neonates

Traumatic Pseudoaneurysm

- History of trauma, healed rib, and other skeletal fractures
- Narrowing of descending thoracic aorta may coexist with pseudoaneurysm

Inferior Rib Notching Differential

- Neurofibromatosis
- Venous collaterals (superior vena cava obstruction)
- Decreased pulmonary blood flow (tetralogy of Fallot, pulmonary atresia)

- Blalock-Taussig shunt (ribs 1 and 2)

PATHOLOGY

General Features

- Etiology
  - Muscular theory
    - Migration of tissue from ductus arteriosus into aortic wall and subsequent contraction
  - Hemodynamic theory
    - Decreased aortic blood flow during fetal development may not allow proper aortic growth
    - Increased incidence of coarctation in disorders in which left ventricular outflow tract obstruction reduces aortic blood flow
    - Decreased incidence of coarctation in disorders in which decreased ductal flow is present (e.g., tetralogy of Fallot)
- Associated abnormalities
  - **Bicuspid aortic valve (reported in 50-85%)**
  - Ventricular septal defect
  - Patent ductus arteriosus
  - Cerebral aneurysms (2.5-10.0%)
  - Variable evidence regarding increased risk of coronary artery disease

Staging, Grading, & Classification

- Classification (controversial)
  - Previously used classifications (e.g., infantile and adult type) discouraged due to overlapping manifestations
- Pathophysiologic classification
  - Preductal: Stenosis proximal to ductus arteriosus
  - Ductal: At insertion of ductus arteriosus
  - Post ductal: Stenosis distal to ductus arteriosus
- **Simple coarctation**
  - Occurs in isolation
- **Complex coarctation**
  - Occurs in presence of other intracardiac anomalies, thus, tends to manifest in infancy
  - Often preductal

Gross Pathologic & Surgical Features

- Obstructing membrane or ridge of tissue near aortic isthmus
- May develop cystic medial necrosis adjacent to coarctation site; predisposes to aneurysm or dissection

CLINICAL ISSUES

Presentation

- Most common signs/symptoms
  - **Neonates**
    - Asymptomatic if coarctation not severe or patent ductus arteriosus
    - If severe coarctation or closed ductus arteriosus, may have heart failure
    - Decreased femoral pulses, associated murmurs
  - **Children and adults**
    - May be asymptomatic
    - Leg claudication
    - Angina pectoris
    - Severe hypertension
- Other signs/symptoms
  - Turner syndrome: Short, webbed neck; broad chest; pigmented facial nevi; short 4th metacarpals

Demographics

- Sex
  - M:F = 2:1
- Ethnicity
  - White:Asian = 7:1
- Epidemiology
  - Incidence: 2-6 per 10,000 births
  - Comprises 5-10% of cases of congenital heart disease

Natural History & Prognosis

- Without repair
  - 75% mortality rate by age 46
- With repair
  - ~ 90% survival rate at 20 years; decreased chance of survival with increased age at repair
  - Recoarctation (2-14%)
  - Postoperative aneurysms (increased risk after patch aortoplasty)
  - Long-term survival rate decreased due to hypertension, coronary artery disease, dissection
- Pregnancy-related issues
  - Untreated coarctation: Increased risk of dissection and intracranial hemorrhage
  - Treated coarctation: Increased rate of miscarriage and preeclampsia

Treatment

- Indications for treatment
  - Infant with severe stenosis and heart failure
  - Longstanding hypertension
  - Hemodynamically significant stenosis (gradient > 20 mmHg)
  - Extensive collateral flow
  - Female patient planning pregnancy
- Surgical correction: 1st-line treatment for infants
- Balloon angioplasty
  - 1st-line treatment for older children and adults for native coarctation or recoarctation
- Stent placement

DIAGNOSTIC CHECKLIST

Consider

- Search for subtle signs of coarctation in any young patient with hypertension

Image Interpretation Pearls

- Enlarged collaterals imply significant stenosis

SELECTED REFERENCES

1. Chetan D et al: Challenges in diagnosis and management of coarctation of the aorta. Curr Opin Cardiol. 37(1):115-22, 2022
2. Saran N et al: Management of coarctation and aortic arch anomalies in the adult. Semin Thorac Cardiovasc Surg. 33(4):1061-8, 2021
3. Karaosmanoglu AD et al: CT and MRI of aortic coarctation: pre- and postsurgical findings. AJR Am J Roentgenol. 204(3):W224-33, 2015
4. Muzzarelli S et al: Prediction of hemodynamic severity of coarctation by magnetic resonance imaging. Am J Cardiol. 108(9):1335-40, 2011

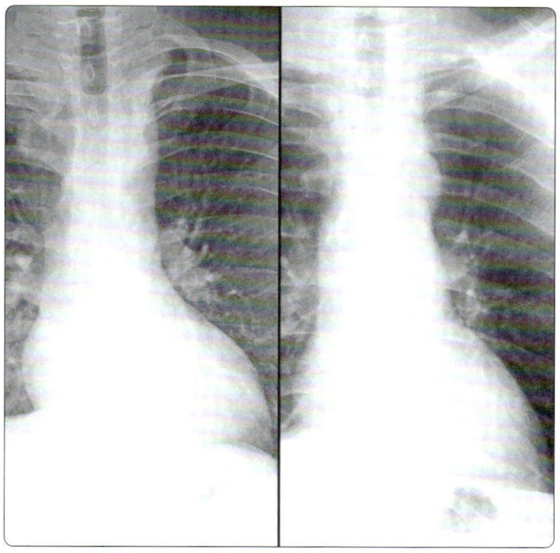

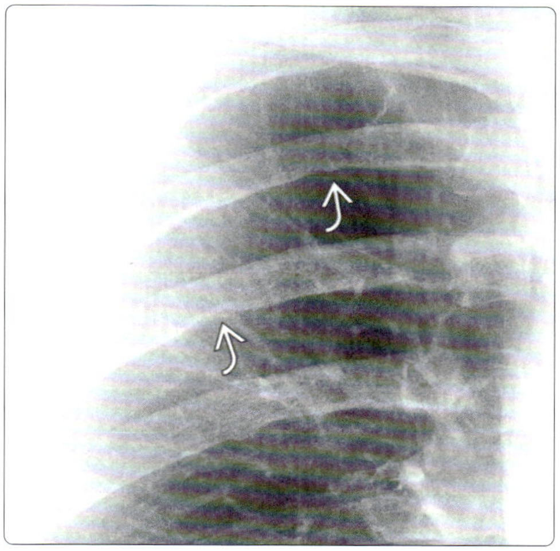

(Left) *PA chest radiographs in 2 different patients with aortic coarctation show an ill-defined mediastinal widening on the left and mediastinal contour abnormality on the right. Visualization of the classic figure 3 sign is often obscured by the presence of mediastinal collaterals.* **(Right)** *PA chest radiograph shows an inferior rib notching, the so-called Roesler sign, a classic radiographic sign of aortic coarctation produced by dilation of collateral vasculature. (Courtesy L. Heyneman, MD.)*

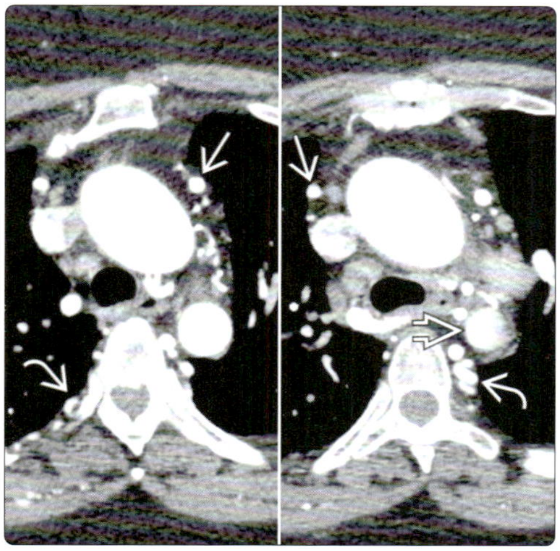

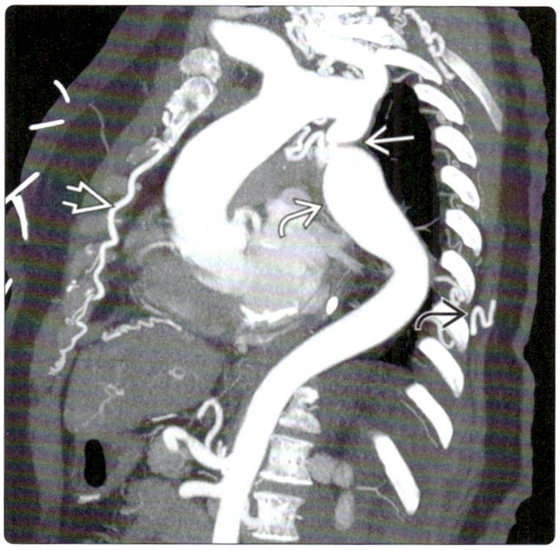

(Left) *Axial CTA images at the prestenotic level (left) and the coarctation site (right) show characteristic focal narrowing due to the coarctation and dilated internal mammary and intercostal arteries that serve as collateral pathways.* **(Right)** *Oblique CTA MIP reformation in the same patient better delineates the coarctation, poststenotic dilatation of the descending thoracic aorta, tortuous and dilated internal mammary artery, and intercostal collateral arteries.*

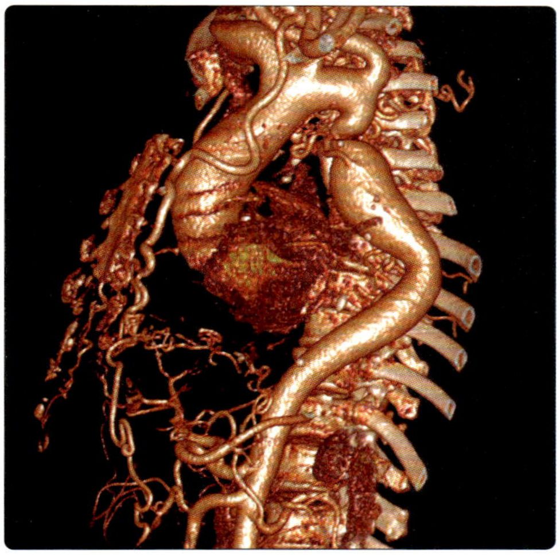

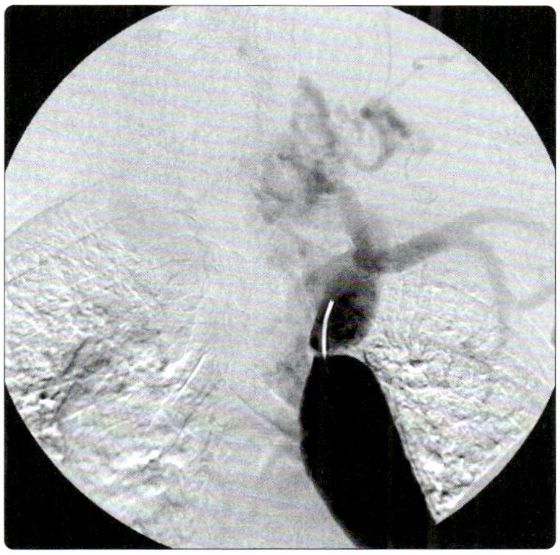

(Left) *Volume-rendered 3D CTA in a patient with aortic coarctation allows for morphologic assessment of the coarctation and provides an overall appreciation of the extent of collateralization. 3D reformations are most helpful for clinicians/surgeons to get the overall picture of the 3D configuration of the pathology.* **(Right)** *DSA in a patient undergoing angiography for subarachnoid hemorrhage shows the catheter tip proximal to an incidentally detected tight aortic coarctation.*

(Left) *Short-axis SSFP MR through the aortic valve shows a bicuspid aortic valve in a patient with aortic coarctation. Note that the aortic valve has only 2 cusps ➡. This is a common association in patients with aortic coarctation.* **(Right)** *Axial SSFP MR through the area of aortic coarctation shows an ascending aorta ➡ normal in diameter, a diminutive proximal descending aorta in the area of coarctation ➡, and a relatively normal diameter of the more distal descending aorta ➡.*

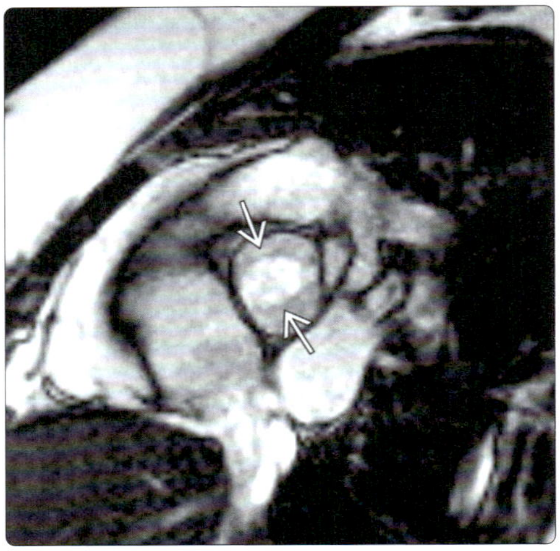

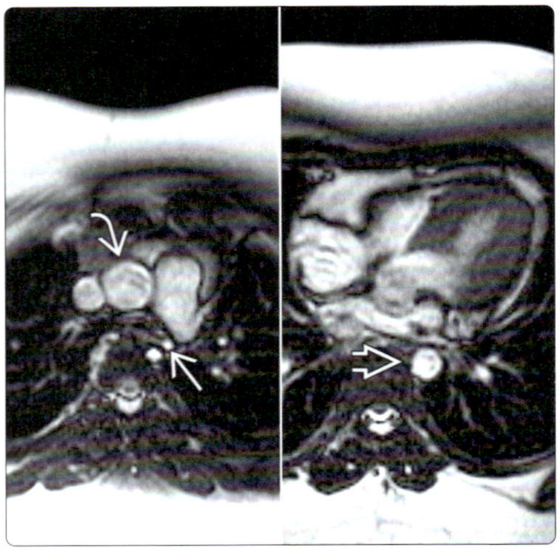

(Left) *Sagittal SSFP MR images in a patient with aortic coarctation show a well-defined long-segment area of stenosis in the proximal descending aorta ➡.* **(Right)** *Oblique aortic MRA MIP reformation in the same patient shows marked stenosis ➡ with extensive regional collaterals resulting from a hemodynamically significant obstruction. MRA is useful (as is CT) for determining the minimal aortic cross-sectional area and for evaluating the pressure gradients and flow volumes.*

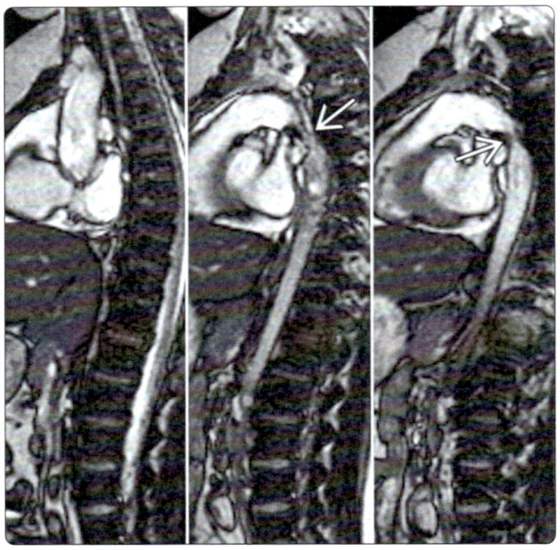

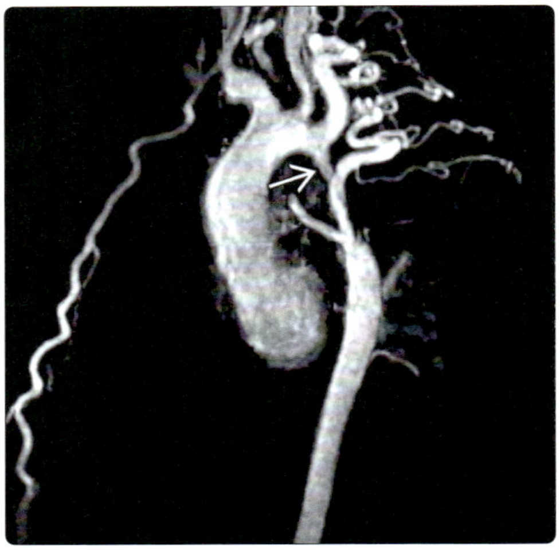

(Left) *Candy cane view from MRA of the thoracic aorta in a patient with repaired aortic coarctation shows mild residual narrowing ➡ at the aortic isthmus.* **(Right)** *4D-flow image of the same patient shows mild increased velocity ➡ at the repaired coarctation site, indicated in red. 4D flow images allow for quantification of flow at multiple levels, including valve levels, and also visually demonstrate flow patterns.*

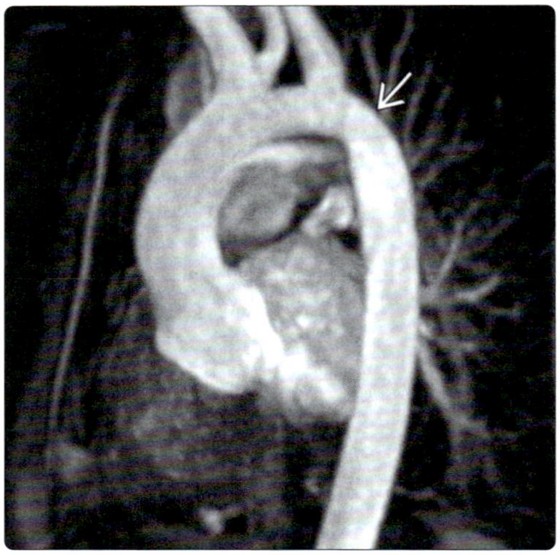

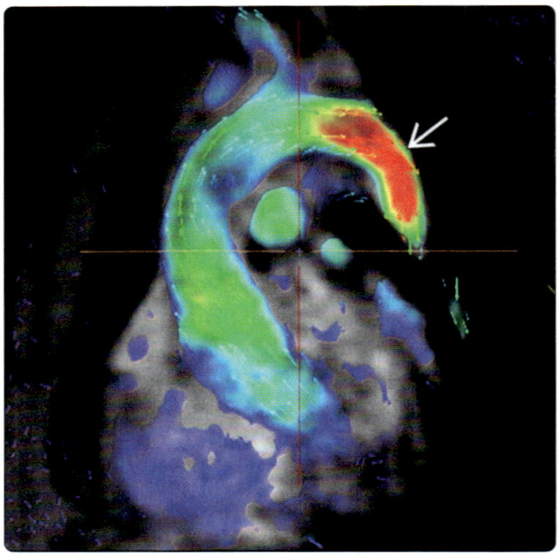

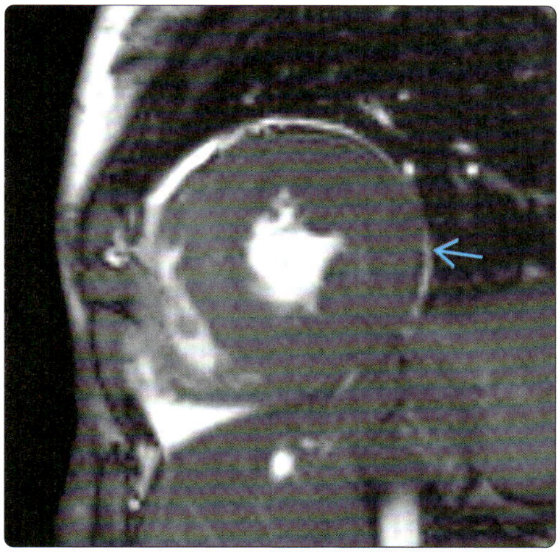

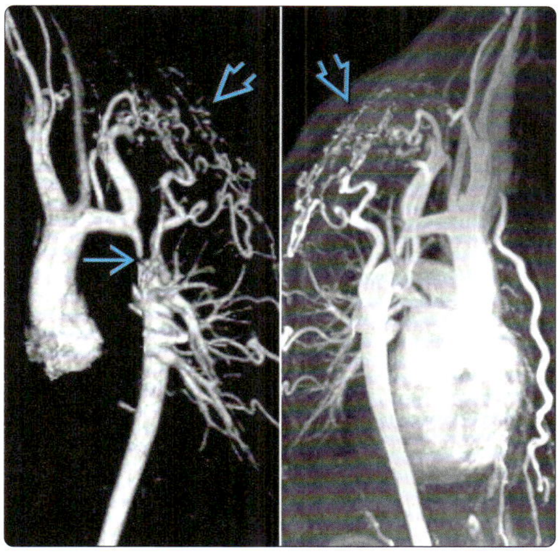

(Left) *Short-axis SSFP cine MR in this patient with coarctation shows concentric thickening of the left ventricular myocardium, consistent with left ventricular hypertrophy. This is a sequela from longstanding upper body arterial hypertension.* **(Right)** *Anterior and posterior MIP views of sagittal aortic MRA demonstrate coarctation and extensive chest wall and mediastinal collaterals. Collateral vessels are better characterized when thin-slice images (e.g., MRA) are reformatted to MIPs.*

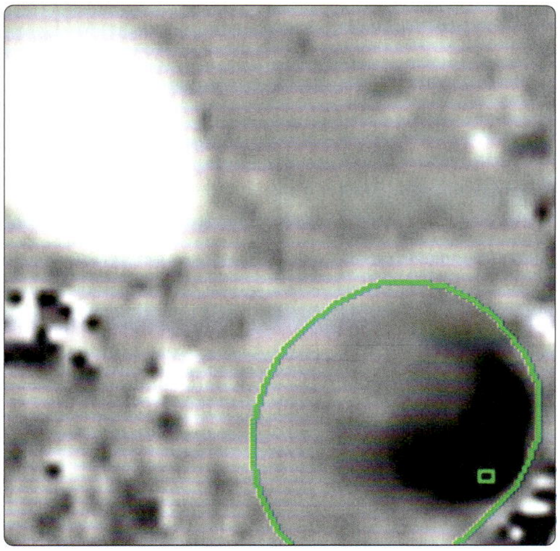

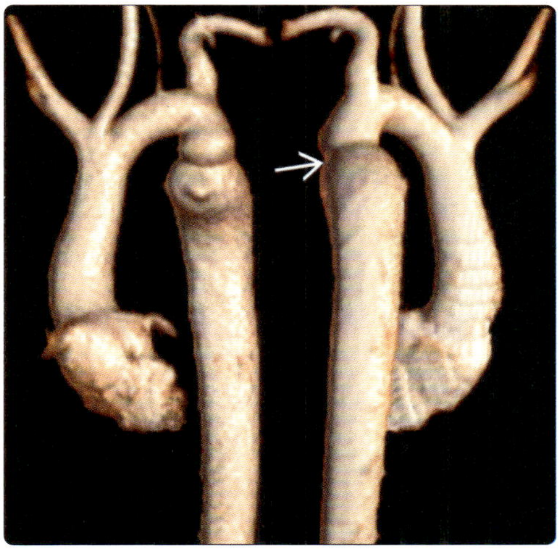

(Left) *This axial phase-contrast MR is from a patient with Shone complex that includes coarctation. While this sequence does not provide good morphologic correlation, it allows calculation of flow velocities and volumes over time, which may be used to quantify heart rate-corrected deceleration time.* **(Right)** *3D volume-rendered MRA in the same patient shows coarctation with poststenotic dilatation. Shone complex includes coarctation, supravalvular mitral ring, parachute mitral valve, and subaortic stenosis.*

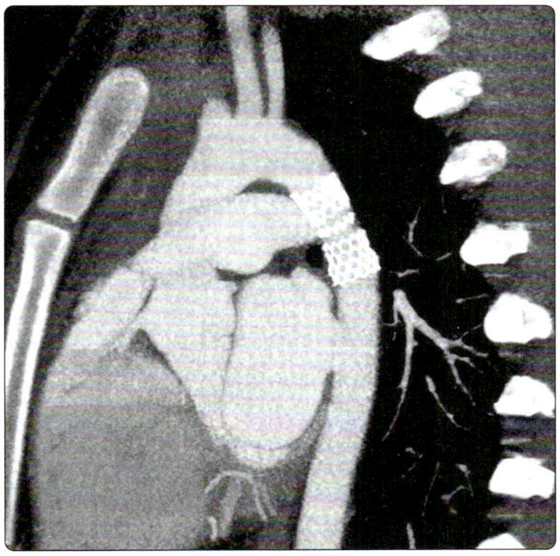

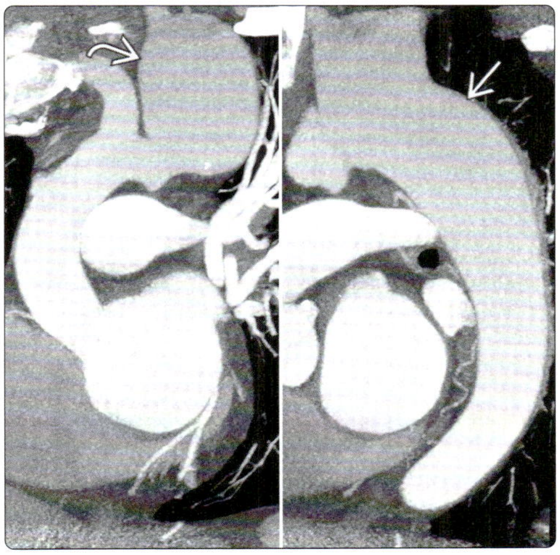

(Left) *This oblique sagittal CTA of the aorta is from a patient with coarctation who underwent successful endovascular stent placement after a failed treatment with angioplasty. CT and MR allow for follow-up and assessment of stent complications.* **(Right)** *Oblique sagittal CTA images in a patient with remote history of surgically corrected aortic coarctation show aneurysmatic dilatation of the left subclavian artery and the proximal descending aorta, a known complication after this type of surgery.*

Interrupted/Hypoplastic Aorta

KEY FACTS

TERMINOLOGY

- Interrupted aortic arch
  - Complete luminal and anatomic wall discontinuity between ascending aorta and descending aorta
- Hypoplastic aortic arch
  - Tubular narrowing without luminal discontinuity

IMAGING

- CTA
  - Best noninvasive modality to assess aortic arch and supraaortic vessels pattern
- US
  - 1st-line modality to assess aortic arch abnormalities
- Best diagnostic clue
  - Interrupted aortic arch
    - Blind ends in distal ascending aorta and proximal descending aorta with luminal discontinuity in between
  - Hypoplastic aortic arch
    - Tubular narrowing of aortic arch; proximal aortic arch < 60% &/or distal aortic arch < 50% of diameter of ascending aorta

TOP DIFFERENTIAL DIAGNOSES

- Coarctation of aorta

PATHOLOGY

- Type A (13%)
  - Interruption distal to left subclavian artery
- Type B (84%)
  - Interruption between left common carotid artery and left subclavian artery
- Type C (3%)
  - Interruption between brachiocephalic trunk and left common carotid artery

CLINICAL ISSUES

- Rare condition
  - 1% of congenital heart disease

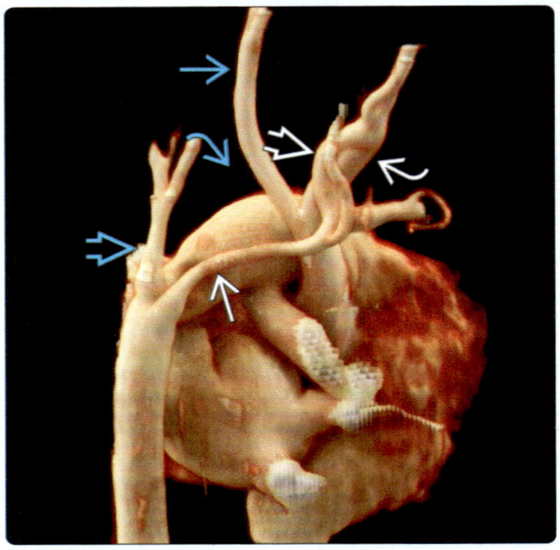
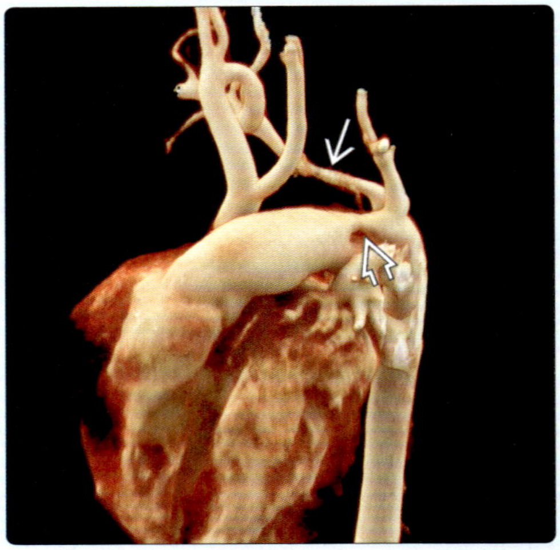

(Left) *Posterior oblique CTA cinematic rendering shows type B interrupted aortic arch with an aberrant right subclavian artery. Also note the collateral vessel with right carotid artery. Left carotid artery and left subclavian artery (LSA) are also shown.* **(Right)** *Anterosuperior oblique CTA cinematic rendering shows type B interrupted aortic arch (IAA) with aberrant right subclavian artery. Patent ductus arteriosus (PDA) provides blood flow to both subclavian arteries and the distal descending aorta (DA).*

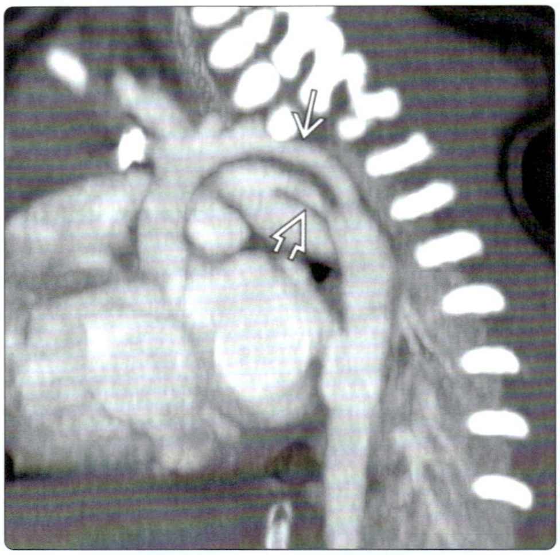
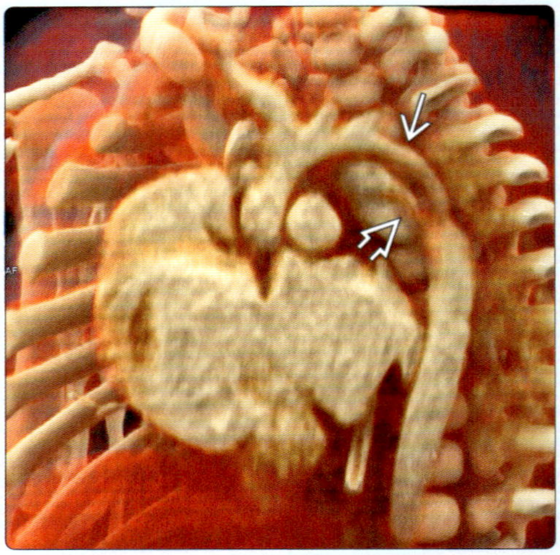

(Left) *Sagittal oblique MIP CTA shows a hypoplastic aortic arch and PDA.* **(Right)** *Sagittal oblique CTA cinematic rendering in the same patient shows a hypoplastic aortic arch and PDA. CT is the best noninvasive imaging modality to assess aortic arch and supraaortic vessel patterns as well as to measure vessel diameters.*

TERMINOLOGY

Abbreviations

- Interrupted aortic arch (IAA)
- Hypoplastic aortic arch (HAA)

Synonyms

- Atresia of aortic arch

Definitions

- IAA
  - Complete luminal discontinuity between ascending aorta and descending aorta
    - Not true interruption, as there is fibrotic continuity between blind ends
- HAA
  - Tubular narrowing of aortic arch without luminal discontinuity

IMAGING

General Features

- Best diagnostic clue
  - IAA
    - Blind-ending distal ascending aorta and proximal descending aorta with luminal discontinuity in between
  - HAA
    - Tubular narrowing of aortic arch
      - Proximal arch < 60% &/or distal aortic arch < 50% of diameter of ascending aorta
      - Transverse aortic arch z-score usually < -3
- Location
  - Aortic arch: Proximal or distal
- Size
  - Variable
- Morphology
  - IAA: Complete anatomic discontinuity between ascending aorta and descending aorta
  - HAA: Tubular narrowing of aortic arch

CT Findings

- CTA
  - Interruption: Blind ending ascending and descending aorta without luminal opacification of arch
    - Type, site, and length of interruption
    - Type A: Distal to left subclavian artery
    - Type B: Between left common carotid and subclavian arteries
    - Type C: Between right brachiocephalic and left common carotid arteries
  - Hypoplasia: Small caliber of aortic arch
    - Best modality for measuring vessel diameters
  - Best noninvasive modality to assess aortic arch and supraaortic vessels pattern
  - New-generation scanners provide faster acquisition without sedation or ECG gating
  - High-resolution 3D reconstructions provides roadmap for surgery

MR Findings

- MRA
  - High-resolution images of aorta without radiation; can be performed ± contrast
  - Types of interrupted arch
  - Shows diameters of each aortic segment and length of HAA
    - Hypoplasia: External diameter of proximal arch, distal arch, or isthmus measuring < 60%, < 50%, or < 40% of that of ascending aorta
    - Transverse aortic arch z-score usually < -3
    - This assumes that ascending aorta diameter is normal
  - Dynamic MRA shows multiple vascular phases, providing information about aorta, pulmonary arteries and veins, and systemic venous return pattern with single gadolinium injection
  - Associated anomalies can be evaluated
- MR cine
  - Biventricular function assessment, including ejection fraction, end-diastolic, and end-systolic volumes
  - Wall motion abnormalities
  - Evaluation of additional intracardiac abnormalities (such as septal defects)

Ultrasonographic Findings

- 1st modality to assess aortic arch abnormalities in children
- Define true interruption or HAA and type of IAA by looking at pattern of supraaortic trunks
- Associated patent ductus arteriosus (PDA)
  - Size, flow, aortic and pulmonary ostial diameters
- Associated cardiac abnormalities: Atrial septal defect (ASD), ventricular septal defect (VSD), left ventricular outflow tract (LVOT) obstruction, aorticopulmonary window defect

Imaging Recommendations

- Best imaging tool
  - CTA or MRA
- Protocol advice
  - Newborn and infants: Contrast injection based on body weight
  - Bolus tracking position and HU threshold are variable and depend on scanner speed to start acquisition
  - Newborn and infants: Acquisition can be started immediately after contrast injection

DIFFERENTIAL DIAGNOSIS

Coarctation of Aorta

- Focal narrowing at aortic isthmus
  - Same location as type A interruption
- Usually short segment of luminal narrowing
- No complete loss of continuity, like interruption
  - Occasionally, extremely tight stenosis may be seen
- More pronounced poststenotic dilation
  - In interruption, arch is smaller caliber, and branch vessels are straighter than normal
- With advanced cases, distinguishing features may disappear

Focal Atresia of Aortic Arch

- Most common at aortic isthmus, similar to type A interruption
- Lumen is interrupted, but aortic wall is present
- Fibrous strand between ascending and descending aorta

PATHOLOGY

General Features

- Etiology
  - Type A
    - Abnormal regression of left 4th aortic arch late in development after left subclavian artery is in position
      - Reduced blood flow through 4th aortic arch during embryologic phase
      - Insufficient development of aortic arch with spectrum from coarctation to atresia to IAA
      - Conal septum not malaligned or deviated; no subaortic stenosis
  - Type B
    - High association with chromosome 22q11.2 microdeletion
    - Abnormal regression of left 4th arch, early in development, before cephalad migration of left subclavian artery
    - Malalignment of infundibular septum with muscular septum → LVOT narrowing → decreased growth, hypoplasia, and interruption of arch due to absolute decrease in cardiac output
  - Type C
    - Abnormal regression of ventral portion of left 3rd and 4th arches
- Genetics
  - 50% of patients with IAA have chromosome 22q11.2 deletion
  - 42% of patients with DiGeorge syndrome have IAA
- Associated abnormalities
  - IAA
    - PDA is essential for life in all patients (seen in 97% of cases)
    - VSD in 90% of IAA
    - Other congenital heart abnormalities are present in 98%
      - Subaortic stenosis
      - Bicuspid aortic valve
      - Truncus arteriosus
      - Aortopulmonary window
      - Transposition of great arteries
      - Double-outlet right ventricle
      - Functional single ventricle
      - Persistent 5th arch
      - Anomalous origin of subclavian artery
  - HAA
    - ASD
    - VSD
    - PDA

Staging, Grading, & Classification

- Type A (13%)
  - Interruption distal to left subclavian artery
- Type B (84%)
  - Interruption between left common carotid artery and left subclavian artery
- Type C (3%)
  - Interruption between right brachiocephalic trunk and left common carotid artery
- In any of these types, 3 subtypes may be seen depending on origin of right subclavian artery
  - Subtype 1: Normal subclavian artery origin
  - Subtype 2: Aberrant right subclavian artery distal to origin of left subclavian artery
  - Subtype 3: Isolated right subclavian artery originating from right ductus arteriosus

CLINICAL ISSUES

Presentation

- Most common signs/symptoms
  - Differential cyanosis (ductal right-to-left shunt)
    - Type A
      - Normal saturation in both arms and head, desaturated legs
    - Type B
      - Normal saturation in right arm and head, desaturated left arm and legs
    - Type C
      - Normal saturation in right arm and right carotid artery, desaturated left carotid artery, left arm and legs
- Other signs/symptoms
  - When ductus arteriosus begins to close, neonate develops signs of hypoperfusion and cardiogenic shock
  - Death usually occurs 4-10 days after closure of ductus arteriosus
    - By 1 month, 76% of untreated infants are dead; by 1 year, > 90% are dead

Demographics

- Age
  - Neonates
- Sex
  - Male patients: 59%
  - Female patients: 41%
- Epidemiology
  - Rare condition
    - 1% of congenital heart disease
  - 2/100,000 live births

Natural History & Prognosis

- When untreated and ductus arteriosus closes, distal hypoperfusion leads to renal failure, lactic acidosis, and eventually death in few days

Treatment

- Surgical correction is only treatment; goal is to establish continuity in aortic arch
- Prostaglandin E_1 is given to maintain patency of ductus arteriosus until neonate is stable for surgical correction

SELECTED REFERENCES

1. LaPar DJ et al: Surgical considerations in interrupted aortic arch. Semin Cardiothorac Vasc Anesth. 22(3):278-84, 2018
2. Hanneman K et al: Congenital variants and anomalies of the aortic arch. Radiographics. 37(1):32-51, 2017
3. Ramos-Duran L et al: Developmental aortic arch anomalies in infants and children assessed with CT angiography. AJR Am J Roentgenol. 198(5):W466-74, 2012
4. Hellinger JC et al: Congenital thoracic vascular anomalies: evaluation with state-of-the-art MR imaging and MDCT. Radiol Clin North Am. 49(5):969-96, 2011

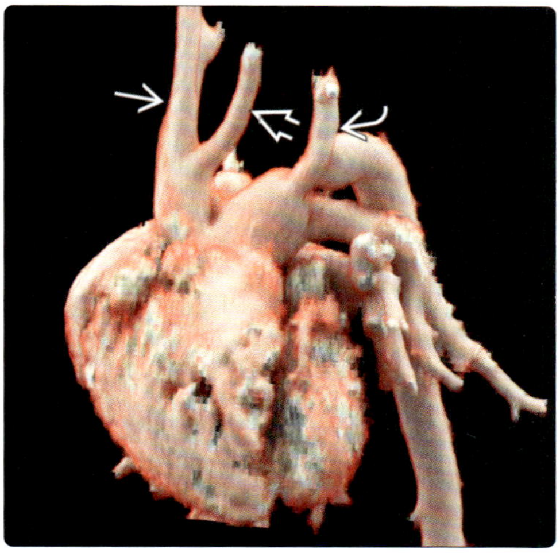

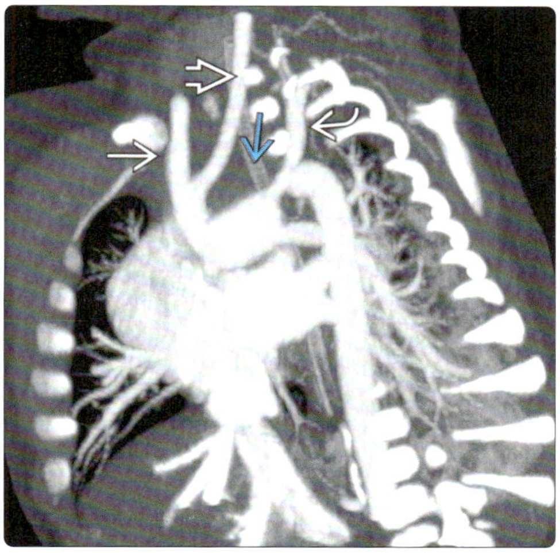

(Left) *Anterosuperior oblique CTA cinematic rendering shows type B IAA. The brachiocephalic trunk (BCT) and left carotid artery originate from the proximal aorta. The LSA originates from the ductal arch.* **(Right)** *Sagittal oblique MIP CTA shows type B IAA. The BCT and left common carotid artery (LCC) originate from the proximal aorta. The LSA originates from the ductal arch.*

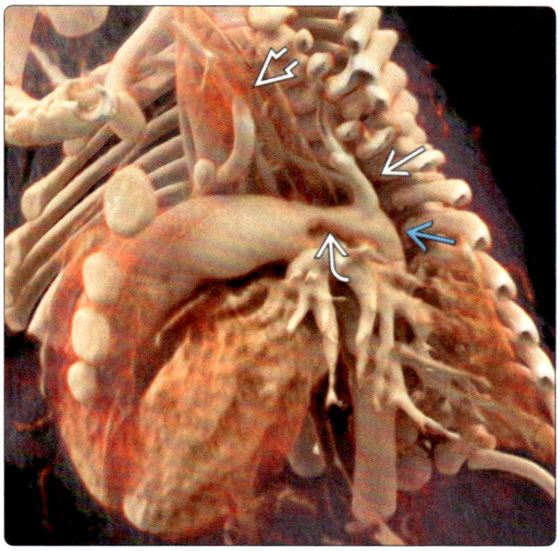

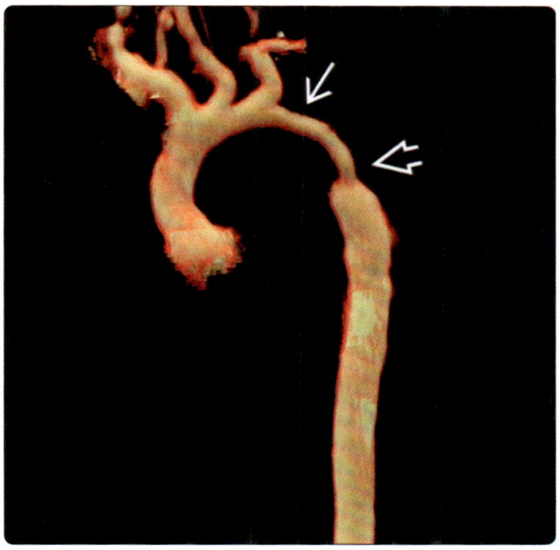

(Left) *CTA cinematic rendering demonstrates type B IAA. The LSA originates from the DA. The BCT and LCC originate from the proximal ascending aorta (AA). The PDA provides blood flow to both the LSA and DA.* **(Right)** *Sagittal oblique CTA cinematic rendering shows a hypoplastic distal aortic arch involving the isthmus and proximal DA.*

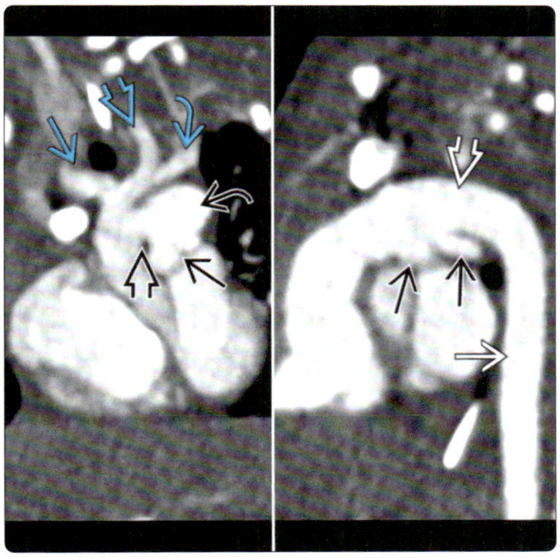

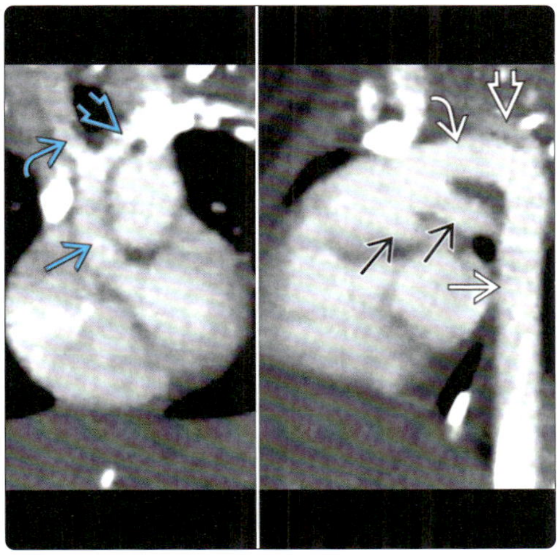

(Left) *Neonate with type A IAA shows AA terminating as the BCT, LCC, and LSA (left). Notice the AP window defect between the AA and main pulmonary artery (MPA). A PDA supplies the DA. PA branches are visible.* **(Right)** *Coronal (left) and sagittal (right) images in a neonate with type B IAA show the AA terminating as the BCT and LCC. The LSA and DA are supplied by a PDA. PA branches arise from the MPA. (Courtesy S. Kligerman, MD.)*

Double Aortic Arch

KEY FACTS

TERMINOLOGY

- Double aortic arch (DAA)
  - Persistent right and left aortic arches, each one giving rise to separate ipsilateral subclavian and carotid arteries

IMAGING

- Chest radiography
  - Frontal projection: Bilateral paratracheal opacities, bilateral tracheal indentations
  - Lateral projection: Posterior tracheal indentation
- CTA
  - Right aortic arch
    - Larger and higher in most patients (right dominant)
  - Left aortic arch
    - Often smaller than right aortic arch
  - 4-artery sign: Symmetric take-off of 4 aortic branches on axial image at thoracic inlet (2 ventral carotids and 2 dorsal subclavians)
  - 1 descending aorta, usually contralateral to dominant arch (i.e., left)
- Airway CT
  - Tracheomalacia: Tracheal collapse adjacent to vascular ring during expiration
  - Bronchomalacia: Left main bronchus collapse adjacent to midline descending aorta during expiration

CLINICAL ISSUES

- Most common symptomatic vascular ring
- Typically manifests in neonates
- Children
  - Dyspnea, often during feeding
  - Stridor and wheezing (exacerbated by crying)
  - Tachypnea, apnea
- Adults
  - May be asymptomatic
- Treatment: Surgical division of smaller or atretic aortic arch and ligamentum arteriosus

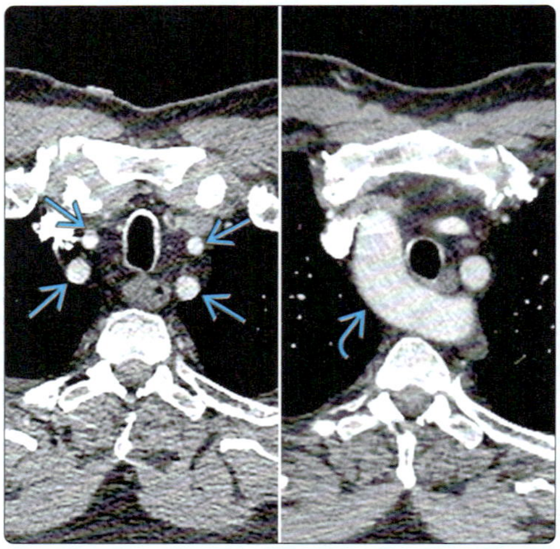

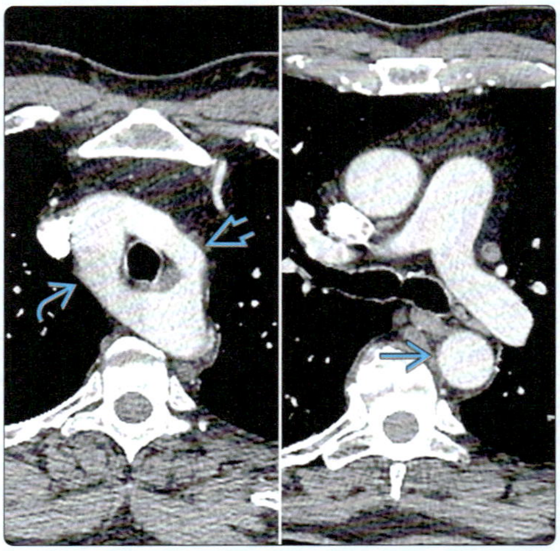

(Left) *Composite axial CTA at contiguous levels in a patient with a double aortic arch (DAA) shows symmetric take-off of 4 aortic branches at thoracic inlet (i.e., 2 carotids and 2 subclavian arteries), the so-called 4-artery sign. This sign has been described in the setting of DAA. Note the right aortic arch (RAA).* **(Right)** *Composite axial CTA in the same patient shows the larger RAA and smaller left aortic arch. Note the left descending thoracic aorta, which is typically contralateral to the dominant arch.*

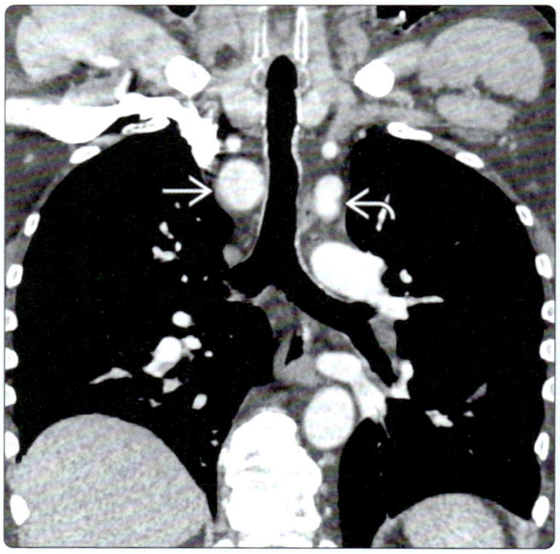

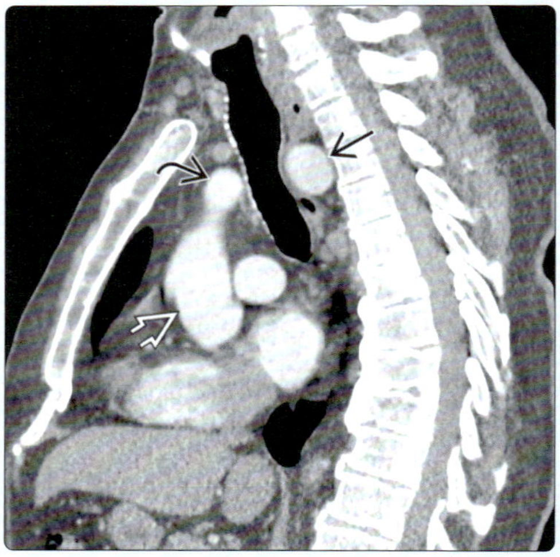

(Left) *Coronal CTA in the same patient shows a cephalad, larger RAA and a more caudal, smaller left aortic arch. Note the mild tracheal impression of the RAA. A larger RAA is the most common variant seen in DAA.* **(Right)** *Sagittal CTA in the same patient shows the distal RAA causing a posterior indentation of the trachea. Also note the ascending aorta (with slab artifact) and the proximal left aortic arch.*

TERMINOLOGY

Abbreviations

- Double aortic arch (DAA)

Definitions

- Persistent right and left aortic arches, each one giving rise to separate ipsilateral subclavian and carotid arteries

IMAGING

General Features

- Best diagnostic clue
  - Chest radiography: Bilateral paratracheal opacities with concentric midtracheal narrowing

Radiographic Findings

- Radiography
  - Frontal projection
    - Bilateral paratracheal opacities
  - Lateral
    - Posterior tracheal indentation

Fluoroscopic Findings

- Esophagram
  - Frontal projection: S-shaped, bilateral indentations on contrast-filled esophagus, right higher and larger than left
  - Lateral view: Large posterior indentation, often oblique

CT Findings

- CTA
  - Right aortic arch
    - Larger in most patients (right dominant)
    - More cephalad than left
    - Courses behind esophagus
  - Left aortic arch
    - Often smaller than right aortic arch
    - Left aortic arch atresia can be confused with right aortic arch
      - Inferior tethering of left subclavian artery
      - ± aortic diverticulum
  - **4-artery sign**: Symmetric take-off of 4 aortic branches on axial image at thoracic inlet (2 ventral carotids and 2 dorsal subclavians)
  - 1 descending aorta, usually contralateral to dominant arch (i.e., left)
- Airway CT
  - Inspiration and expiration CT may help differentiate tracheomalacia from tracheal stenosis
  - Tracheomalacia: Tracheal collapse adjacent to vascular ring during expiration

MR Findings

- As accurate as CT in assessing vascular anatomy and tracheal stenosis
- Of value in young individuals due to lack of ionizing radiation

Imaging Recommendations

- Best imaging tool
  - MR and CT are equally accurate in assessing vascular and tracheal anatomy
- Protocol advice
  - Multiplanar reformations are helpful in delineating arch anatomy and tracheal abnormalities

DIFFERENTIAL DIAGNOSIS

Right Aortic Arch With Aberrant Left Subclavian Artery and Kommerell Diverticulum

- Kommerell diverticulum may mimic left aortic arch on frontal chest radiograph
- Tracheal indentation on lateral chest radiograph
- Differentiation usually requires cross-sectional imaging

Right Aortic Arch With Mirror Image Branching and Aortic Diverticulum

- Lack of inferior tethering of left subclavian artery
- Aortic diverticulum is more common in DAA with atretic left aortic arch

Left Pulmonary Artery Sling

- Anterior esophageal and posterior tracheal indentations
- May be associated with tracheomalacia

PATHOLOGY

General Features

- Etiology
  - Persistence of right and left 4th aortic arches
- Associated abnormalities
  - 20% associated with congenital heart disease
    - Tetralogy of Fallot (most common)
  - Tracheobronchomalacia

Gross Pathologic & Surgical Features

- Tight vascular ring with tracheal and esophageal compression
- Dominance: Right (~ 70%) > left (~ 20%) > codominant (~ 5%)

CLINICAL ISSUES

Presentation

- Most common signs/symptoms
  - Children
    - Dyspnea, often during feeding
    - Stridor and wheezing (exacerbated by crying)
    - Tachypnea, apnea
  - Adults
    - May be asymptomatic
    - Esophageal obstruction (i.e., dysphagia)

Demographics

- Most common symptomatic vascular ring
- Typically manifests in neonates

Treatment

- Surgical division of smaller or atretic aortic arch and ligamentum arteriosus

SELECTED REFERENCES

1. Li S et al: Congenital abnormalities of the aortic arch: revisiting the 1964 Stewart classification. Cardiovasc Pathol. 39:38-50, 2018
2. Hanneman K et al: Congenital variants and anomalies of the aortic arch. Radiographics. 37(1):32-51, 2017

(Left) *Frontal radiograph in the same patient shows mild concentric narrowing* → *of the midtrachea with more prominent right paratracheal nodular opacity.* **(Right)** *Lateral radiograph in the same patient shows the posterior tracheal indentation* → *from retrotracheal course of the RAA, a classic finding in DAA. This narrowing is often related to the distal portion of the RAA, as it courses posterior to the esophagus to join the RAA.*

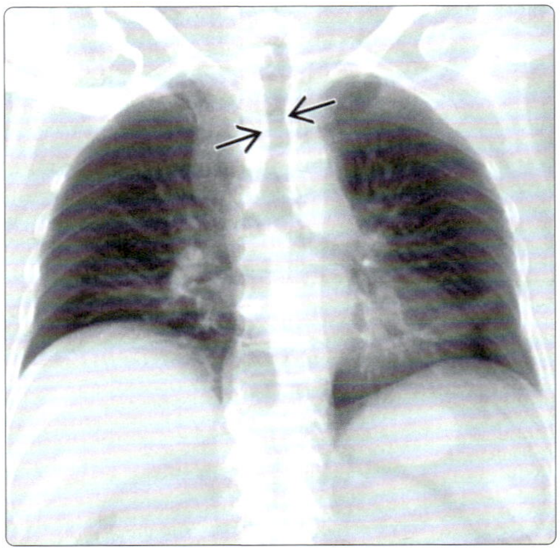

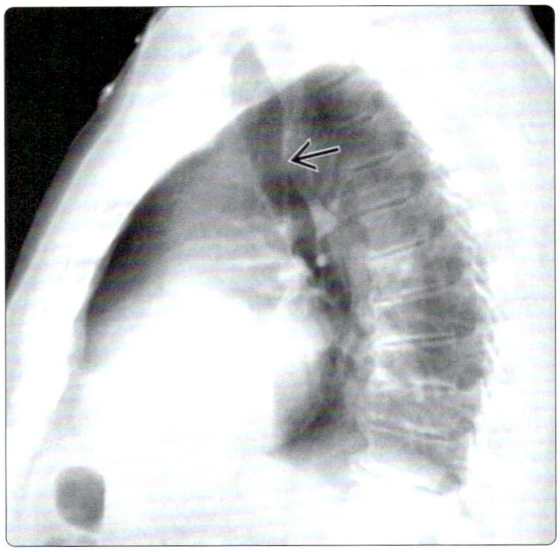

(Left) *Sagittal 3D reformation of chest CTA shows a patent RAA* → *and smaller left aortic arch* →. *There are 4 major symmetrical branches (2 ventral carotids and 2 dorsal subclavian arteries), each set arising form each aortic arch. This is known as the 4-artery sign. The trachea and esophagus (not shown) are completely surrounded by the vascular ring.* **(Right)** *Graphic shows a DAA with a complete vascular ring encircling and compressing the trachea and esophagus.*

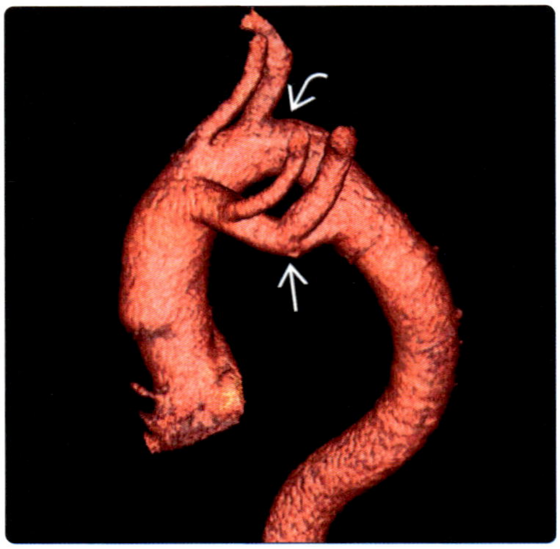

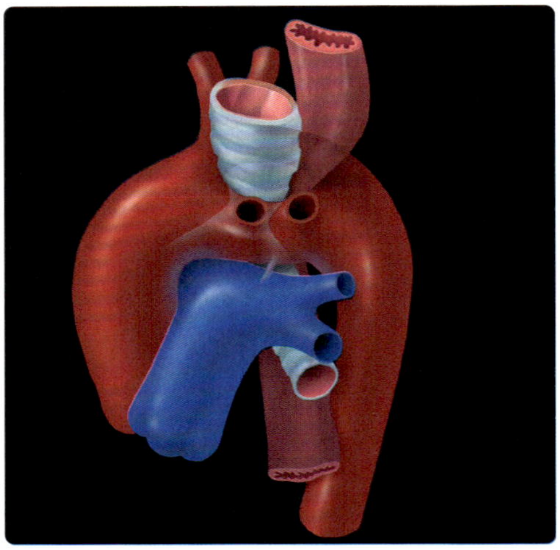

(Left) *Esophagram in a neonate with stridor shows right* → *and smaller left* → *indentations of the esophagus on frontal view due to a DAA. There is posterior indentation* → *in the lateral view related to the RAA.* **(Right)** *Frontal 3D reformation from a chest CT in an asymptomatic patient with a DAA shows higher and larger right* → *vs. left* → *tracheal indentations on the AP reformation. Note posterior indentation* → *related to the RAA in the lateral reformation.*

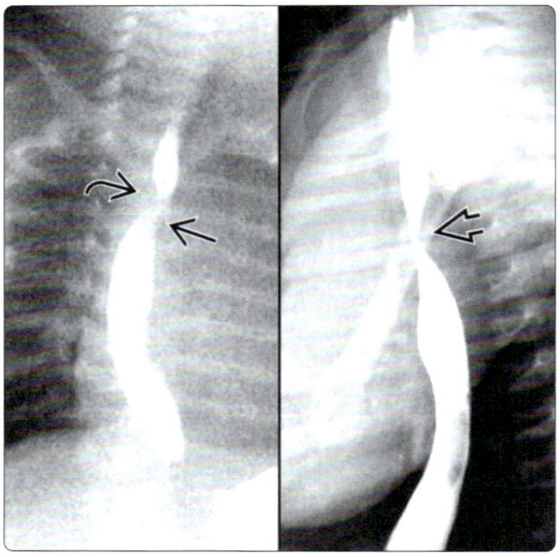

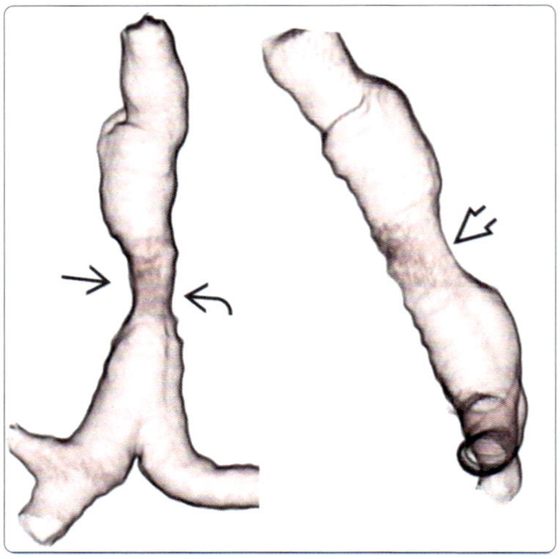

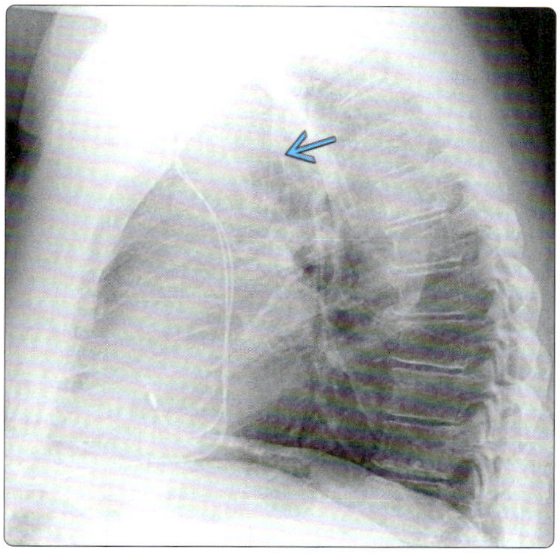

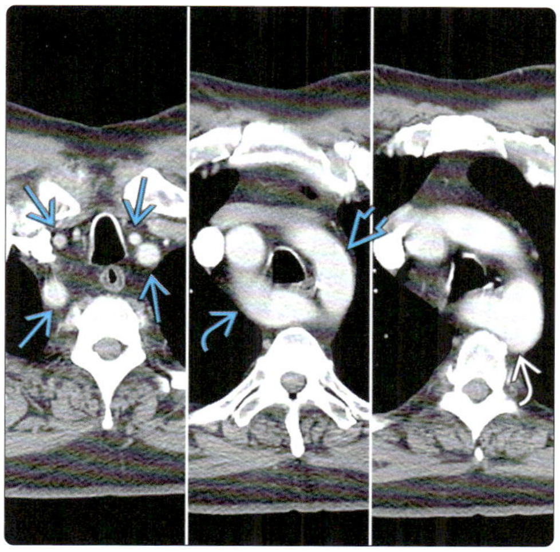

(Left) *Lateral chest radiograph in a patient with a DAA shows abnormal posterior tracheal indentation. This can also be seen in the setting of other vascular rings, such as those with diverticulum of Kommerell or pulmonary artery sling.* **(Right)** *Composite axial CTA at contiguous levels shows the RAA and left aortic arch similar in size. Note, however, the lack of the 4-artery sign (i.e., lack of symmetry of the 4 head/neck vessels at the thoracic inlet). There is a left descending thoracic aorta.*

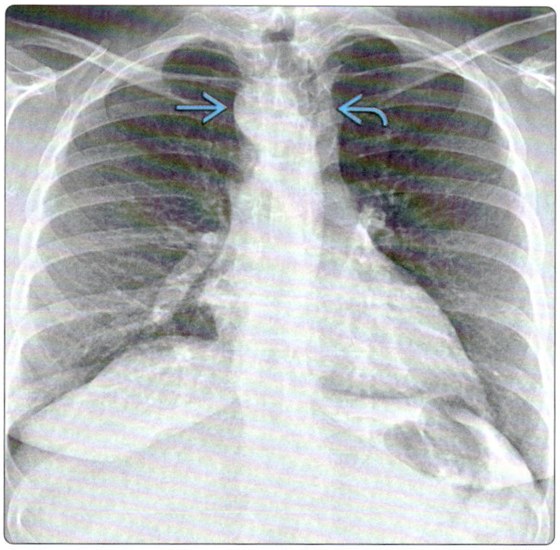

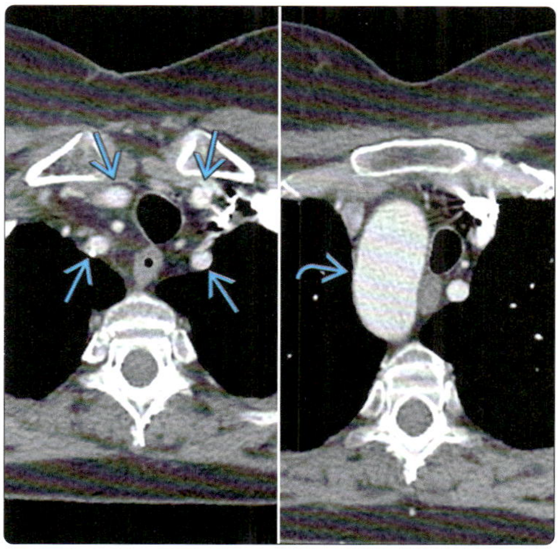

(Left) *Frontal chest radiograph in a patient with a DAA with an atretic left arch shows right paratracheal opacity related to the RAA with marked tracheal indentation. The same imaging finding can also be seen in an isolated RAA.* **(Right)** *Composite axial CTA at contiguous levels in the same patient shows symmetric take-off of 4 aortic branches at the thoracic inlet (i.e., 4-artery sign). Note the presence of a large RAA, which is mildly deviating the trachea to the left.*

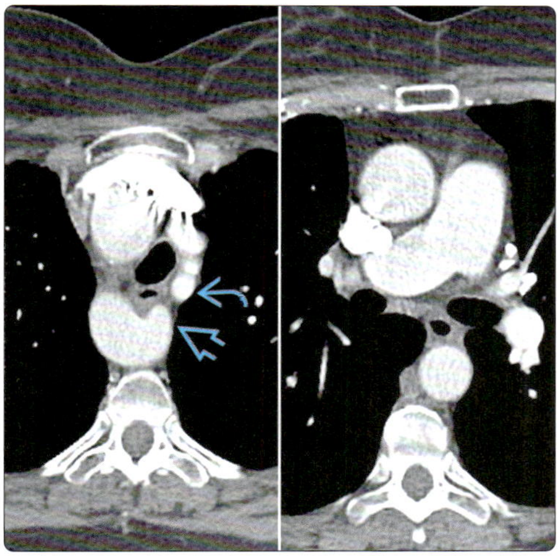

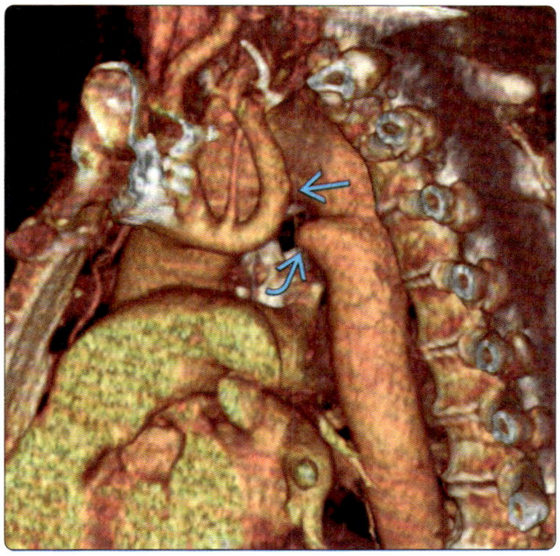

(Left) *Composite axial CTA at contiguous levels in the same patient shows an atretic left aortic arch with a posteriorly tethered left subclavian artery. The later is helpful to differentiate from an RAA with mirror image branching in which the take-off of the left subclavian artery tends to be more anterior.* **(Right)** *Sagittal oblique SSD CTA in the same patient shows the posterior tethering of the left subclavian artery and the atretic left aortic arch, resulting in a vascular ring.*

KEY FACTS

TERMINOLOGY

- Right aortic arch (RAA)
  - Aortic arch located to right of trachea
- Common variations
  - RAA with aberrant left subclavian artery (ALSA) ± Kommerell diverticulum (KD)
  - RAA with mirror-image branching

IMAGING

- Radiography
  - Right paratracheal nodular opacity and indentation of right tracheal margin on frontal chest radiograph
  - KD: Retroesophageal opacity with indentation of posterior tracheal margin on lateral chest radiograph
- CT
  - RAA with ALSA with retroesophageal course ± KD
  - RAA with mirror-image branching
  - RAA with left descending aorta with retroesophageal aortic segment

TOP DIFFERENTIAL DIAGNOSES

- Double aortic arch
- Mediastinal mass

CLINICAL ISSUES

- RAA with ALSA
  - Most patients are asymptomatic
  - Some patients with KD may have dysphagia or stridor
- RAA with mirror-image branching
  - Cyanotic congenital heart disease
- RAA with left descending aorta (circumflex aorta)
  - Ductus ligament between pulmonary artery and ALSA constitutes vascular ring
- Treatment
  - Symptomatic RAA with ALSA/KD may require division of ligamentum via left thoracotomy

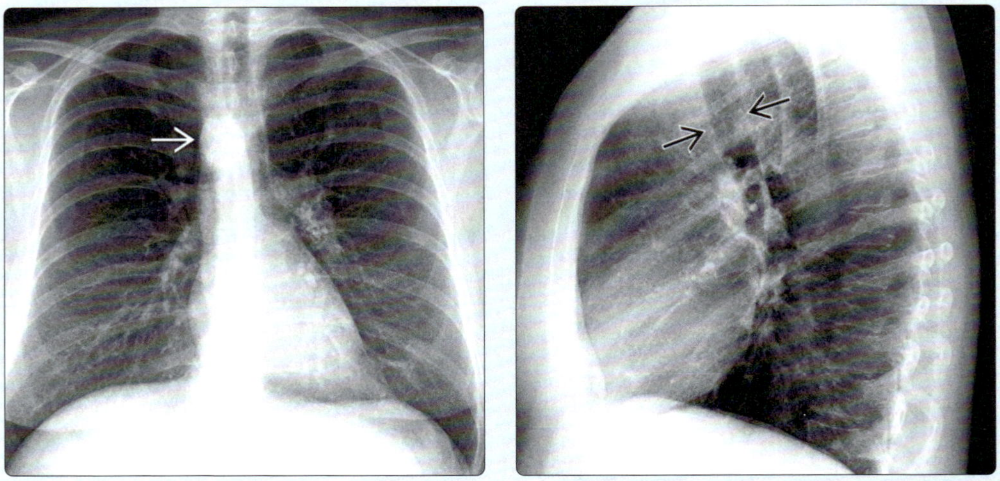

(Left) *PA chest radiograph in a patient with right aortic arch (RAA) and aberrant left subclavian artery (ALSA) without Kommerell diverticulum (KD) shows RAA ➡ as a right paratracheal nodular opacity with right tracheal indentation.* **(Right)** *Lateral chest radiograph in the same patient shows the normal configuration of the trachea ⇨. ALSA with KD can show indentation of posterior tracheal margin; however, differentiation from ALSA without KD is not always possible.*

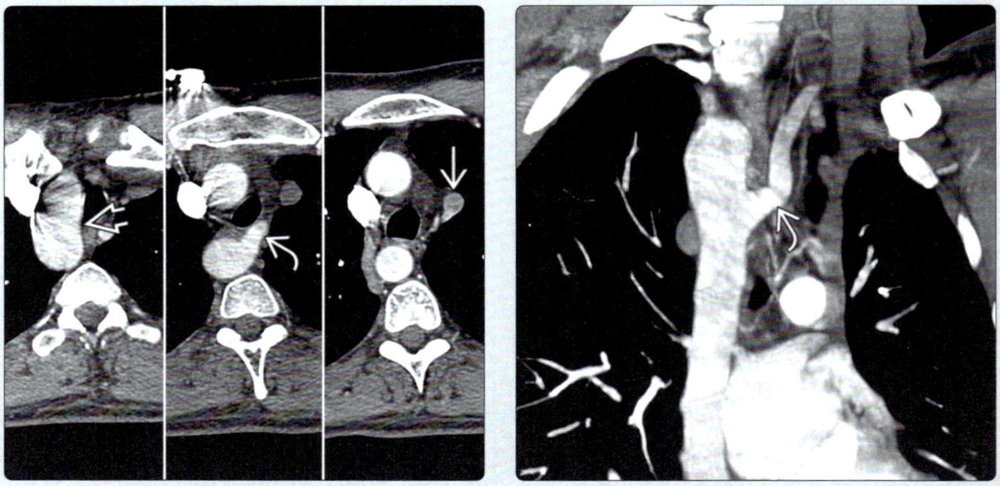

(Left) *Axial chest CTA in an asymptomatic patient with RAA ➡, ALSA ➡, and descending thoracic aorta on the right reveals an incidentally noted persistent left superior vena cava ➡ draining into the coronary sinus.* **(Right)** *Coronal reformation CTA in the same patient shows ALSA ➡ arising as the last aortic branch. There is no KD. The lack of KD usually indicates absence of a ductus ligament on the side of the anomalous subclavian artery (SCA); therefore, this does not constitute a vascular ring.*

TERMINOLOGY

Abbreviations

- Right aortic arch (RAA)

Definitions

- Aortic arch located to right of trachea, crossing right main stem bronchus
- Common variations
  - RAA with mirror-image branching
  - RAA with aberrant left subclavian artery (ALSA) ± Kommerell diverticulum (KD)
    - Saccular dilatation at level of ALSA
    - Implies left-sided ligamentum arteriosum and vascular ring
- Uncommon variations
  - RAA with left descending aorta (circumflex aorta)
  - RAA with isolation of left subclavian artery
  - RAA with aberrant brachiocephalic artery
  - RAA with unilateral absence of pulmonary artery

IMAGING

General Features

- Best diagnostic clue
  - Indentation of right tracheal margin due to paratracheal mass

Radiographic Findings

- Radiography
  - General features for different variations
    - Right paratracheal opacity
    - Indentation of right tracheal margin
  - RAA with ALSA
    - + KD
      - Retroesophageal nodular opacity
      - Indentation of posterior tracheal margin
      - Can simulate left aortic arch (LAA) on frontal projection
  - RAA with mirror-image branching
    - ± dextrocardia
    - High association with congenital heart disease
  - RAA with unilateral absence of pulmonary artery
    - Hypoplastic ipsilateral hemithorax with contralateral hyperinflation
    - Absent or grossly ↓ pulmonary vascular markings

CT Findings

- RAA with ALSA (most common)
  - 4 great vessels from left to right in following order: Left common carotid, right common carotid, right subclavian, ALSA
  - ALSA with retroesophageal course
  - ± KD (bulbous dilatation at origin of ALSA)
- RAA with mirror-image branching
  - 3 great vessels from left to right in following order: Left brachiocephalic, right common carotid, right subclavian
  - Rarely, blind aortic diverticulum (similar to KD)
- RAA with left descending aorta (circumflex aorta)
  - Retroesophageal aortic segment
- RAA with isolation of left subclavian artery
  - 3 great vessels from left to right in following order: Left carotid, right carotid, right subclavian
  - Left subclavian artery is blind ended, connected to aortic arch by ductus ligament

MR Findings

- Same accuracy as CT to assess for variations of vascular anatomy
- Absence of ionizing radiation is significant advantage, especially in younger patients

DIFFERENTIAL DIAGNOSIS

Double Aortic Arch

- Differentiation on radiography may be not possible, as KD can simulate LAA
- CT and MR are diagnostic
  - Patent RAA and LAA with larger RAA and smaller LAA
  - Double aortic arch (DAA) with atretic LAA
    - Inferior tethering of left subclavian artery
    - Aortic diverticulum more common in DAA

Mediastinal Mass

- Right paratracheal lymphadenopathy and esophageal neoplasm can simulate RAA on chest radiography

PATHOLOGY

General Features

- Etiology
  - Embryologic considerations
    - RAA with ALSA develops from interruption between left common carotid and left subclavian arteries
    - RAA with mirror-image branching develops from interruption distal to left subclavian artery
- Associated abnormalities
  - RAA with ALSA ± KD: Low incidence of congenital heart disease
  - RAA with mirror-image branching: High incidence of congenital heart disease (~ 98%)
    - RAA in 25% of patients with tetralogy of Fallot
    - RAA in 25-50% of patients with truncus arteriosus

CLINICAL ISSUES

Presentation

- Most common signs/symptoms
  - RAA with ALSA
    - Presence of KD constitutes vascular ring, often loose
    - Patients with KD may have dysphagia or stridor

Natural History & Prognosis

- Determined mostly by coexisting congenital heart disease

Treatment

- Symptomatic RAA with ALSA/KD
  - Requires division of ligamentum via left thoracotomy
- RAA with mirror-image branching
  - Treatment of associated congenital heart disease

SELECTED REFERENCES

1. Prabhu S et al: Anatomic classification of the right aortic arch. Cardiol Young. 30(11):1694-701, 2020

(Left) *PA chest radiograph in an asymptomatic patient with RAA, ALSA, and KD shows RAA as a right paratracheal nodular opacity* ➡ *with an indentation of the right tracheal margin.* **(Right)** *Lateral chest radiograph in the same patient shows an indentation of the posterior tracheal margin* ↪*, which relates to the presence of a KD. This suggests that mirror-image branching is not present. Note that KD implies the presence of a vascular ring, which may or may not be symptomatic.*

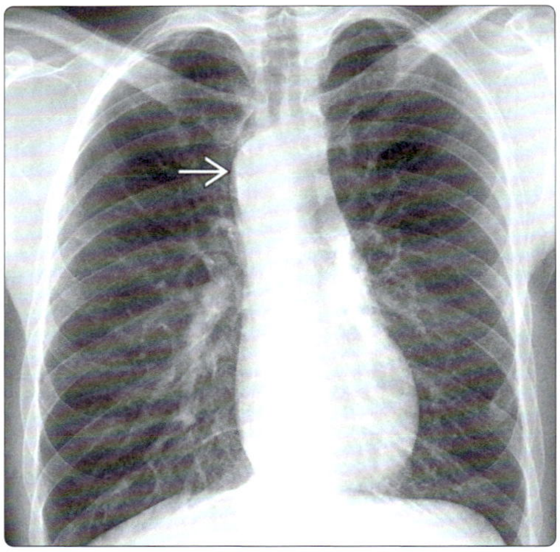

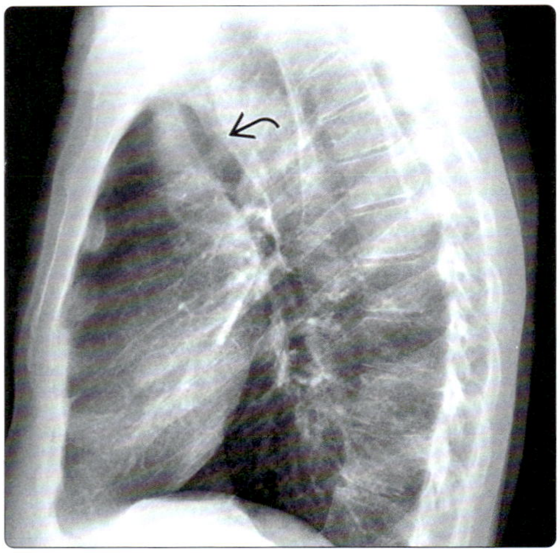

(Left) *Composite axial chest CTA in a patient with RAA, ALSA, and KD demonstrates RAA* → *and ALSA/KD* ↪ *with mild dilatation of the proximal esophagus* ➡ *superior to the KD.* **(Right)** *Sagittal chest CTA reformation in the same patient shows posterior tracheal indentation by the KD* →*. KD implies the presence of a ductus ligament contralateral to the arch and, hence, constitutes a vascular ring. KD predisposes to dysphagia when present (dysphagia lusoria).*

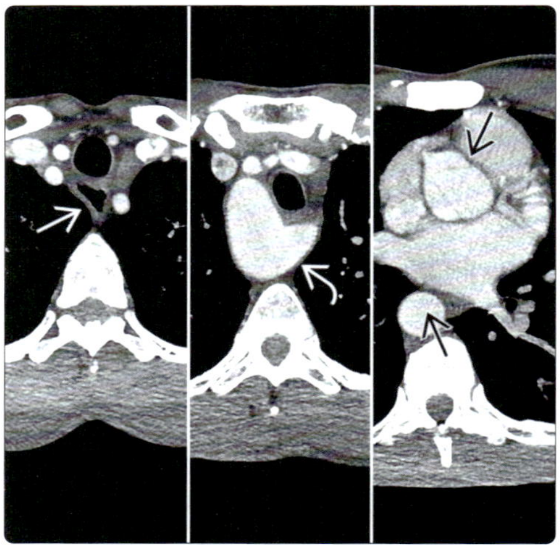

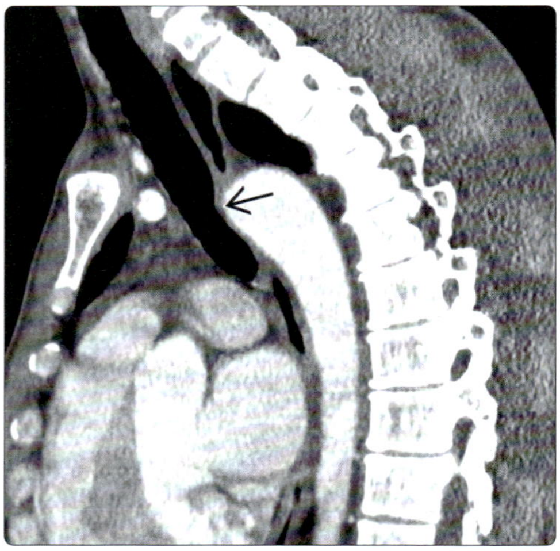

(Left) *Oblique coronal chest CTA reformation in the same patient shows a bulbous configuration* → *of the origin of the ALSA, a classic feature of KD. KD is a consequence of the presence of a ductus arteriosus on the side of the SCA. Pathophysiologically, patients with KD may have symptoms (e.g., dysphagia lusoria) related to a vascular ring completed by the ligamentum arteriosum.* **(Right)** *Anterior and posterior CTA 3D reformations in the same patient with RAA, ALSA* ➡*, and KD* ↪ *show the bulbous appearance of the KD.*

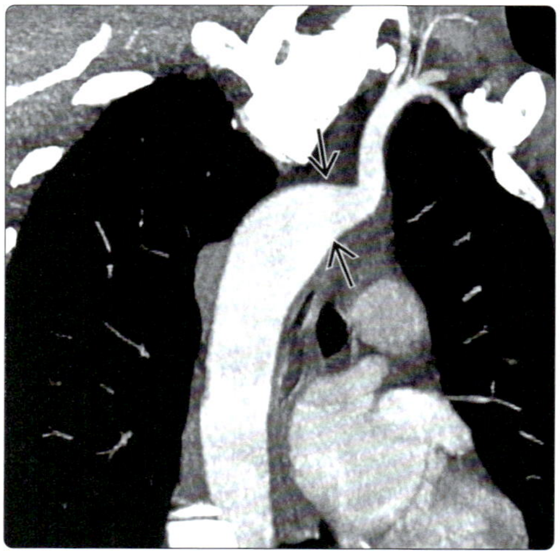

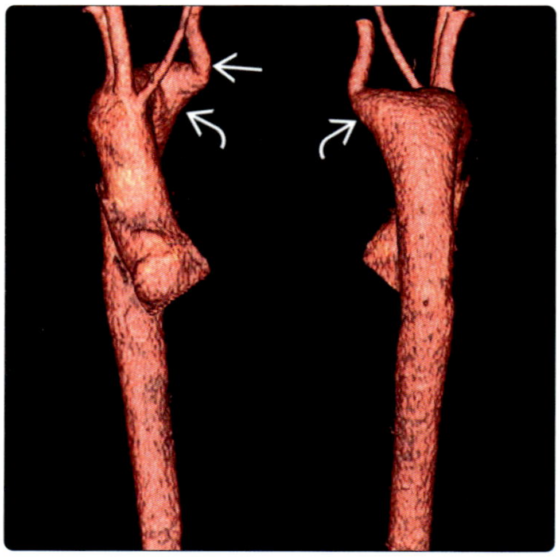

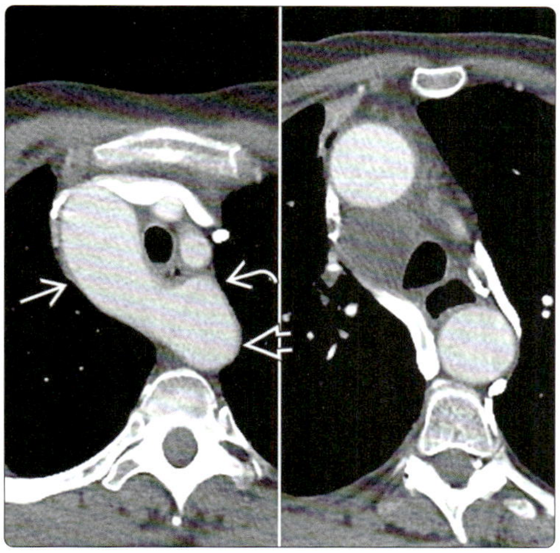

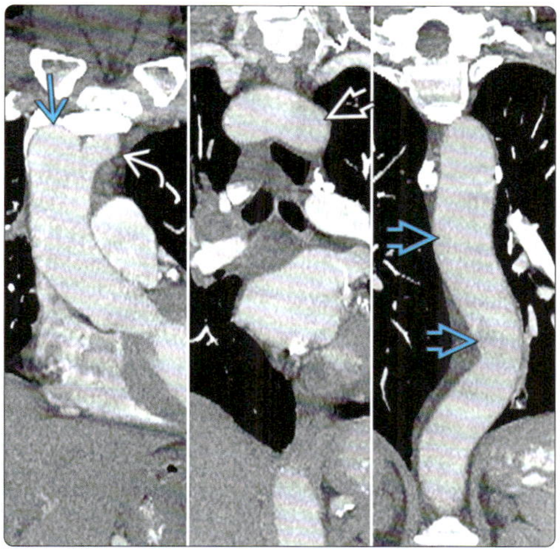

(Left) *Composite axial chest CTA shows RAA with a retroesophageal left descending aorta (circumflex aorta), blind aortic diverticulum, and mirror-image branching.* **(Right)** *Composite chest CTA coronal reformation in the same patient shows RAA, left brachiocephalic trunk, blind aortic diverticulum, and left descending aorta. The circumflex aorta implies a vascular ring, which often is loose and occasionally symptomatic.*

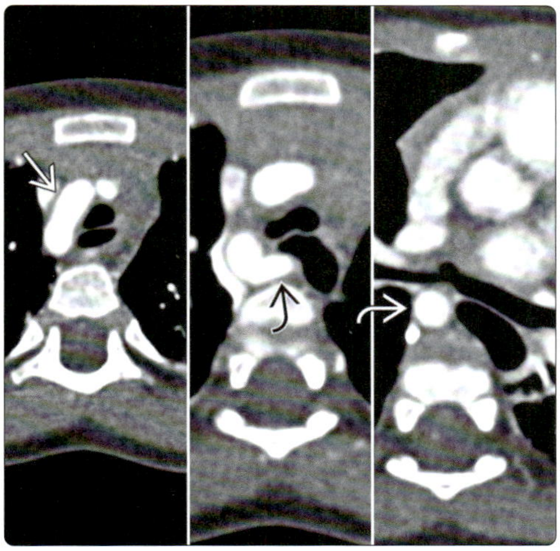

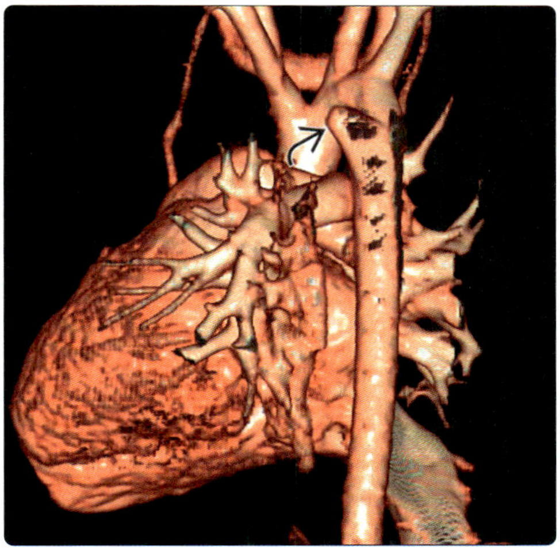

(Left) *Axial chest CTA in an infant with RAA with mirror-image branching and aortic diverticulum with stridor shows a right-sided descending thoracic aorta.* **(Right)** *Posterior 3D CTA in the same patient is shown. Despite the presence of a blind aortic diverticulum, this case represents an RAA, not a double aortic arch (DAA) with atretic left aortic arch (LAA), given the lack of inferior tethering of the left SCA. (Courtesy R. Reina, MD.)*

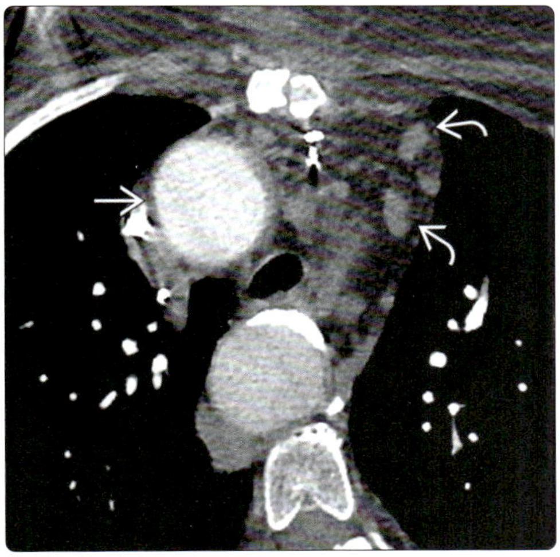

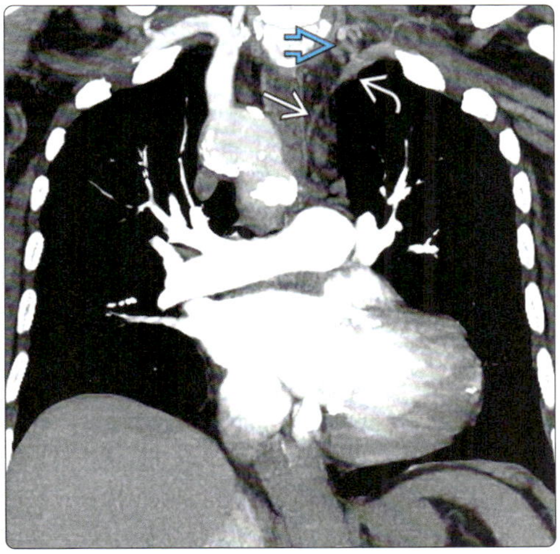

(Left) *Axial chest CECT shows RAA with isolation of the SCA. Note the presence of prominent arterial collaterals.* **(Right)** *Coronal chest CECT in the same patient shows the blind origin of the left SCA with a cord-like structure extending from it to the aortic wall representing a ductus ligament, which can clinically represent a loose ring. Note extensive arterial collaterals, which supply the left SCA.*

Persistent Fifth Arch

KEY FACTS

TERMINOLOGY

- Rare congenital vascular anomaly
- May be isolated or associated with other abnormalities
  - Complex congenital cardiac heart disease
  - Vascular anomalies
  - Skeletal anomalies
- 2 distinct forms
  - **Systemic-to-systemic connection**: 5th arch arises at brachiocephalic trunk and reconnects at descending aorta
  - **Systemic-to-pulmonary connection**: 5th arch connects with embryologic remnant of 6th aortic arch, which is usually left pulmonary artery

IMAGING

- Contrast-enhanced MRA most appropriate in children with suspected persistent 5th arch
- Short segment of duplication aortic arch with 2 parallel distinct lumina in systemic-to-systemic connection
- Abnormal vessel connecting aorta with isolated pulmonary artery in systemic-to-pulmonary connection

CLINICAL ISSUES

- Presentation depends on which type of connections exists and on associated cardiac and vascular anomalies
- Associated cardiovascular anomalies
  - Ventricular septal defect (most common)
  - Pulmonic valve or artery stenosis/atresia
  - Interruption of aortic arch
  - Coarctation of aorta
  - Transposition of great arteries
  - Pentalogy of Fallot
  - Patent ductus arteriosus
  - Tricuspid atresia
- In case of coarctation/obstruction, surgical patching or conduit interposition may be indicated

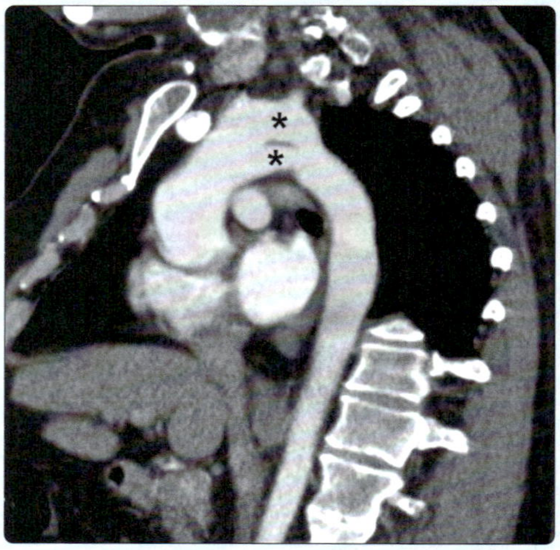
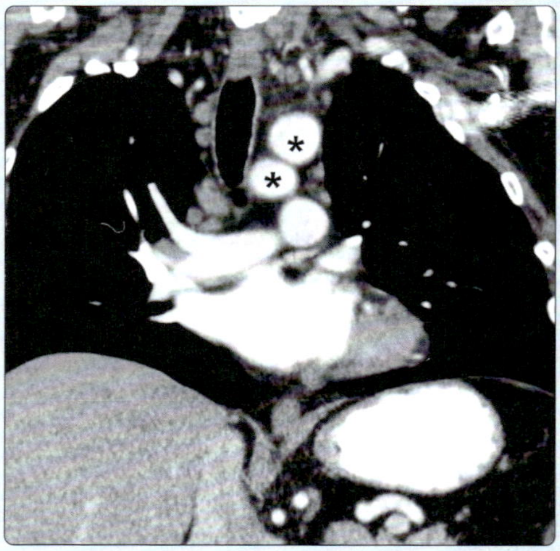

(Left) *Aortic arch "candy cane" view of CTA shows separation of the aortic arch into 2 distinct vessels (*). The superior is the normal 4th aortic arch giving rise to the arch vessels. The inferior is the persistent 5th aortic arch.* **(Right)** *Coronal CTA in the same patient shows the short axis of aortic arches with a double-barrel appearance (*). The 4th and persistent 5th arch have a figure of 8 configuration in the short axis, which allows differentiation from dissection.*

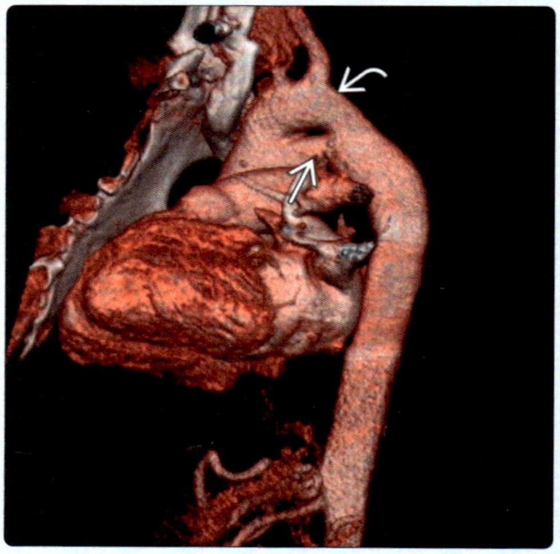
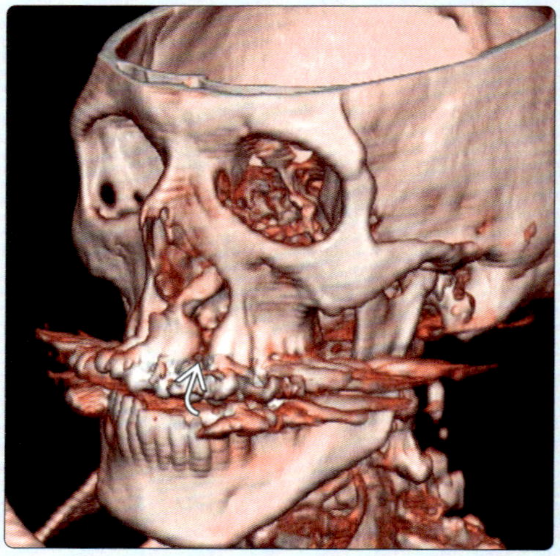

(Left) *Oblique 3D volume-rendered reconstruction shows the relationship of the 4th arch ➔ with the arch vessels. Note the abnormal persistent 5th arch ➔ arising from the aorta at the level of the brachiocephalic trunk and reentering into the descending thoracic aorta at its isthmus.* **(Right)** *Oblique 3D reconstruction of the skull in the same patient shows a cleft palate ➔. Other skeletal anomalies in this patient include fused ribs and hemi vertebra (not shown).*

TERMINOLOGY

Synonyms

- Ipsilateral double aortic arch
- Double lumen aortic arch

Definitions

- Rare congenital vascular anomaly of aortic arch
  - May be isolated
  - Often associated with other congenital cardiac, vascular, or skeletal anomalies
- 2 distinct forms
  - Systemic-to-systemic connection
    - 5th arch arises at brachiocephalic trunk and reconnects at descending aorta
  - Systemic-to-pulmonary connection
    - 5th arch connects with embryologic remnant of 6th aortic arch, which is usually left pulmonary artery

IMAGING

General Features

- Best diagnostic clue
  - Short segment of duplication of aortic arch with 2 parallel distinct lumina
    - May have interrupted arch
  - Abnormal vessel connecting aorta with pulmonary artery
- Location
  - Aortic arch
    - Cephalad of arches is 4th arch, which gives rise to arch vessels
    - Lower arch is persistent 5th arch

Radiographic Findings

- Radiography
  - May demonstrate associated findings, such as vertebral anomalies

CT Findings

- CTA
  - 2 distinct left aortic arches with what may appear as septation separating them
  - Double-barrel appearance on coronal oblique short-axis views
  - May have interrupted arch
  - May show anomalous connection between aorta and isolated left pulmonary artery
  - May demonstrate associated cardiovascular and skeletal abnormalities

MR Findings

- Same as CTA findings
- Superior to echocardiography due to acoustic window restrictions near aortic arch

Imaging Recommendations

- Best imaging tool
  - CTA or MRA
- Protocol advice
  - Contrast-enhanced MRA most appropriate in children with suspected persistent 5th arch

DIFFERENTIAL DIAGNOSIS

Aortic Dissection

- Easily differentiated by double-barrel appearance of persistent 5th arch: 2 round lumina form "figure of 8" on arch short-axis views

Patent Ductus Arteriosus

- Systemic-to-pulmonary connection may mimic large PDA
- PDA would communicate distally to arch arteries

Aortopulmonary Window

- Abnormal connection between proximal aorta and pulmonary trunk

CLINICAL ISSUES

Presentation

- Most common signs/symptoms
  - Often present after birth due to associated cardiac or vascular defects
    - Ventricular septal defect (most common), pulmonic valve or artery stenosis/atresia, tricuspid atresia
    - Interruption of aortic arch, coarctation of aorta, transposition of great arteries, persistent truncus arteriosus, PDA
  - Could be hemodynamically beneficial
    - Systemic-to-systemic connection; if associated with coarctation of aorta or interrupted aortic arch
    - Systemic-to-pulmonic connection; when associated with pulmonary or tricuspid atresia
- Clinical profile
  - Association with intrauterine thalidomide exposure and chromosomal disorders
  - Weinberg classification defines 3 types (A,B,C)
    - Type A: Double-lumen aortic arch (arch vessels arise from upper 4th; lower is 5th arch)
    - Type B: Single-lumen arch; 4th arch is interrupted; 5th arch originates from ascending and connects to descending aorta
    - Type C: 5th originates from proximal brachiocephalic artery off of ascending aorta and connecting to pulmonary artery via 6th arch

Demographics

- Epidemiology
  - Extremely rare congenital malformation

Treatment

- In case of coarctation/obstruction, surgical patching or conduit interposition may be indicated

DIAGNOSTIC CHECKLIST

Consider

- May have obstruction due to associated coarctation
  - Check BP difference between upper and lower extremities (BP in both arms)

SELECTED REFERENCES

1. Shan H et al: Persistent fifth aortic arch: a comprehensive literature review. Front Pediatr. 11:1183345, 2023
2. Liu Y et al: Persistent fifth aortic arch: a single-center experience, case series. Transl Pediatr. 10(6):1566-72, 2021

Aberrant Right Subclavian Artery

KEY FACTS

TERMINOLOGY

- Aberrant right subclavian artery (ARSA) as last branch of left-sided aortic arch, isthmus, or proximal descending aorta
- Course: Retroesophageal 80%; intertracheoesophageal 15%; pretracheal 5%

IMAGING

- Barium esophagogram shows persistent esophageal narrowing at level of extrinsic compression with oblique course
- CTA or MRA help to understand origin and course of supraaortic trunks
- No vascular ring formed by left aortic arch and ARSA
- Loose vascular ring if ARSA originates from Kommerell diverticulum
- Complete vascular ring if ARSA with circumflex right descending thoracic aorta with right ductus

TOP DIFFERENTIAL DIAGNOSES

- Major aortopulmonary collateral arteries (MAPCAs)
- Right arch with aberrant left subclavian artery
- Retroesophageal diverticulum

PATHOLOGY

- Regression of right 4th arch between right subclavian and right common carotid arteries, including right ductus arteriosus

CLINICAL ISSUES

- Most common congenital aortic arch abnormality (0.5-2.0%)
- 90-95% asymptomatic; incidental imaging finding
- Adults: Dysphagia (lusoria), dyspnea, back pain
- Infants: Cough, stridor, aspiration pneumonia
- Surgery for symptoms, aneurysm, or large diverticulum

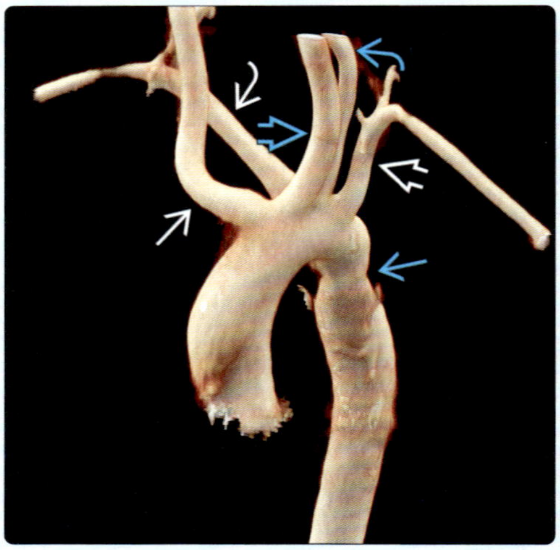

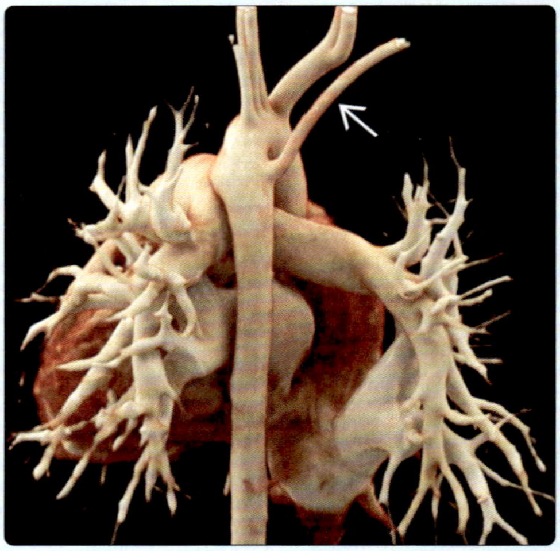

(Left) *CTA cinematic rendering reconstruction shows 5 branches from the aortic arch. From the proximal to distal, the branches are: Right common carotid artery, left internal carotid artery, left external carotid artery, left subclavian artery, and aberrant right subclavian artery (ARSA). Mild aortic coarctation is also noted.* **(Right)** *CTA cinematic rendering reconstruction shows ARSA that originates as the last branch from the aortic arch and courses behind the esophagus to reach the right.*

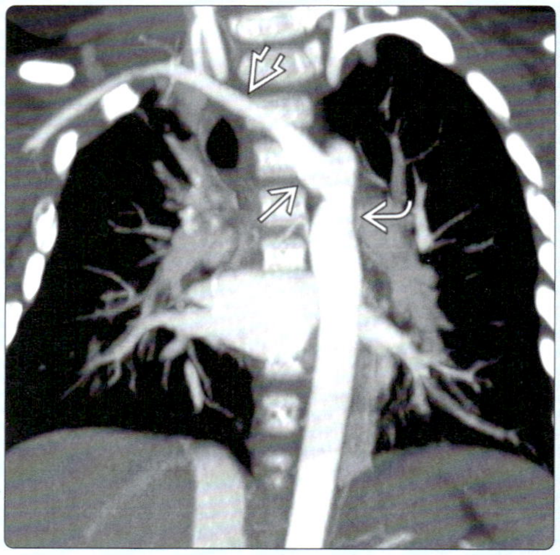

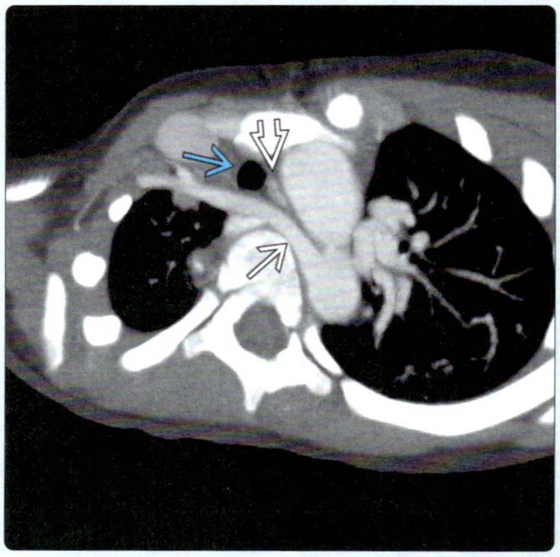

(Left) *Coronal oblique MIP CTA shows a prominent Kommerell diverticulum, which is a dilatation of a proximal ARSA that originates in the proximal descending aorta.* **(Right)** *Axial oblique MIP reconstruction from a CTA shows an ARSA with retroesophageal course causing esophageal compression between aortic arch, trachea, and ARSA.*

TERMINOLOGY

Abbreviations

- Aberrant right subclavian artery (ARSA)

Definitions

- Aberrant origin of right subclavian artery as last branch of left-sided aortic arch or proximal descending aorta

IMAGING

General Features

- Best diagnostic clue
  - Retroesophageal/retrotracheal course of ARSA
- Location
  - ARSA takeoff from distal aortic arch, isthmus, or proximal descending aorta
  - Course: Retroesophageal 80%; intertracheoesophageal 15%; pretracheal 5%
- Size
  - Usually normal vessel caliber
  - Dilated proximal segment in Kommerell diverticulum
  - Aneurysm may be present
- Morphology
  - No vascular ring formed by left aortic arch and ARSA
  - Loose vascular ring if ARSA originates from Kommerell diverticulum
    - Right ductus/ligamentum arteriosum completes ring
    - Seen in 15-30% of ARSA
  - Complete vascular ring if ARSA with circumflex right descending thoracic aorta and right ductus
    - Arch itself crosses midline, posterior to esophagus
    - Right ductus extends from descending aorta to right pulmonary artery, completing vascular ring

CT Findings

- CTA
  - Excellent modality to demonstrate aortic arch configuration and branching pattern
  - Evaluates esophageal and tracheal compression
- NECT: May be seen incidentally
- 4D CT: May show dynamic esophageal compression during cardiac cycle due to distension of ARSA during systole

MR Findings

- MRA
  - Arch vessel branching pattern is (from right to left): Right common carotid artery; left common carotid artery; left subclavian artery; right subclavian artery (RSA)
  - Course: Obliquely from caudal left to cranial right
  - Aneurysm of ARSA: 1.5x d of distal subclavian artery
  - Left ductus may be seen; no vascular ring
  - Posterior esophageal compression in 10%
    - Usually in 4th or 5th decade
    - Stretching, sclerosis/calcification, aneurysm of ARSA
  - Complete vascular ring may be seen if
    - Kommerell diverticulum: Dilation of origin of ARSA
    - Circumflex right descending thoracic aorta with arch behind esophagus

Imaging Recommendations

- Best imaging tool
  - CTA or MRA
- Protocol advice
  - ECG gating is not necessary if only evaluation of vascular ring is desired
    - High-pitch helical mode of dual source CT scanner (Flash) mode, provide anatomic information

DIFFERENTIAL DIAGNOSIS

Major Aortopulmonary Collateral Arteries

- Collateral vessels arising from descending aorta that end in lungs in patients with pulmonary artery atresia

Right Arch With Aberrant Left Subclavian Artery

- Mirror image of left arch with ARSA
- 90% have left ductus vascular ring

Retroesophageal Diverticulum

- Outpouching at origin of aberrant left subclavian artery in right aortic arch; seen in 60% of these cases

PATHOLOGY

General Features

- Etiology
  - Right 4th arch regresses between RSA and right common carotid artery, including ductus arteriosus
    - Distal right dorsal aorta forms proximal RSA
    - Distal portion from 7th right intersegmental artery
- Associated abnormalities
  - ARSA is present in 35% of patients with Down syndrome
  - Kommerell diverticulum: 14.9%
  - Aneurysm of distal RSCA: 12.8%
  - Others: Coarctation; patent ductus arteriosus; ventricular septal defect; truncus bicaroticus; type B interrupted arch

CLINICAL ISSUES

Presentation

- Most common signs/symptoms
  - 90-95% asymptomatic; usually incidental finding in imaging studies
- Other signs/symptoms
  - Adults: Dysphagia (lusoria), dyspnea, back pain, arm claudication, abnormal chest x-ray
  - Infants: Cough, stridor, occasionally aspiration pneumonia
  - Rare: Ruptured diverticulum; dissection

Demographics

- Sex: F:M = 3:1
- Epidemiology
  - Most common congenital aortic arch abnormality
  - Prevalence 0.5-2.0% of population

Treatment

- Surgery for symptoms, aneurysm, or large diverticulum

SELECTED REFERENCES

1. Robb CL et al: Subclavian artery: anatomic review and imaging evaluation of abnormalities. Radiographics. 42(7):2149-65, 2022

Pseudocoarctation

KEY FACTS

TERMINOLOGY

- Aortic arch elongation with kinking of thoracic aorta distal to origin of left subclavian artery at level of ductus arteriosus

IMAGING

- Frontal chest radiograph
  - Mass-like opacity in left superior mediastinum; may mimic mediastinal mass
  - Double left aortic arch and reverse 3 sign
  - No rib notching
- Lateral chest radiograph
  - Redundant aortic arch buckled forward at isthmus
- Best imaging tool: Contrast-enhanced 3D CT and MR angiography, phase-contrast CMR
  - Elongated distal aortic arch and proximal descending thoracic aorta with kinking and buckling
  - Evaluate for complications: Aneurysm formation, subclavian steal syndrome
- Pseudocoarctation of aorta (PCOA) distinguished from coarctation of aorta (COA) by
  - No hemodynamically significant aortic narrowing by MR or catheter angiography
  - No collateral arteries or significant poststenotic dilatation
  - No left ventricular hypertrophy

TOP DIFFERENTIAL DIAGNOSES

- Coarctation of aorta
- Aortic aneurysm
- Mediastinal mass

PATHOLOGY

- Elongation of distal aortic arch due to abnormal growth of preductal aorta

DIAGNOSTIC CHECKLIST

- Sagittal views for CTA and MRA are most useful for demonstrating PCOA

(Left) *Coronal oblique graphic in a patient with pseudocoarctation of the aorta (PCOA) demonstrates an elongated, kinked, and buckled aortic arch ➡ distal to the origin of left subclavian artery ➡ at the level of the ductus arteriosus.* **(Right)** *Sagittal oblique volume-rendered CTA shows kinking and mild narrowing ➡ of the proximal descending aorta at the level of the ligamentum arteriosum, consistent with pseudocoarctation. No enlarged collateral bronchial, intercostal, or internal mammary arteries are present.*

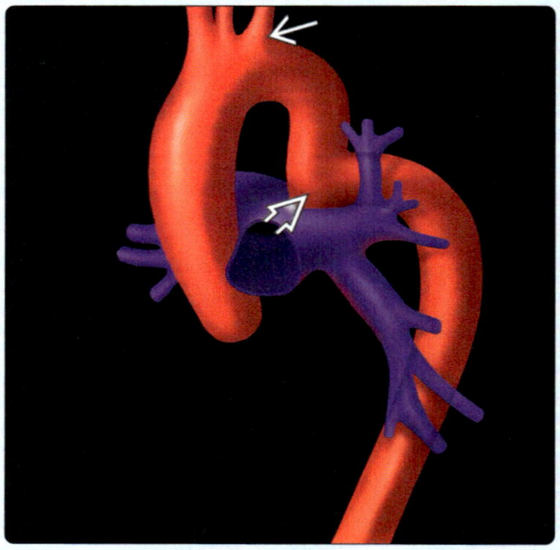

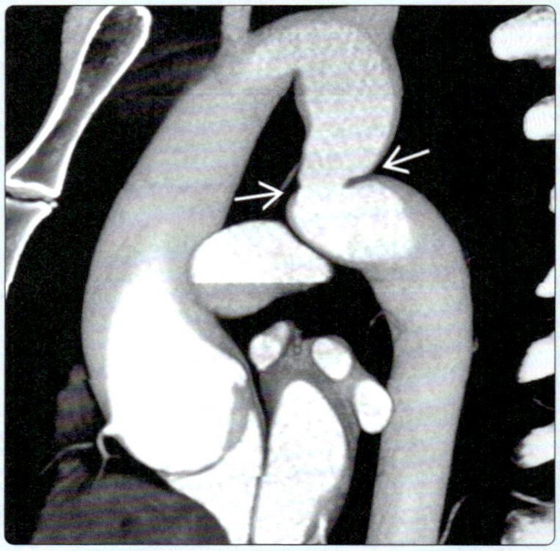

(Left) *Posteroanterior chest radiograph shows a prominent and high-riding aortic arch ➡. The normal heart size and absence of rib notching due to collateral vessels distinguish PCOA from coarctation of the aorta (COA).* **(Right)** *Lateral chest radiograph in the same patient demonstrates forward buckling of the aortic arch ➡ at the isthmus. The aorta ➡ is enlarged proximal to the narrowed segment ➡.*

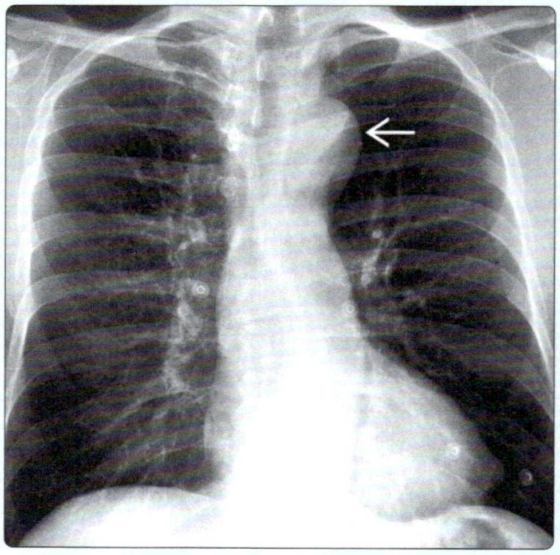

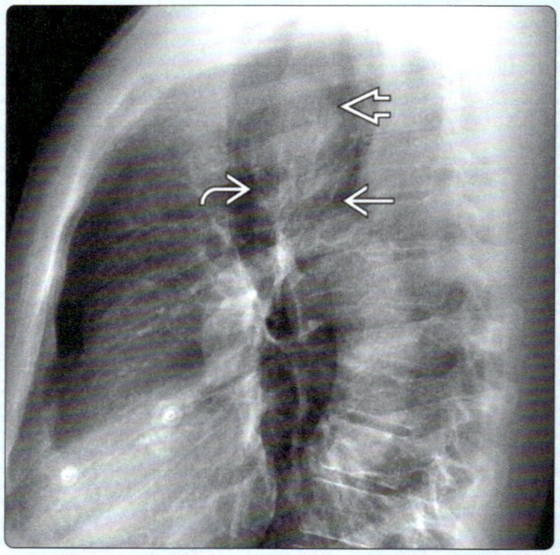

TERMINOLOGY

Abbreviations

- Pseudocoarctation of aorta (PCOA)

Synonyms

- Aortic buckling
- Aortic kinking
- Atypical coarctation
- Nonobstructive coarctation
- Redundant aortic arch

Definitions

- Elongation and kinking of aortic arch and proximal thoracic aorta distal to origin of left subclavian artery (SCA) at level of ductus arteriosus
- Distinguished from coarctation of aorta (COA) by lack of hemodynamically significant stenosis

IMAGING

General Features

- Best diagnostic clue
  - Kinking and buckling of aorta at level of ductus arteriosus with pressure gradient < 25 mmHg
- Location
  - Aortic isthmus at site of attachment of ligamentum arteriosum distal to origin of left SCA
- Size
  - Normal caliber or dilatation > 4 cm, or, occasionally, stenotic at site of aortic buckling
- Morphology
  - Elongation of distal aortic arch (AA) and proximal descending thoracic aorta (DTA); acute anterior angulation of AA at level of ligamentum arteriosum without significant obstruction

Imaging Recommendations

- Best imaging tool
  - CTA or MRA
- Protocol advice
  - 3D CTA in sagittal orientation with MIP and MPR reconstructions
  - 3D high-resolution MRA in sagittal view with MIP and volume rendering
  - Time-resolved MRA for evaluation of flow patterns and collateral pathways
  - Phase-contrast velocity-encoded sequence for measurement of peak velocities and pressure gradients
  - 4D flow MR for flow patterns and quantification

Radiographic Findings

- Frontal chest radiograph
  - Mediastinal widening, mass-like opacity in left superior mediastinum mimicking mediastinal mass or aneurysm
  - Double left AA sign
    - Aorta proximal to kinking appears higher than normal AA
    - Aorta distal to kinking appears lower than normal with tortuous AA course, producing S-shaped figure
  - Reverse 3 sign: Outlines medial side of aortic indentation in DTA and E sign in esophagogram
  - No rib notching
- Lateral chest radiograph
  - AA is buckled forward at isthmus

CT Findings

- NECT
  - Elongated and tortuous distal AA and proximal DTA
  - Anterior and medial displacement of distal AA
  - Kink in posterior and lateral margins of aorta at isthmus
- CTA
  - Elongated redundant distal AA and proximal DTA with kinking and buckling
  - Minimal or no luminal narrowing of distal transverse arch at attachment of ligamentum arteriosum
  - High AA extending into left supraclavicular region (children)
  - Bicuspid aortic valve may be present
  - Aortic aneurysm may be present
  - Poststenotic dilatation ± depending on hemodynamic significance
  - Abnormal origins of arch arteries; dilatation of brachiocephalic arteries
- General
  - Distinguished from COA based on absent hemodynamically significant aortic narrowing, poststenotic dilatation, collateral arteries, and left ventricular hypertrophy

MR Findings

- MRA
  - Contrast-enhanced 3D MRA
    - Kinking and buckling of elongated and tortuous distal AA and proximal DTA
    - May be associated with aortic aneurysms due to altered hemodynamics
  - Time-resolved MRA
    - May show steal phenomenon in presence of SCA stenosis as reversal of flow in vertebral artery
  - Phase-contrast flow MR
    - No elevation of velocity; normal/minimal increased pressure gradient (peak pressure gradient < 25 mmHg) across kink
    - Flow reversal in steal phenomenon
  - 4D flow CMR/4D phase-contrast CMR
    - Quantification of flow volume, retrograde flow/fraction in aorta, peak velocity and gradient at site of maximum kinking
    - 3D flow visualization of highly disrupted flow patterns in tortuous aorta
    - Elevated wall shear stress (WSS) in PCOA may contribute to aorta dilatation or pseudoaneurysm due to its correlation with blood flow velocity
    - Elevated flow velocity and elevated peak WSS seen in kinked aorta/ PCOA
    - Aneurysm sacs associated with PCOA shows vortex flow during systole with lower peak WSS

Angiographic Findings

- High position of AA
- Reverse 3 sign: Notch in descending aorta at attachment of short ligamentum arteriosum

- Gold standard for accurate pressure gradient measurement before intervention planning or if diagnostic uncertainty

DIFFERENTIAL DIAGNOSIS

Coarctation of Aorta

- Congenital narrowing of aorta at isthmus distal to left SCA origin
  - Diffuse hypoplasia of AA distal to origin of innominate artery may be associated
- Chest radiograph with rib notching or reverse E or 3 sign from pre- and poststenotic dilatation
- Hemodynamically significant stenosis
  - Elevated peak pressure gradient > 20 mmHg
  - Poststenotic aortic dilation
  - Collateral vessels: Internal mammary, intercostal, parascapular, epigastric arteries
    - Rib notching on chest XR
  - Left ventricular hypertrophy
- Both COA and PCOA associated with bicuspid aortic valve

Hypoplastic Aortic Arch

- Mostly in children; commonly seen in patients with COA
- If external diameter of distal arch segment is < 50% of ascending aorta; z-score of 2 or lower, no pressure gradient across narrowed portion

Aortic Aneurysm

- Usually seen in atherosclerotic aorta with calcified intimal plaque
- Saccular or fusiform dilatation with mural thrombus often present within periphery of aneurysm
- Commonly seen in older adult patients; may rupture or result in aortic dissection

Mediastinal Mass

- Mass-like opacity on chest radiograph
- CT and MR angiography can differentiate soft tissue mass from PCOA

PATHOLOGY

General Features

- Etiology
  - Elongated distal AA and proximal DTA due to failed compression of 3rd-7th dorsal aortic segments causing longer AA that kinks at ductus arteriosum level
  - Short taut ligamentum arteriosum or patent ductus arteriosus
- Associated abnormalities
  - Aberrant SCA; cervical AA; left superior vena cava, left vertebral artery origin from AA, aneurysmal dilatation of SCA
  - Aortic stenosis; sinus of Valsalva aneurysm; coarctation of distal descending aorta
  - Bicuspid aortic valve; aortic valve incompetence; mitral valve prolapse
  - Left-to-right shunts; atrial septal defect; ventricular septal defect; patent ductus arteriosus
  - Aortic aneurysm leading to sudden aortic rupture or aortic dissection

Microscopic Features

- Aneurysms associated with PCOA result from cystic medial necrosis rather than atherosclerosis

CLINICAL ISSUES

Presentation

- Most common signs/symptoms
  - Usually asymptomatic or resistant or difficult to treat hypertension

Demographics

- Epidemiology
  - Very uncommon congenital anomaly occurring in isolation or with other congenital heart diseases

Natural History & Prognosis

- Typically asymptomatic
  - Aneurysmal dilatation may develop; may result in rupture or dissection
    - Necessitates annual surveillance of thoracic aorta for early diagnosis and intervention of aortic aneurysm

Treatment

- Conservative management in asymptomatic and mildly symptomatic patients
- Surgical treatment for complications
  - Aneurysm formation
    - Open repair: Artificial or biologic grafts
    - Closed repair: Endovascular stent graft
  - Aortic dissection
    - Stanford type A: Surgery due to involvement of ascending aorta
    - Stanford type B: Medical control of hypertension is standard; surgery or endovascular stenting in complicated cases
  - Subclavian steal syndrome
    - Angioplasty/stenting of SCA
    - Common carotid artery-to-SCA bypass, innominate artery-to-SCA bypass, or axillary artery-to-axillary artery bypass

DIAGNOSTIC CHECKLIST

Image Interpretation Pearls

- Sagittal views for CTA and MRA are most useful for demonstrating PCOA
  - 3D CTA with MIP and MPR reconstructions
  - 3D MRA with MIP and volume rendering
- No hemodynamically significant aortic narrowing, poststenotic dilatation, left ventricular hypertrophy, or collateral arteries
  - Allows differentiation from COA

SELECTED REFERENCES

1. Mahadevappa M et al: Pseudocoarctation of the arch and the abdominal aorta: a review. Curr Cardiol Rev. 19(5):73-82, 2023
2. Ito H et al: Assessment of pseudocoarctation of the aorta with saccular aneurysms by four-dimensional flow magnetic resonance imaging and histological analysis. Ann Vasc Dis. 15(4):348-51, 2022
3. Dyverfeldt P et al: 4D flow cardiovascular magnetic resonance consensus statement. J Cardiovasc Magn Reson. 17:72, 2015
4. Singh S et al: Hypoplasia, pseudocoarctation and coarctation of the aorta - a systematic review. Heart Lung Circ. 24(2):110-8, 2015

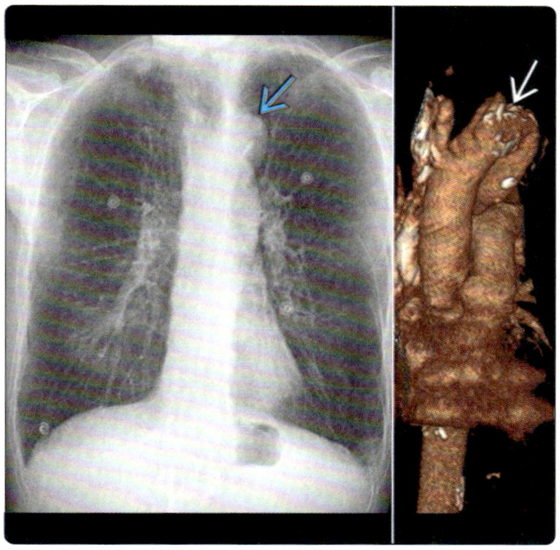

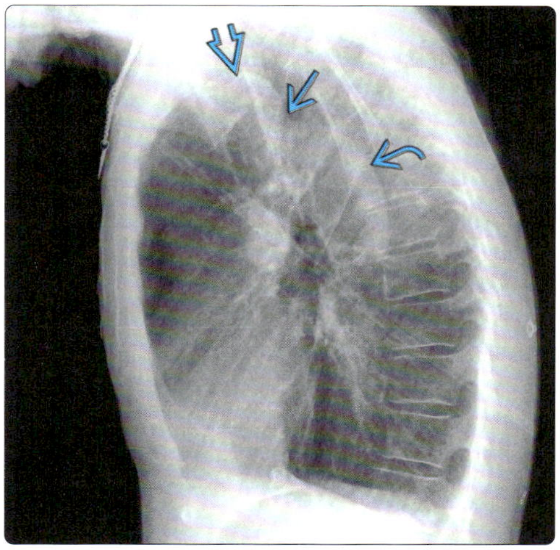

(Left) *PA radiograph with bone subtraction (left) in a 67-year-old man shows abnormal elongation of the proximal descending thoracic aorta (DTA), which can be visualized in coronal 3D volume-rendered image (right).* **(Right)** *Lateral radiograph shows elongation and superior extension of the aortic arch, which then courses inferiorly with kinking before taking its normal course. These findings are highly suggestive of pseudocoarctation.*

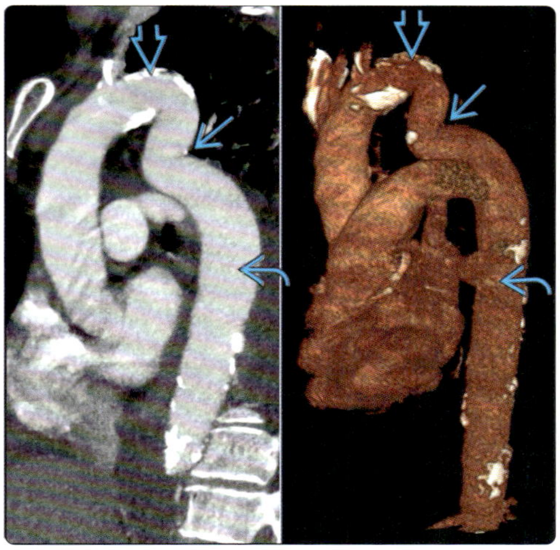

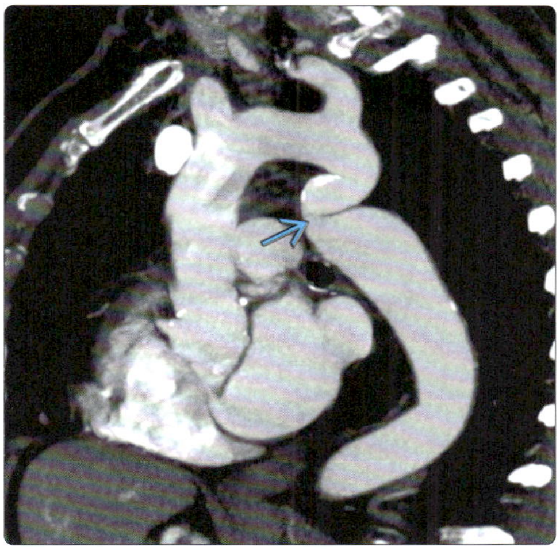

(Left) *MIP (left) and volume-rendered (right) images in the same patient show aortic PCOA with elongation and superior extension of the proximal DTA, which then extends inferiorly with kinking before taking its normal course.* **(Right)** *PCOA in an asymptomatic 72-year-old woman shows elongation and kinking of the proximal DTA. There was no gradient across the lesion on phase-contrast MR. The aorta is aneurysmal distal to PCOA, measuring 3.5 cm.*

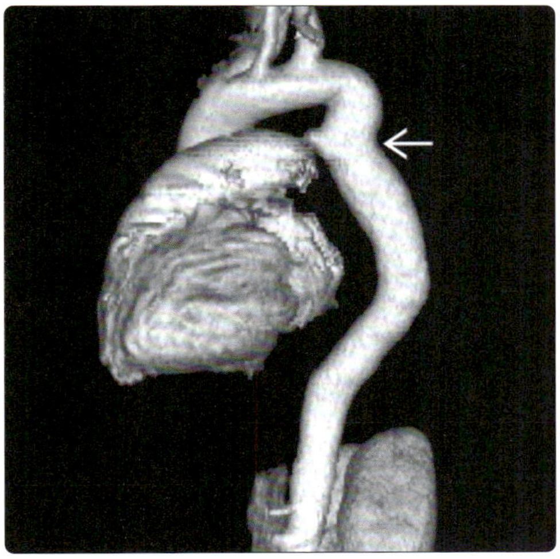

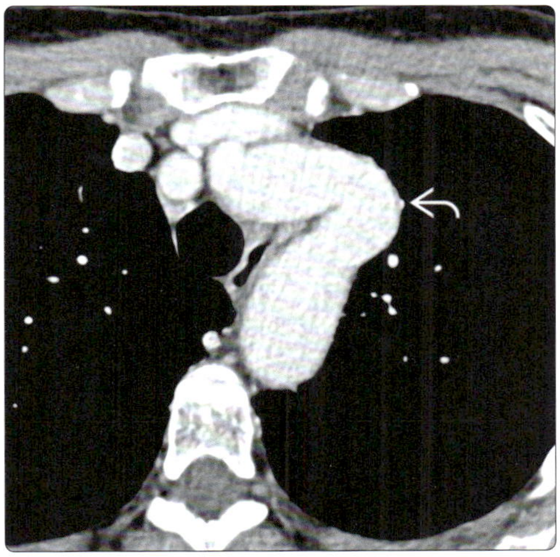

(Left) *Sagittal 3D volume-rendered CTA in a patient with PCOA demonstrates kinking and mild narrowing of the proximal descending aorta at the level of the ligamentum arteriosum.* **(Right)** *Axial CECT in a patient with PCOA shows marked kinking and buckling of the aortic arch. No enlarged collateral bronchial, intercostal, or internal mammary arteries are identified.*

Ductus Diverticulum

KEY FACTS

TERMINOLOGY

- Smooth focal bulge along anteromedial aspect of aortic isthmus at site of obliterated ductus arteriosus

IMAGING

- Chest radiography
  - Frontal: Opacity in aortopulmonary window
  - Lateral: Small, bump-like opacity at distal transverse aortic arch
- Contrast-enhanced CTA or MRA
  - Differentiate between typical and atypical appearances
  - Evaluate for aneurysmal dilatation
  - Differentiate from traumatic pseudoaneurysm
- Ductus diverticulum aneurysm
  - Saccular dilatation along anterior inferior margin of aortic isthmus
  - Superior margin of aneurysm extends to left subclavian artery
- Differentiate from traumatic pseudoaneurysm
  - Presence of smooth, uninterrupted margins of diverticulum
  - No dissection flap
  - Absence of mediastinal or periaortic hematoma

TOP DIFFERENTIAL DIAGNOSES

- Aortic isthmus (traumatic) pseudoaneurysm
- Aortic ulcerated atherosclerotic plaque
- Aortic aneurysm
- Kommerell diverticulum
- Patent ductus arteriosus

CLINICAL ISSUES

- Typically incidental finding
  - Most patients are asymptomatic
- Aneurysmal dilatation of ductus diverticulum necessitates intervention if > 3 cm
  - Endovascular stent graft or conventional open surgical repair

(Left) *Graphic demonstrates normal anatomy of the great vessels and the presence of a ductus diverticulum (DD) →, part of the remnant of the embryologic ductus arteriosus that connected the pulmonary arteries and the aorta in utero. The rest of the ductus becomes the ligamentum arteriosum →.* **(Right)** *Axial (left) and sagittal oblique (right) images in a 85-year-old woman show a broad-based DD → with rim calcification. This is a common finding in patients of all ages and should not be confused with pathology.*

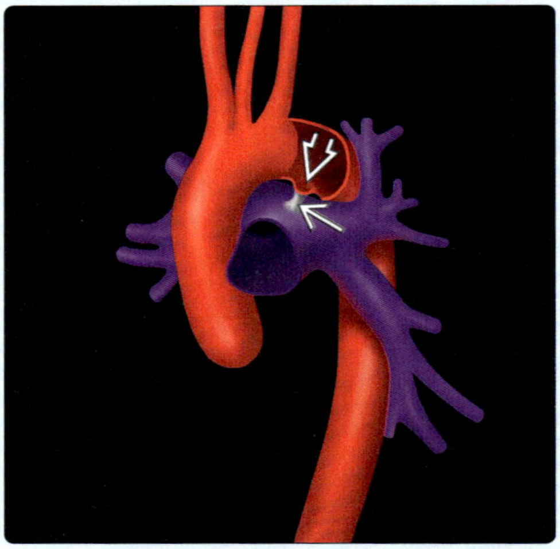

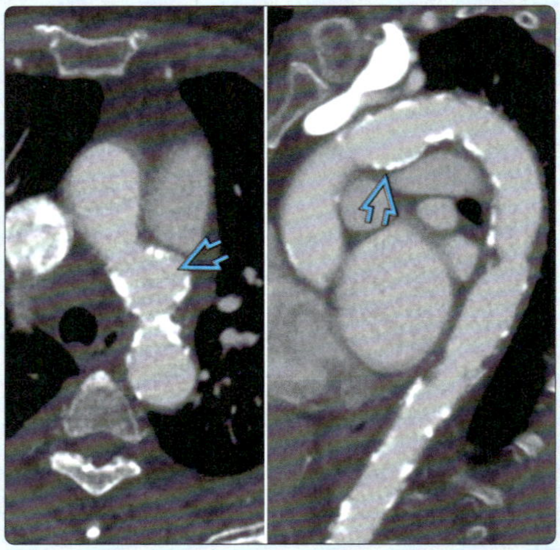

(Left) *Axial CECT shows a typical DD → arising from the very proximal portion of the descending thoracic aorta (DTA), just distal to the left subclavian artery.* **(Right)** *Coronal reformatted CECT demonstrates a typical DD →. The close proximity of the DD to the pulmonary trunk reflects its underlying etiology as the remnant of the infundibular part of the ductus arteriosus that connected the pulmonary artery to the aortic arch in utero.*

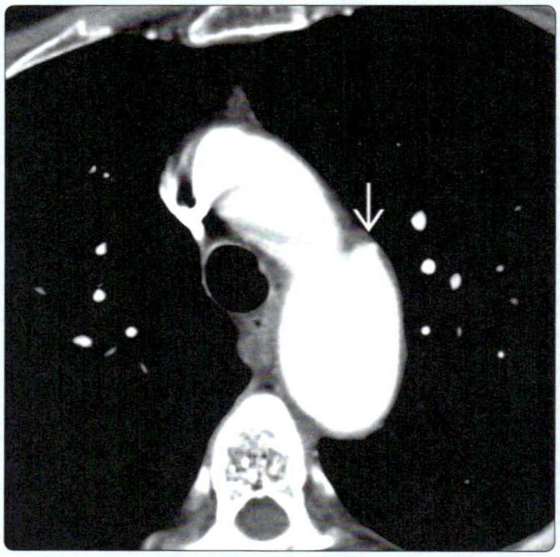

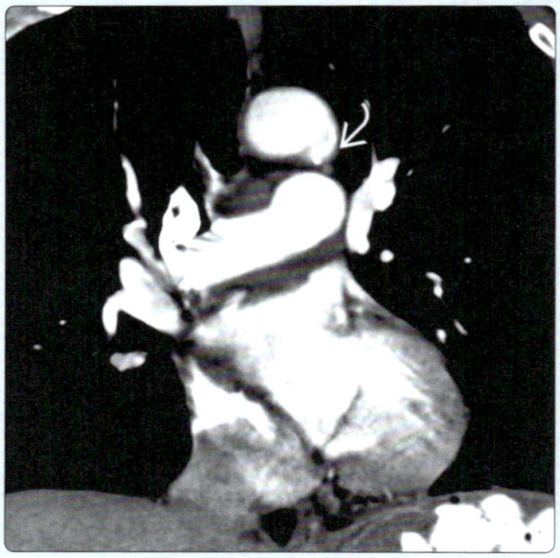

TERMINOLOGY

Synonyms

- Ductus bulge; ductus bump

Definitions

- Smooth focal bulge along anteromedial aspect of aortic isthmus at site of obliterated ductus arteriosus/ligamentum arteriosum

IMAGING

General Features

- Best diagnostic clue
  - Well-defined, smooth, broad-based outpouching from anteromedial aspect/lesser curvature of aortic isthmus with obtuse angle with aorta
  - Mediastinum and aorta are otherwise unremarkable
- Location
  - Along anteromedial aspect of aortic isthmus
- Size
  - Usually small bulge
  - May increase aortic diameter by average of 4.3 mm
  - Unusually enlarged ductus referred to as aneurysm
    - Aneurysmal dilatation of ductus diverticulum > 3 cm needs surgical intervention
- Morphology
  - Smooth bulging of aortic side of ductus arteriosus

Imaging Recommendations

- Best imaging tool
  - 3D CT or MR angiography (CTA, MRA)
- Protocol advice
  - Contrast-enhanced CTA
    - Sagittal oblique thin-slice (≤ 1 mm) reconstructed images
      - □ Essential to identify and assess relationship of ductus with pulmonary artery (PA), aortic arch, and subclavian artery (SCA)
      - □ Visualize smooth shoulders of ductus diverticulum
    - Volume-rendering technique (VRT)
      - □ To convey 3D anatomic relationships with adjacent vessels and structures than MIP
  - Noncontrast 3D slap MRA or contrast-enhanced MRA
    - Sagittal oblique and coronal thin reconstructed MIP
    - Consider sagittal oblique and axial black-blood imaging

Radiographic Findings

- Frontal chest radiograph
  - May manifest as opacity in aortopulmonary window
- Lateral chest radiograph
  - Small, bump-like opacity at distal arch/isthmus

CT Findings

- General
  - Best visualized on sagittal oblique reconstructed images
  - May be difficult to identify ductus diverticulum on axial due to partial volumining from oblique orientation
- Typical appearance
  - Broad-based, contrast-filled outpouching at anteromedial aortic isthmus extending blindly inferiorly toward main PA
    - Best clue: Smooth, uninterrupted margins; gently sloping, symmetric shoulders; obtuse angles with aorta at its superior and inferior margins
  - Increase in aortic lumen ≤ 1 cm
  - Smaller vertical height diameter (5.5 mm vs. 11.2 mm) and broader base (14.9 mm vs. 8.8 mm) compared with traumatic pseudoaneurysm
- Atypical appearance
  - Steep and asymmetric sloping
  - Acute angles at superior margin with loss of gentle superior angle
  - Ductus may fold back against aorta and result in pseudointimal flap
- Ductus diverticulum aneurysm
  - Saccular dilatation along inferior margin of aortic isthmus opposite origin of left SCA
  - Superior margin of aneurysm extends to left SCA
  - Axial CTA images may show typical 3-star sign at aortopulmonary window
    - Proximal arch, descending aorta, and saccular aneurysm of diverticulum appear as hook-shaped structure
  - Detection of small pedicle/fibrotic portion of ductus linking aneurysm to PA differentiate ductal aneurysm from aneurysm of aorta
  - Partial thrombosis of ductus diverticulum aneurysm can be FDG avid on 18F-FDG PET/CT due to inflammation of wall

MR Findings

- MRA
  - MRA and postcontrast GRE images help exclude pseudoaneurysm from atypical ductus diverticulum
  - Findings similar to those on CTA
    - Smooth outpouching at anteromedial aspect of aortic isthmus
    - No dissection flap

Angiographic Findings

- Contrast-filled, well-defined smooth outpouching arising from anterior inferior margin of aortic isthmus
- No dissection flap
  - Pseudodissection flap may be seen with diverticulum that is folded over
- Contrast retention is rarely seen in atypical ductus diverticulum on delayed angiogram views
  - Typically occurs in traumatic pseudoaneurysm
- Aneurysm of ductus diverticulum
  - Saccular dilatation along anterior inferior margin of aortic isthmus
  - Superior margin of aneurysm extends to left SCA

DIFFERENTIAL DIAGNOSIS

Pseudoaneurysm at Aortic Isthmus (Pseudoductus)

- Due to partial or complete aortic transection
  - Contrast-filled, irregular outpouching
    - Varying size/shape; relatively longer vertical diameter
    - Due to focal disruption of intima and media

- Narrow base and acute angles at cranial and caudal ends
- Intimal flap in underlying aorta
- Mediastinal or periaortic hematoma
- May compress aortic lumen
- Delayed clearance of contrast on angiography

Ulcerated Atherosclerotic Plaque at Aortic Isthmus

- Contrast-filled, irregular outpouching
- Commonly associated with mural thickening and Ca^{++}
- Solitary or multifocal
- Typically seen in older adult patients

Aortic Aneurysm

- Typically atherosclerotic in etiology, seen in older adults
- Not usually localized to region of ductus
- Saccular aneurysm involves anterolateral aorta
- Absence of small fibrotic pedicle seen with ductal aneurysm

Kommerell Diverticulum

- Dilatation/aneurysm of aberrant right/ left SCA origin
- May be associated with right aortic arch and vascular ring

Patent Ductus Arteriosus

- Beyond 3 months after birth
- Left-to-right shunt via funnel, tubular or window-type connection

PATHOLOGY

General Features

- Etiology
  - In developing fetus, ductus arteriosus connects PA to descending aorta for right-to-left shunt
    - Allows most of blood from right ventricle to bypass fetal lungs in utero
    - Normally closes after birth, functionally within 24 to 48 hours and anatomically in 1 week to 2 months
  - Ductus diverticulum is embryologic remnant of infundibular part of ductus arteriosus or remnant of right dorsal aortic root
    - Located at transition from aortic arch to descending aorta called aortic isthmus
      - Aortic isthmus is slightly constricted part of proximal descending thoracic aorta immediately distal to left SCA at attachment point of ductus arteriosus
      - Aortic spindle is small, circumferential bulge just below aortic isthmus
- Associated abnormalities
  - Aneurysm of ductus diverticulum
  - Patent ductus arteriosus
  - Ductus diverticulum common (21%) in acute type B aortic dissection (TBAD)
  - Primary entry tears in acute TBAD located at ductus diverticulum orifice

Staging, Grading, & Classification

- Classification based on appearance
  - Typical, atypical
- Classification of aortic isthmus
  - Type I: Concave contour of aortic isthmus with parallel walls and uniform diameter; most common type
  - Type II: Mild straightening or convexity of aortic isthmus without discrete bulge
  - Type III: Ductus diverticulum: Discrete focal bulge of aortic isthmus least common type (8-26%)

CLINICAL ISSUES

Presentation

- Most common signs/symptoms
  - Asymptomatic
  - Typically incidental finding

Demographics

- Age: More common in children than in adults
- Dissection patients with ductus diverticulum were relatively younger than TBAD alone
- Sex: M = F
- Epidemiology
  - 33% of infants
  - 9-26% of adults in angiography study

Natural History & Prognosis

- Diverticulum usually shrinks over time
  - Small, residual bump at isthmus
- Rarely ductus aneurysm formation in
  - Hypertensive and older adults with atherosclerotic aorta
  - Behçet disease, Marfan and Ehlers-Danlos syndromes
  - Following surgical closure of patent ductus arteriosus
  - Rupture, dissection, thromboembolism, phrenic nerve compression, and infection of aneurysm may occur
- Ligamentum arteriosum (fibrous band) develops from obliteration of ductus arteriosus at aortic isthmus and can develop linear calcification

Treatment

- Usually no treatment required
- Aneurysmal dilatation of ductus diverticulum → intervention if > 3 cm, or enlarging or symptomatic
  - Endovascular stent graft repair
  - Conventional open surgical repair
  - Endovascular coil embolization if standard thoracic endovascular aortic repair (TEVAR) method is unsuccessful

DIAGNOSTIC CHECKLIST

Image Interpretation Pearls

- Best imaging tool: 3D CT or MR angiography (CTA, MRA)
- Best visualized on sagittal oblique reformatted CTA/MRA/angiography images
- Differentiate from traumatic pseudoaneurysm
  - Smooth, uninterrupted margins, broad base with aorta, smaller vertical height
  - Absence of dissection flap
  - Absence of mediastinal or periaortic hematoma

SELECTED REFERENCES

1. Chen D et al: Association of ductus diverticulum and acute type B aortic dissection. Acad Radiol. 30(11):2541-7, 2023
2. Celik E et al: The aortic ductus diverticulum-innocent bystander or potential source of thromboembolic stroke? J Comput Assist Tomogr. 46(3):392-6, 2022

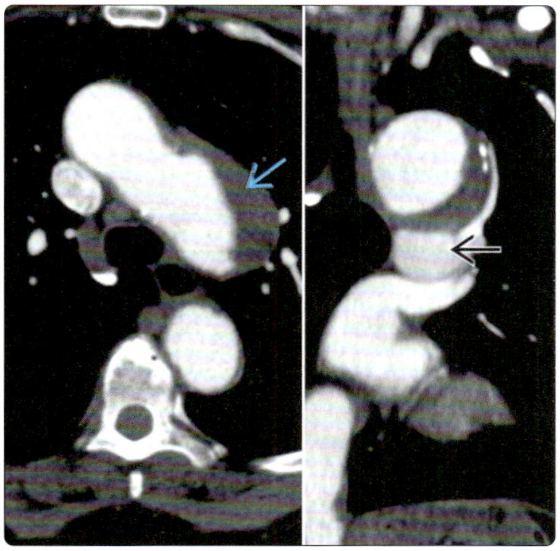

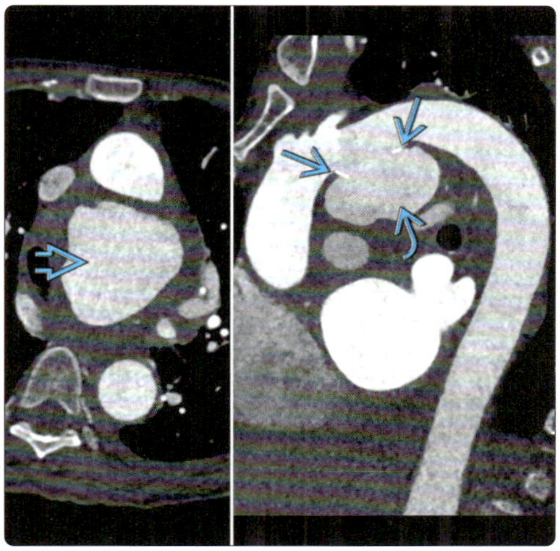

(Left) *CECT though the inferior aspect of the proximal DTA shows a partially thrombosed 4.8-cm ductal aneurysm (DA) ➔ with compression of the left pulmonary artery ➔ on coronal oblique image.* **(Right)** *Axial CECT (left) shows spontaneous contained rupture of a 6 x 4 cm DA ➔ with surrounding hematoma. Sagittal oblique CECT (right) shows the large DA ➔ with small calcifications ➔ along its edge, which are common. There is no aortic atherosclerotic disease. (Courtesy S. Kligerman, MD.)*

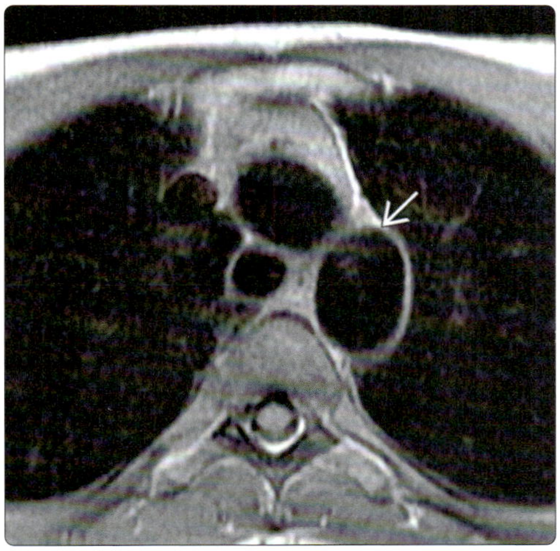

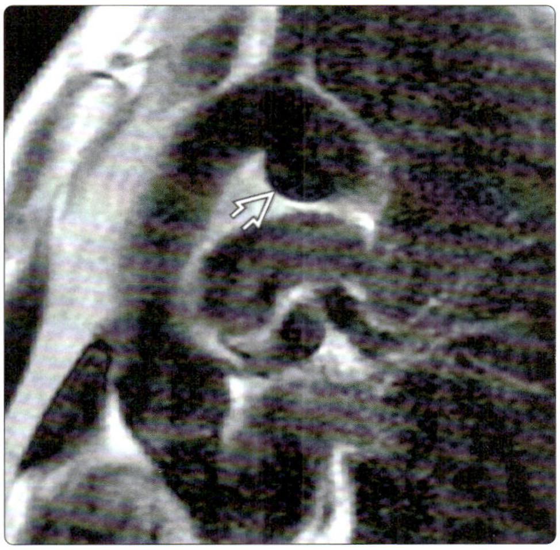

(Left) *Axial black-blood MR of an asymptomatic patient demonstrates focal outpouching ➔ of the anterior wall of aortic isthmus.* **(Right)** *Sagittal black-blood MR in the same patient shows smooth outpouching ➔ from the anteromedial wall of aortic isthmus. These findings are classic for a DD. The absence of an intimal flap and the lack of mediastinal or periaortic hematoma essentially exclude the possibility of a traumatic pseudoaneurysm.*

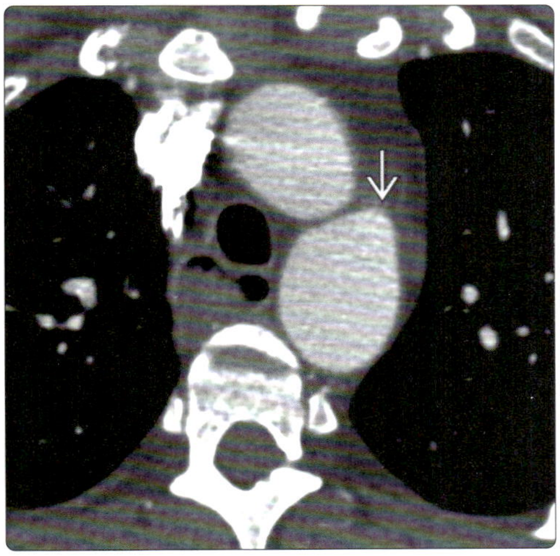

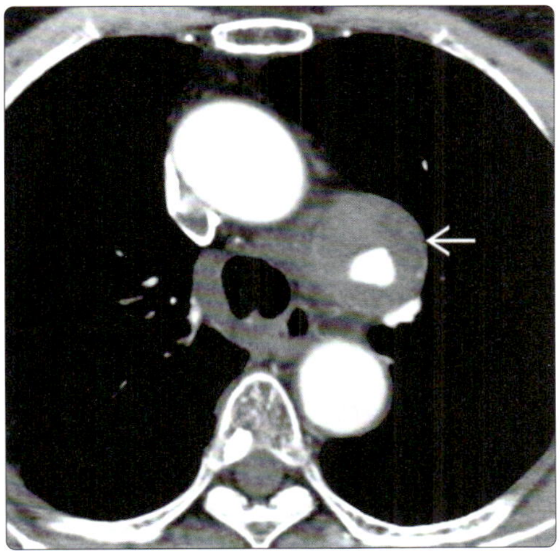

(Left) *Axial CECT demonstrates focal outpouching ➔ from the anterior wall of the aortic isthmus, consistent with a typical DD.* **(Right)** *Axial CECT shows a partially thrombosed DD aneurysm ➔. Although most patients are asymptomatic and require no treatment, the presence of aneurysmal dilatation > 3 cm necessitates endovascular stent graft or open surgical repair.*

KEY FACTS

TERMINOLOGY

- Aortic dilatation > 50% of normal diameter
- Etiology
  - Heritable syndromes with multisystem features
  - Heritable but nonsyndromic
  - Congenital [more common in aortic aneurysm (AA) in younger patients]
  - Degenerative [more common in descending thoracic aorta (DTA) in older patients]
  - Inflammatory; infectious

IMAGING

- Radiography
  - Ascending AA: Curvilinear density along right aspect of mediastinum but often absent
  - Aortic arch aneurysm: Enlarged/obscured aortic arch
  - DTA aneurysm: Focal or diffuse abnormality of left paraaortic interface
- CT
  - High spatial resolution allows for precise measurements
  - AA often has no or limited atherosclerotic disease and more common in heritable and congenital cases
  - DTA aneurysm commonly degenerative and associated with calcified and noncalcified atherosclerotic disease, often with mural thrombus
- MR
  - Excellent for assessment of aortic wall
  - Evaluation of aortic valve and cardiac function
- PET/CT can help diagnose and monitor vasculitis

PATHOLOGY

- Variable depending on cause

CLINICAL ISSUES

- Repair of AA or DTA if ≥ 5.5 cm or smaller if rapid growth or symptomatic
- Repair criteria different based on syndromic and nonsyndromic heritable aneurysms or bicuspid aortic valve

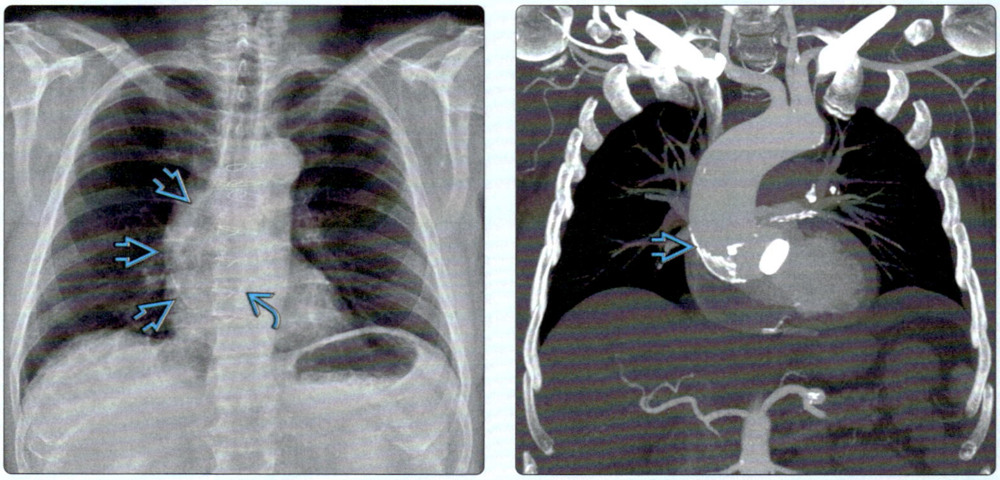

(Left) *PA radiograph in a 73-year-old man with a history of bicuspid valve status post repair shows abnormal right-sided convexity along the superior cardiomediastinal silhouette, suggestive of an ascending aortic (AA) aneurysm. In this case, atherosclerotic calcifications allow for partial visualization of the AA.* **(Right)** *Coronal CECT MIP in the same patient shows the AA atherosclerosis. The AA is aneurysmal with a maximum diameter of 5 cm.*

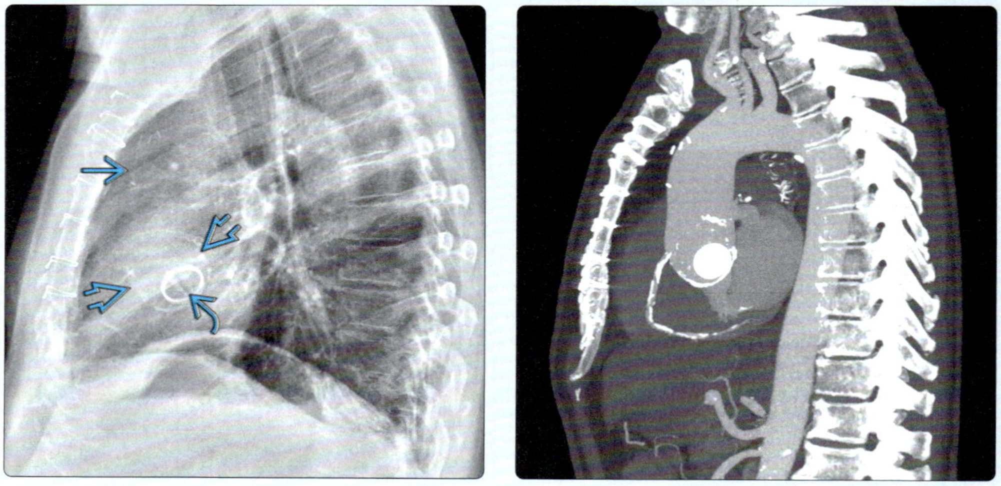

(Left) *Lateral radiograph shows a prosthetic aortic valve with surrounding calcification of the aortic root and AA. A portion of the more superior AA can be partially visualized due to atherosclerosis and adjacent surgical clips from prior aortotomy.* **(Right)** *Sagittal CECT MIP shows the contours of the AA in related to the sternum and other mediastinal structures. While the AA is aneurysmal with a maximum transverse diameter of 5 cm, the aortic arch and descending thoracic aorta (DTA) are normal in size.*

TERMINOLOGY

Abbreviations

- Thoracic aortic aneurysm (TAA)

Definitions

- Aortic dilatation **> 50% of normal diameter**
  - > 2 standard deviations (SDs) above mean
- Per 2022 American College of Cardiology (ACC)/American Heart Association (AHA) Guideline for Diagnosis and Management of Aortic Disease
  - "Aneurysm" should be used when ascending aorta (AA) measures ≥ 4.5 cm due to significant increased risk of dissection
    - For descending thoracic aorta (DTA), aneurysm would be classified at 1.5x mean diameter, which is ~ 4 cm
  - "Dilated" should be used when AA diameter < 4.5 cm but > 2 SDs above mean for age, sex, and body surface area (BSA)
- Aneurysm definition is variable as "normal" size varies depending on age, sex, and associated conditions
  - Diameter of aorta increases with age
    - In one study of patients undergoing lung cancer screening, average and SDs of ascending aortic diameter was 3.21 ± 0.38, 3.35 ± 0.37, and 3.46 ± 0.35 for patients in age groups 55-59, 60-64, and 65-74 years, respectively
  - Diameter is larger in men than women
    - Men (wall-to-wall measurement)
      - □ In 3 large studies, AA mean ranged from 34.1-36 mm
      - □ In Framingham heart study, 41.9 mm was 2 SDs above mean
      - □ For DTA [measured at level of main pulmonary artery (PA)] mean diameter was 25.8 ± 3.0 mm
    - Women
      - □ In 3 large studies, AA mean ranged from 31.9-33.5 mm
      - □ In Framingham heart study, 38.9 mm was 2 SDs above mean
      - □ For DTA (measured at level of main PA) mean diameter was 23.1 ± 2.6 mm
  - Diameter will be larger if measuring entire wall-to-wall diameter vs. measuring only intraluminal area (IA)
    - Men
      - □ In one large study, wall-to-wall diameter > 2 SDs: 40.2, 42.9, and 45.0 mm in age groups 20-40, 41-60, > 60 years, respectively
      - □ IA diameter > 2 SDs: 37.8, 40.5, and 42.6 mm in age groups 20-40, 41-60, > 60 years, respectively
    - Women
      - □ Wall-to-wall diameter > 2 SDs: 38, 40.7, and 42.4 mm for women in age groups 20-40, 41-60, > 60 years, respectively
      - □ > 2 SDs for IA diameter: 35.6, 38.3, and 40 mm in age groups 20-40, 41-60, > 60 years, respectively
  - Diameter is larger if measuring on axial image vs. MPR to get true transverse diameter
    - In one study
      - □ Men: Mean diameter decreases from 3.48 ± 0.36 to 3.41 ± 0.37 between axial and MPR measurements, respectively
      - □ Women: Mean diameter decreases from 3.27 ± 0.36 to 3.22 ± 0.38 between axial and MPR measurements, respectively
  - Diameter increases with increasing BSA
    - e.g., in Framingham Heart Study for men > 65 years of age, mean AA diameter increased from 35.3 to 36.3 to 38.3 with BSA < 1.9, 1.9-2.09, and ≥ 2.1, respectively
    - Similarly, for women 45-54 years of age, mean AA diameter increased from 29.7 to 31.5 to 32.5 with BSA < 1.9, 1.9-2.09, and ≥ 2.1, respectively
    - Similar trends were seen across nearly all age groups and BSAs

Causes of Thoracic Aortic Aneurysms

- Heritable syndromes with multisystem features
  - ~ 20% of TAAs due to genetic or heritable condition
  - Marfan syndrome
    - Aortic root dilation and type A dissection are major causes of morbidity and mortality in these patients
  - Loeys-Dietz syndrome
  - Vascular Ehlers-Danlos syndrome
  - Smooth muscle dysfunction syndrome
  - Others
- Heritable but nonsyndromic
  - Mutations in *ACTA2*, *MYH11*, *PRKG1*, *MYLK*, and others
  - Familial TAAs without identified pathogenic genetic variant known to cause heritable syndrome
- Congenital (more common in AA in younger patients)
  - Bicuspid aortic valve (BAV)
  - Turner syndrome
  - Coarctation of aorta
  - Complex congenital heart disease
- Degenerative (more common in DTA in older patients)
  - Atherosclerosis
  - Hypertension
- Inflammatory
  - Vasculitis
    - Giant cell arteritis
    - Takayasu arteritis
    - Behçet disease
  - IgG4-related disease
  - ANCA-related disease
  - Sarcoidosis
- Infectious (pseudoaneurysm common)
  - Bacterial
  - Fungal
  - Syphilitic
- Posttraumatic (pseudoaneurysm common)

IMAGING

Radiographic Findings

- Radiography
  - **May not be visible (frequent)**
  - Contour abnormality along aortic interface
  - Aortic ascending aneurysm
    - Abnormal convexity along superior right cardiomediastinal silhouette in frontal radiograph

- Fullness of retrosternal space in lateral radiograph
- Rightward tracheal &/or esophageal deviation
- Hilum overlay sign (in distal arch and descending aortic aneurysm)
- Lateralization of left paraaortic interface (in descending aortic aneurysm)
- Ruptured aneurysm
  - Mediastinal widening compared with prior studies
  - Pleural effusions

CT Findings

- Contrast-enhanced CT is excellent tool for aortic assessment
  - ECG-gated preferred for AA assessment
- Aorta measured using multiplanar reconstructions as axial measurements overestimate size
  - Typical landmarks include sinuses of Valsalva, sinotubular junction, maximum AA (often near level of main PA), distal AA, aortic arch, proximal DTA, mid-DTA, distal DTA near diaphragmatic hiatus
- Commonly used terms and definitions
  - Aneurysm
    - AA: ≥ 4.5 cm
      - More commonly encountered in younger patients with little degenerative changes to AA, even with sporadic cases
    - DTA: ≥ 4 cm
      - Most common encountered in older patients with prominent atherosclerotic disease
  - Dilation or ectasia
    - AA: ≥ 4cm, < 4.5cm
- Morphology
  - Fusiform
    - Symmetric dilation of aorta
    - Most common
  - Saccular
    - Asymmetric bulging of aorta
    - Can be seen with both true aneurysm and pseudoaneurysm
    - Often encountered in arch or proximal DTA
  - Annuloaortic ectasia (AAE)
    - Conspicuous dilation of aortic root and AA leading to effacement of sinotubular junction
    - Associated with heritable syndromes
- Specific patterns and associations
  - Marfan, vascular Ehlers-Danlos, Loeys-Dietz: AAE
    - Marked tortuosity of vertebral arteries in Loeys-Dietz
  - BAV: Variable morphology
    - Root phenotype (20%)
      - BAV with aortic regurgitation: Diffuse dilatation of aorta from root to arch
    - Ascending phenotype (70%)
      - BAV with aortic stenosis: Dilatation in tubular AA most common
      - More common in Sievert type 1 BAV (fused raphe)
    - Extended phenotype
      - Dilation from aortic root through proximal half of aortic arch
      - More common in Sievert type 0 BAV (true bicuspid without fused raphe)
  - Degenerative: Most commonly affects DTA with calcified and noncalcified atherosclerotic disease
    - Often associated with mural thrombus
      - Can be crescentic or circumferential
    - Contrast can invaginate between areas of mural thrombus and can mimic penetrating atherosclerotic ulcer
      - However, contrast does not extend beyond confined of aortic wall with irregular mural thrombus
  - Turner syndrome: Coarctation with aneurysm being less common
  - Vasculitis: Aortic wall thickening with associated areas of aneurysmal dilation and stenosis; aortic wall enhancement may be present
  - Infectious
    - Bacterial and fungal: Saccular aneurysm with paraortic soft tissue stranding, fluid, or mass
      - Often with rapid progression and pseudoaneurysm formation
      - Signs of infection in adjacent structure
      - Enhancement in aortic wall
    - Syphilitic: Calcified ascending aortic aneurysm with circumferential wall thickening; wall can enhance on delayed imaging
    - Rupture: Ill-defined aortic wall with surrounding mediastinal hematoma &/or hemothorax

MR Findings

- Similar findings as CT
  - Obtained without use of radiation
  - Similar specific patterns as described above
  - Gated MRA should be performed if possible for root assessment
- Can measure aorta during different phases of cardiac cycle
  - Aortic measurements will be larger during systole
- Additional value
  - T2W imaging to assess for wall edema and plaque characterization
  - T1W/T1W+ imaging to assess for wall enhancement and plaque characterization
  - Delayed enhancement: Assess wall fibrosis (not commonly used)
  - 4D flow: Assess aortic flow patterns

Nuclear Medicine Findings

- PET/CT
  - Excellent tool for differentiating aortic inflammation or infection from other causes of TAA
  - Helpful in monitoring for active disease

Imaging Recommendations

- Best imaging tool
  - CT or MR for evaluation of aneurysm location and size, relationship to major branch vessels, and complications [e.g., dissection, mural thrombus, intramural hematoma (IMH), free rupture]
- Protocol advice
  - ECG gating for anatomic and functional aortic valve assessment
  - MR angiography can be performed with contrast and noncontrast techniques

DIFFERENTIAL DIAGNOSIS

Tortuosity (Aging) of Aorta

- Diffuse aortic redundancy
- May require cross-sectional imaging for assessment

Mediastinal Mass

- Radiographic differentiation from neoplasm may be challenging and at times not possible
- Hilum overlay classic in anterior mediastinal masses
- Curvilinear calcification typical of vascular lesions

Pseudoaneurysm

- Contained rupture of aorta contained by piece of adventitia
  - Extends beyond normal aortic wall
- Can mimic saccular aneurysm
- Common after previous aortic surgery, trauma, or infection
- Can have narrow or wide neck but extends beyond regular confines of aortic wall
- Often has surrounding inflammatory changes
- Disruption of intimal calcification with pseudoaneurysm

Acute Aortic Syndrome

- Aortic dissection (AD), IMH, and penetrating aortic ulcer (PAU) often occur in setting of TAA
- Acute aortic syndrome (AAS) is often symptomatic, whereas TAA is often asymptomatic unless ruptured or causing compression
- During acute stage, imaging findings of AAS can mimic certain findings seen with TAA
  - Mural thrombus in TAA can mimic IMH in some instances
    - In IMH, blood in wall of aorta will often have smooth crescentic shape but can be circumferential
    - Contour is more irregular with mural thrombus
    - Intramural blood in IMH is often more dense that layering mural thrombus in TAA
      - Best seen on noncontrast imaging
  - PAU can be difficult to differentiate from aneurysm with mural thrombus
    - PAU extends beyond confines of aortic wall
    - Discontinuity of atherosclerotic calcification often seen
    - Surrounding hematoma may be present
- Additionally, imaging findings with healed AAS can also mimic findings seen with TAA
  - False lumen of AD can thrombose and mimic aneurysm with mural thrombus
    - Thrombosed false lumen usually has crescentic shape
    - False lumen may be patent elsewhere along aorta

PATHOLOGY

General Features

- **True aneurysm**: Contains all 3 aortic wall layers
- **Atherosclerotic aortic aneurysm**
  - Degenerative process, most common (75%)
    - Old age, smoking, hypertension
  - Shape: Fusiform > saccular
  - Location: Most common in DTA
- **Infectious (mycotic) aneurysm**: Saccular; any location
  - Predisposing causes: IV drug abuse, valvular disease, congenital aortic/cardiac disease, prior aortic/cardiac surgery, adjacent pyogenic infection, immunocompromise
  - Most common pathogens: *Salmonella* spp. and *S. aureus*
  - Shape: Saccular
  - Often pseudoaneurysms
- **Cystic medial necrosis**
  - Degeneration of aortic media with medial necrosis
    - Degeneration and fragmentation of elastic fibers, loss of smooth muscle cells, and interstitial collections of basophilic-staining ground substance
  - Most commonly associated with syndromic and nonsyndromic heritable aneurysms
    - However, also occurs in normal aging and accelerated by hypertension
  - Shape: Fusiform
  - Location: AA most common

Gross Pathologic & Surgical Features

- **Saccular**: Focal, mass-like aortic dilatation
  - May result from remodeling of penetrating aortic ulcer
- **Fusiform**: Diffuse, elongated aortic dilatation

CLINICAL ISSUES

Presentation

- Most common signs/symptoms
  - Atherosclerotic aortic aneurysm: Asymptomatic (most common), chest pain, compression (hoarseness, dysphagia, atelectasis, superior vena cava syndrome)
  - Infectious (mycotic) aneurysm: Fever, leukocytosis
  - Acute chest pain: Rupture, dissection

Demographics

- Age
  - Atherosclerotic aortic aneurysms often free from significant atherosclerotic disease and more common in heritable and congenital cases
  - Descending TAA more commonly degenerative and associated with calcified and noncalcified atherosclerotic disease
- Sex
  - M > F
- Prevalence
  - Increased from 3.5-7.6 per 100,000 persons between 2002-2014, primarily due to increased imaging

Treatment

- Risk reduction: Hypertension control, smoking cessation
- Indications for surgical or interventional aortic repair
  - Sporadic or degenerative aneurysms
    - **AA ≥ 5.5 cm**
      - ≥ 5.0 cm reasonable if patient scheduled to undergo repair of trileaflet aortic valve
    - **Descending aorta ≥ 5.5 cm**; smaller diameter threshold for repair include
      - Symptomatic aneurysms
      - Saccular aneurysm morphology
      - Female

- Thoracic endovascular aortic repair (TEVAR) reasonable for patients who do not have syndromic aneurysm
  - **Rapid growth**
    - ≥ 0.5 cm in 1 year
    - ≥ 0 .3 cm a year for 2 consecutive years
- Marfan syndrome
  - Repair of any part of aorta if diameter > 5cm
  - Repair of aortic root if diameter ≥ 4.5 cm is reasonable if there are high-risk features
    - Family history of dissection
    - Rapid growth
    - Diffuse aortic root and AA dilation
    - Marked vertebral artery tortuosity
    - Cross-sectional aortic root area:patient height ratio ≥ 10 cm^2/m
- Loeys-Dietz syndrome
  - Prophylactic repair of aortic root and AA
  - Size threshold, which ranges ≥ 4 cm to ≥ 5 cm based specific genetic variant, phenotypic features, patient age, aortic growth rates, and family history
- Vascular Ehlers-Danlos
  - No specific guidelines due to increased surgical risk from vascular fragility and increased bleeding
  - Decision should involve multidisciplinary team
- Heritable but nonsyndromic
  - Diameter ≥ 5.0 cm in absence of high-risk features
  - ≥ 4.5 cm in presence of high-risk features
    - Family history of dissection at aortic diameter < 5.0 cm
    - Unexplained sudden death at age < 50 years
    - Rapid aortic growth defined as ≥ 0.5 cm in 1 year or ≥ 0.3 cm per year in 2 consecutive years
- BAV
  - Aortic diameter ≥ 5.5 cm
  - Repair of aortic root if diameter 5-5.4 cm is reasonable if there are high-risk features
    - Family history of dissection
    - Growth rate > 0.3 cm per year
    - Aortic coarctation
    - Root phenotype with isolated root dilation
  - Aortic diameter ≥ 4.5 cm at time of aortic valve replacement or repair
  - Recommend screening of all 1st-degree relatives via echocardiogram
- Surgical repair
  - Open repair: Artificial or biologic grafts
  - Closed repair: Endovascular stent graft

Imaging Follow-Up

- Nonsyndromic: Annual CTA or MRA
- Marfan syndrome: Yearly CT/MR if stable; more frequently if > 4.5 cm/growth
- Loeys-Dietz: Yearly MRA
- Turner syndrome: Every 5-10 years if no risk factors; yearly if abnormalities

DIAGNOSTIC CHECKLIST

Consider

- Ruptured aneurysm in patients with acute chest pain, wide mediastinum, and pleural effusion on radiography
- Normal radiography does not exclude aneurysm or dissection
  - Cross-sectional imaging is used for diagnosis

Reporting Tips

- AAE (blunt sinotubular junction) suggests Marfan syndrome; affects surgical procedure
- Assess coronary arteries and great vessels in cases with associated dissection

SELECTED REFERENCES

1. Rodríguez-Palomares JF et al: Mechanisms of aortic dilation in patients with bicuspid aortic valve: JACC state-of-the-art review. J Am Coll Cardiol. 82(5):448-64, 2023
2. Isselbacher EM et al: 2022 ACC/AHA Guideline for the Diagnosis and Management of Aortic Disease: A Report of the American Heart Association/American College of Cardiology Joint Committee on Clinical Practice Guidelines. Circulation. 146(24):e334-482, 2022
3. Wang J et al: Aortic dilatation in patients with bicuspid aortic valve. Front Physiol. 12:615175, 2021
4. Kallianos KG et al: Imaging thoracic aortic aneurysm. Radiol Clin North Am. 58(4):721-31, 2020
5. Rooprai J et al: Thoracic aortic aneurysm growth in bicuspid aortic valve patients: role of aortic stiffness and pulsatile hemodynamics. J Am Heart Assoc. 8(8):e010885, 2019
6. McComb BL et al: Normative reference values of thoracic aortic diameter in American College of Radiology Imaging Network (ACRIN 6654) arm of National Lung Screening Trial. Clin Imaging. 40(5):936-43, 2016
7. Erbel R et al: 2014 ESC guidelines on the diagnosis and treatment of aortic diseases: document covering acute and chronic aortic diseases of the thoracic and abdominal aorta of the adult. The Task Force for the Diagnosis and Treatment of Aortic Diseases of the European Society of Cardiology (ESC). Eur Heart J. 35(41):2873-926, 2014
8. Goldfinger JZ et al: Thoracic aortic aneurysm and dissection. J Am Coll Cardiol. 64(16):1725-39, 2014
9. Rogers IS et al: Distribution, determinants, and normal reference values of thoracic and abdominal aortic diameters by computed tomography (from the Framingham Heart Study). Am J Cardiol. 111(10):1510-6, 2013
10. Mao SS et al: Normal thoracic aorta diameter on cardiac computed tomography in healthy asymptomatic adults: impact of age and gender. Acad Radiol. 15(7):827-34, 2008
11. Guo D et al: Familial thoracic aortic aneurysms and dissections: genetic heterogeneity with a major locus mapping to 5q13-14. Circulation. 103(20):2461-8, 2001
12. Feigl D et al: Mycotic aneurysms of the aortic root. A pathologic study of 20 cases. Chest. 90(4):553-7, 1986

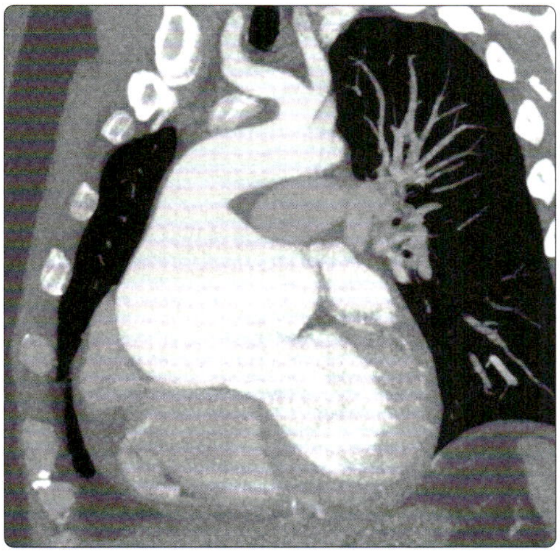

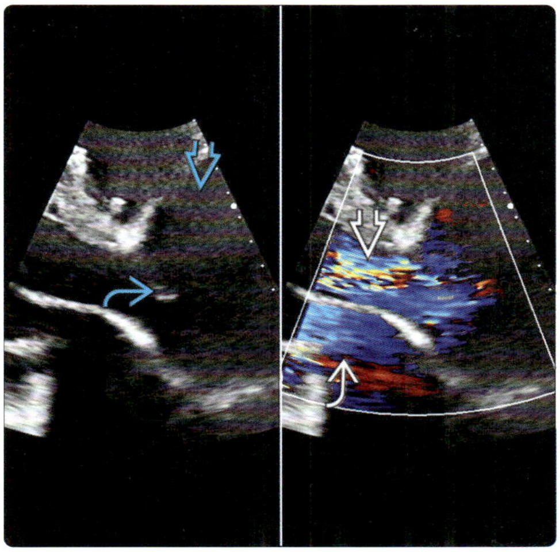

(Left) *Coronal oblique arterial-phase CECT in a 38-year-old with annuloaortic ectasia shows balloon-like AA dilation and effacement of the sinotubular junction. There is rapid tapering of the AA in its midportion. Subsequent work-up diagnosed Marfan syndrome.* **(Right)** *Coned down 3-chamber echocardiogram in a 36-year-old with Marfan syndrome shows balloon-like dilation of the AA above the aortic valve. During diastole, there is severe aortic regurgitation with flow paralleling adjacent mitral inflow.*

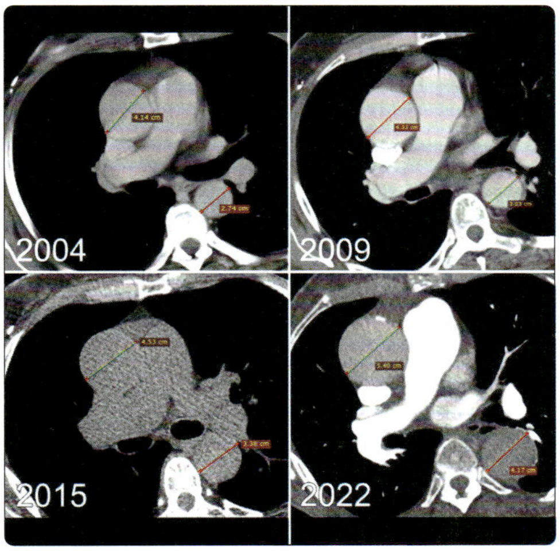

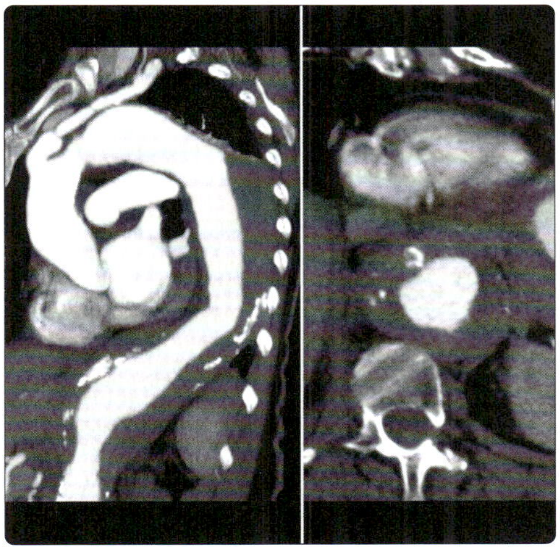

(Left) *Axial CECT images from the years 2004, 2009, 2015, and 2022 are shown. The AA grew from 4.1 cm to 4.3 cm to 4.5 cm to 5.4 cm, respectively. Similarly, the DTA grew from 2.7 cm to 3 cm to 3.4 cm to 4.2 cm.* **(Right)** *Parasagittal (left) and coronal oblique (right) images through the aorta in a 79-year-old show diffuse fusiform atherosclerotic aneurysm of the DTA with extensive layering mural thrombus with areas of calcification due to degenerative changes. The maximum aortic diameter was 6.8 x 6.3 cm. The AA is normal.*

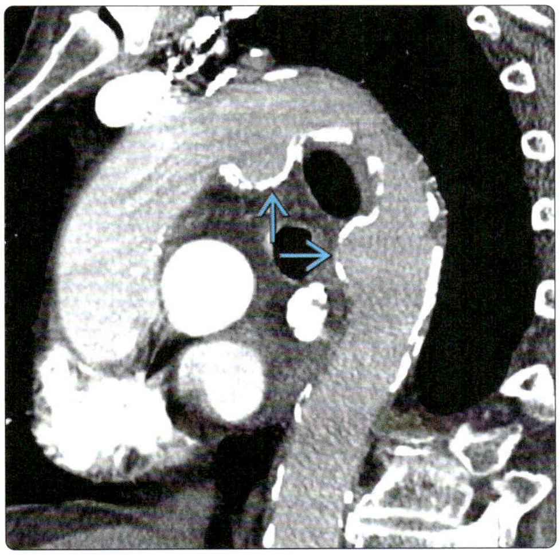

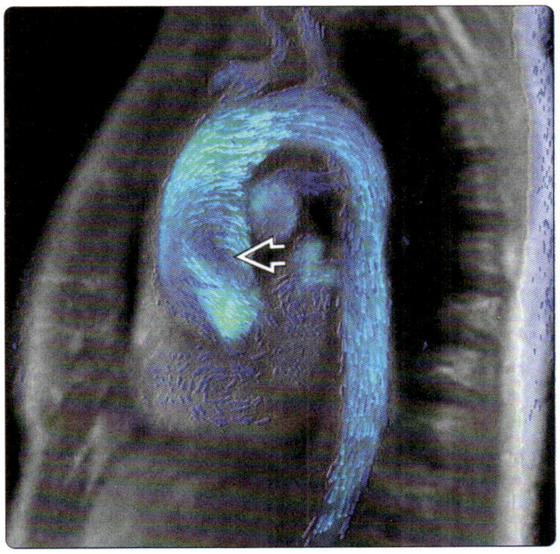

(Left) *Oblique sagittal chest CECT in the same patient shows 2 saccular aneurysms with rather extensive atherosclerotic changes of the thoracic aorta.* **(Right)** *4D flow MR in a patient with a Sievert type 1 bicuspid aortic valve and aortic regurgitation shows vortical flow in the aneurysmal AA. The entire AA is enlarged.*

(Left) *Coronal 5-mm MIP (left) shows circumferential thickening of the AA, which is irregularly dilated to 4.8 cm, not including the wall thickening . Sagittal image (right) shows the AA wall thickening as well as areas of wall thickening and mild stenosis in the abdominal aorta .* **(Right)** *Axial images from a CTA (left) and PET/CT (right) show intense FDG uptake in the wall of the AA . The patient was diagnosed with large vessel vasculitis.*

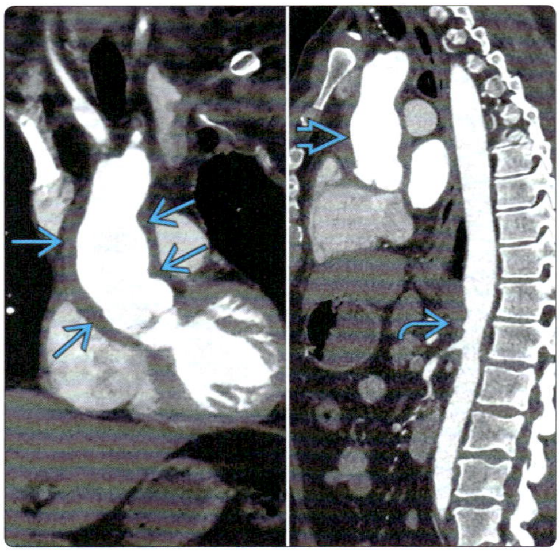

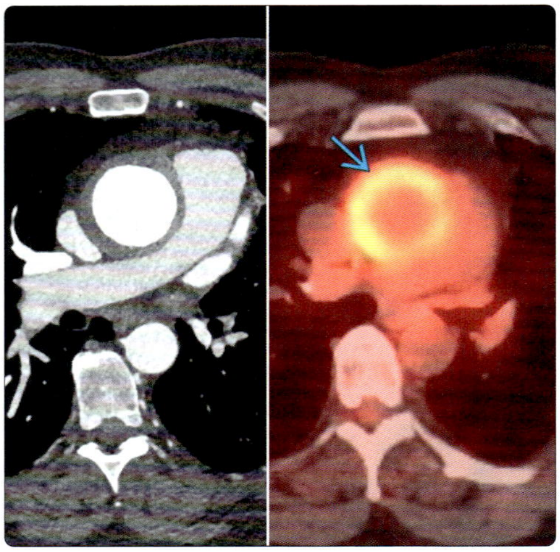

(Left) *AP chest x-ray in a 58-year-old man admitted for deteriorating mental status over 2 months shows prominence of aortic contour . It was unclear if this was related to tortuosity or aneurysm.* **(Right)** *Subsequent CTA shows circumferential wall thickening and aneurysmal dilation of the AA measuring 5 cm. Wall thickening extends into the DTA but is more mild without dilation. Thickening extends around the ostia of the arch vessels with severe stenosis or the left common carotid artery .*

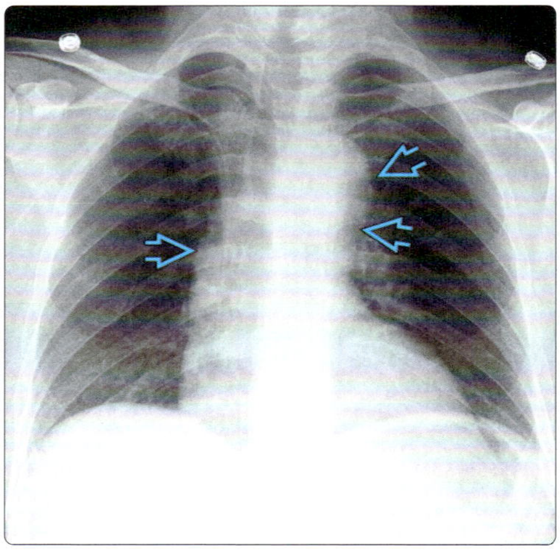

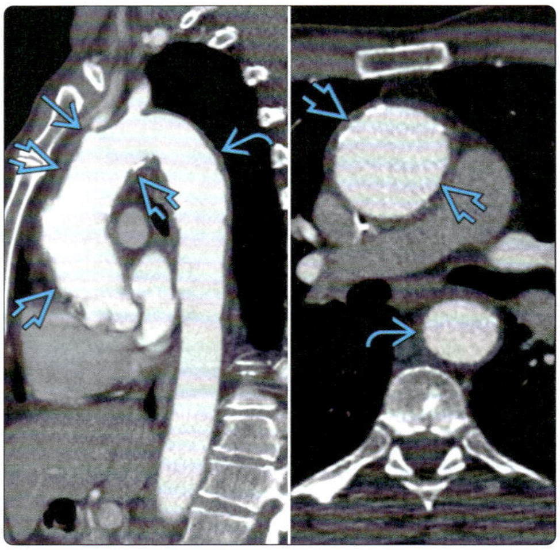

(Left) *Sagittal T1W (L), T1W+ (R), and axial T1W+ (inset) spine MR images show diffuse aortic wall enhancement . CFS-VDRL was 1:1024, diagnosing neurosyphilis. Aorta has a typical appearance for syphilitic aortitis.* **(Right)** *Coronal (L) and sagittal oblique (center) images show a penetrating atherosclerotic ulcer (PAU) with hematoma extending beyond the aorta wall . Adjacent intimal calcification is absent in PAU region. Six years later (R), PAU has increased in size, representing a pseudoaneurysm.*

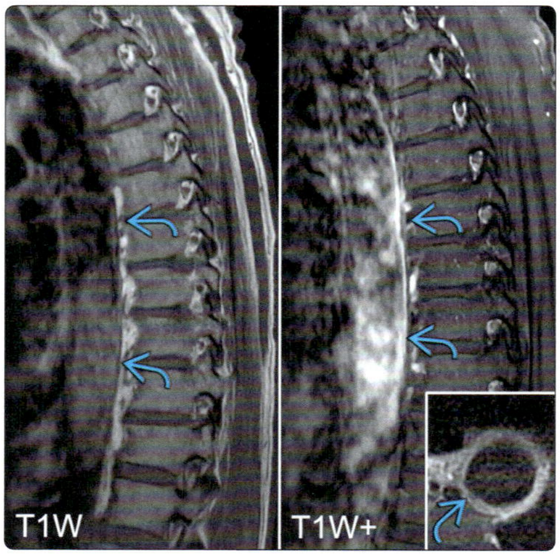

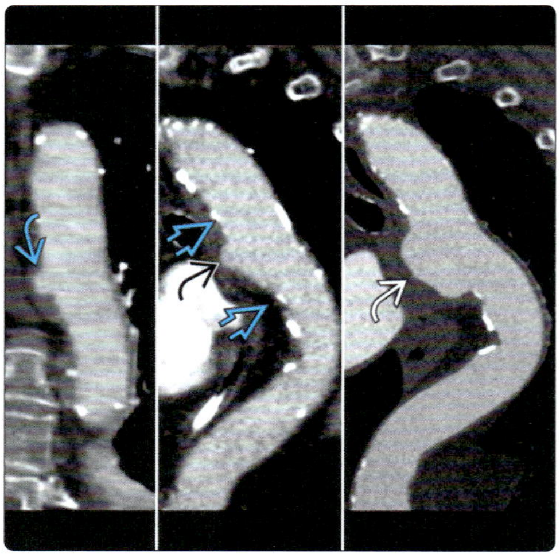

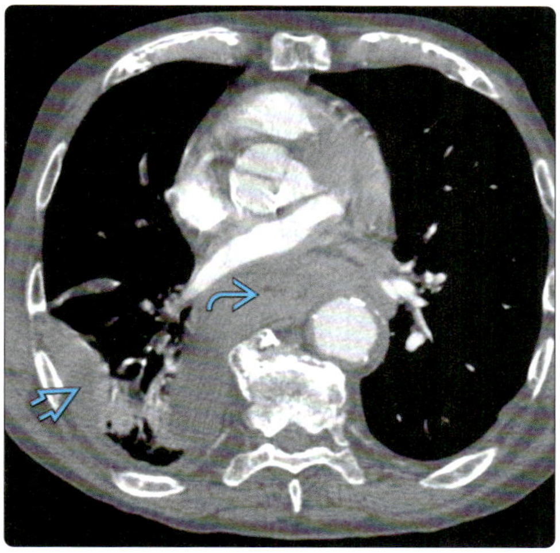

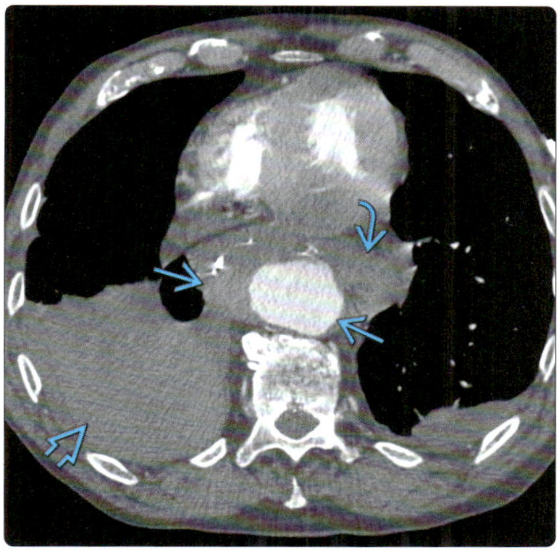

(Left) *Axial CT in a 74-year-old man with chest pain shows a large volume of mediastinal hematoma* *compressing the left atrium. Hemothorax* *is also present. The DTA is aneurysmal with calcified and noncalcified atherosclerotic disease.* **(Right)** *Image more inferiorly in the same patient shows mediastinal hematoma* *and large right hemothorax* *. The DTA is aneurysmal with atherosclerotic disease and mural thrombus* *. Focal rupture of the DTA in this region was confirmed on catheterization.*

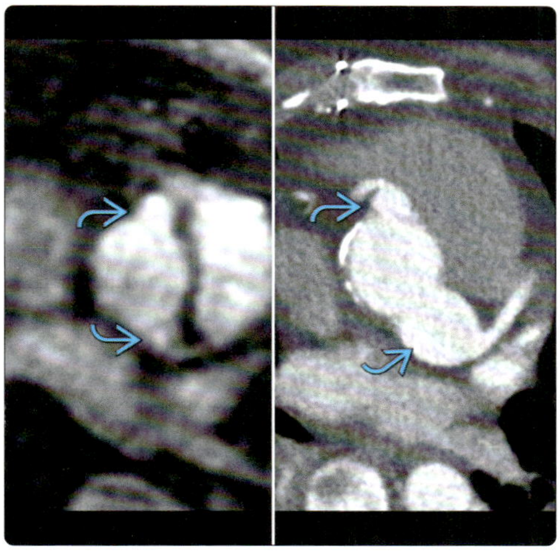

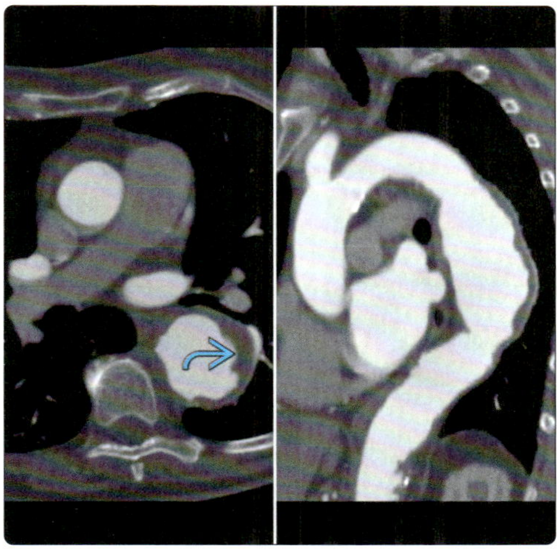

(Left) *Aortic root images in a patient with Marfan syndrome and AA graft repair show aneurysmal dilation of the coronary artery button grafts (BGs)* *, which have increased in size between the years 2004 and 2020. The BGs are from the native aorta and thus susceptible to aneurysm formation.* **(Right)** *Axial (left) and sagittal oblique (right) CECT images of the thoracic aorta in a 73-year-old show extensive fusiform aneurysmal dilation of the DTA measuring up to 5.3 cm with diffuse layering mural thrombus* *.*

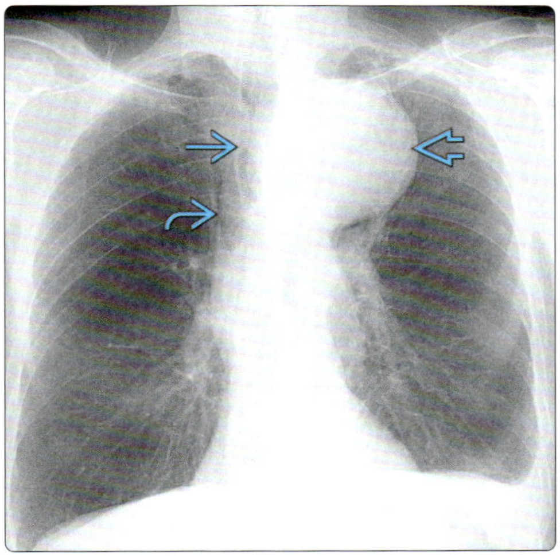

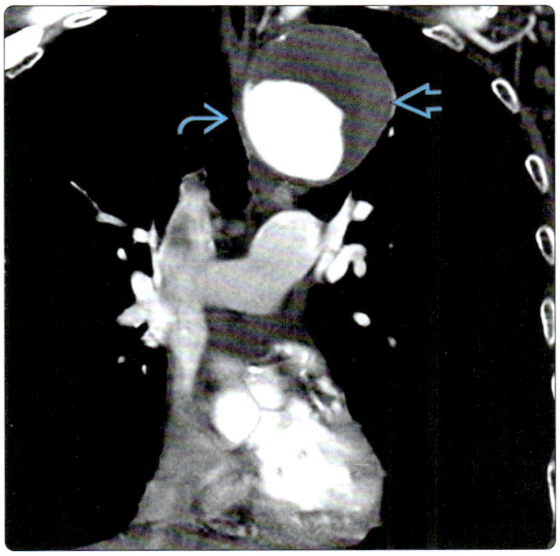

(Left) *PA radiograph in a patient with severe emphysema and small left effusion shows a large mass in the superior mediastinum* *displacing the trachea* *and esophagus* *rightward. The location and rounded appearance could be due to an aneurysm.* **(Right)** *Coronal CTA in the same patient shows a large fusiform aneurysm of the proximal DTA* *displacing the esophagus* *rightward.*

KEY FACTS

TERMINOLOGY

- Aneurysm arising from infection of arterial wall, usually bacterial

IMAGING

- Rapidly growing focal saccular aneurysm arising eccentrically from aortic wall
- Periaortic soft tissue stranding, edema, and fluid
- Adjacent vertebral body or psoas abnormalities due to spread of infection
- Increased uptake of labeled leukocytes at site of aneurysm

TOP DIFFERENTIAL DIAGNOSES

- Atherosclerotic aneurysm
- Inflammatory aneurysm
- Contained rupture
- Aortoenteric fistula

PATHOLOGY

- Bacterial aortitis most commonly caused by *Salmonella* or *Staphylococcus aureus*
- Primary mycotic aneurysm arises from distant, unknown, or remote source of infection
- Secondary mycotic aneurysm arises from specific source of infection

CLINICAL ISSUES

- Fever, signs of sepsis
- Positive blood cultures in most cases
- Surgical resection/grafting following antibiotic therapy

DIAGNOSTIC CHECKLIST

- Contrast-enhanced CTA or MRA with delayed images for evaluation
- Labeled leukocyte scan if indeterminate CTA and MRA

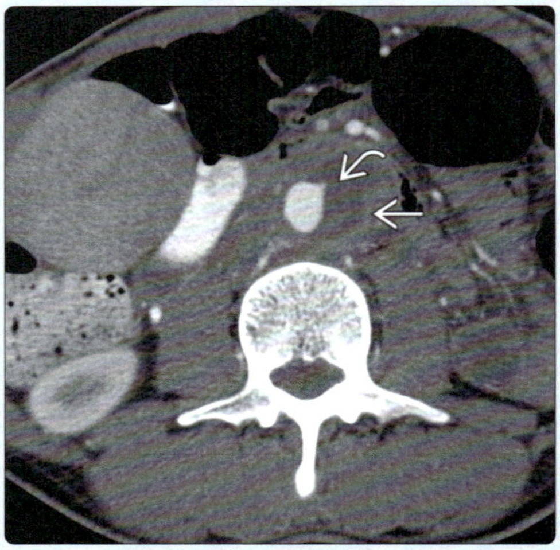

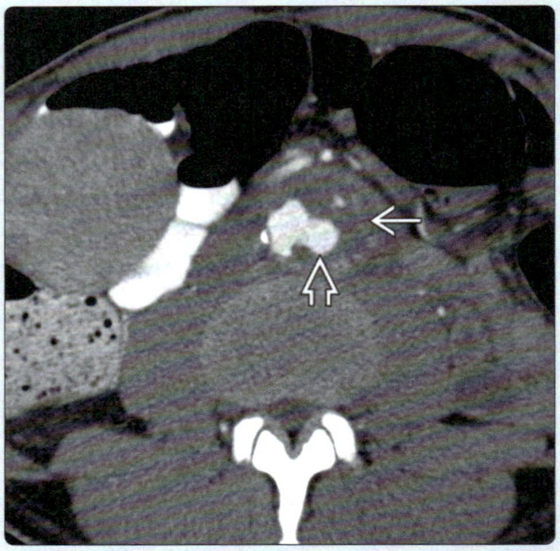

(Left) *Axial CECT of the abdominal aorta shows periaortic, low-density soft tissue ➡ with rim enhancement ➡ of the aortic wall, which is consistent with an infected aortic wall and periaortic abscess.* **(Right)** *Axial CECT of the aorta in the same patient shows an area of focal, small luminal outpouching (pseudoaneurysm) ➡ of the left lateral wall of the aorta with associated periaortic soft tissue swelling ➡, consistent with a mycotic aneurysm.*

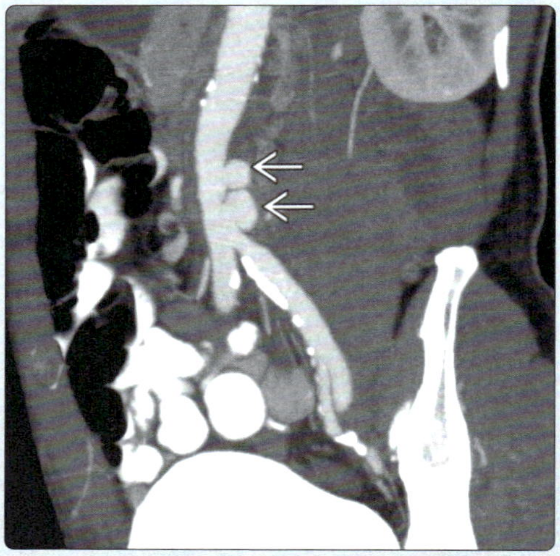

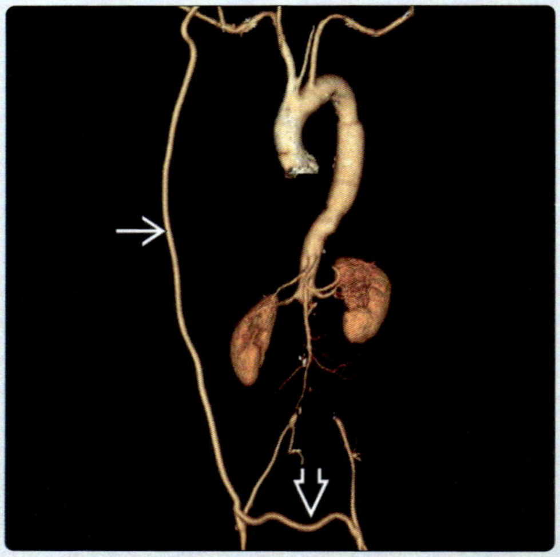

(Left) *Oblique CTA reconstruction in the same patient shows 2 focal contrast outpouchings consistent with mycotic pseudoaneurysms ➡ affecting the lateral wall of the abdominal aorta.* **(Right)** *Coronal CTA of the aortoiliac arteries in the same patient following infrarenal aortic resection shows that the lower extremities are now perfused via a right axillary-femoral artery bypass graft ➡ and cross-femoral bypass graft ➡. Note the absence of resected infrarenal aorta.*

TERMINOLOGY

Synonyms

- Infectious aneurysm (more appropriate term)

Definitions

- Aneurysm arising from infection of arterial wall, usually bacterial

IMAGING

General Features

- Best diagnostic clue
  - Rapidly growing saccular aneurysm arising eccentrically from aortic wall
- Location
  - Anywhere in aorta or other vessels
    - Tends to occur at major branch points of aorta
- Size
  - Variable
- Morphology
  - Usually saccular with focal involvement of artery
  - Periaortic inflammation, abscess, mass
  - Periaortic gas
  - Adjacent vertebral body abnormalities due to spread of infection

Radiographic Findings

- Radiography
  - May reveal increased size of aorta
  - Lytic or sclerotic areas in adjacent bone

CT Findings

- NECT
  - Periaortic soft tissue stranding, edema, and fluid are frequent
  - Periaortic gas
  - Adjacent vertebral body or psoas abnormalities due to spread of infection
  - Periaortic, high-attenuation fluid if ruptured
  - Bacterial aortitis is rarely calcified
  - Syphilitic aortitis shows curvilinear calcifications
- CECT
  - ≥ 1 saccular aneurysm(s) arising from aortic wall, usually focal
  - Lobular contours of aneurysm
  - Enhancement of periaortic soft tissue
  - Rim enhancement in case of abscess
- CTA
  - Saccular, eccentric aneurysms of variable size
  - Enhancing periaortic soft tissue or abscess

MR Findings

- T1WI
  - Periaortic low signal intensity in nonenhanced MR
  - Aortic and periaortic enhancement following gadolinium, especially evident on fat-suppressed images
  - Rim enhancement in case of abscess
  - Adjacent bone abnormality if contiguous infection
- T2WI
  - Periaortic high signal intensity on fat-suppressed T2WI
- Contrast-enhanced MRA
  - ≥ 1 saccular aneurysm(s) arising from aortic wall
  - Effacement of wall with possible leakage at rupture site
  - In addition to MRA, delayed source images need to be analyzed to identify areas of enhancement

Ultrasonographic Findings

- Grayscale ultrasound
  - Useful in children or if superficial arteries are involved
  - Focal, eccentric pseudoaneurysm
  - Perivascular soft tissue or abscess
- Color Doppler
  - Flow within aneurysm with typical yin-yang configuration

Echocardiographic Findings

- Echocardiogram
  - Used to rule out endocarditis as potential source of septic emboli

Angiographic Findings

- Conventional
  - Focal, saccular aneurysm
  - Irregularity of luminal surface

Nuclear Medicine Findings

- Labeled leukocyte scintigraphy
  - Increased uptake at site of aneurysm

Imaging Recommendations

- Best imaging tool
  - Contrast-enhanced CT/CTA
  - Labeled leukocyte scintigraphy
- Protocol advice
  - Obtain delayed images during contrast-enhanced CTA or MRA
  - Review adjacent bones

DIFFERENTIAL DIAGNOSIS

Atherosclerotic Aneurysm

- Slow growing
- More often fusiform
- Often calcified
- No enhancement of aortic wall

Inflammatory Aneurysm

- Distal aorta and iliac involvement
- Thick rind of soft tissue around aorta
- Uniform, rim-like aortic wall enhancement on contrast CT/MR
- Fusiform aneurysm
- Retroperitoneal fibrosis

Contained Rupture

- Focal disruption or gap in aortic wall
- High attenuation in wall or in periphery of aneurysm
- Lack of enhancement

Aortoenteric Fistula

- Most involve duodenum
- Periaortic soft tissue with periaortic gas
- Active contrast material extravasation or pseudoaneurysm
- Presents as gastrointestinal bleed

Surgical material

- History of prior surgery
- Hyperdense on NECT

PATHOLOGY

General Features

- Etiology
  - Bacterial aortitis most commonly caused by *Salmonella* or *Staphylococcus aureus*
  - Syphilitic aortitis involves ascending aorta but spares aortic sinus: Ascending aorta most common location
  - Routes of infection
    - Most often caused by seeding of existing lesion (atheroma or aneurysm) via vasa vasorum
    - Direct extension from infection in vessel wall, i.e., bacterial endocarditis
    - Invasion of aortic wall by extravascular contiguous infection, such as spinal infection or intraabdominal abscess
    - Lymphatic spread
  - *Burkholderia pseudomallei* (causing melioidosis), endemic in Southeast Asia and Northern Australia, is increasingly recognized as agent causing aortitis and mycotic aneurysms
- Associated abnormalities
  - Endocarditis
  - Spinal or retroperitoneal infection
  - Intraabdominal infection

Staging, Grading, & Classification

- Classification system
  - Primary mycotic aneurysm arises from distant, unknown, or remote source of infection
  - Secondary mycotic aneurysm arises from specific source of infection
    - Bacterial endocarditis (intravascular spread)
    - Tuberculosis (contiguous spread)

Gross Pathologic & Surgical Features

- Bacterial aneurysm
  - Noncalcified saccular aneurysm
  - Thinning of aortic wall with periaortic inflammatory changes
- Syphilitic aneurysm
  - Calcified lesion
  - Tree bark appearance when atheroma develops in infected areas

Microscopic Features

- Loss of intima and destruction of internal elastic lamina
- Varying degrees of destruction of media
- Bacteria present on histology
- Common bacteria: *Pseudomonas, Clostridium, Salmonella, Streptococcus, Aspergillus*

CLINICAL ISSUES

Presentation

- Most common signs/symptoms
  - Fever, signs of sepsis
- Symptoms vary greatly
- Nonspecific findings
- Low-grade fever
- Localized pain
- Positive blood cultures
  - Blood cultures are negative in 25% of cases

Demographics

- Epidemiology
  - 0.7-2.6% of all aortic aneurysms
  - Increased risk in
    - Intravenous drug abusers
    - Patients with history of bacterial endocarditis
      - Occurs in 2% of patients with infective endocarditis
      - Most common location is intracranial
      - Rupture more easily and associated with poor prognosis
    - Immunocompromised patients
    - Patients with vascular prostheses (valves, grafts)

Natural History & Prognosis

- Nearly always fatal if untreated
- Acute rupture/hemorrhage seen in 75%
- Mortality rate estimated at 67%

Treatment

- Surgical resection/grafting following antibiotic therapy
- May need extraanatomic bypass grafting
- Endovascular repair in some cases

DIAGNOSTIC CHECKLIST

Consider

- Contrast-enhanced CTA or MRA with delayed images for evaluation
- Labeled leukocyte scan if CTA and MRA are indeterminate

Image Interpretation Pearls

- Focal, eccentric aneurysm of aorta
- Enhancing periaortic soft tissue
- Rim enhancement of periaortic abscess

Reporting Tips

- Include location, size, and involvement of branch vessels
- Check for and report extent of contiguous infection

SELECTED REFERENCES

1. Calderón-Parra J et al: Epidemiology and risk factors of mycotic aneurysm in patients with infective endocarditis and the impact of its rupture in outcomes. Analysis of a national prospective cohort. Open Forum Infect Dis. 11(3):ofae121, 2024
2. Wyss TR et al: Infective native aortic aneurysm: a Delphi consensus document on treatment, follow up, and definition of cure. Eur J Vasc Endovasc Surg. 67(4):654-61, 2024
3. Wu H et al: Mycotic aneurysm secondary to melioidosis in China: a series of eight cases and a review of literature. PLoS Negl Trop Dis. 14(8):e0008525, 2020
4. Haidar GM et al: "In situ" endografting in the treatment of arterial and graft infections. J Vasc Surg. 65(6):1824-9, 2017
5. Sörelius K et al: Endovascular treatment of mycotic aortic aneurysms: a paradigm shift. J Cardiovasc Surg (Torino). 58(6):870-4, 2017
6. Deipolyi AR et al: Imaging findings, diagnosis, and clinical outcomes in patients with mycotic aneurysms: single center experience. Clin Imaging. 40(3):512-6, 2016
7. Murphy DJ et al: Cross-sectional imaging of aortic infections. Insights Imaging. 7(6):801-18, 2016

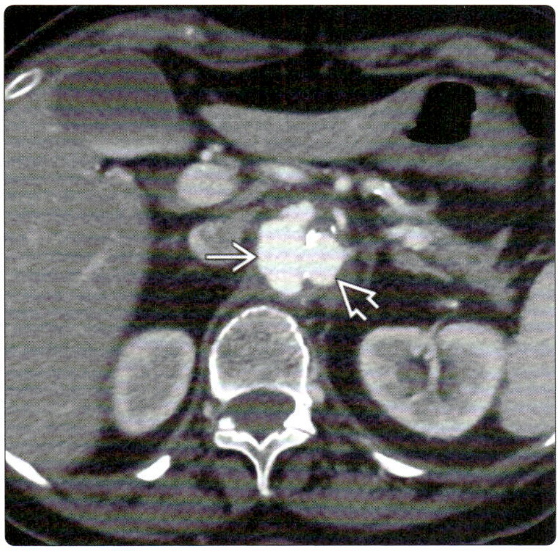

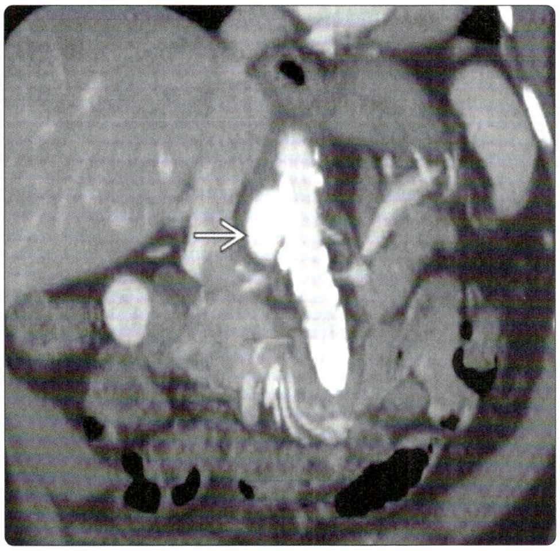

(Left) *Axial CTA of the abdominal aorta shows a focal, eccentric pseudoaneurysm affecting the juxtarenal abdominal aorta. Note the minimal periaortic soft tissue.* **(Right)** *Oblique CTA of the abdominal aorta in the same patient shows a focal, eccentric pseudoaneurysm. There is no significant soft tissue adjacent to the pseudoaneurysm. This patient had bacteremia and spinal infection (not shown). Surgical resection of the aorta confirmed the mycotic nature of the pseudoaneurysm.*

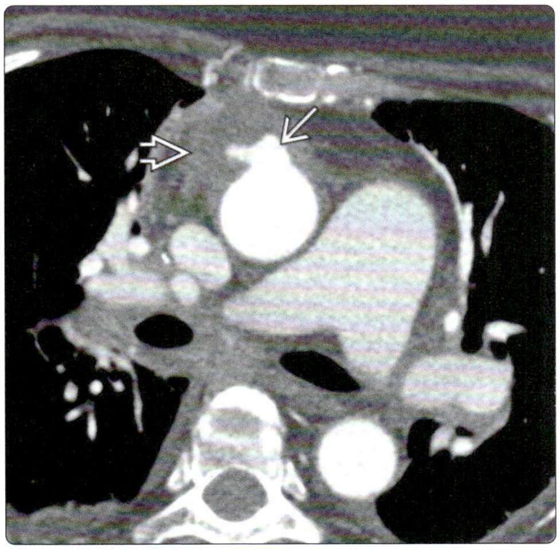

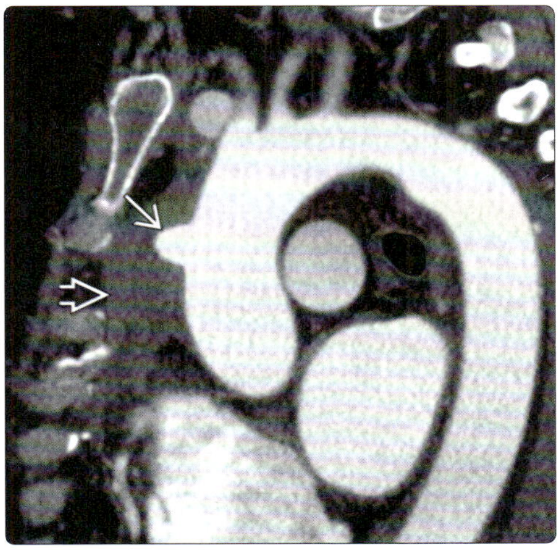

(Left) *Axial CTA of the thoracic aorta shows a focal, eccentric pseudoaneurysm arising from the anterior wall of the ascending aorta with associated periaortic soft tissue.* **(Right)** *Oblique CTA of the thoracic aorta in the same patient shows a focal, eccentric pseudoaneurysm along the anterior wall of the ascending aorta with associated low-density soft tissue. These features are consistent with a mycotic aneurysm.*

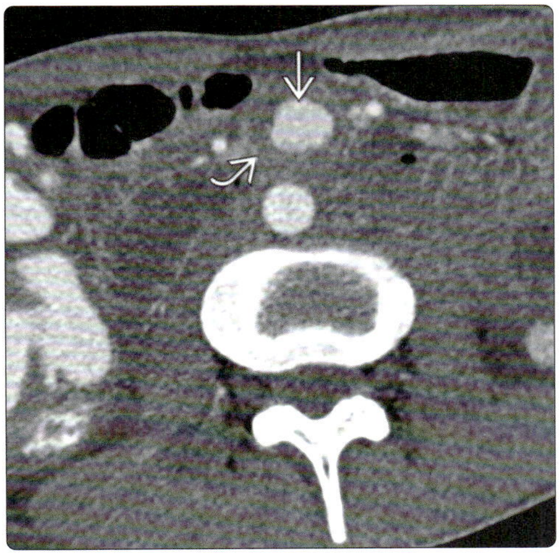

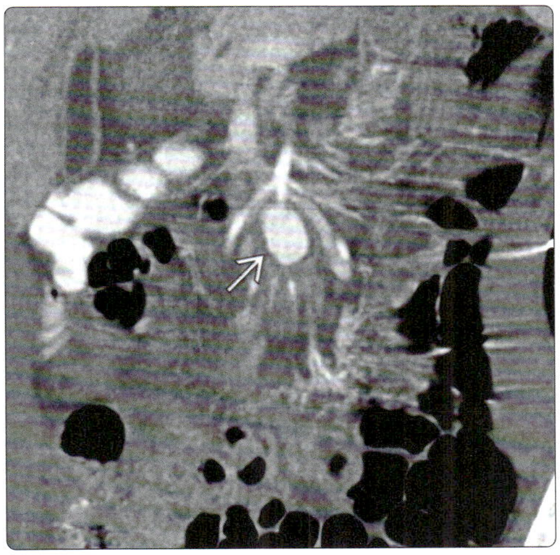

(Left) *Axial CTA of the abdomen shows a pseudoaneurysm arising from a branch of the superior mesenteric artery. Note the perianeurysmal soft tissue.* **(Right)** *Coronal CTA in the same patient confirms the pseudoaneurysm arising from a branch of the superior mesenteric artery. This was secondary to a septic embolus from valvular vegetations in a 30-year-old man with endocarditis secondary to intravenous drug abuse.*

KEY FACTS

TERMINOLOGY

- Congenital systemic connective tissue disorder; skeletal, cardiovascular, and ocular abnormalities

IMAGING

- Radiography
  - Ascending aortic aneurysm
  - Cardiomegaly
  - Pectus deformity, scoliosis, scalloped vertebrae
  - Pneumothorax, apical bullae
- CT
  - Annuloaortic ectasia, aneurysm
  - Aortic rupture: Crescent sign, hematoma
  - Dissection: Intimal flap, true/false lumen
- Echocardiography
  - At diagnosis to assess ascending aorta and 6 months thereafter to determine rate of enlargement
- MR: Similar to CT in sensitivity

TOP DIFFERENTIAL DIAGNOSES

- Familial thoracic aortic aneurysm
- Ehlers-Danlos syndrome
- Bicuspid aortic valve

PATHOLOGY

- Mutation in *FBN1* gene encoding for fibrillin 1
- Autosomal dominant; 25% de novo mutations
- Microscopy: Cystic medial necrosis

CLINICAL ISSUES

- Cardiac/vascular abnormalities
- Pulmonary abnormalities
- Thoracic skeletal abnormalities

DIAGNOSTIC CHECKLIST

- Consider Marfan syndrome in young patients with ascending aortic aneurysm &/or aortic dissection

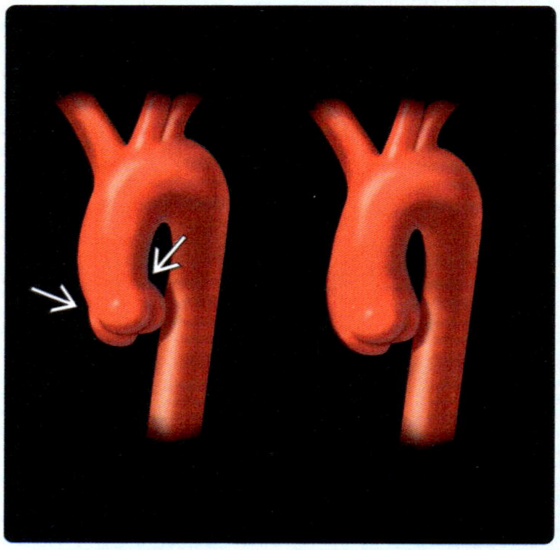
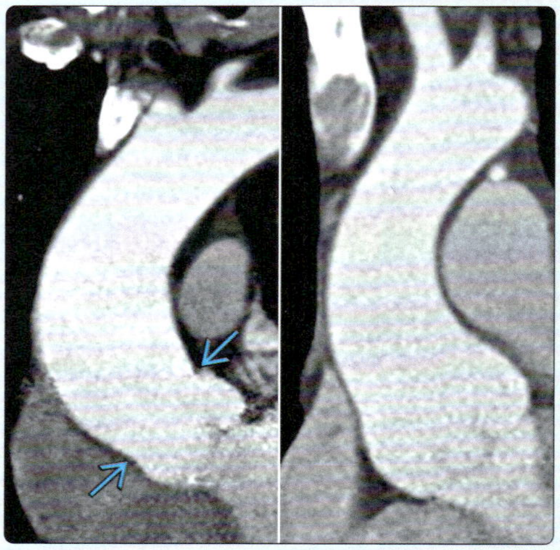

(Left) *Graphic compares a normal ascending aorta (left) with a well-defined sinotubular junction ➡ and annuloaortic ectasia with sinotubular junction effacement (right).* **(Right)** *Coronal oblique CECT shows aneurysms associated with bicuspid aortic valve (left) and Marfan syndrome (MFS) (right) to exemplify annuloaortic ectasia. Note that a sinotubular junction is still identifiable in dilatation due to bicuspid aortic valve ➡ but is effaced in MFS due to dilated aortic root.*

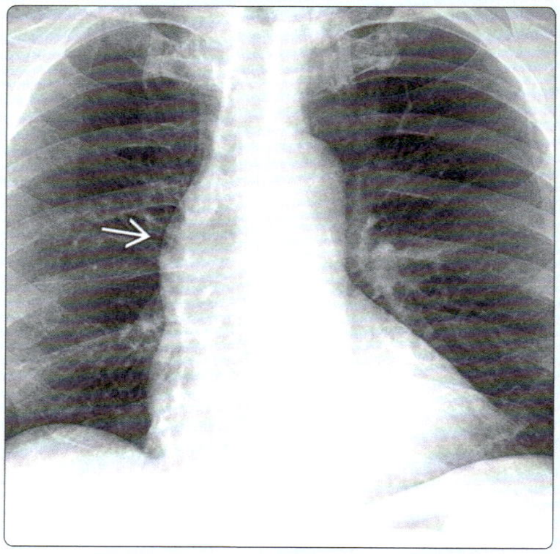
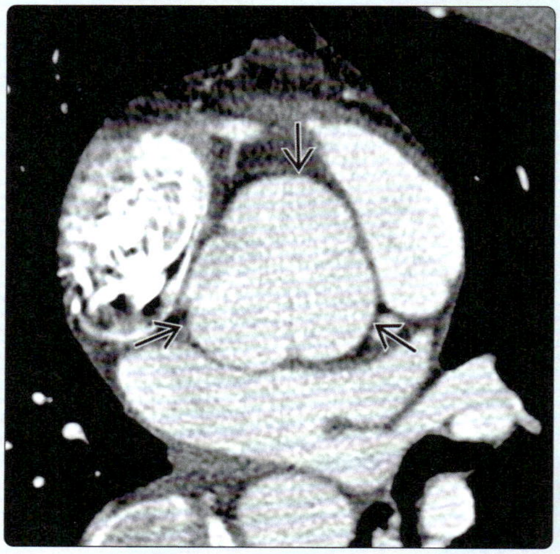

(Left) *PA radiograph of the chest in a patient with MFS shows an abnormal convexity ➡ along the right superior cardiac silhouette. This finding is often associated with a dilated ascending aorta. In young patients, it is commonly associated with bicuspid aortic valve and MFS.* **(Right)** *Axial chest CTA in the same patient shows dilatation of the sinuses of Valsalva ➡ (4.7.x 5.0 x 5.0 cm). Three measurements bisecting each sinus are usually obtained at this level.*

TERMINOLOGY

Definitions

- Marfan syndrome (MFS): Congenital systemic connective tissue disorder characterized by **skeletal**, **cardiovascular**, and **ocular** abnormalities

IMAGING

Radiographic Findings

- **Ascending aortic aneurysm**: Mediastinal widening, right superior cardiomediastinal contour abnormality
- **Cardiomegaly**: Aortic/mitral regurgitation, cardiomyopathy
- Pectus deformity (excavatum, carinatum), scoliosis, scalloped vertebral bodies
- Pneumothorax, apical bullae

CT Findings

- NECT
  - **Annuloaortic ectasia/aneurysm**: Effacement of sinotubular junction (60-80% of patients)
    - Lack of normal transition between aortic root and tubular portion of ascending aorta
    - Indication for surgery: Diameter > 4.5 cm
  - **Aortic rupture**, often contained
    - **Crescent sign**: Crescentic eccentric aortic high-attenuation area
    - **Hematoma**: Mediastinal high attenuation, hemothorax, hemopericardium
- CTA
  - More sensitive than radiography
  - Direct visualization
    - Dissection: Intimomedial defect, true/false lumen
    - Rupture: Active extravasation

MR Findings

- Equivalent to CT, similar accuracy
- Direct visualization of aortic aneurysm and dissection
- Cine MR and phase-contrast imaging are optimal for valve assessment: Aortic &/or mitral regurgitation
- 4D flow MRA provides detailed hemodynamic assessments, including pulse wave velocity (PWV) and peak systolic velocity, to predict future aortic events

Echocardiographic Findings

- Initial assessment of aortic size and 6 months thereafter to determine rate of enlargement

Imaging Recommendations

- Protocol advice
  - Annual imaging is recommended after initial echocardiography

DIFFERENTIAL DIAGNOSIS

Familial Thoracic Aortic Aneurysm

- Sinus of Valsalva aortic aneurysm

Ehlers-Danlos Syndrome

- Aneurysm/rupture: Medium/large muscular arteries
- Systemic: Joint hypermobility, atrophic scars, easy bruising, hernias, hollow organ rupture

Bicuspid Aortic Valve

- Ascending aortic aneurysm; bicuspid aortic valve

Homocystinuria

- Cardiac: Mitral valve prolapse
- Vascular: Intravascular thrombosis
- Systemic: Tall stature, ectopia lentis, long bone overgrowth, intellectual disability

Loeys-Dietz Syndrome

- Cardiac: Patent ductus arteriosus, atrial septal defect, bicuspid aortic valve
- Vascular: Sinus of Valsalva aneurysm, arterial tortuosity, aneurysms in other arteries
- Hypertelorism, cleft palate, broad or bifid uvula, exotropia, craniosynostosis, malar hypoplasia, blue sclerae, dolichostenomelia, arachnodactyly, pectus deformity, scoliosis, joint laxity, rare developmental delay

Shprintzen-Goldberg Syndrome

- Vascular: Rare sinus of Valsalva aneurysm
- Systemic: Hypertelorism, craniosynostosis, arched palate, arachnodactyly, pectus deformity, scoliosis, joint laxity, developmental delay

MASS (Mitral, Aortic, Skin, and Skeletal Manifestations) Syndrome

- Cardiac: Mitral valve prolapse
- Vascular: Borderline/nonprogressive aortic root enlargement
- Systemic: Nonspecific skin and skeletal findings, myopia

PATHOLOGY

General Features

- Etiology
  - Mutation in *FBN1* gene encoding for **fibrillin 1**
  - *TGFBR2* and *TGFBR1* responsible for 10% of all cases
- Genetics
  - Autosomal dominant; 25% de novo mutations

Microscopic Features

- **Cystic medial necrosis**
  - Accumulation of basophilic ground substance in media with cyst-like lesions; no overt cystic or necrotic changes are normally identified
  - Can occur in MFS, Ehlers-Danlos syndrome, and annuloaortic ectasia

CLINICAL ISSUES

Presentation

- Clinical profile
  - **Cardiac abnormalities**
    - Mitral valve regurgitation
      - Children: Mitral regurgitation and heart failure, pulmonary hypertension, death in infancy
      - > 50% auscultatory/echocardiographic evidence of mitral valve dysfunction, typically prolapse
      - Progression of mitral valve prolapse to mitral regurgitation by adulthood
    - Aortic valve regurgitation: Late occurrence from aortic anulus stretching

- Tricuspid valve prolapse
- Dilated cardiomyopathy (uncommon)
- **Vascular abnormalities**: Most common life-threatening manifestations
  - **Annuloaortic ectasia** and **aortic aneurysm**
  - **Aortic dissection**
    - Often type A
    - Acute-onset heart failure typically from severe aortic insufficiency
    - Extension to coronary arteries; myocardial infarction or sudden cardiac death
    - Dilatation/dissection of descending thoracic/abdominal aorta
  - Dilatation of pulmonary trunk
- **Pulmonary abnormalities**
  - Bullae: Predisposed to spontaneous pneumothorax
- **Thoracic skeletal abnormalities**
  - Pectus deformity; can contribute to restrictive lung disease
- **Revised Ghent nosology (Ghent 2)**
  - **Goals**: Identification of patients with higher risk for aortic aneurysm or dissection; simplicity of use of diagnostic criteria; allowance for early diagnosis; consideration of availability and costs of diagnostic tests; better definition of entities, such as familial ectopia lentis, MASS phenotype, and mitral valve prolapse syndrome; and delineation of triggers for alternative diagnoses, such as Loeys-Dietz syndrome
  - **5 major changes** (in comparison with Ghent 1)
    - More diagnostic emphasis on aortic root aneurysm/dissection and ectopia lentis
    - More prominent role of molecular genetic testing (i.e., *FBN1*; *TGFBR1* and *TGFBR2*)
    - Complete removal of some clinical criteria (e.g., dilatation of main pulmonary artery, dilatation or dissection of descending thoracic or abdominal aorta, increased axial length of globe and abnormally flat cornea, hypoplastic iris or hypoplastic ciliary muscle causing decreased miosis, joint hypermobility, spondylolisthesis, highly arched palate, and recurrent or incisional hernia, calcification of mitral anulus, apical blebs of lung), or mitigation of diagnostic relevance of dural ectasia, or adding or modifying clinical criteria, such as myopia > 3 diopters, hindfoot valgus, and thoracolumbar kyphosis
    - Provision of discriminating features of alternative diagnoses, such as Loeys-Dietz syndrome
    - Provision of context-specific recommendations for patient counseling and follow-up
  - **Absence of family history**
    - Aortic root diameter (Z-score ≥ 2) and ectopia lentis = MFS
    - Aortic root diameter (Z-score ≥ 2) and causal *FBN1* mutation = MFS
    - Aortic root diameter (Z-score ≥ 2) and systemic score ≥ 7 points = MFS
    - Ectopia lentis and causal *FBN1* mutation with known aortic root dilatation = MFS
  - **In presence of family history**
    - Ectopia lentis and family history of MFS = MFS
    - Systemic score ≥ 7 points and family history of MFS = MFS
    - Aortic root diameter (Z-score ≥ 2 above 20 years old, ≥ 3 below 20 years) and family history of MFS = MFS
  - **Scoring of systemic features** (maximum total score 20 points)
    - Wrist and thumb sign = 3 points (wrist or thumb sign = 1 point)
    - Pectus carinatum deformity = 2 points (pectus excavatum or chest asymmetry = 1 point)
    - Hindfoot deformity = 2 points (plain pes planus = 1 point)
    - Protrusio acetabuli = 2 points
    - Reduced upper segment:lower body segment ratio and increased arm/height and no severe scoliosis = 1 point
    - Scoliosis or thoracolumbar kyphosis = 1 point
    - Reduced elbow extension = 1 point
    - Facial features (3/5) = 1 point (dolichocephaly, enophthalmos, downslanting palpebral fissures, malar hypoplasia, retrognathia)
    - Pneumothorax = 2 points
    - Skin striae = 1 point
    - Myopia > 3 diopters = 1 point
    - Mitral valve prolapse (all types) = 1 point
    - Dural ectasia = 2 points

Demographics

- Sex
  - M = F
- Epidemiology
  - Incidence: 1 in 3,000-5,000 individuals

Natural History & Prognosis

- Improved prognosis with annual imaging, medical/surgical intervention
- Higher aortic dissection risk during pregnancy

Treatment

- β-adrenergic receptor blockade
- Restriction of vigorous exercise
- Surgical reconstruction: Elective according to aortic diameter or if dissection or rupture
  - Indications for surgery
    - Ascending aorta
      - Diameter ≥ 4.5 cm
      - Diameter ≥ 4.5 cm in family history of early dissection, rapid growth defined as ≥ 0.5 cm/year, and significant aortic regurgitation
    - Aortic arch
      - Diameter > 5.0 cm
    - Descending thoracic aorta
      - Diameter > 5.0 cm

SELECTED REFERENCES

1. Geiger J et al: Longitudinal evaluation of aortic hemodynamics in Marfan syndrome: new insights from a 4D flow cardiovascular magnetic resonance multi-year follow-up study. J Cardiovasc Magn Reson. 19(1):33, 2017
2. von Kodolitsch Y et al: Perspectives on the revised Ghent criteria for the diagnosis of Marfan syndrome. Appl Clin Genet. 8:137-55, 2015

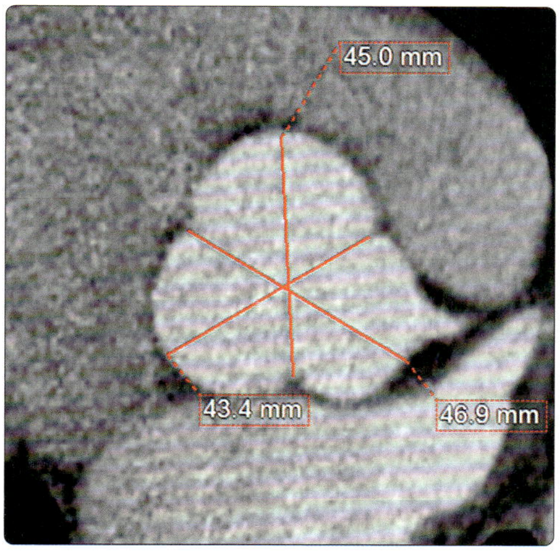

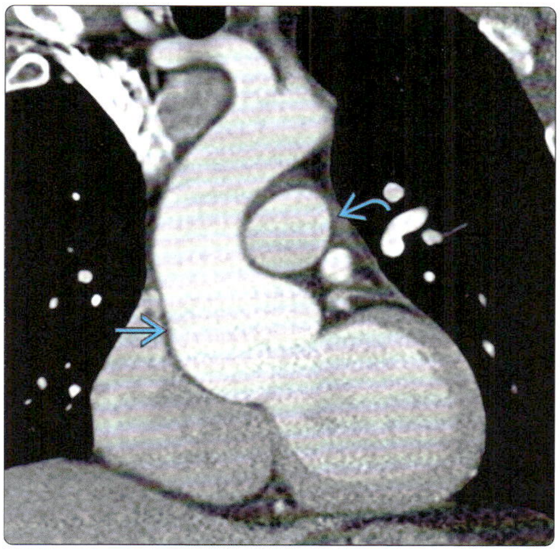

(Left) *Axial CECT in a young patient with MFS shows symmetric dilation of all sinuses of Valsalva.* **(Right)** *Coronal CECT in the same patient shows effacement of the sinotubular junction* ➔, *which is characteristic of MFS. Note diffuse dilatation of the entire ascending thoracic aorta, demonstrating a morphology often referred to as the tulip bulb sign. The pulmonary trunk* ➔ *appears smaller than the aorta. Normally, the pulmonary artery is of the same size as the ascending aorta.*

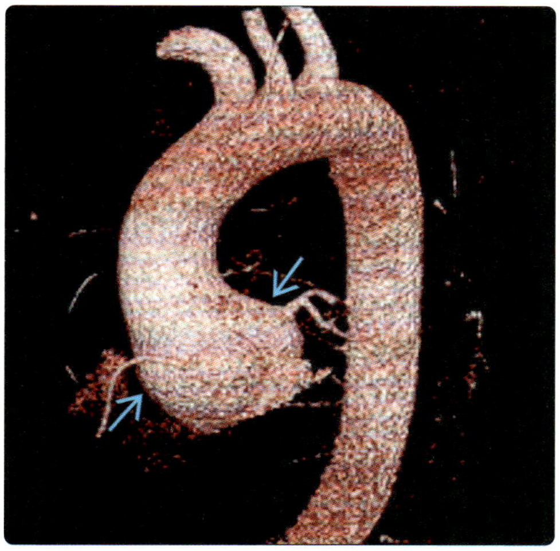

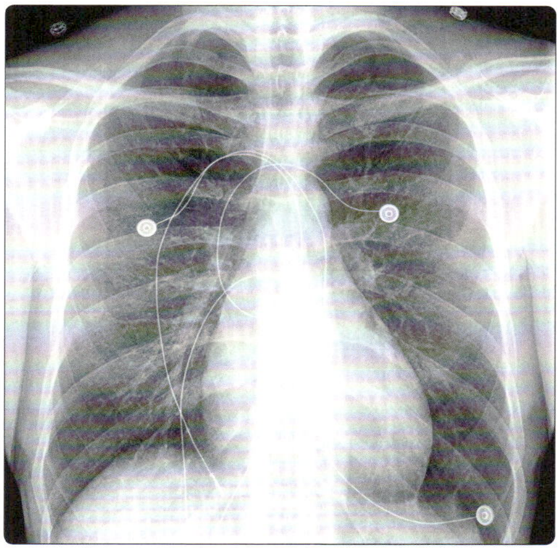

(Left) *Coronal CECT 3D surface rendering in the same patient shows the so-called tulip bulb configuration* ➔ *of the ascending thoracic aorta characteristically seen in MFS due to dilatation of the aortic root with normal appearance of the arch and descending thoracic aorta.* **(Right)** *PA chest radiograph in a patient with MFS and acute aortic syndrome shows no specific cause of the symptoms reported in this individual. A normal radiograph does not exclude aortic dilatation or dissection.*

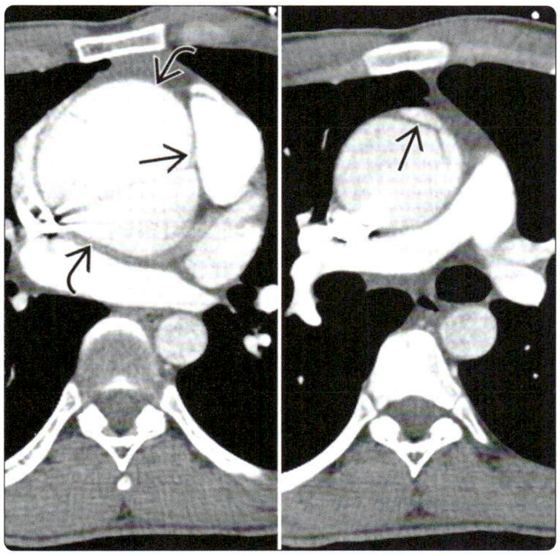

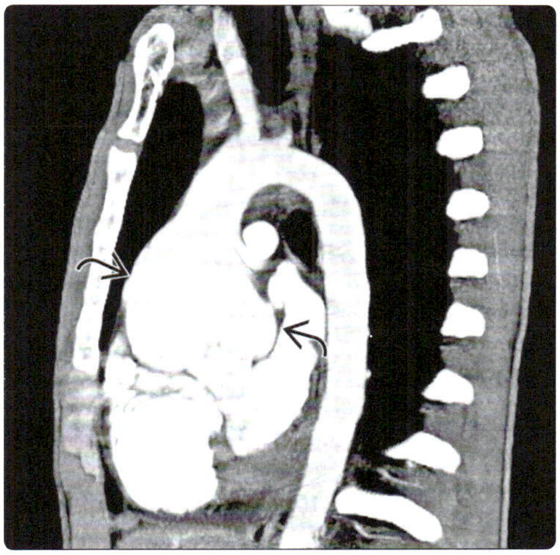

(Left) *Axial CECT in the same patient shows marked aortic root dilatation* ➔. *Note disproportion in the diameter of the pulmonary trunk, which should typically be the same size as the ascending aorta. At the higher level, there is an intimomedial defect representing ascending aortic dissection* ➔. **(Right)** *Oblique sagittal CECT in the same patient shows the classic tulip bulb appearance* ➔ *due to annuloaortic ectasia.*

(Left) *Axial CECT in a young pregnant woman with MFS with acute chest pain shows an intimomedial defect ascending into the descending aorta . Note dilation of the ascending thoracic aorta.* **(Right)** *Coronal oblique CECT in the same patient shows an intimomedial defect extending along the entire ascending aorta. Note effacement of the sinotubular junction , completely absent in this case, a very characteristic feature seen in MFS involving the ascending aorta.*

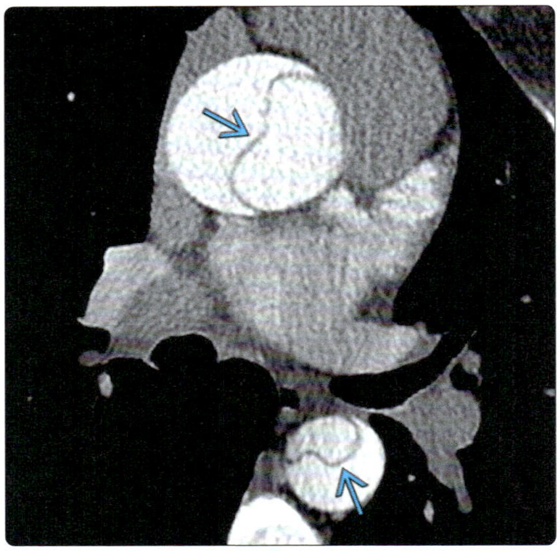

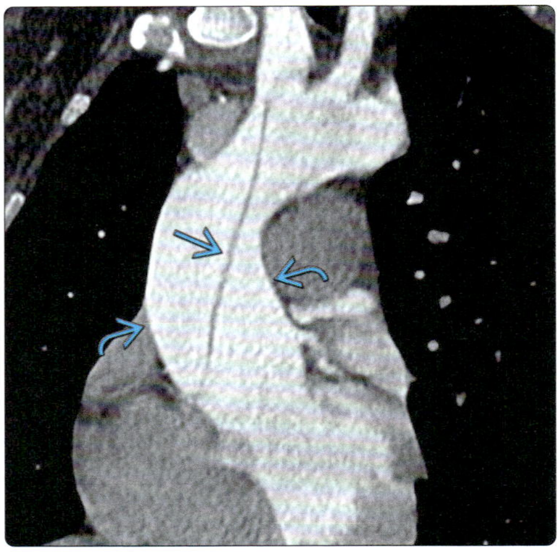

(Left) *Sagittal oblique CECT in the same patient shows an extensive Stanford type A intimomedial defect involving the entire thoracic aorta. Dissection is a known complication of MFS, and pregnant individuals are under particular risk to develop such a complication.* **(Right)** *Axial chest CTA MIP reformation in a patient with MFS shows dilatation of the pulmonary trunk and central pulmonary arteries. (Courtesy L. Heyneman, MD.)*

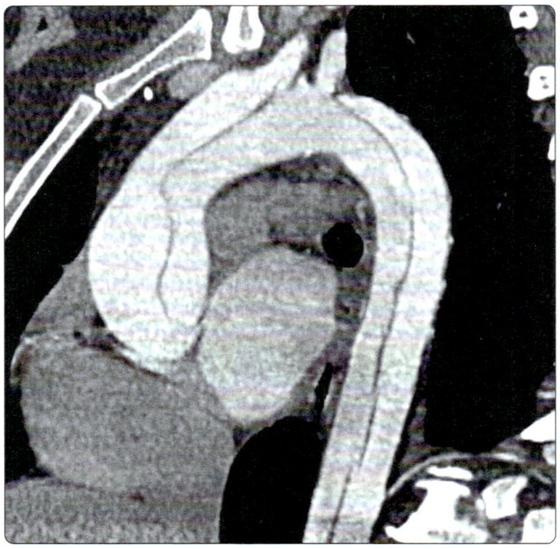

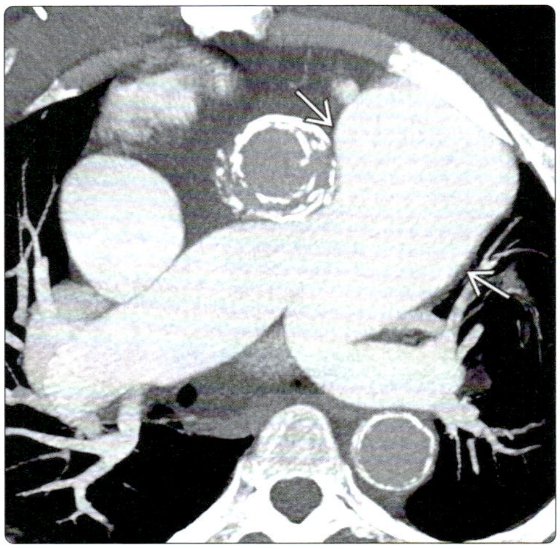

(Left) *Axial CTA in a patient with MFS shows marked dilatation of the aortic root and pectus excavatum deformity . These are major diagnostic criteria for MFS. (Courtesy L. Heyneman, MD.)* **(Right)** *Axial NECT in the same patient shows bilateral apical bullae . This may lead to secondary spontaneous pneumothorax in patients with MFS. (Courtesy L. Heyneman, MD.)*

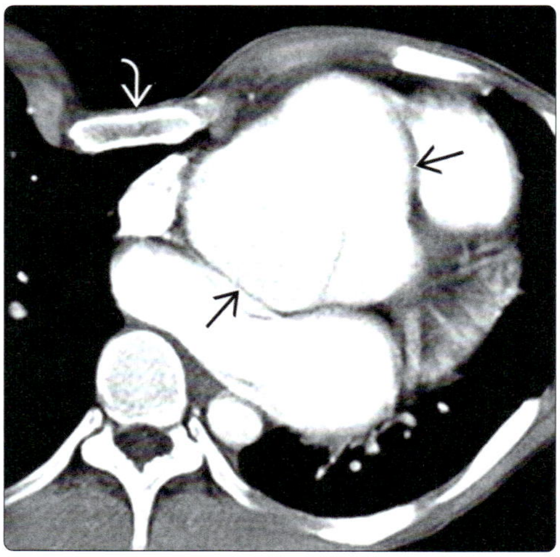

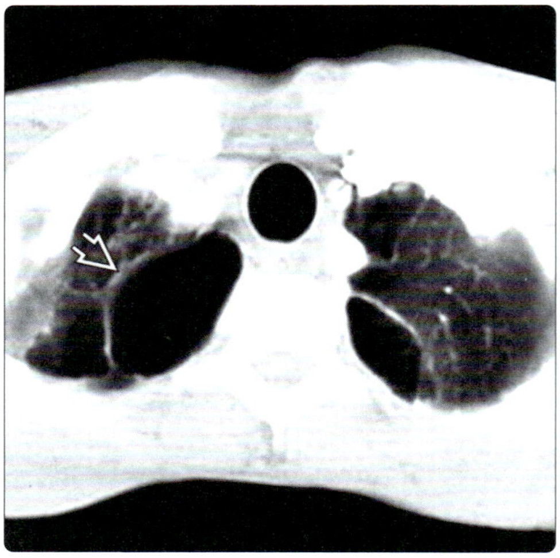

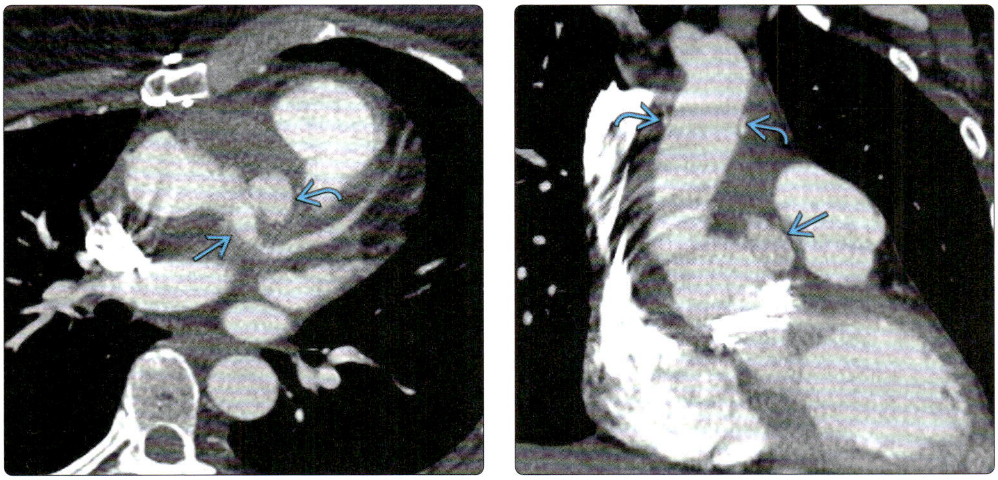

(Left) *Axial CECT in a patient with MFS who underwent a modified Bentall reconstruction of the ascending aorta shows pseudoaneurysm of the left coronary button .* **(Right)** *Coronal oblique CECT in the same patient shows an abnormal contract collection adjacent to the proximal aspect of the graft. Note distal anastomotic felts . Pseudoaneurysm of the coronary buttons is overall an uncommon complication that occurs more frequently in patients with MFS.*

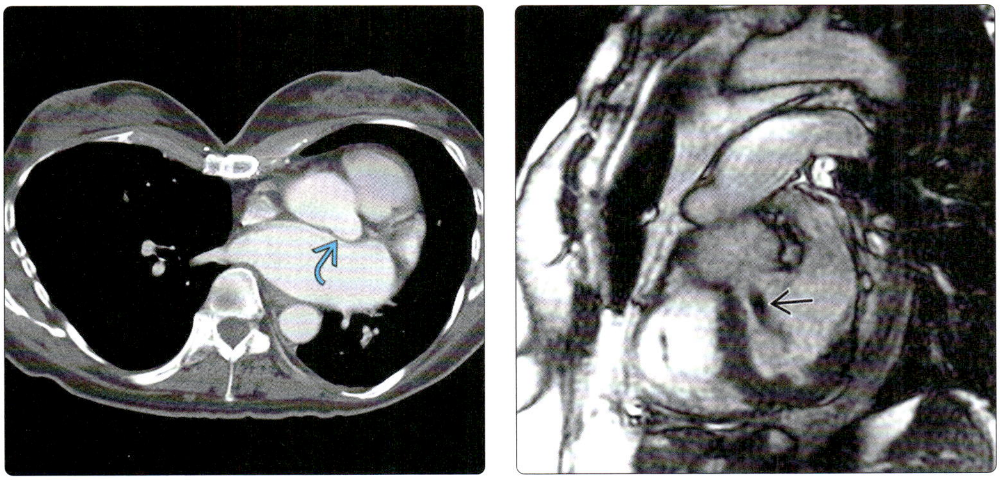

(Left) *Axial CECT in a patient with MFS who underwent a modified Bentall reconstruction of the aorta shows bulb-like dilatation of the left coronary button . Patients with MFS are more prone to develop dilation &/or pseudoaneurysm of the coronary buttons.* **(Right)** *Oblique sagittal SSFP MR in a patient with MFS and ascending aortic aneurysm shows a diastolic jet across the aortic valve, which constitutes one of the major cardiovascular criteria for MFS.*

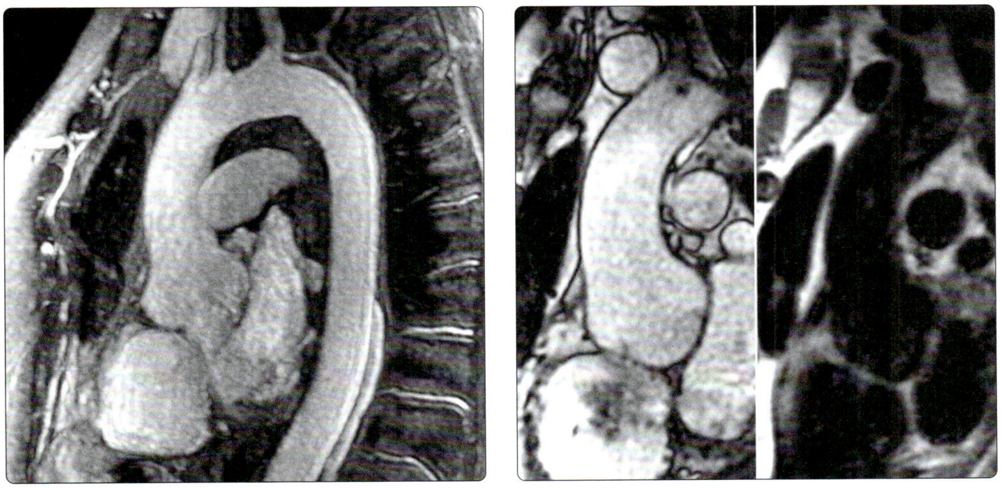

(Left) *Oblique gadolinium-enhanced MRA in the same patient shows dilatation of the aortic root with tulip bulb-like morphology. Volumetric acquisition and postprocessing reformations are some of the advantages of MRA over other sequences.* **(Right)** *Oblique sagittal SSFP and dark blood (HASTE) MR in a patient with MFS show dilatation of the proximal ascending aorta with effacement of the sinotubular junction. Both sequences are suitable to depict ascending aortic morphology.*

Introduction

Although acute aortic syndrome (AAS) may be caused by a variety of differing disease processes that affect the integrity of the aortic wall, they usually manifest with similar clinical symptoms, including acute chest &/or back pain. In the widely accepted basic classification, there are 3 diseases that make up AAS, namely aortic dissection, intramural hematoma (IMH), and penetrating aortic ulcer (PAU). Some authors have proposed including 3 additional entities: Aortitis, intraluminal aortic thrombus, and intimal tear from trauma. For the purposes of this introduction, we will focus on the 3 original entities.

Knowledge of normal aortic wall anatomy is central to understanding the different disease processes that make up AAS. The aortic wall is composed of 3 layers: The tunica intima, tunica media, and tunica externa or tunica adventitia. These are commonly referred to as the intima, media, and adventitia. The intima is the innermost layer; it is composed of thin endothelial cells on a basement membrane. The media is the thickest layer and is composed of smooth muscle cells bounded by an internal and external elastic lamina. The media is responsible for giving the aorta its elastic properties. The adventitia is the thin outermost layer of the aorta; it is composed of collagen fibers and nerves. The aortic wall blood supply comes from small vessels called the vasa vasorum that travel within the adventitia and outer aspect of the media.

Aortic Dissection

Aortic dissection is the most common and deadly AAS with an overall incidence of 0.2-0.8% of the population. Early diagnosis and treatment are critical, as 75% of patient deaths occur in the first 2 weeks following presentation. Aortic dissection is caused by an intimal tear within an already weakened aortic wall. Blood enters through the defect into the medial layers and propagates (or dissects) caudally and cranially, causing the formation of a "false" lumen. The term " rue lumen" is used to differentiate the false lumen from the original aortic lumen.

Risk factors for aortic dissection include age, hypertension, cocaine use, pregnancy, aortic coarctation, aortitis, or other disease processes that weaken the aortic wall, such as Marfan syndrome, Loeys-Dietz syndrome, Ehlers-Danlos syndrome, bicuspid aortic valve, or other connective tissue diseases.

The classic clinical presentation is chest pain radiating to the back, although patients may also present with chest pain without radiation, dyspnea, &/or syncope. Historically, acute aortic dissection is defined by symptoms lasting < 2 weeks, whereas chronic aortic dissection is defined by symptoms lasting > 2 weeks. The time course of aortic dissection is classified as acute (< 14 days), subacute (15-90 days), and chronic (> 90 days), based on pathologic responses and remodeling.

Intramural Hematoma

IMH is uncommon, accounting for ~ 10-20% of patients with AAS. It is characterized by hemorrhage within the media of the aortic wall that is usually caused by spontaneous bleeding from the vasa vasorum. In contradistinction to aortic dissection, there is no intimal tear with IMH and no flow-containing false lumen. Hypertension is the leading risk factor for developing an IMH, and, similar to aortic dissection, patients present with severe chest pain radiating to the back. IMH is classified using the Stanford system (type A IMH and type B IMH) with similar risk profile and management.

Penetrating Aortic Ulcer

PAU is an ulceration of an atheromatous plaque that has eroded through the inner intima to reach the media of the aortic wall. There is often associated IMH. Ninety percent of PAUs occur in the descending thoracic aorta. The ascending aorta is likely relatively "protected" from atherosclerosis due to rapid blood flow from the left ventricle. Some authors hypothesize that further enlargement of the PAU and extension beyond the adventitia is responsible for many thoracic aortic pseudoaneurysms. PAU is most commonly seen in older men with hypertension. Presentation is similar to that of aortic dissection or IMH with severe chest pain that often radiates to the back.

Diagnosis

Chest radiograph is the initial imaging test performed in the majority of patients presenting with acute chest pain. The most reliable radiographic signs of aortic pathology include a widened mediastinum, interval displacement of intimal calcification (with the ring sign indicating > 5-mm displacement of the aortic lumen past the calcified intima), and abnormal aortic contour. Unfortunately, the chest radiograph is neither sufficiently sensitive nor specific for excluding aortic pathology. Chest radiography in AAS can reveal secondary findings, such as left apical cap, tracheal and esophageal deviation, left mainstem bronchus depression, loss of paratracheal stripe, pericardial effusion, pleural effusion, and hemothorax, or help identify alternative causes of chest pain.

Currently, multidetector CT (MDCT) has superseded MR and transesophageal echocardiography as the test of choice for patients with suspected aortic pathology because of its rapid image acquisition, widespread availability, and easier monitoring of unstable patients. MDCT has the added benefit of diagnosing nonaortic pathology, which also may lead to chest pain.

Aortic dissection is diagnosed by direct visualization of the dissection flap separating a true and false lumen. Several features are useful to differentiate true from false lumina. The true lumen is generally smaller than the false lumen, more densely opacified, and located along the posterolateral aspect of the descending thoracic aorta. The false lumen in an aortic dissection generally has a larger cross-sectional area and is characterized by slower blood flow, which results in lower contrast attenuation on arterial-phase imaging, or it may show no enhancement if thrombosed. It can contain linear "cobweb" strands of tissue with a similar density to the intimal flap and may display the beak sign, where the false lumen wedges around the true lumen. Windsock appearance in aortic dissection refers to the complete dissection of the entire intima, creating a circumferential intimal flap. This results in a narrow, filiform-shaped true lumen, which may lead to intimointimal intussusception, where one part of the aorta slides into another due to the intimal dissection. The Mercedes-Benz sign may appear in cases of triple-channel dissection, where a secondary dissection occurs within one of the existing channels, resulting in 3 distinct lumina.

IMH is best diagnosed on the noncontrast scan, as the high-density lesion is often obscured when there is intraluminal contrast. The most common imaging appearance is a crescentic high-density lesion within the aortic wall. The hematoma may displace intimal calcification inward. The aortic lumen is often of normal caliber, but it may be narrowed. It is important to document the location (Stanford type A or B) and the extent of involvement.

PAU is a contrast-filled outpouching extending into the media of the aortic wall. The lesion is usually associated with extensive atherosclerotic plaque. It is important to distinguish PAU from an aortic pseudoaneurysm caused by trauma or infection. Consider a mycotic pseudoaneurysm when there is periaortic fat stranding and leukocytosis. Consider a traumatic pseudoaneurysm in the setting of trauma or when the outpouching occurs at a location predisposed to traumatic injury (e.g., ligamentum arteriosum, aortic root, or diaphragmatic hiatus). PAU often enlarges over time and may extend beyond the aortic wall to become a pseudoaneurysm.

Photon-counting CT (PCCT) offers promising advantages in imaging for AAS by providing higher spatial resolution, improved image quality, and reduced radiation exposure compared to conventional CT. These features allow PCCT to better detect subtle aortic wall abnormalities, such as intimal tears and IMHs, and it minimizes artifacts that can obscure crucial details.

MR is often used when CT angiography (CTA) is contraindicated or unavailable for evaluating aortic dissection or for surveillance to reduce radiation exposure in young patients. MR effectively demonstrates the intimal flap, true and false lumina, and the extent of dissection into branch vessels, and it is also useful for assessing end-organ perfusion. IMHs cannot be detected with MR angiography (MRA); however, on T1-weighted imaging, IMH appears isointense in acute stages and hyperintense in subacute cases. Steady-state free precession (SSFP) cine MR can reveal the intimal flap with an intermediate signal, while the reentry site shows low-signal turbulent flow. The false lumen, whether containing blood flow or thrombus, presents medium to low signal intensity. MR can also assess complications, such as aortic insufficiency and pericardial rupture.

Phase-contrast MR allows for the quantification of blood flow velocities, particularly at sites of aortic dissection or aneurysm. It helps to measure flow in both the true and false lumina, which is critical for understanding the hemodynamic consequences of aortic dissection. This technique also helps in identifying turbulent flow patterns, which may suggest areas of high risk for further aortic wall damage.

4D flow MR enhances phase-contrast MR by adding a temporal component, allowing for the visualization of blood flow in 3 spatial dimensions over time. This technique provides additional data on hemodynamic properties, such as wall shear stress, vorticity, and kinetic energy, and it evaluates flow or thrombosis in the false lumen more reliably. It also reveals distinct flow patterns, including bidirectional flow, retrograde flow in the true lumen, and helical flow in the false lumen, which are associated with aortic expansion.

Nuclear medicine, particularly FDG PET/CT, has promising applications in AAS that extend beyond identifying aortic wall disease as incidental, nononcologic findings. It highlights inflammation and metabolic activity in the aortic wall, correlating with risk factors, such as aneurysm instability and potential rupture. Increased F-18 FDG uptake indicates heightened inflammation and can help differentiate between acute and stable dissection. This promising technique is useful for assessing the severity of acute aortic dissection, determining the age of the dissection, and predicting rupture risk by tracking metabolic activity.

Classification

There are 2 classification systems currently in use: DeBakey and Stanford. The systems are based on the location of the intimal tear/hematoma and the extent of aortic involvement. The Stanford system is favored and has replaced the original DeBakey classification, as it dictates proper patient management and prognostic consequences. The Stanford system is not based on the location of the intimal tear but rather on whether the ascending aorta is involved by the disease process. Stanford type A involves the ascending aorta and usually requires immediate surgery or endovascular therapy, whereas Stanford type B does not involve the ascending aorta and is generally managed medically. Lesions involving the aortic arch but not the ascending aorta are classified as Stanford type B. The DeBakey classification is divided into 3 groups: Type 1 lesions originate in the ascending aorta and extend into the descending thoracic aorta (Stanford A), type 2 lesions originate in and involve only the ascending aorta (Stanford A), and type 3 lesions originate in and involve only the descending aorta (Stanford B).

Suggested MDCT Protocol for Suspected Aortic Dissection

The imaging protocol usually encompasses a noncontrast low-dose acquisition to detect IMH and to differentiate calcification from contrast on enhanced scans. Thicker slices are usually reconstructed to limit noise.

The arterial-phase imaging is best performed with bolus tracking and ECG gating or triggering if ascending aortic pathology is suspected to avoid pulsation artifact that can mimic dissection (pseudoflaps). The use of high-pitch dual-source acquisition or whole-heart axial acquisition is most useful if scanner technology allows this because motion-free images can be acquired at low radiation doses. Alternatively, the entire aorta can be scanned without gating, immediately followed by a gated acquisition that is limited to the aortic root, which minimizes the net radiation dose. Thin-section reconstructions are recommended for arterial-phase CTA.

Delayed (1-minute) low-dose acquisitions can be helpful to differentiate a thrombosed false lumen from slow flow within a false lumen, and they may aid in demonstrating extravasation in some circumstances. Thicker slices are usually reconstructed to limit noise.

Reporting

The pathology type (dissection, IMH, or PAU), location, entrance tear site, maximal aortic diameter, presence of atheroma or thrombus, extension into branch vessels, secondary signs of end-organ ischemia or malperfusion, and signs of aortic rupture (e.g., mediastinal or pericardial blood, contrast extravasation, or hemothorax) should be reported.

Pitfalls in Diagnosis

There are multiple imaging artifacts that mimic the intimal flap of aortic dissection. The most widely seen is pulsation artifact caused by movement of the ascending aorta during end-systole and end-diastole. This artifact is lessened through the use of ECG gating or a 180° linear interpolation reconstruction algorithm. Too much contrast in the superior vena cava may cause streak artifact, which may mimic aortic dissection. Too little arterial enhancement may lead to a false-negative examination. The major pitfall in diagnosing IMH is lack of a noncontrast examination.

Report Elements for Aortic Dissection

Stanford type (A or B)
Location of the initiating primary intimal tear
Extent, termination, and length of dissection
Which lumen is true and false (matters for endovascular therapy)
Maximum size of the affected aorta at its largest caliber and the size of the false lumen
Presence of thrombus in false lumen
Complications, such as aortic rupture, hemopericardium and tamponade, coronary artery occlusion or dissection, cervical branch occlusion or stenosis, and visceral organ infarcts
Compare with prior exams for any changes

Prognosis

The mortality rate for type A aortic dissection is high, reaching 90% in untreated patients with an early mortality rate of ~ 1-2% per hour. Mortality decreases substantially, to 40%, in treated individuals. Type B aortic dissection is much more favorable with ~ 85% of patients being alive at 1 year with appropriate medical management.

Complications

There are 4 common life-threatening complications of Stanford type A dissections caused by propagation of the intimal flap: Pericardial hemorrhage with tamponade, aortic valve rupture with severe aortic regurgitation, coronary artery dissection with resultant myocardial infarction, and carotid artery dissection with stroke. Aortic dissection can also be fatal by causing end-organ ischemia in the abdominal vasculature. There are 2 main mechanisms that lead to end-organ hypoperfusion: Direct dissection flap extension into the mesenteric vasculature and dynamic occlusion due to a dissection flap acting like a curtain in front of the mesenteric or renal artery. Aortic dissection and PAU can also rupture into the mediastinum or pleural space, leading to rapid exsanguination.

Treatment

There are 3 accepted treatment options for the AAS: Surgery, endovascular therapy, and medical management with blood pressure control. All patients receive medications (e.g., β-blockers) directed at reduction of blood pressure to limit disease progression. Emergent surgery is the mainstay treatment option for most Stanford type A lesions due to its survival benefit over medical management. The goals of surgery are to excise and obliterate the entry point to the false lumen and to reconstitute the aorta by placement of an interposition graft into the aorta. Aortic valve replacement or repair is considered in the setting of aortic valve insufficiency.

Medical therapy is the gold standard for uncomplicated type B lesions. It consists of aggressive blood pressure control. Endovascular therapy with stent grafting is being increasingly utilized in the setting of complicated type B aortic dissection (i.e., mesenteric, renal, or lower extremity ischemia; enlarging PAU; or persistent pain refractory to medical therapy).

Surveillance

Follow-up imaging is typically required to exclude complications from therapy or document disease progression. Surveillance of the aorta is ideally performed with either CTA or MR depending on patient age. Patients with treated acute aortic dissection or IMH may be imaged at 1 and 6 months and yearly thereafter if stable. Patients with chronic dissection are imaged at discharge and yearly for up to 3 years or when symptoms occur. Imaging follow-up in patients with PAU who underwent repair should follow the same guidelines as for those who had thoracic aortic aneurysm repair. If treated with thoracic endovascular aortic repair, surveillance imaging with CT is recommended after 1 month, at 12 months, and then annually if stable. MR is a reasonable alternative to CT. If open repair of PAU was performed, CT or MR within 1 year and then every 5 years is appropriate in the absence of residual aortopathy; annual imaging is recommended if residual aortopathy or abnormal findings are present on surveillance imaging. In patients with PAU managed medically, CT is reasonable after 1 month and, if stable, every 6 months for 2 years and then based on patient age and PAU characteristics.

Selected References

1. Higashigaito K et al: CT angiography of the aorta using photon-counting detector CT with reduced contrast media volume. Radiol Cardiothorac Imaging. 5(1):e220140, 2023
2. Ramaekers MJFG et al: A clinician's guide to understanding aortic 4D flow MRI. Insights Imaging. 14(1):114, 2023
3. Zanon C et al: Advantages of photon-counting detector CT in aortic imaging. Tomography. 10(1):1-13, 2023
4. Writing Committee Members et al: 2022 ACC/AHA guideline for the diagnosis and management of aortic disease: a report of the American Heart Association/American College of Cardiology Joint Committee on Clinical Practice Guidelines. J Am Coll Cardiol. 80(24):e223-393, 2022
5. Ko JP et al: Chest CT angiography for acute aortic pathologic conditions: pearls and pitfalls. Radiographics. 41(2):399-424, 2021
6. Murillo H et al: Aortic dissection and other acute aortic syndromes: diagnostic imaging findings from acute to chronic longitudinal progression. Radiographics. 41(2):425-46, 2021
7. Vilacosta I et al: Acute aortic syndrome revisited: JACC state-of-the-art review. J Am Coll Cardiol. 78(21):2106-25, 2021
8. Bossone E et al: Acute aortic syndromes: diagnosis and management, an update. Eur Heart J. 39(9):739-749d, 2018
9. Sakalihasan N et al: (Tissue PET) vascular metabolic imaging and peripheral plasma biomarkers in the evolution of chronic aortic dissections. Eur Heart J Cardiovasc Imaging. 16(6):626-33, 2015
10. Reeps C et al: Imaging of acute and chronic aortic dissection by 18F-FDG PET/CT. J Nucl Med. 51(5):686-91, 2010

Acute Aortic Syndrome

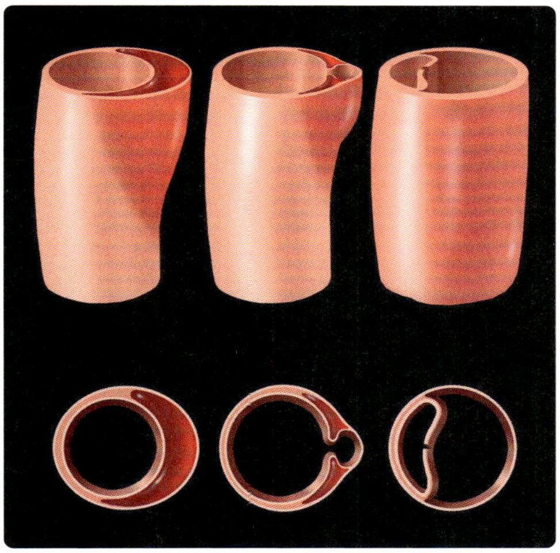

Intramural Hematoma

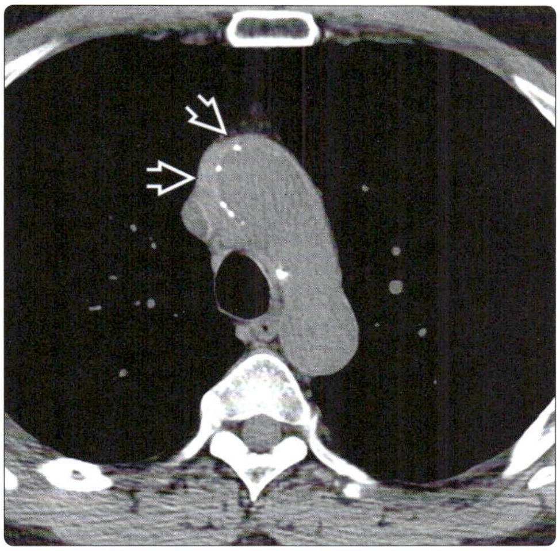

(Left) *Graphic depicts the 3 diseases that traditionally encompass the acute aortic syndrome. On the left, an intramural hematoma without intimal tear is illustrated; in the middle is a penetrating aortic ulcer (PAU) with adjacent focal hematoma, and on the right is a classic aortic dissection with intimal tear.* **(Right)** *Axial NECT shows thickening → of the ascending aortic wall with associated high density (Stanford type A intramural hematoma). The calcification marks the location of the aortic wall intima.*

Intramural Hematoma

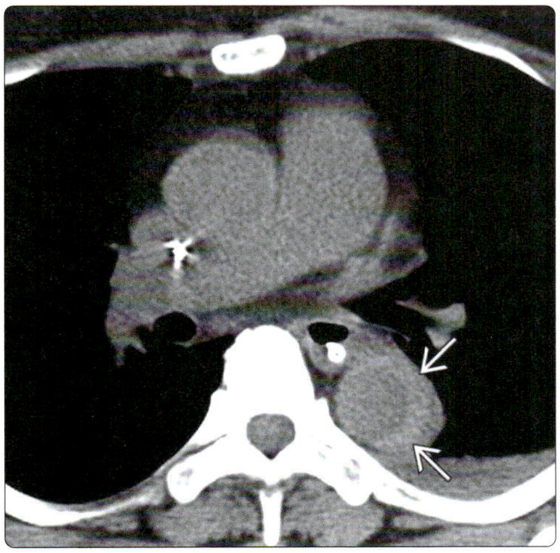

Intramural Hematoma

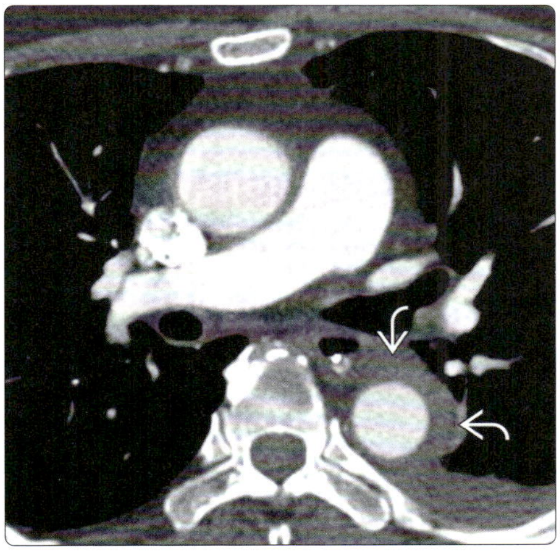

(Left) *Axial NECT shows a nearly complete circumferential crescent → of high density within the descending thoracic aorta (Stanford type B intramural hematoma).* **(Right)** *Axial CECT in the same patient shows thickening → of the descending thoracic aortic wall from intramural hematoma. Note that contrast within the aortic lumen makes it difficult to appreciate the high density within the aortic wall, explaining why noncontrast CT is a required part of the protocol.*

Penetrating Aortic Ulcer

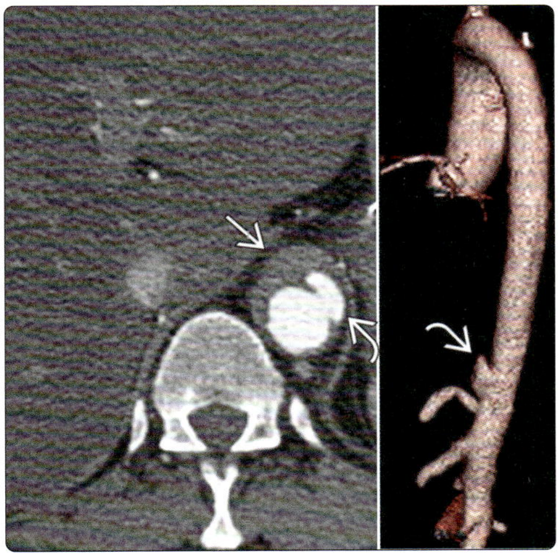

Penetrating Aortic Ulcer

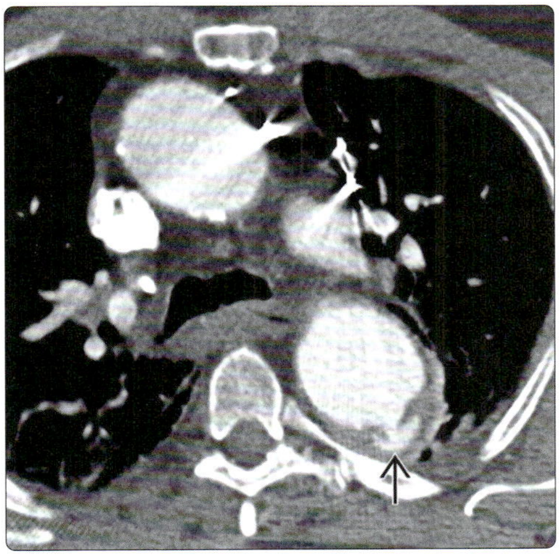

(Left) *Axial and volume-rendered CTA images show a saccular outpouching → of contrast from the descending thoracic aorta (penetrating aortic ulcer). There is associated intramural hematoma →.* **(Right)** *Axial CTA shows an outpouching of contrast → with a narrow neck from the proximal descending thoracic aorta (penetrating aortic ulcer), which does not extend beyond the aortic wall. There is associated atheroma and thickening of the aortic wall, likely intramural hematoma.*

Intramural Hematoma

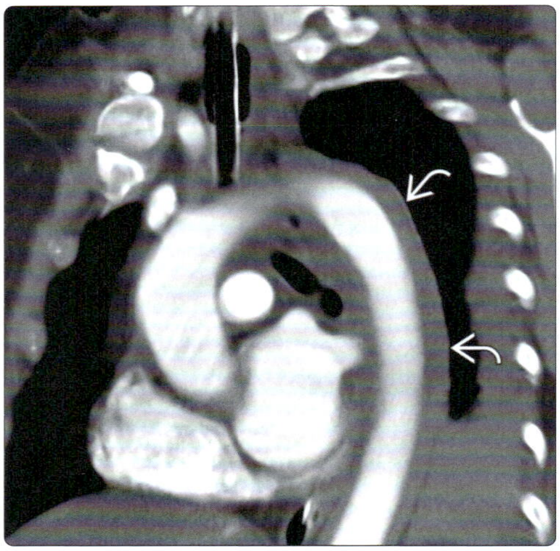

Stanford and DeBakey Dissection Classifications

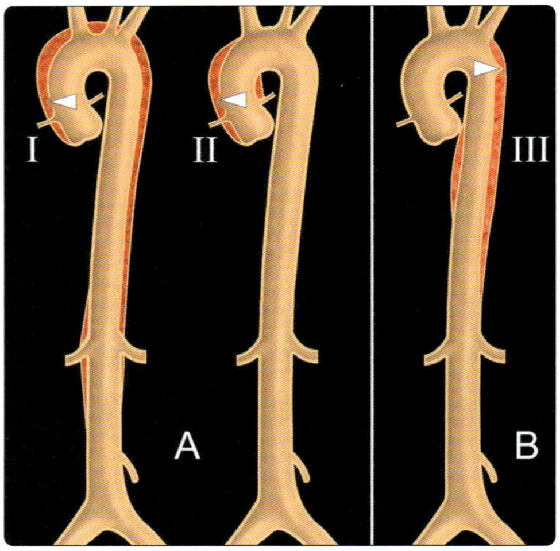

(Left) *Sagittal CECT shows thickening of the descending thoracic aortic wall from an intramural hematoma.* **(Right)** *Graphic depicts the Stanford and DeBakey classification systems used in aortic dissection. DeBakey type 1 involves both the ascending and the descending segments of thoracic aorta, type 2 only the ascending aorta, and type 3 only the descending aorta. The Stanford system divides lesions into those that involve the ascending aorta (type A) and those that do not (type B).*

Stanford Type B

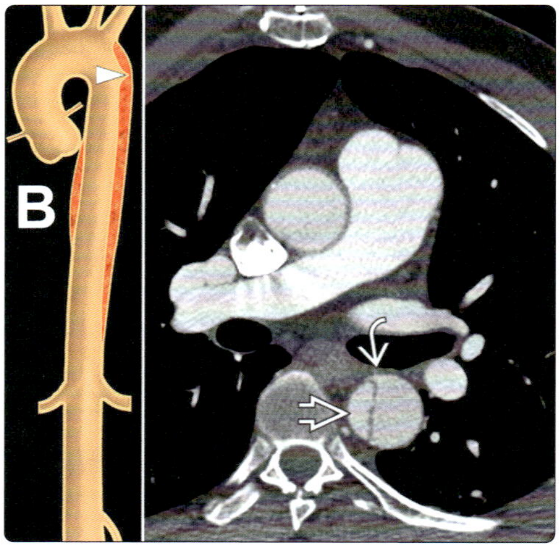

Stanford Type A

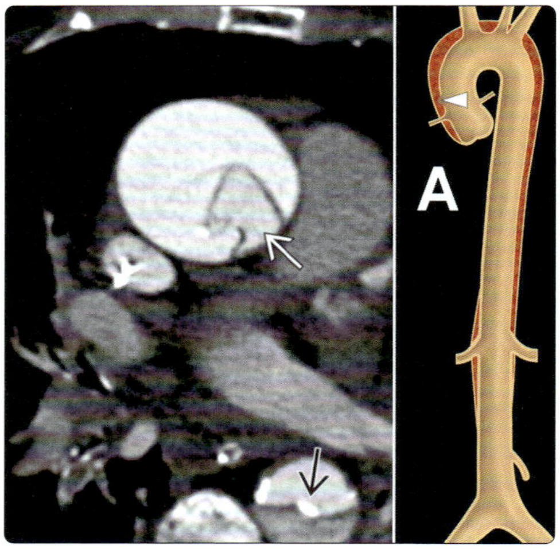

(Left) *Axial CECT demonstrates aortic dissection of the descending thoracic aorta but normal ascending aorta (Stanford type B). Note the larger false lumen with a beak sign and smaller true lumen.* **(Right)** *Axial CTA shows type A dissection with a thin flap within the dilated ascending aorta delineating the smaller true lumen. Note the displaced intimal calcification in the flap within the descending thoracic aorta.*

Pseudodissection

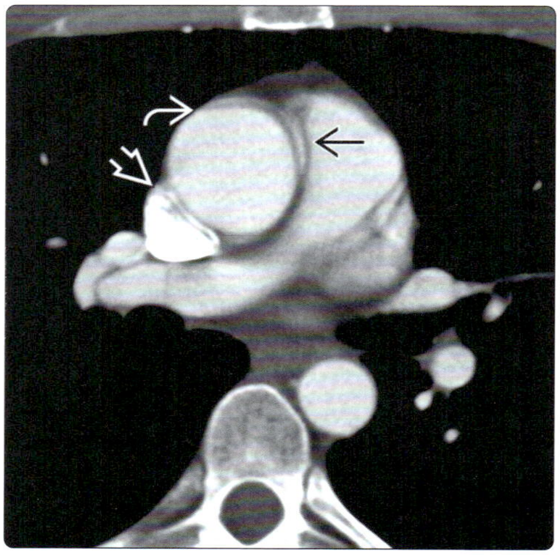

Pseudodissection

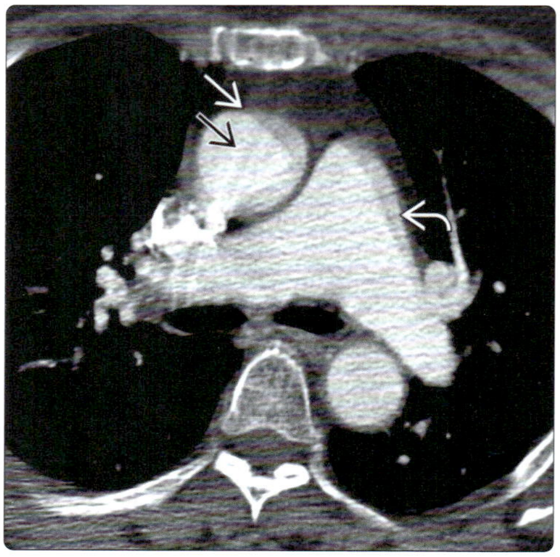

(Left) *Axial nongated CTA shows a dilated ascending aorta with pseudodissection from a pulsation artifact. Note the similar pulsation artifacts in the superior vena cava and main pulmonary artery.* **(Right)** *Axial CECT shows a beam-hardening streak artifact from high-density contrast within the superior vena cava and a pulsation artifact causing pseudodissection in the ascending aorta. A similar pulsation artifact is noted in the main pulmonary artery.*

Dissection Extent

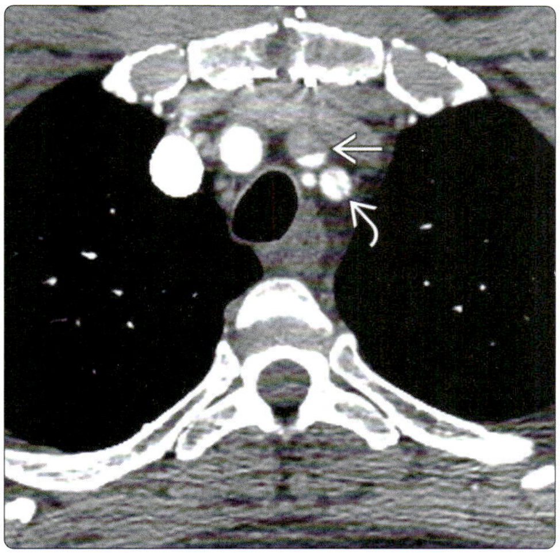

Embolic Infarction

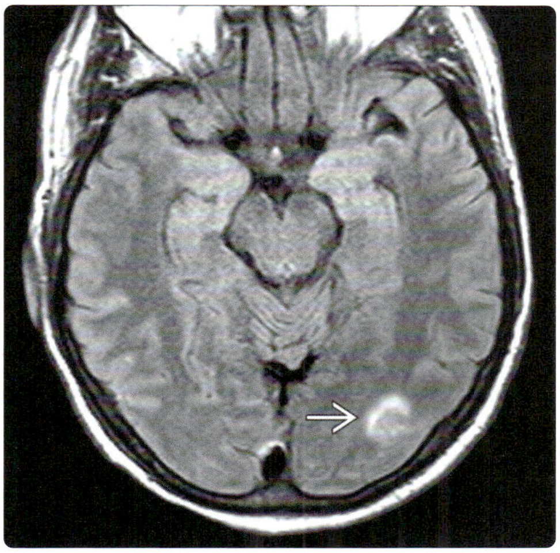

(Left) *Axial CTA shows intimal flaps from a Stanford type A aortic dissection extending into the left common carotid → and left subclavian → arteries. The false lumen of the left common carotid artery is void of contrast, which may be due to slow flow or thrombosis. Enhancement on delayed imaging would prove slow flow.* **(Right)** *Axial FLAIR MR in the same patient shows high signal intensity → within the left parietooccipital lobe due to embolic infarction.*

Stanford Type A and Hemopericardium

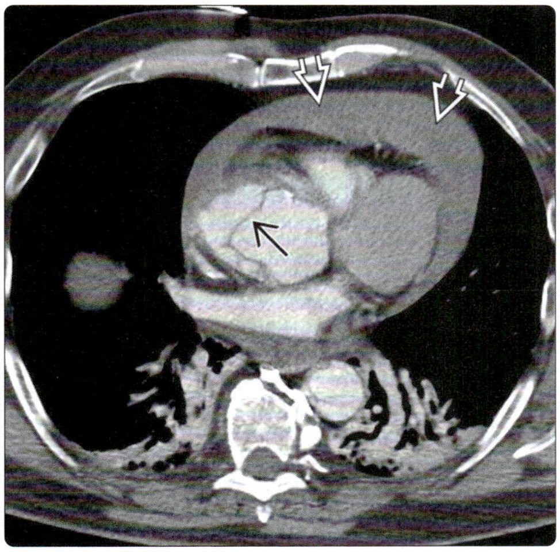

Dissection With Pericardial Tamponade

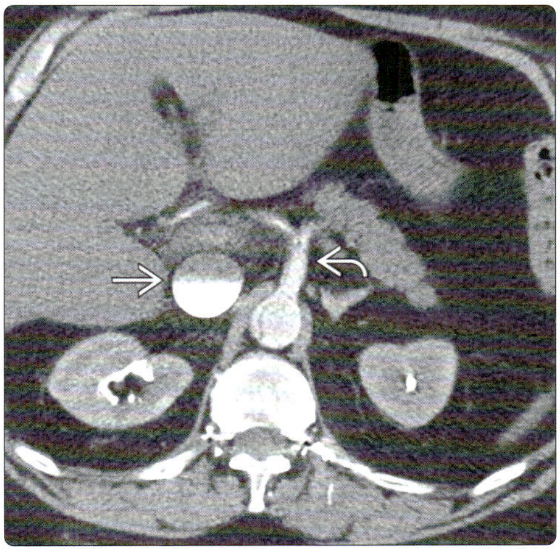

(Left) *Axial CTA shows a Stanford type A dissection → within the ascending aorta and high-density pericardial fluid indicative of hemopericardium →. A descending aortic dissection flap is also present.* **(Right)** *Axial CTA in the same patient shows the dissection extending into the abdominal aorta and superior mesenteric artery →. Note the dense contrast refluxed and layering in the superior vena cava → due to pericardial tamponade.*

Torn Intimal Flap Prolapse

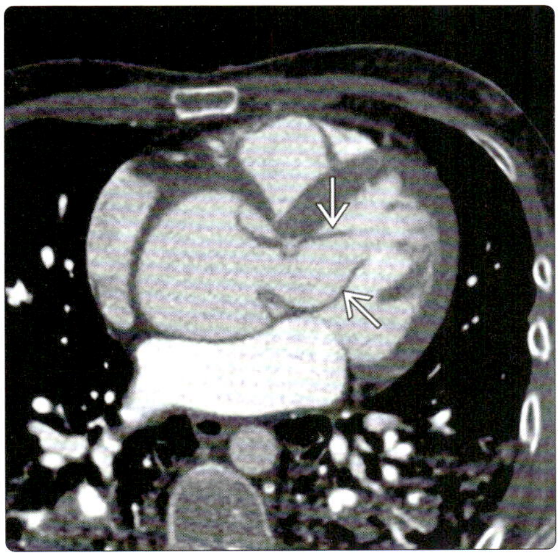

Stanford Type A Dissection

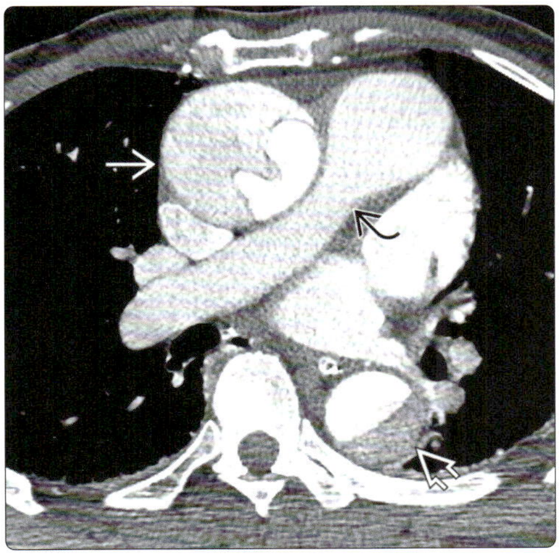

(Left) *Axial CTA shows a Stanford type A aortic dissection with the torn intimal flap → prolapsing through the aortic valve, leading to severe aortic regurgitation. The 4 life-threatening complications include myocardial infarction, stroke, pericardial tamponade, and severe aortic insufficiency.* **(Right)** *Axial CTA shows a Stanford type A dissection involving the ascending → and descending → segments of the thoracic aorta. Ascending aorta dilation narrows the right pulmonary artery →.*

(Left) *Axial CECT shows a traumatic aortic transection* ➡ *with pseudoaneurysm of the proximal descending thoracic aorta. It is important to differentiate this entity from a penetrating aortic ulcer. Most traumatic aortic injuries occur at the isthmus and may have an associated pseudoaneurysm, intraluminal filling defect, or active contrast extravasation.* **(Right)** *Oblique aortogram in the same patient shows a traumatic pseudoaneurysm* ⇨ *at the ligamentum arteriosum.*

Traumatic Aortic Transection

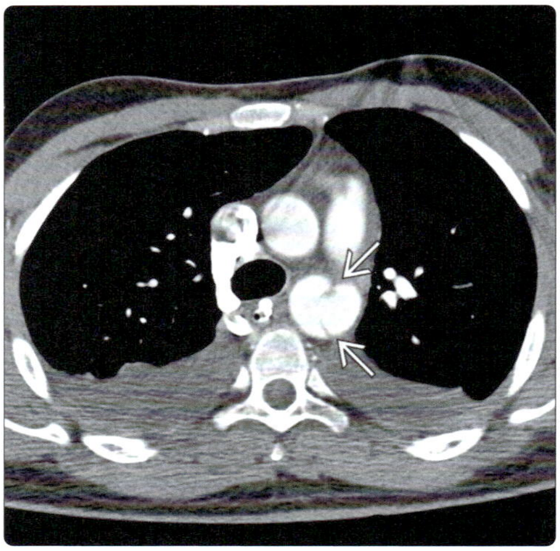

Traumatic Aortic Transection

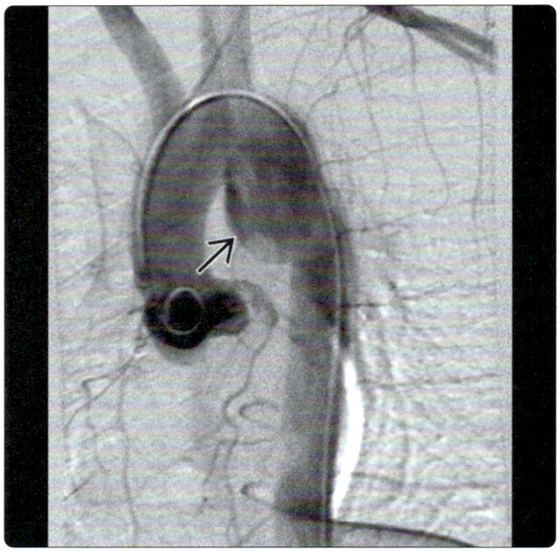

(Left) *Oblique catheter aortogram shows an intimal flap* ➡ *that originates in the descending thoracic aorta and extends into the abdomen (Stanford type B dissection).* **(Right)** *Oblique catheter aortogram in the same patient shows repair of the dissection by placement of an endoluminal stent graft* ➡ *within the aorta.*

Stanford Type B Dissection

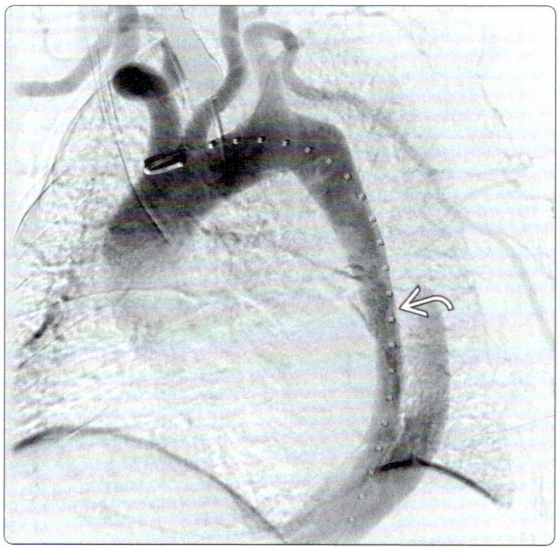

Repaired Type B Dissection

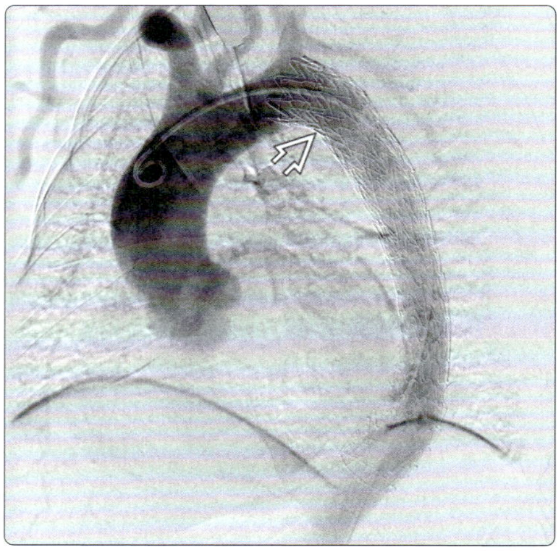

(Left) *Axial CTA shows the typical postoperative appearance of an interposition graft within the ascending thoracic aorta. The high-density outer ring* ➡ *is part of the graft. Note the persistent dissection* ➡ *in the descending thoracic aorta.* **(Right)** *Sagittal CTA shows thoracic endovascular aortic repair for a complicated type B aortic dissection. There is contrast* ⇨ *along the inferior aspect of the proximal stent graft, which indicates a type Ia endoleak.*

Interposition Graft Repair

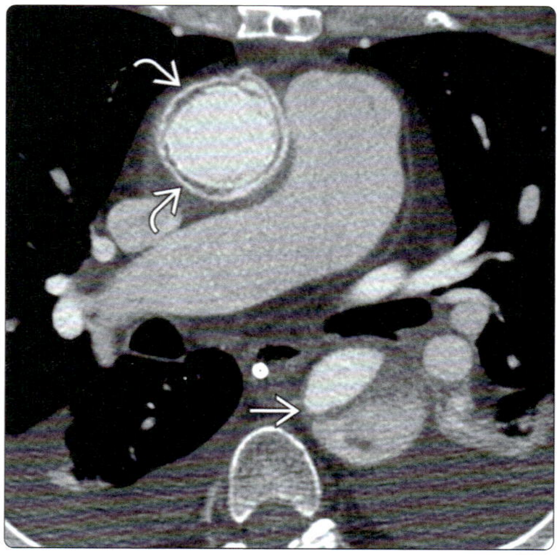

Endovascular Aortic Repair

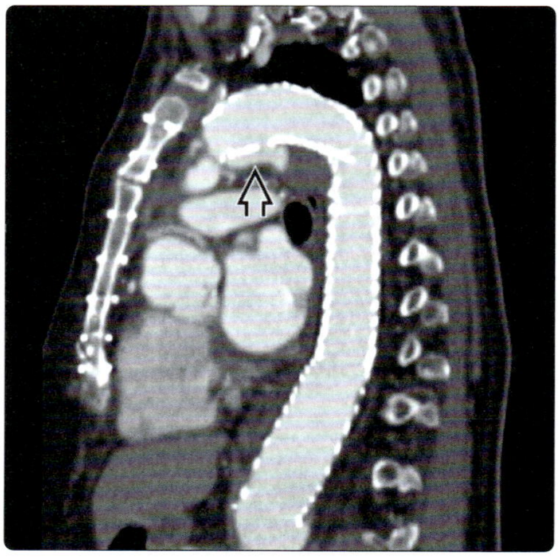

Partially Thrombosed False Lumen

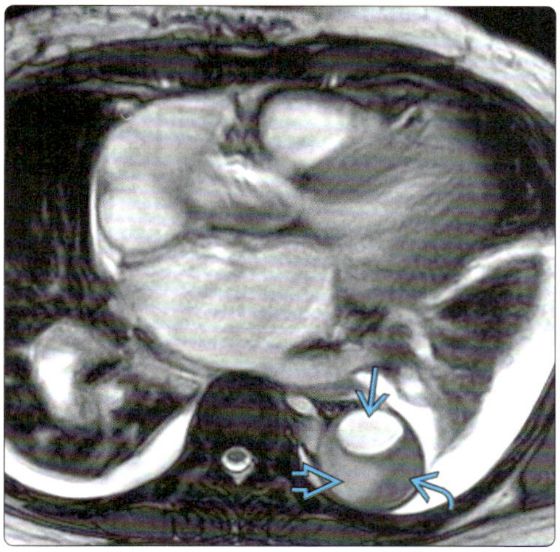

Flow in False and True Lumen

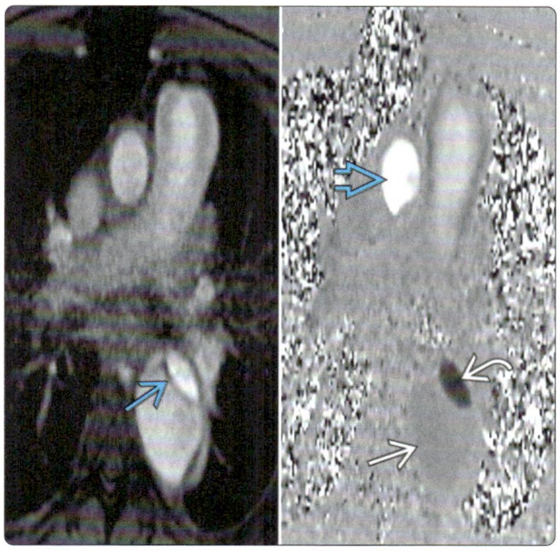

(Left) *Axial SSFP cardiac MR shows differential signal intensities in a known aortic dissection with high signal in the true lumen →, intermediate signal in the false lumen ⇒, and low signal in the mural thrombus ↪.* **(Right)** *Axial phase-contrast MR shows flow direction with low descending flow in the large false lumen ➡ compared to the smaller true lumen ➦ (dark flow indicates caudal flow, phase-sensitive sequence). Note the dissection flap → and bright cephalad forward flow in the ascending aorta ⇒.*

Intramural Hematoma

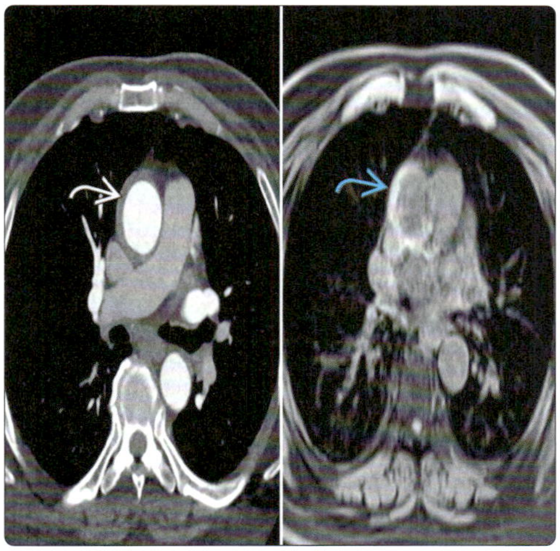

Thrombosed False Lumen

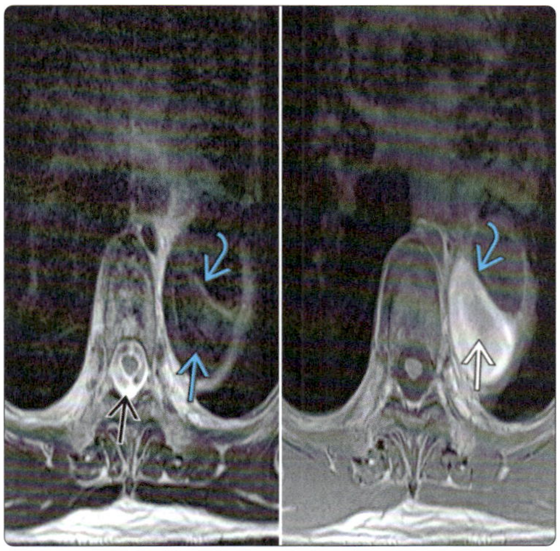

(Left) *Axial CT and fat-saturated T1 MR show eccentric thickening within ascending aortic wall on CT ➦, while T1 MR shows eccentric hyperintense signal ↪, indicating blood within the wall and confirming intramural hematoma.* **(Right)** *Axial T2 (note bright CSF signal ➡) and noncontrast T1 images show an intimal flap → in the descending thoracic aorta with a thrombus-filled large false lumen (iso- to hypointense on T2 → and hyperintense on T1 ➡).*

Thrombosed False Lumen

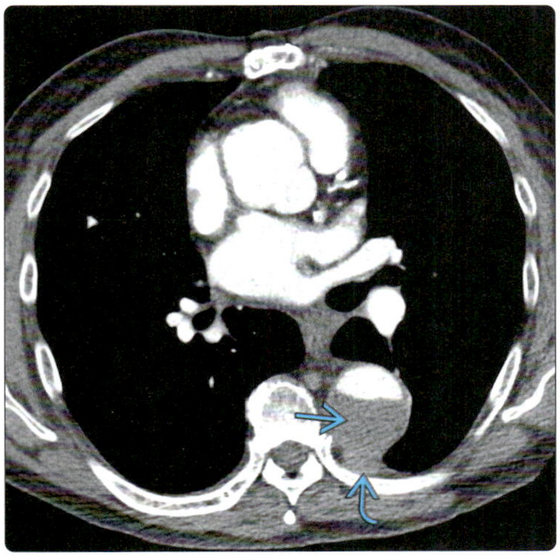

Thrombosed False Lumen

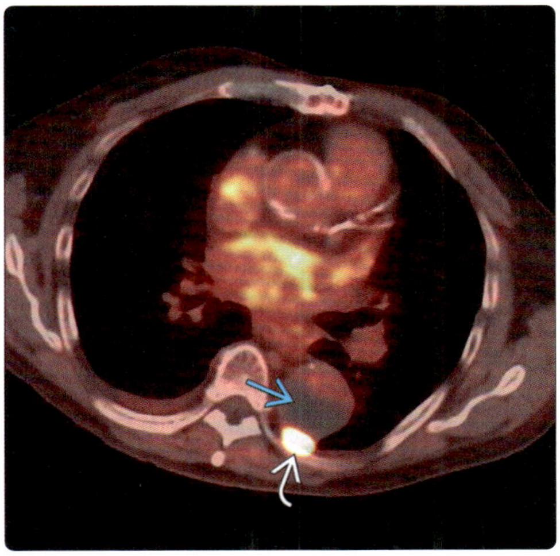

(Left) *Axial CTA shows dissection in the descending thoracic aorta with a thrombosed false lumen → and a focal saccular outpouching in the posterior aortic wall ↪.* **(Right)** *Fused FDG PET/CT in the same patient shows differential blood pool tracer in the descending aorta from dissection with no tracer in the thrombosed false lumen →. Intense FDG uptake at the posterior focal saccular outpouching ➦ suggests significant inflammatory activity and potential progression.*

Aortic Dissection

KEY FACTS

TERMINOLOGY

- Blood enters media of aortic wall through intimal defect and splits wall longitudinally

IMAGING

- 2 distinct lumina (false and true) with interposed intimal flap
  - False lumen: Larger cross-sectional area, beak sign, cobweb sign, thrombosis, and delayed enhancement
  - True lumen: Continuity with undissected portion of aorta and smaller cross-sectional area
- Radiograph: Progressive aortic enlargement, widened mediastinum (> 8 cm), and abnormal (blunted) aortic knob
- CT: Highly accurate
  - Slightly less accurate for ascending aorta unless ECG-gated study
- MR: Well-suited for follow-up
- Transesophageal echocardiography: Operator dependent and with limited field of view

TOP DIFFERENTIAL DIAGNOSES

- Thrombosed aneurysm
- Aortic wall hematoma
- Syndromes associated with aortic dissection

PATHOLOGY

- Media degeneration associated with many diseases and syphilitic aortitis, crack cocaine use, and iatrogenic (catheter angiography, cardiac surgery, valve replacements)
- Tear in intimal layer leading to formation and propagation of subintimal hematoma

CLINICAL ISSUES

- Type A: Surgery due to involvement of aortic root
- Type B: Medical control of hypertension is standard
- Percutaneous therapy for complicated nonsurgical patients with type B dissections

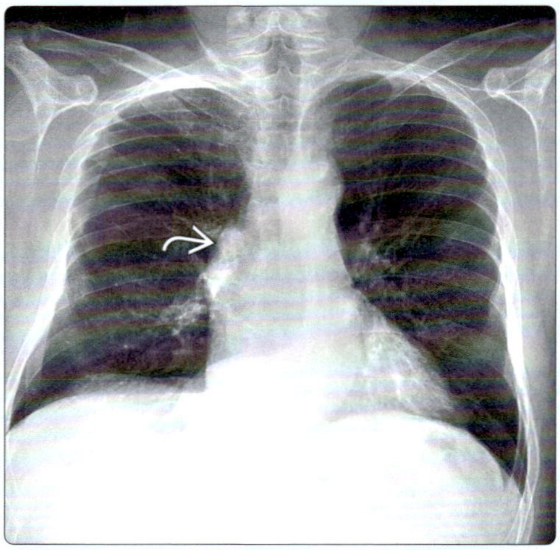
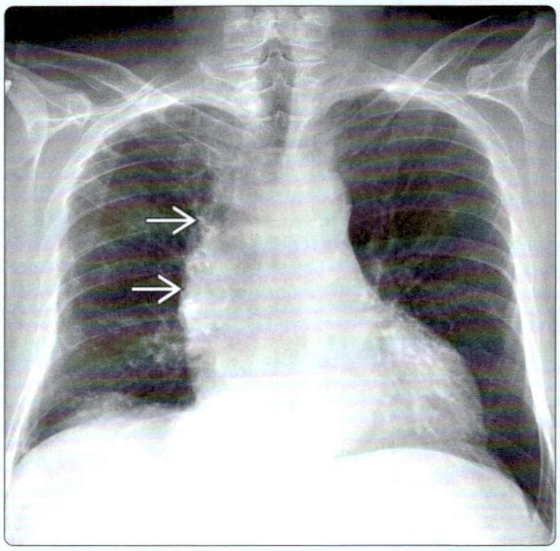

(Left) *Frontal chest radiograph shows subtle abnormal contour of the ascending aorta, suggestive of ascending aortic aneurysm ➦, but this finding is nonspecific. The descending aorta is tortuous, which can be seen in systemic hypertension.* **(Right)** *Frontal radiograph in the same patient presenting a few months later with acute chest pain shows increased abnormal contour and abnormal widening of the mediastinum ➡, suggestive of aortic dissection.*

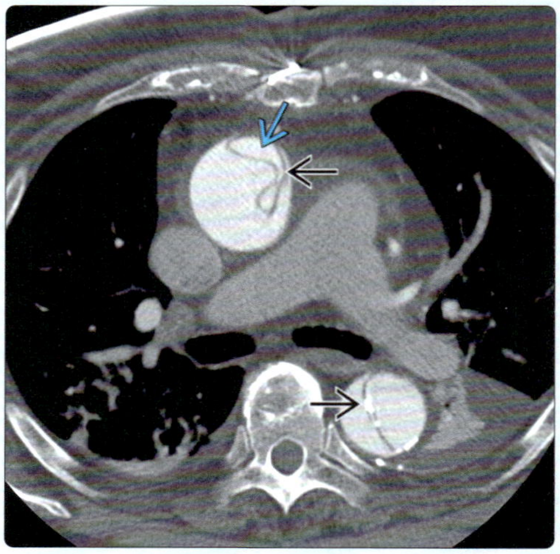
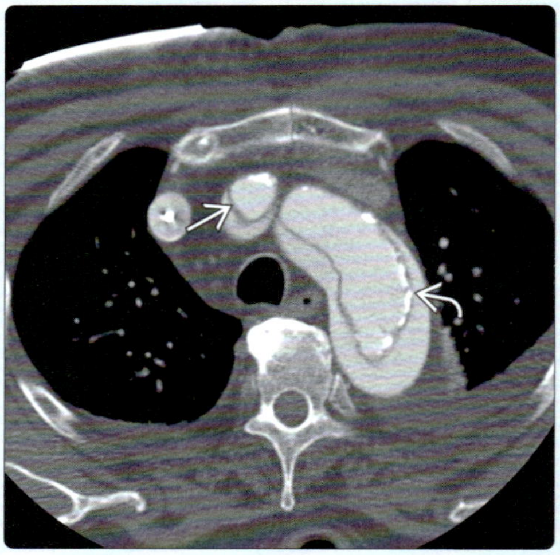

(Left) *Axial CTA through the thorax in a patient with Stanford type A dissection shows a nearly circumferential dissection flap ➡ involving the ascending and descending aortas. Note the small true lumen in the ascending aorta ➡. The intimal flap can be quite mobile on gated cine imaging.* **(Right)** *Axial CTA at the level of arch in the same patient shows extension of the dissection flap into the right brachiocephalic artery ➡. Note the displaced intimal calcification in the descending aorta ➦.*

TERMINOLOGY

Abbreviations

- Aortic dissection (AD)

Definitions

- Blood enters media of aortic wall through intimal defect and splits wall longitudinally

IMAGING

General Features

- Best diagnostic clue
  - 2 distinct lumina with interposed intimal flap: Double-barrel aorta
  - Displacement of intimal calcification or compression/distortion of aortic lumen
- Location
  - Stanford classification
    - Type A (60%): Involves ascending aorta
    - Type B (40%): Does not involve ascending aorta
  - DeBakey classification
    - Type I: Originates in ascending aorta, involves at least aortic arch, and may involve descending aorta
    - Type II: Originates in and confined to ascending aorta
    - Type III: Originates in descending aorta; IIIa: Limited to descending aorta; IIIb: Extends below diaphragm

Radiographic Findings

- Radiography
  - Often abnormal CXR but nonspecific
    - 25% are normal
  - Widened mediastinum (> 8 cm)
  - Abnormal (blunted) aortic knob in 66%
  - Ring sign: > 5-mm displacement of aortic lumen past calcified aortic intima
    - Apparent displacement of intimal calcification may be projectional artifact
  - Left apical cap, tracheal deviation, depression of left mainstem bronchus, esophageal deviation, loss of paratracheal stripe, pericardial effusion, and hemothorax
  - Progressive aortic enlargement on serial images

CT Findings

- NECT
  - Widening of aorta, irregularity of aortic wall, and intramural or periaortic acute thrombus
  - Hyperattenuating mediastinal, pericardial, or pleural fluid (blood)
  - Internally displaced intimal calcification
- CECT
  - Intimal flap separates true and false lumina
  - True vs. false lumen
    - False lumen is larger than true lumen
    - False lumen wedges around true lumen, beak sign
    - Cobweb sign of false lumen due to collagenous media remnants
  - False lumen contrast attenuation
    - Usually, slower flow with lower contrast attenuation on arterial phase
    - Thrombosis leads to nonenhancement
      - ◻ Complete thrombosis/reduced flow in false lumen decreases risk of aortic dilatation
  - Windsock appearance: Dissection of entire intima leads to circumferential intimal flap
    - Filiform-shaped, narrow true lumen
    - Leads to intimointimal intussusception
  - Triple-channel dissection: Secondary dissection within 1 channel (Mercedes-Benz sign)
  - Complications of AD
    - Rupture into pericardium, left pleural cavity, mediastinum, right ventricle, left atrium, vena cavae, pulmonary arteries
    - Pericardial tamponade
    - Acute aortic regurgitation
    - Major aortic branch obstruction
    - Visceral or extremity malperfusion
      - ◻ Compression of true lumen by false lumen
      - ◻ Intimal flap in renal, celiac, mesenteric, or extremity arteries
      - ◻ Renal: Absence of nephrographic effect in late phase of CT
  - Retrograde dissection into aortic arch
    - In 27% of type B dissections; higher mortality (43%)

MR Findings

- T1WI
  - Site of intimal tear; type and extent of dissection
  - Signal intensity within false lumen is variable
    - Depends on blood flow; thrombus: Presence, age, composition; and pulse sequence
    - Usually signal is seen due to slow flow
      - ◻ Flow void in true lumen
  - Useful in abdominal arterial involvement and monitoring of progression of dissection and aneurysm formation
- MRA
  - Demonstrates flap, true and false lumen
  - Extent of flap into branch vessels can be seen
  - End-organ perfusion can be evaluated
- SSFP cine
  - Intimal flap: Intermediate signal
  - Reentry site: Low-signal turbulent flow between lumina
  - False lumen with blood flow/thrombus: Medium to low signal
  - Aortic insufficiency and pericardial rupture
- Phase-contrast imaging
  - Flow dynamics of lumina can be evaluated
  - 4D flow MR
    - Detailed evaluation of hemodynamics
      - ◻ Flow/thrombosis of false lumen evaluated more reliably than CT
      - ◻ Retrograde flow is less in true than false lumen
      - ◻ Helical flow in false lumen is sign of aortic expansion
- Progressive aortic enlargement evaluated by MR/cardiac CT
  - Features predictive of descending aortic enlargement
    - > 10-mm primary intimal tear in descending aorta
    - Descending aorta > 35 mm
    - False lumen > 22 mm in proximal descending aorta
    - False lumen > 2/3 of total descending aorta
    - Partially thrombosed distal false lumen

   - Distal suture line leak
   - Helical flow in false lumen
- Remodeling: 10% volumetric difference of aorta
  - Favorable remodeling: > 10% decrease in false lumen or > 10% increase in true lumen diameter
  - Unfavorable remodeling: Increased diameter of false and decreased diameter of true lumen
    - Due to persistent refilling of false lumen

Imaging Recommendations

- CT: Highly accurate and rapid; imaging procedure of choice
  - ECG gating or high-pitch helical mode is necessary to avoid risk of false-positives in aortic root
- MR: Better suited in nonemergent setting: Anatomic information; flow dynamics of false and true lumen

DIFFERENTIAL DIAGNOSIS

Thrombosed Aneurysm

- Large aorta and aortic lumen size

Intramural Hematoma

- Hemorrhage within wall with no identifiable intimal tear, flap, or false lumen
- Caused by bleeding from vasa vasorum into media

Penetrating Aortic Ulcer

- Perforation of aortic wall in region of ulcerated atherosclerotic plaque
- Most common in descending aorta

PATHOLOGY

General Features

- Etiology
  - Medial degeneration is associated with many diseases that predispose to dissection
    - Hypertension (70%), atherosclerosis
    - Structural collagen disorder (Marfan or Ehlers-Danlos syndrome)
    - Congenital disease (aortic coarctation; bicuspid or unicuspid valve); pregnancy
  - Syphilitic aortitis, crack cocaine use, and iatrogenic (catheter angiography, cardiac surgery, valve replacements)
- Dissections almost exclusively originate in thoracic aorta and secondarily involve abdominal aorta

Gross Pathologic & Surgical Features

- Intimal tear: Formation/propagation of subintimal hematoma
  - 5-10% are without intimal tear; dissection is attributed to rupture of aortic vasa vasorum
- Diseases that weaken aortic wall predispose to AD

CLINICAL ISSUES

Presentation

- Most common signs/symptoms
  - Sudden onset of ripping or tearing chest pain
  - Anterior chest pain: Ascending AD
  - Neck or jaw pain: Aortic arch dissection
  - Back tearing or ripping pain: Descending AD
  - Myocardial infarction
  - 50% of AD: Women < 40 years, related to pregnancy
- Sudden onset of aortic insufficiency, neurologic deficits in 20% of cases, and ischemic extremity

Demographics

- Age
  - 75% in 40-70 years; peak at 50-65 years
- Sex
  - M:F = 3:1
- Ethnicity
  - Black > White > Asian patients

Natural History & Prognosis

- Acute AD: < 2 weeks from initial onset of symptoms; subacute: 2 weeks to 3 months; chronic: > 3 months
- Complications: Rupture, cardiac tamponade, aortic insufficiency with acute heart failure, occlusion of coronary or supraaortic vessels
- 21% of patients die before hospital admission
- If untreated, 33% die within 24 hours; 50% within 48 hours

Treatment

- Type A: Surgery due to involvement of aortic root
  - Ascending aorta only: Supracoronary ascending aorta replacement, intimal resection, aortic valve repair/replacement
  - Arch/hemiarch: Antegrade thoracic endovascular aortic repair (TEVAR), elephant trunk, frozen elephant trunk, or multibranched arch graft
  - Bentall procedure: If valve cusps are dissected or with Marfan syndrome with preexisting root aneurysm
- Type B: Conservative treatment is standard (Rx of hypertension)
  - Surgery in complicated cases
    - Mesenteric, renal, extremity ischemia
    - Rupture, aneurysmal enlargement of false lumen; descending aorta > 6 cm
    - Hemodynamic instability, pseudocoarctation syndrome, distal embolization
  - Percutaneous therapy (aortic stent graft or fenestration of flap) for complicated nonsurgical patients with type B dissections
    - Visceral malperfusion, dilated aortic arch or proximal descending aorta (≥ 4.5 cm), impending rupture
- DISSECT classification system for endovascular decision making
  - Based on 6 features: **D**uration, **i**ntimal tear, **s**ize of dissected aorta, **s**egmental **e**xtent of involvement, **c**linical complications, **t**hrombosis of false lumen
- TEVAR in subacute/chronic setting
  - Descending aorta > 5.5 cm, > 5-mm growth/6 months, refractory pain, impending aortic rupture

SELECTED REFERENCES

1. Writing Committee Members et al: 2022 ACC/AHA Guideline for the Diagnosis and Management of Aortic Disease: a report of the American Heart Association/American College of Cardiology Joint Committee on Clinical Practice Guidelines. J Am Coll Cardiol. 80(24):e223-393, 2022
2. Ko JP et al: Chest CT angiography for acute aortic pathologic conditions: pearls and pitfalls. Radiographics. 41(2):399-424, 2021
3. Murillo H et al: Aortic dissection and other acute aortic syndromes: diagnostic imaging findings from acute to chronic longitudinal progression. Radiographics. 41(2):425-46, 2021

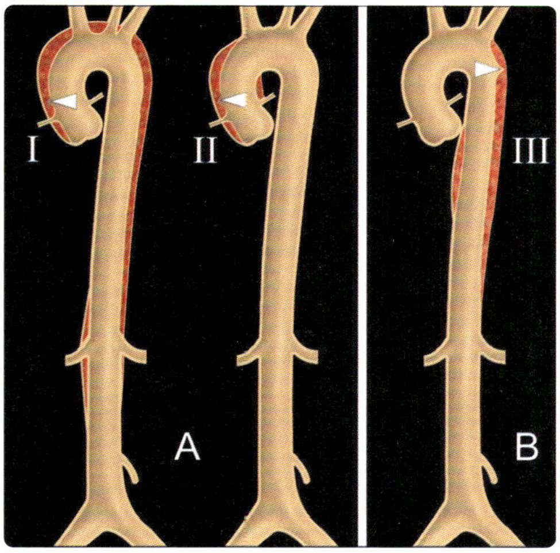

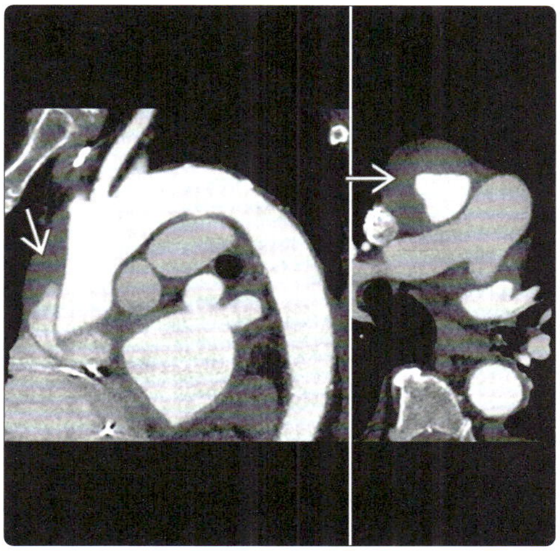

(Left) *DeBakey type I and Stanford class A include dissections that involve the ascending aorta. DeBakey type II is confined to the ascending aorta, and type I extends beyond. DeBakey type III dissections are confined to the descending aorta. Stanford class B includes all dissections not involving the ascending aorta (involving arch &/or descending aorta).* **(Right)** *"Candy cane" sagittal oblique (left) and axial (right) CTA views show Stanford type A aortic dissection with partially thrombosed false lumen.*

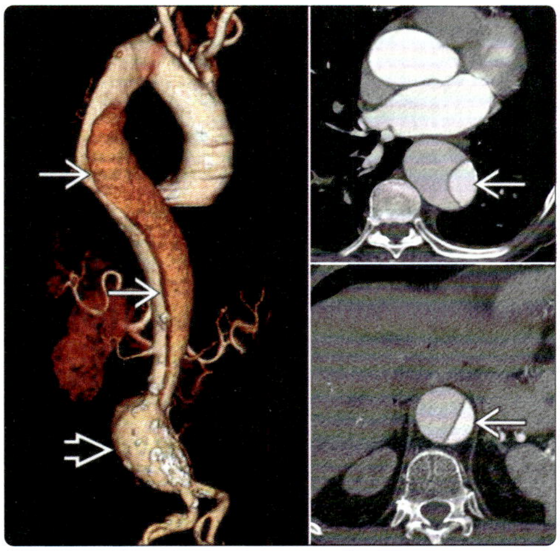

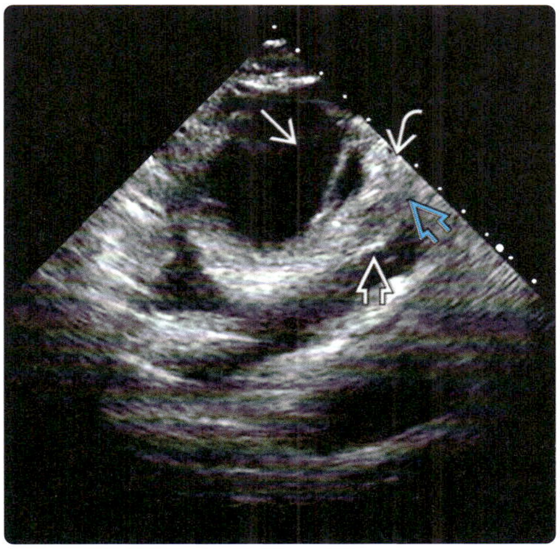

(Left) *Axial and VR CTA show Stanford type B aortic dissection involving descending thoracic and abdominal aorta. The true lumen is smaller and located laterally. Note the infrarenal abdominal aortic aneurysm.* **(Right)** *Transthoracic echocardiogram shows ascending aortic dissection with dissection flap (white interface) separating true and false lumina. Most of the false lumen is hyperechoic, suggesting thrombosis. The small, anechoic portion corresponds to a patent false lumen.*

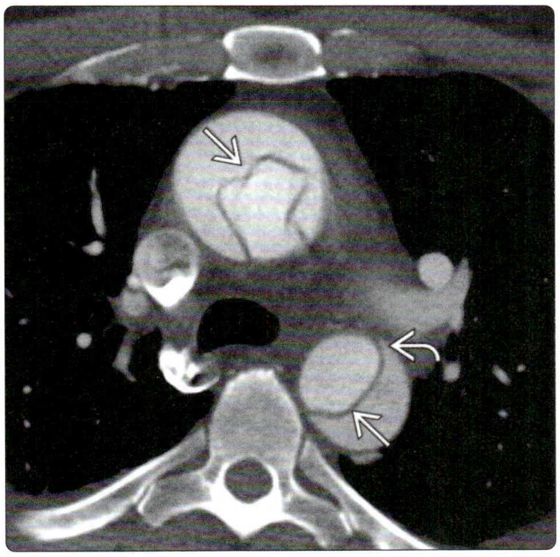

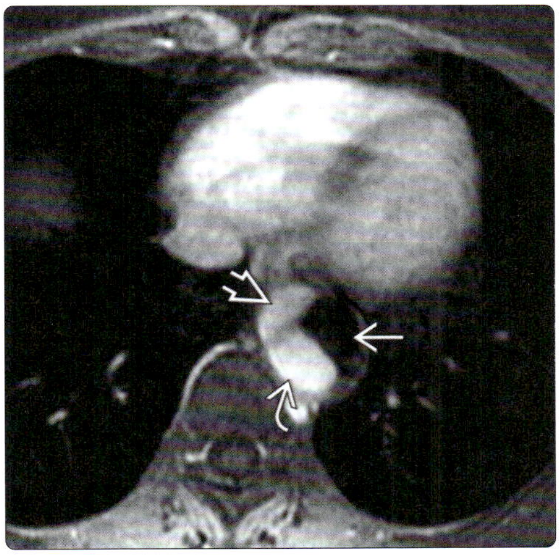

(Left) *Axial CECT shows acute type A aortic dissection with flap that is convex toward false lumen. Note that a beak sign is present in the false lumen. The appearance of a beak sign is attributed to the higher systolic pressure in the true lumen.* **(Right)** *Axial MRA shows chronic type B aortic dissection with partial thrombosis of the false lumen (hypointense area). Compared with the false lumen, the true lumen is relatively small. Note the perfused portion of the false lumen.*

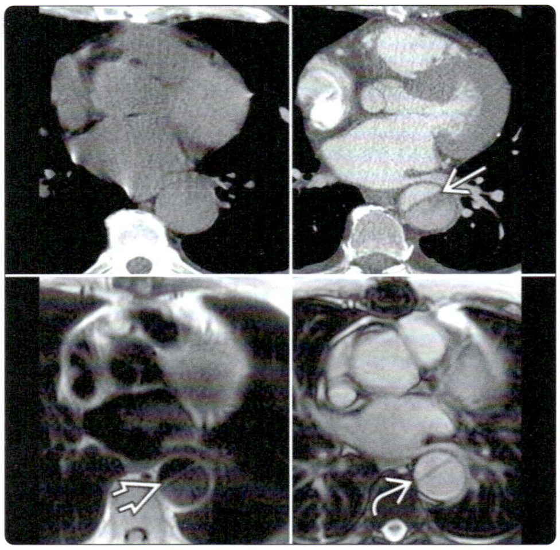

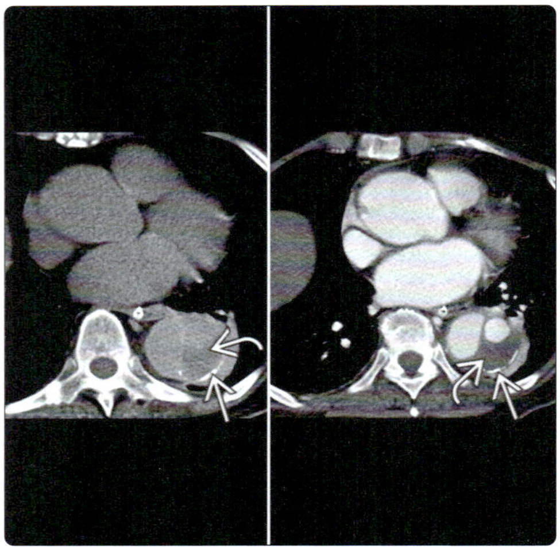

(Left) *Axial NECT, CTA, and MR in a patient with type B aortic dissection are shown. The aortic dissection is not seen on NECT. Axial unenhanced MR shows aortic dissection on HASTE (dark blood) and SSFP (bright blood), an advantage over NECT.* **(Right)** *Axial NECT and CTA show chronic descending thoracic aortic dissection with a flat dissection flap. Outer wall calcification and thrombus are present in the false lumen.*

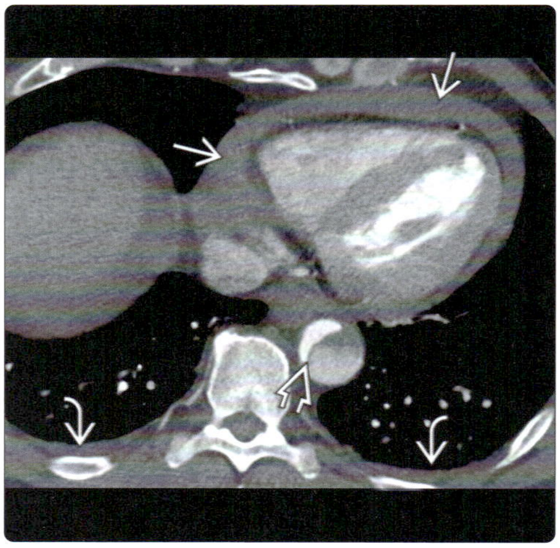

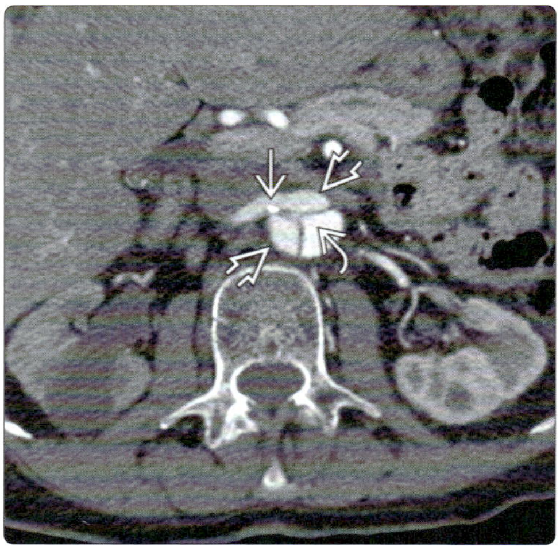

(Left) *Axial CECT shows a high-attenuation pericardial effusion, consistent with a hemopericardium, as well as bilateral trace pleural effusions. The dissection flap is clearly visible in the descending thoracic aorta.* **(Right)** *Axial CTA shows abdominal aortic dissection with Mercedes-Benz sign relating to a triple-channel dissection resulting in 2 false lumina. One of the 2 intimal flaps extends to the origin of the right renal artery.*

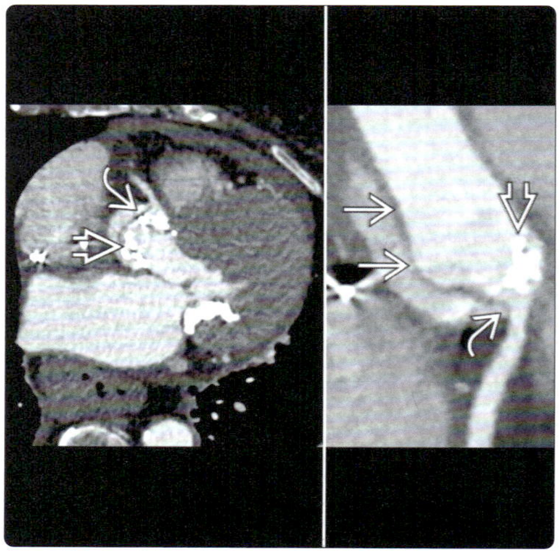

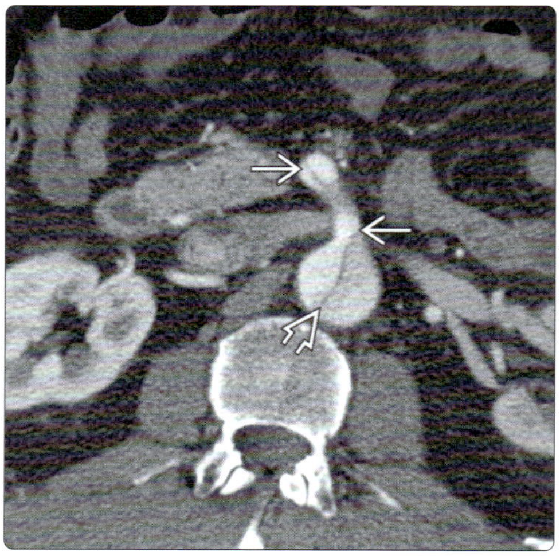

(Left) *Axial (left) and oblique (right) CTA demonstrate a type A aortic dissection involving the right coronary artery ostium in a patient status post percutaneous aortic valve implantation/replacement (TAVI/R).* **(Right)** *Axial CTA shows an abdominal aortic dissection. Note that the dissection flap does extend into the superior mesenteric artery, which remains well perfused.*

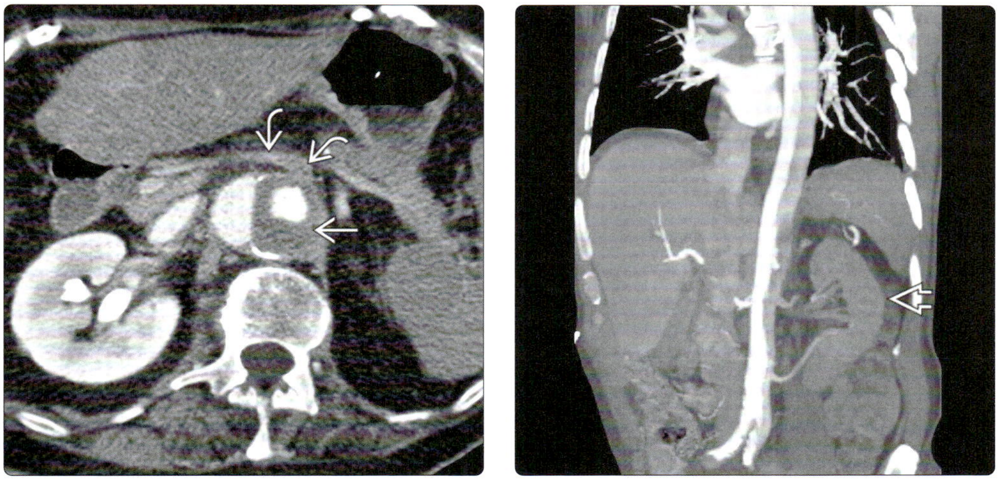

(Left) *Axial CTA shows partial eccentric thrombosis of the false lumen in a chronic aortic dissection. The celiac artery ↷ arises from the false lumen → and is thrombosed.* **(Right)** *Oblique MIP CTA shows dissection of the descending thoracic and abdominal aorta. Note main and accessory renal arteries arising from the partially thrombosed false lumen and a subtotal infarct of the left kidney ⇨. Main and accessory renal arteries demonstrate partial flow.*

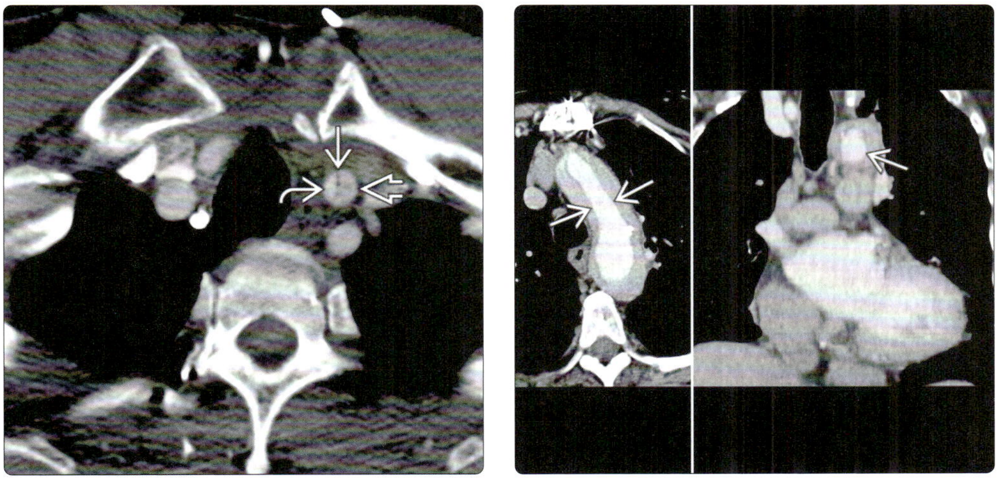

(Left) *Axial CTA shows a dissection flap extending into the left common carotid artery →. The true lumen ↷ is smaller and enhances more than the false lumen ⇨.* **(Right)** *Axial (left) and coronal (right) CTA show atypical appearance of an aortic dissection involving the entire intima → of the thoracic aorta circumferentially. This phenomenon may subsequently lead to intimointimal intussusception.*

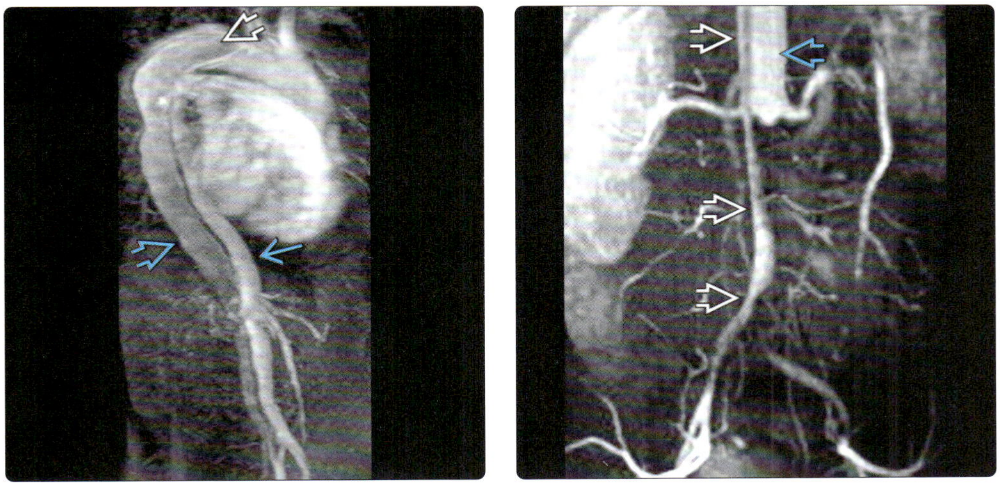

(Left) *Sagittal MRA shows an aortic dissection, which is seen starting from the arch distal to the origin of the left subclavian artery ⇨, and extends into the abdominal aorta, extending into the iliac arteries. The true lumen → enhances more than the false lumen ↷.* **(Right)** *Coronal MR cine shows the false lumen ⇨ supplying the left renal artery. The small, compressed true lumen ⇨ supplies the right renal artery. The false lumen is thrombosed in the infrarenal area.*

KEY FACTS

TERMINOLOGY

- Complete circumferential intimal tear in type A > type B aortic dissection
- Delaminated intima then rolls upon itself

IMAGING

- Best visualized with ECG-gated CTA
- Circumferential intimal tear → unidirectional or bidirectional intimointimal intussusception (IIIS)
  - Anterograde (43%): Intima superior circumferential intimal tear delaminates upward
    - Intimal often folded upon itself in aortic arch
  - Retrograde (56%): Intima inferior to circumferential tear delaminates inferiorly
    - Intimal may prolapse into LV during diastole
  - Bidirectional (1%): IIIS both anterograde and retrograde
- Between delaminated intima that has intussuscepted superiorly &/or inferiorly, portion of aorta appears "normal" but actually lacks intima
  - Missing flap or naked aorta sign

CLINICAL ISSUES

- Diagnosis not prospectively made before surgical intervention in 49% of anterograde IIIS and 16% of retrograde IIIS
- Anterograde
  - Chest pain
  - Neurologic symptoms (62%)
  - Asymmetric blood pressure (57%)
- Retrograde
  - Myocardial infarction (26.5%)
  - Severe aortic regurgitation
- Mean age: 54 years
- M > F
- Overall mortality: 24%
- Treatment is surgical repair

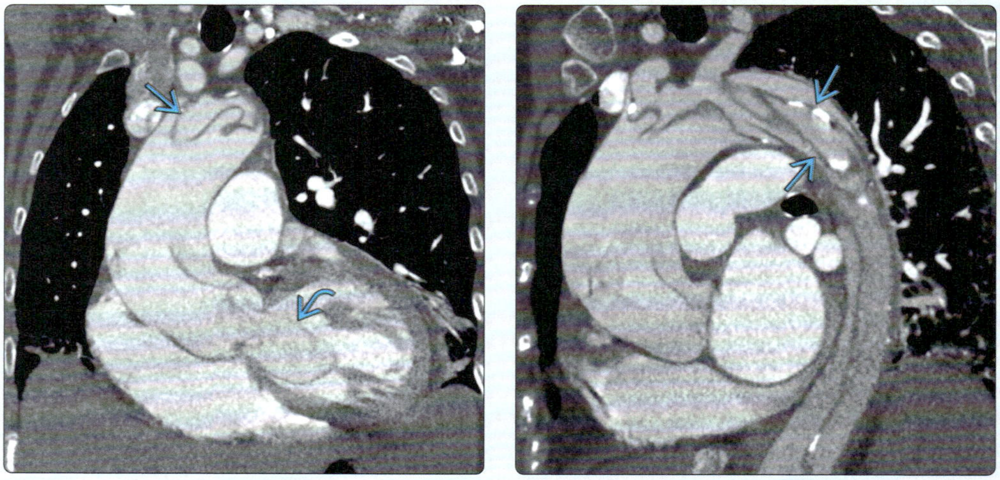

(Left) *Type A aortic dissection with bidirectional intimointimal intussusception (IIIS) is shown. At the point of circumferential intimal tear, the delaminated intima rolls anterograde ➔ into the aortic arch and retrograde ➔ into the left ventricle.* **(Right)** *Sagittal oblique CECT shows the anterograde IIIS folded upon itself in the proximal descending thoracic aorta ➔. Intimal calcifications can be seen.*

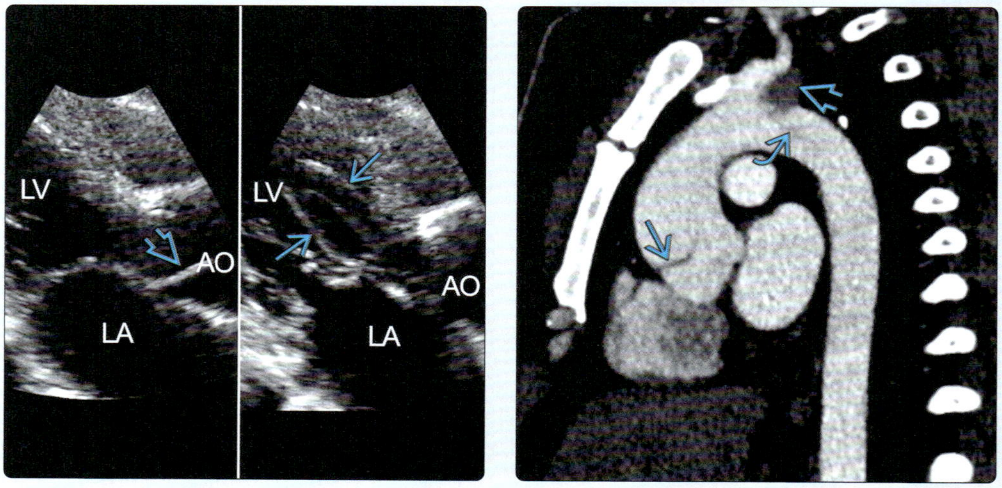

(Left) *Echo image during systole (left) shows a portion of the delaminated intima in the ascending aorta ➔. During diastole (right), there is retrograde IIIS into the left ventricle ➔.* **(Right)** *CTA in a 31-year-old man with chest and arm pain shows a type A dissection with a circumferential intimal tear and flap ➔ in the aortic root. The anterograde IIIS has lodged into and occluded the left subclavian artery ➔. Only a small portion of intima is in the aortic arch ➔.*

TERMINOLOGY

Abbreviations

- Intimointimal intussusception (IIIS)

Definitions

- Complete circumferential intimal tear in type A aortic dissection; delaminated intima then rolls upon itself like tube sock; given this is circumferential tear, intima can intussuscept anterograde (upward) into aortic arch (AA)/descending thoracic aorta (DTA) &/or retrograde (downward) into aortic root and left ventricle (LV)

IMAGING

General Features

- Best diagnostic clue
  - Type A dissection where layers of intimal are folded in on itself within ascending &/or DTA
- Location
  - Ascending aorta or AA (98%)
  - DTA (2%)

Radiographic Findings

- No specific radiographic findings are visible other than findings associated with type A dissection

CT Findings

- Best visualized with ECG-gated CTA
- Findings of type A dissection in most cases
- Circumferential intimal tear leads to either unidirectional or bidirectional IIIS
  - Anterograde (43%): Intima superior to level of circumferential intimal tear delaminates upward into AA and DTA
    - Intimal is often seen folded upon itself in AA or DTA
    - Intima may obstruct arch vessels leading to neurologic sequela
  - Retrograde (56%): Intima inferior to level of circumferential tear delaminates inferiorly into aortic root and may prolapse into LV during diastole
  - Bidirectional (1%): IIIS both anterograde and retrograde
- Between delaminated intima that has intussuscepted superiorly &/or inferiorly, there is portion of aorta that appears normal, i.e., free of dissection flap
  - This portion of aorta lacks intima
  - Sometimes called missing flap or naked aorta sign
- Anterograde IIIS can involve entire thoracic aorta and extend into abdominal aorta or into iliac arteries
  - IIIS occluding superior mesenteric artery (SMA) can lead to mesenteric ischemia

MR Findings

- Few case reports of IIIS visualized with MR
- Best seen with bright-blood imaging, such as gated SSFP imaging or contrast-enhanced MRA
- Similar findings to CT with unidirectional or bidirectional intima that has rolled upon itself superiorly &/or inferiorly

Echocardiographic Findings

- May see portion of intimal flap prolapsing into LV
  - 71% in retrograde IIIS
- Intimal flap in aortic root
- Aortic regurgitation; often severe
  - 84% in retrograde IIIS

Imaging Recommendations

- Best imaging tool
  - ECG-gated CTA

DIFFERENTIAL DIAGNOSIS

Type A Dissection Without Intimointimal Intussusception

- Will not see delaminated intimal folded on itself in aortic lumen

CLINICAL ISSUES

Presentation

- Most common signs/symptoms
  - Anterograde
    - Chest pain
    - Neurologic symptoms (62%)
      - Cerebrovascular accident
      - Syncope
    - Asymmetric blood pressure (57%)
      - Likely due to subclavian artery occlusion
  - Retrograde
    - Chest and back pain
    - Dyspnea
    - Myocardial infarction (26.5%)
    - Aortic regurgitation (84%); often severe

Demographics

- Mean age: 54 years
- M > F

Natural History & Prognosis

- Overall mortality: 24%
  - Preoperative and postoperative mortality of 14% and 9%, respectively
  - Similar mortality for anterograde and retrograde IIIS

Treatment

- Diagnosis not prospectively made before surgical intervention in 49% of anterograde IIIS and 16% of retrograde IIIS
- Aortotomy and surgical repair
  - Various techniques, including Bentall repair, ascending aortic and arch replacement
  - Intussuscepted intima may be retracted upward &/or downward and tacked down to aorta

SELECTED REFERENCES

1. Dokollari A et al: Aortic intimo-intimal intussusception in Stanford type A acute aortic dissection. Eur Heart J. 42(34):3410, 2021
2. Wu ZY et al: Aortic Intimo-intimal intussusception: a pooled analysis of published reports. Ann Vasc Surg. 75:471-8, 2021
3. Sanders LH et al: Radiological diagnosis and classification of antegrade and retrograde Stanford type A intimal intussusception. Int J Cardiovasc Imaging. 23(5):659-65, 2007

Aortic Intramural Hematoma

KEY FACTS

TERMINOLOGY

- Intramural hematoma (IMH) (literally blood in wall) in its broadest sense refers to fresh thrombus/clot within aortic wall; term IMH is used clinically (and somewhat confusingly) for 2 different meanings
  - IMH as aortic dissection (AD) variant such as AD with thrombosed false lumen or AD with small entry and absent reentry tear
  - IMH as purely descriptive term referring to often localized hematoma ("bruise") in aortic wall, which can be associated with broad range of acute aortic pathologies, including penetrating aortic ulcer, limited intimal tear, traumatic aortic injuries, rupturing aneurysms, iatrogenic dissections, etc.

IMAGING

- NECT: Crescentic or eccentric aortic wall hyperdensity
- CECT
  - Crescentic or eccentric aortic wall thickening
  - Ulcer-like projections (ULP): Outpouching of contrast with wide intimal opening (i.e., > 3 mm), limited to intima
  - Intramural blood pool (IBP)
    - Pool of contrast with small luminal communication (1-2 mm)

TOP DIFFERENTIAL DIAGNOSES

- Aortitis (Takayasu and giant cell arteritis)
- Aortic aneurysm with mural thrombus

PATHOLOGY

- Stanford classification
  - Type A (~ 40%): Ascending ± descending aorta
  - Type B (~ 60%): Descending aorta

CLINICAL ISSUES

- Abrupt onset of severe chest or back pain, hypertension
- Treatment
  - Type A IMH: Surgical treatment
  - Type B IMH: Medical treatment and close follow-up

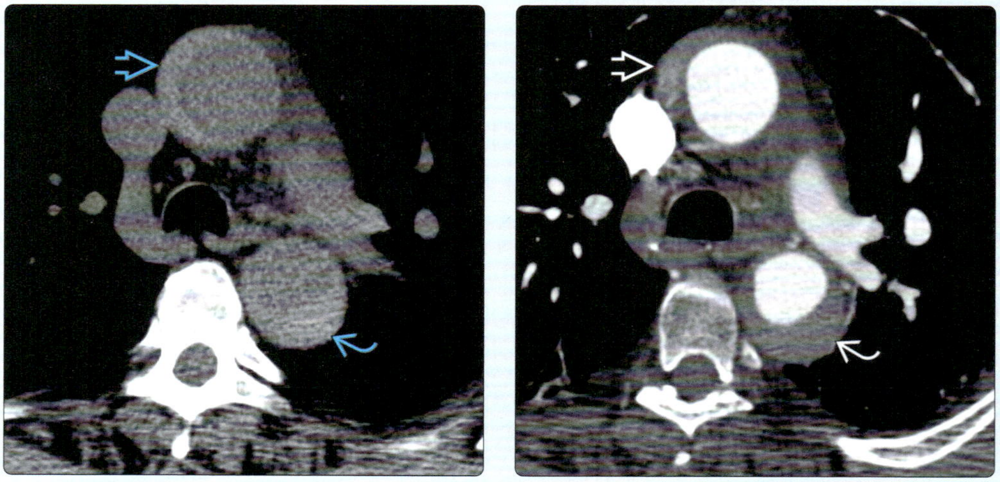

(Left) *Axial NECT in a patient with Stanford type A intramural hematoma (IMH) shows crescent-shaped wall hyperdensity at the ascending and descending aorta.* **(Right)** *Axial CT angiography shows crescentic aortic wall thickening in the ascending and descending aorta. Type A IMH is typically treated surgically.*

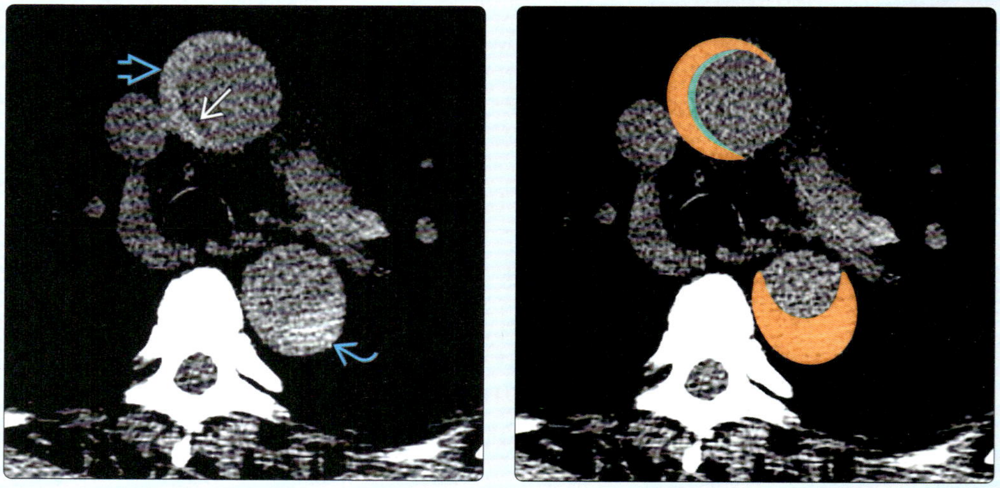

(Left) *Narrow window settings can improve the visibility of the hyperattenuated, crescent-shaped ascending and descending aortic wall. A hypoattenuating, crescent-shaped thickened intima is also notable due to atherosclerosis.* **(Right)** *The orange overlay represents the hyperattenuating IMH. The light green overlay marks the thickened, atherosclerotic intima.*

TERMINOLOGY

Abbreviations

- Intramural hematoma (IMH), aortic dissection (AD)

Definitions

- IMH (literally: blood in wall) in its broadest sense refers to fresh thrombus/clot within aortic wall; term IMH is used clinically (and somewhat confusingly) for 2 different meanings
  - IMH as AD variant
    - AD thrombosed false lumen or AD with small entry and absent reentry tear
  - IMH as purely descriptive term referring to often localized hematoma ("bruise") in aortic wall

IMAGING

General Features

- Best diagnostic clue
  - Aortic wall hyperdensity on NECT can be focal, crescentic, elongated, &/or circumferential

CT Findings

- NECT
  - Focal, crescentic, elongated, &/or circumferential aortic wall hyperattenuation
    - Narrow window width and level settings helpful to recognize hyperattenuating IMH
- CTA
  - Crescentic or eccentric aortic wall thickening, smooth lumen-wall interface
  - Often, no discrete intimomedial flap seen on CT but can be identified surgically or pathologically in nearly all cases
  - Common features of IMH (dissection variant)
    - Intramural blood pool (IBP)
      - Pool of contrast with no obvious or very small luminal communication (1-2 mm)
      - Usually not associated with worse prognosis [unlike ulcer-like projection (ULP)]
    - ULP
      - Contrast outpouching with wide (> 3 mm) connection to flow lumen
      - New intimal injury in area of high shear stress w/o atherosclerosis
      - Highest risk: ULP > 20-mm diameter, > 15-mm depth, or in ascending aorta/arch
      - Differentiation from penetrating aortic ulcer (PAU): Lack of irregular intima/atherosclerosis, no IMH, not seen initially; can be indistinguishable
  - PAU: Intramural blood can be associated with acute PAU
    - Intimal disease in severe atherosclerosis; ulcer-like plaque burrows through intima into media
    - May be associated with focal or segmental IMH
  - Limited intimal tear (LIT): Intramural blood can be associated with LIT

DIFFERENTIAL DIAGNOSIS

Aortitis (Takayasu and Giant Cell Arteritis)

- Inflammation of large and medium-sized arteries
- Scattered areas of stenosis ± aneurysm
- Parietal thickening simulates IMH on CTA
  - Not hyperdense on NECT
- Mural enhancement on MR or delayed CT with contrast

IgG4 and Erdheim-Chester Disease Aortitis or Periaortitis

- Circumferential enhancing aortic or periaortic soft tissue
  - Hyperintense on NECT
- Aneurysmal dilation or lumen stenosis less common
- Infiltrating periaortic soft tissue

Aortic Aneurysm With Mural Thrombus

- Mural thrombus in lumen of dilated aorta and not in wall

PATHOLOGY

General Features

- Etiology
  - Medial degeneration with isolated intimal tear (small, usually undetectable by CT), contained hemorrhage in vessel media, no exit tear

Staging, Grading, & Classification

- Stanford classification
  - Type A (~ 40%): Ascending aorta ± descending aorta
  - Type B (~ 60%): Excludes ascending aorta

CLINICAL ISSUES

Presentation

- Most common signs/symptoms
  - Abrupt onset of severe chest or back pain
  - Hypertension

Natural History & Prognosis

- Evolution patterns of IMH
  - Spontaneous resolution (~ 10%)
  - Evolution or coexistence with AD (28-47%)
  - Aortic rupture (20-45%)
  - Stability over time (rare)
- Predictors of poorer prognosis and ↑ mortality
  - Dilated aorta: ascending 48-55 mm, descending 40-41 mm
  - IMH thickness > 10-11 mm
    - PAU in acute phase: ↑ incidence of progression
- Stanford type A

Treatment

- Type A IMH: Surgical treatment
- Type B IMH: Medical treatment and close follow-up
- PAU should be treated early (e.g., endovascular or surgery)
- IBP usually observed and follow-up CTA

SELECTED REFERENCES

1. Ko JP et al: Chest CT angiography for acute aortic pathologic conditions: pearls and pitfalls. Radiographics. 41(2):399-424, 2021
2. Murillo H et al: Aortic dissection and other acute aortic syndromes: diagnostic imaging findings from acute to chronic longitudinal progression. Radiographics. 41(2):425-46, 2021
3. Moral S et al: Clinical implications of focal intimal disruption in patients with type B intramural hematoma. J Am Coll Cardiol. 69(1):28-39, 2017

(Left) *Axial black-blood MR in a patient with type B IMH shows the presence of hyperintense crescentic IMH along the descending thoracic aorta. This intensity behavior is consistent with acute hemorrhage.* **(Right)** *Axial SSFP MR in the same patient shows that the IMH is iso- to slightly hyperintense when compared with adjacent muscles. MR is as efficient as CT in determining and characterizing the presence of IMH and may be used when CT is unavailable or contraindicated.*

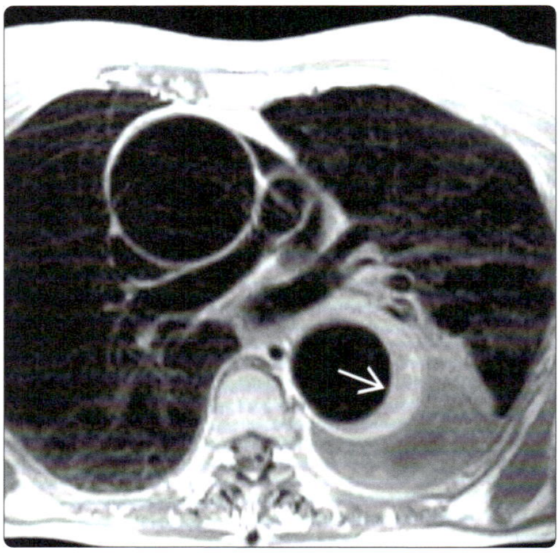

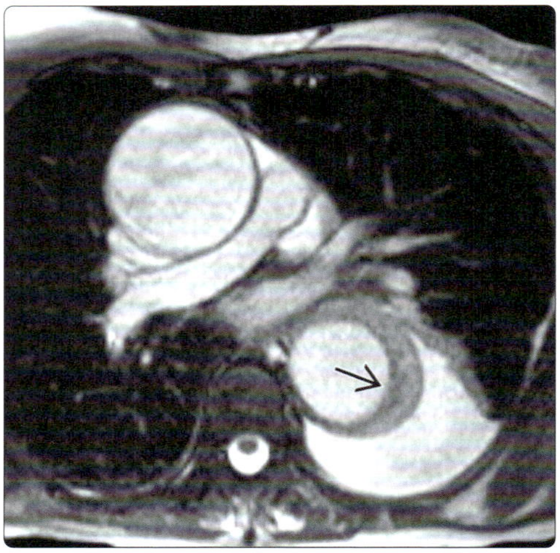

(Left) *Sagittal oblique CTA shows type B IMH. Note decreased diameter of the aortic lumen along the area of IMH. This is a helpful finding to differentiate from aortitis, which usually does not exhibit such features.* **(Right)** *Axial chest CTA in a patient with IMH shows a large penetrating aortic ulcer (PAU) with a broad neck along the distal thoracic aorta, likely the primary cause of the IMH. Note also an ulcer-like projection (ULP) along the aortic arch.*

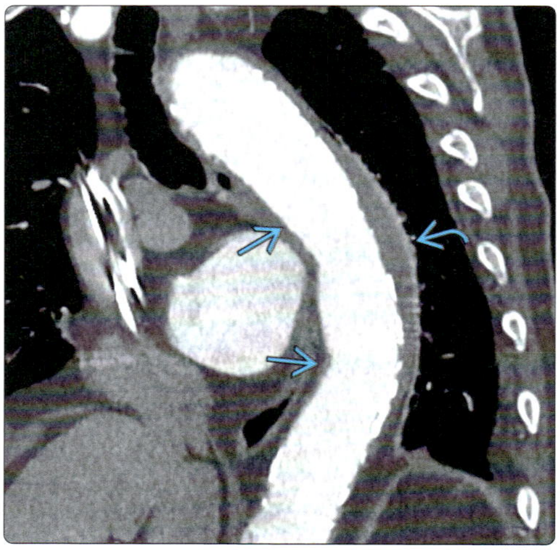

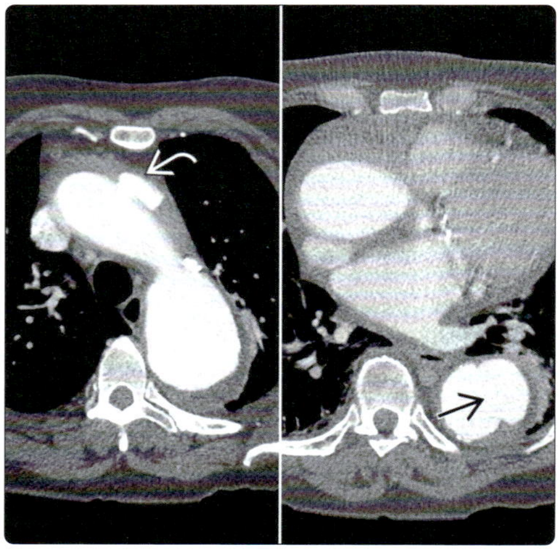

(Left) *Axial CECT in a patient with type B IMH shows focal aortic projection consistent with ULP. This collection was not present on the baseline CTA but developed on follow-up imaging.* **(Right)** *Axial CECT in the same patient shows interval enlargement of ULP and new aortic dissection. ULP are characterized by absence on baseline, development on follow-up imaging, and wide communication with the aortic lumen. ULP implies a poorer prognosis with evolution into aortic dissection or aneurysm.*

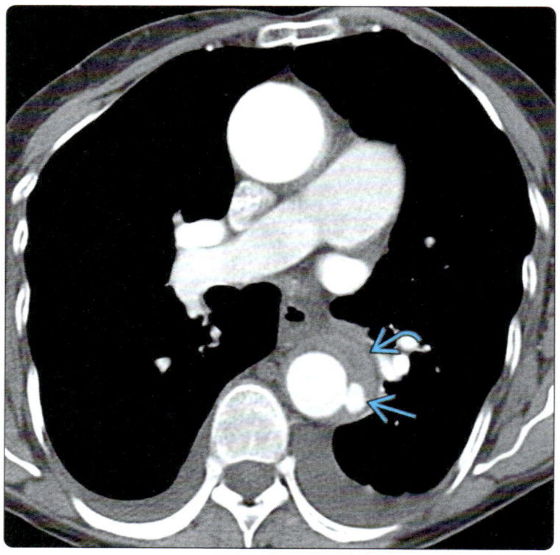

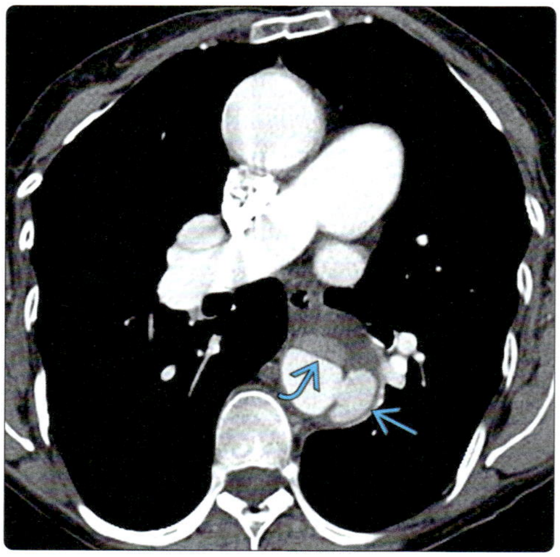

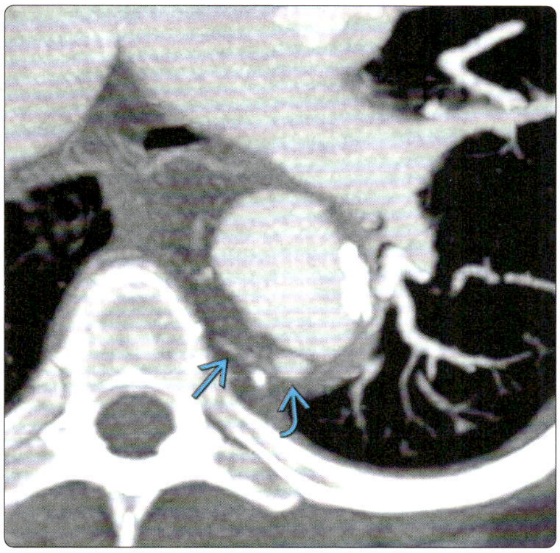
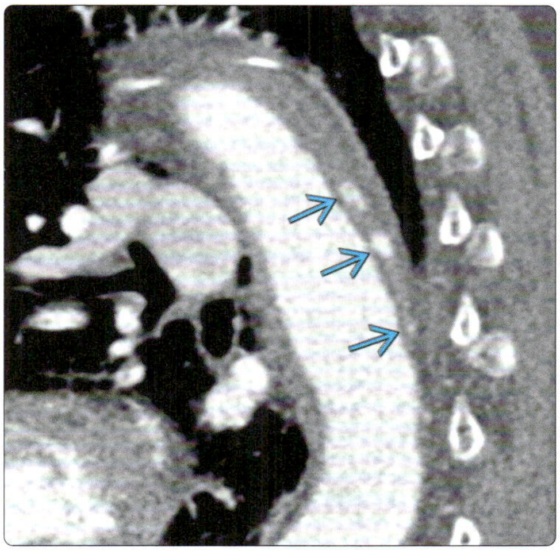

(Left) *Axial MIP CTA in a patient with type B IMH shows an intramural blood pool (IBP) ➔. There is no clear communication with the aortic lumen, but there is visible communication with an adjacent intercostal artery ➔.* **(Right)** *Sagittal oblique CTA in the same patient shows multilevel IBP ➔ related to contiguous intercostal arteries. This appearance is often referred to as Chinese ring-sword sign. Overall, IBP (as opposed to ULP) can be closely observed with follow-up imaging (i.e., CTA), as they will typically resolve.*

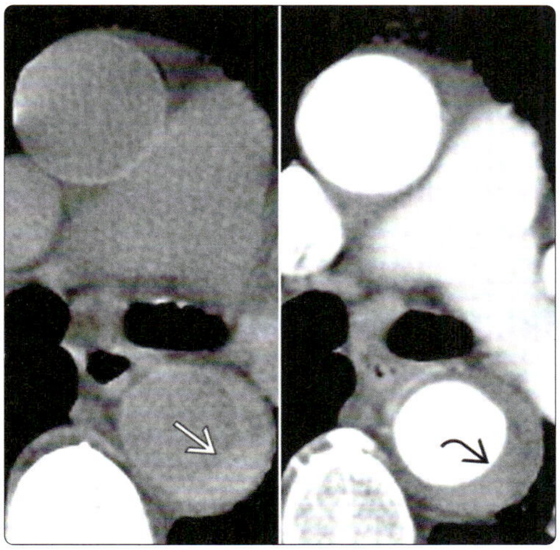
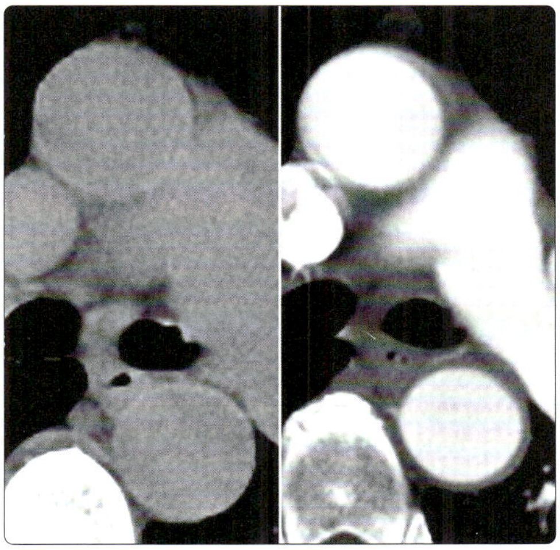

(Left) *Axial chest NECT in a patient with type B IMH treated clinically shows the classic crescentic aortic wall hyperdensity ➔. CTA demonstrates the classic crescentic wall thickening ➔.* **(Right)** *Axial NECT and CTA in the same patient show complete resolution of the IMH. IMH can resolve, remain stable, or progress to a variety of complications, including aortic dissection and rupture. CT remains the best follow-up tool for patients with type B IMH.*

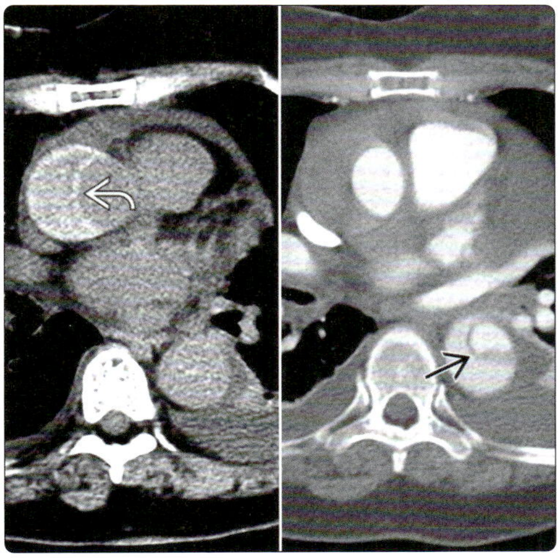
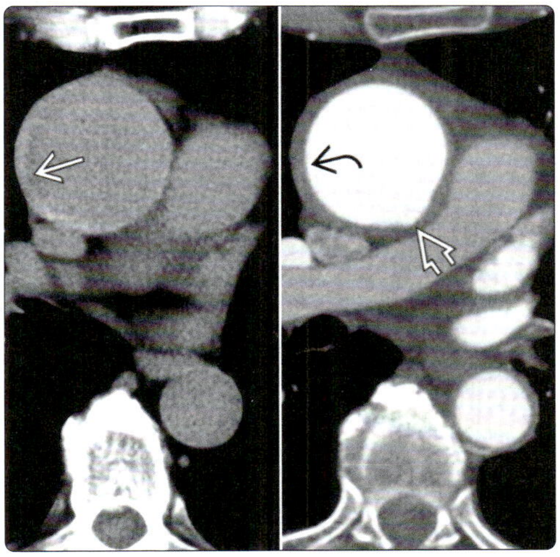

(Left) *Axial chest NECT and CTA in a patient with type A IMH ➔ show a coexistent descending thoracic aortic dissection ➔.* **(Right)** *Axial chest NECT and CTA in a patient with incomplete dissection show crescentic hyperdensity ➔ and thickening ➔ along the ascending aorta, findings identical to those seen in IMH. Note the discrete bulging ➔ along the posterior ascending thoracic aorta, distal to the origin of the left coronary artery. This characteristic finding is classically seen in incomplete aortic dissection.*

Penetrating Atherosclerotic Ulcer

KEY FACTS

TERMINOLOGY

- Ulceration of atherosclerotic plaque that penetrates internal elastic lamina into media with variable amount of intramural hematoma (IMH)

IMAGING

- NECT: Abnormal aortic contour if penetrating atherosclerotic ulcer (PAU) has penetrated beyond adventitia; possible IMH if acute
- CTA: Contrast outpouching extending beyond expected depth of aortic intima ± IMH
- MR: Similar sensitivity and findings to CTA, but less practical in emergent evaluation of acute aortic syndrome

TOP DIFFERENTIAL DIAGNOSES

- Ulcerated atherosclerotic plaque (nonpenetrating ulcer)
- Intimomedial disruptions in IMH (focal intimal disruption, intramural blood pool)
- Chronic healed PAU
- Mycotic pseudoaneurysm

CLINICAL ISSUES

- Acute: Chest/back pain in thoracic aorta, abdominal/back/flank pain in abdominal aorta
- Chronic: Common incidental finding, asymptomatic, never associated with IMH
- Older adults (typically 7th decade or later), M > F
- Risk factors: Hypertension, tobacco use, coronary artery disease, chronic obstructive pulmonary disease, and renal insufficiency
- Concomitant aortic aneurysm is common
- Acute PAU (symptomatic ± IMH) are more likely to progress to perforation or aortic rupture
- Chronic healed PAU (asymptomatic without IMH) are unlikely to progress
- Consider treatment if symptomatic, complicated, or large

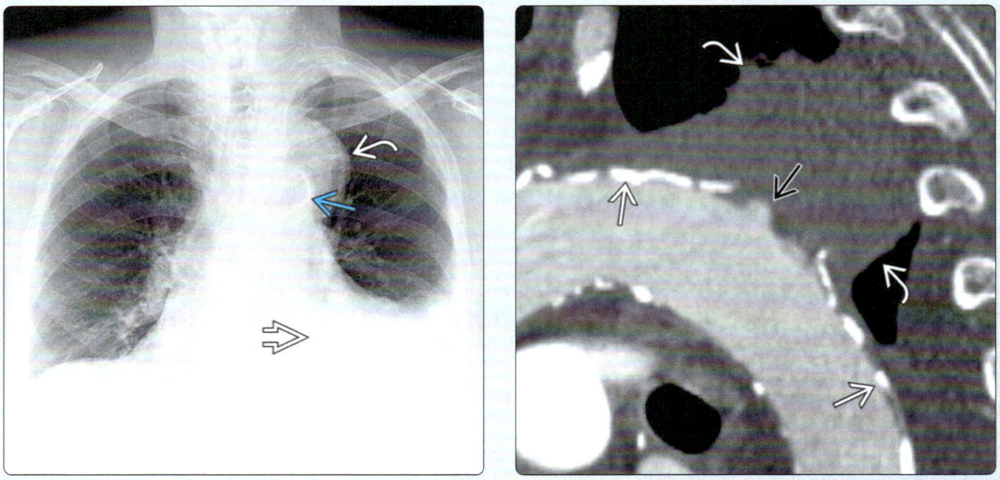

(Left) *PA chest radiograph in a patient with penetrating aortic ulcer (PAU) of the aortic arch shows a mediastinal mass ➔ lateral to the aortic arch from associated hematoma and a left pleural effusion ➔. Note the aortic intimal calcification ➔.* **(Right)** *Sagittal oblique CTA in the same patient shows extensive atherosclerosis of the aorta ➔ with a small, penetrating ulcer ➔ and a large focal mural hematoma ➔. PAUs are associated with a variable degree of intramural hematoma (IMH), either focal (as in this case) or diffuse.*

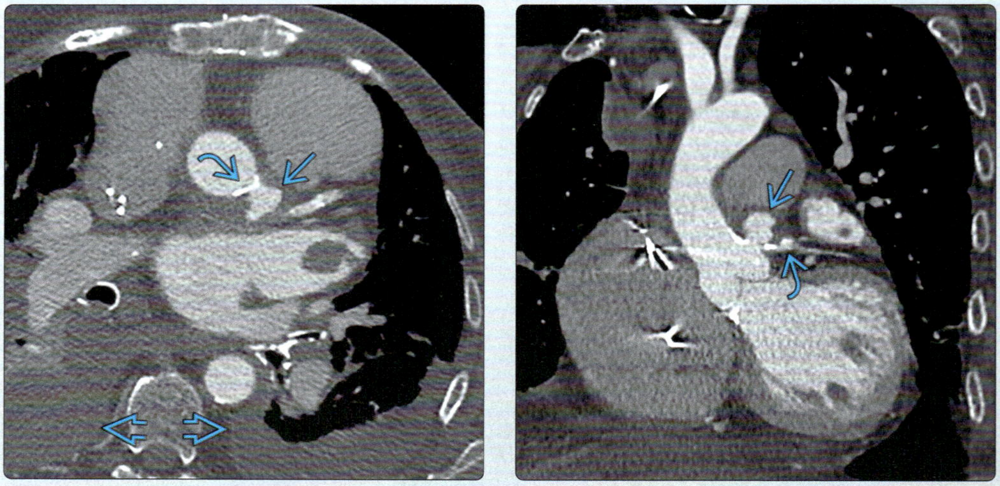

(Left) *Axial CECT of the chest in a patient with PAU at the proximal ascending thoracic aorta shows an outpouching extending beyond the aortic wall ➔, adjacent atherosclerosis ➔, and bilateral pleural effusions ➔.* **(Right)** *Coronal oblique CECT in the same patient shows the relationship of PAU ➔ with the ascending aorta and left coronary artery ➔. Location in the ascending aorta and acute chest pain are the most important factors that determine emergent treatment due to high risk of rupture.*

TERMINOLOGY

Abbreviations

- Penetrating atherosclerotic ulcer (PAU)

Definitions

- Ulceration of atherosclerotic plaque penetrating through internal elastic lamina into media or beyond

IMAGING

General Features

- Best diagnostic clue
  - Contrast extending beyond expected depth of intima in setting of atherosclerosis
- Location
  - Most commonly involves mid- to distal descending thoracic aorta
  - Patients with acute PAU commonly have chronic atherosclerotic ulcers and aneurysms

Radiographic Findings

- Chest radiography is insensitive and often normal
- Pleural effusion is common when acute

CT Findings

- NECT
  - ± focally abnormal aortic contour if PAU extends beyond adventitia
  - ± adjacent concentric or crescentic hyperattenuating intramural hematoma (IMH) (if acute)
  - Associated calcified atherosclerotic plaques
- CTA
  - Intraluminal contrast extending beyond expected depth of intima; ± focal adjacent IMH if acute
  - Often better appreciated on NECT
  - Adjacent hemorrhage (i.e., contained rupture or pseudoaneurysm); may progress to aortic rupture

MR Findings

- MRA
  - Similar findings and sensitivity to CTA, but is less cost-effective and less practical in emergent acute aortic syndrome (AAS) evaluation

Imaging Recommendations

- Protocol advice
  - Obtain NECT before CTA to help identify IMH

DIFFERENTIAL DIAGNOSIS

Ulcerated Atherosclerotic Plaque

- Ulceration confined to aortic intima; does not extend beyond expected depth of intima
- Ulcerated plaques (a.k.a. ruptured plaques) in side branches of aorta cause most of acute cardiovascular events
  - Myocardial infarct if in coronary arteries; stroke if in cerebral vasculature

Intimomedial Disruptions in Intramural Hematoma

- Focal intimal disruption: > 0.3-cm orifice, representing isolated entry tear, more likely to progress
  - Additional terms used in literature include ulcer-like projection and isolated primary intimal tear
- Intramural blood pool (IBP): < 0.3-cm orifice, representing avulsed branch vessel (therefore descending aorta only), more likely to spontaneously resolve
  - Additional terms used in literature include natural fenestrations, branch artery pseudoaneurysms, and focal puddles (corresponding to IBP)

Chronic Healed Penetrating Atherosclerotic Ulcer

- Asymptomatic and no IMH = unlikely to progress

Traumatic Aortic Injury

- History of trauma/additional traumatic findings; not associated with atherosclerosis

Mycotic Pseudoaneurysm

- Clinical evidence of infection; not associated with atherosclerosis; can be morphologically similar to PAU

PATHOLOGY

General Features

- Etiology
  - Manifestation of advanced atherosclerosis

Gross Pathologic & Surgical Features

- Variable presence/degree of IMH

CLINICAL ISSUES

Presentation

- Most common signs/symptoms
  - Acute-onset sharp chest/back pain in thoracic aorta, abdominal/back/flank pain in abdominal aorta

Demographics

- Epidemiology
  - M > F; PAU represents 2-7% of all AASs
  - Classic atherosclerosis risk factors, established atherosclerotic diseases
- Age: Older adults (typically 7th decade or later)

Natural History & Prognosis

- Evolution of PAU
  - Acute PAU (symptomatic ± IMH) can → aortic rupture
  - If associated with IMH, CT attenuation of mural thrombus decreases and becomes isodense to blood pool within 7-10 days on NECT
- High-risk features: Diameter ≥ 13-20 mm, depth ≥ 10 mm, significant growth, associated saccular aneurysm, or increasing pleural effusion

Treatment

- Medical management if uncomplicated
- Open or endovascular surgical intervention if complicated
  - Rupture (impending), malperfusion, uncontrollable pain/hypertension

SELECTED REFERENCES

1. Isselbacher EM et al: 2022 ACC/AHA guideline for the diagnosis and management of aortic disease: a report of the American Heart Association/American College of Cardiology joint committee on clinical practice guidelines. Circulation. 146(24):e334-482, 2022
2. Vilacosta I et al: Acute aortic syndrome revisited: JACC state-of-the-art review. J Am Coll Cardiol. 78(21):2106-25, 2021

(Left) *Axial NECT of the chest in a patient with PAU at the aortic arch with aortic rupture shows an anterior mediastinal mass due to mediastinal hematoma →, indicating rupture. Note that PAU can simulate the presence of an anterior mediastinal mass, and contrast remains critical for appropriate differentiation.* **(Right)** *Axial CTA of the chest in the same patient shows a large ulceration along the anterior proximal aortic arch → with surrounding mediastinal hemorrhage → and extensive atherosclerosis →.*

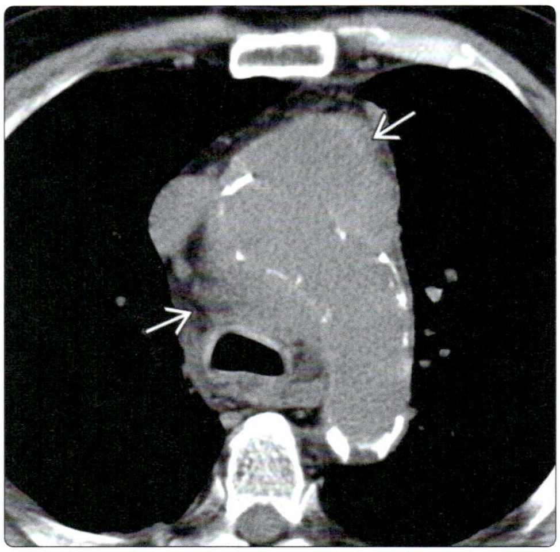

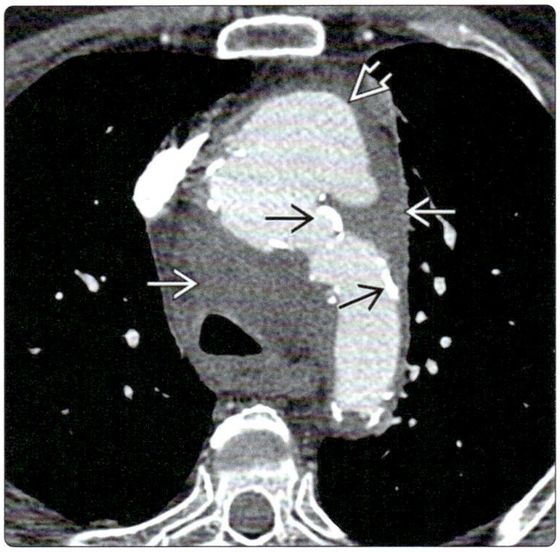

(Left) *Sagittal oblique reformation in the same patient depicts the ulceration → and large pseudoaneurysm → along the proximal arch. Note extensive calcific atherosclerosis →.* **(Right)** *Volume-rendered CTA in the same patient shows the large pseudoaneurysm →, which is compressing the proximal left carotid artery →. Volume renderings may be helpful to thoracic surgeons for surgical planning.*

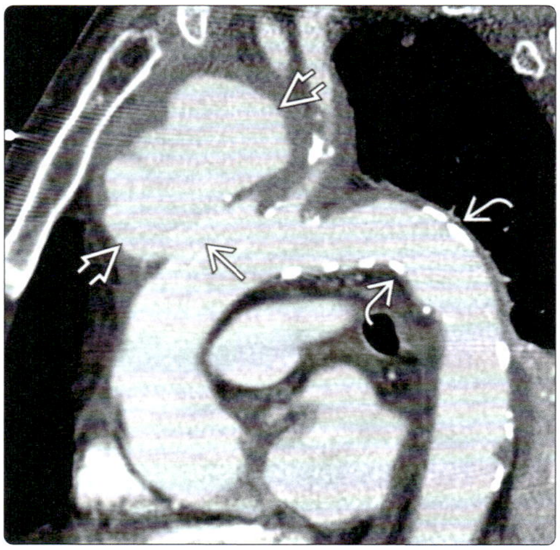

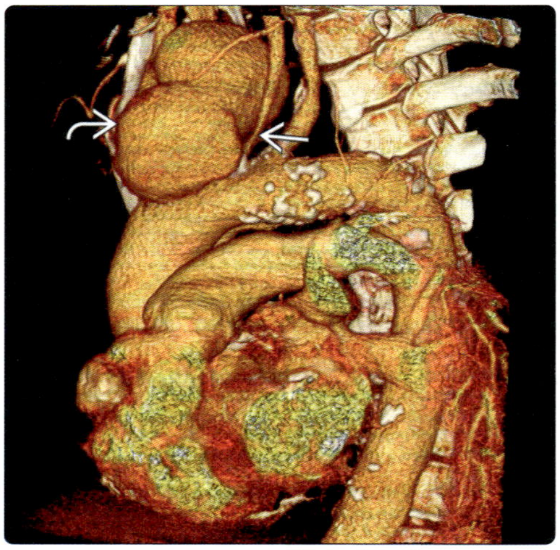

(Left) *SSFP (left) and T1W (middle) MR images in a 67-year-old woman with chest pain and history of anaphylaxis with iodinated contrast shows a small PAU in the descending thoracic aorta → with surrounding IMH →. Angiogram prior to stent placement (right) shows the PAU →. (Courtesy S. Kligerman, MD.)* **(Right)** *CTA in a man with chest pain shows extensive atherosclerotic disease and a small PAU → with surrounding IMH →. (Courtesy S. Kligerman, MD.)*

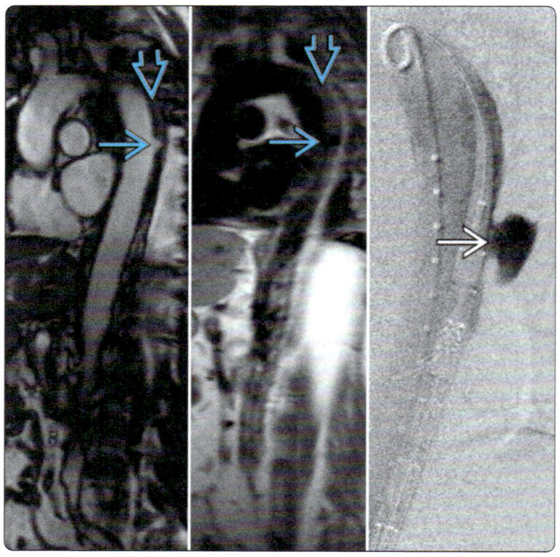

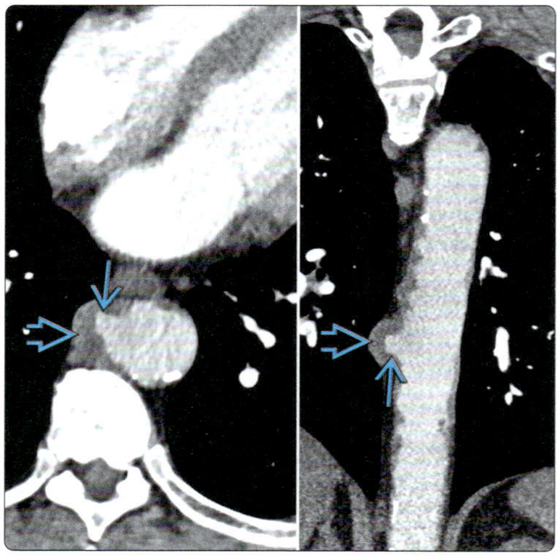

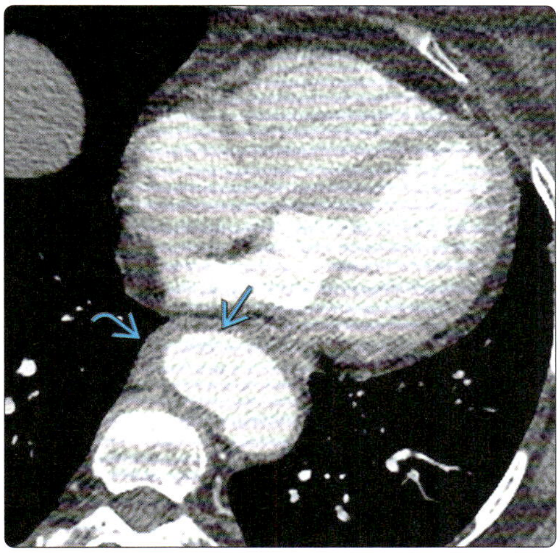

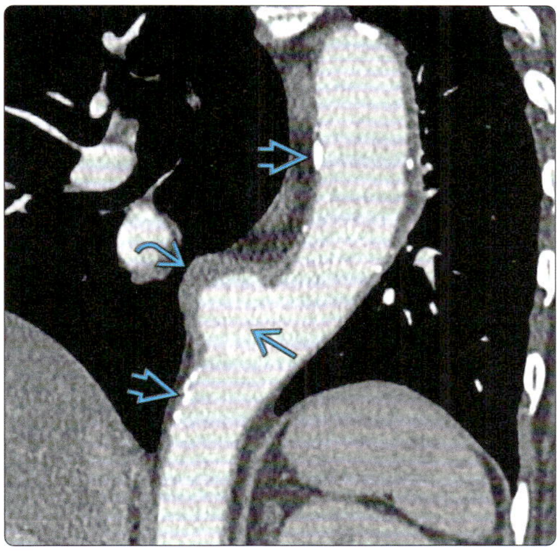

(Left) *Axial CECT of the chest in a patient with PAU at the descending thoracic aorta shows lobulation of the right lateral wall of the aorta with a variable amount of adjacent IMH. The most common location of PAU is the descending aorta, followed by the abdominal aorta, and, rarely, the ascending aorta.* **(Right)** *Coronal oblique CECT in the same patient shows focal outpouching from PAU with a small amount of adjacent IMH. Also note scattered atherosclerosis.*

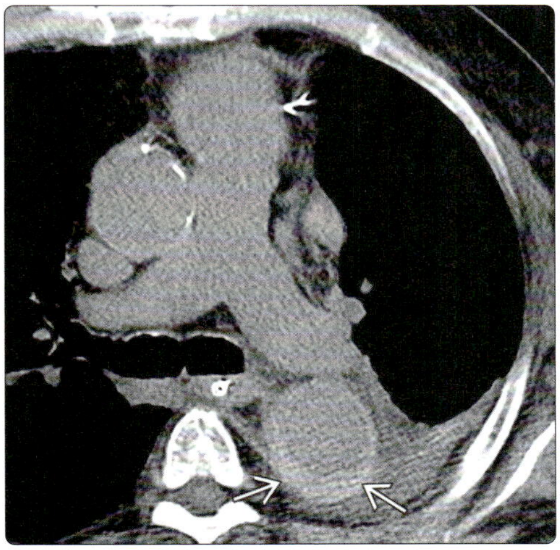

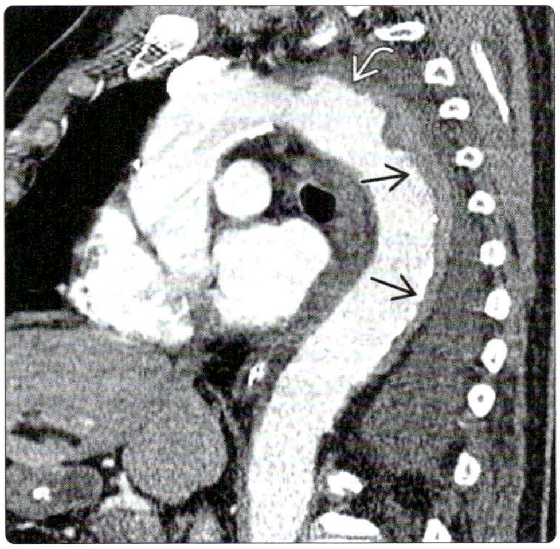

(Left) *Axial NECT of the chest in a patient with IMH secondary to PAU shows crescentic hyperdensity along the descending aorta, consistent with IMH. NECT is helpful in differentiating PAU with IMH from arteritis, which is not hyperdense.* **(Right)** *Sagittal CTA of the chest in a patient with IMH secondary to PAU shows a large, relatively shallow ulceration extending beyond the expected aortic margin. Note also the aortic wall thickening from IMH.*

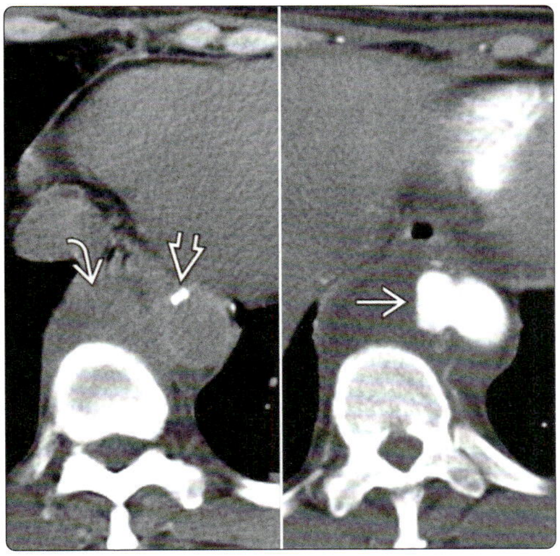

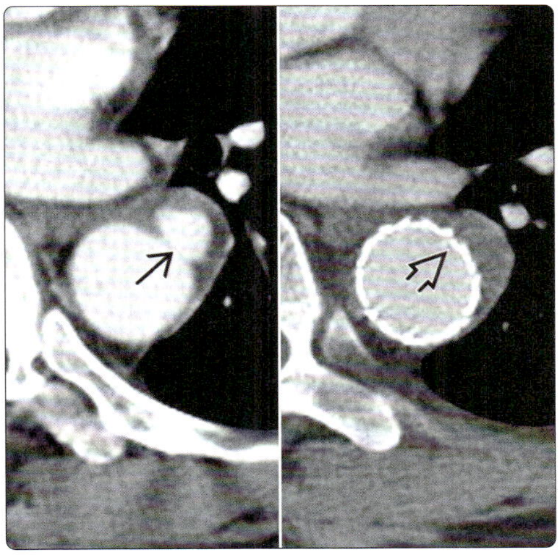

(Left) *Axial NECT (left) and CTA (right) in a patient with contained rupture of a descending aortic PAU show retrocrural hemorrhage and atherosclerosis with contrast extending beyond the expected aortic margin.* **(Right)** *Axial CTA of the chest before (left) and after (right) treatment shows a PAU along the descending thoracic aorta, which is excluded after placement of an endovascular stent. Endovascular therapy has become the treatment of choice whenever feasible.*

Limited Intimal Tear

KEY FACTS

TERMINOLOGY

- Limited tear, incomplete dissection, partial thickness tear, limited dissection
- Limited tears of aorta are rare cause of acute aortic syndromes (AASs), representing ~ 5% of AASs

IMAGING

- In general, limited intimal tears (LITs) appear as intimal irregularity or defect, often associated with undermined edge (reminiscent of localized dissection), which may contain small amount of thrombus, and bulging of corresponding outer wall of aorta
- Actual **tear** can be subtle and difficult to delineate, as it can be linear or have more complex shapes
- **Edges** of tear can be subtle, unexpected contour irregularity of inner surface of aorta; edges can be lifted or rolled off remainder of wall, reminiscent of dissection; undermined edges can contain intramural thrombus

CLINICAL ISSUES

- **Natural history** of acute LITs is poorly understood
- LITs are **treated similar to aortic dissections**
- Stanford type A LITs (affecting ascending aorta) typically undergo open surgical replacement of aorta
- In Stanford type B LITs (not involving ascending aorta), medical management is appropriate unless complications occur; anatomically suitable type B LITs can undergo endovascular aortic repair
- All patients with LITs require **life-long follow-up** and imaging surveillance

DIAGNOSTIC CHECKLIST

- Key to diagnosing LITs is being aware of existence of these relatively rare lesions
- Contour irregularities of inner surface of aorta, which cannot be explained by motion artifacts or other cause, should raise suspicion of LIT

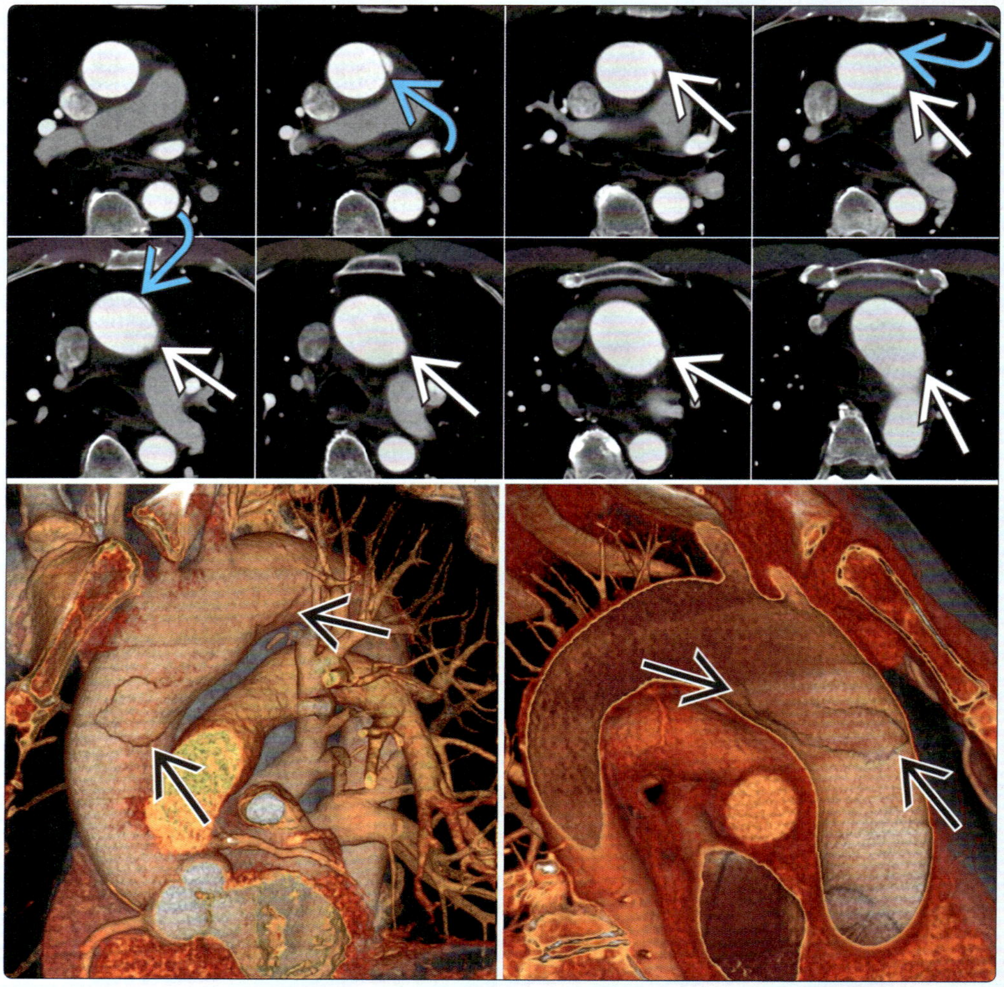

CT images (top) show a linear filling defect and contour irregularity in the ascending and transverse aorta. Note undermined edges of the tear ⇨ and the bulging wall ➡. 3D images (bottom) show a longitudinally oriented limited tear ⇨ seen from the outside (left) and inside (right). (Courtesy Chin et al.)

TERMINOLOGY

Abbreviations

- Limited intimal tear (LIT)

Synonyms

- Limited tear, incomplete dissection, partial thickness tear, limited dissection

Definitions

- Limited tears of aorta are rare cause of acute aortic syndromes (AASs), representing ~ 5% of AASs
- Limited tears fall under spectrum of diseases characterized pathologically by degeneration of media layer of aortic wall

IMAGING

General Features

- Best diagnostic clue
  - Intimal irregularity or defect, often associated with undermined edge, which may contain small amount of thrombus; bulging of delaminated and exposed outer wall of aorta
- Location
  - LITs occur more commonly in ascending aorta than in arch or descending aorta
  - LITs are oriented longitudinally, or are circumferentially relative to aortic axis
- Size
  - Tear itself can range from few millimeters to several centimeters in length; width can range from few mm to few centimeters
- Morphology
  - Actual tear can be subtle and difficult to delineate
    - Can be linear or have more complex shapes (figure 8 shape)
  - Edges of tear can be subtle
    - Can appear as unexpected contour irregularity of inner surface of aorta
    - Edges can also be undermined with portion of intimomedial tissue lifted off remainder of wall, reminiscent of dissection, but without fully formed false lumen
  - Outer wall of aorta at level of LIT may show subtle focal bulging
    - Outer wall of aorta only consists of residual adventitia, equivalent to outer wall of false lumen in aortic dissection

CT Findings

- Aortic luminal contour abnormality in shape of linear or complex-shaped tear
  - Edge of tear is better visualized if it is lifted off, giving appearance of focal dissection flap, or accompanied by small amount of intramural thrombus
  - Exposed and delaminated remainder of (outer) aortic wall bulges outward
- Associated findings may be similar to those seen in aortic dissection
  - Pericardial fluid or hemopericardium (in type A lesions)
  - Pulmonary artery subadventitial hematoma
  - Periaortic mediastinal stranding (in type B lesions)

Ultrasonographic Findings

- LITs have been described on transesophageal and transthoracic echocardiography

Imaging Recommendations

- Best imaging tool
  - CTA, ideally with ECG gating
- Protocol advice
  - CT scans without motion artifacts in ascending aorta can be achieved with fast scanning techniques (fast gantry rotation, high-pitch, wide detector), and, most reliably, by ECG gating
    - If ECG gating is not routinely performed, or if suspicious aortic lesion is detected (e.g., on pulmonary embolism CT study), repeat injection and ECG gated scan can be performed
  - Multiplanar reformations are essential and increase confidence for presence or absence of subtle LIT
  - 3D volume-rendered images with "transparent blood" display are most helpful to see shape and extent of lesion

DIFFERENTIAL DIAGNOSIS

Artifacts

- Motion artifacts from transmitted cardiac pulsation (double contours of aortic wall on CT) can simulate or obscure subtle LITs
- Motion artifacts are often visible on both opposing aortic walls, whereas true aortic lesions usually affect only 1 side
- Repeat scan with ECG gating usually allows accurate diagnosis

Intramural Hematoma

- There is overlap between spectrum of LITs and spectrum of intramural hematomas (IMHs)
  - LITs can be associated with localized intramural blood, notably at undermined edges of tear, but predominant finding is intimal tear and defect
- It would not be fundamentally wrong to consider some LITs as IMH with large entry tears
  - Main task for radiologist is to recognize lesion as acute aortic pathology
  - Treatment is dictated by location and presence of complications rather than by specific type or classification of lesion

Penetrating Atherosclerotic Ulcer

- LITs are sometimes mislabeled as PAUs, most notably if LIT is small and has small hematoma associated with it
- Pathology of PAUs is very different though, since PAUs are atherosclerotic lesions, whereas LITs are under spectrum of diseases characterized by media degeneration

PATHOLOGY

General Features

- LITs fall under spectrum of aortic diseases characterized pathologically be degeneration of aortic media
  - Formerly, but incorrectly, termed cystic media necrosis
- Other diseases characterized by media degeneration are classic aortic dissection and IMH (dissection variant)

- Of note, media degeneration can precede acute event for years; loss of coherence between layers of aortic wall can go unnoticed for long time until entry tear allows physical separation and delamination of wall layers
- Media degeneration is prerequisite for aortic dissection and its variants, IMH, and LIT; conversely, normal aorta does not dissect
- Causes of media degeneration are
  - Severe, untreated hypertension
    - Most common cause of media degeneration
  - Aging: Normal aging results in media degeneration
  - Genetic diseases: Marfan syndrome, Ehlers-Danlos IV syndrome, familial aortic aneurysms and dissections

Staging, Grading, & Classification

- Limited tears are anatomically categorized similar to aortic dissections
  - Stanford type A for ascending aortic lesions
  - Stanford type B for all other lesions that do not affect ascending aorta
- Similar to classic dissection, LITs are considered hyperacute (24 hours), acute (< 14 days), subacute, or chronic (> 3 months)

Gross Pathologic & Surgical Features

- Intimal-medial tear; limited or focal medial layer dissection plane, medial degeneration

CLINICAL ISSUES

Presentation

- Most common signs/symptoms
  - Clinical presentation of acute LITs is similar to other acute diseases of aorta, summarized under clinical term acute AASs
    - AAS symptoms: Acute, sharp, severe chest or back pain
    - AAS can be caused by number of aortic diseases other than LITs, such as classic dissection, IMH, PAU, and also rupturing aneurysms
- Other signs/symptoms
  - LITs may cause little or no symptoms, evidenced by occasional incidental detection of chronic LITs in patients who do not remember specific event

Demographics

- Patients with LITs are on average slightly older than patients with classic aortic dissection and patients with IMH

Natural History & Prognosis

- Natural history of acute LITs is poorly understood
- **Acute phase**: Similar to aortic dissection, first 14 days are considered acute phase of disease
- **Subacute phase** (15-90 days): LITs seem to evolve with any IMH component receding and disclosing depth of undermined edges; tear may become more visible if edges become thicker and less mobile, and exposed adventitial bulge may become deeper (similar to false lumen increase during subacute phase in dissection)
- **Chronic phase**: Delaminated portion of aortic wall that is exposed to systemic pressure will continue to dilate and can become aneurysmal; since less wall is exposed in LITs than in classic dissection, changes over time may be less
  - Chronic LITs are occasionally detected in asymptomatic patients, suggesting that they may present with less conspicuous symptoms in some cases
- All patients with LITs require life-long follow-up and imaging surveillance

Treatment

- LITs are treated similar to aortic dissections
  - Stanford type A LITs (affecting ascending aorta) typically undergo open surgical replacement of aorta
  - In Stanford type B LITs (not involving ascending aorta), medical management is appropriate unless complications occur, such as rupture and malperfusion
    - Anatomically suitable type B LITs requiring intervention will undergo thoracic endovascular aortic repair

DIAGNOSTIC CHECKLIST

Consider

- Key to diagnosing LITs is being aware of existence of these relatively rare lesions

Image Interpretation Pearls

- Contour irregularities of inner surface of aorta, which cannot be explained by motion artifacts or other causes, should raise suspicion of LIT
- If associated with undermined edge or with subtle intramural blood, this should prompt further visualization with multiplanar reformats, and, ideally, with volume-rendered 3D images, which can more clearly demonstrate characteristics of this lesion

Reporting Tips

- LITs are aortic emergency and need to be reported and communicated urgently, similar to acute aortic dissection
- Distinction between type A lesions (ascending aorta involved) vs. type B lesions is critical, since former usually undergo urgent surgical repair
- Presence of complications, such as pericardial fluid, hemopericardium, tamponade; signs of rupture, branch vessel compromise

SELECTED REFERENCES

1. Madani MH et al: Limited aortic intimal tears: CT imaging features and clinical characteristics. Radiol Cardiothorac Imaging. 4(6):e220155, 2022
2. Chin AS et al: Acute limited intimal tears of the thoracic aorta. J Am Coll Cardiol. 71(24):2773-85, 2018
3. Svensson LG et al: Intimal tear without hematoma: an important variant of aortic dissection that can elude current imaging techniques. Circulation. 99(10):1331-6, 1999
4. Murray CA et al: Spontaneous laceration of ascending aorta. Circulation. 47(4):848-58, 1973

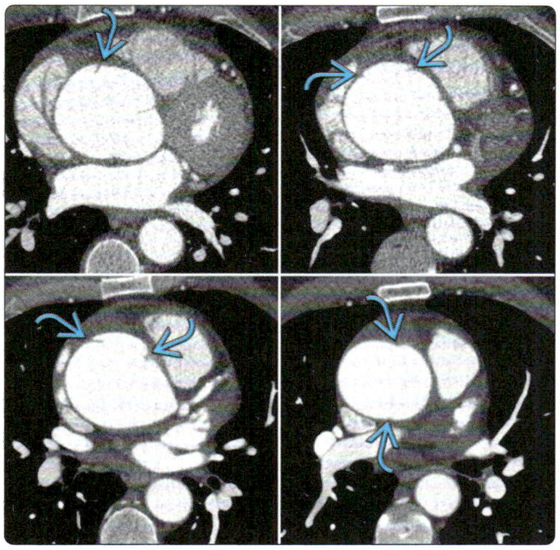

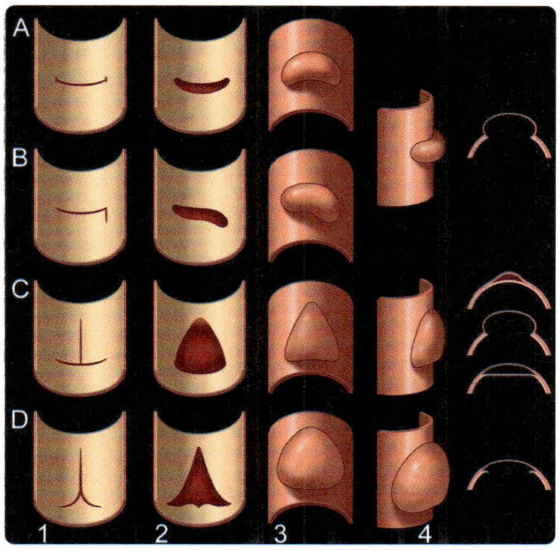

(Left) *Axial ECG gated images of a limited intimal tear (LIT) show contour irregularities in the ascending aorta, which correspond to the undermined edges of a large LIT. (Courtesy Chin et al.)* **(Right)** *Schematic shows the luminal view of intimomedial tear shapes (column 1), their stretched open luminal appearance in a pressurized aorta (column 2), external bulges (column 3), and side view (column 4). Schematic also illustrates linear (A), L-shaped (B), T-shaped (C), and star/complex shaped (D) tears. (Courtesy Madani et al.)*

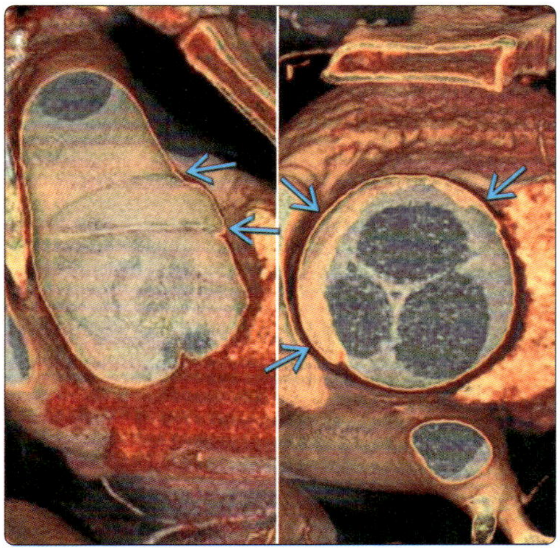

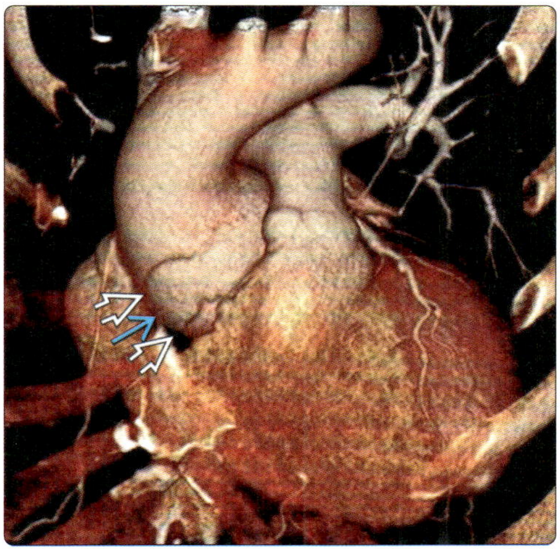

(Left) *Inner/luminal view of a semicircumferential LIT in the ascending aorta is shown. Note that the tear is stretched open in vivo (left). The edge of the tear is viewed from above (right).* **(Right)** *External view of the semicircumferential LIT shows a band or stripe of bulging tissue in the ascending aorta with sharp, undermined edges.*

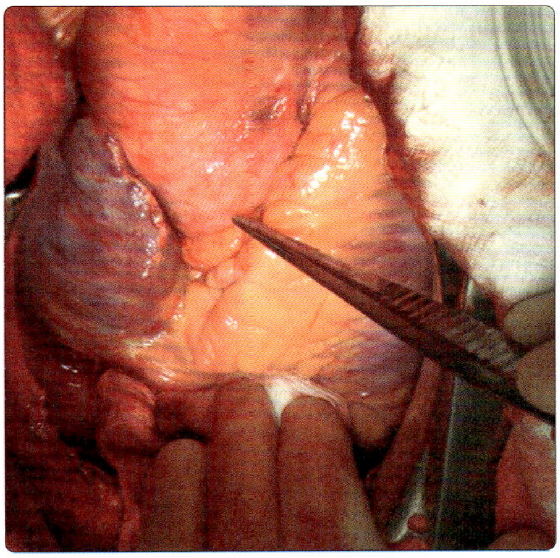

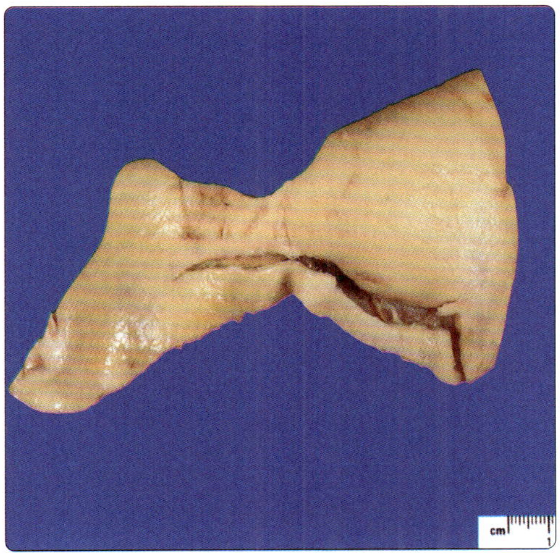

(Left) *Corresponding intraoperative photograph shows a very thin aortic wall only consisting of residual adventitia. The normal aortic wall is thicker with a more yellow hue due to the underlying intact media, which contains elastin.* **(Right)** *Photograph of the LIT in a resected aortic wall is shown. Note that in vitro, the shape of the tear is mostly linear with a small "L" on the right end. In vivo, in a pressurized aorta, that tear appears stretched open, and exposed underlying adventitial will bulge out (as shown on CT images).*

(Left) *CECT shows contour abnormality with a filling defect representing a limited aortic intimal tear* ➡*. An associated periaortic and mediastinal hematoma is consistent with impending rupture.* **(Right)** *The proximal end of the LIT shows the undermined edge, reminiscent of a dissection, seen on the left aspect of the ascending thoracic aorta* ➡*. (Courtesy S. Kligerman, MD.)*

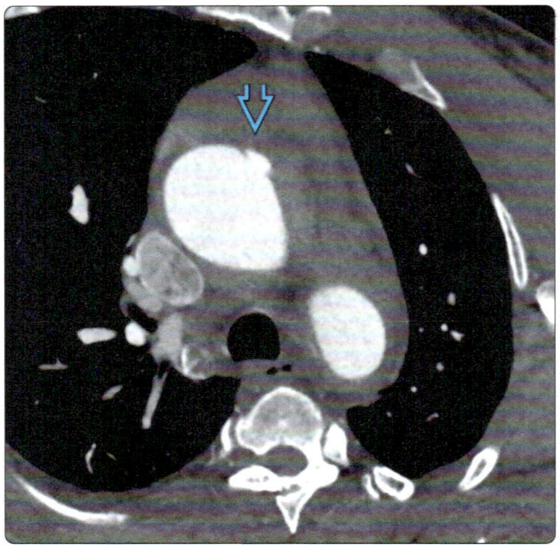

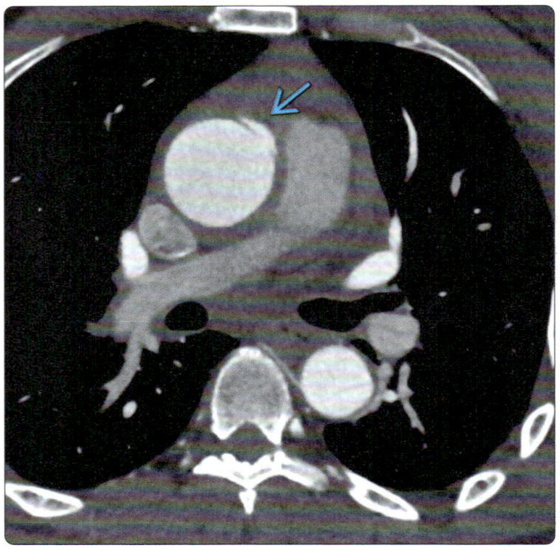

(Left) *Chronic LITs show slightly thicker* ➡*, undermined edges, no periaortic stranding, and no associated intramural blood.* **(Right)** *Corresponding oblique sagittal CECT in the same patient shows a focal tissue flap consistent with an undermined edge of a LIT* ➡*. (Courtesy S. Kligerman, MD.)*

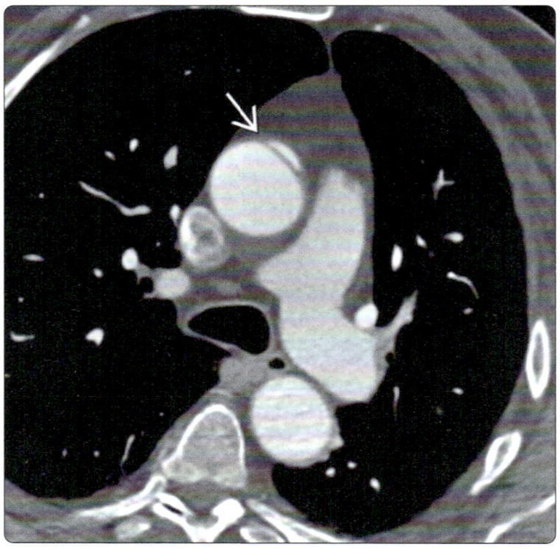

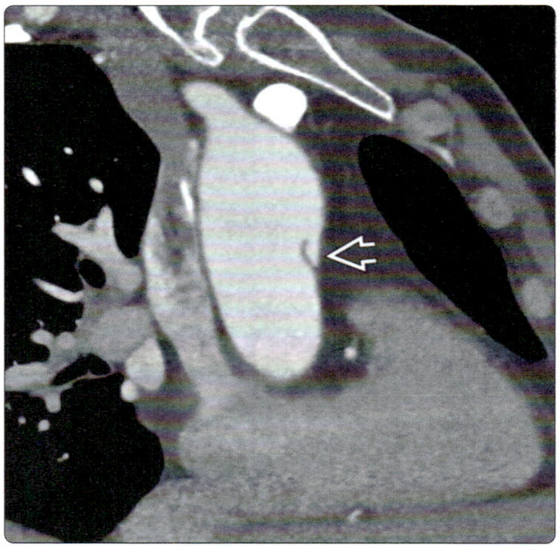

(Left) *The classic appearance of a LIT in the aortic arch with a wide, stretched open tear with undermined edges* ➡ *and bulging of the outer aortic wall* ➡ *is shown.* **(Right)** *Corresponding oblique coronal view shows a LIT with a small, undermined edge/flap* ➡ *and a mild bulge of the outer aortic contour* ➡*. (Courtesy S. Kligerman, MD.)*

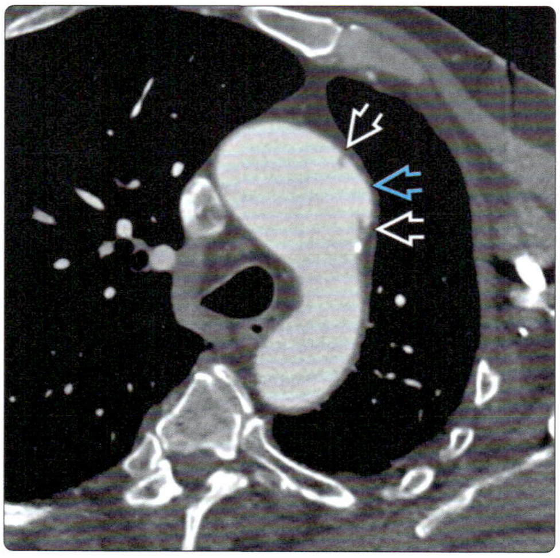

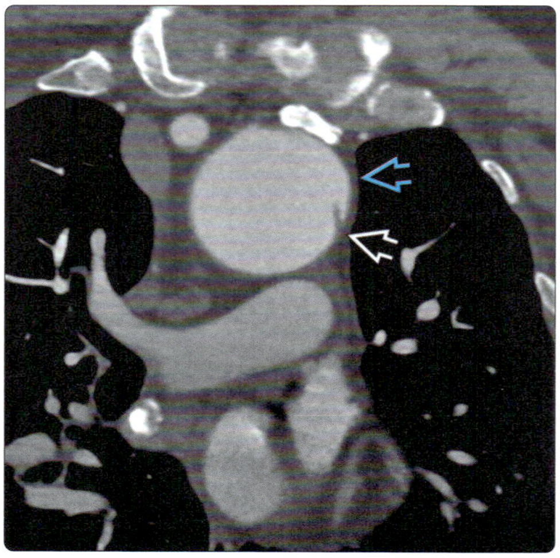

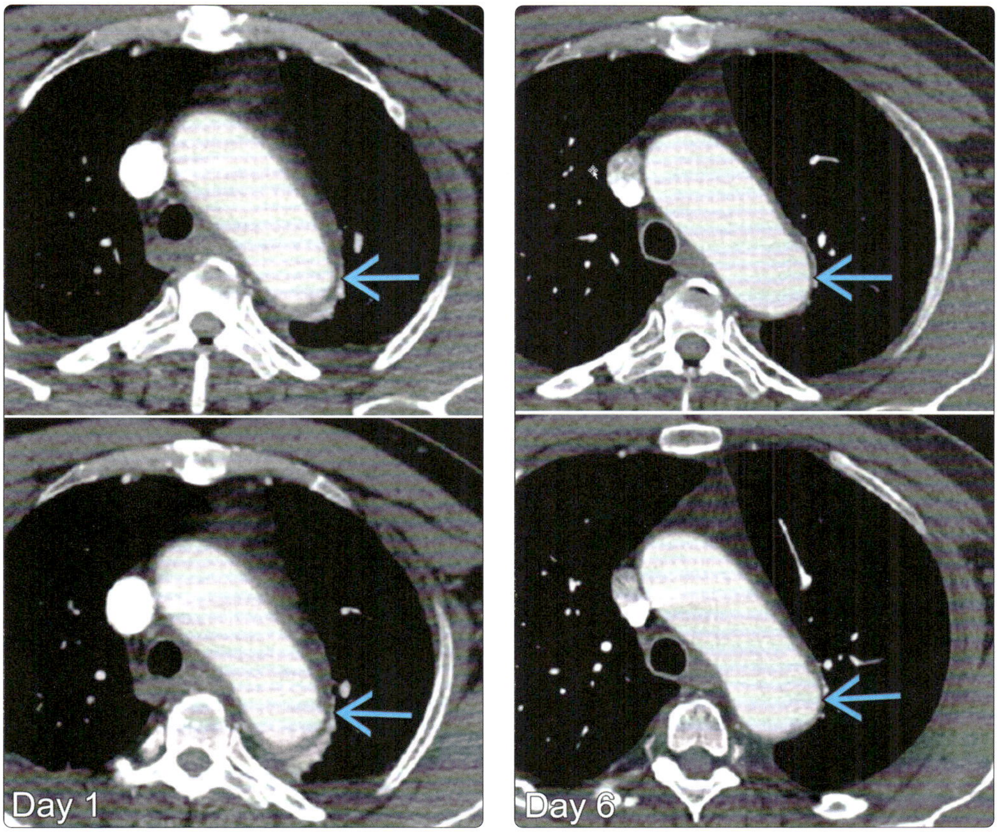

(Left) *Very subtle contour irregularity in the proximal descending thoracic aorta is seen, which was initially missed on day 1 of hospitalization when only axial images were reviewed.* **(Right)** *Follow-up imaging (day 6) again shows only very subtle bulging of the descending thoracic aorta with contour irregularities at the edge. Only the side-by-side comparison raises the suspicion of an aortic abnormality.*

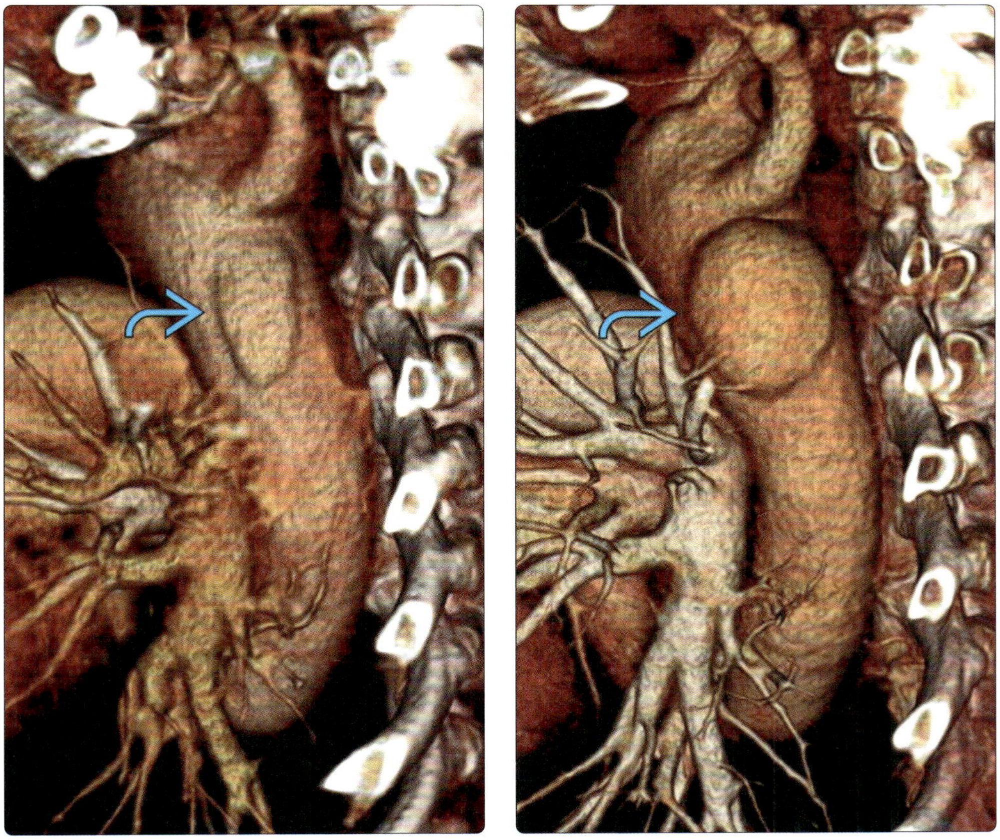

(Left) *3D volume-rendered view of the proximal descending aorta clearly shows the LIT is apparent even on day 1.* **(Right)** *3D volume-rendered image on day 6 clearly shows the LIT and that it has grown and expanded over just a few days.*

Aortic Aneurysm: Rupture

KEY FACTS

TERMINOLOGY

- Dilated aorta with disruption through all 3 layers of aortic wall leading to extravasation of blood into surrounding structures
- May occur in setting of acute aortic syndrome where intimal injury is precipitating factor that leads to disruption of wall containing residual medial and adventitia

IMAGING

- Risk of rupture or dissection often linked to aneurysm size, morphology, and rate of growth
- Ascending aortic aneurysms (AAs), asymptomatic
  - In patients with sporadic root and ascending AAs, repair considered with aneurysm size ≥ 5 cm
  - In patients with genetic aortopathy, repair considered if AA diameter is ≥ 4 cm
- Descending thoracic aorta, asymptomatic
  - In patients with intact descending thoracic aneurysm, repair recommended if diameter ≥ 5.5 cm
  - In patients with high risk of rupture, repair recommended if diameter ≥ 5 cm
- Abdominal aortic aneurysm (AAA), asymptomatic
  - Elective repair with AAA diameter of ≥ 5.5 cm and ≥ 5 cm in men and women, respectively
- Symptomatic patients should undergo repair regardless of size
- Depending on rate of growth, repair recommended with
  - Sporadic thoracic aneurysms and growth rate ≥ 0.5 cm in 1 year or ≥ 0.3 cm per year in 2 consecutive years
  - Genetic aortopathy or bicuspid aortic valve and growth ≥ 0.3 cm in 1 year
  - AAA growing ≥ 1 cm in 1 year
- CTA findings of rupture
  - Hemomediastinum, hemopericardium, or hemothorax, hemoperitoneum depending on site
  - Focal discontinuity in aneurysm wall or disruption of otherwise circumferential aortic calcifications

(Left) *PA CXR in a 63-year-old man with severe chest and abdominal pain in Mexico 3 weeks earlier (who underwent CTA at that time and was told he had a significant problem, but no surgeon would operate) shows increased density in middle mediastinum extending into the abdomen ➔ with a partially loculated right pleural effusion ➔.* **(Right)** *CTA in the same patient after he traveled to the USA shows rupture of a large thoracoabdominal aortic aneurysm ➔ with right hemothorax ➔ and blood in the mediastinum ➔.*

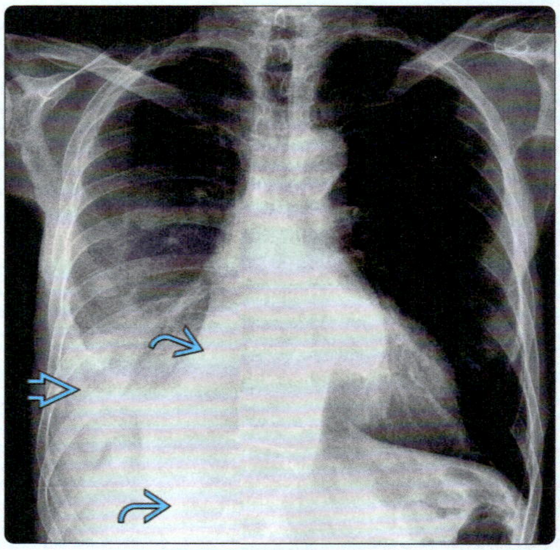

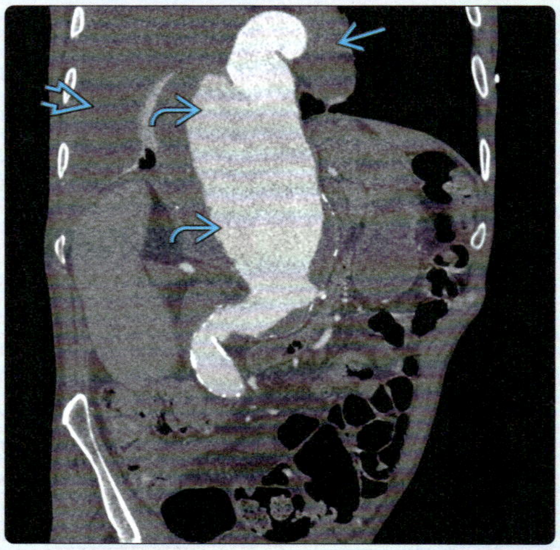

(Left) *Delayed phase from the CTA in the same patient better shows complex loculated fluid collections in right pleural space ➔ and mediastinum ➔ due to blood products. The aneurysm ➔ is again seen.* **(Right)** *Axial oblique CTA (L) after branch fenestrated endovascular thoracoabdominal aortic aneurysm repair for a ruptured aneurysm shows both type III endoleak at left renal artery and superior mesenteric artery origin ➔. The left kidney is infarcted ➔. DWI image (R) 1 day after repair shows a large PCA territory infarct ➔.*

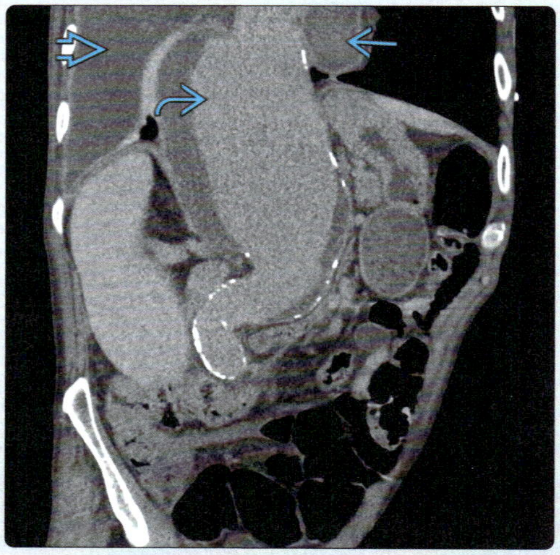

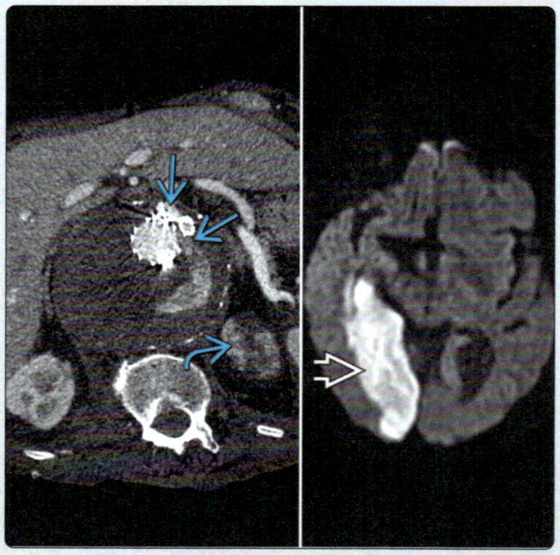

TERMINOLOGY

Definitions

- Dilated aorta with disruption through all 3 layers of aortic wall leading to extravasation of blood into surrounding structures
- May occur in setting of acute aortic syndrome where intimal injury is precipitating factor that leads to disruption of wall containing residual medial and adventitia

IMAGING

General Features

- Best diagnostic clue
  - Enlarged thoracic aorta with associated hemomediastinum, hemopericardium, or hemothorax is highly suggestive of ruptured thoracic aortic aneurysm (TAA)
- Location
  - Abdominal aortic aneurysm (AAA) > TAA
  - TAA most common in ascending thoracic aorta
  - However, most ruptures involve AAA descending TAA
- Size
  - Risk of rupture or dissection often linked to aneurysm size, morphology, and rate of growth
  - Thoracic aneurysms
    - Aneurysm ≥ 6 cm was significantly associated with risk of rupture or dissection
      - Yearly rate of rupture or dissection ≥ 6 cm ranges from 10-15%
      - At ≥ 7 cm, rate dramatically increases to > 40%
    - Ascending aortic aneurysms (AAs)
      - For sporadic aortic root and ascending AAs, repair now recommended in certain patients with aneurysm size ≥ 5 cm
      - Patients with genetic disorders, such as Marfan syndrome, Ehlers-Danlos syndrome, Loeys-Dietz syndrome, and familial TAA &/or dissection, repair should be considered if AA diameter is 4.0-5.0 cm
    - Descending thoracic aorta
      - In patients with intact descending thoracic aneurysm, repair recommended if diameter ≥ 5.5 cm
      - In patients with high risk of rupture, repair recommended if diameter ≥ 5 cm
      - Risk of rupture includes genetic aortopathy, aneurysm causing symptoms, saccular aneurysm, female sex, concern for mycotic aneurysm/pseudoaneurysm, and growth rate ≥ 0.5 cm in 1 year
  - AAA
    - Risk of 5-year rupture 20-40% with aneurysms > 5 cm
    - Elective repair for asymptomatic patients with AAA diameter of ≥ 5.5 cm and ≥ 5 cm in men and women, respectively
    - For symptomatic patients, should be repaired regardless of size
- Morphology
  - May be fusiform or saccular with former being more common and latter associated with increased risk of rupture
  - Wall calcification and mural thrombus are common and may be extensive
  - Aortic tortuosity may complicate surgical approach and should be described
- Rate of growth
  - Repair recommended for those with sporadic thoracic aneurysms and growth rate ≥ 0.5 cm in 1 year or ≥ 0.3 cm per year in 2 consecutive years
  - Repair recommended for those with heritable thoracic aortic disease or bicuspid aortic valve and growth ≥ 0.3 cm in 1 year
  - Repair recommended if AAA is rapidly expanding ≥ 1 cm in 1 year

Radiographic Findings

- Mediastinal widening may be seen in ruptured or unruptured TAA but is often difficult to appreciate
- Pleural effusion (hemothorax) if ruptured into pleural space
- Pericardial effusion (hemopericardium) if ruptured into pericardial space
- Following thoracic endovascular aortic repair (TEVAR), endograft migration, kinking, or fracture may be identified

CT Findings

- NECT
  - In patients unable to receive contrast, TAA morphology and diameter may be assessed on NECT
  - Signs of frank or impending rupture, such as hemomediastinum and intramural hematoma, are both evident on NECT
  - Following TEVAR, NECT is also useful for distinguishing calcified mural thrombus from endoleak
- CTA
  - Impending, contained, or frank rupture
    - Hemomediastinum, hemopericardium, or hemothorax depending on location of rupture
    - Focal discontinuity in aneurysm wall or disruption of otherwise circumferential aortic calcifications
    - Dense crescent sign: Intramural hematoma or dissection of acute blood into mural thrombus
    - Lysis of thrombus with expansion of contrast-enhanced flow lumen

MR Findings

- Can provide much of same information as CTA without ionizing radiation
- Following TEVAR, MR is most useful in setting of nickel titanium (nitinol) grafts, which do not produce susceptibility artifacts
- LGE of excluded aneurysm sac is sensitive for detecting endoleaks
- Time-resolved MR angiography and 4D phase-contrast MR (4D flow) are useful in further characterizing endoleaks

Echocardiographic Findings

- Transthoracic echocardiography can evaluate aortic root and proximal ascending thoracic aorta as well as complications, such as aortic regurgitation, pericardial effusion, and pericardial tamponade, but is limited by acoustic windows and operator dependence

- Transesophageal echocardiography can evaluate entire thoracic aorta with exception of portion of distal ascending aorta and proximal arch, which may be obscured by tracheobronchial tree

Imaging Recommendations

- Best imaging tool
  - NECT + CTA
- Protocol advice
  - CTs should be reconstructed using thin (submillimeter) slices to allow for high-quality multiplanar reconstruction (MPRs)
  - NECT is useful for identifying blood products, and, following endovascular repair, for distinguishing calcified mural thrombus from endoleak
  - ECG gating is crucial for accurate evaluation aortic root and ascending aorta
  - Delayed imaging is useful for fully opacifying flow lumen in very large aneurysms and for identifying endoleaks occult on arterial phase

DIFFERENTIAL DIAGNOSIS

Aortic Aneurysm Without Rupture

- AAs are not uncommon, especially in older patients
- Coexistent pericardial and pleural effusions are not uncommon in patients with TAA due to underlying cardiovascular disease
- In some patients, TAAs with complex ulcerated plaque with coexistent simple transudative pleural and pericardial effusions could potentially mimic rupture

Acute Aortic Syndrome With Rupture

- Aortic dissection, intramural hematoma, or penetrating atherosclerotic ulcer can all lead to aortic rupture
- Presence of intimal injury is characteristic of AAS
  - If rupture occurs in AAS, it is due to disruption of residual media and overlying adventitia
- In AAs with rupture, rupture is through all 3 layers of aortic wall

Aortic Pseudoaneurysm

- Aortic dilation contained by overlying adventitia due to vascular injury
- Commonly secondary to trauma, surgery, or infection
- More likely to be saccular, able to expand, and change shape rapidly

Large Vessel Vasculitis or Inflammatory Aortitis (IgG4 or Erdheim-Chester Disease)

- Patients often symptomatic with chest/back pain, weight loss, and elevated inflammatory markers
- Areas of stenosis often with coexistent aneurysm
- Circumferential wall thickening in areas, often associated with enhancement
- Inflammation in periaortic fat could mimic rupture

PATHOLOGY

General Features

- Cystic medial degeneration results in progressive loss of elastin in tunica media
- Aortic wall stress increases with aortic diameter (governed by Laplace's Law)
- Rupture may occur in TAA with disruption of all 3 layers of aortic wall
- Rupture may also occur in setting of acute aortic syndrome
  - Intimal injury is precipitating cause
  - Rupture occurs through residual media and adventitia
- Recognition of rupture is more important than differentiating between etiologies, although different etiologies may lead to different methods of repair

CLINICAL ISSUES

Presentation

- Most common signs/symptoms
  - Chest pain, hemorrhagic shock, tamponade
  - Unruptured TAAs are usually asymptomatic and identified incidentally on imaging

Demographics

- TAA occurs in 5-10 per 100,000 person-years
- Risk factors for TAA rupture include
  - Large diameter (especially > 6.0 cm)
  - Rapid aneurysm growth (≥ 0.5 cm/year)
  - Saccular morphology
  - Female sex
  - Hereditary or infectious etiology

Natural History & Prognosis

- Once ruptured, usually fatal without repair
- Rate of growth and risk of rupture are highly dependent upon underlying etiology as aforementioned

Treatment

- Ascending AA with rupture
  - Open repair
- Arch aneurysm with rupture
  - Open repair with arch replacement
- Descending thoracic or AAA with rupture
  - TEVAR or open surgical repair
  - TEVAR showed lower mortality and reduced risk of paraplegia, stroke, and hypovolemic shock compared to open repair

SELECTED REFERENCES

1. Writing Committee Members et al: 2022 ACC/AHA guideline for the diagnosis and management of aortic disease: a report of the American Heart Association/American College of Cardiology Joint Committee on clinical practice guidelines. J Thorac Cardiovasc Surg. 166(5):e182-331, 2023
2. Isselbacher EM et al: 2022 ACC/AHA guideline for the diagnosis and management of aortic disease: a report of the American Heart Association/American College of Cardiology Joint Committee on clinical practice guidelines. Circulation. 146(24):e334-482, 2022
3. Bhave NM et al: Multimodality imaging of thoracic aortic diseases in adults. JACC Cardiovasc Imaging. 11(6):902-19, 2018
4. Kim JB et al: Risk of rupture or dissection in descending thoracic aortic aneurysm. Circulation. 132(17):1620-9, 2015

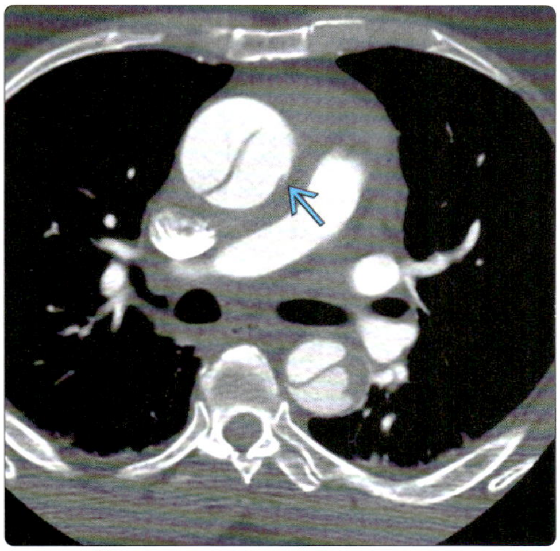

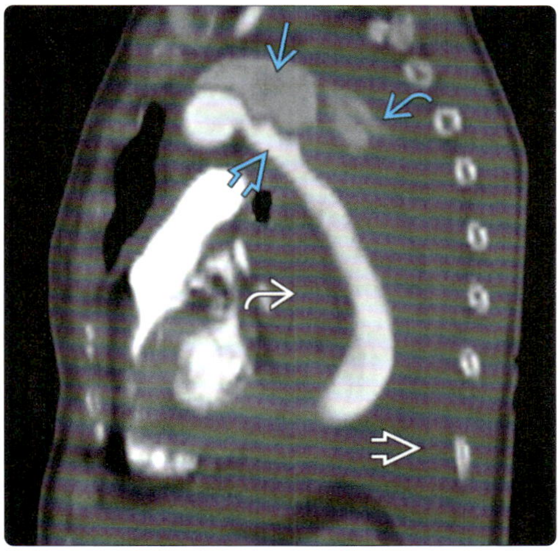

(Left) *CTA in a 71-year-old man with chest pain shows an aneurysmal ascending aorta with type A dissection. Mediastinal and pericardial hematoma indicate rupture. The only potential rupture site seen on CTA was a slight contour irregularity, which was confirmed surgically.* **(Right)** *CTA in a 76-year-old woman with severe chest pain shows an aneurysmal aorta with a type B dissection with true and false lumens. The false lumen has ruptured, leading to extensive mediastinal hematoma and hemothorax.*

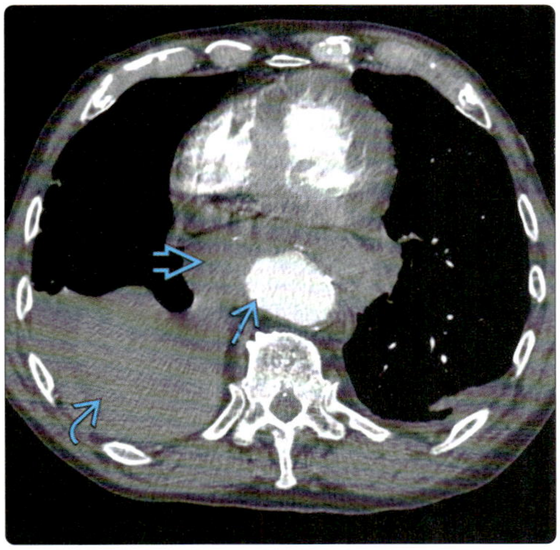

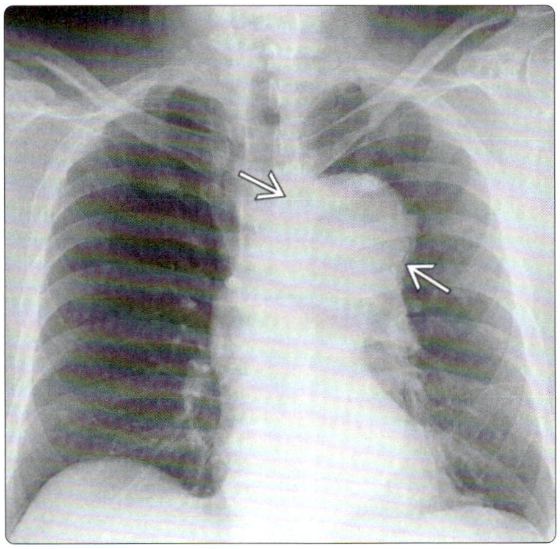

(Left) *Axial CT in an 83-year-old man with severe chest pain shows a thoracic aortic aneurysm with mild irregularity of the right wall with surrounding mediastinal hematoma and large right hemothorax. Rupture was confirmed surgically.* **(Right)** *PA radiograph in a man in his '80s who presented with streptococcus pneumonia bacteremia and left shoulder pain demonstrates an enlarged aortic contour concerning for thoracic aortic aneurysm. CTA was recommended.*

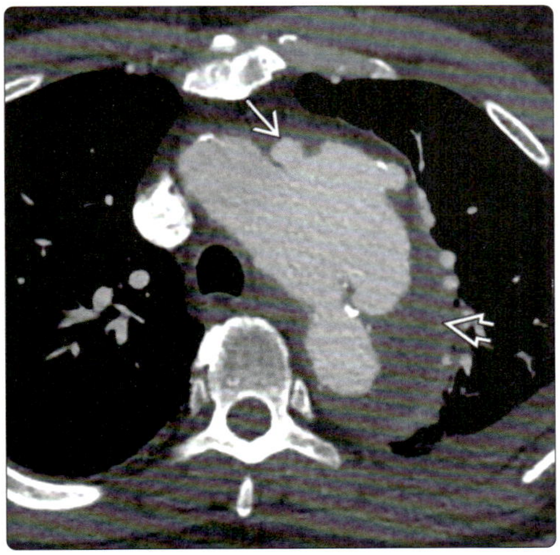

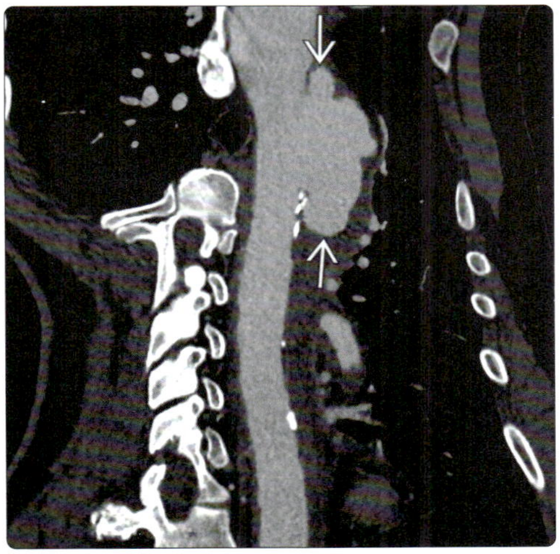

(Left) *CTA in the same patient shows a large, multilobulated saccular pseudoaneurysm arising from the lateral aspect of the aortic arch with surrounding soft tissue, concerning for mycotic aneurysm given the known bacteremia.* **(Right)** *Curved planar reconstruction of the aorta in the same patient shows the size and extent of the large, lobulated saccular mycotic pseudoaneurysm. Differentiation between a mycotic pseudoaneurysm and ruptured aneurysm can be difficult without appropriate history.*

Takayasu Arteritis

KEY FACTS

TERMINOLOGY

- Pulseless disease
- Chronic granulomatous vasculitis of large vessels

IMAGING

- Best diagnostic clue: Wall thickening of large vessels
  - Thoracic aorta and branches
  - Pulmonary artery involvement is less common
- NECT: Aortic wall thickening
- CECT: Aortic wall thickening and enhancement
  - Stenosis, occlusion, aneurysm
- MRA: Aortic narrowing, dilatation
- Angiography: 4 types classified by location
- PET/CT is used for treatment monitoring
- Complications
  - Stenosis > occlusion
  - Aneurysm
  - Dissection

TOP DIFFERENTIAL DIAGNOSES

- Giant cell arteritis
- Aortic coarctation

PATHOLOGY

- Autoimmune etiology is suspected
- Specific types of human leukocyte antigen are common among patients

CLINICAL ISSUES

- Disease stages
  - Early or prepulseless phase
  - Vascular inflammatory phase
  - Late quiescent occlusive or pulseless phase
  - Triphasic disease in minority of patients
- F:M = 8:1
- Heart failure is most common cause of death
- Treatment
  - Corticosteroids, angioplasty, surgical bypass

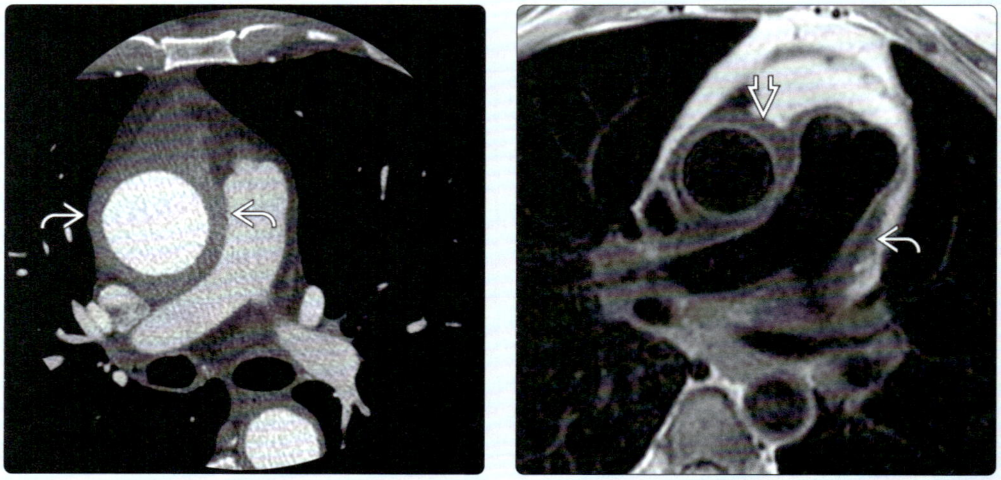

(Left) *Axial CECT in a patient with Takayasu arteritis (TA) shows marked thickening of the wall of the ascending thoracic aorta ➡. The thoracic aorta and its branches, particularly the left subclavian artery, are the most commonly affected vessels in TA.* **(Right)** *Axial T1 MR in a patient with TA demonstrates thickening of the wall of the ascending thoracic aorta ➡ and the pulmonary trunk ➡. Vessel stenosis, occlusion, and aneurysm formation may complicate cases of TA.*

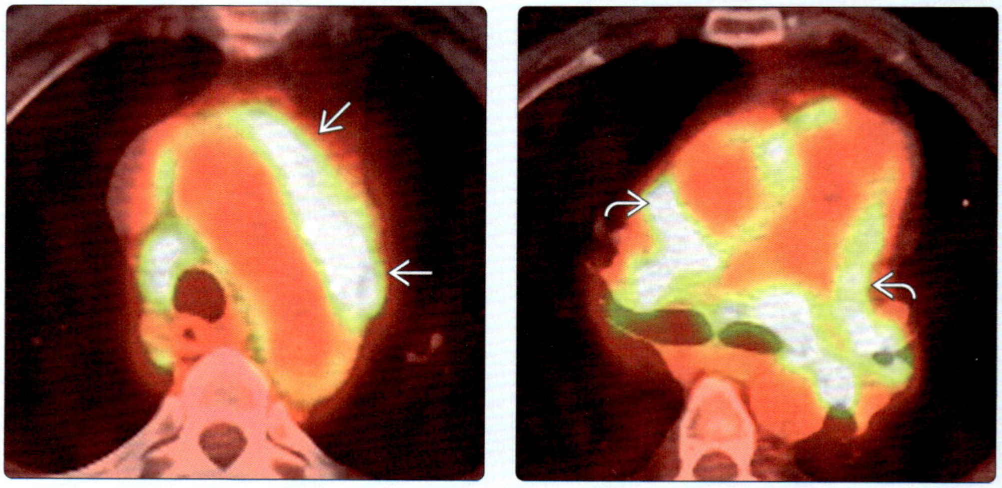

(Left) *Axial fused PET/CT in a patient with active TA demonstrates intense FDG uptake within the mediastinum adjacent to the aortic arch ➡ in a region of soft tissue attenuation that was present on the localization CT.* **(Right)** *Axial fused PET/CT in the same patient shows intense FDG uptake within the mediastinum adjacent to the ascending aorta and pulmonary arteries ➡. FDG uptake may be low grade to intense in TA, and PET/CT is an effective way of monitoring treatment response.*

TERMINOLOGY

Abbreviations

- **Takayasu arteritis (TA)**

Synonyms

- **Pulseless disease**

Definitions

- Chronic granulomatous vasculitis of large vessels

IMAGING

General Features

- Best diagnostic clue
  - Wall thickening of large vessels
- Location
  - **Thoracic aorta and branches**
    - **Left subclavian artery** is most commonly affected
    - Ostial stenoses or occlusion of arch vessels
  - Pulmonary artery (PA) involvement is less common
- Evidence of medium or large vessel involvement on imaging is absolute requirement for diagnosis of TA

CT Findings

- NECT
  - Vessel wall thickening, iso-/hyperdense to muscle
- CECT
  - **Vessel wall thickening and enhancement**
  - **Stenosis, occlusion, aneurysm**
  - 95% sensitivity and 100% specificity for diagnosis of TA
  - Delayed/venous phase: Double ring enhancement pattern
    - Hyperenhanced outside ring: Active inflammation of media and adventitia
    - Poor enhancing inside ring: Swelling of intima
    - Can be used to assess treatment response

MR Findings

- T1WI
  - **Wall thickening: Aorta and branches**
  - Wall edema can be seen in STIR images
- T1WI C+
  - **Enhancement of thickened vessel wall**
- MRA
  - Focal/diffuse narrowing of aorta and branches
  - Aortic dilatation (ascending > descending)
  - Stenosis > occlusion
  - Aortic regurgitation, dissection, aneurysm
- Disease activity
  - Active disease: Wall edema and delayed enhancement can be seen
    - Poor and inconsistent correlation with disease activity
  - Development of new lesion in previously unaffected vascular territory is evidence of active disease/progression
    - Evaluate for new lesions in other territories

Ultrasonographic Findings

- Grayscale ultrasound
  - Vascular wall thickening, dilation, stenosis
    - Diffuse arterial wall thickening: Macaroni sign
    - Carotid intima-media thickness > 1 mm is considered to be inflammatory vascular disease
- Color Doppler
  - Luminal stenosis, change in blood flow patterns
  - 81% sensitivity and 100% specificity for diagnosing TA

Angiographic Findings

- Early: Aortic wall thickening, rarely, stenosis
- Late: Stenosis, occlusion, aneurysm; 4 types
  - I: Aortic arch branches
  - II: Thoracic aorta (a: Ascending, B: Descending) and branch vessels
  - III: Descending thoracic and abdominal aorta ± renal arteries; may have atypical coarctation
  - IV: Abdominal aortic ± renal arteries
  - V: Entire aorta and its branches

Nuclear Medicine Findings

- PET
  - FDG uptake; ranges from low grade to intense
  - Treatment monitoring: Multiple qualitative and quantitative methods

DIFFERENTIAL DIAGNOSIS

Giant Cell Arteritis

- Affects large vessels in older patients (> 50 years)

Vasculitis Mimics

- Infections (tuberculosis, syphilis, HIV, bacterial)
- Atherosclerosis; thromboembolism
- Genetic disorders: Marfan, Ehlers-Danlos IV, Loeys-Dietz, Grange
- Congenital: Coarctation, Turner syndrome, Williams syndrome
- Unknown etiology: Fibromuscular dysplasia, segmental arterial mediolysis

Behçet Disease

- Large vessel vasculitis seen in 30% of these patients
- Proximal PA aneurysms are common

Other Causes of Aortitis

- Ankylosing spondylitis, rheumatoid arthritis, Cogan syndrome, relapsing polychondritis, IgG4-related disease

PATHOLOGY

General Features

- Etiology
  - Autoimmune etiology is suspected
  - Infectious triggers suspected: Mycobacterium tuberculosis
    - Suspected association with active or latent TB
- Genetics
  - Specific types of human leukocyte antigen are common
    - Strong association with HLA-B52

Gross Pathologic & Surgical Features

- Wall thickening of large vessels

Microscopic Features

- Granulomatous inflammation of arterial wall
  - Intimal proliferation; fibrosis of media and adventitia

Classification Criteria for Takayasu Arteritis: 2022 ACR/EULAR

Absolute Requirements	
Age ≤ 60	
Evidence of vasculitis on imaging	
Additional Clinical Criteria	
Female sex	+1
Angina or ischemic cardiac pain	+2
Claudication	+2
Vascular bruit	+2
Diminished pulse in upper extremity	+2
Carotid artery abnormality	+2
Systolic BP difference in arms ≥ 20 mmHg	+1
Additional Imaging Criteria	
Number of affected artery territory	
1 arterial territory	+1
2 arterial territories	+2
3 or more arterial territories	+3
Symmetric involvement of paired arteries	+1
Abdominal aorta involvement with renal or mesenteric involvement	+3
Score of ≥ 5 points = Takayasu arteritis	

Adapted from 2022 American College of Rheumatology/EULAR classification criteria for Takayasu arteritis, 2022.

CLINICAL ISSUES

Presentation

- Most common signs/symptoms
  - **Early or prepulseless phase**
    - Low-grade fever, malaise, weight loss, fatigue
  - **Vascular inflammatory phase**
    - Vascular insufficiency
    - Symptoms are minimized by collateral formation
  - **Late quiescent occlusive or pulseless phase**
    - Diminished/absent pulses, vascular bruits, claudication
    - Blood pressure discrepancies in upper extremity
    - Subclavian steal syndrome
    - Hypertension, aortic regurgitation
    - Neurologic symptoms: Headache, dizziness, seizures, stroke
      - Ocular symptoms (ranging 8-68%): Hypertensive retinopathy or Takayasu retinopathy (due to hypoperfusion)
  - Triphasic pattern is seen in minority of patients
    - Disease is usually recurrent; phases may coexist
    - Interval between early and late phases is variable
  - **Cardiac involvement**
    - Myocardial ischemia: 84% of asymptomatic patients
    - Can cause angina, myocardial infraction, or sudden cardiac death
    - Coronary involvement is independent predictor of poor long-term outcomes
      - Type 1 (most common): Stenosis or occlusion of coronary ostia and proximal coronary artery
      - Type 2: Diffuse or focal coronary arteritis (skip lesions)
      - Type 3: Coronary aneurysms
- Other signs/symptoms
  - Pulmonary hypertension when PA is involved
    - Increases risk of early mortality

Demographics

- Age
  - Most common in 2nd and 3rd decades of life
- Sex
  - F:M = 8:1
- Epidemiology
  - Most common in Asia
  - Affects 6 out of 1,000 persons worldwide
  - Annual incidence in USA: 2-3

Natural History & Prognosis

- Congestive heart failure is most common cause of death
- Hypertension is poor prognostic factor

Treatment

- Corticosteroids are 1st-line treatment; cyclophosphamide and methotrexate are 2nd line
- Angioplasty, surgical bypass, or stent placement for stenosis and occlusion

SELECTED REFERENCES

1. Somashekar A et al: Updates in the diagnosis and management of Takayasu's arteritis. Postgrad Med. 135(sup1):14-21, 2023
2. Grayson PC et al: 2022 American College of Rheumatology/EULAR classification criteria for Takayasu arteritis. Arthritis Rheumatol. 74(12):1872-80, 2022
3. Jia S et al: Application progress of multiple imaging modalities in Takayasu arteritis. Int J Cardiovasc Imaging. 37(12):3591-601, 2021
4. Chatterjee S et al: Clinical diagnosis and management of large vessel vasculitis: Takayasu arteritis. Curr Cardiol Rep. 16(7):499, 2014

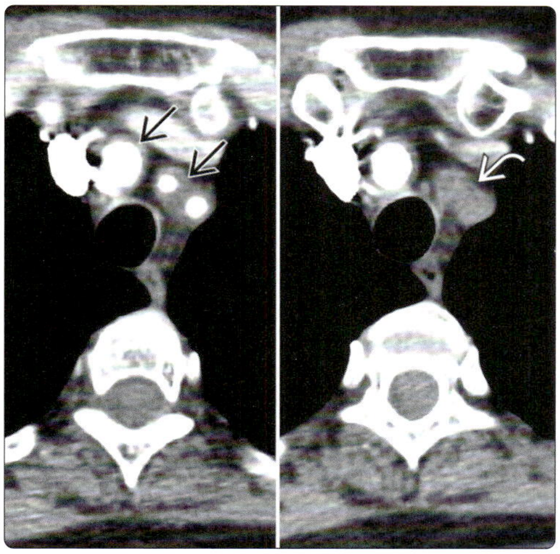

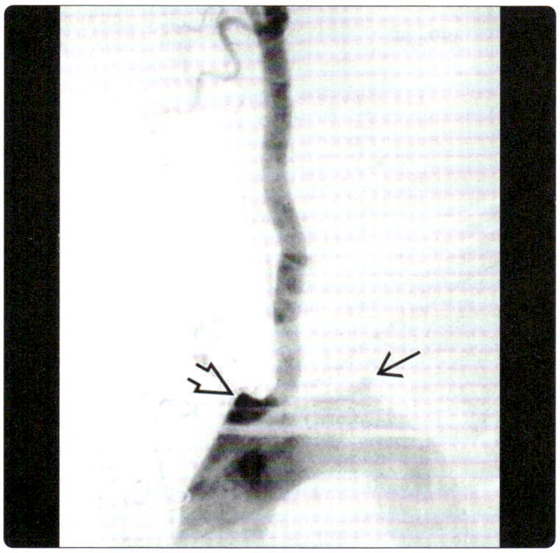

(Left) *Composite image with axial CECT shows wall thickening ⇨ of the proximal right brachiocephalic, left common carotid, and left subclavian arteries. There is more distal occlusion ➡ of the left common carotid and left subclavian arteries. The left subclavian artery is the most common branch vessel affected in patients with TA.* **(Right)** *Sagittal oblique DSA in another patient with TA shows patency of the left common carotid artery with occlusion of the right brachiocephalic ⇨ and left subclavian arteries ⇨.*

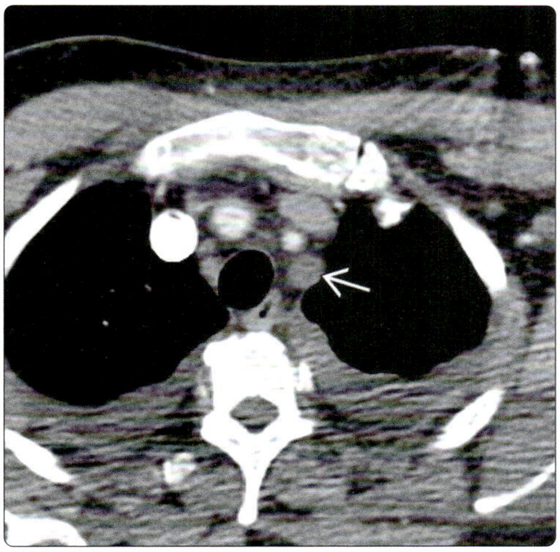

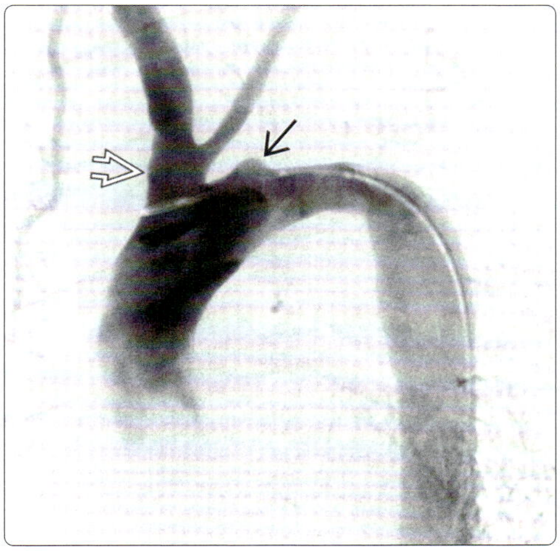

(Left) *Axial CECT in a patient with TA shows soft tissue attenuation and no contrast opacification within the left subclavian artery ➡, consistent with occlusion.* **(Right)** *Sagittal oblique DSA in the same patient with TA shows occlusion of the left subclavian artery ⇨. Note the common origin ➡ of the right brachiocephalic and left common carotid arteries.*

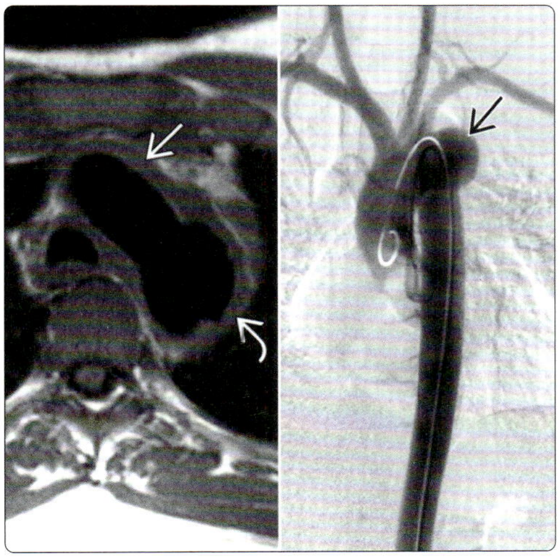

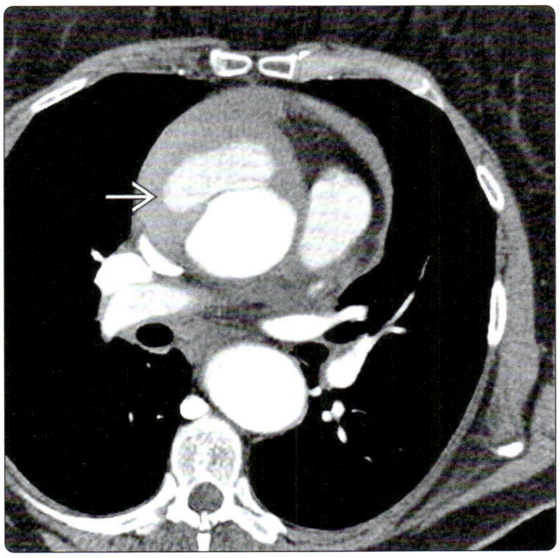

(Left) *Composite image with axial T1 MR (left) and DSA (right) shows aortic wall thickening ➡ and a focal aneurysm ↷ confirmed on subtraction aortic DSA ⇨.* **(Right)** *Axial CECT in a patient with TA shows an aortic dissection with marked intramural hemorrhage surrounding the false lumen ➡. TA was confirmed on pathologic examination of the resected specimen.*

Giant Cell Arteritis

KEY FACTS

TERMINOLOGY

- Chronic, systemic, large or medium-sized, often granulomatous vasculitis
  - Often involves thoracic aorta and major branches
  - Often involves temporal artery

IMAGING

- CTA
  - Concentric aortic thickening (> 2 mm)
  - Aortic aneurysm; classically ascending aorta
  - Aortic dissection: Intimomedial flap
- MR
  - Assessment of active inflammation
  - Delayed enhancement after gadolinium
- Ultrasonography
  - High specificity and sensitivity; operator dependent
  - Hypoechoic halo temporal &/or axillary arteries
- PET
  - Active inflammation demonstrates ↑ FDG uptake

TOP DIFFERENTIAL DIAGNOSES

- Takayasu arteritis
  - May be identical to GCA
  - Extremely rare in patients > 50 years
- Atherosclerotic disease
  - May be difficult to differentiate radiographically, though clinical symptoms often facilitate process
  - Similar age group

CLINICAL ISSUES

- Headache, visual disturbances, jaw claudication
- Polymyalgia rheumatica
- Serologic markers
  - ↑ sedimentation rate
  - ↑ C-reactive protein
  - Thrombocytosis
- Treatment
  - Corticosteroids

(Left) *Axial CTA of the chest in a patient with giant cell arteritis (GCA) shows soft tissue ➡ density material surrounding the great vessels. (Courtesy C. S. Restrepo, MD.)* **(Right)** *Axial chest CTA in the same patient shows concentric thickening of the thoracic aorta, which is a common finding in patients with GCA but is indistinguishable from Takayasu arteritis. GCA is more common in patients > 50 years old. Concomitant NECT is recommended to help differentiate from intramural hematoma. (Courtesy C. S. Restrepo, MD.)*

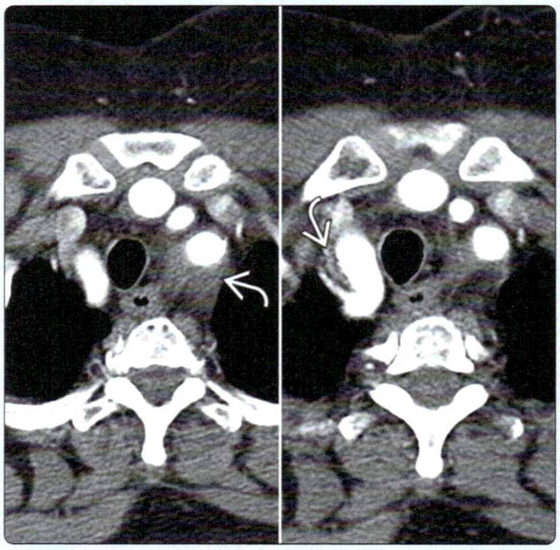

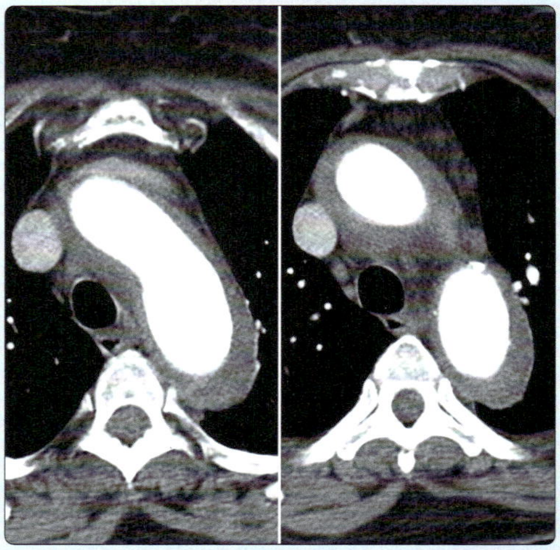

(Left) *Coronal FDG PET/CT in the same patient shows marked uptake of FDG along the ascending aortic wall ➡. FDG PET has excellent sensitivity and specificity for the diagnosis of GCA and may be used when clinical or serological discrepancies arise during or after treatment of this condition.* **(Right)** *Coronal FDG PET/CT in a patient with GCA shows diffuse uptake along the ascending aortic wall ➡ as well as along the subclavian and axillary arteries bilaterally ➡.*

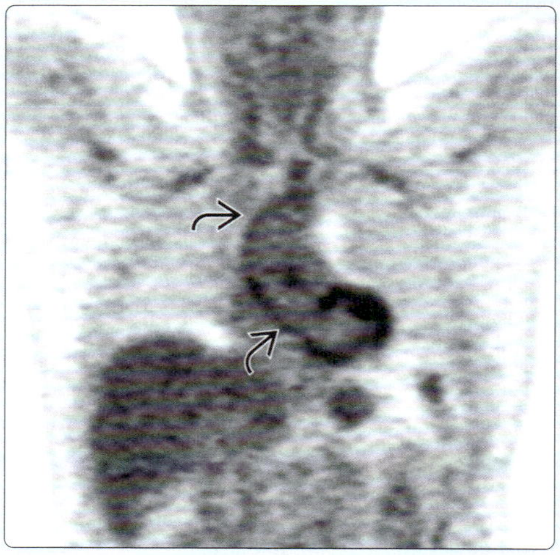

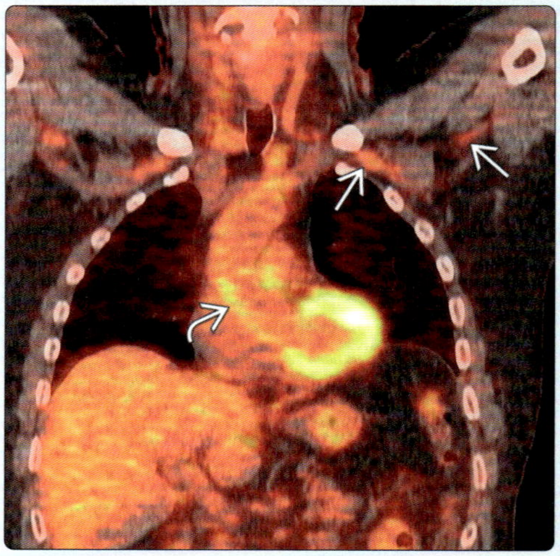

TERMINOLOGY

Abbreviations

- Giant cell arteritis (GCA)

Synonyms

- Temporal arteritis
  - Cranial GCA (C-GCA) often referred to as temporal arteritis; terminology not longer recommended, as sparing of temporal artery is not uncommon and because disease may involve large vessels
  - Horton disease

Definitions

- Granulomatous autoimmune vasculitis affecting larger arteries and aorta
  - C-GCA: Often involves temporal artery and other head/neck vessels, but may also involve aorta and major branches
  - Large-vessel GCA (LV-GCA): Often involves thoracic aorta and major branches
  - Frequently associated with polymyalgia rheumatica (PMR)
    - Aching and morning stiffness in shoulders, hip girdle, and neck

IMAGING

General Features

- Location
  - Temporal artery
  - Aorta and aortic branches

CT Findings

- NECT
  - Typically, GCA involving aorta is not as apparent or dense as intramural hematoma; however, there can be hyperdensity if associated with hemorrhage or calcification
  - Transmural calcification is often similar to calcified atherosclerotic plaques (common)
- CTA
  - Concentric aortic thickening (> 2 mm)
  - Aortic stenosis
  - Aortic aneurysm; classically ascending aorta
  - Aortic dissection: Intimomedial flap
  - Limited role in C-GCA

MR Findings

- Equally accurate as CT for morphologic assessment on several sequences (e.g., T1WI, T2WI, HASTE, SSFP, etc.)
- Contrast-enhanced MRA is more accurate to assess areas of stenosis and aneurysm
- Assessment of active inflammation
  - Contrast-enhanced sequences: Delayed enhancement (i.e., $\uparrow$ signal) of vessel wall after gadolinium
  - Fat-saturated STIR sequence: High signal of thickened vessel wall
- Cranial (temporal artery) involvement
  - High sensitivity and specificity
  - Mural thickening (> 0.5 mm)
  - Mural high T2 signal and contrast enhancement

Angiographic Findings

- Stenosis (often long, regular, and smooth-walled)
- Occlusion
- Aneurysm
- Limited in diagnosis of early vasculitis

Nuclear Medicine Findings

- PET
  - LV-GCA: Active inflammation demonstrates $\uparrow$ FDG uptake
    - Subclinical inflammation of large vessels in 80% with GCA and ~ 30% PMR
    - Response to treatment correlates with $\downarrow$ FDG uptake
  - Limited role in C-GCA, not recommended

Imaging Recommendations

- Best imaging tool
  - MR
    - STIR: Thickening and high signal of aortic wall
    - Contrast-enhanced MR: Thickening and enhancement of aortic wall
    - MRA is helpful to detect areas of stenosis and aneurysm
- Protocol advice
  - Consider concomitant NECT to differentiate from intramural hematoma
    - Caveat: GCA can occasionally be hyperdense
- PET
  - Recognized role in patient with fever &/or inflammation of unknown origin
  - Unclear role in follow-up, especially asymptomatic patients without elevated inflammatory markers

DIFFERENTIAL DIAGNOSIS

Takayasu Arteritis

- May have similar imaging appearance to GCA
- Rare in patients > 50 years old

Other Systemic Vasculitides

- e.g., polyarteritis nodosa, syphilitic aortitis
- Occurs most often in small and medium-sized arteries
- Biopsy and pattern of distribution often help differentiation

Fibromuscular Dysplasia

- Most often affects renal arteries
  - Can also involve carotid arteries
- Results in stenoses; occasional spontaneous dissection

Atherosclerotic Disease

- May be difficult to differentiate radiographically, though clinical symptoms often facilitate process
- Similar age group

PATHOLOGY

Staging, Grading, & Classification

- Temporal artery biopsy remains diagnostic gold standard for C-GCA
- Predictors of positive temporal artery biopsy
  - Jaw claudication
  - Neck pain

- C-reactive protein > 2.45 mg/dL
- Sedimentation rate > 47 mm/h
- Thrombocytosis
- Pallid optic disc edema
- Temporal artery abnormalities
- Temporal artery biopsy can be negative (10-15%)

Gross Pathologic & Surgical Features

- Involvement of aorta (65.0%)
- Involvement of main aortic tributaries (57.5%)
  - Brachiocephalic trunk (47.5%)
  - Subclavian arteries (42.5%)
  - Carotid arteries (35.0%)
  - Femoral arteries (30.0%)
  - Splanchnic arteries (22.5%)
  - Axillary arteries (17.5%)
  - Iliac arteries (15.0%)
  - Renal arteries (7.5%)

Microscopic Features

- Focal chronic inflammatory cell infiltrates
  - Granulomas in vessel wall formed by CD4(+) T cells and macrophages
- Focal areas of intimal hyperplasia
  - Proliferation of smooth muscle cells, which leads to narrowing of arterial lumen and eventually ischemia
- Focal areas of fragmentation of inner elastic lamina
- Focal concentric scars around inner elastic lamina

CLINICAL ISSUES

Presentation

- Most common signs/symptoms
  - Headache
  - Visual disturbances
  - Jaw claudication
- Other signs/symptoms
  - PMR
    - Present in 50% of patients at diagnosis of GCA
    - 20% of PMR will develop GCA
    - Clinical manifestations
      - Morning stiffness
      - Pain (shoulder > hip or neck)
      - Synovitis and bursitis
      - Swelling and tenosynovitis
      - ↓ range of motion
      - Muscle tenderness
      - Subjective weakness
      - Systemic signs and symptoms (e.g., malaise, fatigue, depression, anorexia, weight loss, fever)
- Clinical profile
  - Clinical phenotypes
    - C-GCA (temporal arteritis with headache and visual disturbance)
    - LV-GCA (arm/limb claudication, chest pain)
    - PMR
    - Phenotypes can overlap
  - Serologic markers
    - ↑ erythrocyte sedimentation rate
    - ↑ C-reactive protein
    - Thrombocytosis
  - Association with HLA-DRB1*04
  - LV-GCA linked to other systematic diseases, such as Behçet disease or hyper-IgG4 syndrome
  - Factors for aneurysm formation
    - Aortic insufficiency
    - Murmur at time of diagnosis
    - Hyperlipemia
    - ↑ eritrosedimentation in combination with polymyalgia symptoms
    - ↑ levels of IL-2

Demographics

- Age
  - Patients > 50 years old
  - Incidence ↑ steadily with age
- Sex
  - Women > men
- Ethnicity
  - More common in people of Northern European and Scandinavian descent
- Epidemiology
  - Lifetime risk of developing GCA in USA: 1% in women and 0.5% in men

Natural History & Prognosis

- Prognosis for visual recovery is poor
- ↑ risk aortic aneurysm formation and dissection: 17-fold and 2.5x higher risk of thoracic and abdominal aortic aneurysms
  - ↓ survival rate
- Involvement of coronary arteries may result in myocardial infarction or congestive heart failure
- Bowel necrosis (uncommon)
- 15-30% of PMR cases eventually develop GCA

Treatment

- GCA and PMR: Corticosteroids
- Aspirin
- Other (2nd-line therapy)
  - Methotrexate
  - Azathioprine
  - Tocilizumab (IL-6 receptor alpha inhibitor)

DIAGNOSTIC CHECKLIST

Consider

- Annual surveillance to assess for aneurysm and dissection

SELECTED REFERENCES

1. Pepper K: Giant cell arteritis. Postgrad Med. 135(sup1):22-32, 2023
2. Braun J et al: The role of 18F-FDG positron emission tomography for the diagnosis of vasculitides. Clin Exp Rheumatol. 36 Suppl 114(5):108-14, 2018
3. Dejaco C et al: The spectrum of giant cell arteritis and polymyalgia rheumatica: revisiting the concept of the disease. Rheumatology (Oxford). 56(4):506-15, 2017
4. Buttgereit F et al: Polymyalgia rheumatica and giant cell arteritis: a systematic review. JAMA. 315(22):2442-58, 2016

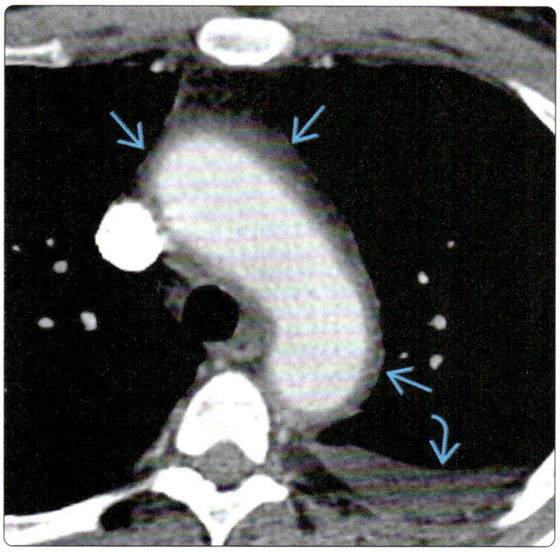

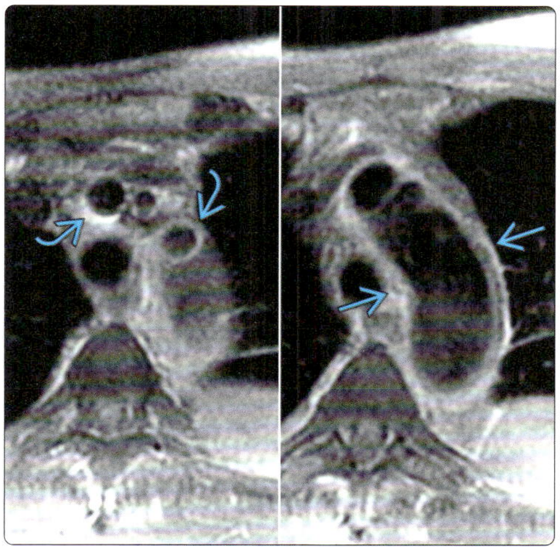

(Left) *Axial CTA in a patient with GCA shows diffuse arterial wall thickening* ➡ *and stranding of the periaortic fat. Note the reactive left pleural effusion* ➦*.* **(Right)** *Axial double inversion recovery FS MR in the same patient at different levels shows diffuse high signal of the aortic wall* ➡ *as well as head and neck vessels* ➦*. MR is the preferred method to assess for active inflammation also seen in the form of vessel parietal enhancement after intravenous gadolinium.*

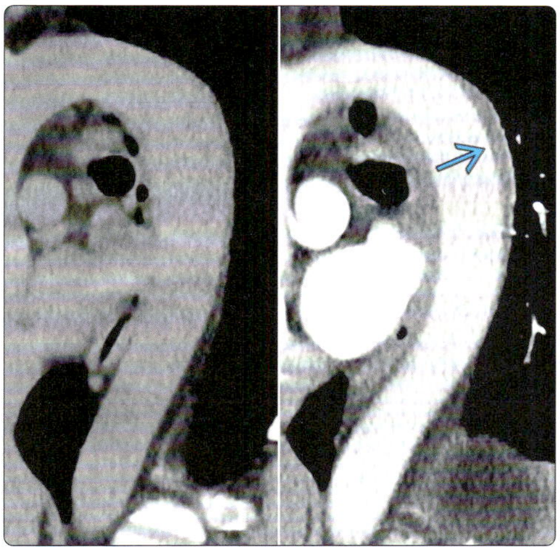

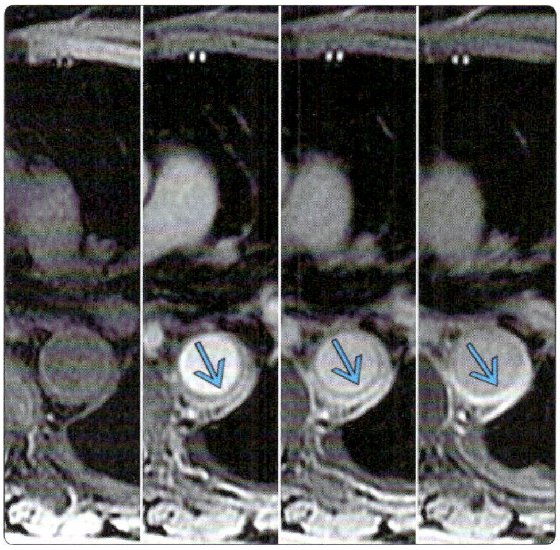

(Left) *Sagittal reformat CECT in a patient with GCA before and after contrast shows focal parietal thickening along the posterior descending thoracic aorta, only evident on CECT* ➡*. Typically, vasculitis is not hyperdense on NECT as opposed to intramural hematoma.* **(Right)** *3D GRE MR (unenhanced and post contrast) at the same level shows progressive enhancement of the aortic wall after administration of intravenous contrast* ➡*.*

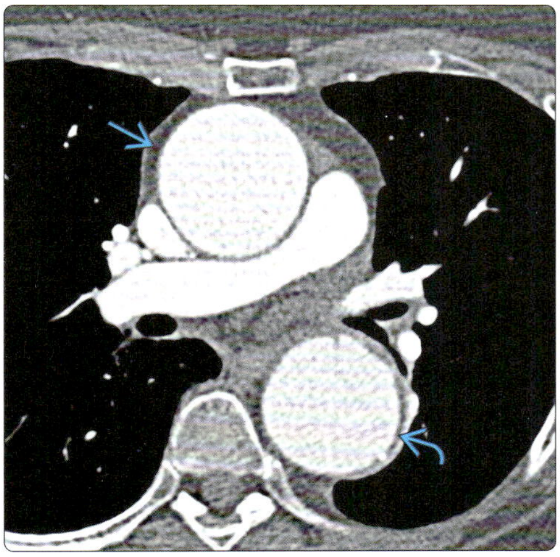

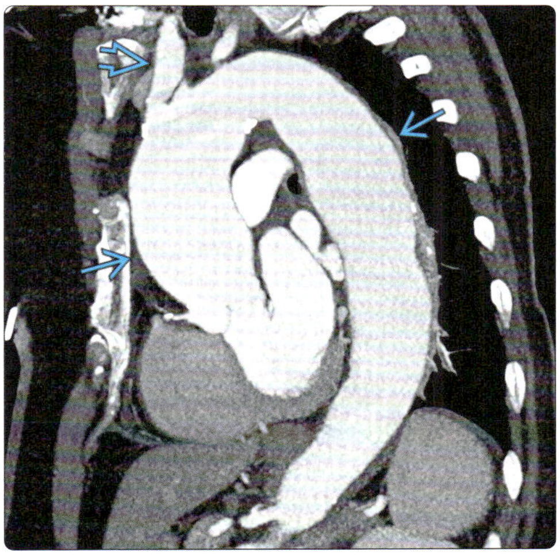

(Left) *Axial CTA in a patient with unsuspected GCA who underwent reconstruction of the ascending aorta due to aneurysm is shown. Note the aneurysmal ascending* ➡ *and descending aorta* ➦*.* **(Right)** *Sagittal CECT MIP in the same patient shows diffuse aneurysmal thoracic aorta* ➡*. Note also the aneurysmal right brachiocephalic trunk* ⇨*. Aneurysm is a very common complication of undiagnosed and untreated GCA only evident after resection.*

Traumatic Aortic Injury

KEY FACTS

TERMINOLOGY

- Traumatic injury of aorta (TAI) as result of motor vehicle collision (MVC), fall, or, less commonly, penetrating trauma
- Synonyms: Acute TAI, blunt traumatic aortic rupture, blunt aortic trauma, blunt aortic injury, aortic transection, traumatic aortic pseudoaneurysm
- Minimal aortic injury (MAI)

IMAGING

- Radiography
  - Wide mediastinum: Hematoma, exclusion of TAI
  - 1st rib fracture: Severe trauma, possible TAI
- CTA: Imaging modality of choice
  - Aortic isthmus (90%); commonly on inferomedial aspect
  - Direct: Intramural hematoma; intimal flap; pseudoaneurysm
  - Indirect: Periaortic hematoma; irregular aortic contour; sudden aortic caliber change
  - Sensitivity 98%; specificity 80%

TOP DIFFERENTIAL DIAGNOSES

- Wide mediastinum of other etiology
- Mediastinal hematoma: Other causes
- Ductus diverticulum (type III)
- Infundibulum of bronchial-intercostal trunk
- Atherosclerotic ulceration
- Fusiform enlargement proximal descending aorta

CLINICAL ISSUES

- No specific or sensitive signs or symptoms until hemodynamic instability ensues
- Urgent diagnosis; 50% die within 24 hours if untreated
- Cause of death in 20% of high-speed MVCs
- Treatment
  - Surgical repair: 70-85% survival (up to 20% surgical mortality)

(Left) *AP chest radiograph in a young man struck by a car shows widening of the superior mediastinum, a left apical cap, a right tracheal/endotracheal and enteric tube deviation, thick paratracheal stripes, and loss of the aortic arch and the AP window.* **(Right)** *Axial CTA in the same patient shows active contrast extravasation from the ruptured descending aorta and a large mediastinal hematoma that produces mass effect on the esophagus, airways, and pulmonary arteries.*

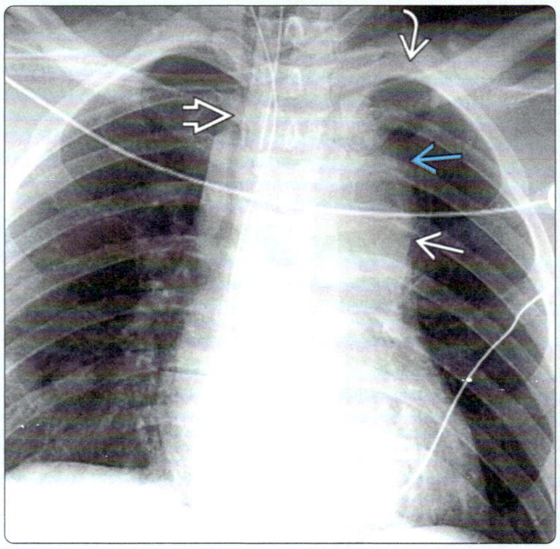

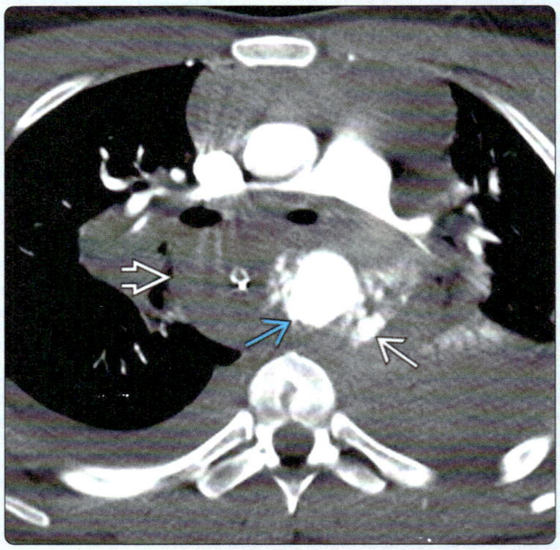

(Left) *Axial CTA in a 23-year-old man with a stab wound to the anterior chest shows mediastinal hemorrhage and laceration of the anteromedial ascending aorta with adjacent intramural hematoma.* **(Right)** *Sagittal oblique aortogram following blunt chest trauma shows a large pseudoaneurysm at the aortic isthmus. CTA has largely replaced conventional angiography for the diagnosis of traumatic aortic injury (TAI) but still plays an important role in TAI treatment with endovascular stent graft placement.*

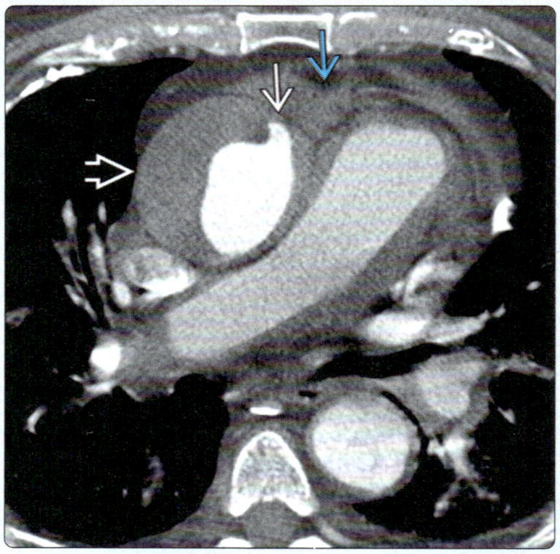

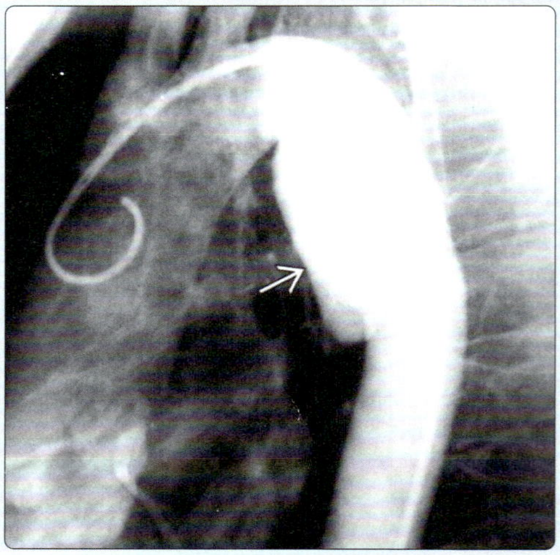

TERMINOLOGY

Abbreviations

- Traumatic aortic injury (TAI)

Synonyms

- Minimal aortic injury (MAI)
- Significant aortic injury (SAI)

Definitions

- Traumatic injury of aorta as result of motor vehicle collision (MVC), fall or, less commonly, penetrating trauma

IMAGING

General Features

- Best diagnostic clue
  - **Widened mediastinum** on AP chest radiography
  - **Intramural hematoma (IMH), intimal flap, pseudoaneurysm or rupture** on CTA
- Location
  - **Aortic isthmus (90% of initial survivors)**; commonly along inferomedial aspect at level of left pulmonary artery
  - Ascending aorta (5-14% of initial survivors)
    - Most die at scene of accident
  - Diaphragmatic hiatus (1-12%)
    - May be associated with diaphragmatic injury
  - Multiple sites rarely affected

Radiographic Findings

- Radiography
  - **Indirect signs** related to mediastinal hemorrhage
  - Signs of TAI: Sensitive but not specific
  - Most signs present in 30-70% of patients
    - **Widened superior mediastinum** (> 8 cm or > 25% of transthoracic diameter)
    - **Left apical pleural cap**
    - Abnormal aortic arch contour
    - Obscuration of AP window
    - Right tracheal &/or endotracheal tube shift
    - Right enteric tube shift
    - Wide paravertebral stripe
    - Wide right paratracheal stripe
    - Inferior displacement of left mainstem bronchus
  - 1st rib fracture indicates severe trauma and possible TAI
    - 1st rib protected by clavicle and scapula, requires considerable force to break
    - Frequency of TAI is 15-30%
  - Any of aforementioned signs requires further investigation to exclude aortic transection
  - Normal chest radiograph (7%)
  - Chronic pseudoaneurysm (2% of survivors)
    - Peripherally calcified mass at aorticopulmonary window

CT Findings

- NECT
  - Often shows mediastinal hematoma, rarely shows site of tear
- CTA
  - Imaging modality of choice
    - Direct visualization of aortic tear, markedly reducing need for aortography
    - Sensitivity: 98%, specificity: 80%
  - **Direct signs**
    - IMH
    - **Intimomedial flap ± thrombus**
    - **Pseudoaneurysm or contained rupture**
    - Rarely complete rupture with active extravasation
    - Aortic dissection
  - Indirect signs
    - Periaortic/mediastinal hematoma
    - Irregular aortic contour
    - Sudden aortic caliber change; pseudocoarctation: Best seen on MPR
  - MAI: Absent contour abnormality
    - 10% of acute TAI (ATAI)
    - Increased diagnosis due to improved spatial resolution of CT
    - Intimal flap (small < 1 cm; large > 1 cm) ± thrombus; IMH without contour abnormality
    - May remain stable or resolve
  - SAI: Contour abnormality present
    - IMH + contour abnormality; pseudoaneurysm (< or > 1 cm); aortic rupture
  - More severe injuries: Have both direct and indirect findings
  - Pitfalls of TAI
    - Pulsation or streak artifact, especially at aortic root
      - ECG gating required
    - Ambiguous findings
      - Use different slice thickness, imaging plane, reconstruction kernel, or different phase of cardiac cycle
  - Mimics of TAI
    - Ductus diverticulum; infundibulum; other causes of mediastinal hematoma; atherosclerotic plaque
  - Chronic traumatic pseudoaneurysm
    - Develop in undiagnosed or untreated injuries
    - At isthmus; with extensive peripheral calcification; ± thrombus
    - Calcification protects against rupture

MR Findings

- MR generally has no role in evaluation of acute trauma
  - Limited by issues related to transportation and monitoring of critically injured patients

Imaging Recommendations

- Best imaging tool
  - **CTA is imaging modality of choice**
- Protocol advice
  - Thin slices, MPR, and 3D volume rendering essential for treatment planning
  - ECG gating required for evaluation of aortic root and ascending aorta

DIFFERENTIAL DIAGNOSIS

Widened Mediastinum on Chest Radiograph

- False-positives: Rotation, supine positioning, expiratory imaging, mediastinal fat

Mediastinal Hematoma: Other Causes

- Caused by injury to mediastinal veins, great vessels, pulmonary arteries, or vertebral body fractures
- Arterial injury not identified
- Hematoma usually away from aorta with intact fat plane

Ductus Diverticulum (Type III)

- Remnant of closed or partially closed ductus arteriosus
- Inferomedial outpouching of aortic isthmus
- Smooth, gently sloping shoulders with obtuse angle with aortic wall
- Often calcified; no intimal flap

Infundibulum of Bronchial-Intercostal Trunk

- Takeoff may show bump in aortic contour
- Cone-shaped, smooth walled, with artery at its apex

Atherosclerotic Ulceration

- More common in older patients
- Other coexisting aortic plaques

Normal-Variant Fusiform Dilation of Proximal Descending Aorta

- No intimomedial flap

PATHOLOGY

General Features

- Etiology
  - Theories of pathogenesis
    - Rapid deceleration injury with shearing forces greatest at levels of aortic immobility: Ligamentum arteriosum, aortic root, and diaphragmatic hiatus
    - Osseous pinch: Aorta compressed between anterior chest wall (manubrium, medial clavicles, 1st rib) and spine; transverse tear at aortic isthmus
    - Water hammer effect: Sudden marked increase in intravascular pressure during aortic compression; transverse tear at isthmus
    - Multivariate hypothesis likely: Shearing, torsion, stretching, hydrostatic forces

Gross Pathologic & Surgical Features

- 90% at aortic isthmus
  - From origin of left subclavian artery to ligamentum arteriosum, often anteromedially
- 7-8% involve aortic root; 2% involve descending aorta at diaphragmatic hiatus
- Ascending aortic tear: 20% of coroner cases; rarely survive long enough to reach hospital
- In abdominal aorta: Infrarenal segment is commonly affected
  - Lap belt compression
  - Associations: Lumbar spine fracture, pelvic fracture, injury to bowel, solid organs, spleen
- Range: Intimal hemorrhage to complete transection
- Transverse tears: Segmental (55%) or circumferential (45%); partial (65%) or transmural (35%)
- Noncircumferential tears more common posteriorly
- May involve aortic layers to varying degrees
  - Survivors: Pseudoaneurysm usually contained by adventitia, or, occasionally, mediastinal structures
  - Adventitial injuries occur in 40% of cases and are almost always fatal due to rapid exsanguination

CLINICAL ISSUES

Presentation

- Most common signs/symptoms
  - No specific or sensitive signs or symptoms until hemodynamic instability ensues
  - May have chest pain or dyspnea
- Other signs/symptoms
  - Acute coarctation syndrome rare
- **Urgent diagnosis needed**, as 50% expire within 24 hours if untreated
- Multiple associated injuries: Diaphragm rupture, lung contusion, rib fracture (1st rib), sternal fracture head injury, injury to heart, spleen, and liver

Demographics

- Epidemiology
  - Cause of death in 20% of high-speed MVCs

Natural History & Prognosis

- **85% die at site of trauma**, most often from MVC
- Survival depends on time from injury to intervention
- 2% long-term survival

Treatment

- Surgical repair
  - For aortic root, ascending aorta, and arch
  - Delayed repair may be acceptable in many cases
  - Paraplegia in 10%; directly related to cross-clamp time
- β-adrenergic blocking agents decrease wall stress
- Endovascular stent graft repair
  - Typically for isthmus, descending thoracic aorta, or abdominal aorta
  - Less invasive than surgical repair
  - Feasible in patients with multiple comorbid injuries
- Isolated injuries to intima (10%) may require no treatment and have been shown to resolve
  - Limited data on optimal management

DIAGNOSTIC CHECKLIST

Consider

- Careful evaluation of chest radiograph in trauma for indirect signs of aortic transection

Image Interpretation Pearls

- Consider chronic pseudoaneurysm in any patient with vascular calcification at aorticopulmonary window

SELECTED REFERENCES

1. Kapoor H et al: Minimal aortic injury: mechanisms, imaging manifestations, natural history, and management. Radiographics. 40(7):1834-47, 2020
2. Nagpal P et al: Advances in imaging and management trends of traumatic aortic injuries. Cardiovasc Intervent Radiol. 40(5):643-54, 2017
3. Cullen EL et al: Traumatic aortic injury: CT findings, mimics, and therapeutic options. Cardiovasc Diagn Ther. 4(3):238-44, 2014
4. Kaiser ML et al: Risk factors for traumatic injury findings on thoracic computed tomography among patients with blunt trauma having a normal chest radiograph. Arch Surg. 146(4):459-63, 2011

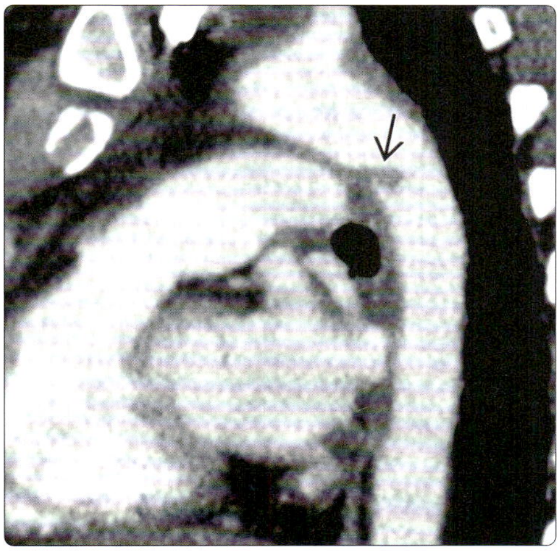

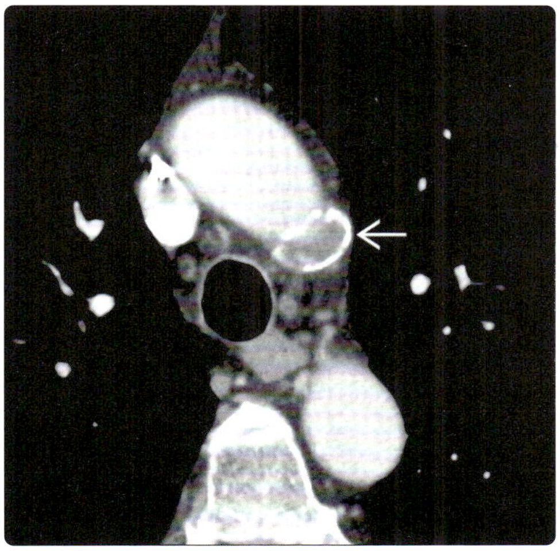

(Left) *Sagittal CECT in a patient involved in a motor vehicle collision shows a transverse segmental tear at the aortic isthmus → without a surrounding mediastinal hematoma, consistent with MAI. The patient had no additional chest injuries, was treated conservatively, and was followed annually with CT.* **(Right)** *Axial CTA in the same patient 5 years following trauma shows calcification and thrombus ➡ within a chronic posttraumatic aortic pseudoaneurysm.*

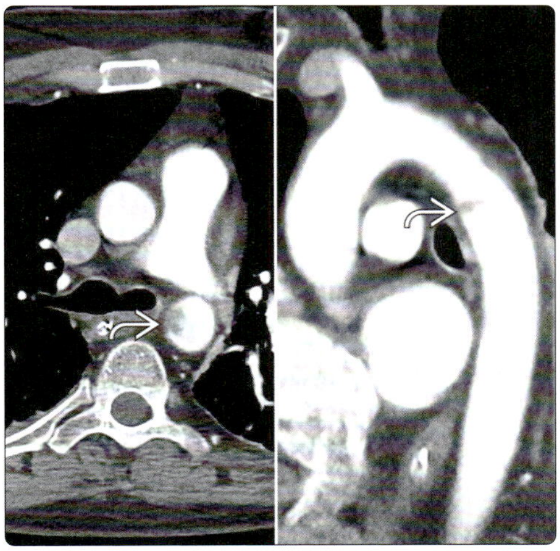

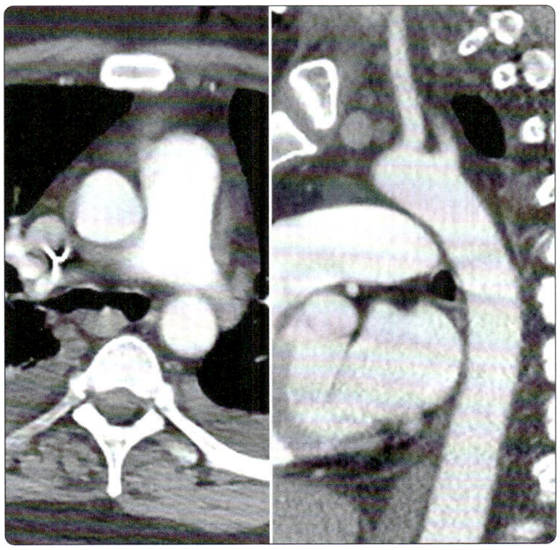

(Left) *Axial (left) and sagittal (right) CTA in a patient with blunt chest trauma show a minimal aortic injury manifesting with a focal intimal flap ➡ in the descending aorta without mediastinal hemorrhage.* **(Right)** *Axial (left) and sagittal (right) CECT in the same patient 9 days later show resolution of the aortic abnormalities. Although minimal aortic injuries are often observed and usually resolve, there is limited data on their optimal management.*

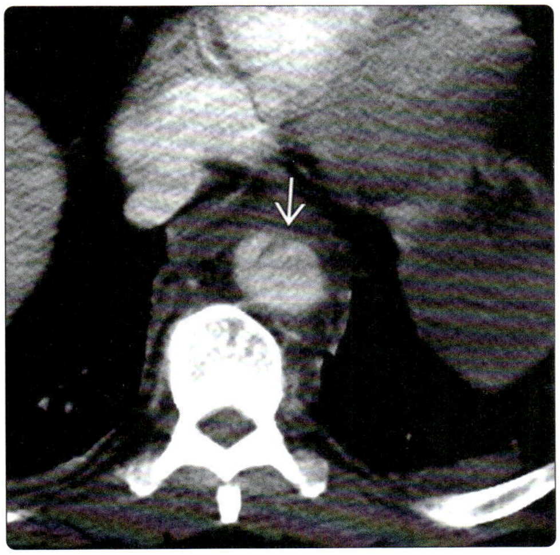

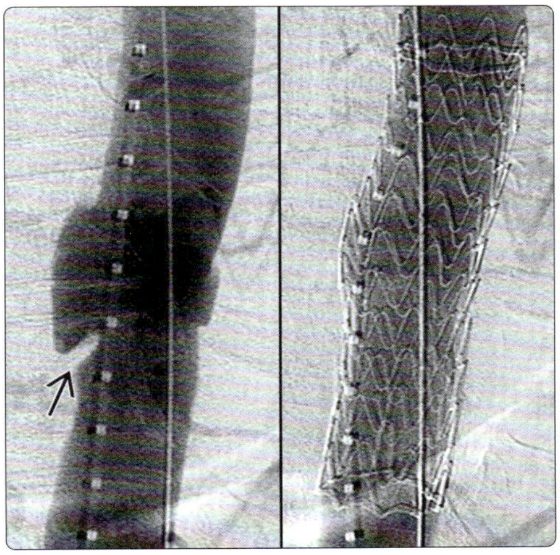

(Left) *Axial CTA of the chest in a 60-year-old unrestrained man following a high-speed motor vehicle collision shows a linear tear from the anterior aspect of the descending aorta at the level of the diaphragm ➡. The patient was hemodynamically unstable and was brought to the operating room.* **(Right)** *AP DSA performed intraoperatively (left) in the same patient shows the aortic injury →, which was successfully treated with an endovascular stent graft (right).*

Chronic Posttraumatic Pseudoaneurysm

KEY FACTS

TERMINOLOGY

- Traumatic disruption of aortic wall that goes undiagnosed in acute setting
- Chronic traumatic aortic injury (CTAI)

IMAGING

- Radiography
  - AP window mass
  - Curvilinear calcification typically lining caudad portion of aortic arch
- CTA
  - Saccular dilatation at isthmus arising from inferior aspect of aortic arch
  - Curvilinear mural calcification along saccular dilatation
- Ancillary findings of remote trauma
  - Healed rib, clavicular or scapular fractures
  - Thoracic vertebral body wedge fractures

TOP DIFFERENTIAL DIAGNOSES

- Nontraumatic aortic aneurysm
  - In atherosclerosis, calcification often lines superoexternal portion of aortic arch and other locations
  - Mycotic aneurysm often lacks calcifications
  - Penetrating aortic ulcer is not common at isthmus; often with extensive atherosclerosis
- Mediastinal mass
- Ductus aneurysm
  - Often indistinguishable from CTAI on imaging

CLINICAL ISSUES

- Asymptomatic; incidental finding on imaging
- 1/3 of CTAI may rupture and cause death if untreated
- Preferred treatment: Endovascular repair, if anatomically suitable (often complex with arch involvement, may need branched device)
- Alternative treatment: Open surgical repair.

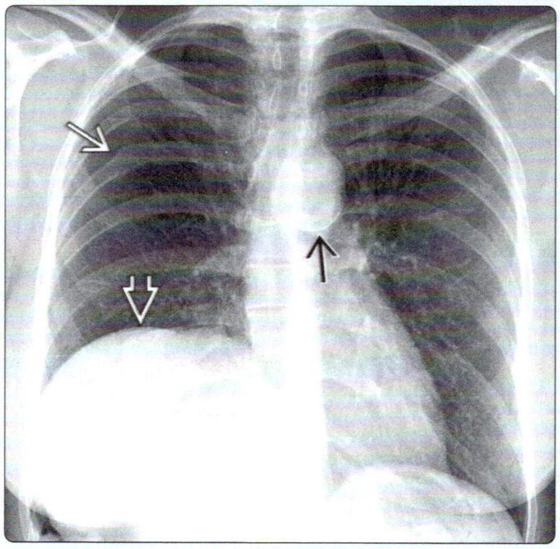

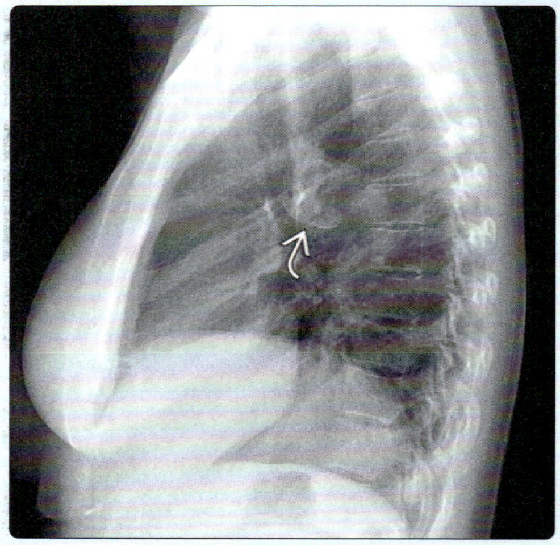

(Left) *PA radiograph of the chest in a young asymptomatic patient with chronic traumatic aortic injury (CTAI) and right diaphragmatic hernia shows curvilinear calcification lining the caudad part of the aortic arch. There is elevation of the right hemidiaphragm form chronic undiagnosed right diaphragmatic hernia. Note remote rib fractures.* **(Right)** *Lateral radiograph of the chest in the same patient shows aortic bulging with intrinsic mural calcification at the isthmus.*

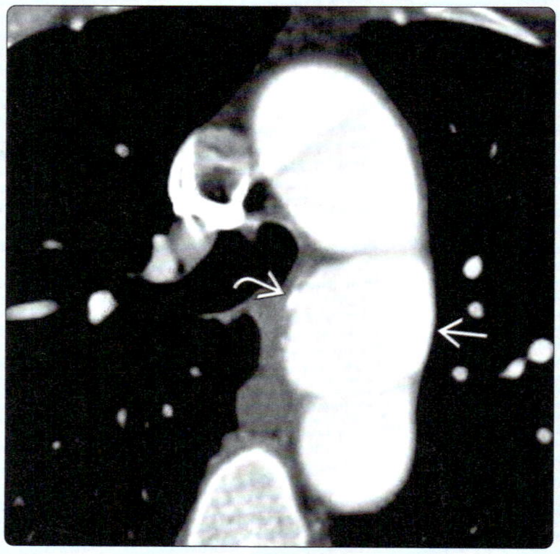

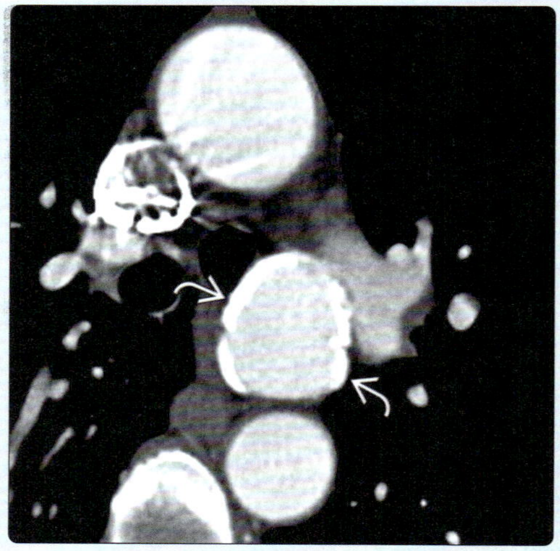

(Left) *Axial chest CTA in the same patient demonstrates saccular isthmic aortic dilatation with some mural calcifications in continuity with the aortic lumen.* **(Right)** *Axial chest CTA in the same patient reveals extensive calcifications along the wall of the pseudoaneurysm. This constitutes the most common imaging appearance of CTAI. The presence of other stigmata of trauma is often helpful to differentiate from ductus aneurysm.*

TERMINOLOGY

Synonyms

- Chronic traumatic aortic injury (CTAI)
- Late or unsuspected posttraumatic pseudoaneurysm

Definitions

- Traumatic disruption of aortic wall
- Not containing 3 vascular wall layers
- Contained by adventitia or thrombus and fibrous tissue

IMAGING

General Features

- Best diagnostic clue
  - Saccular aneurysm with wall calcification at level of aortic isthmus
- Location
  - Near aortic isthmus, typical location of acute traumatic aortic injury; e.g , at undersurface of distal aortic arch, or proximal descending thoracic aorta
- Morphology
  - Saccular, acute margins with aorta

Imaging Recommendations

- Best imaging tool
  - CTA
- Protocol advice
  - Use of multiplanar reformations on CTA or MRA may be helpful; 3D processing for treatment planning (TEVAR)

Radiographic Findings

- Radiography
  - Frontal projection
    - AP window mass
    - Curvilinear calcification typically lining distal portion aortic arch/proximal descending aorta
    - Rightward tracheal deviation
  - Lateral projection
    - Curvilinear calcified convexity (mass) at aortic isthmus

CT Findings

- CTA
  - Saccular dilatation near aortic isthmus
  - Curvilinear mural calcification at saccular dilatation
  - May contain low-density thrombus
  - May cause extrinsic compression of left main bronchus
  - Ancillary findings of remote trauma
    - Healed rib, clavicular or scapular fractures
    - Thoracic vertebral body wedge fractures
    - Traumatic diaphragmatic hernia

MR Findings

- MRA
  - Contrast-filled saccular dilatation at aortic isthmus in continuity with aorta
  - Intraluminal thrombus appears hypointense
- Black-blood and bright-blood (e.g., SSFP) are as accurate as CTA

Angiographic Findings

- Rarely required (often part of endovascular treatment)

DIFFERENTIAL DIAGNOSIS

Nontraumatic Aortic Pseudoaneurysm

- May be secondary to infection (i.e., mycotic), atherosclerosis/penetrating aortic ulcer (PAU), surgery
- There is history of remote trauma in CTAI, and calcifications are limited to saccular dilatation
- May be impossible to differentiate from pseudoaneurysm [i.e., acute traumatic aortic injury (ATAI) or CTAI] on imaging

Ductus Aneurysm

- May be difficult to distinguish from CTAI on imaging
- Smooth obtuse margins, wide ostium

Mediastinal Mass

- e.g., lung cancer, bronchogenic cyst
- CT with contrast is often diagnostic

PATHOLOGY

General Features

- Etiology
  - Posttraumatic
- Associated abnormalities
  - Osseous fractures (rib, clavicle, sternum, thoracic spine)
  - Diaphragmatic hernia

CLINICAL ISSUES

Presentation

- Most common signs/symptoms
  - Asymptomatic; incidental finding on imaging
  - Chest pain, dysphagia, dyspnea, cough, hoarseness

Demographics

- Epidemiology
  - Unknown incidence
  - Small minority of ATAI cases remain undiagnosed and may become CTAI

Natural History & Prognosis

- 1/3 of CTAI rupture and cause death if untreated
  - May rupture even years after acute injury

Treatment

- Small, asymptomatic aneurysms > 2 years after trauma can followed with CT imaging surveillance
- Traditional treatment: Open surgical repair
- Alternative treatment: Endovascular repair, if anatomically suitable

SELECTED REFERENCES

1. Authors/Task Force Members et al: EACTS/STS guidelines for diagnosing and treating acute and chronic syndromes of the aortic organ. Ann Thorac Surg. 118(1):5-115, 2024
2. Recicarova S et al: Comprehensive multi-modality treatment of thoracic aorta pseudoaneurysms: a single-center experience. Gen Thorac Cardiovasc Surg. 72(6):387-94, 2024
3. Abed H et al: Very late rupture of a post-traumatic abdominal aortic pseudoaneurysm. BMJ Case Rep. 2017, 2017
4. Nizet C et al: Chronic false aneurysm after a healed rupture of the aortic isthmus: TEVAR, hybrid surgery, or open arch repair? Ann Vasc Surg. 31:205.e11-6, 2016

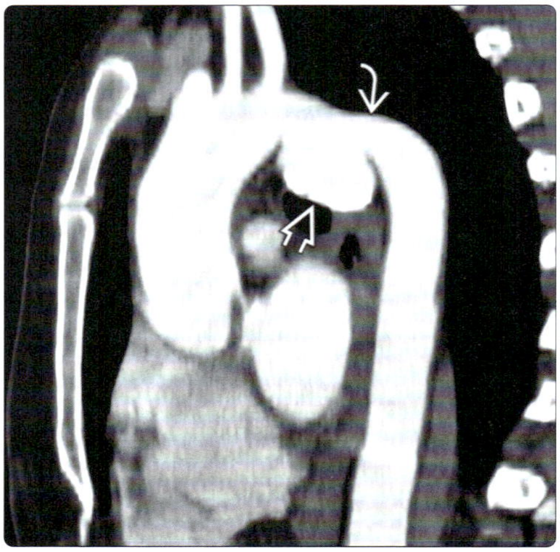

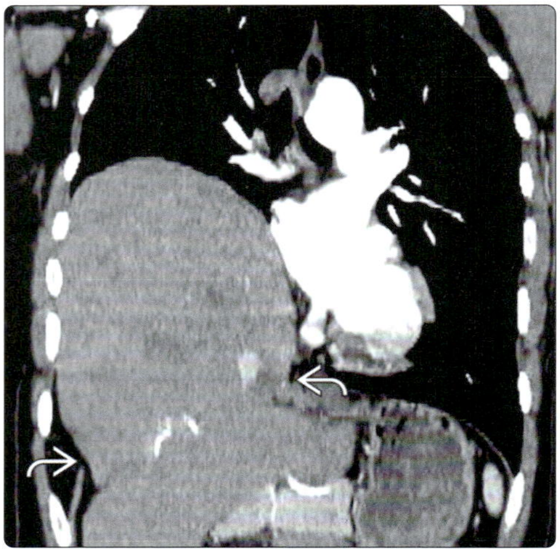

(Left) *Oblique sagittal chest CTA in an asymptomatic patient with CTAI and right diaphragmatic hernia shows a well-defined aortic pseudoaneurysm at the aortic isthmus. Note characteristic sudden change in caliber of the aorta distally, a common finding.* **(Right)** *Coronal chest CTA in the same patient demonstrates characteristic right diaphragmatic rupture with the hourglass sign of the liver and a frank hemidiaphragmatic defect.*

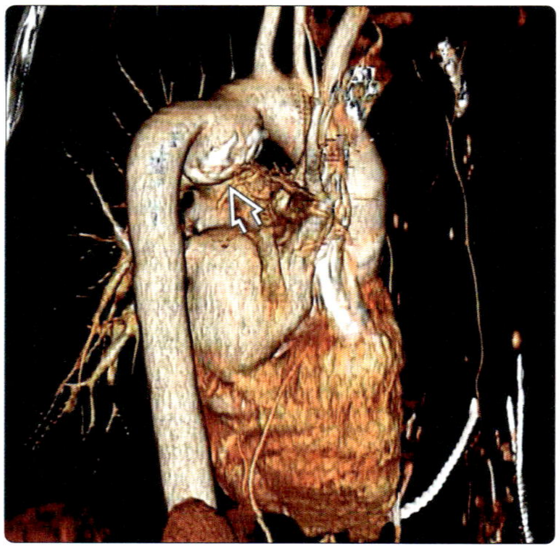

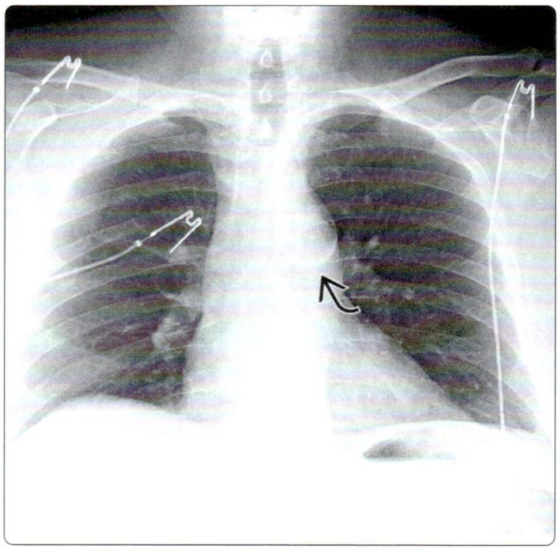

(Left) *Posterior sagittal chest 3D reformation in the same patient demonstrates the aortic pseudoaneurysm and its relationship with the pulmonary artery and the left atrium. 3D reformations may be helpful for better anatomic understanding and appropriate surgical planning.* **(Right)** *PA chest radiograph in an asymptomatic patient with CTAI and a pseudoaneurysm shows curvilinear calcifications along the inferior aspect of the aortic arch.*

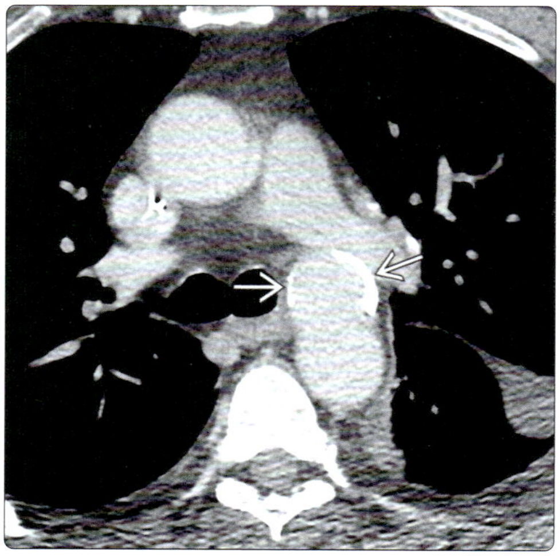

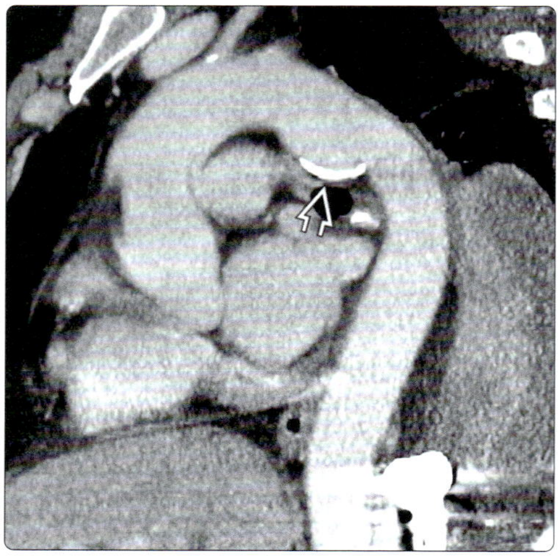

(Left) *Axial chest CTA in the same patient demonstrates well-marginated saccular dilatation of the aorta at the level of the isthmus.* **(Right)** *Oblique sagittal reformation chest CTA in the same patient shows an isthmic pseudoaneurysm with intrinsic curvilinear wall calcifications. A ductus aneurysm can be difficult to differentiate from a CTAI on imaging. However, they both have similar clinical and prognostic considerations as well as treatment.*

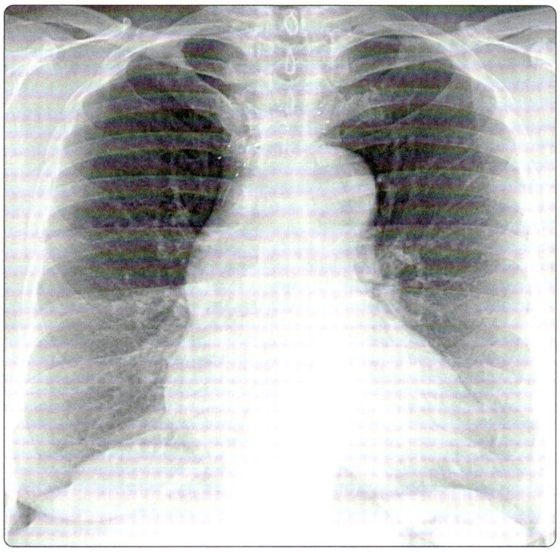

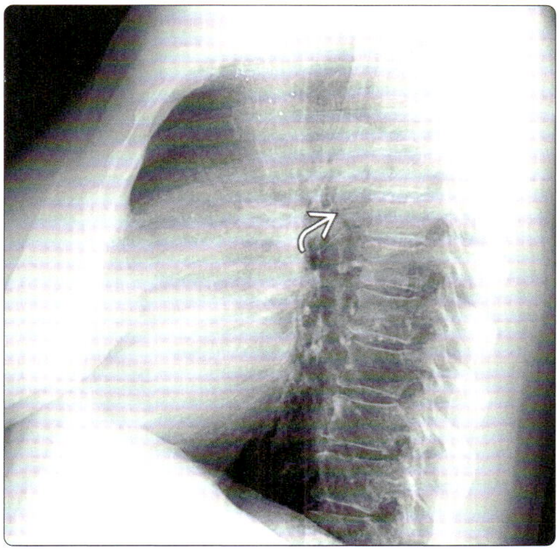

(Left) *PA chest radiograph in an asymptomatic patient with CTAI shows mild widening of the mediastinum.* **(Right)** *Lateral chest radiograph in the same patient demonstrates that, given a lack of significant amount of wall calcification, the abnormality (i.e., the pseudoaneurysm) ➡ is difficult to appreciate on chest radiography. While surgery has traditionally been the preferred treatment for CTAI, conservative treatment may be used in asymptomatic individuals with densely calcified pseudoaneurysms.*

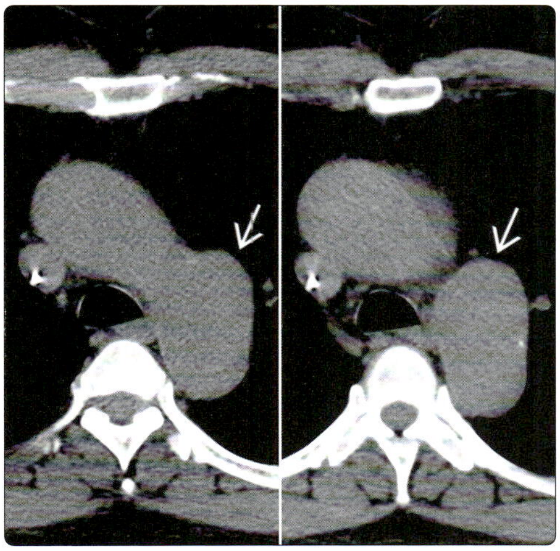

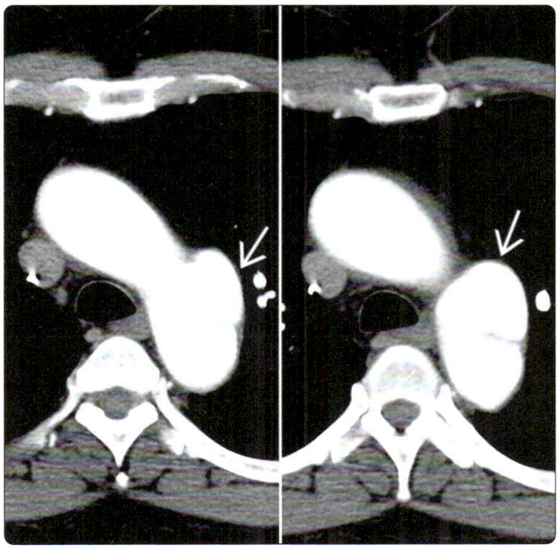

(Left) *Axial NECT in the same patient reveals contour abnormality ➡ at the level of the aortic isthmus.* **(Right)** *Axial CTA in the same patient shows a saccular aneurysm ➡ at the level of the aortic isthmus. In general, some clues that support the diagnosis include a positive clinical history of significant trauma, lack of atherosclerotic changes elsewhere, location of abnormalities at the level of the aortic isthmus, and stigmata of trauma (e.g., healed fractures, diaphragmatic hernia, etc.).*

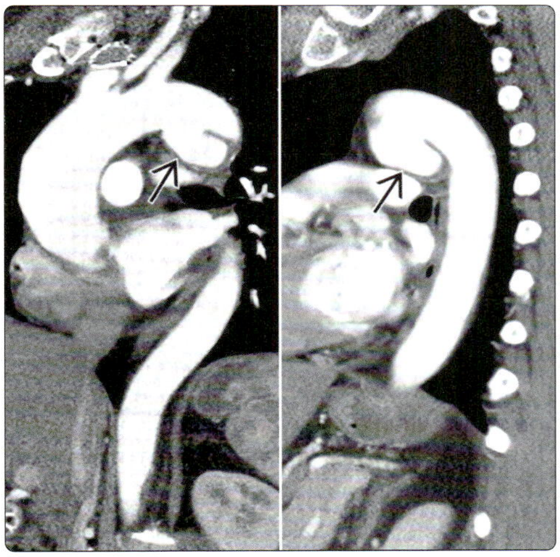

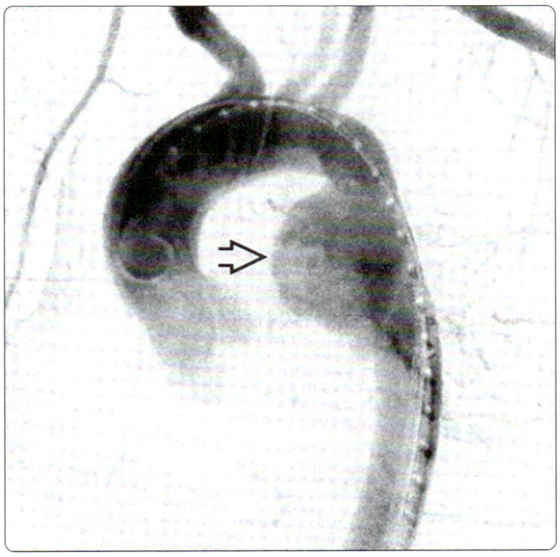

(Left) *Oblique CTA candy cane reformations in the same patient make the identification of the saccular aneurysm ⇨ easier. The lack of mediastinal hemorrhage and other associated injuries support the chronicity of the finding.* **(Right)** *Oblique sagittal DSA in a patient with CTAI shows contrast filling the saccular outpouching ⇨. The CT and angiographic features, along with the patient's history, are consistent with a posttraumatic thoracic aortic pseudoaneurysm.*

Introduction

Diseases affecting the thoracic aorta (TA) often require surgical &/or endovascular intervention to treat acute or chronic conditions or to prevent future aortic life-threatening events, such as aortic rupture and death. It is important for the radiologist to understand the pathology and imaging appearance of aortic lesions requiring intervention. It is also important to understand not only the principles and treatment goals of aortic interventions but also the sufficient details of surgical and endovascular interventions to interpret normal and abnormal postsurgical findings.

Open Surgical, Endovascular, and Hybrid Procedures

Open Surgical Procedures

The 1st successful open thoracic aortic surgeries were performed in the mid-20th century and have substantially evolved since. Modern surgical techniques include the use of cardiopulmonary bypass (for aortic root and ascending aorta surgery) and may require deep hypothermic cardiac arrest with antegrade cerebral perfusion for surgery involving the aortic arch (AA), making these one of the most complex cardiovascular procedures. The basic principle of open surgical procedures is to either repair (valve resuspension, branch reimplantation) or replace a diseased aortic segment with a synthetic graft (e.g., Dacron grafts), autologous tissue (e.g., valve-sparing aortic root repair, Ross procedure), or bioprosthetic tissue [cadaveric homograft; Freestyle graft (pig root)].

Thoracic Endovascular Aortic Repair

The 1st thoracic endovascular aortic repair (TEVAR) of the TA was performed in the late 1990s. The principle is to percutaneously (typically via femoral artery) introduce a **stent graft** (now referred to as **endografts**) into the aorta to either exclude an aneurysm by sealing the endograft proximally and distally within normal aortic tissue (landing zones) or to cover an entry tear and redirect blood flow into the true lumen in aortic dissection. Specific indications for TEVAR are continuing to evolve and expand, not without controversy. A detailed discussion is beyond the scope discussed here.

Hybrid Procedures

Open surgical procedures may be combined with endovascular procedures to achieve the most durable and least invasive treatment of a patient's aortic condition. Examples include arch debranching, carotid to subclavian bypass, and "frozen" elephant trunk grafts.

Indications and Acuity for Open and Endovascular Aortic Repair

Elective Procedures

A wide range of procedures are used to electively treat thoracic aortic diseases.

Prophylactic aortic root &/or ascending aortic replacement in patients with connective tissue diseases: Patients with Marfan syndrome, Loeys-Dietz syndrome, and Ehlers-Danlos IV disease and patients with familiar aneurysms and dissections commonly have aortic root and ascending aortic aneurysms with a high risk of aortic dissection and rupture. Preventive replacement of the aortic root and ascending aorta is considered at a diameter of 4.5 cm. Valve-sparing aortic root replacement (VSARR) (e.g., Tyrone David VSARR) are favored, if possible, to avoid anticoagulation [required with mechanical valve composite valve graft (CVG)] and to delay reoperation, which would be expected in young individuals with bioprosthetic valves.

In aortic aneurysms in nonsyndromic patients, e.g., in patients with atherosclerotic aneurysms of the TA, the indication for surgery is typically 5.5 cm (USA), 6.0 cm (EU), or even larger (7 cm) in patients with high surgical risk. Again, ascending aortic disease and AA aneurysms typically require open surgical replacement of the aneurysm, whereas descending aneurysms may be suitable for endovascular repair (TEVAR).

Emergency Indications and Procedures

Several acute, life-threatening conditions of the aorta require immediate intervention to save a patient's life. Many of these pathologies present clinically with the symptoms of an acute aortic syndrome (AAS).

Type A aortic dissection: Emergency surgical replacement of the ascending aorta is indicated to save these patients' lives. Depending on the extent of the disease, an ascending replacement may need to be combined with (1) aortic root repair and valve resuspension, (2) replacement of the entire aortic root, if the valve cannot be saved and the coronary ostia are involved. Distal extension may include (3) concomitant hemiarch replacement or, rarely, (4) a total arch replacement.

Complicated type B aortic dissection: Patients with acute aortic dissection without involvement of the ascending aorta (type B) can be medically managed with blood pressure and pain control ("uncomplicated type B dissection"). If complications occur, most importantly aortic rupture and branch vessel malperfusion, open or, more commonly, endovascular intervention is indicated.

Traumatic aortic injury: More than minimal traumatic aortic injuries are typically treated with TEVAR.

Common Surgical Procedures of Thoracic Aorta I: Aortic Root

CVG: This is a surgical graft that comes with an incorporated mechanical aortic valve. A CVG replacement of the aortic root consists of surgical resection of the aortic root, including the valve down to the level of the aortic anulus. The CVG with its included mechanical valve is anastomosed to the aortic anulus proximally and connected distally to the ascending aorta. The coronary arteries are reimplanted into the CVG, typically using the button technique. Patients with a CVG need life-long anticoagulation because of the mechanical valve.

VSARR: The basic concept of this procedure is to replace the aortic root with a graft, while sparing the native aortic valve; therefore, this does not require anticoagulation. The 2 basic approaches for VSARR are (1) Yacoub technique (the proximal anastomosis follows the resection edges into the sinuses of Valsalva around the commissures of the aortic valve) and (2) Tyrone David technique [2 proximal suture lines: First, the graft is anastomosed to the aortic anulus (around the valve insertion), then the valve and its commissures are resuspended on the inside of the graft with a 2nd suture line running along the sinuses and around the commissures.] The main advantage of this technique is that the aortic anulus is also secured and cannot continue to dilate over time, which is not unlikely, e.g., in patients with connective tissue disease.

Ross procedure: This procedure replaces a patient's aortic root with their own pulmonary artery and valve (autograft).

The pulmonary artery and valve are then replaced by another graft, typically a homograft.

Homograft root: These are human aortic root grafts harvested from heart transplant recipients. Homografts are used when synthetic graft material needs to be avoided, e.g., after graft infection.

Freestyle graft: This is a commercial graft made of a porcine aortic root. The "pig root" can be used to replace the root, but it can also be implanted into a root [e.g., to replace the valve and a portion of 1 or more sinus(es) of Valsalva].

Note that the **aortic root** extends from the aortic anulus and the 3 sinuses of Valsalva to the sinotubular Junction. The aortic root houses the aortic valve and its apparatus, i.e., cusps, commissures, and the ostia of the coronary arteries. Surgical procedures of the aortic root are therefore more complex than replacing the tubular portion of the ascending aorta.

Coronary Reimplantation and Revascularization in Aortic Root Replacement

Button Bentall procedure: If the aortic root is replaced with synthetic or bioprosthetic graft material, the coronary arteries need to be reimplanted to provide blood supply to the myocardium. This technique consists of excising the coronary ostia with a surrounding rim of tissue ("button") from the native aorta. These coronary buttons are then sutured onto the root graft after a corresponding hole has been cut into the graft, thus enabling blood flow to the coronary arteries.

Cabrol procedure: This is a small-caliber graft (compared to the aortic graft), which is sutured end to end to the coronary ostium on the inside of the aorta. The other end is likewise sutured to the inner orifice of the coronary ostium within the native aortic root. Finally, the Cabrol graft is anastomosed in a side-to-side fashion to the aortic root/ascending aortic graft. Blood flow to the coronaries is therefore from the left ventricle, through the aortic valve, into the root graft, and from there into the Cabrol graft in both directions to the left and right coronary arteries. The aneurysm sac can then be wrapped around the aortic root graft as a final step. Cabrol grafts are rarely used today but can be helpful if the native coronary arteries cannot be mobilized enough to be anastomosed to a graft without tension or in redo procedures.

Coronary artery bypass graft (CABG): Occasionally, short or standard vein grafts or arterial grafts are needed to revascularize the coronary arteries using CABG techniques, e.g., if the coronary ostia cannot be repaired in an aortic dissection.

Common Surgical Procedures of Thoracic Aorta II

Ascending aorta replacement: Synonyms include interposition graft repair, tube graft repair, and supracoronary replacement of the ascending aorta.

Ascending aorta + hemiarch replacement: The term hemiarch typically refers to the extension of the ascending graft, which is cut obliquely, into the undersurface of the AA.

Aortic root and ascending ± hemiarch replacement: Often, the ascending aorta is replaced together with the aortic root &/or a hemiarch. It is important to know where the proximal and distal anastomoses are when interpreting a postoperative CT, as the anastomoses are the most likely sites of complications.

Principles: AA surgery is among the most complex cardiothoracic surgical procedures and is typically performed in aortic centers. Replacement of the AA requires several measures to maintain cerebral blood flow when the AA is clamped for repair. Typically, the AA requires antegrade (or retrograde) cerebral perfusion and deep hypothermic cardiac arrest.

Island technique and peninsula style arch replacement: These techniques refer to the method of reimplantation of the supraarch vessels into a tubular graft and involve reimplanting the segment of native aortic tissue that contains the supraaortic branch vessel origins. This "island" of aortic tissue is anastomosed to the synthetic arch graft. Peninsula style refers to a technique where the patch or native aorta containing the supraarch branch origins remains connected to the descending aorta, similar to a peninsula.

Branched grafts: Most arch replacements are now performed using a synthetic graft that comes prefabricated with 4 side branches. Three side branches can be anastomosed to the 3 arch vessels, whereas the 4th branch is used to temporarily perfuse the brain during the surgical procedure after which this branch is tied off.

Elephant trunk graft: This graft is typically placed at the time of AA replacement. The elephant trunk only has a proximal anastomosis (corresponding to the distal arch graft anastomosis) but no distal anastomosis. The graft floats freely in the descending TA. The presence of an elephant trunk graft in the descending aorta substantially facilitates the surgical or endovascular repair of a diseased descending TA, typically performed as a 2nd stage from a lateral thoracotomy.

Frozen elephant trunk: In contrast to a traditional elephant trunk consisting of soft surgical graft material, a frozen elephant trunk contains a stent graft as well. The endograft can be placed into the surgical elephant trunk at the time of the open arch procedure. Commercial frozen elephant trunks are also available, which are essentially arch grafts (for open repair) with a built-in endograft, which can be deployed into the descending aorta.

Descending aorta replacement: Diseases affecting only the tubular portion of the descending TA are mostly treated by thoracic TEVAR. Complex aneurysms or dissections that are not anatomically suitable for TEVAR as well as aortic aneurysms or dissection in patients with connective tissue diseases typically undergo open surgical repair.

Thoracoabdominal aortic (TAA) replacement: This refers to complex procedures requiring surgical access and clamping of both the thoracic and abdominal aorta. TAA aneurysms are categorized using the Crawford classification (I-IV), which describes from where to where the aorta is diseased and needs to be replaced. The proximal anastomosis can be anywhere in the TA, and the distal anastomosis can be anywhere in the abdominal aorta; thus, the extent can vary substantially. The principle of TAA repair is to assure that all the important aortic branch vessels are reimplanted, including visceral arteries (celiac artery, superior mesenteric artery), renal arteries, and at least 1 (or a patch of) intercostal arteries to prevent spinal chord ischemia.

Post-Stent-Graft Complications: Endoleaks

Type	Description	Treatment and Comments
Type I (Attachment Site Leaks)		
A	Proximal	Emergent treatment as aneurysm or dissection exposed to systemic arterial pressure
B	Distal	Distal flow into distal aortic dissection is common and mostly inconsequential unless outlet is present, which requires emergent treatment
Type II (Collaterals Vessels Leak)		
A	Simple	If arising from intercostal or small branches, can be observed; if arising from big branches, such as head/neck vessels, often results in rapid aneurysmal or false lumen growth and requires emergent treatment
B	Multiple	
Type III (Midgraft or Component Leak)		
Examples	Fracture	Wire fracture with tear in endograft fabric: Needs relining
	Component Leak	Discontinuity of device components (e.g., disengaging of device limb from connecting gate): Needs relining
	Fabric Tear	Tear in endograft, e.g., related to suture breaks, or material fatigue

Imaging Approach to Postsurgical Aorta

Imaging Technique

CT is the imaging modality of choice due to its rapid acquisition time, optimal image quality, and capability for multiplanar and 3D image reconstructions. The imaging protocol should include an initial noncontrast acquisition, followed by a contrast-enhanced acquisition in the arterial phase, possibly with ECG gating for the aortic root and delayed phase imaging after TEVAR.

Normal Postsurgical Findings

Grafts and Surgical Material

The graft anastomosis can be identified by noting felt pledgets, rings, or strips. Rings and strips are almost invariably present along the entire circumference of the anastomosis. The position of the graft can be identified by noting an abrupt caliber and contour change between the graft and the native aorta. Furthermore, a false intimomedial flap (pseudoflap) is often seen where there is graft angulation and should not be mistaken for a dissection. These findings are best seen on multiplanar reformatted images, which allow visualization along the long axis of the vessel.

Perfusion ("Chimney") Grafts

Some surgical procedures require temporary perfusion of the brain via the axillary artery, which can be performed via a surgical graft (chimney graft or perfusion graft) that is anastomosed end to side (rather than direct cannulation). Perfusion grafts can also be sutured to the innominate artery or to the common femoral artery (for TAA repair). These grafts are oversewn after surgery, and the remaining graft stumps can be confused with small pseudoaneurysms.

Surgical Complications

Clinically, the most important complications are stroke, paraplegia, bleeding, infections, and death. The role of postoperative imaging is to document the accomplishments of the surgical goals and the identification of unexpected complications.

Anastomotic Leaks/Dehiscence/Pseudoaneurysms

The most common location for a breach of aortic wall integrity is at the site of a surgical anastomosis, both in the acute setting as well as months or many years after a procedure. It is therefore critical to know where anastomoses have been placed (e.g., any aorta-to-graft anastomosis, coronary buttons, branch graft anastomoses). Early leaks or dehiscence usually require surgical repair. Small chronic pseudoaneurysms may stay remarkably stable over many years but require life-long surveillance.

Graft Complications and Infection

Rarely, surgical grafts can be redundant and twisted, resulting in unintentional graft stenoses. Over many years, the native aorta becomes longer, and grafts may become redundant, resulting in graft kinking and folding, which can result in graft stenosis, which in turn can result in hemolysis.

Thoracic Endovascular Aortic Repair Complications

Device-Related Complications

Post-TEVAR imaging can demonstrate the correct or incorrect position, expansion, and sealing of an endograft.

Complications include endograft collapse or migration, dissection, or pseudoaneurysm. Endograft infection/fistula formation is a rare, but often fatal complication often identified by the presence of air/fluid around the graft, soft tissue thickening, and irregular enhancement adjacent to the graft.

Stent graft-induced new entry (SINE) refers to a new entry tear in the dissection membrane or aortic wall caused by the proximal or distal end of the endograft exerting a force against the adjacent aortic tissue.

Endoleaks

Endoleaks are characterized by persistent perfusion of the excluded portion of the aorta following endovascular stent placement (originally intended for aneurysmal sac exclusion). Five main types of endoleaks are generally recognized, in addition to a mixed type. Type I or type III endoleaks usually require prompt intervention for repair, whereas low-pressure type II endoleaks can be managed conservatively with serial imaging surveillance. In the setting of aortic dissection, the treatment goal is not necessarily complete occlusion of the false lumen but coverage of the entry tear and redirecting blood flow into the true lumen. A good proximal seal is required, but retrograde perfusion distally is an expected finding. Instead of the term endoleak, this setting is better described as persistent perfusion, which, hopefully, over time, leads to false lumen thrombosis.

Distal Anastomosis on NECT and CTA

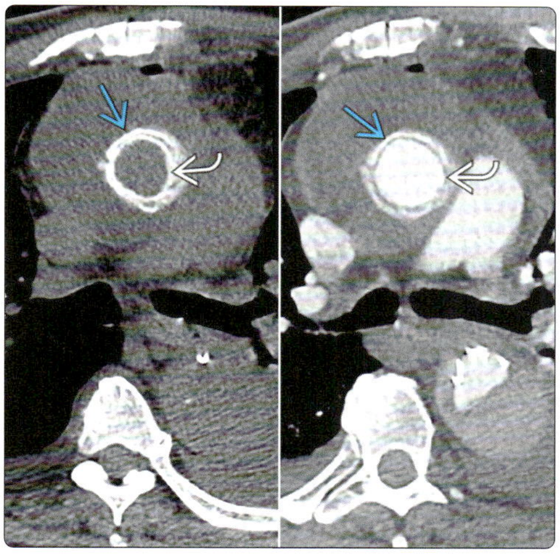

Supracoronary Repair

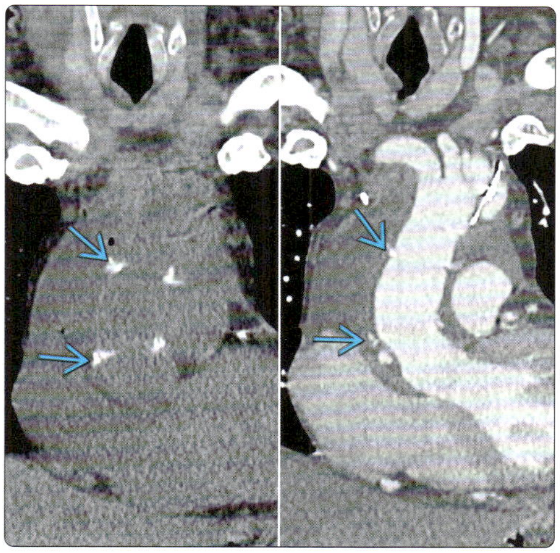

(Left) *NECT and CTA at the level of the distal anastomosis following supracoronary reconstruction are shown. Note the hyperdense appearance of the anastomotic felt on NECT and CTA* ➔*. The graft is also hyperdense on NECT but is isodense relative to blood pool on CTA* ➔*.* **(Right)** *NECT and CTA following supracoronary repair are shown. Note the hyperdense anastomotic felt at the anastomoses* ➔*. This may mimic a pseudoaneurysm if noncontrast images are not obtained.*

Inclusion-Type Supracoronary Graft

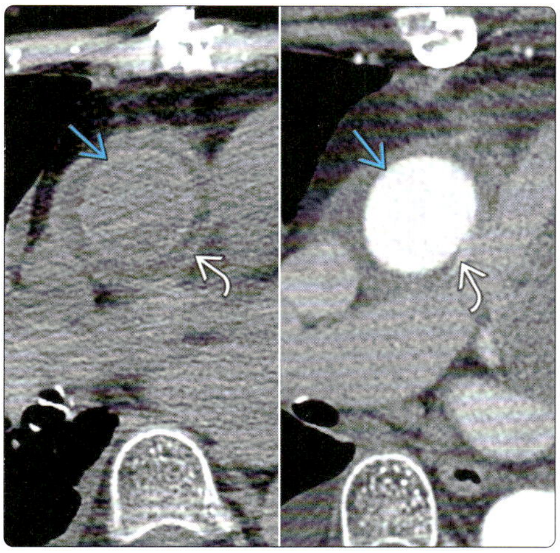

Sagittal NECT Post Wheat Procedure

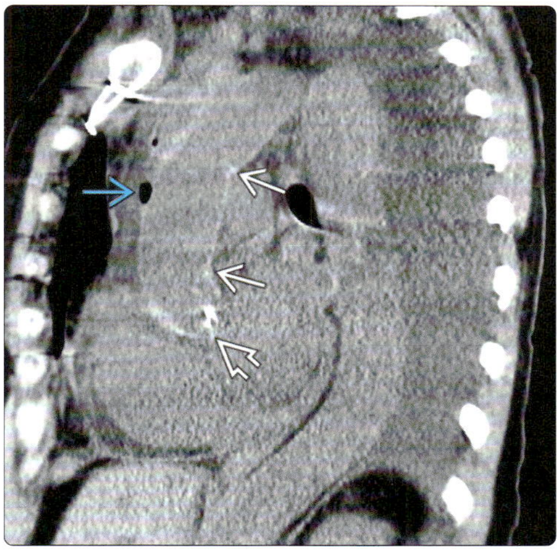

(Left) *NECT and CTA demonstrate an inclusion-type supracoronary graft. Note the native aorta* ➔ *wrapped around the graft* ➔ *with an intervening fluid-filled space.* **(Right)** *Sagittal NECT shows changes following a Wheat procedure. A prosthetic aortic valve* ➔ *is present as well as a hyperdense graft with abrupt change in contour at the anastomosis* ➔*. A small amount of perigraft fluid and air are present, a common postsurgical finding* ➔*.*

Pseudoflap on CTA

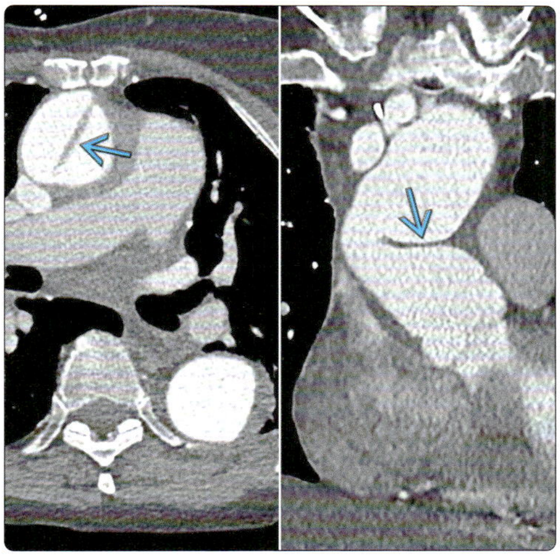

Wheat Procedure

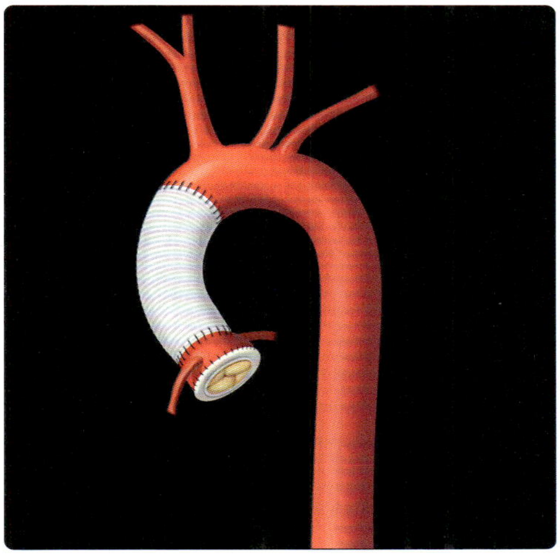

(Left) *Axial and coronal CTA show a pseudoflap within a supracoronary graft distal to the proximal anastomotic site* ➔ *mimicking an intimomedial flap. Coronal reformatted image better demonstrates the pseudoflap within the graft with kinking of the graft wall and excluding of an intimomedial dissection flap.* **(Right)** *Graphic shows a Wheat procedure with a supracoronary synthetic aortic graft sparing the aortic root, including the coronary ostia and a separate aortic valve prosthesis.*

(Left) *Axial CTA following a Wheat procedure shows a large perigraft fluid collection with mild rim enhancement secondary to seroma. However, when present, collections > 1.5 cm in the early postoperative period are associated with a higher risk of pseudoaneurysm formation.* **(Right)** *Graphic shows a modified Bentall procedure, which consists of a composite prosthetic aortic valve and synthetic graft. The coronary arteries are sutured onto the graft with a rind of native aortic tissue composing the "buttons".*

Perigraft Fluid Collection Post Wheat Procedure

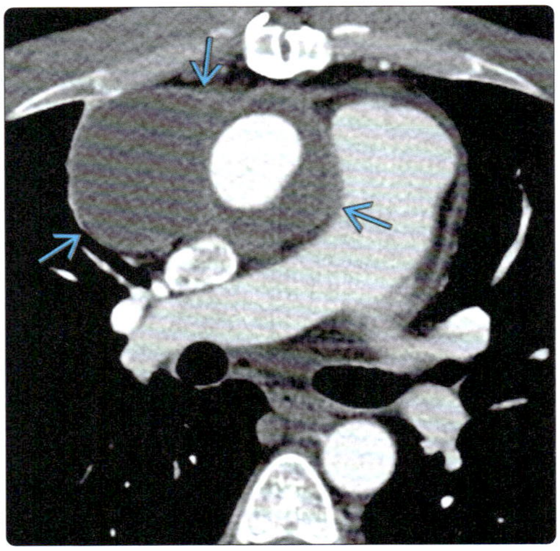

Modified Bentall Procedure

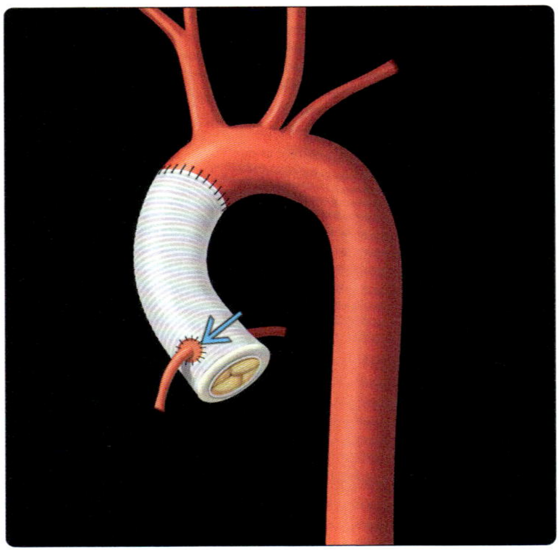

(Left) *Axial CTA shows the appearance of the coronary "buttons" at the modified Bentall procedure. Note the hyperdense felts indicating the coronary anastomosis and bulbous appearance of the proximal coronary arteries, which should not be mistaken for pseudoaneurysm.* **(Right)** *Coronal CTA of the same patient shows the hyperdense anastomotic felts, abrupt caliber change between the graft and native aorta, and a prosthetic aortic valve.*

Coronary "Buttons"

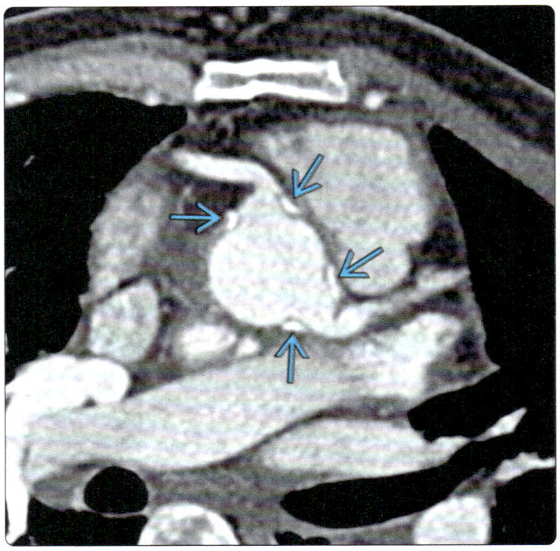

Hyperdense Anastomotic Felts

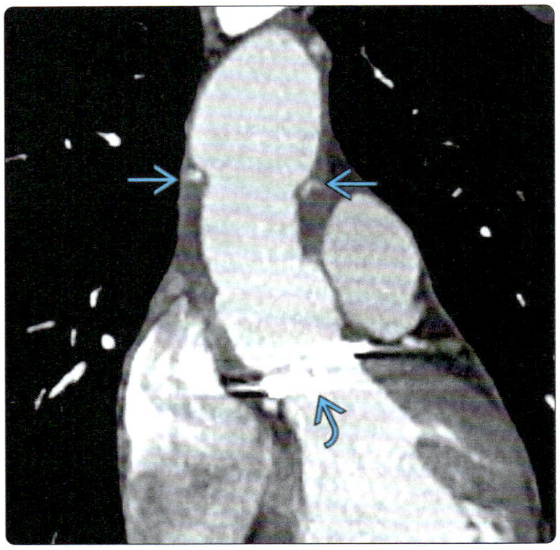

(Left) *Axial CTA after modified Bentall repair shows a complex pseudoaneurysm at the distal anastomotic site with an associated perigraft fluid collection. An intimomedial dissection flap is also visualized in the descending thoracic aorta.* **(Right)** *Coronal CTA in the same patient shows a large pseudoaneurysm at the proximal anastomotic site and an associated perigraft fluid collection. Pseudoaneurysms typically occur along the anastomosis, often identified as hyperdense pledgets on CT.*

Pseudoaneurysm Post Modified Bentall Repair

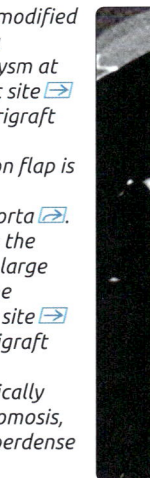

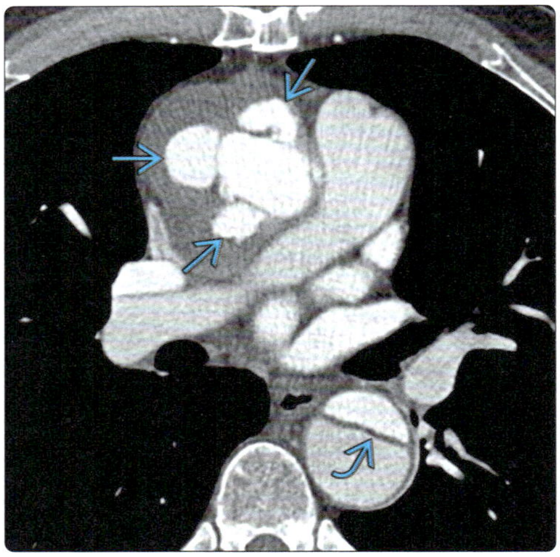

Large Pseudoaneurysm

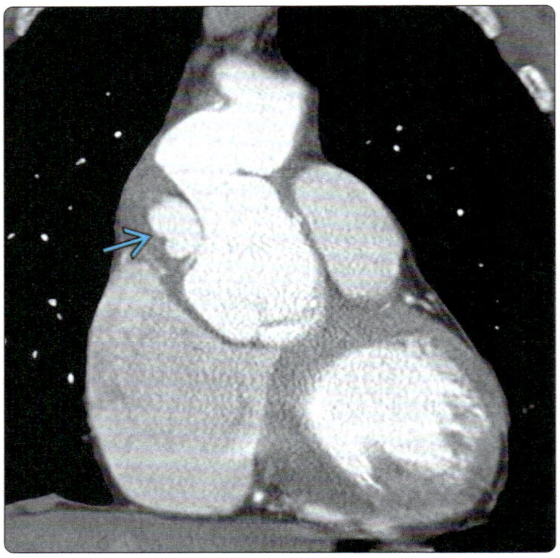

CTA Post Modified Bentall Repair

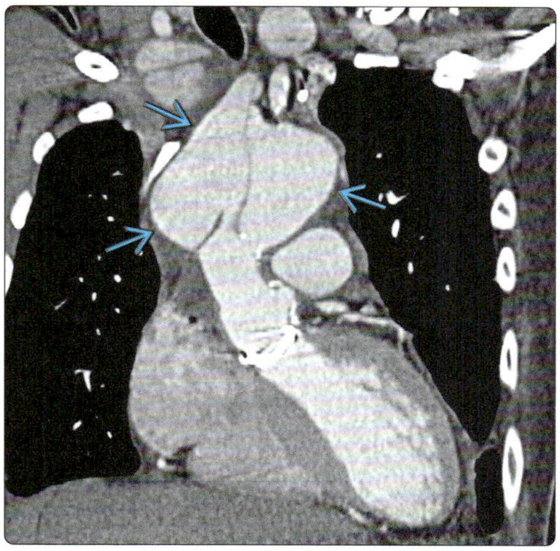

Pseudoaneurysms

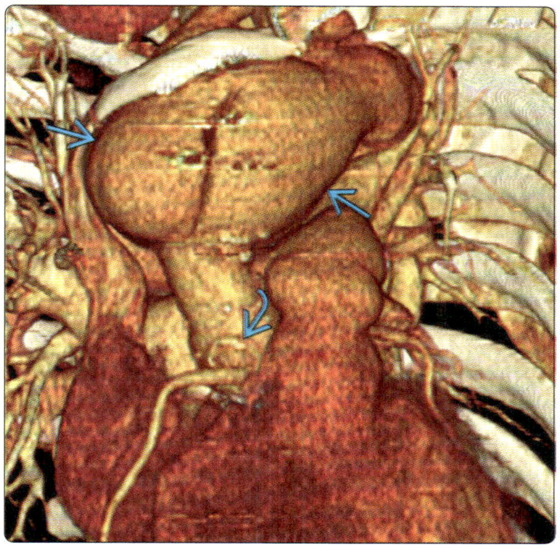

(Left) *Coronal CTA after a modified Bentall procedure in a patient with Marfan syndrome shows a large pseudoaneurysm at the distal anastomosis →.* **(Right)** *3D volume-rendered CECT in the same patient following a modified Bentall procedure again shows a large pseudoaneurysm at the distal anastomosis →. Pseudoaneurysms may or may not be associated with graft infection. They are more common in patients with Marfan syndrome. Note a right coronary button of a modified Bentall reconstruction →.*

Cabrol Procedure

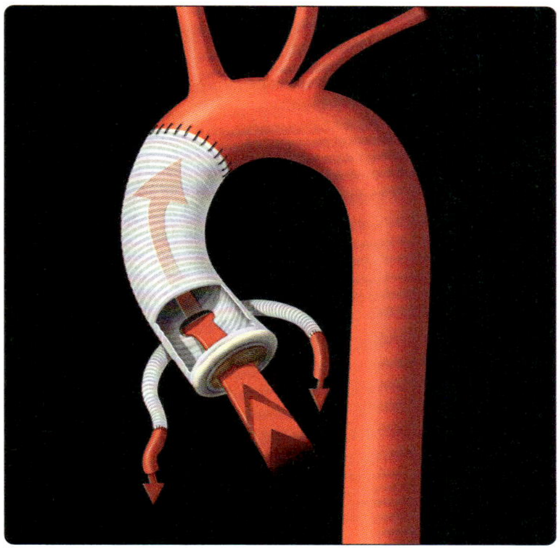

Normal Cabrol Procedure

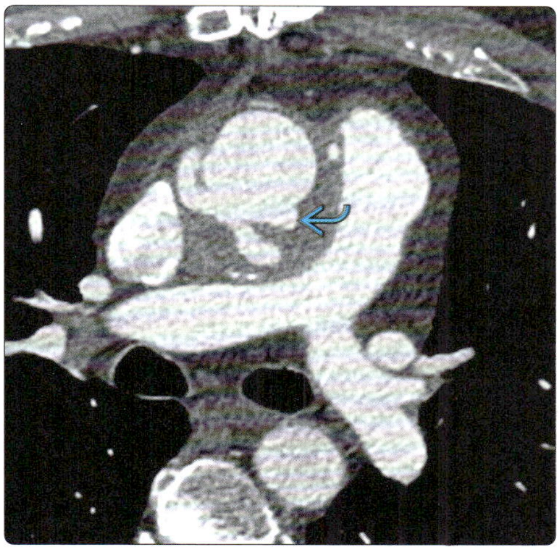

(Left) *Graphic shows a Cabrol procedure composed of a composite synthetic graft and prosthetic aortic valve. The coronary arteries are sutured onto prosthetic conduits, which are attached to the graft.* **(Right)** *Axial CTA demonstrates a normal appearance following a Cabrol procedure. The coronary artery conduits are widely patent. Note the hyperdense appearance of surgical felt, which may be misinterpreted as a pseudoaneurysm →.*

Obstructed Left Coronary Artery Conduit

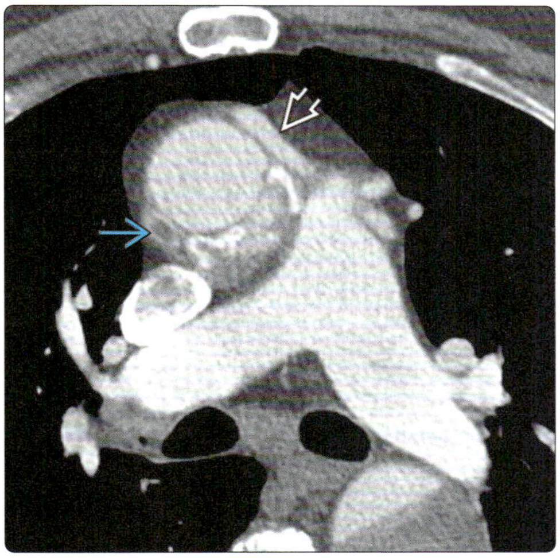

Cabrol Procedure on MIP

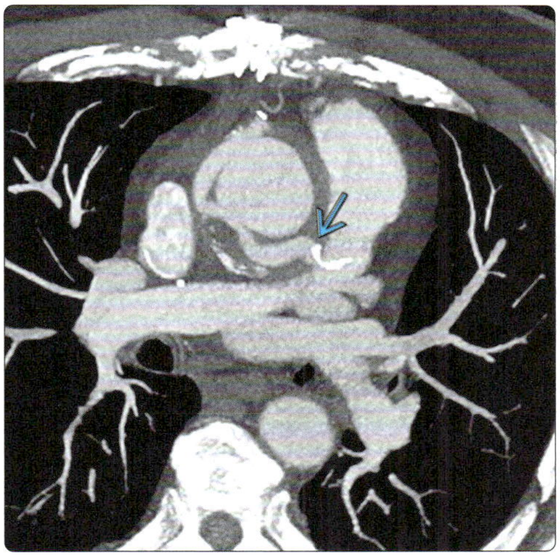

(Left) *Axial CTA after a Cabrol procedure shows an obstructed left coronary artery conduit → likely related to intimal hyperplasia. The right coronary artery conduit is widely patent →.* **(Right)** *Axial CTA maximum intensity projection (MIP) following a Cabrol procedure shows kinking → within a coronary artery conduit near the anastomosis with the densely calcified native coronary artery. The Cabrol procedure is seldom used given the frequency of complications of the coronary limbs.*

(Left) *Axial CTA following a Ross procedure shows aneurysmal dilatation of the aortic root (note the adjacent pulmonary trunk that is normally about the same size as the adjacent ascending aorta), a common complication in the setting of this surgery, which results in aortic valve insufficiency.* **(Right)** *Coronal reformat CTA in the same patient following a Ross procedure shows aneurysmal dilatation of the aortic root. The Ross procedure is used in young individuals and does not require anticoagulation.*

Ross Procedure

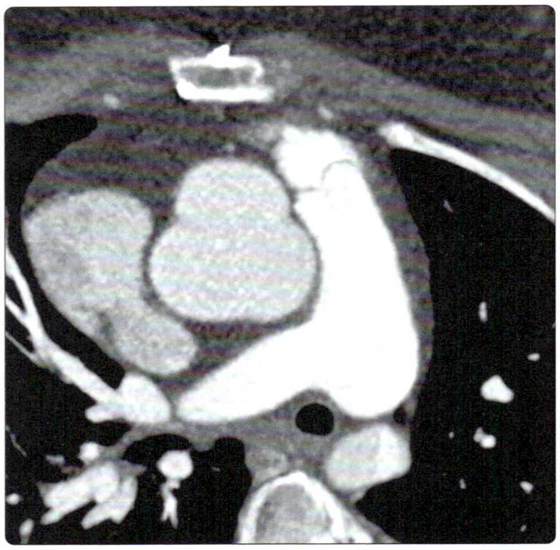

Aneurysmal Dilatation of Aortic Root

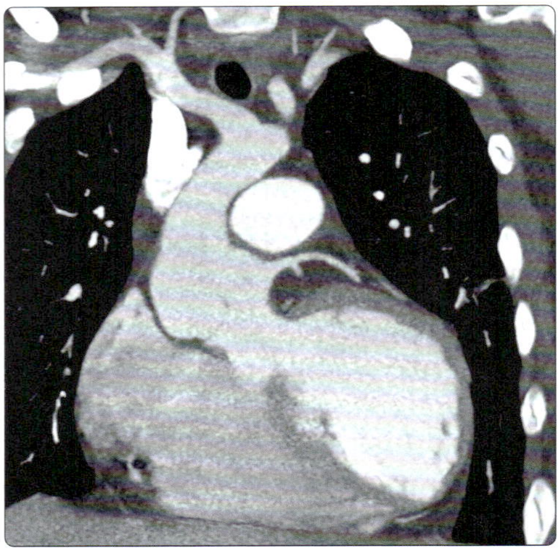

(Left) *Graphic demonstrates the elephant trunk procedure (stage 1), composed of a composite synthetic graft involving the aortic arch and extending into the descending thoracic aorta, where it lies freely .* **(Right)** *Axial CTA following stage 1 of an elephant trunk procedure is shown. The free-floating edge of the graft is seen with the lumen of the aneurysmal native descending the thoracic aorta. This is the normal appearance and should not be mistaken as a true intimomedial defect seen in aortic dissection.*

Elephant Trunk Procedure

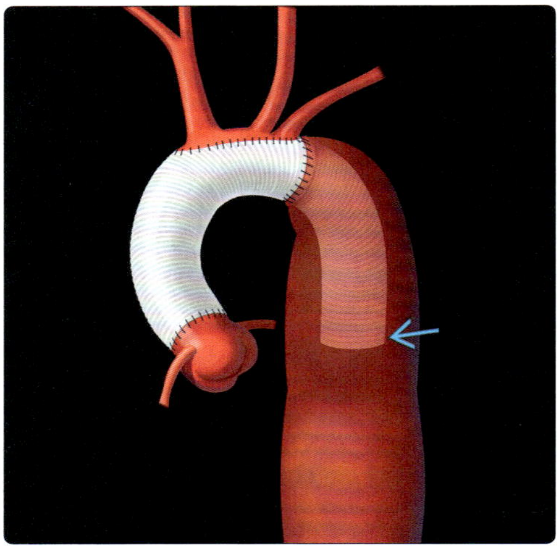

Stage 1 Elephant Trunk Procedure

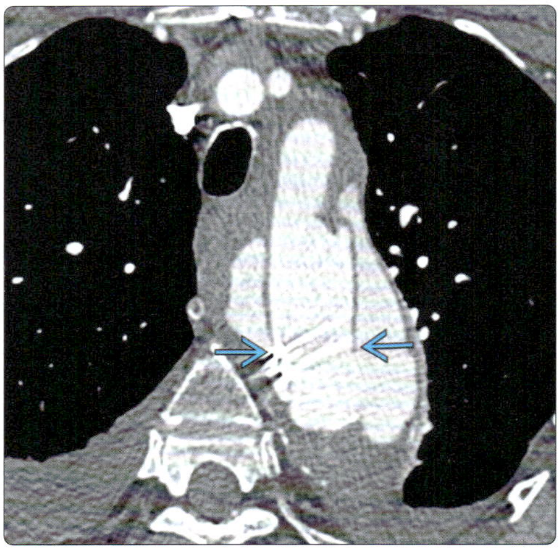

(Left) *Sagittal CTA in the same patient following stage 1 of an elephant trunk procedure shows the free-floating end of the graft within the aneurysmal descending aortic lumen. Note the proximal anastomosis at the ascending thoracic aorta .* **(Right)** *Sagittal CTA in the same patient after a stage 2 hybrid elephant trunk procedure is shown. Note the reconstruction of the ascending aorta with a conventional synthetic graft and an endograft along the arch and descending thoracic aorta .*

Free-Floating End of Graft

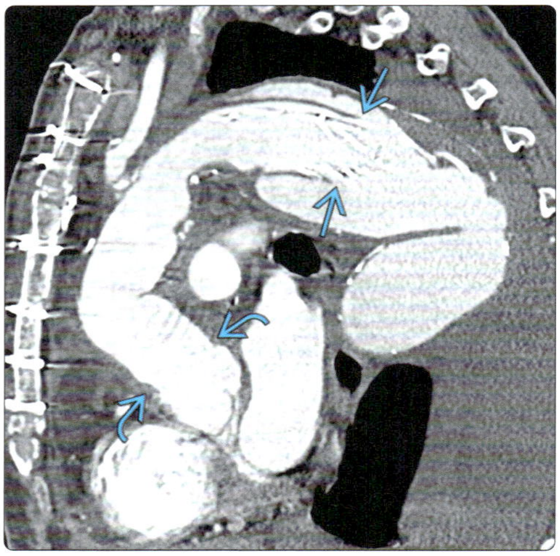

Stage 2 Hybrid Elephant Trunk Procedure

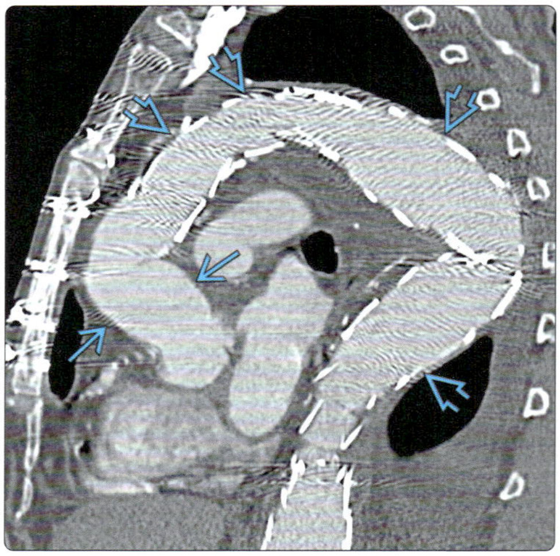

Type I Endoleak Following Thoracic Endovascular Aortic Repair

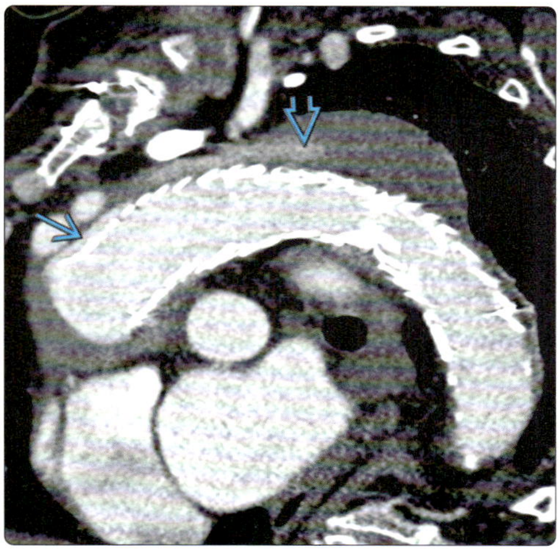

Type IB Endoleak Following Thoracic Endovascular Aortic Repair

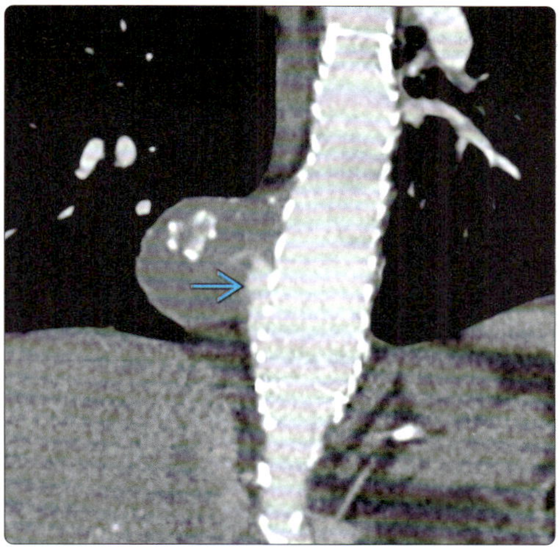

(Left) *Sagittal CTA demonstrating a type I endoleak following thoracic endovascular aortic repair (TEVAR) is shown. Contrast material undermines the proximal landing zone of the stent graft and communicates with the excluded aneurysm sac.* **(Right)** *Coronal CTA shows a type IB endoleak following a TEVAR. Contrast extends cephalad from the distal landing zone and communicates with the aneurysm sac.*

Type II Endoleak Post Thoracic Endovascular Aortic Repair

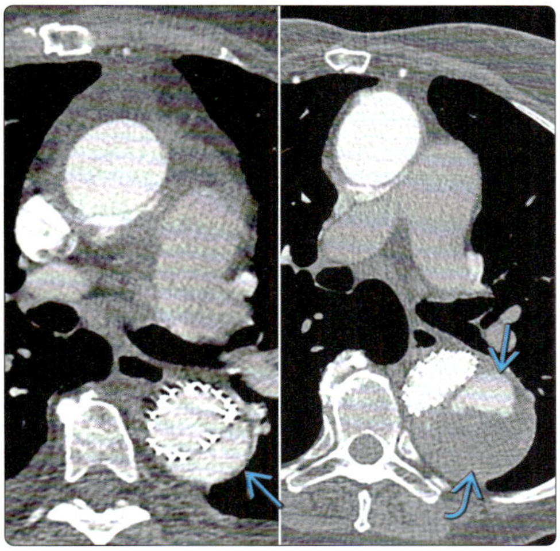

Contrast Filling False Lumen

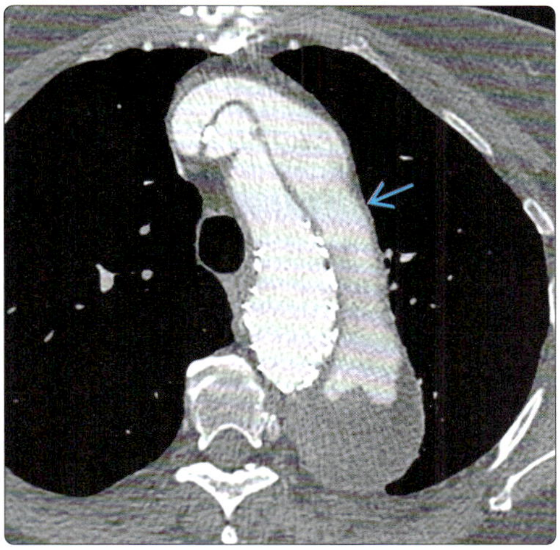

(Left) *Composite image from axial CTA at different levels shows a type II endoleak after a TEVAR within the descending thoracic aorta for dissection. Contrast opacifies the false lumen with similar attenuation to blood pool. Thrombus is also present in the false lumen.* **(Right)** *Axial CTA in the same patient shows contrast filling the false lumen arising from the right brachiocephalic trunk. Type II endoleaks are often benign when arising from small branches but require treatment when arising from large vessels, as in this case.*

Lumbar Collateral Vessels

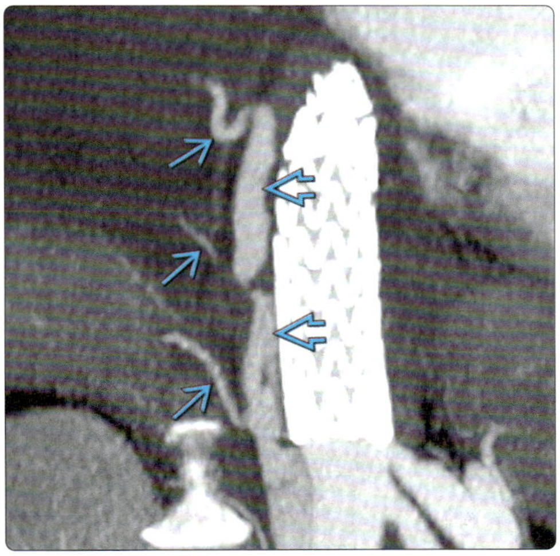

Collapse of Proximal Stent

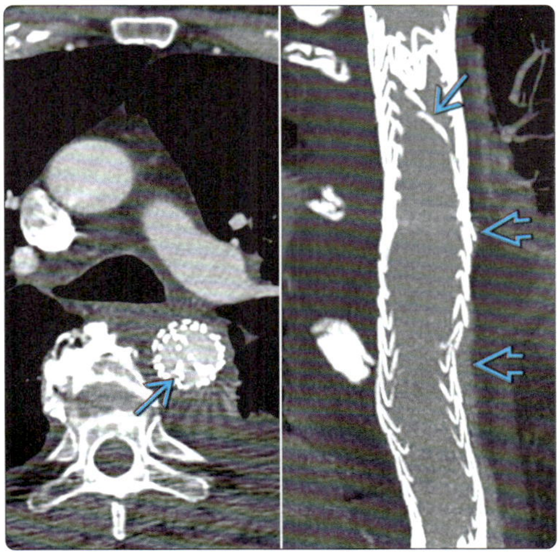

(Left) *Coronal CTA MIP shows a type IIB endoleak. Multiple lumbar collateral vessels supply the excluded false lumen with contrast opacification similar to a blood pool.* **(Right)** *Composite axial and curved MIP reformat CTA in a patient treated with 2 overlapped stents along the descending aorta shows collapse of the proximal stent with subsequent contrast material undermining the overlapped stent grafts propagating distally, consistent with associated type IIIB junctional endoleak.*

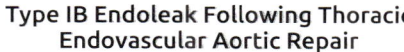

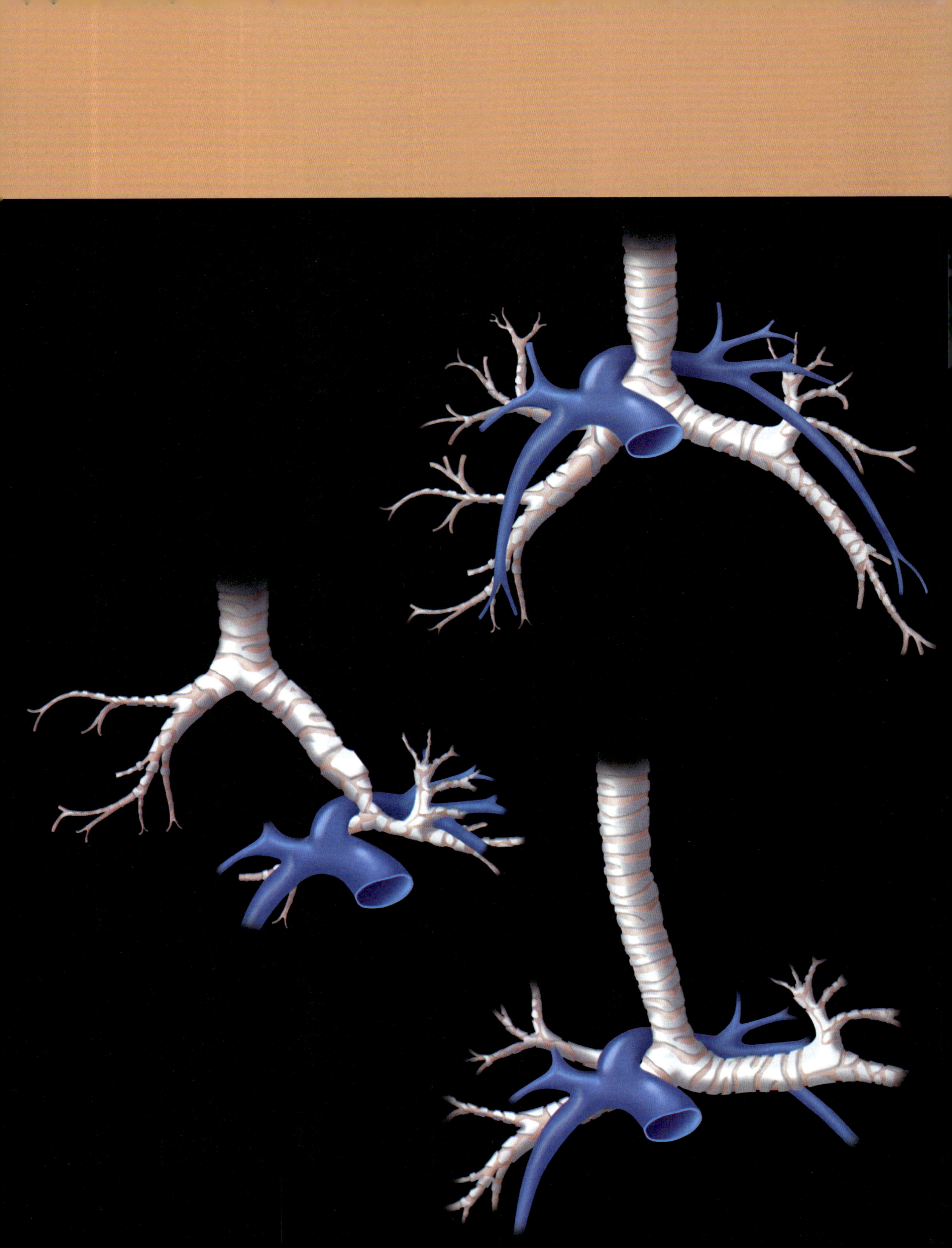

SECTION 10

Pulmonary Arteries

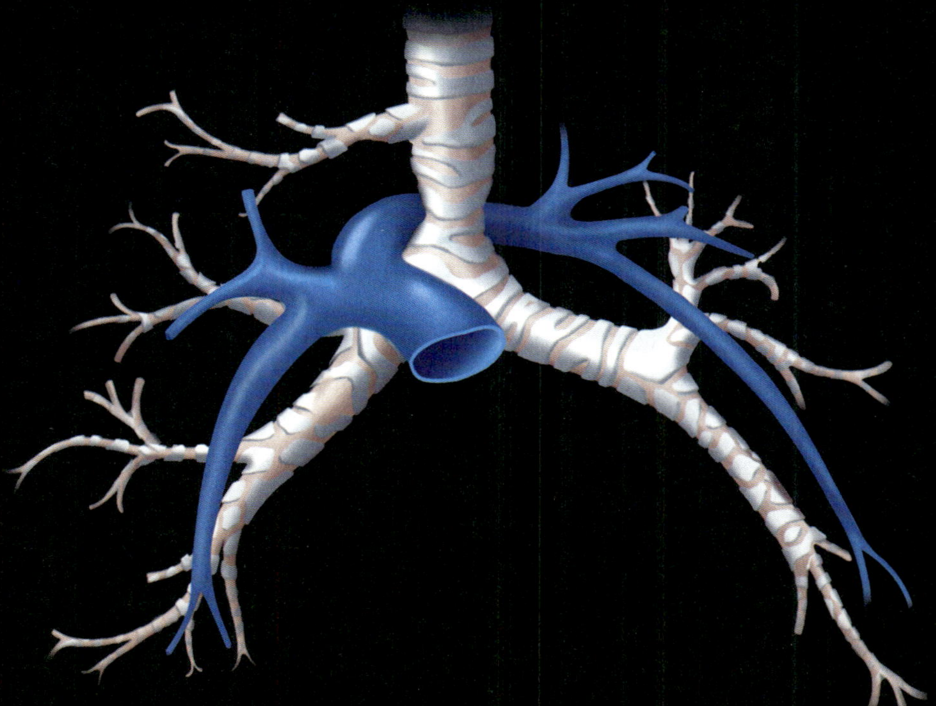

Introduction

The pulmonary arteries (PAs) transport deoxygenated blood from the right ventricle to the lungs, where gas exchange occurs through the capillary-alveolar membrane. The pulmonary veins (PVs) return oxygenated blood to the left atrium. Pathologies of the pulmonary vasculature often result in symptoms, such as dyspnea, chest pain, or a decrease in exercise tolerance, but can also be asymptomatic and incidentally detected on imaging. The main abnormalities of PAs and PVs detected on cross-sectional imaging include abnormal diameters and filling defects. Congenital structural abnormalities of the pulmonary vasculature also occur.

Imaging Protocols

The PAs are most often imaged by multidetector CT using CT pulmonary angiography (CTPA) protocols. CTPA is routinely used to evaluate pulmonary embolism (PE) and can be used to assess other structural abnormalities of the PAs. Optimal PA contrast enhancement can be achieved by using an automated bolus-tracking technique or a small test bolus injection by monitoring a region of interest placed within the main PA or right ventricle. Protocols may use fixed or weight-based IV contrast dosing with an injection rate of 4-5 mL/sec. Reduced tube voltage allows greater contrast attenuation while maintaining spatial resolution. A multiphase IV contrast injection with a primary bolus followed by a more dilute saline contrast mixture can decrease beam hardening artifact from concentrated contrast in the superior vena cava and right heart.

The PVs are best opacified by contrast in a more delayed phase compared to the PAs. The PVs are well opacified by most routine contrast-enhanced chest CT protocols.

MR pulmonary angiography can be performed in selected patient populations. High temporal resolution images of flow through the pulmonary vascular system can be achieved using time-resolved MRA sequences. Noncontrast sequences can also be used to evaluate pulmonary vasculature, including steady-state free precession (SSFP), fresh blood imaging with double-inversion fast spin-echo sequence, and time-of-flight or phase-contrast techniques.

Abnormalities of lung perfusion can be evaluated using iodine maps from dual-energy CT (DECT). DECT is often used to characterize the extent of abnormal pulmonary perfusion in chronic PE and can be used to increase the sensitivity of CTPA for acute PE.

Imaging Anatomy

Pulmonary Arteries

The main PA (or pulmonary trunk) arises from the right ventricle and courses anterior and to the left of the ascending aorta. It bifurcates into the right and left PAs. The right PA then bifurcates into the truncus anterior, which supplies the right upper lobe, and the right interlobar PA, which further divides into the right middle and right lower lobar branches. Similarly, the left main PA bifurcates into the left upper lobar PA and left descending or interlobar PA, which divides into the lingular and left lower lobar branches. There are 10 segmental branches of the right lung and 8 segmental branches of the left lung. Segmental and subsegmental anatomy is extremely variable. PAs course adjacent to the bronchi and bronchioles. Within the lungs, the pulmonary arterioles are centrilobular in location.

Pulmonary Veins

In ~ 70% of individuals, 4 separate PVs (a superior and an inferior PV on each side) are present, each with a separate left atrial ostium. A common ostium for the superior and inferior PVs most frequently occurs on the left side. Supernumerary PVs can also be seen, most commonly an accessory ostium for the right middle lobe vein or a "top" PV draining the posterior segment of the right upper lobe or superior segment of the right lower lobe. Within the lungs, the PVs run along the periphery of the secondary pulmonary lobules with the pulmonary lymphatics.

Abnormalities in Vascular Diameter

Dilated Pulmonary Artery

Pulmonary hypertension is one of the most common causes of dilatation of the central PAs. Depending on the cause, distal branches may be either dilated or pruned. For instance, in some cases of idiopathic pulmonary arterial hypertension (PAH), pruning of the distal PA branches is often present, whereas, in cases of genetic PAH due to *BMPR2* mutation, distal vasculature is often dilated and tortuous. In PAH secondary to left-to-right shunt, the segmental and subsegmental PA branches are often dilated. When a dilated main PA is seen with findings of pulmonary edema and lymphadenopathy in the setting of a normal-sized left atrium, pulmonary venoocclusive disease/pulmonary capillary hemangiomatosis should be considered. A dilated right atrium along with right ventricular dilation and hypertrophy can be seen in any cause of PH.

A dilated pulmonary trunk with asymmetric dilatation of the left PA is seen in the setting of pulmonic valve stenosis, caused by the leftward direction of the flow jet through the stenotic valve.

Less common causes of PA dilatation include PA aneurysms and pseudoaneurysms. Aneurysms tend to be fusiform in shape and are often secondary to congenital heart disease with large left-to-right shunts are seen with connective tissue disorders, such as Marfan syndrome. Pseudoaneurysms tend to be more saccular in shape and are commonly iatrogenic, due to infection, or posttraumatic. Behçet disease and Hughes-Stovin syndrome can also lead to segmental and subsegmental pseudoaneurysms, which can appear similar in appearance, although signs of surrounding hemorrhage or frank hemoptysis often suggests pseudoaneurysms. Neoplasms can also erode in PA branches and lead to pseudoaneurysms.

A dilated and often tortuous PA branch can be seen feeding a pulmonary arteriovenous malformation, which will be associated with a dilated draining PV.

Narrowing of Pulmonary Artery

PA stenosis with focal or tubular narrowing of the involved PA can be congenital or acquired. Congenital PA stenosis, often detected in pediatric patients, is usually associated with congenital heart disease or clinical syndromes, such as Noonan or Williams syndrome. In adults, PA stenosis can be related to chronic PA thromboembolism, vasculitis, fibrosing mediastinitis, and sarcoidosis. External compression by primary or metastatic cancer or lymphadenopathy is also a common cause of narrowing of the PA.

Dilated Pulmonary Vein

Pulmonary varix refers to localized dilatation of a PV and is usually asymptomatic. It most commonly occurs near a PV ostium, which may be atretic.

Narrowing of Pulmonary Vein

PV stenosis is a rare condition. The congenital form is usually detected in childhood and can be associated with congenital heart disease. In adults, PV stenosis is most frequently secondary to complications for ablation therapy for atrial fibrillation.

PV narrowing or occlusion can also be due to external compression by neoplasm or fibrosing mediastinitis.

Intravascular Filling Defects

Filling Defects in Pulmonary Arteries

Acute PEs are the most common cause of PA filling defects. An acute PE can be occlusive or nonocclusive. An occlusive acute clot will often distend the vessel and will be associated with a perfusion defect on DECT and V/Q scan. Occlusive emboli can lead to pulmonary infarction, which typically appears as a peripheral wedge-shaped opacity, often with central, bubbly-appearing ground glass with surrounding consolidation. An nonocclusive acute clot will often be centrally located with the vessel and should not lead to a perfusion defect or infarct. A large clot burden, even if nonocclusive, can cause elevated PA and right heart pressures, with dilation of the right ventricle with flattening or inversion of the interventricular septum. Similarly, elevated right atrial pressures can lead to leftward displacement of the interatrial septum. Right ventricle hypertrophy should be absent in acute disease unless some other cause of pulmonary hypertension is present.

A small percentage of acute PEs fail to resolve; chronic thromboemboli have variable appearances. Similar to acute PE, a chronic PE can be nonocclusive or occlusive. Nonocclusive chronic PEs appear as intravascular peripheral linear bands or crisscrossing webs. Unless there is more distal complete occlusion, these defects will show no perfusion defects on DECT or V/Q scan. With complete occlusion, involved vessels contract and rapidly attenuate rather than expand, as seen with an acute PE. These defects can be hard to detect, especially if the occlusion is ostial. However, due to complete occlusion, defects will be present on perfusion imaging. If the burden of a chronic PE is great enough, the patient can develop chronic thromboembolic pulmonary hypertension (CTEPH), which is the main cause of group 4 pulmonary hypertension.

A wide variety of malignancies, including renal cell carcinoma, hepatocellular carcinoma, melanoma, and sarcomas, can embolize to PA branches and subsequently grow. Initially, these can be difficult to differentiate from bland acute PE, although tumor emboli may cause the vessel to have a beaded appearance. PA sarcoma (PAS) is a primary tumor arising from the intima of the PAs and can mimic a acute or chronic PE. It most commonly arises in the right, left, or main PA, but can arise in segmental or subsegmental vessels as well. It is usually unilateral, and evidence of distal acute or chronic embolism contralateral to the affected side should be absent. The best clue to the diagnosis of intravascular tumor is continued growth despite appropriate anticoagulation. MR is often superior in detection of contrast enhancement within these lesions as enhancement is often minimal or absent during pulmonary arterial phase of imaging. FDG PET is an excellent tool to help differentiate as most PAS and tumor emboli will be hypermetabolic.

In situ thrombus is a mimic of chronic PE and represents lining thrombus that can occur due to either slow PA flow or due to PA atherosclerosis. Both tend to occur with severe pulmonary hypertension, most often related to group 1 pulmonary hypertension, especially in the setting of uncorrected congenital heart disease. The presence of intimal calcification associated with the in situ thrombus can help differentiate, but it is not always present. In situ thrombus can also be seen within a PA stump after pneumonectomy or lobectomy.

Flow-related artifact from incomplete mixing of IV contrast with nonopacified blood can mimic a PE; these artifacts can be caused by early bolus timing, parenchymal lung disease with resulting regional flow variations, inflow from nonopacified bronchial artery collaterals that can develop in pulmonary hypertension, or inflow of nonopacified blood from the inferior vena cava due to transient decrease in intrathoracic pressure with deep inspiration.

Filling Defects in Pulmonary Veins

Filling defects in the PVs, especially in protocols performed in the early phase of contrast injection, such as CTPA, are often related to flow-related artifact rather than pathology. Extension of tumor into the PVs can occur in primary thoracic malignancy or metastasis. PV thrombosis can also occur, usually as an iatrogenic complication or ablation for atrial fibrillation, lung resection, or transplantation. Interlobular septal thickening, ground-glass opacity, and consolidation can be seen in the affected lobe due to pulmonary edema or venous infarct.

Radiographic Findings

Although multidetector CT is the imaging modality of choice for the pulmonary vasculature, chest radiography remains the most common initial imaging study. The main PA corresponds to a small convexity along the left mediastinal border inferior to the aortic convexity on the frontal chest radiograph. Mild prominence of the main PA can be normal, especially in young women. Dilatation of the main PA and left PA, but not the right PA, should raise suspicion for pulmonic valve stenosis. Dilatation of the main PA and central PAs bilaterally is usually related to pulmonary hypertension. In the setting of acute or chronic central or lobar PE, the proximal and involved PA may be visibly distended. Underperfusion or oligemia distal to the involved vessel may cause the Westermark sign, which is rarely observed prospectively.

Selected References

1. de Jong CMM et al: Modern imaging of acute pulmonary embolism. Thromb Res. 238:105-16, 2024
2. Moore J et al: Chronic thromboembolic pulmonary hypertension: clinical and imaging evaluation. Clin Chest Med. 45(2):405-18, 2024
3. Vlahos I et al: Dual-energy CT in pulmonary vascular disease. Br J Radiol. 95(1129):20210699, 2022
4. AlNuaimi D et al: Pulmonary venous varix associated with mitral regurgitation mimicking a mediastinal mass: a case report and review of the literature. Radiol Case Rep. 13(2):404-7, 2018
5. Aluja Jaramillo F et al: Approach to pulmonary hypertension: from CT to clinical diagnosis. Radiographics. 38(2):357-73, 2018
6. Goerne H et al: Imaging of pulmonary hypertension: an update. Cardiovasc Diagn Ther. 8(3):279-96, 2018
7. Hassani C et al: Comprehensive cross-sectional imaging of the pulmonary veins. Radiographics. 37(7):1928-54, 2017
8. Taslakian B et al: CT pulmonary angiography of adult pulmonary vascular diseases: technical considerations and interpretive pitfalls. Eur J Radiol. 85(11):2049-63, 2016

Enlarged Pulmonary Arteries on Radiography

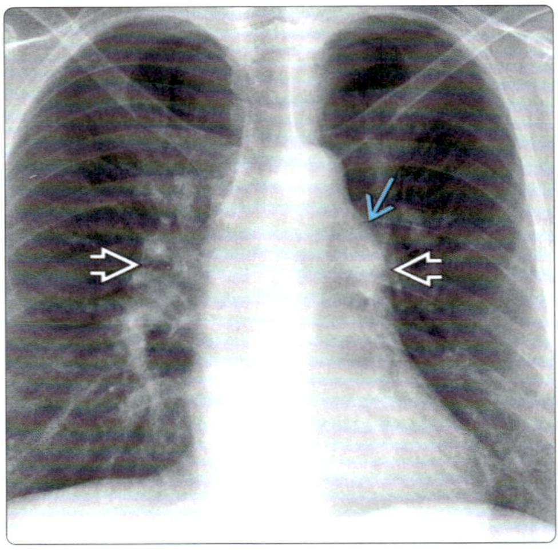

Enlarged Pulmonary Artery on CT

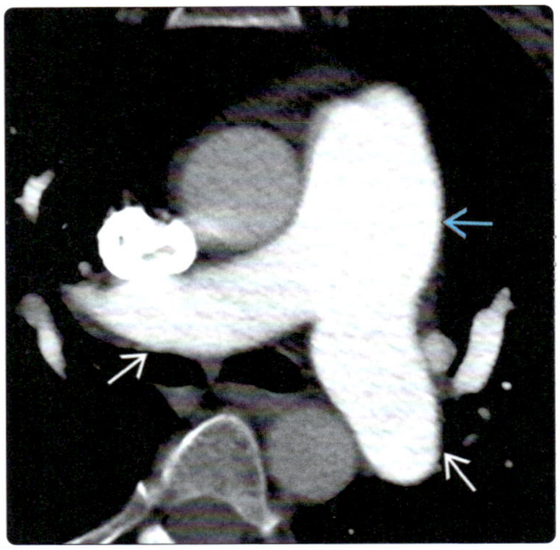

(Left) *PA radiograph in a patient with primary pulmonary hypertension shows bilateral hilar enlargement corresponding to dilated central pulmonary arteries (PAs)* → *and relatively small caliber of the more distal PAs ("pruning"). Convexity inferior to the aortic contour of the left mediastinal border* → *represents dilated main PA.* **(Right)** *Axial CT of the same patient shows a dilated main PA* → *and dilated right and left PAs* →.

Pulmonary Venoocclusive Disease

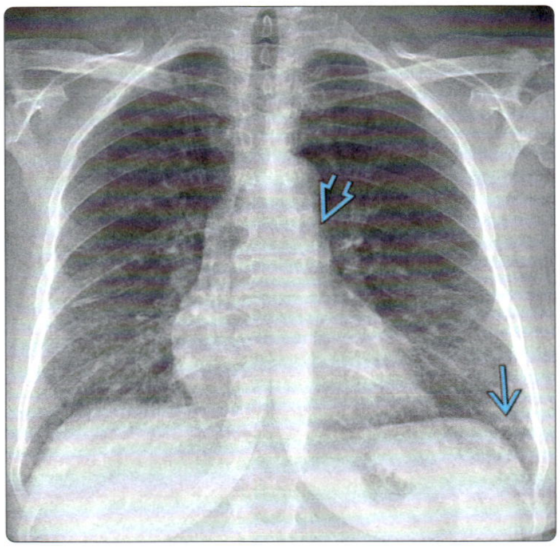

Pulmonary Venoocclusive Disease

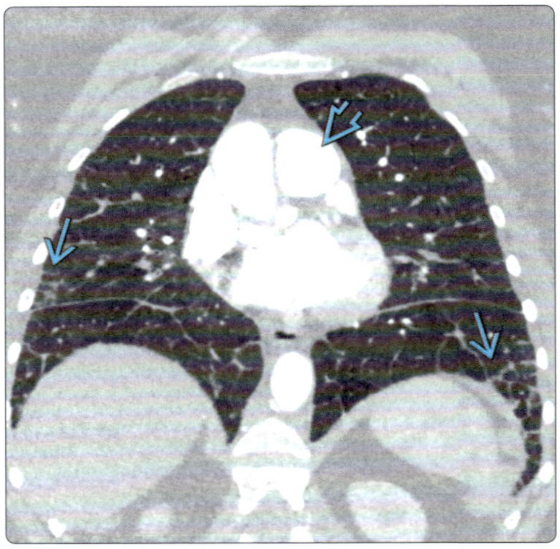

(Left) *PA radiograph in a 41-year-old woman with severe pulmonary hypertension and a mean PA pressure of 55 mmHg shows mild enlargement of the main PA* → *and extensive bilateral septal thickening* →. *Pulmonary wedge pressures and left ventricular function were normal.* **(Right)** *CECT shows extensive bilateral septal thickening* → *without pleural effusions. The main PA measured 3.6 cm* → *and was wider than the adjacent ascending aorta. Findings were suspicious for PVOD, which was confirmed after left lung transplant.*

Pulmonary Artery Narrowing due to Lung Cancer

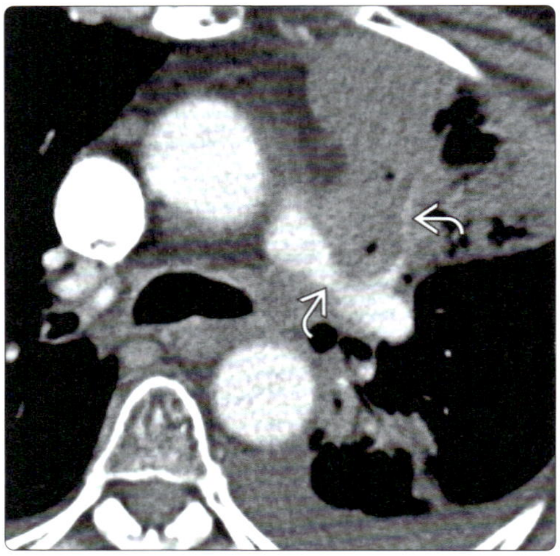

Pulmonary Artery Pseudoaneurysm in Hugh-Stovin Syndrome

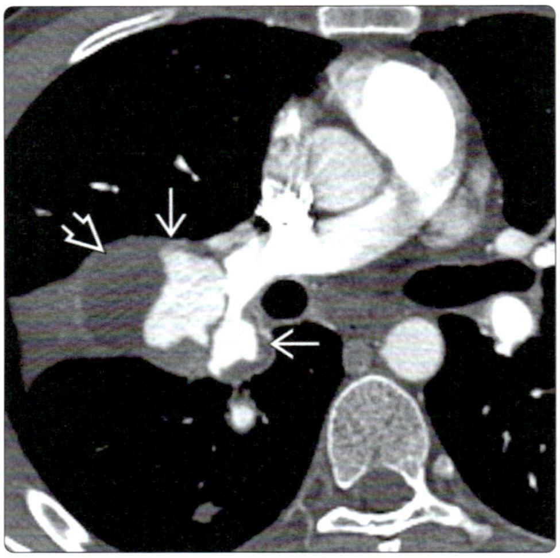

(Left) *Axial CECT in a patient with lung cancer shows narrowing of the left upper lobe PA* → *due to external compression by a lung mass and lymphadenopathy.* **(Right)** *Axial CECT in a patient with Hughes-Stovin syndrome shows focal saccular dilatation of PA branches* →, *representing PA aneurysms or pseudoaneurysms. Intraluminal filling defects represent in situ thrombus* →.

Pulmonary Artery Sarcoma

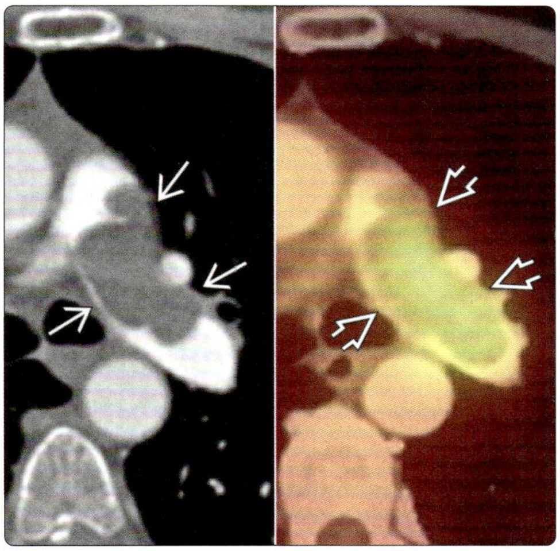

Pulmonary Vein Varix

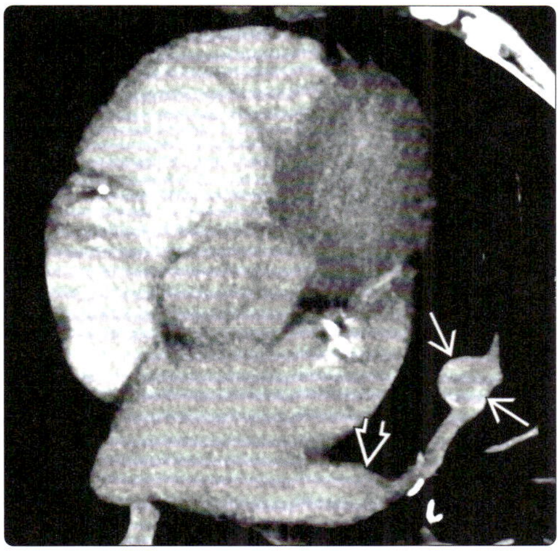

(Left) *Axial CECT (left) and fused FDG PET/CT (right) show a filling defect in the main and left PAs with associated FDG uptake. Endovascular biopsy revealed primary PA sarcoma.* **(Right)** *Axial oblique CECT MIP reformat shows focally dilated segmental pulmonary vein in the lingula, representing a pulmonary vein varix, draining to the left superior pulmonary vein.*

Pulmonary Vein Thrombosis

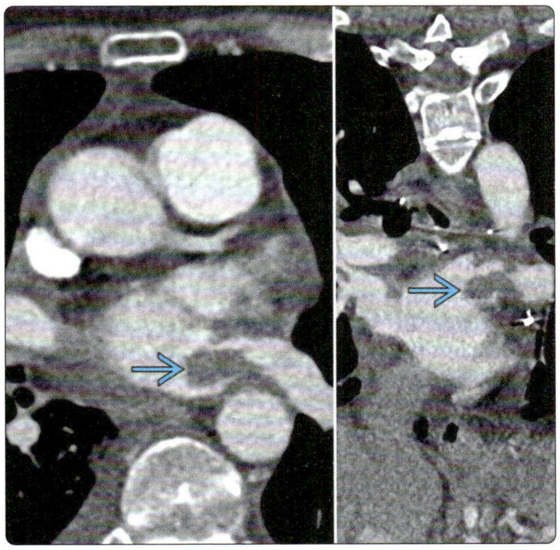

Pulmonary Vein Flow Artifact

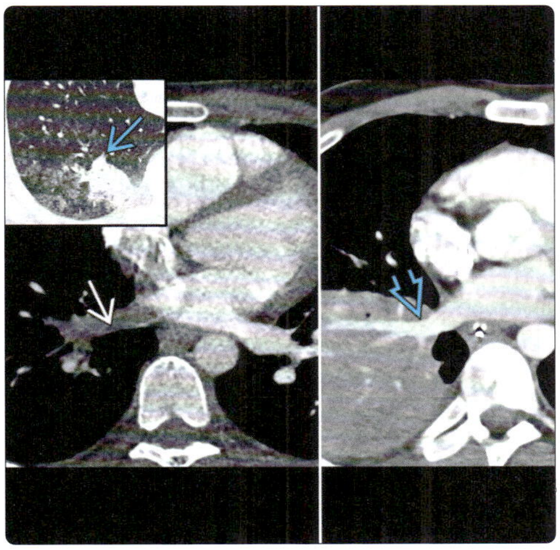

(Left) *Axial and coronal oblique CECT MPR of a patient after bilateral lung transplant show thrombus extending from the left inferior pulmonary vein to the left atrium near the pulmonary venous anastomosis.* **(Right)** *Axial pulmonary CTA of a patient with right lower lobe consolidation representing streptococcal pneumonia shows a filling defect with indistinct borders in the right inferior pulmonary vein, representing flow artifact, not present on a venous-phase CT performed the next day (right).*

Fibrosing Mediastinitis With Pulmonary Vein Occlusion

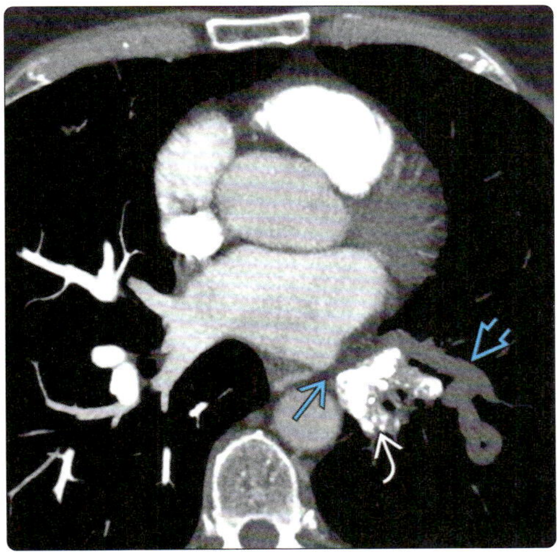

Iatrogenic Pulmonary Vein Stenosis

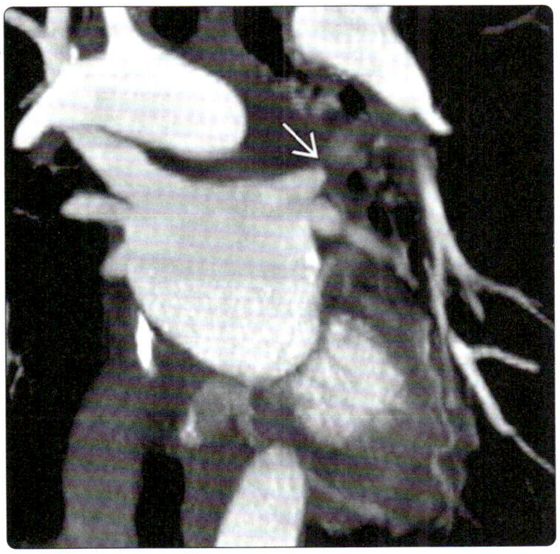

(Left) *Axial CECT MIP shows occlusion of the left inferior pulmonary vein in a patient with fibrosing mediastinitis. Calcified perihilar lymph nodes and a tortuous venous collateral draining to the left superior pulmonary vein are shown. The left lower lobe PA was also occluded.* **(Right)** *Coronal oblique cardiac CT MIP reformat of a patient after pulmonary venous ablation shows severe left superior pulmonary vein occlusion. Note that the patient has 3 pulmonary vein ostia on the right, a normal variant.*

Proximal Interruption of Pulmonary Artery

KEY FACTS

TERMINOLOGY

- Proximal interruption of pulmonary artery (PIPA)
- Failed development of proximal pulmonary artery

IMAGING

- Radiography
  - Small ipsilateral lung and hilum
  - Aortic arch usually contralateral to interrupted pulmonary artery
- CT
  - Absence or early termination of proximal pulmonary artery
  - Enlarged ipsilateral collateral intercostal, bronchial, internal mammary, and subclavian arteries
  - Contralateral aortic arch
  - Normal bronchial branching pattern
  - Small ipsilateral lung with subpleural fibrosis, cystic change
  - Compensatory hyperinflation of contralateral lung

TOP DIFFERENTIAL DIAGNOSES

- Swyer-James-McLeod syndrome
- Scimitar syndrome

PATHOLOGY

- Left PIPA: Higher incidence of congenital cardiovascular anomalies

CLINICAL ISSUES

- Signs/symptoms
  - Recurrent pulmonary infection
  - Hemoptysis
  - Pulmonary arterial hypertension
  - Can be asymptomatic if isolated
- Prognosis
  - Determined by associated cardiac anomalies and pulmonary arterial hypertension

(Left) *AP chest radiograph shows proximal interruption of the right pulmonary artery (PIPA) with small right hemithorax and right hilum, and hyperinflation of the left lung with enlarged left pulmonary artery (PA). The aortic arch is typically contralateral to the interrupted PA.* **(Right)** *Axial pulmonary CTA MIP in the same patient shows interruption of the right PA at its expected origin. Dilated and tortuous bronchial arteries contribute to systemic collateral arterial supply to the right lung.*

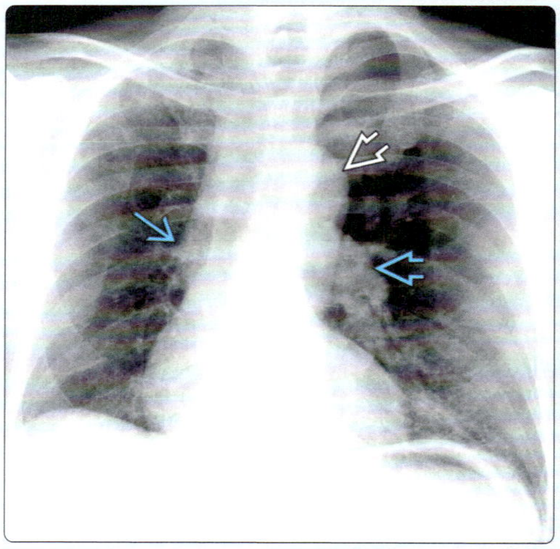

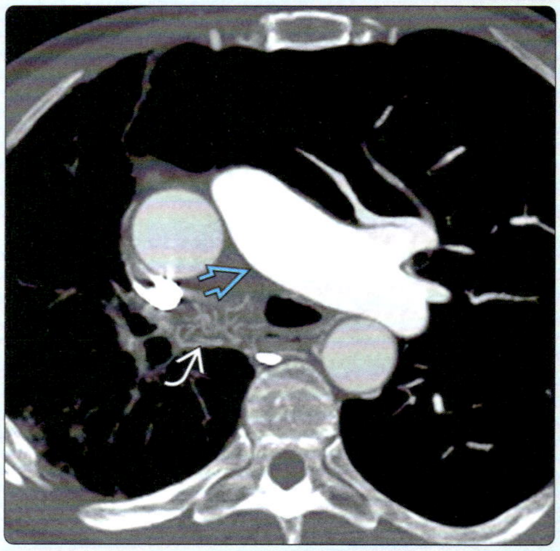

(Left) *Oblique coronal pulmonary CTA MIP in the same patient shows decreased vascularity of the right lung and dilated left PA. Dilated systemic arteries from the abdominal aorta contribute to collateral perfusion of the right lung.* **(Right)** *Coronal pulmonary CTA in the same patient at lung windows shows a small right hemithorax with right apical scarring and bronchiectasis and hyperinflated left lung. Thickened septa and fissures in the right lung represent transpleural collateral vessels.*

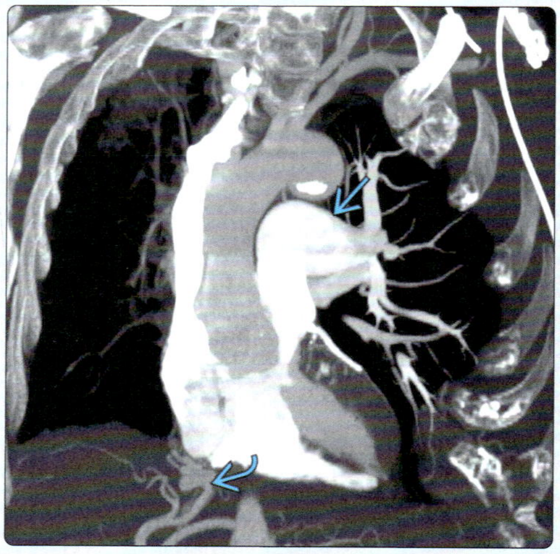

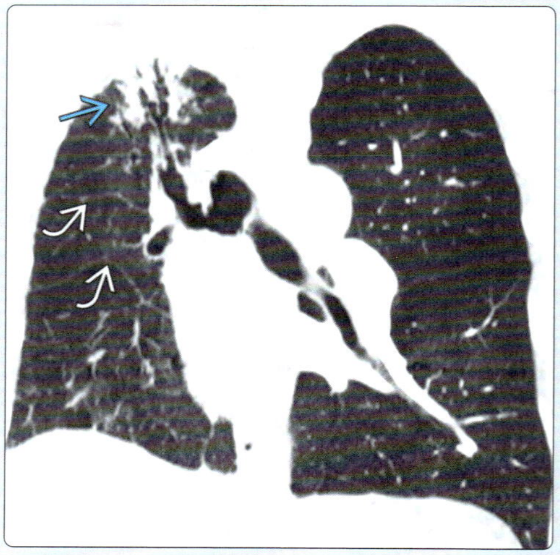

TERMINOLOGY

Abbreviations

- Proximal interruption of pulmonary artery (PIPA)

Synonyms

- Numerous terms for this entity
- Unilateral "absence," "atresia," or "agenesis" of pulmonary artery (PA)
  - "Interruption" preferred as intrapulmonary PAs intact

Definitions

- Failed development of proximal PA

IMAGING

General Features

- Best diagnostic clue
  - Small hilum with small ipsilateral lung
  - Aortic arch almost always contralateral to PIPA
- Location
  - Right > left

Radiographic Findings

- Radiography
  - Affected hemithorax
    - **Volume loss with ipsilateral mediastinal shift and hemidiaphragm elevation**
    - **Small or indistinct hilum**
    - Fine subpleural reticulation or cyst
  - Unaffected hemithorax
    - Hyperinflation, relative hyperlucency, enlarged PA
  - Aortic arch typically on opposite side of interrupted PA
  - ± cardiomegaly due to associated cardiac anomalies and pulmonary hypertension (PH)

CT Findings

- CECT
  - **Proximal PA may be completely absent or terminate within 1 cm of origin**
  - Normal bronchial branching pattern
  - Affected lung
    - Small in size
    - Often subpleural reticulation ± bronchiectasis
    - Cystic change common
    - Small PA branches with hypoperfusion
      - Reduced iodine density on iodine map
    - Enlarged ipsilateral collateral arteries (internal mammary, bronchial, intercostal, subclavian)
      - Anastomose with intrapulmonary PA branches
  - Unaffected lung
    - Large in size
    - Enlargement of PA branches with hyperperfusion
      - All right heart output goes to this lung
      - Patients may develop PH
  - Numerous potential congenital cardiovascular anomalies
    - Associated with unilateral interruption of PA on left

MR Findings

- Similar to CT findings; can be used to assess associated congenital cardiac abnormalities

Imaging Recommendations

- Best imaging tool
  - CECT for evaluation of PAs and collaterals
  - MR for evaluation of associated cardiac abnormalities

DIFFERENTIAL DIAGNOSIS

Swyer-James-McLeod Syndrome

- Unilateral small hyperlucent lung and small ipsilateral PA
  - Expiratory air-trapping
  - PAs present

Scimitar Syndrome

- Right lung hypoplasia
- Anomalous pulmonary vein descends vertically, usually drains into inferior vena cava
- PA present

Developmental Anomalies of Primitive Lung Bud

- Type 1: Agenesis: Complete absence of lung, bronchus, and vascular supply
- Type 2: Aplasia: Absence of lung and vasculature; rudimentary bronchus
- Type 3: Hypoplasia: Small PA and bronchus; rudimentary lung

PATHOLOGY

General Features

- Etiology
  - Involution of proximal 6th primitive arch with intact intrapulmonary vessels
- Associated abnormalities
  - Left PIPA has higher incidence of associated congenital cardiovascular anomalies
    - Tetralogy of Fallot, patent ductus arteriosus, atrial septal defect, arteriovenous canal defect, etc.

CLINICAL ISSUES

Presentation

- Most common signs/symptoms
  - May be asymptomatic
  - Recurrent pulmonary infections
  - Dyspnea; PH
  - Hemoptysis

Demographics

- Epidemiology
  - Estimated prevalence of 1 in 200,000

Natural History & Prognosis

- Determined by associated cardiac anomalies, PA hypertension, or frequency of recurrent infections

Treatment

- Revascularization of interrupted artery in infancy
- Embolization of systemic collaterals for hemoptysis

SELECTED REFERENCES

1. Zhang MJ et al: Proximal interruption of the pulmonary artery: a review of radiological findings. Front Pediatr. 10:968652, 2022
2. Williams EA et al: Proximal interruption of the pulmonary artery. J Thorac Imaging. 34(1):56-64, 2019

(Left) *PA chest radiograph in an asymptomatic patient with left PIPA shows a small left lung, a small left hilum, a right aortic arch, and a shift of the mediastinal structures to the left.* **(Right)** *Lateral chest radiograph in the same patient demonstrates absence of the left PA. The mediastinum is shifted posteriorly due to rotation of the mediastinum and anterior extension of the hyperinflated right lung.*

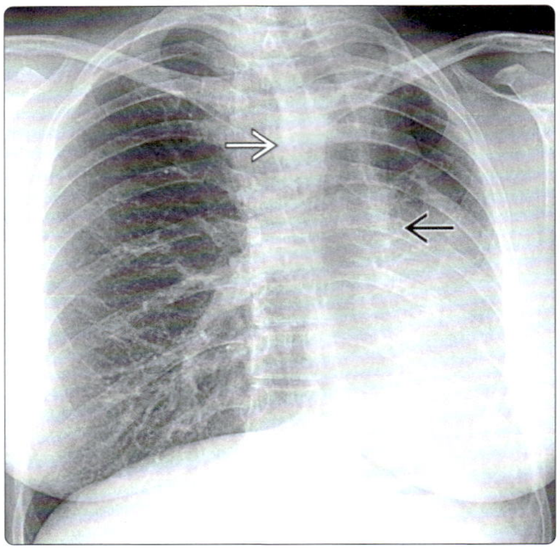

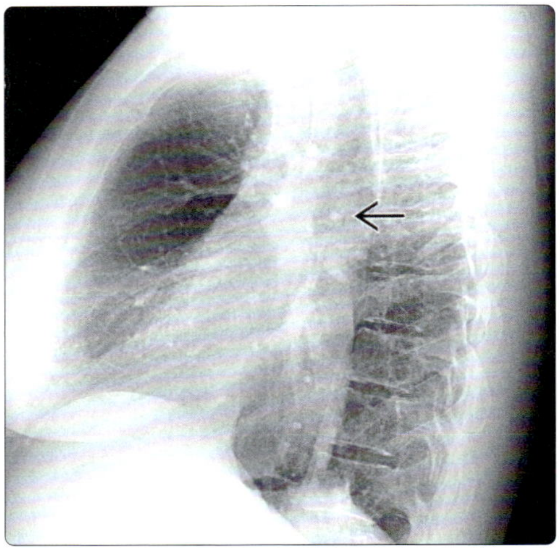

(Left) *Coronal CECT MIP in a nonsmoking 31-year-old woman shows left PIPA with a right aortic arch. There is no significant volume loss on the left.* **(Right)** *There is diffuse cystic change in the left lung, which is why there is no mediastinal shift. The right-sided PA branches are enlarged as it received all the right heart output. Moderate pulmonary hypertension was present on echo. Although congenital heart disease is often seen with left PIPA, it was absent in this case. (Courtesy S. Kligerman, MD.)*

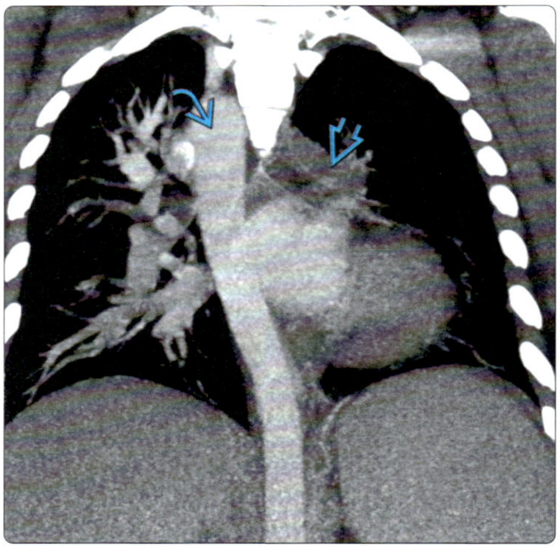

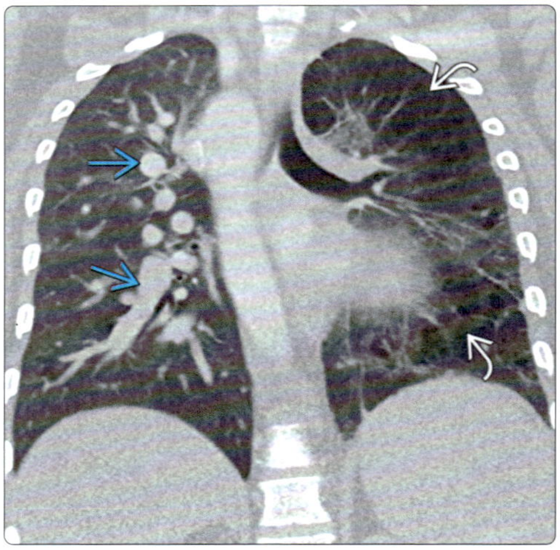

(Left) *Coronal CECT MIP in a patient with right PIPA shows extensive bronchial, phrenic, and intercostal artery collateralization with the right lung. There is rightward mediastinal shift.* **(Right)** *Coronal CECT shows extensive right-sided subpleural cystic change with scattered nodular scarring. It is unclear if these changes are the result of systemic arterial pressures supplying the right lung, prior infarcts, prior infections, or some combination. (Courtesy S. Kligerman, MD.)*

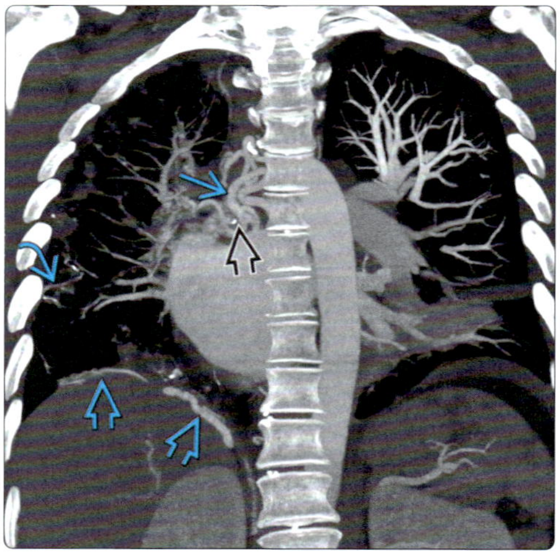

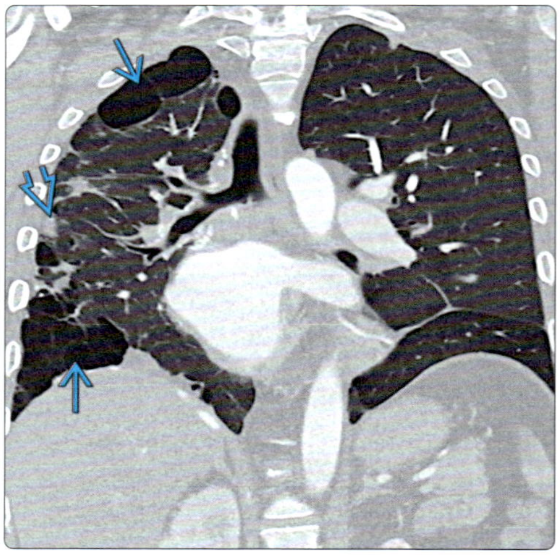

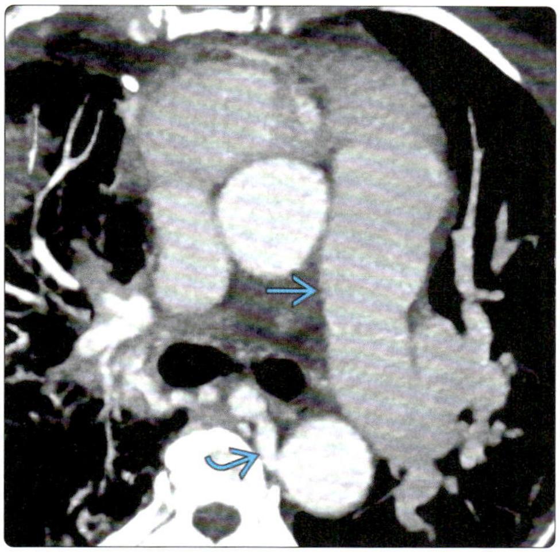

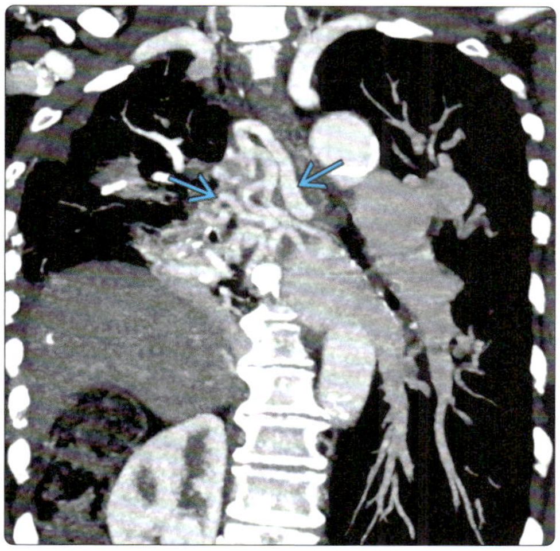

(Left) *Axial CECT MIP shows right PIPA at its expected origin. Dilated bronchial arteries arising from the descending aorta contribute to systemic arterial supply to the right lung.* **(Right)** *Coronal oblique CECT MIP in the same patient shows additional markedly dilated and tortuous bronchial arteries providing systemic arterial supply to the right lung.*

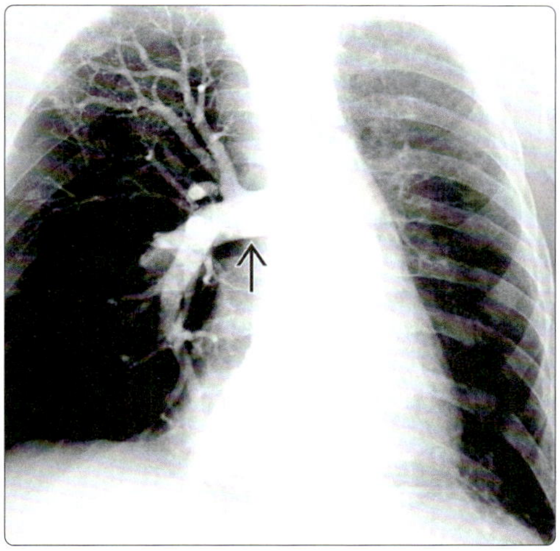

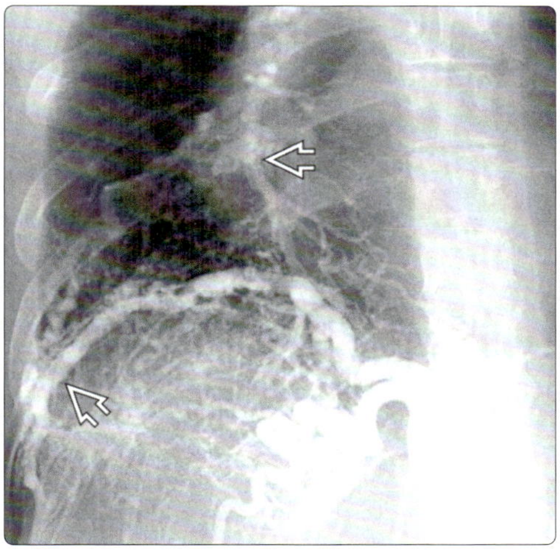

(Left) *Frontal pulmonary artery angiography in a patient with left PIPA shows an enlarged right PA and nonvisualization of the left PA.* **(Right)** *Frontal angiography in a patient with hemoptysis and interrupted right PA shows multiple enlarged systemic collateral arteries supplying the right lung. Angiography and embolization may be required to treat recurrent or severe hemoptysis.*

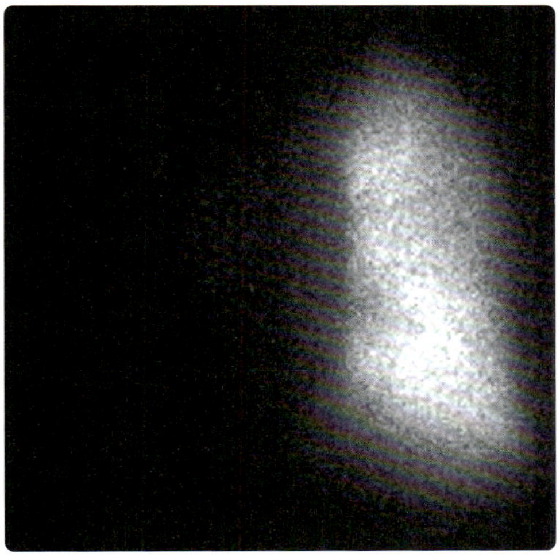

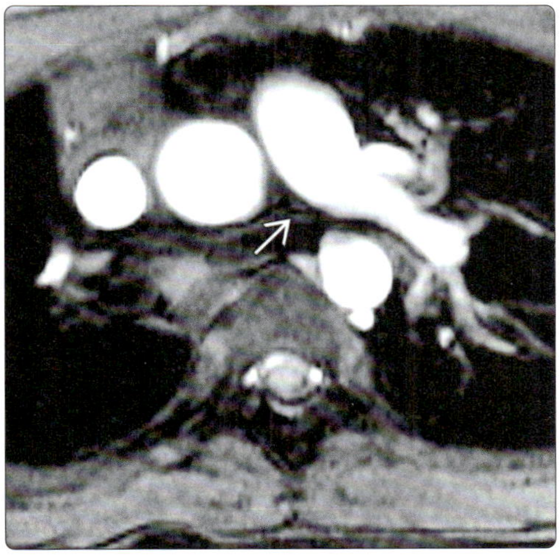

(Left) *Anterior projection from a perfusion scintigram shows absence of activity/perfusion to the right lung secondary to right PIPA.* **(Right)** *Axial T2 MR shows a normal main PA, normal left PA, and right PIPA. MR may be obtained in patients with PIPA to define the PA anatomy and evaluate associated congenital cardiac abnormalities.*

Pulmonary Sling

KEY FACTS

TERMINOLOGY

- Left pulmonary artery sling (LPAS)
- LPA arising from posterior aspect of right PA (RPA), forming "sling" around distal trachea as it courses leftward between trachea and esophagus
- 5% of vascular rings

IMAGING

- Radiography
  - Soft tissue mass between distal trachea and esophagus on lateral radiograph
- CTA
  - LPAS arising from superior aspect of proximal RPA
  - LPAS passes between esophagus and trachea
  - Tracheal narrowing ranges from mild to severe
- MRA
  - Similar findings on MRA compared to CTA
  - Evaluation of lungs limited with MR
- Low inverted T pseudocarina to left of midline
- Complete tracheal rings

TOP DIFFERENTIAL DIAGNOSES

- Double aortic arch and right aortic arch with diverticulum
- Middle mediastinal mass
- Distinction made using CT or MR

CLINICAL ISSUES

- Infants: Stridor, recurrent pneumonia
- Adults: Often incidental finding
- LPAS type II: ↑ morbidity and mortality due to associated anomalies
- Treatment
  - Asymptomatic LPAS type I: No treatment required
  - LPAS type I with respiratory symptoms: LPA reimplantation, patent ductus arteriosus, or ductus ligament ligation
  - LPAS type II: LPA reimplantation and sliding tracheoplasty

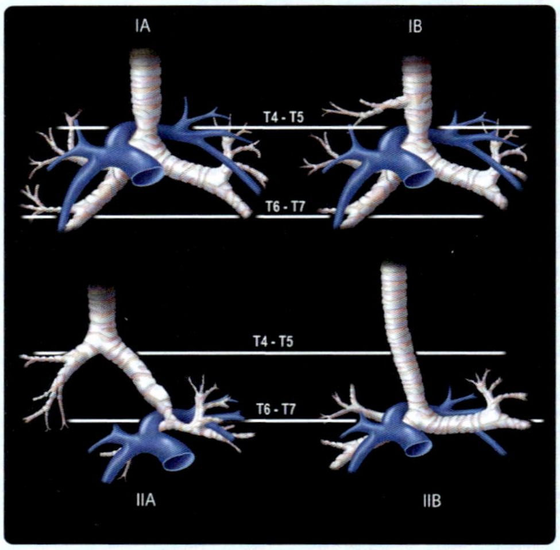

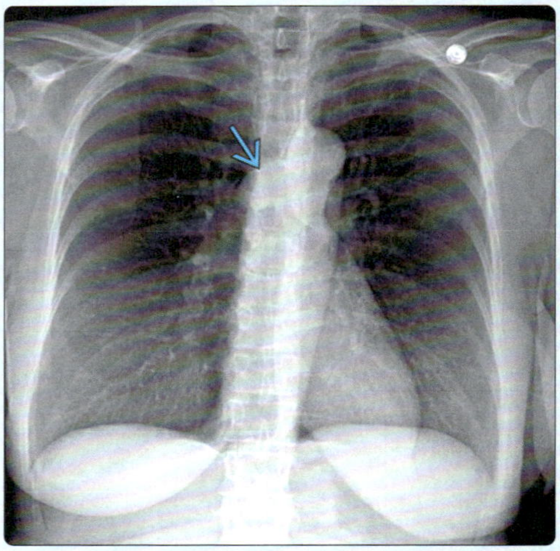

(Left) *Graphic depicts left pulmonary artery sling (LPAS) type I (IA = normal tracheal branching; IB = tracheal bronchus) and type II, which has a low-level, inverted T-shaped carina (IIA = tracheal bronchus at usual carinal level; IIB = low pseudocarina).* **(Right)** *AP radiograph in a 67-year-old-woman who presented to the emergency department with chest pain shows an abnormal linear structure in the mediastinum inferior and to the right of the aortic arch* ⇒.

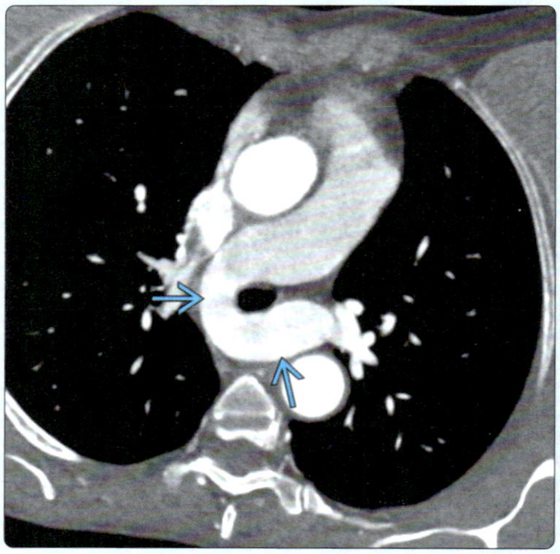

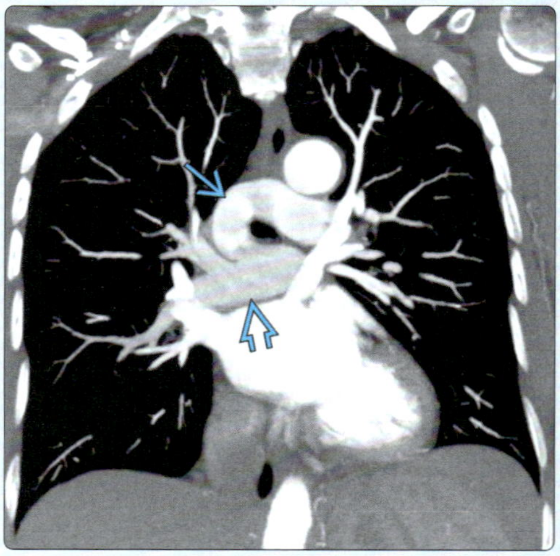

(Left) *Axial oblique CECT shows the LPA* ⇒ *to the right of the trachea and coursing posterior in the mediastinum before extending leftward to supply left lung. The trachea is surrounded by > 270° and mildly compressed.* **(Right)** *Coronal oblique MIP shows the LPA* ⇒ *arising from the superior aspect of the right (RPA)* ⇒. *LPAS type IA has a superior and posterior course before extending leftward to supply the left lung. This correlates with the abnormal mediastinal structure on radiograph.*

TERMINOLOGY

Abbreviations

- Left pulmonary artery sling (LPAS)

Definitions

- LPA originates from posterior aspect of right pulmonary artery (RPA), forming "sling" around distal trachea as it courses toward left between trachea and esophagus
- 5% of vascular rings

IMAGING

Radiographic Findings

- Radiography
  - LPAS type I
    - Right-sided hyperinflation (due to bronchomalacia)
    - Occasional left-sided hyperinflation
    - Occasional tracheal stenosis
    - Newborn period
      - Prolonged opacification of right lung due to retained fluid on frontal radiograph
      - Right-sided indentation of carina and right main stem bronchus on frontal radiograph
    - In adults, may be able to detect abnormal vascular structure to right of distal trachea, superior to RPA
  - LPAS type II
    - Bilateral hyperinflation
    - Right-sided volume loss
    - Long-segment tracheobronchial stenosis
    - Poorly defined trachea with leftward shifted pseudocarina and horizontal main bronchi
  - LPAS types I and II: Soft tissue mass between midtrachea and esophagus on lateral radiograph

Fluoroscopic Findings

- Esophagram
  - Variable positivity and specificity
  - Unnecessary if clinical suspicion of LPAS
  - Anterior and posterior esophageal indentation on lateral projection

CT Findings

- CTA
  - LPAS arising from superior aspect of proximal RPA
  - LPAS passes between esophagus and trachea
  - Variable degree of tracheal narrowing
    - Narrowing can be exacerbated by tracheobronchomalacia
    - Consider dynamic expiratory scan
  - Complete tracheal rings may be present
    - Hard to detect on CT
  - LPAS type I
    - LPAS abutting distal trachea and right main bronchus at T4-T5 level
    - Airway branching pattern differentiates types IA and IB
      - LPAS type IA: Normal branching
      - LPAS type IB: Tracheal bronchus
  - LPAS type II
    - LPAS abutting distal trachea at level T5-T6
    - Long-segment tracheobronchial stenosis
      - Typically from tracheal bronchus to abnormally low pseudocarina
      - Segment often referred to as intermediate left bronchus
    - Other tracheobronchial branching abnormalities
      - Right bridging bronchi (i.e., crossing midline from origin in medial left main bronchus)
      - Low inverted T pseudocarina to left of midline with bridging and left main bronchi
    - Pulmonary abnormalities
      - Right pulmonary hypoplasia and agenesis with small or absent RPA
      - Occasional left lung hypoplasia

MR Findings

- Equally accurate to assess anatomic abnormalities
- Main advantage: Lack of ionizing radiation
- Disadvantages: Lungs and airways are suboptimally assessed
  - Longer scan times may require anesthesia and sedation
- Cardiac gated and respiratory gated techniques are recommended
- Consider multiplanar black-blood (e.g., HASTE) and white-blood (e.g., SSFP) sequences

Ultrasonographic Findings

- Can occasionally be diagnosed on prenatal ultrasound

Echocardiographic Findings

- Echocardiogram
  - Distorted anatomy can make evaluation very limited
  - Absence of normal PA bifurcation
  - Anomalous origin of LPA from proximal RPA
  - Useful in associated congenital heart disease

Imaging Recommendations

- Best imaging tool
  - CTA faster and more available, especially in critically ill patients
- Protocol advice
  - Thin-slice imaging (< 1 mm) to best display anatomy for surgical planning

DIFFERENTIAL DIAGNOSIS

Double Aortic Arch and Right Aortic Arch With Aortic Diverticulum

- Both can cause obstructive symptoms (e.g., stridor, dyspnea, apnea, recurrent pneumonia)
- Cross-sectional imaging exhibits typical findings of LPAS

Middle Mediastinal Mass

- e.g., lymphadenopathy bronchogenic cyst, esophageal duplication cyst
- Cross-sectional imaging exhibits typical findings of LPAS

Congenital Lobar Emphysema (or Overinflation)

- Hyperlucent (hyperinflated) lung similar to hyperinflation from LPAS on radiography
- Cross-sectional imaging exhibits typical findings of LPAS

PATHOLOGY

General Features

- Etiology
  - Embryology
    - Abnormal obliteration or failure of development of left 6th aortic arch
      - Left postbranchial PA vessels cannot connect with left 6th branchial arch
      - Secondary connection is acquired to right 6th branchial arch through embryonic peritracheal primitive mesenchymal vessels
  - Severe stridor
    - May be associated with tracheobronchomalacia (often LPAS type I)
    - May be associated with intrinsic airway narrowing (often LPAS type II)
    - Compression of distal trachea and main stem bronchi may lead to hyperinflation and atelectasis
- Genetics
  - Occasional descriptions in twins raise concern of some genetic influence
- Associated abnormalities
  - Congenital heart disease and vascular anomalies
    - Atrial septal defect (ASD)
    - Ventricular septal defect
    - Patent ductus arteriosus (PDA)
    - Tetralogy of Fallot
    - Aortic coarctation
    - Persistent superior vena cava ± coronary sinus ASD
    - Interrupted aortic arch
    - Double aortic arch
    - Scimitar syndrome
    - Partial anomalous venous return
  - Tracheal
    - Tracheal stenosis
    - Right tracheal bronchus
    - Right bridging bronchus
    - Tracheobronchomalacia
    - Complete tracheal rings
  - Lung
    - Pulmonary sequestration
    - Horseshoe lung
  - Gastrointestinal
    - Imperforate anus
    - Biliary atresia
    - Absent gallbladder
    - Meckel diverticulum
    - Hirschsprung disease
  - VACTERL (vertebral anomalies, anal atresia or imperforate anus, cardiac anomalies, tracheoesophageal fistula, renal and limb defect)

Staging, Grading, & Classification

- LPAS type I: Sling at T4-T5 (just above usual carina level); occasional tracheal stenosis
  - LPAS type IA: Without tracheal bronchus
  - LPAS type IB: With tracheal bronchus
- LPAS type II: Sling at T5-T6 (lower than usual carina level) and low, T-shaped carina; long-segment tracheal stenosis with complete cartilaginous rings
  - Type IIA: Right tracheal bronchus (at usual carina level)
  - Type IIB: Low pseudocarina with right bridging bronchus

Gross Pathologic & Surgical Features

- LPA forms "sling" around trachea as it passes leftward between trachea and esophagus
- Vascular ring
- LPAS hilum lies posteriorly to left main stem bronchus
- Right lung hypoplasia and agenesis
- Severe distal tracheal and right main bronchial stenosis
- Main stem bronchi have abnormal horizontal course (inverted T) with abnormal branching patterns to upper and lower lobes (types IIA and IIB)
- Often associated with complete tracheal cartilaginous rings (50%)

CLINICAL ISSUES

Presentation

- Most common signs/symptoms
  - Infants: Stridor, wheezing, recurrent pneumonia
  - Adults: Often incidental finding
- Other signs/symptoms
  - Noisy breathing, "seal bark" cough, apnea, recurrent pneumonia

Demographics

- Age
  - Young children who are symptomatic
  - In adults, most often asymptomatic

Natural History & Prognosis

- LPAS type I: ↓ morbidity and mortality
- LPAS type II: ↑ morbidity and mortality due to associated anomalies
  - Intrinsic tracheobronchial anomalies
  - Congenital heart disease
  - Pulmonary and systemic anomalies

Treatment

- Asymptomatic LPAS type I: No treatment required
- LPAS type I with respiratory symptoms: LPA reimplantation, PDA, or ductus ligament ligation
- LPAS type II: LPA reimplantation and sliding tracheoplasty

SELECTED REFERENCES

1. Bennett S et al: Fetal diagnosis and management of pulmonary artery sling: a case series. Prenat Diagn. 44(6-7):868-75, 2024
2. Liu Y et al: Management strategies for congenital heart disease comorbid with airway anomalies in children. J Pediatr. 264:113741, 2024
3. K Rahmath MR et al: Pulmonary artery sling: an overview. Pediatr Pulmonol. 58(5):1299-309, 2023
4. Hirsig LE et al: Congenital pulmonary artery anomalies: a review and approach to classification. J Clin Imaging Sci. 8:29, 2018
5. Bueno J et al: Congenital anomalies of the pulmonary arteries: spectrum of findings on computed tomography. Radiologia. 59(3):209-17, 2017
6. Leonardi B et al: Imaging modalities in children with vascular ring and pulmonary artery sling. Pediatr Pulmonol. 50(8):781-8, 2015

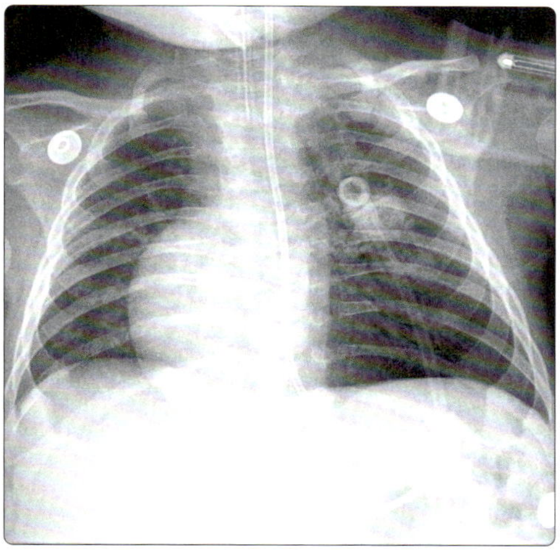

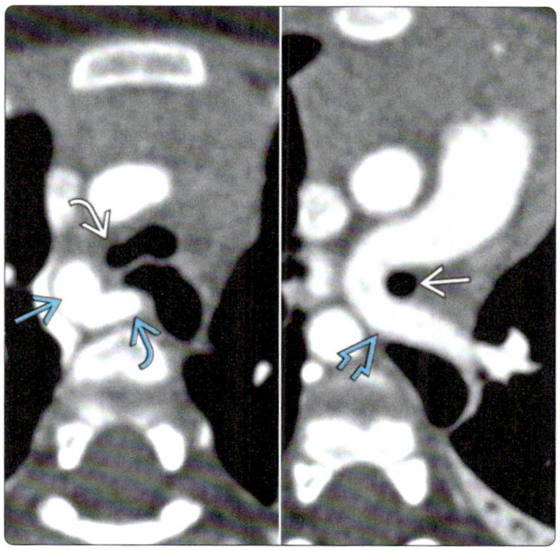

(Left) *AP CXR in a patient with LPAS type IIA shows right lung volume loss with rightward cardiomediastinal shift secondary to tracheal stenosis.* **(Right)** *Axial CECT in the same patient shows multiple abnormalities: Right aortic arch, Kommerell diverticulum, right tracheal bronchus, and anomalous origin of the LPA coursing behind a lower than normal trachea, often referred to as intermediate left bronchus. (Courtesy R. Reyna, MD.)*

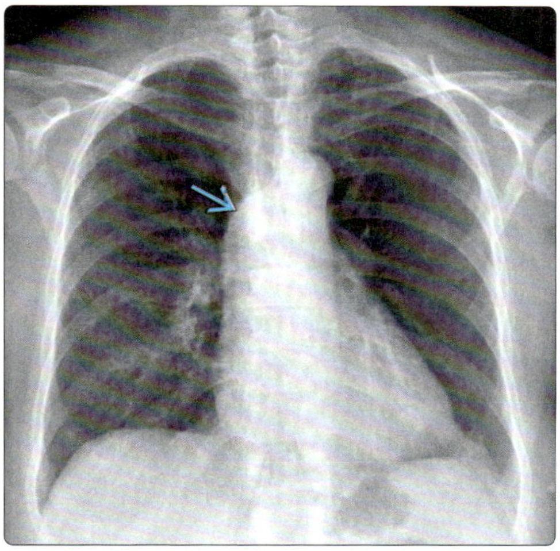

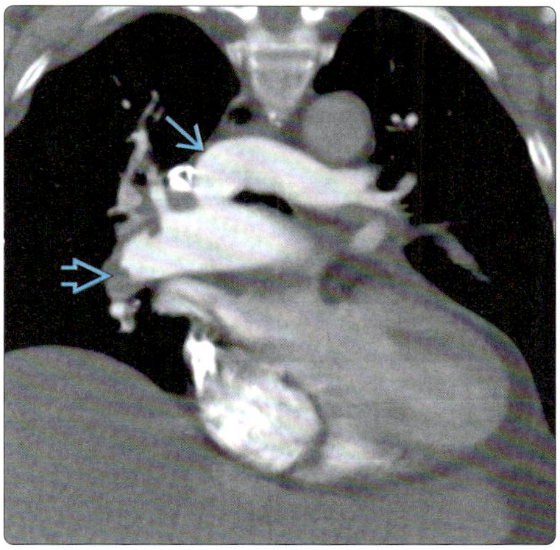

(Left) *PA CXR in a 67-year-old woman with chest pain shows slightly atypical mediastinal soft tissue contour outlining right aspect of the tracheal wall. The ascending aortic contour should be lower and in the anterior mediastinum, which should not outline the right tracheal wall.* **(Right)** *The abnormal density on PA CXR is from LPAS type IA, which arises from the superior aspect of the RPA and courses superiorly and laterally, surrounding the trachea, which is narrowed. The patient also has bilateral pulmonary emboli.*

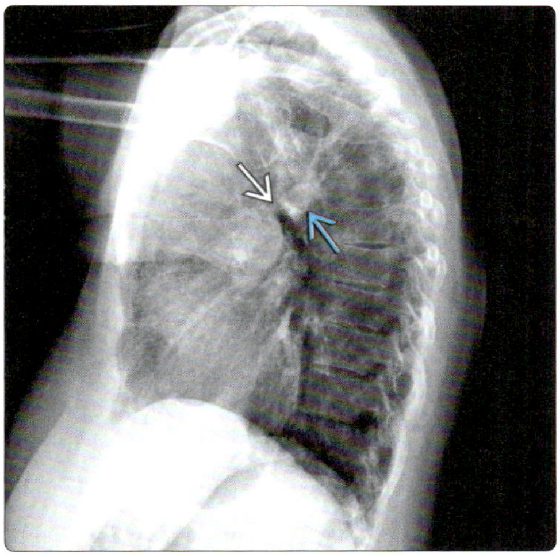

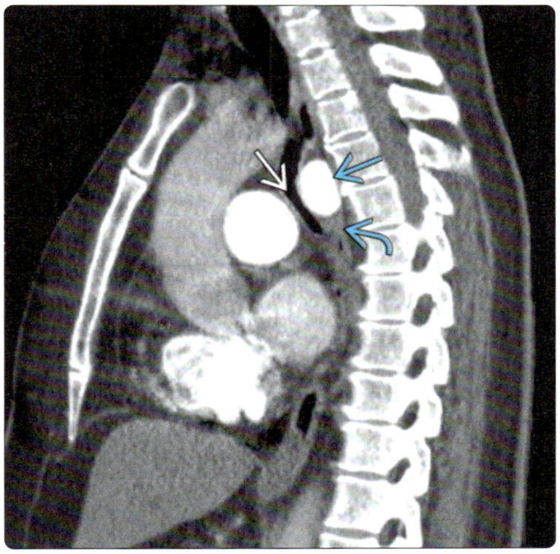

(Left) *Lateral CXR shows anomalous retrotracheal LPA associated with narrowing of the trachea. The esophagus is posterior to this anomaly. Other vascular anomalies, such as a diverticulum of Kommerell, are located behind the esophagus.* **(Right)** *Sagittal CECT shows the retrotracheal LPA from LPAS type I with associated moderate tracheal narrowing. Although not well seen on this image, the esophagus is posterior to the LPA.*

Pulmonary Arteriovenous Malformation

KEY FACTS

TERMINOLOGY

- Abnormal communication between pulmonary artery and vein

IMAGING

- Radiography
  - Nodule with feeding artery(ies) and draining vein(s)
- CT/MR
  - Sharply defined, round or oval nodule with feeding artery(ies) and draining vein(s)
    - Simple: ≥ 1 feeding arteries from same segmental artery
    - Complex: Multiple feeding arteries from different segmental arteries
  - Hepatopulmonary syndrome (HPS)
    - Dilated subpleural vessels extend to pleural surface
    - Cirrhotic liver
  - Glenn or Fontan circuit
    - Similar findings to HPS
    - Usually limited to right lung due to hepatic venous blood flow to left lung
- Contrast echocardiography: Late bubbles in left atrium due to intrapulmonary shunts

TOP DIFFERENTIAL DIAGNOSES

- Pulmonary artery aneurysm/pseudoaneurysm
- Meandering pulmonary vein
- Venous varix
- Veno-venous collaterals
- Metastases
- Solitary pulmonary nodule

PATHOLOGY

- Multiple PAVMs associated with hereditary hemorrhagic telangiectasia

DIAGNOSTIC CHECKLIST

- Consider PAVM in lung nodule with associated tubular opacities representing feeding artery and draining vein

(Left) *PA and lateral chest radiographs demonstrate a well-defined, lobular opacity ➡ in the left perihilar region representing the feeding artery and draining vein of a pulmonary arteriovenous malformation (PAVM).* **(Right)** *Coronal CT in the same patient shows the feeding artery ➡ and draining vein ➡. This is an example of a simple PAVM, which is characterized by 1 or more feeding arteries arising from the same segmental pulmonary artery.*

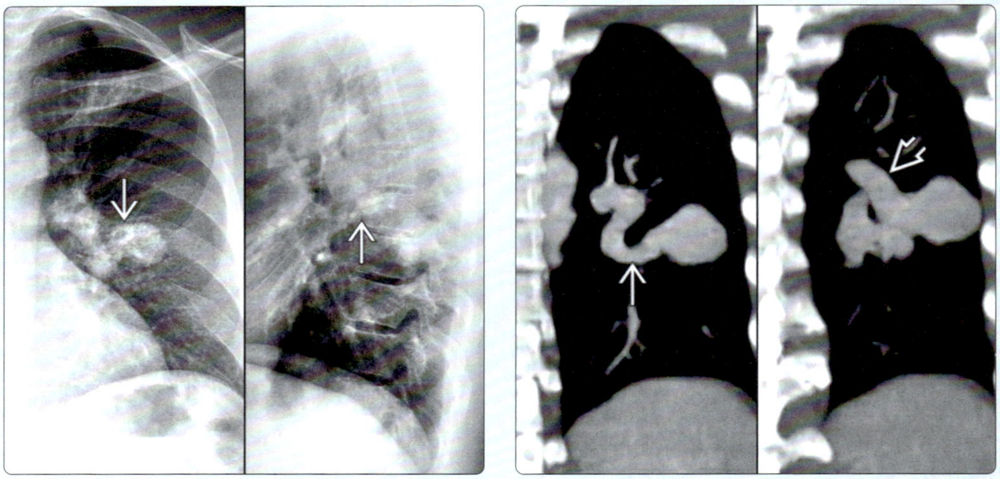

(Left) *Axial oblique CECT MIP in a 47-year-old woman with HHT shows a simple AVM in the right upper lobe with a single feeding artery ➡ supplying the nidus ➡ with a single draining vein ➡, which is slightly larger than the artery.* **(Right)** *60-mm CECT MIP in the same patient shows numerous coils in the left lung from prior coil embolizations ➡. Numerous smaller PAVMs in the right lung ➡, many of which are diminutive in size, remain untreated. Numerous additional treated and untreated PAVMs were present bilaterally.*

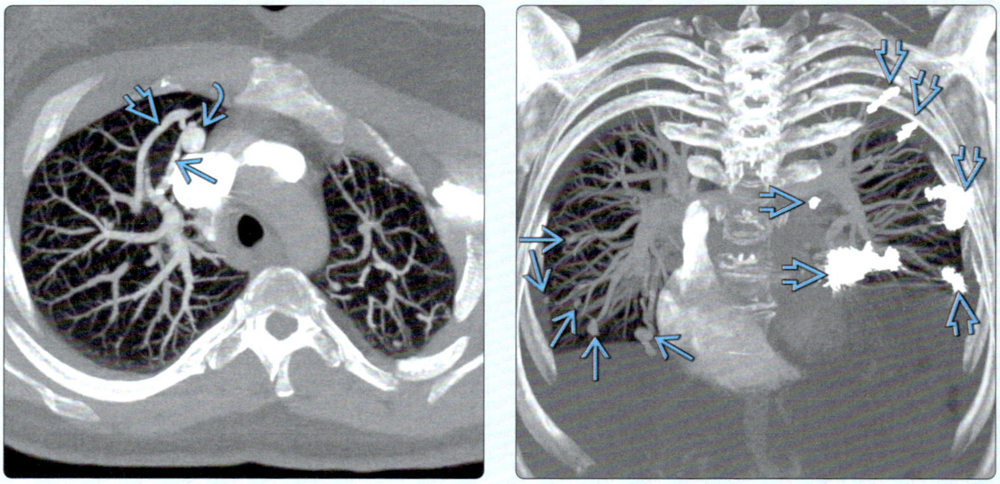

TERMINOLOGY

Abbreviations

- Pulmonary arteriovenous malformation (PAVM)

Definitions

- Abnormal communication between pulmonary artery and vein; direct right-to-left shunt
  - **Congenital**
    - Hereditary hemorrhagic telangiectasia (HHT)
    - Sporadic (rare)
  - **Acquired**
    - Hepatopulmonary syndrome (HPS)
      - Liver disease
      - Dilated peripheral pulmonary vasculature
      - Increased alveolar-arterial oxygen gradient on room air
    - Post correction of complex congenital heart disease (CHD)
      - Glenn or Fontan circuits

IMAGING

General Features

- Best diagnostic clue
  - Nodule(s) with feeding artery(ies) and draining vein(s)
- Location
  - Peripheral lower lobes (50-70%): Medial 1/3 of lung
- Size
  - Variable

Radiographic Findings

- Radiography
  - Sensitivity for PAVMs: 50-70%
  - Round, oval, or lobulated well-defined nodule with enlarged feeding and draining vessels

CT Findings

- PAVMs most numerous in mid- and lower lung zones
- Sharply defined round or oval nodule (nidus) with feeding artery(ies) and draining vein(s)
  - **Simple (90%)**
    - 1 or more feeding arteries from same segmental artery
    - 1 or more draining veins
      - Veins usually often larger than feeding arteries
    - Aneurysm sac is simple and not septated
    - Ground-glass opacity near nidus likely due to volume average of microscopic telangiectasias
  - **Complex (10%)**
    - Multiple feeding arteries from different segmental arteries
    - May have multiple draining veins
    - Aneurysm sac is septated or plexiform
    - Complex AVM subtypes
      - Diffuse (5% of complex PAVMs): Disseminated involvement of multiple segments or lobes with numerous, variably sized lesions
      - Telangiectatic: Seen in children and can appear as focal ground-glass opacity; feeding and draining vessels may be absent
- Measurement of feeding artery for embolization planning
  - No set guidelines and varies based on publication
    - Some suggest measuring 2-3 mm from nidus
    - Other suggest measuring just distal to last artery distal to noninvolved branches
      - Often 2-3 cm proximal to nidus
- HPS
  - Type 1: Distal vascular dilatation with subpleural telangiectasia (type 1)
    - Dilated subpleural vessels extending to pleural surface
  - Type 2: AVMs
    - Nodular dilated or peripheral pulmonary vasculature
  - Cirrhotic liver
- Glenn or Fontan circuit in corrected CHD
  - Similar findings to HPS
  - More common on R > L

MR Findings

- MRA: Similar to CT for detection
  - Good accuracy
  - No radiation
- Adjunct in preembolization planning
- Time-resolved MRA: Noninvasive evaluation of patency

Echocardiographic Findings

- With contrast, bubbles seen in left heart after venous injection
  - Delay of 3-8 cardiac cycles for bubbles to appear in left atrium for extracardiac shunt
    - With intracardiac shunt, bubbles appear in ≤ 2 cycles

Angiographic Findings

- Usually enlarged pulmonary artery(ies) supplying rounded nidus with enlarged draining vein(s)
- Used primarily for treatment and not for diagnosis

Nuclear Medicine Findings

- Tc-99m MAA: Right-to-left shunt evaluation

Imaging Recommendations

- Best imaging tool
  - CT with MIP images
- Protocol advice
  - Thin-slice imaging < 1 mm
  - CTA for initial screening
  - Screen for PAVM with CT every 3-5 years
    - Low-dose noncontrast CT can be used
      - Risk of paradoxical air embolism from contrast IV injection
      - Filters to remove air bubbles should be used

DIFFERENTIAL DIAGNOSIS

Pulmonary Artery Aneurysm/Pseudoaneurysm

- Usually at branching points
- No draining vein

Pulmonary Vein Varix

- Congenital
  - Intrapulmonary vein bypasses atretic segment of normal pulmonary vein
  - Rarely associated with HHT
- Acquired

- Mitral valve disease-related pulmonary hypertension
- End-stage liver disease
- No arterial connection

Pulmonary Vein to Pulmonary Vein Collaterals

- Often seen in central pulmonary vein obstruction
- Network of pulmonary veins connect to bypass obstruction

Systemic to Pulmonary Vein Collaterals

- Seen after Fontan procedure
- Major cause of shunting

Meandering Pulmonary Vein

- Tortuous pulmonary vein with circuitous course but drains into left atrium
- Multiple pulmonary veins often seen draining into meandering pulmonary vein
- Not associated with central obstruction

Solitary Pulmonary Nodule

- Lung cancer, granuloma, hamartoma

Bronchial Atresia, Mucocele

- Can be high attenuation and mimic PAVM
- Surrounding hyperlucent lung in bronchial atresia

Hypervascular Metastases

- No dilated feeding artery or draining vein

PATHOLOGY

General Features

- Etiology
  - HHT caused by variety of genetic mutations
  - HPS
    - Unclear cause
    - Possibly from excessive vasodilator production
  - Glenn or Fontan circulation in complex CHD
    - Liver may play role in PAVM development
    - PAVMs in lung not receiving hepatic venous flow
      - In many, superior vena cava flow directed toward right lung and inferior vena cava flow directed toward left
      - Right lung does not receive hepatic flow
- Genetics
  - HHT: Autosomal dominant disorder
    - *ENG*: Higher risk of pulmonary and brain AVMs
    - *ACVRL1*: Higher risk of hepatic AVMs
    - *SMAD4*: Associated with juvenile polyposis
    - Other rarer and unknown mutations

Gross Pathologic & Surgical Features

- Draining veins usually larger than feeding arteries
- HPS: Dilated precapillary vasculature and pleural vessels with direct arteriovenous communication

CLINICAL ISSUES

Presentation

- Most common signs/symptoms
  - May be asymptomatic
    - However, other findings and symptoms associated with HHT often present
      - Epistaxis
      - Anemia
      - GI bleeding
  - Patients with multiple or large PAVMs
    - Hemoptysis
    - Shortness of breath may be multifactorial
      - Blood that transits PAVM does not participate in alveolar gas exchange
      - Could be due to shunting in liver or anemia
  - Cerebral abscess
    - Pulmonary capillaries remove circulating bacteria
  - Systemic emboli
    - Blood transiting PAVM not filtered by capillaries
    - Thrombi can pass into systemic circulation

Demographics

- Age
  - 10% are diagnosed in infancy or childhood
- Sex
  - M:F = 1:2

Natural History & Prognosis

- PAVM growth during childhood and pregnancy
  - Growth also occurs in pulmonary hypertension
- Most smaller PAVMs do not grow over time
- Risk of stroke independent of size

Treatment

- Complications can occur independent of feeding artery size
  - Treatment decisions based on feasibility vs. risk rather than feeding vessel size
- Coil embolotherapy via interventional approach
  - Feeding vessel diameter of 2 mm considered treatable
  - Recanalization in up to 20%

DIAGNOSTIC CHECKLIST

Consider

- Consider PAVM in lung nodule with associated tubular opacities representing feeding artery and draining vein

Diagnosis

- Blood test for identification of mutation (80% of patients)
- Genetic screening
- Screening of at-risk patients with contrast echocardiography
- Clinical diagnosis (Curacao criteria)
  - Brain, lung, or liver AVMs
  - Epistaxis
  - Family history of HHT
  - Telangiectases

SELECTED REFERENCES

1. Raptis DA et al: CT appearance of pulmonary arteriovenous malformations and mimics. Radiographics. 42(1):56-68, 2022
2. Yap CW et al: The role of interventional radiology in the diagnosis and treatment of pulmonary arteriovenous malformations. J Clin Med. 11(21):6282, 2022
3. Faughnan ME et al: Second international guidelines for the diagnosis and management of hereditary hemorrhagic telangiectasia. Ann Intern Med. 173(12):989-1001, 2020
4. Müller-Hülsbeck S et al: CIRSE standards of practice on diagnosis and treatment of pulmonary arteriovenous malformations. Cardiovasc Intervent Radiol. 43(3):353-61, 2020

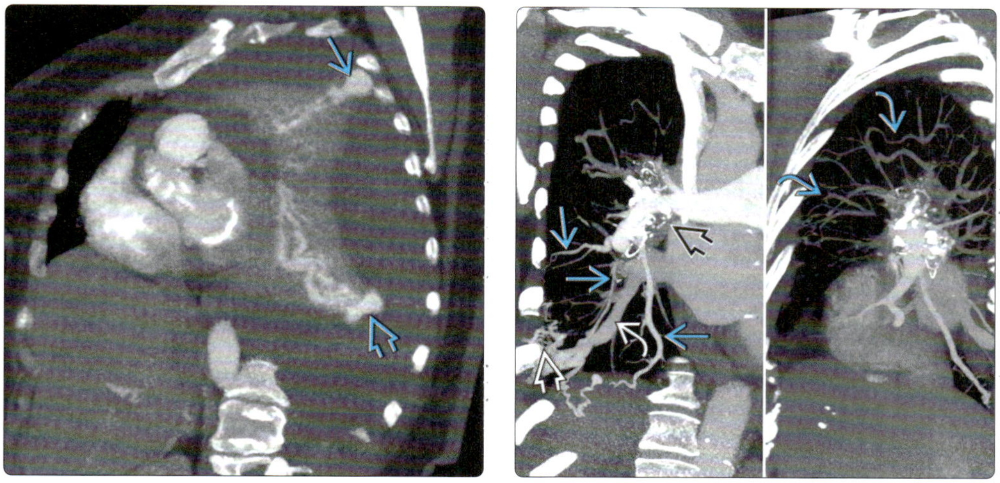

(Left) *A woman with HHT and a large hemothorax has a simple left upper lobe PAVM ➡ that has bled into the pleural space. The complex left lower lobe bilobed PAVM ➡ is supplied by 2 basilar segments.* **(Right)** *Coronal (left) and sagittal (right) oblique CECT MIPs in a 58-year-old woman with HHT and fibrosing mediastinitis (FM) show a complex RLL AVM ➡ fed by 3 segmental arteries ➡ with a large draining vein ➡. FM occludes the right superior pulmonary vein (PV) ➡. Numerous PV to PV collaterals ➡ bypass the occlusion.*

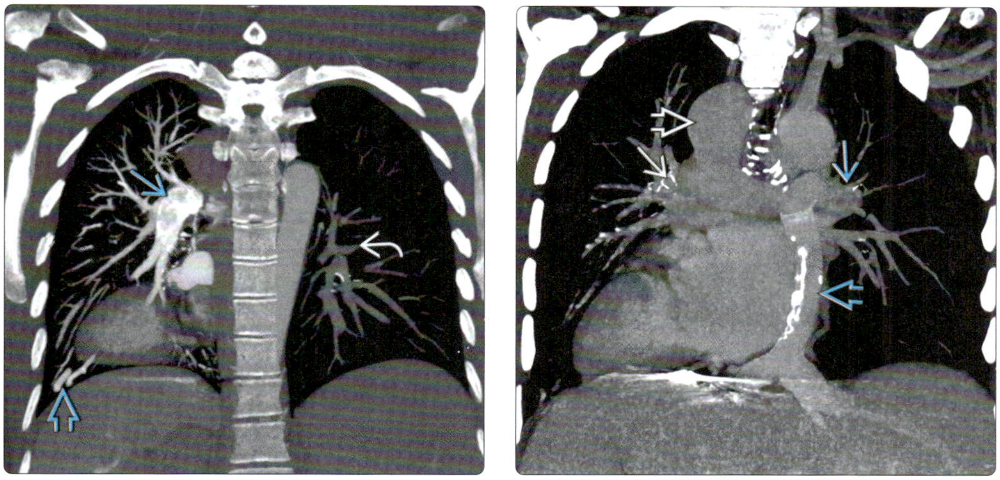

(Left) *Patient with polysplenia, situs inversus, and complex congenital heart disease status post bidirectional Glenn is shown. Pulmonary arterial phase shows unilateral right lung enhancement ➡ from SVC flow. The left lung, which receives IVC flow, is unopacified ➡. A right basilar PAVM ➡ is seen.* **(Right)** *10-mm CECT MIP shows the IVC ➡, which received hepatic venous flow, feeding the left pulmonary artery ➡. The SVC ➡, which is enlarged due to azygous continuation, supplies the right pulmonary artery ➡.*

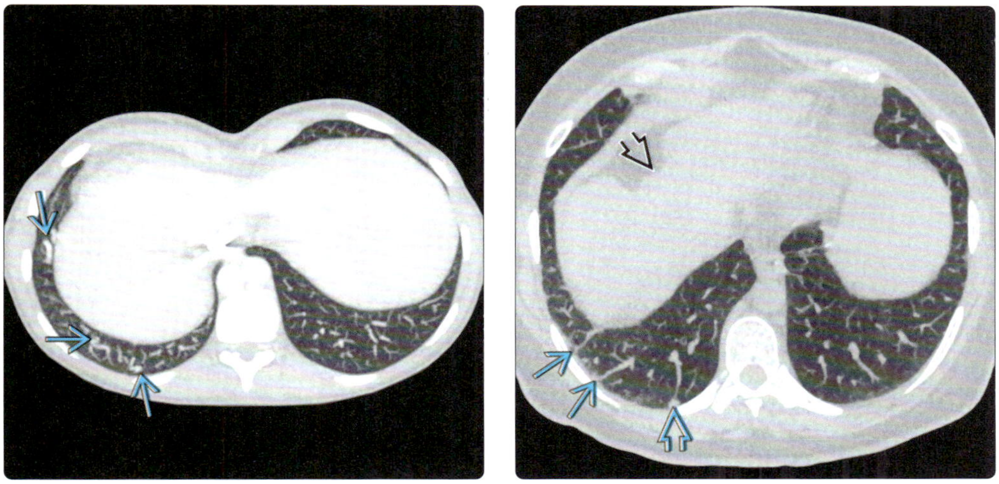

(Left) *Three-mm CECT MIP shows multiple right PAVMs ➡ with diffuse enlargement of the peripheral vasculature. This is secondary to the right lung receiving no hepatic blood. The left lung, which receives hepatic blood flow from the IVC, is normal.* **(Right)** *CT in a 63-year-old man with liver cirrhosis ➡ and portal hypertension shows dilated peripheral pulmonary arteries touching the pleural surface ➡. One of the dilated vessels has an peripheral nodular appearance ➡, consistent with type II hepatopulmonary syndrome.*

Pulmonary Aneurysm

KEY FACTS

TERMINOLOGY

- Focal dilatation of pulmonary artery involving all 3 layers of arterial wall

IMAGING

- Chest radiography
  - Round perihilar opacity
  - Nonspecific pulmonary nodule or consolidation
- CT
  - Marked dilation of main pulmonary artery or central pulmonary arteries common in pulmonary hypertension, congenital cases, and syndromic causes of aneurysm
  - Focal or long-segment dilation of more peripheral pulmonary vasculature more common in vasculitis, infection, and trauma
  - Associated mural thrombosis may be present
  - Vessel may be occluded distal to aneurysm
  - Adjacent hemorrhage or saccular shape concerning for pseudoaneurysm

TOP DIFFERENTIAL DIAGNOSES

- Pulmonary artery pseudoaneurysm
  - Pseudoaneurysms and aneurysms may coexist in certain etiologies, such as Behçet disease and Hughes-Stovin syndrome
  - Surrounding ground-glass opacity due to hemorrhage and saccular shape concerning for pseudoaneurysms
- Pulmonary arteriovenous malformation
  - Direct connection between pulmonary artery and vein, sometimes with intervening capillary network

CLINICAL ISSUES

- Presentation: Hemoptysis, dyspnea, chest pain, incidental
- Treatment
  - Endovascular intervention (focal aneurysms): Embolization, stent-graft
  - Surgical resection
  - Immunosuppression for Behçet disease and Hughes-Stovin syndrome

(Left) *PA radiograph in a 12-year-old boy with a history of Behçet disease and new-onset hemoptysis shows multiple rounded pulmonary lesions with patchy right basilar opacity.* **(Right)** *Coronal CECT MIP shows bilateral pulmonary artery aneurysms (PAAs) and pseudoaneurysms, which are difficult to differentiate based on appearance alone. Many of the aneurysms show peripheral mural thrombus, and the lower lobe branches are occluded distal to the lesions. (Courtesy E. Weihe, MD.)*

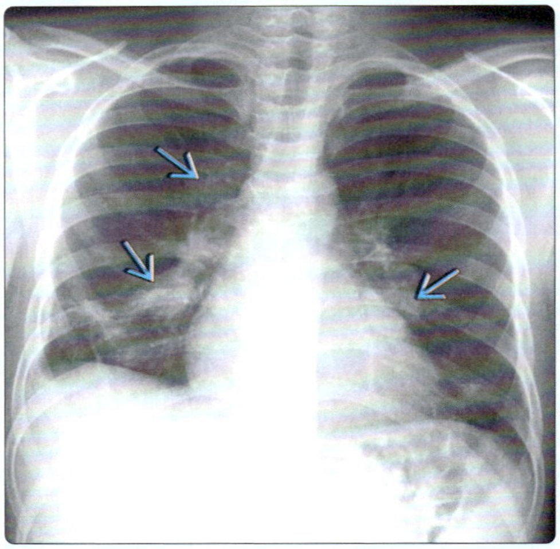

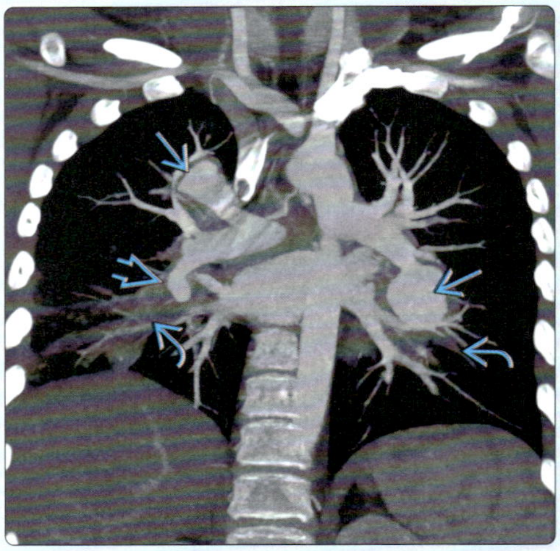

(Left) *CT shows a partially thrombosed pseudoaneurysm. Air in the pseudoaneurysm is due to fistulation with adjacent bronchus, causing the hemoptysis. Adjacent pulmonary hemorrhage is present. There is evidence of prior aneurysm resection.* **(Right)** *Five-mm CECT MIP (left) shows aneurysmal dilation of the main and left pulmonary artery (PA). The right PA is normal. Two-mm minIP (right) shows a thickened bicuspid pulmonic valve. Pulmonic stenosis was confirmed on echocardiogram.*

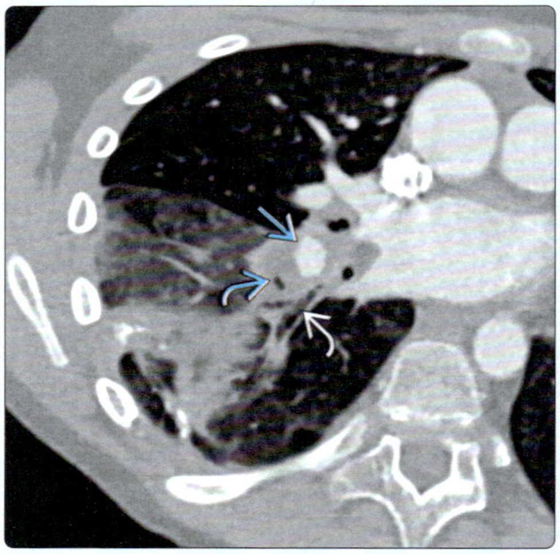

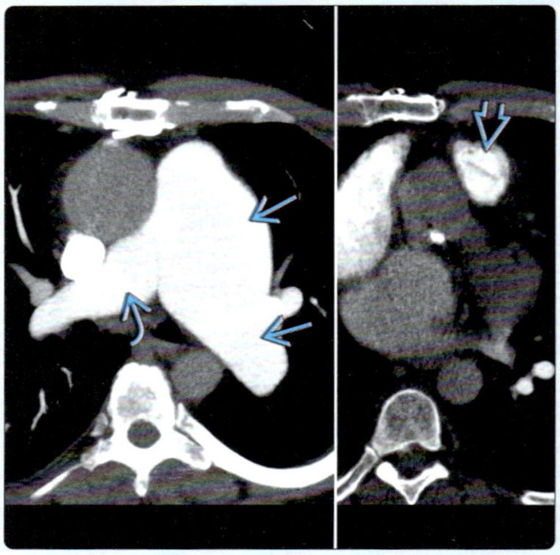

TERMINOLOGY

Abbreviations

- Pulmonary artery aneurysm (PAA)

Definitions

- Dilatation of pulmonary artery (PA) involving all 3 layers of arterial wall

IMAGING

General Features

- Best diagnostic clue
  - Dilatation of PA
- Location
  - Main, hilar, lobar, segmental, or subsegmental PAs
  - Peripheral PAA is less common

Radiographic Findings

- Radiography
  - Central (main or lobar) PAA
    - Lobulated contour of PA
    - Round hilar or perihilar opacity
    - Hilar enlargement depending on size
  - Peripheral (segmental or subsegmental) PAA
    - Nonspecific pulmonary nodule(s)

CT Findings

- Dilatation of PA
  - Usually fusiform in shape but can be saccular
  - Saccular aneurysms may be partially thrombosed
  - Peripheral segmental/subsegmental PAA may be small and subtle
    - Sometimes better visualized in lung window
- Adjacent ground-glass opacity or consolidation may represent hemorrhage due to rupture or leakage
- Pulmonary hypertension (PH)
  - PA dilation secondary to increased pulmonary pressures
- Congenital
  - Congenital heart disease associated with increased pulmonary blood flow
    - Patent ductus arteriosus
    - Atrial > ventricular septal defects
    - Tetralogy of Fallot
  - Congenital pulmonary valvular abnormalities
    - Valvular pulmonary stenosis
      - □ Enlarged main and left PAs
      - □ Thickening of pulmonary valve, which is often inconspicuous on CT
    - Subvalvular or supravalvular stenosis
      - □ Band or web above or below valve
  - Sequela of repair
    - More commonly leads to pseudoaneurysm
- Syndromic causes of aneurysm
  - Commonly associated with ascending aortic aneurysms or annuloaortic ectasia
    - Marfan syndrome
    - Loeys-Dietz syndrome
    - Vascular Ehlers-Danlos syndrome
- Vasculitis
  - Behçet disease
    - Pseudoaneurysms more common than aneurysms
      - □ ± vascular wall thickening and enhancement
      - □ Surrounding ground-glass opacity due to hemorrhage
    - PA filling defect more often in situ thrombi than emboli
    - Often areas of stenosis associated with dilation
    - Pulmonary infarct can be present
    - Deep venous thrombosis (vena cava, innominate, and subclavian veins)
    - Intracardiac thrombus (particularly in right ventricle)
  - Hughes-Stovin syndrome (HSS)
    - Single or multiple PAA or pseudoaneurysms
    - Systemic arterial aneurysms, including bronchial artery aneurysm
    - Thrombosis of vena cava, jugular vein, or cardiac chambers
  - Large vessel vasculitis
    - Giant cell and Takayasu arteritis
      - □ Indistinguishable on imaging
      - □ PAA uncommon but can occur
      - □ Associated areas of circumferential wall thickening and stenosis
      - □ Associated systemic vascular involvement
- Infection
  - Can lead to both aneurysm and pseudoaneurysm formation
    - Numerous etiologies, including bacterial, viral, and fungal
  - May be associated with sepsis or septic emboli
- Malignancy
  - Leads to pseudoaneurysm formation more frequently than PAA
  - May be result of tumor invasion, embolism, or associated treatment
  - Signs or history of malignancy
- Trauma or iatrogenic
  - Lead to pseudoaneurysm formation
    - Swan-Ganz
    - Transthoracic or endobronchial biopsy
    - Ablation therapy
    - Surgery
    - Penetrating > blunt trauma
  - History or imaging findings of trauma or recent intervention

MR Findings

- MR angiographic findings similar to that of CT
- Wall thickening and enhancement often better seen than on CT
- Better evaluation of congenital heart disease

Angiographic Findings

- Depicts focal dilation of PA
- In Behçet disease, vascular puncture may lead to aneurysm formation; therefore, CTA is preferable for diagnosis

Imaging Recommendations

- Best imaging tool
  - CTA with multiplanar reformations is most sensitive, particularly for small, peripheral PAAs

DIFFERENTIAL DIAGNOSIS

Pulmonary Artery Pseudoaneurysm

- Does not involve all 3 layers of vessel wall
- Saccular or irregular instead of fusiform shape
- More often related to iatrogenic or noniatrogenic trauma or infection
- More likely to rupture
- More often peripheral (involving smaller PA branches)
- Can coexist with PA true aneurysms

Pulmonary Arteriovenous Malformation

- Enhancing nodular nidus on CT
- Dilated feeding PA and draining vein

PATHOLOGY

General Features

- Genetics
  - Behçet disease: HLA-B51

Gross Pathologic & Surgical Features

- Behçet disease
  - Inflammation of vasa vasorum → ischemia/weakening of vessel wall → true and pseudoaneurysms
  - Adventitial fibrosis and thrombus formation can occur
- HSS
  - Diffuse dilatation and partial occlusion of PAA

Microscopic Features

- Behçet disease
  - Neutrophilic infiltration with endothelial swelling and fibrinoid necrosis
- HSS
  - Perivascular lymphomonocytic infiltration with sclerosis

CLINICAL ISSUES

Presentation

- Most common signs/symptoms
  - Usually asymptomatic
  - Hemoptysis, sometimes severe
  - Dyspnea
- Other signs/symptoms
  - Chest pain
- Behçet disease
  - Behçet triad: Oral ulcerations, genital ulceration, uveitis
  - Skin findings: Folliculitis, erythema nodosum
  - Venous thrombophlebitis
  - Fever

Demographics

- Age
  - Behçet disease and HSS: Mean age: 34 years
- Sex
  - Behçet disease and HSS: M:F = 3:1
- Ethnicity
  - Behçet disease
    - Ancient Silk Road: Far East, Middle East, eastern Mediterranean
- Epidemiology
  - Behçet disease
    - Turkey: 4 cases per 1,000
    - Asia: 2-30 cases per 100,000
    - USA: < 1 case per 100,000

Natural History & Prognosis

- Behçet disease
  - Rupture of aneurysm or pseudoaneurysm can lead to life-threatening hemoptysis
    - Better survival rate in more recent reports due to better treatment
  - PAA can be present at time of diagnosis or develop years after initial presentation
- HSS
  - Aneurysm rupture and hemoptysis is main cause of death
  - Small aneurysm can stabilize or regress with immunosuppression

Treatment

- Peripheral PAA
  - Intravascular coil or balloon embolization
  - Surgical resection of involved lung segment or lobe if limited disease
- Main PAA
  - Surgical repair
    - Excision of aneurysm and prosthetic patch replacement
    - Pneumonectomy
    - High morbidity and mortality
- Behçet disease and HSS
  - Corticosteroids, cyclophosphamide, or other immunosuppressants
  - Anticoagulation is generally not recommended

DIAGNOSTIC CHECKLIST

Consider

- Possible underlying cause
  - Pulmonary hypertension
  - Congenital
  - Syndromic causes of aneurysm
  - Vasculitis
  - Infection, malignancy, trauma; iatrogenic more likely to be pseudoaneurysms

SELECTED REFERENCES

1. Emad Y et al: Pulmonary embolism versus pulmonary vasculitis in Hughes-Stovin syndrome: characteristic computed tomography pulmonary angiographic findings and diagnostic and therapeutic implications. HSS International Study Group. Thromb Res. 239:109040, 2024
2. Doi A et al: Surgical management of giant pulmonary artery aneurysms in patients with severe pulmonary arterial hypertension. J Card Surg. 37(4):1019-25, 2022
3. Gupta M et al: Pulmonary artery aneurysm: a review. Pulm Circ. 10(1):2045894020908780, 2020
4. Kalra-Lall A et al: Brief review: pulmonary artery aneurysms and pseudoaneurysms. Int J Cardiovasc Imaging. 35(7):1357-64, 2019
5. Nuche J et al: Frequency, predictors, and prognostic impact of pulmonary artery aneurysms in patients with pulmonary arterial hypertension. Am J Cardiol. 123(3):474-81, 2019
6. Mehdipoor G et al: Imaging manifestations of Behcet's disease: key considerations and major features. Eur J Radiol. 98:214-25, 2018

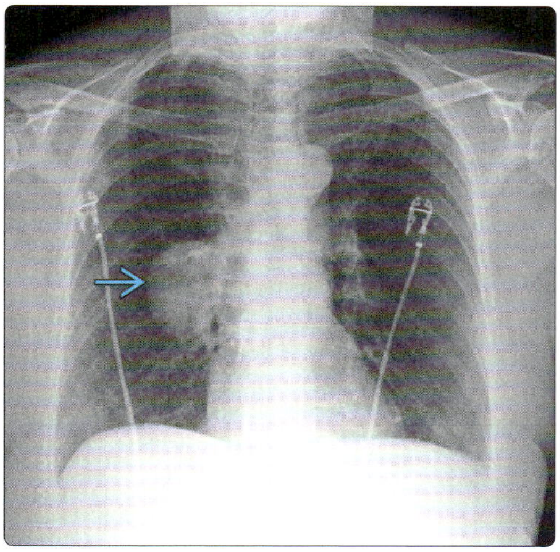

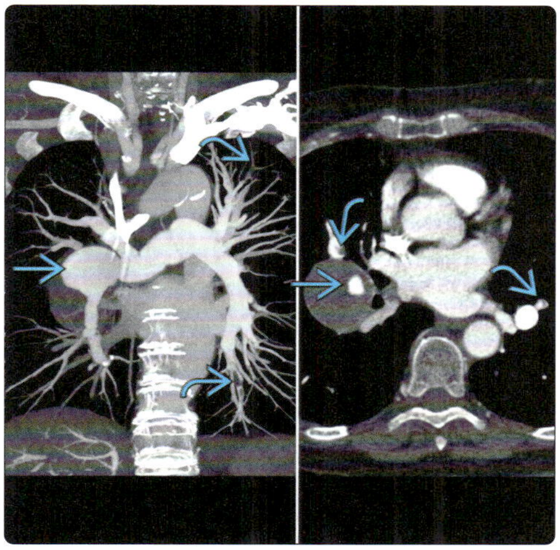

(Left) *AP radiograph in a 59-year-old woman with history of repeated deep venous thrombosis shows a rounded mass in the right hilum .* **(Right)** *Coronal MIP (left) and axial (right) images from a CTPA show a large, partially thrombosed PAA involving the right interlobar PA . Numerous bilateral pulmonary emboli ranging from acute to chronic are present. This constellation of findings were thought to be secondary to Hughes-Stovin syndrome.*

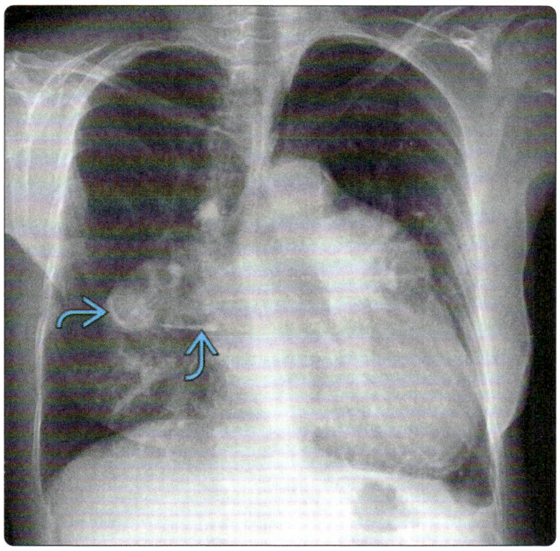

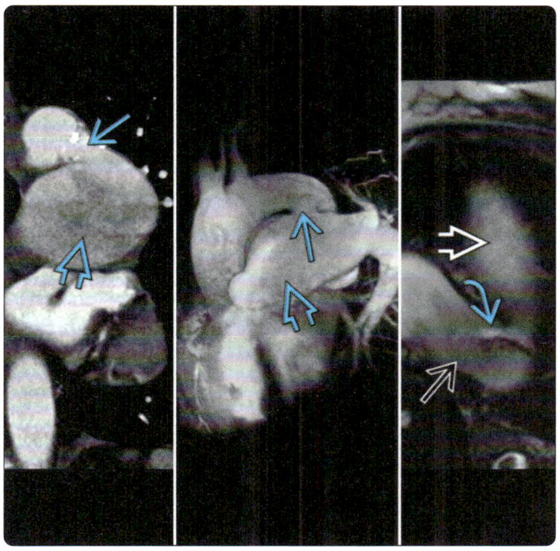

(Left) *PA CXR in a 48-year-old woman from Turkmenistan shows massive enlargement of the PAs. Calcification along the PAs is seen , suggestive of severe pulmonary hypertension.* **(Right)** *Coronal CT (left) and 3D MIP MRA (center) show a large patent ductus arteriosus with an aneurysmal main PA measuring 7.2 cm. SSFP cardiac MR (right) shows right-to-left flow from the main PA into the descending aorta due to Eisenmenger physiology.*

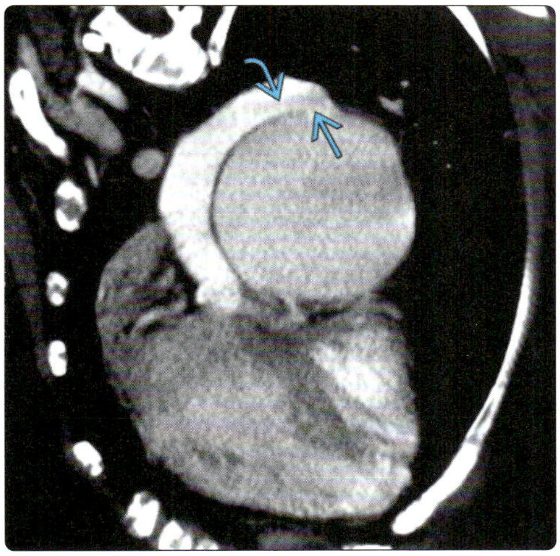

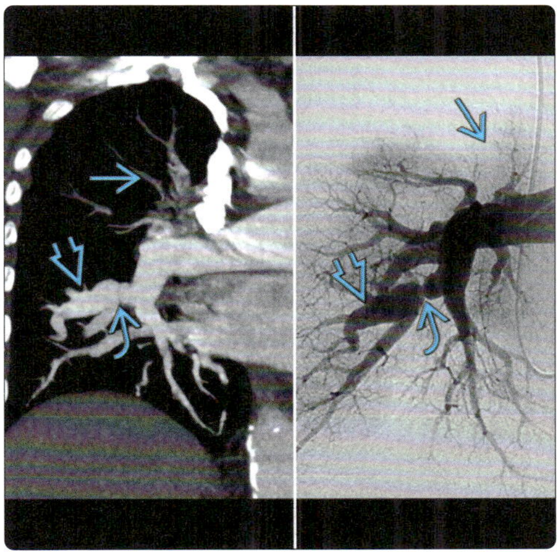

(Left) *CECT in a 51-year-old man shows a large patent ductus arteriosus with a massive main PA measuring 9.2 cm. Lower attenuation contrast from the PA is seen in the adjacent descending aorta due to Eisenmenger physiology.* **(Right)** *Coronal CECT MIP (left) and corresponding angiogram (right) show a ring stenosis of the right lower lobe anterior segment PA with fusiform poststenotic dilation . The right upper lobe PA is chronically occluded . Findings are due to a large vessel vasculitis.*

Pulmonary Artery Pseudoaneurysm

KEY FACTS

TERMINOLOGY

- Pulmonary artery pseudoaneurysm (PAP)

IMAGING

- Radiography
  - Focal consolidation
  - Nodule or mass
  - Previous pulmonary artery catheter in distal position
- CT
  - Enhancing nodule arising from pulmonary artery branch
  - Ground-glass halo suggests hemorrhage
  - Mycotic pseudoaneurysms can be associated with cavity, consolidation, septic emboli
- MDCT with pulmonary angiography protocol is optimal for detection of PAP

TOP DIFFERENTIAL DIAGNOSES

- Pulmonary artery aneurysm
- Pulmonary arteriovenous malformation

PATHOLOGY

- Etiology
  - Iatrogenic: Pulmonary artery catheter, surgery, lung biopsy
  - Trauma (penetrating or blunt)
  - Infection: TB, bacterial or fungal infection
  - Vasculitis: Hughes-Stovin, Behçet

CLINICAL ISSUES

- Signs and symptoms: Hemoptysis, chest pain, incidental imaging finding
- Mortality rate: Up to 50% in untreated patients
- Treatment
  - Embolization, stent graft
  - Surgical ligation of vessel or resection of involved portion of lung
  - Reported cases of regression after treatment of infection or neoplasm

(Left) *Coronal oblique CECT MPR shows an irregular, rounded contrast collection → arising from a subsegmental pulmonary artery in the left lower lobe →, representing a pseudoaneurysm in the setting of necrotizing pneumonia with cavitary consolidation →.* **(Right)** *Axial oblique CECT MPR of the same patient shows the left lower lobe pseudoaneurysm → within cavitary consolidation →.*

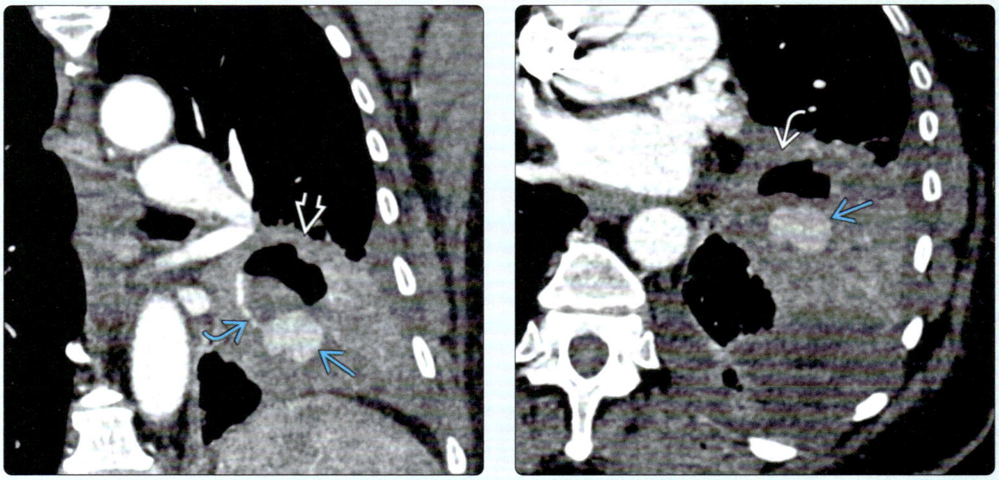

(Left) *Oblique selective catheter angiogram shows a focal irregular collection of contrast → with a narrow neck → arising from a left lower lobe subsegmental pulmonary arterial branch. The pseudoaneurysm continues to fill with contrast → on subsequent images of the same series.* **(Right)** *Oblique selective catheter angiogram from the same patient shows coils within the feeding pulmonary artery → after endovascular treatment.*

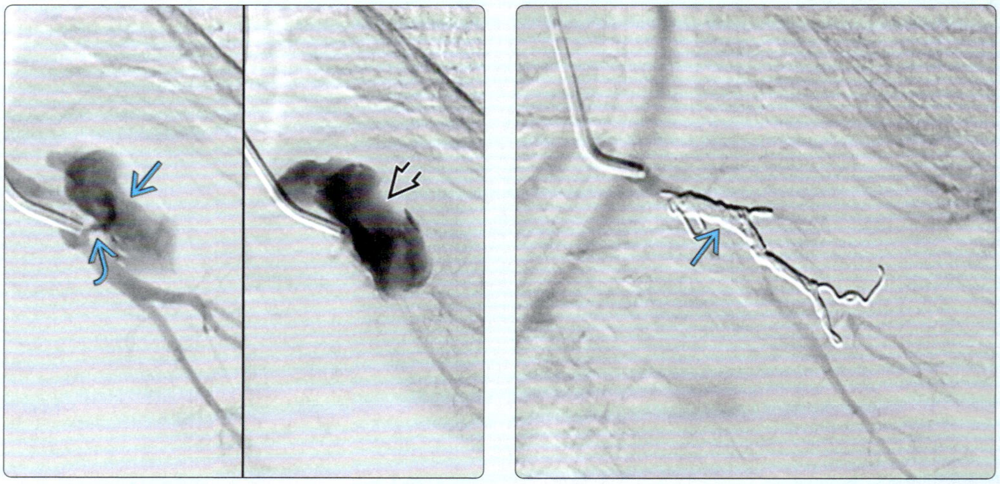

TERMINOLOGY

Abbreviations

- Pulmonary artery pseudoaneurysm (PAP)

Definitions

- Focal dilation/outpouching of pulmonary artery (PA)
  - Does not involve all 3 layers of vessel wall
  - Mostly saccular &/or irregular in shape

IMAGING

Radiographic Findings

- Focal nodule or mass
- Surrounding hazy opacities or consolidation from hemorrhage
- Pleural fluid hemothorax

CT Findings

- Enhancing nodule or mass (saccular aneurysm) arising from PA branch
  - Peripheral branches > proximal artery
  - Multiple in endocarditis, vasculitis, or metastases
- Eccentric in situ thrombus within dilated PA
- Surrounding hemorrhage
- Mycotic PAP: cavity, consolidation, septic emboli
- Bronchial or intercostal arteries may be dilated
- Best seen on CTA; delayed-phase imaging may be helpful

MR Findings

- Time-resolved MRA (TWIST, TRIX) or repeated MRA (VIBE, LAVA, THRIVE) sequences helpful
- Enhancing lesion adjacent to or arising from PA branch

Imaging Recommendations

- Best imaging tool
  - MDCT with pulmonary angiography protocol
    - Helps identify source of bleeding in hemoptysis
    - Provides road map for endovascular interventions

Angiographic Findings

- Focal saccular outpouching arising from PA branches

DIFFERENTIAL DIAGNOSIS

Pulmonary Artery Aneurysm

- Difficult to distinguish from PAP based on imaging
  - Certain etiologies, such as vasculitis, can have combination of pulmonary artery aneurysm and PAP
- Fusiform dilatation of PA is more suggestive of aneurysm

Pulmonary Arteriovenous Malformation

- Nidus with feeding artery and 1 or more draining veins
- Feeding PA may be enlarged
  - In contrast, PA proximal to PAP is usually of normal size

Hypervascular Neoplasm

- Carcinoid tumor or metastasis from renal cell carcinoma, thyroid cancer, melanoma, etc.
  - Enhancing nodule &/or mass
  - ± ground-glass halo due to perilesional hemorrhage

PATHOLOGY

General Features

- Etiology
  - Iatrogenic
    - PA catheter causing perforation
      - Incidence: ~ 0.2%
      - Risk factors: Pulmonary arterial hypertension, age > 60 years, anticoagulation
    - Surgery, biopsy, chest tube, etc.
  - Trauma: Penetrating or blunt
  - Vasculitis
    - Behçet disease, Hughes-Stovin, Takayasu
    - Often multiple
    - Can coexist with true PA aneurysms
  - Infection
    - Pneumonia, bacterial abscesses, septic emboli
      - *Staphylococcus aureus, Pseudomonas*
    - Tuberculosis (TB)
      - Rasmussen aneurysm: 4% of chronic TB
      - Common in upper lobes, associated with cavitary disease
    - Aspergillosis, mucormycosis
    - Mycetoma complicating chronic TB or sarcoidosis
  - Neoplasm
    - Lung cancer, sarcoma metastases; erode into PAs
  - Chronic inflammatory lung diseases
    - Cystic fibrosis, bronchiectasis, sarcoidosis
  - Congenital
    - Deficient wall, valvular/postvalvular stenosis, left-to-right shunts

CLINICAL ISSUES

Presentation

- Most common signs/symptoms
  - Hemoptysis
  - Chest pain, dyspnea
  - Incidental imaging finding

Demographics

- Sex: M > F
- Up to 11% of patients undergoing bronchial angiography for massive hemoptysis

Natural History & Prognosis

- If untreated, can enlarge and rupture, leading to hemorrhage and death
- High mortality rate without treatment

Treatment

- Coils or particle embolization
- Endovascular stent graft
- Surgery
  - Ligation of involved PA
  - Wedge resection or lobectomy
- Treatment of underlying etiology

SELECTED REFERENCES

1. Kalra-Lall A et al: Brief review: pulmonary artery aneurysms and pseudoaneurysms. Int J Cardiovasc Imaging. 35(7):1357-64, 2019

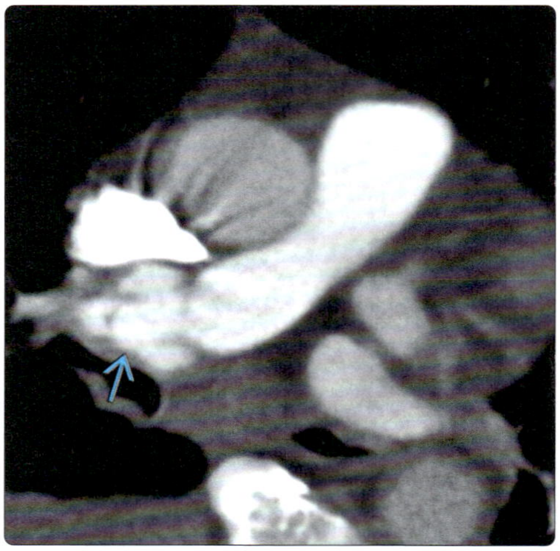

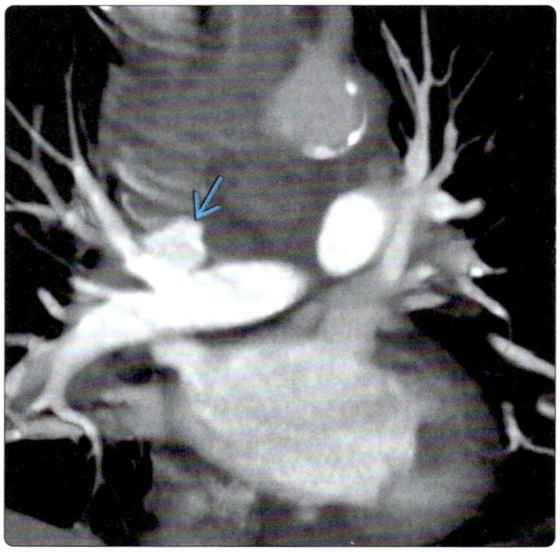

(Left) *Volume-rendered axial oblique CECT in a patient after mediastinoscopy shows irregular contrast outpouching* ➙ *of the proximal right upper lobe pulmonary artery, representing a pseudoaneurysm.* **(Right)** *Coronal oblique volume-rendered CECT of the same patient shows the irregular, saccular pseudoaneurysm* ➙ *arising from the proximal right upper lobe pulmonary artery.*

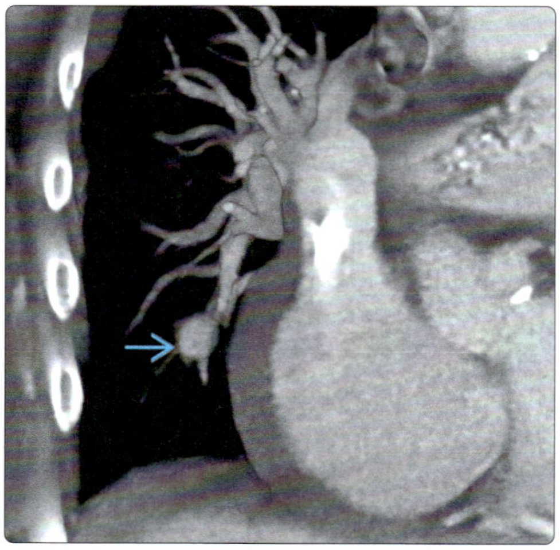

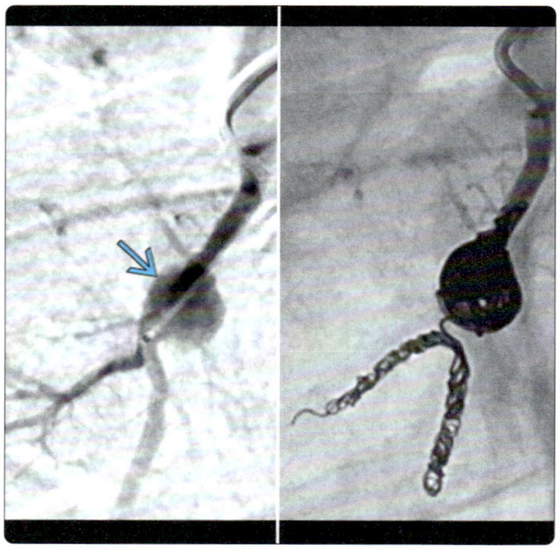

(Left) *Coronal oblique volume-rendered CECT shows a pseudoaneurysm* ➙ *secondary to recent pulmonary artery catheter.* **(Right)** *Catheter angiogram (left) from the same patient shows the saccular pseudoaneurysm* ➙ *arising from a subsegmental right middle lobe pulmonary artery. Posttreatment image (right) shows subsequent embolization with microcoils.*

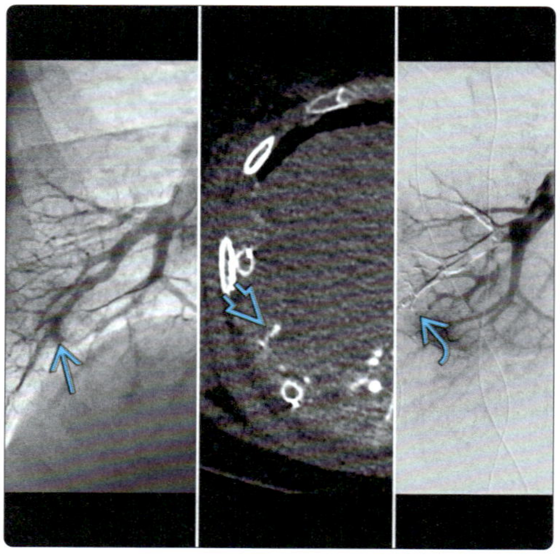

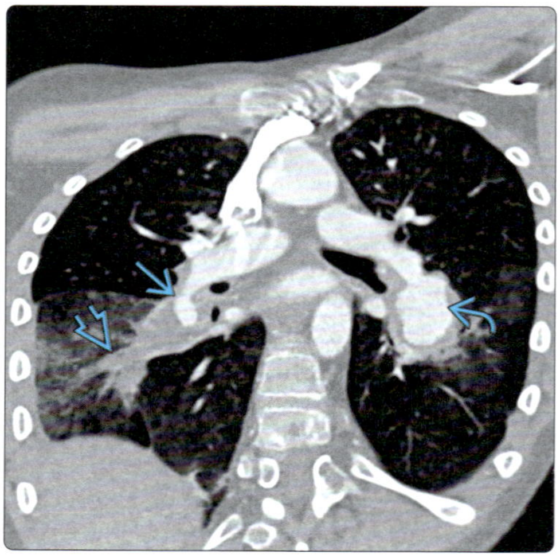

(Left) *PA balloon angioplasty for chronic thromboembolic pulmonary hypertension shows a distal right lower lobe subsegmental branch rupture (left)* ➙ *with active extravasation on subsequent CTA (middle)* ➙*. Patient then undergoes embolization (right)* ➙*.* **(Right)** *CTA in a patient with Behçet disease and hemoptysis shows a right lower lobe pseudoaneurysm* ➙ *with endobronchial hematoma* ➙ *and surrounding hemorrhage. A left lower lobe aneurysm vs. pseudoaneurysm* ➙ *is also seen.*

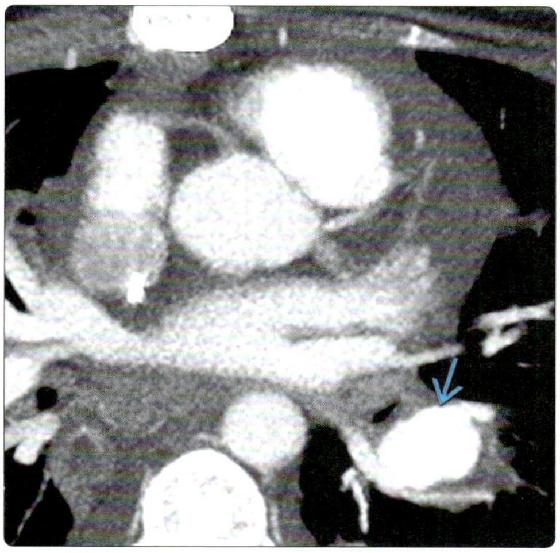
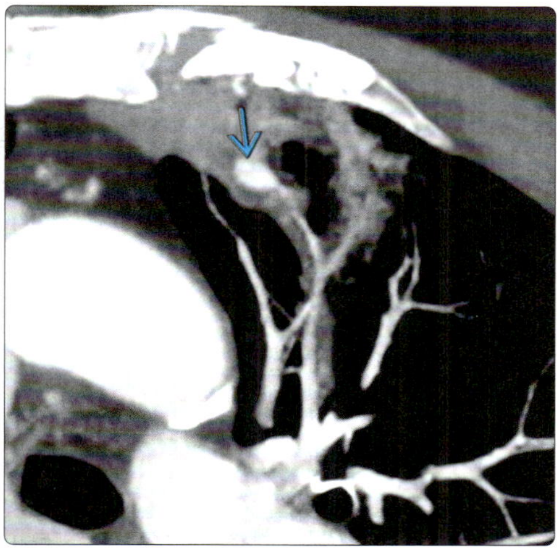

(Left) *Axial CECT MIP in a patient with endocarditis shows a saccular collection of contrast arising from left lower lobe pulmonary artery, representing a pseudoaneurysm in the setting of septic emboli.* **(Right)** *Axial oblique CECT MIP in a patient after radiotherapy of left upper lobe lung cancer shows an ovoid collection of contrast arising from a subsegmental pulmonary artery, representing a pseudoaneurysm within an area of radiation change.*

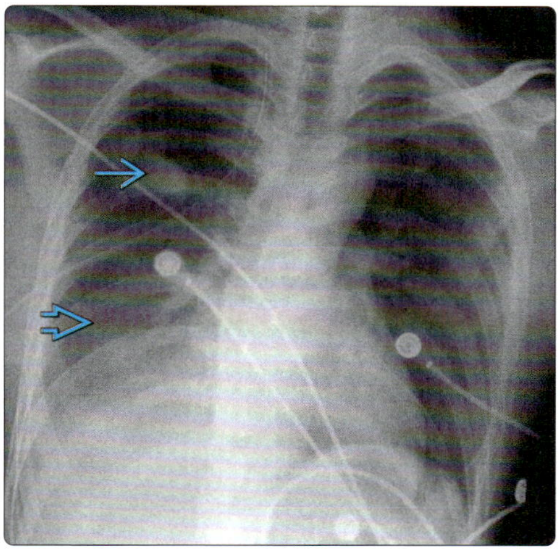
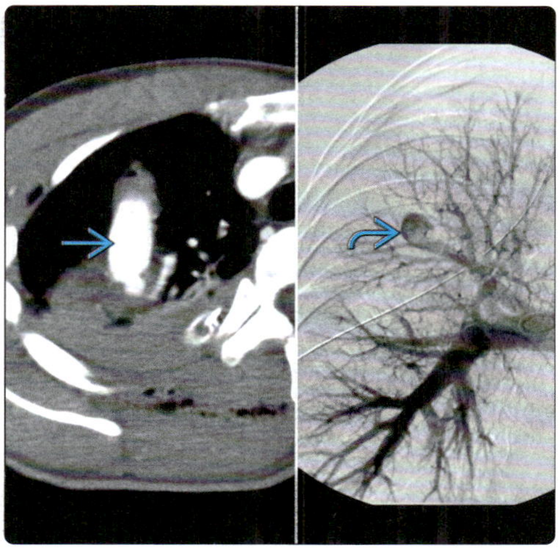

(Left) *AP chest radiograph in a man who was stabbed in the back shows a right upper lung nodule. Mid- and lower lung ground-glass opacity and consolidation are due to hemorrhage.* **(Right)** *CTA (left) shows a large area of contrast extravasation from a right upper lobe pulmonary artery branch from the stab wound. Anterior angiogram (right) shows the pseudoaneurysm, which was embolized.*

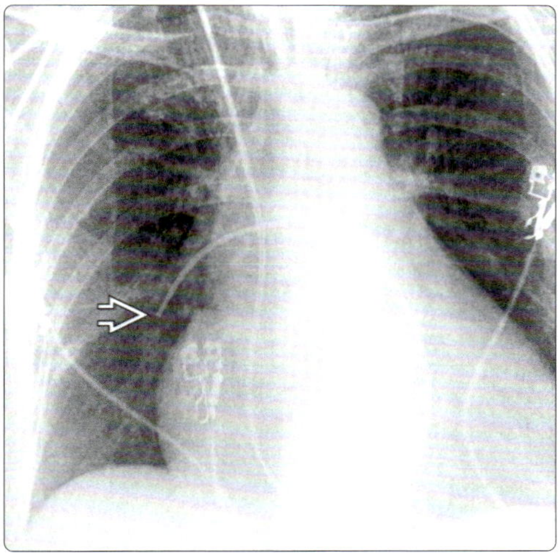
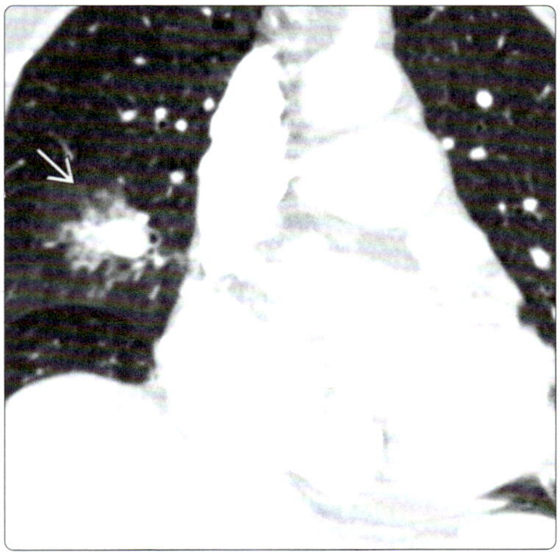

(Left) *AP chest radiograph in a patient with hemoptysis shows a pulmonary artery catheter coursing distal to the right interlobar pulmonary artery with tip in the right middle or lower lobe pulmonary artery.* **(Right)** *Coronal reformat CECT (lung window) in the same patient shows a ground-glass halo surrounding a pseudoaneurysm, consistent with perilesional parenchymal hemorrhage.*

KEY FACTS

TERMINOLOGY

- Acute obstruction of pulmonary arteries secondary to systemic venous clot

IMAGING

- CXR
  - Most often normal
  - Hampton hump due to peripheral infarct with associated ipsilateral pleural effusion
  - Westermark sign: Focal oligemia due to proximal pulmonary artery (PA) obstruction
- Ventilation/perfusion scan: Mismatched perfusion defects
- Pulmonary CTA
  - Imaging modality of choice: Filling defect(s) in pulmonary arterial system
  - Typically central filling defect; may distend artery
  - Right ventricular:left ventricular diameter ratio > 1 suggests right heart strain; poor prognosis
- Dual-energy pulmonary CTA
  - Iodine maps increase sensitivity for small, peripheral pulmonary emboli

TOP DIFFERENTIAL DIAGNOSES

- Flow artifact
- Chronic thromboembolic pulmonary hypertension
- Tumor thrombus/embolus
- Primary PA sarcoma

PATHOLOGY

- 70% of patients with pulmonary embolism (PE) have lower extremity deep vein thrombosis

CLINICAL ISSUES

- Symptoms: Dyspnea, chest pain, tachycardia
- Risk factors: Immobilization, pregnancy, malignancy
- Treatments
  - Anticoagulation [vitamin K antagonists (warfarin), low-molecular-weight heparin, novel oral anticoagulants]
  - Thrombolysis; embolectomy

(Left) *Axial NECT as part of a dissection CT protocol in a 28-year-old woman who passed out during the Baltimore marathon shows high-density filling defects in the pulmonary arteries (PAs).* **(Right)** *Axial CECT at the level of the main PA (MPA) shows acute dilation of the MPA measuring 3.4 cm, which is larger than the adjacent ascending aorta, which measures 2.7 cm. Massive bilateral acute pulmonary emboli (PE) are again seen.*

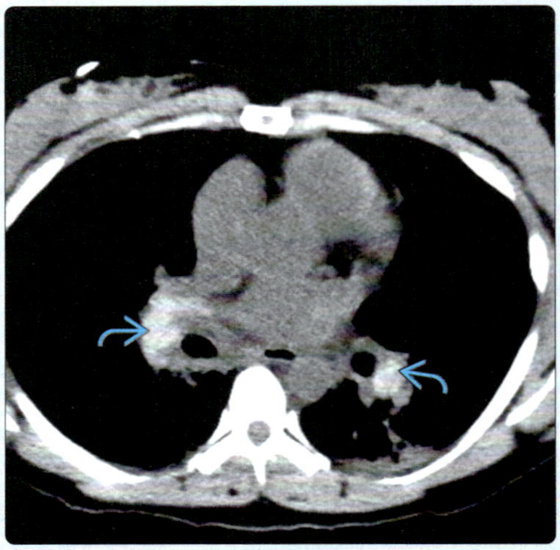

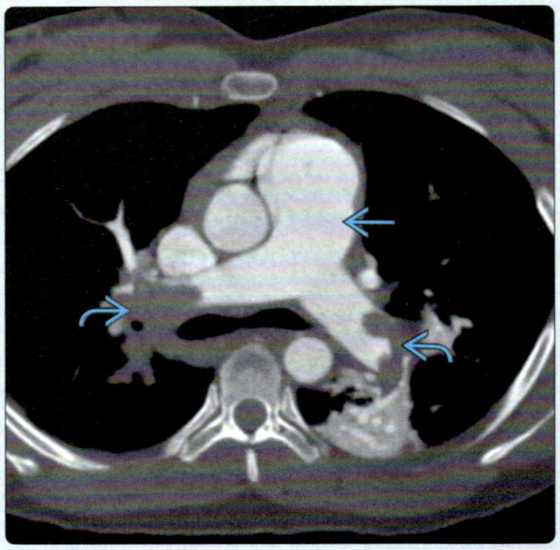

(Left) *Contrast-enhanced portion of the dissection protocol CT shows massive acute PE bilaterally.* **(Right)** *Four-chamber arterial-phase CECT shows findings of right heart strain, including right ventricular (RV) and right atrial (RA) dilation and flattening of the interventricular septum.*

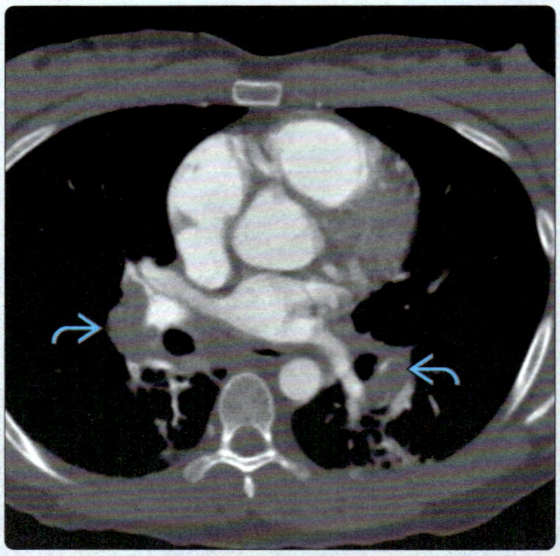

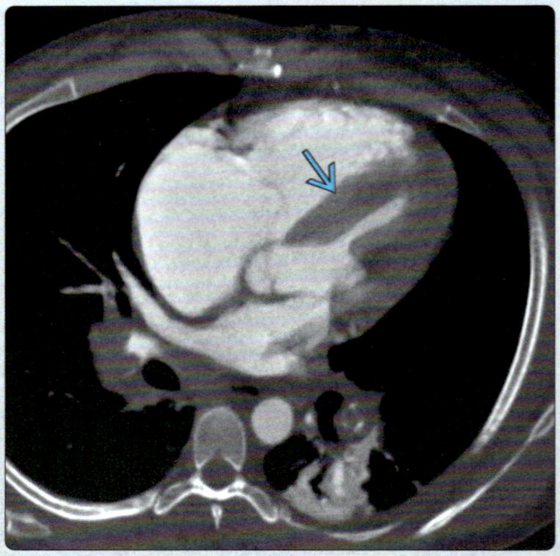

TERMINOLOGY

Abbreviations

- Pulmonary embolism (PE)

Definitions

- Acute obstruction of pulmonary arteries (PAs) most often secondary to systemic venous clot

IMAGING

General Features

- Best diagnostic clue
  - Filling defect within PAs on imaging
- Location
  - PAs
- Size
  - Variable
- Morphology
  - Located centrally within vessel
  - May occlude and expand vessel
  - Sharp interface with intravascular contrast material
  - Saddle embolus: Large embolus that straddles main PA bifurcation

Radiographic Findings

- Radiography
  - Most often normal or nonspecific findings
    - Primarily exclude other causes of symptoms
  - Signs of vascular alteration
    - Westermark sign: Segmental, lobar, or multilobar lucency (oligemia) distal to obstructed PA
      - Can be seen with acute or chronic PE
      - Can occur due to hypoxic vasoconstriction from small airways disease
  - Signs of pulmonary infarct
    - Hampton hump: Peripheral, wedge-shaped opacity with apex pointing toward hilum
      - Usually in lower lungs
      - < 15% of embolic events result in infarction
      - Gradually decrease in size over weeks to months with residual linear scar or pleural thickening
    - Pleural effusion ipsilateral to Hampton hump

CT Findings

- CT pulmonary angiography (CTPA) is examination of choice
  - Highly sensitive and specific with high interobserver agreement
  - Directly demonstrates clot (filling defect) in PA and helps to assess overall clot burden
    - Occlusive
      - Fills entire lumen and may expanded vessel diameter
    - Nonocclusive
      - Filling defect within center of vessel surrounded by contrast
      - Subacute or chronic clot commonly along periphery of vessel
  - Most common in lower lobes, given blood flow
  - Other findings
    - Right heart strain
      - Good predictor of mortality
      - Increased right ventricular:left ventricular (RV:LV) diameter ratio (> 1 in axial plane; > 0.9 in 4-chamber reconstruction)
      - Straightening or bowing of interventricular septum toward LV
      - Reflux of contrast material into distended inferior vena cava (IVC) and hepatic veins
      - RV should not be hypertrophied in acute PE
      - If RV is hypertrophied, findings may be related to acute on chronic PE or other underlying cause of longstanding pulmonary hypertension (PH)
      - Reversal of blood flow across patent foramen ovale (PFO), if present, may lead to systemic embolization of PE
    - Visualization of clot elsewhere
      - Clot in superior vena cava (SVC), internal jugular or subclavian veins
      - RV clot
      - IVC clot often difficult to see due to nonopacified blood flow
      - Right atrial clot may be difficult to differentiate from IVC inflow
      - Clot attached to central venous catheter or device
    - Pulmonary infarct
      - Peripheral, wedge-shaped opacity, often with surrounding ground-glass opacity
      - May have "bubbly" central lucencies due to necrosis
      - Ipsilateral pleural effusion common
  - Negative CTPA outcomes are good (< 1% subsequent embolic rate), as negative study should essentially exclude PE
    - However, errors in diagnosis are not uncommon
      - Errors due to lack of radiologist detection with isolated or distal PE
      - Errors due to technical shortcomings, i.e., bad bolus, incorrect parameters, etc.
      - Errors due to patient factors, i.e., respiratory motion, morbid obesity
    - Artificial intelligence may help detection of PE
- Dual-energy, spectral, or photon-counting CTPA
  - Iodine maps or pulmonary blood volume images show peripheral, wedge-shaped perfusion defects in distribution of PE
    - Improves detection for peripheral PEs
      - Using narrow window on lung windows can create iodine map-like image without dual energy
    - Correlates with other signs of RV dysfunction and PA obstruction
    - Ventilation/perfusion (V/Q) scan, PE must be occlusive for perfusion defect on iodine map
    - Iodine map does not differentiate between hypoperfusion secondary to vascular occlusion vs. hypoxic vasoconstriction

MR Findings

- MRA
  - Prospective Investigation of PE Diagnosis III (PIOPED III): Gadolinium-enhanced MRA
    - Considered only in patients with contraindications to standard tests in experienced centers
    - Technically inadequate study in 25% of patients

  - Sensitivity 78%, specificity 99% in adequate studies
- Filling defect(s) in PA system similar to CTPA
- MR cine
  - Paradoxical systolic motion of interventricular septum if RV pressure is elevated
  - Dilated right heart chambers and PAs

Ultrasonographic Findings

- Doppler US with compression is helpful when lower or upper extremity deep venous thrombosis (DVT) is suspected

Echocardiographic Findings

- Echocardiogram
  - Useful in assessing RV dysfunction and other parameters
    - RV dysfunction: RV hypokinesia, paradoxical septal systolic motion, or RV dilatation
    - PA systolic pressure (PASP) > 25 mmHg at rest is indicative of pulmonary arterial hypertension
    - Tricuspid annular systolic plane excursion (TAPSE) ≤ 15 mm identifies patients with increased risk of 30-day acute PE mortality or rescue thrombolysis

Angiographic Findings

- Now primarily performed for catheter-directed thrombectomy or thrombolysis and for right heart and PA pressure measurements
- 25% false-negative for small subsegmental emboli
- Poor interobserver agreement (30%) for subsegmental emboli

Nuclear Medicine Findings

- V/Q scan findings
  - Abnormal perfusion and normal ventilation result in "mismatched" perfusion defect in PE
  - High sensitivity but poor specificity
    - Normal perfusion scan typically excludes embolus
    - Matched defect can occur with pulmonary infarct
    - Other causes of V/Q mismatch include vasculitis, external compression of PA, PH, and fibrosing mediastinitis
  - Modified PIOPED II criteria
    - Defect size
      - Large defect: Occupies > 75% of segment
      - Moderate defect: Occupies 25-75% of segment
      - Small defect: Occupies < 25% of segment
    - High probability of PE
      - ≥ 2 large segmental mismatched defects (2 moderate defects = 1 large defect)
    - No evidence of PE
      - Normal perfusion
      - 1-3 small, segmental defects
      - Perfusion defect smaller than corresponding CXR finding
      - Solitary triple-matched defect in mid- and upper lung zone confined to single segment
      - Stripe sign around perfusion defects
      - Pleural effusion ≥ 1/3 of pleural cavity with no other perfusion defects in either lung
      - ≥ 2 matched V/Q defects with regionally normal CXR and areas of normal perfusion elsewhere in lung
    - Nondiagnostic
      - All other findings, including intermediate or indeterminate probability
  - Prospective Investigative Study of Acute Pulmonary Embolism Diagnosis (PISAPED) (when no ventilation performed)
    - Increased use of perfusion only scans, especially during and after COVID-19 pandemic
    - Normal
      - No perfusion defects
    - Near normal
      - Perfusion defects ≤ size and shape to following CXR abnormalities: Enlarged cardiovascular, mediastinal, and hilar structures; elevated diaphragm; blunting of costophrenic angle &/or pleural thickening; fissural fluid
    - Abnormal, PE positive
      - Single or multiple wedge-shaped perfusion defects ± matching CXR abnormalities
    - Abnormal, PE negative
      - Single or multiple perfusion nonwedge-shaped perfusion defects ± matching CXR abnormalities

Imaging Recommendations

- Best imaging tool
  - CTPA is study of choice for suspected acute PE
    - V/Q scan for patients with iodinated contrast allergy or renal failure
    - V/Q still recommended as first study for evaluation of chronic thromboembolic PH (CTEPH)
  - In pregnant patients without leg symptoms
    - V/Q scan is preferred if normal CXR
    - CTPA is preferred if abnormal CXR
- Protocol advice
  - Usually performed with bolus tracking with scan triggered automatically at preset attenuation in region of interest
    - Bolus tracker region of interest usually placed in main PA
    - In patients with known right heart failure, consider placement in left atrium to ensure complete transit of contrast through PA system
  - Thin collimation, ≤ 1 mm, with coronal/sagittal ± MIP reformats
  - Consider reduced kV protocols for nonobese patients
    - Try to avoid 140 kV unless using photon-counting CT due to decreased contrast attenuation
  - Fixed or weight-based IV contrast dosing, usually at rate of at least ≥ 4 mL/sec
    - Consider higher rate with obese patients
  - Scanning in caudal to cranial direction may decrease motion artifact at bases, where most PE occur
    - High-pitch helical acquisition, if available, can reduce respiratory and cardiac motion artifacts
  - Use multienergy CT if available

DIFFERENTIAL DIAGNOSIS

Chronic Thromboembolic Pulmonary Hypertension

- Often misdiagnosed as acute PE
- Contraction of vessels with occlusion
- Webs and bands

- RV hypertrophy
- May coexist with acute PE

Flow Artifact

- Low-attenuation filling defect with ill-defined margins; may be higher attenuation than PE
- Main causes
  - Early bolus, often in setting of right heart failure
  - Bronchial artery inflow from chronic vascular or lung disease
  - Slow flow related to parenchymal lung disease, usually chronic, such as fibrosis, emphysema, etc.
  - Congenital heart disease with Fontan circuit
    - SVC flow directed toward one PA, and IVC flow directed toward other
    - CPTA often shows intense opacification of PA branches in one lung and no to minimal opacification of other
  - Slow flow related to pulmonary vein stenosis
- Clues
  - No or little opacification of left atrium is clue to incomplete contrast circulation through pulmonary system
  - Filling defect localized to areas of severe lung disease should raise possibility of flow artifact
- Very important to recognize; otherwise, people may be put on lifelong anticoagulation

Tumor Embolism

- Common primaries include renal cell and hepatocellular carcinoma
- Can demonstrate enhancement; iodine uptake is seen in dual-energy CT; bland thrombus can coexist
- Grow despite anticoagulation
- Dilated, beaded PAs

Pulmonary Artery Sarcoma

- Irregular, lobulated, and wall adherent; may extend across wall
  - Consider PA sarcoma in any clot in main PA, especially if extending across pulmonary valve into RV outflow tract
- May enhance; iodine uptake in dual-energy CT scans; bland thrombus can coexist
- Persistent and grows despite anticoagulation

PATHOLOGY

General Features

- Etiology
  - 70% of patients with PE have lower-extremity DVT

Gross Pathologic and Surgical Features

- Hemodynamic effects: > 50% vascular bed reduction causes PH &/or right heart failure

Microscopic Features

- Pulmonary infarct: Focal necrosis, hemorrhage, and edema involve alveolar wall, bronchi, and vessels

CLINICAL ISSUES

Presentation

- Most common signs/symptoms
  - Dyspnea, chest pain, tachycardia
- Clinical profile
  - Decision support tool, such as Wells criteria, is helpful to determine pretest likelihood of PE
  - Negative high-sensitivity D-dimer test and absence of high pretest probability effectively exclude PE

Demographics

- Age
  - All groups; increased incidence in older patients
- Epidemiology
  - Risk factors
    - Immobilization
      - Hospitalization &/or surgery; long distance air travel
    - Pregnancy or contraceptive medications
    - Malignancy (4% with incidental PE at routine CT)
    - Obesity
    - Congenital hypercoagulable state
    - Indwelling central venous catheters
    - Trauma

Natural History and Prognosis

- 15-30% mortality without appropriate anticoagulation
- Unknown outcomes for untreated subsegmental PE

Treatment

- Anticoagulation is mainstay of treatment
  - Hemorrhagic complications in 2-15%
- Thrombolysis for severely symptomatic patients
- Catheter or surgical embolectomy in selected high-risk patients

SELECTED REFERENCES

1. de Jong CMM et al: Modern imaging of acute pulmonary embolism. Thromb Res. 238:105-16, 2024
2. Hahn LD et al: Multidisciplinary approach to chronic thromboembolic pulmonary hypertension: role of radiologists. Radiographics. 43(2):e220078, 2023
3. Ahuja J et al: Pitfalls in the imaging of pulmonary embolism. Semin Ultrasound CT MR. 43(3):221-9, 2022
4. Expert Panel on Cardiac Imaging et al: ACR Appropriateness Criteria® suspected pulmonary embolism: 2022 update. J Am Coll Radiol. 19(11S):S488-501, 2022
5. Freund Y et al: Acute pulmonary embolism: a review. JAMA. 328(13):1336-45, 2022
6. Derenoncourt PR et al: Ventilation-perfusion scan: a primer for practicing radiologists. Radiographics. 41(7):2047-70, 2021
7. Soffer S et al: Deep learning for pulmonary embolism detection on computed tomography pulmonary angiogram: a systematic review and meta-analysis. Sci Rep. 11(1):15814, 2021
8. Henry TS et al: Smoke: how to differentiate flow-related artifacts from pathology on thoracic computed tomographic angiography. J Thorac Imaging. 34(5):W109-20, 2019

(Left) *This 41-year-old man presented with sharp left-sided chest pain. PA CXR (left) shows a nodular opacity in the left lower lobe (LLL) ➔ with an associated small effusion. The possibility of a pulmonary infarct with Hampton hump was raised. Coronal CT obtained soon after (right) shows the acute PE in the lateral segment of the LLL ➔ with an associated infarct ➔.* **(Right)** *Axial CT show infarcts in the lateral and anteromedial segments ➔. Central "bubbly" lucencies are related to necrosis. A small left effusion ➔ is seen.*

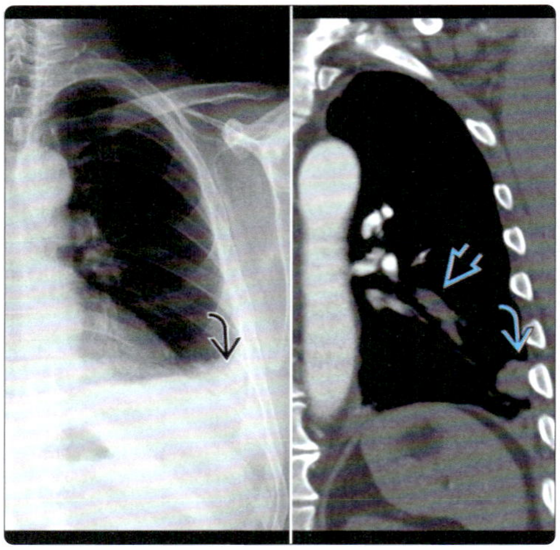

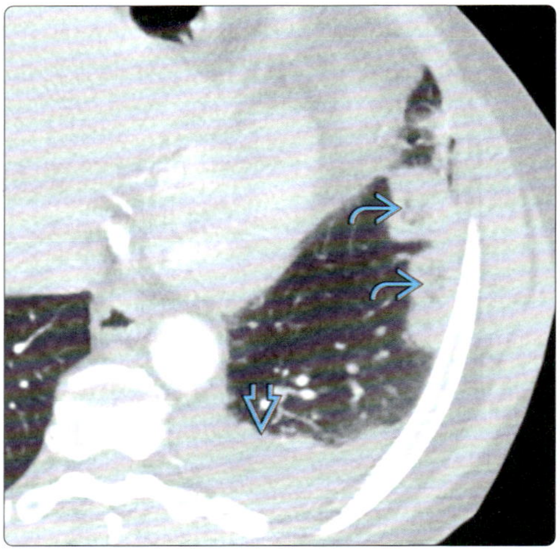

(Left) *Dual-energy CTPA shows occlusion of the right middle lobe PA ➔ (left). This is associated with complete hypoperfusion of the right middle lobe on iodine map (center). However, creating a narrow lung window (right) can also show the hypoperfusion due to PE.* **(Right)** *Axial image in the same patient shows a nonocclusive PE in the LLL ➔. Because the clot is nonocclusive, there will be no perfusion defects on the iodine map.*

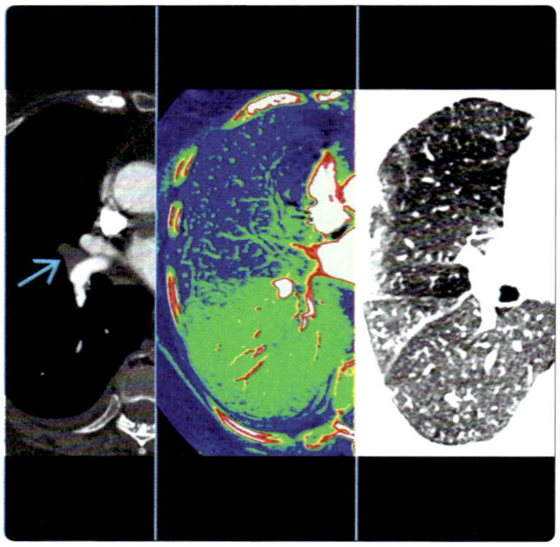

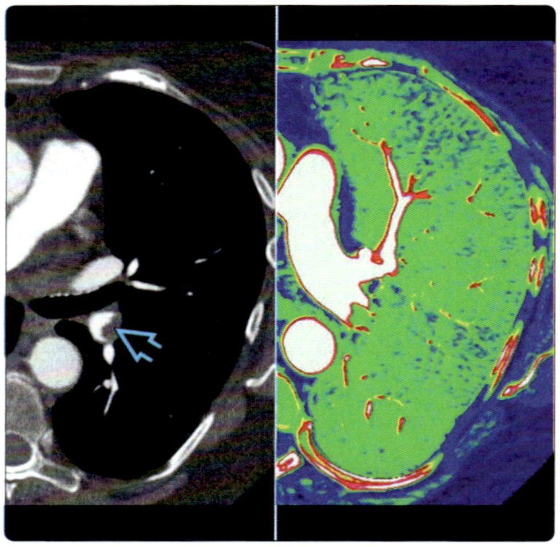

(Left) *Image shows clot in the right PA (RPA) ➔ and multiple areas of pulmonary infarct ➔. There is right-to-left flow across the patent foramen ovale (PFO) ➔. Additionally, there is systemic embolization of clot in the descending thoracic aorta ➔.* **(Right)** *Four-chamber image obtained during systole shows marked dilation of the right heart with inversion of the interventricular septum ➔ and right-to-left flow of blood across a small PFO ➔. There are extensive bilateral acute PE, some ➔ of which is visualized on the right.*

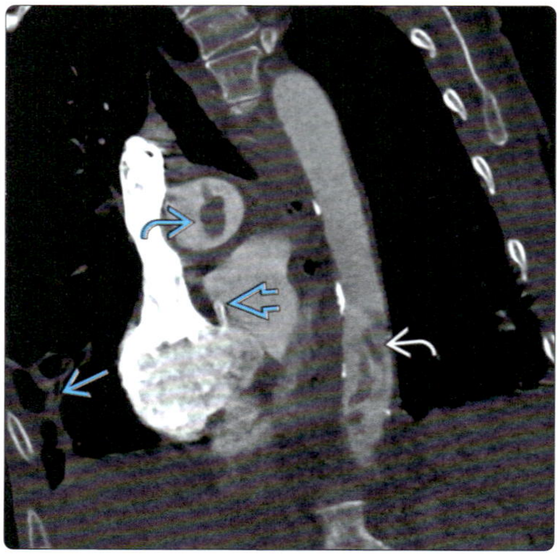

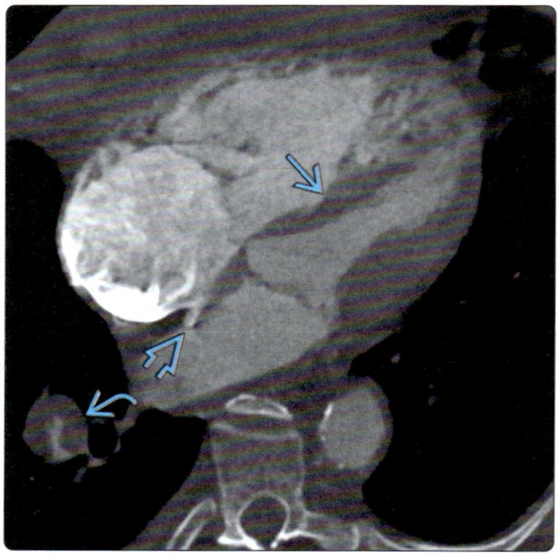

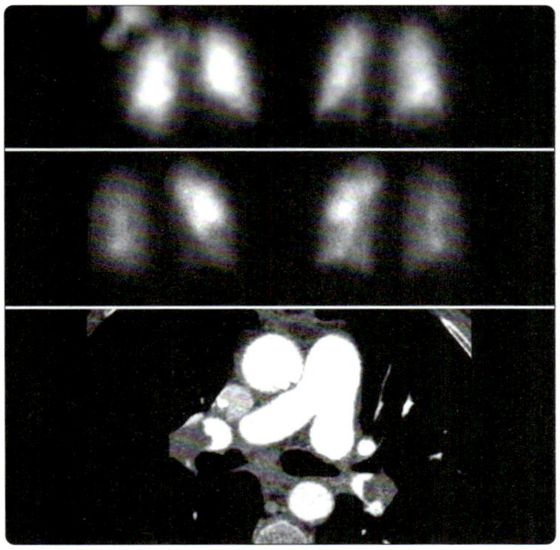

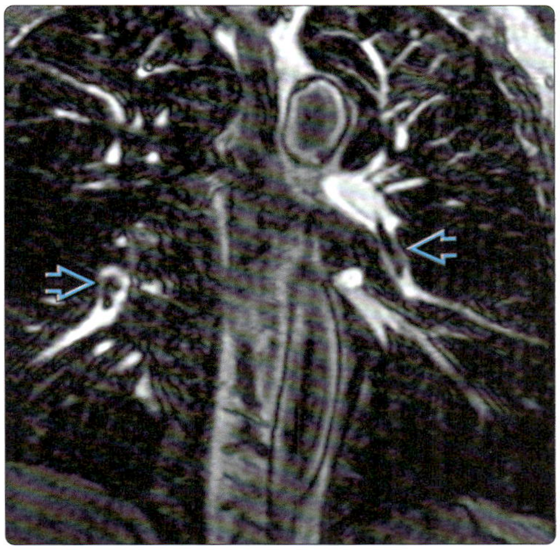

(Left) *Ventilation (V, top) and perfusion (Q, middle) images show normal V with multiple bilateral segmental and subsegmental perfusion defects. Numerous other defects were seen on additional views. Image from a CTA obtained 1 day later shows extensive bilateral PE.* **(Right)** *Gadolinium-enhanced MRA shows bilateral endoluminal signal voids (black) surrounded by a gadolinium-enhanced blood pool, consistent with acute PE →.*

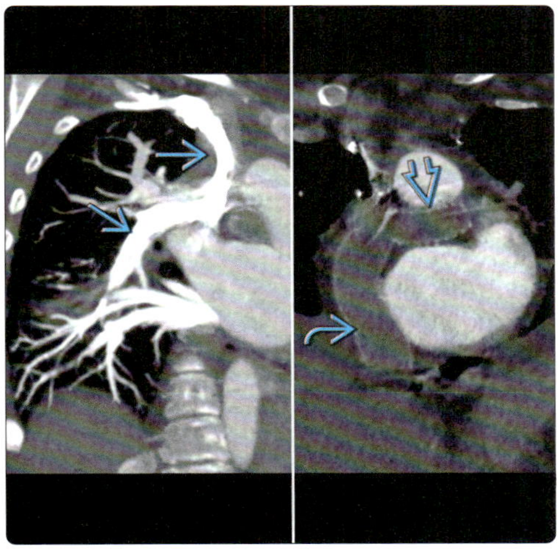

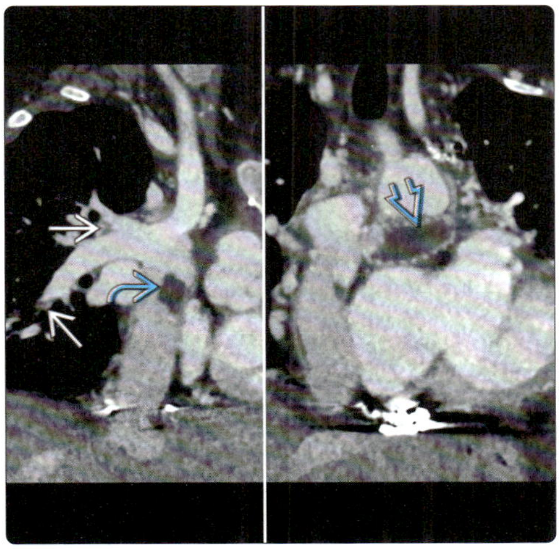

(Left) *Images in a patient s/p Fontan show high-attenuation contrast in the superior vena cava (SVC) directed into the RPA →, obscuring the vasculature. Blood in the inferior vena cava (IVC) →, which supplies the left PA (LPA) →, is unopacified. One cannot diagnose or exclude PE on the left.* **(Right)** *Repeat study done with a modified injection protocol shows homogeneous PA opacification and chronic PE → on the right. There is adherent thrombus in the Fontan → with occlusion of the LPA graft →.*

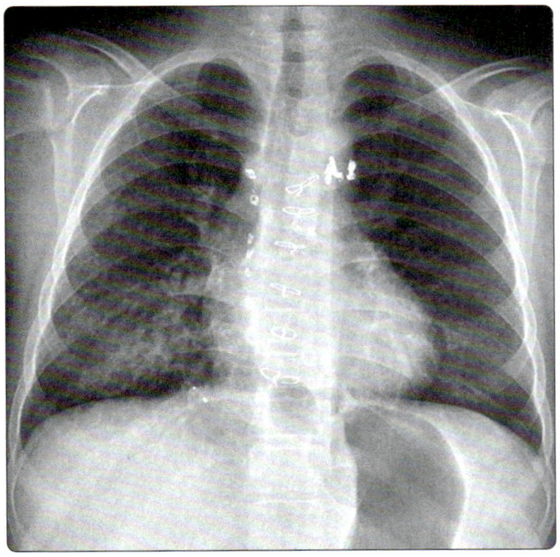

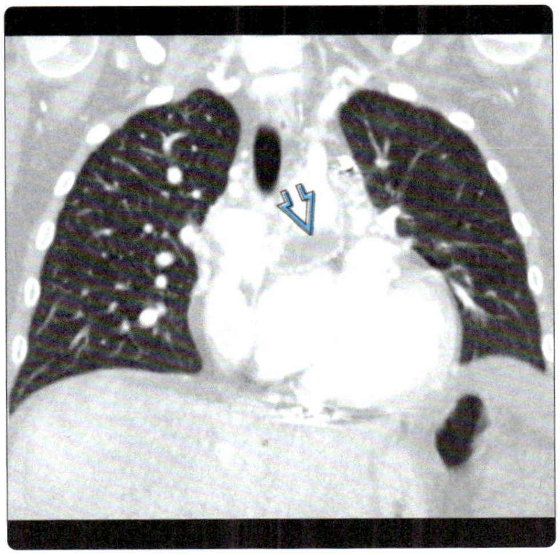

(Left) *PA radiograph in the patient with hypoplastic left heart s/p Fontan shows marked oligemia in the left lung (Westermark sign) compared to the right lung.* **(Right)** *Coronal image from a CTA shows the diffuse oligemia in the left lung compared to the right secondary to occlusion of the LPA graft →.*

(Left) *This 82-year-old presented with stroke and dyspnea. Cardiac CT shows bilateral acute PE with a worm-like thrombus in the RA prolapsing into the RV. The clot crosses a PFO leading to the stroke. Right heart strain is present.* **(Right)** *Short-axis image though the atria in an 82-year-old woman with massive bilateral PE and a stroke shows a large, worm-like RA clot extending through a PFO into the left atrium.*

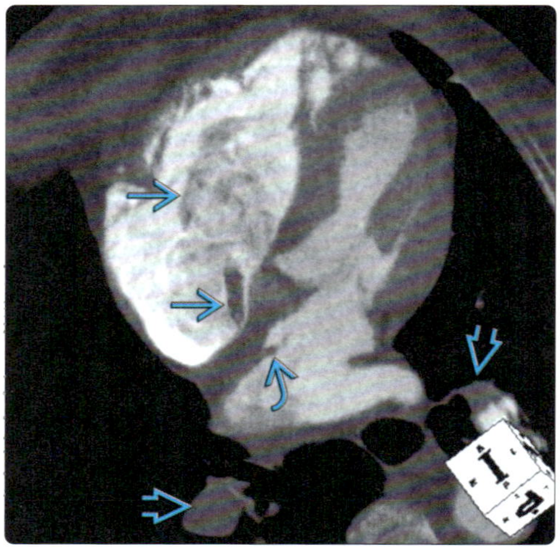

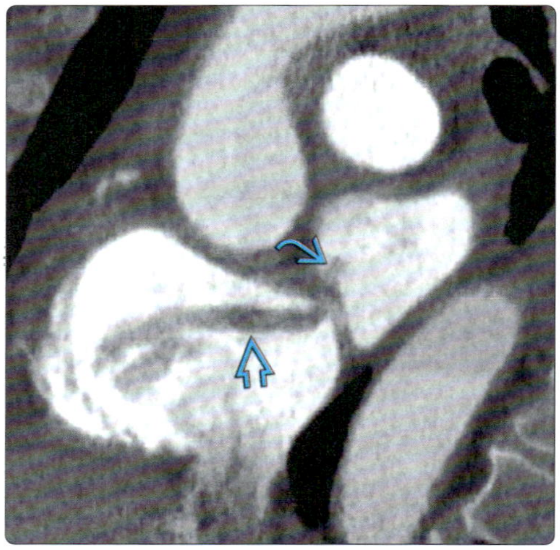

(Left) *Image obtained during surgery shows the RA clot extending through the PFO.* **(Right)** *MRA angiography shows 1 of many acute PEs in a 32-year-old woman with dyspnea and a history of anaphylaxis with iodinated contrast.*

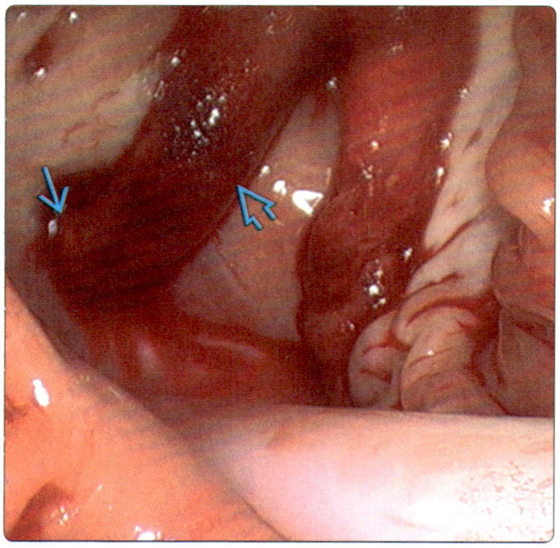

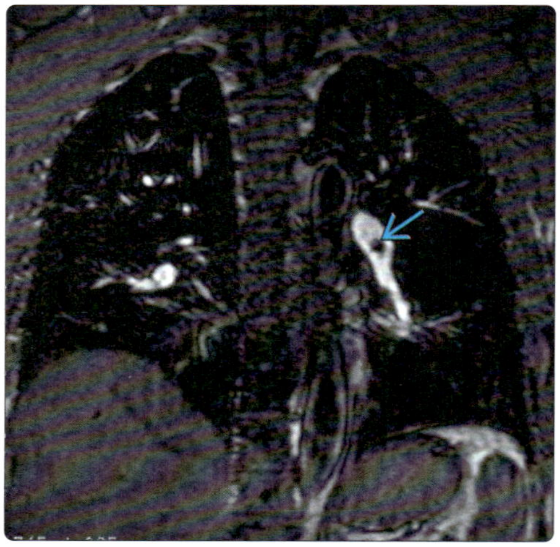

(Left) *CT in a man with dyspnea shows a large expansile unilateral filling defect in the left main PA. There was no PE on the right. While findings are concerning for PA sarcoma, lower-extremity US showed a DVT. Patient was treated with anticoagulation (A/C).* **(Right)** *CTA 6 weeks later shows significant decrease in the size of the PE, which has concave margins. A PA sarcoma will not decrease in size after A/C. The patient underwent thromboendarterectomy, which removed bland thrombus (inset).*

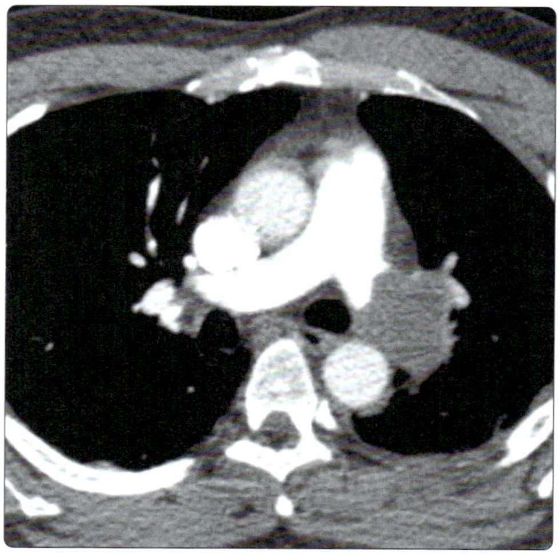

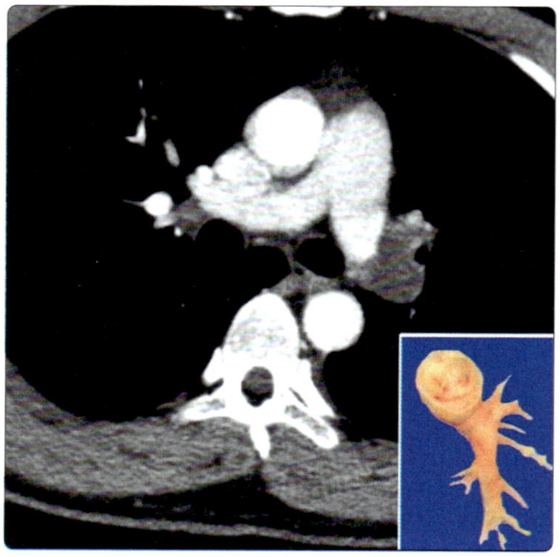

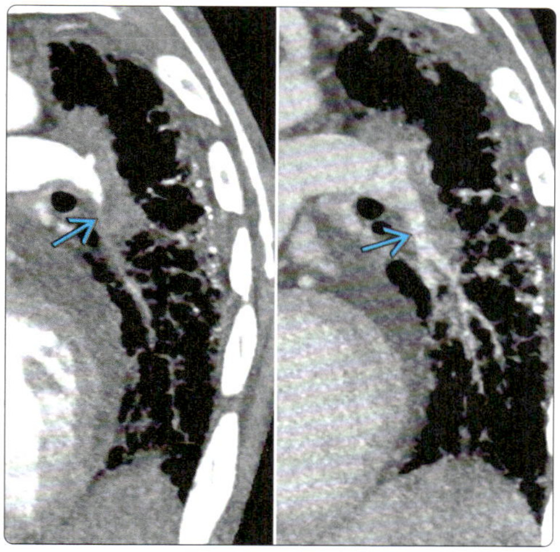

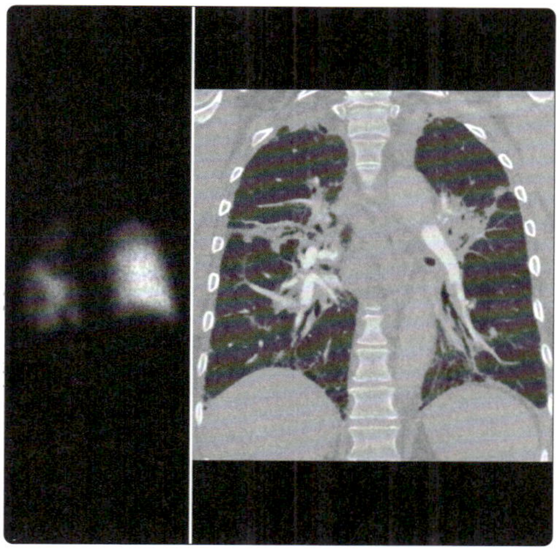

(Left) *Patient with idiopathic pulmonary fibrosis underwent CTPA. Overnight, the exam is interpreted as positive due to apparent LLL basilar branch occlusion upstream from severe fibrosis. Recognizing this as likely artifact, the patient returned for repeat portal venous-phase study (right), which showed no PE.* **(Right)** *V/Q perfusion image (left) shows multiple large left-sided perfusion defects with high probability of PE. Ventilation was normal. CTPA (right) shows no PE. Perfusion defects were from vascular compression from sarcoid.*

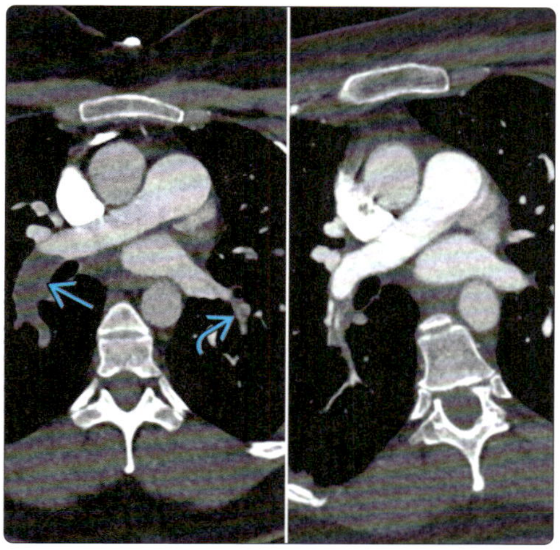

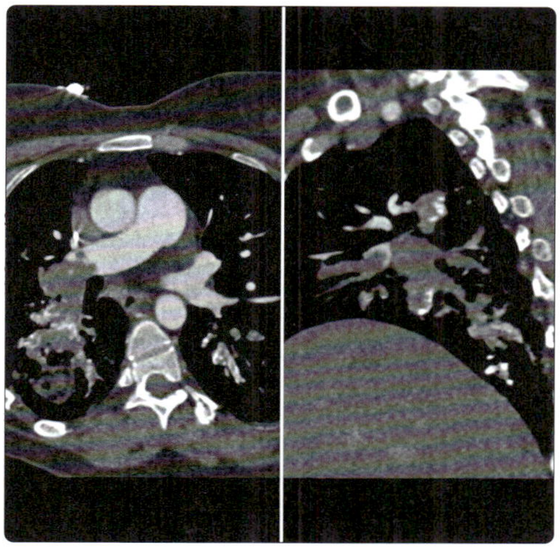

(Left) *CT (L) shows acute PE with the occlusive right lower lobe (RLL) embolus causing vascular distension and central location of nonocclusive filling defects elsewhere. CT 6 months later (R) shows evolution to chronic PE in RLL with the vascular contraction with webs and bands. Left-sided PEs resolved.* **(Right)** *Axial oblique (L) and sagittal (R) CTPA images in a patient with osteosarcoma show bilateral, RPA > LPA filling defects, some of which are ossified. Tumor emboli can mimic acute PE but will grow despite A/C.*

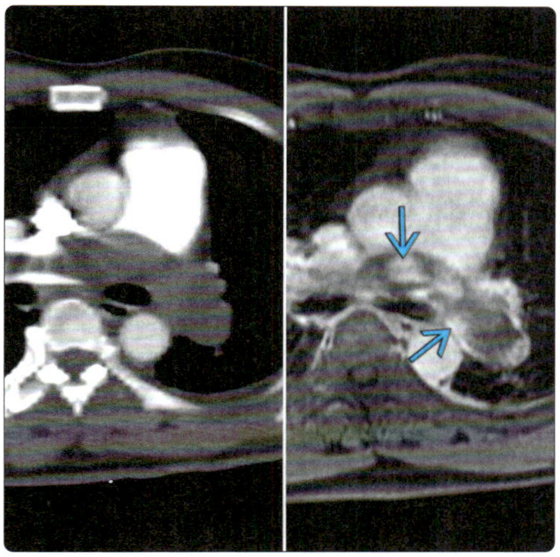

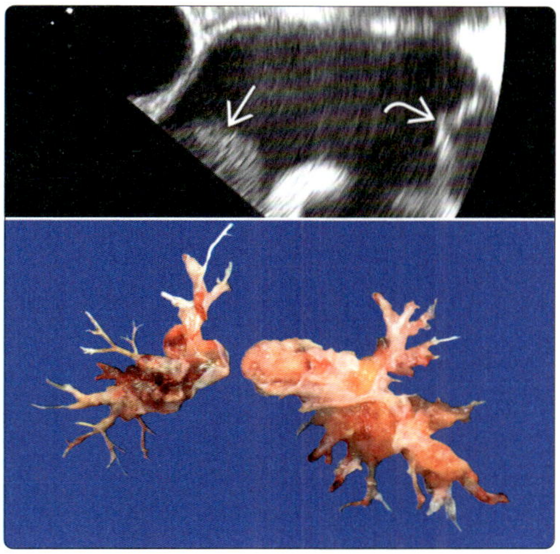

(Left) *CT image (left) shows a large saddle embolus with complete occlusion and expansion of the left MPA. Although this could be a large PE, the filling defect grew despite A/C. Follow-up MR (right) shows enhancement within the filling defect, which is a PA sarcoma.* **(Right)** *Intraoperative echocardiogram (top) shows the mass in the LPA. Pulmonary valve is shown. Bottom image shows the endarterectomy specimen, which was a poorly differentiated sarcoma.*

Pulmonary Hypertension: General Imaging Findings

KEY FACTS

TERMINOLOGY

- Pulmonary hypertension (PH)
- Mean pulmonary artery pressure (mPAP) > 20 mmHg

IMAGING

- Fleischner Society thresholds for suggestion of PH
  - Patients with high risk (> 10% chance of PH)
    - PA diameter of > 30 mm
    - PA:Ao ratio > 0.9
  - Patients at intermediate risk (1-10% chance of PH)
    - PA diameter of > 32 mm
    - PA:Ao ratio > 1
  - Patients at low risk (< 1% chance of PH)
    - PA diameter of > 34 mm
    - PA:Ao ratio > 1.1
- CT findings
  - RV hypertrophy (RVH) often with dilation
    - RV:LV diameter > 1 is considered abnormal
    - Systolic flattening or leftward bowing of interventricular septum (IVS)
  - RA dilation
  - Peripheral pulmonary vasculature
    - Segmental and subsegmental PA branches will be larger than adjacent bronchus
- MR findings
  - RVH and RA dilation
    - Systolic flattening or leftward bowing of IVS
    - Often secondary tricuspid regurgitation (TR)
  - LGE at right ventricular insertion points
  - Phase contrast imaging
    - Min PA area
    - PA flow, velocity, and vortical flow
    - Assessment of IVC and SVC retrograde flow
- Echocardiogram
  - Indirectly estimate PA pressures on TR jet velocity and TR gradient
- Right heart catheterization is gold standard

(Left) *Frontal (left) CXR shows pulmonary artery (PA) and right atrium (RA) dilation. Enlargement of the left heart border may be due to right or left ventricular (RV or LV) enlargement. On lateral CXR (right) decrease in the retrosternal airspace (RAS) suggests RV enlargement. Left atrium (LA) and LV are normal in size.* **(Right)** *Coronal (left) and sagittal (right) CECT show PA and RA dilation. RV dilation decreases the RAS. Chronic thromboembolic disease (CTEPH) is present.*

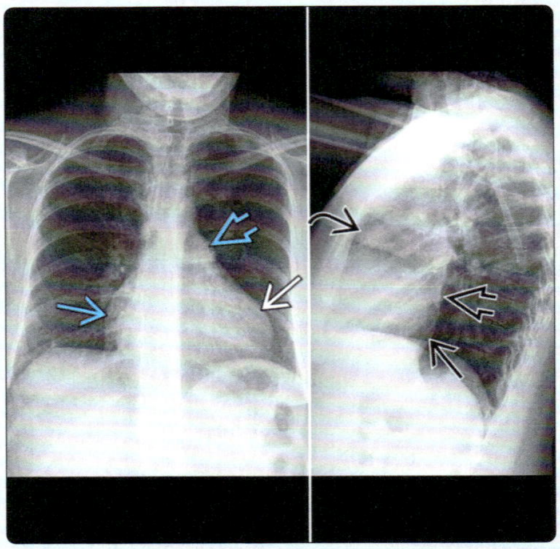

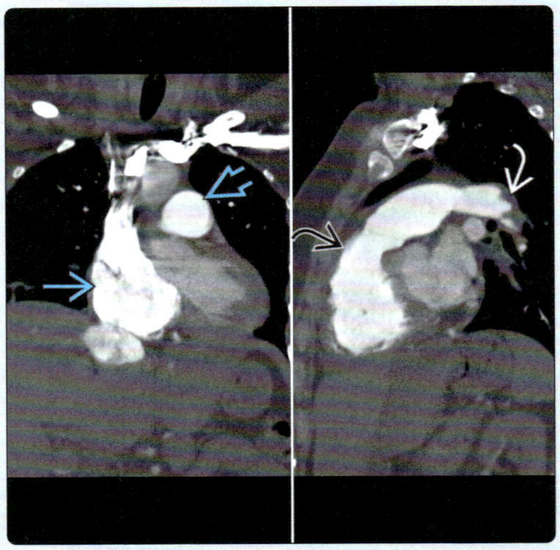

(Left) *Four-chamber view (L) shows RV dilation and hypertrophy (RVH). RV:LV ratio is 1.4. Note CTEPH findings. Axial CT (R) shows ↑ RA diameter of 8 cm. Septal flattening is due to ↑ RV pressures given systolic phase (closed tricuspid valve).* **(Right)** *PA diameter is only 2.7 cm but > aorta, suggesting pulmonary hypertension (PH) (L). Two-mm MIP (R) shows oligemia and hypoperfusion in areas with PA occlusion and adjacent hyperperfusion and dilated PA branches in preserved lung, which helps differentiate PH etiologies.*

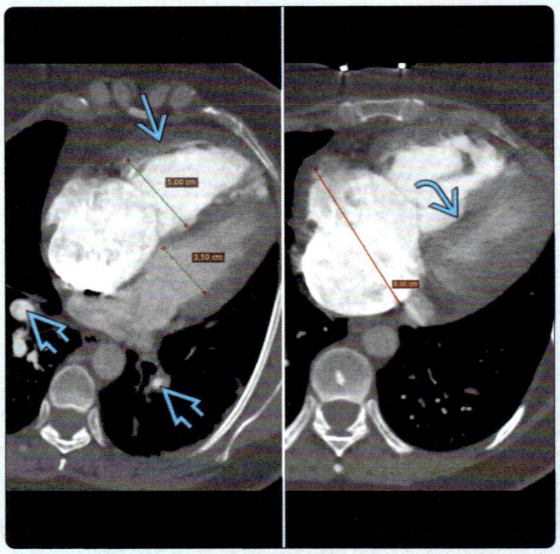

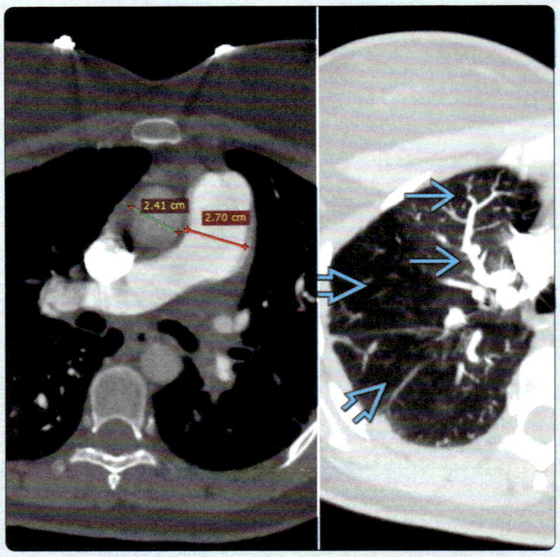

TERMINOLOGY

Abbreviations

- Pulmonary hypertension (PH)

Definitions

- Mean pulmonary artery pressure (mPAP) > 20 mmHg

IMAGING

General Features

- Best diagnostic clue
  - Enlarged main pulmonary artery (PA)
    - PA diameter > aortic diameter
  - Right ventricle (RV) hypertrophy
  - Dilated PA branches

Radiographic Findings

- Enlarged central PAs
- Dilation of RV and right atrium (RA)
  - Reduced retrosternal airspace on lateral
  - Prominent RA contour to right of spine on frontal
  - Difficult to differentiate RV from left ventricle (LV) enlargement on frontal
- Lung parenchyma and peripheral pulmonary vasculature can have variable appearance depending on etiology
  - Group 1 PH: Diffuse peripheral pruning or enlarged vessels extend to pleural surface
  - Group 2 PH: Dilated central vessels with cephalization and septal thickening
  - Group 3 PH: Upper lung oligemia in emphysema; reticulation and bronchiectasis in fibrosis
  - Group 4 PH: Regional areas of oligemia due to proximal vascular obstruction (Westermark sign)
  - Group 5 PH: Variable due to heterogeneity of causes
- Calcification of PAs may be present
  - May be difficult to see on radiograph

CT Findings

- Nonspecific findings of PH
- PA enlargement
  - Please note that majority of papers correlated findings using old definition of PH as > 25 mmHg
  - Ratio of main PA (MPA) to aorta (Ao) diameter >1
    - Specificity of 96% and positive predictive value of 95%
    - For patients < 50 years of age, PA/Ao ratio > 1 more closely correlated with PA pressures than PA size
  - PA diameter ≥ 29 mm
    - Average sensitivity and specificity of 71.9%
      - Near 100% if associated with segmental artery to bronchus ratio is > 1:1 in at least 3 pulmonary lobes
    - For patients > 50 years of age, enlarged PA diameter more closely correlated with PA pressures than PA:Ao ratio
  - Fleischner Society thresholds for suggestion of PH
    - Patients with high risk (> 10% chance of PH)
      - PA diameter of > 30 mm
      - PA:Ao ratio > 0.9
      - Conditions include left heart disease, chronic obstructive pulmonary disease, interstitial lung disease, obstructive sleep apnea, systemic sclerosis (SSc), chronic kidney disease requiring dialysis, congenital heart disease, sickle cell disease
    - Patients at intermediate risk (1-10% chance of PH)
      - PA diameter of > 32 mm; PA:Ao ratio >1
      - Conditions include connective tissue disease (excluding SSc systemic sclerosis), portal hypertension, prior pulmonary embolism, HIV infection, thalassemia, schistosomiasis
    - Patients at low risk (< 1% chance of PH)
      - PA diameter of > 34 mm
      - PA:Ao ratio > 1.1
- Findings of increased right heart pressures
  - Best assessed with ECG-gated cardiac CT with retrospective gating
    - If RV assessment is primary need, can set ROI for bolus tracker in left atrium or main PA
    - If biventricular assessment is desired, may need to adjust contrast injection technique
  - RV hypertrophy
    - RV free-wall thickness ≥ 6 mm
      - Can be measured along free wall or RV outflow tract (RVOT)
      - Sensitivity and specificity of 81% and 92% for PH, respectively
      - Can be difficult to assess on nongated study
  - RV dilation
    - RV:LV diameter > 1 is considered abnormal
      - Best measured on 4-chamber reconstruction
      - Ratio of ≥ 1.28 has sensitivity and specificity of 86% and 86% for PH, respectively
  - Flattening or leftward bowing of interventricular septum (IVS)
    - Best evaluated with ECG-gated cardiac CTA with retrospective gating
      - Systolic flattening due to elevated RV pressures
      - May be accompanied by diastolic flattening due to volume overload
    - On nongated studies, atrioventricular valves closed during systole and open during diastole
  - RA dilation
    - Due to increased RV pressures
    - Functional tricuspid valve (TV) regurgitation due to RV dilation
    - Subsequent superior vena cava and inferior vena cava (SVC and IVC) dilation
    - Threshold for RA enlargement
      - Transverse RA measurement parallel to TV plane
      - Men: ≥ 67 mm (AUC, 0.83)
      - Women: ≥ 64 mm (AUC, 0.93)
- In situ thrombus
  - Most common in pulmonary arterial hypertension (PAH)
  - Must differentiate from chronic thromboembolic pulmonary hypertension (CTEPH)
    - In situ thrombus does not typically lead to vascular occlusion
- Bronchial artery collaterals
  - Variable size depending on etiology

- Typically ↑ in CTEPH or patients with coronary artery disease
- PA calcifications
  - Most common in PAH
  - Most likely related to PA pressures rather than etiology
- Peripheral pulmonary vasculature
  - Segmental and subsegmental PA branches will be larger than adjacent bronchus
  - PA to bronchus ratio > 1 in 3 or 4 lobes has specificity of near 100% for PH
  - May not be accurate in CTEPH given proximal occlusions
- Parenchymal findings (please refer to dedicated PH chapters)
  - Parenchymal findings can help differentiate between etiologies of PH
  - Associated findings include
    - Group 1 PH: Periarteriolar and peribronchovascular ground-glass opacity (GGO) or centrilobular GG nodules
    - Group 2 PH: Septal thickening, perihilar predominant GGO due to pulmonary edema
    - Group 3 PH: Findings of smoking-related lung disease, pulmonary fibrosis, etc.
    - Group 4 PH: Mosaic perfusion with well-defined areas of oligemia directly adjacent to areas of normal or increased size in pulmonary vasculature
    - Group 5 PH: Variable depending on underlying etiology
- Pericardial effusion
  - Portends poor prognosis in PAH
  - Associated with severity of RV failure
  - Correlated best with mean RA pressures
  - Further compromises hemodynamics
    - Worsens inversion of IVS septal motion
    - Impairs LV filling and reduces cardiac output

MR Findings

- Helpful in making diagnosis of PH
- Morphologic changes in RA and RV better seen with MR
  - RV hypertrophy ± dilation; RA dilation
  - Assess RV and RA volumes and RV ejection fraction
- Systolic flattening or inversion of interventricular septum toward LV
  - Due to elevated RV pressures
  - Can see associated with diastolic flattening from increased RV volume
- LGE
  - LGE in RV insertion points in IVS
    - Need to differentiate from RV blood pool
    - Best seen on short-axis plane
- TR common
  - Often secondary to TV annular dilation
- Phase contrast imaging
  - PA area (A)
    - End-systolic area (Amax) and end-diastolic area (Amin)
    - Amin ≥ 6.6 cm^2 with sensitivity and specificity of PH diagnosis of 93% and 88%, respectively
    - Amin ≥ 6 cm^2 detected pulmonary vascular resistance > 3 Woods units (WU) with sensitivity/specificity of 96%/85%
  - PA distensibility
    - Relative cross-section area change (RAC) between Amax and Amin
    - Reduced in PH due to stiffness of vessel
    - Reduced RAC associated with increased mortality
  - PA flow
    - Reduced PA velocities associated with PH
    - Associated with PA dilation
    - Vortical flow in MPA associated with PH
      - Best evaluated with 4D flow imaging
  - IVC and SVC assessment
    - Retrograde flow in SVC and IVC during atrial contraction
    - Average mean velocity best associated with pulmonary vascular resistance
  - Please note that nearly all papers define PH as mPAP > 25 mmHg (older definition)

Echocardiographic Findings

- Similar to MR, echocardiogram is very powerful tool in helping make diagnosis of PH
- Can measure RV and RA volumes and function
- Can indirectly estimate PA pressures based on
  - TR jet velocity (TRV)
    - Measured at tricuspid valve
    - TRV > 2.8 m/s associated with PH
  - TR gradient (TRG)
    - TRG = 4 x TRV^2
    - TRV > 2.8 m/s = TRG > 31 mmHg
    - Using new definition, one large study recommends using TRG > 31 mmHg as cutoff for PH
      - Cutoff is same as with previous definition with PH of > 25 mmHg; however, lower accuracy
  - If TR jet absent, cannot measure

Angiographic Findings

- Right heart catheterization is gold standard for diagnosis of PH
- Normal values
  - Mean RA pressure = 1-5 mmHg
  - RV systolic pressure = 15-30 mmHg
  - RV diastolic pressure = 1-7 mmHg
  - PA systolic pressure = 15-30 mmHg
  - PA diastolic pressure = 4-12 mmHg
  - Mean PA pressure ~ 15 mmHg (> 20 mmHg defines PH)
  - Pulmonary capillary wedge pressure = 4-12 mmHg

Imaging Recommendations

- Best imaging tool
  - Echocardiogram is best initial tool for assessment of PH
  - CT and MR are complementary tools
  - Right heart catheterization is gold standard

SELECTED REFERENCES

1. Baranga L et al: In situ pulmonary arterial thrombosis: literature review and clinical significance of a distinct entity. AJR Am J Roentgenol. 221(1):57-68, 2023
2. Gall H et al: Validity of echocardiographic tricuspid regurgitation gradient to screen for new definition of pulmonary hypertension. EClinicalMedicine. 34:100822, 2021

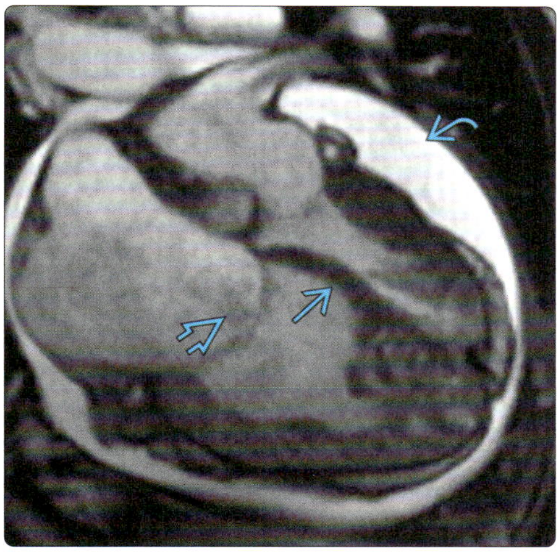

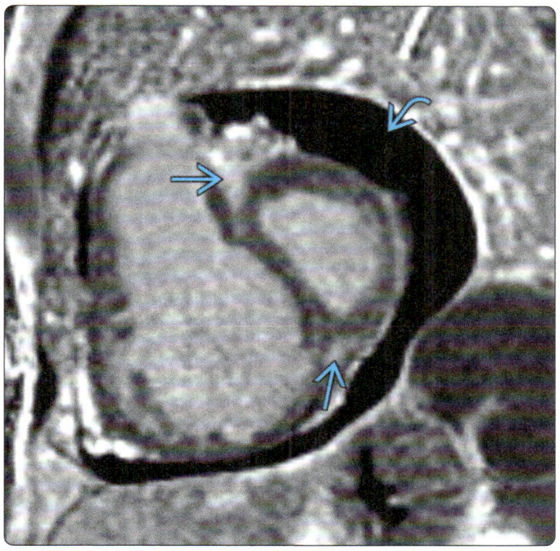

(Left) *Four-chamber view at end-systole (ES) in a 68-year-old woman with severe pulmonary arterial hypertension due to scleroderma shows marked enlargement of the RA and RV with RVH. There is inversion of the interventricular septum (IVS) to the left. A tricuspid regurgitant (TR) jet is partially visualized. A moderate pericardial effusion (PEff) is seen.* **(Right)** *There is pronounced LGE at the ventricular insertion points due to severe PH. Moderate PEff is low signal.*

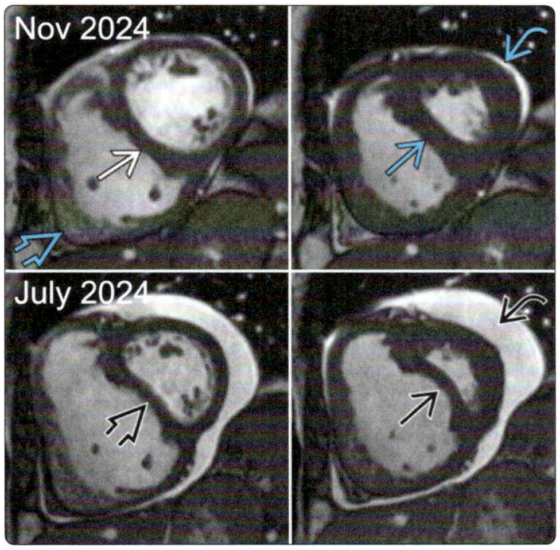

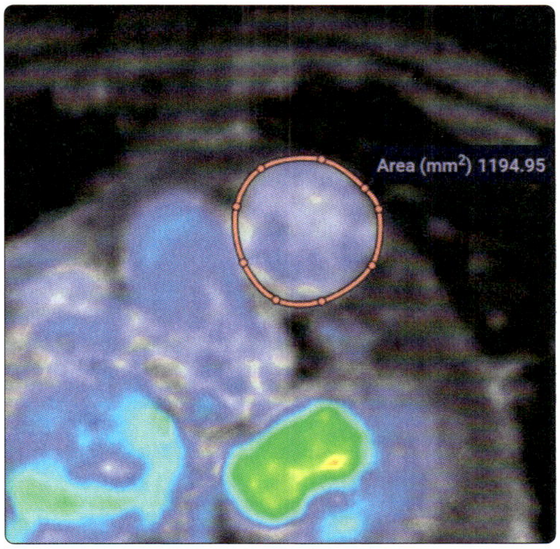

(Left) *MR from Nov 2023 (top row) shows RVH and dilation. The IVS is normal during end diastole (ED) and mildly flattened at ES. There is a small PEff. MR 7 months later (bottom) shows IVS inversion during ED and ES, some of which is related to the now moderate PEff. RV ejection fraction ↓ from 35% to 24%, and ED volume ↑ from 130 to 230 mL/m² in 7 months.* **(Right)** *Cross-section PA diameter and area at ED are 3.7 cm and 12 cm². Average PA velocity is 8 cm/sec. All metrics suggest PH.*

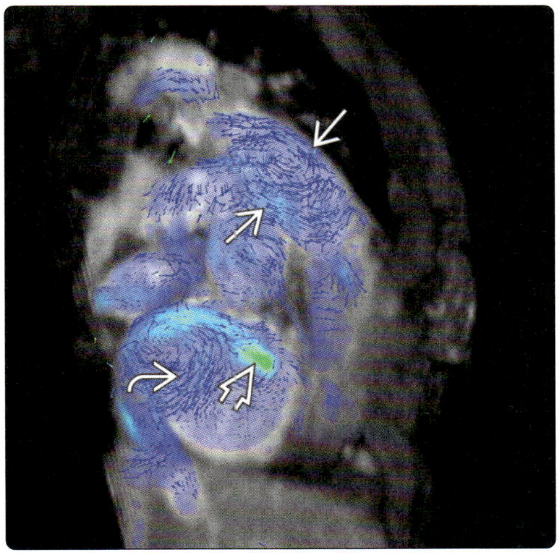

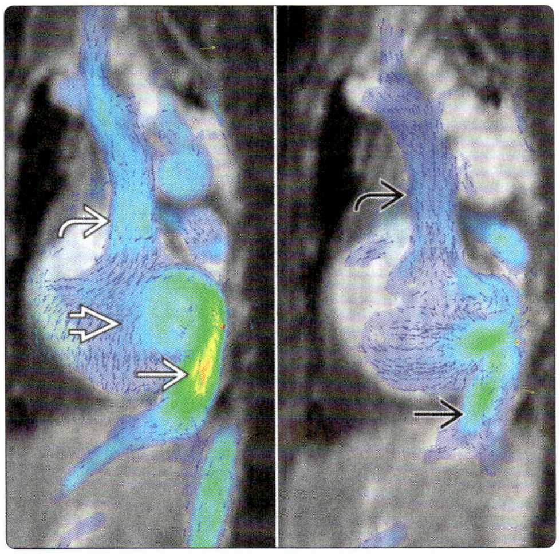

(Left) *Late systolic image shows vortical flow in the MPA and RA. A TR jet is partially visualized.* **(Right)** *With mitral valve opening, there is anterograde flow of blood from the superior vena cava (SVC) and inferior vena cava (IVC) into the RA, where there is vortical flow. During atrial contraction, there is conspicuous retrograde flow from the RA into the SVC and IVC. This finding is seen with PH.*

Group 1 Pulmonary Arterial Hypertension With Overt Features of Venous/Capillary Involvement

KEY FACTS

TERMINOLOGY

- Group 1.6 pulmonary arterial hypertension (PAH)
- Pulmonary venoocclusive disease (PVOD) and pulmonary capillary hemangiomatosis (PCH) previously considered distinct entities
- Recent studies suggest that majority of PCH cases are angioproliferative reaction to postcapillary venous obstruction rather than separate disease
- Similar to groups 1.1, 1.2, 1.3, 1.4 PAH, PVOD/PCH has idiopathic, genetic, and secondary causes

IMAGING

- Typical findings of PH, usually severe with superimposed
  - Symmetric mediastinal and hilar lymphadenopathy
  - Septal thickening
  - Ground-glass centrilobular nodularity: More well defined, smaller than periarteriolar ground glass seen in other causes of PAH
  - Normal left heart size; pleural effusions often absent
- Some cases indistinguishable from other causes of PAH

TOP DIFFERENTIAL DIAGNOSES

- Other causes of group 1 PAH
- Left heart failure with fluid overload in patient with underlying pulmonary hypertension
- Excipient lung disease (IV talcosis)
- Hypersensitivity pneumonitis
- Sarcoidosis

PATHOLOGY

- Venous fibrosis and obstruction (PVOD)
- Associated alveolar wall capillary proliferation (PCH)

CLINICAL ISSUES

- Equal sex distribution
- Poor prognosis
- Survival rates at 1, 3, and 5 years were 86%, 50%, and 27%, respectively
- Lung transplant is only treatment that can prevent death

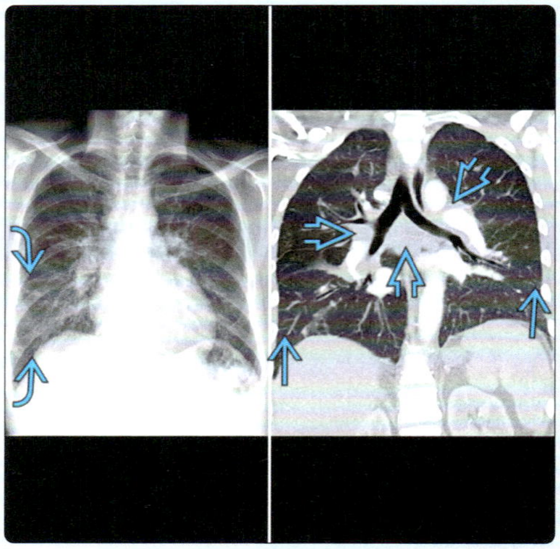

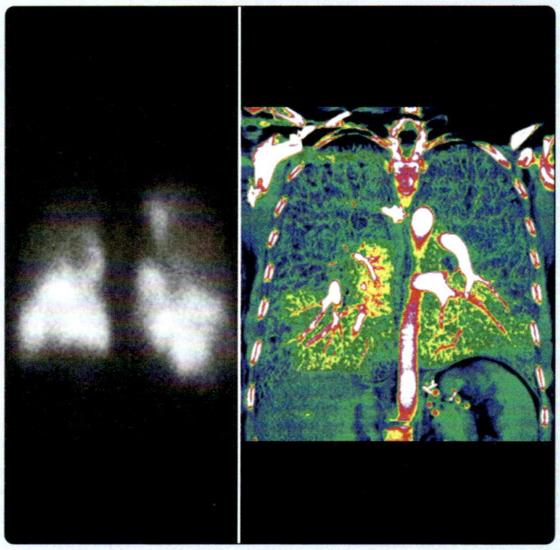

(Left) *PA CXR (L) in a 46-year-old woman shows pulmonary artery and hilar enlargement, bilateral septal thickening ➔, and absent pleural effusion. CTPA (R) showed no thromboembolic disease. Note lymphadenopathy ➔ and septal thickening ➔. No effusions are present. There is lower lobe-predominant ground-glass opacity.* **(Right)** *V/Q scan (L) and dual-energy CPTA (R) show diffuse upper lung hypoperfusion and lower lung hyperperfusion. Perfusion findings would be atypical for chronic thromboembolic pulmonary hypertension.*

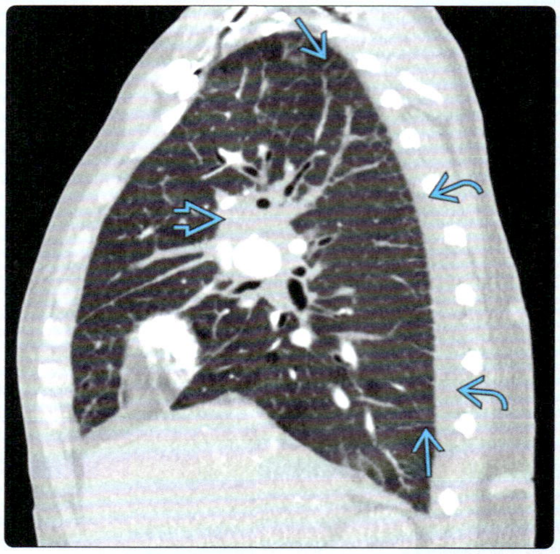

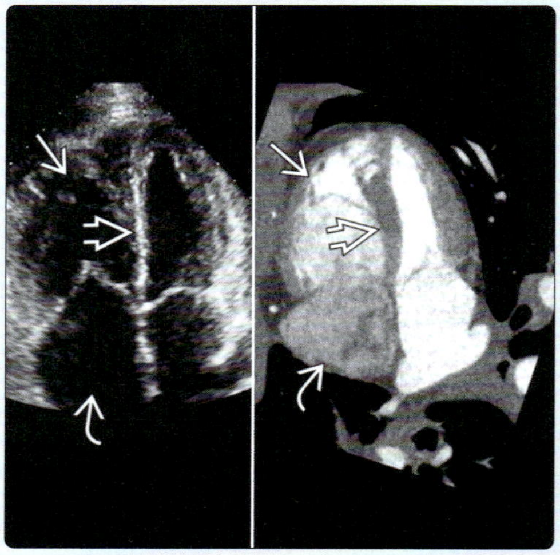

(Left) *Sagittal CECT in a patient after a controlled trial of epoprostenol (vasodilator) with worsening of dyspnea shows ↑ lymphadenopathy ➔, septal thickening ➔, and new bilateral effusions ➔, findings that are highly suggestive of pulmonary venoocclusive disease (PVOD).* **(Right)** *Echocardiogram (L) and coronary CTA (R) at end-systole show right ventricular dilation and hypertrophy ➔, right atrial dilation ➔, and leftward inversion of septum ➔. Left ventricular (LV) ejection fraction was 65%, further supporting PVOD.*

TERMINOLOGY

Abbreviations

- Pulmonary arterial hypertension (PAH)

Synonyms

- Pulmonary venoocclusive disease (PVOD); pulmonary capillary hemangiomatosis (PCH)

Definitions

- Group 1.6 PAH with overt features of venous/capillary involvement
- Previously classified as 1' PAH
- PVOD and PCH previously considered distinct entities
  - Recent studies suggest that majority of PCH cases are angioproliferative reaction to postcapillary venous obstruction rather than separate disease
- PVOD/PCH has primary and secondary causes
  - Idiopathic
    - 10% of cases of idiopathic PAH are PVOD/PCH pathologically
  - Hereditable
    - *EIF2AK4* mutation most common
  - Secondary causes
    - Drug induced
      - Chemotherapy regiments, most commonly alkylating agents
      - Risk increased when combined with radiation or allogenic stem cell transplantation
    - Radiation induced
    - Occupational exposure
      - Organic solvents, such as trichloroethylene
    - Connective tissue disease (CTD)
      - In one small study, 75% of CTD patients with group 1 PAH had findings of PVOD usually associated with PCH
    - HIV infection
    - PVOD/PCH can occur in cases of group 5 PAH, such as sarcoid and pulmonary Langerhans cell histiocytosis

IMAGING

General Features

- Best diagnostic clue
  - Septal thickening, lymphadenopathy, small centrilobular ground-glass nodules, and absent or small pleural effusions associated with general findings of pulmonary hypertension (PH) in patient with normal left ventricular (LV) systolic and diastolic function
- Location
  - Distal pulmonary veins
  - Alveolar walls

Radiographic Findings

- Radiographic findings of PH
- Septal thickening, lymphadenopathy, and absence of pleural effusions
- Normal left heart size

CT Findings

- Various CT findings recognized in PVOD/PCH
- In some instances, parenchymal findings are indistinguishable from other cases of group 1 PAH
  - Diagnosis made only after patient develops acute pulmonary edema after trial of vasodilator therapy
- Image findings of PVOD and PCH can overlap
- Classic findings, best evaluated on CTPA or cardiac gated CTA of chest
  - General findings of PH usually severe
  - Bilateral symmetric mediastinal and hilar lymphadenopathy
    - Likely related to fibrosis of small veins with increased central draining of fluid and lymph
  - Septal thickening
    - Often prominent feature
    - More classically associated with PVOD than PCH
    - Related to septal edema and fibrosis
  - Ground-glass opacity
    - Lower lobe predominant or random distribution
  - Ground-glass centrilobular nodularity
    - Smaller and more well defined than typical periarteriolar and centrilobular ground glass seen in other forms of PAH
      - Both patterns of ground-glass nodularity/opacity can be present in PVOD/PCH
    - Can be predominant finding
      - More classically associated with PCH but usually coexistent with PVOD
    - Usually lower lobe predominant
    - Often more pronounced in hereditary forms
  - Pruning of peripheral vasculature
  - Pleural effusions often absent
    - Small effusions can be seen in minority of patients
  - Normal left heart size
  - Given association with scleroderma, assess for
    - Esophageal dilation
    - Nonspecific interstitial pneumonia > usual interstitial pneumonia pattern of fibrosis
  - Dual-energy CT or spectral imaging
    - Most cases have no perfusion abnormality or hypoperfusion that is not in vascular territory
    - In some cases, perfusion defects can mimic those seen with chronic thromboembolic disease
      - However, no evidence of arterial occlusion on CTA

MR Findings

- Excellent noninvasive tool for assessment of PH
- Limited ability to distinguish between various groups of PAH
- Not currently used as method to diagnose group 1.6 PAH, although diagnosis could be suggested in setting of PH with
  - Symmetric mediastinal and hilar adenopathy
  - Normal LV function
  - Septal thickening
  - Absence of pleural effusions
- Unclear if MR can adequately assess typical centrilobular nodularity seen in many cases of PVOD/PCH

Echocardiographic Findings

- General findings of PH
- Normal LV function

Nuclear Medicine Findings

- Ventilation/perfusion scan
  - In most cases, V/Q scan is normal
  - May show diffuse upper lobe or peripheral hypoperfusion
  - Segmental filling defects are reported in minority of cases and can mimic acute or chronic thromboemboli
    - No evidence of arterial occlusions on CTA

Imaging Recommendations

- Best imaging tool
  - CT pulmonary angiography
- Protocol advice
  - Dual-energy CT with iodine maps could be helpful

DIFFERENTIAL DIAGNOSIS

Other Causes of Group 1 Pulmonary Arterial Hypertension

- In some instances, imaging findings of PVOD/PCH are indistinguishable from other causes of group 1 PAH
- Diagnosis is only suggestive after patient develops acute pulmonary edema after vasodilator therapy

Left Heart Failure With Fluid Overload in Patient With Underlying Pulmonary Hypertension

- Patients with PH can also have coexistent systolic or diastolic left heart failure
- Can lead to imaging picture similar to PVOD/PCH
- Left atrium usually enlarged

Excipient Lung Disease (IV Talcosis)

- Diffuse centrilobular nodularity and PH in setting of normal LV function
- Centrilobular nodules usually diffuse and solid
- History of IV drug abuse
- Septal thickening and lymphadenopathy often less pronounced in excipient lung disease

Hypersensitivity Pneumonitis

- Centrilobular nodularity and ground-glass opacities seen in nonfibrotic hypersensitivity pneumonitis (HP)
- Coexistent severe PH not common in HP
- Septal thickening and lymphadenopathy uncommon in HP
  - Can be seen with acute HP, which is rare
- Clinical history is different

Sarcoidosis

- Symmetric lymphadenopathy and septal thickening can occur in sarcoid
- Septal thickening in PVOD/PCH usually smooth
- Perilymphatic nodules in sarcoid vs. centrilobular nodules in PVOD/PCH

PATHOLOGY

General Features

- Venous fibrosis and obstruction (PVOD)
- Often association with capillary proliferation within alveolar walls (PCH)
- Coexists with typical arterial findings seen in types 1.1-1.4 PAH but less pronounced

Microscopic Features

- PVOD
  - Diffuse intimal fibrosis and obliteration of venules and septal veins
    - More moderate venous fibrosis can occur in longstanding increase in pulmonary venous pressures seen in group 2 disease
  - Intimal remodeling of veins and venules ranges from loose fibrous tissue to dense sclerotic lesions
  - Septal edema and fibrosis with dilated lymphatics
  - Coexistent secondary arterial changes seen in types 1.1-1.4 PAH often present
- PCH
  - Capillary proliferation within alveolar walls
  - Thickening of alveolar septa
  - Coexistent secondary arterial changes seen in types 1.1-1.4 PAH often present

CLINICAL ISSUES

Presentation

- Most common signs/symptoms
  - Dyspnea, fatigue, cough, exertional syncope
- Other signs/symptoms
  - Reduced diffuse capacity of lungs for carbon monoxide

Demographics

- Age
  - Wide age range from pediatric patients to older adults
    - Younger age in patients with *EIF2AK4* mutation
- Sex
  - Equal distribution

Natural History & Prognosis

- Poor prognosis
  - Worse than most forms of PAH
- In study of 327 patients from French PH registry, survival rates at 1, 3, and 5 years were 86%, 50%, and 27%, respectively

Treatment

- Lung transplant is only treatment that can prevent death
- No drugs have proven efficacy for treatment

DIAGNOSTIC CHECKLIST

Consider

- PVOD/PCH in cases of severe PH with septal thickening, lymphadenopathy, small centrilobular ground-glass nodules, and absent or small pleural effusions in patient with normal LV systolic and diastolic function

SELECTED REFERENCES

1. Boucly A et al: Outcomes and risk assessment in pulmonary veno-occlusive disease. ERJ Open Res. 10(1):00612-2023, 2024
2. Simonneau G et al: Haemodynamic definitions and updated clinical classification of pulmonary hypertension. Eur Respir J. 53(1):1801913, 2019
3. Szturmowicz M et al: Pulmonary veno-occlusive disease: pathogenesis, risk factors, clinical features and diagnostic algorithm - state of the art. Adv Respir Med. 86(3), 2018
4. Montani D et al: Pulmonary veno-occlusive disease. Eur Respir J. 47(5):1518-34, 2016
5. Lantuejoul S et al: Pulmonary veno-occlusive disease and pulmonary capillary hemangiomatosis: a clinicopathologic study of 35 cases. Am J Surg Pathol. 30(7):850-7, 2006

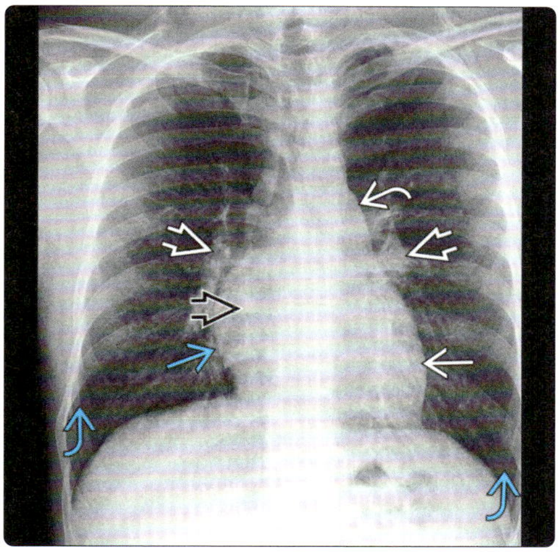

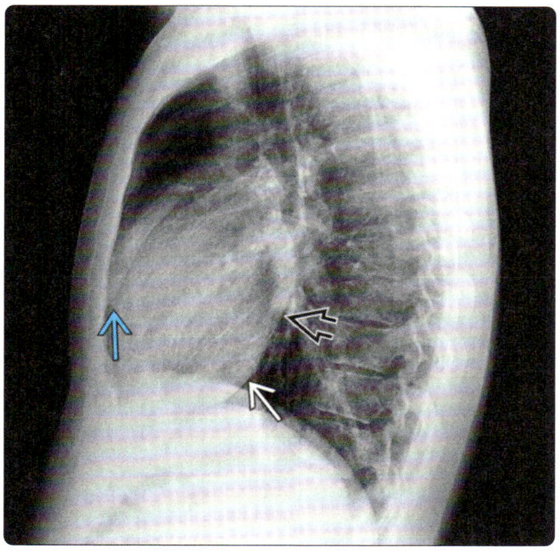

(Left) *PA CXR in a 25-year-old man shows enlargement of the main pulmonary artery , and prominence of the hila , which may be due to pulmonary artery enlargement vs. lymphadenopathy. Right atrial contour is mildly prominent , but the left atrial (LA) and LV contours are normal. Mild septal thickening is present, but there are no pleural effusions.* **(Right)** *Lateral radiograph shows a normal size of the LA and LV . Mild septal thickening is present. There are no effusions.*

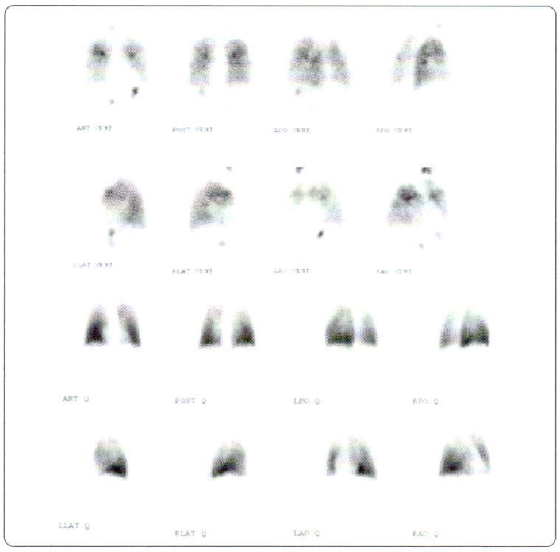

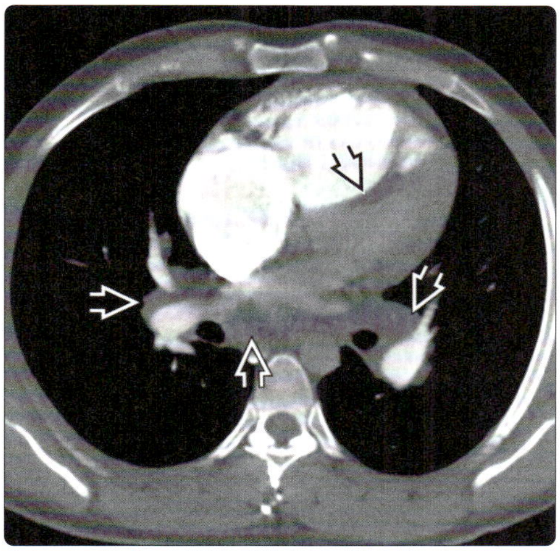

(Left) *Ventilation (top) and perfusion (bottom) scans are normal. Increased perfusion is noted in the lower lobes.* **(Right)** *CT pulmonary angiography shows conspicuously enlarged mediastinal and hilar lymphadenopathy (LAD) . The right ventricle is dilated and hypertrophied with inversion of the interventricular septum to the left due to ↑ right ventricle pressures. The right atrium is mildly dilated. The LA and LV are small in size.*

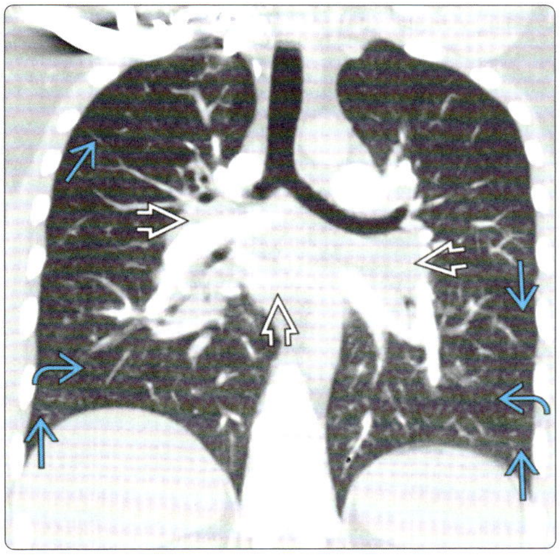

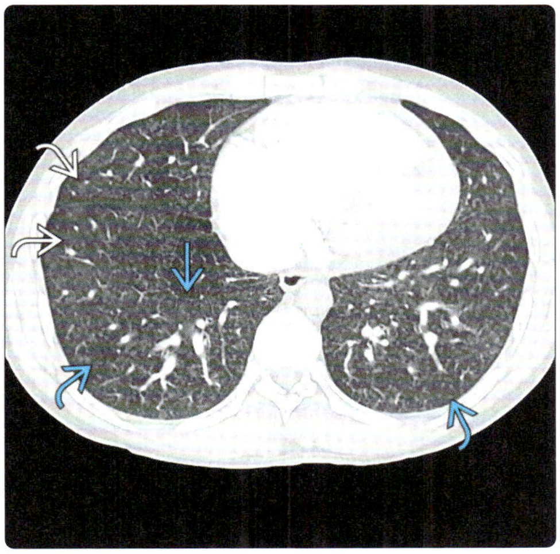

(Left) *Coronal CECT shows LAD , mild septal thickening , and lower lobe-predominant small centrilobular ground-glass nodules (CLGGN) , which are smaller and well defined compared to periarteriolar areas of ground glass (PAGG) seen in cases of pulmonary arterial hypertension (PAH).* **(Right)** *Mixture of well-defined CLGGN superimposed on PAGG is often seen with other forms of PAH and septal thickening without pleural effusions. Explant showed PVOD and pulmonary capillary hemangiomatosis.*

Group 1 Pulmonary Arterial Hypertension

KEY FACTS

TERMINOLOGY

- 1.1 idiopathic pulmonary arterial hypertension (PAH)
- 1.2 hereditable PAH
- 1.3 drug- and toxin-induced PAH
- 1.4 PAH associated with connective tissue disease, HIV, portal hypertension, congenital heart disease, or schistosomiasis
- 1.5 PAH in long-term responders to calcium channel blockers
- 1.6 PAH with overt features of venous/capillary involvement
- 1.7 persistent pulmonary hypertension of newborn

IMAGING ANATOMY

- Findings suggestive of PAH
  - Perivascular and centrilobular ground-glass opacity along peripheral pulmonary arteries
  - In situ thrombus
    - Must be differentiated from CTEPH
  - Pulmonary artery calcifications
  - Coexistent findings of uncorrected congenital heart disease or connective tissue disease

PATHOLOGY

- Combination of features lead to distal pulmonary artery and arteriolar obstruction
  - Endothelial dysfunction and increased contractility of small pulmonary arteries
  - Intimal fibrosis and medial thickening
  - In situ thrombus

CLINICAL ISSUES

- Idiopathic and heritable PAH common in women (79%)
- NIH Registry patients with ≈ 50% mortality rate at 3 years
- Recent clinical trial study groups suggest better outcomes
- PAH-specific medications can improve symptoms, progression, and survival
- Lung transplant for refractive and progressive cases

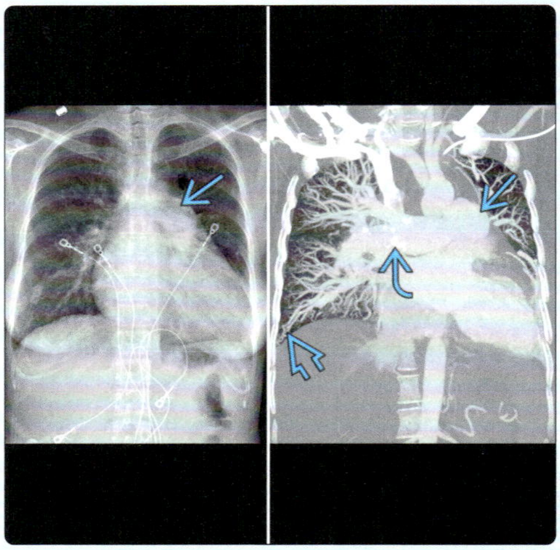
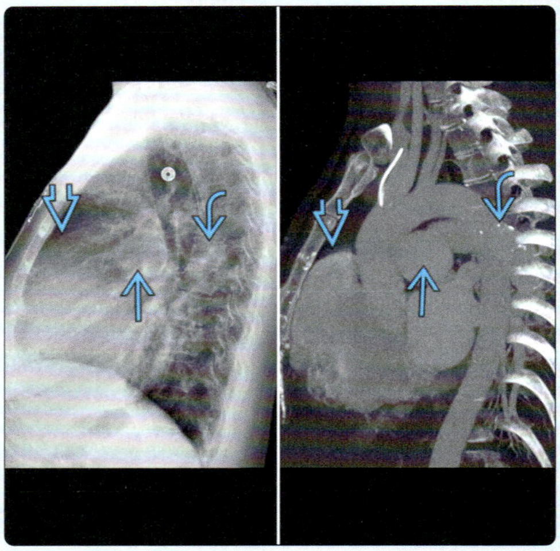

(Left) *CXR (L) and coronal MIP CT (R) in a 45-year-old woman with BMPR2 mutation and pulmonary arterial hypertension (PAH) show PA enlargement →. PA calcification → is due to atherosclerosis from near systemic pressures. PA branches are dilated, tortuous, and reach pleural surface. Areas of neovascularity → can occur with this mutation.* **(Right)** *Lateral CXR (L) and sagittal MIP (R) show PA enlargement → and left PA calcifications →. Right atrium (RA) and ventricle (RV) fill retrosternal space →.*

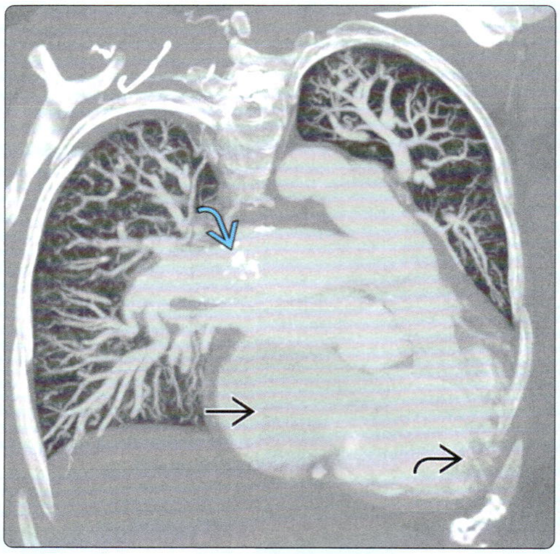
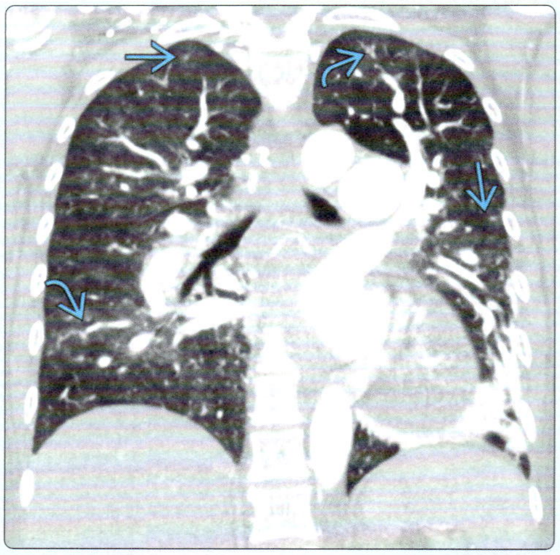

(Left) *MIP CT shows PA calcifications → with dilated, tortuous PA branches extending to the lung periphery. There is RA dilation → and RV hypertrophy →.* **(Right)** *Periarteriolar ground-glass (GG) opacity extends along the PA branches →, which, in cross section, can appear as centrilobular GG nodules →. This is a common finding in PAH but rare in other causes of pulmonary hypertension (PH).*

TERMINOLOGY

Abbreviations

- Pulmonary arterial hypertension (PAH)

Synonyms

- Idiopathic PAH, precapillary pulmonary hypertension (PH), primary PH, associated PAH, hereditable PAH

Definitions

- PH not secondary to
  - Left heart disease (group 2)
  - Parenchymal lung disease (group 3)
  - Pulmonary artery (PA) obstruction (group 4)
  - Multifactorial causes (group 5)
- 1.1 idiopathic PAH
- 1.2 hereditable PAH
  - 1.21 *BMPR2*
  - 1.22 *ALK-1, ENG, SMAD9, CAV1, KCNK3*
  - 1.23 unknown
- 1.3 drug- and toxin-induced PAH
- 1.4 PAH associated with
  - 1.4.1 connective tissue disease (CTD)
  - 1.4.2 HIV infection
  - 1.4.3 PH
  - 1.4.4 congenital heart disease (CHD)
  - 1.4.5 schistosomiasis
- 1.5 PAH in long-term responders to calcium channel blockers (CCB)
  - Small percentage (< 10%) of patients with PAH show
    - Acute vasodilation of pulmonary vasculature in response to inhaled nitrous oxide challenge
    - Improvement in New York Heart Association function class to class I or II
    - Unchanged or improved hemodynamics at 1 year when treated with CCB alone
- 1.6 PAH with overt features of venous/capillary involvement [pulmonary venoocclusive disease (PVOD)/pulmonary capillary hemangiomatosis (PCH)]
- 1.7 persistent PH of newborn (PPHN)

IMAGING ANATOMY

General Features

- Best diagnostic clue
  - Imaging findings of PH
    - Enlarged PA
      - PA diameter > aortic diameter
    - Right ventricular hypertrophy
    - Dilated PA branches
  - Absence of findings that would suggest groups 2-5 as etiology
- Location
  - Precapillary arteries and arterioles

Radiographic Findings

- Difficult to differentiate between etiologies of PH on radiograph in most instances
- Enlarged central pulmonary arteries
- Dilation of right ventricle (RV) and right atrium (RA)
- Pruning of peripheral vasculature seen in some cases
- Calcification of PAs present in some cases
- Shunt vascularity in cases of uncorrected CHD

CT Findings

- Findings suggestive of types 1.1, 1.2, 1.3, and 1.4 PAH
  - Perivascular and centrilobular ground glass (GG)
    - Perivascular GG coursing along long axis of peripheral PAs
    - In cross section, appear as large GG centrilobular nodules
      - Many etiologies suggested
      - Not well validated with radiologic-pathologic correlation
    - In some cases, GG can fill large portion of secondary pulmonary lobule
    - Commonly reported in certain hereditable causes of PAH, such as *BMPR2* mutations
      - Can be seen in various causes of PAH
    - Typically larger than centrilobular GG nodules seen in some cases of PVOD/PCH
    - Not commonly reported in groups 2-5 PH
    - Finding may be absent in less severe disease
  - Morphology of peripheral PAs
    - Peripheral pruning
    - Tortuous and dilated peripheral PAs extending to pleural surface
      - Commonly seen in *BMPR2* mutations
      - Can mimic small arteriovenous malformations
    - Vascular changes different in group 3 and group 4 PH
      - Pruning in areas of parenchymal disease in group 3
      - Pruning in areas of vascular occlusion in group 4
    - Findings may be minimal or absent in less severe disease
  - PA calcifications
    - Related to atherosclerosis of PAs due to systemic or near-systemic pressures
    - Most likely related to PA pressures rather than etiology
    - While uncommon, it is more common in PAH than other causes of PH
      - More common in CHD than idiopathic and hereditable forms
  - In situ (mural) thrombus
    - While uncommon, most common in PAH vs. other causes of PH
      - Can be seen in idiopathic, hereditable, drug-induced, or CHD-related PAH
    - Must differentiate from chronic thromboembolic pulmonary hypertension (CTEPH) as treatments are different
      - In situ thrombus found layering in central PAs and does not typically lead to vascular occlusion
  - Bronchial artery collaterals
    - Can be seen in any cause of PH
    - Typically smaller or absent in cases of idiopathic PAH when compared to CTEPH
    - Collaterals can be large, especially in cases of CHD and *BMPR2* mutations
  - Pericardial effusion
    - Common finding in PAH
      - Wide range from 13-44%

  - Higher incidence in patients with CTD
  - Associated with worse prognosis
- Findings that may point to specific subtype of PAH
  - 1.4.1 CTD
    - Esophageal dilation and nonspecific interstitial pneumonia (NSIP) > usual interstitial pneumonia (UIP) pattern of pulmonary fibrosis in patients with scleroderma
    - Between 7-26% of patients with scleroderma develop PH
    - Pleural &/or pericardial thickening and effusions in patient with SLE
    - Combination of various patterns of fibrosis and extraparenchymal findings in patients with mixed CTD
  - 1.4.4 CHD
    - Uncorrected or late corrected CHD
    - Atrial septal defect, ventricular septal defect, partially anomalous pulmonary venous return, total anomalous pulmonary venous return, atrioventricular septal defect, patent ductus arteriosus, aortopulmonary window, transposition of great arteries, common arterial trunk
    - Depending on cause, CHD can fall under group 2, group 4, or group 5 PH

MR Findings

- Helpful in making diagnosis of PH
- Excluding CHD, not commonly used to distinguish PAH from other causes of PH
  - Can help make diagnosis of groups 2, 4, and 5 PH

Echocardiographic Findings

- Similar to MR, echo is helpful in making diagnosis of PH and assessing for complications
- Excluding CHD, echo is limited in differentiating between causes of PH

Imaging Recommendations

- Best imaging tool
  - CTA is best; no perilymphatic nodularity seen in sarcoid modality to help differentiate between subtypes of PH
  - Certain vascular and parenchymal imaging findings highly suggestive of PAH
- Protocol advice
  - Consider timing off of left atrium due to RV dysfunction in patients with PH
  - Recommend dual-energy imaging as it can help differentiate between CTEPH and other causes of PH
  - Consider cardiac gating to better assess right heart and potentially exclude causes of group 2 PH

DIFFERENTIAL DIAGNOSIS

Group 1.6 Pulmonary Arterial Hypertension With Overt Features of Venous/Capillary Involvement (Pulmonary Venoocclusive Disease and Pulmonary Capillary Hemangiomatosis)

- Imaging features of PVOD/PCH overlap with other types of group 1 PAH
  - In some cases, imaging appears identical to other causes of group 1
- Findings suggestive of PVOD/PCH
  - Septal thickening with normal left ventricular function in PVOD/PCH
  - Symmetric mediastinal and hilar lymphadenopathy common
    - No perilymphatic nodularity seen in sarcoid
  - Centrilobular GG nodules tend to be smaller
- Patients often develop acute pulmonary edema after vasodilator therapy

Pulmonary Hypertension Due to Left Heart Disease (Group 2)

- Most common cause of PH
- Associated with mitral valve disease, heart failure with preserved ejection fraction (diastolic failure), and heart failure with reduced ejection fraction (systolic failure)
- Usually diagnosed with echocardiography &/or cardiac MR

Pulmonary Hypertension Due to Parenchymal Disease (Group 3)

- 2nd most common cause of PH
- Secondary to parenchymal lung disease &/or chronic hypoxia
  - Smoking-related lung disease (SRLD)
  - Pulmonary fibrosis (PF)
  - Obstructive sleep apnea
- SRLD and PF-related PH can be differentiated from other causes of PH based on CT findings
- Obstructive sleep apnea can be suggested in obese patients with PH, but needs further testing to confirm

Pulmonary Hypertension Due to Pulmonary Artery Obstruction (Group 4)

- Most commonly secondary to chronic thromboembolic disease
- Macroscopic vascular occlusions cause mosaic perfusion with vascular distribution
- Chronic thrombus should be recognized on CTA
  - Thrombus may also be seen in right heart
- In situ thrombus in PAH can occasionally mimic CTEPH
  - However, in situ thrombus does not usually lead to vascular occlusion
  - Iodine map from dual-energy CT or perfusion portion of V/Q will not show perfusion defects
- Calcification in chronic clot in CTEPH, which is rare, needs to be differentiated with intimal calcifications due to PA atherosclerosis
- Bronchial artery collaterals usually larger in patients with CTEPH compared to most patients with PAH

Pulmonary Hypertension Due to Multifactorial or Unknown Causes (Group 5)

- Numerous etiologies
- Many causes can be elucidated by characteristic imaging findings
  - Bilateral symmetric adenopathy with perihilar-predominant perilymphatic nodularity and fibrosis in sarcoidosis
  - Large mass in mediastinum or hilum leading to pulmonary vascular obstruction in fibrosing mediastinitis
  - Upper lobe-predominant, bizarrely shaped cysts and nodules in pulmonary Langerhans cell histiocytosis

PATHOLOGY

General Features

- Combination of features cause distal PA and arteriolar obstruction leading to increased pulmonary artery pressures, RV hypertrophy and failure, and eventual death
  - Endothelial dysfunction and increased contractility of small PAs
  - Proliferation and remodeling of endothelial and smooth muscle cells of PAs and arterioles
  - In situ thrombosis
    - Can occasionally be predominant finding

Gross Pathologic & Surgical Features

- Dilation of proximal PAs
- Visible atherosclerotic changes

Microscopic Features

- Plexiform lesions often considered hallmark lesion in severe PAH
  - Represent complex vascular lesions from remodeled PAs and arterioles
    - No contribution from bronchial arteries
  - Glomeruloid-like vascular structures originating like those seen in glioblastomas
  - Most commonly seen at branch point of axial arteries but also occur in interlobular arteries associated with bronchioles and more distal intraacinar arterioles unassociated with airways
  - Exact etiology not well understood
  - Unclear if plexiform lesion is cause of PAH or merely indicator of its presence
  - Seen in 90% of patients with PAH
  - Much higher number of plexiform lesions in women with PAH than in men
- Remodeling of intima and media of small PAs and arterioles
  - Varying degrees of endothelial cell proliferation, muscular hypertrophy, and intimal fibrosis
    - Degree of medial hypertrophy associated with mean PA pressure
- Associated areas of thrombosis &/or arteritis
- Associated findings of interstitial inflammation and fibrosis in patients with CTD
- Patients with PAH who are long-term responders to CCB show more mild disease pathologically

CLINICAL ISSUES

Presentation

- Most common signs/symptoms
  - Exertional dyspnea
  - Fatigue
  - Dizziness
  - Syncope

Demographics

- Wide age range
- Idiopathic and heritable PAH more common in women (79%)
- Consider PAH in patient with imaging findings of PH with history of methamphetamine abuse if other causes have been excluded

Natural History & Prognosis

- NIH Registry patients had ≈ 50% mortality rate at 3 years
- Recent clinical trial study groups suggest better outcomes in modern management era
  - Mortality rates of 20-30% at 3-5 years in French Registry
  - Mortality rates of 10-30% at 1-3 years in REVEAL Registry
- Part of this improvement may be related to patients with less severe disease being enrolled in modern trials as well as other forms of bias

Treatment

- PAH specific medications
  - Endothelin receptor antagonists (ERAs)
  - Phosphodiesterase type 5 (PDE5) inhibitors
  - Soluble guanylate cyclase agonists
  - Prostacyclin analogs
  - Prostacyclin receptor agonists
  - Lung transplant for refractive and progressive cases

DIAGNOSTIC CHECKLIST

Consider

- Consider PAH in young or middle-aged women with imaging findings of severe PH with periarteriolar GG opacity on CT and no clear other explanation for disease

SELECTED REFERENCES

1. Tsoi SM et al: Defining the typical course of persistent pulmonary hypertension of the newborn (PPHN): when to think beyond reversible causes. J Pediatr. 273:114131, 2024
2. Baranga L et al: In situ pulmonary arterial thrombosis: literature review and clinical significance of a distinct entity. AJR Am J Roentgenol. 221(1):57-68, 2023
3. Condliffe R et al: Clinical-radiological-pathological correlation in pulmonary arterial hypertension. Eur Respir Rev. 32(170):230138, 2023
4. Jin Q et al: Medical management of pulmonary arterial hypertension: current approaches and investigational drugs. Pharmaceutics. 15(6):1579, 2023
5. Jone PN et al: Pulmonary hypertension in congenital heart disease: a scientific statement from the American Heart Association. Circ Heart Fail. 16(7):e00080, 2023
6. Kolaitis NA: Lung transplantation for pulmonary arterial hypertension. Chest. 164(4):992-1006, 2023
7. Tamura Y et al: Case report: pathological differences in pulmonary arterial hypertension in long-term responders to calcium channel blockers. Front Cardiovasc Med. 10:1295718, 2023
8. Zhao Q et al: Imaging features in BMPR2 mutation-associated pulmonary arterial hypertension. Radiology. 307(5):e222488, 2023
9. Arano T et al: Heritable pulmonary arterial hypertension complicated by multiple pulmonary arteriovenous malformations. Respir Med Case Rep. 32:101352, 2021
10. Badlam JB et al: United States Pulmonary Hypertension Scientific Registry: baseline characteristics. Chest. 159(1):311-27, 2021
11. Remy-Jardin M et al: Imaging of pulmonary hypertension in adults: a position paper from the Fleischner Society. Eur Respir J. 57(1):2004455, 2021
12. Lee JY et al: A cancer amidst us: the plexiform lesion in pulmonary arterial hypertension. Am J Physiol Lung Cell Mol Physiol. 318(6):L1142-4, 2020
13. Zanatta E et al: Pulmonary arterial hypertension in connective tissue disorders: pathophysiology and treatment. Exp Biol Med (Maywood). 244(2):120-31, 2019
14. Orcholski ME et al: Drug-induced pulmonary arterial hypertension: a primer for clinicians and scientists. Am J Physiol Lung Cell Mol Physiol. 314(6):L967-83, 2018
15. Rajaram S et al: CT features of pulmonary arterial hypertension and its major subtypes: a systematic CT evaluation of 292 patients from the ASPIRE Registry. Thorax. 70(4):382-7, 2015
16. Tio D et al: Risk factors for hemoptysis in idiopathic and hereditary pulmonary arterial hypertension. PLoS One. 8(10):e78132, 2013
17. Stacher E et al: Modern age pathology of pulmonary arterial hypertension. Am J Respir Crit Care Med. 186(3):261-72, 2012

WHO Classification of Pulmonary Arterial Hypertension

1.1 Idiopathic	1.2 Hereditable	1.3 Drug- and Toxin-Induced	1.4 Associated With	1.5 Pulmonary Arterial Hypertension in Long-Term Responders to Calcium Channel Blockers	1.6 Overt Features of Pulmonary Venoocclusive Disease/Pulmonary Capillary Hemangiomatosis	1.7 Persistent Pulmonary Hypertension of Newborn Syndrome
No known cause	1.2.1 *BMPR2*, 80%	**Definite**	1.4.1 CTD	Small percentage of patients with PAH show:	PVOD and PCH previously classified as primary PAH	No transition from intrauterine to extrauterine circulation at birth
Most common cause	1.2.2 *ALK-1, ENG, SMAD9, CAV1, KCNK3*, 5%	Aminorex (weight loss drug pulled from market)	Scleroderma, 75%	Acute vasodilation of pulmonary vasculature in response to inhaled NO challenge	Capillary proliferation in PCH likely related to postcapillary obstruction and not separate disease	Elevated PVR, low PBF, and R → L shunting across PDA and PFO, severe hypoxemia
	1.2.3 unknown, 15%	Fenfluramine (weight loss drug pulled from market)	Mixed CTD, 8%	Improvement in New York Heart Assoc. function class to class I or II	Hereditable cases of PVOD/PCH seen with *EIF2AK4* mutation	Can be idiopathic or secondary Secondary causes divided into perinatal and developmental etiologies
		Benfluorex (related to fenfluramine; appetite suppressant, reduce insulin resistance; still on market)	SLE, 8%	Unchanged or improved hemodynamics at 1 year when treated with CCB alone	Up to 10% of cases of idiopathic, CTD-associated, and drug-induced PAH show PVOD/PCH pathologically	Perinatal etiologies: Meconium aspiration syndrome, respiratory distress syndrome, infection
		SSRIs (maternal use after 20 weeks associated with persistent PH of newborn)	Other CTD, 10%			Developmental etiologies: Pulmonary hypoplasia, CDH, CHD, foregut/GI anomaly, genetic syndrome, vein of Galen malformation; ILD
		Likely	1.4.2 HIV infection			Overall 7.6% 1-year mortality; perinatal causes have improved survival vs. developmental causes
		Methamphetamines, amphetamines	1.4.3 PH			
		L-tryptophan	1.4.4 CHDs			
		Possible	1.4.5 Schistosomiasis			
		Cocaine, phenylpropanolamine, St. John's wort, chemotherapeutic agents, interferon-α, -β				

CCB = calcium channel blockers; CDH = congenital diaphragmatic hernia; CHD = congenital heart disease; CTD = connective tissue disease; ILD = interstitial lung disease; PH = pulmonary hypertension; PAH = pulmonary arterial hypertension; PBF = pulmonary blood flow; PCH = pulmonary capillary hemangiomatous; PDA = patent ductus arteriosus; PFO = patent foramen ovale; PVR = pulmonary vascular resistance; PVOD = pulmonary venoocclusive disease; NO = nitrous oxide; SSRIs = selective serotonin reuptake inhibitors.

18. Jonigk D et al: Plexiform lesions in pulmonary arterial hypertension composition, architecture, and microenvironment. Am J Pathol. 179(1):167-79, 2011
19. Remy-Jardin M et al: Systemic collateral supply in patients with chronic thromboembolic and primary pulmonary hypertension: assessment with multi-detector row helical CT angiography. Radiology. 235(1):274-81, 2005
20. Sitbon O et al: Long-term response to calcium channel blockers in idiopathic pulmonary arterial hypertension. Circulation. 111(23):3105-11, 2005

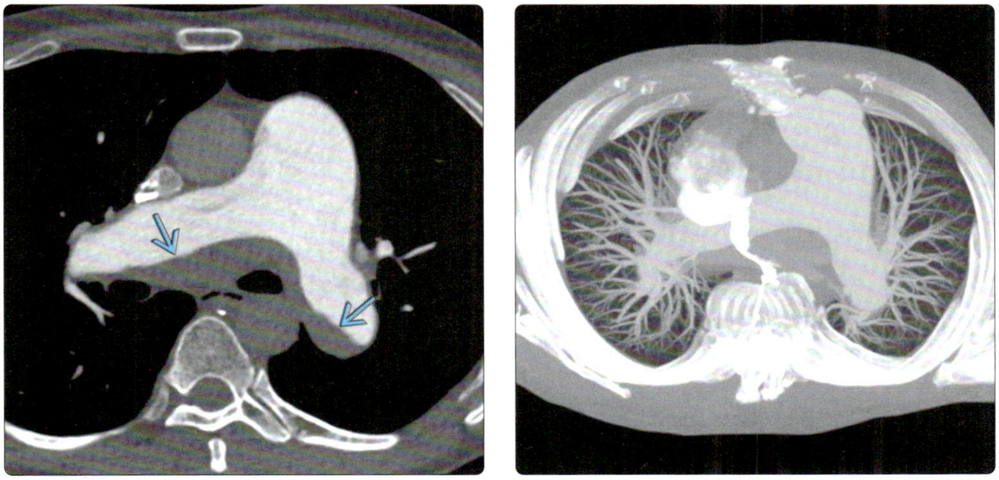

(Left) *Dual-energy CTPA in a 42-year-old man with a long history of methamphetamine abuse shows a large amount of layering in situ thrombi (IST) in the main PAs →. There was no downstream vascular obstruction.* **(Right)** *MIP image shows no evidence of PA occlusion.*

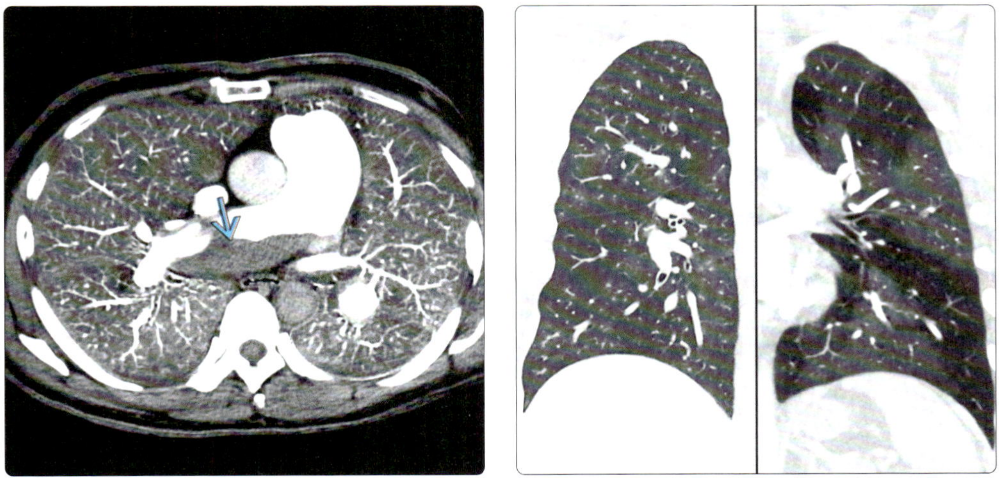

(Left) *Iodine map shows no perfusion defects. The IST → is seen. It is important to differentiate IST from CTEPH, as treatments differ.* **(Right)** *Image of the right lung in a 33-year-old woman with idiopathic PAH and the left lung in a 25-year-old man with show different perfusion patterns. In PAH, perivascular and centrilobular GG opacity is common, while in CTEPH, hypoperfusion in a vascular territory occurs, often with compensatory hyperperfusion of spared regions.*

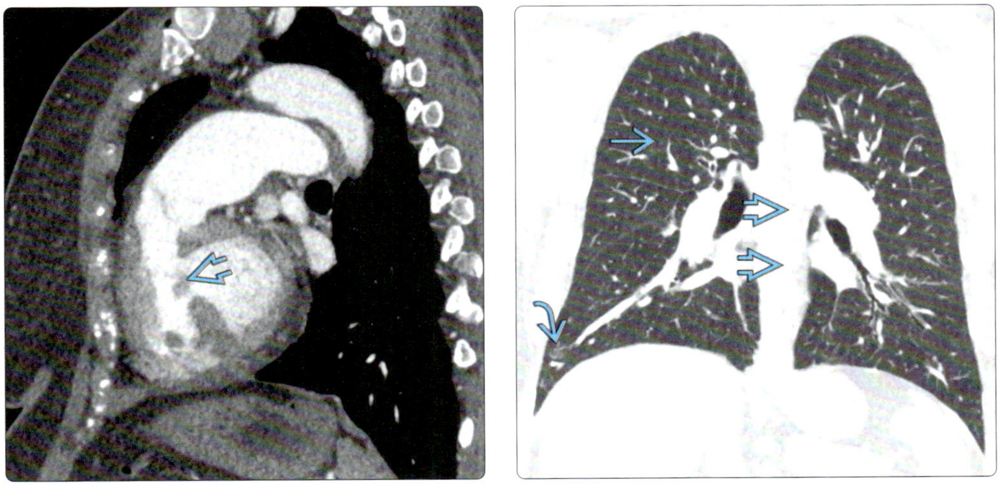

(Left) *CTA in a 52-year-old woman shows a large membranous ventricular septal defect (VSD) →. The main PA measures 3.9 cm, and the RV is hypertrophied. Bidirectional flow across the VSD was seen on echocardiogram.* **(Right)** *Coronal image in the patient with the VSD shows subtle diffuse increase in lung attenuation, centrilobular GG nodularity →, and neovascularity →. Enlarged bronchial artery collaterals → are seen, which are less common in PAH than other causes of PH.*

Group 2 Pulmonary Hypertension

KEY FACTS

TERMINOLOGY

- Pulmonary hypertension (PH) due to left heart disease
  - Isolated postcapillary PH
  - Combined precapillary and postcapillary PH
- Most common cause of PH
  - Accounts for 65-80% of cases
  - 50% of patients with left ventricular failure have PH
- Classification
  - 2.1 PH due to heart failure with preserved left ventricular ejection fraction (HFpEF)
  - 2.2 PH due to heart failure with reduced LVEF (HFrEF)
  - 2.3 valvular heart disease
  - 2.4 congenital lesions with postcapillary PH
    - Congenital left-heart inflow obstructions
    - Congenital left-heart outflow obstruction
    - Congenital cardiomyopathies

IMAGING

- Echocardiogram is best tool for group 2 PH evaluation
- Enlarged left atrium (LA) and findings of PH in absence of other causes
  - Imaging findings of PH may be absent as many cases have only mild PH on right heart catheterization
- CT, MR, and echocardiography (echo) findings
- LA dilation
  - LA measurements vary on age and sex
  - Hard to assess on CT without contrast and ECG gating
- Valvular abnormalities
  - Mitral and aortic valve thickening/calcification in stenosis
  - Subvalvular or supravalvular lesions best seen with echo and MR
  - Valvular flows and gradients measured on MR and echo
- LA and RV pressure measurements estimated on echo
- Right heart catheterization is gold standard for pressure measurements

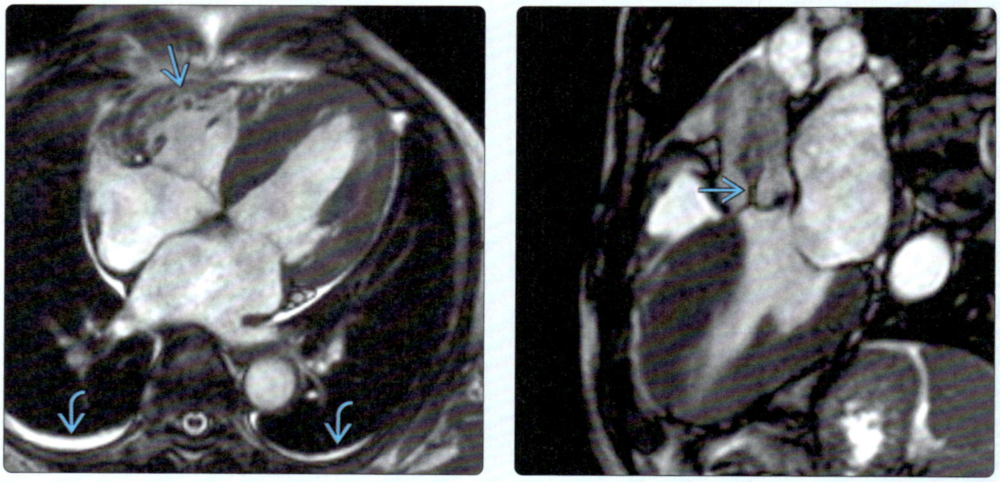

(Left) *End-diastolic cine SSFP MR in a 61-year-old man with heart failure with preserved ejection fraction (HFpEF, EF = 54%) shows left and right → ventricular hypertrophy. Small bilateral pleural effusions → and biatrial dilation are present.* **(Right)** *Systolic MR shows findings of severe aortic stenosis →. Left atrial (LA) volume was 42 mL/m², which is mildly enlarged. Echocardiogram estimated LA pressure at 24 mmHg, and right heart catheterization calculated pulmonary artery (PA) pressures at 41 mmHg.*

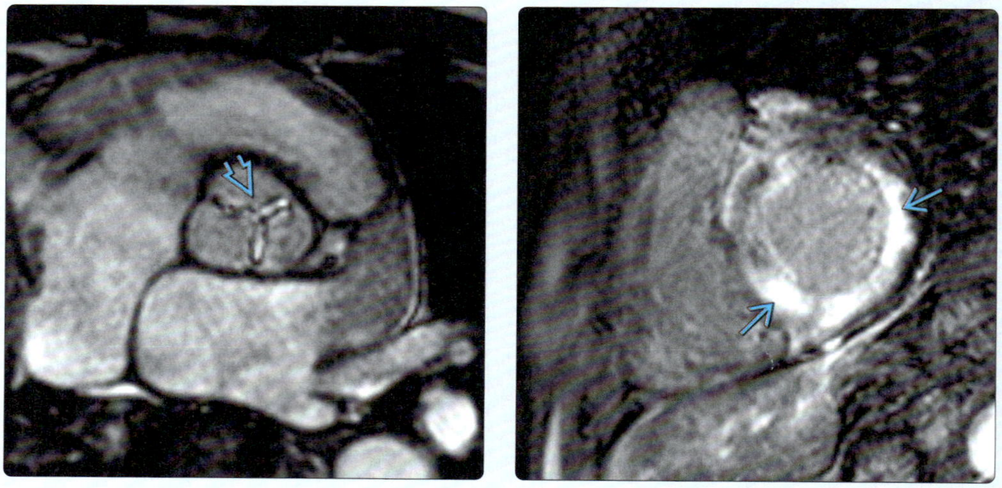

(Left) *Cine MR of the aortic valve at end-systole shows severe aortic stenosis with an aortic valve opening area of 0.9 cm² →.* **(Right)** *LGE MR shows extensive left ventricle (LV) delayed enhancement →. Amyloid was confirmed with endomyocardial biopsy. The group 2 pulmonary hypertension in this patient could be considered multifactorial due to the restrictive cardiomyopathy and severe aortic stenosis.*

TERMINOLOGY

Abbreviations

- Pulmonary hypertension (PH)

Synonyms

- Postcapillary PH; PH due to left heart disease

Definitions

- Most common cause of PH
- PH due to left heart disease
  - 2.1: PH due to heart failure with preserved left ventricular ejection fraction (HFpEF)
    - Diastolic dysfunction
  - 2.2: PH due to heart failure with reduced LVEF (HFrEF)
  - 2.3: Valvular heart disease
    - Aortic stenosis
    - Mitral stenosis
    - Aortic regurgitation
    - Mitral regurgitation
  - 2.4: Congenital cardiovascular conditions leading to postcapillary PH
    - Congenital left-heart inflow obstructions
      - Congenital pulmonary vein stenosis
      - Cor triatriatum with obstruction
      - Supravalvular mitral ring
      - Congenital mitral stenosis or hypoplasia
    - Congenital left-heart outflow obstruction
      - Supravalvular, valvular, or subvalvular aortic stenosis
      - Hypoplastic left heart syndrome (HLHS)
    - Shone syndrome
      - Supravalvular mitral ring, parachute mitral valve, subvalvular aortic stenosis, aortic coarctation
    - Congenital cardiomyopathies

IMAGING

General Features

- Best diagnostic clue
  - Enlarged left atrium (LA) and general findings of PH in absence of other identifiable etiologies
  - Imaging findings may be absent in mild cases of PH

Radiographic Findings

- General findings of PH
  - Imaging findings of PH may be absent
- Associated LA dilation
- Left ventricle (LV) may be enlarged
- Difficult to differentiate between etiologies of PH on radiograph
  - Valvular or LA wall calcification hard to see
- Pulmonary edema and pleural effusions may be present
- Absence of findings to suggest another cause

CT Findings

- Cardiac gated CTA
  - No detailed studies outlining findings associated with group 2 PH
  - General findings of PH may be more mild or absent in mild PH
  - Difficult to see many findings without ECG gating or contrast
- Left atrium
  - Dilation
    - Left atrial measurements vary on age and sex
      - Men have larger absolute LA volumes than women
      - Values similar when adjusted for body surface area
    - LA volumes increase with age
    - For all patients, regardless of age
      - Absolute (indexed) LA end-diastolic volume is 74 ± 18 mL (41 ± 10 mL/m^2), 86 ± 21 mL (40 ± 9 mL/m^2), 80 ± 20 mL (41 ± 9 mL/m^2) for women, men, and all patients, respectively
      - Absolute (indexed) LA end-diastolic diameter (measured in 3-chamber plane) is 35 ± 5 mm (17 ± 2 mm), 35 ± 4 mm (18 ± 4 mm), 35 ± 4 mm (18 ± 3 mm) for women, men, and all patients, respectively
  - Calcification
    - LA wall calcifications rare
      - Most commonly seen in severe mitral stenosis
  - Cor triatriatum
    - LA partially dividing into 2 chambers by thick fibromuscular band
      - Can be horizontal or transverse in orientation
    - Associated with other congenital defects in pediatric patients
      - Secundum atrial septal defect and partial anomalous pulmonary venous return most common
    - Often incidental finding in adult patients
- LV
  - Hypertrophied with LA dilation in some cases of HFpEF
  - Dilated with LA dilation in some cases of HFrEF
- Valvular abnormalities
  - Mitral valve
    - Thickening and calcified in mitral stenosis
      - Must differentiate from mitral annular calcification
    - Supravalvular mitral ring is difficult to recognize on CT
  - Aortic valve
    - Thickening and calcification in aortic stenosis
      - Calcification well assessed on noncontrast CT
      - May be bicuspid
    - Subvalvular stenosis
      - Band or web of soft tissue below aortic valve
      - Narrowing of LV outflow track due to hypertrophied basilar septum
    - Supravalvular stenosis
      - Focal narrowing with hourglass morphology is most common
      - Focal narrowing due to web or soft tissue band
      - Diffuse aortic hypoplasia
- Nonspecific findings of pulmonary edema and pleural effusions common

MR Findings

- Qualitative assessment of LV systolic and diastolic function
  - HFpEF and HFrEF diagnosis
- Myocardial tissue characterization
  - Diagnosis of ischemic or nonischemic cardiomyopathies
- Atrial diameter and volume measurement

  - Absolute (indexed) LA end-diastolic volume is 68 ± 14.9 mL (40 ± 6.7 mL/m²), 77 ± 14.9 mL (39 ± 6.7 mL/m²), 73 ± 14.9 mL (40 ± 6.7 mL/m²) for women, men, and all patients, respectively
  - Absolute (indexed) LA end-diastolic diameter (measured in 3-chamber plane) is 31 ± 0.5 mm (18 ± 0.3 mm), 33 ± 0.5 mm (17 ± 0.3 mm), 32 ± 0.5 mm (17 ± 0.3 mm) for women, men, and all patients, respectively
- Valvular pathology and flow
  - Anatomic assessment for mitral and aortic stenosis
  - Measurement of velocities with phase contrast (PC)
  - Quantification of aortic and mitral regurgitation
- Congenital heart disease
  - Morphology of obstruction well evaluated with MR
  - Can measure velocities across obstruction with PC

Echocardiographic Findings

- Robust assessment of mitral and aortic valves
  - Transesophageal better than transthoracic MV evaluation
  - Can measure jet velocity in cases of stenosis
  - Methods to measure regurgitant volume and valve area
  - Can assess for congenital anomalies
- Left atrial function and volume evaluation
  - Absolute (indexed) LA end-diastolic volume is 46.2 ± 11.8 mL (28 ± 6.7 mL/m²), 53.4 ± 15.1 mL (28.1 ± 7.1 mL/m²), 49.9 ± 14.1 mL (28.1 ± 6.9 mL/m²) for women, men, and all patients, respectively
- Left atrial pressure estimation
- Right ventricular systolic pressure estimation
  - Estimated from tricuspid regurgitant jet velocity using modified Bernoulli equation
- LV systolic and diastolic function evaluation

Imaging Recommendations

- Best imaging tool
  - Echocardiogram

DIFFERENTIAL DIAGNOSIS

Left Heart Inflow or Outflow Obstruction Without Pulmonary Hypertension

- Classic imaging findings of PH may be absent in group 2
  - PA may be normal in size
  - Right heart may be normal
- Similarly, left heart dilation and increase in left atrial pressure does not equate to PH
  - Need right heart catheterization to make diagnosis of PH

Group 1 Pulmonary Arterial Hypertension

- Degree of PH usually much more severe in PAH than in group 2 PH
  - Greater RV dilation and hypertrophy in PAH
- Left heart often normal in PAH
- No periarteriolar ground glass opacity in group 2 PH

Group 3 Pulmonary Hypertension

- In isolated group 3 PH, parenchymal abnormalities are predominant finding
  - However, some patients will have both group 2 and group 3 PH
- Left heart often normal in isolated group 3 PH

Group 4 Pulmonary Hypertension

- Absence of pulmonary arterial filling defect in group 2 PH
- Left cardiac chambers often normal in group 4 PH
- Mosaic attenuation pattern in group 4 PH

Group 5 Pulmonary Hypertension

- Left cardiac chambers usually normal in most cases of group 5 PH
- Characteristic mediastinal and parenchymal findings in group 5 PH

PATHOLOGY

General Features

- Most common cause of PH, accounting for 65-80% of cases
  - 50% of patients with left ventricular failure have PH

Staging, Grading, & Classification

- Begins as isolated postcapillary PH but can progress to combined precapillary and postcapillary PH
- Isolated postcapillary PH
  - Elevated LA pressures (LAP) lead to LA dilation
  - Reduced LA compliance and fibrosis further increased LAP
  - Passive transmission of increased LAP to pulmonary vasculature
  - Pressure measurements
    - Mean pulmonary artery pressure > 20 mmHg
    - Pulmonary artery wedge pressure > 15 mmHg
    - Pulmonary vascular resistance (PVR) < 3 Woods units
- Combined precapillary and postcapillary PH
  - Increase in LAP may cause alterations in pulmonary arteries, including medial hypertrophy and intimal fibrosis
  - Pressure measurements
    - Mean pulmonary artery pressure > 20 mmHg
    - Pulmonary artery wedge pressure > 15 mmHg
    - Pulmonary vascular resistance > 3 Woods units

CLINICAL ISSUES

Demographics

- Most patients are older

Treatment

- Correction of underlying cause, if possible
- Sildenafil (phosphodiesterase-5 inhibitors)
  - Improved quality of life and pulmonary hemodynamics
- Riociguat (soluble guanylate cyclase stimulator)
  - No change in mPAP

SELECTED REFERENCES

1. Moles VM et al: Pulmonary hypertension in heart failure with preserved ejection fraction. Cardiol Clin. 40(4):533-40, 2022
2. Singh A et al: Normal values of left atrial size and function and the impact of age: results of the World Alliance Societies of Echocardiography Study. J Am Soc Echocardiogr. 35(2):154-64.e3, 2022
3. Guazzi M et al: Pulmonary hypertension in HFpEF and HFrEF: JACC review topic of the week. J Am Coll Cardiol. 76(9):1102-11, 2020
4. Vachiéry JL et al: Pulmonary hypertension due to left heart disease. Eur Respir J. 53(1), 2019
5. Stojanovska J et al: Reference normal absolute and indexed values from ECG-gated MDCT: left atrial volume, function, and diameter. AJR Am J Roentgenol. 197(3):631-7, 2011

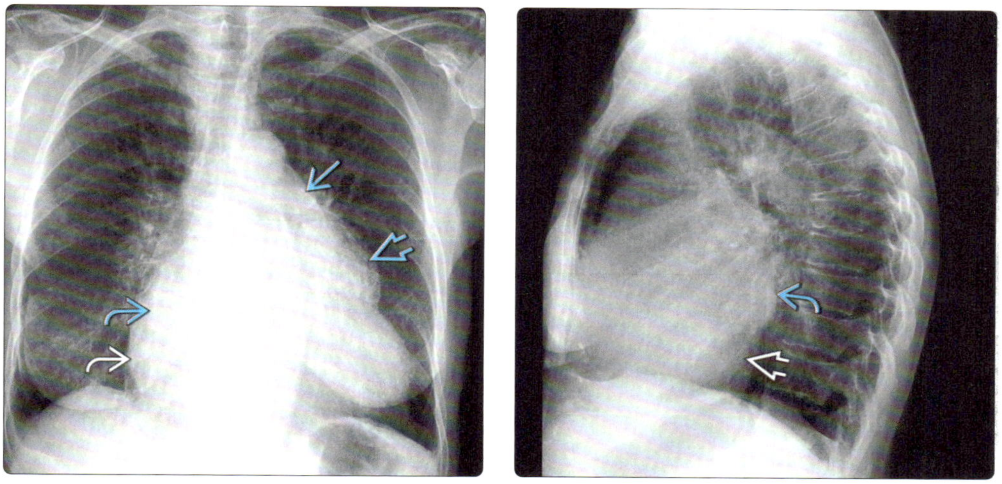

(Left) *PA radiograph in a 71-year-old woman shows LA enlargement with a double density sign and an enlarged LA appendage. The main PA is dilated. The right atrium is also enlarged.* **(Right)** *Lateral radiograph shows LA enlargement with more mild left ventricular and right ventricle enlargement. Echocardiogram confirmed rheumatic heart disease with mitral and aortic valve stenosis and tricuspid regurgitation. Mean PA pressure was 39 mmHg on right heart catheterization.*

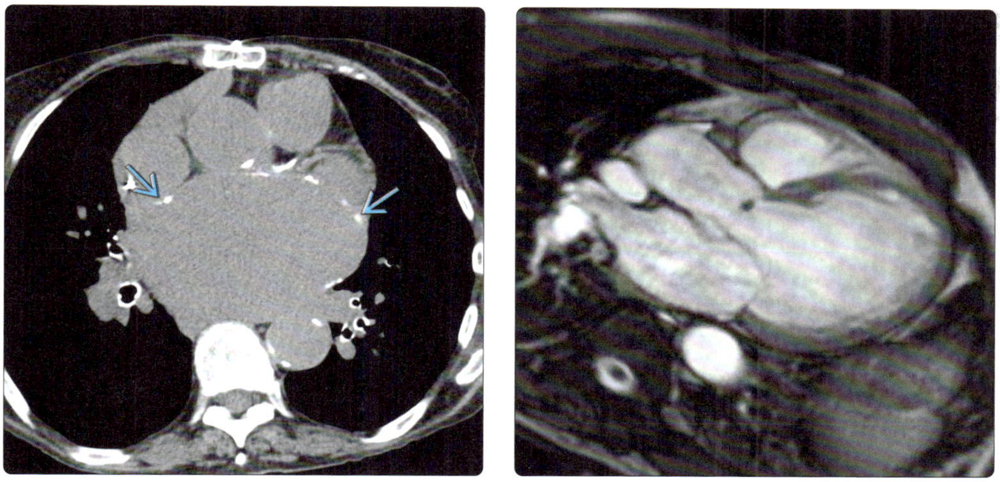

(Left) *CT performed soon after mitral and tricuspid valve replacement shows linear left atrial wall calcifications due to prolonged elevated LA pressures.* **(Right)** *Cardiac MR in a 22-year-old man with heart failure with reduced ejection fraction (HFrEF) secondary to a nonischemic dilated cardiomyopathy shows LV dilation. Ejection fraction was 16%. Left and right heart catheterization showed normal coronary arteries and an elevated PA pressure of 28 mmHg, consistent with mild pulmonary hypertension.*

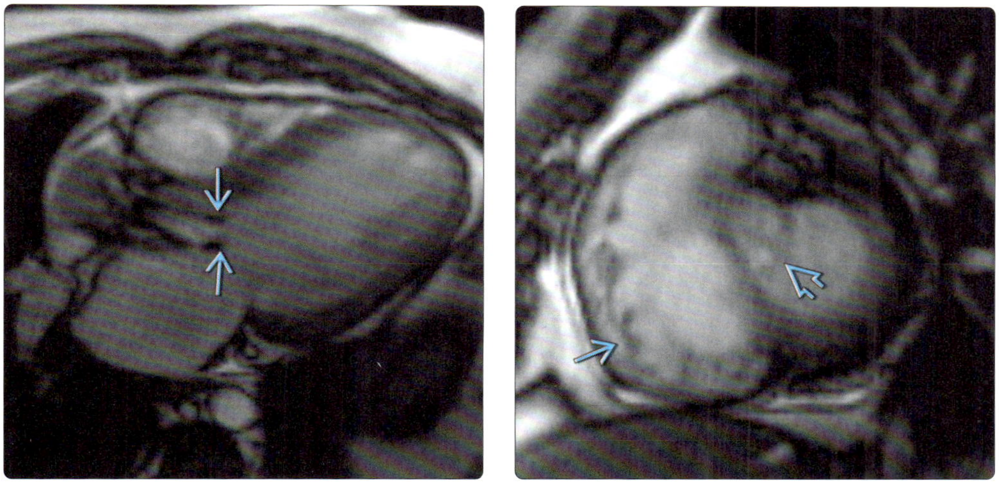

(Left) *MR in 53-year-old man with dyspnea shows a high-velocity dephasing jet originating below the aortic valve from a web causing severe subaortic stenosis. The LV and LA are dilated. The LV ejection fraction was 34%.* **(Right)** *Diastolic short-axis cine MR shows right ventricular dilation and hypertrophy. The web can be partially visualized in the LV outflow track. The longstanding subaortic stenosis led to both increased LV and LA pressures, subsequent HFrEF, and group 2 PH.*

Group 3 Pulmonary Hypertension

KEY FACTS

TERMINOLOGY

- Pulmonary hypertension (PH) associated with lung disease or chronic hypoxia
  - Airway, parenchymal, &/or interstitial lung disease
  - Hypoventilation syndromes (arterial partial pressure of CO_2 > 45 mmHg)
    - Obesity hypoventilation syndrome (OHS)
    - Chest wall deformities
    - Neuromuscular disorders
    - Central alveolar hypoventilation syndrome
    - Congenital central hypoventilation syndrome
  - Sleep-disordered breathing (sleep apnea)
  - Chronic hypoxia without lung disease (high altitude)
  - Lung developmental abnormalities
- 2nd most common cause of PH

IMAGING

- General imaging features of PH
- Superimposed findings of parenchymal or airways disease
- Superimposed findings suggestive of hypoventilation syndrome
  - Obesity
  - Atrophy of chest wall musculature
  - Chest wall deformity
  - Diaphragmatic elevation
- CT best modality for help elucidate cause of group 3 PH

PATHOLOGY

- Mechanism of group 3 PH is multifactorial
  - Hypoxic vasoconstriction
  - Parenchymal destruction
  - Vascular injury with remodeling and inflammation

CLINICAL ISSUES

- Patients tend to be older men
- Survival in group 3 PH worse than group 1 PAH, even when controlled for age, sex, and comorbidities
- Treatment of underlying lung disease if possible

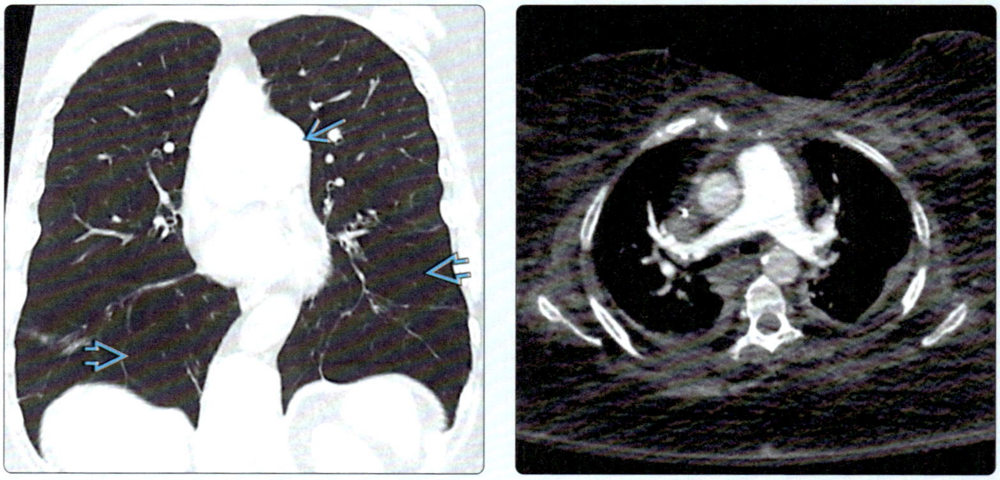

(Left) *NECT in a 55-year-old man with history of alpha-1 antitrypsin deficiency shows lower lobe panlobular emphysema ➡. The 3.8-cm main pulmonary artery (PA) ➡ is larger than the adjacent ascending aorta (AA). Mean PA pressure (PAP) on right heart catheter was 31 mmHg.* **(Right)** *Main PA diameter measures 4.2 cm in this patient with BMI of 70, obesity hypoventilation syndrome, sleep apnea, and severe pulmonary hypertension (PH). Diffuse atrophy of chest wall musculature also contributes to hypoventilation.*

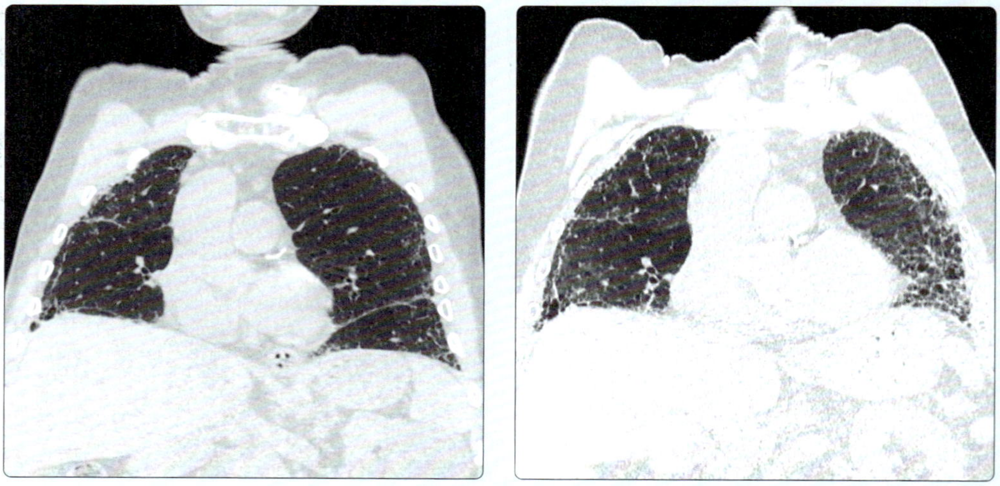

(Left) *NECT in a 67-year-old man with idiopathic pulmonary fibrosis (IPF) shows lower lobe-predominant subpleural reticulation with volume loss. The main PA measured 3.1 cm in transverse diameter, and right heart catheterization (RHC) showed a mean PAP of 24 mmHg.* **(Right)** *NECT in the same patient 5 years later shows progression of lower lobe-predominant fibrosis. The main PA measured 3.6 cm in transverse diameter, and mean PAP on RHC was 32 mmHg.*

TERMINOLOGY

Abbreviations

- Pulmonary hypertension (PH)

Definitions

- PH associated with lung disease or chronic hypoxia
  - Airway, parenchymal, &/or interstitial lung disease
    - Obstructive lung disease
    - Restrictive lung disease
      - In interstitial lung disease, PH is present in 3.5-15%, 30-50%, and 60-90% of patients with early disease, advanced disease, and at time of transplant, respectively
    - Mixed obstructive and restrictive lung disease
  - Hypoventilation syndromes (arterial partial pressure of CO_2 > 45 mmHg)
    - Obesity hypoventilation syndrome (OHS)
      - Nearly 90% of patients with OHS have obstructive sleep apnea (OSA)
    - Chest wall deformities caused by
      - Pectus excavatum
      - Kyphosis &/or scoliosis
      - Severe trauma
      - Ankylosing spondylitis
    - Neuromuscular disorders
      - Inherited, such as muscular dystrophy, neurologic motor dysfunction, metabolic myopathy, etc.
      - Acquired, such as amyotrophic lateral sclerosis, inflammatory myopathy, myasthenia gravis, etc.
    - Central alveolar hypoventilation syndrome
      - Secondary to underlying neurologic disease or drugs
    - Congenital central hypoventilation syndrome
    - Chronic obstructive pulmonary disease (COPD)
      - Chronic hypoventilation common in patients with severe COPD
  - Sleep-disordered breathing
    - OSA
    - PH is uncommon in OSA in absence of other coexistent conditions, such as OHS or COPD
  - Chronic hypoxia without lung disease
    - High altitude
      - People living above 2,500 m are at risk of developing PH
  - Lung developmental abnormalities
- 2nd most common cause of PH
  - Group 2 most common

IMAGING

General Features

- Best diagnostic clue
  - General imaging features of PH with
    - Superimposed findings of parenchymal or airways disease
    - Superimposed findings that may suggest hypoventilation syndrome
      - Obesity
      - Atrophy of chest wall musculature
      - Chest wall deformity
      - Diaphragmatic elevation
    - Superimposed findings that may suggest OSA
      - Nearly 70% of patients with OSA are obese
      - However, many patients with OSA are overweight or have BMI < 25

Radiographic Findings

- General imaging features of PH
- Secondary findings of conspicuous parenchymal, interstitial, or airways disease
- Secondary findings of chest wall deformity, obesity, diaphragmatic elevation, etc.

CT Findings

- General imaging findings suggestive of PH
  - Assessment of right heart and vasculature better after administration of intravenous contrast
- Secondary findings, such as
  - Emphysema
  - Pulmonary fibrosis in
    - Radiologic usual interstitial pneumonia (UIP) pattern
    - Radiologic nonspecific interstitial pneumonia (NSIP) pattern
    - Fibrotic hypersensitivity pneumonitis (fHP)
      - Can appear as radiologic UIP pattern
    - Desquamative interstitial pneumonia
    - Sequelae of healed acute lung injury
  - Lymphangioleiomyomatosis
    - Usually mild PH
    - Associated with degree of involvement
  - Primary and secondary causes of airways disease
    - Smoking related
    - Asthma
    - Bronchiectasis
      - Congenital or acquired
    - Constrictive bronchiolitis
    - Cystic fibrosis
  - Findings that may lead to hypoventilation
    - Obesity
    - Congenital or acquired chest wall deformities
    - Chest wall muscular atrophy
    - Diaphragmatic elevation

MR Findings

- General findings of PH
- Not typically used for diagnosis of group 3 PH

Echocardiographic Findings

- Excellent noninvasive tool for assessment of PH
- Cannot assess lung parenchyma
- Accuracy of echocardiography in patients with advanced lung disease is low
  - Tendency to overestimate pulmonary pressures

Imaging Recommendations

- Best imaging tool
  - CT is best noninvasive tool for assessment of etiology of group 3 PH
  - Diagnosis of PH requires right heart catheterization

DIFFERENTIAL DIAGNOSIS

Group 1-4 Pulmonary Hypertension

- Presence of coexistent lung disease in patients with PH is common
  - May be minor finding in patients with groups 1-4 PH and may have little contribution toward PH
    - For instance, mild interstitial lung abnormality or emphysema in patient with extensive chronic thromboembolic disease
  - However, patients can have multifactorial causes of PH, which may be related to a single risk factor
    - For instance, emphysema and ischemic heart disease in heavy smoker leading to both group 2 and group 3 PH
    - Or components of group 1 and group 3 PH related to PAH (NSIP pattern of fibrosis) and OHS in obese patients with scleroderma
- Detailed clinical and physiologic assessments needed to help make these diagnoses
  - Spirometry moderately to severely impaired in patients with group 3 PH and lung disease
  - Different hemodynamic response during cardiopulmonary exercise testing in group 3 patients compared with other types of PH
    - Exercise limitations related to ventilation
      - Reduced breathing reserve
      - Normal O2 pulse
      - Normal CO/VO2 slope
      - Mixed venous oxygen saturation above lower limit
      - Increase in PaCO2 during exercise

Group 5 Pulmonary Hypertension

- Sarcoid can lead to fibrotic lung disease but is classified as group 5
  - Characteristic imaging findings of sarcoid often with superimposed symmetric mediastinal and hilar lymphadenopathy
- Pulmonary Langerhans cell histiocytosis (PLCH) is now classified as group 5 PH
  - Associated with smoking and thus findings of smoking-related lung disease often coexistent

Findings Associated With Group 3 Pulmonary Hypertension but Without Pulmonary Hypertension

- Imaging findings associated with group 3 PH very common, do not always cause PH
- Right heart catheterization needed to make diagnosis of PH

PATHOLOGY

General Features

- Mechanism of group 3 PH is multifactorial
  - Hypoxic vasoconstriction
  - Parenchymal destruction
  - Vascular injury with remodeling and inflammation

Microscopic Features

- Most data from explants or autopsies in patients with advanced UIP or COPD
  - Destruction of parenchyma with loss of microvasculature and capillaries
  - Compression of peripheral vasculature due to alveolar and secondary lobular collapse in UIP
  - Thickening of media and intima from chronic hypoxia
    - Hypoxia induces endothelial cell damage and smooth muscle proliferation
      - Can lead to irreversible arteriolar intimal thickening, medial hypertrophy, and adventitial collagen deposition
    - Morphologic vascular lesions in COPD related to severity of PH

CLINICAL ISSUES

Presentation

- Most common signs/symptoms
  - Dyspnea and fatigue during exercise eventually progressing to rest
  - Respiratory failure
  - Lower extremity edema

Demographics

- Given association with IPF and COPD, patients tend to be older than those with group 1 PH
- More common in men than women

Natural History & Prognosis

- Survival in group 3 PH worse than group 1 PH, even when controlled for age, sex, and comorbidities
- Even nonsevere PH (pulmonary vascular resistance < 5 Woods units) in patients with group 3 associated with decreased quality of life and increased morbidity

Treatment

- Treatment of underlying lung disease if possible
- Supplemental oxygen therapy
- Weight loss treatments in those with OHS
- Treatment of sleep apnea
- Lung transplant if necessary
- Medications in PAH not shown to be effective in treating group 3 PH although certain classes of medications still being studied

DIAGNOSTIC CHECKLIST

Consider

- Group 3 PH in patients with imaging findings suggestive of PH with coexistent lung disease

SELECTED REFERENCES

1. Danhaive O et al: Pulmonary hypertension in developmental lung diseases. Clin Perinatol. 51(1):217-35, 2024
2. Arslan A et al: Evolution of pulmonary hypertension in interstitial lung disease: a journey through past, present, and future. Front Med (Lausanne). 10:1306032, 2023
3. Humbert M et al: 2022 ESC/ERS guidelines for the diagnosis and treatment of pulmonary hypertension. Eur Heart J. 43(38):3618-731, 2022
4. Singh N et al: Group 3 pulmonary hypertension: from bench to bedside. Circ Res. 130(9):1404-22, 2022
5. Wenninger S et al: Hypoventilation syndrome in neuromuscular disorders. Curr Opin Neurol. 34(5):686-96, 2021
6. McGettrick M et al: Group 3 pulmonary hypertension: challenges and opportunities. Glob Cardiol Sci Pract. 2020(1):e202006, 2020

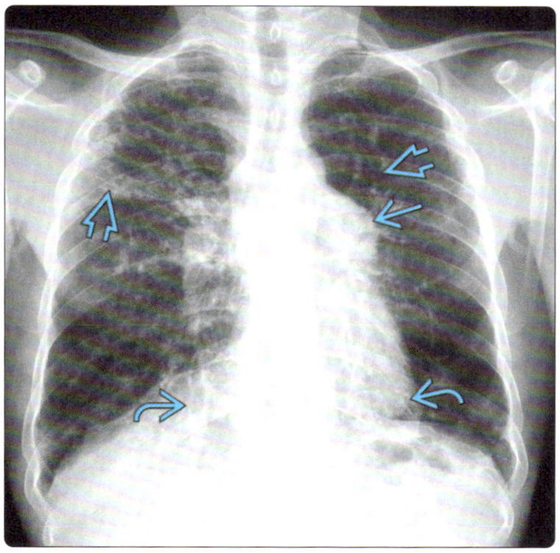

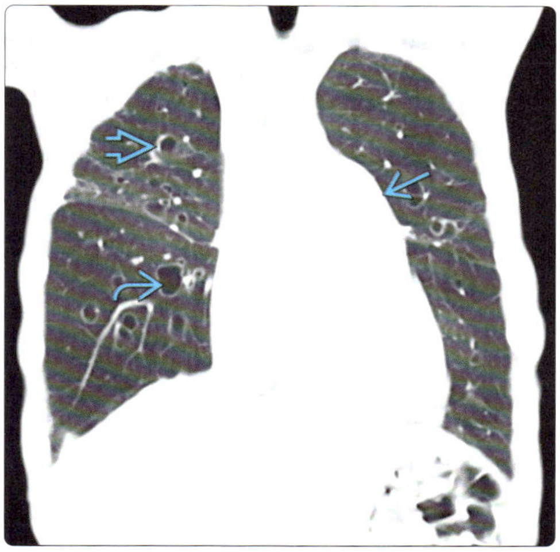

(Left) *PA radiograph in a 40-year-old man with common variable immunodeficiency (CVID) shows enlargement of the main PA →, lower lobe ↪ greater than upper lobe ⇨ bronchiectasis, and patchy areas of nodularity and consolidation.* **(Right)** *CECT more anteriorly shows main PA enlargement →, lower lobe ↪ greater than upper lobe ⇨ bronchiectasis, and conspicuous mosaic attenuation. Mean PAP via RHC was 38 mmHg.*

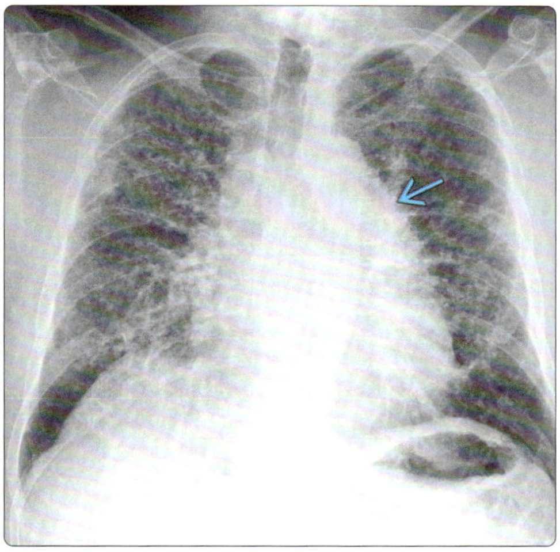

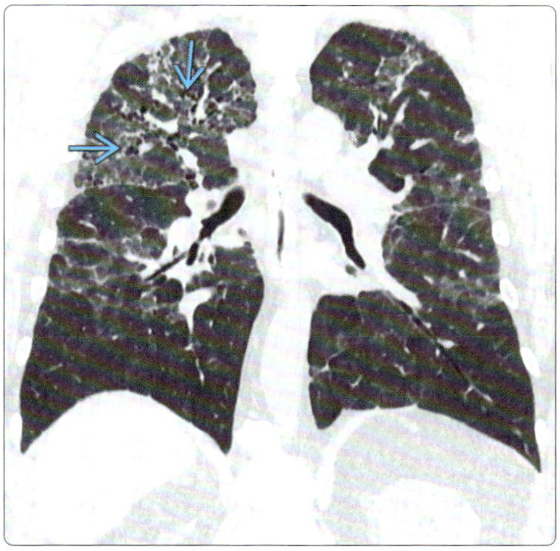

(Left) *Radiograph in a 59-year-old parrot owner shows an enlarged PA → with mid and upper lung-predominant peribronchovascular fibrosis and ground-glass opacity (GGO) extending to the lung periphery with associated subpleural reticulation.* **(Right)** *NECT shows upper lobe-predominant fibrosis with GGO and traction bronchiectasis →. A 3-density sign is present in areas of hypoattenuation, normal lung, and increased attenuation, consistent with fibrotic hypersensitivity pneumonitis (fHP).*

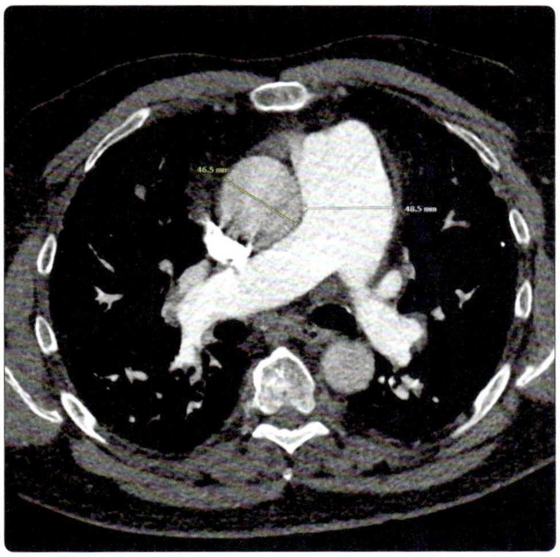

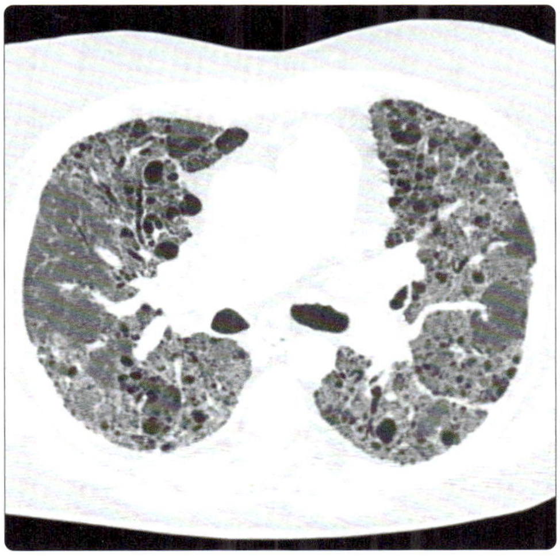

(Left) *CTPA study in a patient with fHP shows PA enlargement measuring 4.9 cm, while the ascending aorta measures 4.7 cm; however, the patient's mean PAP was only mildly elevated at 27 mmHg on RHC.* **(Right)** *NECT in a heavy smoker with pathologically proven desquamative interstitial pneumonia, and emphysema with airspace enlargement with fibrosis shows diffuse GGO with areas of cystic change and mild bronchiectasis. The main PA is enlarged. Mean PAP on RHC was 40 mmHg.*

Group 4 Pulmonary Hypertension

KEY FACTS

TERMINOLOGY

- Pulmonary hypertension (PH) due to pulmonary artery (PA) occlusion
  - Chronic thromboembolic disease PH (CTEPH)
  - Other PA obstructions
  - PA sarcoma (PAS)
  - Metastatic tumor emboli to PA
  - Arteritis without connective tissue disease
  - Congenital PA stenosis; parasitic infection

IMAGING

- High rate of radiologist misdiagnosis of CTEPH
- CT pulmonary angiography (CTPA), ideally performed with dual-energy, spectral, or photon-counting technology
  - Chronic endoluminal filling defects that lead to complete or partial occlusion of PA branch
    - Partial filling defects usually more eccentric compared to central filling defects in acute pulmonary embolism (PE)
  - Complete occlusion
    - Vessels with CTEPH often contracted due to organized thrombus and intimal fibrosis
      - Often expanded with acute PE
  - Partial occlusion
    - Bands: Linear filling defects across PA branch
    - Webs: Intertwined bands form webs
  - Mosaic perfusion in vascular distribution very helpful in making diagnosis
  - Iodine maps using multienergy CT can help detect perfusion defects
  - Bronchial artery collaterals often large in CTEPH
- Ventilation/perfusion (V/Q) scan
  - Still recommended as 1st study used for assessment of CTEPH
  - Negative V/Q scan has high specificity

CLINICAL ISSUES

- CTEPH is only form of PH that can be cured surgically

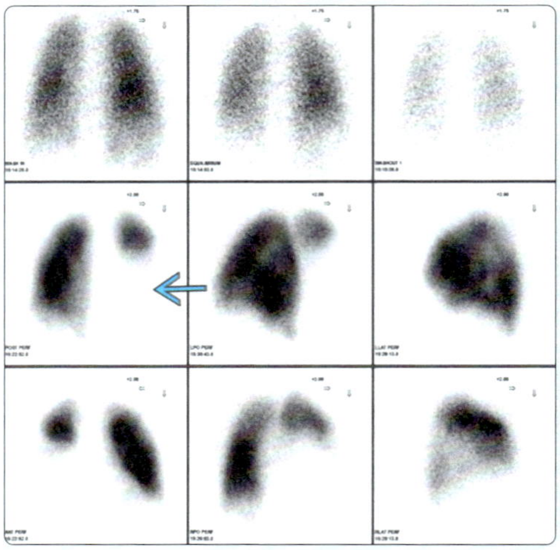

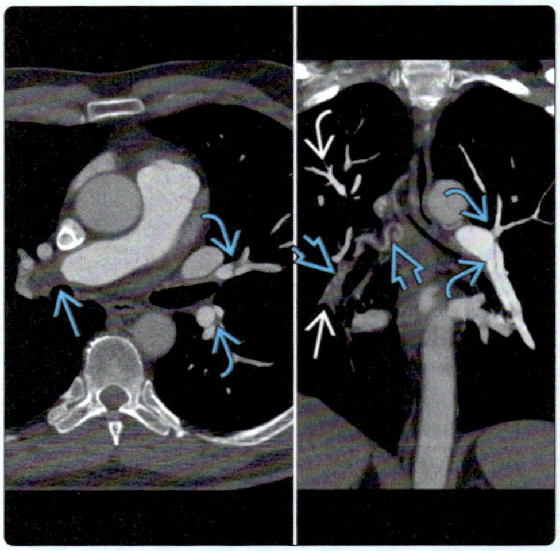

(Left) *V/Q scan shows extensive perfusion defects in the right lung. Very mild perfusion defects are present on the left.* **(Right)** *Axial (right) and coronal MIP (left) images show large chronic thrombus in the right pulmonary artery (RPA) just distal to the apical segment, which is partially patent. The RPA is contracted distally. Although the V/Q showed only minimal defects on the left, extensive nonocclusive webs and bands are present. Large right bronchial collaterals are seen.*

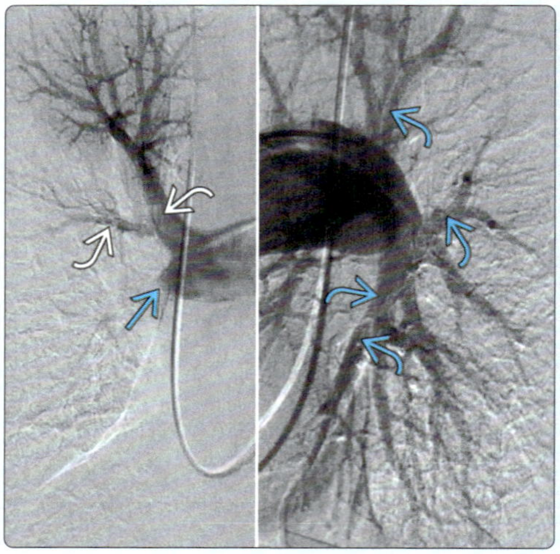

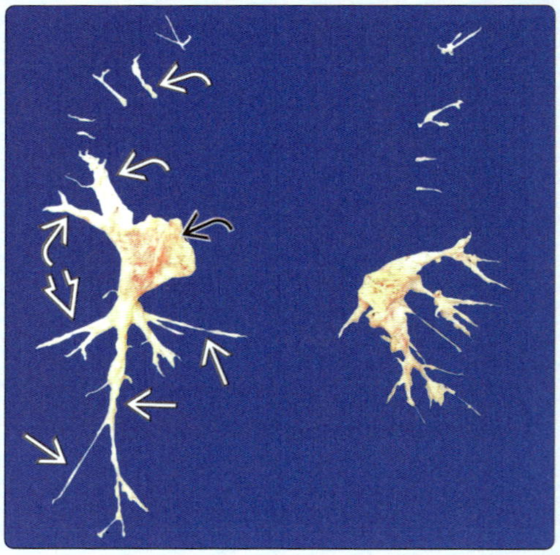

(Left) *DSA of RPA (left) shows RPA occlusion with a pouch defect. Only apical segment is patent with associated linear webs and bands. There are numerous linear webs and bands in all left lobes.* **(Right)** *Pulmonary thromboendarterectomy (PTE) specimen shows intima with associated chronic thrombus removed from RPA, right upper, right middle, and right lower lobes. There are similar specimens from left PA. Patients mean PA pressure ↓ from 46 mmHg to 22 mmHg after PTE.*

TERMINOLOGY

Definitions

- Pulmonary hypertension (PH) due to pulmonary artery (PA) occlusion
  - Chronic thromboembolic disease PH (CTEPH)
  - Other PA obstructions
    - PA sarcoma (PAS)
    - Metastatic tumor emboli to PA
      - Renal cell carcinoma
      - Uterine and germ cell testicular tumors
      - Other tumors
    - Arteritis without connective tissue disease
    - Congenital PA stenosis
    - Parasitic infection
      - PA hydaticosis
- Chronic thromboembolic pulmonary disease (CTEPD)
  - Chronic pulmonary emboli without resting PH

General Comments

- Cardiac sarcomas are not covered here; refer to specific chapter

IMAGING ANATOMY

General Features

- Best diagnostic clue
  - General findings of PH
  - Intravascular filling defects of varying size, number, and morphology depending on underlying cause
  - Mosaic perfusion defects in vascular distribution
- Location
  - PAs
- Size
  - Variable
- Morphology
  - Variable depending on etiology

Radiographic Findings

- General findings of PH
- Difficult to make diagnosis of CTEPH based on radiograph alone
  - Westermark sign
    - Can be difficult to recognize
    - Focal area of oligemia due to upstream PA occlusion
  - Subpleural scarring due to prior infarct

CT Findings

- CT pulmonary angiography (CTPA), ideally performed with dual-energy, spectral, or photon-counting technology
- CTEPH
  - Imaging findings of CTEPH can be variable
  - High rate of radiologist misdiagnosis of CTEPH
    - Lack of awareness of imaging findings
    - Poor protocols limit diagnosis of distal disease
  - Chronic endoluminal filling defects that lead to complete or partial occlusion of PA branch
    - Involves lower lobes greater than upper lobes
  - Complete occlusion
    - Vessels with CTEPH often contracted due to organized thrombus and intimal fibrosis
      - Vessel often expanded with acute disease
      - Vessel can appear "absent" with ostial disease
    - Filling defects often more eccentric in CTEPH and CTEPD
      - Typically more central in acute pulmonary embolism (PE)
  - Partial occlusion
    - Bands: Linear filling defects across PA branch
    - Webs: Intertwined bands form webs
    - Eccentric thrombi: Chronic clot along long axis of vessel that do not transverse vessel
  - Acute on chronic disease
    - Many patients with CTEPH and CTEPD have hypercoagulable disorders
    - Presence of acute disease does not exclude presence of associated chronic disease
    - Interventional therapies intended for acute disease can lead to severe vascular injury and death in patients with chronic disease
  - Parenchymal findings
    - Mosaic perfusion in vascular distribution very helpful in making diagnosis
      - Areas of hypoperfusion often well delineated and correspond to vascular territory with visible proximal occlusion
      - Need occlusive thrombus for perfusion defects
    - Iodine maps using dual-energy CT, spectral CT, or photon-counting CT can help detect subtle perfusion abnormalities
      - Should correlate with anatomic occlusion, as not all perfusion defects are related to vascular etiology
      - Hypoxic vasoconstriction or oligemia from small airway or parenchymal abnormality will also cause hypoperfusion
      - Need to assess lung parenchyma and airway morphology to help differentiate
    - In severe cases, unobstructed vessels will appear engorged with surrounding parenchymal ground-glass opacity due to compensatory hyperperfusion
      - All of right heart output being directed to small number of patent vessels
  - Additional vascular findings
    - Bronchial artery collaterals often conspicuous in CTEPH
      - Will provide systemic arterial supply to lung with pulmonary arterial occlusion
      - Not as common or pronounced in many other causes of PH
    - Chronic clot in inferior vena cava or right heart
  - Uncommon vascular findings
    - Unilateral CTEPH
      - Rare
    - CTEPH starting in main PA (mPA) proximal to bifurcation
      - Rare
      - Should consider other causes, such as sarcoma
    - Calcified CTEPH
      - Need to differentiate intimal calcification seen with any cause of severe PH from calcified clot
- Metastatic tumor emboli to PAs

- Often mimics acute pulmonary emboli with vascular expansion
- Usually localized in segmental and subsegmental vasculature
  - Can be more central
- Vessels filled with tumor emboli may have beaded shape
- Tumor emboli will continue to grow despite anticoagulation
- Look for associated tumor in inferior vena cava or right heart
- Enhancement often subtle or absent, especially during pulmonary arterial phase of imaging
  - Consider additional portal venous-phase imaging if suspected
  - Enhancement may be conspicuous with renal cell carcinoma, melanoma, thyroid, etc.

- Arteritis without connective tissue disease
  - Inflammatory, often circumferential wall thickening of central > peripheral PAs
  - Morphologic appearance of vessels is abnormal
    - Long-segment concentric narrowing with poststenotic dilation
    - Vessels may be obstructed and can mimic CTEPH
  - Distribution of disease may be atypical compared to CTEPH
    - Upper lobe predominance may be seen in vasculitis; very rare with CTEPH
  - Best clue is associated findings of vasculitis involving systemic vasculature
    - May be absent
  - Enhancement of arterial walls may be seen on portal venous-phase imaging
- PA hydatidosis
  - Hydatid disease can rarely involve PAs
  - Presents as chronic low-attenuation filling defects expanding PAs
    - PA filling defects may have septations due to multilocular hydatid cysts
  - Wall enhancement of PAs often present
  - Associated findings
    - Classic multilocular cystic lesion in liver
    - Parenchymal hydatid cysts may be present

MR Findings

- CTEPH
  - Disadvantages to CTPA
    - Less sensitive for distal segmental and subsegmental disease
    - Longer imaging time
  - Advantages
    - No ionizing radiation
    - Assessment of right heart function and morphology
    - Assessment pulmonary perfusion
    - Assessment of pulmonary flow and velocities
- Metastatic tumor emboli
  - MR not routinely used for diagnosis of tumor emboli
  - Certain tumors, such as renal cell carcinoma and melanoma, may show intense enhancement
- Arteritis not due to connective tissue disease
  - MR and MRA are excellent tools for assessing arteritis involving pulmonary or systemic vasculature
  - Similar to CT, shows wall thickening of involved vasculature with varying degrees of smooth concentric stenosis and aneurysmal dilation
  - Wall thickening often enhances post contrast
  - With active inflammation, increased signal in wall on T2W imaging
- PA hydatidosis
  - Intravascular hydatid disease is low signal on T1W imaging and high signal on T2W imaging
  - Can see septations within PA filling defects better with MR than CT
  - Associated T2W high-signal cystic lesions in liver ± lungs

Echocardiographic Findings

- Echocardiogram is excellent, noninvasive tool for assessing PH
- Cannot diagnose CTEPH
  - May visualize clot in right heart or in mPA
- May be able to see PAS when central or crossing pulmonary valve

Angiographic Findings

- Right heart catheterization (RHC) with digital subtraction pulmonary angiography (DSPA)
  - Gold standard for assessing pulmonary pressures and hemodynamics
    - Precapillary PH
      - Mean PA pressure (mPAP) > 20 mmHg
      - PA wedge pressure (PAWP) ≤ 15 mmHg
      - Pulmonary vascular resistance (PVR) ≥ 240 dynes/sec/cm^{-5} or ≥ 3 Wood units
  - DSPA
    - Some surgeons still prefer DSPA to CTPA
    - Advantages
      - Traditionally higher spatial resolution than CTPA
      - Newer photon-counting CT has spatial resolution as low as 0.2 mm
      - Can assess pulmonary perfusion
      - Excellent for visualizing concentric, long-segment narrowing with poststenotic dilation common seen in vasculitis
    - Limitations
      - Invasive
      - Vessels overlap and can obscure subtle defects, especially during pulmonary venous filling
      - Higher radiation than CTPA
      - Layering thrombus can be missed
      - Cannot accurately differentiate between CTEPH and other chronic filling defects, such as PAS and intravascular tumor emboli

Nuclear Medicine Findings

- PET/CT
  - Can help differentiate PAS and intravascular tumor emboli from CTEPH
    - Nearly 90% of PAS show FDG uptake
    - Tumor emboli commonly FDG avid as well
  - PET/CT can help diagnosis of large vessel vasculitis
    - Increased FDG uptake in involved vasculature
- Ventilation/perfusion (V/Q) scan
  - Still recommended as 1st study used for assessment of CTEPH

- Negative V/Q scan has high specificity
- Positive scan requires additional evaluation with cross-sectional imaging or DSPA
  - Cannot differentiate between CTEPH from other causes of filling defects

Imaging Recommendations

- Best imaging tool
  - CTPA with dual-energy, spectral, or photon-counting technology
- Protocol advice
  - In nearly all cases, CTEPH and CTEPD can be visualized on CTPA in setting of correct protocol
  - Need < 1-mm slice thickness at minimum
  - Iodine maps can help visualize areas of vascular hypoperfusion
    - Should correlate with anatomic occlusion
  - Monoenergetic imaging can help improve attenuation of contrast bolus if necessary
  - Importance of breath hold should be explained to patient
  - Contrast should be injected at rate of at least 5 cc/sec, especially in obese patients
  - Can consider additional portal venous phase of imaging if tumor is suspected

DIFFERENTIAL DIAGNOSIS

Acute Pulmonary Embolism

- Acute PE more common than CTEP
  - Estimated that just over 3% of patients with acute PE develop CTEPH
- Acute PE with coexistent chronic PE not uncommon
- Both present with intraluminal filling defects
  - Acute PE tends to be more central and will distend vessel
- Clinical scenarios are usually different

In Situ Thrombus in Pulmonary Arterial Hypertension

- Forms longitudinally along walls of PAs
  - Can mimic CTEPH
- Tends not to occlude PA branches, unlike CTEPH
- Mosaicism seen in pulmonary arterial hypertension (PAH) and CTEPH often appear different

Differentiating Between Etiologies of Group 4 Pulmonary Hypertension

- Can be difficult to differentiate between CTEPH, PAS, tumor emboli, and vasculitis
- Above describes methods of differentiation

PATHOLOGY

General Features

- CTEPH
  - Occlusion of PA branches leads to increased PA pressures
  - Microvasculopathy, similar to what is seen in PAH, occurs in patients with CTEPH
    - Occurs in both regions with proximal occlusion unobstructed vascular beds
      - Increased blood flow with increased endothelial sheer stress may lead to microvasculopathy in unobstructed regions
      - Systemic to pulmonary circulation collaterals through hypertrophied bronchial arteries and vasa vasorum exposes vascular bed to systemic pressures and development of arteriopathy distal to obstructed vasculature

Staging, Grading, & Classification

- University of California, San Diego CTEPH surgical classification
  - Level 0: No disease
  - Level 1: Disease starting in MPA from pulmonary valve to takeoff of upper lobe branch
    - Level 1C: Level 1 disease with complete occlusion of PA
  - Level 2: Disease starting distal to takeoff of upper lobe branches to segmental ostia
  - Level 3: Disease starting in segmental vasculature
  - Level 4: Disease starting in subsegmental vasculature
- Jamieson surgical classification
  - Type 1: Fresh (acute) thrombus in main lobar PAs
  - Type 2: Intimal thickening and fibrosis ± organized thrombus proximal to segmental arteries
  - Type 3: Fibrosis, intimal webbing, and thickening ± organized thrombus within segmental arteries only
  - Type 4: Microscopic distal arteriolar vasculopathy without visible thromboembolic disease

CLINICAL ISSUES

Presentation

- Most common signs/symptoms
  - Usually present with signs of right heart failure
    - Peripheral edema, dyspnea, syncope, and exertional chest pain

Demographics

- CTEPH
  - Wide age range of patients
  - Most have had recorded history of PE or deep venous thrombosis
    - Up to 25% of patients with CTEPH have no history of PE
  - Risk factors for developing CTEPH
    - Characteristics of acute PE
      - Unprovoked PE
      - Diagnostic delay of > 2 weeks
      - Right ventricular dysfunction at time of acute PE
    - Patient characteristics
      - Antiphospholipid syndrome
      - Factor VIII or von Willebrand factor elevation
      - Abnormal fibrinogen variants
      - History of malignancy or hypothyroidism
      - Splenectomy
      - Indwelling catheters or ports
- Tumor embolism
  - Patients with underlying malignancy
- Arteritis
  - Most common in patients with Takayasu arteritis (TA)
    - In one large study, PA involvement in ~ 6% of patients with TA
  - Primarily seen in young women

- PA hydatidosis
  - Reported in younger patients but can occur in anyone with hydatid disease

Natural History & Prognosis

- CTEPH
  - Surgery significantly improves survival
    - Survival in patients who do not undergo surgery improved compared to years past
      - Significantly worse than those that undergo pulmonary thromboendarterectomy (PTA)
- Tumor embolism
  - Poor prognosis
- Arteritis
  - Can lead to PH if PAs are involved
  - Overall 1-, 3-, and 5-year survival rates in patients with TA-associated PH were 94.0%, 83.2%, and 77.2%, respectively
- PA hydatidosis
  - No studies on long-term outcomes

Treatment

- CTEPH
  - Only form of PH that can be cured surgically
  - PTA or pulmonary endarterectomy (PEA)
    - Complex surgical procedure with circumferential resection of intima and chronic thrombus along longitudinal plane
      - Only done at several specialized surgical centers
      - Mortality at best centers is < 1% but > 24% at centers with less experienced surgeons
      - Expert surgeons can remove subsegmental clot with good clinical outcomes
      - Required lifelong anticoagulation
    - PH can persist after successful removal of clot
      - May be related to PAH-like microangiopathy that can occur in CTEPH
      - In other cases, rethrombosis may occur, requiring repeat PTE or balloon angioplasty (BPA)
  - BPA
    - Wire passed across partially occluded vessel and inflated to break apart chronic clot
      - Wire cannot pass across complete occlusion
      - Initially, procedure had very high mortality but is now similar to PTE mortality when performed at specialized centers
      - PA branches can rupture due to relatively thinner media compared to systemic muscular arteries
      - Only several vessels can undergo BPA during single session so requires numerous sessions
    - In most institutions in USA, main indications for BPA include
      - Patient not good surgical candidate, refuses PTE, has recurrent or residual disease after PTE
      - Some centers with perform repeat PTE surgeries for patients with residual or recurrent disease
      - Predominantly nonobstructive lesions limited to segmental and subsegmental vasculature
    - In Japan, BPA is more frequently performed
  - Medical therapy
- Metastatic pulmonary emboli
  - Treatment of underlying primary neoplasm
- Arteritis
  - Medical therapy of underlying vasculitis
  - Some centers have performed BPA of stenotic lesions with promising results
- PA hydatidosis
  - Even with appropriate antiparasitic medications, can be very difficult to treat
  - Few centers in world will perform surgical removal of intravascular hydatid disease

DIAGNOSTIC CHECKLIST

Consider

- CTEPH in setting of PH with intraluminal filling defects that contract PAs

Image Interpretation Pearls

- Imperative to closely assess distal segmental and subsegmental vasculature
  - Patients with isolated subsegmental disease can undergo PTE with good clinical outcomes

SELECTED REFERENCES

1. Chin K et al: Long-term Survival and Quality of Life: Results From the United States Chronic Thromboembolic Pulmonary Hypertension Registry. CHEST Pulmonary. Vol 1, Issue 2. Science Direct. Elsevier, 2023
2. Hahn LD et al: Multidisciplinary approach to chronic thromboembolic pulmonary hypertension: role of radiologists. Radiographics. 43(2):e220078, 2023
3. Yang J et al: Evaluation and management of chronic thromboembolic pulmonary hypertension. Chest. 164(2):490-502, 2023
4. Yang J et al: Outcomes Associated With Catheter-Directed Therapies in Chronic Thromboembolic Pulmonary Hypertension: Cautionary Tales From a Single-Center Case Series. CHEST Pulmonary. Vol 1, Issue 2. Science Direct. Elsevier, 2023
5. Brookes JDL et al: Pulmonary thromboendarterectomy for chronic thromboembolic pulmonary hypertension: a systematic review. Ann Cardiothorac Surg. 11(2):68-81, 2022
6. Erkilinç A et al: Is there any role of pulmonary endarterectomy in pulmonary arterial hydatidosis? Ann Thorac Surg. 114(6):2093-9, 2022
7. Huang Z et al: Long-Term outcomes after percutaneous transluminal pulmonary angioplasty in patients with takayasu arteritis and pulmonary hypertension. Front Immunol. 13:828863, 2022
8. Jansa P et al: Epidemiology of chronic thromboembolic pulmonary hypertension (CTEPH) in the Czech Republic. Pulm Circ. 12(1):e12038, 2022
9. Jiang X et al: Clinical features and survival in Takayasu's arteritis-associated pulmonary hypertension: a nationwide study. Eur Heart J. 42(42):4298-305, 2021
10. Kligerman S et al: Optimizing the diagnosis and assessment of chronic thromboembolic pulmonary hypertension with advancing imaging modalities. Pulm Circ. 11(2):20458940211007375, 2021
11. Ropp AM et al: Intimal sarcoma of the great vessels. Radiographics. 41(2):361-79, 2021
12. Simonneau G et al: Haemodynamic definitions and updated clinical classification of pulmonary hypertension. Eur Respir J. 53(1), 2019
13. Yang J et al: Pulmonary artery involvement in Takayasu's arteritis: diagnosis before pulmonary hypertension. BMC Pulm Med. 19(1):225, 2019
14. Almutairi A et al: Case report of hydatid cyst in the pulmonary artery uncommon presentation: CT and MRI Findings. Case Rep Radiol. 2018:1301072, 2018
15. Thistlethwaite PA et al: Operative classification of thromboembolic disease determines outcome after pulmonary endarterectomy. J Thorac Cardiovasc Surg. 124(6):1203-11, 2002

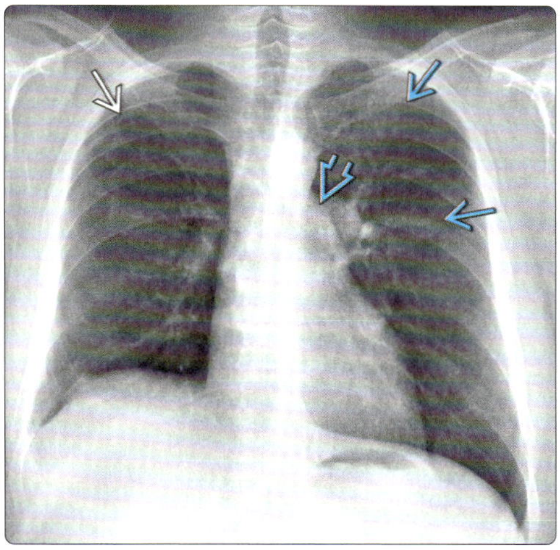
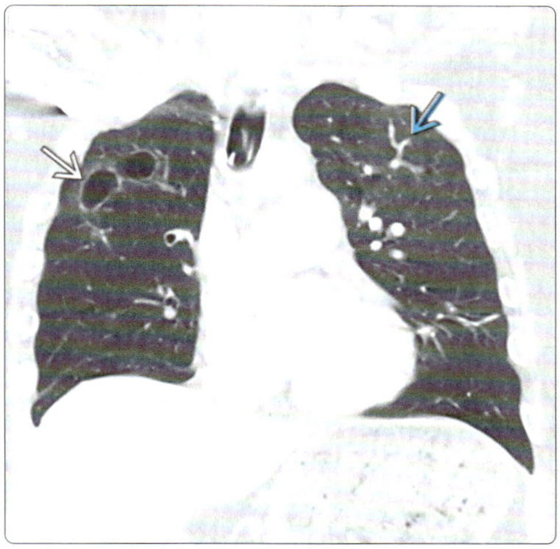

(Left) *Chest x-ray in a 35-year-old man shows PA enlargement* ⇨ *with right lung contraction, scarring, and cystic change* ➡. *The right lung, lingula, and left lower lobe (LLL) oligemia are present (Westermark sign). Only the left upper lobe (LUL) has normal vasculature* ➡. **(Right)** *Coronal CT shows diffuse right lung oligemia with peripheral scarring and cystic change* ➡ *from prior infarct. Oligemia is also present in the lingula and LLL. Only the LUL has normal vasculature* ➡.

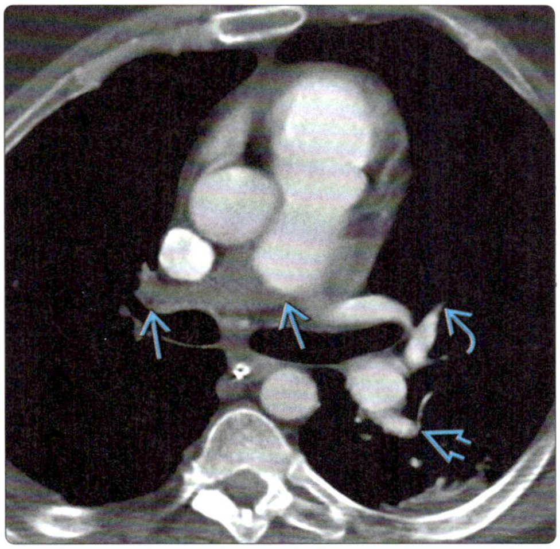
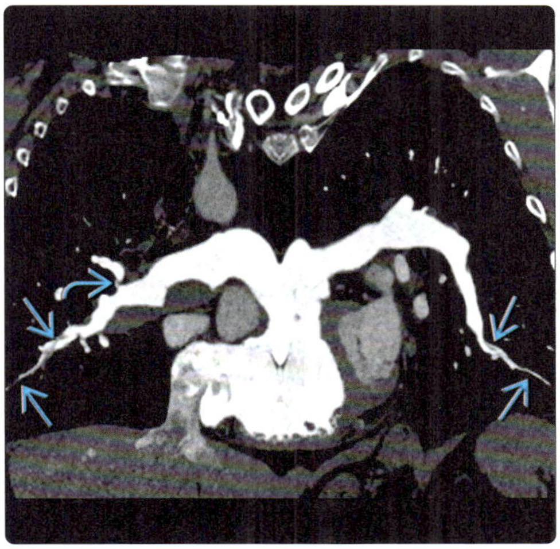

(Left) *CTPA with 3-mm slice thickness shows complete occlusion and contraction of the RPA* ➡ *due to chronic clot. Abrupt lingular* ➡ *and superior segment* ⇨ *occlusions are difficult to detect with 3-mm slices. At a minimum, slices < 1 mm should be used to diagnose CTEPH.* **(Right)** *CTPA in a 63-year-old with CTEPH performed on a photon-counting CT (PCT) with 0.4-mm slice thickness shows a few segmental (S)* ➡ *and subsegmental (SS)* ➡ *clots in this patient with extensive bilateral S (UCSD level 3) and SS (UCSD level 4) disease.*

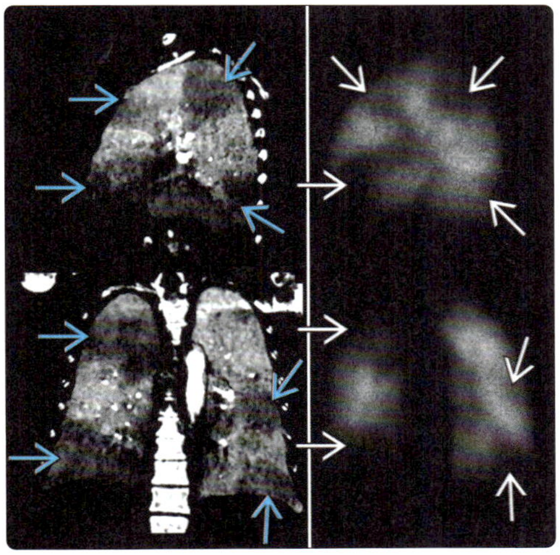
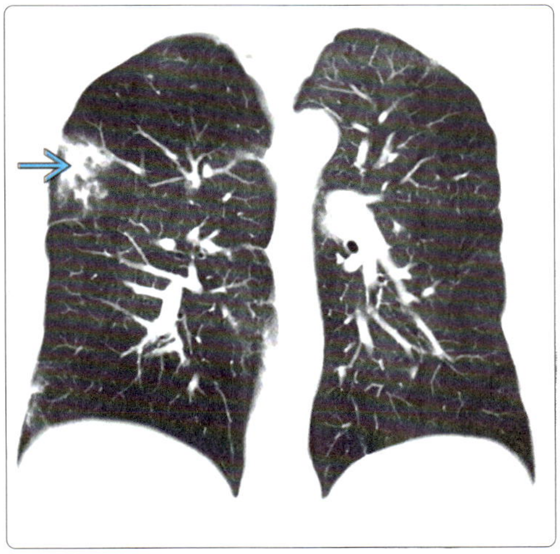

(Left) *Right sagittal and coronal iodine map images from PCT CTPA (right) show extensive bilateral perfusion defects* ➡, *which correlate with perfusion defects from V/Q scan* ➡. **(Right)** *Coronal CECT shows bilateral, well-defined areas of peripheral hypoattenuation with decreased vascularity from proximal occlusions. Only the central vasculature and the LUL apicoposterior segment have normal-appearing vessels. A subacute infarct* ➡ *is seen. The mosaic perfusion correlates with the coronal iodine map image.*

(Left) *CTPA in a patient with severe pulmonary hypertension (PH) due to CTEPH shows numerous bilateral segmental and subsegmental chronic clots . The inferior vena cava is dilated due to severely elevated right heart pressures .* **(Right)** *PTE specimen shows bilateral segmental and subsegmental clot and intima. A fibrin sheathe from an indwelling catheter is seen centrally. Patient's mPAP ↓ from 56-33 mmHg after PTE. Persistent PH is likely related to a microangiopathy that can develop in CTEPH patients.*

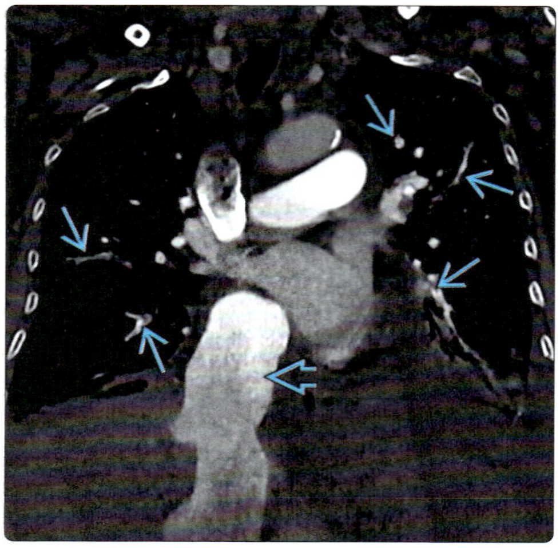

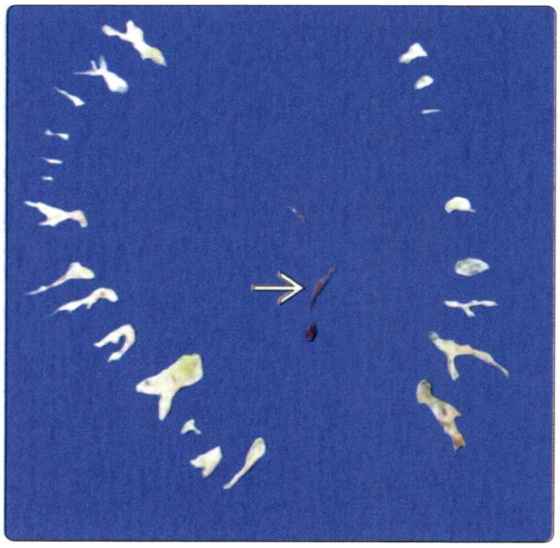

(Left) *Axial oblique CTPA in a 31-year-old woman with PH shows a large, sausage-shaped mass in the LPA with an appearance concerning for a PA sarcoma. Note extensive segmental and subsegmental chronic pulmonary emboli (PE) . Given the presence of chronic PE on the right, the diagnosis of CTEPH was made.* **(Right)** *Coronal image in the same patient shows bilateral mosaic perfusion with well-delineated areas of hypoperfusion and vascular attenuation , supporting the diagnosis of CTEPH.*

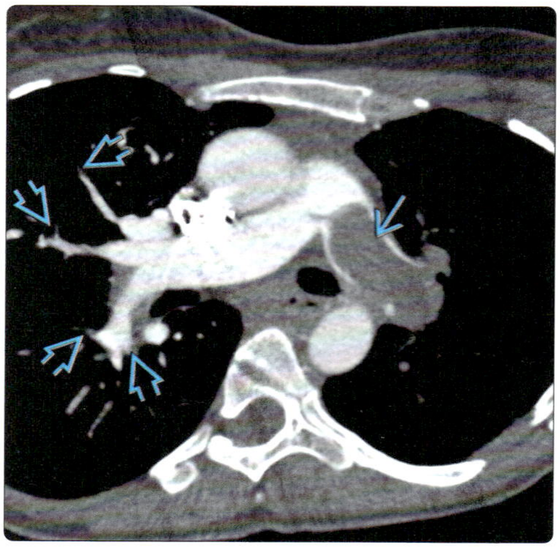

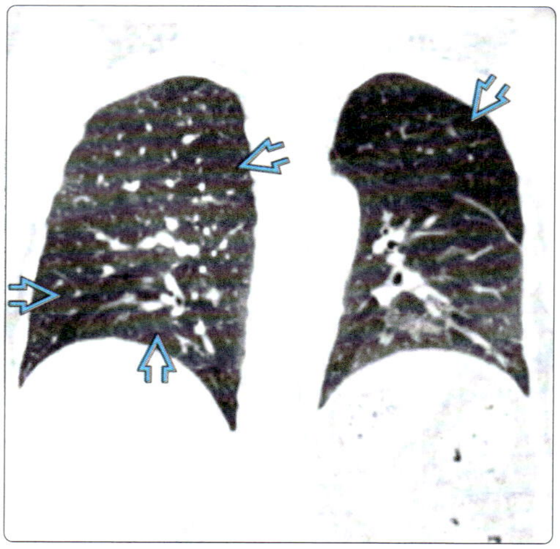

(Left) *Repeat CTPA 2 months after the start of anticoagulation in the same patient shows the decreased size of the previous LPA mass, which now has a concave border . Chronic PE is again seen on the right.* **(Right)** *20-mm thick MIP image shows an isolated LLL descending pulmonary artery chronic clot (UCSD level 2) and hypertrophied bronchial arteries . The left inferior pulmonary vein is unopacified due to the lack of blood flow to the LLL. Unilateral CTEPH is uncommon but does occur.*

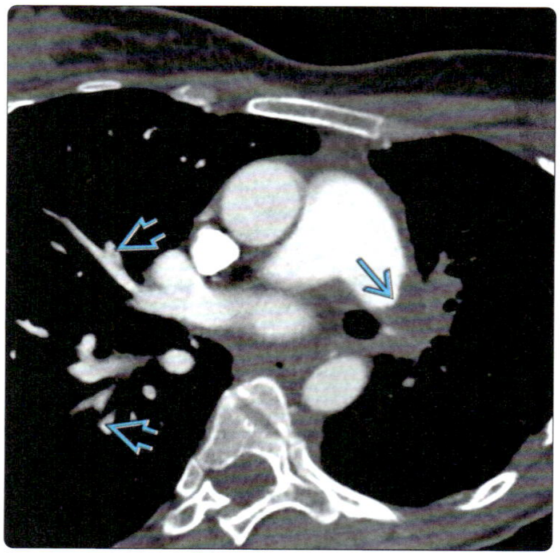

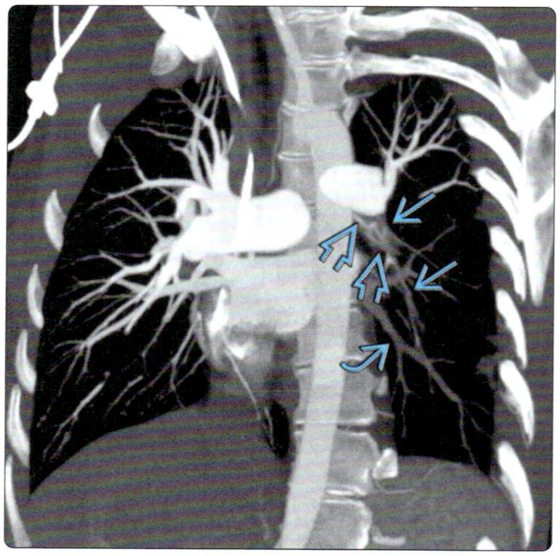

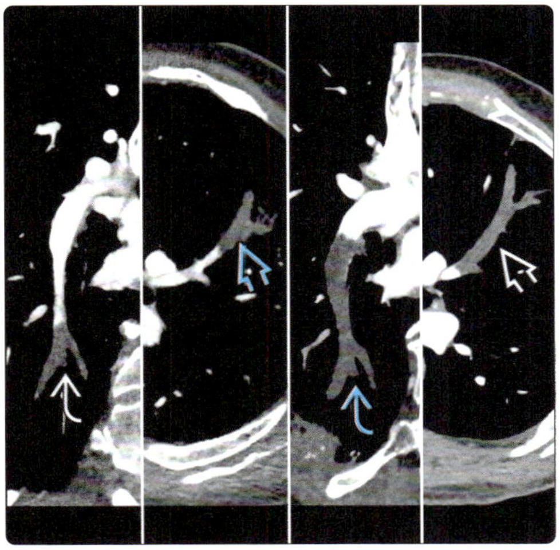

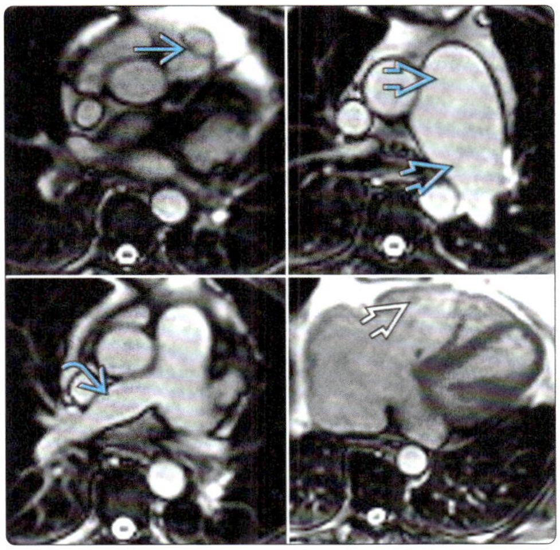

(Left) *CTPA (left) in a man with a sacral chordoma shows bilateral filling defects ➔, ➔, thought to be acute PE. Despite anticoagulation, repeat CTPA 4 months later (right) shows growth and proximal extension of the filling defects now recognized as tumor emboli ➔, ➔.* **(Right)** *Images show pulmonary valve thickening ➔, main PA and left PA dilation ➔, normal RPA ➔, and hypertrophy of the right ventricle ➔ with septal flattening in a patient with congenital pulmonary stenosis and PH.*

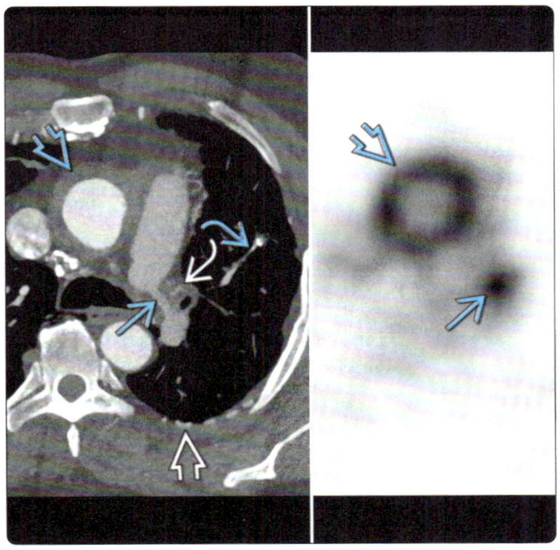

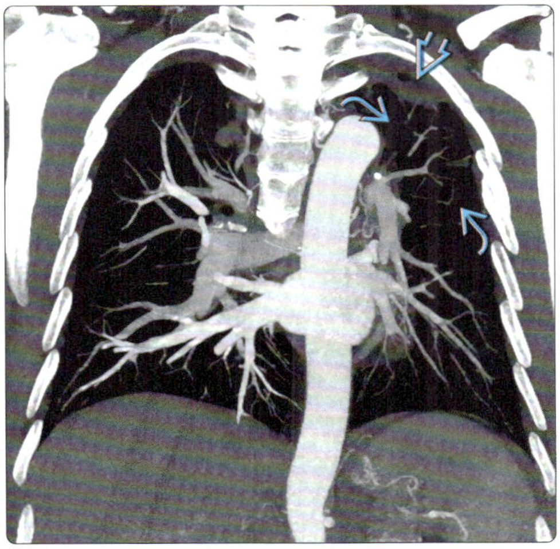

(Left) *CTA (left) and 18 FDG PET (right) in a man with Takayasu arteritis with mild PH show wall thickening of the aorta ➔ and narrowing of the left PA ➔, both of which show FDG uptake. The LUL PA branches are occluded centrally ➔ and peripherally ➔. Intercostal ➔ collaterals are present.* **(Right)** *There is a paucity of LUL PA branches ➔ and left apical scarring from prior infarct ➔. PAs elsewhere are nearly completely normal. The distribution is atypical for CTEPH.*

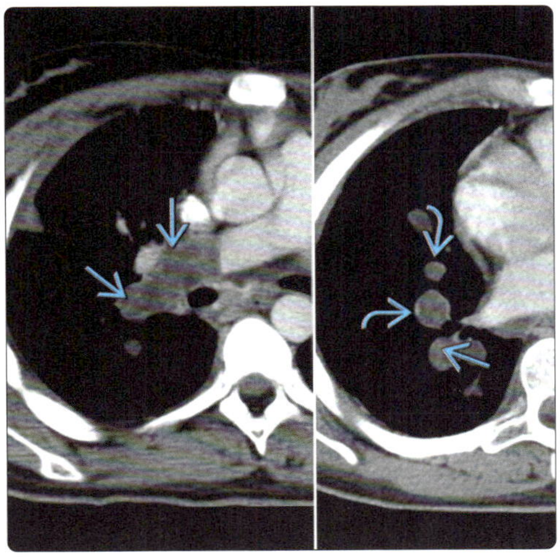

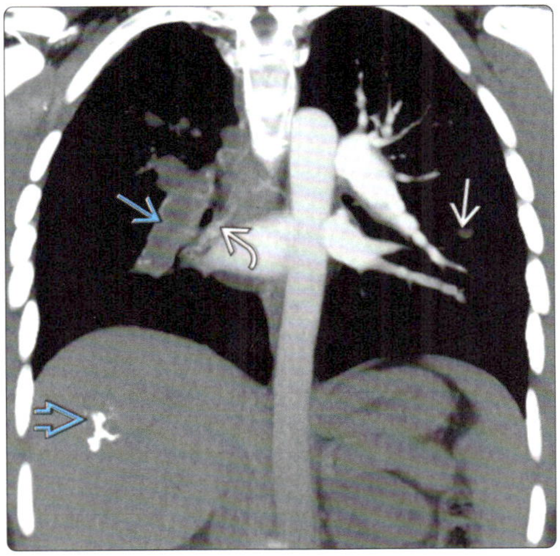

(Left) *Image in an 18-year-old woman from Kuwait shows an expansile, hypoattenuating filling defect with internal septations ➔ in the right main PA (left), extending into all of the right middle and lower lobe branches (right). The PA walls ➔ enhance.* **(Right)** *Image in the same patient 3 years later shows persistent filling defects on the right ➔ > left ➔. Bronchial artery collaterals ➔ and a partially calcified hydatid cyst in the liver ➔ are seen. The patient had moderate PH due to intravascular hydatid disease.*

KEY FACTS

TERMINOLOGY

- Pulmonary hypertension (PH) due to unclear or multifactorial mechanisms
  - 5.1: Hematologic disorders
    - Myeloproliferative disorders
      - Chronic myelogenous leukemia, chronic eosinophilic leukemia, chronic neutrophilic leukemia
      - Polycythemia vera, essential thrombocythemia, primary myelofibrosis
    - Chronic hemolytic anemias
      - Sickle cell disease
      - β-thalassemia
  - 5.2: Systemic and metabolic disorders
    - Sarcoidosis
    - Pulmonary Langerhans cell histiocytosis (PLCH)
    - Neurofibromatosis
    - Gaucher disease
    - Glycogen storage disease (GSD)
  - 5.3: Other
    - Fibrosing mediastinitis
    - Chronic kidney disease (CKD)
  - 5.4: Complex congenital heart disease (CHD)
    - Segmental PH
      - Unilateral absence of a pulmonary artery (UAPA)
      - Isolated pulmonary artery (PA) of ductal origin
      - Hemitruncus
      - Pulmonary atresia with ventricular septal defect (VSD) and major aortopulmonary collateral arteries
      - Other
  - Single ventricle
  - Scimitar syndrome
- Changes compared to prior classification of group 5 PH
  - Splenectomy and thyroid disorders removed from group 5 PH
  - LAM reclassified as group 3 PH

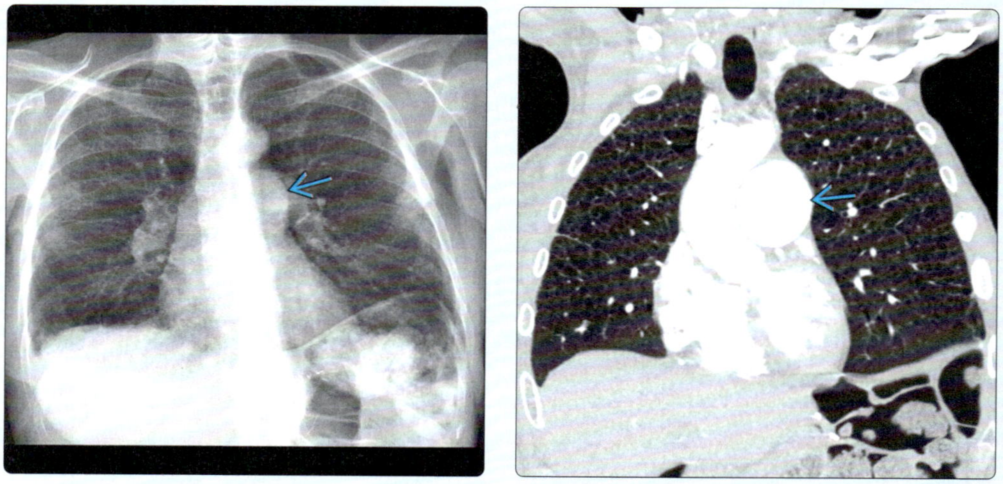

(Left) *CXR in a 32-year-old woman with a heavy smoking history and schizophrenia shows main pulmonary artery (MPA) → enlargement and dilation of the left and right lower lobe (LLL, RLL) branches. The lungs show diffuse but upper lobe-predominant reticulation without fibrosis.* **(Right)** *CT shows MPA enlargement → of 4.9 cm. The lungs show diffuse but upper lobe-predominant, bizarrely shaped cysts with scattered emphysema, consistent with advanced pulmonary Langerhans cell histiocytosis.*

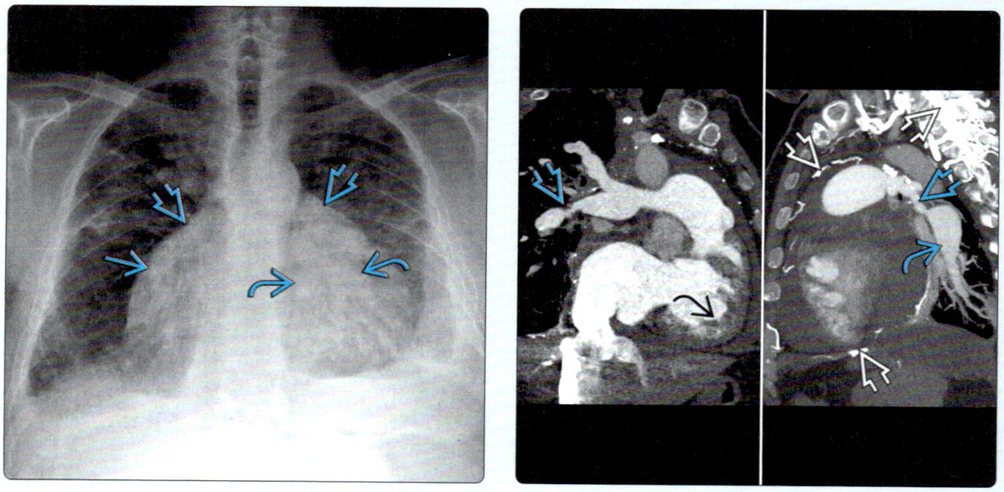

(Left) *CXR shows globular cardiac enlargement. Mediastinal and hilar calcifications are present ⇒. The MPA is enlarged as are the LLL ⇗ and RLL → PAs.* **(Right)** *Right PA image (left) and left PA MIP (right) show hilar calcification associated with severe PA stenoses ⇒ with poststenotic dilation ⇗ due to fibrosing mediastinitis. Right ventricle (RV) hypertrophy ⇗ with MPA and IVC dilation is noted. Venous collaterals ⇒ are from SVC obstruction. Mean PA pressure (mPAP) was 86 mmHg. A moderate pericardial effusion is seen.*

TERMINOLOGY

Abbreviations

- Pulmonary hypertension (PH)

Definitions

- PH due to unclear or multifactorial mechanisms
- 5.1: Hematologic disorders
  - Myeloproliferative disorders
    - Disorders with primary expression of myeloid phenotype: Lower rate of PH, near 11%
      - Chronic myelogenous leukemia, chronic eosinophilic leukemia, chronic neutrophilic leukemia
      - High rate of transformation into acute leukemia
      - PH may be drug induced (dasatinib), pulmonary venoocclusive disease (PVOD) from bone marrow transplant, tumor microembolism
    - Disorders with erythroid or megakaryocytic hyperplasia: High rate of PH
      - Polycythemia vera (PH in 8-77%), essential thrombocythemia (PH in 48%), primary myelofibrosis (PH in 12-14%)
      - Low rate of transformation into acute leukemia
      - PH may be due to chronic thromboembolic pulmonary hypertension (CTEPH), portal hypertension, PVOD from bone marrow transplant, tumor microembolism, ↑ vascular endothelial growth factor levels
  - Chronic hemolytic anemias
    - Sickle cell disease (SCD): PH in 6% by right heart catheterization (RHC)
      - PH due to CTEPH, left heart disease, altered blood viscosity, endothelial dysfunction, and elevated carbon monoxide
    - β-thalassemia: PH in 1.1-4.8% by RHC
      - PH due to chronic hemolysis, iron overload from transfusion, hypercoagulability, splenectomy, hypoxemia, and changes to circulating cells
- 5.2: Systemic and metabolic disorders
  - Sarcoidosis: PH in 6.4% by RHC
    - Parenchymal lung disease, granulomatous vasculopathy, extrinsic compression of vessels, myocardial involvement
  - Pulmonary Langerhans cell histiocytosis (PLCH): PH in ~ 10%
    - Due to parenchymal and vascular involvement
      - Pulmonary vascular lesions most pronounced in venules
  - Neurofibromatosis: Exact incidence unknown but low
    - Related to parenchymal and vascular disease
  - Gaucher disease: PH in 30% untreated, 7% treated
    - Glucocerebroside in the interstitium, vasculopathy due to pulmonary alveolar capillary occlusions, bone marrow microembolism
  - Glycogen storage disease (GSD)
    - 11 types of GSD
    - PH primarily described in GSD type 1 (von Gierke disease)
      - Exact incidence unknown
- 5.3: Other
  - Fibrosing mediastinitis: PH in as many as 50% of patients seeking medical attention
    - Obstruction of pulmonary arteries &/or pulmonary veins
  - Chronic kidney disease (CKD) ± hemodialysis (HD): Wide ranges of PH: stage 5 CKD, 9-39%; on HD, 19-69%, on peritoneal dialysis, 0-42%
    - Numerous factors, including LV dysfunction, volume overload, liver disease, arteriovenous fistula, exposure to dialysis membranes, hypertension and ↑ arterial rigidity, lung disease, endothelial dysfunction, sleep-disordered breathing
- 5.4: Complex congenital heart disease (CHD)
  - Segmental PH
    - In most cases, causes of segmental PH are recognized early in life and can be corrected; if left uncorrected, severe PH can develop
    - In segmental PH, high-pressure and high-velocity blood flow from systemic circulation leads to PH in one lung while PH develops in contralateral lung as it receives all right heart outflow
      - Unilateral absence of a pulmonary artery (UAPA): PH in 20-44%
      - Isolated pulmonary artery (PA) of ductal origin
      - Hemitruncus (anomalous origin of right PA from aorta)
      - Pulmonary atresia with ventricular septal defect (VSD) and major aorticopulmonary collaterals (MAPCAs); segmental PH is bilateral
      - Other
  - Single ventricle
    - Cause of PH in single ventricle morphology very complex and often does not meet classic criteria for PH
      - Unoperated
      - Operated
  - Scimitar syndrome (SS)
    - PH more common in patients diagnosed with infantile form of SS (22-64%) vs. adult form (0-25%)
    - Associated right lung hypoplasia
    - Associated cardiac anomalies in 75%, most commonly secundum atrial septal defect
- Changes compared to prior classification of group 5 PH
  - Splenectomy and thyroid disorders removed from group 5 PH
  - LAM reclassified as group 3 PH

IMAGING

General Features

- Best diagnostic clue
  - Imaging features are heterogeneous given variety of underlying conditions classified under group 5 PH
- Location
  - Variable

Radiographic Findings

- General findings of PH plus variable imaging features depending on underlying condition

CT Findings

- General findings of PH plus variable imaging features depending on underlying condition

MR Findings

- General findings of PH plus variable imaging features depending on underlying condition

Echocardiographic Findings

- Echocardiogram is best initial study if there is concern for PH

Angiographic Findings

- RHC is gold standard for diagnosis of PH

Imaging Recommendations

- Best imaging tool
  - Echocardiogram is best initial tool for assessment of PH when there is concern for Group V PH
  - RHC is gold standard

DIFFERENTIAL DIAGNOSIS

Group 1 Pulmonary Arterial Hypertension

- Many forms of complex CHD are classified as group 1 pulmonary arterial hypertension (PAH)
  - However, segmental PH, single ventricle morphology, and scimitar syndrome are classified as group 5
- Classic parenchymal findings in PAH not seen in group 5 PAH
- Hematologic conditions with group 5 PH may mimic PAH in certain situations
  - Splenic abnormalities (autoinfarction, splenomegaly, splenectomy) may point toward group 5 PH

Groups 2-4 Pulmonary Hypertension

- Because etiologies of group 5 PH are often multifactorial, findings associated with groups 2, 3, or 4 PH may coexist
  - For instance, in sarcoidosis, there may be findings of group 2 PH due to cardiac involvement and group 3 PH due to parenchymal fibrosis
  - Similarly, patients with SSD may have findings of group 2 PH due to cardiac involvement and group 4 PH due to CTEPH
- However, other factors associated with PH in these cases are not visible on imaging in most cases
  - While macroscopic compression of vessels can sometimes be seen with sarcoidosis, microscopic granulomatous pulmonary vasculopathy that is often present cannot be visualized
  - One cannot easily assess altered blood viscosity, endothelial dysfunction, and elevated carbon monoxide that also lead to PH in SSD

Disorders Associated With Group 5 Pulmonary Hypertension but Without Pulmonary Hypertension

- In general, minority of patients with disorders and diseases associated with group 5 PH will have PH on RHC
- If there is concern for PH, echocardiogram should be 1st study ordered for right heart pressure assessment

PATHOLOGY

General Features

- Various pathologies associated with group 5 PH

CLINICAL ISSUES

Presentation

- Most common signs/symptoms
  - Clinical issues are complex and variable given heterogeneity of conditions that lead to group 5 PH

Demographics

- Variable depending on cause

Natural History & Prognosis

- Variable depending on cause
- In general, patients with group 5 PH have worse outcomes than those with same condition without PH

Treatment

- Treatment is variable depending on cause

SELECTED REFERENCES

1. Zeder K et al: Pulmonary hypertension and chronic kidney disease: prevalence, pathophysiology and outcomes. Nat Rev Nephrol. 20(11):742-54, 2024
2. Montani D et al: Clinical phenotype and outcomes of pulmonary hypertension associated with myeloproliferative neoplasms: a population-based study. Am J Respir Crit Care Med. 208(5):600-12, 2023
3. Seymour E et al: Surgical and cardiac catheterization outcomes of scimitar syndrome patients: a three decade single-center experience. Pediatr Cardiol. 44(3):579-86, 2023
4. Ghazarian A et al: Pulmonary hypertension in an adult with unilateral absence of left pulmonary artery. SAGE Open Med Case Rep. 10:2050313X221127667, 2022
5. Wang A et al: Pulmonary hypertension caused by fibrosing mediastinitis. JACC Asia. 2(3):218-34, 2022
6. Wang K et al: Treatment and prognosis of scimitar syndrome: a retrospective analysis in a single center of East China. Front Cardiovasc Med. 9:973796, 2022
7. Radzikowska E: Update on pulmonary Langerhans cell histiocytosis. Front Med (Lausanne). 7:582581, 2021
8. Song IC et al: Pulmonary hypertension in patients with chronic myeloid leukemia. Medicine (Baltimore). 100(33):e26975, 2021
9. Stempel JM et al: Pulmonary arterial hypertension in hospitalized patients with polycythemia vera (from the National Inpatient Database). Am J Cardiol. 143:154-7, 2021
10. Zhang S et al: Prevalence of sarcoidosis-associated pulmonary hypertension: a systematic review and meta-analysis. Front Cardiovasc Med. 8:809594, 2021
11. Lopez-Mattei J et al: Prevalence of pulmonary hypertension in myelofibrosis. Ann Hematol. 99(4):781-9, 2020
12. Austin M et al: Prevalence and effect on survival of pulmonary hypertension in myelofibrosis. Clin Lymphoma Myeloma Leuk. 19(9):593-7, 2019
13. Rosenzweig EB et al: Paediatric pulmonary arterial hypertension: updates on definition, classification, diagnostics and management. Eur Respir J. 53(1), 2019
14. Sha JM et al: Repair of hemitruncus with irreversible pulmonary hypertension. Ann Thorac Surg. 108(1):e35-6, 2019
15. Simonneau G et al: Haemodynamic definitions and updated clinical classification of pulmonary hypertension. Eur Respir J. 53(1), 2019
16. Jutant EM et al: Pulmonary hypertension associated with neurofibromatosis type 1. Eur Respir Rev. 27(149), 2018
17. Fraidenburg DR et al: Pulmonary hypertension associated with thalassemia syndromes. Ann N Y Acad Sci. 1368(1):127-39, 2016
18. Parent F et al: A hemodynamic study of pulmonary hypertension in sickle cell disease. N Engl J Med. 365(1):44-53, 2011
19. Vida VL et al: Scimitar syndrome: a European Congenital Heart Surgeons Association (ECHSA) multicentric study. Circulation. 122(12):1159-66, 2010
20. Altintas A et al: Pulmonary hypertension in patients with essential thrombocythemia and reactive thrombocytosis. Leuk Lymphoma. 48(10):1981-7, 2007

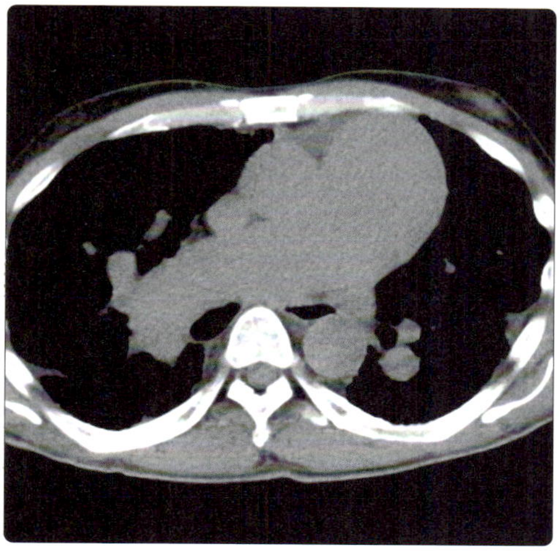

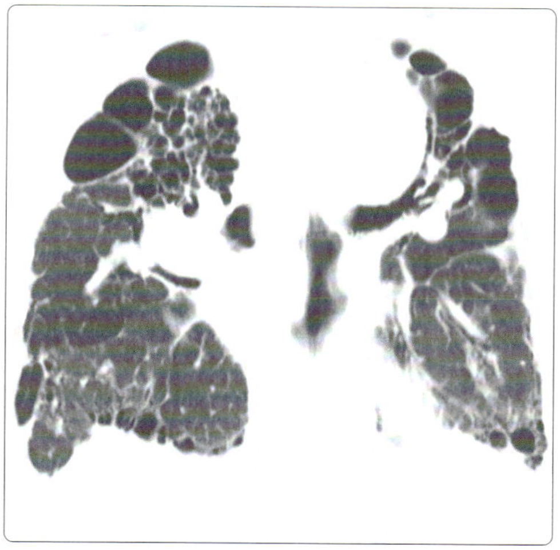

(Left) *Axial NECT in a patient with known sarcoidosis shows massive enlargement of the MPA compared to the adjacent ascending aorta. No lymphadenopathy was present.* **(Right)** *Coronal NECT in the same patient shows perihilar and upper lobe-predominant fibrosis with traction bronchiectasis and upper lobe-predominant peribronchovascular and cystic change due to sarcoid. The mPAP on right heart catheterization was 43 mmHg.*

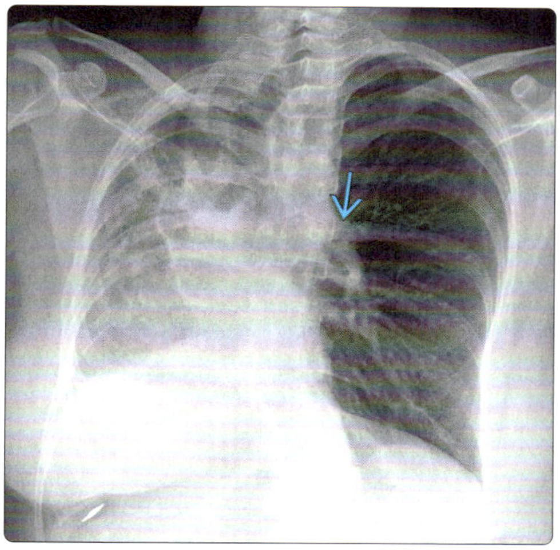

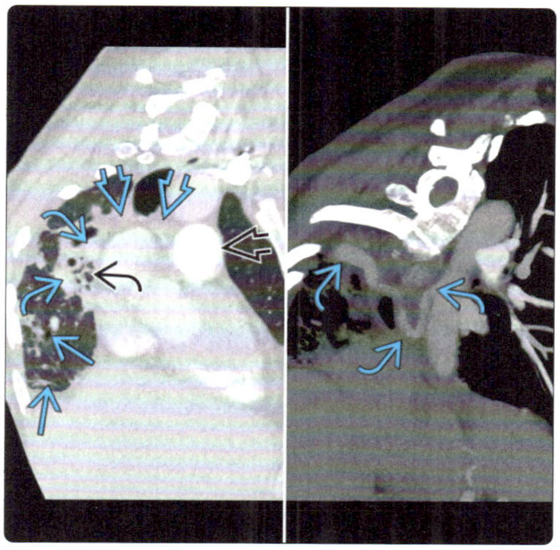

(Left) *CXR in an 39-year-old woman shows right-sided mediastinal shift. There is hazy opacity in the mid and lower left lung, which is hypoplastic. LPA branches are present.* **(Right)** *MPR (left) shows unilateral absence of the RPA. Tortuous vessel in the right lung is a large systemic collateral from the aorta, best seen on MIP (right). Scarring with bronchiectasis and cystic change on the right is due to longstanding systemic arterial supply. The MPA measures 3.2 cm, and mPAP is 28 mmHg.*

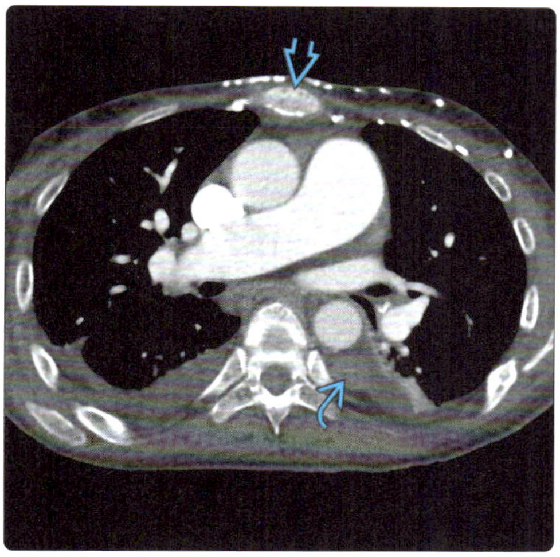

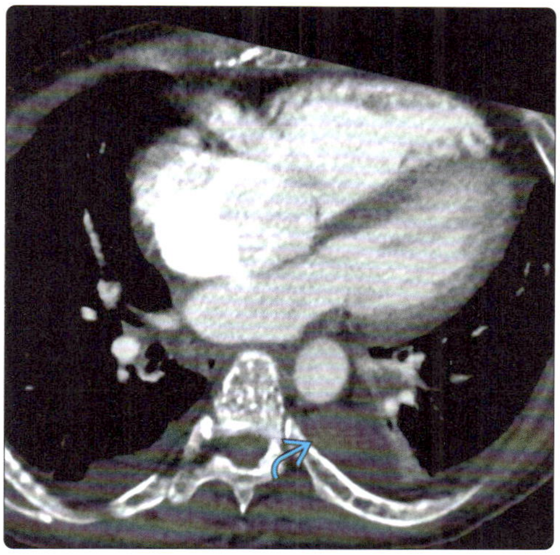

(Left) *Axial CECT in a 36-year-old man with β-thalassemia major shows an enlarged PA, osteopenia with expansion of multiple bones, and one of many paraspinous masses due to extramedullary hematopoiesis (EH).* **(Right)** *Four-chamber reconstruction shows dilation and hypertrophy of the right ventricle. The right atrium is also enlarged. Another focus of EH is seen, as is severe osteopenia and bony expansion.*

Pulmonary Artery Sarcoma

KEY FACTS

IMAGING

- Pulmonary artery sarcoma (PAS) most frequently discovered on CT pulmonary angiography (CTPA)
- CT findings
  - Large mass often with convex margins most commonly found in left pulmonary artery (LPA), right PA (RPA), or main PA
    - Can show contralateral growth into opposite side
  - Invasion through arterial wall can occur but often absent
  - Increased vascularity within PAS often absent on pulmonary arterial-phase imaging
  - May have noncontiguous filling defects distal to main tumor due to tumor emboli
  - If soft tissue mass is unilateral (centered in RPA or LPA), does not cross midline, and there are contralateral intravascular filling defects, findings may be due to chronic thromboembolic pulmonary hypertension (CTEPH)
- MR findings
  - Variable signal on T1W and T2W but usually hypointense and hyperintense to muscle, respectively
  - 1st-pass perfusion may be absent or subtle
  - Enhancement on T1W+ imaging often present
  - Restricted diffusion often present but variable
- PET/CT
  - Even in absence of vascular enhancement, nearly 90% of PAS should show FDG uptake

PATHOLOGY

- Diverse histologic patterns
- Undifferentiated pleomorphic sarcomas most common

CLINICAL ISSUES

- Overall poor survival
- Median survival 14-26 months
- Pulmonary thromboendarterectomy often performed but only to improve clinical symptoms

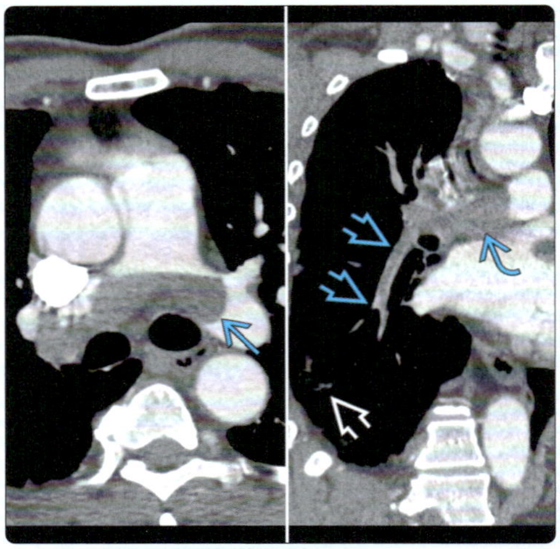

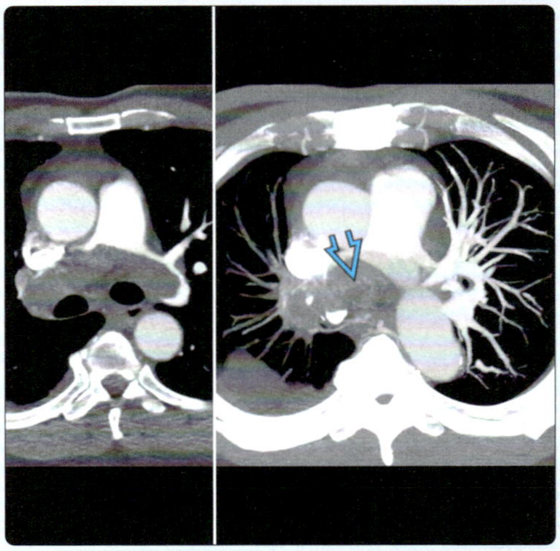

(Left) *Axial CTPA shows a mass-like filling defect in the right pulmonary artery (RPA) extending into the left PA (LPA) with a convex margin. Coronal CTPA shows contraction of the interlobar PA distal to the filling defect with a subpleural infarct mimicking CTEPH.* **(Right)** *CECT 5 wks later (same patient) shows growth of the mass despite anticoagulation. MIP image shows no filling defects distal to the LPA, which would be atypical for CTEPH. Neovascularity in the mass further supports the diagnosis of PA sarcoma (PAS).*

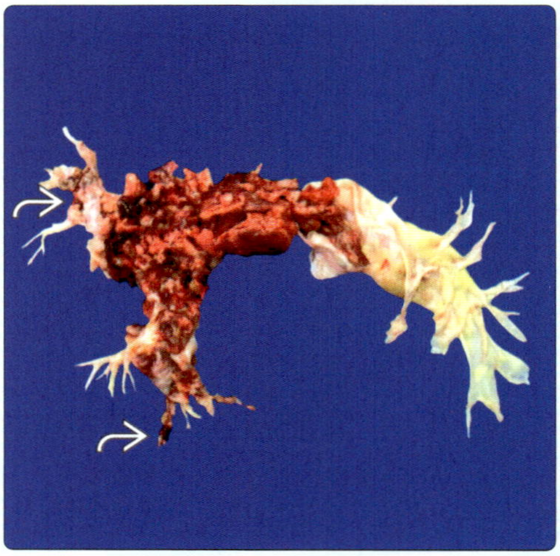

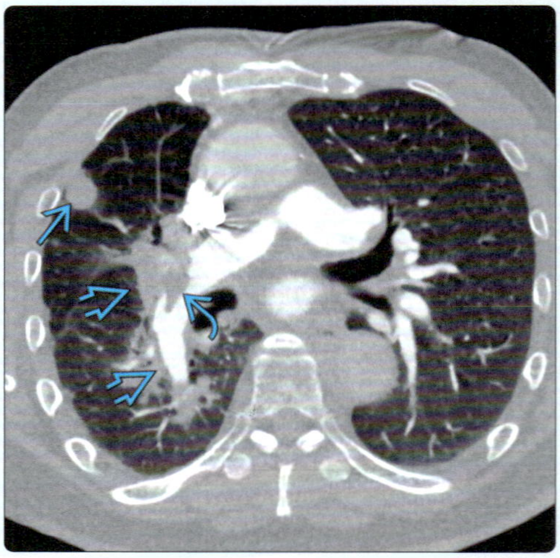

(Left) *Photograph of the PAS specimen from the same patient shows areas of tumor along the distal resection margin. Although the majority of the PAS was poorly differentiated, a few foci of osteosarcoma were present on histopathology.* **(Right)** *CTPA in the same patient 11 months after resection shows postradiation changes in the right lung and a new right upper lobe metastases. Intravascular soft tissue in the interlobar PA had grown over many studies, consistent with recurrent PAS.*

TERMINOLOGY

Abbreviations

- Pulmonary artery sarcoma (PAS)

Definitions

- Primary sarcoma arising from intima of pulmonary arteries (PAs)

IMAGING

General Features

- Best diagnostic clue
  - Large, often sausage-shaped mass most commonly found in left PA (LPA), right PA (RPA), or main PA (MPA)
- Location
  - PAs
- Size
  - Variable, but usually large
- Morphology
  - Variable appearance and shape

Radiographic Findings

- General findings of pulmonary hypertension (PH)
- Difficult to make diagnosis of PAS on radiograph
  - Westermark sign
    - Uncommon and difficult to recognize
    - Localized oligemia due to upstream PA occlusion
  - Potential pulmonary metastases

CT Findings

- PAS most frequently discovered on CT pulmonary angiography (CTPA)
- Often large, expansile mass in MPA, LPA, or RPA
  - While convex margins creating sausage-shaped mass filling PA is common, concave or flat margins can occur
  - May show contralateral growth into opposite side
  - Can mimic acute or chronic pulmonary embolus
    - Vasculature distal to mass can be contracted due to proximal obstruction, mimicking chronic thromboembolic PH CTEPH)
- Large filling defect in MPA extending across pulmonary valve should be considered sarcoma until proven otherwise
- Invasion through arterial wall can occur but often absent
- Subtle intimal thickening proximal or distal to tumor usually due to intimal spread of tumor
  - Diffuse intimal spread of tumor remote to primary mass is usually present
- Increased vascularity within PAS often not visible on pulmonary arterial phase
  - Add additional delayed-phase imaging if PAS is suspected
- May have noncontiguous filling defects distal to main tumor due to tumor emboli
  - If soft tissue mass is unilateral (centered in RPA or LPA), does not cross midline, and there are contralateral intravascular filling defects, findings may be due to CTEPH
- Rounded pulmonary nodules in setting of lesion suggestive of PAS are metastases until proven otherwise
- Due to potential differentiation of PAS, chondroid and osteoid matrix present in primary PA chondrosarcoma and osteosarcoma, respectively
- Bronchial artery collaterals often smaller than in CTEPH
- If sarcoma is suspected, can perform PET/CT, MR, or even short-term interval follow-up CTA after anticoagulation attempt
  - Although there may be thrombus intermixed with tumor, use of anticoagulation does not change size of PAS
  - However, in CTEPH, initial use of anticoagulation will almost always shrink or change morphology of clot

MR Findings

- PAS
  - Excellent tool for helping distinguish PAS from CTEPH
  - Most sarcomas are hypointense to mildly hyperintense to muscle on T1W and isointense to hyperintense on T2W imaging
  - 1st-pass perfusion may be absent or subtle
  - Enhancement on T1W+ imaging often present but heterogeneous
    - Should acquire postcontrast imaging during arterial- and venous-phase imaging
    - Enhancement may not be present on early systemic arterial-phase imaging
    - Lack of enhancement does not entirely exclude PAS
    - Mild peripheral enhancement can be seen with chronic thrombus
  - Restricted diffusion often present but variable

Echocardiographic Findings

- Excellent noninvasive tool for assessing PH
- Cannot diagnose PAS
- May be able to detect soft tissue in MPA, potentially crossing pulmonary valve

Nuclear Medicine Findings

- PET/CT
  - Can help differentiate PAS from CTEPH
    - Even in absence of vascular enhancement, nearly 90% of PAS should show FDG uptake
- Ventilation/perfusion (V/Q) scan
  - Cannot differentiate between impaired perfusion from CTEPH, PAS, or other filling defects

Imaging Recommendations

- Best imaging tool
  - PAS often 1st detected on CTPA
    - Diagnosis can often be made or strongly suggested on initial imaging
  - In cases where diagnosis is uncertain, MR or PET should be considered after initiation of anticoagulation (unless contraindicated)
    - Short-term repeat CTPA, potentially with portal venous-phase imaging, could be performed after initiation of anticoagulation if MR or PET difficult to obtain or unavailable
- Protocol advice
  - CTPA
    - Consider dual-energy, spectral, or photon-counting CT if available to assess for subtle tumor enhancement

- Can consider additional portal venous phase of imaging if tumor is suspected
- Recommend submillimeter slice thickness
- MR
  - Cardiac and respiratory gated
  - Variable T1W and T2W precontrast imaging
  - 1st-pass perfusion through mass
  - Multiple runs of T1W+ imaging through mass
  - LGE imaging with high TI time (500-600 msec) could be used to help differentiate tumor from thrombus

DIFFERENTIAL DIAGNOSIS

Chronic Thromboembolic Disease

- CTEPH is main differential for PAS
- Can be very difficult to differentiate
  - Vasculature is contracted distal to occlusion in both CTEPH and PAS
- Sausage-shaped mass in LPA or RPA should raise concern for PAS but can be seen with CTEPH as well
  - Any mass-like filling defect in MPA, especially if crossing pulmonary valve, should be PAS until proven otherwise
- Distal emboli contralateral to unilateral mass-like filling defect is more suggestive of CTEPH
- Bronchial artery collaterals often larger with CTEPH than PAS
- PET or MR can be used to differentiate, as can short-term interval CTPA after initiation of anticoagulation
  - CTEPH should decrease in size if patient has not previously received anticoagulation
  - PAS will remain unchanged or grow

Acute Pulmonary Embolism

- Uncommon for acute PE to fill the majority of MPA, LPA, or RPA
- Clinical presentations often different

In Situ Thrombus

- Extends longitudinally along walls of central PAs
- May be circumferential but does not tend to fill and obstruct PA
- Usually coexistent findings of PAH

PATHOLOGY

General Features

- Arise from intima of elastic PAs
  - Often referred to as intimal sarcomas because of site of origin
- Variety of histologic types similar to those seen with soft tissue sarcoma

Gross Pathologic & Surgical Features

- Most have bilateral involvement, although one side predominates
- Gelatinous soft tissue masses that fill PA
- Cut surface is soft unless tumor has osteosarcomatous or chondrosarcomatous elements

Microscopic Features

- Diverse histologic patterns
- Undifferentiated pleomorphic sarcomas and myxofibrosarcoma are most and 2nd most common, respectively
  - Numerous less common subtypes include rhabdomyosarcoma, leiomyosarcoma, synovial sarcoma, angiosarcoma, and epithelioid hemangioendothelioma
- 1/6 will show elements of osteosarcoma or chondrosarcoma
- Rare subtype is inflammatory myofibroblastic tumor
  - Acellular tumor with good prognosis

CLINICAL ISSUES

Presentation

- Most common signs/symptoms
  - Nonspecific findings of PH
- Other signs/symptoms
  - Weight loss and hemoptysis

Demographics

- Average age of 53 years with wide age range
- Occurs in women slightly more frequently than men

Natural History & Prognosis

- Overall poor survival
  - Median survival 14-26 months
  - Inflammatory myofibroblastic tumor has improved survival

Treatment

- Surgical options
  - Pneumonectomy if tumor localized to lobar or segmental vessels
  - Intrapericardial pneumonectomy can remove intrapericardial portion of 1 PA and entire lug
    - Even if tumor appears respectable, intimal spread of tumor throughout central PAs is common
  - Full-thickness resection occasionally performed where central PAs are removed and replaced with Dacron graft
  - Pulmonary thromboendarterectomy often performed but only to improve clinical symptoms
- Chemotherapy and radiation are often given
  - Various regimens, most with little survival benefit

DIAGNOSTIC CHECKLIST

Consider

- PAS in any case of mass-like filling defect with convex margins in LPA, RPA, or MPA

SELECTED REFERENCES

1. Kronzer E et al: Primary pulmonary artery sarcoma versus pulmonary thromboembolism: a multimodal imaging comparison. J Thromb Thrombolysis. 52(4):1129-32, 2021
2. Ropp AM et al: Intimal sarcoma of the great vessels. Radiographics. 41(2):361-79, 2021
3. Liu MX et al: Differential diagnosis of pulmonary artery sarcoma and central chronic pulmonary thromboembolism using CT and MR images. Heart Lung Circ. 27(7):819-27, 2018
4. Boland MB et al: Pulmonary sarcomas. In practical thoracic pathology: Diseases of the heart, lung, and thymus. Wolters Kluwer, 2017

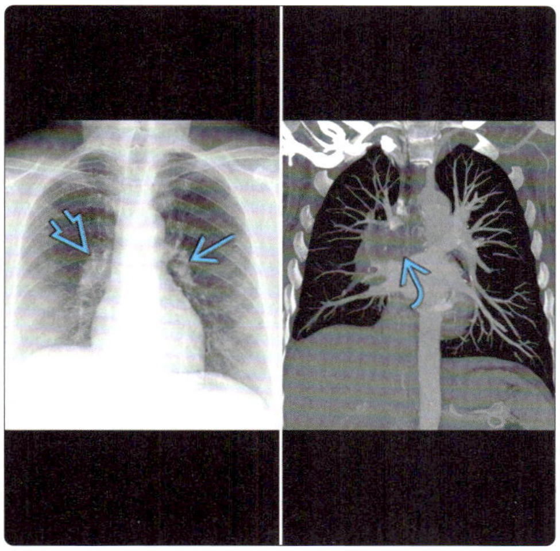

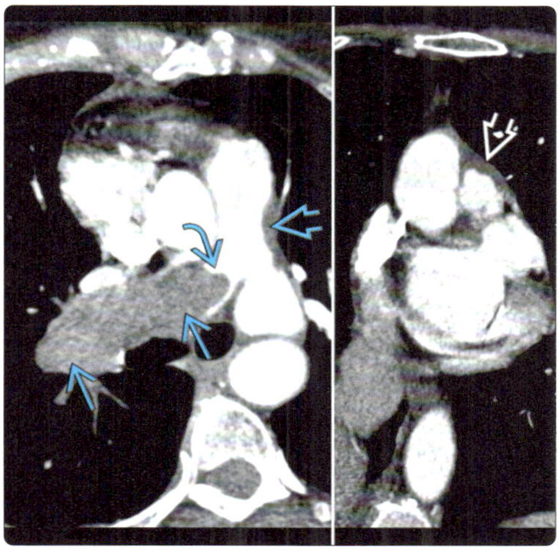

(Left) *PA radiograph (left) in a 61-year-old woman shows enlargement of the RPA ➡ compared to the LPA ➡. The right lung is small in size with oligemia. Coronal CT shows a large filling defect in the RPA ➡ with near-complete distal occlusion. The LPA and distal branches are normal, making CTEPH unlikely.* **(Right)** *CTPA in the same patient shows the large expansile mass in the RPA ➡ with a convex margin ➡, suggestive of PAS. Close inspection reveals asymmetric intimal thickening of the MPA ➡ extending near the level of the pulmonic valve ➡.*

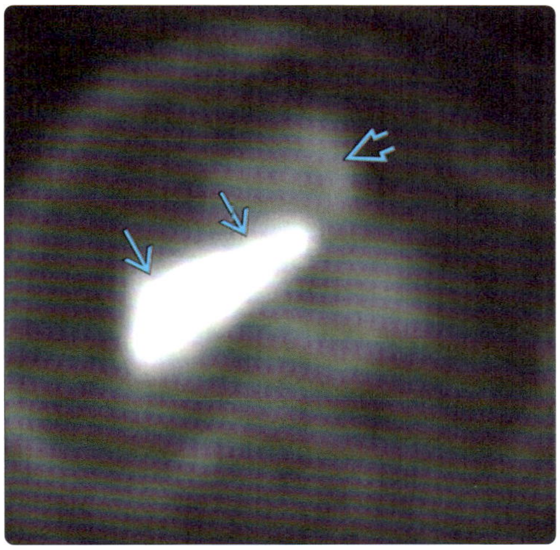

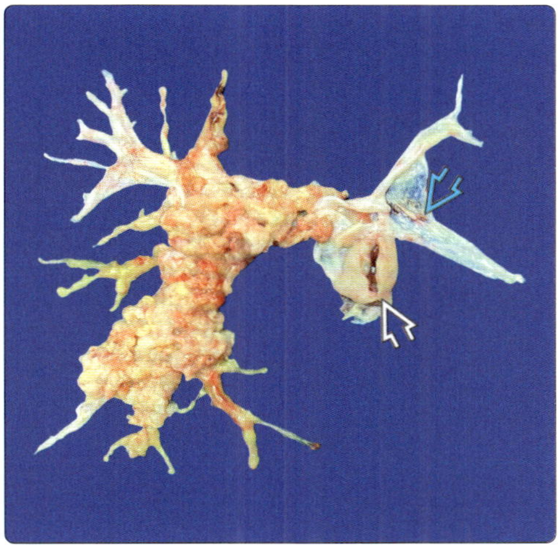

(Left) *Axial oblique FDG PET in the same patient shows intense uptake ➡ in the main portion of the PAS. However, there is also subtle asymmetric uptake in the MPA near the pulmonic valve ➡.* **(Right)** *Gross specimen shows the large right undifferentiated pleomorphic PAS. Tumor is present along the distal resection margin. Circumferential endarterectomy specimen ➡ from the MPA near the level of the pulmonic valve is seen. A small amount of tumor was present in the LPA ➡.*

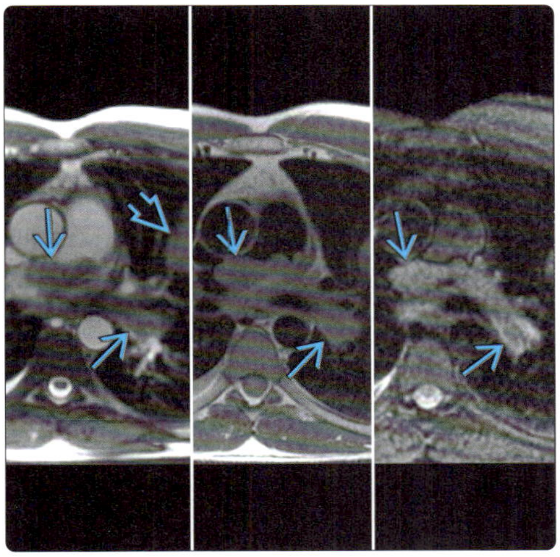

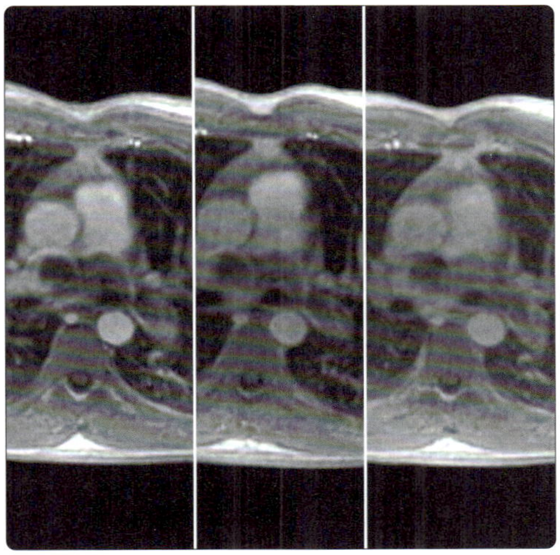

(Left) *Axial SSFP (left), T1W (middle), and STIR (right) MR images in a 38-year-old man with poorly differentiated PAS show a mass filling the LPA extending across midline into the RPA ➡. The mass is iso- to hypointense to muscle on SSFP, isointense to muscle on T1W, and hyperintense on T2W sequences. A pulmonary metastasis ➡ is partially visualized.* **(Right)** *Axial T1 C+ MR images at 1 minute (left), 2 minutes (center), and 5 minutes (right) post contrast show mild progressive enhancement of the PAS.*

Branch Pulmonary Artery Stenosis

KEY FACTS

TERMINOLOGY

- Stenosis of pulmonary artery (PA) branches

IMAGING

- Focal, web-like or long-segment tubular narrowing of PA branches
- CTA or MRA: Best imaging tool
  - Used to assess severity, length, and distribution of stenosis and underlying cause
- Conventional angiography: ↑ pressure gradient within pulmonary arterial system is diagnostic

TOP DIFFERENTIAL DIAGNOSES

- Vasculitis
- Chronic thromboembolism
- Pulmonary atresia
- Pulmonary valve stenosis
- Pulmonary vein stenosis

PATHOLOGY

- Most commonly congenital in etiology
  - Associated with congenital heart disease
  - Component of clinical syndromes
- Acquired
  - Sequela of surgery or radiation
  - Fibrosing mediastinitis

CLINICAL ISSUES

- Much more commonly encountered and described in pediatric population
- Children: Symptoms related to congenital heart disease
- Adults: Progressive dyspnea and fatigue
- Treatment
  - Surgical revascularization for proximal PA stenosis/atresia associated with congenital heart disease
  - Percutaneous balloon angioplasty ± stent in select cases

(Left) *3D reformation demonstrates a central posterior stenosis ➡ in a patient with a Blalock-Taussig shunt ➡. Although branch pulmonary stenosis (PS) is typically congenital, revascularization procedures may result in acquired branch pulmonary artery (PA) stenosis.* **(Right)** *Angiography demonstrates multiple stenoses ➡ and dilatation ➡ involving the left segmental and subsegmental PAs. PA stenosis may manifest as focal, web-like or long-segment tubular narrowing of the PAs.*

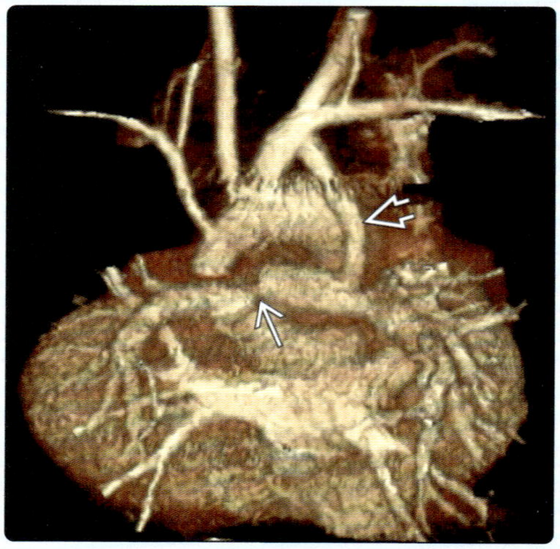

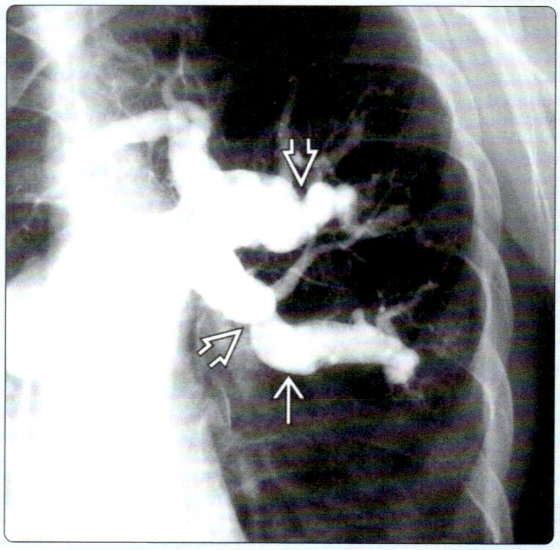

(Left) *CTA images in a 22-year-old woman with Alagille syndrome show hypoplasia of the right ➡ and left ➡ PAs with associated stents due to branch PS. The patient also has a unicuspid aortic valve ➡ (inset).* **(Right)** *In addition to more central branch PS, there is severe hypoplasia of a few peripheral branches, such as the apicoposterior segment of the left upper lobe ➡ (left) with associated perfusion defect ➡.*

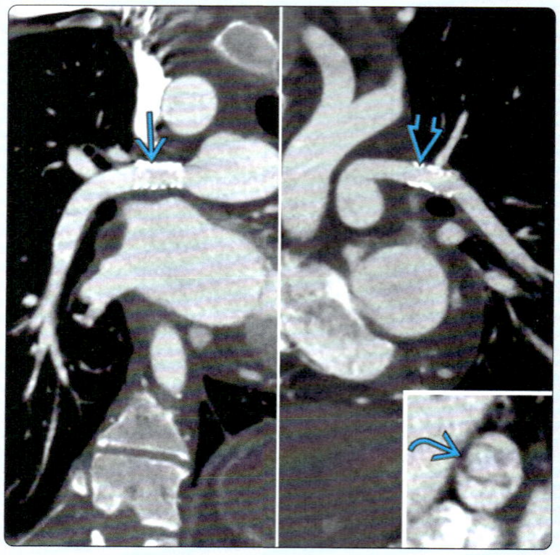

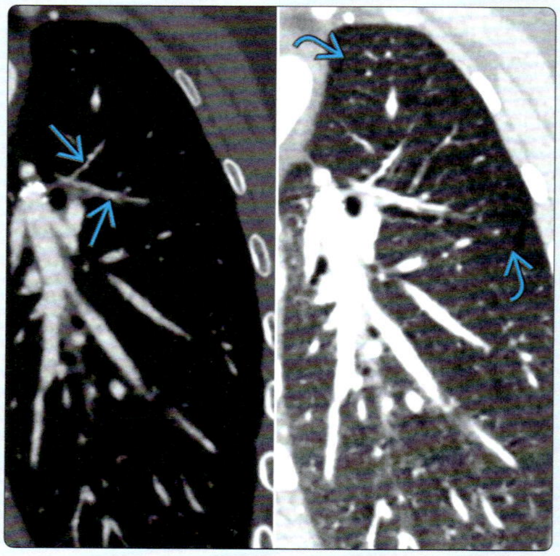

TERMINOLOGY

Definitions

- Stenosis of pulmonary artery (PA) branch

IMAGING

General Features

- Best diagnostic clue
  - Focal, web-like or long-segment tubular narrowing of PA branches
  - Collateral aortopulmonary circulation to lung in chronic branch pulmonary stenosis (PS)

Radiographic Findings

- Radiography
  - Heart size is typically normal
  - Right heart enlargement may be seen in severe chronic PA stenosis
    - Filling of retrosternal clear space in lateral view
  - Pulmonary vascularity is usually normal
    - ↓ in severe PA stenosis
  - Poststenotic dilatation may occasionally be evident

CT Findings

- NECT
  - Calcification may be seen in setting of mediastinal fibrosis
  - Right heart dilation in longstanding severe obstruction due to pulmonary hypertension
  - Parenchymal findings variable depending on location and severity of stenosis
    - Mild stenosis may show no abnormality
    - Severe stenosis or occlusion → hypoattenuation in affected parenchyma due to ↓ flow
- CTA
  - Focal narrowing or diffuse ↓ in caliber of affected vessel(s)
  - Associated congenital heart disease in congenital cases of branch PS
    - Aortopulmonary collateral vessels can occur but more commonly with pulmonary atresia or severe central PS rather than branch PS
  - In acquired branch stenosis, lesion(s) causing compression can be assessed
  - Narrowing of corresponding pulmonary veins may be seen in setting of extrinsic compression

MR Findings

- T1WI
  - Evaluate soft tissue anatomy of mediastinum or lesions surrounding stenosed PAs
- T2WI
  - Can characterize lesion(s) causing extrinsic compression in acquired branch PS
- MRA
  - Assess severity and extent of branch PS
    - Focal narrowing/occlusion vs. long-segment narrowing
    - Single vessel or multivessel
  - Assess other congenital cardiovascular anomalies
- SSFP cine
  - Evaluation of anatomy and associated cardiovascular anomalies
    - Flow acceleration through stenosis
- Phase-contrast MR
  - Assess flow across branch PS
  - Peak systolic velocity > 1.5 m/s implies hemodynamically significant stenosis

Echocardiographic Findings

- Echocardiogram
  - Limited acoustic window for branch PS
  - May demonstrate associated cardiac abnormalities
  - Access pulmonary valve
- Pulsed Doppler
  - Parasternal and subcostal views to assess central PA flow velocities
  - Peripheral stenosis not directly visualized

Angiographic Findings

- Conventional
  - Defines location, length, number, and severity of stenotic segments
  - Elevated pressure gradient within pulmonary arterial system is diagnostic
  - Balloon angioplasty in select cases only
    - Proximal and well-localized severe stenosis
    - Possible stent placement

Nuclear Medicine Findings

- V/Q scan
  - Tc-99m macroaggregated albumin
    - Segmental and subsegmental perfusion defects in cases of obstruction

Imaging Recommendations

- Best imaging tool
  - CTA or MRA

DIFFERENTIAL DIAGNOSIS

Adult-Acquired Pulmonary Artery Stenosis

- Chronic pulmonary embolism
- Vasculitis
  - Takayasu arteritis
    - Young to middle-aged women
    - PAs affected in > 50% of cases
    - Usually bilateral and multifocal
    - Predilection for upper lobe branches
  - Connective tissue disorders
    - Scleroderma
    - Rheumatoid arthritis
    - Systemic lupus erythematosus
  - Behçet disease
  - Wegener granulomatosis
  - Eosinophilic granulomatosis with polyangiitis (Churg-Strauss syndrome)

Pulmonary Atresia

- Congenital malformation characterized by failed development of pulmonary valve orifice
- 2 distinct types based on status of interventricular septum

- Pulmonary atresia with ventricular septal defect and major aortopulmonary collateral arteries (MAPCAs)
  - Hypoplastic/absent PAs
  - MAPCAs supply 1 or both lungs
- Pulmonary atresia with intact ventricular septum
  - Normal-sized PAs supplied by ductus arteriosus and patent foramen ovale
- Best diagnostic clue: Right ventricular outflow tract (RVOT) ± pulmonary valve atresia
- Boot-shaped configuration of heart on chest radiography

Pulmonary Valvular Stenosis

- Congenital obstruction of RVOT and pulmonary valve
- Enlargement of pulmonary trunk and left PA

Pulmonary Vein Stenosis

- Typically postprocedural in etiology
  - Postradiofrequency ablation of ectopic atrial foci in pulmonary vein sleeves
  - Following reanastomosis of anomalous pulmonary vein

PATHOLOGY

General Features

- Etiology
  - Congenital
    - Most common cause of branch PA stenosis
    - Associated with congenital heart disease
      - Tetralogy of Fallot (TOF)
      - Pulmonary atresia
      - Truncus arteriosus
      - Pulmonary valve stenosis
      - Patent ductus arteriosus
    - Component of clinical syndromes
      - Alagille, Cutis laxa, Ehlers-Danlos, Noonan, Russell-Silver, Williams
    - Congenital rubella infection
    - PA coarctation
      - Discrete, severe PA stenosis or occlusion, usually left sided, directly adjacent to ductus
      - Similar to aortic coarctation, due to invasion of ductal tissue around PA
      - Patent ductus arteriosus supplies blood to PA distal to stenosis/occlusion
      - Associated with right-sided obstructive lesions, such as TOF
  - Acquired
    - Following pulmonary revascularization procedures
      - Fontan and Blalock-Taussig shunt
      - Arterial switch
    - Fibrosing mediastinitis
    - Sequela of thoracic surgery or radiation

Staging, Grading, & Classification

- PA stenosis may be divided into 4 types
  - Type 1: Isolated stenosis of pulmonary trunk or left main or right main PA
  - Type 2: Stenosis at truncal bifurcation and extending into main PAs
  - Type 3: Multiple peripheral stenosis
  - Type 4: Combination of central and peripheral stenosis

Gross Pathologic & Surgical Features

- Proximal to or at site of stenosis
  - Thickening of PA wall
  - Hardened stenotic regions
  - Narrowing of PA branches
- Distal to site of stenosis
  - Poststenotic dilatation of PA branches
  - Thinning of PA wall
- Aortopulmonary collateral circulation through bronchial arteries

Microscopic Features

- Children
  - Fibrous intimal proliferation
  - Medial hypoplasia/dysplasia
  - Loss of elastic fibers in affected segments
  - Nonparallel arrangement of smooth muscles
- Adults
  - ↑ in smooth muscle cells and disorganized elastic fibers in media
    - Luminal encroachment

CLINICAL ISSUES

Presentation

- Most common signs/symptoms
  - Children
    - Symptoms related to congenital heart disease
  - Adults
    - Progressive dyspnea and fatigue
    - Symptoms related to pulmonary hypertension

Demographics

- Age
  - Much more commonly encountered and described in pediatric population

Natural History & Prognosis

- Serious and long-term complication of congenital heart disease
- Noncardiac comorbidities often determine course and prognosis
- Variable prognosis depending on etiology

Treatment

- Surgical revascularization for proximal PA stenosis/atresia associated with congenital heart disease
- Percutaneous balloon angioplasty ± stent in select cases

SELECTED REFERENCES

1. Vadher AB et al: Stenotic lesions of pulmonary arteries: imaging evaluation using multidetector computed tomography angiography. Clin Imaging. 69:17-26, 2021
2. Escalon JG et al: Congenital anomalies of the pulmonary arteries: an imaging overview. Br J Radiol. 92(1093):20180185, 2019
3. Hirsig LE et al: Congenital pulmonary artery anomalies: a review and approach to classification. J Clin Imaging Sci. 8:29, 2018
4. Carter BW et al: Congenital abnormalities of the pulmonary arteries in adults. AJR Am J Roentgenol. 202(4):W308-13, 2014

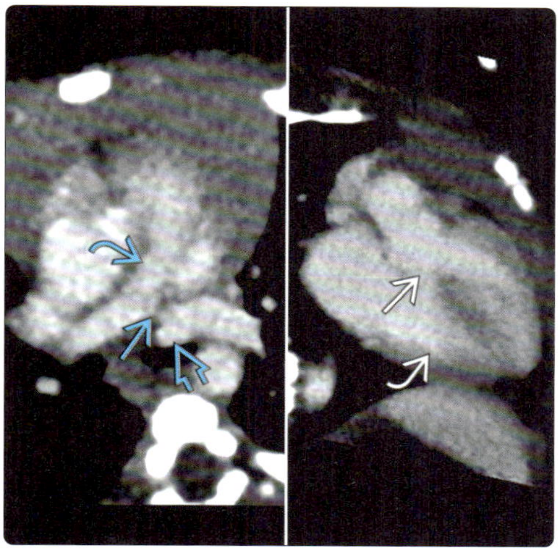

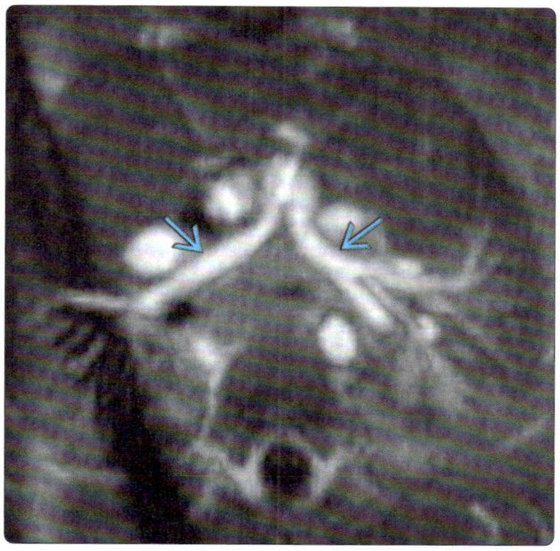

(Left) *Axial CTA (left) in a newborn shows severe focal proximal left PA (LPA) stenosis → due to a pulmonary coarctation, which can be seen in complex congenital heart disease. A patent ductus arteriosus supplies the LPA distal to the stenosis →. The main PA is small in size →. Image of the heart (right) shows an overriding aorta with VSD → and RV hypertrophy → from tetralogy of Fallot.* **(Right)** *MR angiogram in a newborn with Williams syndrome shows severe diffuse hypoplasia of the PAs →.*

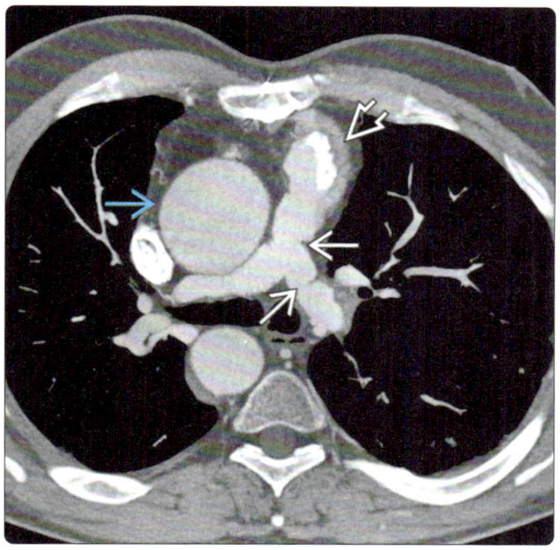

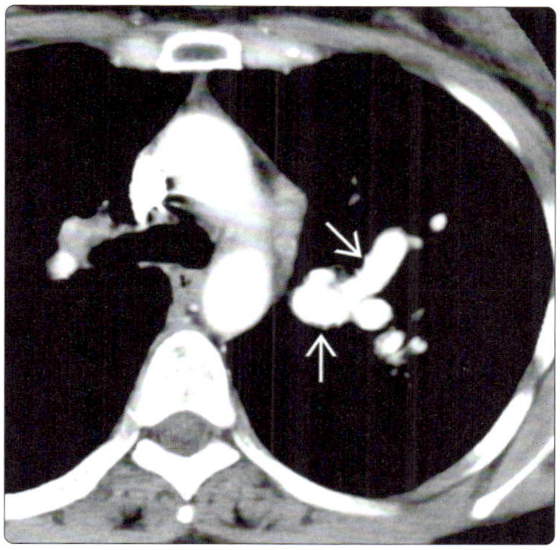

(Left) *Axial CECT in a patient with Tetralogy of Fallot shows multiple web-like PA stenoses →. Note patch repair of RV outflow tract obstruction → and right-sided descending thoracic aorta →.* **(Right)** *Axial CECT demonstrates poststenotic dilatation of peripheral PA branches → extending into the left lung. Multiple peripheral PA stenosis represent type 3 PA stenosis.*

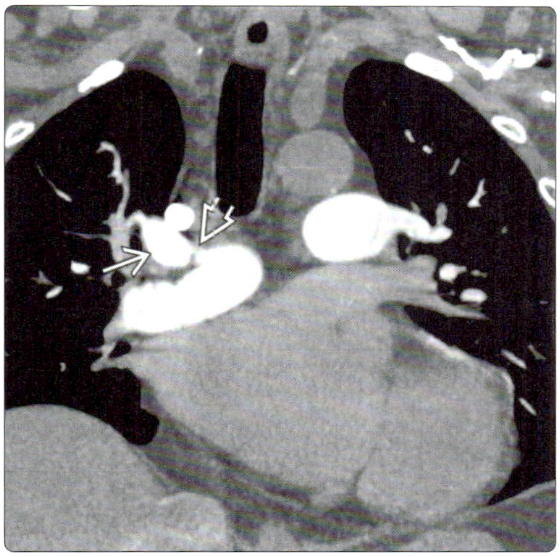

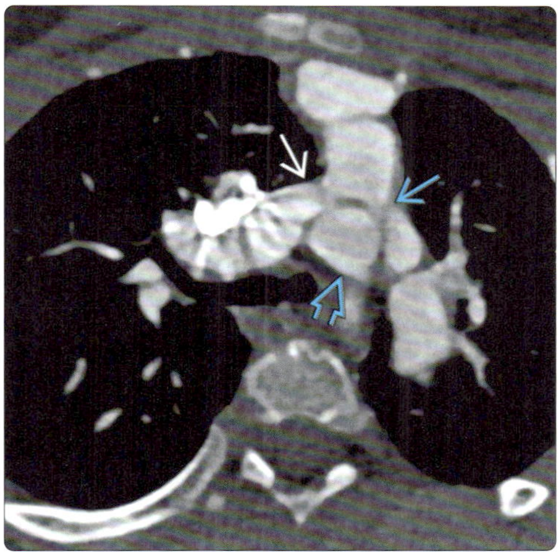

(Left) *Coronal reformat CTA shows focal stenosis of the truncus anterior branch → of the right PA. Note the poststenotic dilatation →.* **(Right)** *Axial reconstructed MPR CTA in a patient with D-transposition of great arteries status post arterial switch shows the PAs draped over the aorta →. Moderate narrowing of the right PA → and LPA → branches is seen.*

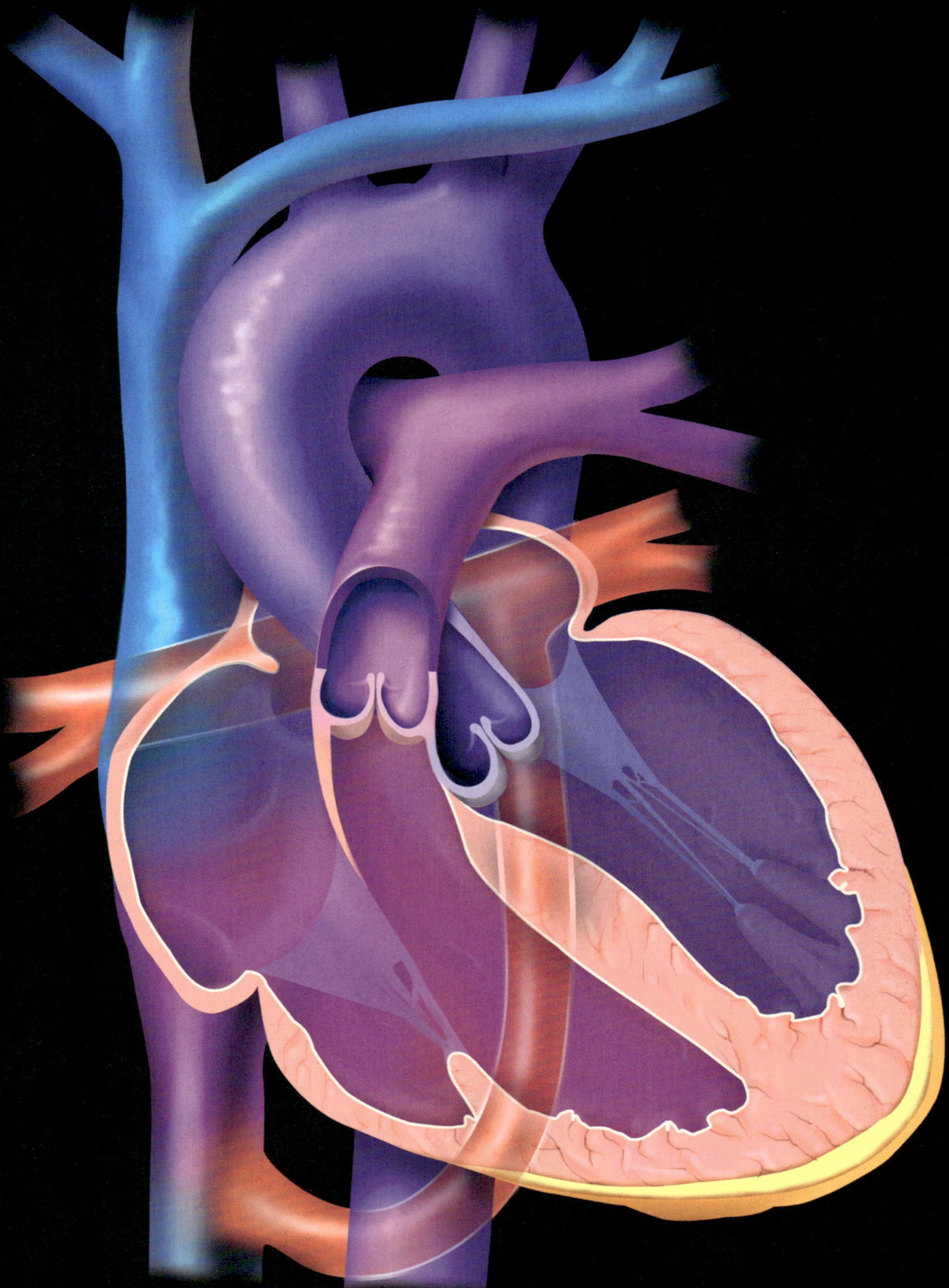

SECTION 11

Veins

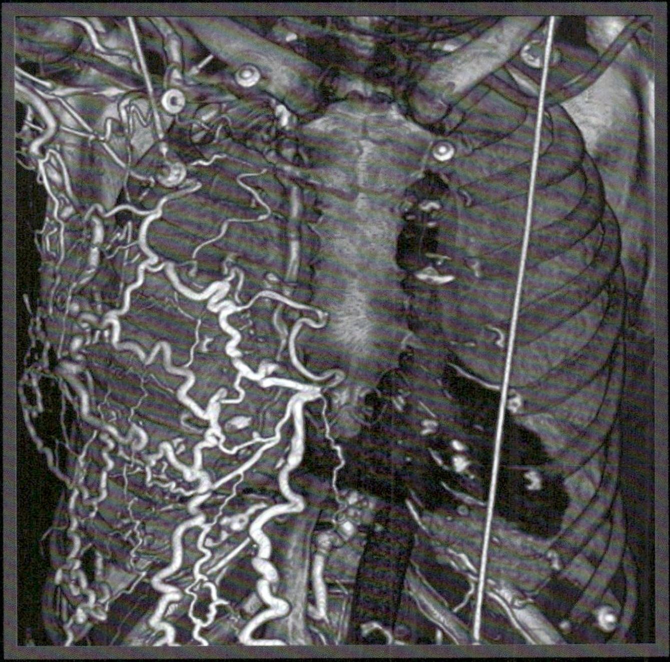

Anatomy-based Imaging Issues

Imaging venous diseases requires a thorough understanding of venous anatomy, pathophysiology, clinical aspects, differential diagnosis, and available therapeutic options. Noninvasive imaging techniques have replaced catheter-based venography as the 1st imaging modality of choice in venous diseases. Extremity veins are assessed with ultrasound (US) and color Doppler US. Intraabdominal and intrathoracic veins are challenging to assess with US and require CT venography/MR venography (CTV/MRV) for comprehensive visualization. Catheter-based venography is rarely used only for diagnostic purposes, but useful to assess flow dynamics, collateral flow, intravascular pressure, and posttreatment changes. Intravascular US (IVUS) as part of catheter venography is useful in assessing intraluminal and mural abnormalities.

Pathologic Issues

Venous disorders can be categorized into venoocclusive diseases, venous insufficiency (or valvular incompetence), venous aneurysms, abnormal arteriovenous communications, venolymphatic malformations, and congenital anomalies.

Pathology-based Imaging Issues

Venoocclusive Disease

Venoocclusive disease includes acute and chronic thrombosis, webs, neoplastic invasion (primary, secondary), and extrinsic compression. Acute thrombosis in the veins is associated with vessel expansion and perivenous edema. On grayscale US, an acute thrombus is anechoic or hypoechoic within an expanded vein, which may be challenging to detect. An acutely thrombosed vein is noncompressible, and flow is absent on color Doppler US. CTV demonstrates an intraluminal filling defect, rim-like enhancement of the vein wall, and perivenous fat stranding. MRV ± intravenous contrast shows findings comparable to CTV. T2-weighted images are helpful in assessing perivenous inflammation. Chronic deep venous thrombosis results in scarring of the vein with complete occlusion or partial recanalization of the vein. US may show a partially compressible, small-caliber vein with multiple flow channels within the lumen. CTV or MRV show filling defects in a small-caliber vein with associated collateral veins. Intravenous tumor extension or primary venous tumor (such as leiomyomatosis) appear similar to that of acute deep venous thrombosis (intraluminal filling defect on CTV/MRV and noncompressible vein on US); however, contrast-enhanced studies demonstrate enhancement of the intravenous tumor that is not observed in bland (nontumor) thrombus. Extrinsic venous compression is readily apparent on CTV/MRV.

Venous webs are usually congenital; however, acquired webs can result from chronic deep venous thrombosis and extrinsic venous compression. Congenital webs occur in large veins, such as the inferior vena cava (IVC) and hepatic veins, and are best observed on US, high-resolution double inversion recovery T1-weighted MR, CTV, catheter venography, and IVUS. The webs appear as thin, transverse, linear soft tissue structures, and, depending on the severity of obstruction, may be associated with venous dilation or collateral formation. Acquired webs are usually multiple and of varied thickness. Calcifications, commonly observed with chronic deep vein thrombosis, are well seen on CT. Acquired webs are best visualized on IVUS, but catheter venography can detect flow limiting webs, especially when there is flow between the webs.

Extrinsic venous compression can occur from normal or normal variant adjacent arteries, muscles, and bones, or from pathologic entities, such as tumors and enlarged lymph nodes. CT and MR are helpful in detecting pathologic causes of venous compression. Dynamic extrinsic compression of the veins by bones, ligaments, and other soft tissues (e.g., thoracic outlet syndrome, May-Thurner syndrome, popliteal venous compression) can be assessed on color Doppler US and MRV/CTV. Catheter venography can provide a definitive diagnosis in indeterminate cases. Color Doppler US of the peripheral veins may allow detection of secondary effects of central venous occlusion by demonstrating absence of respiratory phasicity in the venous flow. Extrinsic venous compression may also lead to development of collateral veins depending on the severity of obstruction, peripheral venous thrombosis, and peripheral venous valvular insufficiency. Chronic repetitive compression of the veins by arteries (as seen in May-Thurner syndrome) may lead to chronic endothelial injury, mural spurs, chronic webs, and occlusion. CTV/MRV are useful in assessing extrinsic compression with catheter venography and IVUS providing definitive diagnosis. Time-of-flight (TOF) MRV may be helpful in the assessment of the hemodynamic significance of such extrinsic venous compression through detection of flow reversal or collateral flow. Following endovascular therapy, venous flow assessment can be performed with color Doppler US, CTV/MRV, and catheter angiography. MRV is not useful in assessing patency of venous stents.

Venous Insufficiency

Venous insufficiency results from the failure of venous valvular function as a result of primary venous wall/valve disease or secondary to chronic deep venous thrombosis or chronic venous hypertension from a central venous obstruction. Chronic venous insufficiency of the lower extremities may lead to varicose veins in the legs, pedal edema, dermatitis related to chronic venous stasis, lipodermatosclerosis, and venous ulcerations. Patients usually present with cosmetic embarrassment from varicose veins, leg pain, fatigue, heaviness or discomfort, leg swelling, skin discoloration, or ulcer. Imaging allows accurate identification of the location and severity of valvular incompetence. Color Doppler US evaluation is the best imaging test to assess venous insufficiency of the extremities. Valve closure times are assessed during a stress maneuver (e.g., Valsalva or squeeze-release technique). The normal valve closure times are as follows: 0.5 second for saphenous veins and 1.0 second for deep veins. Chronic venous insufficiency affecting the perforator veins is often difficult to assess, but dilated (> 3.5 mm in diameter) perforator veins are usually considered abnormal. MRV/CTV have shown promise in detecting dilated perforator veins. Chronic venous insufficiency may also affect the gonadal veins leading to varicocele in men and pelvic varices in women. These could be detected on multiphase contrast-enhanced MRV/CTV and catheter venography.

Venous Aneurysms

Venous aneurysms are rare and defined as a focal area of venous dilatation communicating through a single channel with the main venous structure, excluding pseudoaneurysm, arteriovenous communication, and varicose vein. Venous aneurysms are usually congenital or occur as a result of valvular insufficiency or abnormal arteriovenous communication. Congenital venous aneurysms are either incidentally detected or identified during a work-up of a pulmonary embolism. Venous aneurysms affecting the extremity veins can be well assessed on US, whereas those involving the chest and abdomen are best assessed on CTV or MRV. Catheter venography may sometimes be false-negative if the aneurysm is thrombosed.

Vascular Malformations

Malformations are nonneoplastic vascular abnormalities that are classified by the International Society for the Study of Vascular Anomalies (ISSVA) as simple, combined malformations of major named vessels and those associated with anomalies. An arteriovenous malformation is associated with direct arteriovenous communication. Arteriovenous communication is also seen in an arteriovenous fistula (congenital, traumatic, or iatrogenic) and arteriovenous tumoral shunting. Such communications can result in localized venous hypertension, valvular insufficiency, and enlarged primary and collateral veins. The presence of arterialized waveforms in the veins during color Doppler US evaluation indicates an arteriovenous communication. Multiphasic MRV/CTV are often the initial noninvasive imaging tests to assess arteriovenous communications, demonstrating the communication between arteries and veins without interposition of a capillary bed. Feeding arteries and draining veins can be characterized. Catheter venography can be used for accurate and comprehensive characterization.

Slow-flow lesions, particularly venous malformations, are the most common vascular anomaly, which can be type 1, isolated without venous connection; type 2, draining into a normal vein; type 3, draining into dysplastic veins; and type 4, venous ectasia. Doppler US is often the 1st-line imaging test that can demonstrate multiple tubular structures with monophasic venous flow or no flow. MR shows marked T2 hyperintensity from slow flow. Flow voids are not seen, but dysplastic draining or ectatic veins can be seen. CT and MR can show phleboliths. Contrast enhancement is typically slow, but can be rapid, homogeneous, or, heterogenous. No arterial enhancement is seen, but persistent delayed enhancement is.

Congenital Anomalies

Congenital venous anomalies are common but are of clinical significance only if major veins (such as the IVC) are atretic. Duplicated and abnormally persistent veins are of significance when instrumentation or surgical therapy is planned. Major venous anomalies can be well evaluated with CTV/MRV.

Imaging Protocols

Color Doppler US

Extremity veins are best assessed on grayscale US combined with color Doppler US. Each named vein is assessed in transverse and longitudinal planes. A compression technique is applied while imaging the vein in a transverse plane to assess venous patency. Venous flow dynamics are assessed in the longitudinal plane. The veins of the extremities demonstrate a respirophasic flow pattern unless centrally obstructed and show flow augmentation when distally compressed. The abdominal veins may be visualized in thin individuals, but the evaluation is often limited due to bowel gas and body habitus.

CTV

Direct CTV refers to imaging of the veins during the 1st pass of the contrast material in the territory where intravenous contrast material is injected. The contrast material is diluted with normal saline to 10-20% concentration to avoid streak artifacts. This study is not preferred due to lower accuracy than US, but it is occasionally requested for evaluation of extremity veins when US is not conclusive or suboptimal.

Indirect CTV is a common technique where veins are imaged during the venous phase following an intravenously administered bolus of a contrast material. This technique usually requires a large volume (100-150 mL) of normal-strength iodinated contrast material and adequate time delay (90-120 seconds for portomesenteric, hepatic, and renal veins, and 120-180 seconds for extremity veins and iliocaval veins) from contrast material administration until start of scanning. Thin sections (2.5-5.0 mm) are adequate to assess venous thrombosis.

MRV

Noncontrast MRV is useful in the assessment of venous patency (via double inversion recovery T1-weighted, steady-state free precession, TOF sequences) and flow direction (via TOF sequences). Contrast-enhanced MRV is performed as a multiphase examination to capture the various phases of contrast material flow through the arteries, capillaries, and veins. Contrast-enhanced MRV is highly useful in the assessment of venous patency, venous reflux, and detection of collateral flow. Multiphasic/dynamic studies following contrast material administration allow the detection of flow dynamics. MRV could also be performed in various body positions to assess dynamic extrinsic venous compression.

Catheter Venography

Ascending venography refers to the catheterization of a peripheral vein and injection of a large volume of contrast material to assess the proximal vein patency. This study is commonly used to assess the extremity veins by cannulating the hand or foot vein. It is important to position the extremity in an anatomic and dependent position to adequately assess the veins. Images are obtained in 2 orthogonal planes.

Descending venography is performed to assess valvular competence. A catheter is positioned in a vein (common femoral vein if assessing the saphenofemoral junction valve), and contrast material is injected while the patient performs the Valsalva maneuver so that the retrograde flow of contrast material can be detected.

IVUS

IVUS is usually part of catheter venography. The US probe is mounted on a catheter and used to assess the lumen and luminal surface of the venous wall. Images are obtained in both transverse and longitudinal planes. IVUS is also useful in assessing the patency of intravascular stents.

Selected References

1. Ota Y et al: Vascular malformations and tumors: a review of classification and imaging features for cardiothoracic radiologists. Radiol Cardiothorac Imaging. 5(4):e220328, 2023
2. Garcia R et al: Duplex ultrasound for the diagnosis of acute and chronic venous diseases. Surg Clin North Am. 98(2):201-18, 2018
3. Murphy DJ et al: Vascular CT and MRI: a practical guide to imaging protocols. Insights Imaging. 9(2):215-36, 2018
4. Caputo WJ et al: Venous intervention improves patient outcomes. Surg Technol Int. 30:77-9, 2017
5. Lin YT et al: Comprehensive evaluation of patients suspected with deep vein thrombosis using indirect CT venography with multi-detector row technology: from protocol to interpretation. Int J Cardiovasc Imaging. 26(Suppl 2):311-22, 2010

UPPER EXTREMITY VENOUS ANATOMY

Upper Extremity Superficial Veins

- Cephalic vein: Courses along radial aspect of arm
  - Ascends in front of elbow between brachioradialis and biceps brachii muscles
    - Communicates with basilic vein via median cubital (median basilic) vein at level of elbow
    - Located in superficial fascia along anterolateral surface of biceps brachii muscle
  - Passes superiorly between deltoid and pectoralis major muscles in deltopectoral groove
    - Drains into axillary vein in arch-like configuration
- Basilic vein: Courses along ulnar aspect of arm
  - Ascends medially along biceps in upper arm
    - Frequently joins brachial vein in upper arm

Upper Extremity Deep Veins

- Brachial vein: Usually paired
  - Terminate(s) in axillary vein
- Axillary vein: Returns blood from lateral aspect of thorax, axilla, and upper extremity
  - Starts at border of teres major muscle as continuation of brachial vein; ends at outer edge of 1st rib
  - Tributaries include basilic and cephalic veins
- Subclavian vein: Continuation of axillary vein
  - Courses from outer border of 1st rib to medial border of anterior scalene muscle
    - Subclavian vein lies anterior to anterior scalene muscle, whereas artery lies posterior
  - Thoracic duct drains into left subclavian vein
    - Duct enters near subclavian vein junction with left internal jugular vein

CERVICOTHORACIC VENOUS ANATOMY

Cervical Veins

- Internal jugular vein: Formed by union of sigmoid and inferior petrosal sinuses with common facial vein
  - Courses with common carotid artery and vagus nerve inside carotid sheath
    - Provides venous drainage for brain, face, and neck
  - Joins with subclavian vein medially to form brachiocephalic vein
- External jugular vein: Formed by union of posterior retromandibular vein and posterior auricular vein
  - Courses superficial to sternocleidomastoid muscle
    - Drains into subclavian vein more laterally than internal jugular vein
  - Provides venous drainage for exterior of cranium and deep parts of face
- Thyroidal veins: Arise from venous plexus surrounding thyroid gland; often multiple in number
  - Superior and middle thyroidal: Direct tributaries to internal jugular vein
  - Inferior thyroidal: Drain into brachiocephalic veins
- Vertebral vein: Derived from small venous tributaries that form plexus around vertebral artery
  - Plexus ends in single trunk that exits from 6th cervical vertebral transverse foramen
    - Enters brachiocephalic vein posteriorly near origin

Thoracic Veins

- Brachiocephalic (innominate) vein: Formed by union of subclavian and internal jugular veins
  - Veins join at level of sternoclavicular joint
- Superior vena cava (SVC): Formed by union of right and left brachiocephalic veins
  - Courses posterior to manubrium and sternum on right
- Azygos vein: Formed by union of ascending lumbar and right subcostal veins at 12th thoracic vertebral level
  - Ascends in posterior mediastinum; arches over right mainstem bronchus to join SVC
  - Drains posterior thorax and abdomen into SVC
- Hemiazygos vein: Begins in left ascending lumbar or left renal vein
  - Passes upward through left crus of diaphragm to enter thorax on left; mirrors lower azygos vein
    - At ~ 9th thoracic vertebra, courses rightward behind aorta and esophagus to enter azygos vein
- Accessory hemiazygos vein: Courses inferiorly along left side of spine, draining upper posterior thorax
  - Drains 4th-7th posterior intercostal veins
  - Either courses rightward at ~ 8th thoracic vertebra to join azygos vein or ends in hemiazygos vein
- Superior intercostal veins: Right- and left-sided veins that drain 2nd-4th intercostal spaces posteriorly
  - Right superior intercostal vein drains into azygos vein
  - Left drains into left brachiocephalic vein
- Internal thoracic (mammary) vein: Arises from superior epigastric vein; terminates in brachiocephalic vein
  - Paired vein that drains anterior chest and breasts
    - Receives drainage from anterior intercostal veins

LOWER EXTREMITY VENOUS ANATOMY

Lower Extremity Superficial Veins

- Great saphenous vein (GSV): Originates from dorsal venous pedal arch; courses anterior to medial malleolus
  - Ascends medially in lower leg, courses over medial epicondyle of femur at knee level, then runs anteromedially along thigh
    - Joins common femoral vein at saphenofemoral junction (SFJ) in femoral triangle region
  - Anastomoses freely with small saphenous vein (SSV) in calf
  - Has tributaries from medial, lateral, and posterior thigh
    - May form accessory saphenous vein branches that enter GSV at or near SFJ
    - Superficial epigastric, superficial iliac circumflex, and superficial external pudendal veins join GSV at SFJ
- SSV: Originates laterally from dorsal venous pedal arch; courses behind lateral malleolus
  - Ascends along posterior calf alongside sural nerve; passes between gastrocnemius muscle heads
  - Often variable anatomy of SSV drainage
    - Usually enters popliteal vein at saphenopopliteal junction around level of knee joint
    - May not drain into popliteal vein but instead may enter GSV at variable level
    - Main SSV may continue as Giacomini vein

- Giacomini vein (a.k.a. posterior thigh extension): Vein communicating between GSV and SSV; usually is thigh extension of SSV branch
  - Ascends along posterior thigh
  - Typically joins GSV in upper 1/3 of thigh
  - Found in 60-70% of individuals

Lower Extremity Deep Veins

- Calf veins: 3 sets of paired veins draining lower leg
  - Anterior tibial veins: Arise from dorsal pedal veins; run in interosseous membrane between tibia and fibula
    - Join posterior tibial veins to form popliteal vein
    - Drain ankle, knee, and tibiofibular joints along with anterior portion of lower leg
  - Posterior tibial veins: Receive blood from medial and lateral plantar veins
    - Drain posterior calf and plantar surface of foot
    - Receive most important calf perforator veins: Cockett perforators (superior, medial, and inferior)
  - Peroneal (fibular) veins
    - Return blood from lateral compartment of calf
    - Drain into posterior tibial veins
- Popliteal vein: Formed by junction of posterior and anterior tibial veins
  - Courses adjacent to popliteal artery behind knee
    - Returns blood from paired calf veins
- Femoral vein: Continuation of popliteal vein
  - Begins at adductor canal; ends at inguinal ligament
    - Receives drainage of lower extremity via popliteal, profunda femoral, and GSVs
  - Some use term superficial femoral vein for lower segment of femoral vein coursing in adductor canal
    - Differentiates femoral vein segments before and after profunda femoral vein inflow
    - Usage of term is discouraged; causes confusion, as this vein is deep rather than superficial

Lower Extremity Perforator Veins

- Connect superficial and deep veins
  - Valves direct blood from superficial to deep system
  - ~ 150 perforator veins in each leg
- Major lower extremity perforators
  - Foot and ankle perforators: Connect to pedal arches
  - Leg (calf) perforators: Connect saphenous branches with paired deep veins of calf
    - Include posterior tibial perforator veins (formerly termed Cockett perforators)
  - Knee perforators: Connect GSV with popliteal and other deep veins at knee level
    - Include medial knee perforators (formerly termed Boyd perforators); common site for varicose veins
  - Thigh perforators: Connect GSV to femoral vein
    - Include distal thigh perforator (formerly termed Dodd perforator) and medial thigh perforator (formerly termed Hunter perforator)

ABDOMINAL & PELVIC VENOUS ANATOMY

Systemic Abdominal and Pelvic Veins

- Inferior vena cava (IVC) and tributaries: Drain both lower extremities and abdominal and pelvic viscera that are not alimentary tract components
  - External iliac veins: Arise at inguinal ligament; terminate when joined by internal iliac veins
    - Connect femoral veins to common iliac veins
    - Inferior epigastric and deep circumflex iliac veins drain into external iliac veins
  - Internal iliac (hypogastric) veins: Begin near greater sciatic foramen; join with external iliac vein to form common iliac vein
    - Tributaries drain external genitalia, uterus, vagina, prostate, bladder, lower rectum, gluteal muscles
  - Common iliac veins: Formed by union of external and internal iliac veins
    - Outflow drainage for lower extremities and pelvis
  - Both renal veins drain directly into IVC
    - Left gonadal and adrenal veins drain into left renal vein
    - Right adrenal and gonadal veins drain into IVC

Portal Venous System

- Portal vein and tributaries: Responsible for directing blood from components of gastrointestinal tract to liver
  - Normally no connection with systemic venous system

VARIANT VENOUS ANATOMY

Superior Vena Cava and Tributaries

- Left SVC: Most common congenital venous anomaly of thorax
  - Seen in isolation in only 10% of cases; majority accompanied by normal but smaller right SVC
    - Termed SVC duplication if both present
  - Can result in right-to-left shunt in minority of cases
- Left azygos arch: May occur in association with left SVC
  - Left superior intercostal vein forms communication between left SVC and accessory hemiazygos vein

Inferior Vena Cava and Tributaries

- Duplicated IVC: Results from persistence of both supracardinal veins
  - Left IVC typically ends at left renal vein, which crosses anterior to aorta to join right IVC; normal suprarenal IVC
    - Prevalence of 0.2-3.0%
- Left IVC: Results from regression of right supracardinal and persistence of left supracardinal vein
  - Left IVC joins left renal vein, which crosses to unite with right renal vein and form normal suprarenal IVC
    - Prevalence of 0.2-0.5%
- Azygos continuation of IVC: Absence of hepatic IVC
  - IVC receives blood from kidneys and passes posteriorly to enter thorax as azygos vein
    - Azygos vein joins SVC at normal location in chest
- Circumaortic left renal vein: 2 left renal veins
  - Superior renal vein receives left adrenal vein and crosses aorta anteriorly
  - Inferior renal vein receives left gonadal vein and crosses aorta posteriorly
  - Prevalence may be as high as 8.7%
- Retroaortic left renal vein: Single-variant renal vein
  - Passes posterior to aorta
    - May result in "posterior nutcracker" syndrome
  - Prevalence of 2.1%

NORMAL ABDOMINAL SYSTEMIC AND PORTAL VENOUS ANATOMY

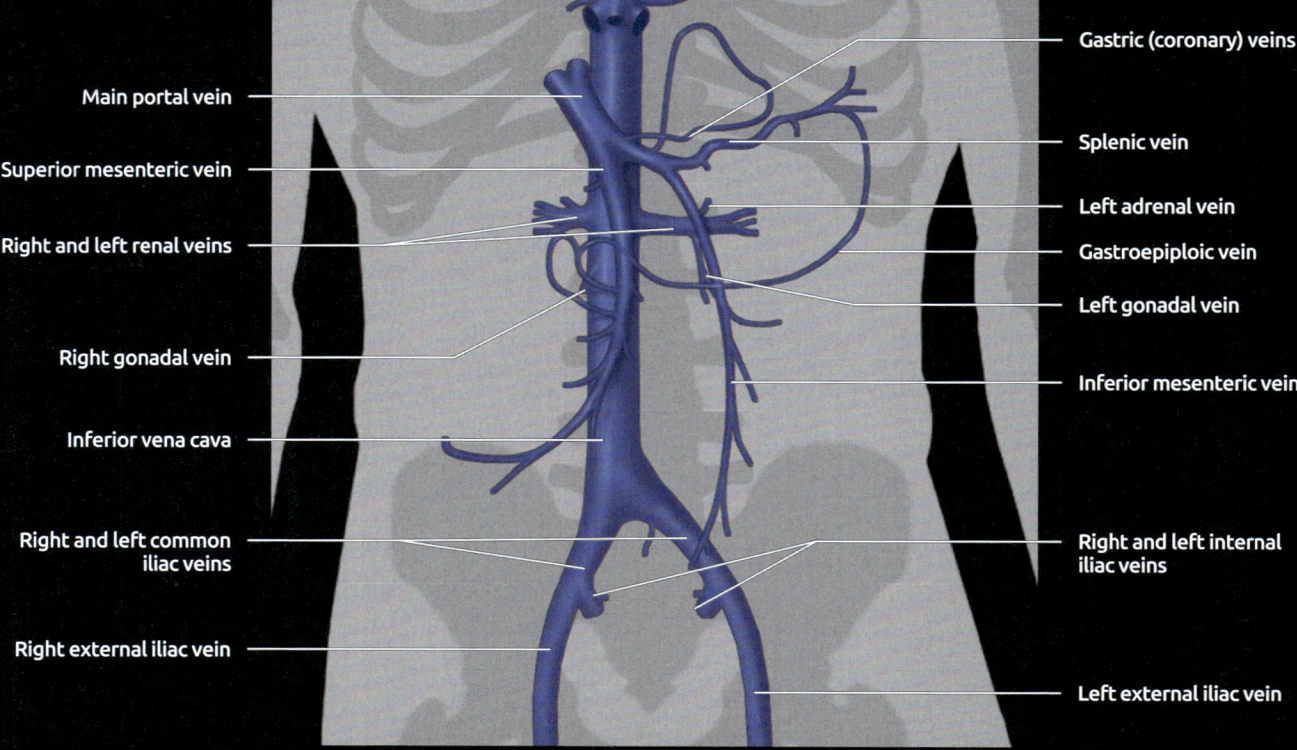

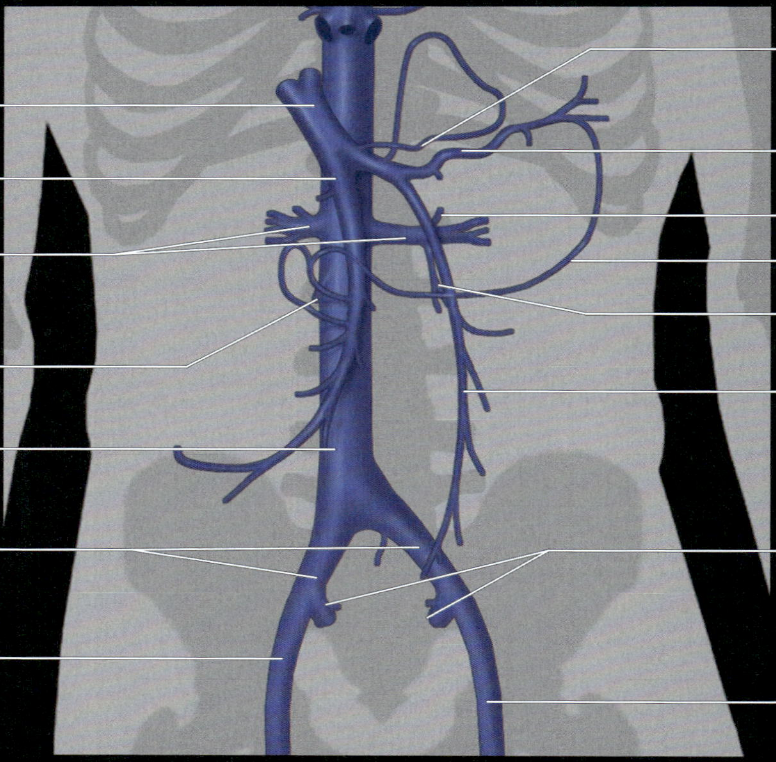

Graphic shows normal systemic and portal venous anatomy of the abdomen and pelvis. The inferior vena cava (IVC) is formed by the confluence of the right and left common iliac veins and, thus, provides central venous return for the lower extremities in addition to the pelvis and abdomen. Because the IVC is located to the right of the midline, there are some normally occurring asymmetries in venous drainage patterns. Gonadal and adrenal veins drain directly into the IVC on right but into renal vein on left. Left and right renal veins both drain directly into the IVC. All lumbar veins and hepatic veins usually drain directly into IVC, which drains into right atrium and also anastomoses in abdomen with azygos venous system. The latter is formed by ascending lumbar veins along right side of lumbar spine. Normally, portal venous system is completely separate from IVC and systemic veins. Portal venous system is responsible for returning blood from various parts of gastrointestinal tract to liver and supplies ~ 70% of liver perfusion. Portal vein is formed by the union of the superior mesenteric and splenic veins. Other important tributaries of portal vein include inferior mesenteric, gastric, and cystic veins.

VENOUS ANATOMY OF NECK, THORACIC INLET, AND UPPER THORAX

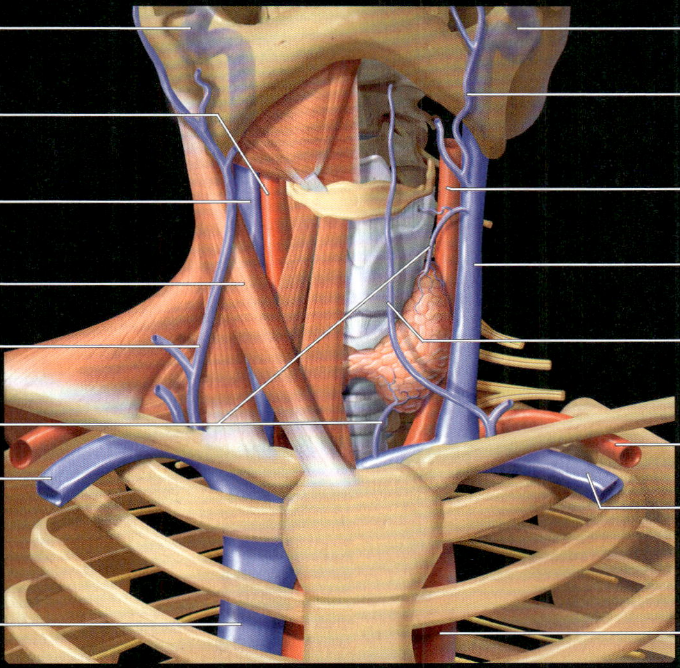

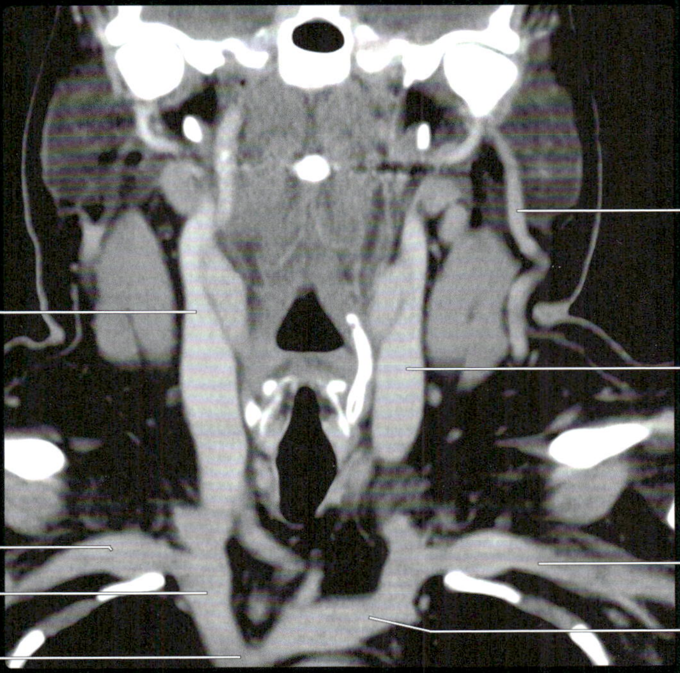

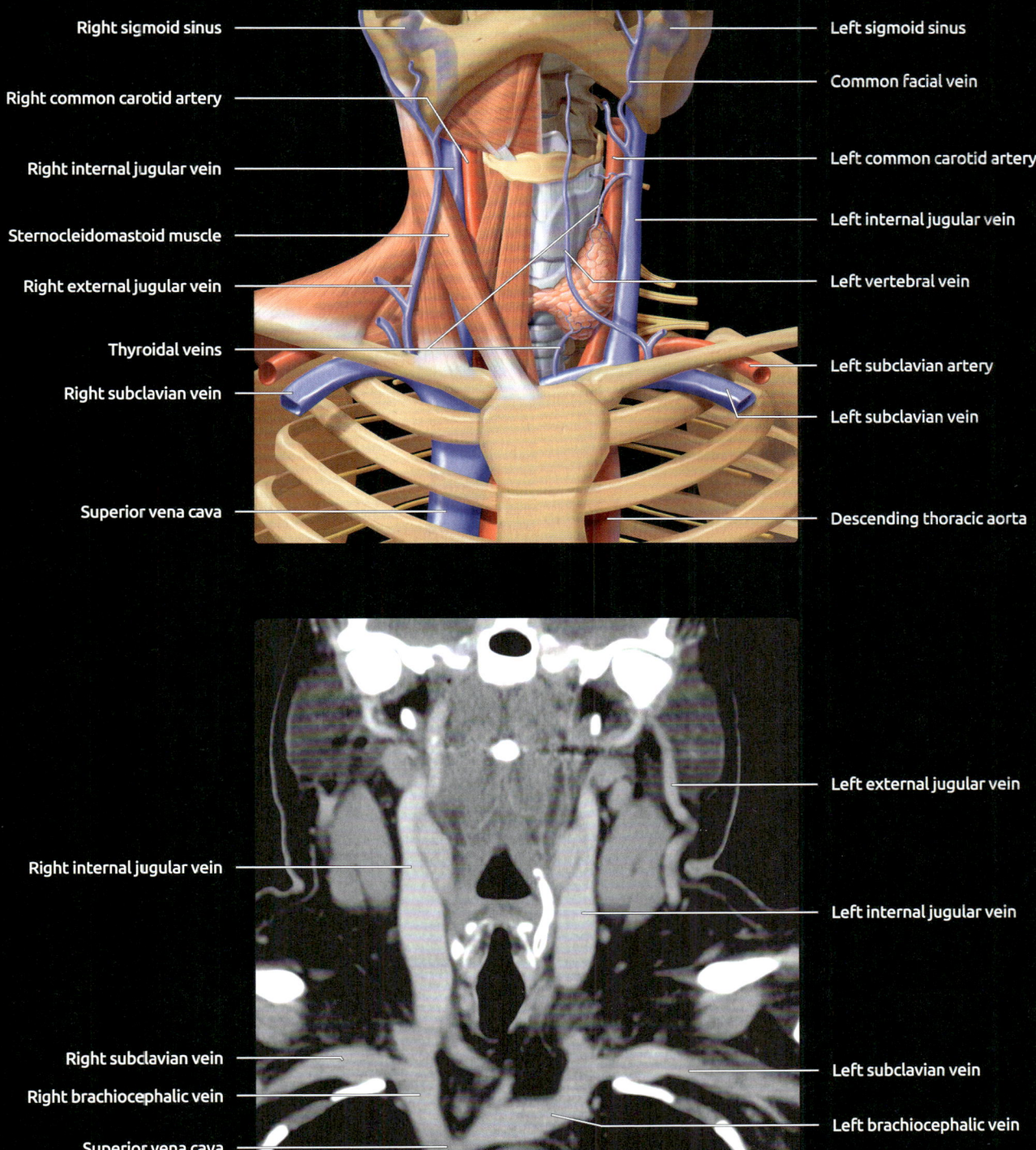

(Top) *Graphic shows the venous anatomy of the neck, thoracic inlet, and upper thorax. Internal jugular vein (IJV) is formed by the union of the sigmoid and inferior petrosal sinuses, which are joined by common facial vein. Right and left IJVs course with the common carotid artery and vagus nerve inside the carotid sheath and provide venous drainage for the brain, face, and neck. They join their subclavian vein counterparts medially to form right and left brachiocephalic veins, which in turn join to form superior vena cava (SVC). The external jugular veins (EJVs) are formed by the union of the posterior retromandibular vein and posterior auricular vein. They course superficial to the sternocleidomastoid muscle and drain into the subclavian vein more laterally than do the IJVs. EJVs provide venous drainage for the exterior of the cranium and deep parts of the face.* **(Bottom)** *Coronal reformatted CT venogram shows the normal cervicothoracic venous anatomy. IJV begins at the jugular foramen at the skull base. Its inferior course is lateral to the carotid arteries. IJVs and EJVs have a relatively superficial course and are thus susceptible to damage but are also easily accessible for venous catheterization.*

ANATOMY OF THORACIC VEINS, SUPERIOR VENA CAVA, AND TRIBUTARIES

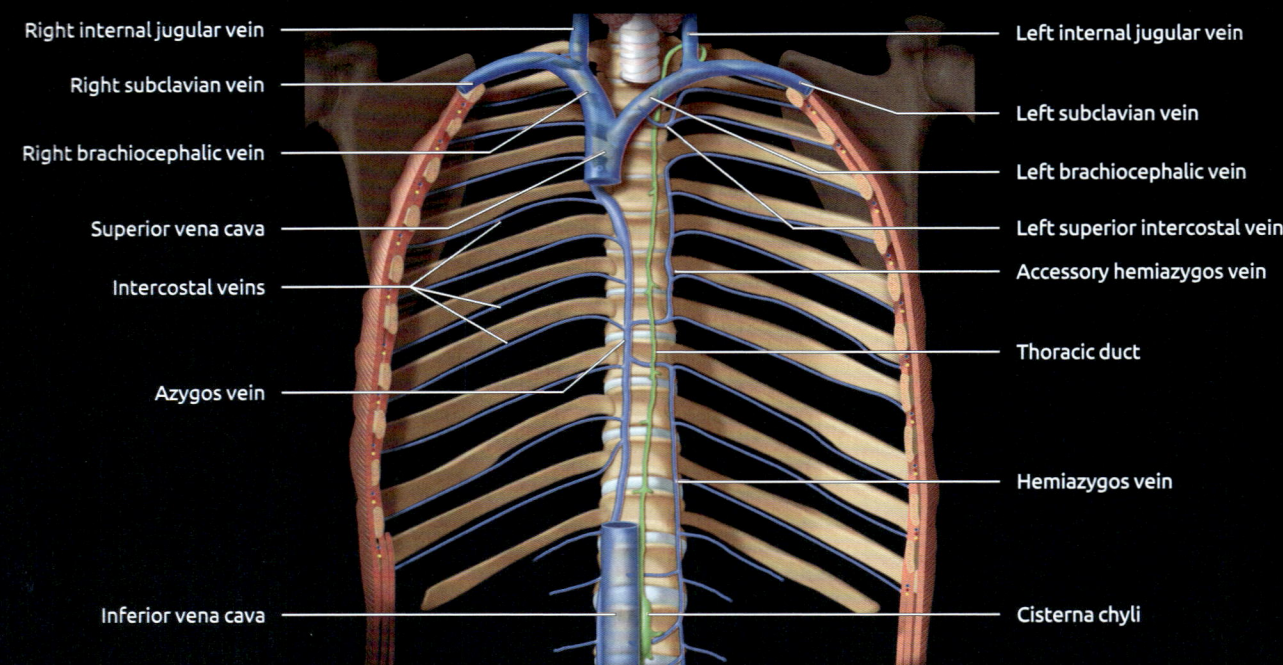

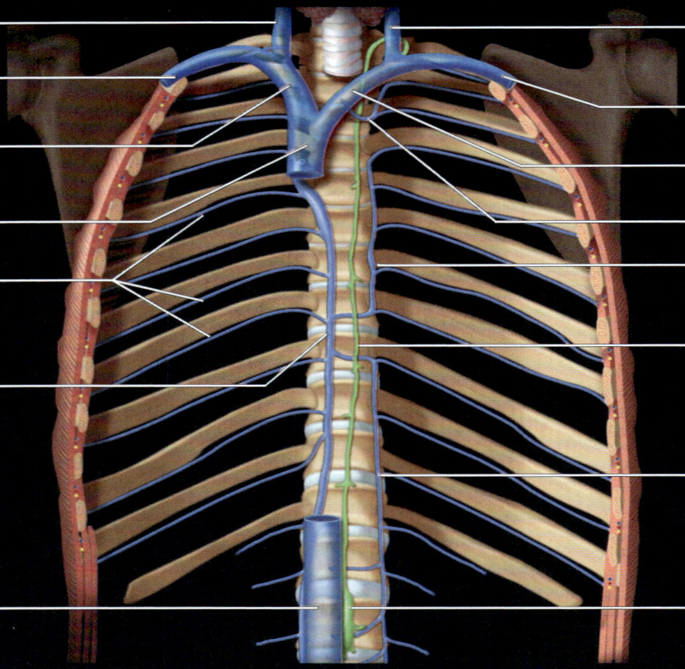

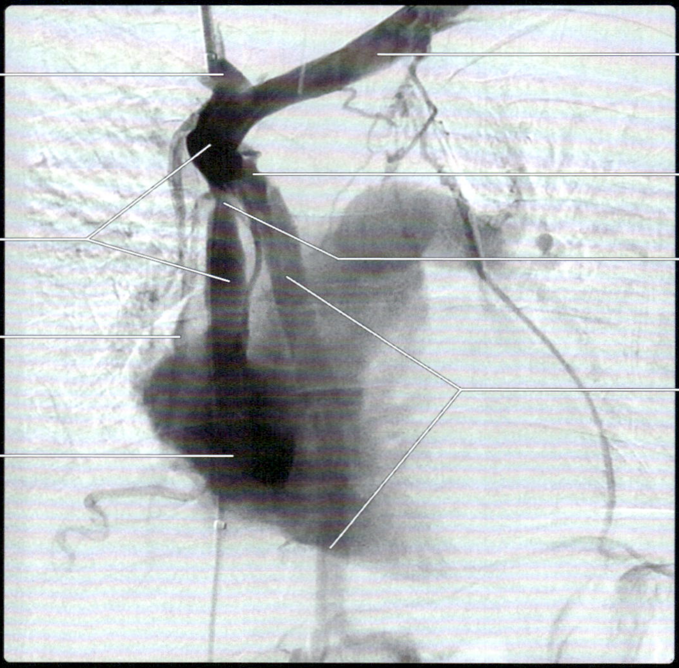

(Top) *Normal anatomy of the thoracic veins is shown. Internal jugular and subclavian veins join bilaterally to form the right and left brachiocephalic or innominate veins that join to form the SVC, which courses behind manubrium and sternum to enter right atrium. The azygos, hemiazygos, and accessory hemiazygos veins connect SVC and IVC. They course along the right and left sides of the upper lumbar and thoracic spine and drain posterior abdomen and thorax. The azygos vein ascends on the right and drains into SVC above the level of the right mainstem bronchus. The hemiazygos vein ascends on the left and crosses to the right, posterior to the aorta, thoracic duct, and esophagus to join the azygos vein. The accessory hemiazygos vein descends on left and may join hemiazygos vein or cross to right to join the azygos vein.* **(Bottom)** *The anatomy of the SVC and some of its tributaries is shown. The right and left brachiocephalic veins join to form the SVC, which drains into the right atrium to return venous blood from the head, neck, and upper extremities. The azygos vein ascends from the abdomen in the posterior mediastinum and arches over the right mainstem bronchus to join the SVC.*

ANATOMIC VARIANTS OF INFERIOR VENA CAVA

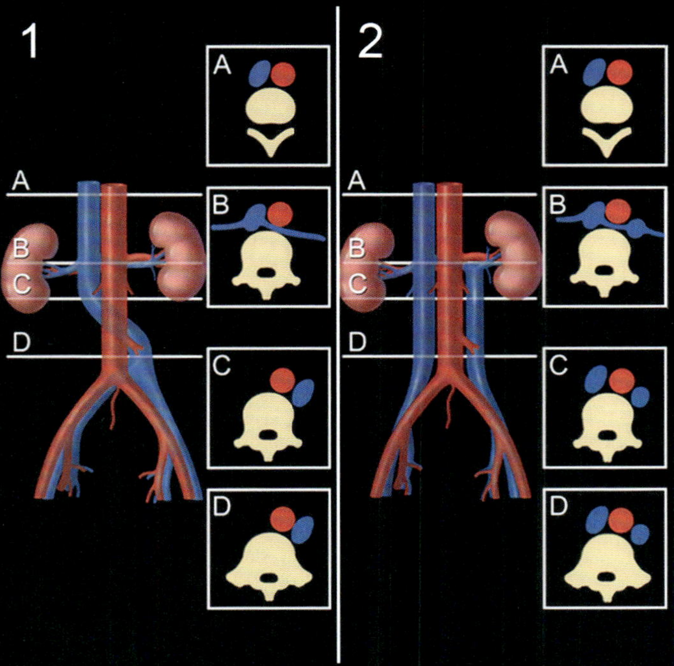

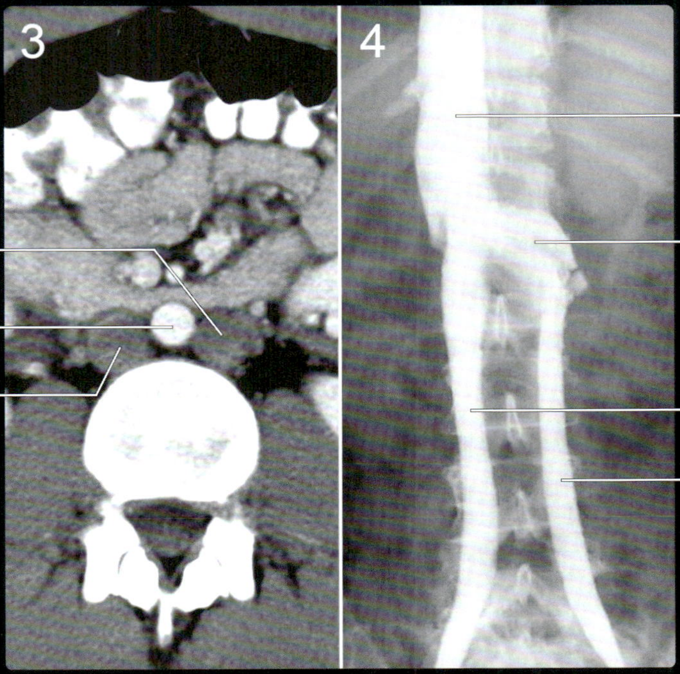

(Top) *Graphic shows 2 anatomic IVC variants with insets demonstrating cross-sectional anatomy at various levels. In panel 1, the infrarenal IVC is completely left-sided (insets C and D) and enters the left renal vein, which then crosses to the right (inset B). The left renal vein may cross anterior to the aorta or may be retroaortic, as in this example. Above the renal veins, the IVC is in a normal right-sided location. Panel 2 shows a duplicated IVC. There is a normal right-sided moiety (insets A-D). The left-sided moiety has the same anatomy as a solitary left-sided IVC as the cava ascends on the left to drain into the left renal vein (inset B). The left renal vein then crosses to the right, and the suprarenal IVC is in a normal right-sided location (inset A).* **(Bottom)** *Duplication of the IVC results from persistence of both supracardinal veins and has a reported prevalence of 0.2-3.0%. Cross-sectional CECT (panel 3) typically shows large venous structures paralleling the abdominal aorta on either side. Contrast venography (panel 4) shows that the left-sided caval moiety drains into the left renal vein, while the right component ascends normally.*

Left Superior Vena Cava

KEY FACTS

TERMINOLOGY

- Persistent left superior vena cava (PLSVC)
- Rare variant venous structure that drains blood from left upper extremity and head and neck region
  - Vast majority drain into right atrium via coronary sinus
  - Small percentage drain into left atrium (right-to-left shunt)
- Failure of regression of left anterior cardinal vein during embryologic development

IMAGING

- Radiography
  - Left-sided central venous catheter courses caudally, parallel to spine along left mediastinal border, into heart
- CT
  - Rounded structure in left mediastinum lateral to aortic arch
  - Courses caudally to left of left main pulmonary artery and left atrium
  - Joins dilated coronary sinus then right atrium
- Echocardiogram
  - Should suspect PLSVC when dilated coronary sinus is visualized

TOP DIFFERENTIAL DIAGNOSES

- Partial anomalous pulmonary venous return from left upper lobe
- Malpositioning of left central venous catheter
  - Left internal mammary vein
  - Left subclavian artery → descending aorta

CLINICAL ISSUES

- Usually asymptomatic, incidental finding on imaging or during central venous catheter placement
- Associated with congenital heart disease and arrhythmia
- Risk for paradoxical thromboembolism and air embolism if PLSVC drains into left atrium

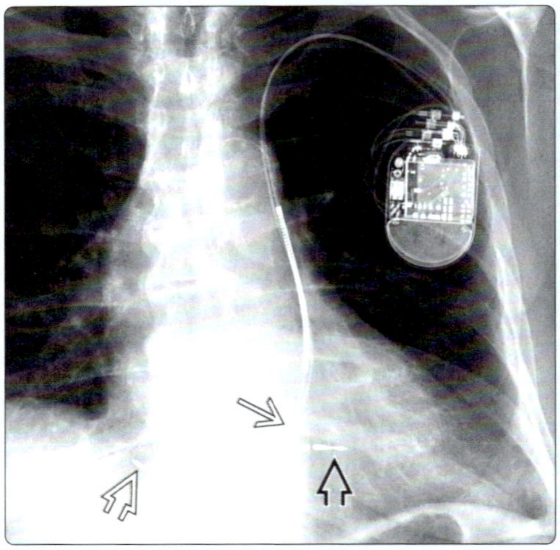

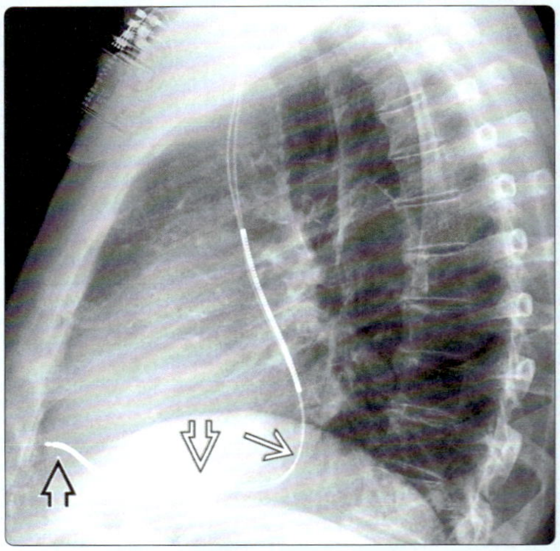

(Left) *PA radiograph in a patient with an implantable cardioverter-defibrillator placed via left subclavian approach shows left mediastinal vertical lead course, which then courses medially into the coronary sinus and right atrium (RA). The right ventricle (RV) lead loops in the RA, crosses the tricuspid valve, and terminates in the RV.* **(Right)** *Lateral radiograph shows the vertical course of the leads posterior to the left ventricle into the coronary sinus, then anteriorly into the RA and RV.*

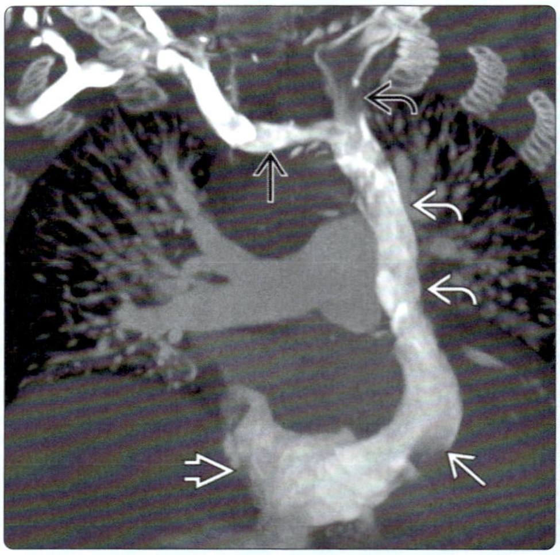

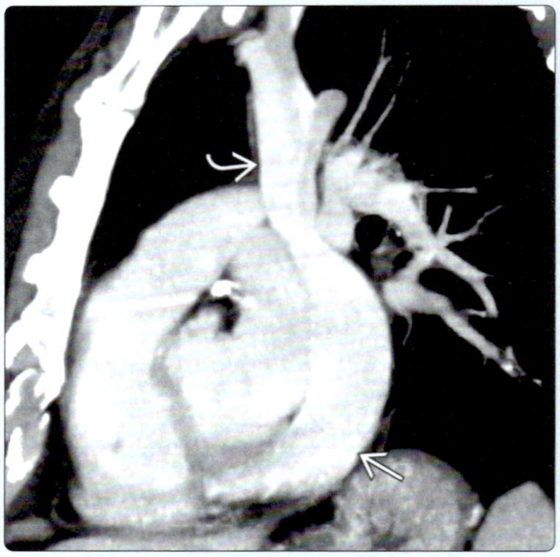

(Left) *Coronal oblique CECT MIP reconstruction in the same patient prior to the implantable cardioverter-defibrillator placement shows a bridging vein connecting the right internal jugular and subclavian veins to the left brachiocephalic vein to form a persistent left superior vena cava (PLSVC), which drains into the coronary sinus and RA.* **(Right)** *Sagittal reformat CECT shows the left superior vena cava (LSVC) coursing posterior to the left heart into the coronary sinus.*

TERMINOLOGY

Abbreviations

- Left superior vena cava (LSVC)

Synonyms

- Persistent LSVC (PLSVC)

Definitions

- Variant venous structure draining venous blood from left upper extremity and head and neck region

IMAGING

General Features

- Size
  - Larger if right SVC is absent
  - Similar in size to right SVC if bilateral SVC present, although variable

Radiographic Findings

- Left-sided central venous catheter courses caudally, parallel to spine along left mediastinal border, into heart
- Usually not visible without device in PLSVC
- Occasionally, opacity lateral to aortic knob and descending aorta

CT Findings

- Axial images: Round or oval structure in left mediastinum lateral to aortic arch
  - Courses lateral to left main pulmonary artery, medial to left superior pulmonary vein, and left of left atrium
- Vast majority drain into right atrium via dilated coronary sinus (no shunt)
- Very small percentage drain into left atrium directly or through unroofed coronary sinus or through left superior pulmonary vein (right-to-left shunt)
- Absent right SVC (10-20%)
  - Bridging vein (right brachiocephalic) drains right jugular and subclavian veins, which joins left brachiocephalic vein to form LSVC
  - Nearly 50% have congenital cardiac abnormalities
- Bilateral SVC (80-90%)
  - May see no communicating vein, normal brachiocephalic vein, or ≥ 1 abnormal venous connections between right and LSVC
  - Left brachiocephalic vein is absent in ~ 65%
  - Right SVC drains into right atrium normally
- Left superior intercostal vein can connect PLSVC with accessory hemiazygos vein to form left-sided azygous arch

MR Findings

- Same findings as CT
- Associated lesions can be characterized, including unroofed coronary sinus
- Quantification of shunt, if present

Ultrasonographic Findings

- Dilated coronary sinus on parasternal long-axis view PLSVC, diameter > 1 cm
- With contrast (agitated saline) injection into left upper extremity vein
  - Enhancement of dilated coronary sinus before right atrium confirms LSVC drains into coronary sinus
  - Enhancement of left atrium instead of right atrium suggests unroofed coronary sinus
- With contrast injection into right upper extremity vein
  - Enhancement of coronary sinus before right atrium: Right SVC is absent

DIFFERENTIAL DIAGNOSIS

Partial Anomalous Pulmonary Venous Return, Left Upper Lobe

- Left upper lobe veins coalesce and drain into left brachiocephalic vein
- No normal left superior pulmonary vein

Malpositioning of Left Central Venous Catheter

- Left mediastinal course of catheter on frontal radiograph also seen with catheter in
  - Left internal mammary vein, left superior intercostal and accessory hemiazygos vein, left subclavian artery to descending thoracic aorta, extravascular placement

PATHOLOGY

General Features

- Etiology
  - Failure of regression of left anterior cardinal vein caudal to left brachiocephalic vein during development
- Associated abnormalities
  - Raghib syndrome: PLSVC draining into left atrium; coronary sinus atrial septal defect, absent coronary sinus

CLINICAL ISSUES

Demographics

- Epidemiology
  - Most common congenital venous anomaly of thoracic systemic venous return
  - 0.3-0.5% of general population
  - 4-12% of patients with congenital cardiac anomalies
  - Associated with arrhythmia and conduction abnormalities
  - Associated with esophageal atresia

Natural History & Prognosis

- Various reported complications when pacemaker leads or catheter are inserted via left subclavian vein
- PLSVC draining into left atrium creates right-to-left shunt
  - Potential for systemic thromboembolism or air embolism
  - Medications delivered through catheter or left upper extremity vein enter systemic circulation

DIAGNOSTIC CHECKLIST

Reporting Tips

- Characterize venous return to right or left atrium and also report right central venous anatomy

SELECTED REFERENCES

1. Azizova A et al: Persistent left superior vena cava: clinical importance and differential diagnoses. Insights Imaging. 11(1):110, 2020

(Left) *Axial CECT shows a round structure in the left lateral paraaortic region, consistent with LSVC. Note the right-sided SVC in the expected region. No bridging vein is noted between the bilateral SVC.* **(Right)** *Composite sagittal CECT images in the same patient show right-sided SVC draining into the RA normally, while the LSVC drains into the coronary sinus. Also note that the coronary sinus is dilated.*

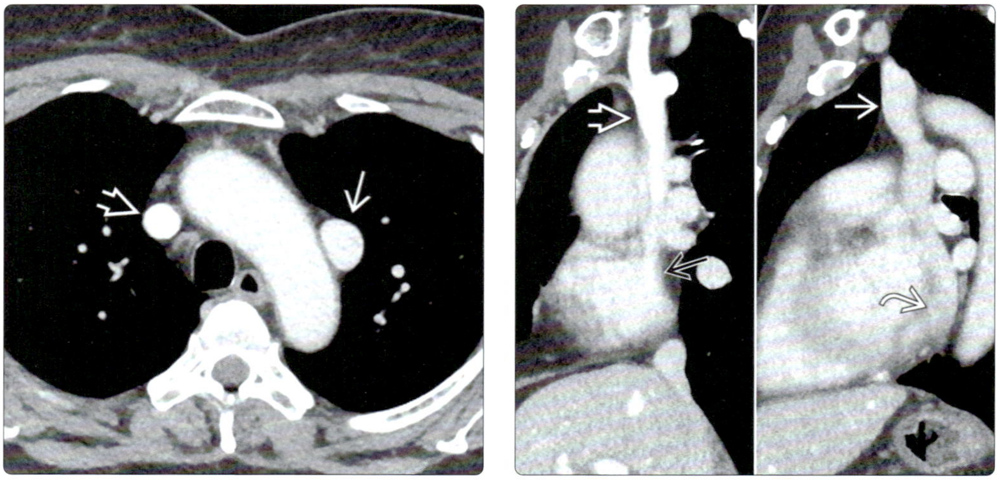

(Left) *Axial CECT shows a rounded vasculature in the left lateral paraaortic region consistent with a LSVC. No right-sided SVC is identified. Also note the catheter within the LSVC.* **(Right)** *Coronal oblique CECT MIP in the same patient shows the LSVC draining into the coronary sinus. There is no right SVC, thus the right brachiocephalic vein joins the left brachiocephalic vein and forms the LSVC. Note that central catheter terminates in the LSVC.*

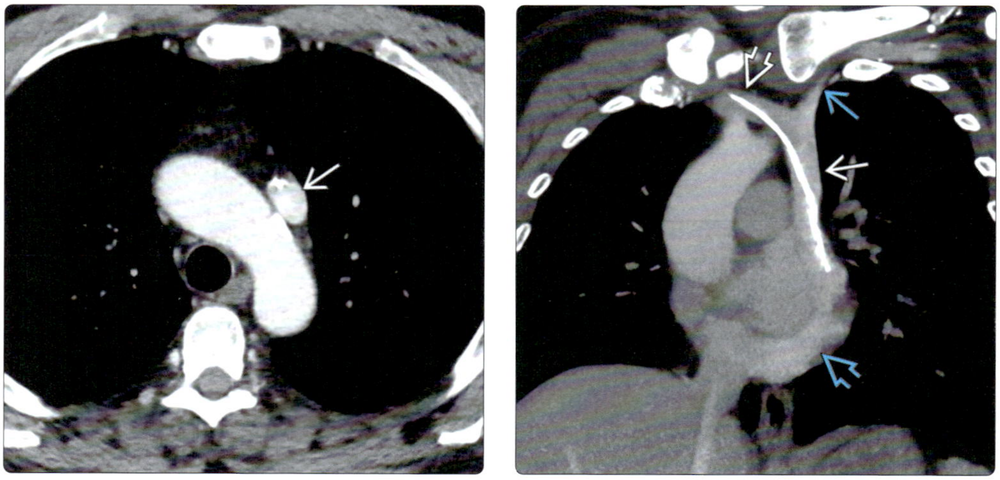

(Left) *Axial T1 C+ FS MR shows the right and LSVC. Note the smaller size of the LSVC due to the presence of a bridging vein (not shown).* **(Right)** *Curved multiplanar MR angiogram reconstruction in the same patient shows the LSVC drains into the coronary sinus. At the superior aspect of the coronary sinus, there is communication between the left atrium and coronary sinus, consistent with a partial unroofed coronary sinus.*

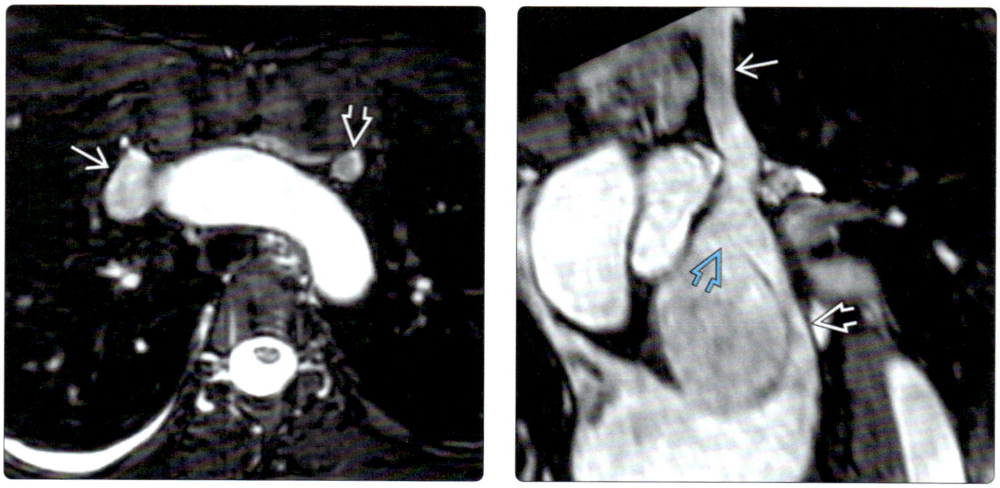

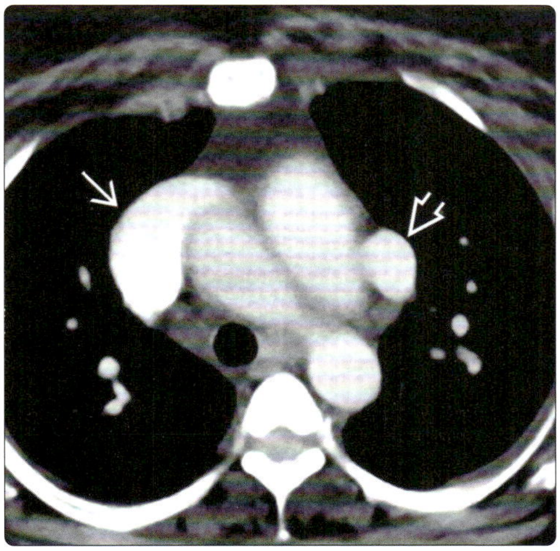

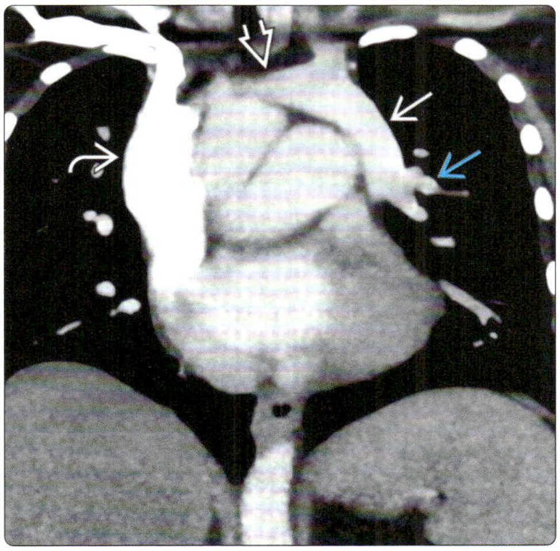

(Left) *Axial CECT shows the normal appearance of the right SVC ➔ and an additional vascular structure in the left paraaortic region ➔.* **(Right)** *Coronal reconstruction in the same patient shows left-sided vasculature ➔ draining into the left innominate vein ➔ and right SVC ➔. Note the communication with small pulmonary veins →, confirming anomalous pulmonary venous return. This is a mimicker of the LSVC and can be diagnosed by identification of communication with pulmonary veins.*

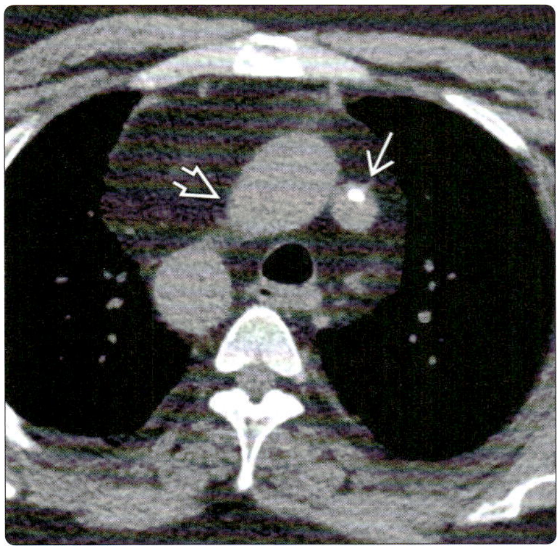

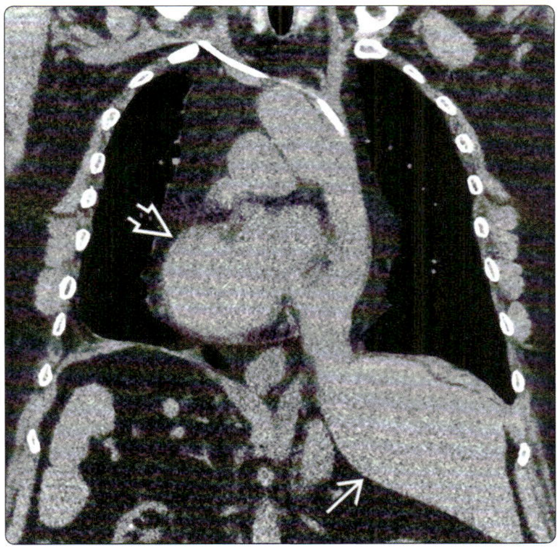

(Left) *Axial NECT in a patient with Kartagener syndrome shows absence of the right SVC in its expected location. There is a left-sided vascular structure ➔ in the left mediastinum. Note the right-sided aortic arch ➔ and descending aorta.* **(Right)** *Coronal oblique reconstruction in the same patient shows situs inversus totalis and dextrocardia ➔. Note the liver ➔ is on the left. The left-sided vasculature corresponds to mirror imaging of the right SVC due to situs abnormality, not an actual persistent LSVC.*

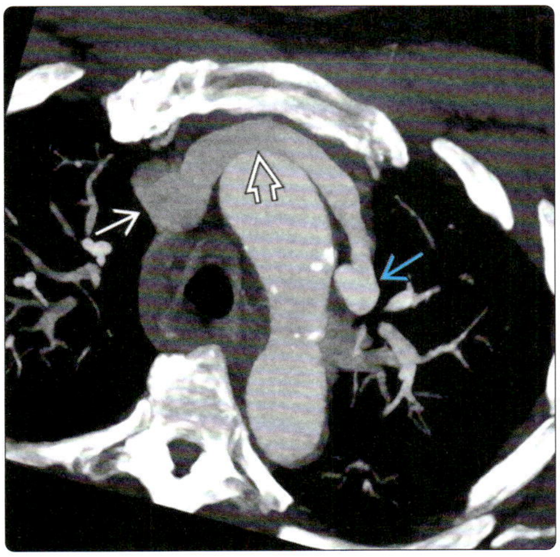

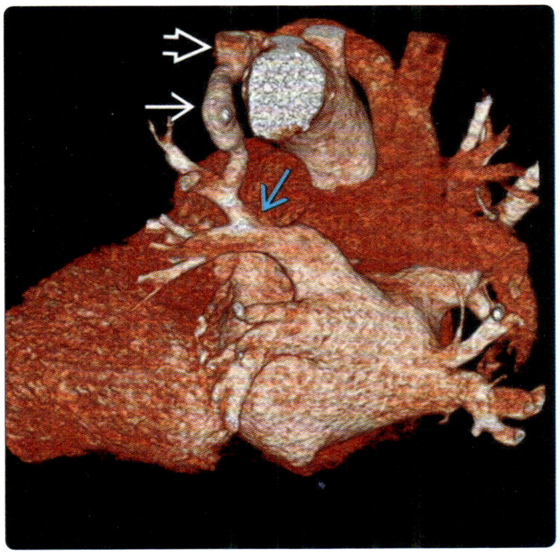

(Left) *Axial oblique CECT MIP reconstruction in a patient with atrial fibrillation shows a right SVC ➔, left innominate vein ➔, and additional vascular structure in the left mediastinum → draining into left innominate vein, which acts as a bridging vein.* **(Right)** *Posterior 3D volume-rendered CECT in the same patient shows an aberrant vessel ➔ communicating with both the left superior pulmonary vein → and left innominate vein ➔. This is a levoatriocardinal vein, which is a rare, persistent vein between pulmonary and systemic venous circulations.*

Azygos Continuation of Inferior Vena Cava

KEY FACTS

TERMINOLOGY

- Inferior vena cava (IVC) interrupted above renal veins
- Azygos vein carries venous return from lower extremities

IMAGING

- Radiography
  - Enlarged azygos arch in right tracheobronchial angle
  - Dilated if > 10-mm diameter in erect position
  - Bilateral left lungs and bronchi with heterotaxy
- CTA or MRA
  - Absent suprarenal and intrahepatic portions of IVC
  - Hepatic veins enter suprahepatic IVC or right atrium
  - Dilated azygos drains into superior vena cava (SVC)
  - Dilated hemiazygos in hemiazygos continuation
  - Polysplenia heterotaxy syndrome
    - Bilateral left sidedness
    - Multiple spleens; situs ambiguus
    - Bilateral hyparterial bronchi with bilobed lungs
  - Congenital heart disease, especially ASD and VSD

TOP DIFFERENTIAL DIAGNOSES

- Azygos enlargement from SVC obstruction, high-volume states, pulmonary hypertension
- Intrahepatic IVC occlusion by tumor/thrombus
- Mimicker of azygos enlargement on radiography
  - Enlargement of azygos region lymph node
  - Double aortic arch

CLINICAL ISSUES

- Often asymptomatic
- Symptoms related to congenital heart disease
- Prognosis related to associated anomalies
- May be lethal if inadvertently ligated at surgery
- Treatment is related to associated anomalies

DIAGNOSTIC CHECKLIST

- Difficulties may arise during catheter-based intervention through IVC, such as right heart catheterization

(Left) *Graphic shows characteristic features of azygos continuation of inferior vena cava (IVC). The hepatic portion of IVC is absent. The azygos vein ➔ is enlarged and provides the main venous drainage below the diaphragm. Identification of azygos continuation is vital in surgical planning to avoid inadvertent surgical ligation of the azygos vein.* **(Right)** *PA chest radiograph shows enlargement of the azygos arch ➔ in the right tracheobronchial angle in a patient with azygos continuation of the IVC.*

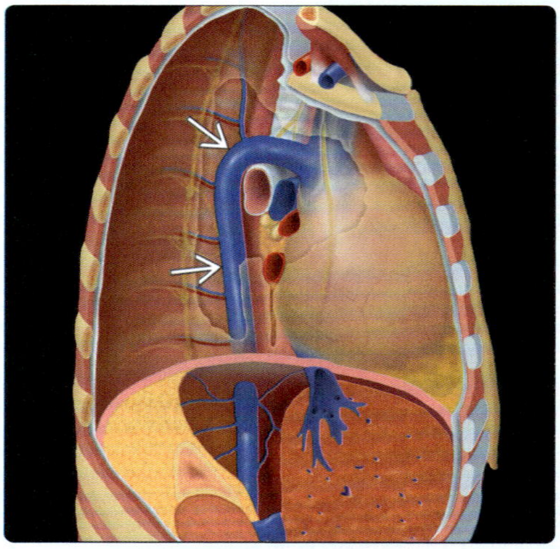

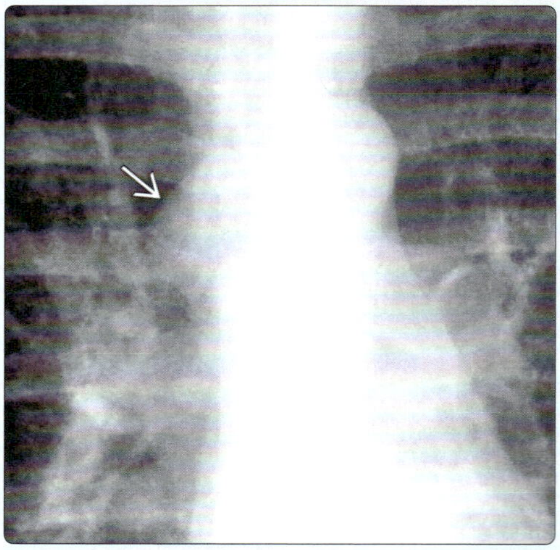

(Left) *Axial CECT in a patient with azygos continuation of the IVC shows an enlarged azygos vein ➔ arching over the right mainstem bronchus and entering the superior vena cava ➔.* **(Right)** *Axial CECT of the abdomen in the same patient shows the enlarged azygous vein ➔ and heterotaxy with a midline liver ➔, a right-sided stomach ➔, and polysplenia ➔. Azygos continuation of the IVC is associated with heterotaxy syndrome.*

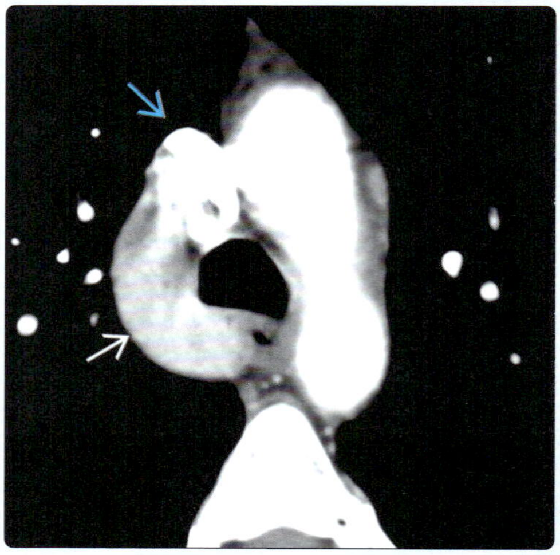

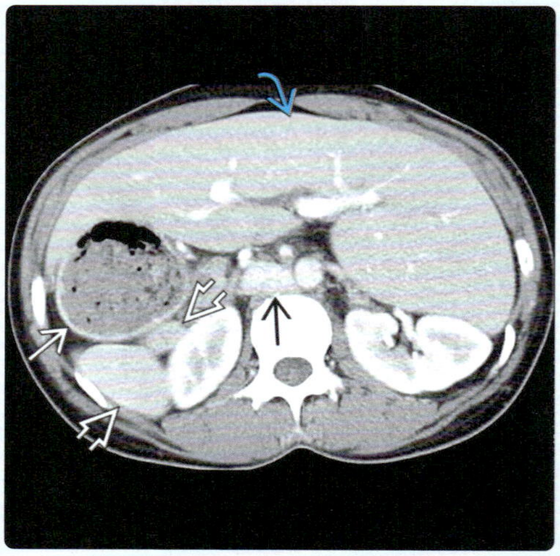

TERMINOLOGY

Synonyms

- Interruption of inferior vena cava (IVC)

Definitions

- Absence of intrahepatic segment of IVC
- Large azygos vein carries venous return from lower extremities
  - With left-sided IVC, large hemiazygos vein carries venous return from lower extremities

IMAGING

General Features

- Best diagnostic clue
  - Absence of intrahepatic segment of IVC with dilated azygos or hemiazygos vein

Radiographic Findings

- Frontal
  - Focal rounded enlargement of azygos arch in right tracheobronchial angle

CT Findings

- CECT
  - Absent suprarenal and intrahepatic portions of IVC
    - Hepatic veins drain in suprahepatic IVC or right atrium
  - Large paraspinal vessel corresponding to azygos (right) or hemiazygos (left) continuation
  - Dilated azygos courses upward and drains into superior vena cava (SVC)
  - Dilated hemiazygos courses upward
  - **Assess for findings of polysplenia (heterotaxy)**
    - Bilateral left sidedness
      - Multiple spleens; situs ambiguus
      - Bilateral bilobed (left-sided morphology) lungs
      - Bilateral hyparterial (left-sided morphology) bronchi
    - Congenital heart disease
      - Especially atrial septal defect (ASD) or ventricular septal defect (VSD)
    - Midline or transposed abdominal viscera, intestinal malrotation or nonrotation, preduodenal portal vein, truncated pancreas

MR Findings

- Same findings as described in CTA in all sequences

Imaging Recommendations

- Best imaging tool
  - CTA or MRA

DIFFERENTIAL DIAGNOSIS

Azygos Enlargement (Other Causes)

- SVC obstruction; high-volume status; pulmonary hypertension
- IVC is normal in all these entities

Azygos Region Lymphadenopathy

- Normal azygos arch, vein, IVC

Occlusion of Intrahepatic Inferior Vena Cava by Tumor/Thrombosis

- Renal cell carcinoma, hepatocellular carcinoma, or bland thrombus
- Intrahepatic IVC present

Double or Right-Sided Aortic Arch

- Venous structures normal

PATHOLOGY

General Features

- Etiology
  - Failure of right subcardinal-hepatic anastomosis → atrophy of right subcardinal vein → blood shunted from suprasubcardinal anastomosis through retrocrural azygos vein, derived from right supracardinal vein
- Genetics
  - Sporadic
- Associated abnormalities
  - **Polysplenia (bilateral left sidedness)**
  - Congenital heart disease
    - ASD, VSD, partially anomalous pulmonary venous return, pulmonary atresia

CLINICAL ISSUES

Presentation

- Most common signs/symptoms
  - Often asymptomatic; discovered incidentally
- Other signs/symptoms
  - Symptoms related to congenital heart disease
  - May be associated with sick sinus syndrome

Demographics

- Age
  - Variable; early in life if associated severe congenital heart defect (CHD)
- Sex
  - No predilection
- Epidemiology
  - Prevalence < 0.6%
  - 0.2-4.3% of cardiac catheterizations for congenital heart disease

Natural History & Prognosis

- Related to associated anomalies, particularly CHD
- May be lethal if inadvertently ligated at surgery

Treatment

- Related to associated anomalies, particularly CHD

DIAGNOSTIC CHECKLIST

Consider

- Difficulties may arise during catheter-based intervention through IVC, such as right heart catheterization

SELECTED REFERENCES

1. Li SJ et al: The inferior vena cava: anatomical variants and acquired pathologies. Insights Imaging. 12(1):123, 2021
2. Kim SS et al: Various congenital anomalies of the inferior vena cava: review of cross-sectional imaging findings and report of a new variant. Abdom Radiol (NY). 43(8):2130-49, 2018

KEY FACTS

TERMINOLOGY

- Specific subtype of partial anomalous pulmonary venous return
- Synonyms: Hypogenetic lung/pulmonary venolobar syndrome

IMAGING

- Scimitar vein = curved anomalous venous trunk resembling Turkish sword, located in right medial costophrenic sulcus near right heart border
- Right lung hypoplasia
- Dextroversion of heart; apex is still directed toward left
- CT or MR is best at showing typical drainage of scimitar vein into inferior vena cava (IVC)
- CT or MR angiography also show anomalous systemic arterial supply and right pulmonary artery and mainstem bronchus hypoplasia
- Phase-contrast MR for shunt flow calculation

TOP DIFFERENTIAL DIAGNOSES

- Meandering pulmonary vein
- Partial anomalous pulmonary venous return
- Isolated right pulmonary hypoplasia
- Pulmonary sequestration
- True dextrocardia with abdominal situs solitus

CLINICAL ISSUES

- Age of presentation depends on degree of right lung hypoplasia, coexistent congenital heart disease, and presence of systemic supply to right lung
  - Older age of presentation, usually milder disease course
  - Large shunt: Development of irreversible pulmonary hypertension
- Treatment
  - Surgical repair when left-to-right shunt > 2:1
  - Baffling of common right pulmonary vein onto left atrium
  - Embolization of systemic arterial supply

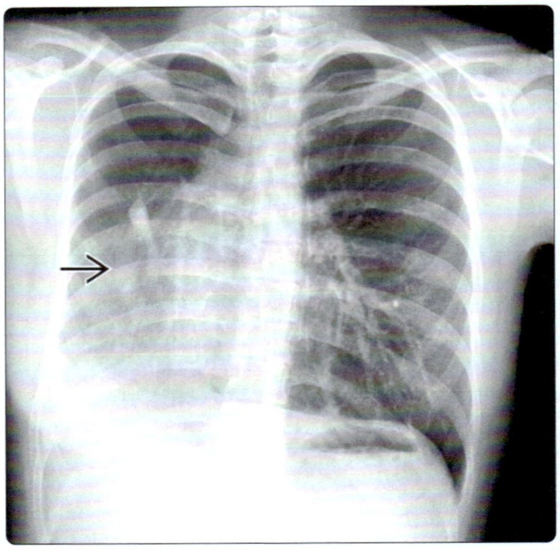

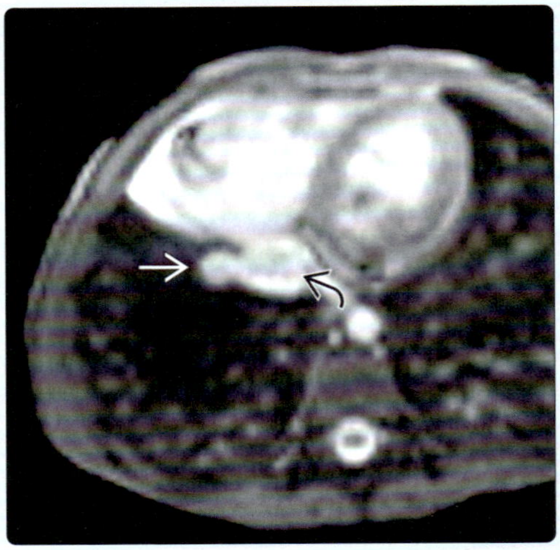

(Left) *Frontal radiograph of the chest shows low right lung volume and rightward mediastinal shift. A tubular density → is seen in the right mid- and lower chest parallel to the right heart border.* **(Right)** *Axial image from an SSFP sequence of a cardiac MR shows an anomalous pulmonary vein → draining into the inferior vena cava (IVC) ↷, consistent with Scimitar syndrome. There is right-sided mediastinal shift but situs solitus. Note the low volume of the right lung.*

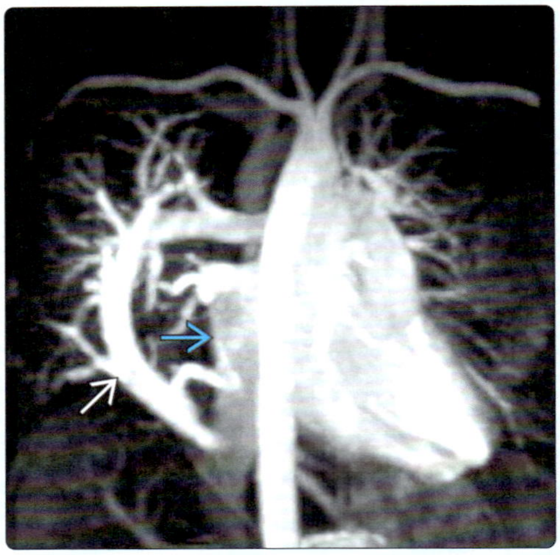

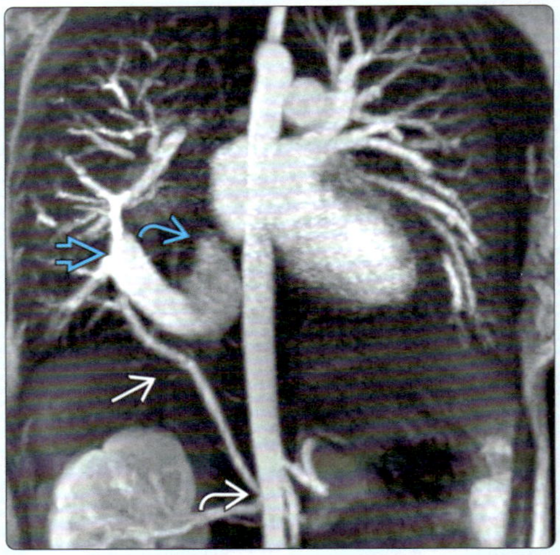

(Left) *Coronal MRA demonstrates a large, abnormal pulmonary vein → draining into the IVC →, consistent with partial anomalous pulmonary venous return. Note the appearance of the anomalous vein resembles a Turkish sword ("scimitar").* **(Right)** *Coronal MIP reconstruction from an MRA shows an anomalous right inferior pulmonary vein → draining into the dilated IVC ↷. There is systemic arterial supply to the right lung → originating from the abdominal aorta adjacent to the right renal artery ↷.*

TERMINOLOGY

Synonyms

- Hypogenetic lung/pulmonary venolobar syndrome

Definitions

- Anomalous right pulmonary venous connection to inferior vena cava (IVC) with right lung hypoplasia
- Often associated: Ipsilateral systemic arterial supply, cardiac dextroposition
- Left-to-right shunt

IMAGING

General Features

- Best diagnostic clue
  - Scimitar vein = curved anomalous venous trunk resembling Turkish sword
    - Right medial costophrenic sulcus near right heart border
    - Increases in caliber in caudal direction
  - Hypoplastic right lung

Radiographic Findings

- Radiography
  - Scimitar vein in right medial costophrenic sulcus
  - Right lung hypoplasia with right-sided mediastinal shift
    - Cardiac dextroversion: Apex still directed left
  - Prominent right atrium (RA), shunt vascularity

CT Findings

- Scimitar vein joins IVC
  - Anomalous vein drains entire right lung in 57%
- Varying degrees of right lung hypoplasia
  - Hypoplasia severity associated with earlier diagnosis
- Right lung systemic arterial supply in 50%
  - Possible associated pulmonary artery hypoplasia
- Congenital heart disease (CHD) in ~ 60%
  - Secundum atrial septal defect (ASD) most common
- Often absent right-sided pulmonary veins draining into left atrium

MR Findings

- MRA: Provides roadmap for surgery/intervention
- Assessment of coexisting CHD
- Phase-contrast MR: Shunt quantification (Qp:Qs ratio)

Imaging Recommendations

- CTA or MRA for comprehensive assessment

DIFFERENTIAL DIAGNOSIS

Meandering Pulmonary Vein

- Anomalous course of single pulmonary vein
- Normal drainage into left atrium; no shunt

Right-Sided Partial Anomalous Pulmonary Venous Return

- Right pulmonary vein(s) to superior vena cava (SVC), azygos vein, RA
- No hypoplasia of right lung
- Often associated with sinus venosus ASD

Isolated Right Pulmonary Hypoplasia

- Normal right pulmonary venous connection to left atrium

Pulmonary Sequestration

- Mass in right lung base, not connected to bronchial tree
- Systemic arterial supply
- Venous drainage: Pulmonary or systemic vein

PATHOLOGY

General Features

- Associated abnormalities
  - In one large study of 485 patients, CHD in 62%
    - ASD in 50% of all patients
      - Ostium secundum most common
    - Ventricular septal defect (VSD) or patent ductus arteriosus (PDA) in 13%
    - Coarctation or pulmonary artery anomalies ~ 2%
    - Tetralogy of Fallot in small percentage
- Embryology
  - Abnormal right lung development with secondary anomalous pulmonary venous connection

Gross Pathologic & Surgical Features

- Anomalous right pulmonary venous drainage to IVC
  - Drains entire right lung in 57% of patients
- Right lung hypoplasia or agenesis
  - Most commonly affects right upper or middle lobes
- Systemic arterialization of right lung base in 50%

CLINICAL ISSUES

Presentation

- Most common signs/symptoms
  - Age of presentation associated with degree of right lung hypoplasia, systemic supply to right lung, and CHD
    - Newborn: Congestive heart failure, right heart volume overload, pulmonary hypertension
    - Young child: Recurrent infections in right lung base
    - Older child and adult: Asymptomatic, incidental imaging finding

Natural History & Prognosis

- Pulmonary arterial hypertension in 32% due to shunting
  - Most common in neonates and young children
- Postoperative mortality 6%, more common in patients with lung resection
- May be asymptomatic for many years with small shunt

Treatment

- Surgical repair is indicated when left-to-right shunt > 2:1
- Baffling of common right pulmonary vein onto left atrium
- Embolization of systemic arterial supply to avoid bleeding
- Partial or complete right lung resection in < 10% of patients
  - Associated with more complications and higher mortality

SELECTED REFERENCES

1. Vida VL et al: The natural history and surgical outcome of patients with scimitar syndrome: a multi-centre European study. Eur Heart J. 39(12):1002-11, 2018
2. Wang H et al: Scimitar syndrome in children and adults: natural history, outcomes, and risk analysis. Ann Thorac Surg. 105(2):592-98, 2018

KEY FACTS

TERMINOLOGY

- Total anomalous pulmonary venous return (TAPVR)
- Embryologic failure of common pulmonary vein (PV) to connect to left atrium (LA)

IMAGING

- CT
  - 3D CT angiography: For pre- and postoperative PV caliber measurements
  - Thickened interlobular septa, peribronchial cuffing, and ground-glass opacity suggest postoperative anastomotic pulmonary venous stenosis
- MR
  - Gadolinium-enhanced MRA: Allows for multiplanar reformations and volume-rendered 3D imaging
  - Cine MR: Used for functional cardiac assessment and visualization of flow jets and valvular regurgitation
  - Phase-contrast MR: Used for detection of PV anastomotic stenosis
- No PVs connecting to LA

TOP DIFFERENTIAL DIAGNOSES

- Cor triatriatum
- Hypoplastic left heart syndrome
- Persistent fetal circulation syndrome, primary pulmonary hypertension

PATHOLOGY

- 3 types
  - Supracardiac TAPVR (type I): Vertical common PV carries blood from both lungs and joins left innominate vein
  - Cardiac TAPVR (type II): Common PV joins coronary sinus or right atrium directly
  - Infracardiac TAPVR (type III): Common PV traverses diaphragm to join portal vein, ductus venosus, or inferior vena cava
  - Mixed TAPVR (type IV): PVs drain to at least 2 different locations

(Left) *Graphic shows pulmonary veins ➡ forming a retrocardiac common vein ➡ that descends below the diaphragm to drain into the inferior vena cava (IVC) (left-to-right shunt). An atrial septal defect (ASD) ➡ allows for right-to-left shunting, resulting in an admixture lesion.* **(Right)** *AP radiograph shows increased vascularity and a curvilinear density overlying the mediastinum ➡, which may be mistaken for a normal thymus. However, this curvilinear structure can be seen extending into the middle mediastinum ➡.*

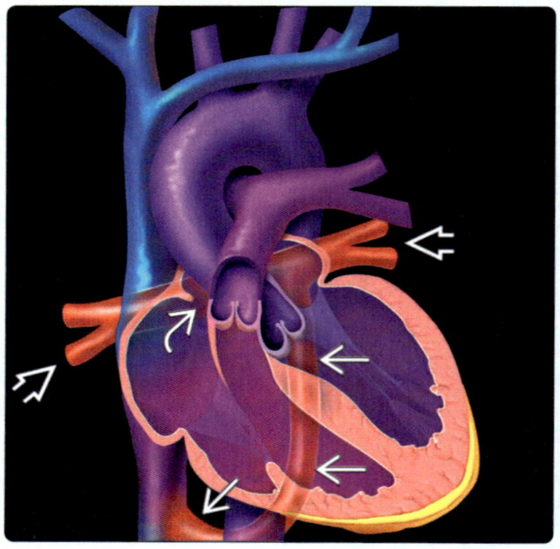

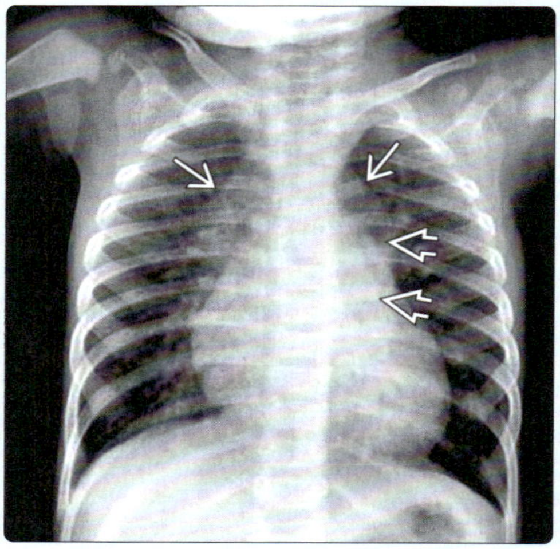

(Left) *Coronal CTA shows multiple pulmonary veins ➡ draining into a vertical vein ➡ in a patient with supracardiac total anomalous pulmonary venous return (TAPVR) (type I), the most common type of TAPVR.* **(Right)** *Coronal CTA MIP in the same patient shows that the large anomalous draining pulmonary vein ➡ empties into an enlarged left brachiocephalic vein ➡, which then drains into the enlarged superior vena cava (SVC) ➡. (Courtesy S. Kligerman, MD.)*

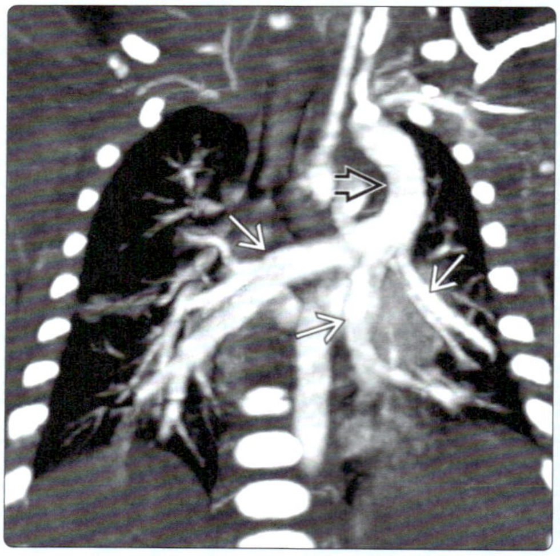

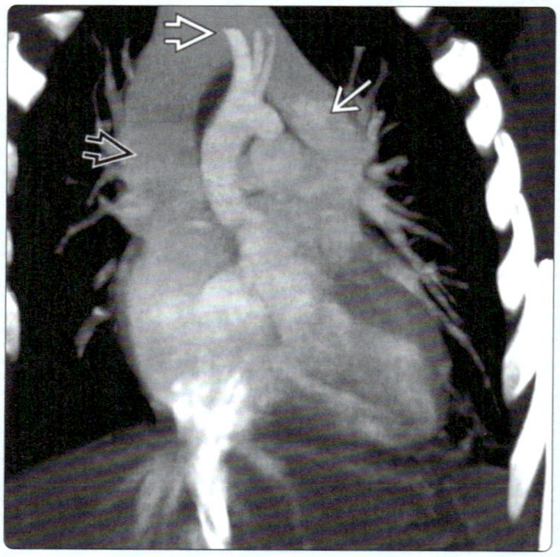

TERMINOLOGY

Abbreviations

- Total anomalous pulmonary venous return (TAPVR)

Synonyms

- Total anomalous pulmonary venous connection (TAPVC)

Definitions

- Embryologic failure of common pulmonary vein (PV) to connect to left atrium (LA)
  - Anomalous connection of PVs to right atrium (RA), coronary sinus, systemic veins, or tributaries leading to left-to-right shunt
  - Atrial septal defect (ASD) of varying size (right-to-left shunt) resulting in admixture lesion

IMAGING

General Features

- Best diagnostic clue
  - No PVs connecting to LA
- Echocardiography provides most information in neonates, infants
  - MR or CT used in select patients with suboptimal echo
    - Poor acoustic window; mixed TAPVR; TAPVR in complex congenital heart disease (CHD)

Radiographic Findings

- Radiography
  - Snowman heart appearance on chest radiograph (type I)
  - Indistinguishable from ASD on chest radiograph (type II)
  - Small heart, reticular pattern in lungs; edema on chest radiograph (type III)
  - Cardiomegaly (types I and II), small heart (type III)
  - Shunt vascularity (types I and II), pulmonary edema (type III)
  - Left vertical vein may be visible in type I

CT Findings

- CT angiography
  - Preoperative determination of anatomy and drainage
    - 3D reconstructions provide surgical road map
  - Used for pre- and postoperative PV measurements
  - Additional defects, including ASD, enlarged RA and ventricle
  - Findings of asplenia heterotaxy (bilateral right sidedness)
    - Aorta ipsilateral to infrarenal inferior vena cava (IVC)
    - Bilateral eparterial bronchi and trilobed lungs
    - Severe CHD
      - □ High percentage of patients with have TAPVR
    - Bilateral right atrial morphology
    - Intestinal malrotation or nonrotation, centrally located liver
- Postoperative venous stenosis: Thick interlobular septa, peribronchial cuffing, and ground-glass opacities

MR Findings

- T1WI
  - Anomalous connection is best seen in axial plane
- Cine MR
  - Demonstrates anomalous connection, flow jets
  - ASD, enlarged RA and ventricle
  - Quantification of ventricular volumes and function
- Gadolinium-enhanced MRA
  - Best pulse sequence to define anatomy
  - Multiplanar reformations and volume-rendered 3D
- Phase-contrast imaging
  - Useful in PV anastomotic stenosis
    - Flow velocities > 100 cm/s are diagnostic

Ultrasonographic Findings

- Abdominal US in type III may demonstrate large infradiaphragmatic vascular channel from thorax with flow towards abdomen
  - Variable intrahepatic or extrahepatic connection
    - Blood eventually drains into IVC, hepatic vein, portal vein, or ductus venosus
  - May demonstrate area of narrowing with flow acceleration

Echocardiographic Findings

- Lack of connection of PVs to LA
- Right-sided chamber enlargement in types I and II
- Patent foramen ovale (PFO)
- Associated cardiac and abdominal situs abnormalities
- Limited assessment of postoperative venous obstruction

Angiographic Findings

- Conventional
  - Seldom required for primary diagnosis
  - After repair: For diagnosis and treatment of anastomotic pulmonary venous stenosis

Imaging Recommendations

- Echocardiography for primary diagnosis
- CT/MR for postoperative anastomotic stenosis

DIFFERENTIAL DIAGNOSIS

Cor Triatriatum

- Pulmonary venous connection has occurred but stenotic
- Membrane divides atrium into 2 chambers

Hypoplastic Left Heart Syndrome

- Pulmonary blood returns to LA; atretic or hypoplastic mitral valve causes shunting via ASD into RA
- Small left ventricle and ascending aorta
- Patent ductus arteriosus (PDA) with retrograde aortic flow toward arch vessels

Persistent Fetal Circulation Syndrome or Primary Pulmonary Hypertension

- Associated with severe hyaline membrane disease, meconium aspiration

PATHOLOGY

General Features

- Genetics
  - No specific genetic defect is found
  - Occasionally associated with other complex cyanotic heart disease, asplenia syndrome, or atrioventricular canal
- 4 types

- Type I: Supracardiac TAPVR (most common)
  - Vertical common PV joins left innominate vein
    - Usually anterior to left pulmonary artery and behind left atrial appendage
    - Occasionally posterior to left pulmonary artery, which may cause venous obstruction from compression between left pulmonary artery and bronchus
  - Narrowing of entrance to left innominate vein can result in obstruction
  - Dilated innominate vein, SVC, and right heart
  - PFO or ASD often present and only source of flow to left heart
- Type II: Cardiac TAPVR
  - Common PV joins RA directly, usually through coronary sinus
    - Can drain to right SVC, directly to RA or azygos vein
  - Dilated PVs and coronary sinus
  - Obstruction is unusual
- Type III: Infracardiac TAPVR
  - Common PV traverses diaphragm to join portal vein (most common) at confluence of superior mesenteric and splenic veins, ductus venosus, hepatic or IVC
  - Confluence is posterior to LA, vertically oriented (inverted fir tree appearance)
  - High (> 90%) prevalence of obstruction
- Type IV: Mixed TAPVR (least common)
  - PVs drain to at least 2 different locations
    - e.g., right PVs to coronary sinus; left PVs to left innominate vein

- Hemodynamics
  - All pulmonary venous return is to right heart (extracardiac left-to-right shunt)
  - Intracardiac right-to-left shunt is through ASD or PFO
  - All types are admixture lesions
- Low systemic blood flow may lead to associated hypoplasia of left-sided cardiac chambers
- Embryology
  - Lack of normal incorporation of primitive common PV into posterior wall of LA
  - Persistence and enlargement of embryologic pathways for pulmonary venous return via umbilicovitelline and cardinal veins
  - Isolated or associated with complex CHD, including asplenia heterotaxy
- Pathophysiology
  - All types have PFO to allow for obligatory right-to-left flow, leading to varying degrees of cyanosis (less severe in types I and II: Pulmonary hypercirculation)
  - Nonobstructive TAPVR (types I and II): ASD physiology, pulmonary plethora, congestive heart failure
  - Obstructive TAPVR (type III): Common PV enters higher pressure portal system → pulmonary venous congestion and edema

Staging, Grading, & Classification

- Category: Cyanotic
  - Heart size and pulmonary vascularity depend on type

Gross Pathologic & Surgical Features

- Corrective surgery connects common PV via window with LA, and all other abnormal pulmonary venous connections are ligated

CLINICAL ISSUES

Presentation

- Symptom severity depends on interatrial connection size and pulmonary resistance
- Types I and II: Initially asymptomatic, followed by congestive heart failure
- Type III: Severe cyanosis at birth
- PDA: Persistent fetal circulation

Demographics

- 1-3% of CHD, more frequent in neonatal period
  - 2% of deaths due to CHD in 1st year of life

Natural History & Prognosis

- Highly variable
- No patient survives without surgical treatment
- Types I and II: Initially asymptomatic with gradual development of congestive heart failure (ASD physiology)
- Type III, obstructive forms: Death within month
- After surgical repair: Determined by associated cardiac anomalies and development of PV anastomotic stenosis

Treatment

- Prostaglandin E1 to improve systemic perfusion in pulmonary hypertension
- Early surgical anastomosis of PV to LA

DIAGNOSTIC CHECKLIST

Consider

- Volume-rendered 3D imaging CT/MR to define anatomy
- Look for anastomotic PV stenoses on postoperative CTA or MRA
- Look for connection with LA to exclude cor triatriatum (if no connection to RA) or unroofed coronary sinus (if coronary sinus collects PVs and drains into RA)

SELECTED REFERENCES

1. Goerne H et al: Total anomalous pulmonary venous return. Radiology. 307(3):e222085, 2023
2. Türkvatan A et al: Multidetector computed tomographic angiography imaging of congenital pulmonary venous anomalies: a pictorial review. Can Assoc Radiol J. 68(1):66-76, 2017
3. Husain SA et al: Total anomalous pulmonary venous connection: factors associated with mortality and recurrent pulmonary venous obstruction. Ann Thorac Surg. 94(3):825-31; discussion 831-2, 2012
4. Vyas HV et al: MR imaging and CT evaluation of congenital pulmonary vein abnormalities in neonates and infants. Radiographics. 32(1):87-98, 2012
5. Molinari F et al: Total anomalous pulmonary venous return with connection to the supradiaphragmatic inferior vena cava: assessment and diagnosis by multidetector computed tomography. Heart Lung Circ. 20(5):341-2, 2011
6. Seale AN et al: Total anomalous pulmonary venous connection: morphology and outcome from an international population-based study. Circulation. 122(25):2718-26, 2010
7. Lakshminrusimha S et al: Use of CT angiography in the diagnosis of total anomalous venous return. J Perinatol. 29(6):458-61, 2009

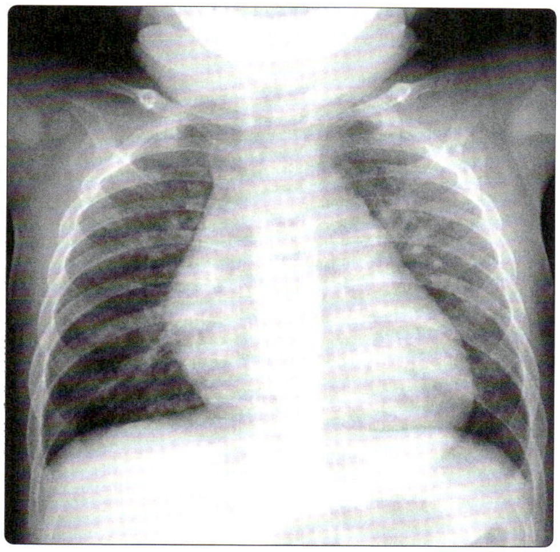

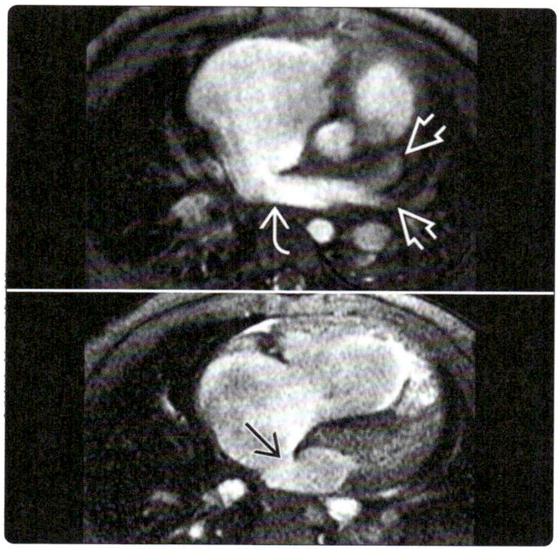

(Left) *AP radiograph shows an enlarged right heart without pulmonary obstruction in a patient with cardiac TAPVR.* **(Right)** *Axial MR cine images show pulmonary veins draining into the posterior common vein, which drains into the right atrium (cardiac TAPVR). Note the enlarged right atrium and ventricle and a large ASD. The ASD provides the systemic blood supply.*

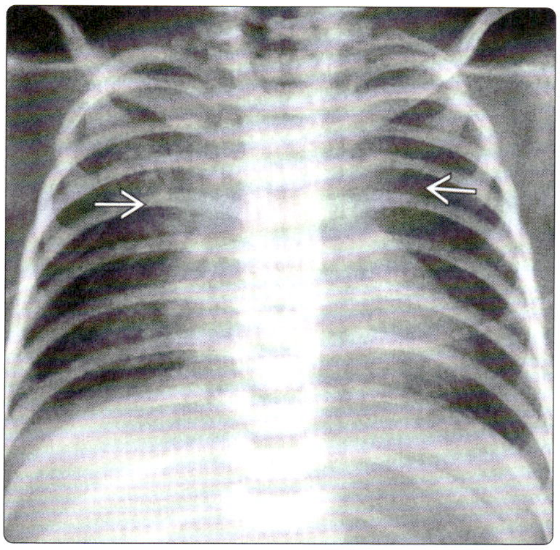

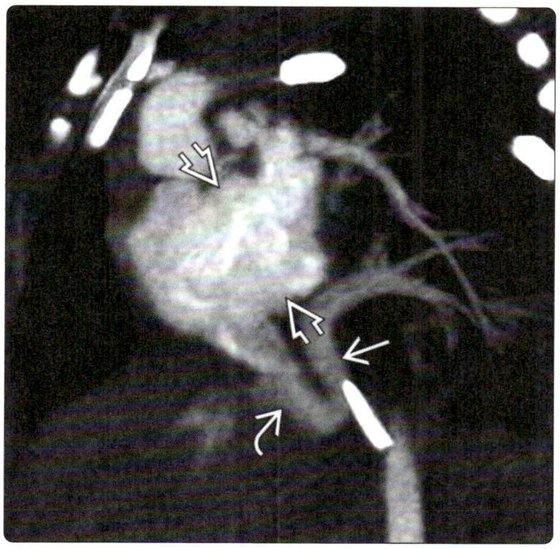

(Left) *AP radiograph shows a normal-sized heart but increased perihilar opacity due to pulmonary edema in a patient with infradiaphragmatic TAPVR (type III). As seen in this case, chest radiographic findings in TAPVR are often nonspecific.* **(Right)** *Sagittal CTA reformation shows the left-sided pulmonary veins draining into a dominant single large vein, which then extends below the diaphragm and into the IVC, consistent with type III TAPVR. There is absence of the atrial septum.*

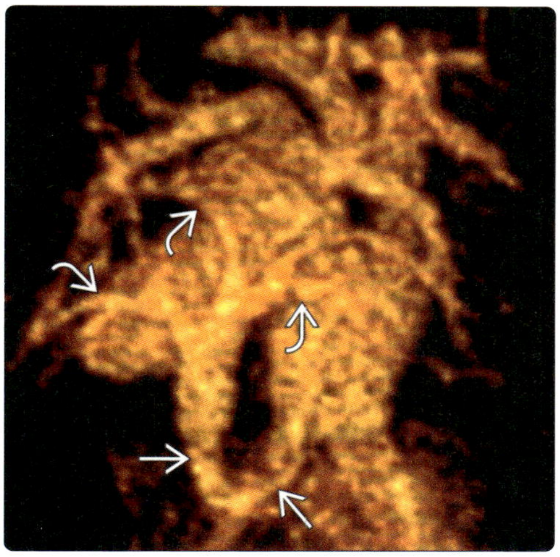

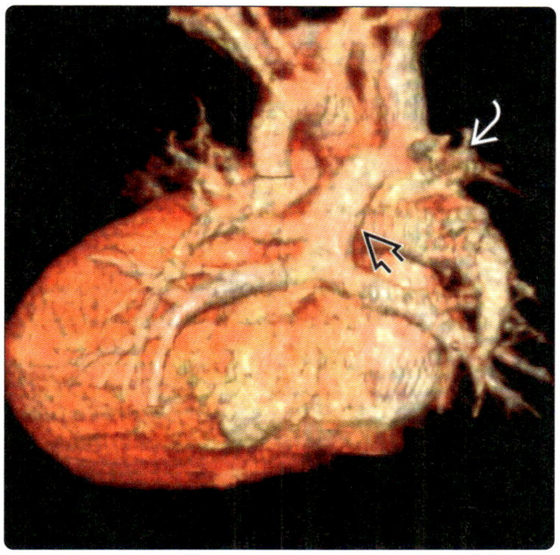

(Left) *3D reconstruction from a cardiac MR shows confluence of all pulmonary veins into an anomalous vein that courses below the diaphragm and eventually drains into the right atrium.* **(Right)** *Volume-rendered 3D CTA shows a common vein draining into the SVC and the right upper pulmonary vein draining directly into the SVC. This is considered "mixed" anomalous pulmonary return.*

Partial Anomalous Pulmonary Venous Return

KEY FACTS

TERMINOLOGY

- Partial anomalous pulmonary venous return (PAPVR)
- Congenital anomaly in which pulmonary veins (PVs) drain into systemic circulation rather than into left atrium

IMAGING

- Radiography
  - Rarely identifies abnormal vein
  - Obstructive venous drainage may cause pulmonary congestion
  - If significant left-to-right shunt: Cardiomegaly and pulmonary plethora
- CT
  - Abnormal drainage of PVs
  - Multiplanar capabilities of isovolumetric acquisition are helpful in identifying abnormal vein
  - Right-sided PAPVR draining into superior vena cava (SVC) associated with sinus venosus atrial septal defect (ASD)
- MR
  - Phase-contrast imaging is helpful in determining shunt volume and fraction

TOP DIFFERENTIAL DIAGNOSES

- Left SVC
- Pulmonary varix
- Left superior intercostal vein

PATHOLOGY

- Persistent embryologic systemic venous connections
- Right-sided PAPVR into SVC is associated with sinus venosus ASD

CLINICAL ISSUES

- Usually incidental radiographic finding
- Usually normal life span if shunt < 2:1
- Consider surgical or percutaneous closure of ASD

(Left) *A 2-month old with multiple PAPVRs is shown. The left-sided pulmonary veins (PVs) and a small accessory right middle lobe PV drain into a common trunk → vertical vein (VV) → left brachiocephalic vein (LBCV). The right upper lobe PV drains into the superior vena cava (SVC). The right inferior PV drains into the left atrium.* **(Right)** *PAPVR with the left superior PV → VV → LBCV is shown. The left inferior and accessory lingula PV drain normally into the left atrium.*

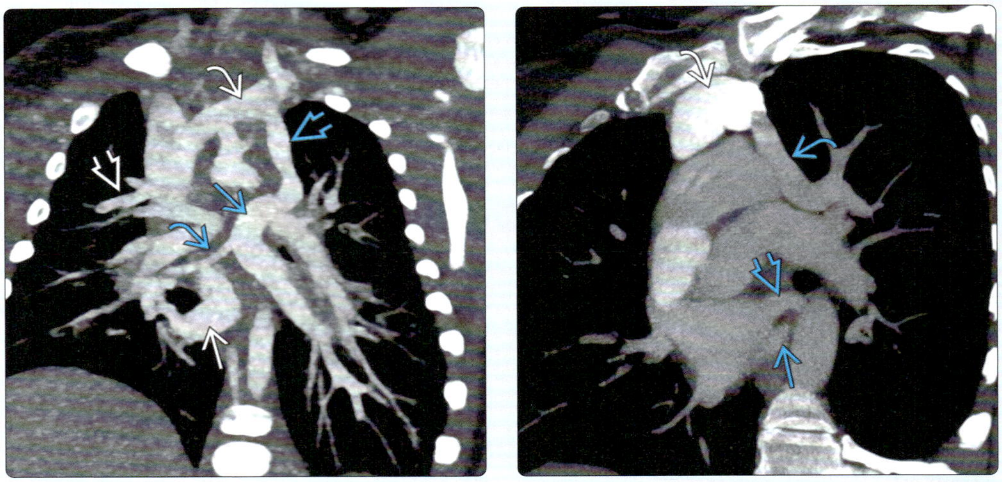

(Left) *RVOT SSFP image (left) shows a right superior PAPVR with flow jet into the SVC and right atrium. Axial oblique image (right) shows a sinus venosus atrial septal defect with a flow from left to right.* **(Right)** *PA radiograph in a young patient with cardiomegaly and pulmonary edema shows an enlarged vascular structure in the left upper lung that represents a PAPVR, which drained the entire left lung. A partially obstructive cor triatriatum was also present.*

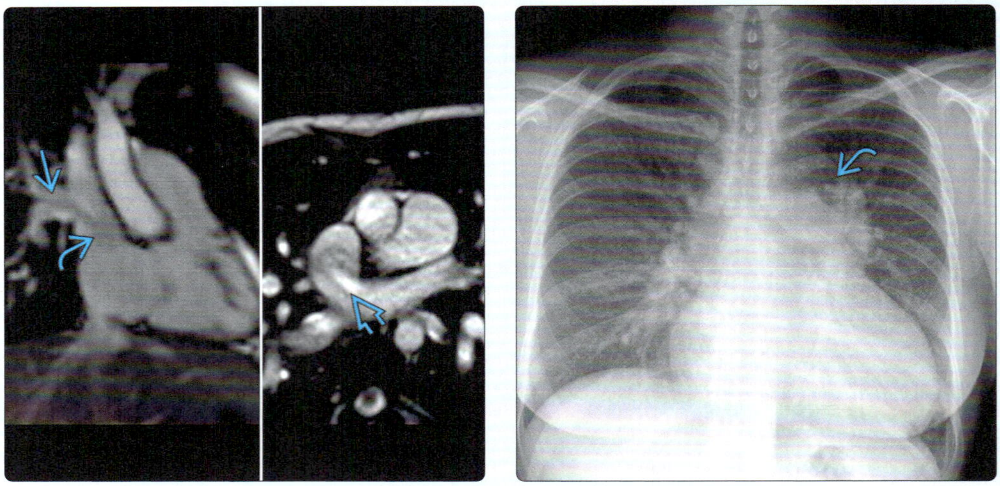

TERMINOLOGY

Abbreviations

- Partial anomalous pulmonary venous return (PAPVR)

Definitions

- Congenital anomaly in which 1-3 pulmonary veins (PVs) drain into systemic venous circulation rather than into left atrium (LA)
  - Scimitar syndrome is right-sided PAPVR draining into inferior vena cava (IVC) accompanied by hypoplasia of right lung and dextroposition of heart

IMAGING

General Features

- Best diagnostic clue
  - Demonstration of abnormal PV drainage on cross-sectional imaging
- Location
  - Right side: Drainage to superior vena cava (SVC), azygous vein, right atrium, coronary sinus, or IVC
  - Left side: Drainage of left superior PV → vertical vein (VV) → left brachiocephalic vein (LBCV)
  - Left upper lobe (47%), right upper lobe (38%), right lower lobe (13%), left lower lobe (2%), bilateral (4%)

Radiographic Findings

- Radiography
  - Abnormal vein is rarely identified
  - Scimitar vein is curvilinear anomalous vein coursing inferiorly from midright lung, usually into IVC
    - Associated with small right lung, cardiac dextroposition, bilateral left-sided bronchial branching
  - Obstructive venous drainage may cause pulmonary congestion
  - If significant left-to-right shunt: Cardiomegaly (right heart)

CT Findings

- CECT
  - Abnormal PV drainage
  - Right-sided PAPVR draining into SVC associated with sinus venosus atrial septal defect (ASD)

MR Findings

- Abnormal PV drainage seen best in MRA or 3D navigator-gated SSFP; also in cine SSFP and DIR FSE
- Associated sinus venosus defect: Defect in wall separating SVC/IVC and LA
- Velocity-encoded phase-contrast MR: Quantifies shunts
- Dilated right atrium and ventricle in large shunt

DIFFERENTIAL DIAGNOSIS

Left Superior Vena Cava

- Drains into dilated coronary sinus
- Right SVC may be absent

Left Superior Intercostal Vein

- Aortic "nipple" on chest radiograph

Meandering Right Pulmonary Vein

- Anomalous course of right PV, draining into LA
  - Meandering PVs: > 1 PV with anomalous course, draining into LA

PATHOLOGY

General Features

- Etiology
  - Persistent embryologic systemic venous connections
- Associated abnormalities
  - Right PAPVR into SVC: Sinus venosus ASD
    - Sinus venosus ASD seen in 42% of those with right upper lobe PAPVR; PAPVR seen in 90% of sinus venosus defect
  - Scimitar syndrome: Hypoplastic right pulmonary artery, systemic blood supply to right lung, extralobar sequestration, horseshoe lung, pulmonary arteriovenous malformation, ASD

CLINICAL ISSUES

Presentation

- Most common signs/symptoms
  - Depends on size of shunt
  - Often incidental finding
    - Left-sided PAPVR more commonly asymptomatic
  - However, significant left-to-right shunt or associated ASD can lead to earlier presentation
  - Scimitar syndrome
    - Infants can have severe congestive heart failure (CHF) and pulmonary hypertension
    - Older children have less severe symptoms

Demographics

- Epidemiology
  - Incidence: 0.5-0.7%

Natural History & Prognosis

- Usually normal life span if shunt < 2:1

Treatment

- Options, risks, complications
  - Reimplantation if significant shunt
    - Closure of ASD if present
  - Inadvertent clipping causes persistent localized pulmonary edema
  - Contralateral pneumonectomy: PAPVR shunt may now account for majority of cardiac output

DIAGNOSTIC CHECKLIST

Image Interpretation Pearls

- If PAPVR is detected, look carefully for ASD

SELECTED REFERENCES

1. Masrani A et al: Anatomical associations and radiological characteristics of scimitar syndrome on CT and MR. J Cardiovasc Comput Tomogr. 12(4):286-9, 2018
2. Hassani C et al: Comprehensive cross-sectional imaging of the pulmonary veins. Radiographics. 37(7):1928-54, 2017
3. Vyas HV et al: MR imaging and CT evaluation of congenital pulmonary vein abnormalities in neonates and infants. Radiographics. 32(1):87-98, 2012

Pulmonary Vein Stenosis

KEY FACTS

TERMINOLOGY

- Congenital stenosis of pulmonary vein (PV) in isolation or associated with congenital heart disease (CHD)
- Acquired stenosis of PV; post intervention [pulmonary vein ablation (PVA) for atrial fibrillation, cardiovascular surgery] or secondary to extraluminal compression/infiltration (fibrosing mediastinitis, sarcoidosis, neoplasm, etc.)

IMAGING

- Any treated PV is susceptible to stenosis
  - Left inferior PV ostium most common
- Preprocedure CTA defines PV anatomy, helps size catheters

TOP DIFFERENTIAL DIAGNOSES

- PV thrombosis
- PV pseudostenosis
- PV varix

PATHOLOGY

- Congenital PV stenosis from failed late incorporation of primitive common PV into left atrium, associated with other CHD
- Acquired PV stenosis most commonly from PVA (iatrogenic); swelling (early) and fibrosis (late)
  - Extraluminal compression/infiltration: Lung cancer, lymphoma, primary cardiac sarcoma, metastases, sarcoidosis, fibrosing mediastinitis, radiation, others

CLINICAL ISSUES

- Congenital PV stenosis rare (0.4% of all CHD)
- Acquired PV stenosis incidence decreasing with modern PVA techniques
- Clinical presentation depends on number of PVs involved and severity of obstruction
- Frequently asymptomatic if single vein is involved

(Left) *Graphic shows the typical appearance of ostial left inferior pulmonary vein (PV) stenosis following radiofrequency ablation.* **(Right)** *Coronal oblique cardiac CT shows discrete narrowing ➡ of the left inferior PV as well as abnormal soft tissue ➡ in the expected region of the left superior PV. The abnormal soft tissue represents the occluded/thrombosed superior PV post radiofrequency ablation.*

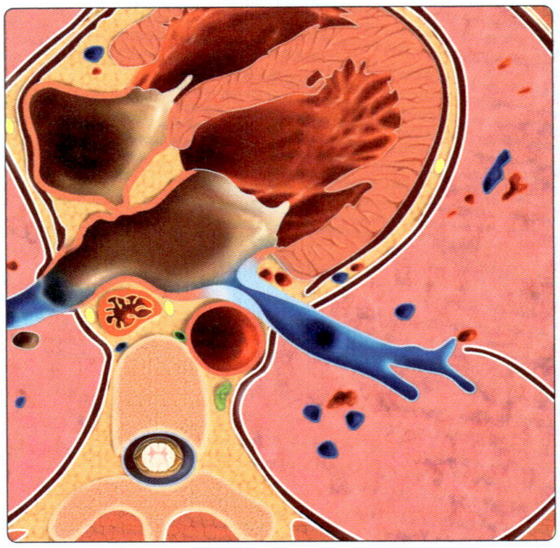

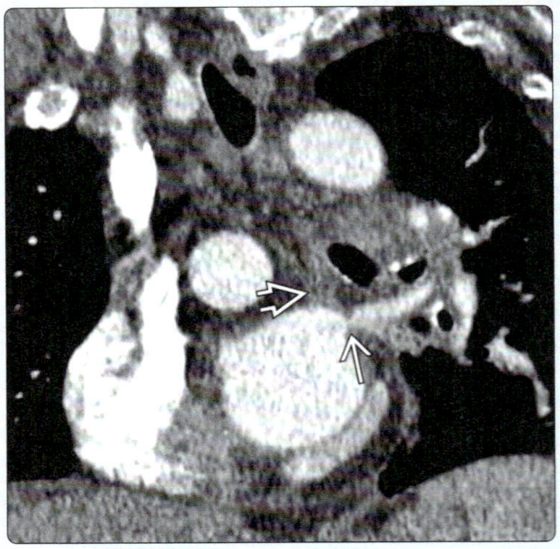

(Left) *Axial CTA shows a focal stenosis of the left inferior PV ostium ➡ following radiofrequency ablation. The left atrium (LA) is enlarged.* **(Right)** *Posteriorly directed oblique MRA in a patient who underwent radiofrequency isolation of the PVs shows a focal, web-like narrowing ⇨ of the left superior PV as it enters the LA.*

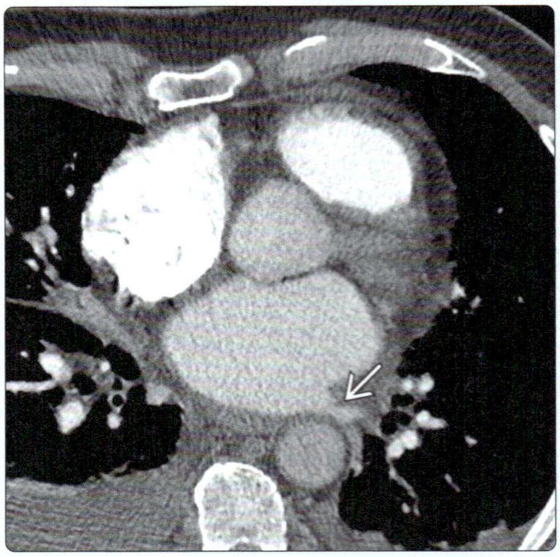

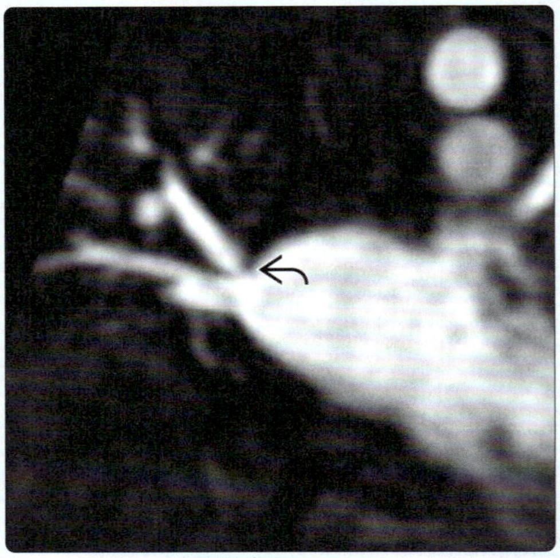

TERMINOLOGY

Definitions

- Congenital stenosis of pulmonary vein (PV) in isolation or associated with congenital heart disease (CHD)
- Acquired stenosis of PV; post intervention [pulmonary vein ablation (PVA) for atrial fibrillation, cardiovascular surgery] or secondary to extraluminal compression/infiltration (fibrosing mediastinitis, sarcoidosis, neoplasm, etc.)

IMAGING

General Features

- Best diagnostic clue: Direct visualization of PV stenosis
- Location: Any treated PV; left inferior PV ostium (LIPV) most susceptible to effects of PVA
- Size: Mild diameter stenosis < 50%, severe > 70%

Radiographic Findings

- Edema in lung drained by stenotic PV
- Posttreatment changes, hilar mass, lymphadenopathy

CT Findings

- CECT: Direct visualization of PV stenosis
  - Pitfall: Normal oval shape may mimic stenosis; comparison with pretreatment images helpful
- Delayed enhancement of affected veins and pulmonary arteries
- Signs of venous hypertension (HTN) in affected lung: Interlobular septal thickening and ground-glass opacity; edema, hemorrhage, or infarction
- Visualization of extraluminal compression and signs of underlying cause
  - Sarcoidosis: Bilateral hilar and mediastinal lymphadenopathy compressing PVs; pulmonary parenchymal findings can be seen
  - Fibrosing mediastinitis: Mediastinal or hilar soft tissue mass causing PV stenosis

MR Findings

- MR (contrast/noncontrast): Direct visualization of stenosis
- Velocity-encoded cine phase contrast to measure velocity, gradient, or flow

Echocardiographic Findings

- Intracardiac echocardiography: Now preferred for ablation procedures; better PV ostial definition; reduced complications, sedation, and fluoroscopic time
- Increased PV velocity, turbulent flow at junction of PV and left atrium (LA)

Angiographic Findings

- Visualize stenosis, measure gradient, pruning of peripheral arteries, delayed contrast arrival in LA

DIFFERENTIAL DIAGNOSIS

Pulmonary Vein Thrombosis

- Visualization of thrombus in lumen of PV, lack of visualization of previously seen vein

Pulmonary Vein Pseudostenosis

- Typically, LIPV, compressed between LA and descending aorta
- Not true fixed stenosis; caliber changes with cardiac cycle in ECG-gated cardiac CT
- Acquisition in prone position eliminates LA compression

Pulmonary Vein Varix

- Fusiform dilation; no narrowing at junction with LA

PATHOLOGY

General Features

- Etiology
  - Congenital: Connective tissue overgrowth, medial hypertrophy, intimal fibrosis within enveloping myocardial sleeve after failed incorporation of primitive PV into LA
  - Acquired: Based on underlying cause

CLINICAL ISSUES

Presentation

- Most common signs/symptoms
  - May be asymptomatic if single vein is involved
  - Dyspnea, cough, hemoptysis, pleuritic pain

Demographics

- Epidemiology
  - Congenital: Rare, 0.4% of all CHD
    - Associated with other CHD (50%) (e.g., anomalous pulmonary venous return, septal defects, TGA)
  - Acquired: Occurs either as result of prior intervention (iatrogenic) or secondary to extraluminal compression or infiltration of PV
    - Iatrogenic: Occurs as complication of pulmonary vein ablation or cardiac surgery (repair of CHD)
      - PVA for atrial fibrillation is most common cause of acquired PV stenosis; 3-6 months after procedure
      - Incidence decreasing with modern PVA techniques (2% vs. 6% in older series)
      - Varies by RF technique, imaging technique, definition of stenosis
    - Secondary to compression/infiltration of PV: Fibrosing mediastinitis, sarcoidosis, neoplasms (lung cancer, primary cardiac sarcomas, lymphoma, metastases)

Natural History & Prognosis

- Post PVA: ~ 10% progress and ~ 10% regress

Treatment

- Angioplasty and stent (~ 50% restenose)
  - Asymptomatic patient: Unknown risk of pulmonary HTN, progression to complete occlusion

SELECTED REFERENCES

1. Feins EN et al: Pulmonary vein stenosis: anatomic considerations, surgical management, and outcomes. J Thorac Cardiovasc Surg. 163(6):2198-207.e3, 2022
2. Suntharos P et al: Treatment of congenital and acquired pulmonary vein stenosis. Curr Cardiol Rep. 22(11):153, 2020
3. Galizia M et al: Radiologic review of acquired pulmonary vein stenosis in adults. Cardiovasc Diagn Ther. 8(3):387-98, 2018
4. Hassani C et al: Comprehensive cross-sectional imaging of the pulmonary veins. Radiographics. 37(7):1928-54, 2017

(Left) *Axial cardiac CTA in a patient with newly diagnosed cor triatriatum to map the anatomy shows persistent membrane in the LA ➡, consistent with cor triatriatum. Note the normal appearance of left inferior PV ➡, which has a close relationship to the persistent membrane at the orifice.* **(Right)** *Axial CECT in the same patient at a higher level shows the normal appearance of the left superior PV ➡.*

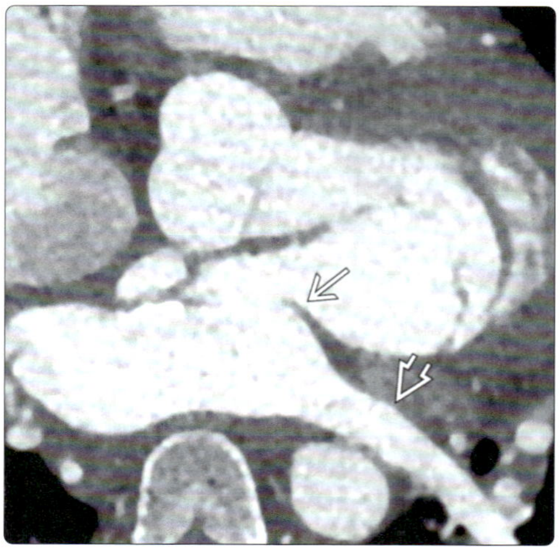

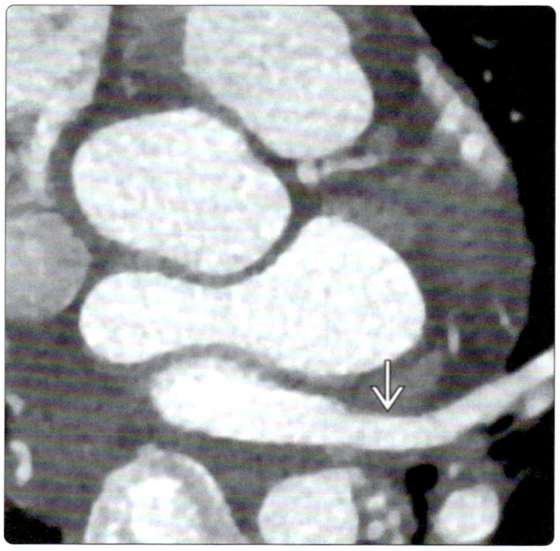

(Left) *Axial oblique MIP CECT in the same patient status post corrective surgery of cor triatriatum shows significant stenosis of the left inferior PV ➡. A few months later, the patient returned with shortness of breath, and a repeat cardiac CT was performed.* **(Right)** *Sagittal oblique CT shows severe stenosis of the left superior PV ➡ near its ostium.*

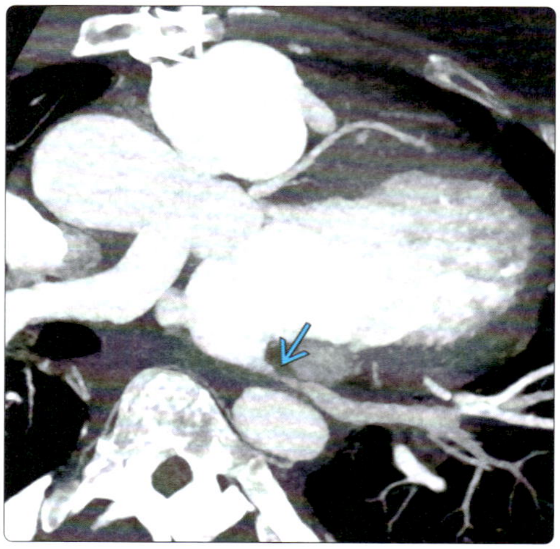

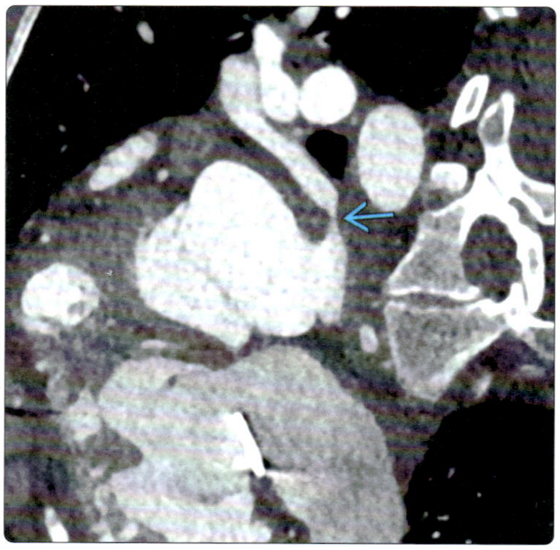

(Left) *Axial lung window CECT in a patient with osteal PV stenosis shows mosaic perfusion ➡ and interlobular septal thickening ➡ due to pulmonary edema secondary to PV stenosis.* **(Right)** *The patient was treated with percutaneous stent placement. Coronal oblique MPR CECT shows kissing stents ➡ in the left superior and inferior PVs, which are widely patent. After stent placement, the patient's symptoms were relieved.*

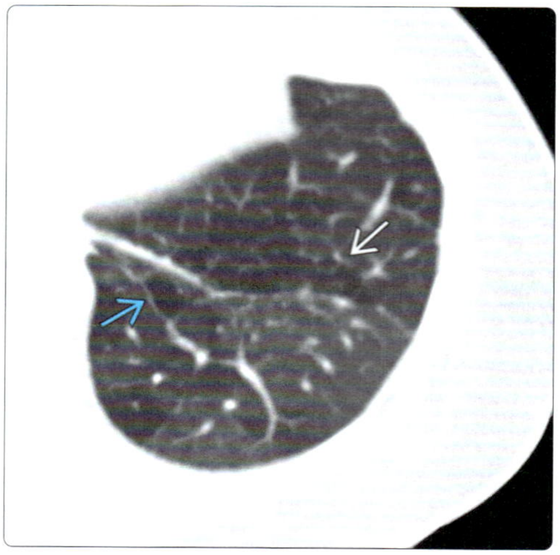

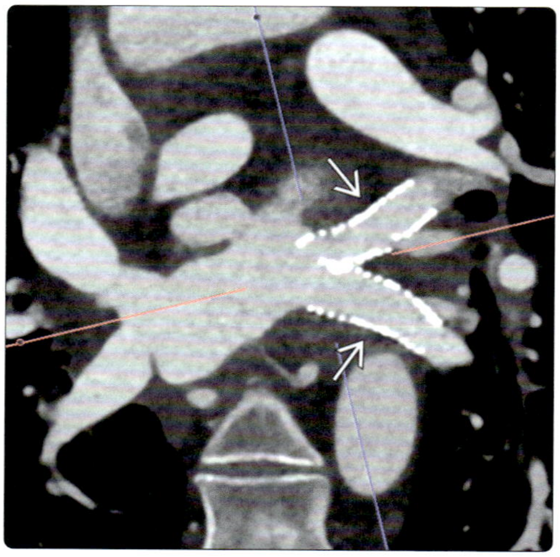

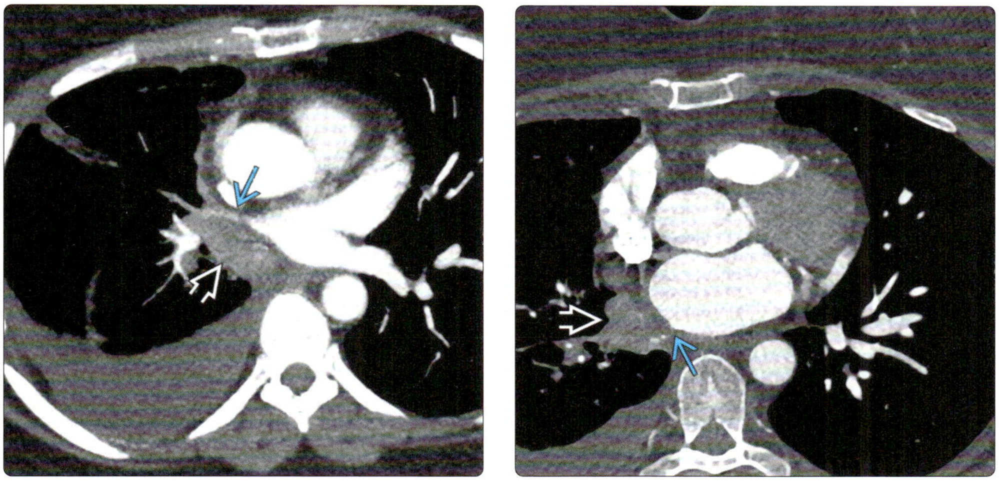

(Left) *Axial MIP CECT in a patient with fibrosing mediastinitis secondary to histoplasmosis shows a right perihilar soft tissue lesion/thickening ⇨ resulting in significant narrowing of the right superior PV →. Also note moderate right pleural effusion.* **(Right)** *Axial image in the same patient at a lower section shows right hilar soft tissue lesion/thickening ⇨ causing complete occlusion of right inferior PV. Note the expected orifice and location of the right inferior PV →.*

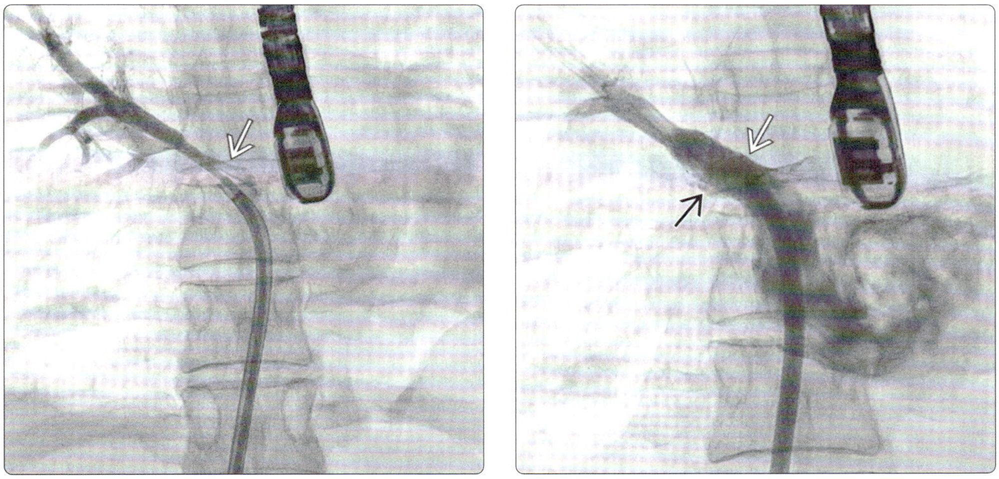

(Left) *The patient underwent catheter angiography of PVs. Selective angiogram of the right superior PV with distal contrast injection demonstrates significant narrowing near the orifice ⇨.* **(Right)** *The stenotic segment was treated with balloon angioplasty and stent placement. Poststent angiogram of the right superior PV shows increased caliber of the contrast passage ⇨ with patent stent →. Note the contrast in the left atrium.*

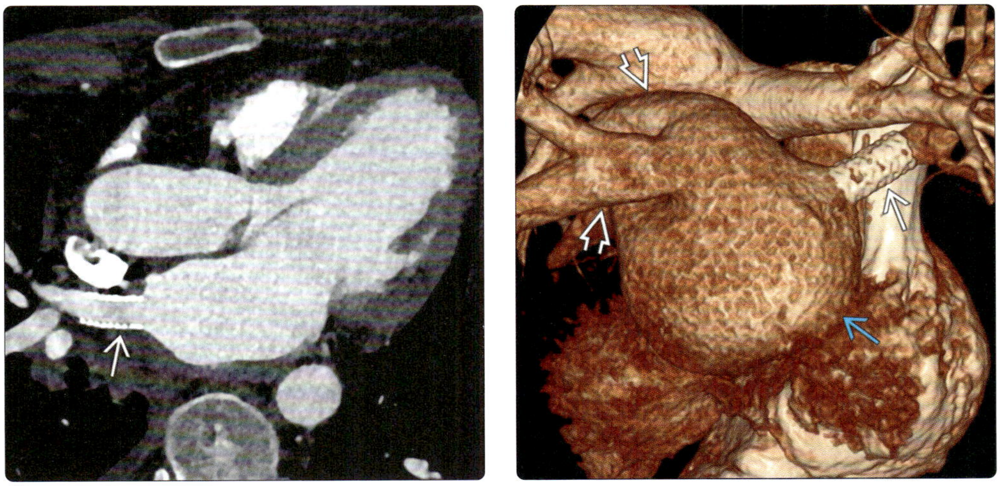

(Left) *Axial oblique cardiac CECT in the same patient shows widely patent stent ⇨ in the right superior PV with increased caliber of the vessel. Note that right perihilar soft tissue thickening persists.* **(Right)** *Posterior oblique volume-rendered CECT in the same patient shows the stented right superior PV ⇨ and normal left-sided PVs ⇨. Note the absence of right inferior PV due to complete occlusion. Note the expected location of the right inferior PV →.*

Superior Vena Cava Syndrome

KEY FACTS

TERMINOLOGY

- Superior vena cava (SVC) obstruction by intraluminal, intramural, or extrinsic disease
- Impaired venous return from head, neck, upper extremities, and trunk to right atrium

IMAGING

- Radiography
  - May be normal
  - Mediastinal widening
  - Mediastinal/paramediastinal mass
- CT and MR
  - Nonopacification of SVC on CT and MR
  - Extrinsic compression by mass or lymphadenopathy
  - Intraluminal filling defect
  - Multiple collateral vessels

TOP DIFFERENTIAL DIAGNOSES

- Thoracic outlet syndrome
- Brachiocephalic vein occlusion or stenosis
- Thrombosis, stenosis, or occlusion of deep upper extremity veins
- Persistent left SVC with absent right SVC

PATHOLOGY

- Malignant etiologies (70%): Lung cancer, metastatic disease, lymphadenopathy, lymphoma
- Benign etiologies (30%): Granulomatous disease, iatrogenic, adjacent compression

CLINICAL ISSUES

- SVC syndrome is clinical diagnosis
- Face, neck, upper trunk, and upper extremity edema are most common symptoms

DIAGNOSTIC CHECKLIST

- Consider SVC syndrome when patient with known malignancy develops typical signs and symptoms

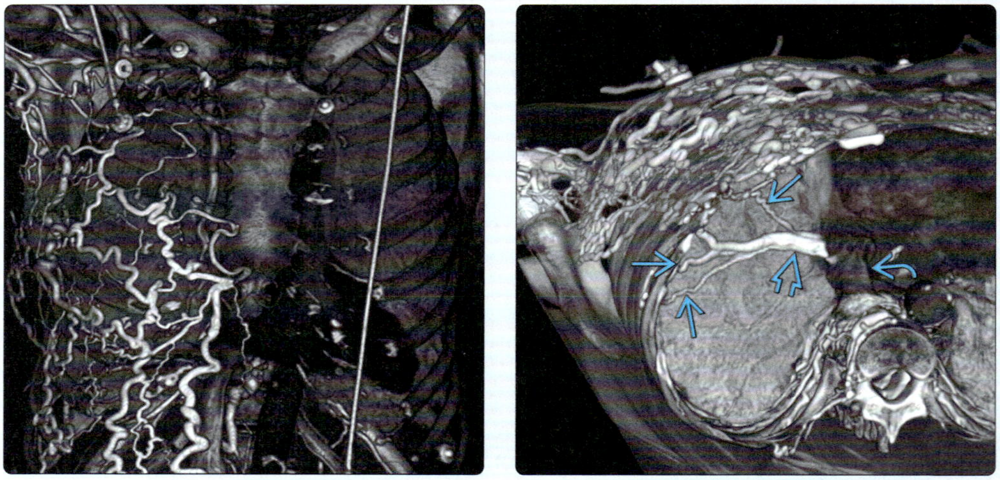

(Left) *Coronal VR image shows innumerable, enlarged, tortuous chest wall, intercostal, internal mammary, and mediastinal collaterals extending below the diaphragm in a patient with known superior vena cava (SVC) obstruction due to lymphoma.* **(Right)** *VR image through the liver shows the innumerable venous collaterals. Some extend through the liver into the portal vein before draining into the inferior vena cava (IVC). This collateral pathway is the cause of the hot quadrate lobe sign.*

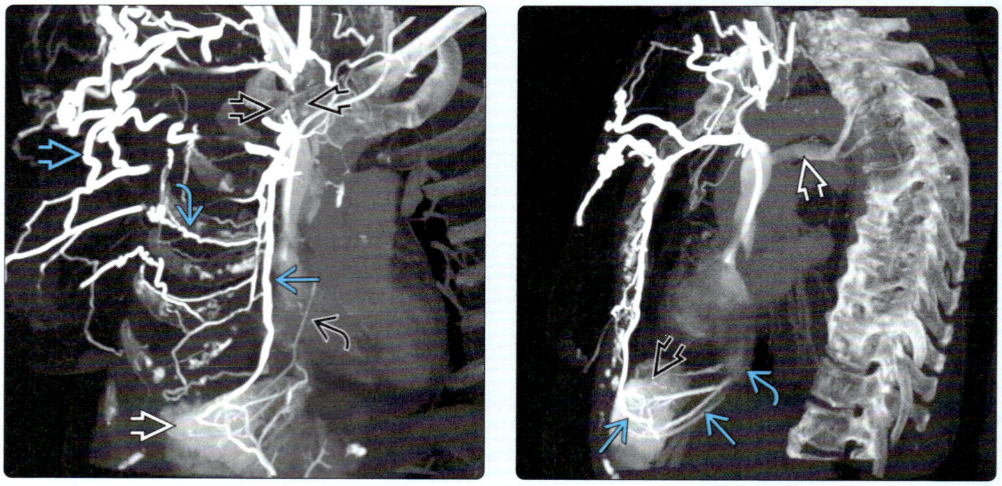

(Left) *MIP image in a woman with metastatic melanoma shows dilated chest wall, intercostal, mediastinal, and internal mammary collaterals from near-complete SVC occlusion superior to the azygous vein (AV). While some collaterals drain into the AV, most drain into the IVC. Notice the hot quadrate lobe sign.* **(Right)** *Collaterals extend through the liver, draining into the IVC. A hot quadrate lobe sign is seen. A small amount of collateral flow is through the azygos system.*

TERMINOLOGY

Abbreviations

- Superior vena cava (SVC)

Definitions

- Obstruction of SVC due to intraluminal, intramural, or extrinsic disease
  - Impaired venous return from head, neck, upper extremities, and trunk to right atrium

IMAGING

General Features

- Best diagnostic clue
  - Nonopacification of SVC
  - Multiple collateral veins coursing through mediastinum and chest wall

Radiographic Findings

- Radiography
  - May be **normal**
    - Most common in mediastinal fibrosis
    - Iatrogenic SVC obstruction
  - **Widened mediastinum**
    - Dilated SVC
    - Mediastinal mass or lymphadenopathy
  - **Right hilar or paramediastinal mass**
  - Enlarged azygos arch and vein

CT Findings

- CECT
  - **Nonopacification of SVC**
    - Obstruction
      - Extrinsic compression or invasion by mass or lymphadenopathy
      - Intraluminal thrombus
      - Scarring from longstanding indwelling catheter
  - **Multiple collateral vessels**
    - Neck, chest wall, mediastinum
  - **Dilated mediastinal vessels, which serve as collaterals**
    - Azygos and hemiazygos system
    - Internal mammary veins
    - Brachiocephalic veins
  - **Cause of obstruction often visible**
  - **Inflow of contrast-enhanced blood into inferior vena cava (IVC)**
    - Can see focal hepatic enhancement in quadrate lobe
  - **Anatomic classification**
    - SVC obstruction localized above azygos vein
      - Some collateral blood flow through azygos and intercostal veins into SVC caudal to obstruction
    - SVC obstruction at azygos vein
      - Collateral blood flow into IVC
    - SVC obstruction localized below azygos vein
      - Collateral blood flow through azygos and hemiazygos system into IVC

MR Findings

- T1WI C+
  - Evaluation of adjacent structures and causes of external SVC compression
- MRV
  - **Nonopacification of SVC**
  - Enlarged azygos arch and vein
  - Multiple collateral vessels
    - Neck, chest wall, and mediastinum

Ultrasonographic Findings

- Grayscale ultrasound
  - **Dilatation of visualized SVC**
    - Stable lumen size with respiration or cardiac cycle
  - Echogenic intraluminal thrombus
  - Potential mass or indwelling catheter
  - Distended subclavian, brachiocephalic, and jugular veins
- Pulsed Doppler
  - Altered subclavian vein spectral waveforms
  - Absent normal transmission of atrial waveform, respiratory phasicity, or response to provocative maneuvers
    - Monophasic antegrade flow
    - Low-velocity flow
- Color Doppler
  - Sluggish or absent blood flow

Angiographic Findings

- DSA
  - Venography is performed when cross-sectional imaging is nondiagnostic
    - Performed superior or peripheral to obstruction
    - Stasis or retrograde flow in subclavian or brachiocephalic veins
      - May mimic subclavian or brachiocephalic vein occlusion
  - Extrinsic compression or invasion by mass or lymphadenopathy
    - Effacement of SVC
  - Indwelling catheters and pacemaker leads
    - Long, smooth narrowing
  - Intraluminal filling defect representing thrombus
  - No intraluminal contrast = occlusion
  - Multiple collateral vessels
  - Azygos arch and vein enlargement

Nuclear Medicine Findings

- Radionuclide uptake in liver
  - **Hot quadrate sign**
  - 1st described with Tc-99m sulfur-colloid scan
- Radionuclide venography with Tc-99m microaggregated albumin
  - Generated time-activity curves can show evidence of SVC obstruction
  - Multiple collateral vessels

Imaging Recommendations

- Best imaging tool
  - CT and MR for optimal demonstration of nonopacification of SVC
    - Evaluation of adjacent mediastinal structures
  - Venography is useful for planning endovascular or surgical procedures
- Protocol advice
  - Thin-slice imaging ($\leq$ 1 mm)

- Coronal and sagittal reformations to visualize site and extent of obstruction
- Consider arterial and delayed phases

DIFFERENTIAL DIAGNOSIS

Thoracic Outlet Syndrome

- Multiple collateral vessels in neck and upper chest
- Focal narrowing at junction of clavicle and 1st rib
- Patent SVC on contrast-enhanced imaging studies

Brachiocephalic Vein Occlusion or Stenosis

- Multiple collateral vessels in neck and upper chest
- Stenosis or occlusion of brachiocephalic vein
- Patent SVC on contrast-enhanced imaging studies

Thrombosis, Stenosis, or Occlusion of Deep Upper Extremity Veins

- Usually from indwelling catheters or pacemaker leads
- Multiple collateral vessels
- Upper extremity swelling may mimic SVC obstruction
- Patent SVC and central veins

Persistent Left Superior Vena Cava With Absent Right Superior Vena Cava

- No collateral vessels
- No SVC in right superior mediastinum
- Vein in left superior mediastinum draining into coronary sinus
  - Coronary sinus dilated

PATHOLOGY

General Features

- Etiology
  - **Malignant causes (70%)**
    - Lung cancer (most common)
    - Lymphoma
    - Metastatic tumor and lymphadenopathy
      - Breast, renal, melanoma, etc.
    - Primary mediastinal mass
  - **Nonmalignant causes (30%)**
    - **Granulomatous infection or sequela**
      - Tuberculosis or histoplasmosis
      - Fibrosing mediastinitis
    - **Noninfectious granulomatous disease**
      - Sarcoid
      - Silicosis
    - **Iatrogenic**
      - Indwelling catheters and pacemaker leads
      - Radiation fibrosis
    - **Benign tumors**
    - **Compression from adjacent structures**

CLINICAL ISSUES

Presentation

- Most common signs/symptoms
  - Facial and arm edema
  - Nonpulsatile distended neck and chest veins
  - Headache or syncope
  - Dyspnea, dysphagia, hoarseness
- Other signs/symptoms
  - Syncope, seizures, visual changes
  - Coma in severe cases

Demographics

- Age
  - Range: 18-76 years
    - Mean: 54 years
  - Malignant etiologies
    - Older (40-60 years)
  - Benign etiologies
    - Younger (30-40 years)
- Sex
  - Malignant etiologies: M > F
  - Benign etiologies: M = F
- Epidemiology
  - **Malignant**: 70%
  - **Benign**: 30%

Natural History & Prognosis

- Gradual, progressive obstruction of SVC
  - Insidious onset of symptoms
- Survival depends on course of underlying disease
- Benign etiologies
  - Rarely fatal
- Malignant etiologies
  - Usually not cause of death
  - Most die from metastatic malignancy
    - Survival correlates with tumor histology

Treatment

- Malignant etiologies
  - Radiation therapy
  - Chemotherapy targeted toward type of neoplasm
- Anticoagulation
- Endovascular therapy
  - Catheter-directed thrombolysis
  - Endovascular stent placement
- Surgical therapy
  - Venous bypass
  - Venous transposition

DIAGNOSTIC CHECKLIST

Consider

- SVC syndrome when patient with known malignancy develops typical signs and symptoms

Image Interpretation Pearls

- Nonopacification of SVC
- Multiple collateral vessels in neck, chest wall, and mediastinum
- Hot quadrate lobe sign

SELECTED REFERENCES

1. Wright K et al: Malignant superior vena cava syndrome: a scoping review. J Thorac Oncol. 18(10):1268-76, 2023
2. Azizi AH et al: Superior vena cava syndrome. JACC Cardiovasc Interv. 13(24):2896-910, 2020
3. Sonavane SK et al: Comprehensive imaging review of the superior vena cava. Radiographics. 35(7):1873-92, 2015

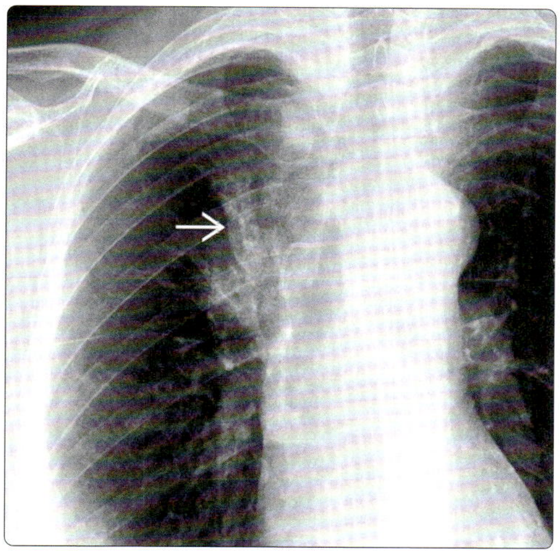

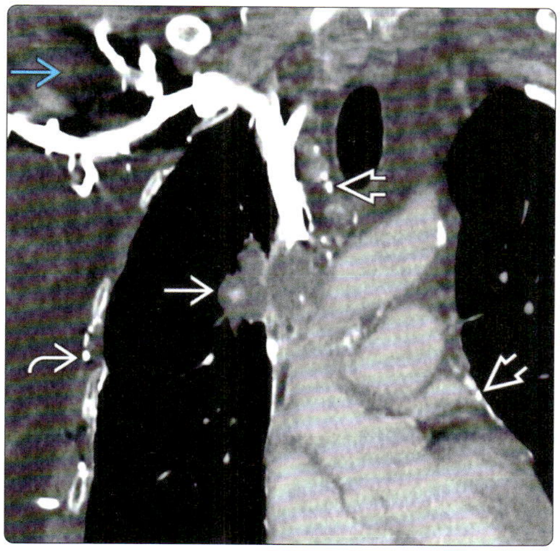

(Left) *PA radiograph shows an irregular, mass-like opacity in the right upper lobe in a patient with small cell lung cancer.* **(Right)** *Coronal CECT of the same patient demonstrates a small cell carcinoma of the right upper lobe invading the mediastinum and SVC. Note the intense opacification of the right brachiocephalic vein with contrast material and the presence of collateral vessels in the mediastinum and right chest wall.*

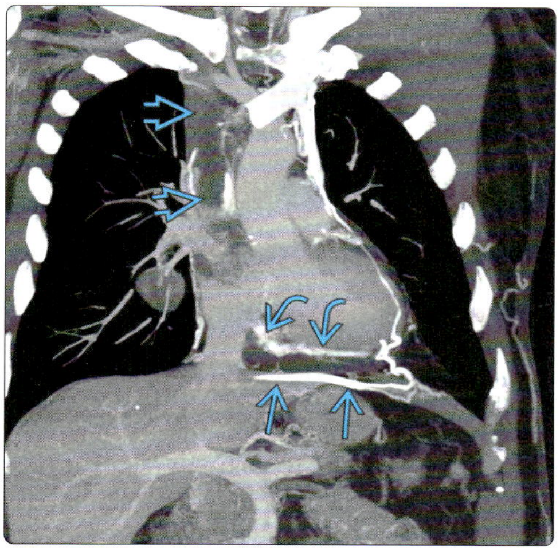

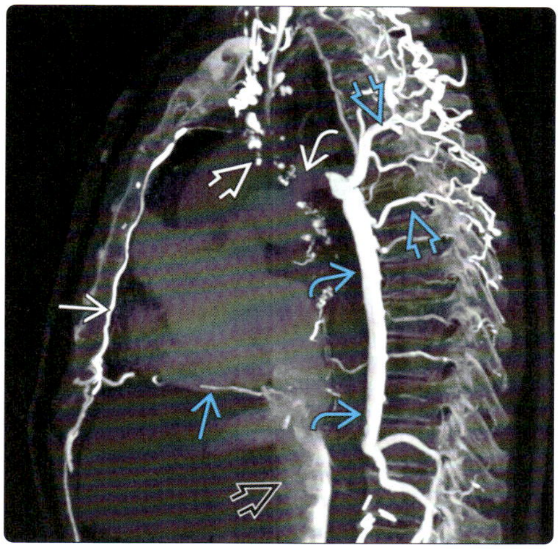

(Left) *This 62-year-old man with metastatic sarcoma has a mass obstructing the entire SVC. Mediastinal collaterals are present, some of which drain into the right atrium via the coronary veins, while others drain into the IVC via phrenic collaterals.* **(Right)** *Sagittal CECT in a 52-year-old woman with fibrosing mediastinitis shows SVC and central AV occlusion. Exuberant paravertebral collaterals will drain into the IVC via the AV. Internal mammary and phrenic collaterals also drain into the IVC.*

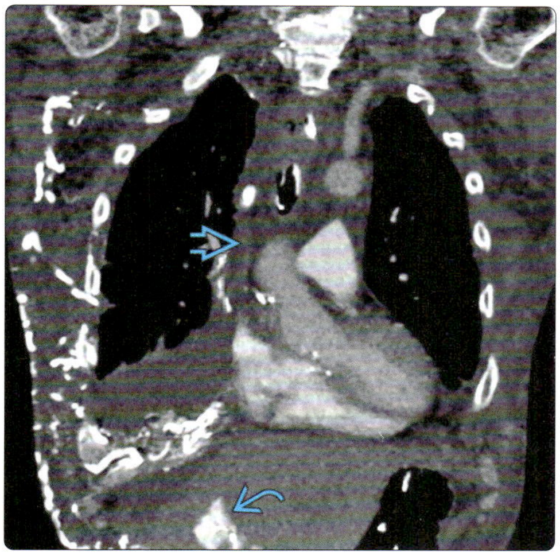

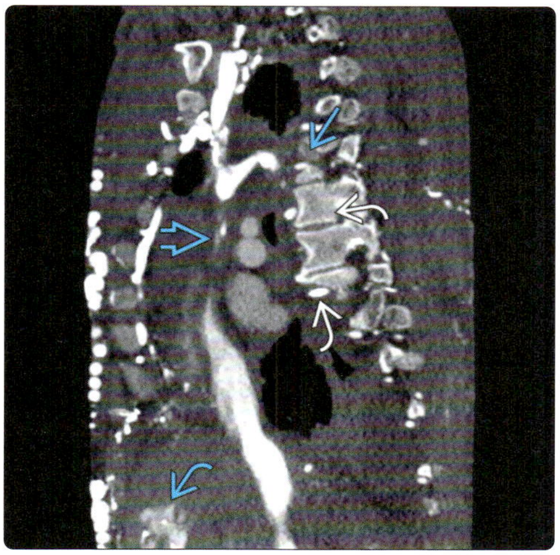

(Left) *Dialysis patient with a catheter related to SVC occlusion inferior to the AV is shown. Numerous chest wall, intercostal, and mediastinal collaterals drain into the IVC. A hot quadrate lobe sign is present.* **(Right)** *Sagittal CT shows SVC occlusion and extensive chest wall, internal mammary, and mediastinal collaterals, which drain into the IVC. A hot quadrate lobe sign is seen. Retrograde flow through the AV, which receives blood for the paravertebral veins, will also drain into the IVC.*

May-Thurner Syndrome

KEY FACTS

TERMINOLOGY

- Compression of left common iliac vein (CIV) by right common iliac artery
- Synonyms: Iliac vein compression syndrome, Cockett syndrome, iliocaval vein syndrome

IMAGING

- Extrinsic compression of left CIV by right common iliac artery
- Presence of collaterals in pelvis crossing midline to join contralateral iliac veins and dilated ascending lumbar vein
- Time-of-flight MRV shows absence of flow in left internal iliac vein due to flow reversal and dilated ascending lumbar vein
- IVUS can determine vessel size and internal wall morphology; may also demonstrate intraluminal spur and assist with treatment planning (stent placement)
- Left common femoral vein Doppler may show absence of respiratory variations, suggesting proximal obstruction

TOP DIFFERENTIAL DIAGNOSES

- Radiation, chemotherapy, and hormonal therapy
- Pelvic tumors
- Chronic deep venous thrombosis

CLINICAL ISSUES

- Unilateral swelling, pain, and aching of left leg
- Venous stasis and ulcers
- Treatment options
  - Standard: Anticoagulation, compression stockings
  - Catheter-directed thrombolysis followed by endovascular intervention (balloon angioplasty and stenting)
  - Surgery: Thrombectomy, direct surgical reconstruction or bypass, vein patch angioplasty

DIAGNOSTIC CHECKLIST

- Consider May-Thurner syndrome in young to middle-aged women with swelling of left lower extremity

(Left) *Coronal graphic depicts the anatomic relationship of iliac vessels. The left common iliac vein lies between the right common iliac artery and the lumbosacral spine where it may be compressed, causing left deep venous thrombosis (DVT).* **(Right)** *Axial oblique TOF MRV shows occlusion ➡ of the left common iliac vein at its confluence with the right common iliac vein. Note normal patent right internal iliac vein ⇨. The left internal iliac vein ↪ is not visualized on this TOF MRV due to flow reversal.*

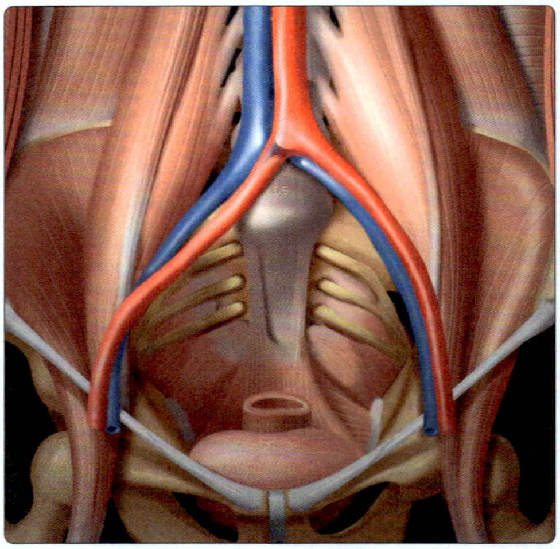

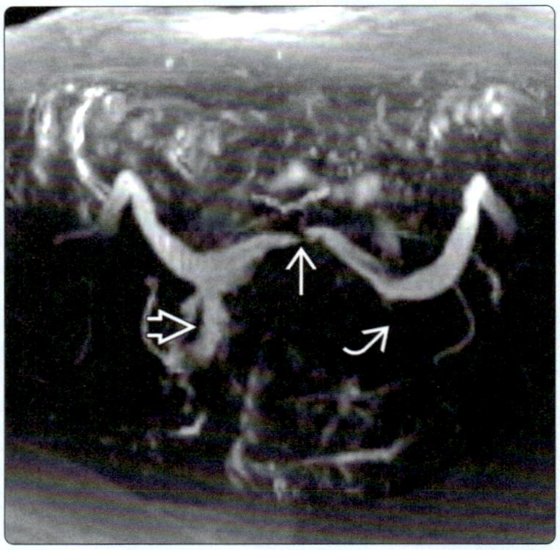

(Left) *Axial CE MRV shows compression of the left common iliac vein ➡ by the right common iliac artery ↪ against the lumbar spine.* **(Right)** *Axial CE MRV shows cross-pelvic collateral veins ↪. Note the patent left internal iliac vein ➡, suggesting that its absence on TOF MRV is secondary to flow reversal and not due to thrombosis. Flow reversal in the left internal iliac vein on TOF MRV and the presence of pelvic collaterals on CE MRV suggest that the venous compression is hemodynamically significant.*

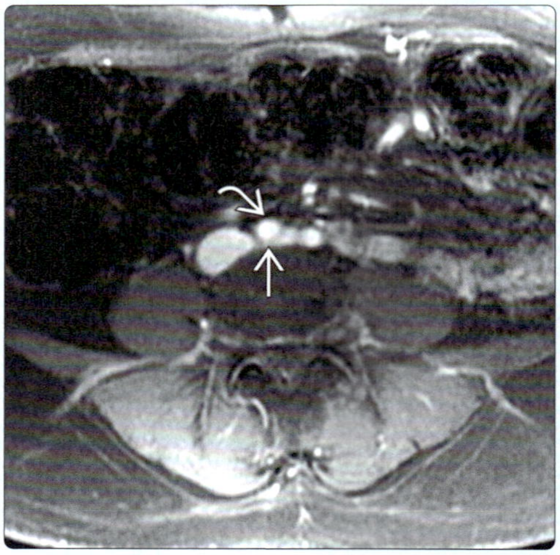

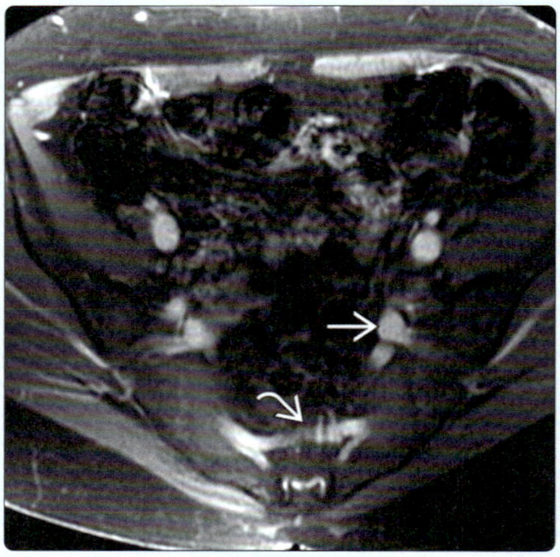

TERMINOLOGY

Synonyms

- Iliac vein compression syndrome (IVCS)
- Cockett syndrome
- Iliocaval vein syndrome

Definitions

- Compression of left common iliac vein (CIV) by right common iliac artery, which crosses over it, with associated secondary left lower extremity deep venous thrombosis (DVT)

IMAGING

General Features

- Best diagnostic clue
  - Young women with persistent left lower leg edema
- Location
  - Left CIV between right common iliac artery and spine

CT Findings

- CECT
  - Extrinsic compression of left CIV by right common iliac artery
  - Diameter of left CIV at site of compression is smaller than normal
  - Presence of collaterals in pelvis crossing midline to join contralateral iliac veins
  - Enlarged ascending lumbar vein with collaterals to vertebral plexus of veins
  - Lower extremity DVT
  - Tortuosity of aortoiliac arteries
  - Mild to moderate degenerative changes in lumbar vertebrae and sacrum

MR Findings

- MRV
  - Time-of-flight (TOF) MRV shows absence of flow in left internal iliac vein due to flow reversal and dilated ascending lumbar vein
  - Contrast-enhanced MRV shows area of compression or obstruction and pelvic collaterals
  - Disadvantages
    - Vascular region above bifurcations has disturbed nonlaminar flow and can present confusing picture mimicking intraluminal filling defects

Ultrasonographic Findings

- Color Doppler
  - Standard test to diagnose lower extremity DVT
  - Difficult visualization of iliac vessels due to bowel gas
  - 20% of iliac vein US studies are nondiagnostic in best vascular laboratories
  - Left common femoral vein Doppler may show absence of respiratory variations of venous flow, suggesting proximal obstruction
  - Collateral veins in groin or pubic area may be seen in some cases

Angiographic Findings

- Venography (femoral, popliteal, or pedal access)
  - Used as diagnostic and therapeutic tool
  - Compression or occlusion of left CIV
  - Cross-pelvic collaterals
  - Dilated ascending lumbar vein with collaterals to vertebral plexus and hemiazygos veins
  - Direct pressure measurement across iliofemoral stenosis during venography
    - Significant stenosis: Difference > 2 mmHg at rest or 3 mmHg with exercise
    - Nondiagnostic pressure gradient does not exclude diagnosis of IVCS
  - Standard amount of dye injected into foot is not sufficient to evaluate iliac veins in pelvis

Other Modality Findings

- Intravascular ultrasound (IVUS)
  - 12.5-MHz or 20 MHz-transducer introduced through sheath into lumen of veins
  - Can determine vessel size and internal wall morphology
  - May demonstrate intraluminal spur and assist with treatment planning (stent placement)
- Air plethysmography
  - Helps investigate and determine cause and severity of venous complaints and find evidence of proximal obstruction
  - May also be nondiagnostic because of collateralization or insufficient narrowing to change flow dynamics

Imaging Recommendations

- Best imaging tool
  - Femoral venography
  - MRV
  - IVUS
- Protocol advice
  - MRV: Include 2D TOF to assess flow direction in left internal iliac vein and ascending lumbar vein

DIFFERENTIAL DIAGNOSIS

Immobilization

- Risk of developing DVT of lower extremities during conventional lower limb immobilization: 4.5-71.4% depending on indication for immobilization and method of diagnosing DVT

Trauma

- Increased risk of developing DVT and pulmonary embolism following polytrauma
- Exact incidence is unknown

Surgery

- Cancer-related surgery increases risk of DVT complications because of frequent venous trauma
- Postsurgical risk of developing DVT ranges from 15-40% (in most surgery patients) to as high as 60% in orthopedic surgery patients

Radiation, Chemotherapy, and Hormonal Therapy

- Patients with malignancies have increased risk of thromboembolism
  - DVT and pulmonary embolism may present as complication after diagnosis of cancer
- Risk factors include radiotherapy, chemotherapy, and hormonal therapy

Catheterization

- Presence of peripheral catheters increases risk of developing DVT in 2-40%

Pelvic Tumors

- Patients with active cancer have 4x increased risk of developing venous thromboembolism compared with individuals without cancer
  - Risk increases to 6.5x with chemotherapy
  - Pelvic tumors or lymph nodes may compress left CIV, thereby mimicking May-Thurner syndrome

Chronic Deep Venous Thrombosis

- Chronic DVT of iliac vein leads to small, narrowed, occluded vein
- Underlying venous compression is difficult to assess in chronic DVT

PATHOLOGY

General Features

- Associated abnormalities
  - DVT
- Physical entrapment of left CIV between right common iliac artery and 5th lumbar vertebra

Staging, Grading, & Classification

- 3 stages
  - Asymptomatic compression at left iliocaval confluence without intrinsic changes or development of venous collateral vessels on venography
  - Development of intraluminal filling defects (spurs)
  - Iliofemoral thrombosis

Gross Pathologic & Surgical Features

- Compression of left iliac veins against lumbar vertebrae can cause chronic irritation of vascular endothelium
  - Leads to endothelial proliferation and hyperplasia

Microscopic Features

- Collagen and elastin deposition result in formation of spurs
  - Spurs: Replacement of normal intima and media of vein by well-organized connective tissue covered with endothelium
  - Spurs create mechanical obstruction to flow and increase risk of left-sided iliofemoral thrombosis

CLINICAL ISSUES

Presentation

- Most common signs/symptoms
  - Unilateral swelling, pain, and aching of left leg
  - Venous stasis and ulcers
- Other signs/symptoms
  - Phlegmasia cerulea dolens

Demographics

- Age
  - 2nd-4th decades
- Sex
  - M < F
- Epidemiology
  - 2-5% of women undergoing evaluation for venous disorder of lower extremities
  - DVT occurs 3-8x more frequently on left side

Natural History & Prognosis

- Progressive disease with long-term disabling complications
- Diagnosis of compression before insurgence of thrombosis and insufficiency is essential for good prognosis

Treatment

- Options, risks, complications
  - Treatment goals
    - With chronic symptoms
      - Resolve, significantly improve, or prevent chronic pain, aching, edema, venous claudication, or ulceration
      - Improve quality of life
    - With acute iliofemoral DVT
      - Prevent pulmonary embolism, restore unobstructed venous return, preserve valve function, prevent recurrence
  - Treatment options
    - Standard: Anticoagulation, compression stockings
    - Catheter-directed thrombolysis followed by balloon angioplasty and stenting
    - Surgery: Thrombectomy, direct surgical reconstruction or bypass, vein patch angioplasty
      - Long-term success is limited as patency of left CIV following surgery is between 40-88%
  - Complications
    - Pulmonary embolism
    - Retroperitoneal hemorrhage

DIAGNOSTIC CHECKLIST

Consider

- May-Thurner syndrome in young to middle-aged women with swelling of left lower extremity

Image Interpretation Pearls

- Venography: Stenosis of left CIV and presence of pelvic venous collaterals crossing midline

SELECTED REFERENCES

1. Poyyamoli S et al: May-Thurner syndrome. Cardiovasc Diagn Ther. 11(5):1104-11, 2021
2. Knuttinen MG et al: May-Thurner: diagnosis and endovascular management. Cardiovasc Diagn Ther. 7(Suppl 3):S159-64, 2017
3. McDermott S et al: May-Thurner syndrome: can it be diagnosed by a single MR venography study? Diagn Interv Radiol. 19(1):44-8, 2013
4. Jones TM et al: Maximal venous outflow velocity: an index for iliac vein obstruction. Ann Vasc Surg. 26(8):1106-13, 2012
5. Wu WL et al: Comprehensive MDCT evaluation of patients with suspected May-Thurner syndrome. AJR Am J Roentgenol. 199(5):W638-45, 2012
6. Raffini L et al: May-Thurner syndrome (iliac vein compression) and thrombosis in adolescents. Pediatr Blood Cancer. 47(6):834-8, 2006
7. Shebel ND et al: Diagnosis and management of iliac vein compression syndrome. J Vasc Nurs. 23(1):10-7; quiz 18-9, 2005
8. Forauer AR et al: Intravascular ultrasound in the diagnosis and treatment of iliac vein compression (May-Thurner) syndrome. J Vasc Interv Radiol. 13(5):523-7, 2002
9. Wolpert LM et al: Magnetic resonance venography in the diagnosis and management of May-Thurner syndrome. Vasc Endovascular Surg. 36(1):51-7, 2002

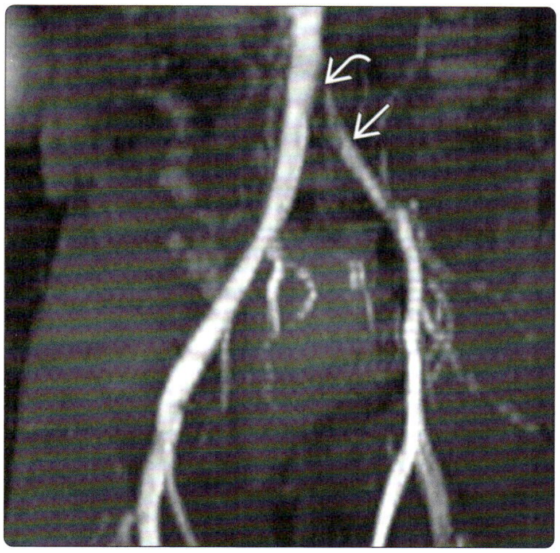

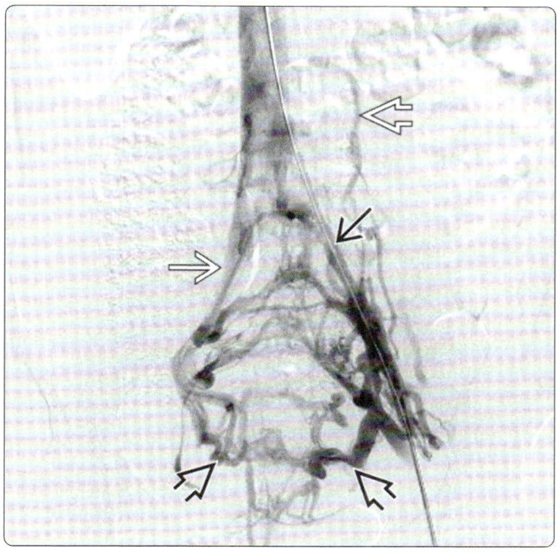

(Left) *Coronal TOF MRV in a patient with left lower extremity DVT shows a small, diffusely narrowed left common iliac vein with occlusion of its proximal-most portion secondary to iliac vein compression by the right common iliac artery.* **(Right)** *AP venography from the left external iliac vein (same patient) shows severe narrowing of the left common iliac vein with dilated cross-pelvic collaterals filling the right common iliac vein. Note the enlarged left ascending lumbar vein.*

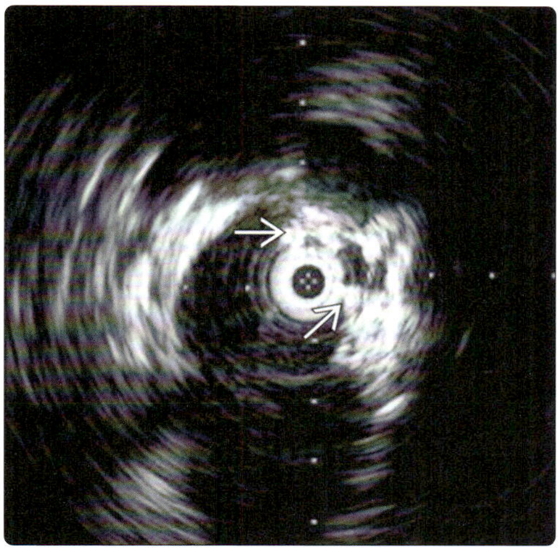

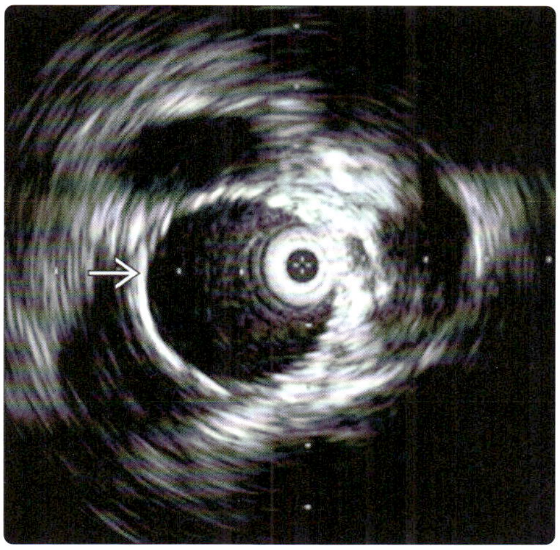

(Left) *Axial IVUS shows multiple mural adherent spurs along the anterior wall of the left common iliac vein in a patient with symptoms of paradoxical embolism and stroke. The patient is known to have a cardiac septal defect. These spurs act as nidi for thrombus formation. Spurs are secondary to chronic venous endothelial irritation, which is itself secondary to the compression caused by the pulsating right common iliac artery.* **(Right)** *Axial IVUS following a metallic stent placement shows patent stent.*

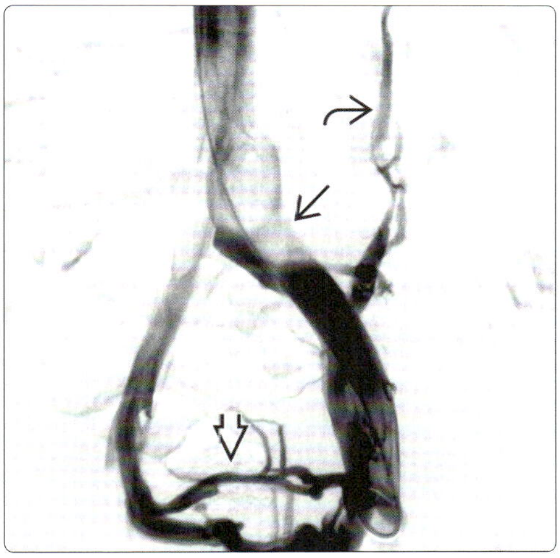

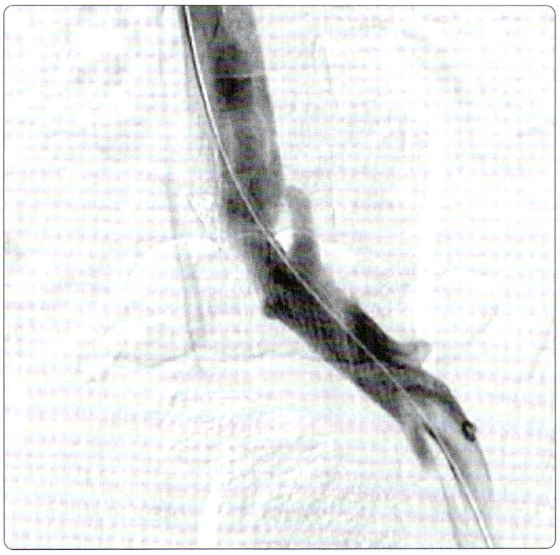

(Left) *AP venography from left external iliac venous injection shows compression of the left common iliac vein with cross-pelvic collaterals, a dilated ascending lumbar vein, and a recurrent left lower extremity DVT. These features are consistent with May-Thurner syndrome.* **(Right)** *AP venography through a left external iliac vein injection following left common iliac vein stent placement shows good flow through the left common iliac vein with absence of pelvic venous collaterals.*

KEY FACTS

TERMINOLOGY

- Compression of left renal vein between aorta and superior mesenteric artery (SMA)
  - Causes left renal venous outflow obstruction

IMAGING

- Initial screening using color Doppler US
  - Peak velocity measurements in renal vein and inferior vena cava (IVC)
- ≥ 50% compression of left renal vein between abdominal aorta and SMA on US/CT/MR
- Catheter confirmation of renal venous hypertension
  - Pressure measurements in left renal vein and IVC
  - Pressure gradient > 3 mmHg is diagnostic

PATHOLOGY

- Venous hypertension leads to development of collaterals with intrarenal and perirenal varicosities
  - Microscopic or gross hematuria can result from rupture of collateral veins into collecting system

CLINICAL ISSUES

- **Presentation (signs and symptoms)**
  - Flank, pelvic, or abdominal pain; often has accompanying hematuria, proteinuria
  - If left ovarian vein reflux and pelvic varicosities occur, may have pelvic congestion syndrome symptoms
  - If left-sided varicocele occurs in male patient, can cause testicular pain, infertility
- **Treatment**
  - Conservative management of mild symptoms; venous hypertension may eventually resolve
  - Recurrent/massive hematuria requires treatment
  - Surgical/endovascular treatment goal: Decrease intrarenal venous pressure by eliminating venous outflow obstruction

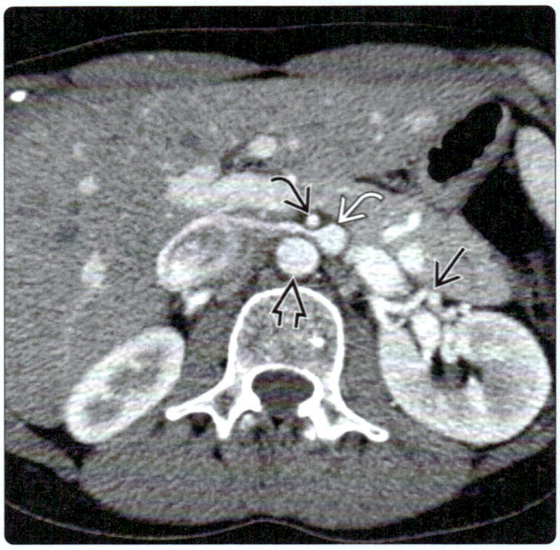

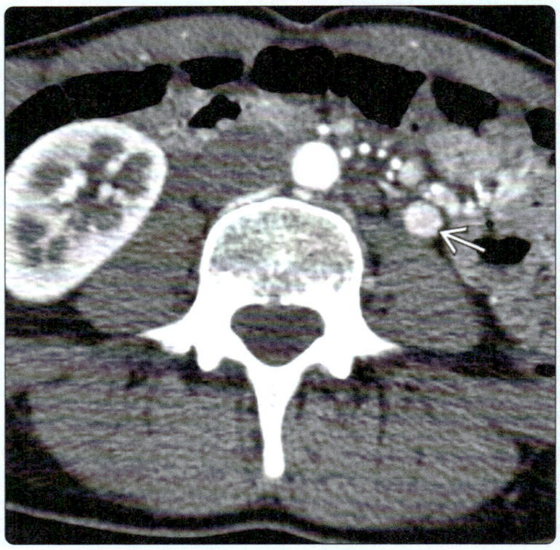

(Left) *Axial CECT in a patient with hematuria accompanied by left flank and pelvic pain shows marked left renal vein ➡ compression as it courses between the SMA ➡ and abdominal aorta ➡. This has caused left renal vein outflow obstruction with formation of numerous perirenal venous collaterals ➡.* **(Right)** *More caudally, a dilated left gonadal vein ➡ is seen. As with the perirenal collaterals, venous outflow obstruction has led to alternative venous drainage routes for the left kidney to decompress the renal venous hypertension.*

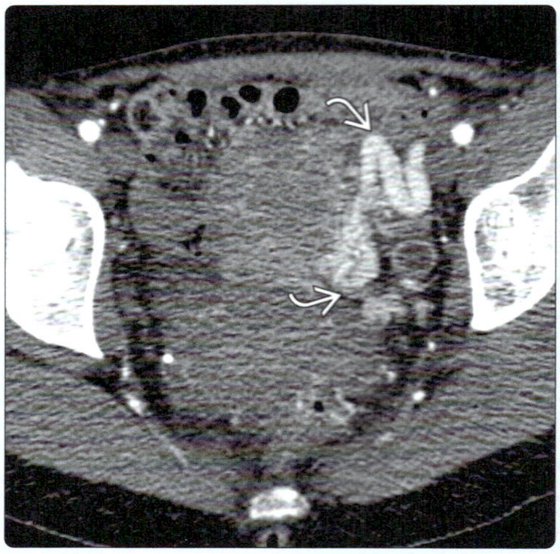

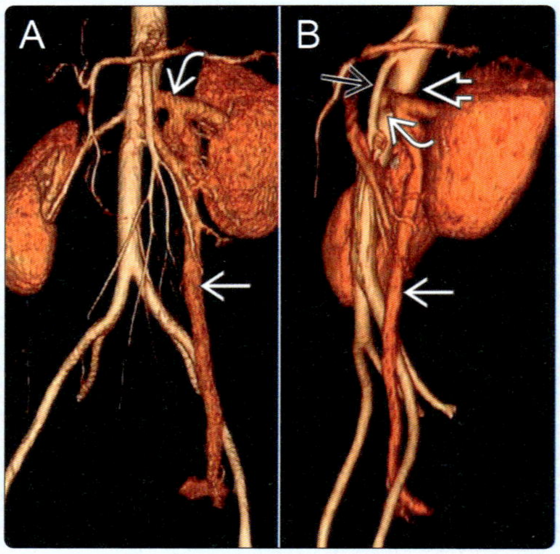

(Left) *Axial CECT shows left-sided pelvic varices ➡ due to retrograde flow in the left gonadal vein. The patient had pelvic congestion symptoms, a known complication of nutcracker syndrome.* **(Right)** *3D reconstructions in (A) coronal and (B) sagittal planes show the dilated left renal vein ➡ that is compressed as it crosses between the SMA ➡ and abdominal aorta ➡. A dilated left gonadal vein ➡ is seen throughout its length into the pelvis. Retrograde flow in the gonadal vein decompresses the left renal vein outflow obstruction.*

TERMINOLOGY

Definitions

- Compression of left renal vein between aorta and superior mesenteric artery (SMA)
  - Causes left renal venous outflow obstruction
    - Results in left renal venous hypertension
      - May have accompanying hematuria
      - May have engorged, edematous left kidney with intrarenal/perirenal varices
    - Secondary pelvic congestion syndrome may occur
      - Due to retrograde flow in left gonadal vein

IMAGING

General Features

- Best diagnostic clue
  - Left renal vein compressed between aorta and SMA
    - Causes dilatation of proximal left renal vein
      - May have associated intrarenal/perirenal varices
    - Enlarged gonadal vein due to reflux/retrograde flow
      - May lead to left varicocele/pelvic varices
    - Best seen on axial CT/MR imaging
- Location
  - Left renal vein courses between anterior aspect of abdominal aorta and dorsal aspect of SMA

Imaging Recommendations

- Best imaging tool
  - Initial screening using color Doppler US
    - Peak velocity measurements in renal vein and inferior vena cava (VC)
  - CECT in arterial and venous phases
    - Look for compressed left renal vein
  - Catheter confirmation of renal venous hypertension
    - Pressure measurements in left renal vein and IVC

Ultrasonographic Findings

- Color Doppler
  - Renal Doppler US is very sensitive initial screening test
  - Peak velocity measurements are used to assess for gradient between left renal vein and IVC
  - May demonstrate left intrarenal and perirenal varicosities and venous collaterals

CT Findings

- CECT
  - ≥ 50% compression of left renal vein between abdominal aorta and SMA
  - Aorta to SMA angle ≤ 35° on sagittal view
  - Beak sign with abrupt narrowing of left renal vein at level of SMA on axial view
    - Sensitivity 91.7%, specificity 88.9%
  - Ratio of left renal vein size at the left hilum and the narrowed segment can also be used; ≥ 4.9 suspicious for nutcracker syndrome
    - Higher ratios are associated with more clinical symptoms
  - Extensive left intrarenal and perirenal varicosities or venous collaterals may be present
  - CT venography findings are similar to those of left renal DSA venography

MR Findings

- MRV
  - Similar findings as on CT venography or DSA

Angiographic Findings

- DSA
  - Left renal venography with measurement of pressure gradient between IVC and left renal vein is used to confirm nutcracker syndrome in selected cases
    - Renal vein is "flattened" due to extrinsic compression by adjacent arterial structures
      - Contrast attenuated in compressed segment
    - Pressure gradient > 3 mmHg is diagnostic
  - May see enlarged, tortuous renal hilar varices draining into retroperitoneal venous collaterals

DIFFERENTIAL DIAGNOSIS

Arteriovenous Fistula

- Rapid flow hemodynamics and high venous pressures within enlarged renal vein
  - May result in perirenal varices

Congenital Venous Malformation

- May be extensive, with numerous points of communication with retroperitoneal veins

Renal Vein Thrombosis

- Acute thrombosis results in renal dysfunction, back pain, and hematuria
- Frequently associated with systemic disease
  - Dehydration
  - Hypercoagulable state
  - Neoplasm
- May be associated with intrinsic renal disease
  - Nephrotic syndrome
  - Glomerulonephritis
  - Tumor

Vascular Renal Tumor

- Arteriovenous shunting within tumor (e.g., renal cell carcinoma) may result in renal vein varices

Spontaneous Splenorenal Shunt

- Relatively infrequent condition occurring in and complicating hepatic cirrhosis and portal hypertension
  - Elevated pressure within splenic vein causes spontaneous decompression into left renal vein
  - Results in pressurized and dilated left renal vein
    - Accompanying renal vein, retroperitoneal varices

Obstructing Renal or Ureteral Calculus

- Obstructive uropathy from calculus causing unilateral flank, pelvic, or abdominal pain, and hematuria
  - Mimics symptoms of nutcracker syndrome

PATHOLOGY

General Features

- Etiology
  - Left renal vein normally courses between aorta and SMA
    - Vein may be compressed between these structures; can result in left renal venous hypertension

    - ◻ Venous hypertension leads to development of collaterals with intrarenal and perirenal varicosities
    - ◻ Microscopic or gross hematuria can result from rupture of collateral veins into collecting system
    - ◻ May be exacerbated in upright position
    - ◻ Suspected correlation with low BMI; symptoms may resolve with increasing BMI
  - If left renal vein is retroaortic, it can be compressed between anterior aorta and posterior vertebral column
  - Rare causes; compression by malignancy, lymphadenopathy, scoliosis, pregnancy, and rapid weight loss
- Associated abnormalities
  - Abdominal &/or left flank pain
  - Hematuria
  - Mild to moderate proteinuria
  - Female pelvic varicosities/pelvic congestion syndrome
  - Male varicoceles
  - Pediatric chronic fatigue syndrome
- Important cause of nonglomerular hematuria to be considered in pediatric age group
- Left renal vein compression and resultant renal venous hypertension can lead to left gonadal vein congestion and pelvis congestion syndrome

Gross Pathologic & Surgical Features

- Fibrosis may be present between aorta and SMA, where left renal vein courses

Microscopic Features

- Renal biopsy shows spectrum from normal to mild or moderate mesangial proliferative nephritis

CLINICAL ISSUES

Presentation

- Most common signs/symptoms
  - Flank, pelvic, or abdominal pain
    - Often has accompanying hematuria, proteinuria
      - ◻ Urine cytology, ureteroscopy, US, and renal biopsy are used in assessing unilateral hematuria etiology
- Other signs/symptoms
  - If left ovarian vein reflux and pelvic varicosities occur, may have pelvic congestion syndrome symptoms
  - If left-sided varicocele occurs in male patient, can cause testicular pain, infertility
- Clinical profile
  - 2 age distributions; different presentations
    - Thin young woman with recent substantial weight loss, new onset of vague flank pain, and hematuria
    - Pediatric patient with microscopic hematuria and associated mild to moderate proteinuria that may be orthostatic or with sudden onset of dark urine

Demographics

- Age
  - Pediatric and young adult
- Sex
  - M = F

Natural History & Prognosis

- Childhood nutcracker syndrome may be transient
  - May spontaneously resolve with growth
  - May resolve as venous collaterals develop
- Extensive venous collateral development may result in female pelvic congestion syndrome or male varicocele

Treatment

- Options, risks, complications
  - Conservatively manage patients with mild symptoms
    - Venous hypertension may resolve as collateral veins develop
  - Persistent, recurrent, or massive hematuria is indication for treatment
  - Surgical and endovascular treatment goal is to lower intrarenal venous pressure by eliminating venous outflow obstruction
    - Various surgical treatment options in severe cases
      - ◻ Autotransplantation of left kidney
      - ◻ Left renal vein reanastomosis to IVC
      - ◻ Nephrectomy
    - Reported endovascular treatments have included angioplasty (PTA) and intravascular stent placement
      - ◻ PTA is usually ineffective; stent typically required
      - ◻ Some operators reluctant to place intravascular stent due to young age of patient and lack of data on long-term effectiveness/outcomes/complications
      - ◻ Currently no consensus on indication for and success of endovascular treatment
    - Gonadal vein embolization is used to decompress pelvic varices if pelvic congestion symptoms present in association with nutcracker syndrome

DIAGNOSTIC CHECKLIST

Consider

- Nutcracker syndrome in pediatric patient with hematuria and proteinuria
- Nutcracker syndrome in differential diagnosis of young female who presents with vague flank, pelvic, or abdominal pain, and hematuria
- Nutcracker syndrome as possible etiology/contributing factor to pelvic congestion syndrome symptoms in female patients or left-sided varicocele in male patients

Image Interpretation Pearls

- Compression of left renal vein between aorta and SMA on US, CECT, or MRV is nondiagnostic for nutcracker syndrome in absence of intrarenal/perirenal varices
  - Unless pressure gradient is demonstrated by Doppler measurements or direct venous manometry

SELECTED REFERENCES

1. Nastasi DR et al: A systematic review on nutcracker syndrome and proposed diagnostic algorithm. J Vasc Surg Venous Lymphat Disord. 10(6):1410-6, 2022
2. Franco-Mesa C et al: Nutcracker syndrome. J Cardiovasc Surg (Torino). 62(5):467-71, 2021
3. Kolber MK et al: Nutcracker syndrome: diagnosis and therapy. Cardiovasc Diagn Ther. 11(5):1140-9, 2021
4. Kim SH: Doppler US and CT diagnosis of nutcracker syndrome. Korean J Radiol. 20(12):1627-37, 2019
5. Wang X et al: Results of endovascular treatment for patients with nutcracker syndrome. J Vasc Surg. 56(1):142-8, 2012
6. Chen S et al: Endovascular stenting for treatment of nutcracker syndrome: report of 61 cases with long-term followup. J Urol. 186(2):570-5, 2011

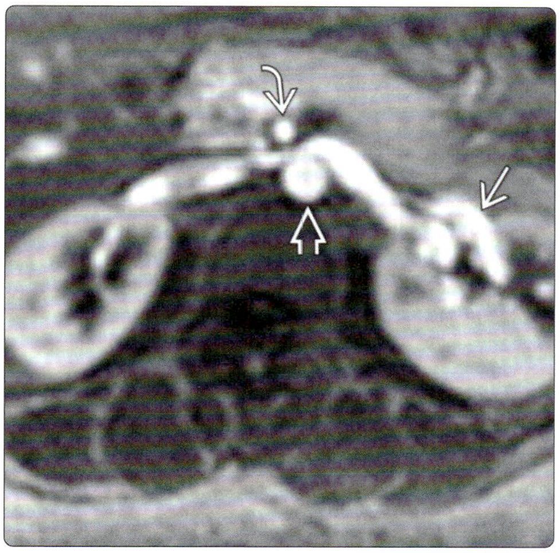

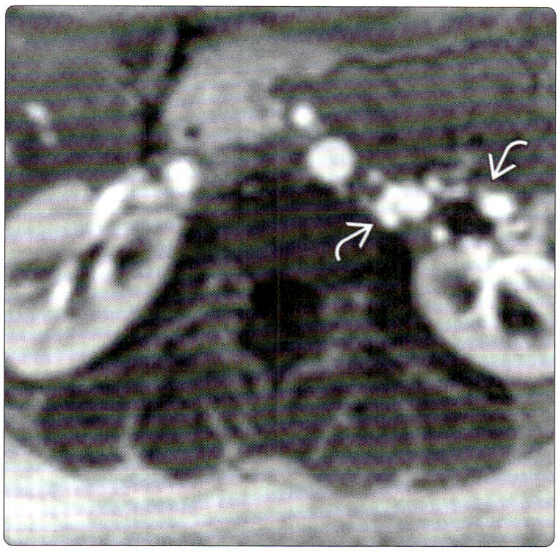

(Left) *Axial MRV in a patient with hematuria and pelvic pain shows marked compression of the left renal vein between the SMA and the anterior aspect of the abdominal aorta. Collateral perirenal varices are also present. Hematuria results when these varicosities rupture into a collecting system.* **(Right)** *More caudal axial MRV shows the extensive retroperitoneal collaterals that have developed as a result of the nutcracker compression of the left renal vein and the associated left renal venous hypertension.*

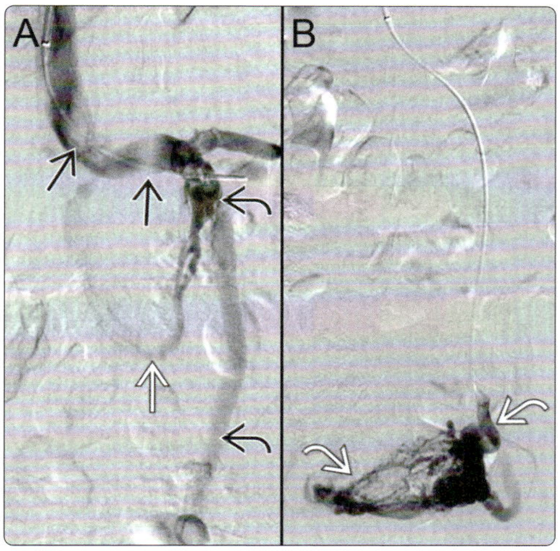

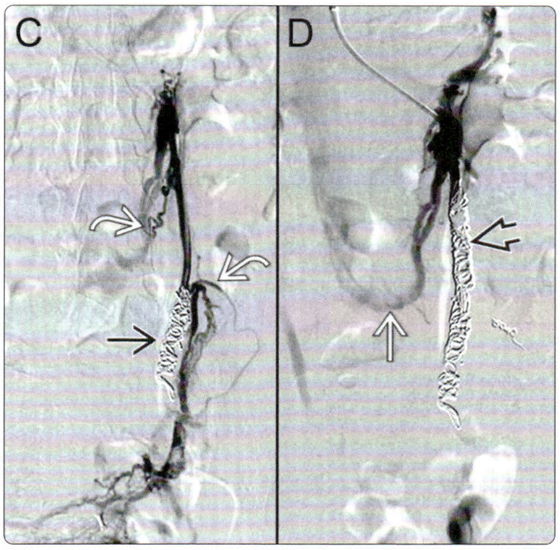

(Left) *(A) DSA after MRV shows contrast attenuation where arterial structures compress the renal vein, with reflux into the gonadal vein and drainage into the IVC via a retroperitoneal collateral. (B) Left gonadal vein DSA shows pelvic varices.* **(Right)** *Gonadal vein coil embolization was performed to decompress the pelvic varices. (C) DSA shows coils distally, but filling of additional channels. (D) Coils were also placed proximally to preserve drainage via the retroperitoneal collateral.*

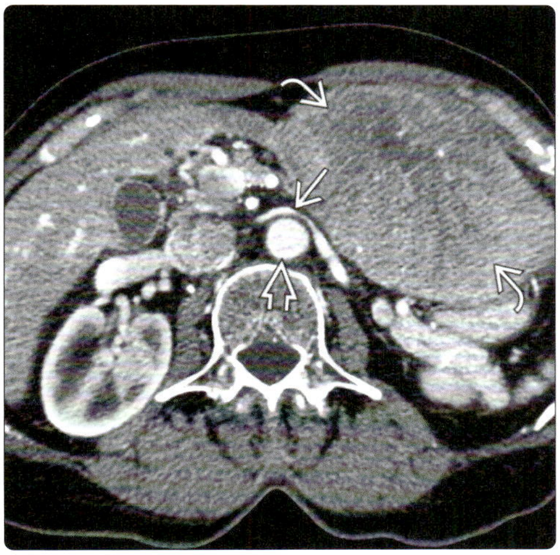

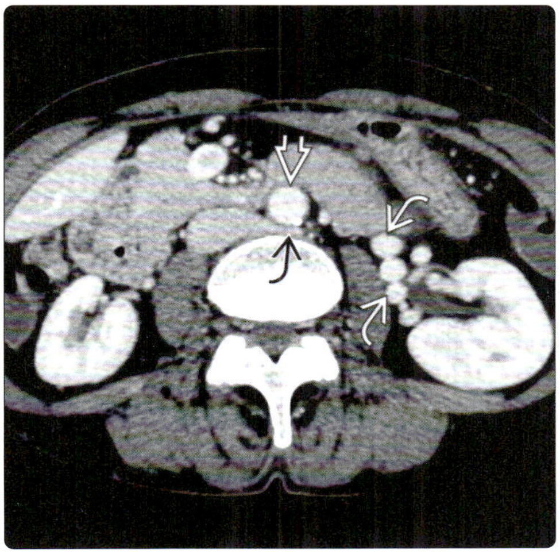

(Left) *Nutcracker syndrome may be mimicked by pathology that causes left renal venous hypertension. Axial CECT shows extrinsic compression of the left renal vein against the aorta by a large mass in the left hepatic lobe.* **(Right)** *In addition to hepatic compression of the main left renal vein, there is a retroaortic left renal vein, a vascular variant. Venous compression against the spine by the aorta further exacerbates left renal venous outflow obstruction. Perirenal varices are present.*

INDEX

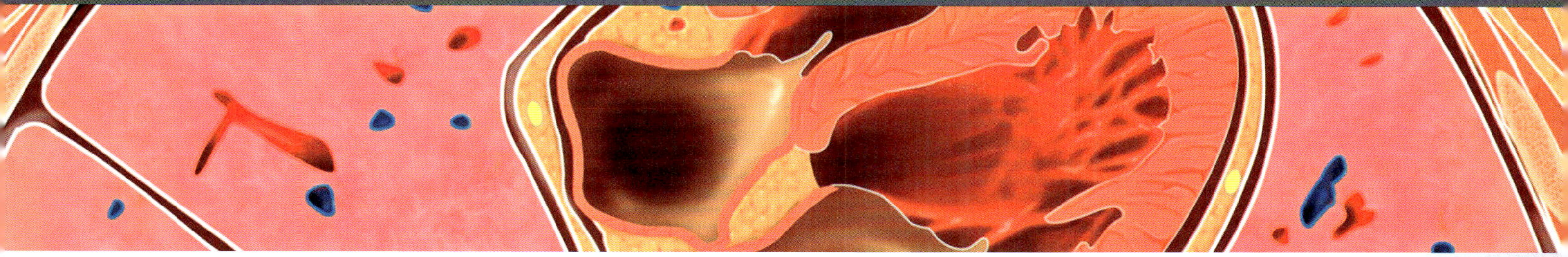

A

INDEX

INDEX

INDEX

INDEX

INDEX

B

C

INDEX

INDEX

INDEX

INDEX

INDEX

INDEX

D

INDEX

E

INDEX

F

G

I

INDEX

INDEX

J

K

L

M

INDEX

INDEX

N

INDEX

INDEX

INDEX

INDEX

Q

R

INDEX

S

T

U

V

INDEX

INDEX

W

X